Guelph Public Library

Health Guide
Canada

Guide canadien de la santé

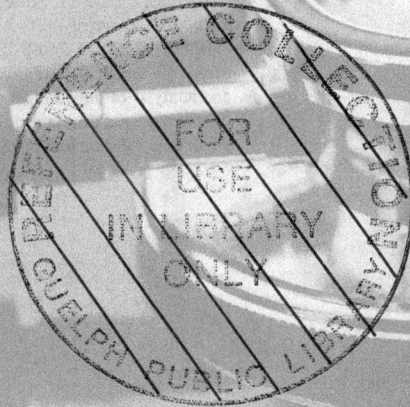

Additional Publications

For more detailed information or to place an order, see the back of the book.

CANADIAN ALMANAC & DIRECTORY 2017
Répetoire et almanach canadien
2,534 pages, 8 1/2 x 11, Hardcover
170th edition, November 2016
ISBN 978-1-61925-953-9
ISSN 0068-8193

A combination of textual material, charts, colour photographs and directory listings, the *Canadian Almanac & Directory* provides the most comprehensive picture of Canada, from physical attributes to economic and business summaries to leisure and recreation.

CANADIAN WHO'S WHO 2017
1,326 pages, 8 3/8 x 10 7/8, Hardcover
December 2016
ISBN 978-1-68217-212-4
ISSN 0068-9963

Published for over 100 years, this authoritative annual publication offers access to over 10,000 notable Canadians in all walks of life, including details such as date and place of birth, education, family details, career information, memberships, creative works, honours, languages, and awards, together with full addresses. Included are outstanding Canadians from business, academia, politics, sports, the arts and sciences, and more, selected because of the positions they hold in Canadian society, or because of the contributions they have made to Canada.

FINANCIAL POST DIRECTORY OF DIRECTORS 2017
Répertoire des administrateurs
1,363 pages, 5 7/8 x 9, Hardcover
70th edition, September 2016
ISBN 978-1-68217-396-1
ISSN 0071-5042

Published biennially and annually since 1931, this comprehensive resource offers readers access to approximately 16,300 executive contacts from Canada's top 1,400 corporations. The directory provides a definitive list of directorships and offices held by noteworthy Canadian business people, as well as details on prominent Canadian companies (both public and private), including company name, contact information and the names of executive officers and directors. Includes all-new front matter and three indexes.

GOVERNMENTS CANADA 2017
Gouvernements du Canada
1,300 pages, 8 1/2 x 11, Softcover
10th edition, January 2017
ISBN 978-1-68217-240-7
ISSN 1493-3918

Governments Canada provides a solution to finding the departments and people that you are searching for within our federal and provincial political system.

CANADIAN PARLIAMENTARY GUIDE 2017
Guide parlementaire canadien
1,332 pages, 6 x 9, Hardcover
151st edition, March 2017
ISBN 978-1-68217-524-8
ISSN 0315-6168

Published annually since before Confederation, this indispensable guide to government in Canada provides information on federal and provincial governments, with biographical sketches of government members, descriptions of government institutions, and historical text and charts. With significant bilingual sections, the Guide covers elections from Confederation to the present, including the most recent provincial elections.

ASSOCIATIONS CANADA 2017
Associations du Canada
2,226 pages, 8 1/2 x 11, Hardcover
38th edition, February 2017
ISBN 978-1-68217-473-9
ISSN 1186-9798

Over 20,000 entries profile Canadian and international organizations active in Canada. Over 2,000 subject classifications index activities, professions and interests served by associations. Includes listings of NGOs, institutes, coalitions, social agencies, federations, foundations, trade unions, fraternal orders, political parties. Fully indexed by subject, geographic location, electronic addresses, executive name, acronym, mailing list availability, conferences and publications.

FINANCIAL SERVICES CANADA 2017-2018
Services financiers au Canada
1,464 pages, 8 1/2 x 11, Softcover
20th edition, April 2017
ISBN 978-1-68217-520-0
ISSN 1484-2408

This directory of Canadian financial institutions and organizations includes banks and depository institutions, non-depository institutions, investment management firms, financial planners, insurance companies, accountants, major law firms, associations, and financial technology companies. Fully indexed.

CANADIAN ENVIRONMENTAL RESOURCE GUIDE 2016-2017
Guide des ressources environnementales canadiennes
880 pages, 8 1/2 x 11, Softcover
21st edition, July 2016
ISBN 978-1-61925-955-3
ISSN 1920-2725

Canada's most complete national listing of environmental organizations, product and service companies and governmental bodies, all indexed and categorized for quick and easy reference. Also included is the Environmental Industry Update, with recent events, maps, rankings, statistics, and trade shows and conferences. The online version features even more content, including associations, special libraries, law firms, and federal/provincial government information.

LIBRARIES CANADA 2016-2017
Bibliothèques Canada
880 pages, 8 1/2 x 11, Softcover
31st edition, August 2016
ISBN 978-1-61925-961-4
ISSN 1920-2849

Libraries Canada offers comprehensive information on Canadian libraries, resource centres, business information centres, professional associations, regional library systems, archives, library schools, government libraries, and library technical programs.

MAJOR CANADIAN CITIES: COMPARED & RANKED
Comparaison et classement des principales villes canadiennes
816 pages, 8 1/2 x 11, Softcover
1st edition, November 2013
ISBN 978-1-61925-260-8

Major Canadian Cities: Compared & Ranked provides an in-depth comparison and analysis of the 50 most populated cities in Canada. Following the city chapters are ranking tables that compare the demographics, economics, education, religion and infrastructure of the cities listed.

2017-2018
3rd Edition

Health Guide Canada

Guide canadien de la santé

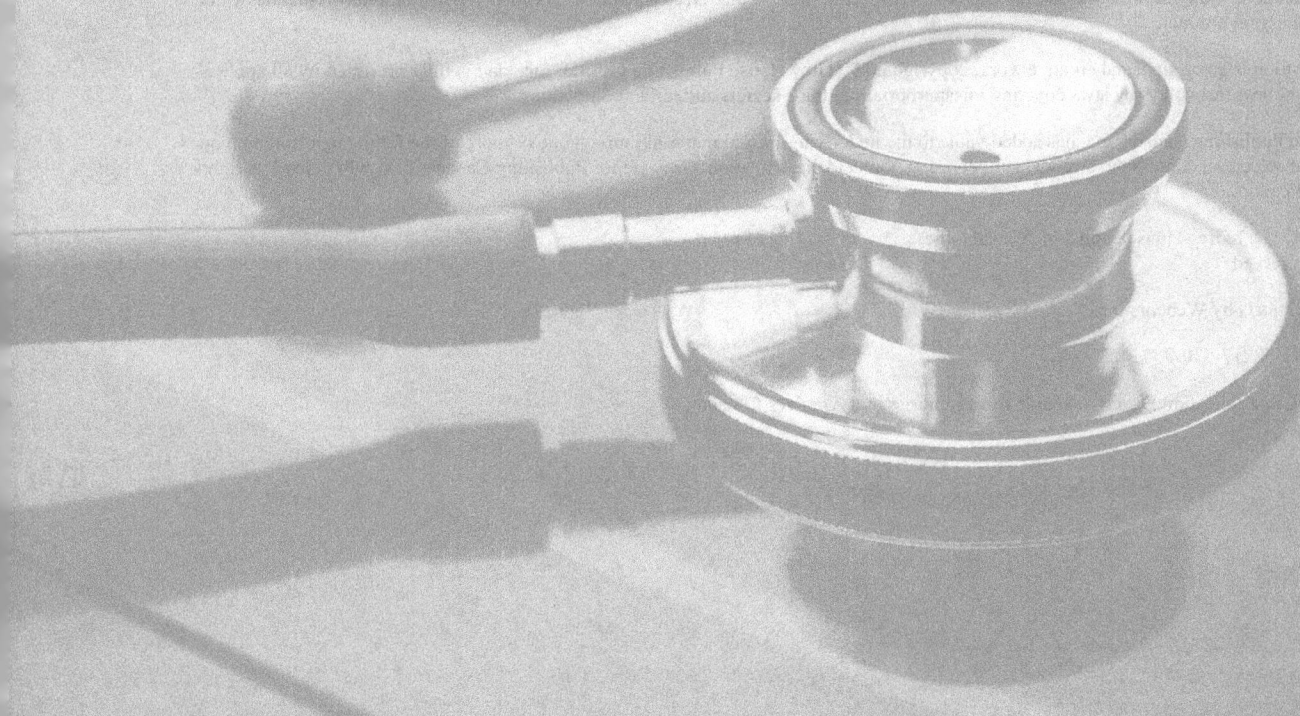

GREY HOUSE
PUBLISHING CANADA

Grey House Publishing Canada
PUBLISHER: Leslie Mackenzie
GENERAL MANAGER: Bryon Moore
MANAGING EDITOR: Stuart Paterson
ASSOCIATE EDITORS: Kathlyn Del Castillo; Laura Lamanna

Grey House Publishing
EDITORIAL DIRECTOR: Laura Mars
MARKETING DIRECTOR: Jessica Moody
PRODUCTION MANAGER: Kristen Hayes
COMPOSITION: David Garoogian

Grey House Publishing Canada
555 Richmond Street West, Suite 512
Toronto, ON M5V 3B1
866-433-4739
FAX 416-644-1904
www.greyhouse.ca
e-mail: info@greyhouse.ca

Grey House Publishing Canada, Inc. is a wholly owned subsidiary of Grey House Publishing, Inc. USA.

Printed in Canada by Webcom Inc.

ISBN: 978-1-68217-530-9

Cataloguing in Publication Data is available from Libraries and Archives Canada.

Table of Contents

Table des matières

According to the World Health Organization, chronic diseases are the leading cause of mortality in the world, representing 60% of all deaths. The Public Health Agency of Canada has calculated that three of every five Canadians aged 20 or older have a chronic illness, and four out of five are at risk. *Health Guide Canada* offers a comprehensive overview of 107 chronic and mental illnesses from Addison's to Wilson's disease, including a new entry this edition on Guillain-Barré Syndrome. Each chapter includes an easy-to-understand medical description, plus a wide range of condition-specific support services and information resources that deal with the variety of issues concerning those with a chronic or mental illness, as well as those who support the illness community.

The word *chronic* comes from the Greek word *chronos,* meaning *time* (the Greek god Chronos is often depicted as Father Time). The World Health Organization defines a chronic disease as one "of long duration and generally slow progression." It is rarely curable and will likely cause significant changes to the person's quality of life. Mental health disorders include a wide variety of psychological illnesses.

Health Guide Canada contains thousands of ways to deal with the many aspects of chronic or mental health disorders. It includes associations, government agencies, libraries and resource centres, educational facilities, hospitals and publications. In addition to chapters dealing with specific chronic or mental conditions, there is a chapter relevant to the health industry in general, as well as others dealing with charitable foundations, death and bereavement groups, homeopathic medicine, indigenous issues and sports for the disabled.

This guide will provide critical information to those dealing for the first time with the stress and crucial need-to-know issues, as well as to those already coping with chronic disease. *How can I connect with others with diabetes? What cancer treatment is best for me? What genetic disorders could my child be at risk of inheriting? What factors are influencing the health of Canadians?* You'll find ways to answer these questions and more in Grey House's newly updated health text.

In addition to patients and families, hospital and medical centre personnel can find the support they need in their work or study. *Health Guide Canada* is full of resources crucial for people with chronic illness as they transition from diagnosis to home, home to work, and work to community life.

Health Guide Canada provides, in one source, comprehensive, critical, immediate information, from national associations to local health centres. Each listing will provide a description, address (including website, email address and social media links, if possible) and executives' names and titles, as well as a number of details specific to that type of organization.

Educational Material

To access information by specific chronic illness, body system or disorder category, the cross-referenced Chronic Illness–Body System chart in the front of the book makes it easy.

Two reports—*Health Status of Canadians 2016* and *A Focus on Family Violence in Canada*—by the Public Health Agency of Canada provide an overview of the factors affecting the health of Canadians.

A Glossary of medical terminology, showing the meanings of prefixes, roots and suffixes follows the reports.

Arrangement

Section I: Chronic & Mental Illnesses contains 107 chronic or mental condition chapters, which are arranged alphabetically by name of the disorder. Each chapter begins with a brief and straightforward description of the illness, showing probable causes, symptoms, prevalence and treatment options.

Following each description are disease-specific resources. Chapters contain the following: associations, publications, government agencies, libraries and resource centres, educational facilities, and hospitals—a total of over 5,000 listings. Listings include the name of the organization or publication, address, phone, fax number, email, website, social media links and executives, as available. Brief descriptions and other details are included depending on the type of listing: an association, for example, may include the year it was founded and yearly dues; while a magazine might include its frequency and number of pages.

Section II: General Resources includes similar categories to Section I, but shows information related to health in general instead of to a specific illness.

Section III: Appendices include charitable foundations, which among other entities lists organizations devoted to granting wishes of chronically and terminally ill individuals; death and bereavement listings showing support services for those who find themselves or a loved one close to death or grieving a loss; homeopathic medicine facilities providing information on where to access more holistic services; organizations devoted to indigenous health issues; and sports groups for the disabled.

Section IV: Statistics contains statistical data drawn from Statistics Canada and the Fraser Institute, showing information on numbers of people with different illnesses in Canada, the performance of the health program and wait times for certain procedures.

Rounding out this directory are the Entry Name and Publication Indexes, which allow users additional access to the information.

Health Guide Canada is also available for subscription on CIRC: Canada's Information Resource Centre. Subscribers to CIRC can access their subscriptions online and do customized searches that make finding information quicker and easier. Visit www.circ.greyhouse.ca for more information.

We acknowledge the valuable contribution of those individuals and organizations who have responded to our information gathering process throughout the year; your help and timely responses to our questionnaires are greatly appreciated.

Every effort has been made to ensure the accuracy of the information included in this edition of *Health Guide Canada*. Do not hesitate to contact us with comments or if revisions are necessary.

Selon l'Organisation mondiale de la Santé, les maladies chroniques constituent la principale cause de mortalité dans le monde alors qu'elles expliquent 60 % des décès. L'Agence de la santé publique du Canada a calculé que 3 Canadiens sur 5 âgés de 20 ans ou plus sont aux prises avec une maladie chronique et que 4 Canadiens sur 5 sont à risque de le devenir. Le *Guide canadien de la santé* donne un aperçu global de 107 maladies chroniques et mentales, de la maladie d'Addison à celle de Wilson, y compris une nouvelle entrée portant sur le syndrome de Guillain-Barré. Chaque chapitre comprend une description médicale facile à comprendre, une vaste gamme de services de soutien particuliers à l'éta et des ressources documentaires qui portent sur diverses questions relatives aux personnes qui sont aux prises avec une maladie chronique ou mentale et à ceux qui soutiennent la communauté liée à cette maladie.

Le terme « chronique » provient du grec « chronos » qui signifie « temps » (le dieu grec Chronos est souvent dépeint en tant que père du temps). Selon l'Organisation mondiale de la Santé, une maladie chronique est de longue durée et progresse habituellement lentement. On peut rarement la guérir et il y a de fortes chances qu'elle modifie grandement la qualité de vie de la personne. Les problèmes de santé mentale couvrent un large éventail de maladies psychologiques.

Le *Guide canadien de la santé* contient des milliers de moyens pour composer avec divers aspects d'une maladie chronique ou d'un problème de santé mentale. Il comprend des associations, des organismes gouvernementaux, des bibliothèques et des centres de documentation, des services d'éducation, des hôpitaux et des publications. En plus des chapitres qui portent sur des états chroniques ou mentaux, un chapitre traite de l'industrie de la santé en général; d'autres abordent les fondations qui réalisent des rêves, les groupes de soutien axés sur le décès et le deuil, la médecine homéopathique, les questions autochtones et les sports pour les personnes handicapées.

Ce guide donne une information cruciale à ceux et celles qui doivent composer, pour la première fois, avec la tension et les enjeux essentiels de même qu'à toute personne aux prises avec une maladie chronique. *Comment puis-je entrer en communication avec d'autres personnes qui souffrent de diabète? Quel traitement du cancer me convient le mieux? Quels troubles génétiques mon enfant risque-t-il d'hériter? Quels facteurs influencent la santé des Canadiens?* Vous trouverez comment répondre à ces questions, entre autres, dans ce document sur la santé de Grey House récemment mis à jour.

Les membres du personnel des hôpitaux et des centres médicaux peuvent trouver, au même titre que parents et familles, le soutien dont ils ont besoin dans le cadre de leur travail ou de leurs études. Le *Guide canadien de la santé* est rempli de ressources capitales pour les personnes qui souffrent d'une maladie chronique alors qu'elles passent du diagnostic au retour à la maison, de la maison au travail et du travail à la vie au sein de la communauté.

Le *Guide canadien de la santé* réunit des renseignements exhaustifs, critiques et immédiats, des associations nationales aux centres de santé locaux. Chaque entrée comprend une description, une adresse (y compris le site Web, le courriel et les liens des médias sociaux, lorsque possible), les noms et titres des directeurs de même que plusieurs détails particuliers à ce type d'organisme.

Matériel didactique

Le tableau à référence croisée Maladie chronique—systèmes et appareils de l'organisme, au début du livre, simplifie l'accès aux renseignements par maladie chronique particulière, système de l'organisme et catégorie de problème.

Deux articles—*État de santé des Canadiens 2016* et *Regard sur la violence familiale au Canada*—publiés par l'Agence de la santé publique du Canada, donnent un aperçu des facteurs qui ont une incidence sur la santé des Canadiens.

Un glossaire de terminologie médicale, montrant les significations des préfixes, des racines et des suffixes, suit les articles.

Plan

La section I contient 107 chapitres portant sur la maladie chronique ou mentale; elle est organisée en ordre alphabétique de nom de maladie. Chaque chapitre commence par une description brève et simple de la maladie, des causes probables apparentes, des symptômes, de la prévalence et des possibilités de traitement.

Des ressources particulières à la maladie accompagnent chaque description. Les chapitres comprennent des associations, des publications, des organismes gouvernementaux, des bibliothèques et centres de documentation, des services d'éducation et des hôpitaux. Cet ouvrage de référence décrit plus de 5 000 entrées. Elles comprennent le nom de l'organisme ou le titre de la publication, son adresse, numéro de téléphone, numéro de télécopieur, adresse électronique, site Web, les liens vers les médias sociaux et les directeurs, lorsque l'information est accessible. Selon le type d'entrée, de brèves descriptions et d'autres détails sont fournis. Par exemple, une association peut indiquer l'année de sa création et le montant de sa cotisation annuelle; une revue peut indiquer son tirage et le nombre de pages qu'elle compte.

La section II, qui porte sur les ressources génériques, comprend les renseignements connexes à la santé en général, sans être reliés à une maladie en particulier.

La section III comprend des annexes comme les œuvres de charité, dont font partie les organismes qui réalisent les rêves de personnes aux prises avec une maladie chronique ou en phase terminale; des entrées portant sur le décès et le deuil comprenant des services de soutien pour ceux et celles qui se préparent à mourir ou dont un être cher se trouve dans cette situation ou qui pleurent une perte; des services de médecine homéopathique qui donnent de l'information sur l'accès à des services plus holistiques; des organismes dédiés aux questions de santé autochtones; des groupes de sport pour les personnes handicapées.

La section IV contient des données statistiques tirées de Statistiques Canada et de Fraser Institute, montrant l'information sur des nombres de personnes avec différentes maladies au Canada, le programme de santé et temps d'attente pour certaines procédures.

Un index de nom et un index des publications complète ce répertoire afin de permettre aux utilisateurs d'accéder autrement à l'information.

Le *Guide canadien de la santé* est également offert par inscription au CDC : Centre de documentation du Canada. Les abonnés au CDC peuvent accéder à leurs inscriptions en ligne et effectuer des recherches personnalisées afin de trouver l'information plus rapidement et plus facilement. Consultez www.circ.greyhouse.ca pour obtenir plus d'information.

Nous tenons à souligner la précieuse contribution des personnes et des organismes qui ont collaboré tout au long de l'année à notre procédé de cueillette d'information; votre aide, vos réponses à nos questionnaires dans les délais impartis sont grandement appréciés.

Tous les efforts ont été faits pour assurer l'exactitude des renseignements compris dans la présente édition de *Guide canadien de la santé*. N'hésitez pas à communiquer avec nous pour nous faire part de vos commentaires ou pour nous demander une révision, le cas échéant.

The following chart lists the illness and its body system(s) or disorder category. Chronic conditions not listed, such as Cancer, Genetic Disorders and Metabolic Disorders, do not fall into a specific system(s). A cross-reference chart follows that lists the information in reverse—body system or disorder categories followed by chronic illnesses.

CHRONIC & MENTAL ILLNESS	BODY SYSTEM/DISORDER CATEGORY
Addison's Disease	Endocrine
Adjustment Disorders	Behavioural
Aging	Cells & Tissues
AIDS/HIV	Immune, Infectious Disease
Allergies	Immune
Alzheimer's Disease	Nervous
Amyotrophic Lateral Sclerosis	Nervous
Anxiety Disorders	Behavioural
Arthritis	Muscular, Skeletal
Asthma	Respiratory
Ataxia	Nervous
Attention Deficit Hyperactivity Disorder	Behavioural, Developmental
Autistic Spectrum Disorders	Behavioural, Developmental
Brain Tumours	Nervous
Blood Disorders	Blood
Carpal Tunnel Syndrome	Muscular, Skeletal, Nervous
Celiac Disease	Gastrointestinal
Cerebral Palsy	Nervous, Muscular
Chronic Fatigue Syndrome	Immune
Chronic Pain	Nervous
Cognitive Disorders	Nervous
Conduct Disorder	Behavioural
Congential Heart Disease	Cardiovascular
Cooley's Anemia (Thalassemia)	Blood
Crohn's Disease	Gastrointestinal
Cystic Fibrosis	Respiratory, Gastrointestinal
Diabetes Mellitus	Endocrine
Down Syndrome	Developmental
Eating Disorders (Anorexia Nervosa, Bulimia)	Behavioural
Endometriosis	Reproductive
Epilepsy	Nervous
Fabry Disease	Gastrointestinal
Fibromyalgia	Muscular, Skeletal
Gastrointestinal Disorders	Gastrointestinal
Gaucher Disease	Gastrointestinal
Gender Dysphoria	Behavioural
Growth Disorders	Developmental
Guillain-Barré Syndrome	Immune, Nervous
Gulf War Syndrome	Nervous
Head Injuries	Nervous
Hearing Loss	Sensory
Heart Disease	Cardiovascular
Hemophilia	Blood
Hepatitis	Infectious Disease
Huntington Disease	Nervous
Hydrocephalus	Nervous
Hypertension	Cardiovascular
Impulse Control Disorder	Behavioural
Incontinence	Urinary
Infertility	Reproductive
Kidney Disease	Gastrointestinal
Leprosy	Dermatologic, Nervous
Liver Disease	Gastrointestinal

Lung Disease	Respiratory
Lupus Erythematosus	Cells & Tissues
Lymphatic Disorders	Lymphatic
Mental Illness: General	Behavioural
Migraine	Cardiovascular, Nervous
Mood Disorders	Behavioural
Multiple Sclerosis	Nervous
Muscular Dystrophy	Nervous
Myasthenia Gravis	Nervous
Neurofibromatosis	Nervous, Dermatologic
Osteogenesis Imperfecta	Skeletal
Osteoporosis	Skeletal
Paget's Disease	Skeletal
Paraphilias	Behavioural
Parkinson's Disease	Nervous
Pediatric Mental Health Issues	Nervous, Behavioural
Personality Disorders	Behavioural
Post-Polio Syndrome	Muscular, Skeletal
Prader-Willi Syndrome	Endocrine
Psychosomatic Disorders	Behavioural
Raynaud's Disease	Cardiovascular
Sarcoidosis	Cells & Tissues, Respiratory
Schizophrenia	Behavioural
Scleroderma	Cells & Tissues, Dermatologic
Scoliosis	Skeletal
Sexual Disorders	Reproductive
Sexually Transmitted Infections	Reproductive, Infectious Disease
Sickle Cell Disease	Blood
Sjogren's Syndrome	Cells & Tissues
Skin Disorders	Dermatologic
Speech Impairments	Developmental, Nervous
Spina Bifida	Nervous, Skeletal
Spinal Cord Injuries	Nervous
Stroke	Nervous
Substance Abuse and Dependence	Behavioural
Tay-Sachs Disease	Nervous
Thyroid Disease	Endorcrine
Tick-Borne Diseases	Infectious Disease
Tourette Syndrome	Nervous
Tuberculosis	Respiratory, Infectious Disease
Tuberous Sclerosis	Nervous, Dermatologic
Turner Syndrome	Endocrine
Ulcerative Colitis	Gastrointestinal
Visual Impairment	Sensory
Wilson Disease	Gastrointestinal

BY BODY SYSTEM/DISORDER CATEGORY

Behavioural
Adjustment Disorders; Anxiety Disorders; Attention Deficit Disorder; Autism; Conduct Disorders; Dissociative Disorders; Eating Disorders; Gender Dysphoria; Impulse Control Disorder; Mental Illness; Mood Disorders; Paraphilias; Pediatric Mental Health Issues; Personality Disorders; Psychosomatic Disorders; Schizophrenia; Substance Abuse and Dependence

Blood
Blood Disorders; Cooley's Anemia; Hemophilia; Sickle Cell Disease

Cardiovascular
Heart Disease; Hypertension; Migraine; Raynaud's Disease

Cells & Tissues
Aging; Lupus Erythematosus; Scleroderma; Sjogren's Syndrome

Dermatologic
Leprosy; Neurofibromatosis; Scleroderma; Skin Disorders; Tuberous Sclerosis

Developmental
Attention Deficit Disorder; Autism; Down Syndrome; Growth Disorders; Speech Impairments

Endocrine
Addison's Disease; Diabetes; Turner Syndrome

Gastrointestinal
Celiac Disease; Crohn's Disease; Cystic Fibrosis; Fabry Disease; Gastrointestinal Disorders; Gaucher Disease; Kidney Disease; Liver Disease; Ulcerative Colitis; Wilson Disease

Immune
AIDS; Allergies; Chronic Fatigue Syndrome; Guillain-Barré Syndrome

Infectious Disease
AIDS; Hepatitis; Sexually Transmitted Diseases; Tick-Borne Diseases; Tuberculosis

Lymphatic
Lymphatic Disorders

Muscular
Arthritis; Carpal Tunnel Syndrome; Cerebral Palsy; Fibromyalgia Syndrome; Post-Polio Syndrome

Nervous
Alzheimer's Disease; Amyotrophic Lateral Sclerosis; Ataxia; Brain Tumours; Carpal Tunnel Syndrome; Cerebral Palsy; Chronic Pain; Cognitive Disorders; Dissociative Disorders; Epilepsy; Guillain-Barré Syndrome; Gulf War Syndrome; Head Injuries; Huntington Disease; Hydrocephalus; Leprosy; Multiple Sclerosis; Muscular Dystrophy; Myasthenia Gravis; Neurofibromatosis; Parkinson's Disease; Pediatric Mental Health Issues; Speech Impairments; Spina Bifida; Spinal Cord Injuries; Stroke; Tay-Sachs Disorder; Tourette Syndrome; Tuberous Sclerosis

Reproductive
Endometriosis; Impotence; Infertility; Sexual Disorders; Sexually Transmitted Infections

Respiratory
Asthma; Cystic Fibrosis; Lung Disease; Tuberculosis

Skeletal
Arthritis; Carpal Tunnel Syndrome; Fibromyalgia Syndrome; Osteognesis Imperfecta; Osteoporosis; Paget's Disease; Post-Polio Syndrome; Scoliosis; Spina Bifida

Sensory
Hearing Loss; Visual Impairment

Urinary
Incontinence

INDIGENOUS POPULATIONS

In 2011, approximately 1.4 million or 4% of Canadians identified themselves as Indigenous. Among these Canadians, 61% self-identified as First Nations, 32% as Métis and 4% as Inuit.[7] Indigenous populations were significantly younger than the general Canadian population with almost 50% being under the age of 25 years compared to 30% of the non-Indigenous population.[7]

4%
OF CANADIANS IDENTIFIED THEMSELVES AS INDIGENOUS

PERCENTAGE OF THAT POPULATION IDENTIFY
as First Nations **61%**
as Métis **32%**

PERCENTAGE OF THE POPULATION WHO ARE UNDER THE AGE OF 25
50% of the Indigenous population
30% of the non-Indigenous population

FOREIGN-BORN POPULATIONS

In 2011, approximately 7 million people living in Canada identified themselves as foreign-born, which represented 21% of the total population.[8] 17% arrived in Canada between 2006 and 2011 with 57% being from Asia and 14% from Europe.[8]

21%
PEOPLE LIVING IN CANADA IDENTIFIED THEMSELVES AS FOREIGN BORN

INTERNATIONAL COMPARISON

Canada's annual population growth rate was the highest among G7 countries in 2012/2014 at 1% .[9] Canada's population is not growing as quickly as in the past.[2]

ANNUAL POPULATION GROWTH RATE IN G7 COUNTRIES, 2012/2014[9]

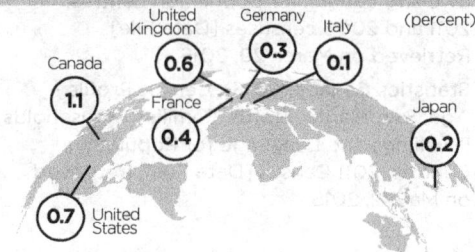

(percent)

Canada **1.1**
United Kingdom **0.6**
Germany **0.3**
Italy **0.1**
France **0.4**
Japan **-0.2**
United States **0.7**

Notes to the reader
- The estimated population represents the number of Canadians whose usual place of residence is in Canada. It also includes any Canadians staying in a dwelling in Canada on Census Day and having no usual place of residence elsewhere in Canada, as well as non-permanent residents (e.g., a person and his or her family who is lawfully in Canada on a temporary basis under the authority of a valid document such as a work permit, study permit, Minister's permit or refugee).[1]
- Indigenous populations consist of First Nations, Métis and Inuit.
- G7 countries include seven of the world's industrialized countries, namely the United States, Japan, Germany, France, the United Kingdom, Italy and Canada that form an informal discussion group and economic partnership

For more information on Canada's population, please see:
- Statistics Canada

References

1. Statistics Canada (2016). Canada's population estimates, fourth quarter 2015. Quarterly Demographic Estimates, 29(4), (91-002-X).

2. Statistics Canada (2015). Table 051-0001 – Estimates of population, by age group and sex for July 1, Canada, provinces and territories. [Data file]. November 18, 2016.

3. Statistics Canada (2016). Population and dwelling counts, for population centres, 2011 and 2006 censuses [Data File]. Retrieved on March 29, 2016.

4. Statistics Canada (2013). Census Profile – Age, Sex, Marital Status, Families, Households, Dwellings and Language for Population Centres, 2011 Census [Data File]. Retrieved on May 12, 2015.

5. Canadian Institute of Health Information (2011). Health Care in Canada, 2011: A Focus on Seniors and Aging. Ottawa ON: Canadian Institute of Health Information.

6. Statistics Canada (2016). Annual Demographic Estimates: Sub-provincial Areas 2015.

7. Statistics Canada (2016). Aboriginal Identity, Age Groups, Registered or Treaty Indian Status, Area of Residence: On Reserve and Sex for the Population in Private Households of Canada, Provinces and Territories, 2011 National Household Survey [Data File]. Retrieved on November 18, 2016.

8. Statistics Canada (2013). 2011 National Household Survey: Immigration, place of birth, citizenship, ethnic origin, visible minorities, language and religion. The Daily.

9. Statistics Canada (2014). Annual Demographic Estimates. Canada, Provinces, and Territories, 2014.

How healthy are we?

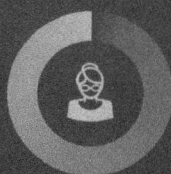

LIFE EXPECTANCY   LOW BIRTH WEIGHT   COMMUNITY BELONGING   PERCEIVED HEALTH   PERCEIVED MENTAL HEALTH

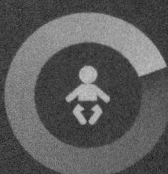

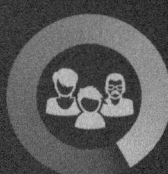

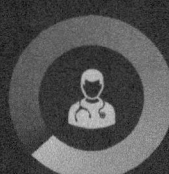

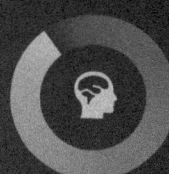

Life expectancy at birth

In 2012, the average life expectancy at birth in Canada was estimated at 82 years.[1]

Life expectancy at birth is the number of years a person is expected to live from birth onwards.[2] It is one measure of a nation's health and is affected by a variety of factors, such as genetics, lifestyle, diet, access to healthcare, education and income, and rates of diseases and conditions.[2-6]

OVER TIME, BY SEX

The average life expectancy at birth has increased since the early 1920s.[1, 7, 8] Women consistently have a higher life expectancy than men.[1, 7, 8]

LIFE EXPECTANCY AT BIRTH OVER TIME AND BY SEX, 1991 AND 2012[1,7]

1991		2012	
Men	Women	Men	Women
75 years	**81** years	**79** years	**84** years

BY INCOME

In urban centres in 2005–2007, life expectancy at birth for Canadians tended to be higher for people living in high-income neighbourhoods.[9]

LIFE EXPECTANCY AT BIRTH BY SEX AND NEIGHBOURHOOD INCOME, 2005–2007[9]

(in years)

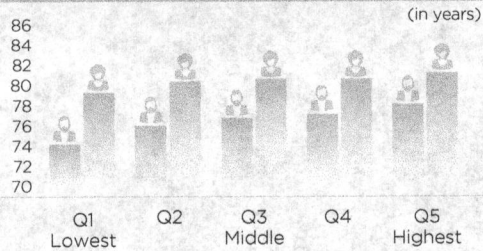

| | Q1 Lowest | Q2 | Q3 Middle | Q4 | Q5 Highest |

Quintiles (Q) are calculated by dividing the Canadian population into five groups of equal size (quintiles) based on neighbourhood income.

INDIGENOUS POPULATIONS

Available data suggest that Indigenous populations have lower life expectancy at birth than non-Indigenous populations.[10] Projections for 2017 suggest this is especially true for Inuit.[11]

LIFE EXPECTANCY AT BIRTH, PROJECTIONS FOR 2017[11]
(in years)

	♂	♀
First Nations	73	78
Métis	74	80
Inuit	64	73
Canada (total)	79	83

INTERNATIONAL COMPARISON

In 2012, life expectancy at birth in G7 countries was highest in Japan at 80 years for men and 86 years for women and lowest in the United States at 76 years for men and 81 years for women. Canada ranked in the middle at 79 years for men and 84 years for women.[12]

LIFE EXPECTANCY AT BIRTH IN G7 COUNTRIES, 2012[11]

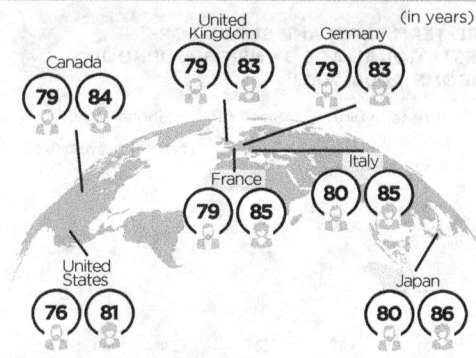

(in years)

Canada: 79 84
United Kingdom: 79 83
Germany: 79 83
France: 79 85
Italy: 80 85
United States: 76 81
Japan: 80 86

Notes to the reader

- Life expectancy is the number of years a person would be expected to live starting at birth if mortality rates stayed the same over his or her lifetime.[3]

- Indigenous populations consist of First Nations, Métis and Inuit.

- G7 countries include seven of the world's industrialized countries, namely the United States, Japan, Germany, France, the United Kingdom, Italy and Canada, that form an informal discussion group and economic partnership.

For more information on life expectancy, please see:

- Statistics Canada

- Organisation for Economic Co-Operation and Development

References

1. Statistics Canada (2016). Table 053-0003 – Elements of the life table, Canada, provinces and territories, annual (number), (CANSIM database)

2. World Health Organization (n.d.). Life expectancy. Retrieved on March 29, 2016.

3. Hertz, E., Hebert, J.R., Landon, J. (1994). Social and environmental factors and life expectancy, infant mortality, and maternal mortality rates: results of a cross-national comparison. Social Science and Medicine, 39(1), 105-114.

4. Rao, V. (1988). Diet, mortality and life expectancy : a cross national analysis. Journal of Population Economics, 1(3), 225-233.

5. Martikainen, P., Makela, P., Peltonen, R., Myrksyla, M. (2014). Income differences in life expectancy: the changing contribution of harmful consumption of alcohol and smoking. Epidemiology, 25(2), 182-190.

6. Manuel, D.G., R. Perez, C. Bennett, L. Rosella, M. Taljaard, M. Roberts et al. (2012). Seven More Years: The Impact of Smoking, Alcohol, Diet, Physical Activity and Stress on Health and Life Expectancy in Ontario. Toronto, ON: Institute for Clinical Evaluative Sciences, Public Health Ontario.

Martel, L. (2013). Mortality: Overview, 2010 and 2011. Report on the Demographic Situation in Canada. Statistics Canada.

7. Statistics Canada (2012). Life expectancy at birth, by sex, by province [Data File]. Retrieved on May 12, 2015.

8. Greenberg, L. & Normandin, C. (2011). Disparities in life expectancy at birth. Health at a Glance, 1. Statistics Canada.

9. Morency, J.D., Caron-Malenfant, E., Coulombe, S., Langlois, S. (2015). Projections of the Aboriginal Population and Households in Canada, 2011 to 2036. Statistics Canada.

10. Statistics Canada (2010). Aboriginal statistics at a glance. Ottawa ON: Statistics Canada.

11. Organisation for Economic Co-operation and Development. (2015). OECD.Stat [Data File].

Low birth weight

In 2013, 24,000 or just over 6% of newborns had a low birth weight.[1]

Low birth weight is defined as a weight of less than 2,500 grams at birth. Being born at a low birth weight increases the risk for short- and long-term impacts on health.[2-6]

OVER TIME

Just over 18,000 or 5.6% of babies born in 2000 and just under 24,000 or 6.3% in 2013 had a low birth weight.[1]

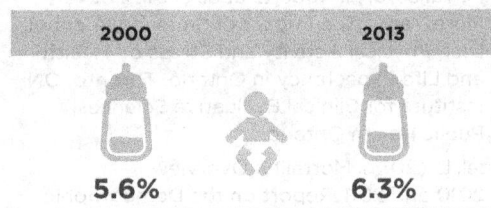

2000	2013
5.6%	6.3%

BY INCOME

National data on low birth weight by income are not available. Data by income are available for pre-term birth and small-for-gestational-age. Pre-term birth and being small for gestational age are conditions associated with low birth weight.[2,3]

In 2006–2007, the proportion of preterm births and babies that were small for their gestational age was higher in low income neighbourhoods than in the highest income neighbourhood.[3]

PRE-TERM BIRTH AND SMALL-FOR-GESTATIONAL-AGE BY NEIGHBOURHOOD INCOME, 2006-2007[3]

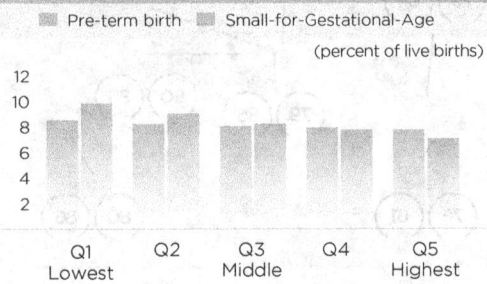

Pre-term birth Small-for-Gestational-Age

(percent of live births)

| | Q1 Lowest | Q2 | Q3 Middle | Q4 | Q5 Highest |

Quintiles (Q) are calculated by dividing the Canadian opulation into five groups of equal size (quintiles) based on neighbourhood income.

BY AGE

A higher proportion of babies with a low birth weight are born to mothers under the age of 20 years and between the ages of 35 to 49 years.[7]

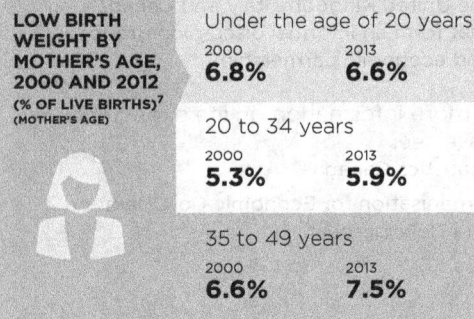

LOW BIRTH WEIGHT BY MOTHER'S AGE, 2000 AND 2012 (% OF LIVE BIRTHS)[7] (MOTHER'S AGE)

	Under the age of 20 years	
	2000	2013
	6.8%	6.6%

	20 to 34 years	
	2000	2013
	5.3%	5.9%

	35 to 49 years	
	2000	2013
	6.6%	7.5%

INDIGENOUS POPULATIONS

Data on low birth weight in Indigenous populations **are not directly comparable** to the data described above.

In First Nations on-reserve in 2008/2010, mothers aged 35 years or older were more likely to report giving birth to a baby with low birth weight than mothers in other age groups.[8]

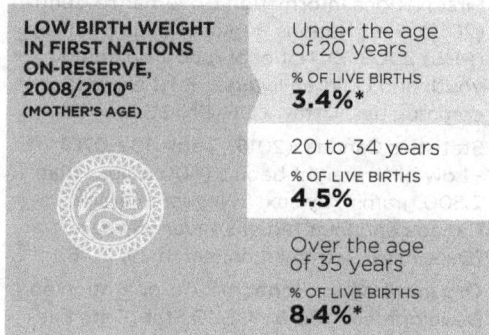

LOW BIRTH WEIGHT IN FIRST NATIONS ON-RESERVE, 2008/2010[8] (MOTHER'S AGE)	Under the age of 20 years % OF LIVE BIRTHS **3.4%*** 20 to 34 years % OF LIVE BIRTHS **4.5%** Over the age of 35 years % OF LIVE BIRTHS **8.4%***

*High sampling variability. Interpret data with caution

In Inuit regions in 2004–2008, the proportion of low birth weights in Nunavut and Nunavik was higher than the overall Canadian population (which included all Inuit regions).[9]

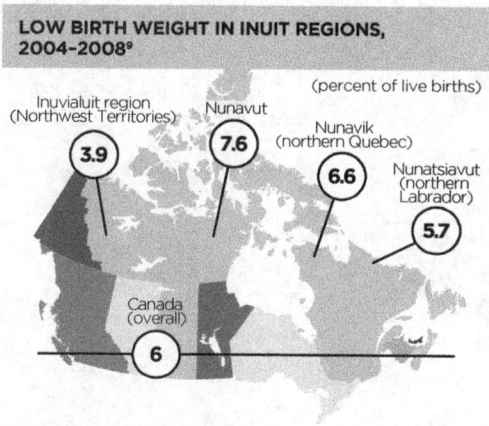

LOW BIRTH WEIGHT IN INUIT REGIONS, 2004-2008[9]

(percent of live births)

Inuvialuit region (Northwest Territories) **3.9**
Nunavut **7.6**
Nunavik (northern Quebec) **6.6**
Nunatsiavut (northern Labrador) **5.7**
Canada (overall) **6**

INTERNATIONAL COMPARISON

In 2011, the proportion of newborns with a low birth weight among G7 countries ranged from 6% to 10%. Canada had the lowest proportion of babies born at a low birth weight at 6%.[10]

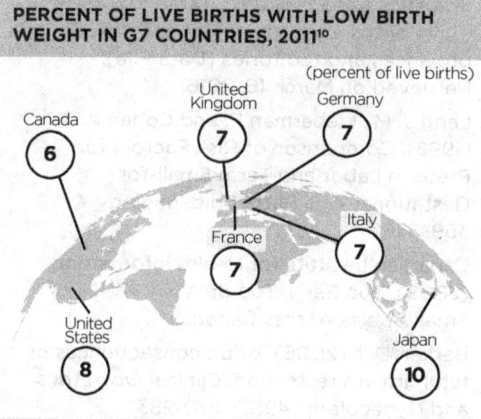

PERCENT OF LIVE BIRTHS WITH LOW BIRTH WEIGHT IN G7 COUNTRIES, 2011[10]

(percent of live births)

Canada **6**
United Kingdom **7**
Germany **7**
France **7**
Italy **7**
United States **8**
Japan **10**

Notes to the reader

- Indigenous populations consist of First Nations, Métis and Inuit.
- Data on First Nations on-reserve are from the First Nations Regional Health Survey (2008/10). Prenatal health data, including information on birth weight, were obtained through the child survey. This survey was completed by the child's primary caregiver.[8]
- G7 countries include seven of the world's industrialized countries, namely the United States, Japan, Germany, France, the United Kingdom, Italy and Canada, that form an informal discussion group and economic partnership.

For more information on children's health and well-being, please see:

- Government of Canada
- Public Health Agency of Canada
- World Health Organization

References

1. Statistics Canada (2016). Table 102-4509 - Live births, by birth weight and sex, Canada, provinces and territories [Data File]. Retrieved on March 16, 2016.

2. Lang J. M., Lieberman E. and Cohen A. A. (1996). Comparison of Risk Factors for Preterm Labor and Term Small-for-Gestational-Age Birth. Epidemiology 7, 369–376.

3. Canadian Institute for Health Information (2009). Too Early, Too Small: A Profile of Small Babies Across Canada.

4. Barker, D.J. (2006). Adult consequences of fetal growth restriction. Clinical Obstetrics and Gynecology, 49(2), 270-283.

5. Barker, D.J. (2007). The original the developmental origins theory. Journal of Internal Medicine, 261(5), 412-417.

6. Calkins, K., Devaskar, S.U. (2011). Fetal origins of adult disease. Current Problems in Pediatric and Adolescent Health Care, 41(6), 158-176.

7. Statistics Canada (2016). Table 102-4511 - Live births, birth weight indicators, by characteristics of the mother and child, Canada (annual) [Data File]. Retrieved on March 16, 2016.

8. First Nations Information Governance Centre (2012). First Nations Regional Health Survey (RHS) 2008/10: National report on adults, youth and children living in First Nations communities. Ottawa ON: FNIGC.

9. Statistics Canada. (2016). Table 102-0701 - Low birth weight babies (500 to less than 2,500 grams), by sex, five-year average, Canada and Inuit regions (every 5 years) [Data File]. Retrieved on March 29, 2016.

10. Organisation for Economic Co-operation and Development. (2015). OECD.Stat [Data File].

Community belonging

In 2014, over 19 million or two thirds of Canadians said they had a somewhat or very strong sense of community belonging.[1]

2 in 3 Canadians said they had a somewhat or very strong sense of community belonging.[1]

SOMEWHAT OR VERY STRONG SENSE OF COMMUNITY BELONGING

2 in 3 Canadians

A sense of community belonging can positively influence a person's long-term physical and mental health.[2-4]

OVER TIME

The proportion of Canadians who consider their sense of community belonging to be somewhat or very strong has remained constant over time.[1]

2003	2014
64%	66%

BY INCOME

In 2014, Canadians living in the lowest income households were less likely to report a somewhat or very strong sense of community belonging than those living in the highest income households.[5]

SENSE OF COMMUNITY BELONGING BY HOUSEHOLD INCOME, 2014[5]

(percent of population)

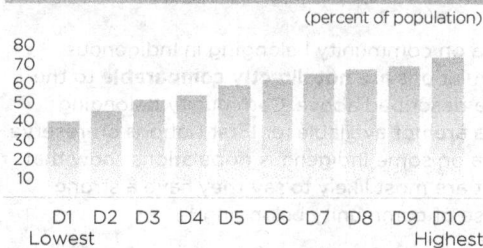

| D1 | D2 | D3 | D4 | D5 | D6 | D7 | D8 | D9 | D10 |
| Lowest | | | | | | | | | Highest |

Deciles (D) are calculated by dividing the Canadian population into ten groups of equal size (deciles) based on household income.

BY SEX

In 2014, 66% of men and 67% of women said they had a somewhat or very strong sense of community belonging.[1]

MEN	WOMEN
66%	67%

BY AGE

Community belonging differs by age. In 2014, younger and older age groups were more likely to say they had a somewhat or very strong sense of community belonging than other age groups. The proportion of Canadians who report a somewhat or very strong sense of community belonging is lowest among those aged 20 to 34 years.[1]

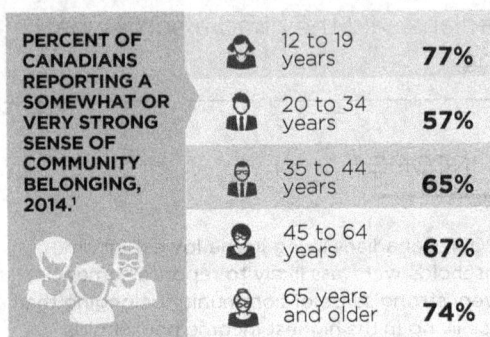

PERCENT OF CANADIANS REPORTING A SOMEWHAT OR VERY STRONG SENSE OF COMMUNITY BELONGING, 2014.[1]		
	12 to 19 years	**77%**
	20 to 34 years	**57%**
	35 to 44 years	**65%**
	45 to 64 years	**67%**
	65 years and older	**74%**

INDIGENOUS POPULATIONS

Data on community belonging in Indigenous populations **are not directly comparable** to the data described above. Community belonging data are not available for First Nations on-reserve. Data on some Indigenous populations show that Inuit are most likely to say they have a strong sense of community belonging.[6]

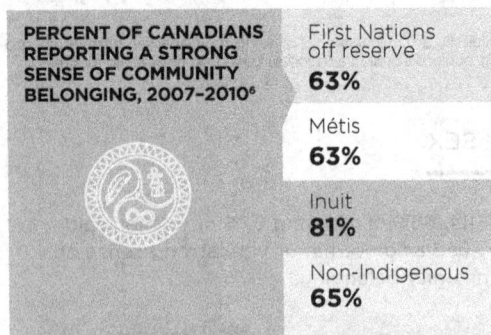

PERCENT OF CANADIANS REPORTING A STRONG SENSE OF COMMUNITY BELONGING, 2007-2010[6]	
	First Nations off reserve **63%**
	Métis **63%**
	Inuit **81%**
	Non-Indigenous **65%**

Data presented in this table are adjusted by age. Indigenous populations tend to be younger than non-Indigenous populations which can affect the ability to compare data across groups.

INTERNATIONAL COMPARISON

Data on community belonging are not collected internationally.

Notes to the reader

- A sense of belonging is based on a person's attachment to and social comfort with their community, friends, family, workplace, or personal interests.[1,2]
- Indigenous populations consist of First Nations, Métis and Inuit.

References

1. Statistics Canada (2016). Table 105-0501 – Health indicator profile, annual estimates, by age group and sex, Canada, provinces, territories, health regions (2013 boundaries) and peer groups, occasional [Data File]. Retrieved on March 30, 2016.

2. Kitchen, P., Williams, A. & Chowhan, J. (2012). Sense of Community Belonging and Health in Canada: A Regional Analysis. Social Indicators Research, 107(1), 103-126.

3. Shields, M. (2008). Community belonging and self-perceived health. Health Reports, 19(2), 1-11.

4. Berkman, L.F., Glass, T. Brissette, I., Seeman, T.E. (2000). From social integration to health: Durkheim in the new millennium. Social Science and Medicine, 51, 843-857.

5. Statistics Canada. Canadian Community Health Survey (2014) [Share Microdata File]. Ottawa, ON: Statistics Canada. All computations on these microdata were prepared by the Public Health Agency of Canada and the responsibility for the use and interpretation of these data is entirely that of the author(s).

6. Gionet, L., Roshananfshar, S. (2013). Select health indicators of First Nations people living off reserve, Métis and Inuit. Health at a Glance, no.82-624-X.

Perceived health

In 2014, 18 million or three in five Canadians said they felt they had very good or excellent health.[1]

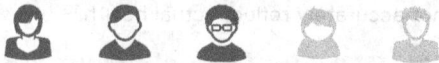

3 in 5 Canadians said they felt they had **very good** or **excellent** health.[1]

HAD VERY GOOD OR EXCELLENT HEALTH

3 in 5 Canadians

Perceived health is a subjective measure of how people feel about their health and can be a good reflection of actual health.[2-4] Health means not only the absence of disease or injury but also physical, mental and social well-being.[1]

OVER TIME

The proportion of Canadians reporting that they felt they had **very good** or **excellent** health has not changed.[1]

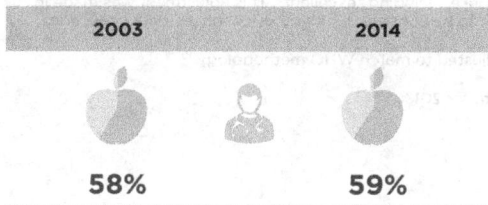

2003	2014
58%	59%

BY INCOME

In 2014, Canadians in the lowest household incomes were less likely to report feeling they had **very good** or **excellent** health than those living in the highest income households.[5]

PERCEPTION OF VERY GOOD OR EXCELLENT HEALTH BY HOUSEHOLD INCOME, 2014[5]

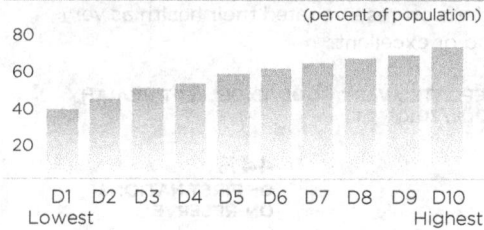

(percent of population)

| D1 | D2 | D3 | D4 | D5 | D6 | D7 | D8 | D9 | D10 |
Lowest   Highest

Deciles (D) are calculated by dividing the Canadian population into ten groups of equal size (deciles) based on household income.

BY SEX

In 2014, the same proportion of men and women rated their health as very good/excellent or fair/poor.[1]

PERCENT OF CANADIAN MEN AND WOMEN REPORTING VERY GOOD/EXCELLENT OR FAIR/POOR HEALTH, 2014[1]

Very good or excellent		Fair or poor	
Men	Women	Men	Women
59%	59%	12%	12%

INDIGENOUS POPULATIONS

Data on perceived health in Indigenous populations **are not directly comparable** to the data described above. In 2008/2010, 44% of First Nations on-reserve rated their health as very good or excellent.[6]

REPORTED VERY GOOD/EXCELLENT HEALTH, 2008/2010[6]

44%
OF FIRST NATIONS ON-RESERVE

In 2007–2010, First Nations off reserve, Métis and Inuit were less likely than non-Indigenous people to report that their health was **very good** or **excellent**.[7]

PERCENT OF CANADIANS REPORTING EXCELLENT/ VERY GOOD HEALTH, 2007-2010[7]	First Nations off reserve	50%
	Métis	54%
	Inuit	55%
	Non-Indigenous	63%

Data presented in this table are adjusted by age. Indigenous populations tend to be younger than non-Indigenous populations which can affect the ability to compare data across groups.

INTERNATIONAL COMPARISON

Perceived health is not measured the same way across all countries, so data were adjusted so that they could be compared. Data presented above represent **very good** or **excellent** health. These data can be reported overtime, by income and by sex. The data below for Canada represent **good**, **very good** and **excellent** health (they include all positive responses) in order to allow for the comparison of perceived health among G7 countries.[8] At 88%, Canada and the United States had the highest proportion of people among G7 countries in 2014 who said that they felt they had good or very good health.[8] It should be noted that perceived health is a subjective measure that can be affected by factors such as culture. This means that for some cultures, perceived health may not accurately reflect actual health.[10]

PERCENT OF PEOPLE REPORTING GOOD/ VERY GOOD* HEALTH IN G7 COUNTRIES, 2014[8]

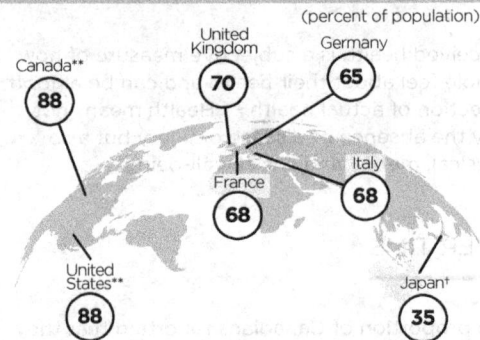

(percent of population)

Canada** 88

United Kingdom 70

Germany 65

France 68

Italy 68

United States** 88

Japan† 35

* For Canada, good/very good data indicate any positive response, including "excellent". This adjustment was made in order to be consistent with other countries' data collection.

**Adjusted to match WHO methodology.[10]

† Data for 2013

Notes to the reader

- To measure perceived health, Canadians 12 years and older were asked if they felt their health was excellent, very good, fair or poor.[1]

- Indigenous populations consist of First Nations, Métis and Inuit.

- G7 countries include seven of the world's industrialized countries, namely the United States, Japan, Germany, France, the United Kingdom, Italy and Canada, that form an informal discussion group and economic partnership.

For more information on health, please see:

- Government of Canada
- Statistics Canada
- World Health Organization

References

1. Statistics Canada (2016). Table 105-0501 - Health indicator profile, annual estimates, by age group and sex, Canada, provinces, territories, health regions (2013 boundaries) and peer groups, occasional [Data File]. Retrieved on March 30, 2016.

2. Shields, M., Shooshtari, S. (2001). Determinants of self-perceived health. Health Reports, 13(1), 35-52.

3. Smith, P.M., Glazier, R.H., Sibley, L.M. (2010). The predictors of self-rate health and the relationship between self-rated health and health service needs are similar across socioeconomic groups in Canada. Journal of Clinical Epidemiology, 63(4), 412-421.

4. Nielsen, T.H. (2015). The relationships between self-rated health and hospital records. Health Economics, 25(4), 497-512.

5. Statistics Canada (2014). Canadian Community Health Survey, 2014 [Share Microdata File]. Ottawa, ON: Statistics Canada. All computations on these microdata were prepared by the Public Health Agency of Canada and the responsibility for the use and interpretation of these data is entirely that of the author(s).

6. First Nations Information Governance Centre (2012). FNIGC Data Online [Data File]. Retrieved on December 3, 2014.

7. Gionet, L., Roshananfshar, S. (2013). Select health indicators of First Nations people living off reserve, Métis and Inuit. Health at a Glance, no.82-624-X.

8. Organisation for Economic Co-operation and Development (2015). OECD.Stat [Data File]. Retrieved on November 12, 2015.

9. Organisation for Economic Co-operation and Development (2016). Health Statistics 2016. Perceived health status. Definitions, Sources and Methods.

10. Jylha, M., Guralink, J.M., Ferrucci, L., Jokela, J., Heikkinen, E. (1998). Is self-rated health comparable across cultures and genders? Journals of Gerontology, Series B, 53B(3), S144-S152.

Perceived mental health

In 2014, 21 million or 7 in 10 Canadians said they felt they had excellent or very good mental health.[1]

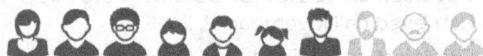

7 in 10 Canadians said they felt they had excellent or very good mental health.[1]

EXCELLENT OR VERY GOOD MENTAL HEALTH

7 in 10 Canadians

Perceived mental health is a subjective measure of how people feel about their mental health and can be a good reflection of actual mental health. Mental health is an important aspect of overall health and well-being.[2-4]

OVER TIME

The proportion of Canadians who consider their mental health to be either very good or excellent has decreased slightly.[1]

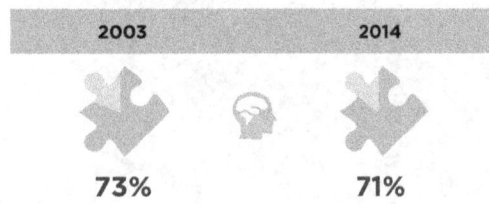

2003	2014
73%	71%

BY INCOME

In 2014, Canadians with the lowest household incomes were less likely than those with the highest income households to report feeling they had very good or excellent perceived mental health.[5]

PERCEPTION OF VERY GOOD OR EXCELLENT MENTAL HEALTH BY HOUSEHOLD INCOME, 2014[5]

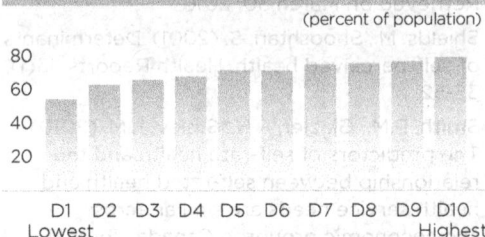

(percent of population)

D1 D2 D3 D4 D5 D6 D7 D8 D9 D10
Lowest   Highest

Deciles (D) are calculated by dividing the Canadian population into ten groups of equal size (deciles) based on household income.

BY SEX

In 2014, 72% of men and 70% of women rated their mental health as very good or excellent.[1]

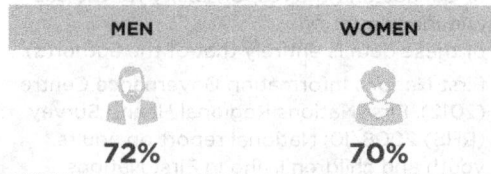

MEN	WOMEN
72%	70%

INDIGENOUS POPULATIONS

Data on perceived mental health in Indigenous populations **are not directly comparable** to the data described above. Data for First Nations on-reserve measured how often people felt they were mentally balanced most or all of the time.[6]

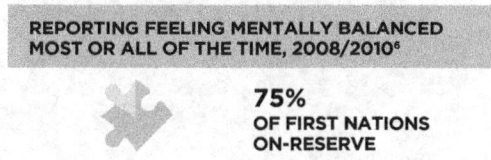

REPORTING FEELING MENTALLY BALANCED MOST OR ALL OF THE TIME, 2008/2010[6]

75%
OF FIRST NATIONS ON-RESERVE

Data on First Nations living off reserve, Métis and Inuit measured how people perceived their mental health. In 2007–2010, Inuit were least likely to rate their mental health as excellent or very good.[7]

PERCENT OF INDIGENOUS PEOPLES REPORTING EXCELLENT/VERY GOOD MENTAL HEALTH, 2007–2010[7]		
	First Nations off reserve	**66%**
	Métis	**67%**
	Inuit	**65%**
	Non-Indigenous	**75%**

Data presented in this table are adjusted by age. Indigenous populations tend to be younger than non-Indigenous populations which can affect the ability to compare data across groups.

INTERNATIONAL COMPARISON

Data on perceived mental health are not collected such that they can be compared across countries.

Notes to the reader
- To measure perceived mental health, Canadians 12 years and older were asked if they felt their health was excellent, very good, fair or poor.[1]
- Indigenous populations consist of First Nations, Métis and Inuit.
- Data on First Nations living on-reserve are from the First Nations Regional Health Survey (2008/10). Self-reported mental balance was measured based on how often people felt mentally balanced ("all of the time," "most of the time," "some of the time" or "none of the time").[8]

For more information on mental health, please see:
- Government of Canada
- Mental Health Commission of Canada

References

1. Statistics Canada. (2016). Table 105-0501 – Health indicator profile, annual estimates, by age group and sex, Canada, provinces, territoies, health regions (2013 boundaries) and peer groups, occasional [Data File]. Retrieved on March 30, 2016.

2. Mental Health Commission of Canada (2012). Changing Directions, Changing Lives: The mental health strategy for Canada. Calgary, AB: Mental Health Commission of Canada.

3. Public Health Agency of Canada (2014). Mental Health Promotion. Retrieved on May 26, 2015.

4. Mawani, F., Gilmour, H. (2010). Validation study on self-rated mental health. Health Reports, 21(3).

5. Statistics Canada (2014). Canadian Community Health Survey, 2014 [Share Microdata File]. Ottawa, ON: Statistics Canada. All computations on these microdata were prepared by the Public Health Agency of Canada and the responsibility for the use and interpretation of these data is entirely that of the author(s).

6. First Nations Information Governance Centre (2012). First Nations Regional Health Survey (RHS) 2008/10: National report on adults, youth and children living in First Nations communities. Ottawa ON: FNIGC.

7. Gionet, L., Roshananfshar, S. (2013). Select health indicators of First Nations people living off reserve, Métis and Inuit. Health at a Glance, no.82-624-X.

8. First Nations Information Governance Centre (2012). FNIGC Data Online [Data File]. Retrieved on December 3, 2014.

What is influencing our health?

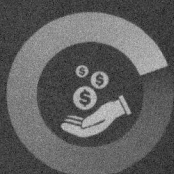

INCOME

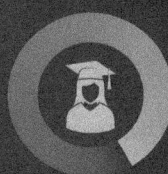

EDUCATION

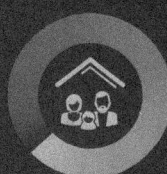

HOUSING

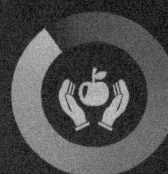

FOOD SECURITY

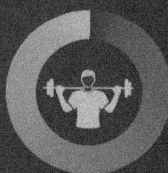

PHYSICAL ACTIVITY

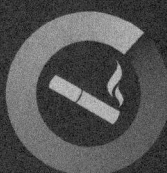

SMOKING

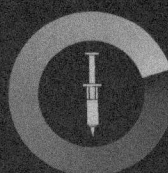

IMMUNIZATION

Income

In 2014, the average household income after taxes was $68,000.[1] Just under 5 million or just over 1 in 10 Canadians were living in low-income households.[2]

Just over 1 in 10 Canadians were living in low-income households.[2]

LIVING IN LOW-INCOME HOUSEHOLDS

just over 1 in 10 Canadians

For this section, low income is considered as any income that is less than half of a country's average income, calculated after taxes and transfers.[2,8] Income influences people's health and is an important predictor of health outcomes, such as life expectancy and risk for some diseases.[3-7]

AVERAGE INCOME (AFTER TAXES) IN THOSE LIVING IN HIGHEST AND LOWEST INCOME LEVELS, 1976–2014[9]

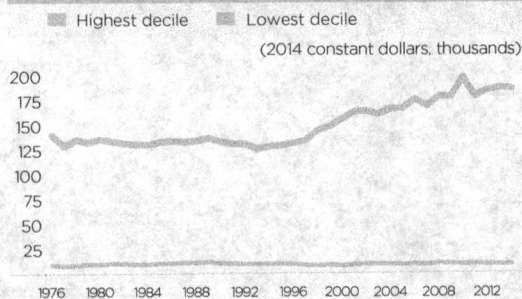

Legend: Highest decile · Lowest decile
(2014 constant dollars, thousands)

Deciles are calculated by dividing the Canadian population into ten groups of equal size (deciles) based on income.

OVER TIME

The proportion of Canadians living in low income has fluctuated from 13% in 1976 to 11% in 1989 and back to 13% in 2014.[8] The gap between those with the highest and lowest incomes has been growing.[9]

BY SEX

In the past, men were less likely to have a low income than women. More recently, men and women were equally likely to have a low income.[2]

PERCENT OF CANADIAN MEN AND WOMEN LIVING WITH A LOW INCOME, 1976 AND 2014[2]

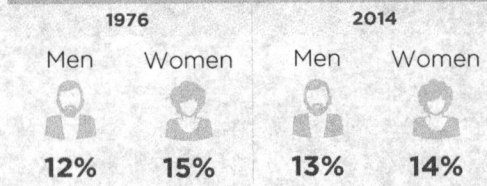

	1976		2014	
	Men	Women	Men	Women
	12%	15%	13%	14%

BY AGE

The proportion of older Canadians who have a low income has decreased from 31% in 1976 to 13% in 2013. Other age groups have seen a slight increase.[2]

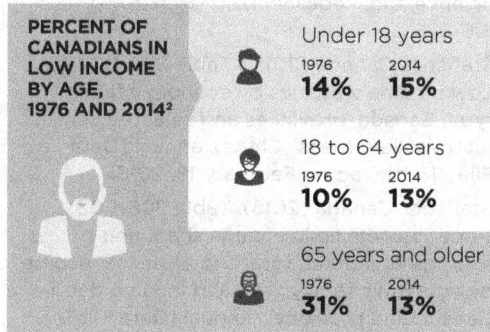

PERCENT OF CANADIANS IN LOW INCOME BY AGE, 1976 AND 2014[2]		
	Under 18 years	
	1976 **14%**	2014 **15%**
	18 to 64 years	
	1976 **10%**	2014 **13%**
	65 years and older	
	1976 **31%**	2014 **13%**

INDIGENOUS POPULATIONS

Data on income in Indigenous populations **are not directly comparable** to the data described above. Comparable data show that Indigenous populations, particularly First Nations at just over 30%, were more likely to have a low income than non-Indigenous populations at just under 15%.[10]

PERCENT OF CANADIANS LIVING IN LOW INCOME, 2011[10]	
First Nations	**30%**
Métis	**20%**
Inuit	**22%**
Total Indigenous	**25%**
Non-Indigenous	**15%**

INTERNATIONAL COMPARISON

In 2013, the proportion of people living in low-income was highest in the United States at just under 18% and lowest in France at 8%. Canada ranked in the middle of G7 countries at just under 13%.[11]

PERCENT OF PEOPLE LIVING IN LOW-INCOME (AFTER TAXES AND TRANSFERS) IN G7 COUNTRIES, 2013[11]

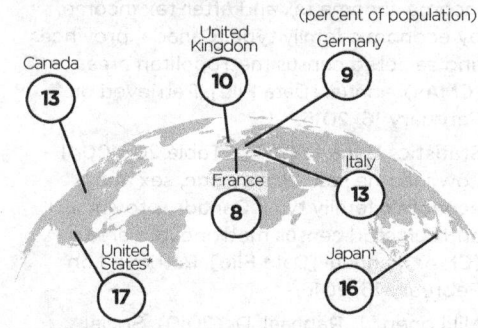

(percent of population)

Canada **13**
United Kingdom **10**
Germany **9**
France **8**
Italy **13**
United States* **17**
Japan† **16**

† data for 2012

For more information on income, please see:
- Statistics Canada
- Organisation for Economic Co-Operation and Development

Notes to the reader
- Indigenous populations consist of First Nations, Métis and Inuit.
- The data on Indigenous populations have not been adjusted for their high cost of living, meaning gaps may not accurately represent reality.
- G7 countries include seven of the world's industrialized countries, namely the United States, Japan, Germany, France, the United Kingdom, Italy and Canada, that form an informal discussion group and economic partnership.

References

1. Statistics Canada (2015). Table 206-0011 – Market income, government transfers, total income, income tax and after-tax income, by economic family type, Canada, provinces and selected census metropolitan areas (CMAs), annual [Data File]. Retrieved on February 16, 2016.

2. Statistics Canada (2015). Table 206-0041 – Low income statistics by age, sex and economic family type, Canada, provinces and selected census metropolitan areas (CMAs), annual [Data File]. Retrieved on February 16, 2016.

3. Mikkonen, J., Raphael, D. (2010). Social Determinants of Health: The Canadian Facts. (Toronto: York University School of Health Policy and Management).

4. Canadian Medical Association. (2013). Canadian Medical Association Submission on Motion 315 (Income Inequality).

5. James, P. D., Wilkins, R., Detsky, A. S., Tugwell, P. et al. (2007). Avoidable mortality by neighbourhood income in Canada: 25 years after the establishment of universal health insurance. Journal of Epidemiology and Community Health, 61(4), 287-296.

6. Lysy, Z., Booth, G. L., Shah, B. R., Austin, P. C. et al. (2013). The impact of income on the incidence of diabetes: A population-base study. Diabetes Research and Clinical Practice, 99(3), 372-379.

7. Pickett, K. E., Wilkinson, R. G. (2015). Income inequality and health: A causal review. Social Science and Medicine, 128(March 2015), 316-326.

8. Statistics Canada (2015). Table 206-0042 – Low income statistics by economic family type, Canada, provinces and selected census metropolitan areas (CMAs), annual [Data File]. Retrieved on February 16, 2016.

9. Statistics Canada (2015). Table 206-0031 – Upper income limit, income share and average of market, total and after-tax income by economic family type and income decile, Canada and provinces, annual [Data File]. Retrieved on February 16, 2016.

10. Statistics Canada (2016). Selected demographic, sociocultural, education and labour characteristics, sex and income status in 2010 for the population in Private Households of Canada, Provinces, Census Metropolitan Areas and Census Agglomerations, 2011 National Household Survey National Household Survey, Statistics Canada Catalogue no. 99-014-X2011043.

11. Organisation for Economic Co-operation and Development (2015). OECD.Stat [Data File]. Retrieved on November 12, 2015.

Education

In 2014, just under 18 million or 90% of Canadians between the ages of 25 to 64 years had completed high school.[1] Just under 13 million or 66% had graduated with a postsecondary certificate or university degree.[1]

90% of Canadians completed high school and 66% graduated with a postsecondary certificate or university degree.[1]

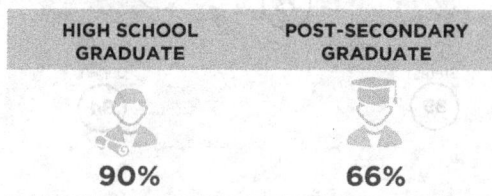

HIGH SCHOOL GRADUATE	POST-SECONDARY GRADUATE
90%	66%

A higher level of education is linked to better health through a variety of factors such as higher income and better health literacy.[2-7]

DID YOU KNOW? In Canada, the ability to read and do math has been getting worse over time.[11,12] In 2012, almost 50% of Canadians aged 25 to 65 years had low scores for literacy skills, 55% had low scores for numeracy skills and 43% had low scores for both.[13]

OVER TIME

The proportion of Canadians aged 25 to 64 years who graduated from high school has been increasing in Canada.[1]

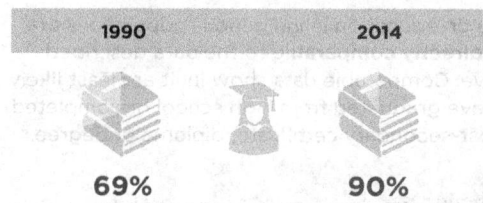

1990	2014
69%	90%

BY INCOME

In 2011, 50% of Canadians in the top 10% income level and 20% of those below that income level had a university degree.[8]

LEVEL OF EDUCATION COMPLETED BY INCOME (HIGHEST LEVEL ACHIEVED), 2011[8]

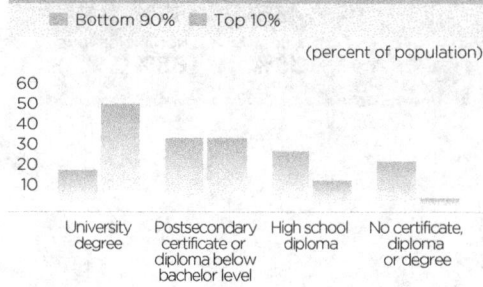

■ Bottom 90% ■ Top 10%

(percent of population)

University degree | Postsecondary certificate or diploma below bachelor level | High school diploma | No certificate, diploma or degree

BY SEX

The proportion of Canadians graduating from a post-secondary institution has increased for both men and women.[1]

PERCENT OF CANADIAN MEN AND WOMEN WHO COMPLETED A POST-SECONDARY CERTIFICATE, DIPLOMA OR DEGREE, 1990 AND 2014[1]

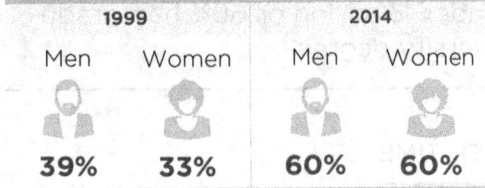

1999		2014	
Men	Women	Men	Women
39%	33%	60%	60%

INDIGENOUS POPULATIONS

Data on education in Indigenous populations **are not directly comparable** to the data described above. Comparable data show Inuit are least likely to have graduated from high school or completed a post-secondary certificate, diploma or degree.[9]

PERCENT OF CANADIANS WHO COMPLETED HIGH SCHOOL OR GRADUATED WITH A POST-SECONDARY CERTIFICATE, DIPLOMA OR DEGREE, 2011[9]

Graduated from high school (or equivalent)

FIRST NATIONS	MÉTIS
67%	79%
INUIT	NON-INDIGENOUS
52%	88%

Completed a post-secondary certificate, diploma or degree

FIRST NATIONS	MÉTIS
45%	55%
INUIT	NON-INDIGENOUS
36%	65%

INTERNATIONAL COMPARISON

In 2012, 89% of Canadians completed high school, which is the same proportion as in the United States. This is the second highest among G7 countries, after Japan, where the proportion of people completing high school was 94%.[10]

PERCENT OF PEOPLE WHO GRADUATED FROM HIGH SCHOOL IN G7 COUNTRIES, 2012[10]

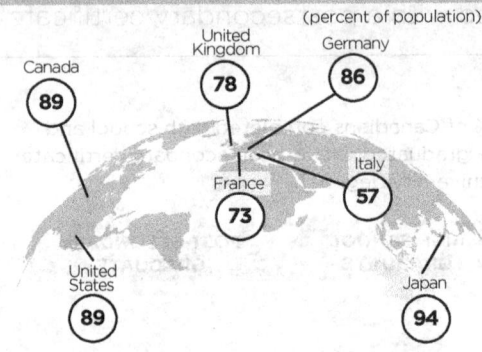

(percent of population)

Canada 89
United Kingdom 78
Germany 86
France 73
Italy 57
United States 89
Japan 94

Notes to the reader
- High school graduates include people who have received a high school diploma or, in Quebec, completed Secondary V or, in Newfoundland and Labrador, completed fourth year of secondary.[1]
- Post-secondary graduates include people who have completed, at minimum, a certificate (including a trade certificate) or diploma from an educational institution beyond the secondary level. This includes certificates from vocational schools, apprenticeship training, community college, Collège d'Enseignement Général et Professionnel (CEGEP), and schools of nursing. Also included are certificates below a bachelor's degree obtained at a university.[1]
- Indigenous populations consist of First Nations, Métis and Inuit.

- For international comparisons, educational attainment represents the number of adults aged 25 to 64 holding at least an upper secondary degree over the population of the same age, as defined by the OECD-ISCED classification.[10]
- G7 countries include seven of the world's industrialized countries, namely the United States, Japan, Germany, France, the United Kingdom, Italy and Canada, that form an informal discussion group and economic partnership.

For more information on education, please see:
- Statistics Canada
- Organisation for Economic Co-Operation and Development

References

1. Statistics Canada (2016). Table 282-0004 - Labour force survey estimates (LFS), by educational attainment, sex and age group, annual (persons unless otherwise noted) [Data File]. Retrieved on February 18, 2016.

2. Mikkonen, J., Raphael, D. (2010). Social Determinants of Health: The Canadian Facts. Toronto, ON: York University School of Health Policy and Management).

3. Feinstein, L., Sabates, R., Anderson, T. M., Sorhaindo, A. et al. (2006). What are the effects of education on health? In Measuring the Effects of Education on Health and Civic Engagement, (pp. 171-382). Copenhagen: Organisation for Economic Co-Operation and Development.

4. World Health Organization (2003). Social Determinants of Health. The Solid Facts, 2nd Edition.

5. Gan, L., Gong, G. (2007). Estimating interdependence between health and education in a dynamic model. NBer Working Paper Series, Working Paper 12830.

6. Cutler, D. M., Lleras-Muney, A. (2006). Education and Health: Evaluating Theories and Evidence. NBer Working Paper Series, Working Paper 12352.

7. Grossman, M., Kaestner, R. (1997). Effects of Education on Health. In The Social Benefits of Education, (pp. 69-124). [Behrman, J.R, Stacey, N. (Eds.)]. Ann Arbor: University of Michigan Press.

8. Statistics Canada (2015) Education and occupation of high-income Canadians. Statistics Canada, NHS in Brief, catalogue no. 99-014-X2011003.

9. Statistics Canada (2015). Aboriginal statistics at a glance: 2nd edition. Ottawa ON: Statistics Canada

10. Organisation for Economic Co-operation and Development (2015). OECD.Stat [Data File]. Retrieved on November 12, 2015.

11. Government of Canada, Council of Ministers of Education (2013). Skills in Canada – First Results from the Programme for the International Assessment of Adult Competencies (PIAAC).

12. Organisation for Economic Co-Operation and Development (2013). OECD Skills Outlook 2013: First Results from the Survey of Adult Skills.

13. Statistics Canada (2014). University graduates with lower levels of literacy and numeracy skills Insights on Canadian Society, Catalogue no. 75-006-X.

Housing

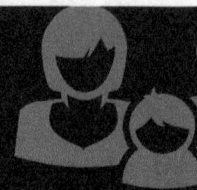

In 2011, almost 2 million or just over 1 in 10 Canadian households reported living in core housing need.[1]

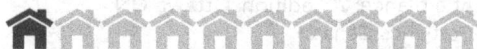

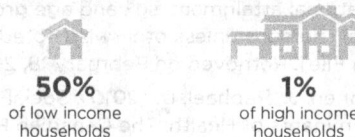

Just over 1 in 10 Canadian households reported living in core housing need.[1]

LIVING IN CORE HOUSING NEED

1 in 10 Canadian households

Poor housing conditions have been linked to poor health and well-being, as well as increased stress and feelings of vulnerability.[2-5] Core housing need is an indicator that measures whether or not Canadians are living in a house that meets Canada Mortgage and Housing Corporation (CMHC)'s housing standards. This includes not meeting at least one standard that assesses adequacy (e.g., does it need repairs?), affordability (e.g., how much does it cost?) or suitability (e.g., does it have enough bedrooms for the number and types of occupants?).[1]

OVER TIME

The proportion of Canadian households in core housing need has remained unchanged.[1]

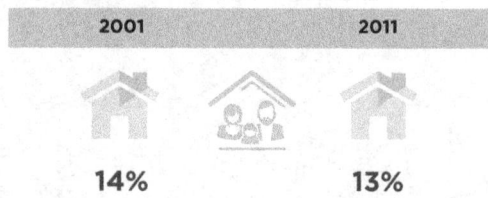

2001	2011
14%	13%

BY INCOME

In 2011, 50% of low income households and less than 1% of high income households were in core housing need.[6]

IN CORE HOUSING NEED

50%	1%
of low income households	of high income households

BY SUBPOPULATION

In 2011, the proportion of Canadians in core housing need differed by sub-population:[6]

- 29% of single parent households where the parent was a woman;
- 27% of people who were renting a place;
- 24% of single woman households;
- 19% of Indigenous households;
- 17% of immigrant households;
- 15% of households whose primary maintainer was between the ages of 15 to 29 years, and;
- 14% of senior households.

INDIGENOUS POPULATIONS

Generally, Indigenous populations have higher rates of core housing need.[1,6-8] Almost 100,000 or 19% of Indigenous households were in core housing need in 2011 compared to 12% of non-Indigenous households.[6]

PERCENT OF HOUSEHOLDS IN CORE HOUSING NEED, 2011[6]	First Nations Status Indian	23%
	First Nations Non-Status Indian	19%
	Métis	15%
	Inuit	34%
	Indigenous (overall)	19%
	Non-Indigenous	12%
	Canada (overall)	13%

For First Nations on-reserve, the definition of housing need differs from CMHC's definition in that it does not include the need to meet affordability standards. **This means the data above are not comparable to the data presented below.** Based on this definition, First Nations on-reserve were more likely to be in core housing need than the overall Canadian population.[8]

PERCENT OF HOUSEHOLDS IN CORE HOUSING NEED, 2011[8]	First Nations on-reserve	33%
	Canada (overall)	4%

INTERNATIONAL COMPARISON

Data on housing are not collected such that they can be compared across countries.

Notes to the reader
- The primary household maintainer is the person in the household responsible for major household payments such as the rent or mortgage.[6]
- Indigenous populations consist of First Nations, Métis and Inuit.

For more information on housing, please see:
- Canada Mortgage and Housing Corporation

References
1. Canada Mortgage and Housing Corporation (2015). Housing in Canada Online (HICO) [Data File]. Retrieved on May 28, 2015.
2. Dunn, J. R., Hayes, M. V., Hulchanski, J. D., Hwang, S. W. et al. (2006). Housing as a socio-economic determinant of health: findings of a national needs, gaps and opportunities assessment. Canadian Journal of Public Health, 97 (Supplement 3), S11-S15.
3. Krieger, J., Higgins, D. L. (2002). Housing and health: time again for public health action. American Journal of Public Health, 92(5), 758-768.
4. Mikkonen, J., Raphael, D. (2010). Social Determinants of Health: The Canadian Facts. Toronto ON: York University School of Health Policy and Management.
5. Waterston, S., Grueger, B., Samson, L., Canadian Paediatric Society. (2015). Housing need in Canada: Healthy lives start at home. Canadian Paediatric Society, 20(7), 403-407.
6. Canada Mortgage and Housing Corporation (2014). Canadian Housing Observer, 2014. Canada: Canada Mortgage and Housing Corporation.
7. Shewchuk, S., Prentice, J. (2015). 2011 Census/National Household Survey Housing Condition Series: Issue 5 Inuit Households in Canada.
8. Prentice, J. (2016). 2011 Census/National Household Survey Housing Condition Series: Issue 8 – Housing Conditions of On-Reserve Aboriginal Households.

Food insecurity

In 2011–2012, more than 1 million or just under 1 in 10 Canadian households were living with moderate to severe food insecurity.[1]

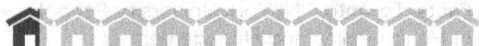

Just under 1 in 10 Canadian households were living with moderate to severe food insecurity.[1]

LIVING WITH MODERATE TO SEVERE FOOD INSECURITY

Just under 1 in 10 Canadian households

Food plays a key role in health and well-being and is a basic human need.[2,3] Food insecurity means not having physical and economic access to enough safe, affordable and nutritious food to meet dietary needs and food preferences for an active and healthy life.[4,5] Parents in food-insecure households may forgo food to ensure their children are fed.[6]

DID YOU KNOW? Food safety is also an important issue. An estimated 4 million Canadians suffer from food-related illnesses every year, with 11,600 hospitalizations and 238 deaths associated with these illnesses.[14]

OVER TIME

From 2007–2008 to 2011–2012, the proportion of Canadian households living with food insecurity remained unchanged at 8%.[1]

BY INCOME

In 2011–2012, 31% of the lowest income households and less than 1% of the highest income households had moderate to severe household food insecurity.[7,8] 21% of households using government benefits as their main source of income and 6% of households with other main sources of income were food insecure.[9]

INDIGENOUS POPULATIONS

Data on food insecurity in Indigenous populations **are not directly comparable** to the data described above. In 2008/2010, 54% First Nations on-reserve households reported being either moderately or severely food insecure.[10]

PERCENT OF FIRST NATIONS ON-RESERVE HOUSEHOLDS WITH MODERATE OR SEVERE FOOD INSECURITY, 2008/2010[10]	Moderately food insecure **40%**
	Severely food insecure **14%**

Food insecurity is significantly higher in Indigenous households. In 2007–2010, 27% of Inuit households reported having low to very low food security.[11] Other surveys suggest that rates of food insecurity in Inuit households may be even higher, reaching over 62%.[12,13]

PERCENT OF HOUSEHOLDS WITH LOW TO VERY LOW FOOD SECURITY, 2007–2010[11]		
First Nations off reserve	**22%**
Métis	**15%**
Inuit	**27%**
Non-Indigenous	**7%**

Data presented in this table are adjusted by age. Indigenous populations tend to be younger than non-Indigenous populations which can affect the ability to compare data across groups.

INTERNATIONAL COMPARISON

Food insecurity is not collected in a systematic fashion for industrialized countries. The United Nations and other international organizations regularly monitor food insecurity in developing regions and countries.[15]

Notes to the reader
• Food insecurity is defined as whether or not households are able to afford the food they need. According to Statistics Canada, levels of food security are defined as: food secure—no difficulty with food access; moderately food insecure—some compromise in quality and/or quantity of food consumed; severely food insecure—food intake is reduced and eating patterns disrupted.
• Indigenous populations consist of First Nations, Métis and Inuit.

For more information on food and health, please see:
• Canada's Food Guide
• Public Health Agency of Canada
• United Nations

References
1. Statistics Canada (2013). Table 105-0546 - Household food insecurity measures, by presence of children in the household, Canada, provinces and territories, occasional (number unless otherwise noted) [Data File]. Retrieved on November 20, 2014.
2. Agudo, A. (2005). Measuring intake of fruit and vegetables. World Health Organization.
3. World Health Organization (2004). Global Strategy on Diet, Physical Activity and Health. World Health Organization.
4. United Nations (1996). Rome Declaration on World Food Security. Retrieved on December 2, 2014.
5. Seligman, H. K., Laraia, B. A., Kushel, M. B. (2010). Food Insecurity is Associated with Chronic Disease among Low-Income NHANES Participants. The Journal of Nutrition, 140(2), 304-310.
6. McIntyre, L., Glanville, N.T., Raine, K.D., Dayle, J.B., et al. (2003). Do low-income lone mothers compromise their nutrition to feed their children? Canadian Medical Association Journal, 168(6), 686-691.
7. Statistics Canada. Canadian Community Health Survey (2011). [Share Microdata File]. Ottawa, ON: Statistics Canada. All computations on these microdata were prepared by the Public Health Agency of Canada and the responsibility for the use and interpretation of these data is entirely that of the author(s).
8. Statistics Canada. Canadian Community Health Survey (2012). [Share Microdata File]. Ottawa, ON: Statistics Canada. All computations on these microdata were prepared by the Public Health Agency of Canada and the responsibility for the use and interpretation of these data is entirely that of the author(s).
9. Roshanafshar, S., Hawkins, E. (2015). Food insecurity in Canada. Statistics Canada, Health at a Glance. Catalogue no. 82-624-X.
10. First Nations Information Governance Centre (2015). FNIGC Data Online [Data File]. Retrieved on March 30, 2016.
11. Gionet, L., Roshananfshar, S. (2013). Select health indicators of First Nations people living off reserve, Métis and Inuit. Health at a Glance, no.82-624-X.

12. Huet, C., Rosol, R., Egeland, G.M. (2012). The prevalence of food insecurity is high and the diet quality poor in Inuit communities. Journal of Nutrition, 142(3), 541-547.

13. Egeland, G.M., Pacey, A., Cao, Z., Sobol, I. (2010). Food insecurity among Inuit pre-schoolers: Nunavut Inuit Child Health Survey, 2007–2008. Canadian Medical Association Journal, 182(3), 243-248.

14. Thomas, M.K., Murray, R., Flockhart, L., Pintar, K., Fazil, A., Nesbitt, A., Marshall, B., Tatryn, J., Pollari, F. (2015). Estimates of foodborne illness-related hospitalizations and deaths in Canada for 30 specified pathogens and unspecified agents. Foodborne pathogens and disease, 12(10), 820-827.

15. United Nations (2015). The State of Food Insecurity in the World 2015. Meeting the 2015 international hunger targets: taking stock of uneven progress. Rome, FAO.

Physical activity

In 2013, just over 2 in 10 adults and 1 in 10 children and youth met the Canadian Physical Activity Guidelines.[1]

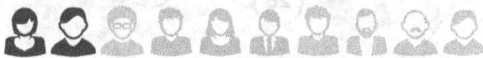

Just over 2 in 10 adults and 1 in 10 children and youth met the Canadian Physical Activity Guidelines.[1]

MET THE CANADIAN PHYSICAL ACTIVITY GUIDELINES

2 in 10 Canadian Adults

1 in 10 Canadian Children and Youth

Physical activity can improve health, lower the risk for many chronic health conditions and contribute to the healthy development of children and youth.[2-5] Physical activity can be measured in many different ways which can make it challenging to report on. In this section, physical activity is measured based on comparisons to the Canadian Physical Activity Guidelines, energy expenditures and amounts of physical activity per day or week.

DID YOU KNOW? Individuals who meet the recommended guidelines for physical activity can still be at risk for developing poor health if a significant amount of their waking hours are spent not being active.[11, 12]

OVER TIME

Data on physical activity related to the Canadian Physical Activity Guidelines are only available for 2009, 2011 and 2013. While rates have fluctuated, there is no evident trend yet.[1]

BY AGE AND SEX

In 2013, the proportion of people who met the Canadian Physical Activity Guidelines differs by age and sex. It is important to note that different age groups have different guidelines.[1]

PERCENT OF CANADIANS MEETING THE CANADIAN PHYSICAL ACTIVITY GUIDELINES BY AGE AND SEX, 2013[1]

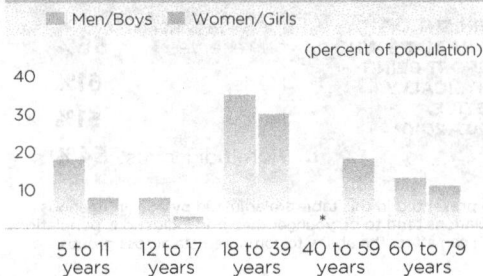

■ Men/Boys   ■ Women/Girls

(percent of population)

40
30
20
10

5 to 11 years | 12 to 17 years | 18 to 39 years | 40 to 59 years | 60 to 79 years

* too unreliable to report

BY INCOME

In 2005, Canadians with a personal income of over $60,000 spent 9% of their leisure time being active while Canadians with a personal income below $30,000 spent 7% of their leisure time being active.[6]

INDIGENOUS POPULATIONS

Data on physical activity in Indigenous populations **are not directly comparable** to the data described above as they are not measured against the Canadian Physical Activity Guidelines and were collected in a different manner. In 2008/2010, First Nations on-reserve were asked about their levels of activity.[7]

- 62% of children aged 6 to 11 years were considered active.
- 49% of youth aged 12 to 17 years were considered active.
- 25% of adults aged 18 years and older were considered active.

In 2007–2010, First Nations off reserve and Métis were more likely to report being active during their leisure time than other groups.[8]

PERCENT OF CANADIANS WHO REPORT BEING PHYSICALLY ACTIVE, 2007–2010[8]		
First Nations off reserve	**56%**
Métis	**61%**
Inuit	**51%**
Non-Indigenous	**54%**

Data presented in this table are adjusted by age. Indigenous populations tend to be younger than non-Indigenous populations which can affect the ability to compare data across groups.

INTERNATIONAL COMPARISON

International comparisons are based on **inactivity** rather than meeting/not meeting specific guidelines. In 2010, Canada ranked as the second least inactive country for people 18 years and older and for youth ages 11 to 17.[9] Different age groups had different definitions of inactivity.[9]

PERCENT OF PEOPLE WHO ARE INACTIVE IN G7 COUNTRIES, 2010[9]
Adults 18 years and older

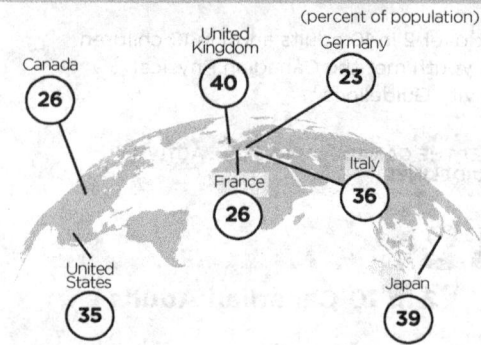

(percent of population)

Canada 26
United Kingdom 40
Germany 23
France 26
Italy 36
United States 35
Japan 39

PERCENT OF PEOPLE WHO ARE INACTIVE IN G7 COUNTRIES, 2010[9]
Youth 12 to 17 years

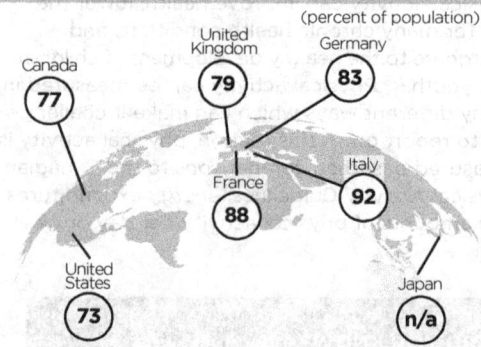

(percent of population)

Canada 77
United Kingdom 79
Germany 83
France 88
Italy 92
United States 73
Japan (n/a)

Notes to the reader

- For the data reported above, meeting <u>Canada's Physical Activity Guidelines</u> is defined as follows: Children and youth (5 to 17 years) should do at least 60 minutes of moderate-to-vigorous activity every day. Adults (18 to 79 years) should do at least 150 minutes of moderate-to-vigorous activity per week in periods of activity that are at least 10 minutes long.[1]

- <u>Indigenous populations</u> consist of First Nations, Métis and Inuit.

- Data on First Nations living on-reserve are from the First Nations Regional Health Survey (2008/10). People were asked to report the frequency and duration of physical activities they had undertaken in the previous year. These activities were reported as a metabolic equivalent value.[13] For all age groups, those with energy expenditures of less than 1.5 kcal/kg/day were considered to be inactive; those with energy expenditures between 1.5 kcal/kg/day and 2.9 kcal/kg/day were considered to be moderately active; and those with energy expenditures of 3 kcal/kg/day or greater were considered to be active.[7]

- Data on First Nations living off-reserve, Métis and Inuit are from Statistics Canada's Canadian Community Health Survey. People were considered to be physically active if they had an average energy expenditure of 3 kcal/kg/day or more, moderately active if they had an average energy expenditure of 1.5-2.9 kcal/kg/day and inactive if they had an average energy expenditure of less than 1.5 kcal/kg/day.[8]

- <u>G7 countries</u> include seven of the world's industrialized countries, namely the United States, Japan, Germany, France, the United Kingdom, Italy and Canada, that form an informal discussion group and economic partnership.

- Internationally, inactvity was measured as less than 150 minutes of moderate intensity or 75 minutes of vigorous-intensity physical activity per week for adults 18 years or older; and less than 60 minutes of moderate- to vigourous-intensity physical activity daily for ages 11 to 17 years.[10]

For more information on physical activity, please see:

- <u>Canadian Physical Activity Guidelines</u>
- <u>World Health Organization</u>

References

1. Statistics Canada (2015). Table 117-0019 – Distribution of the household population meeting/not meeting the Canadian physical activity guidelines, by sex and age group, occasional (percentage) [Data File]. Retrieved on May 26, 2015.

2. Statistics Canada (2015). Directly measured physical activity of adults, 2012 and 2013. Retrieved on October 7, 2015.

3. Canadian Society for Exercise Physiology. (2012). Canadian Physical Activity Guidelines - Scientific Statements.

4. Statistics Canada (2015). Directly measured physical activity of children and youth, 2012 and 2013. Retrieved on March 23, 2015.

5. Janssen, I., Leblanc, A. G. (2010). A systematic review of the health benefits of physical activity and fitness in school-aged children and youth. International Journal of Behavioral Nutrition and Physical Activity, 7(40).

6. Hurst, M. (2007). Who participates in active leisure? Health Reports, Vol. 18, No. 3, Statistics Canada, Catalogue 82-003.

7. First Nations Information Governance Centre (2012). First Nations Regional Health Survey (RHS) 2008/10: National report on adults, youth and children living in First Nations communities. Ottawa ON: FNIGC.

8. Gionet, L., Roshananfshar, S. (2013). Select health indicators of First Nations people living off reserve, Métis and Inuit. Health at a Glance, no.82-624-X.

9. World Health Organization (2015). Global Health Observatory Data Repository [Data File]. Retrieved on November 19, 2015.

10. World Health Organization (2011). WHO Indicator and Measurement Registry. version 1.7.0.

11. Tremblay, M. S., Colley, R. C., Saunders, T. J., Healy, G. N. et al. (2010). Physiological and health implications of a sedentary lifestyle. Applied Physiology, Nutrition, and Metabolism, 35(6), 725-740.

12. Canadian Society for Exercise Physiology. (n.d.). Canadian Physical Activity Guidelines and Canadian Sedentary Behaviour Guidelines. Retrieved on May 7, 2015.

13. Ainsworth, B. E., Haskell, W. L., Whitt, M. C., Irwin, M. L., Swartz, A. M., Strath, S.J., O'Brien W.L., Basser D.R., Jr., Schmitz K.H., Emplaincourt P.O., Jacobs, D.R., Jr., Leon, A. S. (2000). Compendium of physical activities: An update of activity codes and MET intensities. Medicine & Science in Sports & Exercise, 32(Supplement 9), S498–504

Smoking

In 2015, just under 4 million or just over 1 in 10 Canadians smoked regularly or occasionally.[1]

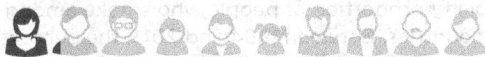

Just over 1 in 10 Canadians smoked regularly or occasionally.[1]

SMOKED REGULARLY OR OCCASIONALLY

Just over 1 in 10 Canadians

Canadians who smoked daily consumed an average of 14 cigarettes a day.[1]

Smoking is a leading cause of preventable disease and premature death. Both smoking and exposure to second-hand smoke have been linked to a number of cardiovascular and respiratory diseases and other chronic conditions.[3-7]

DID YOU KNOW? More Canadians are trying e-cigarettes. In 2015, approximately 3.9 million or 13% of Canadians 15 years and older had tried e-cigarettes compared to 2.5 million or 9% in 2013.[1,2] Young adults are most likely to try e-cigarettes with 31% or 734,000 Canadians aged 20 to 24 years saying they tried them in 2015.[1,2]

OVER TIME, BY SEX

In 1999, 25% of Canadians 15 years and older were daily or occasional smokers. By 2015, this had dropped to 13%.[1,8] In 2015, 16% of men and 10% of women were current smokers.[1] Men smoked an average of 15 cigarettes per day while women smoked 12.[1]

PERCENT OF CANADIANS WHO SMOKED (DAILY OR OCCASIONAL) BY SEX, 1985 TO 2015[1,2,8,9]

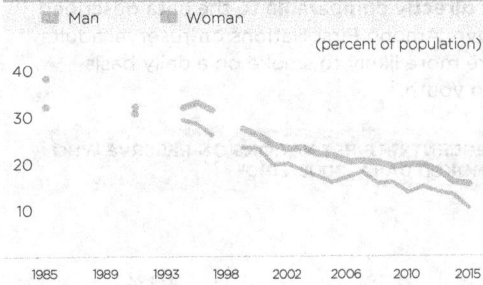

Man   Woman

(percent of population)

40

30

20

10

1985 1989 1993 1998 2002 2006 2010 2015

Data on smoking have not been collected every year since 1985. There are differences in the methods used to collect data and how questions were asked in surveys over this period. Caution should be used when interpreting these results.

BY INCOME

In 2013, 27% of people living in the lowest-income households and 14% of people living in the highest-income households said they smoked.[10]

BY AGE

In 2015, young adults were most likely to smoke compared to other age groups.[1,2] Only adults aged 25 years and older have were less likely to smoke in 2015 than in 2013.[1,2]

PERCENT OF CANADIANS WHO WERE CURRENT SMOKERS, 2013 AND 2015[1,2]

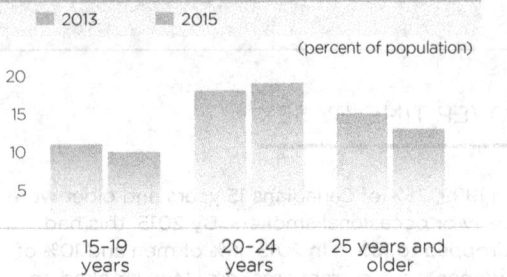

■ 2013   ■ 2015

(percent of population)

| 15-19 years | 20-24 years | 25 years and older |

INDIGENOUS POPULATIONS

Data on smoking in Indigenous populations **are not directly comparable** to the data described above. Among First Nations on-reserve, adults were more likely to smoke on a daily basis than youth.[11]

PERCENT OF FIRST NATIONS ON-RESERVE WHO SMOKED DAILY, 2008/2010[11]

43%
18 years

20%
12 to 17 years

In 2007–2010, Indigenous peoples were more likely to say they smoked daily or occasionally than non-Indigenous people.[12]

PERCENT OF CANADIANS WHO SMOKED DAILY OR OCCASIONALLY, 2007-2010[12]	First Nations off reserve	40%
	Métis	36%
	Inuit	48%
	Non-Indigenous	21%

Data presented in this table are adjusted by age. Indigenous populations tend to be younger than non-Indigenous populations which can affect the ability to compare data across groups.

INTERNATIONAL COMPARISON

Canada continues to have the second lowest smoking proportion of people who smoke among G7 countries. Between 1994 and 2013, the percent of people who smoked daily decreased by 45% in Canada compared to a reduction of 39% in the United States and that of 20% in France.[13]

PERCENT OF PEOPLE WHO SMOKED DAILY IN G7 COUNTRIES, 1994 AND 2014[13]

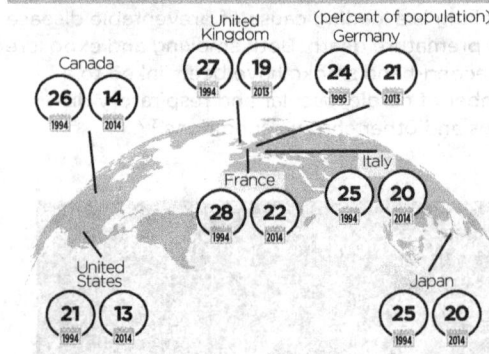

(percent of population)

Canada: 26 (1994), 14 (2014)
United Kingdom: 27 (1994), 19 (2013)
Germany: 24 (1995), 21 (2013)
Italy: 25 (1994), 20 (2014)
France: 28 (1994), 22 (2014)
United States: 21 (1994), 13 (2014)
Japan: 25 (1994), 20 (2014)

Notes to the reader

- Data on smoking are measured among Canadians aged 15 years and over who have identified themselves as current smoker (either daily smokers or occasional smokers).[1]

- Indigenous populations consist of First Nations, Métis and Inuit.

- G7 countries include seven of the world's industrialized countries, namely the United States, Japan, Germany, France, the United Kingdom, Italy and Canada, that form an informal discussion group and economic partnership.

For more information on smoking, please see:

- Government of Canada
- Canadian Tobacco, Alcohol and Drugs Survey
- World Health Organization

References

1. Government of Canada (2016). Table 1. Smoking status and average number of cigarettes smoked per day, by age group and sex, 2015 [Data File]. Retrieved on November 9, 2016.

2. Government of Canada (2015). Table 1. Smoking status and average number of cigarettes smoked per day, by age group and sex, 2013 [Data File]. Retrieved on March 31, 2016.

3. Rehm, J., Baliunas, D., Brochu, S., Fischer, B. et al. (2006). The Costs of Substance Abuse in Canada, 2002. Highlights. Ottawa ON: Canadian Centre on Substance Abuse.

4. Baliunas, D., Patra, J., Rehm, J., Popova, S. et al. (2007). Smoking-attributable mortality and expected years of life lost in Canada 2002: Conclusions for prevention and policy. Chronic Diseases in Canada, 27(4), 154-162.

5. United States Department of Health and Human Services (2014). The Health Consequences of Smoking-50 Years of Progress.
A Report of the Surgeon General. Atlanta: Centers for Disease Control and Prevention, Coordinating Center for Health Promotion, National Center for Chronic Disease Prevention and Health Promotion, Office on Smoking and Health, United States Department of Health and Human Services.

6. Kroon, L. A. (2007). Drugs interactions with smoking. American Journal of Health-System Pharmacy, 64(18), 1917-1921.

7. New South Wales Health (2012). Medication interactions with smoking and smoking cessation.

8. Health Canada (2013). Overview of Historical Data, 1999-2012. Table 1 – Percentage of current smokers, by age group and sex, age 15+ years, Canada 1999 to 2012 [Data File]. Retrieved on December 3, 2014.

9. Gilmore, J. (2000). Report on Smoking Prevalence in Canada, 1985 to 1999. Ottawa ON: Statistics Canada.

10. Statistics Canada (2013). Canadian Community Health Survey, 2013 [Share Microdata File]. Ottawa, ON: Statistics Canada. All computations on these microdata were prepared by the Public Health Agency of Canada and the responsibility for the use and interpretation of these data is entirely that of the author(s).

11. First Nations Information Governance Centre (2012). First Nations Regional Health Survey (RHS) 2008/10: National report on adults, youth and children living in First Nations communities. Ottawa ON: FNIGC.

12. Gionet, L., Roshananfshar, S. (2013). Select health indicators of First Nations people living off reserve, Métis and Inuit. Health at a Glance, no.82-624-X

13. Organisation for Economic Co-operation and Development. (2015). OECD.Stat [Data File]. Retrieved on November 12, 2015.

Immunization

In 2013, 90% of two year old children had received one dose for measles and 77% had received the recommended four doses of vaccine against diphtheria, pertussis (whooping cough), and tetanus (the DPT vaccine).[1] Among seven-year olds, 86% had received the recommended two doses of measles-containing vaccine and 71% had received five doses of the DPT vaccine.[1]

Immunization is one of the greatest public health successes. High immunization rates are important for preventing disease, particularly in those who are most vulnerable such as the very old and the very young.[1] Analysing data on immunization coverage in Canada is challenging because there are large differences in how data are collected.[2] To date, immunization data represent a best available estimate.

DID YOU KNOW? In 2014, 80% of Canadian adults believed that they have received all of the vaccines required for someone their age, but only 6% had the recommended number of pertussis and tetanus vaccine doses in adulthood.[3]

OVER TIME

The proportion of children being vaccinated has remained below national immunization coverage goals of 97% by age two.[1]

PERCENT OF CHILDREN BEING VACCINATED, 2006–2013[1]
Measles vaccine

■ 2 year old   ■ 7 year old

(percent of children)

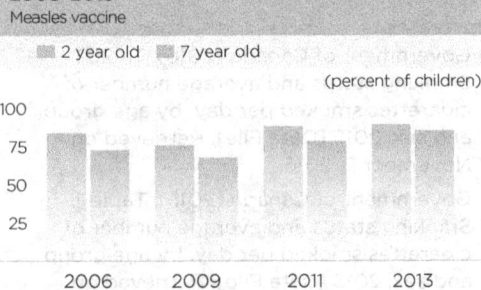

PERCENT OF CHILDREN BEING VACCINATED, 2006–2013[1]
DPT vaccine

■ 2 year old   ■ 7 year old

(percent of children)

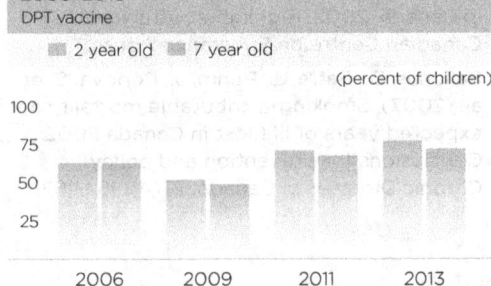

The methods used to estimate immunization coverage have improved over time. Because of significant changes beginning in 2011, **data over time are not directly comparable**.

BY INCOME

National data on immunization rates by income are not available.

INDIGENOUS POPULATIONS

Immunization data have not been reported at a national level for Indigenous populations. Data from program evaluations for Health Canada's First Nations and Inuit Health Branch from 2008 to 2012 suggest that at least 80% of First Nations two year old children living on reserve received the measles, mumps and rubella vaccine in most regions. In First Nations communities, use of this vaccine appears to be increasing.[5]

INTERNATIONAL COMPARISON

In 2015, Canada had the lowest proportion of one year olds vaccinated for DPT among G7 countries.[6] Vaccination schedules, namely at what age children get vaccinated, differ across and within countries, making it challenging to compare data on immunization.

PERCENT OF ONE YEAR OLDS BEING VACCINATED IN G7 COUNTRIES, 1990 AND 2015[6]
Measles vaccine

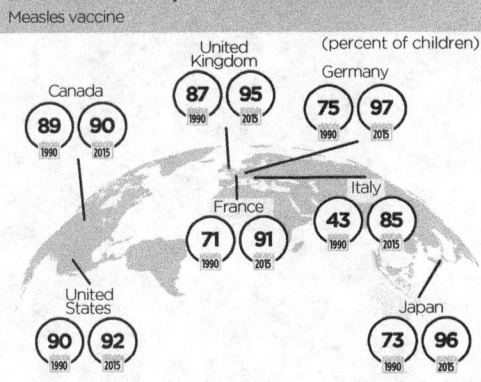

(percent of children)

Canada 89 (1990) 90 (2015)
United Kingdom 87 (1990) 95 (2015)
Germany 75 (1990) 97 (2015)
France 71 (1990) 91 (2015)
Italy 43 (1990) 85 (2015)
United States 90 (1990) 92 (2015)
Japan 73 (1990) 96 (2015)

PERCENT OF ONE YEAR OLDS BEING VACCINATED IN G7 COUNTRIES, 1990 AND 2015[6]
DPT vaccine

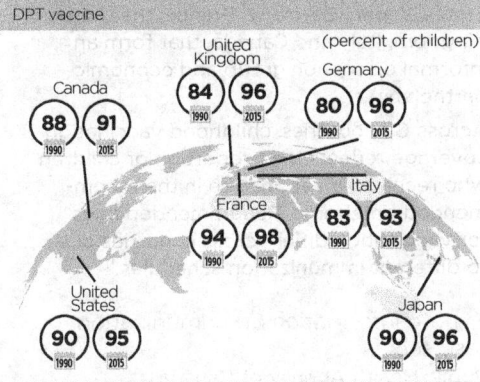

(percent of children)

Canada 88 (1990) 91 (2015)
United Kingdom 84 (1990) 96 (2015)
Germany 80 (1990) 96 (2015)
France 94 (1990) 98 (2015)
Italy 83 (1990) 93 (2015)
United States 90 (1990) 95 (2015)
Japan 90 (1990) 96 (2015)

Notes to the reader

- The Public Health Agency of Canada regularly collects data and monitors immunization coverage in children aged 2, 7 and 17 years, and in girls aged 12-14 years (to assess HPV coverage) by vaccine antigen through the childhood National Immunization Coverage Survey (cNICS). Data from First Nations on reserve are not collected as part of this survey. Starting in 2011, Statistics Canada has been conducting the cNICS on behalf of the Public Health Agency of Canada using a representative sampling method. Data are collected from immunization records held by parents. With parental consent, information is also obtained from health care providers.

- Adult immunization coverage is assessed every two years by the adult National Immunization Coverage survey. Canadians aged 18 years and older are asked about their vaccination history in adulthood.

- Health Canada's First Nations and Inuit Health Branch collects information on immunization coverage through annual community-based reporting to its regional offices.

- Indigenous populations consist of First Nations, Métis and Inuit.

- G7 countries include seven of the world's industrialized countries, namely the United States, Japan, Germany, France, the United Kingdom, Italy and Canada, that form an informal discussion group and economic partnership.

- Across G7 countries, childhood vaccination coverage reflects the proportion of children who received a vaccination in the recommended timeframe. Recommended ages for vaccination differ across countries due to different immunization schedules.[11]

For more information on immunization, please see:
- Public Health Agency of Canada
- World Health Organization

References

1. Public Health Agency of Canada (2015). Canadian Immunization Guide.

2. Busby, C., Chesterley, N. (2015). A shot in the arm: how to improve vaccination policy in Canada. Toronto ON: CD Howe Institute.

3. Public Health Agency of Canada (2008). Final report of outcomes from the National Consensus Conference for Vaccine-Preventable Diseases in Canada, June 12-14, 2005 - Quebec City, Quebec. Canada Communicable Disease Report, 34(Supplement 2), 1-56.

4. Public Health Agency of Canada (2016). Vaccine uptake in Canadian adults: Results from the 2014 adult National Immunization Coverage Survey (aNICS).

5. Health Canada (2015). Evaluation of the First Nations and Inuit Health Branch Communicable Disease Control and Management Programs 2008-2009 to 2013-2014.

6. Organisation for Economic Co-Operation and Development (2016). Child vaccination rates (indicator).

How are we unhealthy?

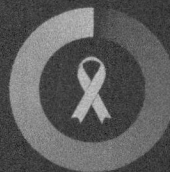
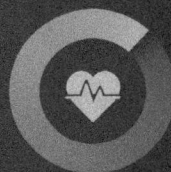
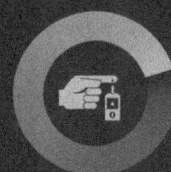
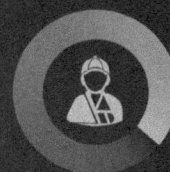

CANCER CARDIOVASCULAR DISEASE DIABETES INJURIES

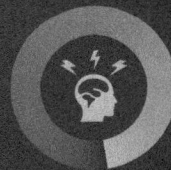
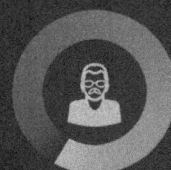
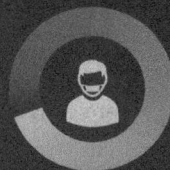

MOOD DISORDERS DEMENTIA TUBERCULOSIS

Cancer

In 2016, more than 200,000 new cases of cancer are expected to be diagnosed.[1] An estimated 2 in 5 Canadians will develop cancer in their lifetime which is most often linked to aging.[1]

2 in 5 Canadians will develop cancer in their lifetime.[1]

DEVELOP CANCER IN THEIR LIFETIME[1]

2 in 5 Canadians

In 2012, cancer was the leading cause of death in Canada at 30% of all deaths. The next leading causes of death are heart disease at 20% of all deaths and cerebrovascular diseases (e.g., stroke) at 5% of all deaths.[2] An estimated 78,800 Canadians are expected to die from cancer in 2016.[1]

OVER TIME, BY SEX

Rates of new cases of cancer have decreased for men and increased slightly for women.[1]

RATE OF NEW CASES OF CANCER BY SEX, 1987–2016[1]

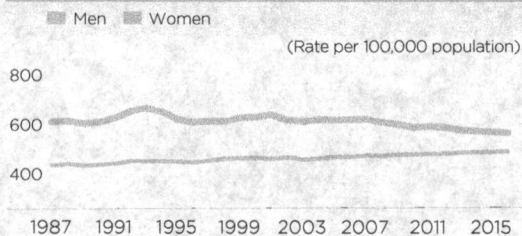

Men   Women

(Rate per 100,000 population)

800	
600	
400	

1987 1991 1995 1999 2003 2007 2011 2015

Data presented in this graph are adjusted by age.

BY INCOME, BY SEX

Data from 1991 to 2006 show that mortality rates for cancer were much higher for those living in the lowest-income households than for those living in the highest-income households.[3]

MORTALITY RATES BY HOUSEHOLD INCOME, 1991–2006

Lowest income quintile		Highest income quintile	
Men	Women	Men	Women
510	**317**	**349**	**244**
per 100,000	per 100,000	per 100,000	per 100,000

Quintiles are calculated by dividing the Canadian population into five groups of equal size (quintiles) based on household income. Data presented in this table are adjusted by age.

BY AGE, BY SEX

Rates of new cases of cancer are higher in older Canadians.[1] Among the oldest Canadians, rates of new cases of cancer are higher in men than women.[1]

RATE OF NEW CASES OF CANCER IN OLDER AGE GROUPS BY SEX, 1990, 2000, 2010 AND 2016[1]
Men

■ 1990 ■ 2000 ■ 2010 ■ 2016

(Rate per 100,000 population)

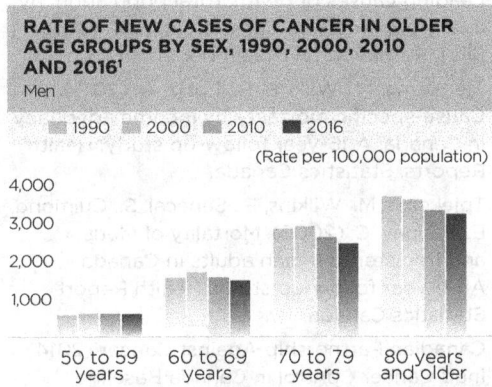

RATE OF NEW CASES OF CANCER IN OLDER AGE GROUPS BY SEX, 1990, 2000, 2010 AND 2016[1]
Women

■ 1990 ■ 2000 ■ 2010 ■ 2016

(Rate per 100,000 population)

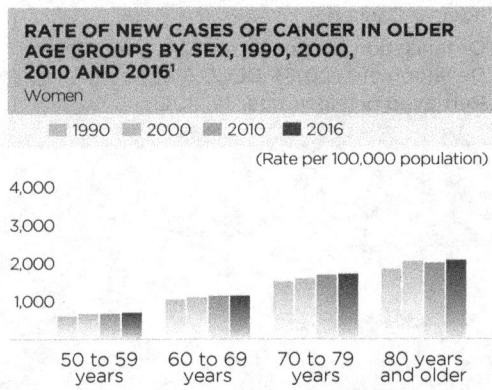

Data presented in these graphs are adjusted by age.

INDIGENOUS POPULATIONS

Data on cancer in Indigenous populations are limited and **not directly comparable to the data** described above. Research on cancer in Indigenous populations has found that:

- Using data from 1991 to 2001, age-standardized mortality rates for all types of cancer were calculated to be 163 per 100,000 for First Nations men, 176 per 100,000 for Métis men and 188 per 100,000 for non-Indigenous men.[4]

- Using data from 1991 to 2001, age-standardized mortality rates for all types of cancer were calculated to be 156 per 100,000 for First Nations women, 180 per 100,000 for Métis women and 134 per 100,000 for non-Indigenous women.[4]

- Rates of cancer are increasing among Inuit in Canada. Using data from 1998 to 2007, the age-standardized rate for new cases of cancers among Inuit was 323 per 100,000 population.[5]

INTERNATIONAL COMPARISON

In G7 countries, the United States had the highest rate of new cases of cancer at 318 cases per 100,000 population in 2012. Japan had the lowest at 217 cases per 100,000 population. Canada had 296 cases per 100,000 population.[6]

RATES OF NEW CASES OF CANCER IN G7 COUNTRIES, 2012[6]

(Rate per 100,000 population)

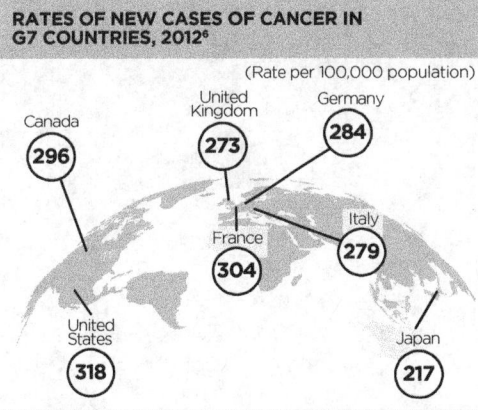

For more information on cancer, please see:

- Public Health Agency of Canada
- Canadian Cancer Society
- World Health Organization
- International Agency for Research on Cancer

Notes to the reader

- Rates are calculated as age-standardized rates per 100,000 population. Age-standardized rates are adjusted so that they account for different age structures in different populations.[3] This allows for comparisons across time. For example, cancer is more common in older age groups. With an aging population, there should be more cases of cancer now than in the past. This would also increase the rate of cancer in the overall population. In order to determine if rates are changing, they need to be adjusted to take out the influence of an aging.

- Indigenous populations consist of First Nations, Métis and Inuit.

- G7 countries include seven of the world's industrialized countries, namely the United States, Japan, Germany, France, the United Kingdom, Italy and Canada, that form an informal discussion group and economic partnership.

References

1. Canadian Cancer Society (2016). Canadian Cancer Society's Advisory Committee on Cancer Statistics. Toronto, ON: Canadian Cancer Society.

2. Statistics Canada (2015). Table 102-0561 – Leading causes of death, total population, by age group and sex, Canada. (annual) [Data File]. Retrieved on December 20, 2015.

3. Tjepkema, M., Wilkins, R., Long, A. (2013). Cause-specific mortality by income adequacy in Canada: A 16-year follow-up study. Health Reports, Statistics Canada.

4. Tpjekema, M., Wilkins, R., Senécal, S., Guimond, E., Penney, C. (2009). Mortality of Métis and Registered Indian adults in Canada: An 11-year follow-up study. Health Report, Statistics Canada.

5. Canadian Partnership Against Cancer (2014). Inuit Cancer Control in Canada Baseline Report. Toronto: Canadian Partnership against Cancer.

6. Organisation for Economic Co-operation and Development (2015). OECD.Stat [Data File]. Retrieved on November 12, 2015.

Cardiovascular disease

In 2014, 6% of Canadians 20 years and older report that they were living with a cardiovascular disease.[1]

Examples of cardiovascular diseases include heart disease and cerebrovascular disease. These two diseases are the second and third most common causes of death in Canada after cancer. High blood pressure is a chronic condition that can increase a person's risk for cardiovascular disease.[2, 3]

OVER TIME

From 2007 to 2014, the proportion of Canadians living with a cardiovascular disease has remained stable at 5%. These rates were adjusted by age so they could be compared over time.[1]

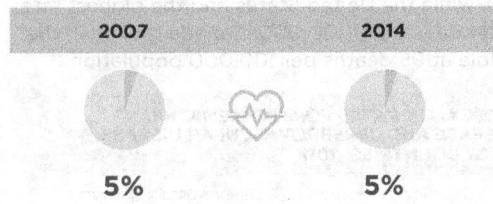

2007	2014
5%	5%

BY INCOME

In 2014, Canadians with the lowest household incomes were more likely than those with the highest household incomes to **report** living with a cardiovascular disease.[4]

PERCENT OF CANADIANS REPORTING LIVING WITH A CARDIOVASCULAR DISEASE BY HOUSEHOLD INCOME, 2014[4]

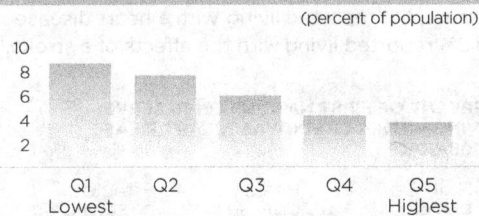

(percent of population)

| Q1 Lowest | Q2 | Q3 | Q4 | Q5 Highest |

Quintiles (Q) are calculated by dividing the Canadian population into five groups of equal size (quintiles) based on household income.

BY SEX

In 2014, 7% of men and 5% of women **reported** living with a cardiovascular disease.[1]

MEN	WOMEN
7%	5%

BY AGE

The proportion of Canadians reporting that they were living with a cardiovascular disease increases with age. A similar pattern was found for high blood pressure.[1]

PERCENT OF CANADIANS LIVING WITH A CARDIOVASCULAR DISEASE BY AGE GROUP, 2014[1]

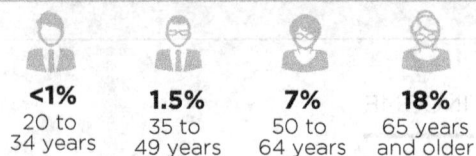

<1%	1.5%	7%	18%
20 to 34 years	35 to 49 years	50 to 64 years	65 years and older

INDIGENOUS POPULATIONS

Data on cardiovascular disease in Indigenous populations **are not directly comparable** to the data described above. In 2008/2010, 22% of First Nations on-reserve reported having high blood pressure, 6% reported living with a heart disease and 2% reported living with the effects of a stroke.[5]

PERCENT OF FIRST NATIONS ON-RESERVE LIVING WITH A CARDIOVASCULAR DISEASE, 2008/2010[5]

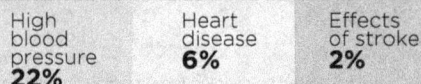

High blood pressure 22%	Heart disease 6%	Effects of stroke 2%

In 2007–2010, First Nations off reserve, Métis and Inuit were less likely to **report** living with a cardiovascular disease or high blood pressure than non-Indigenous people.[6]

PERCENT OF CANADIANS LIVING WITH A CARDIOVASCULAR DISEASE, 2007–2010[6]

	CARDIOVASCULAR DISEASE	HIGH BLOOD PRESSURE
First Nations off reserve	11%	9%
Métis	10%	9%
Inuit	9%*	7%
Non-Indigenous	14%	12%

* High sampling variability. Interpret with caution.

Data presented in this table are adjusted by age. Indigenous populations tend to be younger than non-Indigenous populations which can affect the ability to compare data across groups.

INTERNATIONAL COMPARISON

Data on rates of cardiovascular disease in G7 countries are not collected such that comparisons can be made. Looking at rates of mortality, Japan had the lowest mortality rate from heart disease (ischaemic, meaning reduced blood supply to the heart) at 39 deaths per 100,000 population in 2011, while the United States had the highest rate at 124 deaths per 100,000. Canada ranked in the middle at 95 deaths per 100,000 population.[7]

MORTALITY RATES FOR ISCHAEMIC HEART DISEASE AND CEREBROVASCULAR DISEASE IN G7 COUNTRIES, 2011[7]

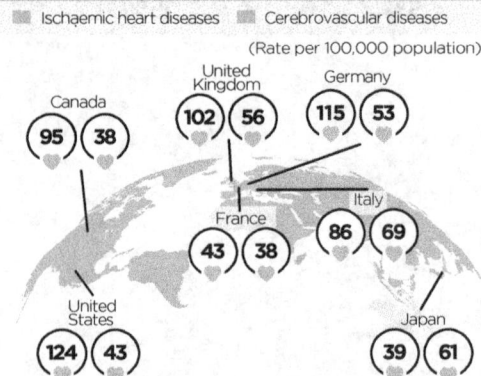

Ischaemic heart diseases   Cerebrovascular diseases

(Rate per 100,000 population)

Country	Ischaemic heart diseases	Cerebrovascular diseases
Canada	95	38
United Kingdom	102	56
Germany	115	53
France	43	38
Italy	86	69
United States	124	43
Japan	39	61

Data presented in this graph are adjusted by age.

Notes to the reader

- Cardiovascular diseases are conditions or diseases of the circulatory system. The four most common types are ischemic heart disease, myocardial infarction or heart attack, congestive heart failure and cerebrovascular disease.[1] Hypertension is a chronic condition that occurs when blood pressure is consistently high for long periods. Hypertension is a leading risk factor for cardiovascular disease.[2]

- Rates are calculated as age-standardized rates per 100,000 population. Age-standardized rates are are adjusted so that they account for different age structures in different populations. For example, cardiovascular diseases are more common in older age groups. With an aging population, there should be more cases now than in the past. In order to determine if rates are changing, they need to be adjusted to take out the influence of an aging population.

- Indigenous populations consist of First Nations, Métis and Inuit.

- G7 countries include seven of the world's industrialized countries, namely the United States, Japan, Germany, France, the United Kingdom, Italy and Canada, that form an informal discussion group and economic partnership.

For more information on cardiovascular diseases, please see:

- Heart and Stroke Foundation
- Public Health Agency of Canada
- Government of Canada

References

1. Public Health Agency of Canada (2016). Chronic Disease and Injury Indicator Framework. Edition 2016, using data from the Canadian Community Health Survey 2014

2. Public Health Agency of Canada, Canadian Institute for Health Information, Canadian Stroke Network, Heart and Stroke Foundation of Canada, Statistics Canada (2009). Tracking Heart Disease and Stroke in Canada, 2009.

3. Public Health Agency of Canada (2010). Report from the Canadian Chronic Disease Surveillance System: Hypertension in Canada, 2010.

4. Statistics Canada. Canadian Community Health Survey (2013). [Share Microdata File]. Ottawa, ON: Statistics Canada. All computations on these microdata were prepared by the Public Health Agency of Canada and the responsibility for the use and interpretation of these data is entirely that of the author(s).

5. First Nations Information Governance Centre (2012). First Nations Regional Health Survey (RHS) 2008/10: National report on adults, youth and children living in First Nations communities. (Ottawa: FNIGC). FNIGC Data Online [Data File].

6. Gionet, L., Roshananfshar, S. (2013). Select health indicators of First Nations people living off reserve, Métis and Inuit. Health at a Glance, no.82-624-X.

7. Organisation for Economic Co-operation and Development (2015). OECD.Stat [Data File]. Retrieved on November 12, 2015.

Diabetes

In 2011, almost 2.7 million or 1 in 10 Canadians 20 years and older were living with diagnosed diabetes (type 1 or type 2) as measured through hospitalizations or physician claims.[1]

1 in 10 Canadians had been diagnosed

BEEN DIAGNOSED WITH DIABETES

1 in 10 Canadians

with diabetes.[1]

Diabetes is one of the most common chronic diseases in Canada and is linked to a variety of complications (e.g., amputations, loss of vision) and other diseases (e.g., cardiovascular disease, kidney disease).[2] Age, obesity and physical inactivity are some of the many risk factors for type 2 diabetes.[2]

OVER TIME

2000	2011
6%	10%

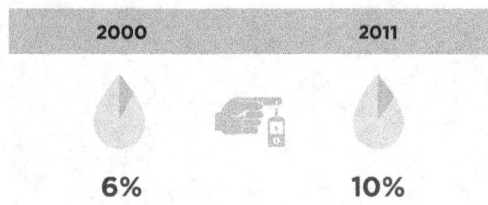

Data adjusted by age and collected from hospitalizations and physicians claims show that:[1]

DID YOU KNOW? Although historically only found in adults, type 2 diabetes has been on the rise globally among children and youth over the past 20 years.[10, 11]

Self-reported data are lower than data collected through hospitalizations and physician claims, but show the same general trend. The proportion of Canadians 12 years and older who **reported** being diagnosed with diabetes (type 1, type 2 or gestational) at some point in their life has been increasing.[3]

Data from hospitalizations and physician claims may be more accurate; however, are not available to make comparisons by sex, income, age and in Indigenous populations. For these analyses (see below), **self-reported** data are used.

BY SEX

In 2014, the proportion of Canadians 12 years and older who **reported** living with diabetes was 6% for men and 5% for women based on age-adjusted data.

PERCENT OF CANADIANS WHO REPORTED BEING DIAGNOSED WITH DIABETES, BY SEX, 2000-2014[3]

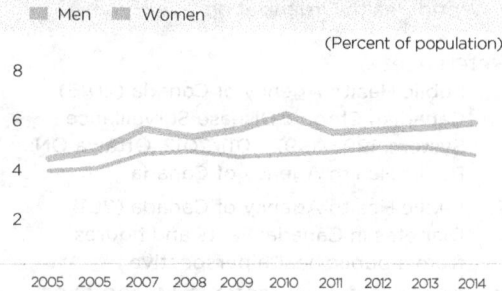

Men   Women

(Percent of population)

2005 2005 2007 2008 2009 2010 2011 2012 2013 2014

Data presented in this graph are adjusted by age.

BY INCOME

From 2003 to 2013, the proportion of Canadians 18 years and older in the lowest income group were more likely to **report** being diagnosed with diabetes (type 1, type 2 or gestational) than those in the highest income group.[4]

PERCENT OF CANADIANS LIVING WITH DIABETES BY INCOME, 2003 AND 2013[4]

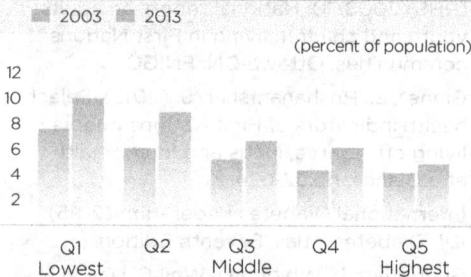

2003   2013

(percent of population)

| Q1 Lowest | Q2 | Q3 Middle | Q4 | Q5 Highest |

Quintiles (Q) are calculated by dividing the Canadian population into five groups of equal size (quintiles) based on income.

BY AGE

The proportion of Canadians 12 years and older **reporting** being diagnosed with diabetes (type 1, type 2 or gestational) increases with age.[5]

PERCENT OF CANADIANS LIVING WITH DIABETES BY AGE GROUP, 2013-2014[5]

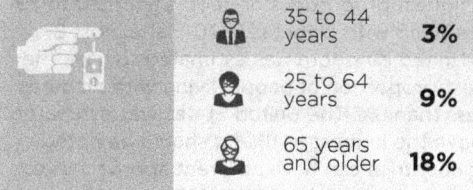

12 to 19 years	**<1%***
20 to 34 years	**1%**
35 to 44 years	**3%**
25 to 64 years	**9%**
65 years and older	**18%**

* High sampling variability. Interpret with caution

INDIGENOUS POPULATIONS

Data on diabetes in Indigenous populations **are not directly comparable** to the data described above. In 2008/2010, 16% of First Nations on-reserve reported they had been diagnosed with diabetes (type 1, type 2 or gestational). Of those reporting being diagnosed with this disease, 81% said they had type 2 diabetes, 9% had type 1 and 6% had gestational diabetes.[6]

PERCENT OF FIRST NATIONS ADULTS ON-RESERVE LIVING WITH DIABETES, 2008/2010[6]	First Nations on-reserve **16%**

In 2007–2010, First Nations off reserve were more likely to be living with diabetes (type 1, type 2 or gestational) than other groups.[7]

PERCENT OF CANADIANS LIVING WITH DIABETES, 2007-2010[7]	First Nations off reserve **6%**
	Métis **4%**
	Inuit **2%***
	Non-Indigenous **4%**

* High sampling variability. Interpret with caution
Data presented in this table are adjusted by age. Indigenous populations tend to be younger than non-Indigenous populations which can affect the ability to compare data across groups.

INTERNATIONAL COMPARISON

International data on diabetes are estimates of diagnosed and undiagnosed diabetes. Among G7 countries, it is estimated that Canada had one of the highest proportions of people aged 20 to 79 years living with diabetes in 2015 at almost 8%. The United Kingdom was estimated to have the lowest proportion of people living with diabetes at less than 5%. The United States was estimated to have the highest at 11%.[8] It should be noted that countries can have different approaches to screening for and diagnosis of diabetes that may affect estimates on how many people are living with diabetes.

PERCENT OF PEOPLE LIVING WITH DIABETES IN G7 COUNTRIES, 2015[8]

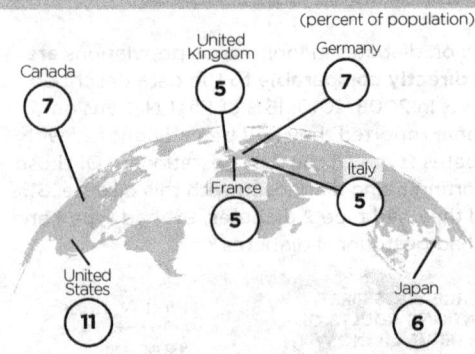

(percent of population)

Canada — 7
United Kingdom — 5
Germany — 7
France — 5
Italy — 5
United States — 11
Japan — 6

Data presented in this graph are adjusted by age.

Notes to the reader

- Diabetes mellitus occurs in several forms with type 1, type 2 and gestational diabetes being the most common types.[2]

- Indigenous populations consist of First Nations, Métis and Inuit.

- Comparing of international rates of diabetes are challenging. The International Diabetes Federation generated age-adjusted estimates for each country by applying the country's age-specific diabetes prevalence estimates to each age-group and standardising the country's population age structure to the global age structure of 2001.[9]

- G7 countries include seven of the world's industrialized countries, namely the United States, Japan, Germany, France, the United Kingdom, Italy and Canada, that form an informal discussion group and economic partnership.

For more information on diabetes, please see:
- Public Health Agency of Canada
- Canadian Diabetes Association
- World Health Organization

References

1. Public Health Agency of Canada (2016). Canadian Chronic Disease Surveillance System, 1996/1997-2011/2012. Ottawa ON: Public Health Agency of Canada.

2. Public Health Agency of Canada (2011). Diabetes in Canada: Facts and figures from a public health perspective.

3. Statistics Canada (2015). Table 105-0503 – Health indicator profile, age-standardized rate, annual estimates, by sex, Canada, provinces and territories, CANSIM

4. Canadian Institutes of Health Information (2015). Trends in Income-Related Health Inequalities in Canada. Technical Report

5. Statistics Canada (2015). Tables 105-0502 – Health indicator profile, two year period estimates, by age group and sex, Canada, provinces, territories, health regions (2013 boundaries) and peer groups.

6. First Nations Information Governance Centre (2012). First Nations Regional Health Survey (RHS) 2008/10: National report on adults, youth and children living in First Nations communities. Ottawa ON: FNIGC.

7. Gionet, L., Roshananfshar, S. (2013). Select health indicators of First Nations people living off reserve, Métis and Inuit. Health at a Glance, no.82-624-X.

8. International Diabetes Federation (2015). IDF Diabetes Atlas, Seventh Edition.

9. Guariguata L, Whiting D, Weil C, Unwin N. (2011). The International Diabetes Federation diabetes atlas methodology for estimating global and national prevalence of diabetes in adults. Diabetes Research and Clinical Practice, 94, 322–32. doi:10.1016/j.diabres.2011.10.040.

10. D'Adamo, E., Caprio, S. (2011). Type 2 Diabetes in Youth: Epidemiology and Pathophysiology. Diabetes Care, 34 (Supplement 2), S161-S165.

11. Pinhas-Hamiel, O., Zeitler, P. (2005). The global spread of type 2 diabetes mellitus in children and adolescents. Journal of Pediatrics, 146(5), 693-700.

Injuries

In 2014, nearly 5 million or just under 2 in 10 Canadians reported experiencing an injury in the previous year that was serious enough to limit their normal activity.[1]

Just under 2 in 10 Canadians reported experiencing an injury in the previous year.[1]

EXPERIENCED AN INJURY IN THE PREVIOUS YEAR

just under 2 in 10 Canadians

Injuries are a leading cause of morbidity and disability for Canadians.[2,3]

OVER TIME

The proportion of Canadians reporting that they experienced an injury in the previous year has increased from 13% in 2003 to 16% in 2014.[1]

DID YOU KNOW? An estimated 20% to 30% of seniors fall each year in Canada.[2] Falls are the leading cause of injury-related hospitalizations for seniors. In 2010-2011, more than 100,000 Canadian seniors were hospitalized due to an injury with 78,000 of these hospitalizations being related to falls.[2,3]

BY INCOME

In 2014, people living in households with the lowest income are less likely to report experiencing an injury than those living in the highest household income.[4]

LOWEST INCOME	HIGHEST INCOME
14%	18%

BY SEX

In 2014, 17% of men and 14% of women reported having experienced an injury in the previous year.[1]

MEN	WOMEN
17%	14%

BY AGE

In 2014, youth were more likely to report having experienced an injury in the previous year than other age groups.[1]

PERCENT OF CANADIANS REPORTING BEING INJURED BY AGE GROUP, 2014[1]		
	12 to 19 years	26%
	20 to 34 years	18%
	35 to 44 years	15%
	45 to 64 years	14%
	65 years and older	10%

INDIGENOUS POPULATIONS

Data on injuries in Indigenous populations are **not directly comparable** to the data described above.

In 2008/2010, 19% of First Nations on-reserve aged 18 years and older reported experiencing an injury in the previous year.[5]

In 2012, 20% of First Nations living off reserve, 21% of Métis and 16% of Inuit aged 19 years and older reported experience an injury in the previous year.[6]

INTERNATIONAL COMPARISON:

Data related to injuries are not collected such that they can be compared across countries.

Notes to the reader
• Data on injuries are reported by Canadians aged 12 years and older as being an injury that occurred in the previous year and was considered to be serious enough to limit normal activities. Repetitive strain injuries are not included.[1] The survey did not ask whether injuries were unintentional and intentional injuries.[1]
• Indigenous populations consist of First Nations, Métis and Inuit.

For more information on injuries, please see:
• Government of Canada
• Public Health Agency of Canada

References
1. Statistics Canada (2016). Table 105-0501 – Health indicator profile, annual estimates, by age group and sex, Canada, provinces, territories, health regions (2013 boundaries) and peer groups, occasional [Data File]. Retrieved on March 30, 2016.

2. Public Health Agency of Canada (2014). Seniors' Fall in Canada: Second Report.

3. Canadian Institute for Health Information 2012). National Trauma Registry Minimum Data Set (NTR MDS), 2010-2011 [Data File]. Retrieved on October 1, 2015.

4. Statistics Canada (2014). Canadian Community Health Survey, 2014 [Share Microdata File]. Ottawa, ON: Statistics Canada. All computations on these microdata were prepared by the Public Health Agency of Canada and the responsibility for the use and interpretation of these data is entirely that of the author(s).

5. First Nations Information Governance Centre (2012). First Nations Regional Health Survey (RHS) 2008/10: National report on adults, youth and children living in First Nations communities. Ottawa ON: FNIGC.

6. Statistics Canada (2012). Aboriginal Peoples Survey, 2012. All computations on these microdata were prepared by the Public Health Agency of Canada and the responsibility for the use and interpretation of these data is entirely that of the author(s).

Mood disorders

In 2014, just over 2 million or just under 1 in 10 Canadians said they had been diagnosed with a mood disorder by a health professional.[1]

Just under 1 in 10 Canadians said they had been diagnosed with a mood disorder.[1]

DIAGNOSED WITH A MOOD DISORDER

just under 1 in 10 Canadians

Mood disorders are among the most common types of psychological disorders in Canada. They can lead to stress, problems at work or with social relationships, as well as poor health and well-being.[2,3]

OVER TIME, BY SEX, BY AGE

The proportion of Canadians who said they had been diagnosed with a mood disorder has been increasing, from 5% in 2003 to 8% in 2014.[1]

PERCENT OF CANADIANS WHO REPORTED BEING DIAGNOSED WITH A MOOD DISORDER, 2003–2014[1]

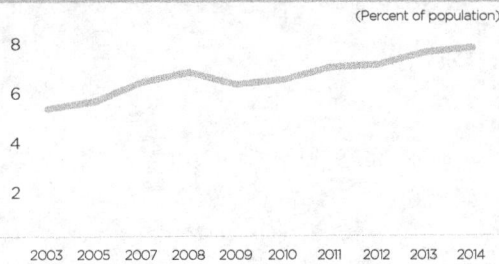

(Percent of population)

2003	2005	2007	2008	2009	2010	2011	2012	2013	2014

The proportion of Canadians who report being diagnosed with a mood disorder is increasing for both men and women. Women are consistently more likely to report being diagnosed with mood disorders than men.[1]

PERCENT OF CANADIANS WHO REPORTED BEING DIAGNOSED WITH A MOOD DISORDER BY SEX, 2003 AND 2014[1]

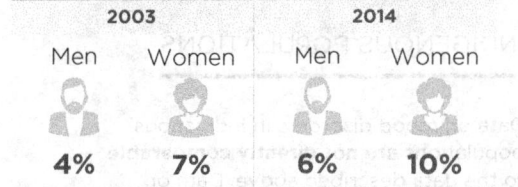

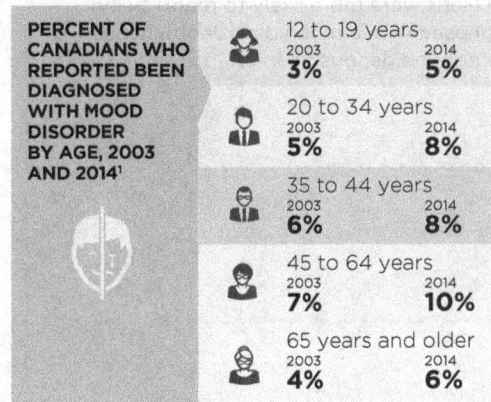

2003		2014	
Men	Women	Men	Women
4%	7%	6%	10%

The proportion of Canadians reporting that they have been diagnosed with a mood disorder has increased in all age groups since 2003.[1]

PERCENT OF CANADIANS WHO REPORTED BEEN DIAGNOSED WITH MOOD DISORDER BY AGE, 2003 AND 2014[1]

Age	2003	2014
12 to 19 years	3%	5%
20 to 34 years	5%	8%
35 to 44 years	6%	8%
45 to 64 years	7%	10%
65 years and older	4%	6%

BY INCOME

In 2014, 14% of Canadians living in the lowest income households and 5% of Canadians living in the highest income households reported having symptoms similar to those of a mood disorder.[4]

PERCENT OF CANADIANS WHO REPORT SYMPTOMS SIMILAR TO THOSE OF A MOOD DISORDER BY HOUSEHOLD INCOME, 2014[4]

(percent of population)

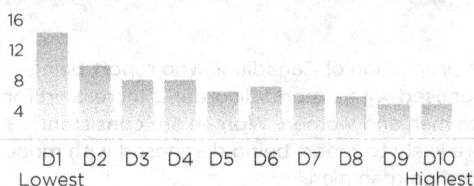

D1	D2	D3	D4	D5	D6	D7	D8	D9	D10
Lowest									Highest

Deciles (D) are calculated by dividing the Canadian population into ten groups of equal size (deciles) based on income.

INDIGENOUS POPULATIONS

Data on mood disorders in Indigenous populations **are not directly comparable** to the data described above. Data on mood disorders have not been collected at a national level for First Nations on-reserve.

In 2007–2010, First Nations living off reserve and Métis were more likely to report being diagnosed with a mood disorder than Inuit and non-Indigenous people.[5]

PERCENT OF CANADIANS REPORTING BEING DIAGNOSED WITH A MOOD DISORDER AT SOME POINT IN THEIR LIFE, 2007-2010[5]

First Nations off reserve	**12%**
Métis	**10%**
Inuit	**5%***
Non-Indigenous	**6%**

* High sampling variability. Interpret with caution

Data presented in this table are adjusted by age. Indigenous populations tend to be younger than non-Indigenous populations which can affect the ability to compare data across groups.

INTERNATIONAL COMPARISON

Data related to mood disorders are not collected such that they can be compared across countries.

Notes to the reader

- Mood disorders are measured in Canadians aged 12 and over. Data presented in this section are based on whether or not people report having been diagnosed by a health professional with a mood disorder (such as depression, bipolar disorder, mania or dysthymia).[1]

- Indigenous populations consist of First Nations, Métis and Inuit.

For more information on mental health, please see:

- Government of Canada
- Mental Health Commission of Canada
- Canadian Mental Health Association

References

1. Statistics Canada (2016). Table 105-0501 – Health indicator profile, annual estimates, by age group and sex, Canada, provinces, territories, health regions (2013 boundaries) and peer groups. (occasional) [Data File]. Retrieved on March 30, 2016.

2. Public Health Agency of Canada (2006). The human face of mental health and mental illness in Canada 2006.

3. Langlois, K.A., Samokhvalov, A.V., Rehm, J., Spence, S.T., Connor Gober, S. (2012). Health state descriptions for Canadians: mental illnesses, no. 4. Ottawa ON: Statistics Canada.

4. Statistics Canada (2014). Canadian Community Health Survey, 2014 [Share Microdata File]. Ottawa, ON: Statistics Canada. All computations on these microdata were prepared by the Public Health Agency of Canada and the responsibility for the use and interpretation of these data is entirely that of the author(s).

5. Gionet, L., Roshananfshar, S. (2013). Select health indicators of First Nations people living off reserve, Métis and Inuit. Health at a Glance, no. 82-624-X.

Dementia

In 2011, an estimated 340,200 or 2% of Canadians aged 40 years and older were living with a diagnosis of dementia.[1]

Alzheimer's disease is the most common form of dementia, representing 60% to 70% of cases.[2] Common symptoms include memory problems, problems with routine tasks and language, impaired judgement and changes in mood and personality. Symptoms become more severe as the disease progresses.[3]

OVER TIME, BY AGE, BY SEX

The number of Canadians living with dementia is expected to double in the next 20 years.[1]

PREDICTED RATES OF CANADIANS 40 YEARS AND OLDER LIVING WITH DEMENTIA, 2011, 2016, 2021, 2026 AND 2031[1]

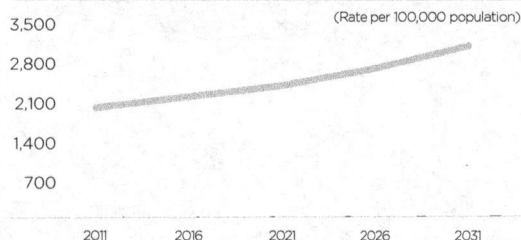

(Rate per 100,000 population)

3,500	
2,800	
2,100	
1,400	
700	

2011   2016   2021   2026   2031

Rates of dementia increase at a similar rate for men and women until 80 years of age, after which they increase more quickly for women than men. The average age of the onset of symptoms is 70 years for men and 74 years for women.[1]

BY INCOME

Data on dementia by income are not available at a national level.

INDIGENOUS POPULATIONS

Limited data are available on dementia for Indigenous populations. Research in 2009 has shown that the age-standardized rate of First Nations living with dementia in Alberta was just under 8 per 1,000 population compared to just under 6 per 1,000 population in non-First Nations Albertans.[4] Dementia also tended to be diagnosed at an earlier age among First Nations than non-First Nations.[4]

INTERNATIONAL COMPARISON

Globally, there are an estimated 47 million people living with dementia. This number is expected to nearly triple by 2050 to almost 132 million people.[5] In 2015, Canada had the second lowest rate of dementia among G7 countries at 14 cases per 1000.[6]

PREDICTED RATE OF PEOPLE LIVING WITH DEMENTIA IN G7 COUNTRIES, 2015 AND 2035[6]

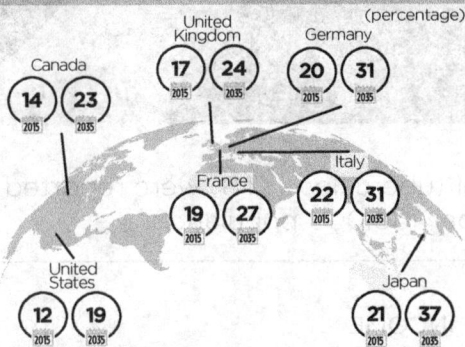

(percentage)

Canada
(14) 2015 (23) 2035

United Kingdom
(17) 2015 (24) 2035

Germany
(20) 2015 (31) 2035

France
(19) 2015 (27) 2035

Italy
(22) 2015 (31) 2035

United States
(12) 2015 (19) 2035

Japan
(21) 2015 (37) 2035

Notes to the reader

- Indigenous populations consist of First Nations, Métis and Inuit.

- G7 countries include seven of the world's industrialized countries, namely the United States, Japan, Germany, France, the United Kingdom, Italy and Canada, that form an informal discussion group and economic partnership.

For more information on Alzheimer's disease and other dementias, please see:

- Government of Canada
- Alzheimer Society of Canada
- World Health Organization

References

1. Public Health Agency of Canada (2014). Mapping Connections: An Understanding of Neurological Conditions in Canada.

2. World Health Organization (2016). Dementia, Fact Sheet No. 362.

3. National Institute on Aging (2014). Alzheimer's Disease Fact Sheet. Retrieved on December 11, 2014.

4. Jacklin, K.M., Walker, J.D., Shawande, M. (2013). The emergence of dementia as a health concern among First Nations populations in Alberta, Canada. Canadian Journal of Public Health, 104(1), e39-e44.

5. Prince, M., Wilmo, A., Guerchet, M., Ali, G.-C. et al. (2015). World Alzheimer Report 2015. The Global Impact of Dementia. An analysis of prevalence, incidence, cost and trends. London: Alzheimer's Disease International.

6. Organisation for Economic Co-operation and Development (2015). Health at a Glance 2015: OECD Indicators.

Tuberculosis

In 2014, 1,568 new and re-treatment cases of tuberculosis (TB) were reported in Canada, resulting in a rate of just over 4 per 100,000 population.[1]

Tuberculosis (TB) is a curable bacterial infection that spreads from person to person primarily through the air.[2]

DID YOU KNOW? Drug-resistant TB is a major global public health issue. Rates of drug-resistant TB are currently low in Canada.[3]

OVER TIME

The number and rates of new TB cases have been decreasing.[1]

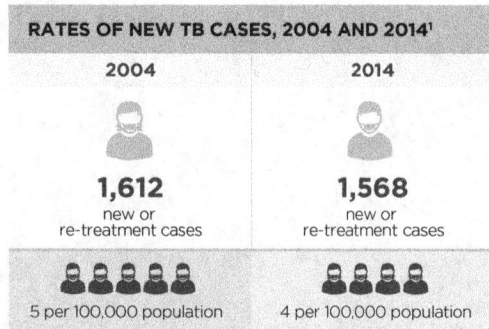

RATES OF NEW TB CASES, 2004 AND 2014[1]	
2004	2014
1,612 new or re-treatment cases	**1,568** new or re-treatment cases
5 per 100,000 population	4 per 100,000 population

BY INCOME

Data at a national level are not available on TB by income. Research has shown that living in a low-income household is one of the risk factors for the transmission of TB.[4]

BY SEX

In 2014, rates of TB were 5 new or re-treatment cases per 100,000 population for men and 4 per 100,000 population for women.[1]

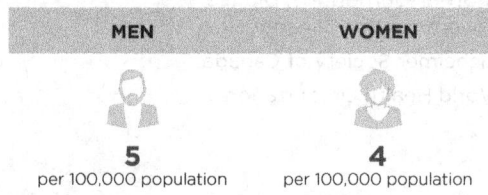

MEN	WOMEN
5 per 100,000 population	**4** per 100,000 population

BY AGE

In 2014, rates of new or re-treated cases of TB were lowest in children and highest in people 75 years and older.[1]

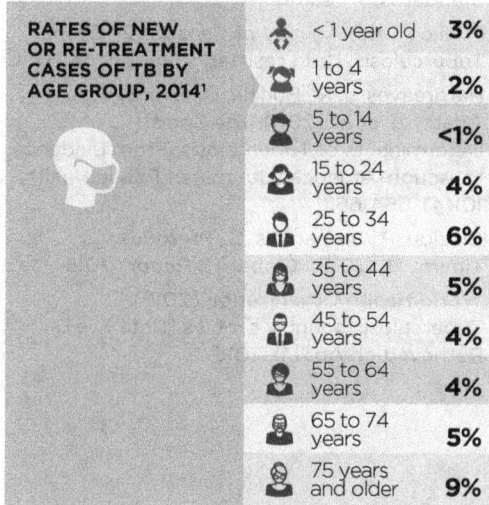

RATES OF NEW OR RE-TREATMENT CASES OF TB BY AGE GROUP, 2014[1]		
	< 1 year old	**3%**
	1 to 4 years	**2%**
	5 to 14 years	**<1%**
	15 to 24 years	**4%**
	25 to 34 years	**6%**
	35 to 44 years	**5%**
	45 to 54 years	**4%**
	55 to 64 years	**4%**
	65 to 74 years	**5%**
	75 years and older	**9%**

INDIGENOUS POPULATIONS

In 2014, Indigenous populations made up 4% of the total Canadian population, but accounted for 21% of reported cases of TB. This resulted in a rate of 20 new or re-treatment cases per 100,000 of the Indigenous population.[1] Rates vary across Indigenous populations. The rate of TB among Inuit is **almost 50 times higher** than the overall Canadian rate.[1]

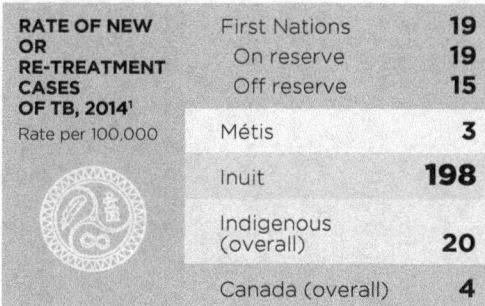

RATE OF NEW OR RE-TREATMENT CASES OF TB, 2014[1] Rate per 100,000		
	First Nations	**19**
	On reserve	**19**
	Off reserve	**15**
	Métis	**3**
	Inuit	**198**
	Indigenous (overall)	**20**
	Canada (overall)	**4**

In 2014, the foreign-born population, which represented approximately 22% of the total Canadian population, accounted for 69% of reported new or re-treatment cases of TB for rate of almost 14 cases per 100,000 population.[1]

INTERNATIONAL COMPARISON

In 2015, there was an estimated 10 million new cases of TB across the world.[5] In G7 countries, Canada had the second lowest rate of new cases of TB at just over 5 cases per 100,000 population.[6] The United States had the lowest rate at 3 per 100,000 population while Japan had the highest at 17 per 100,000 population.[6]

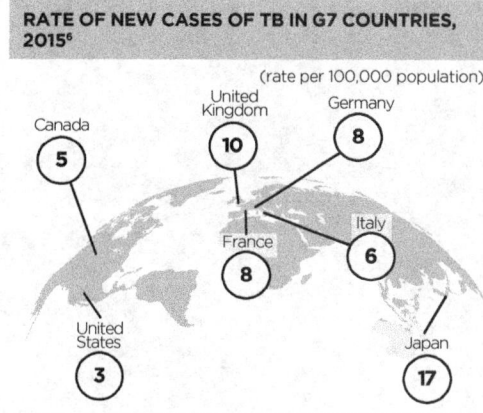

RATE OF NEW CASES OF TB IN G7 COUNTRIES, 2015[6]

(rate per 100,000 population)

Canada **5**
United Kingdom **10**
Germany **8**
France **8**
Italy **6**
United States **3**
Japan **17**

Notes to the reader

- Annual rates of TB are calculated by using the number of new active and re-treatment cases each year. A re-treatment case occurs when a person who was previously diagnosed with TB has a second diagnosis of TB (i.e., reactivated or new infection). To be considered a re-treatment case, the disease must have been inactive for at least six months between the first and second diagnosis.[1]
- Indigenous populations consist of First Nations, Métis and Inuit.

- G7 countries include seven of the world's industrialized countries, namely the United States, Japan, Germany, France, the United Kingdom, Italy and Canada, that form an informal discussion group and economic partnership.

For more information on TB, please see:
- Government of Canada
- Canadian Tuberculosis Standards
- World Health Organization

References

1. Public Health Agency of Canada (2016). Tuberculosis in Canada – Pre-release 2014.

2. Public Health Agency of Canada, the Lung Association and the Canadian Thoracic Society (2014). Canadian Tuberculosis Standards, 7th edition.

3. Public Health Agency of Canada (2015). Tuberculosis: Drug resistance in Canada 2014.

4. Hargreaves, J. R., Boccia, D., Evans, C. A., Adato, M. et al. (2011). The Social Determinants of Tuberculosis: From Evidence to Action. American Journal of Public Health, 101(4), 654-662.

5. Glaziou, P., Sismanidis, C., Pretorius, C., Timimi, H. (2015). Global TB Report 2015 .

6. World Health Organization (2016). Tuberculosis country profiles [Data File]. Retrieved on April 11, 2016.

The Chief Public Health Officer's Report on
the State of Public Health in Canada 2016

A FOCUS ON

FAMILY VIOLENCE IN CANADA

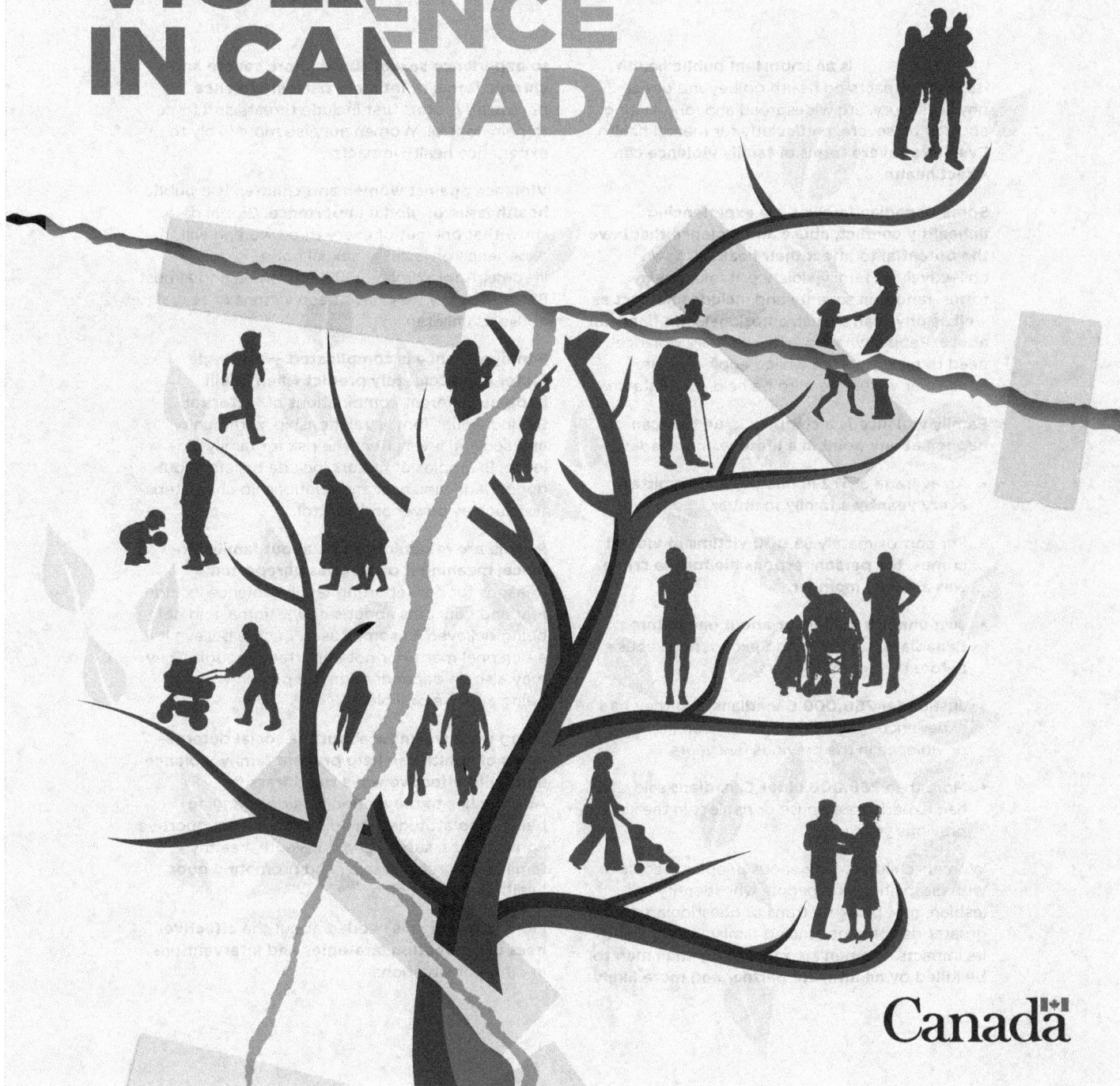

Canada

KEY MESSAGES

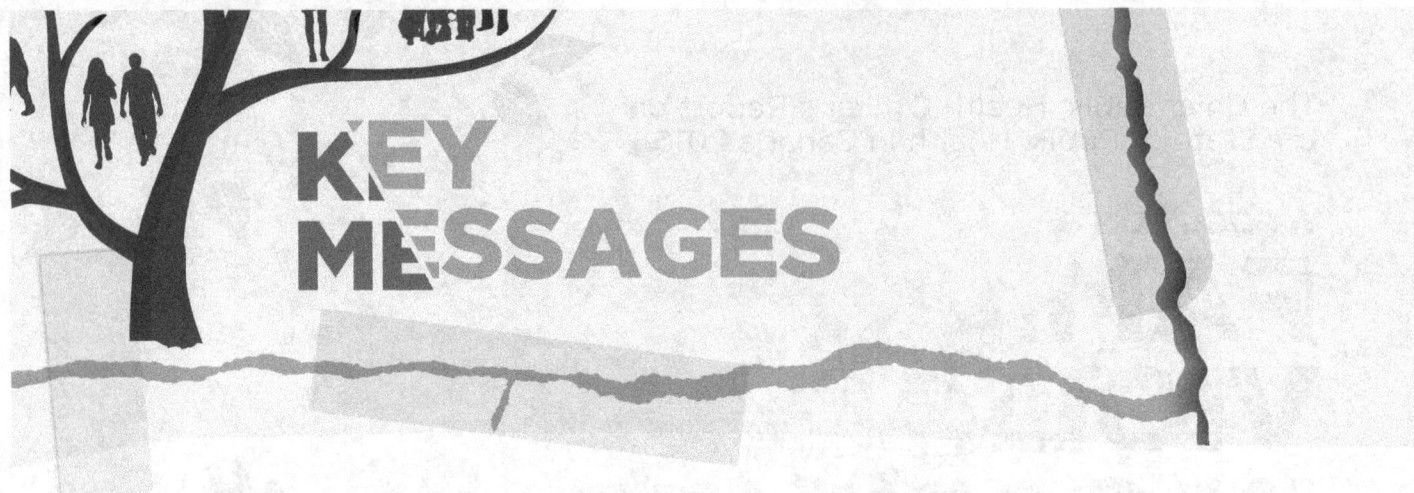

Family violence is an important public health issue. Its impacts on health go beyond direct physical injury, are widespread and long-lasting and can be severe, particularly for mental health. **Even less severe forms of family violence can affect health**.

Some Canadian families are experiencing unhealthy conflict, abuse and violence that have the potential to affect their health. Known collectively as family violence, it takes many forms, ranges in severity and **includes neglect as well as physical, sexual, emotional, and financial abuse**. People who experience family violence need to be supported while people who are abusive or violent need to be held accountable.

Family violence is a complex issue that can happen at any point in a lifetime. In Canada:

- An average of **172 homicides is committed every year by a family member**.

- For approximately **85,000 victims of violent crimes, the person responsible for the crime was a family member**.

- **Just under 9 million, or about one in three Canadians**, said they had experienced abuse before the age of 15 years.

- **Just under 760,000 Canadians** said they had experienced unhealthy spousal conflict, abuse or violence in the previous five years.

- More than **766,000 older Canadians** said they had experienced abuse or neglect in the previous year.

Women, children, Indigenous peoples, people with disabilities, and people who identify as lesbian, gay, bisexual, trans or questioning are at greater risk of experiencing family violence and its impacts. **Women are more likely than men to be killed by an intimate partner and more likely to experience sexual abuse, more severe and chronic forms of intimate partner violence**, particularly forms that include threats and force to gain control. Women are also more likely to experience health impacts.

Violence against women and children is a public health issue of global importance. Global data show that one out of every three women will experience physical or sexual abuse in their lifetime. Approximately 18% of women and almost 8% of men say they have been victims of sexual abuse as children.

Family violence is complicated — no single factor can accurately predict when it will happen. Different combinations of factors at the individual, family, relationship, community and societal level affect the risk for family violence. Examples of factors include beliefs about gender and violence, and relationship characteristics such as power and control.

People are reluctant to talk about family violence, meaning it often goes unreported. Reasons for not reporting family violence include fear and concerns about safety, stigma, and not being believed. In some cases, people believe it is a personal matter or not important enough. They may also be dependent on the person who is being abusive or violent.

Using what we know about the social determinants of health can help prevent family violence and build effective ways to address it. Approaches to prevention include changing beliefs and attitudes, building safe and supportive communities, supporting our youth, healthy families and relationships and promoting good health and well-being.

More knowledge is needed about the **effectiveness of prevention strategies and interventions** in different situations.

Challenges with data on family violence

Statistics Canada regularly reports on family violence in Canada through the analysis of data from police reports and population surveys. These two data sources complement each other, but are not directly comparable. Information from child welfare investigations are collected through the Public Health Agency of Canada's Canadian Incidence Study of Reported Abuse and Neglect.

Collecting and interpreting data on family violence can be challenging for many reasons, including:

People are reluctant to talk about family violence.[1-6]

- They fear for their safety or the safety of their children.
- They depend on the family member who was abusive or violent.
- They have feelings of blame, shame or denial.
- They think that no one will believe them, that they will be blamed or judged or that they will be arrested.
- They do not want anyone to know and feel that it is a personal matter.
- They feel it was minor or not important enough. They addressed it through other means.

There are different definitions of family violence. Not all surveys use the same definition of family violence. Nor do they all measure the same types of family violence.[7,8] Emotional abuse and neglect are the most difficult types to measure because they are hard to define and identify.[7,9]

Family violence is difficult to measure:[7,10-20]

- Police and child welfare data only capture incidents that come to the attention of authorities. Population surveys capture a wider range of incidents, including those that are not reported. Both are important for understanding the scope of family violence in Canada.
- Population surveys do not always measure all forms of family violence or information on how often someone is experiencing it. One piece of data can include a wide range of behaviours.
- Changes in survey data over time can reflect changes in reporting methods or in attitudes that may affect how people answer questions.
- It can be difficult to interpret rates of family violence in small populations. High rates of family violence in small populations can be due to a small number of incidents. In these cases, a small change in the number of incidents can lead to a large change in the rate.
- Data are not always divided into sub-groups. This means there can be limited information for groups at higher risk for family violence, such as Indigenous populations.
- How questions are worded in population surveys can affect the results. This means comparing across different surveys can be a problem.
- Population surveys rely on people's memory of past events. For family violence, these surveys provide reasonably good estimates. If anything, they likely underestimate the issue.

WHO EXPERIENCES FAMILY VIOLENCE IN CANADA?

To understand how many Canadians are at risk for poor health from family violence, we need to know how many Canadians have experienced it.

When Canadians were asked questions about family violence, abuse and conflict, data showed that:

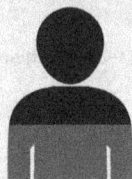

An estimated 9 million or a third of Canadians over the age of 15 years said they had experienced abuse before the age of 15 or 16 years.[2,26,27]

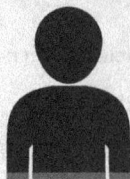

About 760,000 or 4% of Canadians over the age of 15 years said they had experienced intimate partner violence in the previous five years.[10]

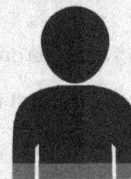

Over 766,000 or 8% of Canadians over the age of 55 years said they had experienced abuse or neglect in the previous year.[27]

Some Canadians are at higher risk for family violence.

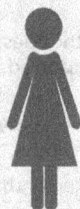

Women are more likely than men to experience more severe and frequent violence from a spouse or someone they are dating.[10]

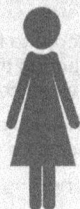

Indigenous women are more likely to experience family violence than non-Indigenous people.[10]

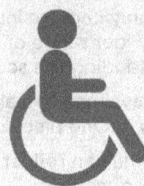

People with disabilities are more likely to experience violence from a spouse, especially more severe types of violence, than people without a disability.[28]

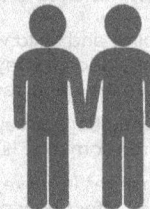

People who identify as lesbian, gay, bisexual, trans or questioning (LGBTQ) are more likely to experience abuse or neglect during childhood, bullying and violence from a spouse or someone they are dating.[10,29-31]

IMPACTS ON CANADIANS

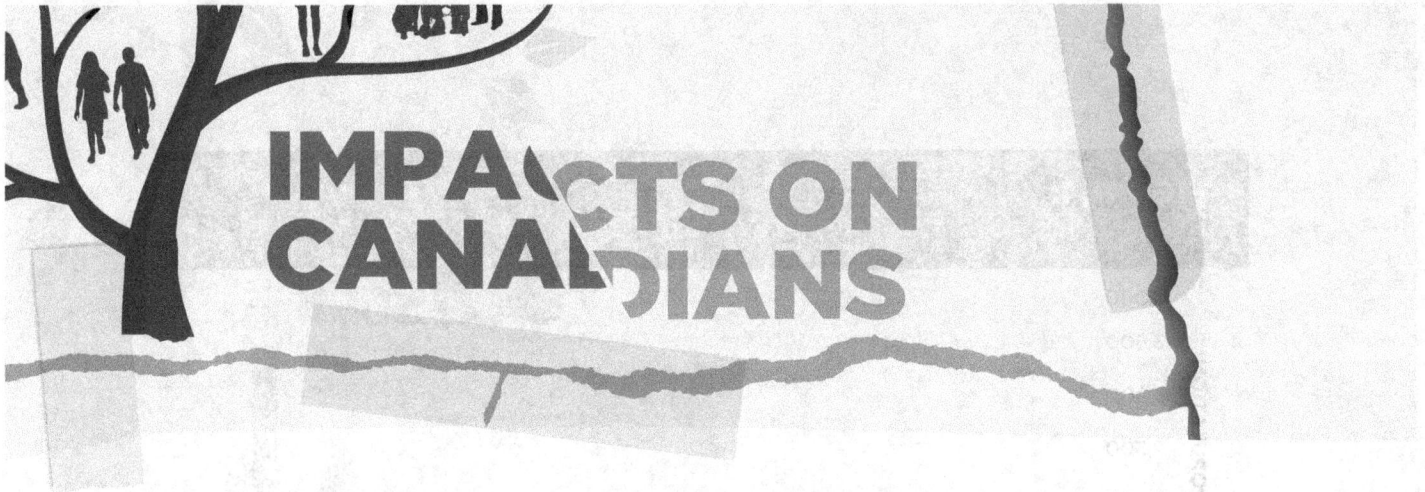

To stop family violence and its effects on health, we need to understand who is experiencing it and how it affects health. Outlined in this section is a snapshot of who in Canada is experiencing family violence, how much it is costing Canadians and how it can lead to early death and poor health.

Family violence in Canada

In 2014, police reports showed that there were over 85,000 victims of family violence in Canada.[10] When dating violence is included, this number increases to 133,920 victims.[10] About 96,000 of these victims were women and almost 20,000 were under the age of 20 years.[10] Like other types of violent crime, family violence reported to the police has decreased across Canada over the past four years (see Figure 1).[10,20]

Recent population survey data show that:

- An estimated 9 million or 30% of Canadians over the age of 15 years said they had experienced abuse before the age of 15 or 16 years.[2,26,27]

- An estimated 760,000 or 4% of Canadians over the age of 15 years said they had experienced spousal conflict, abuse or violence in the previous five years.[10]

- An estimated 4.2 million or 14% of Canadians over the age of 15 years said they had experienced emotional abuse from a spouse or common-law partner at some point in the past.[10]

- An estimated 900,000 or 3% of Canadians over the age of 15 years said they had experienced financial abuse from a spouse or common-law partner at some point in the past.[10]

- An estimated 766,000 or 8% of Canadians over the age of 55 years said they had or neglect from a family member in the previous year.[27]

When Canadians were asked about their experiences of conflict, abuse and violence in their current or population surveys show that rates have decreased in the provinces, but not the territories (see Figure 2). This decrease appears to be mostly due to the fact that severe spousal violence decreasing.[4,5,10]

Why family violence is decreasing is not clear. One reason could be that younger generations are less likely to have experienced family violence than older generations. There are some data to support this idea. In the territories in 2014, 45% of Indigenous peoples between the ages of 45 to 64 years and 26% between the ages of 15 to 34 years said they had experienced abuse or neglect before the age of 15 years.[3] This is not solely related to family violence and may also reflect the residential schools experience. Data from the United States show that women born between 1966 and 1975 were less likely to have experienced intimate partner violence than women born between 1946 and 1955.[91]

FIGURE 1:
POLICE-REPORTED FAMILY VIOLENCE, 2010 AND 2014.[10, 20]

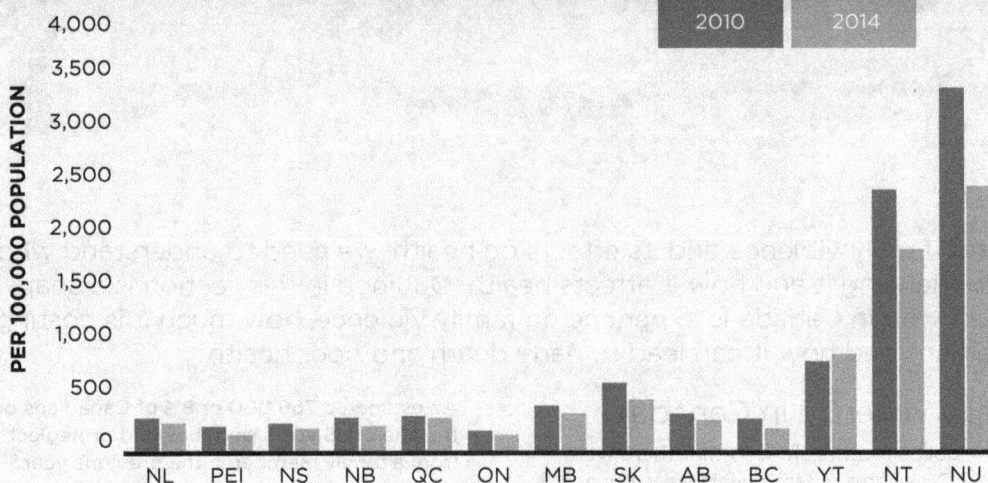

Legend: 2010, 2014

Y-axis: PER 100,000 POPULATION (0 to 4,000)
X-axis: NL, PEI, NS, NB, QC, ON, MB, SK, AB, BC, YT, NT, NU

FIGURE 2:
SELF-REPORTED SPOUSAL VIOLENCE IN CANADA, 2004, 2009 AND 2014.[3, 10, 90]

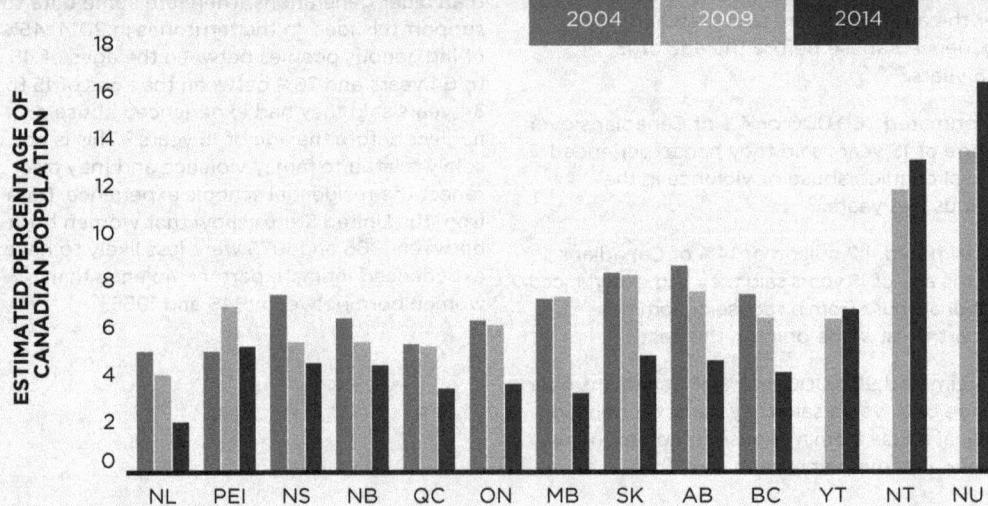

Legend: 2004, 2009, 2014

Y-axis: ESTIMATED PERCENTAGE OF CANADIAN POPULATION (0 to 18)
X-axis: NL, PEI, NS, NB, QC, ON, MB, SK, AB, BC, YT, NT, NU

Notes on the data: Information was collected from Canadians ages 15 years and older and represents spousal violence experienced in the previous five years. Includes legally married, common-law, same-sex, separated and divorced spouses. Information for the territories was not available for all years. For 2009, caution is needed for comparisons of data because data were collected slightly differently in the provinces and territories.

Canadian populations and family violence

Certain populations in Canada are more likely to experience family violence, more severe types and/or more severe impacts. Examples include:

Women: For family violence that is reported to police, women are more likely than men to experience family violence at all ages (see Figure 3).[10] In 2014, 57,835 women and 27,567 men were victims of police-reported family violence.[10]

Population surveys show that in their lifetime, women are more likely to be a victim of family violence than men.[84,85,92] In 2010, global data estimated that 30% of women experience physical or sexual intimate partner violence at some point in their life.[84,85] In high income countries, which included Canada, the proportion was 21%.[85] In 2012, data from two cities in Ontario and Quebec showed the following:[92]

- 29% of women and 15% of men said they had experienced emotional abuse from a family member at least once in their lifetime.

- 15% of women and 6% of men said they had experienced physical abuse from a family member at least once in their lifetime.

Canadian data show that women are two to four times more likely than men to experience sexual abuse in childhood or in their marriage or common-law relationship.[10,26,93] Police reports and child welfare investigations find that girls and boys are equally likely to have experienced other types of abuse.[58,71] Population surveys show that women are more likely than men to say they experienced sexual abuse or were aware of their parents' intimate partner violence in childhood. They were less likely to say they had experienced physical abuse in childhood (see Figure 4).[26]

FIGURE 3:
POLICE-REPORTED FAMILY VIOLENCE, 2014.[10]

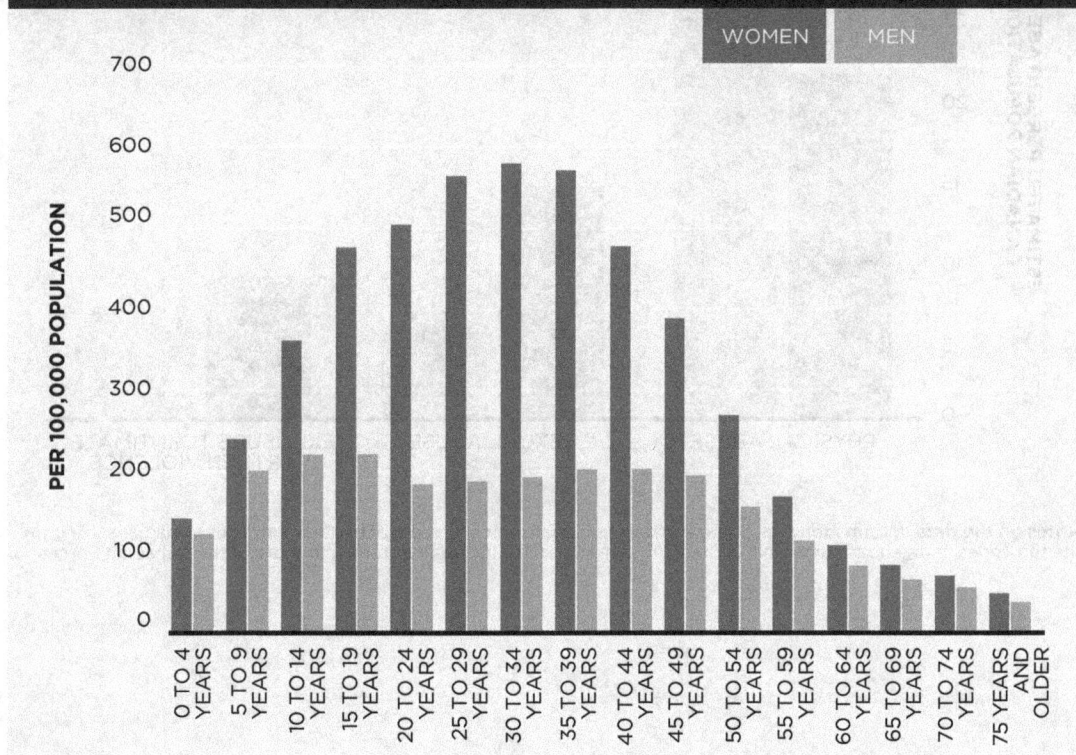

Data from a population survey in 2014 showed that 341,502 or 4% of Canadian women and 418,163 or 4% of Canadian men said they had been a victim of unhealthy conflict, abuse or violence within their marriage or common-law partnership at least once in the previous five years.[10] Women were more likely than men to experience more severe types of intimate partner violence, to experience poor health as a result of intimate partner violence and to be killed by an intimate partner.[4,10]

Indigenous women are also more likely to experience child abuse or violence within their marriage or common-law partnership than Indigenous men. In 2014:[72]

- 14% of Indigenous women and 5% of Indigenous men said they had experienced physical and sexual abuse in childhood.

- 10% of Indigenous women and 8% of Indigenous men said they had experienced violence committed by a spouse or common-law partner in the previous five years.

FIGURE 4:
SELF-REPORTED CHILD ABUSE OR EXPOSURE TO INTIMATE PARTNER VIOLENCE, 2012. [26]

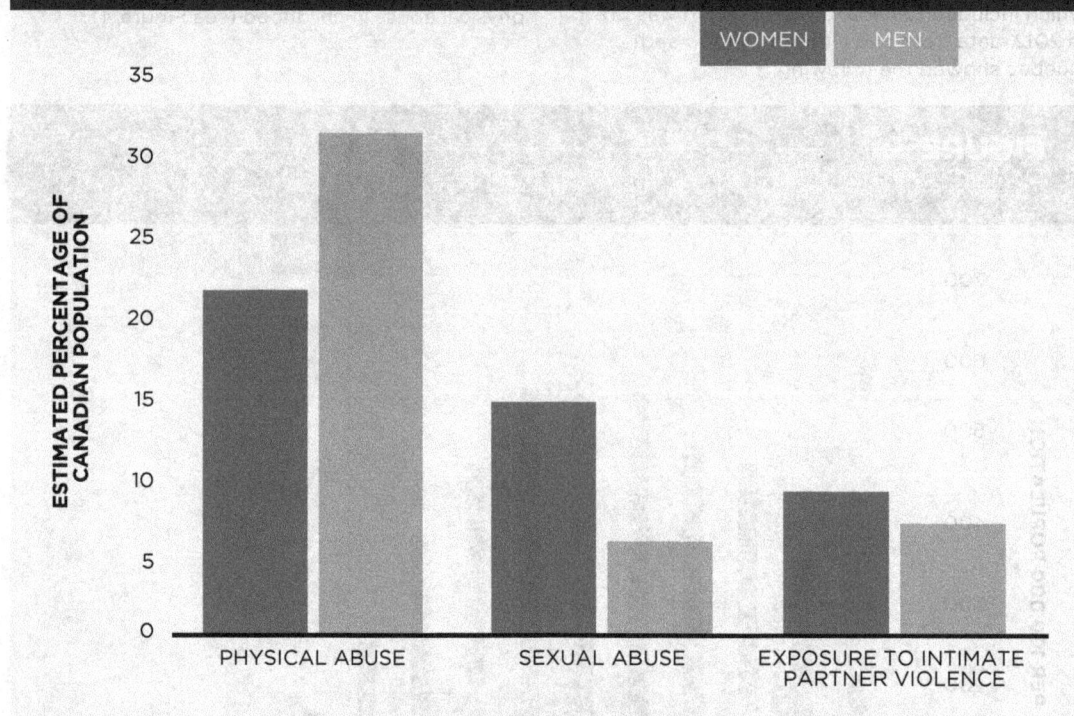

Notes on the data: Information was collected from Canadians ages 18 years and older. Excludes Canadians living in the territories, Indigenous communities or institutions. Does not include full-time members of the Canadian Forces.

Indigenous populations: Indigenous populations are diverse and include First Nations, Métis and Inuit. Family violence in Indigenous communities is the result of many factors including gaps in health and social services, lack of safe places or housing, political and historical context, concerns about the justice system and violence being seen as a normal way to behave. Indigenous women who seek help often need to leave their community. This can mean that they have to leave their sources of support and culture behind.[94] Indigenous peoples may be reluctant to seek help due to the stigma and discrimination they can experience in the health care system.[95]

Indigenous peoples are more likely to experience child abuse and spousal violence than non-Indigenous people. In 2014:[10,72]

- 40% of Indigenous peoples and 29% of non-Indigenous people said they had experienced abuse before the age of 15 years.

- 9% of Indigenous peoples and 4% of non-Indigenous people said they had experienced unhealthy conflict, abuse or violence committed by a spouse or common-law partner in the previous five years.

- 10% of Indigenous women and 3% of non-Indigenous women said they had experienced unhealthy conflict, abuse or violence committed by a spouse or common-law partner in the previous five years.

- Indigenous women were also more likely to report experiencing more severe types of spousal violence and more severe impacts on health than non-Indigenous women.

- Unlike for non-Indigenous women, spousal violence for Indigenous women has not decreased over time.

People with disabilities: People who have a physical disability, health problem or mental health issue that limits their daily activity are more likely to experience spousal violence or sexual violence than people without these types of health issues (see Figure 5).[28,111-113] This is especially true for women.[114]

Intergenerational trauma is a significant issue for some Indigenous communities. For these communities, it is often related to residential schools as well as historical and political contexts.[96-108] Intergenerational trauma happens when a traumatic event not only affects people who experience it, but when it also affects their children and sometimes, grandchildren. For example, children of Indigenous peoples who experienced trauma from residential schools are at higher risk for depression.[100] Other examples of the long-term effects of the residential school experience include loss of traditional knowledge, poor community health, intergenerational stress, disparities in the social determinants of health and disruptions to ethnic and cultural identity.[99,103,109,110]

FIGURE 5:
SELF-REPORTED SPOUSAL VIOLENCE, 2004.[28]

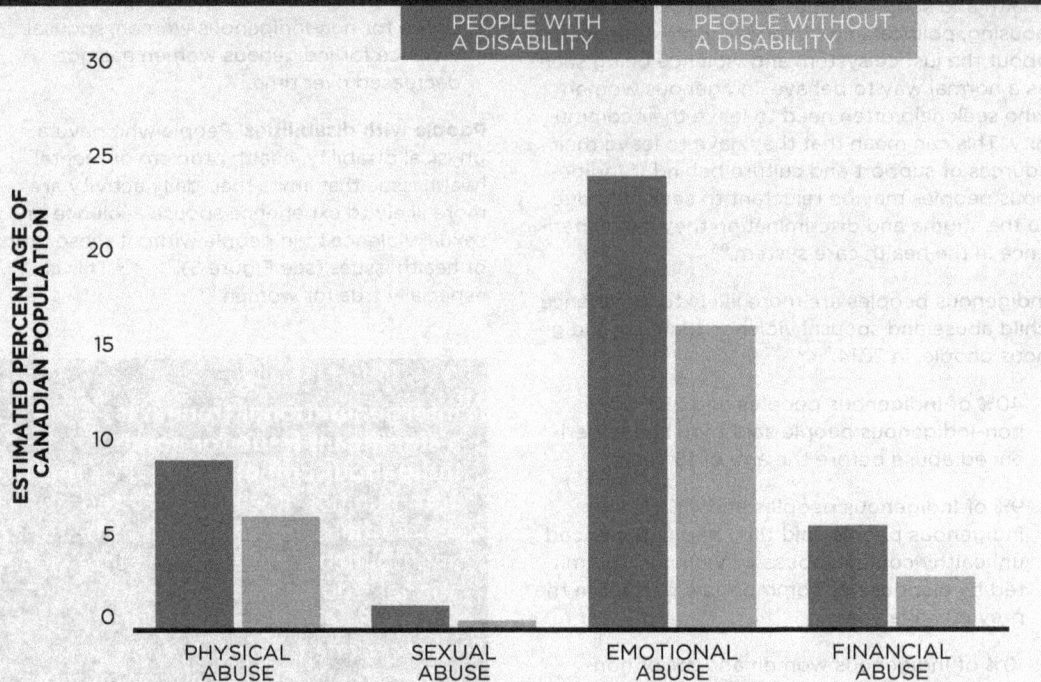

PEOPLE WITH A DISABILITY	PEOPLE WITHOUT A DISABILITY

ESTIMATED PERCENTAGE OF CANADIAN POPULATION

PHYSICAL ABUSE   SEXUAL ABUSE   EMOTIONAL ABUSE   FINANCIAL ABUSE

Notes on the data: A person with a disability is defined as people who said they had difficulty in their daily lives or had a physical disability, health problem or mental health issue that affected their daily activities. Information was collected from Canadians ages 15 years and older and represents spousal violence experienced in the previous five years. Incidents of physical or sexual abuse happened within the previous five years while incidents of emotional or financial abuse happened at any point.

Lesbian, Gay, Bisexual, Transgendered, Queer, Questioning, Intersex and Two-spirited (LGBTQQI2S) community: Data on family violence in the LGBTQQI2S community are limited in Canada, so it is hard to know the full scope of the issue. In 2014, 8% of same-sex partners said they had experienced intimate partner violence in the previous five years compared to 4% of heterosexual partners.[10] For same-sex partners, this is a decrease from 21% in 2004.[10] Research shows that people who identify as LGBTQ are more likely to experience child abuse and neglect, bullying, sexual harassment from peers, dating violence and violence in a marriage or common-law relationship.[10,29-31]

For people who identify as LGBTQ, there are several additional factors that can affect their risk for family violence:[29-31,115-120]

- Family acceptance is a key issue for LGBTQ youth. It can influence self-esteem and social support as well as physical and mental health.

- Lesbian or bisexual women and gay or bisexual men can face challenges related to gender stereotypes. For women, it can be the belief that women are not violent. For men, it can be the belief that men are violent and do not talk about experiencing violence or abuse.

- Other factors include:

  - Stress from being part of a minority group;

  - The threat of being exposed as being LGBTQ;

  - Disclosure of HIV status if relevant;

  - Gender role conflict;

  - Social stigma;

  - Violence external to the relationship, and;

  - Lack of specific support services.

Economic costs of family violence

To date, studies on how much family violence costs Canadians have been limited. Older data suggest that the economic cost of family violence

in Canada is high. It is unclear whether or not these costs have changed over time, as data are not available to make the comparison. Data from 1998 estimate that child abuse and neglect costs Canadians almost $16 billion per year (see Figure 6).[82] Data from 2009 estimate that spousal violence costs Canadians almost $7.4 billion per year (see Figure 6).[83]

For child abuse and neglect, the largest costs are related to lost earnings.[82] For spousal violence, the largest costs are related to intangible costs. These costs include an estimate of how much pain, suffering and loss of life that is caused by spousal violence costs Canadians.[83]

FIGURE 6:
ESTIMATED TOTAL COSTS IN CANADA PER YEAR OF:
A) CHILD ABUSE AND NEGLECT IN 1998;
B) SPOUSAL VIOLENCE IN 2009.[82, 83]

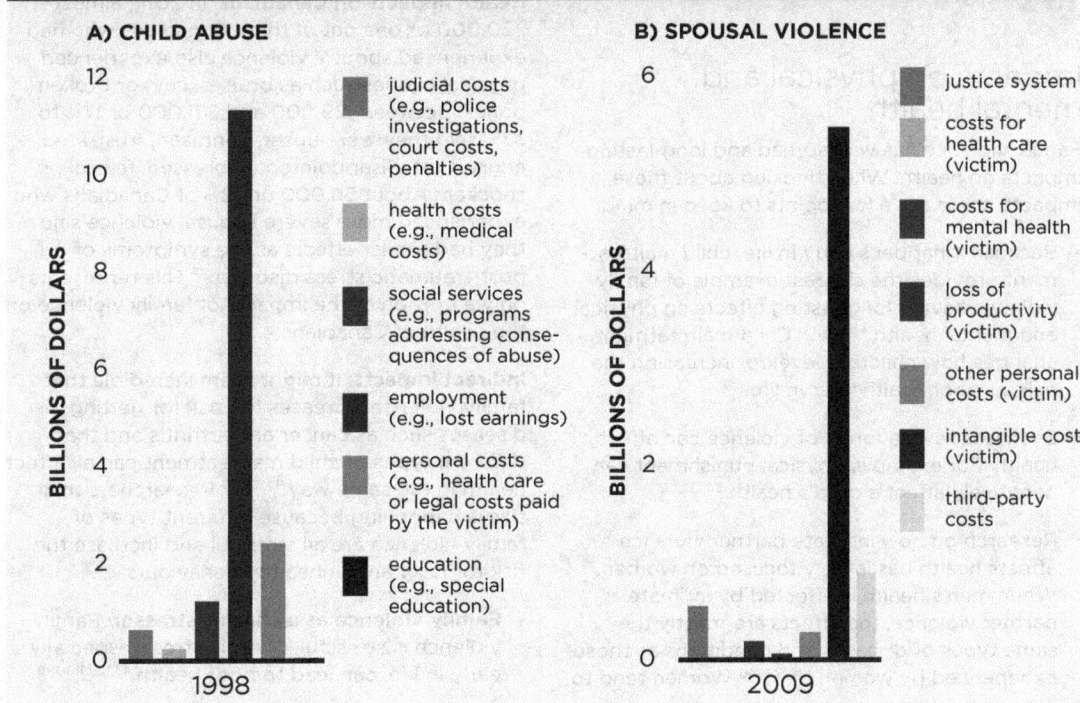

A) CHILD ABUSE

- judicial costs (e.g., police investigations, court costs, penalties)
- health costs (e.g., medical costs)
- social services (e.g., programs addressing consequences of abuse)
- employment (e.g., lost earnings)
- personal costs (e.g., health care or legal costs paid by the victim)
- education (e.g., special education)

1998

B) SPOUSAL VIOLENCE

- justice system
- costs for health care (victim)
- costs for mental health (victim)
- loss of productivity (victim)
- other personal costs (victim)
- intangible costs (victim)
- third-party costs

2009

Mortality

Violence, abuse and neglect increase the risk for early death by homicide and suicide, as well as from diseases and conditions that are related to family violence.[94,121-129] Data on suicides related to family violence, deaths by diseases and conditions related to family violence and deaths due to neglect are limited or lacking.

In 2014, there were 516 homicides in Canada. Of these, 131 or 34% of victims were killed by a family member. Like homicides in general, the number of family homicides have been decreasing, from 229 in 1985 to 131 in 2014.[10,121] Which family member is mostly likely to be accused of a family homicide depends on the age and gender of the victim:

- For infants and children, parents are most likely to be accused of the crime.[130]

- Women are more likely than men to be killed by a spouse, common-law partner or dating partner.[10]

- For older adults, a spouse was most likely to be accused of the crime when older women were victims of family homicide. Adult children were most likely to be accused when older men were victims.[10]

Impacts on physical and mental health

Family violence has widespread and long-lasting impacts on health. When thinking about these impacts, there are a few points to keep in mind:

- Because it happens early in life, child maltreatment provides the clearest example of family violence having long-lasting effects on physical and mental health.[e.g., 59,131] Child maltreatment changes how children develop, increasing the risk for poor health later in life.[129]

- Even less severe forms of violence can affect health. For example, physical punishment can negatively affect a child's health.[34,132,133]

- Research on how intimate partner violence affects health has largely focused on women. When men's health is affected by intimate partner violence, the effects are mostly the same types of diseases and conditions as those experienced by women.[e.g., 73,146] Women tend to experience a wider range of and more severe impacts on their health than men.[4,10,73,147]

- Not much research is available on how the mistreatment of older adults affects their health and well-being.

Outlined in Figure 7 is a simplified picture to show how family violence directly and indirectly affects health.

Can health impacts be 'reversed'?

The English and Romanian Adoptees studies examined neglect in a group of Romanian orphans. These orphans showed many developmental delays and difficulties bonding with caregivers. Adoption in the United Kingdom before the age of six months improved many of these delays in most children. Some children who were adopted at a later age also showed improvement.[134-145]

Health impacts on Canadians: In 2014, almost 250,000 or one out of three Canadians who had experienced spousal violence also experienced physical injuries such as bruises, cuts or broken bones. Between 129,000 and 281,000 or 17% to 37% said they were upset, confused, frustrated, angry, hurt, disappointed, depressed, fearful or shocked. About 59,000 or 32% of Canadians who experienced more severe spousal violence said they had similar effects as the symptoms of post-traumatic stress disorder.[10] This represents only a portion of the impacts of family violence on the health of Canadians.

Indirect impacts: It might seem incredible that family violence increases the risk for getting diseases such as cancer and arthritis and that different types of child maltreatment can all affect health in the same way.[32,61,160] Researchers think this is happening because different types of family violence are all stressful and increase the risk for risky and unhealthy behaviours:

- **Family violence as a chronic stressor**: Family violence is stressful. Chronic stress, especially early in life, can lead to poor health.[43,129,161-199]

FIGURE 7:
A SIMPLIFIED PICTURE OF HOW FAMILY VIOLENCE LEADS TO HEALTH IMPACTS. 26, 32–71, 127, 128, 131, 132, 147–159

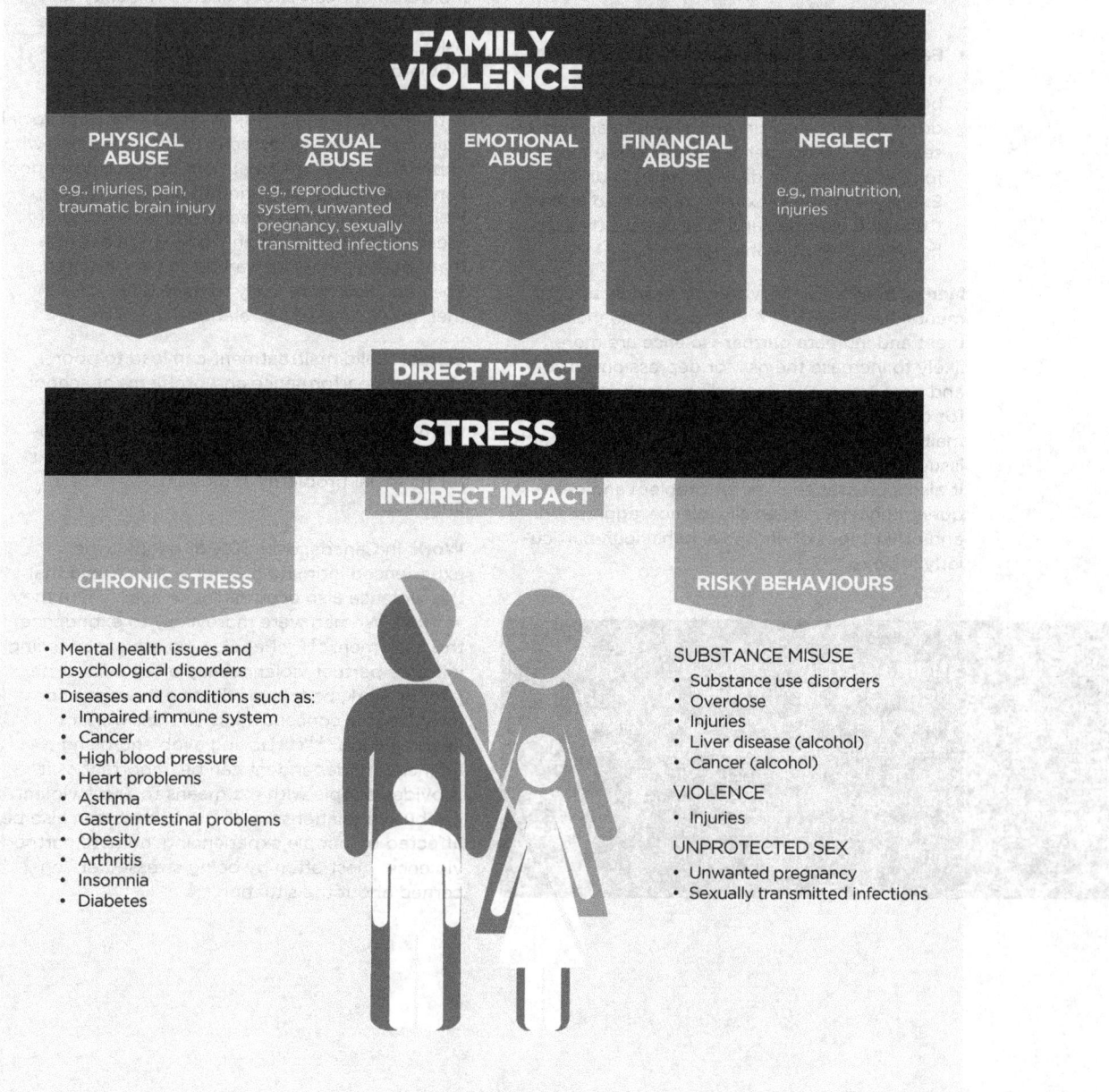

FAMILY VIOLENCE

PHYSICAL ABUSE
e.g., injuries, pain, traumatic brain injury

SEXUAL ABUSE
e.g., reproductive system, unwanted pregnancy, sexually transmitted infections

EMOTIONAL ABUSE

FINANCIAL ABUSE

NEGLECT
e.g., malnutrition, injuries

DIRECT IMPACT

STRESS

INDIRECT IMPACT

CHRONIC STRESS

- Mental health issues and psychological disorders
- Diseases and conditions such as:
  - Impaired immune system
  - Cancer
  - High blood pressure
  - Heart problems
  - Asthma
  - Gastrointestinal problems
  - Obesity
  - Arthritis
  - Insomnia
  - Diabetes

RISKY BEHAVIOURS

SUBSTANCE MISUSE
- Substance use disorders
- Overdose
- Injuries
- Liver disease (alcohol)
- Cancer (alcohol)

VIOLENCE
- Injuries

UNPROTECTED SEX
- Unwanted pregnancy
- Sexually transmitted infections

There are many theories on why this happens. Examples of the effects of chronic stress include changes to how the immune system works and how cells in the human body divide.[129,162,165,200-203] This might explain how experiencing family violence can increase the risk for getting diseases such as heart disease or dementia.[129]

- **Family violence and risky behaviour**: Family violence can lead to risky and unhealthy behaviours such as heavy alcohol consumption, drug use, smoking, unhealthy eating and unsafe sex.[60,204-211] These behaviours increase the risk for a wide range of diseases and conditions. Examples include sexually transmitted diseases through unsafe sex and liver disease through heavy alcohol consumption.[60,206]

Mental health: Family violence strongly affects mental health.[60,73,74,149,206,212] Both child maltreatment and intimate partner violence are more likely to increase the risk for depression, anxiety and post-traumatic stress disorder than the risk for other diseases and conditions.[60,73,149] Child maltreatment increases the risk for mental health issues at any age and for all types of abuse.[131] It also increases the risk for problem and delinquent behaviours such as violence, aggression and other types of antisocial behaviour, particularly in boys.[58,213-215]

Stigma: Family violence can lead to stigma and discrimation, including false ideas that victims are trapped, passive, helpless, depressed, weak or responsible for being a victim.[229-233] The potential for experiencing stigma and discrimination can lead to people being reluctant to seek help.[234]

Other types of impacts

Family violence can affect people's relationships and lives at school and work.

Social relationships: Family violence can affect people's relationships and friendships. Child maltreatment can affect a person's ability to develop healthy relationships and increase the risk for experiencing or being responsible for intimate partner violence. This may be because it also increases the risk for problems dealing with emotions and stress as well as for poor social skills and lower self-esteem.[151,213,217-226] People who experience child maltreatment or harsh parenting can have trouble parenting their own children, which can impact the health and well-being of these children.[227] Women who experience intimate partner violence can be socially isolated. They are also more likely to have difficulties in their family and social relationships.[149,228]

School: Child maltreatment can lead to poor academic performance and problems at school. This is likely due to the fact it affects learning, memory, problem solving, attention and emotion.[129,213,235-241] This can lead to increased risks for financial problems and unemployment in adulthood.[242]

Work: In Canada, over 50% of people who experienced intimate partner violence said that this violence also occurred at or near where they worked. Women were more likely to experience this than men.[243,244] People who are experiencing intimate partner violence may often miss or be late for work, be less productive at work, and have trouble concentrating on their work or keeping a job.[244-248] Having a job and being financially independent can be important as it provides people with the means to end a violent or abusive relationship.[249] Co-workers can also be affected by people experiencing intimate partner violence, most often by being stressed or concerned about the situation.[244]

Factors that affect the health impacts of family violence

Not everyone is at equal risk for poor health from family violence.[250] Outlined below are some examples of factors that affect this risk:

Resilience: Resilience is when someone is able to cope with or recover from a negative experience or stressful situation with little effect to his or her health.[250,251] While family violence affects the health of many people who experience it, some people are resilient.[87,151-154,252-255] Researchers are interested in figuring out why this happens and how this could prevent family violence from leading to poor health.[256]

Genetics and epigenetics: Researchers have found that person's genetic makeup (their genotype) can increase the risk that child maltreatment will lead to depression in adulthood or problem behaviours in adolescence.[257-259] Other genotypes are thought to reduce the risk that child abuse will affect health.[260,261] Epigenetics may also play a role.[129,258,262-269] Stressful experiences in childhood might affect how genes are activated and expressed, which can lead to poor health later in life.[129]

What is 'epigenetics'? Epigenetics is the study of how human biology adapts to a changing environment by altering gene expression and activation. These changes can be passed on to future generations.[270]

Frequency and severity of abuse: There is evidence that the more types of abuse experienced or the more severe and frequent the abuse a child experiences, the higher the risk that child abuse will lead to poor health.[26,50,60,73,75-77,203,271,272] Other stressful or negative events experienced early in life can add to this effect.[78,79] A similar pattern exists for intimate partner violence. The more severe and more frequent the abuse, the more likely intimate partner violence will lead to mental health issues.[74]

Understanding early adversity: Child maltreatment is not the only form of early stress or adversity that leads to impacts on health.[273] The Adverse Childhood Experiences studies were important for showing the link between early adverse experiences and health impacts in adulthood.[273-278]

Age: Whether or not child maltreatment affects later health can depend on what age the abuse or neglect is experienced.[148,224,229,235,236] In some cases, the earlier the maltreatment occurs in childhood, the more likely it will lead to mental health issues.[237]

Gender: Women are more likely than men to experience health impacts from child abuse and intimate partner violence.[10,26,32,73,74,80,87,279,280] In 2014, a Canadian population survey showed that in the previous five years:[10]

- 40% of women and 24% of men said they had experienced physical injuries as a result of spousal violence.

- 22% of women and 9% of men who experienced spousal violence said they had also experienced effects similar to the symptoms of post-traumatic stress disorder.

Women are also more likely than men to be emotionally affected and to experience fear in response to intimate partner violence.[4,10,281-283]

A Concise Guide to Medical Terminology

This Guide is designed to help the reader decipher some unfamiliar terms used in the disorder descriptions. It is helpful to divide medical terms into their basic elements: prefix, root and suffix. Following these examples are 239 commonly used medical prefixes, roots and suffixes.

Example 1: The medical term *microcephaly* is a combination of "micr(o)," meaning small, and "cephal(o)," which means head. Therefore, microcephaly denotes an abnormally small head. In contrast, "macr(o)" means large. Thus, *macrocephaly* indicates an unusually large head.

Example 2: The word *polydactyly* includes "poly," meaning much or many, and "dactyl," which refers to fingers or toes. Thus, the medical term *polydactyly* means the presence of extra fingers or toes. Accordingly, because "brachy" means short, the word *brachydactyly* indicates abnormally short fingers or toes.

Example 3: The term *myositis* is a combination of "my(o)," which denotes muscle, and "itis," meaning inflammation. Therefore, *myositis* means muscle inflammation. When "cardi(o)," meaning heart, is added, forming the term *myocarditis,* the meaning becomes inflammation of heart muscle.

Medical Prefixes, Roots, and Suffixes

A.................absence of, without	cry(o)............cold	hist(o)...........tissue
Ab.................away from	crypt(o).........conceal, hide	hom(o)..........common, same
Acou.............hear	cyan..............blue	hydr(o)..........water
aden(o)..........gland	cyst(o)...........bladder	hyper.............above, beyond, excessive
-algia.............pain	cyt(o)............cell	hypn(o).........sleep
all(o).............other, different	de.................away from, down	hyp(o)...........below, deficient, low
andr(o)..........man	dent(o)..........tooth	hyster(o).......uterus
angi(o).........vessel	dermat(o)......skin	iatr(o)...........physician
ankyl(o).......bent, crooked	di.................two	idi(o)............distinct, separate
ante..............before	dia................apart, through	ili(o)............intestines
anti...............against, counter	digit ....finger or toe	inter ....among, between
arteri(o).........artery	dipl(o)...........double	intra ....inside, within
arthr(o)..........joint	dors(o)..........back	ischi(o)..........hip
audio.............hearing, sound	dys ....abnormal, bad	-itis ....inflammation
auri ....ear	ect(o) ....outside, out of place	kary(o)..........nucleus
aut(o) ....self	-emia.............blood	kilo ....one thousand
bacteri(o) ......bacteria	en..................in, on	kinet(o).........move
bio................life	end(o)...........inside, within	labio..............lips
blast(o)..........bud, early embryonic budding	enter(o).........intestine	lact(o)...........milk
-blast.............formative cell, germinal layer	epi.................above, upon	lapar(o).........flank, loin
blephar(o) .....eyelid	erythr(o)........red	laryng(o).......larynx
brachi(o) ....arm	eso.................inside, within	latero.............side
brachy...........short	esthesi(o) ......feel, perceive	leuc(o) ....white
brady.............slow	eu.................normal, well	leuk(o) ....white
bronch(o)......bronchi	ex..................away from, outside	lien(o)...........spleen
bucc(o)..........cheek	extra..............beyond, in addition, outside of	lingu(o).........tongue
carcin(o) ....cancer	flav(o)...........yellow	lip(o).............fat
cardi(o) ....heart	galact(o)........milk	lith(o)............stone
-cele ....hernia, protrusion, tumor	gastr(o) ....stomach	lymph(o).......water
cent ....one hundred	gen(o) ....gene or reproduction	macr(o) ....large
centr(o) ....centre	gloss(o).........tongue	mal.................abnormal, bad
cephal(o).......head	glyc(o) ....sweet	malac(o)........soft
cerebr(o) ....brain	gnath(o) ....jaw	mamm(o)......breast
cervic ....neck	gram..............draw, record, write	mast(o)..........breast
chole ....bile	graph(o)........record, write	medi..............middle
chondr(o) ......cartilage	gynec(o).......woman	mega ....great, large
circum...........around	hemat(o) ....blood	megal(o) ....great, large
-coele ....body/organ cavity	hemi..............half	melan(o) ....black
contra...........against, counter	hepat(o) ....liver	mening(o) .....membrane
cost(o)..........rib	hex ....six	mes(o)..........middle
crani(o) ....skull	hidr(o)..........sweat	meta..............after, beyond

metr(o)..........uterus	pen...............around	scler(o)..........hard
micr(o)..........small	penia.............abnormal reduction, deficiency	-scope ....instrument for examining
mill(i)............one thousand	pent(a) ....five	semi ....half
mon(o)..........only, single, sole	per................through	sial(o)...........saliva
morph(o)......form, shape, structure	phag(o) ....consume, eat	somat(o).......body
myel(o) ....marrow	pharmaco ......drug, medicine	somn(i) ....sleep
my(o)...........muscle	pharyng(o)....throat	spasm(o).......spasm
myx(o).........mucus	phleb(o) ....vein	spermat(o).....seed
narc(o) ....stupor	phon(o) ....sound	splen(o)........spleen
nas(o)...........nose	phot(o)..........light	spondyl(o) ....vertebra
necr(o) ....corpse, death	physi(o) ....natural, physical	spor(o)..........spore
neo ....new	pil(o).............hair	steat(o)..........fat
nephr(o) ....kidney	-plasia ....development, formation	sten(o)..........compressed, narrow
neur(o)..........nerve	platy..............broad, flat	stomat(o) ......mouth, opening
noci ....pain	pleur(o)..........rib, side	sub ....below, near, under
noso ....disease	-pnea ....breathing	super ....above, beyond, excessive
ocul(o) ....eye	pneumat(o) ...air, breathing	syn ....together, with
odont(o) ....tooth	pneum(o) ......air, breath, lung	tachy ....fast, rapid
-odyn(o).......distress, pain	pod(o)...........foot	tel(o) ....end
olig(o)...........deficient, few, little	poly...............many, much	tetra..............four
-oma.............neoplasm, tumour	post ....after, behind	therm(o)........heat
omphal(o).....navel	pre.................before, in front of	thorac(o) ....chest
onc(o) ....mass, tumour	pro ....before, in front of	thromb(o)......clot
onych(o) ....nail	proct(o).........rectum	-tome ....instrument for cutting
oo.................egg	pseud(o)........false	tox(o)...........poison
ophthalm(o) ..eye	psych(o)........mind	trans ....through, across
orchi(o).........testicle	pulmon(o).....lung	traumat(o).....wound
oro ....mouth	pyel(o) ....pelvis	tri ....three
-osis ....process, disease from	pyr(o)............fire, heat	trich(o).........hair
osse(o) ....bone	quadri............four	troph(o).........food, nourishment
oste(o)..........bone	rachi(o) ....spine	-uria ....urine
ot(o)..............ear	radio ....radiation	vas(o)...........vessel
ovari(o).........ovary	re...................again, back	vertebr(o)......vertebrae
oxy................sharp	ren(o)............kidneys	vesic(o).........bladder or blister
pachy ....thick	retr(o)............backward, behind	xanth(o) ....yellow
pan................whole, all	rheo...............flow	xen(o) ....foreign, different
para...............beside, beyond, resembling	rhin(o)...........nose	xer(o)............dry
path(o) ....disease	sangui ....blood	zyg(o) ....junction, union
ped(o) ....child	sarc(o)...........flesh	

Addison's Disease

Addison's disease, also referred to as adrenal insufficiency, stems from the malfunction of the adrenal glands located on top of the kidneys. In this disease, there is an insufficient amount of cortisol and aldosterone produced by the adrenal cortex, the gland's firm outer layer.

Cause

Most often, Addison's disease results from destruction of the adrenal gland. Patients develop antibodies against their own adrenal tissue (autoimmune reaction). It may also be caused by fungal infections (or other infections such as HIV and tuberculosis), malignant tumours, trauma or blood loss.

Symptoms

The symptoms of Addison's disease usually develop slowly over the course of several months. Signs of the disease may include fatigue, weakness, loss of appetite, nausea and vomiting, low blood pressure (hypotension) and salt cravings. Other symptoms such as darkening of the skin (hyperpigmentation), muscle pain, low blood sugar (hypoglycemia), depression and irritability may also occur. If a person is in acute adrenal failure (Addisonian crisis), there may be a sudden onset of signs and symptoms such as severe vomiting and diarrhea, pain in the lower abdomen, back or legs, low blood pressure, difficulty breathing and loss of consciousness.

Prevalence

Addison's disease is a rare disorder that is diagnosed in about 1 in 100,000 people. It affects men, women and children of all ages.

Treatment Options

Addison's disease is diagnosed after a thorough medical history is taken, and a number of tests are performed. These tests may include a blood test, an ACTH (adrenocorticotropic hormone) test, an insulin-induced hypoglycemia test and imaging tests.

The primary treatment for Addison's disease is hormone replacement therapy. Options to counteract hormonal loss include oral corticosteroids, corticosteroid injections and androgen replacement therapy. During times of illness and surgery, a temporary increase in dosage is usually suggested. Treatment should never be stopped, even for a day, without the advice of a physician. Persons undergoing treatment should wear a medical alert bracelet and carry a medical identification card to let emergency medical providers know of their diagnosis. Immediate treatment—typically through injections of hydrocortisone, saline and sugar—is required during an Addisonian crisis.

People with Addison's disease require lifelong treatment. However, with proper hormone replacement therapy, they are able to lead normal lives.

National Associations

The Canadian Addison Society / La Société canadienne d'Addison
1 Palace Arch Dr., Etobicoke, ON M9A 2S1

Toll-Free: 888-550-5582
Other Communication: newsletter@addisonsociety.ca
e-mail: info@addisonsociety.ca
www.addisonsociety.ca

Overview: A small national charitable organization founded in 1990
Mission: To offer information about Addison's Disease; To assist in the education of the medical society & the public about Addison's Disease
Chief Officer(s):
Harold Smith, President
   president@addisonsociety.ca
Roger Steinmann, Vice-President
   vicepresident@addisonsociety.ca

Rick Burpee, Secretary-Treasurer
   secretary-treasurer@addisonsociety.ca
Publications:
• The Canadian Addison Society Newsletter
Type: Newsletter; *Frequency:* Quarterly
Profile: Society updates & current information regarding Addison's Disease

Adjustment Disorders

Cause

The experience of stress in life is inevitable. Serious life changes such as job loss, divorce and surgery, and more commonplace events like the first day of school and worries about money can all be stressful. When faced with such situations, people usually do their best to cope and move on. However, if a person cannot seem to adjust to these life changes and continues to feel overwhelmed and anxious and have trouble functioning normally, an adjustment disorder—a stress-related mental illness—may be diagnosed. Adjustment disorders are divided into six subtypes: depressed mood; anxiety; mixed anxiety and depressed mood; disturbance of conduct; mixed disturbance of emotions and conduct; and unspecified.

Symptoms

The symptoms of adjustment disorders are both emotional and behavioural, and vary from person to person. However, in all cases, the symptoms begin within three months of experiencing a stressful event. An adjustment disorder may make a person feel sad, nervous, anxious, worried, hopeless or desperate. Physical complaints such as trembling, twitching and skipped heartbeats may also be experienced. People suffering from an adjustment disorder may also exhibit changes in behaviour including social withdrawal, vandalism, truancy, fighting and reckless driving. Adjustment disorders increase the risk of suicidal behaviour, and they also complicate the course of other medical conditions (for example, patients may not take their medication or eat properly). If the symptoms persist for less than six months after the stressor ends, the disorder is considered acute; if symptoms persist for more than six months, the disorder is considered to be chronic.

Prevalence

Men and women of all ages, as well as children, can suffer from this disorder. The chance of having an adjustment disorder is about the same for boys and girls, but among adults, women are twice as likely as men to be affected. In the general population, the prevalence of adjustment disorders is estimated to range from 5 to 20 percent. In the labour market, an adjustment disorder—often referred to as burnout—is one of the most common mental disorders diagnosed in workers.

Treatment Options

The diagnosis of an adjustment disorder is made after a thorough psychiatric evaluation has ruled out other possible diagnoses. For example, symptoms that are part of a personality disorder and become worse under stress are not usually considered to be adjustment disorders unless they are new types of symptoms for the individual. The patient must also meet the criteria for adjustment disorder that are specified in the *Diagnostic and Statistical Manual of Mental Disorders (DSM)*. An emotional or behavioural response that is out-of-proportion to a specific stressor, or that impairs a person's ability to function in social, workplace and school settings meets the criteria, as do symptoms that develop within three months of experiencing a stressful event (other than bereavement).

Anyone who is experiencing one or more stressful events or circumstances, and feels overwhelmed or markedly distressed and cannot function normally, should seek help. The main type of treatment prescribed for adjustment disorder is psychotherapy and, depending on the circumstances, can include individual, couple or family therapy. Medications—most often antidepressants and anti-anxiety agents—are sometimes prescribed for a few weeks or months. In most instances, long-term therapy will not be necessary, and the person can expect significant improvement within 8 to 12 sessions.

National Associations

The Organization for Bipolar Affective Disorder (OBAD)
1019 - 7th Ave. SW, Calgary AB T2P 1A8

Tel: 403-263-7408
Toll-Free: 866-263-7408
e-mail: obad@obad.ca
www.obad.ca

Overview: A medium-sized national charitable organization
Mission: To assist people affected directly or indirectly by bipolar disorder, depression, & anxiety
Chief Officer(s):
Kaj Korvela, Executive Director

International Associations

International Society for Affective Disorders (ISAD)
c/o Caroline Holebrook, Institute of Psychiatry, King's College London, PO72 De Crespigny Park, Denmark Hill, London SE5 8AF UK

Tel: +44 (0) 20 7848 0295; *Fax:* +44 (0) 20 7848 0298
Other Communication: help@isad.org.uk
e-mail: enquiry@isad.org.uk
www.isad.org.uk
twitter.com/ISADTweet

Overview: A large international charitable organization founded in 2001
Mission: To advance research into affective disorders through all relevant scientific disciplines
Chief Officer(s):
Allan Young, President
Anthony Cleare, Treasurer
John Rush, Regional Representative, North America (Canada & the United States)
Caroline Holebrook, Administrator
    caroline.loveland@kcl.ac.uk
Publications:
• Journal of Affective Disorders
Type: Journal; *Editor:* Jair Soares; Paolo Brambilla

Aging

Aging is not a disease, but part of the normal life cycle, and many seniors retain good health and live independently for long past the traditional age of retirement. In time, however, most will develop one or more chronic conditions. In Canada, the number of cases of chronic illness is on the rise among seniors.

Cause
There are a number of reasons why people might be developing age-related disorders more quickly than they did in previous generations. Seniors, and in particular older women, often get little physical activity. In fact, they are the most inactive segment of the population in Canada. In addition, the prevalence of obesity is increasing in the older population. In 2004, the obesity rate for adults aged 75 and over reached 24 percent compared to 11 percent in 1978-79. The risk of injury, chronic disease and poor health increases as a result of being overweight. Smoking is also a factor associated with developing a chronic disease and is implicated in 8 of the 14 top causes of death in people aged 65 years or over in Canada.

Symptoms
Life expectancy for Canadians is longer than it ever has been before—78 years for men, and 83 years for women. However, the number of years spent in good health has been on the decline since reaching a peak in 1996. The types of chronic illness commonly occurring due to aging are chronic pain, diabetes and certain types of cancer. Dementia is also common and currently affects around half a million seniors in Canada. By 2038, it is estimated that more than one million older adults will suffer from this condition.

Prevalence
The elderly population in Canada is growing faster than any other segment of the population, and it is estimated that this trend will continue for the next several decades. In 2015, there were about 5.8 million people in Canada (about one in six Canadians) who were 65 years of age or older, and by 2035 the number of seniors is expected to double. By 2030, it is estimated that almost one in four Canadians will be 65 years of age or older. The 80-plus age category is populated by a far greater number of women than men.

Treatment Options
Treating the elderly requires many medical and non-medical services, integrated to provide a comprehensive continuum of care. Older Canadians can stay healthier and live longer if they adopt healthy eating habits, are physically active, stay socially connected, reduce their risks for falls and refrain from smoking.

See also Alzheimer's Disease

National Associations

Active Living Coalition for Older Adults (ALCOA) / Coalition d'une vie active pour les ainé(e)s
PO Box 143, Stn. Main, Shelburne ON L9V 3L8

Tel: 519-925-1676
Toll-Free: 800-549-9799
Other Communication: Other URL: www.silvertimes.ca
e-mail: alcoa@uniserve.com
www.alcoa.ca
www.facebook.com/726682140748841

Overview: A medium-sized national organization founded in 1993
Mission: To encourage older Canadians to maintain & enhance their well-being & independence through a lifestyle that embraces daily physical activities
Chief Officer(s):
Patricia Clark, Executive Director

Canadian Academy of Geriatric Psychiatry (CAGP) / L'Académie canadienne de psychiatrie gériatrique (ACPG)
#6, 20 Crown Steel Dr., Markham ON L3R 9X9

Tel: 905-415-3917; *Fax:* 905-415-0071
Toll-Free: 855-415-3917
e-mail: cagp@secretariatcentral.com
www.cagp.ca
www.facebook.com/CanadianAcademyofGeriatricPsychiatry

Overview: A small national organization
Mission: To promote mental health for elderly people in Canada
Member of: Council of Academies of the Canadian Psychiatric Association
Chief Officer(s):
Mark Rapoport, President
Maria Kardaris, Manager
Nancy Vasil, Co-Chair, Communications
Publications:
• CAGP [Canadian Academy of Geriatric Psychiatry] E-newsletter
Type: Newsletter; *Frequency:* Quarterly
Profile: CAGP reports, meetings, awards, & statistics
• Canadian Journal of Geriatric Medicine & Psychiatry
Type: Journal
Profile: Peer-reviewed original research on the health & care of older adults, co-sponsored by the Canadian Academy of Geriatric Psychiatry & the Canadian Geriatrics Society

Canadian Alliance for Long Term Care (CALTC)

e-mail: info@caltc.ca
www.caltc.ca

Overview: A medium-sized national organization
Mission: To ensure the delivery fo quality care to vulnerable citizens of Canada

Canadian Association on Gerontology (CAG) / Association canadienne de gérontologie (ACG)

c/o University of Toronto, #160, 500 University Ave., Toronto ON M5G 1V7

Toll-Free: 855-224-2240
www.cagacg.ca
www.linkedin.com/company/canadian-association-on-gerontology
www.facebook.com/CdnAssocGero
twitter.com/cagacg

Overview: A medium-sized national charitable organization founded in 1971
Mission: To develop the theoretical & practical understanding of individual & population aging through multidisciplinary research, practice, education & policy analysis in gerontology; To seek the improvement of the conditions of life of elderly people in Canada
Member of: International Association of Gerontology & Geriatrics
Chief Officer(s):
Verena Menec, Vice-President
Anthony Lombardo, PhD, Executive Director
Alison Phinney, Secretary-Treasurer
Publications:
• Abuse & Neglect of Older Canadians: Strategies for Change
• CAG [Canadian Association on Gerontology] Newsletter / Bulletin d'information de l'ACG
Type: Newsletter; *Frequency:* Quarterly
Profile: Information about conferences, events, students, publications, & CAG news
• Canadian Association on Gerontology Conference Program Books
Frequency: Biennially
• Canadian Association on Gerontology Policy Statements & Issues Papers
• Canadian Journal on Aging [a publication of the Canadian Association on Gerontology]
Frequency: Quarterly; *Accepts Advertising*; *Editor:* Dr. Paul Stolee; *ISSN:* 0714-9808; *Price:* $30student; $71 individual; $115 institution
Profile: A refereed publication with articles about aging concerned with biology, practice, social sciences, & psychology
• National Forum on Closing the Care Gap

Canadian Geriatrics Society (CGS) / Société canadienne de gériatrie (SCG)

#6, 20 Crown Steel Dr., Markham ON L3R 9X9

Tel: 905-415-3917; *Fax:* 905-415-0071
Toll-Free: 855-415-3917
www.canadiangeriatrics.ca
twitter.com/CanGeriSoc

Previous Name: Canadian Society of Geriatric Medicine
Overview: A small national organization founded in 1981
Mission: To promote excellence in the medical care of the elderly; To support high standards of research on geriatrics; To disseminate information about the clinical care of the elderly
Member of: Royal College of Physicians & Surgeons of Canada
Affliation(s): Canadian Association of Gerontology
Chief Officer(s):
Karen Fruetel, President

Canadian Gerontological Nursing Association (CGNA) / Association canadienne des infirmières et infirmiers en gérontologie

www.cgna.net

Overview: A medium-sized national charitable organization founded in 1984
Mission: To promote gerontological nursing practice standards & educational programs in gerontological nursing; To promote the health of elderly persons; To promote networking opportunities; To support & disseminate gerontological nursing research; To represent members to government, education, professional & other appropriate bodies
Affliation(s): Canadian Nurses Association
Chief Officer(s):

Veronique Boscart, RN, MScN, MEd, President
vboscart@conestogac.on.ca
Michelle Heyer, Treasurer
Publications:
• The Canadian Gerontological Nurse [a publication of the Canadian Gerontological Nursing Association]
Type: Newsletter; *Frequency:* Quarterly
• Gerontological Nursing Competencies & Standards of Practice
Type: Document; *Price:* $13 members; $16 non-members
• Perspectives [a publication of the Canadian Gerontological Nursing Association]
Type: Journal; *Frequency:* Quarterly; *ISSN:* 0831-7445

Canadian Rheumatology Association (CRA) / Société canadienne de rhumatologie

#244, 12 - 16715 Yonge St., Newmarket ON L3X 1X4
Tel: 905-952-0698; *Fax:* 905-952-0708
e-mail: info@rheum.ca
rheum.ca

Overview: A small national organization
Mission: To represent Canadian rheumatologists & promote their pursuit of excellence in arthritis care & research in Canada through leadership, education & communication
Affliation(s): Canadian Medical Association, Royal College of Physicians & Surgeons of Canada
Chief Officer(s):
Cory Baillie, President
Jacob Karsh, Sec.-Treas.
Publications:
• Journal of the Canadian Rheumatology Association
Type: Journal; *Frequency:* Quarterly

Canadian Society for the Study of the Aging Male (CSSAM) / Société canadienne pour l'Étude de l'Homme Vieillissant (SCEHV)

71 Dewlane Dr., Toronto ON M2R 2P9
Tel: 416-480-0010; *Fax:* 416-480-0010
e-mail: secretariat@cssam.com
www.cssam.com

Previous Name: Canadian Andropause Society
Overview: A small national organization founded in 1998
Mission: To support research on the physical, medical, sociological, & psychological changes in aging men
Chief Officer(s):
David Greenberg, President

Elder Mediation Canada (EMC)

www.eldermediation.ca

Overview: A medium-sized national organization
Mission: To advance the practice of elder mediation in Canada; to improve the qualifications & effectiveness of mediators
Affliation(s): Elder Mediation International Network; Family Mediation Canada

National Initiative for the Care of the Elderly (NICE) / Initiative nationale pour le soin des personnes âgées

#328, 263 McCaul St., Toronto ON M5T 1W7
Tel: 416-978-0545; *Fax:* 416-978-4771
e-mail: nicenetadmin@utoronto.ca
www.nicenet.ca
facebook.com/NICElderly
twitter.com/NICElderly

Overview: A small national organization
Mission: National network of researchers & practitioners involved in the care of older adults through medicine, nursing & social work
Member of: Network of Centres of Excellence
Chief Officer(s):
Anthony Lombardo, Network Manager

National Pensioners Federation (NPF) / Fédération nationale des retraités
c/o Mary Forbes, Treasurer, 2186 Stanfield Rd, Mississauga ON L4Y 1R5

Tel: 519-359-3221
www.nationalpensionersfederation.ca
www.facebook.com/NPFederation
twitter.com/npfederation
www.youtube.com/user/npfederation

Previous Name: National Pensioners & Senior Citizens Federation
Overview: A large national organization founded in 1945
Mission: To act as an advisory body providing central contacts, facilities for research, surveys, uniform objectives & a national expansion of the pensioners movement; To stimulate public interest in the welfare of senior citizens by means of adequate pensions & social security that will provide comfortable housing & decent living; To protect the rights & interests of pensioners & prospective pensioners; To prevent discrimination & undue delay in granting pensions; To project a social friendly fellowship among the pensioners of Canada
Affliation(s): International Senior Citizens Association
Chief Officer(s):
Herb John, President, 519-350-3221
  herb.john@npfmail.ca
Patrick Brady, Secretary, 604-856-2430
  patbrady@uniserve.com
Mary Forbes, Treasurer, 905-306-1830
  mary.forbes@npfmail.ca

Steelworkers Organization of Active Retirees (SOAR)
234 Eglinton Ave. East, 8th Fl., Toronto ON M4P 1K7

Tel: 416-487-1571; *Fax:* 416-482-5548
Toll-Free: 877-669-8792
e-mail: info@usw.ca
www.usw.ca

Overview: A medium-sized national organization founded in 1985
Mission: To deal with the social, economic, educational, legislative & political developments & concerns of its members & spouses; to fight for the preservation of Social Security, Medicare, better health care protection, as well as for federal laws to better serve the elderly
Affliation(s): United Steelworkers of America
Chief Officer(s):
Doug MacPherson, National Coordinator
  dmacpherson@usw.ca

Provincial Associations

ALBERTA

Alberta Association on Gerontology (AAG)
PO Box 47022, Stn. Edmonton Centre, Edmonton AB T5J 4N1

e-mail: info@albertaaging.ca
www.albertaaging.ca

Overview: A medium-sized provincial charitable organization founded in 1980
Mission: To support persons involved in & concerned with gerontology in their efforts to enhance the lives of the aging population
Member of: Canadian Association on Gerontology
Chief Officer(s):
Vivien Lai, President
Brenda Hannah, Vice-President

Alberta Continuing Care Association (ACCA)
8861 - 75 St. NW, Edmonton AB T6C 4G8

Tel: 780-435-0699; *Fax:* 780-436-9785
e-mail: info@ab-cca.ca
www.ab-cca.ca

Overview: A medium-sized provincial organization founded in 1981 overseen by Canadian Alliance for Long Term Care
Mission: To represent owners & operators of long term care & designated assisted living facilities & home care
Member of: Canadian Alliance for Long Term Care
Chief Officer(s):
Tammy Leach, Chief Executive Officer
  tammy.leach@ab-cca.ca
Heather Aggus, Manager, Communications & Events
  heather.aggus@ab-cca.ca

Alberta Council on Aging
Circle Square Plaza, PO Box 9, #232, 11808 St. Albert Trail, Edmonton AB T5L 4G4

Tel: 780-423-7781; *Fax:* 780-425-9246
Toll-Free: 888-423-9666
e-mail: info@acaging.ca
www.acaging.ca
www.facebook.com/albertacouncilonaging
twitter.com/acaging

Overview: A medium-sized provincial charitable organization
Mission: To define the needs of aging & the aged & to bring the current needs to the attention of government or voluntary agencies & to take action where appropriate; to identify & encourage relevant areas of research & systematic compilation of information affecting aging; to encourage & develop discussion on all problems affecting aging; to inform government at any level on the potential impact of policies & legislation on the aging; to print, publish, distribute & sell publications related to aging; to foster interagency liaison & cooperation

Alberta Gerontological Nurses Association (AGNA)
PO Box 67040, Stn. Meadowlark, Edmonton AB T5R 5Y3

e-mail: info@agna.ca
www.agna.ca
twitter.com/AGNAtweets

Overview: A medium-sized provincial organization founded in 1981 overseen by Canadian Gerontological Nursing Association
Mission: To promote a high standard of nursing care & related health services for older adults; To enhance professionalism in the practice of gerontological nursing
Chief Officer(s):
Lynne Moulton, President
  president@agna.ca
Publications:
• AGNA [Alberta Gerontological Nurses Association] Newsletter
Type: Newsletter; *Frequency:* Quarterly; *Editor:* Debbie Lee

BRITISH COLUMBIA

British Columbia Care Providers Association (BCCPA)
Metrotower I, #738, 4710 Kingsway, Burnaby BC V5H 4M2

Tel: 604-736-4233; *Fax:* 604-736-4266
e-mail: info@bccare.ca
www.bccare.ca
www.linkedin.com/groups/BC-Care-Providers-Association-5003096
www.facebook.com/bccareproviders
twitter.com/BCCareProviders
www.youtube.com/bccareproviders

Also Known As: Care Online
Overview: A small provincial organization founded in 1977 overseen by Canadian Alliance for Long Term Care
Mission: To provide the best possible care for seniors by supporting change, & promoting the growth & success of the association's members
Member of: Canadian Alliance for Long Term Care
Chief Officer(s):
David Cheperdak, President
Daniel Fontaine, CEO

British Columbia Coalition to Eliminate Abuse of Seniors (BCCEAS)
#370, 1199 West Pender St., Vancouver BC V6E 2R1

Tel: 604-688-1927; *Fax:* 604-437-1929
Toll-Free: 866-437-1940; *TTY:* 604-428-3359
e-mail: info@bcceas.ca
www.bcceas.ca
twitter.com/bcceas

Also Known As: BC Centre for Elder Advocacy Support
Overview: A small provincial organization founded in 1994
Mission: To assist & support elderly individuals who are abused or at risk of abuse, or whose rights have been violated
Chief Officer(s):
Sue McIntosh, President
Martha Jane Lewis, Executive Director

British Columbia Psychogeriatric Association (BCPGA)

PO Box 47028, 1030 Denman St., Vancouver BC V6G 3E1
Fax: 888-835-2451
www.bcpga.com
www.facebook.com/pages/BC-Psychogeriatric-Association/138869817
8027128
twitter.com/BCPGA1

Overview: A small provincial organization founded in 1997
Mission: A professional association of clinicians working in the field of mental health and older adults.
Chief Officer(s):
Nancy Jokinen, Co-President, 250-960-5111
  jokinenn@unbc.ca
Dawn Hemingway, Co-President, 250-960-5694
  Dawn.Hemingway@unbc.ca

British Columbia Seniors Living Association (BCSLA)

#300, 3665 Kingsway, Vancouver BC V5R 5W2
Tel: 604-689-5949; *Fax:* 604-689-5946
Toll-Free: 888-402-2722
e-mail: membership@bcsla.ca
www.bcsla.ca

Overview: A small provincial organization
Chief Officer(s):
Marlene Williams, Executive Director
  executivedirector@bcsla.ca
Stuart Bowden, Vice-President, Finance

Family Caregivers of British Columbia

#6, 3318 Oak St., Victoria BC V8X 1R1
Tel: 250-384-0408; *Fax:* 250-361-2660
Toll-Free: 877-520-3267
www.familycaregiversbc.ca
www.facebook.com/FamilyCaregiversBC
twitter.com/caringbc

Previous Name: Family Caregivers' Network Society
Overview: A small provincial charitable organization founded in 1989
Mission: To provide support, education, & information for family caregivers in British Columbia
Chief Officer(s):
Barb MacLean, Executive Director
Alyshia Vogt, President
Publications:
• Caregiver Connection [a publication of the Family Caregivers of British Columbia]
Type: Newsletter; *Frequency:* Quarterly
Profile: Articles about family caregiving issues
• Facilitator's Manual: Educational Activities to Support Family Caregivers
 Price: $75
Profile: Featuring facilitation techniques, outlines for workshops, & learning activities for healthcare provider training programs
• Medical Information Package
 Price: Free with membership in theFamily Caregivers of British Columbia; $3 non-members
Profile: Including a medical information record, information about incapacity planning, plus information from the British Columbia Transplant Society & the Heart & Stroke Foundation
• Network News [a publication of the Family Caregivers of British Columbia]
Type: Newsletter; *Frequency:* Bimonthly; *Price:* Free with membership in the Family Caregivers of British Columbia
Profile: Informative articles about caregiving issues & notices of upcoming events
• Resource Guide for Family Caregivers
Type: Handbook; *Number of Pages:* 160; *Price:* $15 members; $20 non-members
Profile: Practical information to help caregivers make decisions

Gerontological Nursing Association of British Columbia (GNABC)

c/o 328 Nootka St., New Westminster BC V3L 4X4
Tel: 604-484-5698; *Fax:* 604-874-4378
e-mail: gnabc@shaw.ca
gnabc.com

Overview: A medium-sized provincial organization founded in 1981 overseen by Canadian Gerontological Nursing Association

Mission: To promote a high standard of nursing care & related health services for older adults; To enhance professionalism in the practice of gerontological nursing
Chief Officer(s):
Kim Martin, President
  k_martin@shaw.ca

Greater Vancouver Community Services Society (GVCSS)

#500, 1212 West Broadway, Vancouver BC V6H 3V1
Tel: 604-737-4900; *Fax:* 604-737-2922
e-mail: info@gvcss.bc.ca
www.gvcss.bc.ca

Overview: A small provincial organization
Mission: Non-profit provider of in-home health care services to the elderly and individuals with physical and/or developmental disabilities
Chief Officer(s):
Ron McLeod, CEO

MANITOBA

Age & Opportunity Inc.

#200, 280 Smith St., Winnipeg MB R3C 1K2
Tel: 204-956-6440; *Fax:* 204-946-5667
e-mail: info@ageopportunity.mb.ca
www.ageopportunity.mb.ca

Overview: A small provincial organization founded in 1957
Mission: Age & Opportunity Inc. is a not-for-profit, social service agency that offers services and programs to adults aged 55+, living in Manitoba. Services include: legal counselling, housing consultation, therapy dog pairing, crime prevention, settlement & orientation sessions for older immigrants. Programs are numerous, including: language lessons, fitness sessions, arts & crafts, social events.
Chief Officer(s):
Macrae Amanda, CEO

Long Term & Continuing Care Association of Manitoba (LTCAM)

#103, 1483 Pembina Hwy., Winnipeg MB R3T 2C6
Tel: 204-477-9888; *Fax:* 204-477-9889
Toll-Free: 855-477-9888
e-mail: info@ltcam.mb.ca
www.ltcam.mb.ca
www.facebook.com/ltccam
twitter.com/LTCAManitoba
www.youtube.com/LTCAManitoba

Overview: A small provincial organization founded in 1959 overseen by Canadian Alliance for Long Term Care
Mission: To advance long term & continuing care by promoting awareness to government, regional health authorities, health agencies & the community
Chief Officer(s):
Linda Sundevic, President

Manitoba Gerontological Nurses' Association (MGNA)

c/o Leslie Dryburgh, 300 Booth Dr., Winnipeg MB R3J 3M7
Tel: 204-831-2547
e-mail: info@mbgna.com
mbgna.ca

Overview: A medium-sized provincial organization overseen by Canadian Gerontological Nursing Association
Mission: To promote a high standard of nursing care & related health services for older adults; To enhance professionalism in the practice of gerontological nursing
Chief Officer(s):
Poh Lin Lim, President
  plim@vgh.mb.ca

NEW BRUNSWICK

New Brunswick Association of Nursing Homes, Inc. (NBANH) / Association des foyers de soins du Nouveau-Brunswick, inc. (AFSNB)

#206, 1113 Regent St., Fredericton NB E3B 3Z2
Tel: 506-460-6262; *Fax:* 506-460-6253
e-mail: communication@nbanh.com
www.nbanh.com
www.facebook.com/pages/NBANH-AFSNB/347209608754750
twitter.com/NBANH_AFSNB

Overview: A medium-sized provincial organization founded in 1972 overseen by Canadian Alliance for Long Term Care
Mission: To assist members in the provision of quality & efficient care to their residents
Member of: Canadian Alliance for Long Term Care
Chief Officer(s):
Jean-Eudes Savoie, President
Michael Keating, Executive Director
    mkeating@nbanh.com
Robert Stewart, Treasurer

New Brunswick Senior Citizens Federation Inc. (NBSCF) / Fédération des citoyens aînés du Nouveau-Brunswick inc. (FCANB)
#214, 23 - 451 Paul St., Dieppe NB E1A 6W8
Tel: 506-857-8242; *Fax:* 506-857-0315
Toll-Free: 800-453-4333
e-mail: horizons@nbnet.nb.ca
www.nbscf.ca
www.facebook.com/238798849533942
Overview: A medium-sized provincial organization founded in 1968
Mission: To promote the general welfare & leadership of NB's senior citizens regardless of language, race, colour, sex, or creed; to elevate the social, moral, & intellectual standing of NB's senior citizens; to provide information, coordination, communication, & advocating services to members
Chief Officer(s):
Isabelle Arseneault, Director, Operations

New Brunswick Special Care Home Association Inc.
c/o Seely Lodge Inc., 2081 Route 845, Bayswater NB E5S 1J7
Tel: 506-738-8514; *Fax:* 506-738-0892
www.nbscha.com
Overview: A medium-sized provincial organization
Mission: To assist licensed members of the New Brunswick Special Care Home Association Inc. in providing quality, cost effective long term care for seniors and special needs adults in cooperation with the Department of Social Development.
Chief Officer(s):
Jan Seely, President

NEWFOUNDLAND AND LABRADOR

Seniors Resource Centre Association of Newfoundland & Labrador Inc. (SRC NL)
243 Topsail Rd., St. John's NL A1E 2B4
Tel: 709-737-2333; *Fax:* 709-737-3717
Toll-Free: 800-563-5599
e-mail: info@seniorsresource.ca
www.seniorsresource.ca
Previous Name: Seniors Resource Centre
Overview: A small provincial organization founded in 1990
Mission: To promote the independence & well being of older adults in Newfoundland & Labrador through the provision of information as well as various programs & services
Publications:
• Seniors Pride [a publication of the Seniors Resource Centre Association of Newfoundland & Labrador Inc.]
Type: Magazine; *Frequency:* s-a.
• Seniors Resource Centre Association of Newfoundland & Labrador Inc. Newsletter
Type: Newsletter

NORTHWEST TERRITORIES

NWT Seniors' Society (NWTSS)
#102, 4916 - 46th Ave., Yellowknife NT X1A 1L2
Tel: 867-920-7444; *Fax:* 867-920-7601
Toll-Free: 800-661-0878
e-mail: seniors@yk.com
www.nwtseniorssociety.ca
www.facebook.com/nwtseniorssociety
twitter.com/NWTSeniors
Overview: A small provincial organization
Mission: To promote the independence & well-being of older citizens through the provision of programs & services in partnership with responsible government & other organizations; to serve as a consulting

body & advocate for the elderly
Member of: Yukon Council on Aging; Alberta Council on Aging; Saskatchewan Council on Aging
Chief Officer(s):
Barbara Hood, Executive Director
Leon Peterson, President

NOVA SCOTIA

Continuing Care Association of Nova Scotia (CCANS)
c/o Sunshine Personal Home Care, 38A Withrod Dr., Halifax NS B3N 1B1
Tel: 902-446-3140
e-mail: ccans@eastlink.ca
www.ccans.info
Previous Name: Association of Licensed Nursing Homes (ALNH); Associated Homes for Special Care (AHSC)
Overview: A small provincial organization founded in 1964
Mission: To represent continuing care facilities throughout Nova Scotia
Chief Officer(s):
Michael Walsh, President

Federation of Senior Citizens & Pensioners of Nova Scotia (FSCPNS)
c/o Bernie LaRusic, 21 Grandview St., Sydney NS B1P 3N4
Tel: 902-562-1901
Previous Name: Nova Scotia Federation of Senior Citizens & Pensioners
Overview: A medium-sized provincial organization founded in 1973
Mission: To help seniors maintain the health services & pension incomes that they now have
Member of: National Federation of Senior Citizens & Pensioners
Chief Officer(s):
Bernie LaRusic, President
    bernielarusic_392@hotmail.com

Nova Scotia Gerontological Nurses Association (NSGNA)
PO Box 33101, Stn. Quinpool, Halifax NS B3L 4T6
e-mail: ssavage@ssdha.nshealth.ca
www.nsgna.com
Overview: A medium-sized provincial organization founded in 1984 overseen by Canadian Gerontological Nursing Association
Mission: To promote a high standard of nursing care & related health services for older adults; To enhance professionalism in the practice of gerontological nursing
Chief Officer(s):
Sohani Welcher, President, 902-473-8413
    Sohani.welcher@cdha.nshealth.ca
Publications:
• NSGNA [Nova Scotia Gerontological Nurses Association] Newsletter
Type: Newsletter

ONTARIO

Advocacy Centre for the Elderly (ACE)
#701, 2 Carlton St., Toronto ON M5B 1J3
Tel: 416-598-2656; *Fax:* 416-598-7924
www.acelaw.ca
Also Known As: Holly Street Advocacy Centre for the Elderly Inc.
Overview: A small provincial charitable organization founded in 1984
Mission: To provide legal services to low income senior citizens
Chief Officer(s):
Judith Wahl, Executive Director
Publications:
• ACE [Advocacy Centre for the Elderly] Newsletter
Type: Newsletter; *Frequency:* Semiannually; *Price:* Free with membership in the Advocacy Centre for the Elderly
Profile: Articles on legal issues related to seniors
• ACE [Advocacy Centre for the Elderly] Library Reports
Type: Report; *Price:* Free with membership in the Advocacy Centre for the Elderly
Profile: A series of articles on legal issues related to seniors

Concerned Friends of Ontario Citizens in Care Facilities (CFOCCF)
140 Merton St., 2nd Fl., Toronto ON M4S 1A1
Tel: 416-489-0146
Toll-Free: 855-489-0146
e-mail: info@concernedfriends.ca
www.concernedfriends.ca
Overview: A small provincial charitable organization founded in 1980
Mission: To address the issues involving the care & conditions surrounding residents of long-term care facilities; To increase awareness of issues & concerns among the general public & provincial government; To provide information about the rights & responsibilities of residents of long-term care facilities under government legislation
Affliation(s): Self Help Resource Centre of Greater Toronto
Chief Officer(s):
Jordanne Holland, President

Elder Abuse Ontario
#306, 2 Billingham Rd., Toronto ON M9B 6E1
Tel: 416-916-6728
Other Communication: Senior Safety Line: 1-866-299-1011
e-mail: info@elderabuseontario.com
www.elderabuseontario.com
ca.linkedin.com/pub/elder-abuse-ontario/98/b57/a21
www.facebook.com/ElderAbuseOntario
twitter.com/ElderAbuseOnt
www.youtube.com/ElderAbuseOntario
Previous Name: Ontario Network for the Prevention of Elder Abuse
Overview: A small provincial charitable organization founded in 1989
Mission: To carry out The Ontario Strategy to Combat Elder Abuse, as mandated by the Government of Ontario; to create an Ontario that is free from abuse for all seniors
Chief Officer(s):
Joe Bornstein, Chair
Maureen Etkin, Executive Director
maureenetkin@elderabuseontario.com
Mary Mead, Office Manager
admin@elderabuseontario.com
Publications:
• Elder Abuse Newsletter
Type: Newsletter; *Price:* Free with membership in the Ontario Network for the Prevention of Elder Abuse
• Ontario Network for the Prevention of Elder Abuse Annual Report
Type: Yearbook; *Frequency:* Annually

Gerontological Nursing Association of Ontario (GNAO)
PO Box 368, Stn. K, Toronto ON M4P 2E0
e-mail: info@gnaontario.org
www.gnaontario.org
www.facebook.com/811284002323318
twitter.com/GNAOntario
Overview: A medium-sized provincial charitable organization founded in 1974 overseen by Canadian Gerontological Nursing Association
Mission: To promote a high standard of nursing care & related health services for older adults; To enhance professionalism in the practice of gerontological nursing
Affliation(s): Registered Nurses Association of Ontario
Chief Officer(s):
Julie Rubel, President
julie.rubel@gmail.com
Gwen Harris, Treasurer
gcharris@ebtech.net

Older Adult Centres' Association of Ontario (OACAO) / Association des centres pour aînés de l'Ontario
PO Box 65, Caledon East ON L7C 3L8
Tel: 905-584-8125; *Fax:* 905-584-8126
Toll-Free: 866-835-7693
www.oacao.org
Overview: A large provincial charitable organization founded in 1973
Mission: To ensure that seniors in Ontario have opportunities & choices that lead to healthy, active lifestyles
Member of: Federation of Provincial Non-Profit Organizations Working with Seniors; Ontario Community Support Association; Ontario Coalition of Senior Citizens Organizations; United Generations Ontario
Chief Officer(s):

Sue Hesjedahl, Executive Director
sue@oacao.org

The Older Women's Network (OWN) / Réseau des femmes aînées
115 The Esplanade, Toronto ON M5E 1Y7
Tel: 416-214-1518
e-mail: info@olderwomensnetwork.org
olderwomensnetwork.org
Overview: A small provincial charitable organization founded in 1988
Mission: To initiate & support discussion on issues relevant to the well-being of older women; To develop & support legislation to expand opportunities for housing, economic security, & optimum health; To monitor the media in order to encourage a more realistic & positive portrayal of older women; To support the efforts of young women to achieve equal opportunity, freedom from discrimination, abuse & exploitation, & the right to reproductive choice; To support the needs of children; To liaise with movements for social justice in Canada & abroad
Member of: National Action Committee on the Status of Women; Ontario Coalition of Senior Citizens Associations
Affliation(s): One Voice; National Association of Women & the Law; Women's Legal Education & Action Fund

Ontario Association of Non-Profit Homes & Services for Seniors (OANHSS)
#700, 7050 Weston Rd., Woodbridge ON L4L 8G7
Tel: 905-851-8821; *Fax:* 905-851-0744
www.oanhss.org
Previous Name: Ontario Association of Homes for the Aged
Overview: A medium-sized provincial charitable organization founded in 1919 overseen by Canadian Alliance for Long Term Care
Mission: To support members in the provision of quality non-profit long term care, seniors' community services, & housing
Chief Officer(s):
Kevin Queen, Board Chair
Donna A. Rubin, Chief Executive Officer

Ontario Association of Residents' Councils (OARC)
#201, 80 Fulton Way, Richmond Hill ON L4B 1J5
Tel: 905-731-3710; *Fax:* 905-731-1755
Toll-Free: 800-532-0201
e-mail: info@ontarc.com
www.residentscouncils.ca
twitter.com/OARCnews
www.youtube.com/channel/UC9zqu513DgytE8UBLjWo05w
Overview: A small provincial organization founded in 1981
Mission: To represent the views of residents on issues that affect the quality of their lives in long term care facilities & to promote & support the role & development of Residents' Councils
Chief Officer(s):
Dee Lender, Executive Director, 905-731-3710 Ext. 24
dlender@ontarc.com
Julie Garvey, Manager, Administration & Finance, 905-731-3710 Ext. 23
jgarvey@ontarc.com

Ontario Coalition of Senior Citizens' Organizations (OCSCO) / Coalition des organismes d'aînés et d'aînées de l'Ontario (COAAO)
#406, 333 Wilson Ave., Toronto ON M3H 1T2
Tel: 416-785-8570; *Fax:* 416-785-7361
Toll-Free: 800-265-0779
e-mail: ocsco@ocsco.ca
www.ocsco.ca
Also Known As: Ontario Society of Senior Citizens' Organizations
Overview: A large provincial charitable organization founded in 1986
Mission: To improve the quality of life for Ontario's seniors by encouraging seniors' involvement in all aspects of society, by keeping them informed of current issues, & by focusing on programs to benefit an aging population
Chief Officer(s):
Elizabeth Macnab, Executive Director
Jennifer Forde, Specialist, Communications & Program
communications-programs@ocsco.ca

Ontario Community Support Association (OCSA) / Association ontarienne de soutien communautaire

#104, 970 Lawrence Ave. West, Toronto ON M6A 3B6

Tel: 416-256-3010; *Fax:* 416-256-3021
Toll-Free: 800-267-6272
e-mail: reception@ocsa.on.ca
www.ocsa.on.ca
twitter.com/OCSAtweets

Previous Name: Meals on Wheels Ontario Inc.
Overview: A medium-sized provincial charitable organization founded in 1992
Mission: To support & represent the common goals of community-based, not-for-profit health & social service organizations which assist individuals to live at home in their own community
Member of: Canadian Centre for Philanthropy
Chief Officer(s):
Deborah Simon, Chief Executive Officer
    deborah.simon@ocsa.on.ca

Ontario Gerontology Association (OGA) / Association ontarienne de gérontologie

#601, 90 Eglinton Ave. East, Toronto ON M4P 2Y3

Tel: 416-535-6034; *Fax:* 416-535-6907

Overview: A small provincial organization founded in 1981
Affliation(s): Canadian Association on Gerontology

Ontario Home Care Association (OHCA)

PO Box 68018, RPO Blakely, Hamilton ON L8M 3M7

Tel: 905-543-9474
e-mail: info@homecareontario.ca
www.homecareontario.ca
twitter.com/HomeCareOntario

Previous Name: Ontario Home Health Care Providers' Association
Overview: A medium-sized provincial organization founded in 1987
Mission: To service excellence & client satisfaction in the provision of home health & support services in Ontario
Member of: Canadian Home Care Association; Ontario Health Providers' Alliance; Ontario Home & Community Care Council
Chief Officer(s):
Susan D. VanderBent, Chief Executive Officer

Ontario Long Term Care Association (OLTCA)

#500, 425 University Ave., Toronto ON M5G 1T6

Tel: 647-856-3490; *Fax:* 416-642-0635
e-mail: info@oltca.com
www.oltca.com
twitter.com/oltcanews
www.youtube.com/user/OLTCA345

Previous Name: Ontario Nursing Home Association
Overview: A medium-sized provincial licensing organization founded in 1959 overseen by Canadian Alliance for Long Term Care
Mission: Provides professional leadership to the long-term care sector; to empower long-term care facilities to provide high quality & cost-effective health care & accommodation services
Member of: Canadian Alliance for Long Term Care
Chief Officer(s):
Candace Chartier, CEO, 905-470-8995 Ext. 22
    cchartier@oltca.com
Judy Irwin, Senior Manager, Communications, 904-470-8995 Ext. 33
    jirwin@oltca.com

Ontario Rheumatology Association (ORA)

#244, 12 - 16715 Yonge St., Newmarket ON L3X 1X4

Tel: 905-952-0698; *Fax:* 905-952-0708
e-mail: admin@ontariorheum.ca
ontariorheum.ca

Overview: A small provincial organization founded in 2001
Mission: To represent Ontario Rheumatologists and promote their pursuit of excellence in Arthritis care in Ontario.
Affliation(s): Canadian Rheumatology Association
Chief Officer(s):
Arthur Karasik, President
    president@ontariorheum.ca

Saint Elizabeth Health Care (SEHC) / Les soins de santé Sainte-Elizabeth

#300, 90 Allstate Pkwy., Markham ON L3R 6H3

Tel: 905-940-9655; *Fax:* 905-940-9934
Toll-Free: 800-463-1763; *TTY:* 800-855-0511
e-mail: communications@saintelizabeth.com
www.saintelizabeth.com
www.linkedin.com/company/saint-elizabeth-health-care
www.facebook.com/SaintElizabethSEHC
twitter.com/stelizabethSEHC
www.youtube.com/user/SaintElizabethSEHC

Previous Name: Saint Elizabeth Visiting Nurses' Association of Ontario
Overview: A medium-sized provincial charitable organization founded in 1908
Mission: To serve the physical, emotional, & spiritual needs of people in their homes & communities
Member of: Nursing Best Practice Research Unit, through the RNAO & the University of Ottawa
Affliation(s): Canadian Council on Health Services Accreditation
Chief Officer(s):
Noreen Taylor, Chair
Shirlee Sharkey, President & CEO
Heather McClure, Treasurer
Don McCutchan, Secretary
Publications:
• Saint Elizabeth Health Care e-Newsletter
Type: Newsletter
• Saint Elizabeth Health Care Foundation Newsletter
Type: Newsletter
• SEHC [Saint Elizabeth Health Care] Research Activity Report
Type: Report
Profile: Highlights of research achievements

Barrie - North Simcoe Muskoka Service Delivery Centre
#104, 85 Ferris Lane, Barrie ON L4M 6B9

Fax: 877-619-4033
Toll-Free: 888-737-5055
e-mail: info@saintelizabeth.com

Cornwall - Eastern Counties Service Delivery Centre
#5, 1916 Pitt St., Cornwall ON K6H 5H3

Tel: 613-936-8668; *Fax:* 866-619-4059
e-mail: info@saintelizabeth.com

Hamilton - Hamilton, Niagara, Haldimand & Brant Service Delivery Centre
1525 Stone Church Rd. East, Hamilton ON L8W 3P8

Fax: 866-619-4062
Toll-Free: 888-275-2299
e-mail: info@saintelizabeth.com

Kingston - South East Service Delivery Centre
#410, 1471 John Counter Blvd., Kingston ON K7M 8S8

Tel: 613-530-3400; *Fax:* 866-619-4063
e-mail: info@saintelizabeth.com

London - South West Service Delivery Centre
#15, 1100 Dearness Dr., London ON N6E 1N9

Tel: 519-668-2997; *Fax:* 866-619-4065
e-mail: info@saintelizabeth.com

Markham - Central Service Delivery Centre
#201, 90 Allstate Pkwy., Markham ON L3R GH3

Tel: 905-944-1743; *Fax:* 866-619-4074
e-mail: info@saintelizabeth.com

Mississauga - Peel Service Delivery Centre
#5, 6745 Century Ave., Mississauga ON L5N 1V9

Tel: 905-826-0854; *Fax:* 905-826-0854
e-mail: info@saintelizabeth.com

Ottawa - Champlain Service Delivery Centre
#225, 30 Colonnade Rd., Ottawa ON K2E 7J6

Tel: 613-738-9661; *Fax:* 877-619-4038
e-mail: info@saintelizabeth.com

Seaforth - Huron Service Delivery Centre

Chronic & Mental Illnesses

87 Main St. South, Seaforth ON N0K 1W0
Fax: 519-600-0105
Toll-Free: 888-823-1626
e-mail: info@saintelizabeth.com

Thunder Bay - North West Service Delivery Centre
#103, 920 Tungsten St., Thunder Bay ON P7B 5Z6
Tel: 807-344-2002; *Fax:* 807-344-1999
e-mail: info@saintelizabeth.com

Toronto - Toronto Central Service Delivery Centre
#600, 2 Lansing Sq., Toronto ON M2J 4P8
Tel: 416-498-8600; *Fax:* 416-498-0213
e-mail: info@saintelizabeth.com

Whitby - Central East Service Delivery Centre
1549 Victoria St. East, Whitby ON L1N 8R1
Fax: 416-398-3206
Toll-Free: 877-397-1035

Windsor - Erie St. Clair Service Delivery Centre
2473 Ouellette Ave., Windsor ON N8X 1L5
Tel: 519-972-3895; *Fax:* 866-619-4073
e-mail: info@saintelizabeth.com

Woodstock - Oxford County Service Delivery Centre
#5, 695 Canterbury Ave., Woodstock ON N4S 8W7
Tel: 519-539-9807; *Fax:* 866-619-4070
e-mail: info@saintelizabeth.com

United Senior Citizens of Ontario Inc. (USCO)
3033 Lakeshore Blvd. West, Toronto ON M8V 1K5
Tel: 416-252-2021; *Fax:* 416-252-5770
Toll-Free: 888-320-2222
e-mail: office@uscont.ca
www.uscont.ca
www.facebook.com/uscont
Overview: A large provincial organization founded in 1961
Mission: To further the interests & promote the welfare of the senior population in Ontario; To provide for an exchange of ideas for member groups; To assist in the formation of senior citizens clubs
Chief Officer(s):
Bernard Jordan, President
Publications:
• The Voice
Type: Newsletter

PRINCE EDWARD ISLAND

Prince Edward Island Gerontological Nurses Association (PEIGNA)
PE
www.cgna.net/PEIGNA.html
Overview: A medium-sized provincial organization founded in 2004 overseen by Canadian Gerontological Nursing Association
Mission: To promote a high standard of nursing care & related health services for older adults; To enhance professionalism in the practice of gerontological nursing
Chief Officer(s):
Elaine E. Campbell, President
eecampbell@ihis.org

Prince Edward Island Senior Citizens Federation Inc. (PEISCF)
#214, 40 Enman Cres., Charlottetown PE C1E 1E6
Tel: 902-368-9008; *Fax:* 902-368-9006
Toll-Free: 877-368-9008
e-mail: peiscf@pei.aibn.com
www.peiscf.com
Overview: A small provincial organization founded in 1972
Mission: To advance the education opportunities for seniors on PEI; to improve the quality of life for seniors by advising government & other decision making bodies regarding seniors' concerns; to improve the quality of life for seniors; to increase societal understanding of seniors & the aging process through positive role modelling
Chief Officer(s):
Linda Jean Nicholson, Executive Director

QUÉBEC

Association des médecins gériatres du Québec
CP 216, Succ. Desjardins, #3000, 2, Complexe Desjardins, Montréal QC H5B 1G8
Tél: 514-350-5145; *Téléc:* 514-350-5151
Courriel: info@amgq.ca
www.amgq.ca
Aperçu: *Dimension:* petite; *Envergure:* provinciale surveillé par Fédération des médecins spécialistes du Québec
Affliation(s): Fédération des médecins spécialistes du Québec
Membre(s) du bureau directeur:
Maurice St-Laurent, Président
Lillian Plasse, Directrice, Administration
amgq@fmsq.org

Association québécoise de gérontologie (AQG)
6510, rue de Saint-Vallier, Montréal QC H2S 2P7
Tél: 514-387-3612; *Téléc:* 514-387-0352
Ligne sans frais: 888-387-3612
Courriel: info@aqg-quebec.org
www.aqg-quebec.org
www.facebook.com/AQG.Quebec
Aperçu: *Dimension:* moyenne; *Envergure:* provinciale; Organisme sans but lucratif; fondée en 1978
Mission: Promouvoir la qualité des services offerts aux personnes âgées, ainsi que la formation du personnel oeuvrant dans le domaine de la gérontologie; favoriser la recherche; analyser, inspirer et critiquer les politiques et les législations gouvernementales; favoriser la circulation de l'information et provoquer des échanges entre personnes et groupes s'intéressant au vieillissement; sensibiliser la collectivité et les individus à leur vieillissement personnel ainsi qu'au phénomène du vieillissement
Membre de: Association canadienne de gérontologie
Affliation(s): Association canadienne-française pour l'avancement des sciences
Membre(s) du bureau directeur:
Chantal Meessen, Directrice générale

Gustav Levinschi Foundation / La fondation Gustav Levinschi
#110, 1820, av Dr Penfield, Montréal QC H3H 1B4
Tel: 514-932-2595
Overview: A small provincial charitable organization founded in 1967
Mission: To improve physical & mental health & alleviate poverty with special focus on children, adolescents & the elderly, by supporting institutions & organization in this area

Réseau FADOQ / Québec Federation of Senior Citizens
4545, av Pierre-de Coubertin, Montréal QC H1V 0B2
Tél: 514-252-3017
Ligne sans frais: 800-828-3344
Courriel: info@fadoq.ca
www.fadoq.ca
www.facebook.com/reseaufadoq
www.youtube.com/user/ReseauFADOQ
Également appelé: FADOQ
Nom précédent: Fédération de l'âge d'or du Québec
Aperçu: *Dimension:* grande; *Envergure:* provinciale; Organisme sans but lucratif; fondée en 1970
Mission: Promouvoir un concept positif du vieillissement; encourager le maintien et l'amélioration de la qualité de vie et de l'autonomie des aînés; initier et soutenir l'organisation d'activités physiques et de loisirs; redonner aux aînés une nouvelle fierté en les revalorisant à leurs propres yeux comme à ceux de la société; remettre entre les mains des aînés la gestion de leurs affaires
Membre de: Fédération internationale des associations des personnes âgées; Association internationale francophone des aînés; Fédération internationale du vieillissement
Affliation(s): Association québécoise de gérontologie; Conseil canadien de développement social; Réseau canadien des aînés (One Voice); l'Assemblée des aîné(e)s francophones du Canada
Membre(s) du bureau directeur:
Maurice Duport, Président
Danis Prud'homme, Directeur générale

Société québécoise de gériatrie (SQG)
a/s Mme Carole Labrie, 375, rue Argyll, Sherbrooke QC J1J 3H5
Tél: 819-346-9196; *Téléc:* 819-829-7145
Courriel: clabrie.csss-iugs@ssss.gouv.qc.ca
www.sqgeriatrie.org
Aperçu: *Dimension:* petite; *Envergure:* provinciale; Organisme sans but lucratif; fondée en 1985
Membre(s) du bureau directeur:
Tamas Fülöp, Président

YUKON TERRITORY

Elder Active Recreation Association (ERA)
4061 - 4th Ave., Whitehorse YT Y1A 1H1
Tel: 867-456-8252
e-mail: office@elderactive.ca
www.elderactive.ca
Overview: A medium-sized provincial organization
Mission: To enhance the quality of life of Yukon seniors & elders by supporting them in living healthy lives with independence & dignity; to support seniors & elders in helping other seniors & elders to live full, active & healthy lives, & to develop active communities throughout the Yukon where seniors & elders can make positive lifestyle choices, exchange wisdom & connect with others in friendship, recreation & creativity. Physical office address: #302, 309 Strickland St., Whitehorse, YT Y1A 2J9.
Chief Officer(s):
Glen Doumont, Office Coordinator
Jennifer Massie, Program Coordinator
programs@elderactive.ca

Golden Age Society
4061A - 4th Ave., Whitehorse YT Y1A 1H1
Tel: 867-668-5538; *Fax:* 867-633-6944
e-mail: goldenagesociety@gmail.com
www.yukon-seniors-and-elders.org/index.php/ga-home
Overview: A small provincial organization founded in 1976
Mission: To promote & give opportunity for social, recreational activities for seniors in the Yukon
Chief Officer(s):
Deborah Bastien, Office Manager
gas2016@northwestel.net

Yukon Council on Aging (YCOA)
4061B - 4th Ave., Whitehorse YT Y1A 1H1
Tel: 867-668-3383
Toll-Free: 866-582-9707
e-mail: ycoa@yknet.yk.ca
www.yukon-seniors-and-elders.org
Also Known As: Seniors Information Centre
Overview: A small provincial organization founded in 1977
Mission: The YCOA is a volunteer organization of Yukon seniors administered by a Board of Directors elected from its membership
Chief Officer(s):
Connie Dublenko, President

Local Associations

ALBERTA

Calgary Meals on Wheels
3610 Macleod Trail SE, Calgary AB T2G 2P9
Tel: 403-243-2834; *Fax:* 403-243-8438
e-mail: info@mealsonwheels.com
www.mealsonwheels.com
www.facebook.com/calgarymealsonwheels
twitter.com/MealsOnWheelsca
Overview: A small local charitable organization founded in 1965
Mission: To provide nutritious meals as a preventative health measure to individuals in the city of Calgary, to the elderly, to the disabled & to short term convalescents without regard to race, creed or financial status
Chief Officer(s):
Janice Curtis, Executive Director
jcurtis@mealsonwheels.com

Calgary Seniors' Resource Society
3639 - 26 St. NE, Calgary AB T1Y 5E1
Tel: 403-266-6200; *Fax:* 403-269-5183
www.calgaryseniors.org
www.facebook.com/CalgarySeniors
twitter.com/Calgary_Seniors
Previous Name: Senior Citizens' Central Council of Calgary
Overview: A medium-sized local charitable organization founded in 1995
Mission: To enhance the quality of life & human dignity of seniors by supporting their independence through home services & community based programs
Member of: Alberta Council on Aging; Alberta Association on Gerontology
Affiliation(s): Calgary Homeless Foundation
Chief Officer(s):
Mark Kolesar, President

Edmonton Aboriginal Senior Centre (NSC)
Cottage E, 10107 - 134 Ave., Edmonton AB T5E 1J2
Tel: 780-476-6595
e-mail: manager@easc.ca
www.easc.ca
Previous Name: Métis Women's Council of Edmonton
Overview: A small local charitable organization founded in 1986
Mission: To promote welfare, education & interests of Aboriginal seniors within the Edmonton area

Seniors Association of Greater Edmonton (SAGE)
15 Sir Winston Churchill Sq., Edmonton AB T5J 2E5
Tel: 780-423-5510; *Fax:* 780-426-5175
e-mail: info@mysage.ca
www.mysage.ca
www.facebook.com/438132792913806
twitter.com/sageYEG
Previous Name: Society for the Retired & Semi-Retired
Overview: A medium-sized local charitable organization founded in 1970
Mission: To enhance the quality of life of older persons through service, innovation, & advocacy
Affiliation(s): United Way; Imagine Canada
Chief Officer(s):
Barb Burton, President
Karen McDonald, Executive Director

BRITISH COLUMBIA

Abbotsford Social Activity Association
33889 Essendene Ave., Abbotsford BC V2S 2H6
Tel: 604-853-4014; *Fax:* 604-853-4031
e-mail: abbysocialactivityassoc@gmail.com
www.abbysocialactivityassoc.com
Overview: A small local charitable organization founded in 1972
Mission: To provide recreational facilities & activities for seniors in the Abbotsford area of British Columbia
Chief Officer(s):
Jim Curran, Acting President, 604-859-6531

Carefree Society
2832 Queensway St., Prince George BC V2L 4M5
Tel: 250-562-1394; *Fax:* 250-562-1393
e-mail: carefree_society@telus.net
www.carefreesociety.org
Also Known As: handyDART
Overview: A small local charitable organization founded in 1971
Mission: To provide transportation services for the disabled
Affiliation(s): BC Transit

Chown Adult Day Care Centre
Taoist Building, 94 East 15th Ave., Vancouver BC V5T 2R5
Tel: 604-879-0947; *Fax:* 604-879-0121
e-mail: chownadc@shaw.ca
chownadc.com
www.facebook.com/pages/Chown-Adult-Day-Centre/236969846432675
Overview: A small local charitable organization
Mission: The Centre serves frail elders, disabled older & younger adults who need support to maintain health, & live in their community as independently as possible.

Member of: British Columbia Association of Community Care; Health Employers Association of British Columbia

Crossreach Adult Day Centre
3348 West Broadway, Vancouver BC V6R 2B2
Tel: 604-732-1477; *Fax:* 604-732-1430
e-mail: info@crossreachseniors.com
www.crossreachseniors.com
Previous Name: Crossreach Project of Vancouver
Overview: A small local charitable organization founded in 1972
Mission: To provide services to seniors in Vancouver; To support independent living for seniors
Chief Officer(s):
Jessica Malkoske, Executive Director

Finnish Canadian Rest Home Association
2288 Harrison Dr., Vancouver BC V5P 2P6
Tel: 604-325-8241; *Fax:* 604-325-2394
e-mail: info@finncare.ca
finncare.ca
Overview: A small local organization founded in 1958
Mission: To represent a number of Finnish Canadian rest homes & seniors apartments in the Vancouver Area
Chief Officer(s):
Tanya Rautava, Administrator
finnishhome@telus.net

Forever Young Seniors Society (FYSS)
Vancouver BC
Tel: 604-454-9907
e-mail: contact@foreveryoungseniorssociety.com
www.foreveryoungseniorssociety.com
www.youtube.com/user/fysscanada
Overview: A small local organization
Mission: To preserve the Filipino heritage & cultural traditions; To serve Filipino Canadian seniors in the Vancouver area
Chief Officer(s):
Romeo Mercado, President
Juanita Lamothe, Vice-President
Adel Johanson, Secretary
Angie Jimenez, Treasurer
Publications:
• Forever Young Journal
Type: Newsletter
Profile: Society activities, membership news, & forthcoming events

Nelson & District Hospice Society
PO Box 194, Nelson BC V1L 5P9
Tel: 250-352-2337; *Fax:* 250-227-9017
e-mail: nelsonhospice@netidea.com
www.nelsonhospice.org
Overview: A small local charitable organization
Mission: To offer hospice & palliative care in the Nelson & District region
Chief Officer(s):
Jane DiGiacomo, Executive Director

Portuguese Canadian Seniors Foundation
5455 Imperial St., Burnaby BC V5J 1E5
Tel: 604-873-2979; *Fax:* 604-873-2974
www.pcsf.ca
www.youtube.com/user/THEPCSF
Overview: A small local organization founded in 1987
Chief Officer(s):
Maria Viegas Guerreiro, President

ONTARIO

Association of Jewish Chaplains of Ontario
c/o Beth Emeth Bais Yehuda Synagogue, 100 Elder St., Toronto ON M3H 5G7
Tel: 416-633-3838; *Fax:* 416-633-3153
e-mail: info@beby.org
www.beby.org
www.facebook.com/BEBY.Toronto
twitter.com/BethEmeth
Overview: A small local organization

Mission: To draw together those who are active in pastoral care of Jewish people & their families, for fellowship, mutual support & education; to facilitate the understanding of the role & function that a professional performs in the pastoral care of Jewish people in hospitals, seniors' homes, correctional institutions, synagogues & schools; to develop & define standards for Jewish pastoral care providers; to develop & provide training & ensure the availability of competent pastor care where needed
Affiliation(s): Toronto Board of Rabbis
Chief Officer(s):
Bernard Schwartz, President
Pearl Grundland, Executive Director

Association of Jewish Seniors (AJS)
4211 Yonge St., 4th Fl., Toronto ON M2P 2A9
Tel: 416-635-2860; *Fax:* 416-635-1692
e-mail: info@circleofcare.com
www.circleofcare.com
Overview: A medium-sized local organization
Mission: To act as a collective voice for affiliated organizations & members-at-large; To support individual independence among seniors & sustain quality of life in the community
Member of: Circle of Care
Chief Officer(s):
Michael F. Scheinert, President & Chief Executive Officer

Atikokan Native Friendship Centre (ANFC)
PO Box 1510, #307, 309 Main St., Atikokan ON P0T 1C0
Tel: 807-597-1213; *Fax:* 807-597-1473
atikokaninfo.com/business/atikokan-native-friendship-centre
Overview: A small local charitable organization founded in 1983
Mission: To serve as a meeting place for urban, Aboriginal people and also community members regardless of nationality; to provide an Aboriginal Family Support program for families with children up to 6 years old (includes parent relief/ mom/dads & tots, prenatal and postnatal support); to provide health outreach services, healing & wellness services, family violence initiatives, crisis intervention services, seniors care support services, cultural events, educational assistance, food bank, resource library, community support &d assistance for newcomers & community referral services.
Member of: Ontario Federation of Indian Friendship Centres
Chief Officer(s):
Sarah Laurich, Contact
sarahlaurich@gmail.com

Bernard Betel Centre for Creative Living
1003 Steeles Ave. West, Toronto ON M2R 3T6
Tel: 416-225-2112; *Fax:* 416-225-2097
e-mail: reception@betelcentre.org
www.betelcentre.org
Also Known As: Betel Centre
Overview: A small local charitable organization founded in 1965
Mission: To maximize the quality of life for seniors in the community & reflecting Jewish values
Member of: Ontario Community Support Association; Older Adult Centres of Ontario; Association of Ontario Health Centres
Chief Officer(s):
Adam Silver, Executive Director
adams@betelcentre.org

Carefirst Seniors & Community Services Association
#501, 3601 Victoria Park Ave., Toronto ON M1W 3Y3
Tel: 416-502-2323; *Fax:* 416-502-2382
e-mail: info@carefirstseniors.com
www.carefirstseniors.com
www.facebook.com/CarefirstSeniors
twitter.com/CarefirstSenior
Previous Name: Chinese Seniors Support Services Association
Overview: A small local charitable organization
Member of: United Way Greater Toronto, York Region, Peel Region

Mississauga On-Site Drop-In Service
#81, 1177 Central Pkwy W., Mississauga ON L5C 4P3
Tel: 905-270-9988; *Fax:* 905-361-1082
e-mail: mso@carefirstseniors.com

South Toronto Office, Helen Lam Community Service Centre

479 Dundas St. West, Toronto ON M5T 1H1
Tel: 416-585-2013; *Fax:* 416-585-2892
e-mail: sto@carefirstseniors.com
www.carefirstseniors.com

Supportive Housing Services, Alexandra Park
#707, 91 Augusta Ave., Toronto ON M5T 2L2
Tel: 416-603-0909; *Fax:* 416-603-0436
e-mail: shsa@carefirstseniors.com

Supportive Housing Services, Tam O'Shanter
#902, 3825 Sheppard Ave. East, Toronto ON M1T 3P6
Tel: 416-291-1800; *Fax:* 416-291-9586
e-mail: shst@carefirstseniors.com

York Region Community Services Centre
#104A, 420 Hwy 7 East, Richmond Hill ON L4B 3K2
Tel: 905-771-3700; *Fax:* 905-763-3718
e-mail: york@carefirstseniors.com

Catholic Family Services of Hamilton (CFS)
#201, 447 Main St. East, Hamilton ON L8N 1K1
Tel: 905-527-3823; *Fax:* 905-546-5779
Toll-Free: 877-527-3823
e-mail: intake@cfshw.com
www.cfshw.com
www.linkedin.com/company/catholic-family-services-of-hamilton
www.facebook.com/Catholic.Family.Services.Hamilton
twitter.com/CFSHW
www.youtube.com/channel/UCeLsGYd3vHt5PGRkS8JJFjA
Previous Name: Catholic Family Services of Hamilton-Wentworth
Overview: A small local organization founded in 1944 overseen by Ontario Association of Credit Counselling Services
Mission: To provide individual, marriage, family, & credit counselling services in the Hamilton & Burlington communities
Member of: Ontario Association of Credit Counselling Service
Affiliation(s): Ontario Community Support Association; ONTCHILD; Family Services Ontario; Canadian Association for Community Care; Continuing Gerontological Education Cooperative; Older Persons' Mental Health & Addictions Network; Ontario Association on Developmental Disabilities; Ontario Case Managers Association; Ontario Gerontology Association; Ontario Partnership on Aging Development Disabilities
Chief Officer(s):
Linda Dayler, Executive Director & Secretary
Paula Forbes, Associate Director

Community Care for South Hastings
#63, 470 Dundas St. East, Belleville ON K8N 1G1
Tel: 613-969-0130; *Fax:* 613-969-1719
www.ccsh.ca
www.facebook.com/241358299396920
twitter.com/CCSouthHastings
Previous Name: Community Care Belleville
Overview: A small local charitable organization founded in 1980
Mission: To provide programs & services for physically disabled individuals
Member of: Ontario Community Support Association; SEO Community Support Services Network
Affiliation(s): Pensioners Concerned
Chief Officer(s):
Shell-Lee Wert, Executive Director

Deseronto Office
293 Main St., Deseronto ON K0K 1X0
Tel: 613-396-6591; *Fax:* 613-396-6592
Chief Officer(s):
Lisa Murray, Manager, Program

Community Care Peterborough
185 Hunter St. East, Peterborough ON K9H 0H1
Tel: 705-742-7067; *Fax:* 705-745-6011; *TTY:* 705-742-2075
e-mail: centofc@commcareptbo.org
www.commcareptbo.org
www.facebook.com/149883285049420
twitter.com/CommCarePtbo
www.youtube.com/user/CommunityCarePtbo
Overview: A small local charitable organization founded in 1984 overseen by InformOntario

Mission: The association is a network of community offices that provides essential services to seniors & disabled, so they may remain living at home.
Member of: United Way
Chief Officer(s):
Doug Downer, President
Danielle Belair, Executive Director
Publications:
• The Thread
Type: Newsletter

Apsley Office
PO Box 303, 168 Burleigh St., Apsley ON K0L 1A0
Tel: 705-656-4589; *Fax:* 705-656-2542
e-mail: apsley@commcareptbo.org
Chief Officer(s):
Amanda Smith, Program Support

Chemung Office
549 Ennis Rd., Ennismore ON K0L 1T0
Tel: 705-292-8708; *Fax:* 705-292-8750
e-mail: chemung@commcareptbo.org
Chief Officer(s):
Denise Gould, Coordinator

Harvey Office
PO Box 12, 1937 Lakehurst Rd., Buckhorn ON K0L 1J0
Tel: 705-657-2171; *Fax:* 705-657-3457
e-mail: harvofc@commcareptbo.org
Chief Officer(s):
Lynda McKerr, Coordinator

Havelock Office
107 Concession St. North, Havelock ON K0L 1Z0
Tel: 705-778-7831; *Fax:* 705-778-7924
e-mail: havelock@commcareptbo.org
Chief Officer(s):
Tammy Ross, Coordinator

Lakefield Office
PO Box 001, 40 Rabbit St., Lakefield ON K0L 2H0
Tel: 705-652-8655; *Fax:* 705-652-7332
e-mail: lakfield@commcareptbo.org
Chief Officer(s):
Lorri Rork, Coordinator

Millbrook Office
PO Box 257, 22 King St. East, Millbrook ON L0A 1G0
Tel: 705-932-2011; *Fax:* 705-932-4058
e-mail: millofc@commcareptbo.org
Chief Officer(s):
Karen Morton, Coordinator

Norwood Office
PO Box 436, 2281 Hwy. 45, Norwood ON K0L 2V0
Tel: 705-639-5631; *Fax:* 705-639-2511
e-mail: norwood@commcareptbo.org
Chief Officer(s):
Tammy Ross, Coordinator

The Council on Aging of Ottawa (COA) / Le Conseil sur le vieillissement d'Ottawa (CSV)
#101, 1247 Kilborn Pl., Ottawa ON K1H 6K9
Tel: 613-789-3577; *Fax:* 613-789-4406
e-mail: coa@coaottawa.ca
www.coaottawa.ca
www.facebook.com/coaottawa
Previous Name: Ottawa-Carleton Council on Aging
Overview: A small local charitable organization founded in 1975
Mission: To enhance the qualilty of life of all seniors in Ottawa; To work with & for seniors in the community to voice issues & concerns to all levels of government & the general public
Chief Officer(s):
John E. Johnson, President

Council on Aging, Windsor - Essex County (COA)
c/o Centres for Seniors Windsor, 635 McEwan Ave., Windsor ON N9B 2E9

Tel: 519-254-9342; *Fax:* 519-254-1869
e-mail: information@councilonaging.ca
www.councilonaging.ca

Overview: A small local charitable organization founded in 1988
Mission: To enhance the quality of life of seniors in Windsor - Essex County in Ontario; To assist in the development & coordination of services for local seniors
Member of: Provincial Network of Councils
Chief Officer(s):
Deana Johnson, Executive Director

Essex Community Services (ECS)
#7, 35 Victoria Ave., Essex ON N8M 1M4

Tel: 519-776-4231; *Fax:* 519-776-4966
e-mail: ecs@essexcs.on.ca
www.essexcs.on.ca

Previous Name: Community Information - Essex
Overview: A small local charitable organization founded in 1975 overseen by InformOntario
Mission: The organization provides a number of services to members of the community, including door-to-door transporation assistance for seniors, coat collection for children, income tax clinic, job bank, community resource library.
Affiliation(s): Inform Canada
Chief Officer(s):
Kelly Stack, Executive Director
director@essexcs.on.ca

Good Shepherd Refuge Social Ministries
412 Queen St. East, Toronto ON M5A 1T3

Tel: 416-869-3619
www.goodshepherd.ca
www.linkedin.com/company/good-shepherd-ministries
www.facebook.com/goodshepherdTO
twitter.com/goodshepherd_to
www.youtube.com/user/GoodShepherdToronto

Also Known As: Good Shepherd Ministries
Previous Name: Good Shepherd Refuge
Overview: A small local charitable organization founded in 1963
Mission: To provide services to homeless, disadvantaged & marginalized people; To provide the basic necessities of food, shelter & ancillary services, ensuring each client justice, equality, dignity & acceptance; To provide human services that will assist clients in regaining freedom from homelessness
Member of: Ontario Hostels Association
Chief Officer(s):
Werner Zapfe, Chair
David Lynch, Executive Director
Aklilu Wendaferew, Assistant Executive Director
Publications:
• Good Shepherd Journal
Type: Newsletter; *Frequency:* Bi-annually; *Editor:* Adrienne Urquhart; *Price:* Free to supporters
Profile: Provides client, service & donor updates.

Hamilton Niagara Haldimand Brant Community Care Access Centre (HNHB CCAC)
#4, 195 Henry St., Bldg. 4, Brantford ON N3S 5C9

Tel: 519-759-7752
Toll-Free: 800-810-0000
healthcareathome.ca

Overview: A small local organization
Mission: To provide access to community health care services
Chief Officer(s):
Melody Miles, CEO

Hospice of Waterloo Region
298 Lawrence Ave., Kitchener ON N2M 1Y4

Tel: 519-743-4114; *Fax:* 519-743-7021
e-mail: hospice@hospicewaterloo.ca
www.hospicewaterloo.ca
www.facebook.com/hospicewaterloo
twitter.com/hospicewaterloo
www.youtube.com/channel/UCUd8GumvtdxvoGo0WGT2Fog

Overview: A small local charitable organization
Mission: To provide comfort, care & support to people affected by life-threatening illness; To offer services in hospitals, long-term care facilities or in the home
Chief Officer(s):
Judy Nairn, Executive Director
judy@hospicewaterloo.ca

Korean Senior Citizens Society of Toronto (KSCST)
KSCST Centre, 476 Grace St., Toronto ON M6G 3A9

Tel: 416-532-8077; *Fax:* 416-532-9964
e-mail: kscst@hotmail.com
www.kscst.com

Overview: A medium-sized local charitable organization founded in 1973
Mission: To provide social services & programs to Korean senior citizens in the Greater Toronto Area; To promote welfare among members; To promote traditional Korean arts, culture, & values to younger Korean generations
Chief Officer(s):
Bae Kim Jeong, President
Yong Hoo Chung, Chief Director
Kil Yeo Whang, Vice-Chief Director
Kum Suk Hwang, General Manager
Sang-Im Kim, Executive Manager
Hyun-Ju Shin, Coordintor, Programs
Publications:
• Korean Senior Citizens Society of Toronto Newsletter
Type: Newsletter; *Frequency:* Quarterly; *Price:* Free with membership in the Korean Senior Citizens Society of Toronto
Profile: Information & upcoming events for society members

Mid-Toronto Community Services (MTCS)
192 Carlton St., 2nd Fl., Toronto ON M5A 2K8

Tel: 416-962-9449; *Fax:* 416-962-5541
e-mail: admin@midtoronto.com
www.midtoronto.com

Overview: A small local charitable organization founded in 1965
Mission: Provides programs & services to support the independence of seniors & adults with disabilities to continue living in their own homes
Member of: Ontario Community Support Association
Chief Officer(s):
Kaarina Luoma, Executive Director
kluoma@midtoronto.com
Susan Burns, Chair

Mon Sheong Foundation
11211 Yonge St., Richmond Hill ON L4S 0E9

Tel: 905-883-9288; *Fax:* 905-883-9855
Toll-Free: 866-708-0002
e-mail: msf@monsheong.org
www.monsheong.org
twitter.com/MonSheong
instagram.com/monsheong

Overview: A medium-sized local organization founded in 1964
Mission: To recognize the Chinese language & philosophy through caring for the elderly & edifying the young; To provide programs & services which respond to the needs of communities
Member of: Ontario Association of Nonprofit Homes & Services for Seniors
Affiliation(s): Ontario Hospital Association
Chief Officer(s):
Stephanie Wong, CEO

The Olde Forge Community Resource Centre (OFCRC) / Centre de ressources communautaires Olde Forge
2730 Carling Ave., Ottawa ON K2B 7J1

Tel: 613-829-9777
oldeforge.ca

Overview: A small local charitable organization founded in 1970
Mission: To provide an information & referral service; To operate a support service to enable senior citizens to remain in their own homes as long as possible
Member of: Ontario Community Support Association
Chief Officer(s):
Anita Bloom, Executive Director, 613-829-9777 Ext. 224

Scarborough Centre for Healthy Communities (SCHC)
#2, 629 Markham Rd., Toronto ON M1H 2A4
Tel: 416-642-9445
www.schcontario.ca
ca.linkedin.com/company/scarborough-centre-for-healthy-communities
www.facebook.com/ScarboroughCentreforHealthyCommunities
twitter.com/schcont
www.youtube.com/schcont
Overview: A medium-sized local charitable organization
Mission: To offer home support, transportation, medical, & family support programs for individuals & families
Chief Officer(s):
Janice Dusek, Chair & President

Senior Link
3036 Danforth Ave., Toronto ON M4C 1N2
Tel: 416-691-7407; *Fax:* 416-691-8466
e-mail: info@neighbourhoodlink.org
www.neighbourhoodlink.org/seniors
Overview: A small local charitable organization founded in 1975
Mission: To promote the independence & dignity of seniors in their own community
Member of: Ontario Non-Profit Housing Association; Ontario Association of Non-Profit Homes & Services for Seniors; Ontario Community Support Association
Chief Officer(s):
Judith Leon, Contact

Seniors in Need
#102, 40 St. Clair West, Toronto ON M4V 1M2
Tel: 416-550-4850
www.seniorsinneed.ca
www.facebook.com/SeniorsInNeed
twitter.com/seniorsinneed
Overview: A medium-sized local charitable organization founded in 2011
Mission: A grassroots organization that connects concerns Canadians to impoverished seniors; Registered nonprofit sponsors submit the details of a senior in need to a database and donors can find and help a senior of their choosing.
Chief Officer(s):
Peter D. Cook, Founder

Seniors Peer Helping Program
80 Lothian Ave., Toronto ON M8Z 4K5

Tel: 416-239-7252
Also Known As: Peer Helping Centre
Overview: A small local organization founded in 1981
Mission: To provide growth experience for older adults in group setting; to train seniors to help other seniors
Chief Officer(s):
Mary Neale, Chair

The Shepherds' Trust
Catholic Pastoral Centre, #603, 1155 Yonge St., Toronto ON M4T 1W2
Tel: 416-934-3400; *Fax:* 416-934-3444
e-mail: retiredpriests@archtoronto.org
www.shepherdstrust.org
Overview: A medium-sized local charitable organization founded in 1996
Mission: To assist elderly & disabled priests by raising awareness & funds; to provide retired priests with the financial resources to allow them to live a dignified life
Affliation(s): Archdiocese of Toronto
Chief Officer(s):
Brian Clough, Elected Representative, Board of Trustees
Ivan Philip Camilleri, Elected Representative, Board of Trustees
Marisa Rogucki, Coordinator, Retired Diocesan Priests
Publications:
• The Sheperds' Trust Newsletter
Type: Newsletter; *Frequency:* Annual

South West Community Care Access Centre
356 Oxford St. West, London ON N6H 1T3
Fax: 519-472-4045
Toll-Free: 800-811-5147; *TTY:* 519-473-9626
e-mail: info-london@sw.ccac-ont.ca
healthcareathome.ca/southwest
Also Known As: South West CCAC
Overview: A small local charitable organization founded in 1970 overseen by InformOntario
Mission: Online directory of community & social services & resources for citizens of London & area
Affliation(s): London Health Sciences Centre; Middlesex-London Health Unit; St. Joseph's Health Care (London)
Chief Officer(s):
Sandra Coleman, CEO

SPRINT Senior Care
140 Merton St., 2nd Fl., Toronto ON M4S 1A1
Tel: 416-481-0669; *Fax:* 416-481-9829
e-mail: info@sprintseniorcare.org
sprintseniorcare.org
www.linkedin.com/company/sprint-senior-peoples-resources-in-north-to
ro
www.facebook.com/SPRINT.Senior.Care
twitter.com/SPRINT_Sr_Care
www.youtube.com/user/sprintseniorcare
Overview: A small local charitable organization
Mission: To offer community support services to seniors & their families in North Toronto
Chief Officer(s):
Stacy Landau, Executive Director
Publications:
• SPRINT News
Type: Newsletter; *Frequency:* Monthly

Toronto Community Care Access Centre
#305, 250 Dundas St. West, Toronto ON M5T 2Z5
Tel: 416-506-9888; *Fax:* 416-506-0374
Toll-Free: 866-243-0061
e-mail: feedback@toronto.ccac-ont.ca
healthcareathome.ca/torontocentral
ca.linkedin.com/company/toronto-central-community-care-access-centr
e
twitter.com/tcccac
www.youtube.com/torontoccac
Previous Name: Home Care Program for Metropolitan Toronto
Overview: A medium-sized local organization founded in 1964
Mission: To coordinate & deliver health & social care to all people in Metro Toronto who are sick or disabled; to enhance the quality of their lives & enable them to remain at home; to provide & coordinate an appropriate range of services to meet the diverse needs (health & social) of individuals & families
Member of: Canadian Home Care Association; Ontario Home Care Programs Association
Chief Officer(s):
Stacey Daub, CEO
William Yetman, Chair

Toronto Finnish-Canadian Seniors Centre
795 Eglinton Ave. East, Toronto ON M4G 4E4
Tel: 416-425-4134; *Fax:* 416-425-6319
e-mail: reception@suomikoti.ca
www.suomikoti.ca
Also Known As: Suomi-Koti, Toronto
Overview: A small local organization founded in 1982
Mission: To provide multi-lingual care & services, housing & activities for the Finnish community
Chief Officer(s):
Juha Mynttinen, Administrator, 416-425-4134 Ext. 243

VHA Home HealthCare
#600, 30 Soudan Ave., Toronto ON M4S 1V6
Tel: 416-489-2500; *Fax:* 416-482-8773
Toll-Free: 888-314-6622
www.vha.ca
www.facebook.com/VHAHomeHealthCare
twitter.com/VHACaregiving
www.youtube.com/user/VHAHomeHealthCare
Also Known As: Visiting Homemakers Association
Overview: A large local charitable organization founded in 1925
Mission: To be a leading not-for-profit provider of community-based, client-centred health & support services in the Greater Toronto Area
Member of: United Way
Chief Officer(s):
Adwoa K. Buahene, Chair
Carol Annett, President/CEO

QUÉBEC

Association des personnes en perte d'autonomie de Chibougamau inc. & Jardin des aînés
101, av du Parc, Chibougamau QC G8P 3A5
Tél: 418-748-4411
Courriel: jardindesaines@tlb.sympatico.ca
Aperçu: *Dimension:* petite; *Envergure:* locale
Membre(s) du bureau directeur:
Chantal Lessard, Directrice générale

Association pour aînés résidant à Laval (APARL)
#110, 4901, rue St-Joseph, Laval QC H7C 1H6
Tél: 450-661-5252; *Téléc:* 450-661-2497
www.aparl.org
Nom précédent: Aide aux personnes âgées en résidence à Laval inc
Aperçu: *Dimension:* petite; *Envergure:* locale; Organisme sans but lucratif; fondée en 1974
Mission: Offir aux aînés l'intégration sociale, les services et les ressources nécessaires qui brisent leur isolement afin de conserver leur autonomie et leur maintien à domicile; favoriser la participation; encourager
Membre de: Table de concertation; Centre local de services communautaires; Corporation de Développement Communautaire
Membre(s) du bureau directeur:
Sylvie Brunet, Directrice générale

Centre de soutien entr'Aidants (AFSAS)
1688, rue Gustave-Désourdy, Saint-Hubert QC J4T 1Y6
Tél: 450-465-2520; *Téléc:* 250-465-2290
Courriel: info@centredesoutienentraidants.com
www.centredesoutienentraidants.com
Aperçu: *Dimension:* petite; *Envergure:* locale; fondée en 1990
Membre(s) du bureau directeur:
Anyela Vergara, Directrice générale, 450-465-2520 Ext. 205
avergara@centredesoutienentraidants.com

Council for Black Aging / Le Conseil Des Personnes Agées De La Communauté Noire De Montréal
8606, rue Centrale, Montréal QC H4C 1M8
Tel: 514-935-4951
Overview: A medium-sized local organization
Mission: The Council for Black Aging works as an advocate for the needs of Black seniors, undertaking activities designed to advance the interests of Black elders, keeping Black seniors better informed of issues relating to the availability of health and social services, and developing a unique day centre and a nursing home for Black elders.

Partage Humanitaire
#219, 435, boul Curé-Labelle, Laval QC H7V 2S8
Tél: 450-681-1536; *Téléc:* 450-681-3484
Courriel: info@partagehumanitaire.ca
www.partagehumanitaire.ca
Aperçu: *Dimension:* petite; *Envergure:* locale; Organisme sans but lucratif; fondée en 1971
Mission: A pour but de meubler la solitude et valoriser les aînés vivant en établissement et c'est par le biais de loisirs spécialement adaptés à leurs besoins, que sont rejoints ces gens trop souvent oubliés
Membre(s) du bureau directeur:
Gilles Leduc, Président

Marie Bouchart d'Orval, Directrice générale
mariebdorval@partagehumanitaire.ca

SASKATCHEWAN

Saskatoon Senior Citizens Action Now Inc.
310 F Ave. South, Saskatoon SK S7M 1T2
Tel: 306-244-6408
Previous Name: Saskatoon Seniors Action Now Inc.
Overview: A small local charitable organization founded in 1972
Mission: To help develop positive quality of life for seniors & improve community environment for all
Affiliation(s): National Pensioners & Senior Citizens Federation

International Associations

HelpAge Canada / Aide aux aînés Canada
1300 Carling Ave., Ottawa ON K1Z 7L2
Tel: 613-232-0727; *Fax:* 613-232-7625
Toll-Free: 800-648-1111
e-mail: info@helptheaged.ca
www.helptheaged.ca
www.facebook.com/helpagecanada
twitter.com/HelpAgeCanada
www.youtube.com/user/helpage
Previous Name: Help the Aged (Canada)
Overview: A medium-sized international charitable organization founded in 1975
Mission: To meet the needs of poor or destitute elderly people in Canada & the developing world
Affiliation(s): HelpAge International
Chief Officer(s):
Jacques Bertrand, Executive Director
Jack Panozzo, Chair
Ivan Hale, Vice-Chair
Rosalie Gelderman, Secretary
Donald Hefler, Treasurer

HelpAge International (HAI)
PO Box 70156, London WC1A 9GB United Kingdom
Tel: 44-20-7278-7778; *Fax:* 44-207-148-7623
e-mail: info@helpage.org
www.helpage.org
uk.linkedin.com/company/helpage-international
www.facebook.com/HelpAgeInternational
twitter.com/helpage
www.youtube.com/helpage
Overview: A medium-sized international charitable organization founded in 1983
Mission: To campaign on behalf of the world's older population & provide expertise & grants to older people's organizations in 70 developing countries; To assist them to help the most disadvantaged lead independent lives
Affiliation(s): Help the Aged - Canada
Chief Officer(s):
Arun Maira, Chair
Justin Derbyshire, Interim Chief Executive

International Council on Active Aging (ICAA)
3307 Trutch St., Vancouver BC V6L 2T3
Tel: 604-734-4466; *Fax:* 604-708-4464
Toll-Free: 866-335-9777
e-mail: info@icaa.cc
www.icaa.cc
www.linkedin.com/groups?gid=2294475
www.facebook.com/ICAAhome
Overview: A small international organization founded in 2001
Mission: Dedicated to changing the way we age by uniting professionals in the retirement, assisted living, fitness, recreation, rehabilitation, & wellness fields to help dispel society's myths about aging; to help these professionals to empower aging Baby Boomers & older adults to improve their quality of life & maintain their dignity.
Chief Officer(s):
Colin Milner, CEO
colinmilner@icaa.cc
Julie Milner, COO
juliemilner@icaa.cc

International Federation on Aging (IFA) / Fédération internationale du vieillissement (FIV)
Castleview Wichwood Towers, 351 Christie St., Toronto ON M6G 3C3
Tel: 416-342-1655; *Fax:* 416-392-4157
www.ifa-fiv.org
www.facebook.com/378160352195791
twitter.com/IntFedAgeing
Overview: A medium-sized international organization founded in 1973
Mission: To provide a worldwide forum for ageing issues & concerns; to foster the development of associations & agencies that serve or represent older people; to develop a universal charter of rights & responsibilities for the elderly; to advocate for the rights & respect of older people
Affiliation(s): World Health Organization; International Labour Organization; United Nations Educational, Scientific & Cultural Organization
Chief Officer(s):
Bjarne Hastrup, President
Jane Barratt, Secretary General
  jbarratt@ifa-fiv.org

National Publications

Canadian Geriatrics Journal
Previous Name: Geriatrics Today: Journal of Canadian Geriatrics Society
Gordon & Leslie Diamond Health Centre, 2775 Laurel St., 7th Fl., Vancouver, BC V5Z 1M9
Tel: 604-875-4931; *Fax:* 604-875-5696
Circulation: 15,500 *Frequency:* 4 times a year
Official journal of the Canadian Geriatrics Society.
Ken Madden, Editor-in-Chief

Canadian Nursing Home
c/o Health Media Inc., PO Box 45566, 2397 King George Blvd., Surrey, BC V4A 9N3

info@nursinghomemagazine.ca
Circulation: 3,000 *Frequency:* 4 times a year
Agnes Forster, Publisher
Frank Fagan, Editor

Caregiver Solutions
Previous Name: Canada's Family Guide to Home Health Care & Wellness Solutions
Owned By: BCS Communications Ltd.
#803, 255 Duncan Mill Rd., Toronto, ON M3B 3H9
Tel: 416-421-7944; *Fax:* 416-421-8418
Toll-Free: 800-798-6282
Social Media: www.facebook.com/CaregiverSolutions
Circulation: 30,000 *Frequency:* 4 times a year
Caroline Tapp-McDougall, Publisher, caroline@bcsgroup.com
Helmut Dostal, Managing Editor, dostal@bcsgroup.com

Provincial/Local Publications

Long Term Care Today
Ontario Long Term Care Association, #500, 425 University Ave., Toronto, ON M5G 1T6
Tel: 647-256-3490; *Fax:* 416-642-0635
info@oltca.com
Circulation: 5,800 *Frequency:* 2 times a year
Maurice Laborde, Publisher
Roma Ihnatowycz, Editor

Provincial Libraries

Alzheimer Society of Niagara Region
#1, 403 Ontario St., St Catharines, ON L2N 1L5
Tel: 902-687-3914; *Fax:* 905-687-9952
Toll-Free: 877-818-3202
niagara@alzheimerniagara.ca
www.alzheimer.ca/niagara
Social Media: www.youtube.com/user/alzniagara;
twitter.com/alzheimerniagar; www.facebook.com/106624255247
Teena Kindt, CEO
  tkindt@alzheimerniagara.ca

Denise Verreault, Director of Education
  dverreault@alzheimerniagara.ca

The Arthritis Society (Manitoba & Nunavut Division)
#100A, 1485 Buffalo Pl., Winnipeg, MB R3T 1L8
Tel: 204-942-4892; *Fax:* 204-942-4894
Toll-Free: 800-321-1433
info@mb.arthritis.ca
www.arthritis.ca

Baycrest
#2M10, 3560 Bathurst St., 2nd Fl., Toronto, ON M6A 2E1
Tel: 416-785-4224; *Fax:* 416-785-2372
onesearch.library.utoronto.ca/library-info/BAYCREST
Social Media: www.youtube.com/thebaycrestchannel;
twitter.com/baycrest; www.facebook.com/baycrestcentre
Collection: Collection of materials on caring for aging holocaust survivors; 1,000 monographs, 100 journal titles (current, print), and access to over 2000 electronic journals.
Mary McDiarmid, Manager, Library Services
  mmcdiarmid@baycrest.org

Bruyère Continuing Care
60 Cambridge St. North, Ottawa, ON K1R 7A5
Tel: 613-562-6262; *Fax:* 613-569-6734
library@bruyere.org
www.bruyere.org/en/medical-library
Mireille Ethier-Danis, Head of Library
  613-562-6262 ext. 2948

Cambridge Memorial Hospital
700 Coronation Blvd., Cambridge, ON N1R 3G2
Tel: 519-621-2330; *Fax:* 519-740-4938
TTY: 519-621-918
libraryservices@cmh.org
www.cmh.org

Centre d'hébergement Notre-Dame-de-la-Merci
555, boul Gouin ouest, Montréal, QC H3L 1K5
Tél: 514-331-3020; *Téléc:* 514-331-0781

Centre de santé et de services sociaux. Institut universitaire de gériatrie de Sherbrooke
1036, rue Belvédère sud, Sherbrooke, QC J1H 4C4
Tél: 819-780-2220
ctedoc.csss-iugs@ssss.gouv.qc.ca
www.csss-iugs.ca/bibliotheque

Donald Berman Maimonides Geriatric Centre
5795 Caldwell Ave., Montréal, QC H4W 1W3
Tel: 514-483-2121; *Fax:* 514-483-1561
www.donaldbermanmaimonides.net

E.W. Bickle Centre for Complex Continuing Care
130 Dunn Ave., #N234, Toronto, ON M6K 2R7
Tel: 416-597-3422
Jessica Babineau, Information Specialist

Glenrose Rehabilitation Hospital
10230 - 111th Ave., #GE0613, Edmonton, AB T5G 0B7
Tel: 780-735-8823; *Fax:* 780-735-8863
glenroselibrary@albertahealthservices.ca
Donna Gordon, Library Technician
  donna.gordon@albertahealthservices.ca

Institut universitaire de gériatrie de Montréal
4545, ch Queen Mary, Montréal, QC H3W 1W4
Tél: 514-340-2800; *Téléc:* 514-340-2815
www.iugm.qc.ca

Collection: Gériatrie et gérontologie
Audrey Attia, Bibliothécaire
  audrey.attia.iugm@ssss.gouv.qc.ca
Louise Aubut, Technicienne en documentation
  louise.aubut.iugm@ssss.gouv.qc.ca

J.W. Crane Memorial Library of Gerontology & Geriatrics
2109 Portage Ave., Winnipeg, MB R3J 0L3
Tel: 204-831-2152; *Fax:* 204-888-1805
Toll-Free: 855-220-1522
dlclibrary@umanitoba.ca
libguides.lib.umanitoba.ca/deerlodge
Social Media: twitter.com/gerinews
Collection: Clinical, social, and psychological aspects of aging, the administration, organization and operation of long-term care systems, health promotion and outreach programs for seniors, home care and palliative care.
Angela Osterreicher, Librarian
204-831-2107

Kerby Centre
1133 - 7th Ave. SW, Calgary, AB T2P 1B2
Tel: 403-705-3246; *Fax:* 403-705-3211
generaloffice@kerbycentre.com
www.kerbycentre.com
Social Media: www.youtube.com/user/KerbyCentre;
twitter.com/KerbyCentre; www.facebook.com/514905501859242
Collection: Kerby Centre Seniors Directory of Services; materials relating to seniors issues
Luanne Whitmarsh, Chief Executive Officer
403-705-3251

Knowledge Resource Centre 15
#100, 1509 Centre St. South, Calgary, AB T2G 2E6
Fax: 877-747-0295
Toll-Free: 800-432-1845
resource.centre@albertahealthservices.ca
Collection: Journals; Games; Kits; Posters
Deborah Clark, Medical Library Technician
deboraha.clark@albertahealthservices.ca

Meadowood Manor
577 St Anne's Rd., Winnipeg, MB R2M 5B2
Tel: 204-257-2394
info@meadowood.ca
www.meadowood.ca

Princess Elizabeth Guild Library
Princess Elizabeth Bldg, Main Fl., 1 Morley Ave., Winnipeg, MB R3L 2P4
Tel: 204-478-6203
rhcinfo@rhc.mb.ca
www.rhc.mb.ca

Riverview Health Centre
Princess Elizabeth Bldg, 4th Fl., 1 Morley Ave., Winnipeg, MB R3L 2P4
Tel: 204-478-6215
rhcinfo@rhc.mb.ca
www.rhc.mb.ca

St Joseph's Health Care, Parkwood Institute
550 Wellington Rd., London, ON N6C 0A7
Tel: 519-646-6100
www.sjhc.london.on.ca
Collection: Spinal Cord Injury Collection; Heart & Stroke Foundation Collection; Acquired Brain Injury Collection

St. Michael's Health Centre
1400 - 9th Ave. South, Lethbridge, AB T1J 4V5
Tel: 403-382-6400; *Fax:* 403-382-6413
www.covenanthealth.ca

Waterford Hospital
306 Waterford Bridge Rd., St. John's, NL A1E 4J8
Tel: 709-777-3300

National Government

National Seniors Council (NSC) / Conseil national des aînés (CNA)
Phase IV, 8th Floor, Mail Stop 802, 140 Promenade du Portage, Gatineau, QC K1A 0J9
Fax: 819-953-9298
Toll-Free: 800-622-6232
TTY: 800-926-9105
www.canada.ca/en/national-seniors-council.html
The Council, formerly known as the National Advisory Council on Aging, advises the Minister of Employment & Social Development, the Minister of Health, & the Minister of State (Seniors) on issues related to the aging of the Canadian population & the quality of life of seniors. It reviews the needs & problems of seniors & recommends remedial action, liaises with other groups interested in aging, encourages public discussion & publishes & disseminates information on aging.

Chair, Andrew Wister, PhD

Veterans Affairs Canada / Anciens combattants Canada
161 Grafton St., PO Box 7700 Charlottetown, PE C1A 8M9
Tel: 613-996-2242
Toll-Free: 866-522-2122
information@vac-acc.gc.ca
www.veterans.gc.ca
Other Communication: Toll-Free French: 1-866-522-2022; Media Relations: 613-992-7468
twitter.com/veteransENG_ca
www.facebook.com/VeteransAffairsCanada
www.youtube.com/user/VeteransAffairsCa
Provides pensions for disability or death, economic support in the form of allowances, & health care benefits & services to veterans & members of the Canadian Armed Forces, members & ex-members of the RCMP, & their dependents.

Minister, Veterans Affairs, Hon. Kent Hehr, P.C.
Tel: 613-995-1561
Fax: 613-995-1862
Kent.Hehr@parl.gc.ca

Director, Communications & Issues Management, Rob Rosenfeld
Tel: 613-996-4649
Fax: 613-954-1054

Deputy Minister's Office
Deputy Minister, Gen (Ret) Walter Natynczyk
Tel: 902-566-8666
Associate Deputy Minister, Karen Ellis
Tel: 613-944-1710

Service Delivery Branch / Prestation des services
Assistant Deputy Minister, Michel Doiron
Tel: 902-626-2723
Fax: 902-566-8172
Director General, Field Operations, Charlotte Bastien
Tel: 514-496-6413
Fax: 514-496-7303
Director General, Centralized Operations Division, Rick Christopher
Tel: 902-566-8644
Fax: 902-566-8337
Director General, Health Professionals Division & National Medical Officer, Dr. Cyd Courchesne
Tel: 613-945-6939
Fax: 613-864-7471
Director General, Service Delivery & Program Management, Elizabeth Douglas
Tel: 902-566-8808
Fax: 902-314-8897
Director, Planning & Administrative Support, Renate Fournier-Bélanger
Tel: 705-568-4131
Director, VAC Liaison to DND/CAF, Jane Hicks
Tel: 902-995-8248
Director, Health Care, Rehab & Income Support Programs, Carlos Lourenso
Tel: 902-566-8758
Fax: 902-367-7278

Director, Branch Liaison & Strategic Inititatives, Long Term Care Program, Lynne McCloskey
Tel: 902-368-0143
Fax: 902-370-4984
Director, Case Management & Support Services, Anne-Marie Pellerin
Tel: 902-626-2828
Fax: 902-368-0966
Director, Transition, Co-ordination & Integrated Services, Colleen Soltermann
Tel: 902-370-4750
Fax: 902-566-7573
Director, Long Term Care Program, Sandra Williamson
Tel: 902-370-4582
Fax: 902-370-4984

Provincial Government

Alberta Seniors & Housing
PO Box 3100Edmonton, AB T5J 4W3
Tel: 780-644-9992
Fax: 780-422-5954
Toll-Free: 877-644-9992
TTY: 800-232-7215
www.seniors-housing.alberta.ca
Other Communication: Housing Programs: 780-422-0122
Alberta Seniors & Housing is responsible for programming for seniors, as well as housing & community services.

Minister, Hon. Lori Sigurdson
Tel: 780-415-9550
Fax: 780-415-9411
seniors.minister@gov.ab.ca

Deputy Minister, Shannon Marchand
Tel: 780-644-2023
shannon.marchand@gov.ab.ca

Executive Director, Human Resources, Liz Kennedy
Tel: 780-408-8443
liz.kennedy@gov.ab.ca

Director, Communications, Jo-anne Nugent
Tel: 780-638-2978
jo-anne.nugent@gov.ab.ca

Office of the Seniors Advocate
Centre West Bldg., 10035 - 108 St. NW, Main Fl., Edmonton, AB T5J 3E1
Tel: 780-644-0682
Fax: 780-644-9685
Toll-Free: 844-644-0682
TTY: 844-392-9025
seniors.advocate@gov.ab.ca
seniorsadvocateab.ca
The Seniors Advocate provides links to government & community programs & services for seniors, as well as identifying systemic issues & providing policy advice to the Government of Alberta.
Alberta Seniors Advocate, Sheree Kwong See
Tel: 780-644-0678
sheree.kwongsee@gov.ab.ca
Director, Annette Lemire
Tel: 780-415-2751
annette.lemire@gov.ab.ca

Housing Division
44 Capital Blvd., 10044 - 108 St., 3rd Fl., Edmonton, AB T5J 5E6
Tel: 780-422-0122
Other Communication: Rural & Native Mortgage Portfolio, Phone: 780 427-6897
Assistant Deputy Minister, John Thomson
Tel: 780-643-1020
john.thomson@gov.ab.ca
Executive Director, Capital Initiatives, Lynda Cuppens
Tel: 780-422-8474
lynda.cuppens@gov.ab.ca
Executive Director, Housing Funding & Accountability, Robert Lee
Tel: 780-643-1324

Fax: 780-427-0418
robert.lee@gov.ab.ca
Executive Director, Stakeholder Relations & Housing Strategies, Dean Lussier
Tel: 780-427-1751
Fax: 780-422-5124
dean.lussier@gov.ab.ca
Director, Housing Operations & Reporting, Linda Winter
Tel: 780-638-2968
linda.g.winter@gov.ab.ca

Seniors Services Division
Standard Life Centre, 10405 Jasper Ave., 6th Fl., Edmonton, AB T5J 4R7
Assistant Deputy Minister, John Cabral
Tel: 780-422-7270
Fax: 780-644-7602
john.cabral@gov.ab.ca
Executive Director, Seniors Strategic Planning Branch, Kindy Joseph
Tel: 780-644-8613
Fax: 780-422-8762
kindy.joseph@gov.ab.ca
Executive Director, Seniors Program Delivery Branch, Neil McDonald
Tel: 780-422-8522
Fax: 780-422-5954
neil.mcdonald@gov.ab.ca
Director, Strategies & Program Support, Terri Lynn Almeda
Tel: 780-643-3869
terrilynn.almeda@gov.ab.ca
Director, Engagement & Community Initiatives, Jasvinder Chana
Tel: 780-641-9713
jasvinder.chana@gov.ab.ca
Director, Seniors Financial Assistance, Kirsten Ganske
Tel: 780-638-5610
Fax: 780-422-5954
kirsten.ganske@gov.ab.ca
Manager, Alberta Seniors Benefit, Sandy McCrimmon
Tel: 780-422-7262
sandy.mccrimmon@gov.ab.ca

Strategic Services Division
44 Capital Blvd., 10044 - 108 St., 12th Fl., Edmonton, AB T5J 5E6
Assistant Deputy Minister, MaryAnne Wilkinson
Tel: 780-641-9865
Fax: 780-644-5586
maryanne.wilkinson@gov.ab.ca
Chief Information Officer, Chris Kearney
Tel: 780-415-2704
Fax: 780-644-5586
chris.kearney@gov.ab.ca
Executive Director & Senior Financial Officer, Financial Services Branch, Darren Baptista
Tel: 780-422-0927
Fax: 780-644-5586
darren.baptista@gov.ab.ca
Executive Director, Policy, Planning & Legislative Services Branch, Matt Barker
Tel: 780-638-4115
matt.barker@gov.ab.ca

Office of the Seniors Advocate
PO Box 9651 Stn. Prov Govt, Victoria, BC V8W 9P4
Tel: 250-952-3034
Toll-Free: 877-952-3181
info@seniorsadvocatebc.ca
www.seniorsadvocatebc.ca
Seniors Advocate, Isobel Mackenzie
Tel: 250-952-2503
Deputy Seniors Advocate, Nancy Gault
Tel: 250-952-2999
Executive Director, Bruce Ronayne
Tel: 250-952-2998
Director, Communications, Sara Darling
Tel: 250-952-3035
Director, Systemic Review Monitoring, Anita Nadziejko
Tel: 250-952-1177

Manitoba Health, Seniors & Active Living
#100, 300 Carlton St., Winnipeg, MB R3B 3M9

Tel: 204-945-3744
Toll-Free: 866-626-4862
mgi@gov.mb.ca
www.gov.mb.ca/health/index.html

Renamed Health, Seniors & Active Living after the 2016 general election, the department is responsible for the overall quality of the health system in the province, for maintaining the health system, & for ensuring that the health needs of Manitobans are met. Services are provided through regional delivery systems, hospitals & other health care facilities. The Department also makes insured benefits claims payments for residents of Manitoba related to the cost of medical, hospital, personal care, pharmacare & other health services. To lead the way to quality health care, built with creativity, compassion, confidence, trust & respect; empower Manitobans through knowledge, choices & access to the best possible health resources; & build partnerships & alliances for healthy & supportive communities. To foster innovation in the health care system. This is accomplished through: developing mechanisms to assess & monitor quality of care, utilization & cost effectiveness; fostering behaviours & environments which promote health; & promoting responsiveness & flexibility of delivery systems, & alternative & less expensive services.

Minister, Health, Seniors & Active Living, Hon. Kelvin Goertzen
Tel: 204-945-3731
Fax: 204-945-0441
minhsal@leg.gov.mb.ca

Deputy Minister, Karen Herd
Tel: 204-945-3771
Fax: 204-945-4564
dmhlt@leg.gov.mb.ca

Acting Chief Provincial Public Health Officer, Dr. Elise Weiss, M.D., C.C.F.P., F.C.F.P., M.Sc.
Tel: 204-788-6636

Healthy Living & Seniors
c/o Seniors & Healthy Aging Secretariat, #1610, 155 Carlton St., Winnipeg, MB R3C 3H8

Tel: 204-945-6565
Fax: 204-948-2514
Toll-Free: 800-665-6565
seniors@gov.mb.ca
www.gov.mb.ca/healthyliving

Assistant Deputy Minister, Marcia Thomson
Tel: 204-784-3908
Executive Director, Mental Health & Spiritual Health Care, Carly Johnston
Tel: 204-786-7281
Executive Director, Addictions Policy & Support Branch, Tina Leclair
Tel: 204-784-3913
Executive Director, Healthy Living & Healthy Populations, Debbie Nelson
Tel: 204-788-6654
Manager, Tobacco Control & Cessation, Andrew Loughead
Tel: 204-784-3900
Clerk, Healthy Schools & Manitoba in Motion, Stephanie Sawatzky
Tel: 204-788-6661

Service New Brunswick / Service Nouveau Brunswick
Westmorland Pl., PO Box 1998Fredericton, NB E3B 5G4

Tel: 506-457-3581
Fax: 506-444-2850
snb@snb.ca
www.snb.ca

Other Communication: SNB TeleServices Within NB: 1-888-762-8600;
Outside NB: 506-684-7901

Service New Brunswick provides the following services to the public: Service New Brunswick TeleServices (Call Centre); delivery of federal, provincial & municipal government services; Land Registry; Personal Property Registry; Corporate Registry; Property Assessment & Taxation System; & maintaining land information infrastructure.
On Oct. 1, 2015, the new Service New Brunswick was launched, bringing together the former Service New Brunswick, Department of Government Services, FacilicorpNB & New Brunswick Internal Services Agency under one organization.

Minister Responsible, Hon. Ed Doherty
Tel: 506-453-6100
ed.doherty@snb.ca

Chair, Elizabeth Webster

Chief Executive Officer, Roy Alan
Tel: 506-444-2897
alan.roy@snb.ca

Chief Operating Officer, Technology & Health Services, Derrick Jardine
Tel: 506-663-2510
derrick.jardine@snb.ca

Health Services / Services de santé
Tel: 506-457-3581
Fax: 506-444-2850

Vice-President, David Dumont
Tel: 506-663-2510
david.dumont@snb.ca
Executive Director, Clinical Engineering, Charles Beaulieu
Tel: 506-737-5781
Charles.Beaulieu@snb.ca
Executive Director, Strategic Procurement (Health), Ann Dolan
Tel: 506-663-2538
ann.dolan@snb.ca
Executive Director, Supply Chain, Michel Levesque
Tel: 506-869-6140
Michel.Levesque@snb.ca
Executive Director, Laundry & Linen Services, Terry Watters
Tel: 506-674-0058
Terry.Watters@snb.ca
Director, Maintenance - Linen Services, James Belliveau
Tel: 506-457-3581
James.Belliveau@snb.ca
Director, Sourcing Renewal, Nancy Butler-Rioux
Tel: 506-544-2505
Nancy.Butlerrioux@snb.ca
Director, Logistics, Greg Demerchant
Tel: 506-452-5623
greg.demerchant@snb.ca
Director, Procurement (Vitalité), Annick Godin-Bourque
Tel: 506-869-2720
Annick.GodinBourque@snb.ca
Director, Procurement (Horizon), Jana Kirkpatrick
Tel: 506-649-2661
Jana.Kirkpatrick@snb.ca

Technology Services / Services technologiques
435 Brookside Dr., Fredericton, NB E3A 8V4
Tel: 506-444-4600
Fax: 506-444-3784
Toll-Free: 888-487-5050
NBISA-ASINB@gnb.ca

Vice-President, Pam Gagnon
Tel: 506-457-3582
Pam.Gagnon@snb.ca
Executive Director, Health Application Services, Tania Davies
Tania.Davies@snb.ca
Director, Horizon Health Network Application Services, Sharon Jamer
Tel: 506-375-2743
Sharon.Jamer@snb.ca
Director, Provincial Health Services, Dawn O'Donnell
Tel: 506-457-4800
dawn.o'donnell@snb.ca
Director, Vitalité Health Network Application Services, Ghislain Roy
Tel: 506-789-5901
Ghislain.Roy@snb.ca

Seniors & Long Term Care / Aînés et Soins de longue durée
Tel: 506-453-2940
Fax: 506-453-2164
seniors@gnb.ca
www.gnb.ca/seniors

Assistant Deputy Minister, Steven Hart
Tel: 506-453-2181
Steven.Hart@gnb.ca
Director, Long Term Care & Disability Support Services, Joan McGowan
Tel: 506-457-6811
joan.McGowan@gnb.ca
Director, Nursing Homes Services, Janet Thomas
Tel: 506-453-3821
janet.thomas@gnb.ca

Newfoundland & Labrador Department of Children, Seniors & Social Development
PO Box 8700St. John's, NL A1B 4J6

Tel: 709-729-0862
Fax: 709-729-0870
TTY: 855-229-2044
CSSDInfo@gov.nl.ca
www.cssd.gov.nl.ca

In August 2016, the Department of Child, Youth & Family Services & the Department of Seniors, Wellness and Social Development combined to create the Department of Children, Seniors and Social Development. The Department focuses on child protection, youth services, aging, seniors, health promotion, sport & general wellness. The Department is also responsible for the Poverty Reduction Strategy & the Disability Policy Office.

Minister, Hon. Sherry Gambin-Walsh
Tel: 709-729-0659
Fax: 709-729-0662
sherrygambinwalsh@gov.nl.ca

Deputy Minister, Bruce Cooper
Tel: 709-729-0958
brucecooper@gov.nl.ca

Assistant Deputy Minister, Policies & Programs, Rick Healey
Tel: 709-729-0088
rhealey@gov.nl.ca

Assistant Deputy Minister, Corporate Services, Jean Tilley
Tel: 709-729-0656
jeantilley@gov.nl.ca

Assistant Deputy Minister, Services Delivery & Regional Operations, Susan Walsh
Tel: 709-729-3473
swalsh@gov.nl.ca

Director of Communications, Children & Youth, Melony O'Neill
Tel: 709-729-5148
melonyoneill@gov.nl.ca

Director of Communications, Seniors & Wellness, Roger Scaplen
Tel: 709-729-0928
rogerscaplen@gov.nl.ca

Healthy Living Division
Tel: 709-729-6243

Acting Director, Linda Carter
Tel: 709-729-3117
lindacarter@gov.nl.ca
Coordinator, Eat Great & Participate, Stephanie O'Brien
Tel: 709-729-4432
StephanieOBrien@psnl.ca

Poverty Reduction Strategy
Fax: 709-729-5139
Toll-Free: 866-883-6600
povertyreduction@gov.nl.ca

Director, Aisling Gogan
Tel: 709-729-1287
aislinggogan@gov.nl.ca

Recreation & Sport
Tel: 709-729-2829
Fax: 709-729-5293

Director, Michelle Healey
Tel: 709-729-5241
MichelleHealey@gov.nl.ca
Manager, Programs & Strategic Initiatives, Jaime Collins
Tel: 709-729-0855
Jaimecollins@gov.nl.ca

Seniors & Aging Division
Toll-Free: 888-494-2266
Other Communication: Seniors of Distinction Awards: E-mail: seniorsofdistinction@gov.nl.ca

Consultant, Pamela Dawe
Tel: 709-729-4906
Consultant, Henry Kielley
Tel: 709-729-6262

Northwest Territories Department of Health & Social Services (HSS)
5015 - 49th St., PO Box 1320Yellowknife, NT X1A 2L9

www.hss.gov.nt.ca

Other Communication: Media Relations, Phone: 867-920-8927; Health Care Coverage/Vital Statistics: 1-800-661-0830
www.youtube.com/user/HSSCommunications

The Department of Health & Social Services is mandated to provide a broad range of health & social programs & services to the residents of the NWT. Seven regional Health & Social Services Authorities plan, manage & deliver a full spectrum of community & facility-based services for health care & social services. Community health programs include daily sick clinics, public health clinics, home care, school health programs & educational programs. Visiting physicians & specialists routinely visit the communities.

Minister, Health & Social Services; Minister Responsible, Seniors & Persons with Disabilities, Hon. Glen Abernethy
Tel: 867-767-9141 ext: 11135
glen_abernethy@gov.nt.ca

Deputy Minister, Debbie DeLancey
Tel: 867-767-9060 ext: 49005
debbie_delancey@gov.nt.ca

Assistant Deputy Minister, Corporate Services, Derek Elkin
Tel: 867-767-9050 ext: 49001

Assistant Deputy Minister, Health Programs, Kim Riles
Tel: 867-767-9050 ext: 49002

Chief Public Health Officer, Dr. André Corriveau
Tel: 867-767-9063 ext: 49215

Deputy Chief Public Health Officer, Dr. Kami Kandola
Tel: 867-767-9063 ext: 49216

Director, Corporate Planning, Reporting & Evaluation, Lisa Cardinal
Tel: 867-767-9053 ext: 49050
Fax: 867-873-0484

Director, Strategic Human Resource Planning Division, Beth Collinson
Tel: 867-767-9059 ext: 49150

Director, Infrastructure Planning, Perry Heath
Tel: 867-767-9057 ext: 49125

Director, Innovation & Project Management, Dave Nightingale
Tel: 867-767-9058 ext: 49139

Communications Officer, Dorothy Westerman
Tel: 867-767-9052 ext: 49035
Fax: 867-873-0204

Seniors & Continuing Care Services
Fax: 867-920-3088

Director, Victorine Lafferty
Tel: 867-767-9030 ext: 49205

Acting Manager, Continuing Care & Health Systems Planning Unit, Sandra Mann
Tel: 867-767-9030 ext: 49208
Manager, Strategic Initiatives Unit, Stacy Ridgely
Tel: 867-767-9030 ext: 49900

Nova Scotia Department of Seniors
Barrington Tower, 1894 Barrington St., 15th Fl., Halifax, NS B3J 2R8
Tel: 902-424-0770
Fax: 902-424-0561
Toll-Free: 844-277-0770
seniors@NovaScotia.ca
novascotia.ca/seniors
twitter.com/NSSeniors

Committed to ensuring the inclusion, well-being, & independence of seniors in Nova Scotia by facilitating the development of policies on aging & programs for seniors across government & through the provision & coordination of strategic planning, support, services, programs & information.

Minister, Hon. Leo A. Glavine
Tel: 902-424-0770
Fax: 902-424-0561
seniorsmin@novascotia.ca

Deputy Minister, Simon d'Entremont

Executive Director, Faizal Nanji
Tel: 902-424-7933

Ontario Seniors' Secretariat
#601C, 777 Bay St., 6th Fl., Toronto, ON M7A 2J4
Tel: 416-326-7076
Fax: 416-326-7078
infoseniors@ontario.ca
www.ontario.ca/page/ministry-seniors-affairs
The Ontario Seniors' Secretariat supports, develops & delivers public services to improve the quality of life for seniors in Ontario.
Minister Responsible, Seniors Affairs, Hon. Dipika Damerla
dipika.damerla@ontario.ca
Deputy Minister, Accessibility, Francophone Affairs & Seniors Affairs, Marie-Lison Fougère
Tel: 416-212-2320
marie-lison.fougere@ontario.ca
Assistant Deputy Minister, Abby Katz Starr
Tel: 416-326-7069
abby.katzstarr@ontario.ca
Manager, Public Education & Awareness Unit, Deanna Blair
Tel: 416-326-7058
Fax: 416-326-7078
deanna.blair@ontario.ca
Manager, Policy Initiatives, Alan Ernst
Tel: 416-326-8066
alan.ernst@ontario.ca
Acting Manager, Program Policy, Accountability & Agency Relations Unit, Phil Wake
Tel: 416-325-7761
phil.wake@ontario.ca

Prince Edward Island Department of Family & Human Services
Jones Bldg., 11 Kent St., 2nd Fl., PO Box 2000Charlottetown, PE C1A 7N8
Tel: 902-620-3777
Fax: 902-894-0242
Toll-Free: 866-594-3777
www.pe.ca/sss
The Department of Family & Human Services strives to develop healthy & self-reliant individuals & to support vulnerable members of the province. Programs & services are offered to promote social & economic prosperity & the creation of work environments that contribute to a safe, healthy & engaged workforce.

Minister, Hon. Tina M. Mundy
Tel: 902-368-6520
Fax: 902-368-4740
tmmundy@gov.pe.ca

Deputy Minister, Teresa Hennebery

Tel: 902-368-6520
tahennebery@gov.pe.ca

Senior Communications Officer, Darlene Gillis
Tel: 902-620-3409
ddgillis@gov.pe.ca

Corporate Support & Seniors
Corporate Support & Seniors has responsibility for the Senior's Secretariat / the Office of Seniors, records information management, French Language Services, intergovernmental & external relations, & emergency social services.
Manager, Corporate Support & Seniors, Jennifer Burgess
Tel: 902-368-5199
Fax: 902-894-0242
jmburgess@gov.pe.ca
Seniors Policy Advisor, Catherine Freeze
Tel: 902-620-3785
cafreeze@gov.pe.ca
Administrative Support Worker, Leah Baiani
Tel: 902-620-3777
Fax: 902-894-0242
lmbaiani@gov.pe.ca

AIDS/HIV

AIDS, Acquired Immune Deficiency Syndrome, is an infectious disorder that suppresses the normal function of the immune system. AIDS is a result of HIV (Human Immunodeficiency Virus) infection, which destroys the body's ability to fight infections. Specifically, the virus infects and later destroys T-cells, which are a part of the body's immune system that responds to invading organisms. This destructive process is slow and silent, which means that HIV can be contracted years before any symptoms appear. When enough T-cells have been destroyed, the body is invaded by organisms that wouldn't ordinarily be able to cause serious disease.

Cause
HIV transmission requires contact with body fluids (blood, semen, rectal fluid, vaginal fluid or breast milk), and is usually spread from an infected person to a non-infected person by unprotected sexual intercourse, or by sharing needles. Mothers can give the HIV infection to their children before and during childbirth and while breastfeeding.

Symptoms
When first infected with HIV, some people have flu-like symptoms such as a sore throat, fever, and swollen glands, but others have no symptoms at all. In fact, there are people living with HIV who go for years without feeling or looking sick. However, HIV weakens the immune system, so after a number of years the body can no longer fight off infections and weight loss, fever and night sweats are common symptoms. Certain cancers, especially lymphoma and Kaposi's sarcoma, also take advantage of the body's lowered resistance. These diseases—called opportunistic infections—can lead to the onset of AIDS.

Prevalence
In Canada, the first case of AIDS was diagnosed in 1982. Today, an estimated 75,500 Canadians are living with HIV (including AIDS). Of this number, an estimated 6,850 are Aboriginal people, and around 16,880 are women. It is guessed that 25 percent of individuals living with HIV in Canada do not know that they have the infection.

Treatment Options
The only way to diagnose HIV is through a blood test. After infection, it can take some time—three to six months—before HIV antibodies appear in the blood. Therefore, testing should take place at least three months after the last activity that posed a high risk for HIV infection.

Since there is no vaccine to prevent the HIV infection, avoiding contact with the virus is the primary method of prevention. The risk of HIV infection can be reduced by practising safer sex—using a condom during vaginal and anal sex. Injecting drug users should not share needles, and should use new needles and injection equipment each time they inject. The use of needle exchange programs has decreased the spread of HIV infection. When getting a tattoo or body piercing, or having acupuncture or electrolysis, it is important to seek out professionals who follow universal infection-control precautions. Women with HIV who are pregnant should stay on medicine directed against HIV and should not breastfeed. Today, infants born to women who have HIV are treated with a short course of anti-HIV drugs—also known as antiretrovirals—immediately after birth, and this has greatly reduced the incidence of vertical transmission of the infection from mother to child.

Until anti-HIV drugs became available, infected persons usually had a rapid downhill course. Today, combination drug treatment can offer most infected persons a long period of relatively good health. However, the treatment regimen is often complex, involving three or four drugs which must be taken several times a day. Since skipping doses encourages growth of the virus that is resistant to drugs, it is very important to take the drugs exactly as directed. People living with HIV/AIDS must take antiretrovirals every day for life.

Although there is no cure, proper care and treatment can prolong the lives of people with HIV/AIDS, and improve their quality of life.

National Associations

Action Canada for Sexual Health & Rights
251 Bank St., 2nd Fl., Ottawa ON K2P 1X3

Tel: 613-241-4474
Toll-Free: 888-642-2725
Other Communication: Donor inquiries ext 8; Media inquiries ext 7
e-mail: info@sexualhealthandrights.ca
www.sexualhealthandrights.ca
www.facebook.com/actioncanadaSHR
twitter.com/action_canada

Merged from: Canadians for Choice; Canadian Federation for Sexual Health; Action Canada for Population
Overview: A large national charitable organization founded in 2014
Mission: To advance sexual & reproductive health & rights in Canada & abroad through Public education & awareness; Support for the delivery of programs & services in Canada.
Member of: International Planned Parenthood Federation
Chief Officer(s):
Sandeep Prasad, Executive Director
Frédérique Chabot, Health Information Officer
Publications:
• Beyond the Basics: A Sourcebook on Sexual & Reproductive Health Education
Type: Book
Profile: Resource used in schools, public health offices, & community-based health organizations

The AIDS Foundation of Canada
#505, 744 West Hastings St., Vancouver BC V6C 1A5
Tel: 604-688-7294
www.aidsfoundationofcanada.ca
Overview: A medium-sized national organization founded in 1986
Mission: To address the growing problem of HIV disease in Canada; to fund new & innovative ways of assisting infected/affected people with HIV; to support new ways to heighten awareness of HIV disease among the general population

Black Coalition for AIDS Prevention
20 Victoria St., 4th Fl., Toronto ON M5C 2N8
Tel: 416-977-9955; *Fax:* 416-977-7664
e-mail: info@black-cap.com
www.black-cap.com
www.facebook.com/blackcapto

Also Known As: Black CAP
Overview: A medium-sized national organization founded in 1987 overseen by Canadian AIDS Society
Mission: To reduce the spread of HIV infection in Black communities; To enhance the quality of life for Black people living with or affected by HIV/AIDS
Member of: Ontario AIDS Network
Chief Officer(s):
Shannon Thomas Ryan, Executive Director
s.ryan@black-cap.com

Canadian Aboriginal AIDS Network (CAAN)
6520 Salish Dr., Vancouver BC V6N 2C7
Tel: 604-266-7616; *Fax:* 604-266-7612
www.caan.ca
www.facebook.com/CAAN.ca
twitter.com/caan_says

Overview: A medium-sized national organization
Mission: To provide support & advocacy for Aboriginal people living with or affected by HIV/AIDS, TB, aging, mental illness, or other co-morbidity issues
Chief Officer(s):
Emma Palmantier, Chair
Ken Clement, Chief Executive Officer, 604-266-7616 Ext. 227
Merv Thomas, Manager, National Programs Communications, 604-266-7616 Ext. 226
Publications:
• Canadian Journal of Aboriginal Community-Based HIV/AIDS Research (CJACBR)
Type: Journal; *Frequency:* Annually; *Editor:* Renee Masching et al.
Profile: A peer-reviewed journal directed toward Aboriginal HIV/AIDS service organizations, Aboriginal people living with HIV/AIDS, community leaders, policy & decision-makers, & anyone with an interest in HIV/AIDS

Canadian AIDS Society (CAS) / Société canadienne du sida (SCS)
#100, 190 O'Connor St., Ottawa ON K2P 2R3
Tel: 613-230-3580; *Fax:* 613-563-4998
Toll-Free: 800-499-1986
e-mail: casinfo@cdnaids.ca
www.cdnaids.ca
www.facebook.com/aidsida
twitter.com/CDNAIDS
www.instagram.com/cdnaids

Overview: A medium-sized national charitable organization founded in 1988
Mission: To strengthen the response to HIV/AIDS across Canada; To enrich the lives of people living with HIV/AIDS
Chief Officer(s):
Greg Riehl, Chair
gregr@cdnaids.ca
Michael Sangster, Vice-Chair
mikes@cdnaids.ca
Gary Lacasse, Executive Director
gary.lacasse@cdnaids.ca
Gerry Croteau, Secretary
gerryc@cdnaids.ca
Janet MacPhee, Treasurer
janetm@cdnaids.ca
Janne Charbonneau, Officer, Communications
janne.charbonneau@cdnaids.ca
Lynne Belle-Isle, Manager, National Programs
lynne.belle-isle@cdnaids.ca
Tobias Keogh, Manager, Fundraising
tobias.keogh@cdnaids.ca
Publications:
• Canadian AIDS Society Annual Report
Type: Yearbook; *Frequency:* Annually
Profile: Society's achievements, finances, supporters, & volunteers

• InfoCAS
Type: Newsletter; *Frequency:* Quarterly; *Price:* Free
Profile: HIV/AIDS national policy, governmental news, & activities of member groups
• InFocus
Type: Newletter; *Frequency:* Semiannually
Profile: Examination of HIV/AIDS issues, ideas, & information

Canadian AIDS Treatment Information Exchange (CATIE) / Réseau canadien d'info-traitements sida
PO Box 1104, #505, 555 Richmond St. West, Toronto ON M5V 3B1
Tel: 416-203-7122; *Fax:* 416-203-8284
Toll-Free: 800-263-1638
e-mail: info@catie.ca
www.catie.ca
www.linkedin.com/company/canadian-aids-treatment-information-exchange
www.facebook.com/CATIEInfo
twitter.com/CATIEInfo
www.youtube.com/user/catieinfo
Previous Name: Community AIDS Treatment Information Exchange
Overview: A small national charitable organization founded in 1990
Mission: To improve the health & quality of life of all people living with HIV/AIDS (PHAs) in Canada; To provide HIV/AIDS treatment information to PHAs, caregivers & AIDS service organizations who are encouraged to be active partners in achieving informed decision-making & optimal health care; To promote collaboration among affected populations
Member of: Canadian AIDS Society; Ontario AIDS Network; Ontario Hospital Association
Chief Officer(s):
John McCullagh, Chair
  jmccullagh@catie.ca
Laurie Edmiston, Executive Director
  ledmiston@catie.ca
Publications:
• The CATIE [Canadian AIDS Treatment Information Exchange] Exchange
Type: Newsletter; *Editor:* Jim Pollock
Profile: Forum on CATIE & frontline programs
• The Positive Side [a publication of the Canadian AIDS Treatment Information Exchange]
Type: Magazine; *Frequency:* s-a.; *Editor:* Debbie Koenig
Profile: A health & wellness magazine written for people living with HIV

The Canadian Association for HIV Research (CAHR) / L'Association Canadienne de recherche sur le HIV (ACRV)
#744, 1 Rideau St., Ottawa ON K1N 8S7
Tel: 613-241-5785; *Fax:* 613-670-5701
e-mail: info@cahr-acrv.ca
www.cahr-acrv.ca
www.facebook.com/CanadianAssociationforHIVResearch
twitter.com/CAHR_ACRV
Overview: A medium-sized national charitable organization founded in 1991
Mission: Focuses on HIV/AIDS research & education
Chief Officer(s):
Robert Hogg, President
Carol Strike, Secretary
Curtis Cooper, Treasurer
Andrew Matejcic, Executive Director
Shelley Mineault, Project Coordinator
Erin Love, Project Coordinator

Canadian Association of Nurses in HIV/AIDS Care (CANAC) / Association canadienne des infirmières et infirmiers en sidologie
St. Paul's Hospital, #B552, 1081 Burrard St., Vancouver BC V6Z 1Y6
e-mail: admin@canac.org
www.canac.org
Overview: A small national charitable organization founded in 1991
Mission: The Canadian Association of Nurses in AIDS Care (CANAC) is a national professional nursing organization committed to fostering excellence in HIV/AIDS nursing, promoting the health, rights and dignity of persons affected by HIV/AIDS and to preventing the spread of HIV infection.
Affliation(s): Canadian Nurses Association

Chief Officer(s):
Janna Campbell, Executive Assistant
Publications:
• Connection: The Newsletter of the Canadian Association of Nurses in AIDS Care
Type: Newsletter; *Frequency:* 3 pa; *Editor:* Jennifer Shaw
Profile: CANAD / ACIIS news & reports, conference information, events, resources, & employment opportunities

Canadian Foundation for AIDS Research (CANFAR) / Fondation canadienne de recherche sur le SIDA
#602, 200 Wellington St. West, Toronto ON M5V 3C7
Tel: 416-361-6281; *Fax:* 416-361-5736
Toll-Free: 800-563-2873
www.canfar.com
www.facebook.com/canfar
twitter.com/canfar
www.youtube.com/user/CANFAR; www.flickr.com/photos/canfar
Overview: A medium-sized national charitable organization founded in 1987
Mission: To raise awareness in order to fund research into all aspects of HIV infection & AIDS
Chief Officer(s):
Christopher Bunting, President & CEO, 416-361-6281 Ext. 229
  cbunting@canfar.com
Publications:
• CANFAR [Canadian Foundation for AIDS Research] Annual Report
 Frequency: Annually
• Catalyst [a publication of the Canadian Foundation for AIDS Research]
Type: Newsletter
Profile: CANFAR's programs & fundraising events, reports on advances in HIV / AIDS, & updates on research
• Funding Leading-Edge Research: Canada's HIV/AIDS epidemic, the global HIV / AIDS crisis & CANFAR
 Author: S.E. Read, R.S. Remis, J.K. Stewart

Canadian HIV Trials Network (CTN) / Réseau canadien pour les essais VIH
#588, 1081 Burrard St., Vancouver BC V6Z 1Y6
Tel: 604-806-8327; *Fax:* 604-806-8005
Toll-Free: 800-661-4664
e-mail: ctninfo@hivnet.ubc.ca
www.hivnet.ubc.ca
www.linkedin.com/company/2287403
www.facebook.com/CIHR.CTN
twitter.com/CIHR_CTN
www.youtube.com/user/CIHRCTN
Overview: A medium-sized national organization founded in 1990
Mission: To develop treatments, vaccines & a cure for HIV disease & AIDS through the conduct of scientifically sound & ethical clinical trials
Chief Officer(s):
Aslam Anis, National Director
Marina Klein, National Co-Director
Sharon Walmsley, National Co-Director

Atlantic Region
QEII Health Sciences Centre - Victoria General Hospital, 5790 University Ave., Halifax NS B3H 1V7
Tel: 902-473-2700

Ontario Region
University of Ottawa at Ottawa General Hospital, 501 Smyth Rd., Ottawa ON K1H 8L6

Pacific Region
St. Paul's Hospital, John Ruedy Immunodeficiency Clinic, 1081 Burrard St., Vancouver BC V6Z 1Y6

Prairie Region
Southern Alberta HIV Clinic, #3223, 1213 - 4 St. SW, Calgary AB T2R 0X7

Québec Region
Institut thoracique de Montréal, 3650, rue St-Urbain, Montréal QC H2X 2P4

Toronto & Area Office

Sunnybrook Health Science Centre, 2075 Bayview Ave., Toronto ON M4N 3M5

Tel: 416-480-5900

Canadian HIV/AIDS Legal Network / Réseau juridique canadien VIH/sida

#600, 1240 Bay St., Toronto ON M5R 2A7

Tel: 416-595-1666; *Fax:* 416-595-0094
e-mail: info@aidslaw.ca
www.aidslaw.ca
www.facebook.com/CanadianHIVAIDSLegalNetwork
twitter.com/aidslaw
www.youtube.com/aidslaw

Overview: A medium-sized national charitable organization founded in 1992 overseen by Canadian AIDS Society
Mission: To promote the human rights of people living with & vulnerable to HIV/AIDS, in Canada & internationally; through research, legal & policy analysis, education, advocacy & community mobilization
Chief Officer(s):
Richard Elliot, Executive Director, 416-595-1666 Ext. 229
Janet Butler-McPhee, Director of Communications, 416-595-1666 Ext. 228
Publications:
• HIV / AIDS Policy & Law Review
Type: Journal; *Editor:* David Garmaise; *ISSN:* 1712-624X; *Price:* $75 Canada; $125 international
Profile: Analysis & summaries of current developments in HIV/AIDS-related policy and law from an international perspective
• Legal Network News
ISSN: 1488-0997

First Nations Breast Cancer Society

#309, 1333 East 7th Ave., Vancouver BC V5N 1R6

Tel: 604-872-4390; *Fax:* 604-875-0779
e-mail: echoes@fnbreastcancer.bc.ca
www.fnbreastcancer.bc.ca

Overview: A small national organization founded in 1995
Mission: Offers breast cancer education and support to First Nations women.
Chief Officer(s):
Jacqueline Davis, President
jdavis@fnbreastcancer.bc.ca

Prisoners' HIV/AIDS Support Action Network (PASAN)

526 Richmond St. East, Toronto ON M5A 1R3

Tel: 416-920-9567; *Fax:* 416-920-4314
Toll-Free: 866-224-9978
www.pasan.org

Overview: A small national organization founded in 1991
Mission: Prisoners, ex-prisoners, organizations, activists & individuals working together to provide advocacy, education, & support to prisoners on HIV/AIDS, HCV & related issues
Chief Officer(s):
Glen Brown, Interim Executive Director
glen@pasan.org

Red Road HIV/AIDS Network (RRHAN)

#61-1959 Marine Dr., North Vancouver BC V7P 3G1

Tel: 778-340-3388; *Fax:* 778-340-3328
e-mail: info@red-road.org
www.red-road.org
twitter.com/RRHAN

Overview: A small national organization founded in 1999
Mission: The Red Road HIV/AIDS Network works to reduce or prevent the spread of HIV/AIDS; improve the health and wellness of Aboriginal people living with HIV/AIDS; and increase awareness about HIV/AIDS and establish a network which supports the development and delivery of culturally appropriate, innovative, coordinated, accessible, inclusive and accountable HIV/AIDS programs and services
Chief Officer(s):
Kim Louie, Executive Director
klouie@red-road.org
Heidi Standeven, Provincial Coordinator
hstandeven@red-road.org
Publications:
• Bloodlines Magazine
Type: Magazine

Profile: a forum in which Aboriginal Persons Living with HIV/AIDS can share their personal experiences, discuss issues affecting them, offer advice and suggestions to their peers.
• Red Road Aboriginal HIV/AIDS Resource Directory
Type: Directory; *Frequency:* Semi-Annually

2-Spirited People of the First Nations (TPFN)

#105, 145 Front St. East, Toronto ON M5A 1E3

Tel: 416-944-9300; *Fax:* 416-944-8381
www.2spirits.com
www.facebook.com/2spiritsTO
www.instagram.com/2spirits_com

Previous Name: Gays & Lesbians of the First Nations
Overview: A medium-sized national charitable organization founded in 1989
Mission: To create a place where Aboriginal 2-Spirited people can grow & learn together as a community, fostering a positive, self-sufficient image, honouring our past & building a future; to work together toward bridging the gap between the 2-Spirited, Lesbian, Gay, Bisexual & Transgendered community & our Aboriginal identity
Member of: Ontario AIDS Network; Toronto Aboriginal Social Services Association; Canadian Aboriginal AIDS Network
Chief Officer(s):
Art Zoccole, Executive Director Ext. 222
art@2spirits.com

Provincial Associations

ALBERTA

Alberta Reappraising AIDS Society (ARAS)

PO Box 61037, Stn. Kensington, Calgary AB T2N 4S6

Tel: 403-220-0129
e-mail: aras@aras.ab.ca
www.aras.ab.ca

Overview: A small provincial organization founded in 1999
Mission: To provide a science-based alternative information on HIV/AIDS & other infectious diseases; does not provide treatment recommendations
Chief Officer(s):
David Crowe, President, 403-289-6609, Fax: 403-206-7717
david.crowe@aras.ab.ca
Roger Swan, Treasurer

BRITISH COLUMBIA

Positive Living BC

803 East Hastings St., Vancouver BC V6A 1R8

Tel: 604-893-2200; *Fax:* 604-893-2251
Toll-Free: 800-994-2437
e-mail: info@positivelivingbc.org
www.positivelivingbc.org
www.facebook.com/positivelivingbc
twitter.com/pozlivingbc

Previous Name: British Columbia Persons with AIDS Society
Overview: A small provincial charitable organization founded in 1986
Mission: To empower persons in British Columbia who live with HIV/AIDS
Member of: CAS; CAAN; Red Road HIV/AIDS Society; BC Health Coalition; Canadian HIV/AIDS Legal Network
Chief Officer(s):
Neil Self, Chair
Tom McAulay, Vice-Chair
Publications:
• British Columbia Persons with AIDS Society Annual Report
Type: Yearbook; *Frequency:* Annually
• British Columbia Persons with AIDS Society HIV/AIDS eNewslist
Type: Newsletter; *Frequency:* Weekly
• eScoop [a publication of Positive Living BC]
Type: Newsletter; *Frequency:* Bimonthly
• Living+ [a publication of Positive Living BC]
Type: Magazine
Profile: Current issues encountered by those infected & affected by HIV/AIDS
• Positive Living Manual
Type: Manual

Profile: Information for BCPWA members, interested individuals, PWAs, AIDS service organizations, & health care workers

NEW BRUNSWICK

AIDS New Brunswick / Sida Nouveau Brunswick
#G17, 65 Brunswick St., Fredericton NB E3B 1G5

Fax: 888-501-6301
Toll-Free: 800-561-4009
e-mail: info@aidsnb.com
www.aidsnb.com
www.linkedin.com/company/aids-nb
www.facebook.com/aidsnb
twitter.com/aidsnb
www.youtube.com/aidsnb

Overview: A small provincial charitable organization founded in 1987
Mission: To facilitate community-based responses to the issue of HIV/AIDS
Member of: Canadian AIDS Society
Affiliation(s): Atlantic AIDS Network
Chief Officer(s):
Karen Tanner, President
Stephen Alexander, Executive Director, 800-561-4009 Ext. 105
stephen@aidsnb.com

NEWFOUNDLAND AND LABRADOR

AIDS Committee of Newfoundland & Labrador (ACNL)
47 Janeway Pl., St. John's NL A1A 1R7

Tel: 709-579-8656; *Fax:* 709-579-0559
Toll-Free: 800-563-1575
www.acnl.net
www.facebook.com/AIDSCommitteeNL
twitter.com/aidscommitteenl

Previous Name: Newfoundland & Labrador AIDS Committee
Overview: A medium-sized provincial charitable organization founded in 1988 overseen by Canadian AIDS Society
Mission: To prevent new HIV infections through education; to provide support to persons living with HIV/AIDS & their families, friends & partners
Member of: Atlantic AIDS Network
Chief Officer(s):
Gerard Yetman, Executive Director

NOVA SCOTIA

AIDS Coalition of Nova Scotia (ACNS)
#200, 5516 Spring Garden Rd., Halifax NS B3J 1G6

Tel: 902-429-7922; *Fax:* 902-422-6200
Toll-Free: 800-566-2437
Other Communication: Alternate Phone: 902-425-4882
acns.ns.ca
www.facebook.com/AIDSNS
twitter.com/AIDS_NS

Previous Name: Nova Scotia PWA Coalition
Overview: A small provincial charitable organization founded in 1995 overseen by Canadian AIDS Society
Mission: To empower persons living with & affected by HIV/AIDS & those at risk through health promotion & mutual support & to reduce the spread of HIV in Nova Scotia
Member of: Canadian AIDS Society; Canadian HIV/AIDS Legal Network
Chief Officer(s):
Michelle Johnson, Coordinator, Programs, 902-425-4882 Ext. 226
pc@acns.ns.ca

ONTARIO

African & Caribbean Council on HIV/AIDS in Ontario (ACCHO)
20 Victoria St., 4th Fl., Toronto ON M5C 2N8

Tel: 416-977-9955; *Fax:* 416-977-7664
e-mail: administration@accho.ca
www.accho.ca
www.facebook.com/ACCHOntario
twitter.com/ACCHOntario
www.youtube.com/ACCHOntario

Overview: A medium-sized provincial organization

Mission: To provide support & resources to members of the African, Caribbean & Black communities in Ontario who are affected by HIV/AIDS
Chief Officer(s):
Valérie Pierre-Pierre, Director, 416-977-9955 Ext. 292
v.pierrepierre@accho.ca

HALCO
#400, 65 Wellesley St. East, Toronto ON M4Y 1G7

Tel: 416-340-7790; *Fax:* 416-340-7248
Toll-Free: 888-705-8889
e-mail: talklaw@halco.org
www.halco.org

Also Known As: HIV & AIDS Legal Clinic of Ontario
Overview: A small provincial organization founded in 1995
Mission: Community-based legal clinic that provides free legal services to people living with HIV/AIDS in Ontario
Chief Officer(s):
Ryan Peck, Executive Director

Ontario HIV Treatment Network
#600, 1300 Yonge St., Toronto ON M4T 1X3

Tel: 416-642-6486; *Fax:* 416-640-4245
Toll-Free: 877-743-6486
e-mail: info@ohtn.on.ca
www.ohtn.on.ca
www.facebook.com/theOHTN
twitter.com/theOHTN
www.youtube.com/user/OntarioHIVTreatment

Overview: A small provincial organization
Mission: To optimize the quality of life of people living with HIV in Ontario & to promote excellence & innovation in treatment, research, education & prevention through a collaborative network of excellence representing consumers, providers, researchers & other stakeholders
Chief Officer(s):
Sean Rourke, Scientific & Executive Diretor
srourke@ohtn.on.ca

PRINCE EDWARD ISLAND

AIDS PEI
161 St. Peter's Rd., Charlottetown PE C1A 5P7

Tel: 902-566-2437; *Fax:* 902-626-3400
www.aidspei.com
www.facebook.com/pages/AIDS-PEI/156237431556
twitter.com/aidspei

Overview: A small provincial charitable organization founded in 1990 overseen by Canadian AIDS Society
Mission: To provide education & support to Islanders infected or affected by HIV/AIDS; To promote the development of greater understanding & acceptance by the public in relation to persons affected by HIV/AIDS
Member of: Prince Edward Island Literacy Alliance Inc.
Chief Officer(s):
Alana Leard, Executive Director
director@aidspei.com

QUÉBEC

Coalition des organismes communautaires québécois de lutte contre le sida (COCQ-SIDA)
1, rue Sherbrooke Est, Montréal QC H2X 3V8

Tél: 514-844-2477; *Téléc:* 514-844-2498
Ligne sans frais: 866-535-0481
Courriel: info@cocqsida.com
www.cocqsida.com
www.facebook.com/COCQSIDA
twitter.com/COCQSIDA

Aperçu: *Dimension:* moyenne; *Envergure:* provinciale; Organisme sans but lucratif; fondée en 1990
Mission: Représenter les membres afin de favoriser l'émergence et le soutien d'une action concertée dans les dossiers d'intérêt commun; faire reconnaître l'expertise et l'apport des organismes communautaires et non-gouvernementaux dans la lutte contre le sida.
Membre(s) du bureau directeur:
Hélène Légaré, Présidente
Ken Monteith, Directeur général
ken.monteith@cocqsida.com

Coalition sida des sourds du Québec (CSSQ)
Edifice Plessis, #320, 2075, rue Plessis, Montréal QC H2L 2Y4
Ligne sans frais: 877-535-5556
Courriel: info@cssq.org
www.cssq.org

Aperçu: *Dimension:* petite; *Envergure:* provinciale; Organisme sans but lucratif; fondée en 1992 surveillé par Canadian AIDS Society
Mission: Informer et mettre en garde la communauté sourde du Québec contre les risques de contracter le Sida et les ITSS (Infections transmissibles sexuellement par le sang); dispenser des services et activités aux personnes sourdes et malentendantes atteintes du VIH/Sida et de l'ITSS
Affliation(s): Coalition des organismes communautaires québécois de lutte contre le sida
Membre(s) du bureau directeur:
Darren Saunders, Président
Michel Turgeon, Directeur général
direction@cssq.org

Comité des personnes atteintes du VIH du Québec (CPAVIH)
#310, 2075, rue Plessis, Montréal QC H2L 2Y4
Tél: 514-521-8720; *Téléc:* 514-521-9633
Ligne sans frais: 800-927-2844
Courriel: cpavih@cpavih.qc.ca

Aperçu: *Dimension:* moyenne; *Envergure:* provinciale; Organisme sans but lucratif; fondée en 1987
Mission: Informer les personnes vivant avec le VIH/SIDA; promouvoir leurs droits afin d'améliorer leur qualité de vie
Membre de: Canadian AIDS Society

The Farha Foundation / La Fondation Farha
#100, 576, rue Sainte-Catherine Est, Montréal QC H2L 2E1
Tel: 514-270-4900; *Fax:* 514-270-5363
e-mail: farha@farha.qc.ca
www.farha.qc.ca
www.facebook.com/FondationFARHAFoundation
twitter.com/FarhaFoundation
www.youtube.com/user/farhafondation

Overview: A medium-sized provincial charitable organization founded in 1992
Mission: To raise funds to improve the quality of life for persons living with HIV & AIDS throughout Québec
Chief Officer(s):
Nancy Farha, Executive Director Ext. 223
n.farha@farha.qc.ca

Groupe d'action pour la prévention de la transmission du VIH et l'éradication du Sida (GAP-VIES)
3330, rue Jarry Est, Montréal QC H1Z 2E8
Tél: 514-722-5655; *Téléc:* 514-722-0063
Courriel: gapvies@gapvies.ca
www.gapvies.ca

Nom précédent: Groupe haïtien pour la prévention du sida; Groupe d'action pour la prévention du sida
Aperçu: *Dimension:* petite; *Envergure:* provinciale; fondée en 1987 surveillé par Canadian AIDS Society
Mission: Prévenir la transmission du VIH/sida et d'aider les personnes atteintes du virus de l'immunodéficience humaine dans la population en général et dans la communauté haïtienne en particulier; informer et d'éduquer sur les implications de la maladie et les moyens de la prévenir; accompagner les personnes atteintes ainsi que leurs proches
Membre de: Coalition des organismes communautaires québécois de lutte contre le sida
Membre(s) du bureau directeur:
Joseph Jean-Gilles, Directeur général

Mouvement d'information et d'entraide dans la lutte contre le sida à Québec
625, av Chouinard, Québec QC G1S 3E3
Tél: 418-649-1720; *Téléc:* 418-649-1256
Courriel: miels@miels.org
www.miels.org
www.facebook.com/mielsQC

Également appelé: MIELS-Québec
Aperçu: *Dimension:* petite; *Envergure:* provinciale; fondée en 1986 surveillé par Canadian AIDS Society

Mission: Soutenir les personnes vivant avec le VIH/sida et leurs proches; prévenir la transmission du VIH; accueillir et héberger personnes vivant avec le sida
Affliation(s): Société canadienne du sida
Membre(s) du bureau directeur:
Martin Masson, Président
Thérèse Richer, Directrice générale
dgmiels@miels.org

Mouvement d'information, d'éducation et d'entraide dans la lutte contre le sida (MIENS)
CP 723, Chicoutimi QC G7H 5E1
Tél: 418-693-8983; *Téléc:* 418-693-0409
Ligne sans frais: 800-463-3764
Courriel: lemiens@lemiens.com
www.lemiens.com

Aperçu: *Dimension:* petite; *Envergure:* provinciale; Organisme sans but lucratif; fondée en 1988
Mission: Pour fournir des informations sur la prévention du VIH ainsi que de soutenir et d'aider les personnes infectées par le VIH et à leurs proches
Affliation(s): Coalition des organismes québécois de lutte contre le sida

SIDALYS
3702, rue Ste-Famille, Montréal QC H2X 2L4
Tél: 514-842-4439; *Téléc:* 514-842-2284
Courriel: sidasecours@hotmail.com

Nom précédent: Centre des services sida secours du Québec
Aperçu: *Dimension:* petite; *Envergure:* provinciale surveillé par Canadian AIDS Society
Membre de: Coalition des organismes communautaires québécois de lutte contre le sida (COCQ-SIDA)

SASKATCHEWAN

Persons Living with AIDS Network of Saskatchewan Inc.
PO Box 7123, Saskatoon SK S7K 4J1
Tel: 306-373-7766; *Fax:* 306-374-7746
Toll-Free: 800-226-0944
e-mail: plwa@sasktel.net
www.aidsnetworksaskatoon.ca

Also Known As: PLWA Network of Saskatchewan
Overview: A small provincial charitable organization founded in 1987 overseen by Canadian AIDS Society
Mission: To provide & operate support & social activities for persons diagnosed with HIV disease, as well as their families, friends & partners
Member of: Saskatoon Interagency Council on STD's & AIDS; Canadian Centre for Philanthropy

YUKON TERRITORY

Blood Ties Four Directions Centre
307 Strickland St., Whitehorse YT Y1A 2J9
Tel: 867-633-2437; *Fax:* 867-633-2447
Toll-Free: 877-333-2437
e-mail: bloodties@klondiker.com
www.bloodties.ca

Previous Name: AIDS Yukon Alliance
Overview: A small provincial charitable organization founded in 1988 overseen by Canadian AIDS Society
Mission: To acts as an information & support centre; to promote public awareness of AIDS/AIDS & hepatitis C and aid in their prevention; to assist people living with HIV/AIDS & hep C.
Member of: Pacific AIDS Network
Chief Officer(s):
Patricia Bacon, Executive Director
executivedirector@bloodties.ca

Local Associations

ALBERTA

Central Alberta AIDS Network Society (CAANS)
Turning Point, 4611 - 50th Ave., Red Deer AB T4N 3Z9
Tel: 403-346-8858; *Fax:* 403-346-2352
Toll-Free: 877-346-8858
e-mail: info@caans.org
www.caans.org
www.facebook.com/CentralAlbertaAIDSNetwork
twitter.com@CAANSRedDeer
Overview: A small local charitable organization founded in 1988 overseen by Canadian AIDS Society
Mission: To carry out its charitable mission, which includes responsibility for HIV prevention & support, in the David Thompson Health Region, which extends from Drumheller to Drayton Valley & from Nordegg to the Saskatchewan border
Chief Officer(s):
Jennifer Vanderschaeghe, Executive Director
jennifer@caans.org

HIV Community Link (ACAA)
#110, 1603 - 10th Ave. SW, Calgary AB T3C 0J7
Tel: 403-508-2500; *Fax:* 403-263-7358
Toll-Free: 877-440-2437
www.hivcl.org
www.linkedin.com/company/aids-calgary-awareness-association
www.facebook.com/AIDSCalgary
twitter.com/hivcommlink
Also Known As: AIDS Calgary
Previous Name: AIDS Calgary Awareness Association
Overview: A small local charitable organization founded in 1983 overseen by Canadian AIDS Society
Mission: To reduce the harm associated with HIV & AIDS for all individuals & communities in the Calgary region; to provide HIV education & support; to enhance the quality of life & advocate on behalf of people living with HIV; to promote awareness & understanding of HIV issues; to work together with partners in the community to create a caring & compassionate society in the face of HIV & AIDS
Member of: Canadian AIDS Society; Alberta Community Council on HIV/AIDS; Canadian HIV/AIDS Legal Network; Calgary Coalition on HIV & AIDS
Chief Officer(s):
Leslie Hill, Executive Director

HIV Network of Edmonton Society
9702 - 111 Ave. NW, Edmonton AB T5G 0B1
Tel: 780-488-5742; *Fax:* 780-488-3735
Toll-Free: 877-388-5742
www.hivedmonton.com
www.facebook.com/home.php#!/hiv.edmonton?fref=ts
twitter.com/HIVEdmonton
www.youtube.com/user/hivedmontonvideo
Also Known As: HIV Edmonton
Previous Name: AIDS Network of Edmonton Society
Overview: A small local charitable organization founded in 1984
Mission: HIV Edmonton is a community-based, not-for-profit organization that works to reduce HIV/AIDS related stigma & discrimination. It works to educate, support & advocate on behalf of those infected & affected by HIV & related conditions.
Member of: Canadian AIDS Society; Canadian Centre for Philanthropy Canadian HIV/AIDS Legal Network; Canadian Palliative Care Association; Chamber of Commerce
Affliation(s): Alberta Community Council on HIV
Chief Officer(s):
Ken MacDonald, Chair
Shelley Williams, Executive Director
shelley.w@hivedmonton.com

HIV North Society
9607 - 102 St., Grande Prairie AB T8V 2T8
Tel: 780-538-3388; *Fax:* 780-538-3368
www.hivnorth.org
www.facebook.com/106064926090085

Also Known As: HIV North
Previous Name: South Peace AIDS Council of Grande Prairie; Society of the South Peace AIDS Council
Overview: A small local charitable organization founded in 1987 overseen by Canadian AIDS Society
Mission: To provide outreach, education, harm reduction & support programs & services, working collaboratively with other agencies, to fight against HIV/AIDS
Member of: Alberta Community Council on HIV; Canadian AIDS Society; Canadian Society of Association Executives
Chief Officer(s):
Susan Belcourt, Executive Director
director@hivnorth.org

HIV West Yellowhead Society
PO Box 5005, 152 Athabasca Ave., Hinton AB T7V 1X3
Tel: 780-740-0066; *Fax:* 780-740-0060
Toll-Free: 877-291-8811
www.hivwestyellowhead.com
Previous Name: AIDS Jasper Society
Overview: A small local organization founded in 1988 overseen by Canadian AIDS Society
Mission: To promote healthy lifestyles & relationships & prevent the spread of HIV
Member of: Alberta Community Council on HIV
Chief Officer(s):
Lori Phillips, Executive Director
director@hivwestyellowhead.com

Lethbridge HIV Connection (LHC)
1206 - 6th Ave. South, Lethbridge AB T1J 1A4
Tel: 403-328-8186; *Fax:* 403-328-8564
e-mail: info@lethbridgehiv.com
www.lethbridgehiv.com
Previous Name: Lethbridge AIDS Connection Society
Overview: A medium-sized local charitable organization founded in 1986 overseen by Canadian AIDS Society
Mission: To support, educate, advocate & facilitate compassionate & effective community responses to HIV
Member of: Alberta Community Council on HIV; United Way of Southwestern Alberta

Living Positive
#50, 9912 - 106 St., Edmonton AB T5K 1C5
Tel: 780-424-2214
e-mail: living-positive@telus.net
www.facebook.com/LivingPoz
Previous Name: Edmonton Persons Living with HIV Society
Overview: A small local charitable organization founded in 1990 overseen by Canadian AIDS Society
Mission: To provide persons living with HIV infection nurturing, supportive environments in which to develop positive attitudes & self image
Member of: Alberta Community Council on HIV

BRITISH COLUMBIA

AIDS Vancouver (AV)
803 East Hastings St., Vancouver BC V6A 1R8
Tel: 604-893-2201; *Fax:* 604-893-2205; *Crisis Hot-Line:* 604-696-4666
e-mail: contact@aidsvancouver.org
www.aidsvancouver.org
www.facebook.com/aidsvancouver
twitter.com/AIDSVancouver
Also Known As: Vancouver AIDS Society
Overview: A small local charitable organization founded in 1983 overseen by Canadian AIDS Society
Mission: To alleviate individual & collective vulnerability to HIV & AIDS, through care, support, education, advocacy, & research
Member of: Canadian Public Health Association
Chief Officer(s):
Brian Chittock, Executive Director, 604-696-4655
brian@aidsvancouver.org

AIDS Vancouver Island (AVI)
Access Health Centre, 713 Johnson St., 3rd Fl., Victoria BC V8W 1M8
Tel: 250-384-2366; *Fax:* 250-380-9411
Toll-Free: 800-665-2437
e-mail: info@avi.org
www.avi.org
www.facebook.com/aidsvancouverisland?ref=ts
twitter.com/AIDSVanIsle
Overview: A small local charitable organization founded in 1986 overseen by Canadian AIDS Society
Mission: To serve people infected & affected by HIV & Hepatitis C on Vancouver Island & the Gulf Islands, British Columbia; To provide support & combat stigma; To prevent infection
Chief Officer(s):
Katrina Jensen, Executive Director
James Boxshall, Manager, Fund Development & Volunteer Services
Heidi Exner, Manager, Health Promotion & Community Development
George Pine, Manager, Operations
Bryson Hawkins, Director, Finance
Kristen Kvakic, Director, Programs
Publications:
• AVI [AIDS Vancouver Island] Newsletter
Type: Newsletter

Campbell River Office
1371 c. Cedar St., Campbell River BC V9W 2W6
Tel: 250-830-0787; *Fax:* 250-830-0784
Toll-Free: 877-650-8787
Chief Officer(s):
Leanne Cunningham, Contact

Courtenay/Comox Office
355 - 6th St., Courtenay BC V9N 1M2
Tel: 250-338-7400; *Fax:* 250-334-8224
Toll-Free: 877-311-7400
Chief Officer(s):
Sarah Sullivan, Contact

Nanaimo Office
#216, 55 Victoria Rd., Nanaimo BC V9R 5N9
Tel: 250-754-9111; *Fax:* 250-754-9888
e-mail: health.centre@avi.org
avihealthcentre.org
Chief Officer(s):
Dana Becker, Manager

Port Hardy Office
PO Box 52, Port Hardy BC V0N 2P0
Tel: 250-902-2238; *Fax:* 250-949-9953
Chief Officer(s):
Shane Thomas, Manager

ANKORS
West Kootenay Regional Office, 101 Baker St., Nelson BC V1L 4H1
Tel: 250-505-5506; *Fax:* 250-505-5507
e-mail: information@ankors.bc.ca
www.ankors.bc.ca
www.facebook.com/ankors.west
twitter.com/ankorswest
Also Known As: AIDS Network Kootenay Outreach & Support Society
Previous Name: AIDS Network, Outreach & Support Society
Overview: A small local charitable organization founded in 1992
Mission: To provide support, care, outreach & harm reduction services to individuals living with & affected by HIV, AIDS & HepC
Member of: Pacific AIDS Network; Kootenay Pride; Canadian Aids Society; CATIE; Canadian Treatment Action Council; Positive Living BC; Canadian HIV/AIDS Legal Network; HepC BC; Positive Women's Network; Canadian Aboriginial AIDS Network
Affiliation(s): West Kootenay Women's Association; Advocacy Centre; Nelson CARES Society; Nelson Committee on Homelessness
Chief Officer(s):
Cheryl Dowden, Executive Director
cheryl@ankors.bc.ca

Healing Our Spirit BC Aboriginal HIV/AIDS Society
137 East 4 Ave., Vancouver BC V5T 1G4
Tel: 604-879-8884; *Fax:* 604-879-9926
Toll-Free: 866-745-8884
e-mail: info@healingourspirit.org
www.healingourspirit.org
Overview: A medium-sized local charitable organization founded in 1992
Mission: To prevent & reduce the spread of HIV infection in First Nation communities & to support those affected by HIV/AIDS.
Member of: Canadian Aboriginal AIDS Network
Affiliation(s): Red Road HIV/AIDS Network; BC Aboriginal AIDS Awareness Program; AIDS Vancouver; BC Persons with AIDS
Chief Officer(s):
Winston Thompson, Executive Director
winston@healingourspirit.org
Leonard George, President

Living Positive Resource Centre, Okanagan (LPRC)
168 Asher Rd., Kelowna BC V1X 3H6
Tel: 778-753-5830; *Fax:* 778-753-5832
e-mail: info@lprc.ca
www.livingpositive.ca
www.facebook.com/lprcokanagen
Previous Name: ARC, AIDS Resource Centre, Okanagan & Region
Overview: A small local charitable organization founded in 1992
Mission: To educate & inform the public about HIV/AIDS & hepatitis, its transmission, prevention, treatment & care, providing the most accurate & up-to-date information available; to develop & promote community based partnerships for the delivery of education & support; to dispel the myths & misunderstandings & to promote awareness of the discrimination & marginalization of persons infected & affected by HIV/AIDS & hepatitis & to advocate for change; to advocate & lobby for programs & services, necessary to promote wellness & quality of life of persons infected & affected by HIV/AIDS & hepatitis; to facilitate access to emotional, spiritual, social & practical support for persons infected & affected by HIV/AIDS & hepatitis, respectful of their right to determine the direction of their lives; to provide accessible services in non-judgmental, safe, confidential environments; to identify & seek solutions to existing gaps in services
Member of: Canadian AIDS Society; Pacific AIDS Network
Affiliation(s): Central Okanagan Hospice Society; Vernon Hospice; Salmon Arm Hospice; North Okanagan Youth & Family Services; Columbia-Shuswap HIV/AIDS Project; Outreach Health Services
Chief Officer(s):
Clare Overton, Executive Director

Positive Living North: No kheyoh t'sih'en t'sehena Society (PLN)
#1, 1563 - 2nd Ave., Prince George BC V2L 3B8
Tel: 250-562-1172; *Fax:* 250-562-3317
Toll-Free: 888-438-2437
www.positivelivingnorth.ca
www.facebook.com/103410213083441
Previous Name: Prince George AIDS Prevention Program; AIDS Prince George; Prince George AIDS Society
Overview: A small local organization founded in 1992 overseen by Canadian AIDS Society
Mission: To provide services to people live with HIV & their families; 75 per cent of PLN's clients are of Aboriginal descent
Chief Officer(s):
Vanessa West, Executive Director
Publications:
• Common Threads [a publication of Positive Living North]
Type: Newsletter; *Frequency:* Quarterly

Positive Women's Network (PWN)
#614, 1033 Davie St., Vancouver BC V6E 1M7
Tel: 604-692-3000; *Fax:* 604-684-3126
Toll-Free: 866-692-3001
e-mail: pwn@pwn.bc.ca
www.pwn.bc.ca
www.facebook.com/Positivewomensnetwork
twitter.com/pwn_bc
Overview: A small local charitable organization founded in 1989 overseen by Canadian AIDS Society

Mission: Challenging HIV, Changing Women's Lives
Member of: Pacific AIDS Network; Canadian HIV/AIDS Legal Network
Chief Officer(s):
Marcie Summers, Executive Director
   marcies@pwn.bc.ca

MANITOBA

Kali-Shiva AIDS Services
646 Logan Ave., Winnipeg MB R3A 0S7
Tel: 204-783-8565; *Fax:* 204-772-7237
e-mail: kalishiv@mts.net
www.kalishiva.wix.com/shiva
Overview: A small local charitable organization founded in 1987 overseen by Canadian AIDS Society
Mission: To provide community-based support services for persons with HIV/AIDS

NEW BRUNSWICK

AIDS Moncton / SIDA Moncton
80 Weldon St., Moncton NB E1C 5V8
Tel: 506-859-9616; *Fax:* 506-855-4726
e-mail: sidaidsm@nb.aibn.com
www.sida-aidsmoncton.com
twitter.com/AIDSMoncton
Overview: A small local charitable organization founded in 1989 overseen by Canadian AIDS Society
Mission: To improve the quality of life for persons infected & affected by HIV / AIDS; To reduce HIV & other sexually transmitted infections
Chief Officer(s):
Deborah Warren, Executive Director

AIDS Saint John (ASJ)
62 Waterloo St., Saint John NB E2L 3P3
Tel: 506-652-2437; *Fax:* 506-652-2438
e-mail: info@aidssaintjohn.com
www.aidssaintjohn.com
Overview: A small local charitable organization founded in 1987
Mission: To confront HIV & AIDS through providing education, support, prevention & awareness initiatives; to create supportive social environments to people living with & affected with HIV/AIDS; to share our resources & build partnerships to promote the collaborative development of a community-based response to AIDS locally, provincially & regionally
Chief Officer(s):
Leslie Jeffrey, President

NOVA SCOTIA

AIDS Coalition of Cape Breton (ACCB)
150 Bentinck St., Sydney NS B1P 4W4
Tel: 902-567-1766
accb.ns.ca
www.facebook.com/CB.4.harmreduction
Overview: A small local organization founded in 1991 overseen by Canadian AIDS Society
Chief Officer(s):
Christine Porter, Executive Director
   christine.porter@bellaliant.com
Frances Macleod, SANE Project Coordinator
   frances.macleod@bellaliant.com

Healing Our Nations (HON)
31 Gloster Ct., Dartmouth NS B3B 1X9
Tel: 902-492-4255
e-mail: ea@accesswave.ca
www.hon93.ca
www.facebook.com/Healing.Our.Nations
Also Known As: Atlantic First Nations AIDS Task Force
Overview: A small local organization founded in 1991 overseen by Canadian AIDS Society
Mission: To educate First Nation people about HIV/AIDS; to improve the community by elimiating family violence, substance abuse, mental & spiritual malaise leading to depression & suicide.
Member of: Canadian HIV/AIDS Legal Network
Affliation(s): Union of NS Indians; Union of NB Indians; Atlantic Policy Congress; Mawiw Council; Confederacy of Mainland Mi'Kmaq

Chief Officer(s):
Julie Thomas, Program Manager

The Northern AIDS Connection Society (NACS)
33 Pleasant St., Truro NS B2N 3R5
Tel: 902-895-0931; *Fax:* 902-895-3353
Toll-Free: 866-940-2437
e-mail: admin@nhcsociety.ca
www.nhcsociety.ca
www.facebook.com/nhcsns
Previous Name: Truro & Area Outreach Project; Pictou County AIDS Coalition
Overview: A small local organization founded in 1996 overseen by Canadian AIDS Society
Mission: To support & promote the health & well-being of individuals living with HIV & those affected by HIV; To provide prevention education within northern region of Nova Scotia
Affliation(s): Nova Scotia AIDS Coalition
Chief Officer(s):
Albert McNutt, Director
   super@nhcsociety.ca
Dwight Griffiths, Program Coordinator
   programs@nhcsociety.ca
Publications:
• Extreme Reality [a publication of the Northern AIDS Connection Society]
Type: Newsletter; *Frequency:* Quarterly

ONTARIO

AIDS Action Now / Le groupe d'action sida
Toronto ON
e-mail: aidsactionnowtoronto@gmail.com
www.aidsactionnow.org
www.facebook.com/AidsActionNow
twitter.com/AIDSActionNow
vimeo.com/channels/152729
Overview: A small local organization founded in 1989 overseen by Canadian AIDS Society
Mission: To fight for improved treatment, care & support for people living with AIDS & HIV infection

AIDS Committee of Cambridge, Kitchener/Waterloo & Area (ACCKWA)
#203, 639 King St. West, Kitchener ON N2G 1C7
Tel: 519-570-3687; *Fax:* 519-570-4034
Toll-Free: 877-770-3687
www.acckwa.com
www.facebook.com/ACCKWA
twitter.com/AIDSCKW
Overview: A small local charitable organization founded in 1987
Mission: To provide support & education services for people affected by & infected with HIV/AIDS; To mobilize community to respond effectively & with compassion to individuals affected by HIV/AIDS; To advocate on behalf of people infected or affected by HIV
Member of: Canadian Public Health Association
Affliation(s): Ontario AIDS Network; Canadian AIDS Society
Chief Officer(s):
Ruth Cameron, Executive Director
   director@acckwa.com

AIDS Committee of Durham Region (ACDR)
#202, 22 King St. West, Oshawa ON L1H 1A3
Tel: 905-576-1445; *Fax:* 905-576-4610
Toll-Free: 877-361-8750
e-mail: info@aidsdurham.com
www.aidsdurham.com
www.facebook.com/AIDSDurham
twitter.com/AIDSDurham
Overview: A small local charitable organization founded in 1992 overseen by Canadian AIDS Society
Mission: To provide HIV/AIDS related services to the infected, affected & general community in the Region of Durham
Member of: Ontario AIDS Network
Affliation(s): Interagency Coalition on AIDS & Development; Canadian AIDS Treatment Information Exchange; Canadian HIV/AIDS Legal Network; Community Networks; Community Advisory Committee; Local

Planning & Coordinating Group; Feed The Need in Durham; Affrican & Caribbean Council on HIV/AIDS in Ontario
Chief Officer(s):
Margaret McCormack, President
Adrian Betts, Executive Director, 905-576-1445 Ext. 11
director@aidsdurham.com

AIDS Committee of North Bay & Area (ACNBA) / Comité du sida de North Bay et de la région
#201, 269 Main St. West, North Bay ON P1B 2T8
Tel: 705-497-3560; *Fax:* 705-497-7850
Toll-Free: 800-387-3701
e-mail: oaacnba@gmail.com
www.aidsnorthbay.com
www.facebook.com/128216403874712
twitter.com/ACNBA
Overview: A small local organization founded in 1990 overseen by Canadian AIDS Society
Mission: To assist & support all those affected & infected by HIV/AIDS; To limit the spread of the virus through education & awareness strategies
Member of: Ontario AIDS Network
Affiliation(s): Chamber of Commerce Downtown Inprovement Area
Chief Officer(s):
Sal Renshaw, President
Stacey L. Mayhill, Ph.D., Executive Director
acnbaed@gmail.com

AIDS Committee of Ottawa (ACO) / Comité du SIDA d'Ottawa
19 Main St., Ottawa ON K1S 1A9
Tel: 613-238-5014; *Fax:* 613-238-3425
e-mail: info@aco-cso.ca
www.aco-cso.ca
www.linkedin.com/company/1098145
www.facebook.com/acocso
twitter.com/ACOttawa
Overview: A small local charitable organization founded in 1985 overseen by Canadian AIDS Society
Mission: To fight AIDS & HIV infection through advocacy, education & support services
Member of: Ontario AIDS Network
Chief Officer(s):
Khaled Salam, Executive Director, 613-238-5014 Ext. 234
ed@aco-cso.ca

AIDS Committee of Simcoe County (ACSC)
#555, 80 Bradford St., Barrie ON L4N 6S7
Tel: 705-722-6778; *Fax:* 705-722-6560
Toll-Free: 800-372-2272
www.acsc.ca
www.facebook.com/AIDSCommitteeofSimcoeCounty
twitter.com/acsc
Overview: A small local charitable organization overseen by Canadian AIDS Society
Mission: To provide support, education & advocacy to people infected & affected by HIV/AIDS in Simcoe County
Member of: The Canadian AIDS Society; The Ontario AIDS Network; The Greater Barrie Chamber of Commerce
Chief Officer(s):
Gerry L. Croteau, Executive Director
ed@acsc.ca

AIDS Committee of Toronto (ACT)
399 Church St., 4th Fl., Toronto ON M5B 2J6
Tel: 416-340-2437; *Fax:* 416-340-8224
e-mail: ask@actoronto.org
www.actoronto.org
www.facebook.com/ACToronto
twitter.com/ACToronto
www.youtube.com/user/AIDSCommitteeToronto
Overview: A medium-sized local charitable organization founded in 1983 overseen by Canadian AIDS Society
Mission: To provide health promotion, support, education & advocacy for people living with HIV/AIDS & those affected by HIV/AIDS
Member of: Ontario AIDS Network
Chief Officer(s):

John Maxwell, Executive Director, 416-340-2437 Ext. 245
jmaxwell@actoronto.org
Winston Husbands, Director, Research, 416-340-2437 Ext. 454
Jason Patterson, Director, Development, 416-340-2437 Ext. 268
Don Phaneuf, Director, Employment Services, 416-340-2437 Ext. 262
Publications:
• Being Well: The PWA/ACT Wellness Newsletter

AIDS Committee of Windsor (ACW)
511 Pelissier St., Windsor ON N9A 4L2
Tel: 519-973-0222; *Fax:* 519-973-7389
Toll-Free: 800-265-4858
www.aidswindsor.org
www.facebook.com/aidswindsor
Overview: A small local charitable organization founded in 1985 overseen by Canadian AIDS Society
Mission: To mobilize communities to help people affected by HIV/AIDS in the Windsor-Essex & Chatham-Kent areas through advocacy, education & support
Member of: Ontario AIDS Network
Affliation(s): AIDS Support Chatham Kent; Drouillard Road Clinic
Chief Officer(s):
Michael Brennan, Executive Director
mbrennan@aidswindsor.org

AIDS Support Chatham-Kent
Adelaide Place, 67 Adelaide St. South, Chatham ON N7M 4R1
Tel: 519-352-2121; *Fax:* 519-351-7067
Toll-Free: 800-265-4858
Chief Officer(s):
Karyn O'Neil, Associate Director, Development
koneil@aidswindsor.org

AIDS Committee of York Region
#203, 10909 Yonge St., Richmond Hill ON L4C 3E3
Tel: 905-884-0613; *Fax:* 905-884-7215
Toll-Free: 800-243-7717
e-mail: info@acyr.org
www.acyr.org
www.facebook.com/AIDSCommitteeOfYorkRegion
twitter.com/outreachacyr
Overview: A small local organization
Mission: To provide support & education; To promote access to dignified care for people living with HIV/AIDS & those affected by HIV/AIDS
Chief Officer(s):
Vibhuti Mehra, Executive Director

AIDS Niagara
120 Queenston St., St Catharines ON L2R 2Z3
Tel: 905-984-8684; *Fax:* 905-988-1921
Toll-Free: 800-773-9843
e-mail: info@aidsniagara.com
www.aidsniagara.com
www.facebook.com/AIDSNiagara
twitter.com/aidsniagara
Overview: A small local charitable organization founded in 1987
Mission: To improve quality of life for those infected &/or affected by HIV/AIDS & to reduce the spread of HIV
Member of: United Way
Affliation(s): Ontario AIDS Network; Canadian AIDS Society
Chief Officer(s):
Francis Gregotski, Chair
Glen Walker, Executive Director, 905-984-8684 Ext. 112
gwalker@aidsniagara.com

Alliance for South Asian AIDS Prevention (ASAAP)
#315, 120 Carlton st., Toronto ON M5A 4K3
Tel: 416-599-2727; *Fax:* 416-599-6011
e-mail: info@asaap.ca
www.asaap.ca
www.facebook.com/pages/Asaap/262246160480711
twitter.com/ASAAP
www.youtube.com/user/ASAAPTV
Overview: A small local charitable organization founded in 1989 overseen by Canadian AIDS Society
Mission: To prevent the spread of HIV & to promote the health of South Asians infected with & affected by HIV/AIDS.

Member of: Ontario AIDS Network; Council of Agencies Serving South Asians; Interagency Coalition on AIDS & Development
Chief Officer(s):
Rupal Shah, Chair
Vihaya Chikermane, Executive Director
 ed@asaap.ca

Asian Community AIDS Services (ACAS)
#410, 260 Spadina Ave., Toronto ON M5T 2E4
Tel: 416-963-4300; *Fax:* 416-963-4371
Toll-Free: 877-630-2227
e-mail: info@acas.org
www.acas.org
www.facebook.com/AsianCommunityAIDSServices
twitter.com/ACAStoronto
www.youtube.com/user/acasorg
Merged from: Gay Asians Toronto's Gay Asian AIDS Project; Vietnamese AIDS Project; AIDS Alert Project
Overview: A small local charitable organization founded in 1994 overseen by Canadian AIDS Society
Mission: To provide education, prevention & support services on HIV/AIDS to the East & Southeast Asian communities; programs are based on a proactive & holistic approach to HIV/AIDS & are provided in a collaborative, empowering & non-discriminatory manner
Member of: Ontario AIDS Network
Chief Officer(s):
Giovanni Temansja, Chair
Noulmook Sutdhibhasilp, Executive Director, 416-963-4300 Ext. 227
 ed@acas.org

Bruce House
#402, 251 Bank St., Ottawa ON K2P 1X3
Tel: 613-729-0911; *Fax:* 613-729-0959
e-mail: admin@brucehouse.org
www.brucehouse.org
www.facebook.com/MoreThanAHouse
twitter.com/MoreThanAHouse
Overview: A small local charitable organization founded in 1988 overseen by Canadian AIDS Society
Mission: To provide housing, compassionate care & support in Ottawa-Carleton for people living with HIV/AIDS, believing that everyone has the right to live & die with dignity; to operate a 7-bed residence staffed 24-hours a day for people who require extensive support & 34 rent-to-income apartment units for those able to live independently.
Member of: Ontario AIDS Network; Ontario Non-Profit Housing Association
Affiliation(s): City of Ottawa, Province of Ontario, government of Canada, a network of community centers & agencies, local hospitals, physicians, social service agencies, other local charitable agencies & organizations

Casey House Hospice Inc.
9 Huntley St., Toronto ON M4Y 2K8
Tel: 416-962-7600; *Fax:* 416-962-5147
e-mail: heart@caseyhouse.on.ca
www.caseyhouse.com
www.linkedin.com/company/casey-house-foundation
www.facebook.com/CaseyHouseTO
twitter.com/caseyhouseTO
www.youtube.com/caseyhousetv
Overview: A small local charitable organization founded in 1988 overseen by Canadian AIDS Society
Mission: To provide treatment, support & health services for people affected by HIV/AIDS
Member of: Ontario Hospital Association; Canadian Palliative Care Association
Affiliation(s): St. Michael's Hospital
Chief Officer(s):
Joanne Simons, Chief Executive Officer
Ann Stewart, Medical Director

Elevate NWO (ATB)
574 Memorial Ave., Thunder Bay ON P7B 3Z2
Tel: 807-345-1516; *Fax:* 807-345-2505
Toll-Free: 800-488-5840
e-mail: info@elevatenwo.org
www.elevatenwo.org
www.facebook.com/169997633037453
twitter.com/elevatenwo
Previous Name: AIDS Thunder Bay
Overview: A small local charitable organization founded in 1985
Mission: To confront HIV/AIDS infection through prevention, support, education, & advocacy
Member of: Canadian AIDS Society; Ontario AIDS Network
Chief Officer(s):
Dennis Eeles, President
Holly Gauvin, Executive Director
 hgauvin@elevatenwo.org
Publications:
• Front Line
Type: Newsletter; *Editor:* Selly Pajamaki
Profile: Contains association news & important event dates

Fife House
490 Sherburne St., 2nd Fl., Toronto ON M4X 1K9
Tel: 416-205-9888; *Fax:* 416-205-9919
www.fifehouse.org
www.facebook.com/FifeHouse
twitter.com/FifeHouse
Overview: A medium-sized local charitable organization founded in 1988 overseen by Canadian AIDS Society
Mission: To provide secure, affordable, supportive housing & support services to people living with HIV/AIDS
Member of: Ontario AIDS Network; Ontario Non-Profit Housing Association
Chief Officer(s):
Keith Hambly, Executive Director
 khambly@fifehouse.org

Hamilton AIDS Network (HAN)
#101, 140 King St. East, Hamilton ON L8N 1B2
Tel: 905-528-0854; *Fax:* 905-528-6311
Toll-Free: 866-563-0563
www.aidsnetwork.ca
www.facebook.com/TheAIDSNetwork
Previous Name: Hamilton AIDS Network for Dialogue & Support
Overview: A medium-sized local organization founded in 1986 overseen by Canadian AIDS Society
Mission: To help mobilize community-based responses to the needs created & exacerbated by the HIV epidemic in Hamilton & the surrounding community
Member of: Ontario AIDS Network; Canadian AIDS Society
Chief Officer(s):
Tim McClemont, Executive Director
 tmcclemont@aidsnetwork.ca
James Finlay, Director, Finance & Administration
 jfinlay@aidsnetwork.ca
Leanne Parsons, Director, Support & Volunteer Services
 lparsons@aidsnetwork.ca
Karyn Cooper, Director, Community Engagement
 dcep@aidsnetwork.ca

HIV/AIDS Regional Services (HARS)
844A Princess St., Kingston ON K7L 1G5
Tel: 613-545-3698; *Fax:* 613-545-9809
Toll-Free: 800-565-2209
e-mail: hars@kingston.net
www.hars.ca
www.facebook.com/harskingston
Previous Name: Kingston AIDS Project
Overview: A medium-sized local charitable organization founded in 1986
Mission: To prevent spread of Human Immunodeficiency Virus (HIV); To educate people about AIDS & HIV; To support people affected by AIDS & HIV infection
Affiliation(s): Ontario AIDS Network; Canadian AIDS Society; Canadian HIV/AIDS Legal Network
Chief Officer(s):

John MacTavish, Executive Director
Amanda Girling, Coordinator, Education
  amanda@kingston.net

HIV/AIDS Resources and Community Health (ARCH)
#115, 89 Dawson Rd., Guelph ON N1H 1B1
Tel: 519-763-2255; *Fax:* 519-763-8125
Toll-Free: 800-282-4505
e-mail: education@archguelph.ca
www.archguelph.ca
www.facebook.com/archguelph?fref=ts
twitter.com/archguelph
Previous Name: AIDS Committee of Guelph & Wellington County
Overview: A small local charitable organization founded in 1989
Mission: To provide exemplary services, education & support in the area of HIV & AIDS through innovative health promotion strategies & community partnerships
Member of: Ontario AIDS Network; Canadian AIDS Society
Chief Officer(s):
Tom Hammond, Executive Director, 519-763-2255 Ext. 129
  director@archguelph.ca
Tashauna Devonshire, Coordinator, Support Services, 519-763-2255
  Ext. 126
  support@archguelph.ca

John Gordon Home
596 Pall Mall St., London ON N5Y 2Z9
Tel: 519-433-3951; *Fax:* 519-433-1314
e-mail: johngordonhome@lrah.ca
www.johngordonhome.ca
Also Known As: London Regional AIDS Hospice
Overview: A small local organization founded in 1991 overseen by Canadian AIDS Society
Mission: To provide compassionate care to people with AIDS & HIV in a comforting, non-discriminatory, homeike environment; to provide medical, psychosocial, spiritual & personal support
Member of: Ontario AIDS Network; Canadian AIDS Society; Ontario Non-Profit Housing Association
Chief Officer(s):
Bruce Rankin, Executive Director
  brucerankin@lrah.ca

Maggie's: The Toronto Sex Workers Action Project
298A Gerrard St. East, 2nd Fl., Toronto ON M5A 2G7
Tel: 416-964-0150
e-mail: maggiescoord@gmail.com
www.maggiestoronto.ca
www.facebook.com/Maggiestoronto
Also Known As: Maggie's
Previous Name: Maggie's: The Toronto Prostitutes' Community Service Project; Prostitute's Safe Sex Project
Overview: A small local charitable organization founded in 1991
Mission: To provide education & support to assist sex workers in our efforts to live & work with safety & dignity
Member of: Ontario AIDS Network

PARN Your Community AIDS Resource Network (PARN)
#302, 159 King St., Peterborough ON K9J 2R8
Tel: 705-749-9110; *Fax:* 705-749-6310
Toll-Free: 800-361-2895; *TTY:* 705-749-9110
e-mail: getinformed@parn.ca
www.parn.ca
www.facebook.com/PARNStaff
twitter.com/PARN4Counties
Previous Name: Peterborough AIDS Resource Network
Overview: A small local charitable organization founded in 1987 overseen by Canadian AIDS Society
Mission: To support people HIV-infected & HIV-affected
Member of: Canadian AIDS Society; Ontario AIDS Network.
Chief Officer(s):
Kim Dolan, Executive Director
John Lyons, Chair
John Curtis, Treasurer
Publications:
• PARN News
Type: Newsletter; *Frequency:* Quarterly; *Accepts Advertising*

Profile: Thematic issues, such as Hepatitis C, testing, harm reduction, & disclosure

Peel HIV/AIDS Network
#1, 160 Traders Blvd., Mississauga ON L4Z 3K7
Tel: 905-361-0523; *Fax:* 905-361-1004
Toll-Free: 866-896-8700
www.phan.ca
www.facebook.com/PeelHIVAIDSNetwork
twitter.com/phanpeel
www.flickr.com/photos/31432883@N05/
Overview: A small local organization
Chief Officer(s):
Phillip Banks, Executive Director
  phillipb@phan.ca

Positive Youth Outreach (PYO)
399 Church St., 4th Fl., Toronto ON M5B 2J6
Tel: 416-340-8484
e-mail: pyo@actoronto.org
www.actoronto.org/home.nsf/pages/positiveyouthoutreach
Overview: A small local organization founded in 1990 overseen by Canadian AIDS Society
Mission: To provide education, support, advocacy & referral to all youth living with HIV/AIDS regardless of the mode of transmission
Member of: AIDS Committee of Toronto; Ontario AIDS Network

Regional HIV/AIDS Connection
#30, 186 King St., London ON N6A 1C7
Tel: 519-434-1601; *Fax:* 519-434-1843
Toll-Free: 866-920-1601
e-mail: info@hivaidsconnection.ca
www.hivaidsconnection.ca
www.facebook.com/189146047805897
twitter.com/_RHAC
www.youtube.com/user/AIDSLondon
Previous Name: AIDS Committee of London
Overview: A small local organization founded in 1985 overseen by Canadian AIDS Society
Mission: To bring people together in partnership to provide leadership in education, support & advocacy to meet the challenge of HIV/AIDS; To create an atmosphere of trust which enables people living with & affected by HIV/AIDS to make informed choices; To serve the counties of Perth, Huron, Lambton, Elgin, Middlesex, & Oxford.
Member of: Ontario AIDS Network
Chief Officer(s):
Brian Lester, Executive Director, 519-434-1601 Ext. 243
  blester@hivaidsconnection.ca
Mana Khami, President

Regroupement des personnes vivant avec le VIH-sida de Québec et la région
#100, 190 O'Connor St., Ottawa ON K2P 2R3
Tél: 613-230-3580; *Téléc:* 613-563-4998
Courriel: casinfo@cdnaids.ca
www.facebook.com/aidsida
twitter.com/CDNAIDS
Aperçu: *Dimension:* petite; *Envergure:* locale; fondée en 1990 surveillé par Canadian AIDS Society
Mission: Regrouper les personnes vivant avec le VIH/sida

Réseau ACCESS Network
#203, 111 Elm St., Sudbury ON P3C 1T3
Tel: 705-688-0500
Toll-Free: 800-465-2437
e-mail: aaninfo@reseauaccessnetwork.com
www.accessaidsnetwork.com
Also Known As: Réseau ACCESS Network HIV/Hepatitis Health & Social Services Services
Previous Name: AIDS Committee of Sudbury; Access AIDS Committee
Overview: A small local organization founded in 1989 overseen by Canadian AIDS Society
Mission: To serve the needs of HIV positive individuals living in Algoma, Sudbury, & Manitoulin.
Affliation(s): Canada Helps; Ontario Aboriginal HIV/AIDS Strategy; Sudbury Action Centre for Youth; HAVEN Program

The Teresa Group
#104, 124 Merton St., Toronto ON M4S 2Z2
Tel: 416-596-7703; *Fax:* 416-596-7910
e-mail: info@teresagroup.ca
www.teresagroup.ca
www.facebook.com/120076698045376
twitter.com/TheTeresaGroup
Overview: A small local charitable organization founded in 1990 overseen by Canadian AIDS Society
Mission: Serves the needs of children & their families living with or affected by HIV/AIDS
Member of: Ontario AIDS Network; Canadian AIDS Society
Chief Officer(s):
Nicci Stein, Executive Director
Publications:
• Bye-Bye Secrets: A Book About Children Living With HIV or AIDS in their Family
Type: Book; *Number of Pages:* 36; *Price:* $14.95
Profile: The experiences of five girls, aged 8-12 years, who live with HIV/AIDS in their families.
• Early Intervention Programs for Children & Women Living with HIV & AIDS Leaflet
Type: Leaflet
Profile: Descriptions of the following: Pre-Natal, New Moms, Mom & Tots Groups, & The Formula Program
• Hopes, Wishes & Dreams: A Book of Art & Writing by Children Living with HIV/AIDS in their Family
Type: Book; *Number of Pages:* 40; *Price:* $14.95
Profile: Art, poetry & writings by children affected by HIV/AIDS
• How Do I Tell My Kids? A Disclosure Booklet About HIV/AIDS in the Family
Type: Booklet; *Number of Pages:* 48; *Price:* $5.00
Profile: A booklet for adults, designed to help with the process of telling their children that a family member has HIV.
• In Touch [a publication of The Teresa Group]
Type: Newsletter
• Programs & Services Booklet
Type: Brochure
Profile: This brochure outlines what The Teresa Group does.

Toronto PWA Foundation (TPWAF)
200 Gerrard St. East, 2nd Fl., Toronto ON M5A 2E6
Tel: 416-506-1400; *Fax:* 416-506-1404
e-mail: info@pwatoronto.org
www.pwatoronto.org
www.facebook.com/TorontoPWA
twitter.com/TPWA
Also Known As: Toronto People With AIDS Foundation
Previous Name: People with AIDS Foundation
Overview: A small local charitable organization founded in 1987 overseen by Canadian AIDS Society
Mission: To promote the health & well-being of all people living with HIV/AIDS by providing accessible, direct & practical services
Member of: Ontario AIDS Network
Chief Officer(s):
Suzanne Paddock, Interim Executive Director
spaddock@pwatoronto.org

QUÉBEC

Bureau local d'intervention traitant du SIDA (BLITS)
#116, 59, rue Monfette, Victoriaville QC G6P 1J8
Tél: 819-758-2662; *Téléc:* 819-758-8270
Ligne sans frais: 866-758-2662
Courriel: blits@cdcbf.qc.ca
www.blits.ca
www.facebook.com/BLITSvictoriaville
Aperçu: *Dimension:* petite; *Envergure:* locale; Organisme sans but lucratif; fondée en 1989
Membre(s) du bureau directeur:
Gabrielle Bergeron, Présidente
Maryse Laroche, Directrice
blitscoordo@cdcbf.qc.ca
Sylvie Bondon, Agente de bureau
Véronique Vanier, Agente d'éducation
blitsprojet@cdcbf.qc.ca

Bureau régional d'action sida (Outaouais) (BRAS)
#003, 109, rue Wright, Gatineau QC J8X 2G7
Tél: 819-776-2727; *Téléc:* 819-776-2001
Ligne sans frais: 877-376-2727
Courriel: info@lebras.qc.ca
www.lebras.qc.ca
www.facebook.com/bureauregionaldactionsida
Aperçu: *Dimension:* petite; *Envergure:* locale; fondée en 1990
Mission: Développer et promouvoir des actions communautaires vizant l'amelioration de la qualité de vie de la population de l'Outaonais face au VIH/sida
Membre de: Réseau juridique canadien du VIH/Sida; Coalition des organismes communautaires québécois de lutte contre le sida; CATIE, TROCAO, CRIO
Membre(s) du bureau directeur:
Sylvain Laflamme, Directeur général
dg@lebras.qc.ca

Centre d'action sida Montréal (Femmes) (CASMF) / Centre for AIDS Services of Montréal (Women)
1750, rue Saint-André, 3e étage, Montréal QC H2L 3T8
Tél: 514-495-0990; *Téléc:* 514-495-8087
Courriel: casm@netrover.net
www.netrover.com/~casm
Aperçu: *Dimension:* petite; *Envergure:* locale
Mission: Offrir des services aux femmes affectées et infectées par le VIH/SIDA ainsi qu'aux membres de leur famille; ces actions, priorisant les besoins particuliers des femmes, ont pour but d'augmenter leur pouvoir à déterminer la qualité de leur propre vie
Membre de: Canadian AIDS Society; Fédération des femmes du Québec; Conseil des femmes de Montréal; Coalition des organismes communautaires québécois de lutte contre le sida

Centre sida amitié (CSA)
527, rue St-Georges, Saint-Jérôme QC J7Z 5B6
Tél: 450-431-7432; *Téléc:* 450-431-6536
Courriel: csa1@qc.aira.com
twitter.com/Sidaamitie
Aperçu: *Dimension:* petite; *Envergure:* locale; Organisme sans but lucratif; fondée en 1989 surveillé par Canadian AIDS Society

Groupe d'entraide à l'intention des personnes séropositives, itinérantes et toxicomanes (GEIPSI)
1223, rue Ontario est, Montréal QC H2L 1R5
Tél: 514-523-0979; *Téléc:* 514-523-3075
Courriel: info@geipsi.ca
www.geipsi.ca
Aperçu: *Dimension:* petite; *Envergure:* locale; fondée en 1992
Mission: Pour apporter soutien et assistance aux personnes qui sont séropositives
Membre(s) du bureau directeur:
Olivier Lourdel, Président
Yvon Coulliard, Directeur général
Publications:
• Le Sans-Mots

Hébergements de l'envol
6984, rue Fabre, Montréal QC H2E 2B2
Tél: 514-374-1614; *Téléc:* 514-593-9227
Courriel: hebergementlenvol@hotmail.com
pages.infinit.net/lenvol2/
Aperçu: *Dimension:* petite; *Envergure:* locale
Mission: Foyer collectif pour personnes en perte d'autonomie
Affliation(s): Coalition des organismes communautaires québécois de lutte contre le sida

Intervention régionale et information sur le sida en Estrie
505, rue Wellington Sud, Sherbrooke QC J1H 5E2
Tél: 819-823-6704
www.iris-estrie.com
Également appelé: IRIS/Estrie
Aperçu: *Dimension:* petite; *Envergure:* locale; Organisme sans but lucratif; fondée en 1988
Mission: Stimuler et développer une action communautaire pour faire face à la problématique du Sida dans la région de l'Estrie; pour remplir sa mission, l'organisme a regroupé ses actions dans trois programmes spécifiques: Soutien, Prévention, Intervention

Affliation(s): Coalition québécoise des organismes communautaires de lutte contre le sida
Membre(s) du bureau directeur:
Yannick Dallaire, Directeur général
ydallaire.irisestrie@hotmail.com

Maison Amaryllis
1462, rue Panet, Montréal QC H2L 2Z3
Tél: 514-526-3635; *Téléc:* 514-521-9209
Courriel: maison.amaryllis@sympatico.ca
Aperçu: *Dimension:* petite; *Envergure:* locale; Organisme sans but lucratif; fondée en 1990 surveillé par Canadian AIDS Society
Affliation(s): Coalition des organismes communautaires québécois de lutte contre le sida

Maison du Parc
1287, rue Rachel Est, Montréal QC H2J 2J9
Tél: 514-523-6467; *Téléc:* 514-523-6800
Courriel: info@maisonduparc.org
www.maisonduparc.org
Aperçu: *Dimension:* petite; *Envergure:* locale; fondée en 1991 surveillé par Canadian AIDS Society
Membre de: Coalition des Organismes Communautaires Québécois-Sida

Maison Plein Coeur
1611, rue Dorion, Montréal QC H2K 4A5
Tél: 514-597-0554; *Téléc:* 514-597-2788
Courriel: infompc@maisonpleincoeur.org
www.maisonpleincoeur.org
twitter.com/mpleincoeur
Aperçu: *Dimension:* petite; *Envergure:* locale; fondée en 1991
Mission: Contribuer à prévenir le VIH-SIDA, et à promouvoir la santé chez les personnes vivant avec la maladie; offrir des services sans aucune discrimination; favoriser des services communautaires visant à stabiliser la situation des personnes présentant des troubles de santé et d'organisation; améliorer la qualité de vie de la personne en offrant un lieu de partage et d'informations
Membre de: Société canadienne du sida; Coalition des organismes communautaires québécois de lutte contre le sida; Table des Organismes Montréalais de VIH-sida; Centre d'action bénévole de Montréal; Chambre de commerce LGBT du Québec; Conseil canadien de surveillance sur l'accès aux traitements
Membre(s) du bureau directeur:
Elaine Mayrand, Présidente
Chris Lau, Directeur général, 514-597-0554 Ext. 222
chris@maisonpleincoeur.org

Projet d'Intervention auprès des mineurs-res prostitués-ées (PIAMP)
CP 907, Succ. C, 3736, ue St-Hubert, Montréal QC H2L 4V2
Tél: 514-284-1267; *Téléc:* 514-284-6808
Courriel: piamp@piamp.net
piamp.net
Aperçu: *Dimension:* petite; *Envergure:* locale; Organisme sans but lucratif
Mission: Fournit de l'aide et de soutien à la famille et les amis concernés par la prostitution.

RÉZO
CP 246, Succ. C, Montréal QC H2L 4K1
Tél: 514-521-7778; *Téléc:* 514-521-7665
www.rezosante.org
www.facebook.com/REZOsante
twitter.com/rezosante
www.youtube.com/REZOsante
Nom précédent: Action Séro Zéro
Aperçu: *Dimension:* petite; *Envergure:* locale; fondée en 1991
Mission: Développer et coordonner des activités d'éducation et de prévention du VIH-sida et des autres ITSS dans un contexte de promotion de la santé sexuelle auprès des hommes gais, bisexuels et hommes ayant des relations sexuelles avec d'autres hommes de Montréal.
Membre(s) du bureau directeur:
Robert Rousseau, Directeur général, 514-521-7778 Ext. 227
robertrousseau@rezosante.org

Sidaction Mauricie
515, rue Ste-Cécile, Trois-Rivières QC G9A 1K9
Tél: 819-374-5740
Courriel: information@sidactionmauricie.ca
www.sidactionmauricie.ca
Aperçu: *Dimension:* petite; *Envergure:* locale; Organisme sans but lucratif; fondée en 1990 surveillé par Canadian AIDS Society
Mission: Offrir des programmes d'éducation et de prévention au grand public et aux clientèles à risque, en collaboration avec les organismes gouvernementaux et communautaires qui oeuvrent aussi dans le domaine du Sida, et avec les personnes séropositives; l'organisme offre aussi un service de soutien aux personnes atteintes du VIH/Sida et à leurs proches
Membre de: Coalition des organismes communautaires québécois de lutte contre le Sida
Membre(s) du bureau directeur:
Hélène Neault, Adjointe à la coordination

AIDS Programs South Saskatchewan (APSS)
2911 - 5th Ave., Regina SK S4T 0L4
Tel: 306-924-8420; *Fax:* 306-525-0904
Toll-Free: 877-210-7623
e-mail: aidsprograms@sasktel.net
www.aidsprogramssouthsask.com
www.facebook.com/aidsprogramssouthsask
twitter.com/aidsprograms
Previous Name: AIDS Regina, Inc.
Overview: A small local charitable organization founded in 1985 overseen by Canadian AIDS Society
Mission: To meet the needs of people living with AIDS & HIV positive persons; To educate society about HIV & AIDS; To address issues in society which may arise as a result of HIV & AIDS
Member of: Canadian AIDS Society
Chief Officer(s):
Stephanie Milla, Executive Director

AIDS Saskatoon
PO Box 4062, Saskatoon SK S7K 4E3
Tel: 306-242-5005; *Fax:* 306-665-9976
Toll-Free: 800-667-6876
e-mail: admin@aidssaskatoon.ca
www.aidssaskatoon.ca
www.facebook.com/aidssaskatoon
Overview: A small local charitable organization founded in 1986 overseen by Canadian AIDS Society
Mission: To provide support to those affected by AIDS & HIV; to educate & inform the community; to have the community embrace the issues addressed by AIDS Saskatoon
Chief Officer(s):
Dave Moors, President
Danielle Genest, Executive Director

Africans in Partnership Against AIDS (APAA)
526 Richmond St. East, 2nd Fl, Toronto ON M5A 1R3
Tel: 416-924-5256; *Fax:* 416-924-6575
e-mail: info@apaa.ca
www.apaa.ca
www.facebook.com/162063662030
Overview: A small international charitable organization founded in 1993 overseen by Canadian AIDS Society
Mission: To create a stable organization & community response to the impact of HIV/AIDS through capacity development, partnership, growth, & community development & involvement.
Member of: Ontario AIDS Network; Canadian AIDS Society; African Canadian Social Development Council
Chief Officer(s):
Fanta Ongoiba, Executive Director
Publications:
• Kibaru
Type: Newsletter; *Frequency:* Quarterly

International Council of AIDS Service Organizations (ICASO) / Le Conseil international des organisations de lutte contre le SIDA
#311, 120 Carlton St., Toronto ON M5A 4K2
Tel: 416-921-0018
www.icaso.org

Overview: A small international organization founded in 1990
Mission: To promote & support the work of community-based organizations around the world in the prevention of AIDS, & care & treatment for people living with HIV/AIDS, with particular emphasis on strengthening the response in communities with fewer resources; To accomplish these objectives through information sharing, advocacy & network building
Chief Officer(s):
Mary Ann Torres, Executive Director
maryannt@icaso.org
Margaret Quish, Manager, Finance
margaretq@icaso.org
Zhanna Kasperskaya, Coordinator, Program
zhannak@icaso.org

National Libraries

Canadian AIDS Treatment Information Exchange (CATIE)
#505, 555 Richmond St. West, PO Box 1104, Toronto, ON M5V 3B1
Tel: 416-203-7122; *Fax:* 416-203-8284
Toll-Free: 800-263-1638
library@catie.ca
www.catie.ca
Social Media: twitter.com/CATIEInfo; www.facebook.com/CATIEInfo
Tim Rogers, Director, Knowledge Exchange
trogers@catie.ca
416-203-7122 ext. 245
David McLay, Associate Director, Health Information Resources
dmclay@catie.ca
416-203-7122 ext. 232

Provincial Libraries

AIDS Coalition of Nova Scotia
#200, 5516 Spring Garden Rd., Halifax, NS B3J 1G6
Tel: 902-425-4882; *Fax:* 902-422-6200
Toll-Free: 800-566-2437
www.acns.ns.ca

Collection: Resources promoting health & quality of life for persons living with HIV/AIDS & their primary caregivers; Books; Pamphlets; Articles; Reports; Videos; CDS
Shannon Pringle, Executive Director
ed@acns.ns.ca

AIDS Committee of Cambridge, Kitchener/Waterloo & Area
#203, 639 King St. West, Kitchener, ON N2G 1C7
Tel: 519-570-3687; *Fax:* 519-570-4034
Toll-Free: 877-770-3687
support@acckwa.com
www.acckwa.com
Social Media: twitter.com/AIDSCKW; www.facebook.com/ACCKWA
Ruth Cameron, Executive Director
director@acckwa.com
519-570-3687 ext. 304
Carolyn Keays, Coordinator, Youth Sexual Health
education@acckwa.com
519-570-3687 ext. 302

AIDS Committee of North Bay & Area
#201, 269 Main St. West, North Bay, ON P1B 2T8
Tel: 705-497-3560; *Fax:* 705-497-7850
Toll-Free: 800-387-3701
oaacnba@vianet.ca
aidsnorthbay.com
Social Media: twitter.com/ACNBA;
www.facebook.com/128216403874712
Kathleen Jodouin, HIV Education & Outreach Coordinator
jodouink@gmail.com

AIDS Committee of Windsor
511 Pelissier St., Windsor, ON N9A 4L2
Tel: 519-973-0222; *Fax:* 519-973-7389
Toll-Free: 800-265-4858
www.aidswindsor.org

Mark McCallum, President
519-973-0222 ext. 110

AIDS New Brunswick/ SIDA Nouveau-Brunswick
65 Brunswick St., #G17, Fredericton, NB E3B 1G5
Fax: 888-501-6301
Toll-Free: 800-561-4009
info@aidsnb.com
www.aidsnb.com
Social Media: twitter.com/aidsnb; www.facebook.com/AIDSNB;
www.linkedin.com/company/aids-nb
Matthew Smith, Interim Executive Director
matt@aidsnb.com

AIDS Programs South Saskatchewan
2911 - 5th Ave., Regina, SK S4T 0L4
Tel: 306-924-8420; *Fax:* 306-525-0904
www.aidsprogramssouthsask.com
Profile: Supports community health & well-being through sharing HIV/AIDS information & resources
Tom Janisch, Education Coordinator

AIDS Vancouver
803 East Hastings St., Vancouver, BC V6A 1R8
Tel: 604-893-2201; *Fax:* 604-893-2205
contact@aidsvancouver.org
Social Media: www.youtube.com/user/AidsVancouver;
twitter.com/aidsvancouver; www.facebook.com/aidsvancouver
Brian Chittock, Executive Director
brianc@aidsvancouver.org
604-696-4655

AIDS Vancouver Island
Access Health Centre, 713 Johnson St., 3rd Fl., Victoria, BC V8W 1M8
Tel: 250-384-2366; *Fax:* 250-380-9411
Toll-Free: 800-665-2437
info@avi.org
avi.org
Social Media: twitter.com/AIDSVanIsle;
www.facebook.com/aidsvancouverisland
Collection: Research@AVI; publications; statistics; fact sheets; links to other resources
Katrina Jensen, Executive Director
katrina.jensen@avi.org

Blood Ties Four Directions Centre
405 Ogilvie St., Whitehorse, YT Y1A 2S5
Tel: 867-633-2437; *Fax:* 867-633-2447
Toll-Free: 877-333-2437
admin@bloodties.ca
www.bloodties.ca
Patricia Bacon, Executive Director
executivedirector@bloodties.ca

HIV Community Link
#110, 1603 - 10 Ave. SW, Calgary, AB T3C 0J7
Tel: 403-508-2500; *Fax:* 403-263-7358
Toll-Free: 877-440-2437
www.hivcl.org

HIV/AIDS Resources & Community Health
#115, 89 Dawson Rd., Guelph, ON N1H 1B1
Tel: 519-763-2255; *Fax:* 519-763-8125
Toll-Free: 800-282-4505
www.archguelph.ca

Tom Hammond, Executive Director
director@archguelph.ca
519-763-2255 ext. 129

Local Hospitals & Health Centres

MANITOBA

WINNIPEG: Nine Circles Community Health Centre
Affiliated with: Winnipeg Regional Health Authority
705 Broadway, Winnipeg, MB R3G 0X2

Tel: 204-940-6000 *Fax:* 204-940-6003
Toll-Free: 888-305-8647
ninecircles@ninecircles.ca
www.ninecircles.ca
Social Media: www.facebook.com/NineCirclesCommunityHealthCentre;
twitter.com/ninecircleschc; instagram.com/ninecircleschc

Note: Non-profit centre specializing in STI/HIV prevention & care
services
Michael Payne, Executive Director

Allergies

Allergy means altered reactivity. Allergies are usually characterized by a hypersensitivity to substances such as pollens, pet dander, moulds, stinging insects, latex, some medications and certain foods—most commonly, peanuts, tree nuts, milk, egg, shellfish, fish, soy, wheat and sesame. Such substances (allergens) can trigger an allergic response in susceptible individuals.

Cause
The cause of allergies is unclear, although there may be a genetic link: if both parents have allergies, the risk of their children suffering from allergies is estimated at 66 percent. If one parent has allergies, the estimated risk is 60 percent.

Symptoms
Symptoms of allergies usually present in the first few years of life, but they can also develop later, even in adulthood. There is a wide spectrum of allergic symptoms ranging from the mild sneezing, runny nose and congestion of hay fever to life-threatening reactions, known as anaphylaxis. Additional allergic reactions include itchy, watery eyes, skin rashes and asthma. More severe symptoms may include a tingling sensation in the mouth, swelling of the tongue and throat, difficulty breathing, hives, vomiting, abdominal cramps, diarrhea, drop in blood pressure, loss of consciousness and cardiovascular collapse leading to death. Allergic symptoms typically appear within anywhere from a few minutes to two hours after the person has been exposed to the allergen. Allergic symptoms can diminish as children get older, and sometimes even disappear completely.

Prevalence
Seasonal allergic rhinitis, or hay fever, affects more than one in six Canadians, and about one in thirteen Canadians suffer from a food allergy. The prevalence of peanut allergy in the population is estimated to be more than 1 percent, and at least 80 percent of those affected will have the allergy for life.

Treatment Options
Allergies are often diagnosed through skin prick or scratch testing. An allergist puts small drops of certain allergens on the patient's back or arms. Then, the skin under each drop is scratched or pricked to allow the allergen to get under the skin. If the skin becomes red or swollen in any of these spots, an allergy to the antigen that has caused the reaction is confirmed.

Treatment for allergies depends upon the specific substance, beginning with avoidance. For example, during allergy season, hay fever sufferers should limit the amount of time they spend outside in the early morning and late afternoon when pollen counts are high. Keeping windows closed, changing bedding frequently, and choosing hardwood and laminate flooring over carpets can help reduce exposure to allergens such as pollen and spores. The

only way to avoid a food allergy reaction is by strict avoidance of the allergy-causing food. There are no medications that cure food allergies. For non-food allergies, medications such as antihistamines and inhaled bronchodilators, as well as allergy shots to reduce the allergic response, may be prescribed by doctors. Epinephrine, also called adrenaline, is the medication of choice for controlling a severe reaction. Individuals at risk of an anaphylactic reaction should have a bracelet or necklace with that information, and carry and use a pre-filled syringe of epinephrine (EpiPen) for prompt self-treatment.

Most people outgrow their food allergies, although peanuts, tree nuts, fish and shellfish are often considered life-long allergies.

National Associations

AllerGen NCE Inc.
Michael DeGroote Centre for Learning & Discovery, McMaster University, #3120, 1280 Main St. West, Hamilton ON L8S 4K1

Tel: 905-525-9140; *Fax:* 905-524-0611
e-mail: info@allergen-nce.ca
www.allergen-nce.ca
Overview: A medium-sized national organization founded in 2004
Mission: To support research, capacity building activities, & networking regarding allergic disease in Canada; To reduce the mortality & socio-economic impacts of allergy, asthma, & related immune diseases
Chief Officer(s):
Judah Denburg, CEO & Scientific Director
Diana Royce, COO & Managing Director
Kim Wright, Director, Communications & Knowledge Mobilization
April O'Connell, Administrator, Research
Kelly McNagny, Associate Scientific Director
Publications:
• Agenda [a publication of AllerGen NCE Inc.]
Type: Newsletter
Profile: An overview of research, training, partnerships, & networking
• AirWays [a publication of AllerGen NCE Inc.]
Type: Newsletter
Profile: News about training & professional development opportunities
• AllerGen NCE Inc. Annual Report
Type: Yearbook; *Frequency:* Annually
Profile: Highlights of the year & a financial overview
• AllerGen Network Newsletter
Type: Newsletter; *Frequency:* Quarterly
Profile: Information about the management of the network for board & committee members & investigators
• ReAction [a publication of AllerGen NCE Inc.]
Type: Newsletter
Profile: Partnership, training, & networking opportunities

Allergy/Asthma Information Association (AAIA) /
Allergie/Asthme association d'information
#200, 17 Four Season Place, Toronto ON M9B 6E6

Tel: 416-621-4571; *Fax:* 416-621-5034
Toll-Free: 800-611-7011
e-mail: admin@aaia.ca
www.aaia.ca
www.facebook.com/AllergyAsthmaInformationAssociation
Overview: A large national charitable organization founded in 1964
Mission: To create a safer environment for Canadians with allergies, asthma, & anaphylaxis; To assist persons coping with allergies; To act as a national voice for individuals affected by allergy, asthma, & anaphylaxis
Affliation(s): Canadian Society of Allergy & Immunology
Chief Officer(s):
Sharon Van Gyzen, Chair
Sharon Lee, Executive Director
slee@aaia.ca
Louis Isabella, C.A., Treasurer
Publications:
• Allergy Asthma Information Association Newsletter
Type: Newsletter; *Frequency:* Quarterly
Profile: Information for persons affected by allergy, asthma, & anaphylaxis

AAIA BC/Yukon
4730 Redridge Rd., Kelowna BC V1W 3A6
Tel: 250-764-7507; *Fax:* 250-764-7587
Toll-Free: 877-500-2242
e-mail: bc@aaia.ca

Chief Officer(s):
Yvonne Rousseau, Regional Coordinator

AAIA Ontario/Québec/Atlantic
#200, 17 Four Season Pl., Toronto ON M6B 6E6
Tel: 416-621-4571; *Fax:* 416-621-5034
Toll-Free: 800-611-7011

AAIA Prairies/NWT/Nunavut
16531 - 114 St. NW, Edmonton AB T5X 3V6
Tel: 780-456-6651; *Fax:* 780-456-6651
Toll-Free: 866-456-6651
e-mail: prairies@aaia.ca

Chief Officer(s):
Lilly Byrtus, Regional Coordinator

Canadian Society of Allergy & Clinical Immunology (CSACI) / Société canadienne d'allergie et d'immunologie clinique
PO Box 51045, Orléans ON K1E 3W4
Tel: 613-986-5869; *Fax:* 866-839-7501
e-mail: info@csaci.ca
www.csaci.ca
www.facebook.com/471713226291440
twitter.com/csacimeeting

Previous Name: Canadian Society for the Study of Allergy; Canadian Academy of Allergy
Overview: A small national organization founded in 1945
Mission: To ensure optimal patient care by advancing the knowledge & practice of allergy, clinical immunology, & asthma
Chief Officer(s):
Sandy Kapur, President
David Fischer, Vice-President
Harold Kim, Secretary-Treasurer
Publications:
• Allergy, Asthma & Clinical Immunology: Official Journal of the Canadian Society of Allergy & Clinical Immunology
Type: Journal; *Frequency:* Quarterly; *Editor:* Richard Warrington
Profile: Articles to further the understanding & treatment of allergic &immunologic disease
• CSACI [Canadian Society of Allergy & Clinical Immunology] Newsletter / Bulletin CSAIC
Type: Newsletter; *Frequency:* Bimonthly
Profile: CSACI activities, events, & awards

Food Allergy Canada
#507, 505 Consumers Rd., Toronto ON M2J 4V8
Tel: 416-785-5666; *Fax:* 416-785-0458
Toll-Free: 866-785-5660
www.foodallergycanada.ca
www.facebook.com/FoodAllergyCanada
twitter.com/foodallergycan
www.youtube.com/foodallergycanada

Previous Name: Anaphylaxis Canada
Overview: A medium-sized national charitable organization
Mission: To inform, support, educate, & advocate for the needs of individuals & families living with food allergies & those who are at risk from anaphylaxis; To conduct & support research related to anaphylaxis
Affiliation(s): Dare Foods; Enjoy Life; Kellogg Canada; Loblaw Companies Ltd.; Mars Canada; Nestle Canada; Pepsico Canada; Pfizer Canada; Scotiabank Group; TD Securities; TELUS
Chief Officer(s):
Jennifer Gerdts, Chair
Jeff Smith, Vice-Chair
Brian Brennan, Treasurer
Laurie Harada, Executive Director
Beatrice Povolo, Director, Advocacy & Media Relations
Ranjit Dhanjal, Director, Marketing
Tammy White, Office Manager
Publications:
• Food Allergy Canada Brochure
Type: Brochure

• Kids' Club Newsletter [a publication of Food Allergy Canada]
Type: Newsletter
Profile: Information & activities for children living with allergies & anaphylaxis
• The Ultimate Guidebook for Teens with Food Allergies [a publication of Food Allergy Canada]
Type: Book
Profile: Information & advice on food allergies for teenagers

Provincial Associations

ONTARIO

Allergy, Asthma & Immunology Society of Ontario
2 Demaris Ave., Toronto ON M3N 1M1
Tel: 416-633-2215
www.allergyasthma.on.ca

Previous Name: Ontario Allergy Society
Overview: A small provincial organization founded in 1958
Mission: To strive to provide high quality medical services to the public, through consultation by referral from other physicians, as well as through public service education

Environmental Health Association of Ontario (EHA Ontario)
PO Box 33023, Ottawa ON K2C 3Y9
Tel: 613-860-2342
e-mail: helpline@ehaontario.ca
www.ehaontario.ca

Previous Name: Allergy & Environmental Health Association
Overview: A small provincial charitable organization founded in 1975
Mission: To promote awareness of environmental conditions that may be harmful to human health, & advocates less-contaminated sources of food, water, clothing, personal & home care products, home furnishings & building materials
Member of: Human Ecology Foundation of Canada
Affliation(s): EHA Nova Scotia; EHA Québec; EHA Alberta; EHA BC

QUÉBEC

Association des Allergologues et Immunologues du Québec
CP 216, Succ. Desjardins, #3000, 2, Complexe Desjardins, Montréal QC H5B 1G8
Tél: 514-350-5101
Courriel: aaiq@fmsq.org
www.allerg.qc.ca

Aperçu: *Dimension:* moyenne; *Envergure:* provinciale surveillé par Fédération des médecins spécialistes du Québec
Membre de: Fédération des medecins spéialistes du Québec
Membre(s) du bureau directeur:
Sylvie Pelletier, Directrice, Administration

Association québécoise des allergies alimentaires (AQAA)
6020, rue Jean Talon Est, Saint-Léonard QC H1S 3B1
Tél: 514-990-2575
Ligne sans frais: 800-990-2575
allergies-alimentaires.org

Aperçu: *Dimension:* petite; *Envergure:* provinciale; fondée en 1990
Mission: A pour mission d'offrir du support et de l'information, de promouvoir l'éducation et la prévention, ainsi que d'encourager la recherche sur les allergies alimentaires et l'anaphylaxie
Membre de: Food Allergy & Anaphylaxis Alliance
Membre(s) du bureau directeur:
Daniel Lapointe, Directeur général
dlapointe@aqaa.qc.ca

Asthme et allergies Québec
#225, 2590, boul. Laurier, Québec QC G1V 4M6
Tél: 418-627-3141; *Téléc:* 418-627-8716
Ligne sans frais: 877-627-3141
Courriel: info@asthmeallergies.com
asthmeallergies.com
www.facebook.com/171652556213925

Également appelé: Asthmédia
Nom précédent: Association pour l'asthme et l'allergie alimentaire du Québec
Aperçu: *Dimension:* petite; *Envergure:* provinciale; fondée en 1986
Mission: Informer les personnes souffrant d'asthme et d'allergie alimentaire sur leur problème de santé et sur les difficultés vécues par

ces dernières dans leur vie quotidienne
Affliation(s): Desjardins: Caisse populaire de Chalesbourg, GlaxoSmithKline, Sanofi, Paladin
Membre(s) du bureau directeur:
Gervais Bélanger, Directeur général

National Publications

The Chronicle of Skin & Allergy
Owned By: Chronicle Companies
#306, 555 Burnhamthorpe Rd., Toronto, ON M9C 2Y3
Tel: 416-916-2476; *Fax:* 416-352-6199
Toll-Free: 866-632-4766
health@chronicle.org

Circulation: 7,045 *Frequency:* 8 times a year
R. Allan Ryan, Editorial Director
Mitchell Shannon, Publisher

Provincial Libraries

Allergy/Asthma Information Association
#200, 17 Four Season Pl., Toronto, ON M9B 6E6
Tel: 416-621-4571; *Fax:* 416-621-5034
Toll-Free: 800-611-7011
admin@aaia.ca
www.aaia.ca

Collection: Wide range of allergy-related information letters, newsletter with information & tips; restaurant warning cards, allergy alert buttons, anaphylaxis education package.
Sharon Lee, Executive Director

Amyotrophic Lateral Sclerosis

Amyotrophic Lateral Sclerosis (ALS), also called Lou Gehrig's disease, is a fatal neurodegenerative disorder that affects the motor nerves in the brain and spinal cord. It is marked by progressive muscle weakness.

Cause
The cause of ALS is unknown, and in 90 to 95 percent of cases there are no evident risk factors. ALS is inherited in about 5 to 10 percent of cases.

Symptoms
Initial symptoms may be subtle, but early signs of ALS can include twitching and cramping of muscles (particularly in the hands and feet), muscle stiffness or weakness, as well as difficulty in chewing or swallowing. As the disorder progresses, use of legs and arms, breathing, speaking and swallowing become increasingly difficult. Eventually, people with ALS lose control of voluntary movement.

Although the physical symptoms of ALS are most debilitating, the disease does not seem to impair intellectual functioning, although recent research indicates a small number of people with ALS will develop cognitive defects which could progress to a form of dementia. Voluntary eye movement (blinking) and the senses also remain unaffected.

Prevalence
In Canada, there are about 2,500 to 3,000 people living with ALS. Every day, two to three of these people die of the disease. ALS usually strikes people between the ages of 45 and 65, but the disease has also been diagnosed in individuals as young as 16. ALS affects a slightly higher percentage of men than women.

Treatment Options
Since there is no specific test for ALS, the disease is diagnosed by ruling out other diseases with similar symptoms. Tests such as EMG (electromyography), NCV (nerve conduction velocity) and MRI (magnetic resonance imaging) are often ordered. If the results of these tests are negative, and the person's symptoms continue or worsen, ALS is often the diagnosis.

Currently, there is no cure for ALS. Only one medication—riluzole (Rilutek)—has been approved for ALS treatment. Research shows that the drug can prolong the survival of people with ALS by two to three months. Other medications are prescribed to relieve the symptoms of people with ALS. These include drugs to help with pain, depression and insomnia, as well as medications to control drooling and uncontrolled crying or laughing. Patients with swallowing problems sometimes have a feeding tube placed in the stomach to help maintain body weight. People with ALS who have breathing problems might also use an assisted-breathing device, sometimes called a non-invasive ventilation (NIV) device. A regime of physical therapy, occupational therapy, speech and language therapy, and psychological support can also help patients and their families.

The majority of people with ALS—80 percent—live for two to five years after their diagnosis, although up to 10 percent may live for 10 years or more.

National Associations

ALS Society of Canada (ALS) / La Société canadienne de la SLA (SLA)
#200, 3000 Steeles Ave. East, Markham ON L3R 4T9
Tel: 905-248-2052; *Fax:* 905-248-2019
Toll-Free: 800-267-4257
www.als.ca
www.linkedin.com/company/als-society-of-canada
www.facebook.com/ALSCanada1
twitter.com/alscanada

Also Known As: Amyotrophic Lateral Sclerosis Society of Canada
Overview: A large national charitable organization founded in 1977
Mission: To support research towards a cure for ALS; To support ALS partners in their provision of quality care for persons affected by ALS
Member of: Canadian Society of Gift Planners; National Society of Fundraising Executives; International Alliance of ALS/MND Associations; Canadian Centre for Philanthropy; Neuromuscular Research Partnership; Canadian Coalition for Genetic Fairness
Affliation(s): Health Charities Council of Canada
Chief Officer(s):
Tammy Moore, Chief Executive Officer
tm@als.ca
Publications:
• Manual for People Living with ALS [a publication of the ALS Society of Canada]
Type: Manual; *Editor:* Jane McCarthy
• Research News [a publication of the ALS Society of Canada]
Type: Newsletter

Provincial Associations

ALBERTA

ALS Society of Alberta
#250, 4723 - 1 St. SW, Calgary AB T2G 4Y8
Tel: 403-228-3857; *Fax:* 403-228-7752
Toll-Free: 888-309-1111
e-mail: info@alsab.ca
www.alsab.ca
www.facebook.com/ALSALBERTA
twitter.com/ALS_AB

Overview: A small provincial charitable organization overseen by ALS Society Of Canada
Chief Officer(s):
Karen Caughey, Executive Director, 403-228-3857 Ext. 103

Edmonton Chapter
5418 - 97 St. NW, Edmonton AB T6E 5C1
Tel: 780-487-0754; *Fax:* 780-486-3604
Toll-Free: 866-447-0754
e-mail: societynorth@alsab.ca

Chief Officer(s):
Sarah Quinton, Coordinator, Administration & Volunteer Services

BRITISH COLUMBIA

ALS Society of British Columbia
1233-133351 Commerce Pkwy., Richmond BC V6V 2X7
Tel: 604-278-2257; Fax: 604-278-4257
Toll-Free: 800-708-3228
e-mail: info@alsbc.ca
www.alsbc.ca
www.facebook.com/ALSBC
twitter.com/ALS_BC
Overview: A medium-sized provincial charitable organization overseen by ALS Society Of Canada
Mission: The ALS Society of BC is dedicated to providing direct support to ALS patients, along with their families and caregivers
Chief Officer(s):
Wendy Toyer, Executive Director, 604-278-2257 Ext. 222
w.toyer@alsbc.ca

North Central Island Chapter
1233 - 13351 Commerce Parkway, Richmond BC V6V 2X7
e-mail: ncic@alsbc.ca
Chief Officer(s):
Sheldon Cleaves, President, 250-748-8072

Victoria Chapter
PO Box 48038, 3511 Blanshard St., Victoria BC V8Z 7H5
e-mail: victoria@alsbc.ca
Chief Officer(s):
Joyanne Plewes, President

MANITOBA

ALS Society of Manitoba / La societe Manitobaine de la SLA
#2A, 1717 Dublin Ave., Winnipeg MB R3H 0H2
Tel: 204-831-1510; Fax: 204-837-9023
Toll-Free: 866-718-1642
e-mail: HOPE@alsmb.ca
www.alsmb.ca
www.facebook.com/ALSmanitoba
twitter.com/ALSmanitoba
Overview: A small provincial charitable organization founded in 1980 overseen by ALS Society Of Canada
Mission: To improve the quality of life for people with ALS/MND; To invest in research & offer client services
Chief Officer(s):
Diana Rasmussen, Executive Director, 204-837-1291
drasmussen@alsmb.ca

NEWFOUNDLAND AND LABRADOR

ALS Society of Newfoundland & Labrador
Downtown Health Centre, Upper Level, Suite 3, PO Box 844, Corner Brook NL A2H 6H6
Tel: 709-634-9499; Fax: 709-634-9499
Toll-Free: 888-364-9499
e-mail: alssocietyofnfld@nf.aibn.com
www.envision.ca/webs/alsnl
Overview: A small provincial charitable organization overseen by ALS Society Of Canada
Chief Officer(s):
Cheryl Power, Executive Director

NOVA SCOTIA

ALS Society of New Brunswick & Nova Scotia
#113, 900 Windmill Rd., Dartmouth NS B3B 1P7
Tel: 902-454-3636; Fax: 902-453-3646
Toll-Free: 866-625-7257
e-mail: CareandHope@alsnbns.ca
alsnbns.ca
www.facebook.com/ALSNBNS
twitter.com/careandhope
Previous Name: ALS Society of New Brunswick; ALS Society of Nova Scotia
Overview: A small provincial charitable organization overseen by ALS Society Of Canada

Mission: To support people living with ALS
Chief Officer(s):
Kimberly Carter, President & CEO

PRINCE EDWARD ISLAND

ALS Society of PEI
PO Box 1643, Summerside PE C1N 2V5
Tel: 902-439-1600
e-mail: als_society_pei@hotmail.com
www.alspei.ca
www.facebook.com/AlsSocietyOfPei
Overview: A small provincial charitable organization founded in 1984 overseen by ALS Society Of Canada
Mission: To act as a fund-raising and awareness building group for ALS

QUÉBEC

ALS Society of Québec / Société de la SLA du Québec
#200, 5415, rue Paré, Montréal QC H4P 1P7
Tél: 514-725-2653; Téléc: 514-725-6184
Ligne sans frais: 877-725-7725
Courriel: info@sla-quebec.ca
www.sla-quebec.ca
www.facebook.com/slaquebec
twitter.com/SLA_ALS_Quebec
www.flickr.com/photos/slaquebec/collections
Aperçu: *Dimension:* petite; *Envergure:* provinciale; Organisme sans but lucratif; fondée en 1983 surveillé par ALS Society Of Canada
Membre(s) du bureau directeur:
Claudine Cook, Executive Director, 514-725-2653 Ext. 101
ccook@sla-quebec.ca

SASKATCHEWAN

ALS Society of Saskatchewan
90C Cavendish St., Regina SK S4N 5G7
Tel: 306-949-4100; Fax: 306-949-4020
e-mail: alssask@gmail.com
alssask.ca
www.facebook.com/474047055603
Overview: A small provincial charitable organization overseen by ALS Society Of Canada

Local Associations

QUÉBEC

Association Sclérose en Plaques Rive-Sud (ASPRS)
3825, rue Windsor, Saint-Hubert QC J4T 2Z6
Tél: 450-926-5210; Téléc: 450-926-5215
Courriel: info@asprs.qc.ca
www.asprs.qc.ca
www.linkedin.com/company/association-sclérose-en-plaques-rive-sud
twitter.com/asprs2
Aperçu: *Dimension:* petite; *Envergure:* locale; fondée en 1976
Mission: Aider des gens qui a sclérose en plaques de surmonter avec leur maladie en s'engageant dans des activités sociales
Membre(s) du bureau directeur:
Nancy Caron, Directrice générale
nancy.caron@asprs.qc.ca

National Libraries

ALS Society of Canada
#1701, 393 University Ave., Toronto, ON M5G 1E6
Tel: 416-497-2267; Fax: 416-497-8545
Toll-Free: 800-267-4257
www.als.ca
Social Media: twitter.com/alscanada; www.facebook.com/ALSCanada
Tammy Moore, CEO

Anxiety Disorders

It is perfectly normal to feel worried or nervous sometimes, especially if there is an obvious reason: a loved one is late coming home; a yearly evaluation meeting is pending at work; an important social event is looming. Even when you are nervous or anxious with good cause, you continue performing life's functions adequately. Indeed, some anxiety is not only normal, it is necessary, helping us to avoid trouble and danger—like preparing for a test in school, or making sure your child is safely buckled into a car. But if you can't rid yourself of your worry, you worry all the time, and about everything, people close to you comment that you seem bothered and unlike yourself, or if your nervousness is affecting your relationships and your work, it is time to seek help. Without treatment, anxiety disorders can become progressively worse, sometimes causing people who suffer from persistent anxiety to turn to alcohol or other drugs in an effort to seek relief.

There are a number of different anxiety disorders. Several of the most prevalent are discussed in detail below.

Agoraphobia

Agoraphobia usually involves fears connected with being outside the home and being alone. People with agoraphobia also feel anxious about being in places or situations from which it is difficult or embarrassing to escape (such as in the middle seat of a row in a theatre) or in which help may not be immediately available (as in an airplane). People affected by agoraphobia avoid such situations or endure them with distress and fear of having a panic attack. This anxiety significantly interferes with their ability to participate normally in work, domestic and recreational activities. The onset of agoraphobia is usually in late adolescence or early adulthood, but the disorder can develop at any time.

Social Anxiety Disorder

Social anxiety disorder involves the fear of being humiliated or embarrassed in a social situation with strangers, or where other people are watching. Being in these situations causes people with social anxiety disorder intense anxiety, and sometimes they have panic attacks as a result. These individuals realize that their fear is irrational, but they cannot overcome it. Unlike simple shyness, the fear leads to avoidance of important or uncomplicated social situations, and interferes with the ability to function at work or with friends. It is rare to develop social anxiety disorder in adulthood. Usually, the onset is in childhood or early adolescence.

General Anxiety Disorder

General anxiety disorder is characterized by excessive worry and anxiety on most days for at least six months about several events or activities such as work or school performance. People with general anxiety disorder have great difficulty in controlling their exaggerated and unrealistic worries. Their anxiety is connected with at least three of the following: restlessness/feeling on edge, being easily tired, difficulty concentrating, irritability, muscle tension, difficulty falling/staying asleep or restless sleep. Their anxiety or physical symptoms also seriously affect their social lives, work lives or other important areas of functioning. It is most common for general anxiety disorder to develop in childhood or adolescence, but onset in adulthood is also possible.

Phobias

Phobias are characterized by persistent, unreasonable and exaggerated fear of the presence or anticipated presence of a particular object or situation (for example, snake, flying in an airplane, blood). The presence of such an object or situation triggers immediate anxiety which may result in a panic attack. People with phobias know that their fears are exaggerated and unreasonable, but they cannot confront or overcome these fears. Instead, the phobic situation is either avoided or experienced with extreme distress. The avoidance, fearful anticipation, and distress seriously affect their normal routines, work and social activities, and relationships. Specific phobias develop at different ages, depending on the fear. For example, it is more common for animal phobias to begin in childhood, phobias about heights to develop in adolescence, and phobias about enclosed spaces to have their onset in early adulthood. Some phobias (such as blood) are experienced by both men and women, while others are more common in women (spiders).

Panic Disorder

Panic disorder is characterized by panic attacks which come on unexpectedly, and recur over time. These periods of intense fear escalate suddenly, reach a peak within 10 minutes and then diminish. They are accompanied by four or more of the following symptoms: heart palpitations and pounding, rapid heartbeat, sweating, trembling or shaking, shortness of breath, feeling of choking, chest pain, nausea, feeling dizzy or faint, feelings of unreality or detachment, fear of losing control or going crazy, fear of dying, numbness or tingling, and chills or hot flashes. Panic disorder usually develops towards the end of adolescence or at the beginning of adulthood, but can also occur in childhood or later adulthood.

Obsessive Compulsive Disorder

Individuals with obsessive compulsive disorder (OCD) have overwhelming obsessions or compulsions. Obsessions are repeated, intrusive, unwanted thoughts that cause distressing emotions such as anxiety or anguish; a compulsion is a ceaseless urge to do something to lessen the anxiety caused by the obsession. People with OCD have recurrent and persistent thoughts, impulses or images that are experienced as intrusive and inappropriate and that cause marked anxiety or distress. Their thoughts and worries are not simply excessive worries about real-life problems, but can be inflated misinterpretations of the actions and words of others. People with OCD feel driven to perform repetitive behaviours in response to an obsession, or according to rules that must be applied rigidly. They recognize that their obsessions or compulsions are unreasonable, but cannot overcome them. These obsessions or compulsions cause marked distress, are time consuming, or significantly interfere with their normal routine, occupational or academic functioning, or usual social activities. Obsessive compulsive disorder usually begins in adolescence or early adulthood, but may begin in childhood. In males the onset is earlier (between 6 and 15 years old) than for women (between 20 and 29).

Post-Traumatic Stress Disorder

Traumatic events can stay with us for a long time. Such events can range from the rare and horrific, such as severe torture, to more common events such as an automobile accident or a violent crime. Veterans of war often spend years reliving, or trying to forget, the experiences of combat. Effects of some childhood experiences can last well into adulthood.

Post-Traumatic Stress Disorder (PTSD) consists of the psychological and physiological symptoms that arise from experiencing, witnessing or participating in a traumatic event. Three basic types of symptoms occur: re-experiencing, numbing and increased emotional arousal. Re-experiencing includes recurrent and intrusive distressing recollections of the event, including images, thoughts or perceptions; recurrent distressing flashbacks, nightmares or dreams of the event; and acting or feeling as if the traumatic event were recurring. Numbing includes diminished general responsiveness, or desensitization of emotional reactiveness. Increased emotional arousal includes intense psychological distress at exposure to internal or external cues that symbolize or resemble an aspect of the traumatic event; increased physiological reactivity (fast heartbeat or breathing, gastrointestinal distress) on exposure to internal or external cues that symbolize or resemble an aspect of the event; persistent avoidance of stimuli associated with the trauma. Increased emotional arousal includes jumpiness (reacting to ordinary experiences such as loud noises as though they represent danger) and bouts of temper (anger with no or insufficient cause).

The duration of the disturbance is more than one month, and it causes clinically significant distress or impairment in social, occupational or other important settings. If a person survives a life-threatening event, there may also be a profound sense of guilt, particularly if others did not survive the event. These guilty feelings may be exacerbated if the individual perceives his or her survival occurred at the expense of other's safety. People with PTSD often avoid situations that remind them of the traumatic event. This can seriously disrupt normal life, as when, for example, they have to take wide detours in order to go to work, run errands or care for family. People with PTSD may experience a dissociative state when in threatening situations, allowing them to have no recollection afterwards. They may also have somatic physical complaints linked to no discernible anatomic or physiological explanations, and may undergo a profound change of personality. People with PTSD may also suffer from other distinctive mental illnesses brought on by the PTSD: depression, OCD, social phobia or substance abuse. Their anxiety can be acute and intense such as the fear of imminent death in a panic attack, or it can be experienced as the state of chronic nagging worry in generalized anxiety disorder. One might imagine that a person would become resistant to the effects of repeated traumas, but in fact each traumatic event increases the individual's vulnerability to future events. PTSD can occur at any point in a person's life.

Cause
Anxiety disorders are most likely caused by the interplay of biological, genetic, cognitive and psychological factors. If a person has a family history of anxiety disorders, has experienced a traumatic life event, or has suffered from other psychiatric or medical problems, the likelihood of that person developing an anxiety disorder increases.

Symptoms
Although there are specific criteria used to diagnose the different types of anxiety disorders, there are some common symptoms. These include anxious thoughts, beliefs and predictions; avoidance of situations that cause fear or bring about feelings that mimic those experienced when anxious; safety behaviours (for example, always carrying a cell phone or water bottle); and exaggerated physical responses (such as a racing heart, difficulty breathing), often misinterpreted as symptoms of illness, during normal activities. Whatever the intensity or frequency, these symptoms persist over time. One of the hallmarks of anxiety disorders is that the person is unable to control the anxiety, even when he or she knows it is exaggerated and unreasonable. To other people, the person may seem edgy, irritable, to have unexpected outbursts of anger, or to be consumed by an unreasonable fear. For the anxious person, the problem takes up time and effort and becomes a major preoccupation. In addition to the psychological effects (and entangled with them) are the physical effects, that is, a frequent or constant state of physical arousal and tension. This can lead to gastrointestinal upset, headaches and cardiovascular disease. Anxiety disorders negatively affect all aspects of life—family, work and friends.

Prevalence
Anxiety disorders are the most common of all mental illnesses. In any given year, 12 percent of Canadians suffer from anxiety disorders. Anxiety disorders are approximately twice as common in women as in men, and women are hospitalized for anxiety disorders at a higher rate than men in every age category. It is estimated that three out of five people affected by anxiety disorders do not consult a health care practitioner about their condition.

Treatment Options
It is very important to have a full physical examination so that a proper diagnosis of anxiety disorder can be made. The physician needs to rule out general medical conditions that could be causing the signs and symptoms. For example, hyperthyroidism can cause anxiety problems; hypothyroidism can look like depression. Once an anxiety disorder has been diagnosed, medications, psychotherapy or both will be prescribed. Treatment will vary depending on which of the anxiety disorders is diagnosed.

Psychological treatments which have proven helpful in treating anxiety disorders are meditation, stress management, biofeedback and relaxation training. However, cognitive behavioural therapy (CBT) is considered to be the most effective treatment for anxiety disorders. Alone, or in small groups, patients are shown how to identify the thought patterns that cause them anxiety, and then are taught how to challenge them. This is the cognitive aspect of the therapy. In the behavioural portion of the therapy, patients expose themselves bit by bit to the sensations and situations that they are currently avoiding due to their anxieties. Over time, they learn how to control their anxieties.

Pharmacological treatment of anxiety disorders involves the prescription of drugs such as Selective Serotonin Reuptake Inhibitors, or SSRIs, which were originally developed as antidepressants. These drugs have proved to be effective in reducing the symptoms of anxiety, and are now the mainstays of anxiety disorder treatment. To reduce side effects, a low dose of the antidepressant is initially prescribed, and then the dose is slowly increased. Similarly, suddenly stopping an antidepressant can cause rebound symptoms including sleeplessness, headaches and irritability, so the medication should be tapered under the care of a physician. Most patients are prescribed antidepressants for at least six months, and some need to be on them for life. In some cases, Benzodiazepines, or minor tranquilizers, are prescribed for the acute treatment of anxiety symptoms. However, these medications have addictive potential, so they are usually prescribed at low doses for a very short time.

People with anxiety disorders sometimes need to try more than one treatment, or combinations of treatments, before they discover what is most effective for them. Once the proper treatment is determined and provided, most people with anxiety disorders can lead normal lives.

National Associations

Anxiety Disorders Association of Canada (ADAC) / Association Canadienne des Troubles Anxieux (ACTA)
PO Box 117, Stn. Cote-St-Luc, Montréal QC H4V 2Y3
Tel: 514-484-0504
Toll-Free: 888-223-2252
e-mail: contactus@anxietycanada.ca
www.anxietycanada.ca
twitter.com/anxietycanada
Overview: A medium-sized national charitable organization founded in 2002
Mission: To promote the prevention, treatment & management of anxiety disorders, & to improve the lives of people who suffer from them
Chief Officer(s):
Lynn Miller, President

Provincial Associations

BRITISH COLUMBIA

Anxiety Disorders Association of British Columbia
#103, 237 Columbia St. East, New Westminster BC V3L 3W4
Tel: 604-525-7566; *Fax:* 604-525-7586
e-mail: info@anxietybc.com
www.anxietybc.com
www.facebook.com/AnxietyBC
twitter.com/AnxietyBC
www.youtube.com/user/AnxietyBC/
Also Known As: AnxietyBC
Overview: A small provincial organization founded in 1999 overseen by Anxiety Disorders Association of Canada
Mission: To increase awareness of anxiety disorders, including panic disorder, phobias, obsessive-compulsive disorder, and post-traumatic stress disorder; To provide information and resources for individuals wanting to manage their own anxiety
Member of: BC Partners for Mental Health and Addictions Information
Affliation(s): Anxiety BC
Chief Officer(s):
Amir Rasheed, President
Judith Law, Executive Director

MANITOBA

Anxiety Disorders Association of Manitoba (ADAM)
#100, 4 Fort St., Winnipeg MB R3C 1C4
Tel: 204-925-0600; *Fax:* 204-925-0609
Toll-Free: 800-805-8885
e-mail: adam@adam.mb.ca
www.adam.mb.ca
www.facebook.com/anxietydisordersassociationofmanitoba
Overview: A small provincial charitable organization founded in 1986 overseen by Anxiety Disorders Association of Canada
Mission: A peer-led organization for the support of people with anxiety, and to share knowledge and hope with others.
Chief Officer(s):
Richard Shore, Chair

ONTARIO

Anxiety Disorders Association of Ontario (ADAO)
Heartwood House, 404 McArthur Ave., Ottawa ON K1K 1G5
Tel: 613-729-6761
Toll-Free: 877-308-3843
e-mail: info@anxietydisordersontario.ca
www.anxietydisordersontario.ca
www.facebook.com/anxietyottawa
twitter.com/AnxietyOttawa
www.youtube.com/user/anxietyottawa
Overview: A small provincial charitable organization founded in 1997 overseen by Anxiety Disorders Association of Canada
Mission: ADAO's mission is to empower, in an holistic way, the lives of those affected by anxiety through advocacy, education, research support and community programming.
Chief Officer(s):
Joan Riggs, BA, B.S.W., M.S, President

Post Traumatic Stress Disorder Association
93 Dufferin Ave., Toronto ON N6A 1K3
Tel: 604-525-7566; *Fax:* 604-525-7586
e-mail: info@ptsdassociation.com
ptsdassociation.com
Overview: A small provincial charitable organization
Mission: To empower individuals suffering from Post Traumatic Stress Disorder through education, linkages with appropriate services, facilitation of research and discovery into the causation.
Chief Officer(s):
Roméo A. Dallaire, O.C., C.M.M., G, Honorary Chair
Ute Lawrence-Fisher, President & Founder

QUÉBEC

Association/Troubles de l'Humeur et d'Anxiété au Québec (ATHAQ)
QC
Courriel: info@athaq.com
www.athaq.com
Nom précédent: Association/Troubles Anxieux du Québec
Aperçu: *Dimension:* petite; *Envergure:* provinciale; Organisme sans but lucratif; fondée en 1991 surveillé par Anxiety Disorders Association of Cnada
Mission: Formée par un groupe de professionnels oeuvrant dans le domaine des troubles anxieux et de ses comorbidités avec pour but de collaborer au niveau des soins, de l'enseignement, de la recherche, de la formation médicale et de l'information du public
Membre(s) du bureau directeur:
Cédric Aubé, Consultant

Phobies-Zéro
CP 5681, Sainte-Julie QC J3E 1X5
Tél: 450-922-5964; *Téléc:* 450-922-5935
Courriel: admin@phobies-zero.qc.ca
www.phobies-zero.qc.ca
Aperçu: *Dimension:* petite; *Envergure:* provinciale; fondée en 1991
Mission: Aider les gens avec leurs troubles anxieux en leur faisant comprendre leurs problèmes et en leur montrant les moyens de faire face à leur anxiété
Membre(s) du bureau directeur:
Ginette Gonthier, Directrice
ggonthier@phobies-zero.qc.ca

Local Associations

ONTARIO

The Tema Conter Memorial Trust
PO Box 265, King City ON L7B 1A0
Fax: 905-893-1574
Toll-Free: 888-288-8036
e-mail: info@tema.ca
www.tema.ca
www.linkedin.com/groups/Heroes-Are-Human-Tema-Conter-1569977
www.facebook.com/HeroesAreHuman
twitter.com/TEMATrust
www.youtube.com/tematrust
Overview: A small local organization
Mission: To educate emergency care workers about critical incident stress & post-traumatic stress disorder
Chief Officer(s):
Vince Savoia, Executive Director

Arthritis

Arthritis is a nonspecific term meaning inflammation of one or more joints. There are over 100 kinds of arthritis, many of them associated with illnesses of other body systems, such as the skin, gut or liver. Most cases of arthritis are chronic and involve multiple joints. The two most common types are rheumatoid arthritis (RA) and osteoarthritis (OA), sometimes called degenerative joint disease. Juvenile arthritis (JA) affects children and youth.

Cause
Rheumatoid arthritis is an autoimmune disease of the joints, and sometimes other body systems as well, that occurs when the immune system attacks the joint tissues instead of protecting the body from disease and infection as it usually does. The exact reason why the immune system turns on itself in rheumatoid arthritis is still not known. However, it is believed that rheumatoid arthritis develops due to the interaction of genetic, environmental and hormonal factors.

Osteoarthritis is related to repeated wear and tear, most commonly on weight-bearing joints, such as the hip and knee. Being overweight and working at a job that puts repetitive stress on a particular joint are both risk factors for developing osteoarthritis.

Women who have or had a mother or grandmother with osteoarthritis of the hands are more likely to develop osteoarthritis of the hands themselves.

Like rheumatoid arthritis, **juvenile arthritis** is characterized by constant inflammation caused by the inappropriate response of the immune system to something that it mistakenly identifies as an infection.

Symptoms

Although the symptoms of arthritis vary, most people with the disease have painful, stiff and swollen joints.

People with rheumatoid arthritis often have inflammation in the joints of the fingers and wrists, but sometimes other joints or parts of the body like the skin, lungs and eyes are affected, as well. There is a symmetrical pattern to rheumatoid arthritis—if one hand or ankle is affected, the other one will be, too. Other symptoms of rheumatoid arthritis include occasional fevers, fatigue and a sense of not feeling well.

Osteoarthritis is characterized by joint pain and stiffness, most commonly in the hips, knees, lower back, neck and tips of the fingers.

In addition to painful, stiff and swollen joints, children and youth with juvenile arthritis can experience discomfort from irregular growth, and sometimes develop chronic uveitis, an eye inflammation that causes vision loss. Juvenile arthritis is also characterized by flare-ups and remissions of the disease.

Prevalence

In Canada, 4.5 million people aged 15 and older have arthritis, and by 2031, that number is expected to increase to 7 million. Although arthritis can affect anyone at any age, two-thirds of those with arthritis are women.

Rheumatoid arthritis typically begins in the early adult years, and then occurs more frequently as people age. However the disease also strikes children and young adults. Women are much more likely than men to have rheumatoid arthritis.

Osteoarthritis is the most prevalent form of arthritis, affecting more than 10 percent of adults in Canada. Osteoarthritis tends to occur later in life, but often develops earlier in people who have injured their joints in sports. Before the age of 45, this form of arthritis is more common in men, but after the age of 45, more women than men are affected. Juvenile arthritis affects around 61,500 children and youth in Canada.

Treatment Options

There is no single test to diagnose arthritis, so a variety of methods are used to rule out other conditions and confirm diagnosis of the disease. First, the physician takes a medical history, and then performs a thorough physical examination. An X-ray is often ordered to help determine the type of arthritis, and the extent of joint damage. Blood tests are also used, especially to confirm a diagnosis of rheumatoid arthritis.

Depending on the type of arthritis, treatment plans can focus on a combination of the following approaches: physical activity (to strengthen muscles and increase flexibility and joint mobility), rest (to reduce pain and inflammation), weight control (especially for people with osteoarthritis), alternative therapies (massage, acupuncture, local application of heat and cold) and medication. Nonspecific treatment may be used for arthritis of any sort. This includes the nonsteroidal anti-inflammatory drugs (NSAIDs) and acetaminophen. Steroids can be injected into the affected joints in OA and be taken in an oral form for RA. To slow the course of

rheumatoid arthritis, some people take disease-modifying antirheumatic drugs (DMARDs). The newest rheumatoid arthritis medications are biologic response modifiers, genetically engineered medications used to help reduce inflammation. When people with arthritis have severe joint damage, surgery is sometimes recommended.

Although there is no cure for arthritis, with early diagnosis and proper treatment, most people with arthritis can lead normal lives.

National Associations

Arthritis Health Professions Association (AHPA)
#244, 12-16715 Yonge St., Newmarket ON L3X 1X4
e-mail: chardv@yahoo.com
www.ahpa.ca
Overview: A small national charitable organization founded in 1982
Mission: To improve health care standards for people with rheumatic diseases through the promotion of education & support of research among members
Affliation(s): The Arthritis Society
Chief Officer(s):
Leslie Soever, President

Arthritis Society / Société de l'arthrite
#1700, 393 University Ave., Toronto ON M5G 1E6
Tel: 416-979-7228; *Fax:* 416-979-8366
Toll-Free: 800-321-1433
e-mail: info@arthritis.ca
www.arthritis.ca
www.facebook.com/arthritissociety
twitter.com/arthritissoc
Previous Name: Canadian Arthritis & Rheumatism Society
Overview: A large national licensing charitable organization founded in 1948
Mission: To fund & promote arthritis research, programs & patient care. There are division offices in each province & nearly 1,000 community branches throughout Canada
Member of: Canadian Centre for Philanthropy; Coalition of National Voluntary Organizations
Affliation(s): The Bone & Joint Decade
Chief Officer(s):
Drew McArthur, Chair
Janet Yale, President & CEO
Derek Rodrigues, CFO
Publications:
• Impact eNewsletter [a publication of the Arthritis Society]
Type: Newsletter

Alberta/NWT Division
#300, 1301 - 8th St. SW, Calgary AB T2R 1B7
Tel: 403-228-2571; *Fax:* 403-229-4232
Toll-Free: 800-321-1433
e-mail: info@ab.arthritis.ca
www.arthritis.ca/ab
www.facebook.com/TheArthritisSocietyAlberta
Chief Officer(s):
Shirley Philips, Executive Director

British Columbia / Yukon Division
895 West 10 Ave., Vancouver BC V5Z 1L7
Tel: 604-714-5550; *Fax:* 604-714-5555
Toll-Free: 866-414-7766
e-mail: info@bc.arthritis.ca
www.arthritis.ca/bc
Chief Officer(s):
Christine Basque, Executive Director

Manitoba / Nunavut Division
#100A, 1485 Buffalo Pl., Winnipeg MB R3T 1L8
Tel: 204-942-4892; *Fax:* 204-942-4894
Toll-Free: 800-321-1433
e-mail: info@mb.arthritis.ca
www.arthritis.ca/mb
Chief Officer(s):
Donna Wills, Regional Manager

New Brunswick Division
2 - 1010 Hanwell Rd., Fredericton NB E3B 6A4
Tel: 506-452-7191
Toll-Free: 800-321-1433
e-mail: info@nb.arthritis.ca
www.arthritis.ca/nb

Chief Officer(s):
Susan Tilley-Russell, Executive Director, Atlantic Region
stilley-russell@ns.arthritis.ca

Newfoundland & Labrador Division
#220, 31 Peet St., St. John's NL A1B 3W8
Tel: 709-579-8190
Toll-Free: 800-321-1433
e-mail: info@nl.arthritis.ca
www.arthritis.ca/nl

Chief Officer(s):
Susan Tilley-Russell, Executive Director, Atlantic Region
stilley-russell@ns.arthritis.ca

Nova Scotia Division
#210, 3770 Kempt Rd., Halifax NS B3K 4X8
Tel: 902-429-7025; *Fax:* 902-423-6479
Toll-Free: 800-321-1433
e-mail: info@ns.arthritis.ca
www.arthritis.ca/ns

Chief Officer(s):
Susan Tilley-Russell, Executive Director, Atlantic Region
stilley-russell@ns.arthritis.ca

Ontario Division
#1700, 393 University Ave., Toronto ON M5G 1E6
Tel: 416-979-7228; *Fax:* 416-979-8366
Toll-Free: 800-321-1433
e-mail: info@on.arthritis.ca
arthritis.ca/on
www.facebook.com/ArthritisSocietyON
twitter.com/arthritissocON

Chief Officer(s):
Ahmad Zbib, Executive Director

Prince Edward Island Division
Leisure World Bldg., 95 Capital Dr., Charlottetown PE C1E 1E8
Tel: 902-628-2288
Toll-Free: 800-321-1433
e-mail: info@pe.arthritis.ca
www.arthritis.ca/pei

Chief Officer(s):
Susan Tilley-Russell, Executive Director, Atlantic Region
stilley-russell@ns.arthritis.ca

Québec Division
#3120, 380, rue Saint-Antoine ouest, Montréal QC H2Y 3X7
Tél: 514-846-8840; *Téléc:* 514-846-8999
Ligne sans frais: 800-321-1433
Courriel: info@qc.arthrite.ca
www.arthritis.ca/qc

Chief Officer(s):
Eric Amar, Directeur général
eamar@qc.arthritis.ca

Saskatchewan Division
#2, 706 Duchess St., Saskatoon SK S7K 0R3
Tel: 306-244-0045
Toll-Free: 800-321-1433
e-mail: info@sk.arthritis.ca
www.arthritis.ca/sk

Canadian Arthritis Network (CAN) / Le Réseau canadien de l'arthrite
#8-400-6-1, 700 University Ave., Toronto ON M5G 1Z5
Tel: 416-586-4770; *Fax:* 416-586-8395
e-mail: can@arthritisnetwork.ca
www.arthritisnetwork.ca
www.facebook.com/102841629761794
twitter.com/commcan

Overview: A medium-sized national organization founded in 1998
Mission: To improve the quality of life for people with arthritis; To support integrated, trans-disciplinary research & development, with a focus upon inflammatory joint diseases, osteoarthritis, & bioengineering

for restoration of joint function
Member of: Networks of Centres of Excellence
Affliation(s): The Arthritis Society; Canadian Institute of Health Research Institute of Musculoskeletal Health & Arthritis
Chief Officer(s):
Robin Armstrong, Chair
Kate Lee, Managing Director, 416-586-3167
klee2@mtsinai.on.ca
Claire Bombardier, Co-Scientific Director
Monique Gignac, Co-Scientific Director
Publications:
• Annual Report of the Canadian Arthritis Network
Type: Yearbook; *Frequency:* Annually
• Arthritis in Canada
Type: Report
Profile: Impacts of arthritis on Canadians, plus information about ambulatory care, prescription medications, & hospital services
• Research Excellence at the Canadian Arthritis Network
Type: Report; *Number of Pages:* 20

Canadian Rheumatology Association (CRA) / Société canadienne de rhumatologie
#244, 12 - 16715 Yonge St., Newmarket ON L3X 1X4
Tel: 905-952-0698; *Fax:* 905-952-0708
e-mail: info@rheum.ca
rheum.ca

Overview: A small national organization
Mission: To represent Canadian rheumatologists & promote their pursuit of excellence in arthritis care & research in Canada through leadership, education & communication
Affliation(s): Canadian Medical Association, Royal College of Physicians & Surgeons of Canada
Chief Officer(s):
Cory Baillie, President
Jacob Karsh, Sec.-Treas.
Publications:
• Journal of the Canadian Rheumatology Association
Type: Journal; *Frequency:* Quarterly

Provincial Associations

ONTARIO

Ontario Rheumatology Association (ORA)
#244, 12 - 16715 Yonge St., Newmarket ON L3X 1X4
Tel: 905-952-0698; *Fax:* 905-952-0708
e-mail: admin@ontariorheum.ca
ontariorheum.ca

Overview: A small provincial organization founded in 2001
Mission: To represent Ontario Rheumatologists and promote their pursuit of excellence in Arthritis care in Ontario.
Affiliation(s): Canadian Rheumatology Association
Chief Officer(s):
Arthur Karasik, President
president@ontariorheum.ca

Ontario Spondylitis Association (OSA)
18 Long Crescent, Toronto ON M4E 1N6
Tel: 416-694-5493
e-mail: info@spondylitis.ca
spondylitis.ca
www.facebook.com/6562917242

Overview: A small provincial organization
Mission: To provide support, education & public awareness of the disease called Ankylosing Spondylitis
Member of: The Arthritis Society, Canadian Spondylitis Association
Chief Officer(s):
Michael Mallinson, President

QUÉBEC

Association des médecins rhumatologues du Québec (AMRQ)
CP 216, Succ. Desjardins, Montréal QC H5B 1G8
Tél: 514-350-5136; *Téléc:* 514-350-5029
Ligne sans frais: 800-561-0703
Courriel: info@rhumatologie.org
www.rhumatologie.org

Aperçu: *Dimension:* petite; *Envergure:* provinciale surveillé par Fédération des médecins spécialistes du Québec
Mission: La rhumatologie se consacre au diagnostic et au traitement des pathologies qui touchent les articulations, les os, les muscles et tendons et parfois tout organe dans le cadre de maladies systémiques. Ceci regroupe au-delà de 100 conditions pouvant aller de l'arthrite rhumatoïde au lupus érythémateux disséminé en passant par l'arthrose, les vasculites et l'ostéoporose.
Membre de: Fédération des Médecins Spécialistes de Québec (FMSQ)
Membre(s) du bureau directeur:
Frédéric Morin, Président

Local Associations

ONTARIO

Arthritis Research Foundation
R. Fraser Elliott Bldg., 190 Elizabeth St., 5th Fl, Toronto ON M5G 2C4
Tel: 416-340-4975; *Fax:* 416-340-3496
e-mail: info@beatarthritis.ca
www.beatarthritis.ca

Overview: A small local organization
Chief Officer(s):
Joy Davidson, Director, Development
Joy.Davidson@beatarthritis.ca

National Publications

The Journal of Rheumatology
Journal of Rheumatology Publishing Co. Ltd., #901, 365 Bloor St. East, Toronto, ON M4W 3L4
Tel: 416-967-5155; *Fax:* 416-967-7556
jrheum@jrheum.com
Social Media: twitter.com/jrheum
www.facebook.com/journalofrheumatology
Frequency: Monthly
Earl D. Silverman, Editor

Provincial Libraries

The Arthritis Society (Manitoba & Nunavut Division)
#100A, 1485 Buffalo Pl., Winnipeg, MB R3T 1L8
Tel: 204-942-4892; *Fax:* 204-942-4894
Toll-Free: 800-321-1433
info@mb.arthritis.ca
www.arthritis.ca

Holland Orthopaedic & Arthritic Centre Library
#235, 43 Wellesley St. East, Toronto, ON M4Y 1H1
Tel: 416-967-8545

Local Hospitals & Health Centres

ONTARIO

TORONTO: Sunnybrook Health Sciences Centre - Holland Orthopaedic & Arthritic Centre
Affiliated with: Toronto Central Local Health Integration Network
43 Wellesley St. East, Toronto, ON M4Y 1H1
Tel: 416-967-8500 *Fax:* 416-967-8521
www.sunnybrook.ca

Note: Care for complex injuries of the musculoskeletal system, with a focus on traumatic injury management, joint reconstruction & replacement, surgery, sports & activity-related injury management, rehabilitation, & rheumatology. The Clinic has a second location at the main Sunnybrook site, 2075 Bayview Ave., Toronto
Dr. Barry A. McLellan, President & CEO

Asthma

Asthma is a respiratory disorder. In the presence of certain triggers, the sensitive airways of people with this chronic disease become inflamed, fill up with mucus, and then swell and narrow making breathing difficult.

Cause
There are allergic (inflammatory) and non-allergic (symptom) triggers for asthma. Allergic triggers include moulds, pollens, dust mites, animals and cockroaches. Non-allergic triggers include stress, cold air, exercise, smoke, pollutants, chemicals and fumes. Other risk factors for developing asthma include workplace exposure to chemical irritants, a family history of allergic diseases, and exposure to second-hand smoke as a child.

Symptoms
Symptoms of asthma include shortness of breath, wheezing, coughing and chest tightness. These symptoms can come and go, vary in intensity, and differ from person to person.

Prevalence
Approximately three million people in Canada have asthma and the disease accounts for around 80% of the cases of chronic disease in the country. More than 15% of Canadian children have been diagnosed with asthma—it is a leading cause of hospitalization for children. However, some children with asthma will outgrow the disorder by the time they are teenagers or adults. Asthma ranges from mild illness to life-threatening episodes. Each year, about 250 Canadians die from asthma, but if people were better educated about the disease, it is estimated that 80% of these deaths could be prevented.

Treatment Options
To make a diagnosis of asthma, the physician takes a thorough medical history and performs a physical examination of the patient. A spirometer—a machine that measures how much air the patient can inhale and exhale—is also used to determine if there is any obstruction of the airways. The physician may also order chest x-rays, blood and sputum tests, and allergy skin testing.

Treatment of asthma consists of avoiding or minimizing asthma triggers. In addition, medications are used to relieve asthma symptoms. Controllers are long-term medications taken daily to treat inflammation in the airways and prevent symptoms. Relievers are short-term medications used to immediately reduce symptoms such as coughing and wheezing. Some people with asthma also use a peak flow meter—a device that monitors lung function—to determine how well their asthma is being controlled.

Research continues to be directed at finding ways to prevent, treat and cure asthma. Although asthma is a chronic disease, with proper management and medication, most people with asthma can live normal and healthy lives.

See also Lung Disease

National Associations

Allergy/Asthma Information Association (AAIA) /
Allergie/Asthme association d'information
#200, 17 Four Season Place, Toronto ON M9B 6E6
Tel: 416-621-4571; *Fax:* 416-621-5034
Toll-Free: 800-611-7011
e-mail: admin@aaia.ca
www.aaia.ca
www.facebook.com/AllergyAsthmaInformationAssociation
Overview: A large national charitable organization founded in 1964
Mission: To create a safer environment for Canadians with allergies, asthma, & anaphylaxis; To assist persons coping with allergies; To act as a national voice for individuals affected by allergy, asthma, & anaphylaxis
Affliation(s): Canadian Society of Allergy & Immunology
Chief Officer(s):
Sharon Van Gyzen, Chair

Sharon Lee, Executive Director
slee@aaia.ca
Louis Isabella, C.A., Treasurer
Publications:
• Allergy Asthma Information Association Newsletter
Type: Newsletter; *Frequency:* Quarterly
Profile: Information for persons affected by allergy, asthma, & anaphylaxis

AAIA BC/Yukon
4730 Redridge Rd., Kelowna BC V1W 3A6
Tel: 250-764-7507; *Fax:* 250-764-7587
Toll-Free: 877-500-2242
e-mail: bc@aaia.ca

Chief Officer(s):
Yvonne Rousseau, Regional Coordinator

AAIA Ontario/Québec/Atlantic
#200, 17 Four Season Pl., Toronto ON M6B 6E6
Tel: 416-621-4571; *Fax:* 416-621-5034
Toll-Free: 800-611-7011

AAIA Prairies/NWT/Nunavut
16531 - 114 St. NW, Edmonton AB T5X 3V6
Tel: 780-456-6651; *Fax:* 780-456-6651
Toll-Free: 866-456-6651
e-mail: prairies@aaia.ca

Chief Officer(s):
Lilly Byrtus, Regional Coordinator

Asthma Society of Canada (ASC) / Société canadienne de l'asthme
#401, 124 Merton St., Toronto ON M4S 2Z2
Tel: 416-787-4050; *Fax:* 416-787-5807
Toll-Free: 866-787-4050
e-mail: info@asthma.ca
www.asthma.ca
www.facebook.com/AsthmaSocietyofCanada
twitter.com/AsthmaSociety
Overview: A medium-sized national charitable organization founded in 1974
Mission: To optimize the health of people with asthma through education & asthma awareness
Member of: Canadian Network for Asthma Care
Affiliation(s): Family Physicians Asthma Group of Canada; Health Canada Laboratory Centre for Disease Control's National Asthma Control Task Force
Chief Officer(s):
Vanessa Foran, President & CEO, 416-787-4050 Ext. 102
Jenna Reynolds, Director, Programs & Services, 416-787-4050 Ext. 101
Zhen Liu, Office Manager, 416-787-4050 Ext. 105

Canadian Association of Thoracic Surgeons (CATS) / Association canadienne des chirurgiens thoraciques
#300, 421 Gilmour St., Ottawa ON K2P 0R5
e-mail: cats@canadianthoracicsurgeons.ca
www.canadianthoracicsurgeons.ca
Overview: A medium-sized national organization
Mission: To represent thoracic surgeons across Canada
Chief Officer(s):
Drew Bethune, President
Andrew Seely, Secretary-Treasurer & Chair, Programs

Canadian Network for Respiratory Care (CNRC) / Réseau Canadien pour les soins respiratoires (RCSR)
16851 Mount Wolfe Rd., Caledon ON L7E 3P6
Tel: 905-880-1092; *Fax:* 905-880-9733
Toll-Free: 855-355-4672
e-mail: info@cnrchome.net
www.cnrchome.net
Previous Name: Canadian Network for Asthma Care
Overview: A small national charitable organization founded in 1994
Mission: To certify healthcare professionals as asthma & rspiratory educators (CAEs & CREs)
Chief Officer(s):
Cheryl Connors, Executive Director

Canadian Respiratory Health Professionals (CRHP)
c/o Canadian Thoracic Society, #300, 1750 Courtwood Cres., Ottawa ON K2C 2B5
Tel: 613-569-6411; *Fax:* 613-569-8860
e-mail: crhpinfo@lung.ca
crhp.lung.ca
www.facebook.com/334691136607567
Merged from: Cdn Nurses Respiratory, Cdn Physiotherapy Cardio-Respiratory, & Respiratory Therapy Societies
Overview: A small national organization founded in 2004 overseen by Canadian Lung Association
Mission: To promote lung health & the prevention of lung disease
Affliation(s): Canadian Thoracic Society
Chief Officer(s):
Janet Sutherland, Executive Director
Publications:
• Airwaves - The Newsletter of the Canadian Respiratory Health Professionals
Type: Newsletter; *Price:* Free with CRHP membership
Profile: Information for Canadian Respiratory Health Professionals members

Provincial Associations

ONTARIO

Allergy, Asthma & Immunology Society of Ontario
2 Demaris Ave., Toronto ON M3N 1M1
Tel: 416-633-2215
www.allergyasthma.on.ca
Previous Name: Ontario Allergy Society
Overview: A small provincial organization founded in 1958
Mission: To strive to provide high quality medical services to the public, through consultation by referral from other physicians, as well as through public service education

Ontario Respiratory Care Society (ORCS)
#401, 18 Wynford Dr., Toronto ON M3C 0K8
Tel: 416-864-9911; *Fax:* 416-864-9916
e-mail: info@on.lung.ca
www.on.lung.ca
Overview: A medium-sized provincial charitable organization
Mission: To improve lung health through the provision of excellent interdisciplinary respiratory care
Chief Officer(s):
Bruce Cooke, Chair
George Habib, President & CEO
Publications:
• ORCS [Ontario Respiratory Care Society] Update
Type: Newsletter; *Frequency:* 3 pa; *Price:* Free with membership in the Ontario Respiratory Care Society
Profile: ORCS activities & respiratory articles
• Research Review [a joint publication of the Ontario Respiratory Care Society & the Ontario Thoracic Society]
Frequency: Annually; *Price:* Free with membership in the Ontario Respiratory Care Society
Profile: Highlights of researchers & their studies
• RHEIG [Respiratory Health Educators Interest Group] Connections
Frequency: 3 pa; *Price:* Free with membership in the Ontario Respiratory Care Society
Profile: Published by the Respiratory Health Educators Interest Group for members of the group

QUÉBEC

Asthme et allergies Québec
#225, 2590, boul. Laurier, Québec QC G1V 4M6
Tél: 418-627-3141; *Téléc:* 418-627-8716
Ligne sans frais: 877-627-3141
Courriel: info@asthmeallergies.com
asthmeallergies.com
www.facebook.com/171652556213925
Également appelé: Asthmédia
Nom précédent: Association pour l'asthme et l'allergie alimentaire du Québec
Aperçu: *Dimension:* petite; *Envergure:* provinciale; fondée en 1986

Mission: Informer les personnes souffrant d'asthme et d'allergie alimentaire sur leur problème de santé et sur les difficultés vécues par ces dernières dans leur vie quotidienne
Affiliation(s): Desjardins: Caisse populaire de Chalesbourg, GlaxoSmithKline, Sanofi, Paladin
Membre(s) du bureau directeur:
Gervais Bélanger, Directeur général

Réseau québécois de l'asthme et de la MPOC (RQAM)

Institut universitaire de cardiologie et de pneumologie de Québec, #U-3771, 2723, ch Sainte-Foy, Québec QC G1V 4G5
Tél: 418-650-9500; *Téléc:* 418-650-9391
Ligne sans frais: 877-441-5072
Courriel: info@rqam.ca
qww.rqam.ca

Aperçu: *Dimension:* petite; *Envergure:* provinciale
Mission: De fournir un soutien aux professionnels travaillant dans l'asthme dans le secteur de la santé et de leurs patients
Membre(s) du bureau directeur:
Jean Bourbeau, Président

International Associations

American Association for Thoracic Surgery (AARS)

#4550, 500 Cummings Center, Beverly MA 01915 USA
Tel: 978-927-8330; *Fax:* 978-524-0498
www.aats.org
www.facebook.com/AATS1917
twitter.com/AATSHQ
Overview: A medium-sized international organization founded in 1917
Mission: To promote scholarship & scientific research in thoracic & cardiovascular surgery
Chief Officer(s):
Thoralf M. Sundt, President
Publications:
• Journal of Thoracic & Cardiovascular Surgery
Type: Journal; *Editor:* Richard Weisel
Profile: Original articles about the chest, heart, lungs, & great vessels where surgical intervention is indicated
• Operative Techniques in Thoracic & Cardiovascular Surgery: A Comparative Atlas
Editor: J. William Gaynor
Profile: Technique-based articles in cardiovascular & thoracic surgery by renowned surgeons in the field
• Pediatric Cardiac Surgery Annual
Type: Journal; *Frequency:* Annually; *Editor:* Robert D.B. Jaquiss
Profile: Developments in pediatric cardiac surgery
• Seminars in Thoracic & Cardiovascular Surgery
Type: Journal; *Editor:* Harvey Pass; Todd Rosengart
Profile: Topics & issues faced by practising surgeons in clinical practice
• Thoracic Surgery News
Type: Newspaper; *Frequency:* 10 pa; *Editor:* Michael Liptay
Profile: News of general thoracic surgery, adult cardiac surgery, transplantation, & congenital heart disease

Canadian Thoracic Society (CTS) / Société canadienne de thoracologie (SCT)

c/o National Office, The Lung Association, #300, 1750 Courtwood Cres., Ottawa ON K2C 2B5
Tel: 613-569-6411; *Fax:* 613-569-8860
e-mail: ctsinfo@lung.ca
cts.lung.ca
Overview: A medium-sized international charitable organization founded in 1958 overseen by Canadian Lung Association
Mission: To enhance the prevention & treatment of respiratory diseases
Affiliation(s): AllerGen; American College of Chest Physicians; American Thoracic Society; Canadian COPD Alliance; Canadian Respiratory Health Professionals; Canadian Society of Allergy & Clinical Immunology; European Respiratory Society; Guidelines International Network
Chief Officer(s):
Andrew Halayko, President
John Granton, Secretary
Catherine Lemière, Treasurer
Janet Sutherland, Executive Director

Publications:
• Canadian Thoracic Society Annual Report
Type: Yearbook; *Frequency:* Annually
• Canadian Thoracic Society E-Bulletin
Type: Newsletter
Profile: Updates for all members of the Society

International Primary Care Respiratory Group (IPCRG)

c/o Samantha Louw, PO Box 11961, Westhill AB32 9AE Scotland
Tel: 44-1224-743-753; *Fax:* 44-1224-743-753
e-mail: businessmanager@theipcrg.org
www.theipcrg.org
Overview: A medium-sized international organization
Mission: To represent international primary care perspectives in respiratory medicine; To raise standards of care worldwide
Chief Officer(s):
Siân Williams, Executive Officer
execofficer@theipcrg.org
Publications:
• Primary Care Respiratory Journal
Type: Journal
Profile: Original research papers, review, & discussion papers on respiratory conditions commonly found in primary & community settings in countries around the world

Provincial Libraries

Allergy/Asthma Information Association

#200, 17 Four Season Pl., Toronto, ON M9B 6E6
Tel: 416-621-4571; *Fax:* 416-621-5034
Toll-Free: 800-611-7011
admin@aaia.ca
www.aaia.ca
Collection: Wide range of allergy-related information letters, newsletter with information & tips; restaurant warning cards, allergy alert buttons, anaphylaxis education package.
Sharon Lee, Executive Director

Local Hospitals & Health Centres

QUÉBEC

JOLIETTE: CLSC de Joliette
Affiliée à: CISSS de Lanaudière
380, boul Base-de-Roc, Joliette, QC J6E 9J6
Tél 450-755-2111
www.santelanaudiere.qc.ca

Spécialités: Clinique santé; Centre d'enseignement sur l'asthme; Clinique d'enseignement sur le diabète; Services de santé mentale; Cessation tabagique

Ataxia

Ataxia refers to a group of diseases that cause failure of muscular coordination, resulting in a staggered gait, the inability to stand or sit straight and the inability to make smooth, voluntary movements. Most often, ataxia involves deterioration of the cerebellum and the brain and spinal structures that communicate with it.

Cause

Conditions that are associated with ataxia may be hereditary or sporadic. Hereditary ataxias, caused by different gene defects, include spinocerebellar ataxia, episodic ataxia, Friedreich's ataxia, ataxia-telangiectasia, congenital cerebellar ataxia and Wilson's disease. Sporadic cases of ataxia are often a symptom of some other disease, such as multiple sclerosis, syphilis, hypothyroidism, immune system problems or cancers, stroke or vitamin deficiencies. They may also be due to head trauma, exposure to toxins, such as alcohol, or they may be of unknown cause.

Symptoms

Symptoms of ataxia include clumsiness, poor coordination, gait unsteadiness, slurred speech, problems with fine motor tasks and difficulty swallowing. In addition, some people develop sleep disorders, spasticity, stiffness and tremors. Symptoms of ataxia can appear suddenly, or develop gradually over time.

Prevalence

Friedreich's ataxia, the most common hereditary ataxia, affects around one to two people in 40,000 in Canada. Both sexes are affected equally. Symptoms of Friedreich's ataxia typically appear between 5 and 15 years of age, but can also occur in younger children and adults. Other types of hereditary ataxia can develop in childhood, early adulthood or middle age. Sporadic cases of ataxia usually begin in adulthood.

Treatment Options

To diagnose ataxia, the physician performs a physical exam and neurological exam. Blood tests and urine tests are also usually ordered. In addition, magnetic resonance imaging (MRI) or a computerized tomography (CT) scan of the brain can be done to determine the cause of ataxia. Finally, genetic testing is sometimes recommended to determine if a patient has a gene mutation that causes one of the hereditary ataxias.

Sometimes ataxia is resolved by treating the underlying cause. In other cases—when the ataxia is the result of a viral infection, for example—the ataxia will probably get better on its own over time.

There is no specific medication for ataxia, and sometimes the condition is not treatable. In these cases, treatment is usually aimed at improving quality of life through physical, occupational and speech therapy; adaptive devices such as canes, walkers and scooters; psychological support; and career counselling. Genetic counselling is appropriate for those with the hereditary forms of ataxia and their families.

National Associations

Association canadienne des ataxies familiales (ACAF) / Canadian Association for Familial Ataxias (CAFA)
#110, 3800, rue Radisson, Montréal QC H1M 1X6
Tél: 514-321-8684
Ligne sans frais: 855-321-8684
Courriel: ataxie@lacaf.org
www.lacaf.org
www.facebook.com/ataxie.canada
twitter.com/ataxiecanada
www.youtube.com/user/LACAF2010

Également appelé: Ataxie Canada
Nom précédent: Association Canadienne de l'Ataxie de Friedreich
Aperçu: *Dimension:* petite; *Envergure:* nationale; Organisme sans but lucratif; fondée en 1972
Mission: Recueillir des dons du public pour financer les recherches médicales qui se font sur l'Ataxie familial ainsi que d'améliorer la condition de vie des personnes ataxiques (personnes qui sont affligées par la maladie de l'Ataxie de Friedreich)
Membre de: Confédération des organismes de personnes handicapées du Québec
Membre(s) du bureau directeur:
Lucie Gagnon-Ouellet, Présidente
Bianca Guillemette, Vice-Présidente
Isha Bottin, Directrice exécutive
Publications:
• Eldorado [publication of Association canadienne des ataxies familiales]
Type: Journal
Profile: Describes current research on familial ataxia

Central Branch
ON

central.lacaf.org
twitter.com/CAFAcentral

Membre(s) du bureau directeur:
Roger Foley, President
Pam Shortt, Vice-President

Western Branch
Vancouver BC
west.lacaf.org

Membre(s) du bureau directeur:
Brenda Dixon, President
Fiona Jackson, Vice-President

Local Associations

QUÉBEC

Fondation de l'Ataxie Charlevoix-Saguenay / Ataxia of Charlevoix-Saguenay Foundation
#2100, 1000 Sherbrooke ouest, Montréal QC H3A 3G4
Tél: 514-370-3625; *Télec:* 514-370-3615
Courriel: ataxia@arsacs.com
www.arsacs.com
Aperçu: *Dimension:* moyenne; *Envergure:* locale; fondée en 2006
Mission: Financer la recherche scientifique sur l'ataxie récessive spastique autosomique de Charlevoix-Saguenay
Membre(s) du bureau directeur:
Jean Groleau, Président

International Associations

Joubert Syndrome & Related Disoarders Foundation (JSRDF)
c/o Pete Asman, Treasurer, 1415 West Ave., Cincinnati OH 45215 USA
Tel: 614-864-1362
e-mail: president@jsrdf.org
www.jsrdf.org
www.facebook.com/180691234440
twitter.com/jsrdf

Overview: A small international charitable organization founded in 1992
Mission: To serve as an international network of parents who share knowledge, experience & emotional support; to educate physicians & their support teams; to increase awareness & understanding of Joubert Syndrome; to provide support to families who have loved ones diagnosed with Joubert Syndrome
Chief Officer(s):
Karen Tompkins, President
president@jsrdf.org

Attention Deficit Hyperactivity Disorder

Attention Deficit Hyperactivity Disorder (ADHD) is a neurologically based disorder that primarily affects children. ADHD is characterized by distractibility, impulsivity and hyperactivity and is divided into three subtypes based upon the clustering of these symptoms. If all three symptoms are exhibited, the condition is referred to as ADHD combined subtype. If inattention is the only symptom, the classification is ADHD primarily inattentive subtype, formerly known as attention deficit disorder (ADD). If only hyperactivity and impulsivity are displayed, the condition is referred to as ADHD primarily hyperactive-impulsive subtype. The most common of these subcategories is ADHD combined subtype. The primarily hyperactive-impulsive subtype is rare

Cause

Although the exact cause of ADHD is unknown, studies suggest that genetic influences are likely. ADHD is more commonly found in children with a family history of ADHD than in the general population. Research also seems to show that children with ADHD might have a dopamine deficiency in some parts of the brain. Other factors that may lead to the development of ADHD include maternal use of alcohol or nicotine, early exposure to high levels of lead, brain injuries and premature birth.

Symptoms

The three main symptoms of ADHD (inattention, hyperactivity and impulsivity) can vary greatly from day to day, and often change dramatically over the course of a lifetime. Since many children are inattentive, impulsive and rambunctious at times, it is important to note that in ADHD these behaviours are more severe than is typical for a person at a comparable developmental level, often resulting in stress for the child and family.

Possible symptoms of inattention include failing to attend to details, or making careless mistakes in schoolwork, work or other activities; difficulty maintaining attention in tasks or play activities; not listening when spoken to; difficulty following through on instructions and finishing schoolwork, chores or tasks; difficulty organizing tasks or activities; avoiding tasks that demand sustained mental effort, such as schoolwork or homework; losing things needed for tasks or activities, such as toys and school assignments; and being easily distracted or forgetful in daily activities.

Possible symptoms of hyperactivity include fidgeting with hands or feet, or squirming in a chair; leaving a seat in the classroom or other situations where remaining seated is expected; running or climbing about in situations in which it is inappropriate (among adolescents or adults, this may be a feeling of restlessness); difficulty playing or handling leisure activities quietly and being on the go, moving excessively.

Possible symptoms of impulsivity include talking excessively; blurting out answers impulsively before questions are finished; difficulty waiting in turn and intruding impulsively on others' games, activities or conversations.

The consequences of untreated ADHD can be severe. From a young age, people with ADHD tend to experience failure repeatedly. Studies show that 90 percent have academic problems or are underachievers, although these difficulties may not begin until the middle school years. To others, the lack of application and inability to finish tasks may look like laziness or irresponsibility.

Certain behaviours often go along with ADHD. It is common for an affected individual to experience difficulties that can impact peer relations, family life and self-esteem. The person is often frustrated and angry, exhibiting outbursts of temper and bossiness. These difficulties may also manifest themselves through self-imposed social isolation, blaming others, a quickness to fight and a high sensitivity to criticism. Studies show that 50 to 70 percent of people with ADHD have few friends. There may be a higher prevalence of anxiety, depression and learning disorders among people with ADHD. It is estimated that substance abuse problems develop in 52 percent of people with untreated ADHD.

Prevalence
ADHD is the most common mental disorder diagnosed in children in Canada. The prevalence among school-age children is between 5 and 12 percent, with a much greater frequency in boys than girls. While studies suggest that about 50 percent of children with ADHD will improve at puberty, ADHD can exist throughout a lifetime and, in fact, may first be diagnosed in teen or adult years.

Treatment Options
A diagnosis of ADHD is especially difficult to establish in young children, at the toddler and preschool level, because behaviour that is typical at that age is similar to the symptoms of ADHD. Children at that age may be extremely active but not develop the disorder. To identify children with this disorder and to develop the most appropriate treatment plan, parents will need to consult with a psychiatrist, pediatric neurologist or pediatrician.

Initially, a physician may carry out a physical exam, as well as hearing and vision tests in order to rule out other reasons for the symptoms. Often, a psycho-educational assessment is also done to identify co-existing learning disabilities. An interview is usually conducted with the patient and his or her parents, and then symptom rating scales are completed by the patient's parents and

teacher. To confirm a diagnosis of ADHD, the symptoms of impulsivity, hyperactivity and/or inattention need to be observed in two different settings (home and school), be exhibited for at least six months and cause significant impairment to daily life. Also, at least some of the symptoms need to be present before the age of seven.

Treatment of ADHD follows a multimodal, or three-tiered approach which includes education programs with resource or tutorial help; psychological programs (individual, group and family counselling) to improve self-esteem and help families and individuals deal with associated stress; and medical therapy. Treatment must be individualized to address both intrinsic characteristics of the child and relevant environmental factors, and be coordinated with a variety of interventions within the school, home and community.

The person with ADHD has great need for external motivation, consistency and structure. This should be provided by a professional who is familiar with the disorder. For a school-aged child, it is important to enlist the help of the school in designing a treatment plan which should include concrete steps aimed at developing specific competencies (such as handling time, sequencing, problem-solving and social interaction).

Since this condition affects all members of the family, the family needs help in providing consistency and structure, and in changing the role of the person with ADHD as the family member who always gets into trouble. Treatment should be based on an understanding that ADHD is not intentional, and punishment is not a cure.

Stimulant medications, including the new, longer active agents, are the drugs of choice in treating ADHD. For example, newer preparations of medications, such as Concerta and Biphentin, offer once or twice a day dosing, so that children do not need to take medication during the school day. A non-stimulant medication called Strattera is also now available in Canada. This medication stays in the patient's system longer, and is useful for people who experience symptoms of ADHD into the evening.

There is emerging literature concerning adult ADHD, and evidence that some adults can benefit from the same treatments used for children.

Current treatments can have a positive impact and, in some cases, transform behaviours so that a formerly chaotic life becomes one over which the person has much greater control and more frequent experience of success.

National Associations

Canadian ADHD Resource Alliance (CADDRA)
#604, 3950 - 14th Ave., Markham ON L3R 0A9
Tel: 416-637-8583; *Fax:* 416-385-3232
e-mail: info@caddra.ca
www.caddra.ca
Also Known As: Canadian Attention Deficit Hyperactivity Disorder Resource Alliance
Overview: A small national organization
Mission: To take a leadership role in ADHD research in Canada; to develop the Canadian ADHD Practice Guidelines (CAP-G); to facilitate development & implementation of training standards & guidelines; to share information amongst all stakeholder groups; to advocate to governments, teaching environments & employment organizations on ADHD
Chief Officer(s):
Niamh McGarry, Executive Director
niamh.mcgarry@caddra.ca

Canadian Dyslexia Association (CDA) / Association canadienne de la dyslexie

57, rue du Couvent, Gatineau QC J9H 3C8

Tel: 613-853-6539; *Fax:* 819-684-0672
e-mail: info@dyslexiaassociation.ca
www.dyslexiaassociation.ca

Overview: A medium-sized national charitable organization founded in 1991
Affliation(s): Canadian Dyslexia Centre, Heritage Academy

Centre for ADHD Awareness, Canada (CADDAC)

#604, 3950 - 14th Ave., Markham ON L3R 0A9

Tel: 416-637-8584; *Fax:* 905-475-3232
www.caddac.ca
www.facebook.com/pages/CADDAC/420621229045
twitter.com/CentreforADHD

Overview: A small national organization
Mission: The Centre for ADHD Awareness Canada, is a national, non profit, umbrella organization providing leadership in education and advocacy for ADHD organizations and individuals across Canada.
Chief Officer(s):
Heidi Bernhardt, President & Executive Director

Learning Disabilities Association of Canada (LDAC) / L'association Canadienne des troubles d'apprentissage (ACTA)

#20, 2420 Bank St., Ottawa ON K1V 8S1

Tel: 613-238-5721
e-mail: info@ldac-acta.ca
www.ldac-acta.ca
www.facebook.com/ldacacta
twitter.com/ldacacta
www.youtube.com/ldacacta

Overview: A large national charitable organization founded in 1971
Mission: To advance the education, employment, social development, legal rights & general well-being of people with learning disabilities; To create a greater public awareness & understanding of learning disabilities; To promote & develop early recognition, diagnosis, treatment & appropriate educational, social, recreational & career-oriented programs for people with learning disabilities; To promote legislation, research & training of personnel in the field of learning disabilities
Chief Officer(s):
Thealzel Lee, Chair
Claudette Larocque, Executive Director
claudette@ldac-acta.ca
Publications:
• National [a publication of the Learning Disabilities Association of Canada]
Type: Newsletter; *Frequency:* Quarterly

National Literacy & Health Program (NLHP)

c/o Canadian Public Health Association, #404, 1525 Carling Ave., Ottawa ON K1Z 8R9

Tel: 613-725-3769; *Fax:* 613-725-3769
www.cpha.ca/en/portals/h-l/h-l5.aspx

Overview: A small national organization
Mission: To promote awareness among health professionals of the links between literacy and health.
Member of: Canadian Public Health Association
Chief Officer(s):
Greg Penney, Director, National Programs, Canadian Public Health Association

Provincial Associations

ALBERTA

Learning Disabilities Association of Alberta (LDAA) / Troubles d'apprentissage - Association de l'Alberta

PO Box 29011, Stn. Pleasantview, Edmonton AB T6H 5Z6

Tel: 780-448-0360
www.ldalberta.ca
www.facebook.com/185386404841119

Overview: A medium-sized provincial charitable organization founded in 1968 overseen by Learning Disabilities Association of Canada

Mission: To foster public understanding & build support networks to maximize the potential of individuals with learning disabilities; To support children, families, & adults affected by learning disabilities & ADHD
Chief Officer(s):
Ellie Shuster, Executive Director
execdir@ldalberta.ca

Edmonton Chapter
L.Y. Cairns School, 10510 - 45 Ave., Edmonton AB T6H 0A1

Tel: 780-466-1011; *Fax:* 780-466-1095
e-mail: info@ldedmonton.com
www.ldedmonton.ca
www.facebook.com/LDEdmonton
twitter.com/LDEdmonton

Chief Officer(s):
Karen Popal, Programs Coordinator

Red Deer Chapter
3757 - 43 Ave., Lower Level, Red Deer AB T4N 3B7

Tel: 403-340-3885; *Fax:* 403-340-3884
ldreddeer.ca

Chief Officer(s):
Marg Dunlop, Administrative Coordinator

BRITISH COLUMBIA

Learning Disabilities Association of British Columbia (LDAV) / Troubles d'apprentissage - Association de la Colombie-Britannique

#5, 774 Bay St., Victoria BC V8T 5E4

Tel: 250-370-9513
e-mail: info@ldabc.ca
www.ldabc.ca
www.facebook.com/LDABC
twitter.com/LDABC

Overview: A medium-sized provincial organization founded in 1974 overseen by Learning Disabilities Association of Canada
Mission: To advance the education, employment, social development, legal rights & general well-being of people with learning disabilities; To operate as a coordinating body, information centre & provincial representative for chapters within BC
Member of: Learning Disabilities Association of B.C.
Chief Officer(s):
Lynne Kent, Chair
lynne.k@ldabc.ca

MANITOBA

Learning Disabilities Association of Manitoba (LDAM) / Troubles d'apprentissage - Association de Manitoba

617 Erin St., Winnipeg MB R3G 2W1

Tel: 204-774-1821; *Fax:* 204-788-4090
e-mail: ldamb@mts.net
www.ldamanitoba.org

Also Known As: LDA Manitoba
Overview: A medium-sized provincial charitable organization founded in 1966 overseen by Learning Disabilities Association of Canada
Mission: To provide support to all those who are concerned with learning disabilities; To represent individuals & families with learning disabilities
Affliation(s): Learning Disabilities Association of Canada
Chief Officer(s):
Marilyn MacKinnon, Executive Director
ldamanitoba4@mymts.net

NEW BRUNSWICK

Learning Disabilities Association of New Brunswick (LDANB) / Troubles d'apprentissage - Association du Nouveau-Brunswick (TA-ANB)
#203, 403 Regent St., Fredericton NB E3B 3X6
Tel: 506-459-7852; *Fax:* 506-455-9300
Toll-Free: 877-544-7852
e-mail: admin@ldanb-taanb.ca
www.ldanb-taanb.ca
www.facebook.com/LDANBTAANB
twitter.com/LDANB
vimeo.com/user19549796

Also Known As: LDA New Brunswick
Overview: A medium-sized provincial charitable organization founded in 1980 overseen by Learning Disabilities Association of Canada
Mission: Promotes the understanding & acceptance of the ability of persons with learning disabilities to lead meaningful & successful lives. Satellite office in Saint John.
Chief Officer(s):
Deschênes André, Executive Director
Publications:
• Reflexions [a publication of the Learning Disabilities Association of New Brunswick]
Type: Newsletter

Moncton Chapter
63 Peter St., Moncton NB E1A 3W3
Tel: 506-383-5077; *Fax:* 506-383-5077
e-mail: lmleblnc@nbnet.nb.ca

Saint John Chapter (LDASJ)
c/o St. John The Baptist/King Edward School, 223 St. James St., Saint John NB E2L 1W3
Tel: 506-642-4956
e-mail: ldasj@nb.aibn.com
www.ldasj.ca

NEWFOUNDLAND AND LABRADOR

Learning Disabilities Association of Newfoundland & Labrador Inc. (LDANL)
The Board of Trade Bldg., #301, 66 Kenmount Rd., St. John's NL A1B 3V7
Tel: 709-753-1445; *Fax:* 709-753-4747
e-mail: info@ldanl.ca
www.ldanl.ca
www.facebook.com/LearningDisabilitiesNL
twitter.com/LDANL

Also Known As: LDA Newfoundland & Labrador
Overview: A medium-sized provincial charitable organization founded in 2001 overseen by Learning Disabilities Association of Canada
Mission: To work towards the advancement of legal rights, social development, education, employment, & the general well-being of people with learning disabilities
Member of: Learning Disabilities Association of Canada (LDAC)
Chief Officer(s):
David Banfield, Executive Director
david@ldanl.ca
Karen Nelson, Office Manager

NORTHWEST TERRITORIES

Learning Disabilities Association of The Northwest Territories (LDA-NWT)
PO Box 242, Yellowknife NT X1A 2N2
Tel: 867-873-6378; *Fax:* 867-873-6378
e-mail: lda-nwt@arcticdata.ca
Previous Name: The Northwest Territories Association for Children (& Adults) with Learning Disabilities
Overview: A medium-sized provincial organization founded in 1981 overseen by Learning Disabilities Association of Canada
Mission: To help people with learning disabilities achieve their potential in school, the workplace, & in society

ONTARIO

Learning Disabilities Association of Ontario (LDAO) / Troubles d'apprentissage - Association de l'Ontario
#202, 365 Evans Ave., Toronto ON M8Z 1K2
Tel: 416-929-4311; *Fax:* 416-929-3905
e-mail: resource@ldao.ca
www.ldao.ca
www.facebook.com/LDAOntario
twitter.com/ldatschool

Overview: A medium-sized provincial charitable organization founded in 1964 overseen by Learning Disabilities Association of Canada
Mission: To provide leadership in learning disabilities advocacy, research, education & services; To advance the full participation of children, youth & adults with learning disabilities in today's society
Chief Officer(s):
Lawrence Barns, President & CEO
lawrence@ldao.ca
Karen Quinn, Director, Operations
karenq@ldao.ca
Diane Wagner, Senior Manager, Public Policy & Education
dianew@ldao.ca

PRINCE EDWARD ISLAND

Learning Disabilities Association of Prince Edward Island (LADPEI)
#149, 40 Enman Cres., Charlottetown PE C1E 1E6
Tel: 902-894-5032
e-mail: ldapei@eastlink.ca
www.ldapei.ca
www.facebook.com/ldapei
twitter.com/LDAPEI

Overview: A medium-sized provincial charitable organization founded in 1975 overseen by Learning Disabilities Association of Canada
Mission: To advance the interests of people with learning disabilities; To act as a voice for learning disabled people of Prince Edward Island
Member of: Prince Edward Island Literacy Alliance Inc.
Affliation(s): Learning Disabilities Association of Canada (LDAC)
Chief Officer(s):
Martin Dutton, Executive Director
martin@ldapei.ca

SASKATCHEWAN

Learning Disabilities Association of Saskatchewan (LDAS) / Troubles d'apprentissage - Association de la Saskatchewan
221 Hanselman Ct., Saskatoon SK S7L 6A8
Tel: 306-652-4114; *Fax:* 306-652-3220
e-mail: reception@ldas.org
www.ldas.org

Overview: A medium-sized provincial charitable organization founded in 1973 overseen by Learning Disabilities Association of Canada
Mission: To advance the education, employment, social development, legal rights & general well-being of people with learning disabilities. Branches in Regina & Prince Albert.
Member of: The United Way of Saskatoon
Chief Officer(s):
Dale Rempel, Provincial Executive Director
dale.rempel@ldas.org
Laurie Garcea, Director, Psychological Services
Eldeen Kabatoff, Director, Program
Colette Gauthier, Director, Operations

Prince Albert Branch
1106 Central Ave., Prince Albert SK S6V 4V6
Tel: 306-922-1071; *Fax:* 306-922-1073
e-mail: pabranch1@sasktel.net
Chief Officer(s):
Prema Arsiradam, Director

Regina Branch
438 Victoria Ave. East, Regina SK S4N 0N7
Tel: 306-352-5327; *Fax:* 306-352-2260
e-mail: ldas.reginabranch@sasktel.net
Chief Officer(s):
Shelley Kemp, Branch Director

YUKON TERRITORY

Learning Disabilities Association of Yukon Territory (LDAY)
128A Copper Rd., Whitehorse YT Y1A 2Z6

Tel: 867-668-5167; *Fax:* 867-668-6504
e-mail: office@ldayukon.com
www.ldayukon.com

Also Known As: LDA Yukon
Previous Name: Yukon Association for Children & Adults with Learning Disabilities
Overview: A medium-sized provincial charitable organization founded in 1973 overseen by Learning Disabilities Association of Canada
Mission: To provide services & programs for Yukoners with learning disabilities so that they reach their potential & become productive members of society
Chief Officer(s):
Stephanie Hammond, Executive Director
 ed@ldayukon.com
Barb Macrae, President

Local Associations

ALBERTA

CanLearn Society for Persons with Learning Difficulties
#110, 1117 Macleod Trail SE, Calgary AB T2G 2M8

Tel: 403-686-9300; *Fax:* 403-686-0627
Toll-Free: 877-686-9300
e-mail: info@calgarylearningcentre.com
www.calgarylearningcentre.com
facebook.com/pages/canlearn-centre/197617023661313
twitter.com/canlearncentre
www.youtube.com/user/CanLearnSociety

Also Known As: Calgary Learning Centre
Previous Name: Computer Learning & Information Centre Society of Calgary
Overview: A small local charitable organization founded in 1979
Mission: To provide programs & services for learning disabilities, attention deficit / hyperactivity disorder (AD / HD), & literacy issues
Chief Officer(s):
Krista Poole, CEO
Gerry Meek, Chair
Publications:
• CanLearn Society for Persons with Learning Difficulties Annual Report
Type: Yearbook; *Frequency:* Annually
• For the Love of Learning Newsletter
Type: Newsletter
Profile: Information for donors

International Associations

International Dyslexia Association (IDA)
40 York Rd., 4th Fl/, Baltimore MD 21204 USA

Tel: 410-296-0232; *Fax:* 410-321-5069
e-mail: info@interdys.org
eida.org
www.linkedin.com/company/international-dyslexia-association
www.facebook.com/interdys
twitter.com/IntlDyslexia
www.youtube.com/user/idachannel

Overview: A medium-sized international organization
Mission: The IDA actively promotes effective teaching approaches and related clinical educational intervention strategies for dyslexics.

 Ontario Branch
 1785 Foleyet Cres., Pickering ON L1V 2X8

Tel: 416-716-9296
idaontario.com
www.facebook.com/group.php?gid=12300009993
twitter.com/onbida
www.flickr.com/photos/onbida/

Local Schools

ALBERTA

Edmonton: Columbus Academy
#145, 10403 - 172 St., Edmonton, AB T5S 1K9

Tel: 780-440-0708; *Fax:* 780-440-0760
www.upcs.org

Grades: 7-12 *Note:* The school is a special education, private school in Alberta. Students are referred from social service agencies, surrounding school jurisdictions, & parents.
Kathy King, Contact
 kking@upcs.org

Edmonton: **Edmonton Academy**
#2, 810 Saddleback Rd. NW, Edmonton, AB T6J 4W4

Tel: 780-482-5449; *Fax:* 780-482-0902
www.edmontonacademy.com

Grades: 3-12 *Note:* Provides specialized teaching for students with learning disabilities.
Elizabeth Richards, Executive Director
 e.richards@edmontonacademy.com
Laurie Oakes, Principal & Director, Education
 laurie.oakes@edmontonacademy.com

Edmonton: **Phoenix Academy**
#145, 10403 - 172 St., Edmonton, AB T5S 1K9

Tel: 780-440-0708; *Fax:* 780-440-0760
www.upcs.org

Grades: K-12 *Note:* School for students who struggle with behavioural disorders and learning disabilities
Kathy King, Contact
 kking@upcs.org

NOVA SCOTIA

Wolfville: **Landmark East School**
708 Main St., Wolfville, NS B4P 1G4

Tel: 902-542-2237; *Fax:* 902-542-4147
Toll-Free: 800-565-5887
admissions@landmarkeast.org
www.landmarkeast.org
twitter.com/landmarkeast
www.youtube.com/lmeschoolcanada

Grades: 3-12 *Enrollment:* 60 *Note:* The international school serves students with learning disabilities. Landmark East has an overall student-teacher ratio of 3:1.
Jim Sotvedt, Chair
Peter Coll, Headmaster
 pcoll@landmarkeast.org
Glen Currie, Director, Students
 gcurrie@landmarkeast.org

ONTARIO

Belleville: **Sagonaska Demonstration School**
350 Dundas St. West, Belleville, ON K8P 1B2

Tel: 613-967-2830
www.psbnet.ca/eng/schools/sagonaska

Enrollment: 120
Martin Smit, Principal

Milton: **Trillium Demonstration School**
347 Ontario St. South, Milton, ON L9T 3X9

Tel: 905-878-2851
www.psbnet.ca/eng/schools/trillium
TTY: 905-878-7195

Enrollment: 120
Desiree Smith, Principal

Toronto: **Merle Levine Academy**
#318, 4630 Dufferin St., Toronto, ON M3H 5S4

Tel: 416-661-4141; *Fax:* 416-661-4143
merle@merlelevineacademy.com
www.merlelevineacademy.com
www.facebook.com/pages/Merle-Levine-Academy/286041258174405
twitter.com/MLevineAcademy

Grades: Elem.-Sec. *Note:* Private school specializing in areas of learning disabilities, attentional problems (ADD-ADHD) and other disorders affecting academic achievement.
Merle Levine, BA, MEd, Director
  merle@merlelevineacademy.com
Persaud Levine, MA, MEd, Director/Principal
  yuwattee.persaud@merlelevineacademy.com

Provincial Libraries

Learning Disabilities Association of Ottawa-Carleton
160 Percy St., Ottawa, ON K1R 6E5

Tel: 613-567-5864
www.ldaottawa.com

Collection: Factsheets; Audio files; DVDs; Children & young adults' resources
Linda Barbetta, Resource Coordinator

Autism Spectrum Disorders

Autism Spectrum Disorders (ASD) are a distinct group of neurological conditions, characterized by impairment in language and communication skills, which affect about 0.5 percent of the population in Canada. They typically appear during the first three years of life, and are associated with the following risk factors: medical and obstetrical problems such as encephalitis, anoxia (absence of oxygen) during birth and prenatal infections with certain viruses (such as maternal rubella). There is some evidence of genetic transmission. Twin and family studies have shown a genetic predisposition to ASD, but a specific gene has not yet been identified. The siblings of people with the disorder are at increased risk. Some researchers have proposed that the disorder may stem from abnormalities during critical stages of fetal development, including defects in the genes that control and regulate normal brain growth and growth patterns. More recently, environmental toxins and pollutants are being questioned to explain the sharp rise in ASD cases in recent decades, but researchers have been unable to confirm these findings. The disorder is not caused by inappropriate parenting or by routine immunizations.

ASDs affect behaviour, communication, social interaction and other neurological functions in varying degrees of severity, and include the following conditions: Autistic Disorder (AD), Asperger's Syndrome (AS), PDD-NOS (pervasive development disorder — not otherwise specified), Childhood Disintegrative Disorder (CDD) and Rett's Disorder (RD). AD involves cognitive impairments and deficits in social and communication development. AS is similar to AD, but with milder social impairments and no speech or cognitive delays. PPD-NOS describes cases where there is severe impairment in areas such as reciprocal social interaction, but that do not meet the criteria for autistic disorder. CDD involves severe cognitive impairment and loss of social behaviour and language and occurs after three or more years of normal development. RD is a developmental disorder diagnosed mostly in girls after six to 18 months of normal development. Two of the most common ASDs are Autistic Disorder and Asperger's Syndrome.

Autistic Disorder

Cause
Autistic Disorder is a pervasive developmental disorder that affects motor, language, cognitive and social skills. Causes are genetic but undefined, as discussed above.

Symptoms
The symptoms of AD vary widely from person to person and can range from mild to severe. Sometimes, people with this disorder have difficulty sharing something of interest with other people, making eye contact with others or engaging in physical contact.

Some people with AD show little facial expression and find it difficult to make friends. The disorder may not be apparent in early childhood, although parents often sense that there is something wrong because of their child's marked lack of interest in social interaction. Very young children with autism may show no desire for affection and cuddling. Sometimes there is no socially directed smiling or facial responsiveness, and no responsiveness to the voices of parents and siblings. As a result, parents may worry that their child is deaf. Later, the child may be more willing to interact socially, but the quality of interaction varies, and may sometimes be inappropriately intrusive with limited understanding of social rules and boundaries. Children with AD may also focus obsessively on one particular area of interest and engage in ritualistic behaviour (e.g., rocking, spinning, finger flapping).

Autism seems to bring with it an increased risk of other disorders. Seventy-five percent of autistic children have cognitive deficits, and twenty-five percent have cognitive abilities at or above average. Twenty-five percent of individuals with autism also have seizure disorders. The development of intellectual skills is usually uneven. An autistic child may be able to read extremely early, but not be able to comprehend what he or she reads. Other symptoms may include hyperactivity, short attention span, impulsivity, aggressiveness and self-injury, such as head banging, hair pulling and arm biting (particularly in young children). There may be unusual responses to stimuli: less than normal sensitivity to pain but extreme sensitivity to sounds or to being touched. There may be differences in emotional expression, giggling or weeping for no apparent reason, and little or no emotional reaction when one would be expected. Similar unusual responses may be shown in relation to fear; an absence of fear in response to real danger, but great fearfulness in the presence of harmless objects.

In adolescence or adulthood, people with Autistic Disorder may become depressed when they realize their limitations. Follow-up studies suggest that only a small percentage of people with Autistic Disorder live independent adult lives. Even the highest functioning adults may continue to have problems in social interaction and communication, together with greatly restricted interests and activities.

Prevalence
By definition, Autistic Disorder is present before age three. There is a controversy about the observation that autism is much more frequently diagnosed currently than it was in the past. It is not clear whether this is because the condition has actually become more prevalent, or because cases that were missed in the past are now being identified, or because is it being over-diagnosed. There are about 20 cases of the disorder per 10,000 Canadians. Rates of autism are four to five times greater among males than females.

Treatment Options
There are a number of tools used to diagnose Autistic Disorder including the Autism Diagnostic Observation Schedule, the Childhood Autism Rating Scale and the Autism Diagnostic Interview. However, a diagnosis of Autistic Disorder is usually based on the following criteria outlined in the *Diagnostic and Statistical Manual of Mental Disorders*: impairment in the quality of social interaction which may include gross lack of nonverbal behaviour (such as eye contact, facial expression, body postures and gestures), which gives meaning to social interaction and social behaviour; failure to make friends in age-appropriate ways; lack of spontaneously seeking to share interests or achievements with others (not showing things to others, not pointing to, or bringing interesting objects to others); lack of social or emotional give and take (not joining in social play or simple games with others); notable lack of awareness of others and being oblivious of other children (includ-

ing siblings), of their excitement, distress or needs. To be diagnosed with AD, a person must also show a marked impairment in the quality of communication which may include delay in, or lack of, spoken language development. Those who speak cannot initiate or sustain communication with others. There is also a lack of the spontaneous make-believe or imitative play that is common among young children. When speech does develop, it may be abnormal and monotonous. Repetitive use of language may also be demonstrated. The person may also demonstrate restricted repetitive patterns or behaviour such as a restricted range of interests often fixed on one subject and its facts (baseball); a great deal of exact repetition in play (lining up play objects in the same way again and again); resistance and distress if anything in the environment is changed (a chair moved to a different place); insistence on following certain rules and routines (walking to school by the same route each day); repeated body movements (body rocking, hand clapping); persistent preoccupation with details or parts of objects (buttons).

It is difficult or unusual to be able to eradicate all the symptoms of Autistic Disorder, but there are many intervention and education programs which help to improve functioning. It is extremely important, however, that a proper assessment and diagnosis be made as early as possible. Since the disturbance in behaviour is so wide ranging, the diagnosis can require an array of professional skills—psychological, language development, neuropsychological and medical. Such a multiple assessment establishes the presence or absence of other disorders, the level of intellectual functioning, together with individual strengths and weaknesses and the child's capacity for social and personal self-sufficiency. Since the symptoms of Autistic Disorder vary widely, a proper assessment is the foundation for designing and planning an individually tailored intervention program.

The autistic person may benefit from a combination of educational and behavioural interventions, which may reduce many of the behavioural disturbances, and improve the quality of life for the person and his or her family. Many experts believe that applied behavioural analysis (ABA) methods are the most effective. ABA focuses on building social interaction and imitation skills, language skills, appropriate play and attention to social stimuli.

Other treatment may include speech and language therapy, occupational therapy, social and play-related therapy, life skills training and psychological counselling. In some cases, medication may also be prescribed. There is no specific drug to treat the neurological problems associated with AD. Instead, medication may be prescribed to treat the symptoms that sometimes co-exist with AD, including antidepressants for anxiety, stimulant drugs for hyperactivity and attention difficulties, anti-convulsants for seizures and anti-psychotics for extreme behavourial situations.

The diagnosis of Autistic Disorder can be a shattering experience for any family. The outcome of the diagnosis is open-ended and uncertain and includes a lifetime of care. Every member of the family is affected and it is vital to work with and support them.

Asperger's Syndrome

Asperger's Syndrome (AS) is named for Austrian pediatrician Hans Asperger, who in 1944, observed four children who had normal intelligence, but lacked nonverbal communication skills; additionally they did not demonstrate empathy with their peers, and were physically clumsy. Dr. Asperger called the condition Autistic psychopathy and described it as a personality disorder marked by social isolation.

Cause

Causes are genetic but undefined, as discussed above.

Symptoms

The person with Asperger's may not develop age-appropriate relationships or attempt to share interests or pleasures with others. He or she may be unable to reciprocate others' feelings, have difficulty using gestures or facial expressions, be extremely preoccupied with a very narrow area of interest, insist upon very rigid routines, make repetitive movements, and focus on parts of objects rather than the objects as a whole. Asperger's Syndrome does not interfere with the development of language or thinking. However, its symptoms interfere with the individual's social or occupational functioning.

Prevalence

The incidence of Asperger's Syndrome is estimated to be five out of every 10,000 Canadians. Boys are three to four times more likely than girls to have the disorder. Although diagnosed mainly in children, it is being increasingly diagnosed in adults with other mental health conditions such as depression, obsessive-compulsive disorder and attention-deficit hyperactivity disorder.

Treatment Options

Most doctors rely on the presence of a core group of behaviours to diagnose AS.

The two main types of behaviour are problems with social interactions and stereotyped, repetitive patterns of behaviour. Individuals with AS have limited interests and are preoccupied with a particular subject to the exclusion of other activities. Some other characteristics are repetitive routines or rituals; peculiarities in speech and language, such as speaking in an overly formal manner or in a monotone, or taking figures of speech literally; socially and emotionally inappropriate behaviour and the inability to interact successfully with peers; problems with non-verbal communication, including the restricted use of gestures, limited or inappropriate facial expressions, or a peculiar, stiff gaze; clumsy and uncoordinated motor movements.

Treatment for Asperger's Syndrome addresses the core symptoms of the disorder: poor communication skills, obsessive or repetitive routines, and physical clumsiness. No single treatment works best, but the program would include social skills training, cognitive behavioural therapy, medication (to treat co-existing symptoms), occupational/physical therapy and parent training and support.

Although there are no known cures for Autism Spectrum Disorders, there is strong evidence that early diagnosis, early intervention and individualized educational programs provide the opportunity for maximum development for a child with this disorder.

National Associations

Autism Canada / Société canadienne d'autisme
PO Box 366, Bothwell ON N0P 1C0

Tel: 519-695-5858; *Fax:* 519-695-5757
Toll-Free: 866-476-8440
www.autismcanada.org
www.linkedin.com/company/autism-canada
www.facebook.com/autismcanada
twitter.com/autismcanada

Also Known As: Autism Society Canada
Overview: A medium-sized national charitable organization founded in 1976
Mission: To provide support on a national basis to people affected by autism & related conditions through the collective efforts of Canadian provincial & territorial autism societies; To provide information & general referrals to the public regarding autism & related conditions; To promote public awareness of autism & related conditions; To encourage research in fields related or relevant to autism & related conditions; To communicate with government, agencies, & other

organizations on behalf of persons affected by autism & related conditions; To promote actions to ensure people with autism & related conditions live in an environment that supports their well-being & enables them to reach their full potential; To promote & encourage the convening of conferences focused on autism & related conditions
Member of: Autism Society Ontario; World Autism Organization
Chief Officer(s):
Don Blane, Chair
Laurie Mawlam, Executive Director
  laurie@autismcanada.org

Autism Speaks Canada
#120, 2450 Victoria Park Ave., Toronto ON M2J 4A2
Tel: 416-362-6227; *Fax:* 416-362-6228
Toll-Free: 888-362-6227
Other Communication: canadianfamilyservices@autismspeaks.org
www.autismspeaks.ca
www.facebook.com/AutismSpeaksCanada
twitter.com/autismspeaksCAN
Previous Name: National Alliance for Autism Research
Overview: A medium-sized national organization
Mission: To fund & accelerate biomedical research focusing on autism spectrum disorders
Chief Officer(s):
Jill Farber, Executive Director

Canadian National Autism Foundation (CNAF)
PO Box 66512, 38 King St. East, Stoney Creek ON L8G 5E5
Tel: 905-930-8682; *Fax:* 905-930-9744
e-mail: info@cnaf.net
www.cnaf.net
Overview: A small national charitable organization founded in 2000
Mission: To increase autism awareness; To assist families; To raise funds to support Canadian-based autism research
Chief Officer(s):
Tina Fougere, President & Founder

Fragile X Research Foundation of Canada (FXRFC)
167 Queen St. West, Brampton ON L6Y 1M5
Tel: 905-453-9366
e-mail: info@fragilexcanada.ca
www.fragilexcanada.ca
Overview: A small national charitable organization founded in 1997
Mission: To raise public awareness of Fragile X; to raise money for Fragile X research & support services; to establish a support system for those with & affected by Fragile X
Chief Officer(s):
Carlo Paribello, President / Medical Director
  medical@fragilexcanada.ca

Geneva Centre for Autism (GCA)
112 Merton St., Toronto ON M4S 2Z8
Tel: 416-322-7877; *Fax:* 416-322-5894
Toll-Free: 866-436-3829
e-mail: info@autism.net
www.autism.net
www.linkedin.com/company/geneva-centre-for-autism
www.facebook.com/genevacentre
twitter.com/geneva_centre
Overview: A medium-sized national charitable organization founded in 1974
Mission: To provide people with autism & other related disorders with opportunities & resources to fully participate in their communities
Member of: Autism Society of Canada; Autism Society of Ontario; Autism Society of America
Chief Officer(s):
Abe Evreniadis, Interim Chief Executive Officer
Susan Walsh, Chief Operations Officer
Wayne Edwards, Director, Human Resources
Ellie Rusonik, Director, Development

Society for Treatment of Autism / Association canadienne pour l'obtention des services aux personnes autistiques
404 - 94 Ave. SE, Calgary AB T2J 0E8
Tel: 403-253-2291; *Fax:* 403-253-6974
Toll-Free: 888-301-2872
e-mail: intake@sta-ab.com
www.sta-ab.com

Overview: A medium-sized national charitable organization founded in 1988
Mission: To ensure that a comprehensive range of services exists across Canada to meet the needs of individuals with autism & their families, & that autistic people are given the opportunity to achieve maximum independence & productivity within the community
Chief Officer(s):
Peter Johnson, Chair
Dave Mikkelsen, Executive Director

Nova Scotia - Society for Treatment of Autism
PO Box 392, 541 Charlotte St., Sydney NS B1P 6H2
Tel: 902-567-6441; *Fax:* 902-567-0425
e-mail: autism@ns.sympatico.ca
www.nsnet.org/autismns

Saskatchewan - Autism Services
209 Fairmont Dr., Saskatoon SK S7M 5B8
Tel: 306-665-7013; *Fax:* 306-665-7011
www.autismservices.ca
www.facebook.com/pages/Autism-Services-of-Saskatoon/333195500114558
www.youtube.com/user/AutismSaskatoon
Chief Officer(s):
Lynn Latta, Executive Director

Unity for Autism
PO Box 38066, 550 Eglinton Ave. West, Toronto ON M5N 3A8
Tel: 416-414-7726
e-mail: info@unityforautism.ca
www.unityforautism.ca
www.facebook.com/324290850957490
Overview: A medium-sized national charitable organization
Mission: To provide support for individuals with autism & related disorders, as well as their families; To promote research on childhood autism
Chief Officer(s):
Kathy Carsley, Founding Director
  kathy@unityforautism.ca

Provincial Associations

ALBERTA

Autism Society Alberta (ASA)
3639 26 St. NE, Calgary AB T1Y 5E1
Toll-Free: 877-777-7192
e-mail: info@autismalberta.ca
www.autismalberta.ca
www.facebook.com/autismalberta
twitter.com/AutismSocietyAB
Overview: A medium-sized provincial charitable organization founded in 1972 overseen by Autism Society Canada
Mission: To improve the understanding of autism throughout Alberta by the dissemination of information to parents, health care workers, educators, government, private agencies & the public
Affiliation(s): Edmonton Autism Society; Autism Calgary Association; Autism Society Central Alberta
Chief Officer(s):
Deborah Barrett, President
Carole Anne Patenaude, Secretary

BRITISH COLUMBIA

Autism Society of British Columbia
#303, 3701 East Hastings St., Burnaby BC V5C 2H6
Tel: 604-434-0880; *Fax:* 604-434-0801
Toll-Free: 888-437-0880
e-mail: info@autismbc.ca
www.autismbc.ca
www.facebook.com/autismbc
twitter.com/autismbc
Overview: A small provincial charitable organization founded in 1975 overseen by Autism Society Canada
Mission: To promote awareness of autism & the needs of families with a child or adult with autism; To provide advocacy, resources, & referrals to families of people with autism in BC
Chief Officer(s):

Laurie Guerra, President
Anya Walsh, Executive Director

Nanaimo Branch
PO Box 180, Stn. A, Nanaimo BC V9R 5K9
Tel: 250-714-0801; *Fax:* 250-714-0802
www.autismbc.ca/nanaimo.php
twitter.com/autismbcvanisle

Chief Officer(s):
Alexandria Stuart, Coordinator
astuart@autismbc.ca

Prince George Branch
13950 Athabasca Rd., Prince George BC V2N 5X9
Tel: 250-963-0803; *Fax:* 250-963-0804
www.autismbc.ca/prince_george.php

Chief Officer(s):
Heather Borland, Coordinator
hborland@autismbc.ca

MANITOBA

Autism Society Manitoba
825 Sherbrook St., Winnipeg MB R3A 1M5
Tel: 204-783-9563; *Fax:* 204-975-3027
e-mail: info@autismmanitoba.com
www.autismmanitoba.com
www.facebook.com/AutismSocietyOfManitoba
twitter.com/manitobaautism
Overview: A small provincial charitable organization founded in 1977 overseen by Autism Society Canada
Mission: To enhance the quality of life of people with Autism Spectrum Disorder & their families; To promote full inclusion, dignity & development of personal skills & abilities for our members

NEWFOUNDLAND AND LABRADOR

Autism Society Newfoundland & Labrador (ASNL)
PO Box 14078, St. John's NL A1B 4G8
Tel: 709-722-2803; *Fax:* 709-722-4926
e-mail: info@autism.nf.net
www.autism.nf.net
twitter.com/AutismSocietyNL
Overview: A medium-sized provincial charitable organization founded in 1987 overseen by Autism Society Canada
Mission: To promote the diagnosis, treatment, education & integration into the community of all autistic persons; To provide information about autism; To promote research; To promote integrated care for autistic persons; To encourage the formation of parent support groups around the province
Chief Officer(s):
Scott Crocker, Executive Director
scrocker@autism.nf.net

NORTHWEST TERRITORIES

Autism Society Northwest Territories
5204 - 54th St., Yellowknife NT X1A 1W8
Tel: 867-446-0985; *Fax:* 867-873-4124
e-mail: info@nwtautismsociety.org
www.nwtautismsociety.org
www.facebook.com/nwtautismsociety
Overview: A small provincial organization overseen by Autism Society Canada
Mission: To ensure that autistic individuals & their families have access to resources
Chief Officer(s):
Denise McKee, President

NOVA SCOTIA

Autism Nova Scotia (ANS)
5945 Spring Garden Rd., Halifax NS B3H 1Y4
Tel: 902-446-4995; *Fax:* 902-446-4997
Toll-Free: 877-544-4495
e-mail: info@autismns.ca
www.autismnovascotia.ca
www.facebook.com/AutismNovaScotia
twitter.com/autismns

Previous Name: The Provincial Autism Centre
Overview: A small provincial charitable organization founded in 2002 overseen by Autism Society Canada
Mission: To advocate for, educate the public about, & provide support to, persons with autism/pervasive developmental disorders & their families
Affliation(s): Society for Treatment of Autism
Publications:
• Autistics Aloud
Type: Newsletter; *Frequency:* Quarterly
Profile: Displays the many talents amongst the autistic community, explores relevant issues and provides vital insight into autistic life.

ONTARIO

Aspergers Society of Ontario
#231, 3219 Yonge St., Toronto ON M4N 3S1
Tel: 416-651-4037
e-mail: info@aspergers.ca
www.aspergers.ca
www.facebook.com/AspergerOntario
twitter.com/aspergerontario
Overview: A small provincial charitable organization founded in 2000
Mission: To improve public & professional awareness & understanding of Aspergers Syndrome; To promote & support research & the development of diagnoses, treatment, & education programs for those with Aspergers Syndrome; To provide information & referrals for those interested in Aspergers Syndrome; To initiate programs & services which respond to the needs of those affected by Aspergers Syndrome
Chief Officer(s):
Alexandra Prefasi, Executive Director

Autism Ontario
#004, 1179 King St. West, Toronto ON M6K 3C5
Tel: 416-246-9592; *Fax:* 416-246-9417
Toll-Free: 800-472-7789
www.autismontario.com
www.facebook.com/autismontarioprovincial
twitter.com/AutismONT

Also Known As: Autism Society Ontario
Previous Name: Ontario Society for Autistic Citizens
Overview: A medium-sized provincial charitable organization founded in 1973 overseen by Autism Society Canada
Mission: To ensure that individuals with autism spectrum disorders are provided the means to achieve quality of life as respected members of society
Chief Officer(s):
Marg Spoelstra, Executive Director
marg@autismontario.com

PRINCE EDWARD ISLAND

Autism Society of PEI
PO Box 3243, Charlottetown PE C1A 8W5
Tel: 902-566-4844
Toll-Free: 888-360-8681
www.autismsociety.pe.ca
www.facebook.com/autismsocietypei
twitter.com/AutismSocietyPE
Overview: A small provincial organization overseen by Autism Society Canada
Mission: To provide austim resources to families in PEI
Chief Officer(s):
Nathalie Walsh, Executive Director
nathalie@autismsociety.pe.ca

QUÉBEC

Fédération québécoise de l'autisme (FQA) / Québec Federation for Autism
#200, 7675, boul Saint-Laurent, Montréal QC H2R 1W9
Tél: 514-270-7386; *Téléc:* 514-270-9261
Ligne sans frais: 888-830-2833
Courriel: info@autisme.qc.ca
www.autisme.qc.ca
www.facebook.com/autisme.qc.ca
Nom précédent: Société québécoise de l'autisme

Aperçu: *Dimension:* moyenne; *Envergure:* provinciale; Organisme sans but lucratif; fondée en 1976 surveillé par Autism Society Canada
Mission: Promouvoir et défendre les droits et les intérêts de la personne autiste ou ayant un trouble envahissant du développement afin qu'elle accède à une vie digne et à une meilleure autonomie sociale possible; mobiliser tous les acteurs concernés afin de promouvoir le bien-être des personnes, sensibiliser et informer la population sur le trouble du spectre de l'autisme ainsi que sur la situation des familles, et contribuer au développement des connaissances et à leur diffusion
Membre(s) du bureau directeur:
Jo-Ann Lauzon, Directrice générale
  direction@autisme.qc.ca

Miriam Foundation / Fondation Miriam
#620, 8000 boul Décarie, Montréal QC H4P 2S4
Tel: 514-345-1300; *Fax:* 514-345-6904
Toll-Free: 855-365-1300
e-mail: info@miriamfoundation.ca
www.miriamfoundation.ca
www.linkedin.com/company/miriam-foundation
www.facebook.com/FondationMiriamFoundation
twitter.com/FondationMiriam
Overview: A small provincial organization founded in 1970
Mission: To provide services & support for individuals with autism spectrum disorder & intellectual disabilities; To enhance the quality of life for people with autism spectrum disorders & intellectual disabilities; To promote inclusion
Chief Officer(s):
Warren Greenstone, Chief Executive Officer

SASKATCHEWAN

Saskatchewan Families for Effective Autism Treatment (SASKFEAT)
PO Box 173, Shaunavon SK S0N 2M0
e-mail: saskfeat@sasktel.net
www.saskfeat.com
www.facebook.com/SaskFEAT
Previous Name: Saskatchewan Society for the Autistic Inc.
Overview: A small provincial organization founded in 1976 overseen by Autism Society Canada
Mission: To act as a voice for the concerns & needs of parents & families of autistic children & individuals in Saskatchewan; To find the most effective treatment for autistic children & individuals
Affliation(s): Autism Society Canada
Chief Officer(s):
Arden C. Fiala, President
Kathy Chambers, Vice-President
Calvin Fiala, Secretary & Treasurer

YUKON TERRITORY

Autism Yukon
108 Copper Rd., Whitehorse YT Y1A 2Z6
Tel: 867-667-6406
e-mail: info@autismyukon.org
www.autismyukon.org
www.facebook.com/162869033819118
Overview: A small provincial organization overseen by Autism Society Canada
Mission: To provide support for individuals & families affected by autism
Chief Officer(s):
Shirley Chua-Tan, Vice-President

Local Associations

ALBERTA

Autism Calgary Association
#174, 3359 - 27th St. NE, Calgary AB T1Y 5E4
Tel: 403-250-5033; *Fax:* 403-250-2625
e-mail: info@autismcalgary.com
www.autismcalgary.com
www.facebook.com/autismcalgary
twitter.com/autismcalgary
Overview: A small local organization

Mission: Provides support, information and education to families
Chief Officer(s):
Lyndon Parakin, Executive Director, 403-250-5033 Ext. 223
  lyndon@autismcalgary.com
Publications:
• The Autism Echo
Type: Newsletter; *Frequency:* Quarterly

BRITISH COLUMBIA

Child Development Centre Society of Fort St. John & District
10417 - 106th Ave., Fort St John BC V1J 2M8
Tel: 250-785-3200; *Fax:* 250-785-3202
e-mail: info@cdcfsj.ca
www.cdcfsj.ca
Overview: A small local charitable organization founded in 1973
Mission: To promote the treatment & education of children with special needs, to ensure that they & their families are effectively & locally served with dignity & respect.
Member of: BC Association for Child Development & Intervention
Affliation(s): Cerebral Palsy Association of British Columbia
Chief Officer(s):
Andy Ackerman, President
Penny Gagnon, Executive Director

ONTARIO

Kerry's Place Autism Services
34 Berczy St., Aurora ON L4G 1W9
Tel: 905-841-6611; *Fax:* 905-841-1461
e-mail: info@kerrysplace.org
www.kerrysplace.org
www.facebook.com/kerrysplaceautismservices
twitter.com/kerrysplace
Overview: A medium-sized local charitable organization founded in 1974
Mission: To enhance the quality of life of individuals with Autism Spectrum Disorder through support, expertise, collaboration & advocacy
Chief Officer(s):
Isabel Meharry, Interim President & CEO
  imeharry@kerrysplace.org

  Central Region
  38B Berczy St., Aurora ON L4G 1W9
Tel: 905-713-6808
Chief Officer(s):
Tracy Mansell, Regional Executive Director, 905-713-6808 Ext. 318
  tracy.mansell@kerrysplace.org

Eastern Office
189 Victoria Ave., Belleville ON K8N 2B9
Tel: 613-968-5554; *Fax:* 613-967-4555
Chief Officer(s):
Lisa Binns, Regional Executive Director
  lisa.binns@kerrysplace.org

Kerry's Place Toronto
#12A, 219 Dufferin St., Toronto ON M6K 3J1
Tel: 416-537-2000; *Fax:* 416-537-7715
Chief Officer(s):
Kelly West, Regional Executive Director
  kelly.west@kerrysplace.org

Woodview Mental Health & Autism Services
69 Flatt Rd., Burlington ON L7R 3X5
Tel: 905-689-4727; *Fax:* 905-689-2474
e-mail: wcc@woodview.ca
woodview.ca
www.facebook.com/woodviewmha
twitter.com/WoodviewWLC
www.youtube.com/user/WoodviewMHA
Overview: A small local organization
Mission: To provide services & support to youth & adults with Autism Spectrum Disorder, in order to help them live more independently
Chief Officer(s):
Cindy I'Anson, Executive Director
  cianson@woodview.ca

Local Schools

ALBERTA

Calgary: Calgary Quest School
3405 Spruce Dr. SW, Calgary, AB T3C 0A5
Tel: 403-253-0003; *Fax:* 403-253-0025
info@calgaryquestschool.com
www.calgaryquestschool.com
Grades: Pre.-12 *Enrollment:* 160 *Note:* Calgary Quest School offers a program for children with special challenges.
Angela Rooke, Executive Director

Calgary: Janus Academy
2223 Spiller Rd. SE, Calgary, AB T2G 4G9
Tel: 403-262-3333
contact@janusacademy.org
www.janusacademy.org
Other Information: Jr. High & High School Site, Phone: 403-228-5559
Grades: 1-12; Special Education *Enrollment:* 57 *Note:* Janus Academy strives to enhance the lives of children with autism. The program is accredited by Alberta Education & The Association of IndependentSchools & Colleges. Janus Academy is a registered charity.
Stacey Oliver, Principal
Lorie Abernethy, Executive Director
Paige McNeill, Program Director, Elementary School
Koren Trnka, Program Director, Junior & Senior High School

Calgary: New Heights School & Learning Services
4041 Breskens Dr. SW, Calgary, AB T3E 7M1
Tel: 403-240-1312; *Fax:* 403-769-0633
info@newheightscalgary.com
www.newheightscalgary.com
Grades: Pre.-12
Gary Lepine, Chair

Calgary: Third Academy
North Campus
510 - 77th Ave. SE, Calgary, AB T2H 1C3
Tel: 403-288-5335; *Fax:* 403-288-5804
info@thirdacademy.com
www.thirdacademy.com
Grades: 1-12 *Note:* The Third Academy offers an Individualized Program Plan that addresses the needs of students with learning disorders.
Sunil Mattu, LLB (Hons) Law, BEd, Executive Director
S. Lal Mattu, Founder & Ambassador at Large
Rehana Mattu, Principal
Bruce Freeman, Communications Officer & Manager, Transportation
Sabu Alexander, Chief Accountant

Campuses
South Campus
P.O. Box 4
Site 22, RR#8, Calgary, AB T2J 2T9
Tel: 403-201-6335; *Fax:* 403-201-2036

Joe Smith, Principal

Edmonton: Elves Child Development Centre
Elves Special Needs Society
10825 - 142 St., Edmonton, AB T5N 3Y7
Tel: 780-454-5310; *Fax:* 780-454-5889
inquiries@elves-society.com
www.elves-society.com
Grades: Pre.-12 *Note:* The Elves Special Needs Society offers programs for pre-school & older children, youth & adults with disabilities & special needs, as well as outreach to students unable to attend school for extended periods of time.
Barb Tymchak Olafson, Executive Director

BRITISH COLUMBIA

Langley: Whytecliff Agile Learning Centres
Langley School
20561 Logan Ave., Langley, BC V3A 7R3
Tel: 604-532-1268; *Fax:* 604-532-1269
focus@focusfoundation.ca
www.focusfoundation.ca
www.facebook.com/focusfoundationBC
Grades: 8-12 *Enrollment:* 41 *Note:* Whytecliff Agile Learning Centres are provincially accredited, independent schools for boys & girls, aged 13-19, who face personal or behavioural challenges. Many of the students have dropped out of school, or have been excluded or expelled.
Laura Quarin, Principal

Campuses
Whytecliff Agile Learning Centre - Burnaby
3450 Boundary Rd., Burnaby, BC V5M 4A5
Tel: 604-438-4451; *Fax:* 604-438-5572
Grades: 8-12

Richmond: Glen Eden Multimodal Centre
#190, 13151 Vanier Pl., Richmond, BC V6V 2J1
Tel: 604-821-1457; *Fax:* 604-821-1527
glenedenschool@gleneden.org
www.gleneden.org
Grades: K-12 *Note:* Teaches children & adolescents who, because of unique combinations of medical, psychiatric, & developmental problems, are not functioning adequately & have not shown improvement in school based special service programs.
Rick Brennan, Executive Director

Vancouver: PALS Autism School
2409 East Pender St., Vancouver, BC V5K 2B2
Tel: 604-251-7257; *Fax:* 604-251-1627
info@palsautismschool.ca
www.palsautismschool.ca
www.facebook.com/PALSAutismSchool
twitter.com/PALSAutismBC
Grades: K-12; Adult
Andrea Kasunic, Head of School

MANITOBA

Winnipeg: St. Amant School
440 River Rd., Winnipeg, MB R2M 3Z9, Canada
Tel: 204-256-4301; *Fax:* 204-257-4349
inquiries@stamant.ca
www.stamant.mb.ca
www.facebook.com/pages/St-Amant/123434846345
twitter.com/StAmantMB
www.linkedin.com/company/st-amant
www.youtube.com/user/StAmantMB
Grades: K.-12
John Leggat, President & CEO

ONTARIO

Alliston: Above & Beyond Learning Experience
#2, 19 Church St. North, Alliston, ON L9R 1L6
Tel: 705-796-2253; *Toll-Free:* 855-796-2253
able_info@ablearning.org
www.ablearning.org
Grades: 1-12
Mikki White, Principal & Curriculum Developer
Phil White, Vice-Principal

Brant: The Gregory School for Exceptional Learning
1249 Colborne St. West, Brant, ON N3T 5L7
Tel: 519-449-1650
www.kalyanasupportsystems.com/the-gregory-school.html
www.facebook.com/144244872262082
Note: School for children with special needs that require special programming.
Angeline Savard, Principal

Mississauga: Kids CAN Social Centre
Oakwood Academy
2150 Torquay Mews, Mississauga, ON L5N 2M6
Tel: 905-814-0202
info@kidscancentre.com
www.kidscancentre.com
www.facebook.com/kidscan.charity.9
twitter.com/KidsCANCharity
Grades: JK-8 *Note:* Oakwood Academy offers individualized education programs to students with special needs.
Michele Power, Co-Founder & Director, Academic Program
Trillian Taylor, Co-Founder & Director, Transition Program

Oakville: Missing Links Academy
P.O. Box 60026
1515 Rebecca St., Oakville, ON L6L 6R4
Tel: 905-876-0055
info@missinglinks.ca
www.missinglinks.ca
Grades: Pre.-8 *Note:* Missing Links fills the gaps to Autism by delivering unique, individualized programming for the education and treatment of children with Autism Spectrum Disorder (ASD) and other exceptionalities.
Am Badwall, Clinical Director
Mike Daniels, Educational Consultant

Thornhill: Giant Steps Toronto Inc.
School
35 Flowervale Rd., Thornhill, ON L3T 4J3
Tel: 905-881-3104; *Fax:* 905-881-4592
info@giantstepstoronto.ca
www.giantstepstoronto.ca
www.facebook.com/GiantStepsToronto
Note: Giant Steps is a school & therapy centre for elementary school-aged children with Autism Spectrum Disorder (ASD).
Martin Buckingham, President
Colleen Smith, Executive Director
  csmith@giantstepstoronto.ca
Joanne Scott-Jackson, Director, Development
  jscottjackson@giantstepstoronto.ca

Toronto: Bloorview School Authority
150 Kilgour Rd., Toronto, ON M4G 1R8, Canada
Tel: 416-424-3831; *Fax:* 416-425-2981
school@hollandbloorview.ca
www.bloorviewschool.ca
www.facebook.com/HBKRH
twitter.com/#!/bloorviewpr
www.linkedin.com/company/holland-bloorview
www.youtube.com/user/PRBloorview
Note: Bloorview School Authority provides school programs to children & youth with special needs.
Rachee Allen, Chair

Toronto: Brighton School
240 The Donway West, Toronto, ON M3B 2V8
Tel: 416-932-8273; *Fax:* 416-850-5493
contactus@brightonschool.ca
www.brightonschool.ca
twitter.com/brighton_school
Grades: 1-12 *Enrollment:* 60 *Note:* Brighton is a private school for students who learn best in small classes, are one or more years behind academically, have a learning disability or an uneven learning profile.
Kathy Lear, Principal & Executive Director

Toronto: Finding The Way Learning Centre & Bright Start Academy (FTW)
#318, 4630 Dufferin St., Toronto, ON M3H 5S4
Tel: 416-514-1415; *Fax:* 416-514-1410
registration@brightstartacademy.info
www.brightstartacademy.info
www.facebook.com/BSAandFTW
twitter.com/ftwlcautism
Grades: Pre.-9 *Note:* The Academy offers a behaviour & education program for children with autism & learning difficulties.
Allie Offman, Executive Director & Principal

Toronto: Kohai Educational Centre
41 Roehampton Ave., Toronto, ON M4P 1P9
Tel: 416-489-3636; *Fax:* 416-489-3662
kohai@bellnet.ca
www.kohai.ca
www.facebook.com/Kohai.Educational.Centre
www.twitter.com/Kohai41
Grades: Pre.-12 *Note:* Programs & education for students with genetic disorders, behaviour problems, & language disorders.
Barbara Brown, Principal

Toronto: New Haven Learning Centre
301 Lanor Ave., Toronto, ON M8W 2R1
Tel: 416-259-4445; *Fax:* 416-259-2023
info@newhavencentre.com
www.newhavencentre.com
twitter.com/NewHavenCentre
www.linkedin.com/groups/New-Haven-Learning-Centre-3010708
www.youtube.com/user/NewHavenCentre
Note: Centre of Excellence in the treatment and education of children with autism.
Audrey Meissner, Executive Director, 416-259-4445, ext. 12
  ameissner@newhavencentre.com

Toronto: Reach Toronto
#206, 2238 Dundas St. West, Toronto, ON M5R 3A9
Tel: 416-929-1670
www.reachtoronto.ca
www.facebook.com/ReachToronto
twitter.com/reachtoronto
Note: Reach Toronto is a not-for-profit organization, offering unique programs for adults and youth with ASD and Asperger's Syndrome.

Waterloo: KidsAbility School Authority Board
500 Hallmark Dr., Waterloo, ON N2K 3P5, Canada
Tel: 519-886-8886; *Fax:* 519-886-7291
Toll-Free: 1-888-372-2259
info@kidsability.ca
www.kidsability.ca/en/school
www.facebook.com/184568644892738
twitter.com/kidsability
www.youtube.com/user/KidsAbility1957#p/a
Number of Schools: 5 *Note:* KidsAbility School Authority Board serves children with a wide range of special needs. Programs & services include a kindergarten program, individual education plans, composite classes, communication classes, & language classes.
Deirdre Large, Chair - Advisory Council
Linda Rogers, Principal & Secretary to the Board, 519-886-8886, ext. 1225
  lrogers@kidsability.ca
Joanne Cotter, Executive Assistant, 519-886-8886, ext. 1227
  jcotter@kidsability.ca
Cynthia Davis, Chair - Authority Board
  schoolauthoritychair@kidsability.ca

Windsor: John McGivney Children's Centre School Authority
John McGivney Children's Centre
3945 Matchette Rd., Windsor, ON N9C 4C2, Canada
Tel: 519-282-7281; *Fax:* 519-252-5873
school@jmccentre.ca
www.jmccentre.ca
www.facebook.com/243715438993933
Number of Schools: 1 *Note:* The John McGivney Children's Centre School Authority governs the John McGivney Children's Centre School, formerly known as the Children's Rehabilitation Centre School. The school provides a post trauma / post operative rehabilitation program for students from ages four to twenty-one, who live in Windsor / Essex County.
Grant Gagnon, Chair
Elaine Whitmore, CEO, 519-252-7281, ext. 221
Dr. Brenda Roberts-Santarossa, Secretary & Principal
Adelina Irvine, Treasurer

Saint-Laurent: Summit School
École le Sommet
1750, rue Deguire, Saint-Laurent, QC H4L 1M7
Tel: 514-744-2867; *Fax:* 514-744-6410
admin@summit-school.com
www.summit-school.com
Grades: Pre./Elem./Sec.; Spec. Ed.; Eng. *Enrollment:* 600 *Note:*
Educational services for special needs students, from ages 4 to 21,
with developmental disabilities such as autism, behavioural
disturbances & other associated problems.
Herman Erdogmus, Director General
Bena Finkelberg, Vice-Principal
Ron Bergamin, Director, Finance

National Libraries

Geneva Centre for Autism
112 Merton St., 2nd Fl., Toronto, ON M4S 2Z8
Tel: 416-322-7877; *Fax:* 416-322-5894
info@autism.net
www.autism.net/joinus/supporting-membership/reference-library
Social Media: www.youtube.com/user/GenevaCentre4Autism;
twitter.com/geneva_centre; www.facebook.com/genevacentre;
www.linkedin.com/company/geneva-centre-for-autism
Profile: Geneva Centre for Autism focuses on the development and
provision of clinical intervention services and training. The Centre offers
clinical services for individuals with an Autism Spectrum Disorder
(ASD). The Centre's clinical services are supported by
speech-language pathologists, behaviour analysts, therapists, early
childhood educators, occupational therapists, developmental
paediatricians, psychiatrists, psychologists, social workers, and other
professionals. The Centre provides resources for parents,
professionals and those who are affected by Autism Spectrum
Disorders. Over the years, Geneva Centre for Autism has compiled an
extensive collection of resources about ASD and related disorders.
Collection: Reference Library: The Reference Library of Geneva
Centre for Autism offers an extensive collection of autism resources.
The Reference Library access is by appointment only by contacting
info@autism.net or 416-322-7877 ext. 390. Lending Library: Geneva
Centre for Autism's Lending Library houses a collection of autism
related books and DVDs accessible to supporting members of The
Centre.
Abe Evreniadis, Interim Chief Executive Officer
Susan Walsh, Chief Operations Officer

Provincial Libraries

Autism Society of British Columbia
#303, 3701 East Hastings St., Burnaby, BC V5C 2H6
Tel: 604-434-0880; *Fax:* 604-434-0801
Toll-Free: 888-437-0880
info@autismbc.ca
www.autismbc.ca
Social Media: twitter.com/autismbc; www.facebook.com/autismbc
Collection: ASD books, videos and DVDs
Stella Hui, Librarian & Information Officer
shui@autismbc.ca

Local Hospitals & Health Centres

CALGARY: Society for Treatment of Autism (STA)
404 - 94 Ave. SE, Calgary, AB T2J 0E8
Tel: 403-253-2291 *Fax:* 403-253-6974
Toll-Free: 888-301-2872
consultation@sta-ab.com
www.sta-ab.com
Number of Beds: 20 beds
Note: Programs & services for people with autism & other pervasive
developmental disorders
Dave Mikkelsen, Executive Director

AURORA: Kerry's Place Autism Services
38B Berczy St., Aurora, ON L4G 1W9
Tel: 905-713-6808
tmansell@kerrysplace.org
www.kerrysplace.com
Info Line: 905-579-2720
Year Founded: 1974
Note: autistic adults home
Dr. Glenn Rampton, Executive Director
grampton@kerrysplace.org

**FATIMA: Centre de réadaptation en déficience intellectuelle et
troubles du spectre de l'autisme**
Affiliée à: CISSS des Iles
695, ch des Caps, Fatima, QC G4T 2S9
Tél: 418-986-3590
www.cssssdesiles.qc.ca

**LACHINE: Centre de réadaptation de l'Ouest de Montréal
(CROM/WMR)/West Montreal Readaptation Centre**
Affiliée à: CIUSSS de l'Ouest-de-l'Ile-de-Montréal
8000, rue Notre-Dame, Lachine, QC H8R 1H2
Tél: 514-363-3025 *Téléc:* 514-364-0608
infocrom@ssss.gouv.qc.ca
www.crom.ca
Média social: www.facebook.com/CROM.WMRC
Région desservi: CSSS de l'Ouest de l'Ile; CSSS Cavendish; CSSS de
la Montagne
Spécialités: Services spécialisés pour des adultes et enfants
présentant une déficience intellectuelle ou un trouble du spectre
autistique
Dre. Katherine Moxness, Directrice générale

**MONTRÉAL: Centre de réadaptation en déficience
intellectuelle et trouble du spectre de l'autisme**
Affiliée à: CIUSSS du Centre-Sud-de-l'Ile-de-Montréal
**Ancien nom: Centre de réadaptation en déficience
intellectuelle et en troubles envahissants**
Fondation DI-TSA de Montréal, #110, 75, rue de Port-Royal est,
Montréal, QC H3L 3T1
Tél: 514-387-1234
www.ciusss-centresudmtl.gouv.qc.ca

SAINT-JÉRÔME: Centre du Florès
Affiliée à: CISSS de Laurentides
290, rue De Montigny, Saint-Jérôme, QC J7Z 5T3
Tél: 450-569-2970 *Téléc:* 450-569-2961
Ligne sans frais: 877-569-2970
www.centreduflores.com
Fondée en: 1995
Note: Centre de réadaptation

Birth Defects

Birth defects, or congenital abnormalities, are conditions present
at birth that can include structural defects of the heart, major
blood vessels, kidneys, urinary tract, gastrointestinal tract, skeleton and nervous system.

Cause
Although in many instances the cause of the defect is unknown,
in most cases, the complex interaction of genetic and environmental factors is thought to be the cause. Genetic factors may
cause many single malformations and syndromes including Marfan syndrome, Tay-Sachs disease and cystic fibrosis. Some syndromes, such as Down syndrome, result from chromosomal
abnormalities. The risk of this type of birth defect increases with
maternal age. Factors during the pregnancy that can also sometimes result in defects are alcohol abuse, taking certain drugs,
maternal illnesses (such as diabetes) and various infections (rubella, toxoplasmosis, syphilis and cytomegalovirus (CMV)).

Symptoms

More than 4,000 birth defects, ranging from mild to severe, have been identified. The symptoms of some of the more common structural birth defects are described below.

Babies born with a cleft lip or palate have a long opening between the upper lip and the nose or an opening between the roof of the mouth and the nasal cavity. Those with cerebral palsy have difficulty with muscle control and movement and might not be able to speak or swallow. In babies born with clubfoot, there are structural problems with the foot and ankle. In babies born with spina bifida, the spinal column doesn't surround the spinal cord completely, sometimes resulting in loss of bladder and bowel control and paralysis. Congenital heart defects are the result of improper development of parts of the heart.

Prevalence

The incidence of specific abnormalities varies with the type of defect. These defects may be single or several defects may occur together, often known as a syndrome. In Canada, birth defects occur in one in 25 babies. Although they are still one of the leading causes of death in infants in Canada, the rate of infant mortality due to birth defects has been decreasing, likely due to advances in prenatal diagnosis and medical/surgical treatment of birth defects.

Treatment Options

Birth defects can be diagnosed before, at, or after birth, usually during the first year of life. Prior to birth, screening tests such as maternal blood and serum screens and ultrasound evaluation of the fetus can be done to check for potential problems or defects. If an abnormal result is obtained during one of these screening tests, other diagnostic tests are usually offered. These tests can include high resolution ultrasound, chorionic villus sampling (CVS) (where a small piece of the placenta is used to check for genetic or chromosomal disorders) and amniocentesis (where the amniotic fluid surrounding the fetus is tested to identify some defects). If a defect is identified and is serious, parents can decide how or if they wish the pregnancy to proceed.

Other abnormalities may not be identified until birth. Some of these birth defects (such as clubfoot and cleft lip) are easily observed. However, tests such as CT scans, X-rays, tandem mass spectroscopy or hearing tests might be used to detect other birth defects (such as congenital heart defects, congenital hypothyroidism or deafness).

Treatment and outcome vary greatly, depending on the type and severity of the defect. Parents and other family members need honest information and emotional support when caring for a child born with congenital defects. If genetic factors are suspected, the parents should receive genetic counselling.

See also Spina Bifida and Congenital Heart Disease

National Associations

Barth Syndrome Foundation of Canada

#115, 162 Guelph St., Georgetown ON L7G 5X7

Tel: 905-873-2391
Toll-Free: 888-732-9458
www.barthsyndrome.ca
www.facebook.com/barthsyndromecanada

Overview: A medium-sized national charitable organization
Mission: To find research grants into the cause, treatments & cure for Barth Syndrome; To assist Canadian families & physicians dealing with the disease
Affliation(s): Barth Syndrome Foundation Inc.
Chief Officer(s):
Susan Hone, President

Canadian Association of Perinatal & Women's Health Nurses (CAPWHN) / Association canadienne des infirmières et infirmiers en périnatalité et en santé des femmes

2781 Lancaster Rd., Ottawa ON K1B 1A7

Tel: 613-730-4192; Fax: 613-730-4314
Toll-Free: 800-561-2416
e-mail: admin@capwhn.ca
www.capwhn.ca
www.facebook.com/CAPWHN
twitter.com/CAPWHN

Previous Name: Association of Women's Health, Obstetric & Neonatal Nurses Canada
Overview: A medium-sized national organization founded in 2010
Mission: To improve the health of women & newborns; To strengthen the nursing profession in Canada
Chief Officer(s):
Sharon Dore, RN, PhD, President
Fabienne Morton, RN, Treasurer
Rita Assabgui, Executive Director
Publications:
• CAPWHN [Canadian Association of Perinatal & Women's Health Issues] Newsletter
Type: Newsletter; *Frequency:* 3 pa; *Accepts Advertising*
Profile: Activities of CAPWHN & its chapters in the Atlantic provinces, Québec, Ontario, Manitoba & Saskatchewan, & Alberta & British Columbia

Canadian Association of Pregnancy Support Services

#304 - 4820 Gaetz Ave., Red Deer AB T4N 4A4

Tel: 403-347-2827; Fax: 403-343-2847
Toll-Free: 866-845-2151
www.capss.com
www.facebook.com/CanadianAssociationOfPregnancySupportServices
?ref=str
twitter.com/CAPSS_RD

Overview: A small national organization
Mission: A Christian national ministry dedicated to providing support for life and sexual health by partnering with Pregnancy Centres across Canada.
Affliation(s): Evangelical Fellowship of Canada; Canadian Council of Christian Charities
Chief Officer(s):
Lola French, Executive Director, 403-347-2827
  lola@capss.com

Canadian Down Syndrome Society (CDSS) / Société canadienne du syndrome de Down

#103, 2003 - 14 St. NW, Calgary AB T2M 3N4

Tel: 403-270-8500; Fax: 403-270-8291
Toll-Free: 800-883-5608
www.cdss.ca
www.facebook.com/cdndownsyndrome
twitter.com/CdnDownSyndrome
www.youtube.com/user/CdnDownSyndrome

Overview: A medium-sized national charitable organization founded in 1987
Mission: To ensure equitable opportunities for all Canadians with Down Syndrome
Chief Officer(s):
Laura LaChance, Chair
Kirk Crowther, Executive Director
Lynette Gowie, Office Manager
Kaitlyn Pecson, Manager, Communications
Jenny Morrow, Manager, Development
Corrine Grieve, Manager, Resource
Shannon Thomas, Coordinator, Communications & Membership
Publications:
• Canadian Down Syndrome Society Newsletter
Type: Newsletter; *Frequency:* Quarterly
• CDSS [Canadian Down Syndrome Society] Calendar
 Frequency: Annually
• CDSS [Canadian Down Syndrome Society] Information Series
Profile: Topics include Teaching Children with Down Syndrome, Toilet Training Your Child with Down Syndrome, Stubborn Behaviour, Registered Educational Savings Plan, Taxation,Wills & Trusts,

Obstructive Sleep Apnea Syndrome, & Stop Running by Building Skills: Behavioural Approach

Canadian Fanconi Anemia Research Fund / La Fondation canadienne de recherche de l'anémie de Fanconi
PO Box 38157, Toronto ON M5N 3A9
Tel: 416-489-6393; *Fax:* 416-489-6393
e-mail: admin@fanconicanada.org
www.fanconicanada.org

Also Known As: Fanconi Canada
Overview: A small national organization
Mission: To raise money for research into finding a cure &/or treatments for Fanconi anemia; to raise awareness about the disease; to provide support to affected Canadian families

Canadian Foundation on Fetal Alcohol Research (CFFAR) / Fondation canadienne de la recherche dur l'alcoolisation foetale (FCRAF)
#62, 2192 Queen St. East, Toronto ON M4E 1E6
e-mail: info@fasdfoundation.ca
www.fasdfoundation.ca

Overview: A medium-sized national organization founded in 2007
Mission: The Canadian Foundation on Fetal Alcohol Research (CFFAR), is an independent, non-profit foundation created to promote interest and fund research related to the short and long-term bio-medical, psychological and social effects of alcohol consumption during pregnancy, and the prevention of fetal alcohol spectrum disorders (FASD).
Chief Officer(s):
Louise Nadeau, Chair

Canadian Lactation Consultant Association (CLCA) / Association canadienne des consultantes en lactation
4 Innovation Dr., Dundas ON L9H 793
Tel: 905-689-3980; *Fax:* 905-689-1465
e-mail: clca-accl@gmail.com
www.clca-accl.ca
www.linkedin.com/groups/Canadian-Lactation-Consultant-Association-CLCA
www.facebook.com/welcomeback/requests/#!/CLCA.ACCL
twitter.com/cdnlactation

Overview: A small national organization founded in 1986
Affiliation(s): International Lactation Consultant Association
Chief Officer(s):
Lauretta Williams, Administrator

Canadian Marfan Association (CMA) / Association du syndrome de Marfan
PO Box 42257, Stn. Centre Plaza, 128 Queen St. South, Mississauga ON L5M 4Z0
Tel: 905-826-3223; *Fax:* 905-826-2125
Toll-Free: 866-722-1722
e-mail: info@marfan.ca
www.marfan.ca
www.facebook.com/CanadianMarfanAssociation
twitter.com/CanadianMarfan

Overview: A medium-sized national charitable organization founded in 1986
Member of: International Federation of Marfan Syndrome Associations; Thoracic Aortic Disease (TAD) Coalition; Canadian Organization for Rare Disorders
Chief Officer(s):
Barry Edington, Executive Director

DES Action USA
PO Box 7296, Jupiter FL 33468 USA
Toll-Free: 800-337-9288
e-mail: info@desaction.org
www.desaction.org
www.facebook.com/pages/DES-Action-USA/148293015181338

Overview: A small national charitable organization founded in 1979
Mission: To provide public & physician education on special health needs of those exposed to the synthetic estrogen diethylstilbestrol (DES)
Chief Officer(s):
Fran Howell, Executive Director

Down Syndrome Research Foundation (DSRF)
1409 Sperling Ave., Burnaby BC V5B 4J8
Tel: 604-444-3773; *Fax:* 604-431-9248
e-mail: info@dsrf.org
www.dsrf.org
www.linkedin.com/company/down-syndrome-research-foundation
www.facebook.com/DSRFCanada
twitter.com/DSRFcanada
www.instagram.com/dsrfcanada

Overview: A small national charitable organization founded in 1995
Mission: To maximize the ability of people with Down Syndrome to lead independent lives & to participate in the community in which they live; To provide educational programs & services that are guided by foundational research; To collaborate with researchers, professionals & families to empower people with Down Syndrome
Member of: Down Syndrome International
Chief Officer(s):
Geoff Griffiths, Chair
Dawn McKenna, Executive Director
dawn@dsrf.org
Publications:
• Hand in Hand [a publication of the Down Syndrome Research Foundation]
Type: Newsletter; *Frequency:* Quarterly; *Editor:* Glen Hoos

Society of Gynecologic Oncologists of Canada (GOC) / Société des gynécologues oncologues du Canada
780 Echo Dr., Ottawa ON K1S 5R7
Tel: 613-730-4192; *Fax:* 613-730-4314
Toll-Free: 800-561-2416
www.g-o-c.org

Overview: A small national organization founded in 1980
Mission: To improve the care of women with gynecologic cancer; to raise standards of practice in gynecologic oncology & to encourage ongoing research
Chief Officer(s):
Dianne Miller, President
Walter Gotlieb, Sec.-Treas.

Society of Obstetricians & Gynaecologists of Canada (SOGC) / Société des obstétriciens et gynécologues du Canada
780 Echo Dr., Ottawa ON K1S 5R7
Tel: 613-730-4192; *Fax:* 613-730-4314
Toll-Free: 800-561-2416
e-mail: info@sogc.com
www.sogc.org
www.facebook.com/sogc.org
twitter.com/SOGCorg

Overview: A medium-sized national organization founded in 1944
Mission: To promote excellence in the practice of obstetrics & gynaecology; To produce national clinical guidelines for medical education on women's health issues; To promote optimal, comprehensive women's health care
Chief Officer(s):
George Carson, President
Jennifer Blake, Chief Executive Officer
Publications:
• Health News [a publication of the Society of Obstetricians & Gynaecologists of Canada]
Type: Newsletter
Profile: SOGC media reports & health news
• Healthy Beginnings [a publication of the Society of Obstetricians & Gynaecologists of Canada]
Profile: A guide to pregnancy & childbirth
• Journal of Obstetrics & Gynaecology Canada (JOGC)
Type: Journal; *Frequency:* Monthly; *Price:* Free with membership in the Society ofObstetricians & Gynaecologists of Canada
Profile: A peer-reviewed journal of obstetrics, gynaecology, & women's health, featuring original research articles,case reports, & reviews
• Sex Sense [a publication of the Society of Obstetricians & Gynaecologists of Canada]
Profile: A guide to contraception
• SOGC [Society of Obstetricians & Gynaecologists of Canada] News
Type: Newsletter; *Frequency:* 10 pa
Profile: Society work & events, plus information about recent legislation & developments in women's health care

• What You Should Know About The Society of Obstetricians & Gynaecologists of Canada

Sonography Canada / Échographie Canada
PO Box 119, Kemptville ON K0G 1J0

Fax: 613-258-0899
Toll-Free: 877-488-0788
Other Communication: memberinfo@sonographycanada.ca
e-mail: info@sonographycanada.ca
www.sonographycanada.ca

Merged from: Cnd. Assoc. of Registered Diagnostic Ultrasound Professionals & Cnd. Society of Diagnostic Medicial
Overview: A small national organization founded in 2014
Mission: The national voice for diagnostic medical sonographers in Canada
Chief Officer(s):
Tom Hayward, Business Manager
   THayward@sonographycanada.ca
Publications:
• Canadian Journal of Medical Sonography
Type: Journal; *Frequency:* Quarterly
Profile: CJMS is a combination of clinical and scientific content and is distributed to all members of Sonograhy Canada.

Support Organization for Trisomy 18, 13 & Related Disorders
Toronto ON

Tel: 416-805-5736
www.trisomy.org
www.facebook.com/Trisomy18.Trisomy13.Awareness.SOFTrelatedDisorders

Also Known As: SOFT Canada
Overview: A small national licensing charitable organization founded in 1989
Mission: To offer support to families whose children are born with any of the following disorders: Trisomy, Partial Trisomy, Mosaic (not every cell), deletion of all or part of a chromosome, single gene disorders, any other disorder which produces serious, multiple birth defects
Affiliation(s): Easter Seals
Chief Officer(s):
Satinder Sahota, Local Contact
   satinder@sandalwoodpromos.com

Provincial Associations

BRITISH COLUMBIA

British Columbia Ultrasonographers' Society (BCUS)
127 - 62nd Ave. East, Vancouver BC V5X 2E7
www.bcus.org
Overview: A small provincial organization founded in 1981
Mission: To promote & encourage the science & art of diagnostic medical sonography; provide a forum to promote the discussion of matters affecting the field; provide a place for professional growth
Chief Officer(s):
Vickie Lessoway, Executive Director

MANITOBA

Manitoba Down Syndrome Society (MDSS)
#204, 825 Sherbrook St., Winnipeg MB R3A 1M5
Tel: 204-992-2731; *Fax:* 204-975-3027
www.manitobadownsyndromesociety.com
www.facebook.com/ManitobaDownSyndromeSociety
twitter.com/manitobadss
Overview: A small provincial charitable organization founded in 1991
Mission: To provide support, information & opportunities for individuals with Down Syndrome, parents, professionals and other interested persons; To seek resolutions to issues of concern
Affiliation(s): Canadian Down Syndrome Society
Chief Officer(s):
Lorraine Baydack, President
Val Surbey, Vice-President

QUÉBEC

Association des obstétriciens et gynécologues du Québec (AOGQ)
#3000, 2, Complexe Desjardins, Montréal QC H5B 1G8
Tél: 514-849-4969; *Télec:* 514-849-5011
Courriel: info@gynecoquebec.com
www.gynecoquebec.com
Aperçu: *Dimension:* petite; *Envergure:* provinciale; fondée en 1966 surveillé par Fédération des médecins spécialistes du Québec
Mission: Promouvoir l'intérêt professionnel scientifique et économique de ses membres
Membre de: Fédération des médecins spécialistes du Québec
Membre(s) du bureau directeur:
Sylvie Bouvet, Présidente
Marie-Eve Lefebvre, Directrice, Administration

Blood Disorders

Blood disorders, also called hematologic diseases, affect blood plasma, red blood cells, white blood cells or platelets, preventing the blood from doing its job. Some blood disorders are inherited while others may be the result of disease, a side effect of medication, or a diet lacking certain nutrients.

There are three main types of blood disorders: anemia, bleeding disorders and blood cancer.

Anemia
Anemia is the decrease in the number of red blood cells in the blood. Sickle-cell and iron deficiency anemia are two well-known types.

Sickle-cell anemia (SCA) is inherited and can be life threatening. Red blood cells are made rigid and sickle-shaped due to a genetic mutation. As a result, they carry less oxygen to tissues than normal cells and can even adhere to blood vessels, blocking blood flow.

Iron deficiency anemia occurs, as the name suggests, when there is a lack of iron in the blood. Iron is essential for the production of hemoglobin, the protein that carries oxygen from the lungs to the rest of the body.

Cause
Iron deficiency anemia, the most common type, can be caused by blood loss, such as from heavy menstrual bleeding, an ulcer, cancer, a polyp in the digestive system, or prolonged use of aspirin or nonsteroidal anti-inflammatory drugs (NSAIDs). A diet lacking in iron or the inability to absorb iron can also cause anemia.

Sickle-cell anemia occurs when a person inherits the defective form of the sickle-cell gene from both parents. If one normal hemoglobin gene and one defective gene are inherited, a person will carry the sickle-cell trait but remain asymptomatic. However, as a carrier, they can pass on the defective gene to their children.

Symptoms
Although there are specific criteria used to diagnose the different types of anemia, there are some common signs. These include paleness, tiredness, shortness of breath during exercise, unusual food cravings, a rapid heartbeat and dizziness or light-headedness.

In addition to the above, sickle-cell anemia sufferers may also experience a sickle-cell crisis, an episode of sudden, severe pain occurring when sickled red blood cells block blood flow to the limbs and organs.

Prevalence

Approximately 3 percent of Canadians suffer from a form of anemia. About 5,000 Canadians are estimated to have sickle-cell disease.

Treatment Options

Iron deficiency anemia treatments depend on its underlying cause and severity. Where changes to diet alone are not enough, iron injections and even a blood transfusion may be required.

In Canada, screening of all newborn babies for sickle-cell disease is performed in Ontario, British Columbia and Nova Scotia. Prenatal screening for sickle-cell can also be done using a sample of amniotic fluid or tissue from the placenta. Early diagnosis can prevent complications.

Bone marrow and stem cell transplants offer a potential cure but are used infrequently due to the difficulty of finding donors who are genetic matches. Drug treatments for SCD include antibiotics and pain medication. Many sickle-cell patients can experience reasonably good health much of the time and are now living into their forties, fifties and even longer.

Bleeding Disorders

Bleeding disorders are a family of diseases affecting either blood proteins or platelets, which help blood to clot. When these clotting agents are missing or in low number, prolonged bleeding results from a cut or injury. Some examples of bleeding disorders are hemophilia, von Willebrand disease (vWD) and idiopathic thrombocytopenic purpura (ITP).

Hemophilia and vWD are inherited conditions that range from mild to severe, though von Willebrand disease is usually milder than hemophilia.

Idiopathic thrombocytopenic purpura (ITP) is an autoimmune disorder characterized by unusually low levels of platelets. Like hemophilia, it can lead to internal bleeding that can damage joints, organs and tissue over time.

See also Hemophilia

Cause

Hemophilia and von Willebrand disease are usually inherited disorders.

Hemophiliacs carry a genetic defect on their X chromosome, classified as Type A or Type B, depending on which type of clotting factor is lacking (factor VIII in Type A and factor IX in the case of Type B).

Von Willebrand disease is caused by low or malfunctioning von Willebrand factor, a protein essential to clotting.

ITP occurs when the body's immune system is stimulated to attack its own platelets. While the cause of ITP is largely unknown, some cases may be linked to viral or bacterial infections such as HIV, hepatitis C, or Helicobacter pylori (H. pylori).

Symptoms

Bleeding disorders have many symptoms in common, including: bleeding into joints; bleeding into soft tissues and muscles; easy bruising; frequent and prolonged nose bleeds; bleeding from the gums when baby teeth fall out or after dental procedures; abnormal bleeding after surgery, childbirth or trauma; heavy and prolonged menstrual bleeding; bleeding from the umbilical cord stump after birth; and cerebral hemorrhaging.

Prevalence

Hemophilia A and B affect 3,000 Canadians, with the most severe cases occurring almost exclusively in males.

Von Willebrand disease is the most common inherited bleeding disorder with one in 100 Canadians carrying the gene.

There are approximately 6,090 chronic adult ITP cases in Canada.

Treatment Options

The primary treatment for both hemophilia and von Willebrand disease is replacement therapy, whereby a concentrate of clotting factor is introduced intravenously. In the most serious cases of von Willebrand disease, and mild hemophilia, the synthetic hormone desmopressin may be used to stimulate the release of additional clotting factors by the body.

Instances of mild ITP may require no treatment apart from monitoring. Treatment of more serious cases can include the use of corticosteroids to help increase platelet levels. Steroids, however, have side effects and some patients relapse when treatment ends.

Blood Cancers

There are three main types of blood cancer: leukemia, lymphoma and myeloma.

Leukemia is a type of cancer found in the blood and bone marrow and occurs when there is rapid production of abnormal white blood cells.

Lymphoma is the name for a group of over 50 blood cancers that develop in the lymphatic system. It occurs when abnormal lymphocytes (a type of white blood cell that fights infection) multiply and collect in the lymph nodes and other tissues.

Myeloma, also known as multiple myeloma, is a cancer of the plasma cells in the bone marrow.

See also Cancer: Leukemia

Cause

The exact causes of blood cancers are unknown, although research points to genetic predisposition and environment as contributing factors.

Exposure to certain chemicals (e.g., benzene), exposure to radiation, and a weakened immune system may also be risk factors.

Symptoms

Leukemia symptoms can vary depending on the stage of the disease, but typically consist of fatigue, malaise, loss of appetite, weight loss, fever and anemia. There may be few or no symptoms in the early stages of chronic leukemia, which is slow growing. On the other hand, the symptoms of acute leukemia, which is fast growing, can be akin to the flu and come on suddenly within days or weeks.

The most common symptom of lymphoma is a painless swelling in a lymph node, called lymphadenopathy. Some lymphoma patients notice no swelling at all; others may complain of night sweats, weight loss, chills, a lack of energy or itching. There is usually no pain involved in the early stages of lymphoma.

A characteristic symptom of myeloma is pain in the lower back, ribs or sternum. The pain stems from osteolytic lesions that weaken the bone resulting in tiny fractures.

Prevalence

According to 2016 estimates, 5,900 Canadians were diagnosed with leukemia, 8,000 with Non-Hodgkin's lymphoma, 1,000 with Hodgkin's lymphoma, and 2,700 with multiple myeloma. Lymphoma has the fastest rising incidence rate among young adults.

Treatment Options

Chemotherapy, radiation therapy, biological therapy, corticosteroids and bone marrow and stem cell transplants are used to fight leukemia, lymphoma and myeloma.

National Associations

Aplastic Anemia & Myelodysplasia Association of Canada (AAMAC)

#321, 11181 Yonge St., Richmond Hill ON L4S 1L2

Tel: 905-780-0698; *Fax:* 905-780-1648
Toll-Free: 888-840-0039
e-mail: info@aamac.ca
www.aamac.ca

Previous Name: Aplastic Anemia Association of Canada
Overview: A small national charitable organization founded in 1987
Mission: To disseminate information concerning the disease; To form a nation-wide support network for patients, families & medical professionals; To support Canadian Blood Services & their programs; To raise funds for research
Member of: Health Charities Council of Canada
Affliation(s): Network of Rare Blood Disorders
Chief Officer(s):
Pam Wishart, President
Michelle Joseph, Secretary
Janice Cook, Coordinator, British Columbia
Bob Ross, Coordinator, Ontario

Association of Hemophilia Clinic Directors of Canada (AHCDC)

70 Bond St., Toronto ON M5B 1X3

Tel: 416-864-5042; *Fax:* 416-864-5251
e-mail: ahcdc@smh.ca
www.ahcdc.ca

Overview: A small national organization founded in 1994
Mission: To improve the treatment of people with hemophilia
Affiliation(s): Canadian Hemophilia Society
Chief Officer(s):
Annie Kaplan, Contact

Canadian Blood & Marrow Transplant Group (CBMTG) / Société Canadienne de greffe de cellules souches hematopoietiques

#400, 570 West 7th Ave., Vancouver BC V5Z 1B3

Tel: 604-874-4944; *Fax:* 604-874-4378
e-mail: cbmtg@malachite-mgmt.com
www.cbmtg.org

Overview: A small national organization
Mission: To provide leadership in the field of blood & marrow transplantation (BMT); to recognize & promote advances in clinical care; to promote basic, translational & clinical research & education; to represent BMT issues to government agencies, health care organizations & the public; to collaborate with fellow organizations
Chief Officer(s):
Ana Torres, Executive Director
ana.torres@malachite-mgmt.com
Publications:
• CBMTG [Canadian Blood & Marrow Transplant Group] Newsletter
Type: Newsletter; *Frequency:* Quarterly; *Editor:* Nancy Henderson
Profile: Professional news; case studies; clinical papers; questions; letters to the editor; industry news

Canadian Blood Services (CBS) / Societé canadienne du sang

1800 Alta Vista Dr., Ottawa ON K1G 4J5

Tel: 613-739-2300; *Fax:* 613-731-1411
Toll-Free: 888-236-6283
e-mail: feedback@blood.ca
www.blood.ca
www.linkedin.com/company/canadian-blood-services
www.facebook.com/itsinyoutogive
twitter.com/itsinyoutogive
www.youtube.com/18882DONATE

Previous Name: Canadian Red Cross - Blood Services
Overview: A medium-sized national organization founded in 1998
Mission: To manage the blood supply for Canadians; To ensure blood safety
Chief Officer(s):
Leah Hollins, Chair
Graham D. Sher, Chief Executive Officer
Publications:
• BloodNotes [a publication of Canadian Blood Services]
Type: Newsletter
Profile: Information & educational articles for hospital customers
• Canadian Blood Services Annual Report
Type: Yearbook; *Frequency:* Annually

Ancaster
35 Stone Church Rd., Ancaster ON L9K 1S5
Toll-Free: 888-236-6283
Chief Officer(s):
Dunbar Russel, Regional Representative, Ontario

Barrie
#100, 231 Bayview Dr., Barrie ON L4N 4Y5
Toll-Free: 888-823-6283

Brandon
c/o Westman Collection Site, Town Centre, 800 Rosser Ave., Brandon MB R7A 6N5
Toll-Free: 888-236-6283

Burlington
1250 Brant St., Burlington ON L7P 1X8
Toll-Free: 888-236-6283

Calgary
737 - 13th Ave., Calgary AB T2R 1J1
Toll-Free: 888-236-6283
Chief Officer(s):
Mike Shaw, Regional Representative, Alberta, Saskatchewan, Manitoba, Northwest Territories, & Nunavut

Charlottetown
85 Fitzroy St., Charlottetown PE C1A 1R6
Toll-Free: 888-236-6283
Chief Officer(s):
Jeff Scott, Regional Representative, Atlantic

Corner Brook
3 Herald Ave., Corner Brook NL A2H 4B8
Toll-Free: 888-236-6283

Edmonton
8249 - 114th St., Edmonton AB T6G 2R8
Toll-Free: 888-236-6283

Guelph
130 Silvercreek Pkwy. North, Guelph ON N1H 7Y5
Toll-Free: 888-236-6283

Halifax
#252, 7071 Bayers Rd., Halifax NS B3L 2C2
Toll-Free: 888-236-6283
Chief Officer(s):
Jeff Scott, Regional Representative, Atlantic

Kelowna
#103, 1865 Dilworth Dr., Kelowna BC V1Y 9T1
Toll-Free: 888-236-6283

Kingston
850 Gardiners Rd., Kingston ON K7M 3X9
Toll-Free: 888-236-6283

Kitchener-Waterloo

94 Bridgeport Rd. East, Waterloo ON N2J 2J9
Toll-Free: 888-263-3283

Lethbridge
Lethbridge Centre Mall, #220, 200 - 4 Ave. South, Lethbridge AB T1J 4C9
Toll-Free: 888-236-6283

London
820 Wharncliffe Rd. South, London ON N6J 2N4
Toll-Free: 888-236-6283

Chief Officer(s):
Dunbar Russel, Regional Representative, Ontario

Mississauga
#15, 785 Britannia Rd. West, Mississauga ON L5V 2Y1
Toll-Free: 888-236-6283

Moncton
500 Mapleton Rd., Moncton NB E1G 0N3
Toll-Free: 888-236-6283

Oshawa
1300 Harmony Rd. North, Oshawa ON L1K 2B1
Toll-Free: 888-236-6283

Ottawa
1575 Carling Ave., Ottawa ON K1Z 7M3
Tel: 613-560-7440
Toll-Free: 888-236-6283

Chief Officer(s):
Dunbar Russel, Regional Representative, Ontario

Ottawa - Alta Vista Dr. - National Fundraising Office
1800 Alta Vista Dr., Ottawa ON K1G 4J5
Tel: 613-739-2300; Fax: 613-739-2141
Toll-Free: 888-236-6283
campaignforcanadians.ca

Chief Officer(s):
Penny Holmes-Tuor, Manager
penny.holmes-tuor@blood.ca

Peterborough
55 George St. North, Peterborough ON K9J 3G2
Toll-Free: 888-236-6283

Prince George
2277 Westwood Dr., Prince George BC V2N 4V6
Toll-Free: 888-236-6283

Red Deer
#5, 5020 - 68th St., Red Deer AB T4N 7B4
Toll-Free: 888-236-6283

Regina
2571 Broad St., Regina SK S4P 4H6
Toll-Free: 888-236-6283

Chief Officer(s):
Mike Shaw, Regional Representative, Alberta, Saskatchewan, Manitoba, Northwest Territories, & Nunavut

Saint John
405 University Ave., Saint John NB E2L 4G7
Toll-Free: 888-236-6283

Chief Officer(s):
Jeff Scott, Regional Representative, Atlantic

St Catharines
#395, 397 Ontario St., St Catharines ON L2N 4M8
Toll-Free: 888-236-6283

St. John's
7 Wicklow St., St. John's NL A1B 3Z9
Toll-Free: 888-236-6283

Chief Officer(s):
Jeff Scott, Regional Representative, Atlantic

Sarnia
Bayside Mall, 150 Christina St. North, Sarnia ON N7T 7W5
Toll-Free: 888-236-6283

Saskatoon
325 - 20th St. East, Saskatoon SK S7K 0A9
Toll-Free: 888-236-6283

Chief Officer(s):

Mike Shaw, Regional Representative, Alberta, Saskatchewan, Manitoba, Northwest Territories, & Nunavut

Sudbury
235 Cedar St., Sudbury ON P3B 1M8
Tel: 705-674-4003
Toll-Free: 888-236-6283

Chief Officer(s):
Dunbar Russel, Regional Representative, Ontario

Sudbury - National Contact Centre
235 Cedar St., Sudbury ON P3B 1M8
Tel: 705-674-4003; Fax: 705-674-7165
Toll-Free: 888-236-6283

Surrey
15285 - 101 Ave., Surrey BC V3R 8X8
Toll-Free: 888-236-6283

Sydney
850 Grand Lake Rd., Sydney NS B1P 5T9
Toll-Free: 888-236-6283

Toronto - Bay & Bloor
Manulife Centre, 55 Bloor St. West, 2nd Fl., Toronto ON M4W 1A5
Toll-Free: 888-236-6283

Toronto - College St.
67 College St., Toronto ON M5G 2M1
Toll-Free: 888-236-6283

Chief Officer(s):
Dunbar Russel, Regional Representative, Ontario

Toronto - King Street
163 King St. West, Main Fl., Toronto ON M5H 4H2
Toll-Free: 888-236-6283

Vancouver - Oak Street
4750 Oak St., Vancouver BC V6H 2N9
Tel: 604-707-3400
Toll-Free: 888-236-6283

Vancouver - Standard Life
888 Dunsmur St., 2nd Fl., Vancouver BC V6C 3K4
Toll-Free: 888-236-6283

Victoria
3449 Saanich Rd., Victoria BC V8X 1W9
Toll-Free: 888-236-6283

Windsor
3909 Grand Marais Rd. East, Windsor ON N8W 1W9
Toll-Free: 888-236-6283

Winnipeg
777 William Ave., Winnipeg MB R3E 3R4
Toll-Free: 888-236-6283

Chief Officer(s):
Mike Shaw, Regional Representative, Alberta, Saskatchewan, Manitoba, Northwest Territories, & Nunavut

Canadian Hemochromatosis Society (CHS) / Société canadienne de l'hémochromatose
#285, 7000 Minoru Blvd., Richmond BC V6Y 3Z5
Tel: 604-279-7135; Fax: 604-279-7138
Toll-Free: 877-223-4766
e-mail: office@toomuchiron.ca
www.toomuchiron.ca
www.linkedin.com/groups/Canadian-Hemochromatosis-Society-109623
7
www.facebook.com/TooMuchIron
twitter.com/IronOutCanada
www.youtube.com/user/toomuchiron

Overview: A medium-sized national charitable organization founded in 1982
Mission: To increase awareness among the public & medical community with regards to the importance of family screening, early diagnosis & treatment of Hemochromatosis
Member of: International Association of Haemochromatosis Societies
Affliation(s): Haemochromatosis Society of Great Britain; Haemochromatosis Society of Southern Africa; American Hemochromatosis Society Inc.; Association hémochromatose France;

Haemochromatosis Society Australia; Iron Disorders Institute of America

Chief Officer(s):
Patrick Haney, President & Chair
Bob Rogers, Executive Director & CEO

Publications:
• Iron Filings: Newsletter of The Canadian Hemochromatosis Society
Type: Newsletter; *Frequency:* Semiannually; *Price:* Free for members
Profile: Current research, news about hemochromatosis, dietary information, stories, & CHS member information

Canadian Hemophilia Society (CHS) / Société canadienne de l'hémophilie (SCHQ)

#301, 666 Sherbrooke St. West, Montréal QC H3A 1E7
Tel: 514-848-0503; *Fax:* 514-848-9661
Toll-Free: 800-668-2686
e-mail: chs@hemophilia.ca
www.hemophilia.ca
www.facebook.com/CanadianHemophiliaSociety
twitter.com/CHShemophilia
www.youtube.com/user/CanadianHemophilia

Overview: A medium-sized national charitable organization founded in 1953
Mission: To find a cure & to provide services to people with hemophilia or other inherited bleeding disorders; To serve persons infected with HIV or hepatitis through blood & blood products; To enhance the health & quality of life of individuals affected by inherited bleeding disorders
Affliation(s): World Federation of Hemophilia

Chief Officer(s):
David Page, National Executive Director
dpage@hemophilia.ca
Hélène Bourgaize, National Director, Chapter Relations & Human Resources
hbourgaize@hemophilia.ca
Deborah Franz Currie, National Director, Resource Development
dcurrie@hemophilia.ca

Publications:
• All About Carriers
Number of Pages: 133
Profile: Comprehensive guide, for carriers of hemophilia A or B
• All About von Willebrand Disease
Number of Pages: 86
Profile: A comprehensive guide, for persons with the disease
• Canadian Hemophilia Society Annual Report & Financial Statement
Frequency: Annually
• Factor Deficiencies
Profile: A series of publications, with topics such as Factor XI Deficiency, An Inherited Bleeding Disorder, for patients, families, & healthcare providers
• Hemophilia Today
Type: Magazine; *Frequency:* 3 pa; *Editor:* François Laroche
Profile: Current news & relevant issues to inform the hemophilia & bleeding disorders community

Alberta Chapter
PO Box 44171, Edmonton AB T5V 1N6
Toll-Free: 800-668-2686
e-mail: albertachapter@hemophilia.ca
www.hemophilia.ca/en/provincial-chapters/alberta
Chief Officer(s):
Hillary Nemeth, Co-President
Sheri Spady, Co-President

British Columbia Chapter
PO Box 21161, Stn. Maple Ridge Sq., Maple Ridge BC V2X 1P7
Tel: 778-230-9661
e-mail: chsbc@shaw.ca
www.hemophiliabc.ca
Chief Officer(s):
Curtis Brandell, President

Hemophilia Manitoba

944 Portage Ave., Winnipeg MB R3G 0R1
Tel: 204-775-8625; *Fax:* 204-774-9403
Toll-Free: 866-775-8625
e-mail: info@hemophiliamb.ca
www.hemophiliamb.ca
www.facebook.com/186587534783298
twitter.com/HemophiliaMB
www.youtube.com/user/hemophiliamb
Chief Officer(s):
Christine Keilback, Executive Director

Hemophilia Ontario
#10100, 4711 Yonge St., Toronto ON M2N 6K8
Tel: 416-972-0641; *Fax:* 888-958-0307
Toll-Free: 888-838-8846
www.hemophilia.ca/en/provincial-chapters/ontario
Chief Officer(s):
Matthew Maynard, Interim Executive Director
mmaynard@hemophilia.on.ca

Hemophilia Saskatchewan
2366 Ave. C North, Saskatoon SK S7L 5X5
Tel: 306-653-4366
Toll-Free: 866-953-4366
e-mail: hemosask@hemophilia.ca
www.hemophiliask.ca/hemophilia-saskatchewan.html
www.facebook.com/HemophiliaSaskatchewan
twitter.com/HemophiliaSask
Chief Officer(s):
Wendy Quinn, President

New Brunswick Chapter
#173, 337 Rothesay Ave., Saint John NB E2J 2C3
Tel: 506-608-0031
www.hemophilia.ca/en/provincial-chapters/new-brunswick
Chief Officer(s):
Victoria Watts, President
president@chsnb.com

Newfoundland & Labrador Chapter
25 Main Rd., Cavendish NL A0B 1J0
e-mail: chsnlcc@nf.sympatico.ca
hemophilia.ca/en/provincial-chapters/newfoundland-and-labrador
Chief Officer(s):
Jenny Jacobs, President

Nova Scotia Chapter
17 Malcolm Lucas Dr., Enfield NS B2T 1A8
Tel: 902-883-7111
e-mail: nshemophiliasociety@hotmail.com
www.hemophilia.ca/en/provincial-chapters/nova-scotia
Chief Officer(s):
Betty-Anne Hines, President

Prince Edward Island Chapter
PO Box 2951, Charlottetown PE C1A 8C5
www.hemophilia.ca/en/provincial-chapters/prince-edward-island
Chief Officer(s):
Shelley Mountain, President

Section Québec
#514, 2120, rue Sherbrooke Est, Montréal QC H2K 1C3
Tél: 514-848-0666; *Téléc:* 514-904-2253
Ligne sans frais: 877-870-0666
Courriel: info@schq.org
www.hemophilia.ca/fr/sections-provinciales/quebec
www.facebook.com/27424888399
Chief Officer(s):
François Laroche, Président

International Associations

World Federation of Hemophilia (WFH) / Fédération mondiale de l'hémophilie (FMH)
#1010, 1425, boul René-Lévesque ouest, Montréal QC H3G 1T7
Tel: 514-875-7944; *Fax:* 514-875-8916
e-mail: wfh@wfh.org
www.wfh.org
www.facebook.com/wfhemophilia
twitter.com/wfhemophilia
www.youtube.com/user/WFHcommunications
Overview: A medium-sized international licensing organization founded in 1963
Mission: To introduce, improve & maintain care for people with hemophilia & related blood disorders around the world
Affliation(s): World Health Organization; International Society of Blood Transfusion; International Committee on Thrombosis & Haemostasis; International Society of Haematology; Société internationale de chirurgie orthopédique (SICOT)
Chief Officer(s):
Alain Baumann, Chief Executive Officer
Sarah Ford, Director, Strategy & Communications
sford@wfh.org

Brain Tumours

Cause
Brain tumours are either primary (originate in the brain) or metastatic (travel from other cancer sites). Although some primary brain tumours have a genetic basis, and previous radiation treatment to the head is considered a risk factor, in most cases, the cause of a brain tumour is not known. There are many different types of brain tumours, each with a distinctive appearance under the microscope and a characteristic pattern of onset, progression, location and response to treatment. Not all brain tumours are malignant, but benign tumours also can cause serious problems and interfere with normal brain activity.

Symptoms
Depending on the exact site and rate of growth of the tumour, symptoms vary, but seizures and headache are among the most common. Other symptoms may include change in personality, moodiness, impaired vision and hearing, problems with memory, dizziness, confusion, disorientation, nausea, vomiting, lethargy and a varying degree of weakness.

Prevalence
Although the Canadian medical system does not track statistics on primary brain tumours, it is estimated that there are 55,000 Canadians living with a brain tumour, and about 5,000 new cases occur in Canada every year. Malignant brain tumours originating in the brain make up roughly 2 percent of all cancers. They may occur at any age but are most common in early adult and middle life. Metastatic brain tumours occur at some point in 20 to 40 percent of all people with cancer, and their incidence is increasing as cancer patients are living longer.

Treatment Options
Brain tumours are diagnosed with computed tomography (CT) scans and magnetic resonance imaging (MRI).

The treatment of brain tumours, as in many other cancers, consists of a combination of surgical removal, chemotherapy and radiation therapy. Surgery is generally the first step if the tumour is accessible and vital structures will not be disturbed. Radiation is used to stop a tumour's growth or cause it to shrink. Chemotherapy destroys tumour cells that may remain after surgery and radiation. Steroids reduce swelling, and anti-seizure medication is commonly given. If the disease or its treatment has caused damage to the brain's functioning, the patient may also need physical therapy, speech therapy or general supportive care.

The prognosis depends on the patient's age and on the location, extent and precise type of the tumour.

National Associations

Acoustic Neuroma Association of Canada (ANAC) / Association pour les neurinomes acoustiques du Canada
PO Box 1005, 7B Pleasant Blvd., Toronto ON M4T 1K2
Tel: 416-546-6426
Toll-Free: 800-561-2622
www.anac.ca
Overview: A medium-sized national charitable organization founded in 1984
Mission: To provide support & information for those who have experienced acoustic neuromas or other tumors affecting the cranial nerves; To furnish information on patient rehabilitation to physicians & health care personnel; To promote & support research; To educate the public regarding symptoms suggestive of acoustic neuromas, thus promoting early diagnosis & consequent successful treatment
Chief Officer(s):
Carole Humphries, Executive Director

Brain Tumour Foundation of Canada (BTFC) / La Fondation canadienne sur les tumeurs cérébrales
#301, 620 Colborne St., London ON N6B 3R9
Tel: 519-642-7755; *Fax:* 519-642-7192
Toll-Free: 800-265-5106
www.braintumour.ca
www.facebook.com/BrainTumourFoundationofCanada
twitter.com/BrainTumourFdn
www.youtube.com/BrainTumourFdn
Overview: A small national charitable organization founded in 1982
Mission: To find a cure for brain tumors & to improve the quality of life for those affected; To fund brain tumor research; to provide patient & family support services; To educate the public
Member of: North American Brain Tumor Coalition; Canadian Alliance of Brain Tumor Organizations
Chief Officer(s):
Carl Cadogan, CEO
Publications:
• BrainStorm
Type: Newsletter

Canadian Association for Neuroscience (CAN)
c/o DeArmond Management, 2661 Queenswood Dr., Victoria BC V8N 1X6
Tel: 250-472-7644
e-mail: info@can-acn.org
can-acn.org
www.facebook.com/can.acn
twitter.com/CAN_ACN
Overview: A large national organization
Mission: To promote communication among Canadian neuroscientists & encourage research related to the nervous system; To educate about current neuroscience research
Chief Officer(s):
Julie Poupart, Director, Communications

Canadian Association of Electroneurophysiology Technologists Inc. (CAET) / Association canadienne des technologues en electroneurophysiologie inc. (ACTE)
c/o St. Boniface Hospital, 409 Taché Ave., Winnipeg MB R2H 2A6
Tel: 204-233-8563
www.caet.org
Overview: A small national organization founded in 1951
Mission: To advance the knowledge, science, & technology of electroneurophysiology in Canada
Affliation(s): Canadian Board of Registration of Electroencephalograph Technologists Inc. (CBRET)
Chief Officer(s):
Joanne Nikkel, President
joanne.nikkel@caet.org
Bruce Goddard, Vice-President
bruce.goddard@caet.org
Jodi Kent, Secretary & Registrar
jodi.kent@caet.org

Publications:
• Canadian Association of Electroneurophysiology Technologists Inc. Membership Directory
Type: Directory

Canadian Board of Registration of Electroencephalograph Technologists Inc. (CBRET)

c/o Hospital for Sick Children, 555 University Ave., 6th Fl, Atrium 6C, Toronto ON M5G 1X8

Tel: 416-813-6545; *Fax:* 416-813-6709
cbret.org

Overview: A small national licensing organization founded in 1972 overseen by Canadian Association of Electroneurophysiology Technologists, Inc.
Mission: To offer registration & certification procedures for the electroneurodiagnostic profession of electroencephalography (EEG), as regulated by the College of Physicians & Surgeons in each province & territory; To conduct written & oral-practical examinations to determine the knowledge & skills of EEG technologists
Affliation(s): Canadian Association of Electroneurophysiology Technologists (CAET)
Chief Officer(s):
Rohit Sharma, Registrar

Canadian Brain Tumour Consortium (CBTC)

c/o Sunnybrook Health Sciences Centre, #402A, 2075 Bayview Ave., Toronto ON M4N 3M5

Tel: 416-480-4766; *Fax:* 416-480-5054
e-mail: headquarters@cbtc.ca
www.cbtc.ca

Overview: A small national organization founded in 1998
Mission: To act as a national investigator network in the treatment of pediatric & adult patients with brain tumour
Affliation(s): Canadian Congress of Neurological Sciences

Canadian Brain Tumour Tissue Bank

London Health Sciences Centre, University of Western Ontario, 339 Windermere Rd., #C7108, London ON N6A 5A5

Tel: 519-663-3427; *Fax:* 519-663-2930
www.braintumor.ca

Also Known As: Brain Tumor Tissue Bank
Overview: A small national organization
Mission: To supply optimally collected brain tumour tissue to researchers all over the country, internationally & locally in the hopes that some day the cause of & the cure for brain tumours will be found
Affliation(s): The Brain Tumour Foundation of Canada
Chief Officer(s):
Marcela White, Coordinator
marcela.white@lhsc.on.ca

Canadian Neurological Society (CNS) / Société canadienne de neurologie

#709, 7015 Macleod Trail SW, Calgary AB T2H 2K1

Tel: 403-229-9544; *Fax:* 403-229-1661
www.cnsfederation.org

Overview: A medium-sized national organization overseen by Canadian Neurological Sciences Federation
Mission: To promote & encourage all aspects of neurology, including research, education, assessment & accreditation; provide for annual scientific sessions to promote the knowledge & practice of neurology
Chief Officer(s):
Dan Morin, CNSF CEO
dan-morin@cnsfederation.org
Marika Fitzgerald, CNSF Controller
marika-fitzgerald@cnsfederation.org
Publications:
• The Canadian Journal of Neurological Sciences
Type: Journal; *Frequency:* Bimonthly; *Accepts Advertising*; *Editor:* G. Bryan Young; *Price:* Free with CNS membership
Profile: Peer-reviewed original articles

Canadian Society of Clinical Neurophysiologists (CSCN) / Société canadienne de neurophysiologistes cliniques

#709, 7015 Macleod Trail SW, Calgary AB T2H 2K6
Tel: 403-229-9544; *Fax:* 403-229-1661
www.cnsfederation.org

Overview: A small national organization founded in 1990 overseen by Canadian Neurological Sciences Federation
Mission: To promote & encourage all aspects of neurophysiology, including research & education, in addition to assessment & accreditation in the field
Member of: Canadian Neurological Sciences Federation
Affliation(s): Cdn. Brain Tumour Consortium; Cdn. Epilepsy Consortium; Cdn. Stroke Consortium; Cdn. League Against Epilepsy; Cdn. Headache Society; Cdn. Movement Disorders Group; Cdn. Network of MS Clinics; Cdn. Neurocritical Care Group; Amyotrophic Lateral Sclerosis Research Foundation; Consortium of Canadian Centres for Clinical Cognitive Research; Associate Societies: Assn. of Electromyography Technologists of Canada; Canadian Assn. of Electroneurophysiology Technologists; Canadian Assn. of Neuroscience; Canadian Assn. of Neuroscience Nurses; Canadian Assn. of Physical Medicine & Rehabilitation
Chief Officer(s):
Dan Morin, CNSF CEO
dan-morin@cnsfederation.org
Publications:
• Canadian Journal of Neurological Sciences
Type: Journal; *Frequency:* Bimonthly; *Accepts Advertising*; *Editor:* G. Bryan Young
Profile: Peer-reviewed original articles

Neurological Health Charities Canada (NHCC)

c/o Parkinson Canada, #316, 4211 Yonge St., Toronto ON M2P 2A9
Tel: 416-227-9700; *Fax:* 416-227-9600
Toll-Free: 800-565-3000
e-mail: info@mybrainmatters.ca
www.mybrainmatters.ca
www.facebook.com/MyBrainMatters
twitter.com/MyBrainMatters
www.youtube.com/MyBrainMatters

Overview: A large national charitable organization
Mission: To improve quality of life for persons with chronic brain conditions & their caregivers; To increase awareness in the government about neurological issues; To support research
Chief Officer(s):
Joyce Gordon, Chair
Publications:
• Brain Matters [a publication of Neurological Health Charities Canada]
Type: Newsletter; *Frequency:* s-a.

Provincial Associations

ALBERTA

Alberta Neurosurgical Society

c/o Southern Alberta Office, Alberta Medical Association, #350, 708 - 11 Ave. SW, Calgary AB T2R 0E4
Tel: 403-266-3533; *Fax:* 403-269-3538
Toll-Free: 866-830-1274

Overview: A small provincial organization founded in 1947
Affliation(s): Alberta Medical Association
Chief Officer(s):
John H. Wong, President
jwong@ucalgary.ca

BRITISH COLUMBIA

British Columbia Society of Electroneurophysiology Technologists (BCSET)

c/o EEG Department, Penticton Regional Hospital, 550 Carmi Ave., Penticton BC V2A 3G6

Tel: 250-492-1000; *Fax:* 250-492-9037
e-mail: webmaster@bcset.org
www.bcset.org

Overview: A small provincial organization
Mission: A professional non-profit association dedicated to fostering excellence in diagnostic electroneurophysiology, furthering education and providing a forum for discussion and interaction.
Affliation(s): Canadian Association of Electroneurophysiology Technologists
Chief Officer(s):
Tara Cassidy, President

QUÉBEC

Association de neurochirurgie du Québec (ANCQ)
CP 216, Succ. Desjardins, #3000, 2, Complexe Desjardins, Montréal
QC H5B 1G8

Tél: 514-350-5120; Téléc: 514-350-5100
Courriel: ancq@fmsq.org
www.ancq.net

Aperçu: Dimension: petite; Envergure: provinciale; fondée en 1965
surveillé par Fédération des médecins spécialistes du Québec
Mission: Pour représenter les médecins spécialistes et de promouvoir
leurs intérêts
Membre de: Fédération des Médecins Spécialistes de Québec
(FMSQ)
Membre(s) du bureau directeur:
David Mathieu, Président
Manon Gaudry, Directrice, Administration
Publications:
• Interneurone
Type: Newsletter

Association des neurologues du Québec (ANQ)
CP 216, Succ. Desjardins, #3000, 2, Complexe Desjardins, Montréal
QC H5B 1G8

Tél: 514-350-5122; Téléc: 514-350-5172
Courriel: anq@fmsq.org
www.anq.qc.ca
www.facebook.com/109136899239391
twitter.com/assneuroquebec

Aperçu: Dimension: petite; Envergure: provinciale surveillé par
Fédération des médecins spécialistes du Québec
Mission: Représenter des médecins spécialistes qui diagnostique et
traite les maladies affectant le système nerveux central ainsi que le
système nerveux périphérique
Membre(s) du bureau directeur:
Sylvain Chouinard, Président
Anne Lortie, Secrétaire
Ginette Guilbault, Directrice, Administration

Local Associations

BRITISH COLUMBIA

North Okanagan Neurological Association (NONA)
2802 - 34th St., Vernon BC V1T 5X1

Tel: 250-549-1281; Fax: 250-549-3771
e-mail: administration@nona-cdc.com
www.nona-cdc.com
www.facebook.com/NONAChildDevelopmentCentre

Overview: A small local organization founded in 1975
Mission: To provide services for the treatment, education & support of
special needs children & their families
Member of: B.C. Association of Child Development & Rehabilitation
Affiliation(s): Cerebral Palsy Association of British Columbia
Chief Officer(s):
Janice Foster, Executive Director

National Publications

Canadian Journal of Neurological Sciences
c/o Canadian Neurological Sciences Federation, 143N Heritage
Square, #8500 Macleod Trail SE, Calgary, AB T2H 2N1

Tel: 403-229-9544; Fax: 403-229-1661

Circulation: 1,200 Frequency: Bi-monthly
The journal is the official publication of the four member societies of the
Canadian Neurological Sciences Federation: Canadian Neurological
Society (CNS), Canadian Neurosurgical Society (CNSS), Canadian
Association of Child Neurology (CACN), & the Canadian Society of
Clinical Neurophysiologists (CSCN). Peer reviewed articles about the
neurosciences are published in the Canadian Journal of Neurological
Sciences. The journal is circulated to society members, non-members,
& institutions in Canada & around the world.
Lisa Arrington, Managing Editor, larrington@cambridge.org

Provincial Libraries

Montréal Neurological Institute & Hospital
#285, 3801, rue University, Montréal, QC H3A 2B4

Tel: 514-398-1980; Fax: 514-398-5077
library.neuro@mcgill.ca
Social Media: www.facebook.com/MNIHLIB
Collection: Neurosciences collection
Alex Amar, Librarian
alex.amar@muhc.mcgill.ca

Cancer

Cancer is a general term for more than 100 diseases characterized by abnormal or uncontrolled growth of cells. The resulting
mass, or disease, can invade and destroy surrounding normal tissue. Cancer cells from the tumour can also spread (metastasize)
through the blood or lymph (plasmatic fluid) to start new cancers
in other parts of the body. In 2016, about 202,400 new cancer
cases (excluding non-melanoma skin cancer) were diagnosed,
and about 78,800 Canadians died from their disease. Cancer is
the leading cause of death in Canada, and a continued increase
in new cases is expected. Although these figures seem bleak,
most cancers are potentially curable if detected at an early stage.

Cancer, also called a malignancy (from Latin, meaning bad), can
be either a solid tumour (carcinoma), such as lung cancer, or a
disorder of blood cell formation, such as leukemia.

Cancer is caused by an interplay of internal and external factors,
individually or in combination. Abnormal genes can cause multiple changes that affect cell growth. Environmental factors, such
as cigarette smoke (also called a carcinogen-causing cancer)
and exposure to radiation, play a role. Many cancers can be prevented by health awareness. For example, skin cancer could be
drastically reduced by protection from solar rays. Lung cancer,
one of the most prevalent and hazardous cancers, could be drastically reduced by eliminating tobacco use. The Canadian Cancer
Society estimates that 30 percent of all cancer deaths are related
to cigarette smoking.

Cancer treatment may be curative—removes the tumour in the
hope that it will not reoccur, or palliative—prolongs life and mini-
mizes discomfort when a cure is not possible. A treatment program typically includes a combination of surgery, radiation
therapy and chemotherapy. Immunotherapy is the newest form of
treatment and uses agents known as biologic-response modifiers
(BRM), to alter the immune system in its response to malignant
growth. Brief descriptions of the more common cancers follow.

Brain Cancer
The seriousness of brain tumours is determined by their size, location and rate of growth. While brain cancer does not normally
spread to other areas, many other cancers have the propensity of
spreading throughout the nervous system and producing metastatic tumours in the brain. In adults, these tumours are most
commonly from cancer of the lung, breast or skin (melanoma).

Cause
Risk factors for developing brain cancer include previous radiation therapy to the head and certain genetic conditions such as tuberous sclerosis and neurofibromatosis.

Symptoms
Symptoms of brain cancer include headaches, seizures, behaviour problems, changes in eating or sleeping habits, lethargy, dizziness, confusion, memory problems and clumsiness.

Prevalence

Brain cancer occurs at varying rates but overall it comprises approximately 7 cases per 100,000 people in Canada each year. It is most common in people between the ages of 50 and 70. Overall incidence is greater in males than females for most types of brain cancer.

Treatment Options

To diagnose brain cancer, a physician usually takes a complete medical history and performs a physical and neurological exam. Imaging tests such as X-rays, computed tomography (CT) scans or magnetic resonance imaging (MRI) may also be ordered to detect the size of the tumour and to determine if the tumour has spread. To confirm the diagnosis, a biopsy (a procedure where cells are removed from the body and checked to see if they are cancerous) is performed.

Surgery is the most common treatment for brain tumours. In cases where surgery is not possible, part of the tumour still remains after surgery or a tumour has come back, radiation therapy is often also used. Chemotherapy may be given after surgery or in combination with radiation therapy. Steroids may be prescribed to reduce swelling around a brain tumour, and anticonvulsants may be given to patients who are experiencing seizures as a result of a brain tumour.

The five-year net survival rate for patients with brain or spinal cord cancer in Canada is about 24 percent.

See also Brain Tumours

Breast Cancer

Most cases of breast cancer begin in the breast tissue, either in the ducts or the lobules (glands). Ductal carcinoma is the most common type of breast cancer.

Cause

Incidence of breast cancer increases under the following conditions: age (two-thirds of cases develop after age 55), a close relative (mother, sister) with breast cancer, a previous history of breast cancer, a family history of ovarian cancer, exposure to radiation and dense breast tissue. Other risk factors include not having children, early onset of menstruation, late onset of menopause and estrogen replacement therapy. Obesity, drinking alcohol and taking birth control pills may slightly increase the risk of developing breast cancer.

Symptoms

Warning signs that can aid women in detecting breast cancer include lumps, redness, swelling, skin irritation, changes in breast size or shape, tenderness or inversion of the nipple and dimpling of the skin.

Prevalence

Breast cancer is the most common malignant tumour diagnosed in women in Canada. Approximately 25,700 new cases of breast cancer in women were diagnosed in 2016, and 4,900 women died of the disease. As many as one in nine women will develop breast cancer during her lifetime and 1 in 28 will die of it.

Treatment Options

Early detection of breast cancer can be lifesaving. The Canadian Cancer Society recommends that women aged 40 to 49 should talk to a physician about their risks of breast cancer, as well as the benefits and risks of mammography. Women between the ages of 50 and 69 should undergo mammography every two years, and women over 70 should talk to a physician about how often they should have a mammogram.

To confirm diagnosis of breast cancer, a number of tests are usually ordered including a mammogram and other imaging tests such as an ultrasound or computed tomography (CT) scan to detect the size of the tumour and to determine if it has spread. Next, a biopsy (a procedure where cells are removed from the body and checked to see if they are cancerous) is usually performed. In order to identify the type of breast cancer and determine the best treatment option for the patient, laboratory tests such as a hormone receptor status test and a human epidermal growth factor receptor 2 (Her2) test are usually ordered, as well.

Treatments vary, depending on when the cancer is discovered and whether it has spread. Research has shown that the traditional radical mastectomy (removal of the entire breast) can often be replaced by lumpectomy (removal of just the tumour), coupled with radiation therapy. Chemotherapy or hormonal therapy is also prescribed in some cases. Biological therapy (such as Herceptin) may be used for women with invasive breast cancer. The five-year net survival rate for women with breast cancer is 87 percent.

Colorectal Cancer

Colorectal cancer usually begins in the cells that line the rectum or colon, and grows slowly.

Cause

Incidence of colorectal cancer increases in people who are over the age of 50; are male; have a family history of colorectal cancer; are obese; eat low-fiber diets that are high in animal protein, fat and refined carbohydrates; are physically inactive; smoke; drink an excessive amount of alcohol; have inflammatory bowel disease; and have polyps (small growths on the inner wall of the rectum and colon).

Symptoms

Symptoms vary, depending on the location and size of the tumour. Vague signs include weight loss, reduced appetite and general malaise. More specific signs include rectal bleeding, blood in the stool or a change in bowel habits.

Prevalence

In Canada, colon and rectal (colorectal) cancer account for more new cases of cancer per year than any other anatomic site except the lung and prostate. In 2016, an estimated 26,100 Canadians were diagnosed with colorectal cancer, and 9,300 died from it.

Treatment Options

With early diagnosis, colorectal cancer is curable. The Canadian Cancer Society recommends that people over the age of 50 who are at average risk of developing colorectal cancer have a fecal occult blood test (FOBT) or a fecal immunochemical test (FIT) every two years to check the stool for the presence of blood. If the test is positive, flexible sigmoidoscopy in which the doctor inserts a thin, flexible tube into the rectum, or a colonoscopy, performed when a tumour is believed to be higher up the colon, are used to visualize abnormalities and take a tissue sample (biopsy).

Treatment consists of surgical removal of the tumour, followed by radiotherapy or chemotherapy. Biological therapy (drugs made from natural body substances) is now a promising treatment for colorectal cancer at some stages.

The five-year net survival rate for patients with colorectal cancer in Canada is about 64 percent.

Leukemia

Leukemia is a disorder that usually begins in the bone marrow and is characterized by uncontrolled growth of abnormal and immature white or red blood cells. There are two forms of leukemia:

acute, which develops suddenly, worsens quickly and requires immediate treatment, and chronic which develops slowly often with few if any symptoms in the early stages of the disease. Although leukemia is often thought of as a childhood disease, it strikes 10 times as many adults as children.

Symptoms
Warning signs of leukemia are related to the disruption of the different cells in the blood: weakness and fatigue are caused by anemia (decreased red blood cells); easy bruising and hemorrhages (such as nosebleeds) from reduced clotting cells (platelets); and repeated infections from abnormal white cells. Generalized symptoms include weight loss and malaise.

Prevalence
In 2016, 5,900 new cases of leukemia were diagnosed in Canada, and 2,900 people died of the disease.

Treatment Options
To diagnose leukemia, a physician takes a detailed medical history, performs a physical exam and then orders a number of tests to confirm the diagnosis. These tests may include blood tests, a biopsy (a procedure in which a bone marrow sample is removed and checked for leukemia cells) and a lumbar puncture (a procedure in which cerebrospinal fluid is removed and checked for leukemia cells). If tests are positive, cytogenetic tests (chromosome analyses) are done on the bone marrow sample to help identify the type of leukemia.

Treatment for leukemia may include chemotherapy, radiation therapy, biological therapy (for example, monoclonal antibodies and interferon alfa, depending on the type of leukemia) and targeted therapy (for example, cancer growth inhibitors that limit the ability of the cancer cells to grow and divide). Transfusions restore red cells and platelets, and frequent infections are treated with antibiotics. Stem cell transplants, in which new blood cells are provided, are one of the most recent and successful advances in the treatment of this disease.

New treatment, especially for acute leukemia in children, has resulted in dramatic improvements in 5-year survival rates. Today, the 5-year relative survival rate for Canadian children 15 and under with acute leukemia is between 61 and 91 percent.

Liver Cancer
Liver cancer can either be primary, meaning that it started in the cells, bile ducts, blood vessels or tissue of the liver, or secondary, meaning that cancer started somewhere else in the body and then spread to the liver.

Cause
Risk factors for liver cancer include hepatitis B infection, hepatitis C infection, exposure to any agent that causes liver damage (for example, certain industrial chemicals) and cirrhosis of the liver. The remaining patients have no underlying liver disorder.

Symptoms
Symptoms include right upper abdominal pain, weight loss, fatigue, nausea, weakness and a mass on the upper right side of the abdomen.

Prevalence
In 2016, 2,400 new cases of liver cancer were diagnosed in Canada, and 1,200 people died of the disease.

Treatment Options
To diagnose liver cancer, a physician usually takes a detailed medical history and performs a physical exam, looking for signs of fluid buildup or masses in the abdomen or jaundice in the skin

and eyes. To confirm the diagnosis, a series of tests may be ordered including liver function tests (blood tests), a biopsy (a procedure in which a small sample of liver tissue is removed to check for cancerous cells) and imaging tests such as X-rays, computed tomography (CT) scans or magnetic resonance imaging (MRI) to detect the size of the tumour and to determine if the tumour has spread. A laparoscopy, a procedure in which a thin, flexible tube with a tiny camera at the end is inserted through a small cut in the abdomen in order to examine the liver and other nearby organs and take tissue samples, may also be performed.

The most effective treatment for tumours that can be removed and for liver cancer that has not spread is surgery. If the tumours cannot be removed, procedures such as cryosurgery (in which cancer cells are destroyed by freezing them), radiofrequency ablation (where a high-frequency electrical current is used to heat the cancer cells, thereby destroying them) or percutaneous injection (where liquid ethanol is injected into the tumour to kill cancer cells) are sometimes used. Chemotherapy or radiation therapy commonly follows these procedures.

The five-year net survival rate for patients with liver cancer in Canada is about 19 percent.

See also Liver Disease

Lung Cancer
Lung cancer begins in the lung cells, but can spread (metastasize) to other parts of the body. There are two types of lung cancer. Small cell lung cancer (SCLC) develops quickly, often metastasizes and is most commonly diagnosed in smokers. Non-small cell lung cancer develops more slowly and is the most common form of the disease.

Cause
Cigarette smoking and exposure to industrial substances, such as asbestos, are strongly linked to lung cancer. Recent research has shown that exposure to secondhand smoke increases the risk for this disease.

Symptoms
Warning signs of lung cancer are persistent coughing, shortness of breath, sputum streaked with blood, chest pain, fatigue, unexplained weight loss and loss of appetite, and reoccurring pneumonia or bronchitis.

Prevalence
Lung cancer is one of the most prevalent cancers with an estimated 28,400 new cases diagnosed in Canada in 2016. The frequency is increasing rapidly. Originally a disease that primarily affected men older than 60, lung cancer has become the second most common cause of cancer in women. An estimated 20,800 people died of the disease in 2016.

Treatment Options
Early detection is difficult, as symptoms do not appear until the disease is in advanced stages. To diagnose lung cancer, a physician usually takes a detailed medical history, performs a physical examination and orders tests which may include blood tests, imaging tests such as an X-ray, ultrasound, computed tomography (CT) scan or magnetic resonance imaging (MRI), sputum cytology (where phlegm samples are checked for cancer cells) and a biopsy (where a sample of lung tissue is examined for cancer cells).

Treatment for non-small cell lung cancer usually includes surgical removal of the lung if the cancer has not spread (metastasized) or chemotherapy and radiation therapy. Non-small lung cancer that does not respond to chemotherapy or comes back is sometimes treated with targeted therapy (drugs that block the growth and spread of certain types of cancer cells).

Survival rates depend on tumour size, location and whether or not the disease has spread. The five-year net survival rate for patients with lung cancer in Canada is about 17 percent. Because lung cancer is so difficult to treat, public health efforts are focused on prevention.

See also Lung Disease

Oral Cancer

Oral cancer can affect any part of the mouth.

Cause
Risk factors include cigarette, pipe and cigar smoking, as well as the use of chewing tobacco and excessive intake of alcohol. Infection of the mouth with the human papillomavirus (HPV) may also be a risk factor.

Symptoms
Oral cancer symptoms may include a sore that bleeds easily; a lump, thickening or persistent red or white patch in the mouth; pain or bleeding in the lip or mouth; and loose teeth. Difficulties in chewing and swallowing are symptoms of progressive disease.

Prevalence
There were around 4,600 new cases of oral cancer diagnosed in Canada in 2016, and approximately 1,250 people died of the disease. Incidence is more than twice as high in men as in women, and is most frequently found in men over the age of 50.

Treatment Options
Primary care physicians and dentists often detect oral cancer during routine check-ups. To confirm diagnosis, other tests are usually ordered. These may include an X-ray, a computed tomography (CT) scan or magnetic resonance imaging (MRI) of the neck and head, a biopsy (in which a small tissue sample is taken from the mouth to check for cancerous cells) and an endoscopy (a procedure in which a thin, flexible tube with a light at the end is inserted through the mouth or nose to examine the throat, windpipe and lungs and take tissue samples).

Treatment usually consists of surgical removal of the tumour, radiation therapy, chemotherapy or a combination of these therapies. Because oral cancer surgery is frequently disfiguring, reconstructive surgery may be required after the initial surgery.

The five-year net survival rate for patients with oral cancer in Canada is about 63 percent.

Ovarian Cancer

There are three different types of ovarian cancer. The most common is epithelial cell cancer which begins in the cells in the outer surface of the ovary. Germ cell tumours are usually diagnosed in younger women and start in the egg cells in the ovary. Stromal tumours develop in the connective tissue of the ovary.

Cause
Risk factors include a family history of breast cancer or ovarian cancer, a personal history of cancer, being over the age of 50, taking hormone replacement therapy and not having had children. Obesity, smoking, use of fertility drugs and certain types of diet are under investigation as possible risk factors.

Symptoms
Ovarian cancer symptoms usually do not appear until the disease is well developed. The most common sign is an enlarging abdomen from accumulated fluid. Digestive disturbances such as abdominal discomfort, gas and distention, nausea, fatigue, pain during intercourse, abnormal vaginal bleeding and pain in the lower back or leg may also occur.

Prevalence
It is estimated that ovarian cancer develops in 11 in 100,000 women in Canada. In 2016, there were approximately 2,800 new cases of ovarian cancer. Despite its low incidence, it is the cause of more deaths in women than any other female reproductive cancer. In 2016, an estimated 1,750 Canadian women died of the disease.

Treatment Options
Often an abdominal mass is discovered during a routine pelvic examination in women who are symptom-free. Therefore, women age 18 or older, or earlier if they are sexually active, should have annual check-ups. (The Pap smear detects cervical cancer, not ovarian cancer.) To confirm diagnosis, tests including a transvaginal ultrasound (an imaging test of the uterus, vagina, Fallopian tubes and ovaries), blood tests and a biopsy (where a small tissue sample of the ovary is examined for cancerous cells) may be ordered.

Treatment includes surgical removal, usually of one or both ovaries, the Fallopian tubes and the uterus, followed by radiation therapy or varying combinations of chemotherapy. As in all cancers, early detection is the key to effective therapy, however approximately 75 percent of cases of ovarian cancer are diagnosed at advanced stages. If the disease is diagnosed before it has spread to the other parts of the body, the five-year survival rate is 90 percent. For women with advanced stage ovarian cancer, the survival rate is only about 15 to 25 percent.

Pancreatic Cancer

Pancreatic cancer is one of the most dangerous cancers because it is difficult to detect and responds poorly to anticancer therapy. It begins in the cells of the pancreas, most commonly in the pancreatic ducts.

Cause
There is an increased incidence in those who smoke, consume a fatty diet and, to a lesser extent, who are diabetics. Chronic inflammation of the pancreas, especially among alcoholics, is also a predisposing cause.

Symptoms
Pancreatic cancer runs a particularly silent course, with no symptoms until it has significantly advanced. Possible symptoms may include discomfort or pain in the upper abdomen or upper back, weight loss, loss of appetite, nausea and vomiting, and jaundice.

Prevalence
Approximately 5,200 new cases of pancreatic cancer were diagnosed in Canada in 2016, and 4,700 people died of the disease.

Treatment Options
To diagnose pancreatic cancer, a physician takes a detailed medical history and performs a physical examination. To confirm the diagnosis, other tests are usually ordered. These may include blood tests (to check for tumour markers), imaging tests such as a computed tomography (CT) scan or magnetic resonance imaging (MRI) to detect the size of the tumour and to determine if it has spread, a biopsy (a procedure in which a small tissue sample of the pancreas is removed to check for cancerous cells) and an endoscopy (a procedure in which a thin, flexible tube with a light at the end is inserted into the opening of the pancreatic duct to examine the pancreas).

Surgery is the mainstay of therapy; radiation or chemotherapy are often part of treatment.

The five-year net survival rate for patients with pancreatic cancer in Canada is about 8 percent.

Prostate Cancer

Prostate cancer begins in the cells of the prostate gland and, in general, is a slow growing disease.

Cause
Risk factors for prostate cancer may include being older than 65, having a family history of prostate cancer and being of African descent. Obesity, a high-fat, high-calcium diet and physical inactivity are under investigation as possible risk factors for prostate cancer.

Symptoms
Early prostate cancer is symptom free. Pain and difficulty urinating are late signs of prostate cancer. More than 50 percent of patients have a nodule that can be felt by a digital examination.

Prevalence
In Canada, prostate cancer is the most common cancer diagnosed in men. There were approximately 21,600 new cases in 2016, and 4,000 men died of the disease. Incidence rates increase with age; over 80 percent of cases of prostate cancer occur in men over the age of 60.

Treatment Options
The Canadian Cancer Society recommends that men who have a higher risk of prostate cancer because they are of African descent or have a family history of the disease, as well as men who are close to the age of 50, should talk to a doctor about their risk of prostate cancer, as well as the benefits and harms of early detection. The digital rectal examination and PSA (prostatespecific antigen) blood test are used as screening tests for prostate cancer. If these tests are positive, further testing including a transrectal ultrasound (which takes images of the prostrate and rectum) and a biopsy (in which a tissue sample of the prostate is checked for cancerous cells) may be required.

Surgery, radiation, chemotherapy and hormonal therapy (to lower levels of testosterone) are all used to treat prostate cancer, depending on age and health of the patient and how far the disease has progressed.

The five-year net survival rate for patients with prostate cancer in Canada is about 95 percent.

Skin Cancer

The vast majority of skin cancer cases, called basal cell or squamous cell cancers, appear on areas that are most exposed to the sun and are highly curable. Melanoma is the most serious skin cancer.

Cause
Similar to the more benign skin cancers, melanoma develops as the result of excessive exposure to the sun and has a higher incidence among those who work outdoors. Persons with fair complexions are at particular risk.

Symptoms
The warning signs of skin cancer include a persistent skin lesion, especially one that changes in size, colour or shape. Other signs include scaliness, oozing, bleeding, pain or spread of pigmentation.

Prevalence
There were approximately 6,800 new cases of melanoma diagnosed in Canada in 2016, and 1,200 people died of the disease.

Treatment Options
Prevention, especially avoiding the sun's ultraviolet rays between 10 a.m. and 3 p.m., is the most important way to stop the development of melanoma. Sunscreens and protective clothing should be worn by those who spend the majority of their time outside, those who easily sunburn and all children.

To diagnose skin cancer, a physician usually takes a detailed medical history, performs a physical examination and does a biopsy. The biopsy may be excisional (in which the whole lump is removed), incisional (in which a small sample of the lump is removed), shave (where the top layers of skin are removed) or punch (where all the layers of skin are cut to obtain the sample). In all cases, the tissue is then examined for cancerous cells.

Treatment for skin cancer may include surgery to remove the growth, radiation therapy, chemotherapy and biological therapy (drugs made from natural body substances).

Early detection is critical because, despite advances in treatment, melanoma is difficult to cure. For advanced cases of melanoma, the five-year survival rate varies from 13 to 69 percent depending on the risk factors involved.

Stomach Cancer

Stomach cancer usually begins in the cells of the mucosa (the inner layer) of the stomach.

Cause
Diet, smoking and infection are believed to play a role in the development of stomach cancer. It is also more common in persons with vitamin B12 deficiency (pernicious anemia), those who work in rubber processing or lead manufacturing, and those who have had previous stomach surgery or have a family history of stomach cancer.

Symptoms
Symptoms of stomach cancer are usually vague, and include indigestion, abdominal discomfort, bloating, heartburn, fatigue, nausea and weight loss.

Prevalence
There were approximately 3,400 new cases of stomach cancer diagnosed in Canada in 2016, and 2,000 died of the disease. It is more common in men than women and its incidence increases with age.

Treatment Options
To diagnose stomach cancer, a physician usually takes a detailed medical history and performs a physical examination. To confirm the diagnosis, other tests are commonly ordered. These may include blood tests, a fecal occult blood test (FOBT) to check for blood in the stool, imaging tests such as an upper gastrointestinal series (a procedure where the patient swallows a chalky substance called barium which coats the stomach, esophagus and small intestine so that they show up more clearly on an X-ray), a biopsy (in which a small tissue sample is removed to check for cancerous cells) and a gastroscopy (a procedure in which a thin, flexible tube with a light at the end is put down the throat in order to examine the esophagus and stomach).

Removal of the tumour and chemotherapy or radiation is usually the treatment for stomach cancer.

The incidence of stomach cancer is decreasing in both men and women in Canada; however the estimated five-year net survival rate is still only about 25 percent.

Testicular Cancer

Most cases of testicular cancer begin in the germ cells. There are two types of germ cell tumours: seminomas and non-seminomas.

Cause

The cause of testicular cancer is uncertain, but the incidence is increased in men with congenital cryptorchidism (a failure of one or both testes to descend), abnormal development of the testicle or a family history of testicular cancer. Some researchers believe that getting an infection with a virus, such as mumps, may play a role.

Symptoms

Pain in the scrotal sac can occur, but more than 90 percent of patients have a painless, solid testicular swelling.

Prevalence

There were about 1,100 new cases of testicular cancer diagnosed in Canada in 2016. Unlike most cancers, testicular cancer usually occurs in the 15 to 49 age group; the average age at diagnosis is 32 years.

Treatment Options

Fortunately, testicular cancer is one of the most curable of all cancers, In order to discover it early, men must perform self-examination at regular intervals to feel for local abnormal growths such as lumps or nodules.

To diagnose testicular cancer, a physician usually takes a detailed medical history and performs a physical examination. Blood tests, an ultrasound of the testicles and scrotum and an orchiectomy (a procedure in which the testicle is removed to check for cancerous cells) are also often performed.

If the cancer has not spread, an orchiectomy may be the only treatment required. The lymph nodes near the kidney are sometimes removed, as well. In some cases, radiation or chemotherapy is also given.

The estimated five-year net survival rate for testicular cancer is about 96 percent.

Urinary Tract Cancer

The two most common urinary tract cancers are of the bladder and kidney. Bladder cancer usually begins in the lining of the bladder. If it remains there, it is referred to as superficial bladder cancer. If it spreads to the muscle wall of the bladder, it is called invasive bladder cancer.

Cause

Smoking is the greatest risk factor for bladder cancer. Workers exposed to dye, rubber or leather are also at higher risk, as are people who take certain medications such as cyclophosphamide or have a family history of bladder cancer.

The most common type of kidney cancer is renal cell carcinoma. Risk factors for kidney (renal) cancer are cigarette smoking, long-term dialysis and obesity.

Symptoms

Common symptoms of bladder cancer include microscopic or observable blood in the urine and painful, increased and urgent urination. Pain the lower back may also be present. Symptoms of kidney cancer are similar to those in bladder cancer and may also include fatigue, weight loss and a lump in the side of the abdomen.

Prevalence

In Canada, there were about 8,700 new cases of bladder cancer in 2016 and 6,400 new cases of kidney cancer. Approximately 2,300 Canadians died of bladder cancer, and 1,850 died of kidney cancer. Overall, the incidence rate of urinary tract cancer is greater among men than women, and usually occurs in patients who are over 50 years of age.

Treatment Options

To diagnose bladder cancer, a physician usually takes a detailed medical history and performs a physical examination. In most cases, diagnosis is confirmed through blood tests, urine tests and imaging tests such as a computed tomography (CT) scan or magnetic resonance imaging (MRI). Cytoscopy (a procedure in which a thin, flexible tube with a light and tiny camera at the end is passed through the urethra so the inside of the bladder can be examined and a small tissue sample can be obtained for analysis) may also be performed. Bladder cancer may be treated by surgical removal of the tumour combined with chemotherapy, radiation therapy or biological therapy (drugs made from natural body substances).

To diagnose kidney cancer, a physician usually takes a detailed medical history and performs a physical examination. In most cases diagnosis is confirmed through blood tests, urine tests and imaging tests such as a computed tomography (CT) scan or magnetic resonance imaging (MRI).

Total removal of the cancerous kidney is the treatment of choice and is used in nearly 90 percent of cases. Biological therapy (drugs made from natural body substances) and targeted therapies (for example, cancer growth inhibitors that limit the ability of the cancer cell to grow and divide) may also be used.

The five-year net survival rate for kidney cancer is approximately 67 percent; for bladder cancer it is around 73 percent.

Uterine and Cervical Cancer

Cervical cancer begins in the cells of the cervix. Dysplasia is a pre-cancerous condition of the cervix in which cells change and become abnormal. If left untreated, it may lead to cancer. However, most women with dysplasia do not develop cancer.

Cause

Risk factors for cervical cancer include intercourse at an early age, cigarette smoking, multiple sex partners and history of a sexually transmitted disease. Infection with some types of human papillomavirus (HPV) may also lead to cervical cancer. Uterine cancer can start in the cells in the lining of the uterus (endometrial carcinoma) or in the muscle layers of the uterus (uterine sarcoma). Risk factors for uterine cancer include obesity, diabetes, high blood pressure, high dose radiation of the pelvis, late onset of menopause, early onset of menstruation, tamoxifen therapy and estrogen-only hormone replacement therapy.

Symptoms

Warning signs for cervical cancer include bleeding outside the normal menstrual cycle or after menopause, pain in the lower back or pelvis and pain during intercourse. Symptoms of uterine cancer for most women include some form of abnormal bleeding as well as back pain and pain during intercourse.

Prevalence

The overall incidence of cervical cancer has decreased over the past 40 years, due mainly to regular checkups, the use of the Pap smear test for early detection and recently developed vaccines effective against HPV. According to estimates, 1,500 new cases of cervical cancer were diagnosed in Canada in 2016, and 400 women died of the disease. Approximately 6,600 new cases of uterine cancer were diagnosed and 1,100 women died of it.

Treatment Options

The Canadian Cancer Society recommends that all women who are sexually active should start having a Pap test by the age of 21. The test should be performed every one to three years (depending on test results).

In most cases, if a Pap test suggests dysplasia or cervical cancer, a physician will order additional tests which may include a colposcopy (to examine the cervix and vagina and take a small sample of tissue for testing), blood tests and imaging tests such as computed tomography (CT) scans or magnetic resonance imaging (MRI). Cervical cancer in most patients is treated with tissue removal or surgery (depending on the stage of the disease), radiation or chemotherapy, or a combination of these therapies.

Diagnosis of uterine cancer is usually based on a detailed medical history, a physical examination and tests which may include a hysteroscopy (a procedure in which a thin, flexible tube with a light and tiny camera at the end are used to look inside the uterus and take small tissue samples for analysis), blood tests and imaging tests such as computed tomography (CT) scans or magnetic resonance imaging (MRI). Treatment for uterine cancers usually includes surgery, radiation therapy, hormone therapy and, occasionally, chemotherapy.

The five-year net survival rate for cervical cancer is 73 percent; for uterine cancer it is 84 percent.

National Associations

Bladder Cancer Canada (BCC) / Cancer de la vessie Canada
#1000, 4936 Yonge St., Toronto ON M2N 6S3
Toll-Free: 866-674-8889
e-mail: info@bladdercancercanada.org
www.bladdercancercanada.org
www.linkedin.com/company/2599127
www.facebook.com/BladderCancerCanada
twitter.com/BladderCancerCA
www.youtube.com/user/BladderCancerCA
Overview: A medium-sized national charitable organization founded in 2009
Mission: To improve patient support by having a patient to patient support system in place; To offer information about available treatment options; To create greater awareness of bladder cancer
Chief Officer(s):
Ken Bagshaw, Chair
Tammy Northam, Executive Director

Breast Cancer Society of Canada (BCSC) / Société du cancer du sein du Canada
420 East St. North, Sarnia ON N7T 6Y5
Tel: 519-336-0746; *Fax:* 519-336-5725
Toll-Free: 800-567-8767
e-mail: bcsc@bcsc.ca
www.bcsc.ca
www.linkedin.com/company/2260739
www.facebook.com/breastcancersocietyofcanada
twitter.com/bcsctweet
www.youtube.com/user/BreastCancerSociety
Also Known As: Breast Cancer Society
Overview: A large national charitable organization founded in 1991
Mission: To support research into the prevention, detection, & treatment of breast cancer
Member of: Canadian Cancer Research Alliance
Chief Officer(s):
Kimberly Carlson, Chief Executive Officer
kcarson@bcsc.ca
Publications:
• Breast Cancer Society of Canada Newsletter

Type: Newsletter
Profile: Recent information about the society & research endeavours

Canadian Association of Medical Oncologists (CAMO) / Association canadienne des oncologues médicaux (ACOM)
PO Box 35164, Stn. Westgate, Ottawa ON K1Z 1A2
Tel: 613-415-6033; *Fax:* 866-839-7501
e-mail: camo@royalcollege.ca
www.cos.ca/camo
Overview: A small national organization
Chief Officer(s):
Christopher Lee, President
Alexi Campbell, Executive Director
Bruce Colwell, Secretary-Treasurer
Publications:
• Canadian Association of Medical Oncologists Membership Directory
Type: Directory
Profile: Offers access to medical oncologists throughout Canada

Canadian Association of Nurses in Oncology (CANO) / Association canadienne des infirmières en oncologie (ACIO)
#301, 750 West Pender St., Vancouver BC V6C 2T7
Tel: 604-874-4322; *Fax:* 604-874-4378
e-mail: cano@malachite-mgmt.com
www.cano-acio.ca
www.facebook.com/336467099484
twitter.com/CANO_ACIO
www.youtube.com/user/CANOACIO
Overview: A medium-sized national organization founded in 1984
Mission: To advocate for improved cancer care for all Canadians
Affliation(s): Canadian Nurses Association; International Society of Cancer Nurses; Canadian Oncology Societies
Chief Officer(s):
Tracy Truant, President
Jyoti Bhardwaj, Executive Director
Publications:
• Canadian Oncology Nursing Journal
Type: Journal; *Frequency:* Quarterly; *Editor:* Margaret I. Fitch
• CANO [Canadian Association of Nurses in Oncology] Connections
Type: Newsletter

Canadian Association of Pharmacy in Oncology (CAPhO) / L'Association canadienne de pharmacie en oncologie (ACPhO)
c/o Sea to Sky Meeting Management Inc., #206, 201 Bewicke Ave., Winnipeg MB V7M 3M7
Tel: 778-338-4142; *Fax:* 704-984-6434
e-mail: info@capho.org
www.capho.ca
www.facebook.com/109491585819684
twitter.com/CAPhO_ACPhO
Overview: A small national organization
Mission: CAPhO, the national forum for oncology pharmacy practitioners & other health care professionals, promotes the practice of oncology pharmacy in Canada, by providing educational opportunites, upholding professional practice standards, & developing the profession as a specialty area of pharmacy practice.
Chief Officer(s):
Joan Fabbro, President
president@capho.org
Mark Pasetka, President-Elect
presidentelect@capho.org
Lori Emond, Treasurer
treasurer@capho.org
Publications:
• CAPhO [Canadian Association of Pharmacy in Oncology] Newsletter
Type: Newsletter; *Frequency:* 3 pa

Canadian Association of Provincial Cancer Agencies (CAPCA)
#300, 1 University Ave., Toronto ON M5J 2P1
Tel: 416-619-5744; *Fax:* 416-915-9224
e-mail: info@capca.ca
www.capca.ca
Overview: A small national charitable organization founded in 1998
Mission: To support the reduction of the burden of cancer, through effective leadership & collaboration between the provincial cancer agencies

Chief Officer(s):
Eshwar Kumar, Chair
Brent Schacter, Chief Executive Officer, 204-787-2128, Fax:
204-786-0196
brent.schacter@cancercare.mb.ca

Canadian Association of Psychosocial Oncology (CAPO) / Association Canadienne d'oncologie psychosociale (ACOP)
#1, 189 Queen St. East, Toronto ON M5A 1S2
Tel: 416-968-0207; *Fax:* 416-968-6818
e-mail: capo@funnel.ca
www.capo.ca

Overview: A small national charitable organization founded in 1986
Mission: To promote excellence in psychosocial oncology services
Chief Officer(s):
Shane Sinclair, President, 403-220-2925, Fax: 403-284-4803
sinclair@ucalgary.ca
Carole Mayer, Vice-President, 705-522-6237 Ext. 2700
cmayer@hsnsudbury.ca
Doris Howell, Secretary, 416-946-4501 Ext. 3419
doris.howell@uhn.on.ca
Nelson Byrne, Treasurer, 289-848-2039, Fax: 844-457-7683
drbyrne@connectcancersupport.ca
Anthony Laycock, Association Manager
Publications:
• The Emotional Facts of Life with Cancer: A Guide to Counselling & Support for Patients, Families, & Friends
Type: Booklet; *Number of Pages:* 32; *Editor:* Beth Kapusta
Profile: Information about professional support to help people cope with cancer
• Oncology Exchange
Type: Journal; *Price:* Free with membership in the Canadian Association of Psychosocial Oncology
Profile: A Canadian interdisciplinary journal

Canadian Association of Radiation Oncology (CARO) / Association canadienne de radio-oncologie (ACRO)
#6, 20 Crown Steel Dr., Markham ON L3R 9X9
Tel: 905-415-3917; *Fax:* 905-415-0071
Toll-Free: 855-415-3917
e-mail: caro-acro@secretariatcentral.com
www.caro-acro.ca
Previous Name: Canadian Association of Radiation Oncologists
Overview: A small national organization founded in 1986
Mission: To act as the voice of radiation oncology in Canada; To promote high standards of patient care, radiation oncology research, & education
Affiliation(s): Royal College of Physicians & Surgeons of Canada; Canadian Medical Association; Canadian Association of Medical Radiation Technologists; Canadian Organization of Medical Physicists; Canadian Association of Nurses in Oncology
Chief Officer(s):
Eric Vigneault, President
Jacqueline Spayne, Secretary-Treasurer
Publications:
• CARO [Canadian Association of Radiation Oncology] Code of Ethics
• Physician / Industry Relationships Guidelines
Profile: Guidelines established by the Canadian Association of Radiation Oncology to assist physicians
• Radiosurgery Scope of Practice in Canada

Canadian Breast Cancer Foundation (CBCF) / Fondation Canadienne pour le Cancer du Sein
#301, 375 University Ave., Toronto ON M5G 2J5
Tel: 416-596-6773
Toll-Free: 800-387-9816
Other Communication: Blog: findinghope.cbcf.org
e-mail: connect@cbcf.org
www.cbcf.org
www.facebook.com/CanadianBreastCancerFoundation
twitter.com/cbcf_
www.youtube.com/cbcfcentral
Overview: A large national charitable organization founded in 1997
Mission: To support the advancement of breast cancer research, education, diagnosis & treatment
Chief Officer(s):
Valerie Steele, Chair

Publications:
• Canadian Breast Cancer Foundation Newsletter
Type: Newsletter
• Canadian Breast Cancer Foundation Community Reports
Type: Report

Atlantic Region
#240, 230 Brownlow Ave., Dartmouth NS B3B 0G5
Tel: 902-422-5520; *Fax:* 902-422-5523
Toll-Free: 866-273-2223
e-mail: cbcfatl@cbcf.org
www.cbcf.org/atlantic

Chief Officer(s):
Jane Parsons, Executive Director

British Columbia/Yukon Region
#300, 1090 West Pender St., Vancouver BC V6E 2N7
Tel: 604-683-2873; *Fax:* 604-683-2860
Toll-Free: 800-561-6111
e-mail: cbcfbc@cbcf.org
www.cbcf.org/bc
www.youtube.com/user/CBCFcentral

Chief Officer(s):
Bernice Scholten, Executive Director
bscholten@cbcf.org

Ontario Region
20 Victoria St., 6th Fl., Toronto ON M5C 2N8
Tel: 416-815-1313; *Fax:* 416-815-1766
twitter.com/CBCF_Ontario
www.youtube.com/user/CBCFOntario

Prairies/NWT Region
HSBC Bank Place, #1800, 10250 101 St., Edmonton AB T5J 3P4
Tel: 780-452-1166; *Fax:* 780-451-6554
Toll-Free: 866-302-2223
www.youtube.com/user/CBCFPNWT

Chief Officer(s):
Chelsea Draeger, Senior Director, Individual Giving & Mid Market Fundraising
Nancy Melnychuk, Director, Events

Canadian Breast Cancer Network (CBCN) / Réseau canadien du cancer du sein (RCCS)
#602, 331 Cooper St., Ottawa ON K2P 0G5
Tel: 613-230-3044; *Fax:* 613-230-4424
Toll-Free: 800-685-8820
e-mail: cbcn@cbcn.ca
www.cbcn.ca
www.facebook.com/168424759878914
twitter.com/CBCN
www.youtube.com/user/CBCNvideos
Overview: A medium-sized national organization founded in 1994
Mission: To act as the national voice of breast cancer survivors
Chief Officer(s):
Cathy Ammendolea, President
Craig Faucette, Operations Manager
Sharon Young, Vice President
Publications:
• Network News [a publication of the Canadian Breast Cancer Network]
Type: Newsletter; *Accepts Advertising*
• Outreach [a publication of the Canadian Breast Cancer Network]
Type: Newsletter

Canadian Cancer Society (CCS) / Société canadienne du cancer
National Office, #300, 55 St Clair Ave. West, Toronto ON M4V 2Y7
Tel: 416-961-7223; *Fax:* 416-961-4189
Toll-Free: 800-268-8874
e-mail: ccs@cancer.ca
www.cancer.ca
www.facebook.com/canadiancancersociety
twitter.com/cancersociety
www.youtube.com/user/CDNCancerSociety
Overview: A large national charitable organization founded in 1938
Mission: To collect donations to fund cancer research in Canada; to disseminate information on cancer prevention & treatments, advocating for healthy environment & lifestyle to reduce the incidence of cancer; to offer individual & group support programs for caregivers, family &

friends of cancer patients

Affiliation(s): Canadian Breast Cancer Research Alliance; Canadian Prostate Cancer Research Initiative; Canadian Tobacco Control Research Initiative; Canadian Strategy for Cancer Control; Chronic Disease Prevention Alliance of Canada

Chief Officer(s):
Robert Lawrie, Chair
Lynne Hudson, President & CEO
Paula Roberts, Vice President, Marketing & Communications
Arlene Teti, Chief Human Resources Officer

Publications:
• Canadian Cancer Statistics [a publication of Canadian Cancer Society]
Frequency: Annually
Profile: Report of cancer incidence & mortality in Canada

Alberta & Northwest Territories Division
#200, 325 Manning Rd. NE, Calgary AB T2E 2P5
Tel: 403-205-3966; *Fax:* 403-205-3979
Toll-Free: 800-661-2262
e-mail: info@cancer.ab.ca
www.cancer.ca
www.facebook.com/CanadianCancerSocietyABNWT
twitter.com/ccs_AlbertaNWT

Chief Officer(s):
Michael Permack, Chair
Dan Holinda, Executive Director
• Believe
Type: Magazine; *Frequency:* Semiannually; *Editor:* Deanna Kraus;
Price: Free for people living with cancer, & Canadian Cancer Society volunteers & donors
Profile: Support services, cancer information, research, supporters, advocacy, & prevention

British Columbia & Yukon Division
565 West 10th Ave., Vancouver BC V5Z 4J4
Tel: 604-872-4400; *Fax:* 604-872-4113
Toll-Free: 800-663-2524
e-mail: frontdesk@bc.cancer.ca
www.facebook.com/CanadianCancerSocietyBCY
twitter.com/cancersocietybc

Chief Officer(s):
Faye Wightman, Executive Director
Cheryl Swallow, Vice-President, Finance & Administration

Division du Québec
5151, boul de l'Assomption, Montréal QC H1T 4A9
Tél: 514-255-5151; *Téléc:* 514-255-2808
Courriel: webmestre@quebec.cancer.ca
www.facebook.com/sccquebec
twitter.com/SCC_Quebec

Chief Officer(s):
Suzanne Dubois, Directrice générale
André Léger, Directeur, Finances
• Canadian Cancer Society's Annual Report - Québec Division
Type: Yearbook; *Frequency:* Annually
Profile: Financial report & description of society activities submitted to the delegates of the general assembly

Manitoba Division
193 Sherbrook St., Winnipeg MB R3C 2B7
Tel: 204-774-7483; *Fax:* 204-774-7500
Toll-Free: 888-532-6982
e-mail: info@mb.cancer.ca
www.facebook.com/CCSManitoba
twitter.com/CancerSocietyMB

Chief Officer(s):
Elmer Gomes, Chair
Reta Faryon, Contact
rfaryon@mb.cancer
• Community Services Directory
Type: Directory
Profile: Listings of support programs, hair donation programs, home care, transportation, stop smoking programs, & places to find a prosthesis or wig
• Society News
Type: Newsletter

Profile: Volunteer information, upcoming events, & methods of prevention

New Brunswick Division
PO Box 2089, 133 Prince William St., Saint John NB E2L 3T5
Tel: 506-634-6272; *Fax:* 506-634-3808
e-mail: ccsnb@nb.cancer.ca
www.facebook.com/CanadianCancerSocietyNB
twitter.com/CancerSocietyNB

Chief Officer(s):
Michael Costello, Chair
Anne McTiernan-Gamble, Chief Executive Officer

Newfoundland & Labrador Division
Daffodil Place, PO Box 8921, 70 Ropewalk Ln., St. John's NL A1B 3R9
Tel: 709-753-6520; *Fax:* 709-753-9314
Toll-Free: 888-753-6520
e-mail: ccs@nl.cancer.ca

Chief Officer(s):
Matthew Piercey, Chief Executive Officer
mpiercey@nl.cancer.ca
Natasha Denty, Manager, Finance & Operations
• Canadian Cancer Society - Newfoundland & Labrador Division Community Report
Type: Yearbook; *Frequency:* Annually

Nova Scotia Division
5826 South St., Halifax NS B3H 1S6
Tel: 902-423-6183; *Fax:* 902-429-6563
Toll-Free: 800-639-0222
e-mail: ccs.ns@ns.cancer.ca
www.facebook.com/CancerSocietyNS
twitter.com/cancersocietyNS

Chief Officer(s):
David Landrigan, Chair
Kendra Morton, Director, Development
• Canadian Cancer Society - Nova Scotia Division Annual Report
Type: Yearbook; *Frequency:* Annually

Ontario Division
#500, 55 St. Clair Ave. West, Toronto ON M4V 2Y7
Tel: 416-488-5400; *Fax:* 416-488-2872
Toll-Free: 800-268-8874
e-mail: webmaster@ontario.cancer.ca

Chief Officer(s):
Mark Hierlihy, Executive Director
Rowena Pinto, Vice-President, Public Affairs & Strategic Initiatives
Lesley Ring, Vice-President, Development & Marketing
• Hope Blooms
Type: Newsletter; *Frequency:* Monthly
Profile: Cancer research updates, tips to reduce risk of cancer, upcoming events, volunteer profiles

Prince Edward Island Division
#1, 1 Rochford St., Charlottetown PE C1A 9L2
Tel: 902-566-4007; *Fax:* 902-628-8281
e-mail: info@pei.cancer.ca
www.cancer.ca/pei
www.facebook.com/CancerSocietyPE
twitter.com/CancerSocietyPE

Chief Officer(s):
Marlene Mulligan, Executive Director
mmulligan@pei.cancer.ca
• Cancer Quarterly
Type: Newsletter; *Frequency:* Quarterly

Saskatchewan Division
1910 McIntyre St., Regina SK S4P 2R3
Tel: 306-790-5822; *Fax:* 306-569-2133
Toll-Free: 877-977-4673
e-mail: ccssk@sk.cancer.ca
www.facebook.com/jointhefight.sk
twitter.com/jointhefight_sk

Chief Officer(s):
Susan Holmes, Chair
Keith Karasin, Executive Director

Canadian Cancer Society Research Institute
#300, 55 St. Clair Ave. West, Toronto ON M4V 2Y7
Tel: 416-961-7223; *Fax:* 416-961-4189
e-mail: research@cancer.ca
www.cancer.ca/research
Previous Name: National Cancer Institute of Canada
Overview: A medium-sized national organization founded in 2009
Mission: To act as a strong voice in the cancer research community;
To support a broad range of projects that involve Canadian
investigators across the spectrum of cancer research
Chief Officer(s):
Sian Bevan, Vice-President, Research, 416-934-5308
 sian.bevan@cancer.ca
Lori Moser, Manager, Programs, 416-934-5310
 lori.moser@cancer.ca
Publications:
• Research Connection [a publication of the Canadian Cancer Society
Research Institute]
Type: Newsletter
Profile: News for cancer researchers, including information about
research grants

Canadian Cancer Survivor Network (CCSN)
#210, 1750 Courtwood Cres., Ottawa ON K2C 2B5
Tel: 613-898-1871
e-mail: info@survivornet.ca
survivornet.ca
www.facebook.com/CanadianSurvivorNet
twitter.com/survivornetca
Overview: A large national organization
Mission: To help cancer patients & their families cope with their
situation; To educate the public about the costs of cancer
Chief Officer(s):
Jackie Manthorne, President & CEO
 jmanthorne@survivornet.ca

Canadian Hematology Society (CHS) / Société canadienne d'hématologie
#199, 435 St. Laurent Blvd., Ottawa ON K1K 2Z8
Tel: 613-748-9613; *Fax:* 613-748-6392
e-mail: chs@uniserve.ca
www.canadianhematologysociety.org
Overview: A small national organization founded in 1971
Mission: To represent members of the Society & provide information
about hematology
Chief Officer(s):
Aaron Schimmer, President
Publications:
• Canadian Hematology Society Membership Directory
Type: Directory
• Canadian Hematology Society Newsletter
Type: Newsletter; *Frequency:* 3 pa

Canadian Lymphedema Framework (CLF)
#204, 4800 Dundas St. West, Toronto ON M9A 1B1
Tel: 647-693-1083
e-mail: admin@canadalymph.ca
www.canadalymph.ca
Overview: A small national charitable organization founded in 2009
Mission: To advance the treatment of lymphedema & related disorders
in Canada; To promote lymphedema research, practices, & clinical
development
Affliation(s): International Lymphedema Framework
Chief Officer(s):
Anna Kennedy, Executive Director

Canadian Melanoma Foundation (CMF)
c/o Div. of Dermatology, Univ. of British Columbia, 835 - 10th Ave.
West, Vancouver BC V5Z 4E8
Tel: 604-875-4747; *Fax:* 604-873-9919
www.derm.ubc.ca/division/cmf/cmf1.htm
Overview: A small national organization
Mission: A non-profit organization dedicated to improving cancer
prevention and cure.

Canadian Neurological Sciences Federation (CNSF) / Fédération des sciences neurologiques du Canada
143N - 8500 Macleod Trail SE, Calgary AB T2H 2N1
Tel: 403-229-9544; *Fax:* 403-229-1661
www.cnsfederation.org
Previous Name: Canadian Congress of Neurological Sciences
Overview: A medium-sized national organization
Mission: To support the neuroscience professions in Canada,
particularly those members of the CNSF Societies, through education,
advocacy, membership services & research promotion
Chief Officer(s):
Dan Morin, Chief Executive Officer
 dan-morin@cnsfederation.org
Marika Fitzgerald, Manager, Finance & Administration
 marika-fitzgerald@cnsfederation.org
Donna Irvin, Administrator, Membership Services
 donna-irvin@cnsfederation.org
Publications:
• Canadian Journal of Neurological Sciences
Type: Journal; *Frequency:* 6 pa; *Editor:* Dr. Robert Chen
Profile: Published through Cambridge Journals Online, a peer-reviewed
clinical & basic neuroscience research articles, covering neurology,
neurosurgery, clinicalneurophysiology, & pediatric neurology

Canadian Oncology Societies
Fax: 613-247-3511
Toll-Free: 877-990-9044
e-mail: info@cos.ca
www.cos.ca
Overview: A small national organization
Mission: To increase & exchange knowledge in the field of oncology;
To promote the application of such knowledge in the prevention &
diagnosis of cancer & the care of cancer patients & their families; To
promote interdisciplinary approaches to patient care & research in
cancer; To provide a forum for the presentation & discussion of
scientific knowledge & advances in oncology; To further continuing
education for groups & indivduals involved in the care of patients who
require special attention; To support public cancer education programs;
To support & assist the Canadian Cancer Society & the National
Cancer Insitute; To advise government & other agencies on the
provision of health services relevent to oncology
Chief Officer(s):
Charles Pitts, Administrator

Canadian Society for Surgical Oncology (CSSO) / Société canadienne d'oncologie chirurgicale
c/o Jane Hanes, Princess Margaret Hospital, #3-130, 610 University
Ave., Toronto ON M5G 2M9
Tel: 416-946-6583; *Fax:* 416-946-6590
www.cos.ca/csso
Overview: A small national organization founded in 1986
Mission: To encourage optimum cancer patient care through a
multi-disciplinary treatment approach; To promote surgical oncology
training programs in Canadian universities
Affliation(s): Royal College of Physicians & Surgeons of Canada
(RCPSC); Canadian Oncology Societies
Chief Officer(s):
Andy McFadden, President
Jane Hanes, Executive Coordinator

Canadian Urologic Oncology Group (CUOG)
c/o Dr. Fred Saad, CUOG Chairman, 1560 Sherbrooke est, Montréal
QC H2L 4M1
Tel: 514-890-8000
e-mail: fred.saad.chum@ssss.gouv.qc.ca
www.cuog.org
Overview: A small national organization
Mission: Clinical research investigator network committed to furthering
urology research in Canada
Affliation(s): Canadian Urological Association
Chief Officer(s):
Neil Fleshner, Chair

Cancer Advocacy Coalition of Canada (CACC)
#1902, 2 Bloor St. West, Toronto ON M4W 3R1
Tel: 416-642-6472; *Fax:* 416-538-4874
Toll-Free: 855-572-3436
e-mail: cacc@canceradvocacy.ca
www.canceradvocacy.ca
www.facebook.com/CancerAdvocacy
twitter.com/CancerAdvocacy1
canceradvocacy.tumblr.com
Overview: A medium-sized national organization
Mission: To ensure that Canadians receive the best cancer services;
To benefit cancer survivors; To assist in shaping constructive change in
the Canadian cancer system
Chief Officer(s):
Dauna Crooks, Chair
Larry Broadfield, Vice-Chair
Publications:
• Report Card on Cancer in Canada
Frequency: Annually
Profile: Articles about the effectiveness of the cancer system in Canada

Cancer Patient Education Network Canada (CPEN - Canada)
e-mail: info@cancerpatienteducation.org
www.cancerpatienteducation.org
www.linkedin.com/groups?mostPopular=&gid=3300283
www.facebook.com/JoinCPEN
twitter.com/CPEN2014
Overview: A small national organization
Mission: To support cancer care providers in Canada, in the provision
of effective, accurate, & comprehensive patient education; To empower
cancer patients & their families to participate effectively in their care; To
improve health outcomes, through cancer patient, family, & community
education; To develop national standards for best practice in cancer
patient education programs at cancer centres, hospitals, & community
organizations
Chief Officer(s):
Susan Boyko, Chair, CPEN Canada Steering Committee
sboyko@hsnsudbury.ca

Cancer Research Society / Société de recherche sur le cancer
#402, 625, av Président-Kennedy, Montréal QC H3A 3S5
Tel: 514-861-9227; *Fax:* 514-861-9220
Toll-Free: 888-766-2262
e-mail: info@src-crs.ca
www.crs-src.ca
www.linkedin.com/company/cancer-research-society-soci-t-de-recherch
e-s
www.facebook.com/cancerresearchsociety
Overview: A large national charitable organization founded in 1945
Mission: To support basic cancer research through funding & seed
money; To allocate grants & fellowships to universities & hospitals
involved in research across Canada
Chief Officer(s):
Andy Chabot, Executive Director
achabot@src-crs.ca
Nathalie Giroux, Vice-President & Chief Operating Officer
ngiroux@crs-src.ca

Ottawa
#305, 200 Isabella St., Ottawa ON K1S 1V7
Fax: 613-233-1030
Toll-Free: 888-766-2262
e-mail: ottawa@src-crs.ca

Carcinoid NeuroEndocrine Tumour Society Canada
#4103, 3219 Yonge St., Toronto ON M4N 3S1
Tel: 416-628-3189
Toll-Free: 844-628-6788
Other Communication: support@cnetscanada.org
e-mail: info@cnetscanada.org
www.cnetscanada.org
www.facebook.com/cnetscanada
twitter.com/CNETSCanada
www.youtube.com/user/cnetscanada
Also Known As: CNETS Canada
Overview: A large national charitable organization founded in 2007

Mission: To raise awareness about neuroendocrine tumours; to
provide help & support to those suffering from this type of cancer; to
fund research that treats neuroendocrine tumours
Chief Officer(s):
Jacqueline Herman, President & Director, Treatment, Access & Health
Policy
jackie.herman@cnetscanada.org

Childhood Cancer Canada Foundation
#801, 21 St. Clair Ave. East, Toronto ON M4T 1L9
Tel: 416-489-6440; *Fax:* 416-489-9812
Toll-Free: 800-363-1062
e-mail: info@childhoodcancer.ca
www.childhoodcancer.ca
www.facebook.com/ChildhoodCancerCanada
twitter.com/chldhdcancercan
Overview: A large national organization founded in 1987
Mission: To help improve the lives of children suffering from cancer
through family support programs; to fund cancer research
Chief Officer(s):
Glenn Fraser, Chair

British Columbia Childhood Cancer Parent's Association
British Columbia Children's Hospital, #A127A, 4480 Oak St.,
Vancouver BC V6H 3B8
Tel: 604-875-2345

Candlelighters Newfoundland & Labrador
PO Box 5846, St. John's NL A1C 5X3
Tel: 709-745-4448
Toll-Free: 866-745-4448
e-mail: info@Candlelightersnl.ca
www.candlelightersnl.ca
www.facebook.com/CandlelightersNL
twitter.com/CandlelighterNL
Chief Officer(s):
Amananda Kinsman, Coordinator, Provincial Family Program
coordinator@candlelightersnl.ca

Manitoba - Candlelighters Childhood Cancer Support Group
PO Box 350, RR#1, Winkler MB R6W 4A1
e-mail: support@manitobacandlelighters.ca
www.manitobacandlelighters.ca
Chief Officer(s):
Denis Foidart, Chair, 204-737-2684
denlis@wiband.ca

ON - Candlelighters Simcoe
6 Emily Ct., Barrie ON L4N 6B4
Tel: 705-737-4296; *Fax:* 705-737-4836
Chief Officer(s):
Barbara Johnson, Coordinator
albarbjohnson@sympatico.ca

SK - Candlelighters - Prince Albert
350 - 30th St. East, Prince Albert SK S6V 1Z4
Tel: 306-763-7356

SK - Regina Candlelighters
100 cardinal Cres., Regina SK S4S 4Y7
Tel: 306-529-3292
e-mail: sask.candlelighters@sasktel.net
Chief Officer(s):
David Achter, Contact
Tangy Achter, Contact

Children's Tumor Foundation (CTF)
120 Wall St., 16th Fl., New York NY 10005-3904 USA
Tel: 212-344-6633; *Fax:* 212-747-0004
Toll-Free: 800-323-7938
e-mail: info@ctf.org
www.ctf.org
www.linkedin.com/company/children's-tumor-foundation
www.facebook.com/childrenstumor
twitter.com/childrenstumor
Previous Name: National NF Foundation
Overview: A medium-sized national charitable organization founded in
1978
Mission: To sponsor research to find the cause of & cure for both
types of neurofibromatosis - NF1 & NF2; To promote clinical activities

which assure individuals with NF ready access to the highest calibre of medical care; To develop programs to increase public awareness of NF; To provide support services for patients & families, with referrals to qualified healthcare professionals
Member of: International NF Association
Affliation(s): NF Associations worldwide
Chief Officer(s):
Annette Bakker, President & Chief Scientific Officer
Simon Vukelj, Vice-President, Marketing & Communications
Salvo La Rosa, Vice-President, Research & Development

Colon Cancer Canada / Cancer du Colon Canada
#204A, 5915 Leslie St., Toronto ON M2H 1J8
Tel: 416-785-0449; Fax: 416-785-0450
Toll-Free: 888-571-8547
e-mail: info@coloncancercanada.ca
www.coloncancercanada.ca
www.facebook.com/coloncancercda
twitter.com/ColonCancerCda
Previous Name: National Colorectal Cancer Campaign
Overview: A small national organization founded in 1996
Mission: To raise public awareness for the disease of colorectal cancer & to raise money for vital research
Chief Officer(s):
Bunnie Schwartz, President/Co-Founder
hmschwartz@rogers.com
Amy Lerman-Elmaleh, Executive Director/Co-Founder
amy@coloncancercanada.ca

Colorectal Cancer Association of Canada (CCAC)
#204, 60 St. Clair Ave. East, Toronto ON M4T 1N5
Tel: 416-920-4333; Fax: 416-920-3004
e-mail: information@colorectal-cancer.ca
www.colorectal-cancer.ca
www.facebook.com/Colorectal
twitter.com/coloncanada
www.youtube.com/user/ccac1230
Overview: A small national organization
Mission: To support people with colorectal cancer, their families & caregivers; to improve the quality of life of patients & increase awareness of the disease
Chief Officer(s):
Barry D. Stein, President
barrys@colorectal-cancer.ca

DES Action USA
PO Box 7296, Jupiter FL 33468 USA
Toll-Free: 800-337-9288
e-mail: info@desaction.org
www.desaction.org
www.facebook.com/pages/DES-Action-USA/148293015181338
Overview: A small national charitable organization founded in 1979
Mission: To provide public & physician education on special health needs of those exposed to the synthetic estrogen diethylstilbestrol (DES)
Chief Officer(s):
Fran Howell, Executive Director

Kidney Cancer Canada Association
#226, 4936 Yonge St., Toronto ON M2N 6S3
Tel: 416-603-0277; Fax: 416-603-0277
Toll-Free: 866-598-7166
e-mail: info@kidneycancercanada.ca
www.kidneycancercanada.ca
www.linkedin.com/company/kidney-cancer-canada
www.facebook.com/KidneyCancerCanada
twitter.com/KidneyCancer_Ca
www.youtube.com/KidneyCancerCanada
Also Known As: Kidney Cancer Canada
Overview: A medium-sized national charitable organization founded in 2007
Mission: To support & improve the lives of patients & families living with kidney cancer; To raise awareness of kidney cancer treatment options; To promote quality care across Canada; To increase funding for kidney cancer research
Chief Officer(s):

Andrew Weller, Chair
aweller@kidneycancercanada.ca
Heather Chappell, Executive Director
hchappell@kidneycancercanada.ca
Jan Coleman, Coordinator, Administration & Program Development
Publications:
• KCC [Kidney Cancer Canada] Newsletter
Type: Newsletter
• Kidney Cancer Canada Brochure
Type: Brochure

The Leukemia & Lymphoma Society of Canada (LLSC) / Société de leucémie et lymphome du Canada
#804, 2 Lansing Square, Toronto ON M2J 4P8
Tel: 416-661-9541; Fax: 416-661-7799
Toll-Free: 877-668-8326
e-mail: AdminCanada@lls.org
www.llscanada.org
www.linkedin.com/company/5127044
www.facebook.com/LeukemiaandLymphomaSocietyofCanada
twitter.com/llscanada
www.youtube.com/llscanada
Previous Name: Leukemia Research Fund of Canada
Overview: A medium-sized national charitable organization founded in 1955
Mission: To cure leukemia, lymphoma, Hodgkin's disease & myeloma, & to improve the quality of life of patients & their families
Affliation(s): Canadian Centre for Philanthropy
Chief Officer(s):
Shelagh Tippet-Fagyas, President
Ted Moroz, Chair

Atlantic Canada Branch
#H2, 1660 Hollis St., Halifax NS B3J 1V7
Tel: 902-422-5999
Toll-Free: 855-515-5572
www.llscanada.org/atlantic-region
www.facebook.com/llscatlantic
Chief Officer(s):
Joe DiPenta, Regional Director, 905-422-5999 Ext. 7520, Fax: 902-422-5968
joe.dipenta@lls.org

British Columbia/Yukon Branch
#303, 1401 West Broadway, Vancouver BC V6H 1H6
Tel: 604-733-2873
Toll-Free: 866-547-5433
Chief Officer(s):
Donna McLennan, Regional Director
donna.mclennan@lls.org
Sharon Paulse, Manager, Patient Services
sharon.paulse@lls.org
Scott Kehoe, Manager, Fund Development
scott.kehoe@lls.org

Ontario Branch
#804, 2 Lansing Sq., Toronto ON M2J 4P8
Tel: 647-253-5530
Chief Officer(s):
Sandra Harris, Regional Director

Ontario Branch - Ottawa
#701, 116 Albert St., Ottawa ON K1P 5G3
Tel: 613-234-1274

Prairies/Territories Branch - Calgary
#316, 1212 31 Avenue NE, Calgary AB T2E 7S8
Tel: 403-263-5300
www.llscanada.org/prairies-region
Chief Officer(s):
Lauren Atkinson, Regional Director, Fax: 403-263-5303
lauren.atkinson@lls.org

Prairies/Territories Branch - Edmonton
#208, 10240 - 124th St., Edmonton AB T5N 3W6
Tel: 780-758-4261

Prairies/Territories Branch - Saskatoon
#202, 402 - 21st St. East, Saskatoon SK S7K 0C3
Tel: 306-242-6611

Québec Branch
#602, 740, rue St-Maurice, Montréal QC H3C 1L5
Tel: 514-875-1000

Chief Officer(s):
Andy Fratino, Acting Regional Director
andy.fratino@lls.org

Lymphoma Canada
#202, 6860 Century Ave., Mississauga ON L5N 2W5
Tel: 905-858-5967; *Fax:* 905-858-5967
Toll-Free: 866-659-5556
e-mail: info@lymphoma.ca
www.lymphoma.ca
www.linkedin.com/company/lymphoma-foundation-canada
www.facebook.com/LymphomaCanada
twitter.com/lymphomacanada
www.youtube.com/user/LymphomaTV

Previous Name: Lymphoma Foundation Canada
Merged from: Lymphoma Research Foundation of Canada (LRFC); Canadian Lymphoma Foundation (CLF)
Overview: A medium-sized national charitable organization founded in 2000
Mission: To provide education & support for individuals with lymphoma & their support network; To fund medical research to find a cure for lymphatic cancer; To advocate for the best treatment & care for lymphoma patients; To promote further research & new treatments in lymphoma & to promote rapid access to new developments
Chief Officer(s):
Robin Markowitz, Chief Executive Officer
robin@lymphoma.ca
Publications:
• Lymphoma & You: A Guide for Patients Living with Hodgkin's & Non-Hodgkin's Lymphoma
Type: Guide; *Editor:* C. Tom Kouroukis
Profile: Contents include an overview of lymphoma, Non-Hodgkin's & Hodgkin's Lymphoma, new developments in treatment, living withcancer, & a glossary
• Lymphoma Patient Resource
Type: Manual; *Number of Pages:* 146
Profile: A useful resource for patients recently diagnosed with lymphoma

Bureau du Québec
QC
www.lymphoma.ca

Chief Officer(s):
Patricia Gimore, Directrice, Québec
patricia@lymphoma.ca

Myeloma Canada / Myélome Canada
#138, 1800 Le Corbusier, Laval QC H7S 2K1
Tel: 579-934-3885; *Fax:* 514-505-1055
Toll-Free: 888-798-5771
e-mail: contact@myeloma.ca
www.myelomacanada.ca

Overview: A small national organization founded in 2004
Mission: To support persons living with multiple myeloma; To promote clinical research & improved access to drug trials in Canada
Member of: Canadian Cancer Action Network
Affiliation(s): International Myeloma Foundation
Chief Officer(s):
Aldo Del Col, Chair
adelcol@myeloma.ca
Olivier Jerome, Director, Operations
ojerome@myeloma.ca
Martine Elias, Director, Access, Advocacy & Community Relations
melias@myeloma.ca
Josee Rainville, Senior Manager, Communication & Events
jrainville@myeloma.ca
Michelle Oana, Manager, Community Events & Fundraising
moana@myeloma.ca
Publications:
• Multiple Myeloma Patient Handbook
Type: Handbook; *Price:* Free
Profile: Education for myeloma patients & their loved ones, so that they can be an active partner in their care

• Myeloma Canada Newsletter
Type: Newsletter; *Frequency:* Quarterly
Profile: News & developments related to the disease, plus upcoming meetings & fundraisers

Ovarian Cancer Canada (OCC) / Cancer de l'ovaire Canada (COC)
#205, 145 Front St. East, Toronto ON M5A 1E3
Tel: 416-962-2700; *Fax:* 416-962-2701
Toll-Free: 877-413-7970
e-mail: info@ovariancanada.org
www.ovariancanada.org
www.linkedin.com/company/728166
www.facebook.com/OvarianCancerCanada
twitter.com/OvarianCanada
www.youtube.com/OvarianCancerCanada

Previous Name: National Ovarian Cancer Association
Overview: A medium-sized national charitable organization founded in 1997
Mission: To support women & their families living with the disease; To raise awareness in the general public & with health care professionals; To fund research to develop reliable early detection techniques, improved treatments, & a cure
Member of: Canadian Coalition for Genetic Fairness
Chief Officer(s):
Elisabeth Baugh, Chief Executive Officer
ebaugh@ovariancanada.org
Kelly Grover, Vice-President, National Programs & Partners
kgrover@ovariancanada.org
Troy Cross, Vice-President, Development & Marketing
tcross@ovariancanada.org
Sheila Smith, Vice-President, Finance & Administration
ssmith@ovariancanada.org
Janice Chan, Director, Communications
jchan@ovariancanada.org
Roxana Predoi, Director, HR & Operations
rpredoi@ovariancanada.org

Atlantic Regional Office
1542 Queen St., Halifax NS B3J 2H8
Tel: 902-404-7070; *Fax:* 902-404-7071
Toll-Free: 866-825-0788

Chief Officer(s):
Emilie Chiasson, Regional Manager
echiasson@ovariancanada.org

Ontario Regional Office
#205, 145 Front St. East, Toronto ON M5A 1E3
Tel: 416-962-2700; *Fax:* 416-962-2701
Toll-Free: 877-413-7970

Chief Officer(s):
Cailey Crawford, Regional Manager
ccrawford@ovariancanada.org

Pacific-Yukon Regional Office
#330, 470 Granville St., Vancouver BC V6C 1V5
Tel: 604-676-3431; *Fax:* 604-676-3435
Toll-Free: 800-749-9310

Chief Officer(s):
Tracy Kolwich, Regional Manager
tkolwich@ovariancanada.org

Quebec Regional Office
#260, 4950 rue Queen-Mary, Montréal QC H3W 1X3
Tel: 514-369-2972; *Fax:* 514-940-0158
Toll-Free: 888-369-2972

Chief Officer(s):
Monique Beaupré-Lazure, Regional Manager
mbeauprelazure@ovariancanada.org

Western Regional Office
#105B, 1409 Edmonton Trail NE, Calgary AB T2E 3K8
Tel: 403-277-9449; *Fax:* 403-277-9919
Toll-Free: 866-591-6622

Chief Officer(s):
Tracy Kolwich, Regional Manager
tkolwich@ovariancanada.org

Prostate Cancer Canada (PCC) / Fondation canadienne de recherche sur le cancer de la prostate
2 Lombard St., 3rd Fl., Toronto ON M5C 1M1
Tel: 416-441-2131; *Fax:* 416-441-2325
Toll-Free: 888-255-0333
e-mail: info@prostatecancer.ca
www.prostatecancer.ca
www.linkedin.com/company/prostate-cancer-canada
www.facebook.com/prostatecancercanada
twitter.com/ProstateCancerC
www.instagram.com/prostatecancerc
Previous Name: Prostate Cancer Research Foundation of Canada
Overview: A small national organization founded in 1999
Mission: To raise funds for research into the causes, cure & prevention of prostate cancer by engaging Canadians through awareness, education, & advocacy
Member of: Prostate Cancer Alliance of Canada
Affliation(s): Canadian Urological Association
Chief Officer(s):
Ted Nash, Chair
Rocco Rossi, President & Chief Executive Officer
Stuart Edmonds, Vice President, Research, Health Promotion & Survivorship

Rethink Breast Cancer
#570, 215 Spadina Ave., Toronto ON M5T 2C7
Tel: 416-920-0980; *Fax:* 416-920-5798
Toll-Free: 866-738-4465
e-mail: hello@rethinkbreastcancer.com
www.rethinkbreastcancer.com
www.facebook.com/RethinkBreastCancer
twitter.com/rethinktweet
www.youtube.com/user/rethinkbreastcancer1
Overview: A medium-sized national charitable organization
Mission: To help young people concerned about & affected by breast cancer
Chief Officer(s):
Mary-Jo DeCoteau, Executive Director
Publications:
• Upfront
Type: Newsletter; *Frequency:* Quarterly
Profile: Information about upcoming events

Society of Gynecologic Oncologists of Canada (GOC) / Société des gynécologues oncologues du Canada
780 Echo Dr., Ottawa ON K1S 5R7
Tel: 613-730-4192; *Fax:* 613-730-4314
Toll-Free: 800-561-2416
www.g-o-c.org
Overview: A small national organization founded in 1980
Mission: To improve the care of women with gynecologic cancer; to raise standards of practice in gynecologic oncology & to encourage ongoing research
Chief Officer(s):
Dianne Miller, President
Walter Gotlieb, Sec.-Treas.

The Terry Fox Foundation / La Fondation Terry Fox
#150, 8960 University High St., Burnaby BC V5A 4Y6
Tel: 604-200-0541; *Fax:* 604-701-0247
Toll-Free: 888-836-9786
Other Communication: contact@terryfoxrun.org;
international@terryfox.org
e-mail: national@terryfoxrun.org
www.terryfoxrun.org
www.facebook.com/TheTerryFoxFoundation
twitter.com/TerryFoxCanada
www.youtube.com/terryfoxcanada
Also Known As: Terry Fox Run
Overview: A large national charitable organization founded in 1980
Mission: To maintain the vision & principles of Terry Fox while raising money for cancer research through the annual Terry Fox Run, memoriam donations & planned gifts. All money raised by the Foundation is distributed through the National Cancer Institute of Canada
Chief Officer(s):
Bill Pristanski, Chair

Judith Fox, International Director, 604-239-8576
international@terryfoxrun.org

Alberta/NWT/Nunavut Office
#D10, 6115 - 3rd St. SE, Calgary AB T2H 2L2
Tel: 403-212-1336; *Fax:* 403-212-1343
Toll-Free: 888-836-9786
Chief Officer(s):
Wendy Kennelly, Provincial Director
wendy.kennelly@terryfoxrun.org

British Columbia/Yukon Office
2669 Shaughnessy St., Port Coquitlam BC V3C 3G7
Tel: 604-464-2666; *Fax:* 604-464-2664
Toll-Free: 888-836-9786
e-mail: bcyukon@terryfoxrun.org
Chief Officer(s):
Donna White, Provincial Director

International
#150, 8960 University High St., Burnaby BC V5A 4Y6
e-mail: international@terryfoxrun.org
Chief Officer(s):
Rhonda Risenrough, International Director
Rhonda.risebrough@terryfox.org

Manitoba Office
1214 Chevrier Blvd., #A, Winnipeg MB R3T 1Y3
Tel: 204-231-5282; *Fax:* 204-321-5365
Toll-Free: 888-836-9786
e-mail: mb@terryfoxrun.org
Chief Officer(s):
Tammy Ferrante, Provincial Director

New Brunswick/PEI Office
#493, 605 Prospect St., Fredericton NB E3B 6B8
Tel: 506-458-2618; *Fax:* 506-459-4572
Toll-Free: 888-836-9786
e-mail: nbpei@terryfoxrun.org
Chief Officer(s):
Gwen Smith-Walsh, Provincial Director

Newfoundland & Labrador
#202, 835 Topsail Rd., Mount Pearl NL A1N 3J6
Tel: 709-576-8428; *Fax:* 709-747-7277
Toll-Free: 888-836-9786
e-mail: nl@terryfoxrun.org
Chief Officer(s):
Heather Strong, Provincial Director

Nova Scotia Office
#203, 3600 Kempt Rd., Halifax NS B3K 4X8
Tel: 902-423-8131; *Fax:* 902-492-3639
Toll-Free: 888-836-9786
e-mail: ns@terryfoxrun.org
Chief Officer(s):
Barbara Pate, Provincial Director

Ontario Office
#900, 1200 Eglinton Ave. Wast, Toronto ON M3C 1H9
Tel: 416-924-8252; *Fax:* 416-924-6597
Toll-Free: 888-836-9786
e-mail: ontario@terryfoxrun.org
Chief Officer(s):
Martha McClew, Provincial Director

Québec Office
#207, 10 Churchill Blvd., Greenfield Park QC J4V 2L7
Tel: 450-923-9747; *Fax:* 450-923-8468
Toll-Free: 888-836-9786
e-mail: qc@terryfoxrun.org
Chief Officer(s):
Peter Sheremeta, Provincial Director

Saskatchewan Office
1812 - 9th Ave. North, Regina SK S4R 7T4
Tel: 306-757-1662; *Fax:* 306-757-7422
Toll-Free: 888-836-9786
Chief Officer(s):
Heather Mackenzie, Provincial Director
heather.mackenzie@terryfoxrun.org

The 3C Foundation of Canada / Fondation Canadienne des 3c
#200, 1 Hines Rd., Kanata ON K2K 3C7

Tel: 613-237-6690
e-mail: info@3cfoundation.org
www.3cfoundation.org
www.facebook.com/GutTogether

Overview: A medium-sized national charitable organization founded in 1997

Chief Officer(s):
Michele Hepburn, President

Provincial Associations

ALBERTA

Alberta Cancer Foundation (ACF)
#710, 10123 - 99 St. NW, Edmonton AB T5J 3H1

Tel: 780-643-4400; *Fax:* 780-643-4398
Toll-Free: 866-412-4222
e-mail: acfonline@albertacancer.ca
albertacancer.ca
www.facebook.com/albertacancerfoundation
twitter.com/albertacancer
www.youtube.com/user/ABCancerFoundation

Overview: A small provincial charitable organization founded in 1984
Mission: To raise funds to support & enhance the programs & treatment facilities of the Alberta Cancer Board
Member of: Alberta Cancer Board
Chief Officer(s):
Myka Osinchuk, CEO

BRITISH COLUMBIA

British Columbia Cancer Foundation (BCCF)
#150, 686 West Broadway, Vancouver BC V5Z 1G1

Tel: 604-877-6040; *Fax:* 604-877-6161
Toll-Free: 888-906-2873
e-mail: bccfinfo@bccancer.bc.ca
www.bccancerfoundation.com
www.facebook.com/BCCancerFoundation
twitter.com/bccancer

Overview: A medium-sized provincial charitable organization founded in 1935
Mission: To reduce the incidence of cancer, reduce the mortality rate from cancer, & improve the quality of life for those living with cancer, through the acquisition, development, & stewardship of resources
Affiliation(s): British Columbia Cancer Research Centre; British Columbia Cancer Agency
Chief Officer(s):
Douglas Nelson, President & Chief Executive Officer
Luigi (Lou) Del Gobbo, Chief Financial Officer & Vice-President
Patsy Worrall, Vice-President, Marketing & Communications
Cindy Dopson, MBA, CHRP, Director, Human Resources

MANITOBA

CancerCare Manitoba (CCMB)
MacCharles Unit, 675 McDermot Ave., Winnipeg MB R3E 0V9

Tel: 204-787-2197
Toll-Free: 866-561-1026
e-mail: donate@cancercare.mb.ca
www.cancercare.mb.ca
twitter.com/cancercaremb
www.youtube.com/user/CancerCareMB

Also Known As: Action Cancer Manitoba
Overview: A small provincial organization founded in 1930
Mission: To provide exceptional care for patients & their families
Chief Officer(s):
Sri Navaratnam, President & CEO
Valerie Wiebe, Vice-President & Chief Officer, Patient Services
Bill Funk, Interim Chief Operating Officer

Manitoba Tobacco Reduction Alliance
192 Goulet St., Winnipeg MB R2H 0R8

Tel: 204-784-7030; *Fax:* 204-784-7039
e-mail: info@mantrainc.ca
www.mantrainc.ca

Also Known As: ManTRA
Previous Name: Council for a Tobacco-Free Manitoba
Overview: A small provincial organization founded in 1977
Mission: To strive for a tobacco-free society for Manitobans; to encourage & support legislation to restrict smoking in public places & workplaces; to maintain awareness of the hazards of tobacco consumption to identified high-risk target groups
Member of: Canadian Council on Smoking & Health
Chief Officer(s):
Rick Lambert, Chair
Murray Gibson, Executive Director

NEWFOUNDLAND AND LABRADOR

Newfoundland Cancer Treatment & Research Foundation (NCTRF)
300 Prince Philip Dr., St. John's NL A1B 3V6

Tel: 709-777-6484; *Fax:* 709-753-0927

Overview: A medium-sized provincial charitable organization founded in 1971
Mission: To provide excellence in cancer care, including research, cancer prevention, treatment, & support, in Newfoundland & Labrador
Affiliation(s): Canadian Council on Health Services Accreditation

NOVA SCOTIA

Breast Cancer Action Nova Scotia (BCANS)
Mill Cove Plaza, #205, 967 Bedford Hwy., Bedford NS B4A 1A9

Tel: 902-465-2685; *Fax:* 902-484-6436
e-mail: bcans@bcans.ca
www.bcans.ca
www.facebook.com/BreastCancerActionNovaScotia
twitter.com/BCANSBedford

Overview: A medium-sized provincial charitable organization founded in 1994
Mission: To address the obstacles faced by those living with breast cancer; To provide information; To create a support network for those with breast cancer
Affiliation(s): Keller Williams Realty (Harold Shea)
Publications:
• Atlantic Breast Cancer Net E-Newsletter
Type: Newsletter; *Price:* Free with membership in Breast Cancer Action Nova Scotia

ONTARIO

Cancer Care Ontario (CCO)
620 University Ave., Toronto ON M5G 2L7

Tel: 416-971-9800; *Fax:* 416-971-6888
e-mail: info@cis.cancer.ca
www.cancercare.on.ca
www.linkedin.com/company/cancer-care-ontario
www.facebook.com/CCO.Ontario
twitter.com/CancerCare_ON

Overview: A medium-sized provincial organization
Mission: To advise the Ontario government on all aspects of provincial cancer care; To provide information to health care providers & decision makers; To motivate better cancer system performance
Chief Officer(s):
Ratan Ralliaram, Chair
Michael Sherar, President & CEO

Lymphovenous Association of Ontario (LAO)
#203, 4800 Dundas Street West, Toronto ON M9A 1B1

Tel: 416-410-2250; *Fax:* 416-546-8991
Toll-Free: 877-723-0033
e-mail: lymphontario@yahoo.com
www.lymphontario.org

Overview: A small provincial charitable organization founded in 1996
Mission: To educate the public; To promote improved treatments for lymphovenous disorders; To support research for a cure
Affiliation(s): Canadian Disability Organization; Canadian Organization for Rare Disorders
Chief Officer(s):
Denise Lang, President
Anne Blair, Vice-Chair

Wellspring Cancer Support Foundation / Fondation Wellspring pour les personnes atteintes de cancer
4 Charles St. East, Toronto ON M4Y 1T1
Tel: 416-961-1928; *Fax:* 416-961-3721
Toll-Free: 877-499-9904
www.wellspring.ca
wwww.facebook.com/WellspringCAN
twitter.com/wellspringCAN
www.youtube.com/user/WellspringCancer
Overview: A medium-sized provincial charitable organization
Chief Officer(s):
John Philp, Chair
Christina Smith, CEO

QUÉBEC

Association des radio-oncologues du Québec (AROQ)
CP 216, Succ. Desjardins, #3000, 2, Complexe Desjardins, Montréal QC H5B 1G8
Tél: 514-350-5130; *Téléc:* 514-350-5126
Courriel: aroq@fmsq.org
www.aroq.ca
Aperçu: *Dimension:* petite; *Envergure:* provinciale surveillé par Fédération des médecins spécialistes du Québec
Mission: De fournir un forum où ses membres peuvent échanger des idées afin d'aider à améliorer leurs méthodes de traitement
Membre(s) du bureau directeur:
Khalil Sultanem, Président

Conseil québécois sur le tabac et la santé / Québec Council on Tobacco & Health
#302, 4126, rue St-Denis, Montréal QC H2W 2M5
Tél: 514-948-5317; *Téléc:* 514-948-4582
Courriel: info@cqts.qc.ca
www.cqts.qc.ca
twitter.com/cqts
Aperçu: *Dimension:* moyenne; *Envergure:* provinciale; Organisme sans but lucratif; fondée en 1976
Mission: Promouvoir la santé du fumeur et du non-fumeur; faire le lien entre les associations, groupes bénévoles et autres intéressés à la santé publique; trouver des approches et des moyens pour améliorer l'éducation face à l'usage du tabac
Membre de: Conseil canadien pour le contrôle du tabac
Membre(s) du bureau directeur:
Mario Bujold, Directeur général
Claire Harvey, Agente, Communications et relations médias

Fédération québécoise des laryngectomisés / Quebec Federation of Laryngectomees
5565, rue Sherbrooke est, Montréal QC H1N 1A2
Tél: 514-259-5113; *Téléc:* 514-259-8946
Courriel: fqlar@fqlar.qc.ca
www.fqlar.qc.ca
Nom précédent: Association des laryngectomisés de Montréal
Aperçu: *Dimension:* moyenne; *Envergure:* provinciale; Organisme sans but lucratif; fondée en 1979
Mission: Etre la voix de l'ensemble des personnes laryngectomisées, glossectomisées et trachéotomisées du Québec; assurer une meilleure connaissance des besoins particuliers de ces personnes et promouvoir la satisfaction de ces besoins
Affiliation(s): Société canadienne du Cancer; International Association of Laryngectomy
Membre(s) du bureau directeur:
Chantal Blouet, Responsable

Fondation Marie-Éve Saulnier
#102, 3925, Grande-Allée, Saint-Hubert QC J4T 2V8
Tél: 450-926-9000; *Téléc:* 450-766-8843
www.fondationmarieevesaulnier.qc.ca
www.facebook.com/Fondation.Marie.Eve.Saulnier2014
twitter.com/FondationMES
www.youtube.com/channel/UCKSL9-vwaPFPiHGDYXjLs_g
Aperçu: *Dimension:* petite; *Envergure:* provinciale; fondée en 1997
Mission: La Fondation Marie-Éve Saulnier améliore au jour le jour la qualité de vie des enfants atteints de cancer.
Membre(s) du bureau directeur:
Linda Langlois Saulnier, Directrice générale

Fondation québécoise du cancer
2075, rue de Champlain, Montréal QC H2L 2T1
Tél: 514-527-2194; *Téléc:* 514-527-1943
Ligne sans frais: 877-336-4443
Courriel: cancerquebec.mtl@fqc.qc.ca
www.facebook.com/fqcancer
Aperçu: *Dimension:* petite; *Envergure:* provinciale; Organisme sans but lucratif; fondée en 1979
Mission: Vouée à l'amélioration de la condition de la personne atteinte de cancer et de ses proches; offrir des services d'hôtellerie, d'écoute et d'information pour gens atteints du cancer; améliorer la qualité de vie des patients et celle de leurs proches.
Membre(s) du bureau directeur:
Pierre-Yves Gagnon, Directeur général

Hôtellerie de l'Estrie
3001, 12e av nord, Sherbrooke QC J1H 5N4
Tél: 819-822-2125; *Téléc:* 819-822-1392
Courriel: cancerquebec.she@fqc.qc.ca
www.fqc.qc.ca
Membre(s) du bureau directeur:
Marie Toupin, Directrice

Hôtellerie de l'Outaouais
Pavillon Michael J. MacGivney, 555, boul de l'Hôpital, Gatineau QC J8V 3T4
Tél: 819-561-2262; *Téléc:* 819-561-1727
Courriel: cancerquebec.gat@fqc.qc.ca
www.fqc.qc.ca
Membre(s) du bureau directeur:
Corinne Lorman, Directrice

Hôtellerie de la Mauricie
3110, rue Louis-Pasteur, Trois-Rivières QC G8Z 4E3
Tél: 819-693-4242; *Téléc:* 819-693-4243
Courriel: cancerquebec.trv@fqc.qc.ca
www.fqc.qc.ca
Membre(s) du bureau directeur:
Luce Girard, Directrice

Hôtellerie de Montréal
2075, rue de Champlain, Montréal QC H2L 2T1
Tél: 514-527-2194; *Téléc:* 514-527-1943
Ligne sans frais: 877-336-4443
Courriel: cancerquebec.mtl@fqc.qc.ca
www.fqc.qc.ca
Membre(s) du bureau directeur:
Pierre-Yves Gagnon, Directeur

Leucan - Association pour les enfants atteints de cancer / Leucan - Association for Children with Cancer
#300, 550, av Beaumont, Montréal QC H3N 1V1
Tél: 514-731-3696; *Téléc:* 514-731-2667
Ligne sans frais: 800-361-9643
www.leucan.qc.ca
www.linkedin.com/company/1115189
www.facebook.com/leucanpageprovinciale
twitter.com/leucan
instagram.com/leucan
Aperçu: *Dimension:* moyenne; *Envergure:* provinciale; fondée en 1978
Mission: Accroître la confiance en l'avenir des enfants atteints de cancer et de leurs familles
Membre de: Imagine Canada; Association des camps certifiés du Québec; Children's Oncology Camp Association International; Association canadienne des camps pédiatriques en oncologie
Membre(s) du bureau directeur:
Pascale Bouchard, Directeur général
pascale.bouchard@leucan.qc.ca
Publications:
• L'espoir [publication de Leucan - Association pour les enfants atteints de cancer]
Type: Newsletter; *Frequency:* s-a.

Organisation québécoise des personnes atteintes de cancer (OQPAC)

#100, 110 10e rue, Limoilou QC G1L 2M4

Tél: 418-529-1425; *Téléc:* 418-529-9714
Courriel: info@oqpac.com
www.oqpac.com
www.facebook.com/99211283481

Aperçu: *Dimension:* petite; *Envergure:* provinciale; Organisme sans but lucratif; fondée en 1984
Membre(s) du bureau directeur:
Martin Côté, Directeur général

Procure Alliance

#110, 1320 boul. Graham, Mont-Royal QC H3P 3C8

Tel: 514-341-3000
Toll-Free: 855-899-2873
e-mail: info@procure.ca
www.procure.ca
www.facebook.com/PROCURE.ca
twitter.com/procureqc
www.youtube.com/user/procureqc

Also Known As: Alliance Procure
Overview: A medium-sized provincial charitable organization
Mission: To prevent, cure, & raise awareness about prostate cancer by providing research, education, & support
Chief Officer(s):
Laurent Proulx, Executive Director

Société canadienne-française de radiologie (SCFR)

CP 216, Succursdale Desjardins, Montréal QC H5B 1G8

Tél: 514-350-5148; *Téléc:* 514-350-5147
Courriel: courrier@scfr.qc.ca
www.arq.qc.ca

Aperçu: *Dimension:* petite; *Envergure:* provinciale; Organisme sans but lucratif; fondée en 1928
Membre de: Fédération des médecins spécialistes du Québec
Membre(s) du bureau directeur:
Bruno Morin, Président
Vahid Khairi, Secrétaire général

SASKATCHEWAN

Saskatchewan Coalition for Tobacco Reduction (SCTR)

1080 Winnipeg St., Regina SK S4R 8P8

Tel: 306-766-6327; *Fax:* 306-766-6945

Previous Name: Saskatchewan Interagency Council on Smoking & Health
Overview: A small provincial organization founded in 1975
Mission: To advocate, coordinate & educate to ensure a tobacco-free Saskatchewan for all its residents
Member of: Canadian Centre for Tobacco Control
Chief Officer(s):
Lynn Greaves, Contact
   sctr@rqhealth.ca

Local Associations

BRITISH COLUMBIA

Alliance of Cancer Consultants

#206, 2571 Shaughnessy St., Port Coquitlam BC V3C 3G3
Previous Name: International Alliance of Breast Cancer Organizations
Overview: A small local organization
Chief Officer(s):
Tadeusz Slubowski, Director

Vancouver Island Prostate Cancer Research Foundation

#107, 1027 Pandora Ave., Victoria BC V8V 3P6

Tel: 250-920-0772
e-mail: vip@viprostate.org

Overview: A small local charitable organization
Mission: To support prostate cancer patients, by finding better methods of treatment & increasing the quality of life for prostate cancer sufferers
Affliation(s): Canadian Prostate Cancer Network

MANITOBA

Winnipeg Ostomy Association (WOA)

#204, 825 Sherbrook St., Winnipeg MB R3A 1M5

Tel: 204-234-2022
e-mail: woainfo@mts.net
www.ostomy-winnipeg.ca

Overview: A small local charitable organization founded in 1972 overseen by Canadian Ostomy Society
Mission: To assist people with ostomy & related surgeries in Winnipeg and the surrounding area
Chief Officer(s):
Lorrie Pismenny, President
Publications:
• Inside Out
Type: Newsletter; *Frequency:* 6 pa

ONTARIO

Breast Cancer Action (BCA) / Sensibilisation au cancer du sein

#301, 1390 Prince of Wales Dr., Ottawa ON K2C 3N6

Tel: 613-736-5921; *Fax:* 613-736-8422
e-mail: info@bcaott.ca
www.bcaott.ca
www.facebook.com/BCAOttawa
twitter.com/BCAOttawa

Overview: A medium-sized local charitable organization founded in 1993
Mission: To develop programs focused on raising awareness & providing education on breast cancer; To offer support, information & resources for individuals & families affected by breast cancer; To promote the exchange of information among organizations
Chief Officer(s):
Karen Graszat, Executive Director
   executivedirector@bcaott.ca

Candlelighters Childhood Cancer Support Programs, Inc.

#9, 21 Concourse Gate, Ottawa ON K2E 7S4

Tel: 613-715-9157
e-mail: information@candlelighters.net
www.candlelighters.net
www.facebook.com/candlelightersottawa
twitter.com/Candlelighters1
www.flickr.com/photos/candlelighters

Overview: A small local organization
Mission: To help children cope with their cancer diagnosis; to raise awareness about childhood cancer & its effect on the patients
Chief Officer(s):
Jocelyn Lamont, Executive Director
   jocelyn.lamont@candlelighters.net

Mount Sinai Hospital Foundation

#1001, 522 University Ave., Toronto ON M5G 1W7

Tel: 416-586-8203; *Fax:* 416-586-8639
Toll-Free: 877-565-8555
e-mail: foundation@mtsinai.on.ca
www.mshfoundation.ca
www.youtube.com/user/MountSinaiFoundation

Overview: A small local charitable organization founded in 1923
Mission: The Foundation raises & stewards funds to support the Mount Sinai Hospital's patient care, research & education. In 2008, more than $344 million has been raised to fund The Best Medicine Campaign, to support research, innovative programs, improved facilities & technology. Mount Sinai Hospital's Centres of Excellence include: the Samuel Lunenfeld Research Institute, Women's & Infants' Health, Oncology, Acute & Chronic Medicine, & Laboratory Medicine & Infection Control
Chief Officer(s):
Brent S. Belzberg, Chair
Kevin Goldthorp, President
Publications:
• The Best Medicine Matters [a publication of the Mount Sinai Hospital Foundation]
Type: Newsletter; *Frequency:* q.

Ronald McDonald House Toronto
240 McCaul St., Toronto ON M5T 1W5
Tel: 416-977-0458; *Fax:* 416-977-8807
e-mail: info@rmhtoronto.ca
www.rmhtoronto.ca
www.linkedin.com/company/ronald-mcdonald-house-toronto
www.facebook.com/RMHCToronto
twitter.com/RMHToronto
Also Known As: Toronto Children's Care Inc.
Previous Name: Children's Oncology Care of Ontario Inc.
Overview: A small local charitable organization founded in 1981
Mission: To provide a home & support services for out-of-town families whose children are receiving treatment in Toronto hospitals for serious illness
Chief Officer(s):
Sally Ginter, Chief Executive Officer
sginter@rmhctoronto.ca
Anita Price, Office Manager
aprice@rmhctoronto.ca

Zane Cohen Centre for Digestive Diseases Familial Gastrointestinal Cancer Registry (FGICR)
Mount Sinai Hospital, Zane Cohen Centre, PO Box 24, 60 Murray St., Toronto ON M5T 3L9
Tel: 416-586-4800; *Fax:* 416-586-5924
Toll-Free: 877-586-5112
e-mail: zcc@mtsinai.on.ca
www.zanecohencentre.ca
Previous Name: Familial GI Cancer Registry
Overview: A small local organization founded in 1980
Mission: The Registry is an interdisciplinary program dedicated to the specialty care of families affected with rare forms of inherited colorectal cancer.
Publications:
• Network [a publication of the Familial Gastrointestinal Cancer Registry]
Type: Newsletter; *Editor:* Terri Berk

QUÉBEC

A fleur de sein
313 3e Rue, Chibougamau QC G8P 1N4
Tél: 418-748-7914; *Téléc:* 418-748-4422
Aperçu: *Dimension:* petite; *Envergure:* locale; fondée en 1987
Mission: Offrir solidarité, présence, écoute & entraide à ceux & celles qui sont atteints d'un cancer, quel qu'il soit
Membre de: Regroupement Provincial des Organismes et Groupes d'entraide Communautaire en Oncologie; Vie Nouvelle
Affliation(s): Réseau québécoise pour la santé du sein
Membre(s) du bureau directeur:
Suzanne Hamel Migneaul, Présidente, A fleur de sein

Fondation de la greffe de moelle osseuse de l'Est du Québec (FGMOEQ)
1433, 4e av, Québec QC G1J 3B9
Tél: 418-529-5580; *Téléc:* 418-529-4004
Ligne sans frais: 877-520-3466
Courriel: info@fondation-moelle-osseuse.org
www.fondation-moelle-osseuse.org
Aperçu: *Dimension:* petite; *Envergure:* locale; Organisme sans but lucratif; fondée en 1996
Mission: Venir en aide aux personnes greffées et à leurs proches en fournissant des services gratuits ou à coût modique
Membre(s) du bureau directeur:
Pierre Drolet, Président

Institut du cancer de Montréal (ICM) / Montréal Cancer Institute
900, rue St-Denis, Montréal QC H2X 0A9
Tél: 514-890-8213
Courriel: info@icm.qc.ca
www.icm.qc.ca
twitter.com/cancermtl
Aperçu: *Dimension:* petite; *Envergure:* locale; fondée en 1942
Mission: Favoriser la recherche fondamentale et clinique sur le cancer et de préparer la relève dans ce domaine par le biais de l'enseignement et de la formation
Affiliation(s): CHUM, Université de Montréal

Membre(s) du bureau directeur:
André Boulanger, Président
Maral Tersakian, Directrice générale
maral.tersakian@icm.qc.ca

Organisation multiressources pour les personnes atteintes de cancer (OMPAC)
3849, rue Sherbrooke est, Montréal QC H1X 2A3
Tél: 514-729-8833; *Téléc:* 514-729-5390
Ligne sans frais: 866-248-6444
Nom précédent: Organisation montréalaise des personnes atteintes de cancer inc.
Aperçu: *Dimension:* petite; *Envergure:* locale; Organisme sans but lucratif; fondée en 1981
Mission: Apporter aide et assistance aux personnes atteintes de cancer et à leurs proches en offrant des services d'écoute téléphonique, de rencontres individuelles et de groupe, de documentation et de référence, et des activités diverses
Membre(s) du bureau directeur:
Colette Coudé, Directrice générale

International Associations

American Society of Pediatric Hematology / Oncology (ASPHO)
#300, 8735 West Higgins Rd., Chicago IL 60631 USA
Tel: 847-375-4716; *Fax:* 847-375-6483
e-mail: info@aspho.org
www.aspho.org
www.facebook.com/aspho.org
Overview: A medium-sized international organization founded in 1974
Mission: To promote optimal care of children & adolescents with blood disorders & cancer; To advance research, education, treatment, & professional practice
Chief Officer(s):
Amy Billett, President
Sally Weir, Executive Director
Bruce Hammond, Director, Governance & Operations
Judith Greifer, Manager, Marketing & Membership
Publications:
• Pediatric Blood & Cancer
Type: Journal; *Frequency:* Monthly; *Editor:* Peter E. Newburger, MD
Profile: Official journal of the American Society of Pediatric Hematology / Oncology & the International Society of Pediatric Oncology

European Society of Gynaecological Oncology (ESGO)
c/o LOCUS Workspace, Stn. Post Office 1, 1307/22 Krakovska, Prague 110 00 Czech Republic
e-mail: adminoffice@esgomail.org
www.esgo.org
Overview: A medium-sized international organization founded in 1983
Mission: To promote international & cultural communications between gynaecologists, pathologists, surgeons, oncologists, radiotherapists, & other specialists of disciplines related & pertaining to gynaecological oncology; to promote clinical & basic research investigations & spreading of knowledge in gynaecological oncology
Member of: European board & College Obstectrics & Gynecology
Affiliation(s): Federation of European Cancer Societies
Chief Officer(s):
Vesna Kesic, President

International Liver Cancer Association (ILCA)
300, av de Tervueren, Brussels B-1150 Belgium
Tel: +32 (0)2 789 2345; *Fax:* +32 (0)2 743 1550
e-mail: info@ilca-online.org
www.ilca-online.org
www.linkedin.com/groups/International-Liver-Cancer-Association-ILCA-46
www.facebook.com/InternationalLiverCancerAssociation
twitter.com/ILCAnews
Overview: A small international organization
Mission: To advance research in the pathogenesis, prevention, & treatment of liver cancer
Chief Officer(s):
Géraldine Damar, Executive Officer
Peter Galle, President

International Society of Chemotherapy for Infection & Cancer (ISC)

c/o Dept. of Medical Microbiology, Aberdeen Royal Infirmary, Aberdeen AB25 2ZN United Kingdom

Tel: 44 (0) 1224 554 954
www.ischemo.org

Overview: A medium-sized international organization founded in 1961
Mission: To advance the education & science of chemotherapy
Chief Officer(s):
Ian Gould, President
  i.m.gould@abdn.ac.uk
Po-Ren Hsueh, Secretary General
  hsporen@ntu.edu.tw

International Union Against Cancer (IUAC) / Union internationale contre le cancer (UICC)

62, rte de Frontenex, Geneva 1207 Switzerland

Tel: 41-22-809-1811; *Fax:* 41-22-809-1810
e-mail: info@uicc.org
www.uicc.org

Overview: A small international organization founded in 1933
Mission: To advance scientific & medical knowledge in research, diagnosis, treatment & prevention of cancer; To promote all other aspects of the campaign against cancer throughout the world, with emphasis on professional & public education
Affiliation(s): Canadian Cancer Society
Chief Officer(s):
Sanchia Aranda, President
Cary Adams, Chief Executive Officer

Israel Cancer Research Fund (ICRF)

PO Box 29, #616, 1881 Yonge St., Toronto ON M4S 3C4

Tel: 416-487-5246; *Fax:* 416-487-8932
Toll-Free: 866-207-4949
e-mail: research@icrf.ca
www.icrf.ca
www.facebook.com/ICRFToronto
twitter.com/icrftoronto
www.youtube.com/user/ICRFOnline

Overview: A small international charitable organization founded in 1975
Mission: To support scientists who are conducting cancer research in Israel
Chief Officer(s):
Bryna Goldberg, President
Joy Wagner Arbus, Executive Director
  joy.wagner@icrf.ca

Multinational Association for Supportive Care in Cancer (MASCC)

Herredsvejen 2, Hiller3d DK-3400 Denmark

Tel: 45-4820-7022; *Fax:* 45-4821-7022
www.mascc.org
www.linkedin.com/groups/MASCC-ISOO-Supportive-Care-in-5128277
www.facebook.com/589292597781443
twitter.com/CancerCareMASCC
www.youtube.com/user/MASCCorg

Overview: A medium-sized international organization founded in 1990
Mission: To promote research & education in all aspects of supportive care for patients with cancer
Chief Officer(s):
Åge Schultz, Executive Director
  aschultz@mascc.org
Publications:
• MASCC E-News
Type: Newsletter; *Frequency:* Quarterly
Profile: Recent information about organizational changes, deadlines, surveys, & study groups for Multinational Association for Supportive Care in Cancer members
• MASCC Society News
Type: Newsletter; *Frequency:* Monthly; *Editor:* Lisa Schulmeister; Snezana Bosnjak
Profile: Published on the web & in the back of the SCC journal
• Supportive Care in Cancer: The Journal of MASCC
Type: Journal; *Frequency:* Monthly; *Editor:* Fred Ashbury; *Price:* Free with MASCC / ISOO membership

Profile: Original work, reviews, consensus papers, guidelines, & short communications

North American Association of Central Cancer Registries, Inc. (NAACCR, Inc.)

2050 West Iles, #A, Springfield IL 62704-7412 USA

Tel: 217-698-0800; *Fax:* 217-698-0188
www.naaccr.org

Overview: A small international organization
Mission: To develop & promote data standards for cancer registration; To provide certification for population-based registries; To promote the use of cancer surveillance data & systems for cancer control
Chief Officer(s):
Betsy Kohler, Executive Director
  bkohler@naaccr.org
Charlie Blackburn, Chief Operating Officer
  cblackburn@naaccr.org
Recinda Sherman, Manager, Data Use & Research
  rsherman@naaccr.org
Publications:
• NAACCR [North American Association of Central Cancer Registries] Narrative
Type: Newsletter; *Frequency:* Quarterly
Profile: NAACCR updates, reports, & education & training calendar

National Publications

Canadian Oncology Nursing Journal
Owned By: Pappin Communications
c/o Canadian Association of Nurses in Oncology, #301, 750 West Pender St., Vancouver, BC V6C 2T7

Tel: 604-874-4322; *Fax:* 604-874-4378
Frequency: 4 times a year
Margaret I. Fitch, Editor-in-Chief, editor@cano-acio.ca

Oncology Exchange
Owned By: Parkhurst Publishing
400, rue McGill, 3e étage, Montréal, QC H2Y 2G1

Tel: 514-397-8833; *Fax:* 514-397-0228
Circulation: 6,000 *Frequency:* Quarterly
Susan Usher, Editor, usher@parkpub.com

Provincial Libraries

BC Cancer Agency
675 West 10th Ave., Vancouver, BC V5Z 1L3

Tel: 604-675-8000
www.bccancer.bc.ca
François Bénard, Vice-President, Research

Cancer Care Ontario
620 University Ave., Toronto, ON M5G 2L7

Tel: 416-971-9800; *Fax:* 416-971-6888
www.cancercare.on.ca/toolbox/libraries
Profile: An online library consisting of the Health Care Provider Library and archives, Patient Library, and Corporate Library and Archives
Collection: Cancer monographs, reports, workshop proceedings and presentations; Annual reports, financial reports and corporate presentations

CancerCare Manitoba
675 McDermot Ave., Winnipeg, MB R3E 0V9

Tel: 204-787-2197
www.cancercare.mb.ca
Collection: Resources about cancer treatment in languages such as English, French, Chinese, Cree, Filipino, Hindi, Inuktitut, Ojibwe, Oji-Cree, Spanish, Portuguese, Punjabi, & Vietnamese
Sri Navaratnam, President & CEO

Fondation québécoise du cancer
#50, 190 Dorchester sud, Québec, QC G1K 5Y9

Tél: 418-657-5334; *Téléc:* 418-657-5921
Ligne sans frais: 800-363-0063
cancerquebec.que@fqc.qc.ca
fqc.qc.ca
Mèdia social: www.facebook.com/fqcancer
Jacinthe Hovington, Directrice, programmes et services
  jhovington@fqc.qc.ca

Irving Greenberg Family Cancer Centre
#2712B, 3045 Baseline Rd., Level 2, Ottawa, ON K2H 8P4
Tel: 613-737-7700
patientlibrary@ottawahospital.on.ca

London Regional Cancer Centre
790 Commissioners Rd. East, London, ON N6A 4L6
Tel: 519-685-8600

Margaret & Charles Juravinski Cancer Centre
699 Concession St., Hamilton, ON L8V 5C2
Tel: 905-387-9711
jccpfrcentre@hhsc.ca
www.jcc.hhsc.ca

Collection: Books, videos, audio tapes, pamphlets, newsletters &
journals for understanding & coping with cancer
Ralph Meyer, President

Saskatchewan Cancer Agency
4101 Dewdney Ave., Regina, SK S4T 7T1
Tel: 306-766-2213; *Fax:* 306-766-2688
www.saskcancer.ca

Collection: Books; pamphlets & brochures; videos & audiotapes; lists
of relevant websites

Saskatoon Cancer Centre
20 Campus Dr., Saskatoon, SK S7N 4H4
Tel: 306-655-2662; *Fax:* 306-655-2910

Tom Baker Cancer Centre
1331 - 29 St. NW, #CC116, Calgary, AB T2N 4N2
Tel: 403-521-3765; *Fax:* 403-270-8419
krs.libguides.com/aboutus/TBCC

University Health Network
610 University Ave., 5th Fl., Toronto, ON M5G 2M9
Tel: 416-946-4482; *Fax:* 416-946-2084
uhnlibraries@uhn.ca
www.uhn.ca

Bogusia Trojan, Director, Library & Information Services
Ani Orchanian-Cheff, Archivist

Provincial Government

Acute Care / Soins aigus
Tel: 506-444-4128
Fax: 506-453-2958
Other Communication: New Brunswick Cancer Network:
www.gnb.ca/0051/cancer/index-e.asp

Executive Director, Daniel Coulombe
Tel: 506-453-8161
Dan.Coulombe@gnb.ca
Provincial Pharmacy Director, New Brunswick Cancer Network, Erica
Craig
Tel: 506-453-4287
Erica.Craig@gnb.ca
Medical Officer, New Brunswick Cancer Network, S. Eshwar Kumar
Tel: 506-457-7259
Eshwar.Kumar@gnb.ca
Director, Operations, Grlica Bolesnikov
Tel: 506-453-5521

Local Hospitals & Health Centres

ALBERTA

BARRHEAD: Barrhead Community Cancer Centre
Affiliated with: Alberta Health Services
Barrhead Healthcare Centre, 4815 - 51 Ave., Barrhead, AB T7N 1M1
Tel: 780-674-2221 *Fax:* 780-674-6773
www.albertahealthservices.ca

BONNYVILLE: Bonnyville Community Cancer Centre
Affiliated with: Alberta Health Services
Bonnyville Healthcare Centre, 5001 Lakeshore Dr., Bonnyville, AB T9N
2J7
Tel: 780-826-3311 *Fax:* 780-826-6527
www.albertahealthservices.ca

CALGARY: Tom Baker Cancer Centre (TBCC)
Affiliated with: Alberta Health Services
1331 - 29 St. NW, Calgary, AB T2N 4N2
Tel: 403-521-3723 *Fax:* 403-355-3206
Toll-Free: 866-238-3735
calgarypsychosocial@albertahealthservices.ca
www.albertahealthservices.ca

Year Founded: 1958
Note: Programs & services include: medical oncology; surgery (E-mail,
Alberta Radiosurgery Centre: arcinfo@cancerboard.ab.ca); radiation
oncology; radiology; chemotherapy treatments; psychosocial
resources; pathology; genetics; & research.
Teresa Davidson, Executive Director

CANMORE: Bow Valley Community Cancer Centre
Affiliated with: Alberta Health Services
Canmore General Hospital, 1100 Hospital Pl., Canmore, AB T1W 1N2
Tel: 403-678-5536 *Fax:* 403-678-9874
www.albertahealthservices.ca

CANMORE: Camrose Community Cancer Centre
Affiliated with: Alberta Health Services
St. Mary's Hospital, 4607 - 53 St., Canmore, AB T4V 1Y5
Tel: 780-679-6100 *Fax:* 780-679-6196
www.albertahealthservices.ca

DRAYTON VALLEY: Drayton Valley Community Cancer Centre
Affiliated with: Alberta Health Services
Drayton Valley Hospital & Care Centre, 4550 Madsen Ave., Drayton
Valley, AB T7A 1N8
Tel: 780-542-5321 *Fax:* 780-621-4966
www.albertahealthservices.ca

DRUMHELLER: Drumheller Community Cancer Centre
Affiliated with: Alberta Health Services
Drumheller Health Centre, 351 - 9th St. NW, Drumheller, AB T0J 0Y1
Tel: 403-823-6500 *Fax:* 403-823-5076
www.albertahealthservices.ca

EDMONTON: Cross Cancer Institute
Affiliated with: Alberta Health Services
11560 University Ave., Edmonton, AB T6G 1Z2
Tel: 780-432-8771 *Fax:* 780-432-8411
www.albertahealthservices.ca
Social Media: www.facebook.com/179579998746821;
twitter.com/AHS_media; www.youtube.com/AHSChannel
Number of Beds: 56 beds
Note: Cancer prevention, research & treatment program in northern
Alberta.
David Dyer, Executive Director

FORT MCMURRAY: Fort McMurray Community Cancer Centre
Affiliated with: Alberta Health Services
Northern Lights Regional Health Centre, 7 Hospital St., Fort McMurray,
AB T9H 1P2
Tel: 780-791-6161 *Fax:* 780-791-6042
www.albertahealthservices.ca

GRANDE PRAIRIE: Grande Prairie Cancer Centre
Affiliated with: Alberta Health Services
Queen Elizabeth II Hospital, 10409 - 98 St., Grande Prairie, AB T8V
2E8
Tel: 780-538-7588 *Fax:* 780-532-9120
www.albertahealthservices.ca

Note: Programs & services include: cancer treatment & care;
chemotherapy; laboratory; nuclear medicine; pastoral care; pharmacy;
social work; & symptom control & palliative care.

HIGH RIVER: High River Community Cancer Centre
Affiliated with: Alberta Health Services
High River General Hospital, 560 - 9th Ave. West, High River, AB T1V
1B3
Tel: 403-652-2200 *Fax:* 403-652-0199
www.albertahealthservices.ca

HINTON: Hinton Community Cancer Centre
Affiliated with: Alberta Health Services
Hinton Healthcare Centre, 1280 Switzer Dr., Hinton, AB T7V 1V2
Tel: 780-865-3333 *Fax:* 780-865-1099
www.albertahealthservices.ca

LETHBRIDGE: Jack Ady Cancer Centre
Affiliated with: Alberta Health Services
960 - 19th St. South, Lethbridge, AB T1J 1W5
Tel: 403-388-6200
www.albertahealthservices.ca

Note: Programs & services include: cancer treatment & care; chemotherapy; diagnostic imaging; laboratory; palliative care; radiation therapy; & social work.
Dr. Malcolm Brigden, Medical Director

LLOYDMINSTER: Lloydminster Community Cancer Centre
Affiliated with: Alberta Health Services
Lloydminster Hospital, 3820 - 43 Ave., Lloydminster, AB S9V 1Y5
Tel: 306-820-6144 *Fax:* 306-820-6145
www.albertahealthservices.ca

MEDICINE HAT: Margery E. Yuill Cancer Centre
Affiliated with: Alberta Health Services
Medicine Hat Regional Hospital, 666 - 5th St. SW, Medicine Hat, AB T1A 4H6
Tel: 403-529-8000 *Fax:* 403-529-8814
www.albertahealthservices.ca
Year Founded: 1989
Number of Beds: 4 treatment beds
Note: Programs & services include: cancer treatment & care; chemotherapy; colposcopy; diagnostic imaging; laboratory; nuclear medicine; & social work.
Jill Forsyth, Manager

PEACE RIVER: Peace River Community Cancer Centre
Affiliated with: Alberta Health Services
Peace River Community Health Centre, 10101 - 68 St., Peace River, AB T8S 1T6
Tel: 780-624-7500 *Fax:* 780-618-3472
www.albertahealthservices.ca

RED DEER: Central Alberta Cancer Centre
Affiliated with: Alberta Health Services
PO Box 5030, 3942 - 50A Ave., Red Deer, AB T4N 4E7
Tel: 403-343-4422 *Fax:* 403-346-1160
www.albertahealthservices.ca

Note: Programs & services include: cancer treatment & care; chemotherapy; clinical breast health program; nutrition; laboratory; palliative care; pharmacy; radiation therapy; & spiritual care.
Myrna Kelley, Nurse Manager

BRITISH COLUMBIA

KELOWNA: BC Cancer Agency Sindi Ahluwalia Hawkins Centre for the Southern Interior
Affiliated with: Interior Health Authority
Also Known As: Cancer Centre for the Southern Interior
399 Royal Ave., Kelowna, BC V1Y 5L3
Tel: 250-712-3900 *Toll-Free:* 888-563-7773
www.bccancer.bc.ca

Number of Employees: 220
John Larmet, Director, Clinical Operations

VANCOUVER: British Columbia Cancer Agency Vancouver
Affiliated with: Provincial Health Services Authority
600 - 10 Ave. West, Vancouver, BC V5Z 4E6
Tel: 604-877-6000 *Fax:* 604-872-4596
Toll-Free: 800-663-3333
www.bccancer.bc.ca
Social Media: twitter.com/BCCancer_Agency

Note: Cancer prevention, screening, diagnosis, treatment, rehabilitation, & care.

Dr. Malcolm Moore, President
Dr. François Bénard, Vice-President, Research
Brenda Canitz, Acting Vice-President, Patient Experience & Interprofessional Practice
Dr. Lee Ann Martin, Acting Vice-President, Clinical Programs & Quality
Dr. John Spinelli, Vice-President, Population Oncology
Dr. Frances Wong, Vice-President, Medical Affairs & Medical Information

MANITOBA

BRANDON: Western Manitoba Cancer Centre (WMCC)
Brandon Regional Health Centre
Affiliated with: Prairie Mountain Health
300 McTavish Ave. East, Brandon, MB R7A 2B3
Tel: 204-578-2222 *Fax:* 204-578-4991
www.prairiemountainhealth.ca

Year Founded: 2011

WINNIPEG: CancerCare Manitoba
Affiliated with: Winnipeg Regional Health Authority
675 McDermot Ave., Winnipeg, MB R3E 0V9
Tel: 204-787-2197 *Fax:* 204-787-1184
Toll-Free: 866-561-1026
www.cancercare.mb.ca
Social Media: twitter.com/cancercaremb;
www.youtube.com/user/CancerCareMB/videos

Number of Employees: 800
Note: Provides cancer treatment in all areas: prevention, early detection, diagnosis, treatment & care, & end of life care.
Dr. Sri Navaratnam, President & CEO
Nardia Maharaj, Chief Operating Officer
Dr. Piotr Czaykowski, Chief Medical Officer

NEWFOUNDLAND & LABRADOR

ST. JOHN'S: Dr. H. Bliss Murphy Cancer Centre
Dr. H. Bliss Murphy Cancer Care Foundation, 300 Prince Philip Dr., St. John's, NL A1B 3V6
Tel: 709-777-7589

ONTARIO

HAMILTON: Juravinski Cancer Centre
Hamilton Health Sciences
Affiliated with: Hamilton Niagara Haldimand Brant Local Health Integration Network
Former Name: Hamilton Regional Cancer Centre
699 Concession St., Hamilton, ON L8V 5C2
Tel: 905-387-9495
www.jcc.hhsc.ca

Dr. Ralph Meyer, President

KINGSTON: Cancer Centre of Southeastern Ontario
Kingston General Hospital
25 King St. West, Kingston, ON K7L 5P9
Tel: 613-549-6666 *Toll-Free:* 800-567-5722
www.kgh.on.ca

Michael Bell, Program Operational Director

LONDON: London Regional Cancer Program
London Health Sciences Centre
PO Box 5165, 790 Commissioners Rd. East, London, ON N6A 4L6
Tel: 519-685-8600
www.lhsc.on.ca

Note: Specialties: Inpatient & outpatient cancer care; Radiation therapy; Chemotherapy; Syooirt services, such as social work & diet & nutrition counselling
Neil Johnson, Regional Vice-President, Cancer Care

OTTAWA: Ottawa Hospital Cancer Program
General Campus, 501 Smyth Rd., Ottawa, ON K1H 8L6
Tel: 613-737-7700

Note: Specialties: Screening; Early Detection; Diagnosis; Treatment; Supportive Care; Palliative Care; Research
Dr. Jack Kitts, President & CEO

TORONTO: Marvelle Koffler Breast Centre

J. & W. Lebovic Health Complex, Mount Sinai Hospit, 600 University Ave., 12th Fl., Toronto, ON M5G 1X5

Tel: 416-586-8799
www.mountsinai.on.ca/care/mkbc

Year Founded: 1995
Note: Specialties: Outpatient facility for breast health & disease; mammography / breast imaging; pathology; surgery; psychiatry; nutrition; boutique addressing the needs of women who have experienced breast cancer; palliative medicine
Dr. Christine Elser, Head, Familial Breast Cancer Clinic

TORONTO: Princess Margaret Hospital
University Health Network
Affiliated with: Toronto Central Local Health Integration Network
Also Known As: Princess Margaret Cancer Centre

610 University Ave., Toronto, ON M5G 2M9

Tel: 416-946-2000
www.theprincessmargaret.ca
Social Media: www.facebook.com/UniversityHealthNetwork;
twitter.com/UHN_News; www.youtube.com/UHNToronto;
www.linkedin.com/company/university-health-network

Year Founded: 1952
Number of Beds: 202 beds
Number of Employees: 3000
Note: A teaching hospital of the University of Toronto, & a top cancer treatment & research centre. Programs & services include: allied health; dental oncology, ocular & maxillofacial prosthetics; laboratory medicine; medical imaging; medical oncology & hematology; oncology nursing; patient education & survivorship; pharmacy; psychosocial oncology & palliative care; radiation medicine; & surgical oncology. The Ontario Cancer Institute comprises the research wing of the hospital.

TORONTO: Sunnybrook Health Sciences Centre - The Odette Cancer Centre
Affiliated with: Toronto Central Local Health Integration Network

2075 Bayview Ave., Toronto, ON M4N 3M5

Tel: 416-480-5000 *Fax:* 416-217-1338
www.sunnybrook.ca

Note: Comprehensive cancer care, multidisciplinary, evidence-based approach; research, education & community outreach
Dr. Barry A. McLellan, President & CEO

Carpal Tunnel Syndrome

Carpal tunnel syndrome, CTS, is a painful, often debilitating condition caused by compression of the median nerve as it passes through the wrist (carpal tunnel) to the hand.

Cause

While job-related movement—holding vibrating tools or gripping tools tightly, keeping the hands in an awkward position, or engaging in repetitive hand motions—is the most common cause of CTS, people with underlying conditions, such as diabetes, gout, rheumatoid arthritis, obesity and pregnancy, are more prone to experience symptoms. Although less common, the onset of CTS can stem from trauma, such as a blow to the hand or wrist. Some studies also suggest that stress can play a part in the development of carpal tunnel syndrome.

Symptoms

An initial indication of CTS is a feeling that the hand is asleep. Typically, the patient wakes at night with numbness and tingling of the affected hand, usually in the thumb, index, middle and ring finger. The most serious functional problem occurs when numbness and weakness make it difficult to move the thumb into a grasping or pinching position with the other fingers. Everyday activities such as fastening a button, unscrewing a bottle top or turning a key can become next to impossible. In advanced cases, pain associated with CTS may radiate up the arm to the shoulder.

Prevalence

In Canada, around 10 percent of adults are estimated to have a risk of developing carpal tunnel syndrome at some point in their lives. CTS most commonly occurs in women aged 30 to 50 years. The incidence is highest among keyboard users, musicians, assembly-line workers, and others who engage in repetitive hand work.

Treatment Options

Certain tests are conducted to diagnose CTS. In Phalen's test, the hands are placed together, back to back, and the wrist is flexed for one minute. This maneuver generally produces tingling of the hand in a patient with CTS. In Tinel's test, the median nerve is tapped at the wrist. If this results in tingling in one or more fingers, damage to the median nerve is suspected. Electromyography is also used to determine whether there is damage to the median nerve. Electrodes are put on the forearms, and an electric current is passed through the patient. Measurements are then taken to determine how quickly the impulse is transmitted along the median nerve to the muscles.

Certain workplace changes may assist in preventing CTS. Keyboard users, and those engaged in similar activities, can adjust their seats and backrests to assure that their arms are positioned comfortably during work sessions. Employers can rotate jobs among workers, encourage workers to take frequent rest breaks and develop ergonomic programs.

For mild cases of CTS, a lightweight brace, especially worn at night, can decrease symptoms by holding the wrist stable. Marked improvement may arise from wearing a brace for a week or two. However, in many cases, it is recommended that the sufferer cease working until symptoms have improved. Exercises and deep-tissue massage can strengthen the wrist and hand. Over-the-counter anti-inflammatory medications, such as ibuprofen and aspirin, can also reduce symptoms of mild CTS. In more acute conditions, cortisone injections may be administered.

When symptoms are severe and persistent, surgery may be required to reduce pressure on the nerves. The most common surgery is an open incision technique called open carpal tunnel release, which usually improves the condition dramatically. A newer and less invasive procedure is endoscopic carpal tunnel release, which uses a smaller incision and visualizes the operative field using a fiber optic camera. Although it often takes months, most people fully recover from surgery, and do not experience recurrence of carpal tunnel syndrome.

National Associations

Canadian Alliance of Physiotherapy Regulators (CARP) / Alliance canadienne des organismes de réglementation de la physiothérapie (ACORP)
#501, 1243 Islington Ave., Toronto ON M8X 1Y9

Tel: 416-234-8800; *Fax:* 416-234-8820
e-mail: email@alliancept.org
www.alliancept.org

Overview: A large national organization founded in 1987
Mission: To facilitate the sharing of information & build consensus on national regulatory issues in order to assist member regulators in fulfilling their mandate of protecting the public interest
Chief Officer(s):
Katya Masnyk, Chief Executive Officer
Publications:
• Canadian Alliance of Physiotherapy Regulators Annual Report
Type: Report; *Frequency:* Annually; *Price:* Free

Physiotherapy Education Accreditation Canada (PEAC) / Agrément de l'enseignement de la physiothérapie au Canada (EPAC)
#26, 509 Commissioners Rd. West, London ON N6J 1Y5
Tel: 226-636-0632; *Fax:* 778-724-0669
e-mail: info@peac-aepc.ca
www.peac-aepc.ca
Previous Name: Accreditation Council for Canadian Physiotherapy Academic Programs
Overview: A medium-sized national licensing organization founded in 2000
Mission: To provide leadership in maintaining the quality of physiotherapy education in Canada through a comprehensive accreditation program
Member of: Association of Accrediting Agencies of Canada (AAAC); The Canadian Council of Physiotherapy University Programs
Affiliation(s): Accreditation of Interprofessional Health Education (AIPHE)
Chief Officer(s):
Sharon Switzer-McIntyre, President
Kathy Davidson, Executive Director
  kathy.davidson@peac-aepc.ca
Publications:
• Peer Review Team Handbook
Type: Handbook; *Number of Pages:* 49
Profile: Includes the responsibilities of the peer review team members, a detailed schedule for the on-site accreditation review, & information about the final meeting & the written report
• Program Accreditation Handbook
Type: Handbook; *Number of Pages:* 50
Profile: Information about the accreditation of physiotherapy education programs in Canada, for physiotherapy education program faculty & staff who are preparing for accreditation review, members of the accreditation Peer Review Team teams, university administrators, & members of the public

Provincial Associations

ALBERTA

Physiotherapy Alberta - College + Association
Dorchester Bldg., #300, 10357 - 109 St., Edmonton AB T5J 1N3
Tel: 780-438-0338; *Fax:* 780-436-1908
Toll-Free: 800-291-2782
e-mail: info@physiotherapyalberta.ca
www.physiotherapyalberta.ca
www.linkedin.com/company/physiotherapy-alberta—-college-association
www.facebook.com/PTAlberta
twitter.com/PTAlberta
www.youtube.com/user/PTAlberta
Previous Name: College of Physical Therapists of Alberta
Overview: A medium-sized provincial licensing organization founded in 1985 overseen by Canadian Alliance of Physiotherapy Regulators
Mission: To protect the public by the regulation of the practice of physical therapy
Member of: Canadian Alliance of Physiotherapy Regulators; Canadian Physiotherapy Association
Affiliation(s): Alberta Federation of Regulated Health Professions
Chief Officer(s):
Dianne Millette, Registrar, 780-702-5353
  dmillette@physiotherapyalberta.ca
Publications:
• PT Alberta [a publication of Physiotherapy Alberta - College + Association]
Type: Newsletter

BRITISH COLUMBIA

College of Physical Therapists of British Columbia (CPTBC)
#1420, 1200 West 73rd Ave., Vancouver BC V6P 6G5
Tel: 604-730-9193; *Fax:* 604-730-9273
Toll-Free: 877-576-6744
e-mail: info@cptbc.org
www.cptbc.org
Overview: A medium-sized provincial organization founded in 1994 overseen by Canadian Alliance of Physiotherapy Regulators

Mission: To serve and protect the public by ensuring that Physical Therapists provide high quality, competent and ethical services.
Member of: Canadian Alliance of Physiotherapy Regulators
Chief Officer(s):
Brenda Hudson, Registrar
  brenda_hudson@cptbc.org

Physiotherapy Association of British Columbia (PABC)
#402, 1755 West Broadway, Vancouver BC V6J 4S5
Tel: 604-736-5130; *Fax:* 604-736-5606
Toll-Free: 888-330-3999
e-mail: office@bcphysio.org
www.bcphysio.org
www.facebook.com/bcphysio
twitter.com/bcphysio
www.youtube.com/user/BCPhysio
Overview: A medium-sized provincial organization founded in 1927 overseen by Canadian Physiotherapy Association
Mission: To provide leadership & direction to the physiotherapy profession; To foster excellence in practice, education & research
Member of: Canadian Physiotherapy Association
Chief Officer(s):
Kevin Evans, Chief Executive Officer
  kevin@bcphysio.org
Emira Mears, Director, Strategic Communications
  communications@bcphysio.org
Tracy Stewart, Manager, Communications
  tracy@bcphysio.org
Fiona Chiu, Manager, Knowledge
  librarian@bcphysio.org
Sheana Lehigh, Manager, Education
  education@bcphysio.org
Kimberley Payne, Office Administrator

MANITOBA

College of Physiotherapists of Manitoba (CPM)
#211, 675 Pembina Hwy., Winnipeg MB R3M 2L6
Tel: 204-287-8502; *Fax:* 204-474-2506
e-mail: info@manitobaphysio.com
www.manitobaphysio.com
Overview: A small provincial licensing organization founded in 1957 overseen by Canadian Alliance of Physiotherapy Regulators
Mission: To protect the public by ensuring quality physiotherapy is provided to the public
Member of: Canadian Alliance of Physiotherapy Regulators
Chief Officer(s):
Tanya Kozera, Chair
  cpmchair@manitobaphysio.com
Brenda McKechnie, Registrar/Executive Director
Publications:
• In Touch Newsletter [a publication of the College of Physiotherapists of Manitoba]
Type: Newsletter

Manitoba Physiotherapy Association (MPA)
145 Pacific Ave., Winnipeg MB R3B 2Z6
Tel: 204-925-5701; *Fax:* 204-925-5624
Toll-Free: 877-925-5701
e-mail: ptassociation@mbphysio.org
www.mbphysio.org
www.facebook.com/MBPhysiotherapy
twitter.com/MBPhysiotherapy
Overview: A medium-sized provincial organization overseen by Canadian Physiotherapy Association
Mission: To provide leadership & direction to the physiotherapy profession; To foster excellence in practice, education & research
Member of: Canadian Physiotherapy Association
Chief Officer(s):
Allison Guerico, President

NEWFOUNDLAND AND LABRADOR

New Brunswick Physiotherapy Association (NBPA)
PO Box 28117, St. John's NL A1B 4J8
Tel: 709-765-1096
e-mail: atlanticbranches@physiotherapy.ca

Overview: A medium-sized provincial organization overseen by Canadian Physiotherapy Association
Mission: To provide leadership & direction to the physiotherapy profession; To foster excellence in practice, education & research
Member of: Canadian Physiotherapy Association
Chief Officer(s):
Lisa Pike, Executive Director
Colin Hood, President

Newfoundland & Labrador College of Physiotherapists (NLCP)
PO Box 21351, St. John's NL A1A 5G6
Tel: 709-753-6527; *Fax:* 709-753-6526
e-mail: collegept@nf.aibn.com
nlcpt.com
Overview: A small provincial licensing organization founded in 1972 overseen by Canadian Alliance of Physiotherapy Regulators
Mission: To regulate the profession of physiotherapy in Newfoundland & Labrador
Member of: Canadian Alliance of Physiotherapy Regulators
Affliation(s): Canadian Physiotherapy Association
Chief Officer(s):
Ryan Johnston, Chair
Josephine Crossan, Executive Director/Registrar
Publications:
• Newfoundland & Labrador College of Physiotherapists Newsletter
Type: Newsletter

Newfoundland & Labrador Physiotherapy Association (NLPA)
St. John's NL
www.physiotherapy.ca/Atlantic-Branches/Newfoundland
www.facebook.com/NLPhysioAssoc
twitter.com/nlphysioassoc
Overview: A medium-sized provincial organization overseen by Canadian Physiotherapy Association
Mission: To provide leadership & direction to the physiotherapy profession; To foster excellence in practice, education & research
Member of: Canadian Physiotherapy Association
Chief Officer(s):
Lisa Pike, Executive Director
Sherry Lythgoe, President

NORTHWEST TERRITORIES

Northwest Territories & Nunavut Council of the Canadian Physiotherapy Association (NWTNC)
Yellowknife NT
Tel: 867-669-4117; *Fax:* 867-669-4137
Overview: A medium-sized provincial organization overseen by Canadian Physiotherapy Association
Member of: Canadian Physiotherapy Association

NOVA SCOTIA

Nova Scotia College of Physiotherapists (NSCP)
PO Box 309, Stn. Main, Dartmouth NS B2Y 3Y5
Tel: 902-454-0158; *Fax:* 902-484-6381
Toll-Free: 866-225-1060
e-mail: office@nsphysio.com
www.nsphysio.com
Overview: A small provincial licensing organization founded in 1958 overseen by Canadian Alliance of Physiotherapy Regulators
Mission: To assure that the interests of the public are upheld through the regulation & promotion of safe & effective physiotherapy services; To communicate effectively with the membership & thereby affect change on issues of concern to the public
Member of: Canadian Alliance of Physiotherapy Regulators
Chief Officer(s):
Joan Ross, Registrar, 902-454-0158 Ext. 1, Fax: 902-245-3134
registrar@nsphysio.com
Patrick King, Executive Director, 902-454-0158 Ext. 2, Fax: 902-484-6381

Nova Scotia Physiotherapy Association (NSPA)
PO Box 33013, Halifax NS B3L 4T6
Tel: 902-223-0141
e-mail: info@physiotherapyns.ca
www.physiotherapyns.ca

Overview: A medium-sized provincial organization overseen by Canadian Physiotherapy Association
Mission: To provide leadership & direction to the physiotherapy profession; To foster excellence in practice, education & research
Member of: Canadian Physiotherapy Association
Chief Officer(s):
Morah MacEachern, Executive Director
ed@physiotherapyns.ca
Alison McDonald, President
president@physiotherapyns.ca

ONTARIO

College of Physiotherapists of Ontario (CPO) / Ordre des physiothérapeutes de l'Ontario
#901, 375 University Ave., Toronto ON M5G 2J5
Tel: 416-591-3828; *Fax:* 416-591-3834
Toll-Free: 800-583-5885
e-mail: info@collegept.org
www.collegept.org
twitter.com/CollegeofPTs
www.youtube.com/user/CollegeofPts
Overview: A medium-sized provincial organization founded in 1994 overseen by Canadian Alliance of Physiotherapy Regulators
Mission: To protect & serve the public interest by ensuring that physiotherapists provide high quality, competent & ethical services
Member of: Canadian Alliance of Physiotherapy Regulators
Affliation(s): Federation of Health Regulatory Colleges of Ontario; Canadian Physiotherapy Association; Ontario Physiotherapy Association; Federation of State Boards of Physical Therapy; World Confederation of Physical Therapy
Chief Officer(s):
Rod Hamilton, Associate Registrar, Policy Ext. 232
rhamilton@collegept.org
Shenda Tanchak, Registrar & CEO
Lisa Pretty, Communications Director

Ontario Physiotherapy Association (OPA)
#210, 55 Eglinton Ave. East, Toronto ON M4P 1G8
Tel: 416-322-6866; *Fax:* 416-322-6705
Toll-Free: 800-672-9668
e-mail: physiomail@opa.on.ca
www.opa.on.ca
www.linkedin.com/company/2385075
www.facebook.com/OntarioPT
twitter.com/ONTPhysio
www.youtube.com/user/OntarioPhysiotherapy
Overview: A medium-sized provincial organization founded in 1964 overseen by Canadian Physiotherapy Association
Mission: To act as a voice for the physiotherapy profession in Ontario; To ensure the provision of quality physiotherapy services to residents of Ontario
Member of: Canadian Physiotherapy Association
Chief Officer(s):
Dorianne Sauvé, Chief Executive Officer
dsauve@opa.on.ca
Wendy Smith, President
president@opa.on.ca
Sara Pulins, Manager, Marketing & Communications
spulins@opa.on.ca
Publications:
• Ontario Physiotherapy Association Annual Report
Type: Yearbook; *Frequency:* Annually
• Physiotherapy Today [a publication of the Ontario Physiotherapy Association]
Type: Newsletter; *Frequency:* Bimonthly; *Price:* Free with Ontario Physiotherapy Association membership

PRINCE EDWARD ISLAND

Prince Edward Island College of Physiotherapists (PEICP)
PO Box 20078, Charlottetown PE C1A 9E3
Fax: 902-739-3051
e-mail: contact@peicpt.com
www.peicpt.com
Overview: A small provincial licensing organization overseen by Canadian Alliance of Physiotherapy Regulators

Mission: To regulate the practice of physiotherapy on Prince Edward Island, in accordance with the provincial legislation, "Physiotherapy Act"; To protect the public by ensuring competent & ethical practice
Member of: Canadian Alliance of Physiotherapy Regulators

Prince Edward Island Physiotherapy Association (PEI CPA)
PE

www.physiotherapy.ca/Atlantic-Branches/Prince-Edward-Island
Overview: A medium-sized provincial organization overseen by Canadian Physiotherapy Association
Mission: To provide leadership & direction to the physiotherapy profession; To foster excellence in practice, education & research
Member of: Canadian Physiotherapy Association
Chief Officer(s):
Trish Helm Neima, Contact

QUÉBEC

Ordre professionnel de la physiothérapie du Québec (OPPQ)
#1000, 7151, rue Jean-Talon est, Anjou QC H1M 3N8
Tél: 514-351-2770; *Téléc:* 514-351-2658
Ligne sans frais: 800-361-2001
Courriel: physio@oppq.qc.ca
www.oppq.qc.ca
Nom précédent: Ordre professionnel des physiothérapeutes du Québec; Corporation professionnelle des physiothérapeutes du Québec
Aperçu: *Dimension:* moyenne; *Envergure:* provinciale; fondée en 1973 surveillé par Canadian Alliance of Physiotherapy Regulators
Mission: Assurer la protection du public en surveillant l'exercice de la physiothérapie par ses membres et en contribuant à leur développement professionnel
Membre de: Alliance canadienne des organismes de réglementation de la physiothérapie; Association canadienne de physiothérapie
Membre(s) du bureau directeur:
Denis Pelletier, Président
dpelletier@oppq.qc.ca
Claude Laurent, Directeur général et secrétaire
claurent@oppq.qc.ca

SASKATCHEWAN

Saskatchewan Physiotherapy Association (SPA)
#118, 1121 College Dr., Saskatoon SK S7N 0W3
Tel: 306-955-7265; *Fax:* 306-955-7260
www.saskphysio.org
www.facebook.com/saskphysio
twitter.com/saskphysio
Overview: A medium-sized provincial organization overseen by Canadian Physiotherapy Association
Mission: To provide leadership to the physiotherapy profession; To foster excellence in practice, education & research; To promote high standards of health in Saskatchewan
Member of: Canadian Physiotherapy Association
Chief Officer(s):
Chris Wiechnik, President
Lorna MacMillan, Executive Director

YUKON TERRITORY

Physiotherapy Association of Yukon (PAY)
Whitehorse YT
Overview: A medium-sized provincial organization overseen by Canadian Physiotherapy Association
Mission: To unite members of the profession
Member of: Canadian Physiotherapy Association
Chief Officer(s):
Liris Smith, President
smithco@northwestel.net
Publications:
• Yukon Council of Canadian Physiotherapy Association Newsletter
Type: Newsletter; *Frequency:* a.

Provincial Libraries

Holland Orthopaedic & Arthritic Centre Library
#235, 43 Wellesley St. East, Toronto, ON M4Y 1H1
Tel: 416-967-8545

Local Hospitals & Health Centres

ONTARIO

TORONTO: Sunnybrook Health Sciences Centre - Holland Orthopaedic & Arthritic Centre
Affiliated with: Toronto Central Local Health Integration Network
43 Wellesley St. East, Toronto, ON M4Y 1H1
Tel: 416-967-8500 *Fax:* 416-967-8521
www.sunnybrook.ca

Note: Care for complex injuries of the musculoskeletal system, with a focus on traumatic injury management, joint reconstruction & replacement, surgery, sports & activity-related injury management, rehabilitation, & rheumatology. The Clinic has a second location at the main Sunnybrook site, 2075 Bayview Ave., Toronto
Dr. Barry A. McLellan, President & CEO

Celiac Disease

Celiac disease, also called celiac sprue or gluten-sensitive enteropathy, is a chronic disease in which the small bowel cannot adequately absorb nutrients such as iron, folate, Vitamin D, calcium and fat. This inability, called malabsorption, is caused by inflammation of the bowel triggered by a sensitivity to gluten, a cereal protein found in wheat and rye, and less so in barley and oats.

Cause
Family incidence is a valuable clue. For people who have a first degree relative with celiac disease, the risk of developing the disease is 20 times greater. However, studies suggest that both genetic and environmental factors are implicated in the development of the disease. Celiac disease is more common in people with Type I diabetes and certain forms of thyroid and skin disease.

Symptoms
There is no typical presentation of celiac disease. The symptoms vary from person to person, but are often gastrointestinal. Painful abdominal distention, constipation, diarrhea and passage of large, oily, loose stools are common symptoms. Affected children will fail to grow normally and might show signs of malnutrition or developmental delay. Adults may lose weight despite a voracious appetite, and can be affected by iron deficiency anemia and vitamin deficiencies. Other symptoms such as mouth ulcers, arthritis, osteoporosis, joint pain, fatigue, irritability and depression may develop, as well. Close to 10 percent of people with celiac disease also have dermatitis herpetiformis, an itchy, burning skin rash that erupts into blisters on the elbows, buttocks and knees.

Prevalence
In Canada, it is estimated that 1 in 133 people have celiac disease. The disease may appear when a child is first given wheat products, generally in the second year of life. However, close to 30 percent of Canadian children affected by celiac disease are misdiagnosed at first. Some cases of celiac disease do not appear until a person is in their twenties, or later, with women usually showing symptoms 10 to 15 years earlier than men. No matter when the onset of symptoms, it typically takes at least a year to get a diagnosis of celiac disease, and in some cases, it can take as long as 12 years.

Treatment Options
Blood screening tests are helpful in making the diagnosis of celiac disease, but the most definitive test is examination of a small sample of the inflamed bowel.

There is no medication for celiac disease, so withdrawal of dietary gluten is the only current treatment. Vitamins and minerals may also have to be supplemented. Since eating even small amounts of gluten-containing foods can prevent remission or cause relapse, it is important to adhere to a gluten-free diet for life. The earlier a person is diagnosed with celiac disease and treated with a gluten-free diet, the better the chance of preventing long-term complications of the disease such as osteoporosis, liver disease and intestinal cancer.

See also Gastrointestinal Disorders and Crohn's Disease

National Associations

Canadian Celiac Association (CCA) / L'Association canadienne de la maladie coeliaque
Bldg. 1, #400, 5025 Orbitor Dr., Mississauga ON L4W 4Y5
Tel: 905-507-6208; *Fax:* 905-507-4673
Toll-Free: 800-363-7296
e-mail: info@celiac.ca
www.celiac.ca
twitter.com/gfbri

Also Known As: Celiac Canada
Previous Name: Canadian Celiac Sprue Association
Overview: A large national charitable organization founded in 1972
Mission: To increase awareness of celiac & dermatitis herpetiformis among government institutions, health care professionals & the public; to provide information about the disease & a gluten-free diet, & encourges research through the establishment of the J.A. Campbell Research Fund
Chief Officer(s):
Anne Wraggett, President
Leo Turner, Treasurer
Publications:
• Acceptability of Food & Food Ingredients for the Gluten Free Diet
Type: Dictionary; *Price:* Free for new members of the Canadian Celiac Association; $10 non-members
• Celiac News
Type: Newsletter; *Frequency:* 3 pa; *Price:* Free with CCA membership
Profile: Up-to-date information about the diesease & a gluten-free diet

Belleville & Quinte Chapter
c/o Karen Y. Brooks, PO Box 293, Bloomfield ON K0K 1G0
e-mail: chapter.on.bellville.quinte@celiac.ca
Chief Officer(s):
Karen Brooks, President
karenybrooks@sympatico.ca

Calgary Chapter
#1A, 2215 - 27 Ave. NE, Calgary AB T2E 8J2
Tel: 403-237-0304; *Fax:* 403-269-9626
e-mail: info@calgaryceliac.ca
calgaryceliac.com
www.facebook.com/155433831171925
Chief Officer(s):
Cindy Casper, Coordinator, Events
• Calgary Chapter Newsletter
Type: Newsletter; *Frequency:* Quarterly

Edmonton Chapter
#220, 5615 - 101 Ave. NW, Edmonton AB T6A 3Z7
Tel: 780-485-2949; *Fax:* 780-485-2940
e-mail: info@celiacedmonton.ca
www.celiacedmonton.ca
www.facebook.com/296692389521
twitter.com/edmontonceliac
Chief Officer(s):
Don Briggs, President
• Celiac Circular
Type: Newsletter; *Frequency:* Bimonthly; *Price:* Free for members of the Canadian Celiac Association Edmonton Chapter; $20 non-members

Fredericton Chapter
#226, 527 Beaverbrook Ct., Fredericton NB E3B 1X6
e-mail: fred.celiac@gmail.com
Chief Officer(s):
Angela Welch, President, 506-454-3222

Hamilton/Burlington Chapter

PO Box 65580, Stn. Dundas, Dundas ON L9H 6Y6
Tel: 905-572-6775
e-mail: hamiltonceliacchapter@gmail.com
www.glutenfreehamilton.ca
Chief Officer(s):
Laura Harrison, President
Wendy Stewart, Treasurer
• Hamilton Celiac News
Type: Newsletter; *Frequency:* Quarterly; *Accepts Advertising; Editor:* Laura Harrison
Profile: Upcoming events, meeting reports, celiac friendly restaurants, & recipes

Kamloops Chapter
2672 Qu'Appelle Blvd., Kamloops BC V2E 2H7
Tel: 250-319-9978
www.kamloopsceliac.org
www.facebook.com/275537332507738
Chief Officer(s):
Eileen Gordon, Secretary, 250-374-6185
• Canadian Celiac Association Kamloops Chapter Newsletter
Type: Newsletter

Kelowna Chapter
PO Box 21031, Stn. Orchard Park, Kelowna BC V1Y 9N8
Tel: 250-763-7159
kelownaceliac.org
www.facebook.com/pages/kelowna-celiac/205146224439
twitter.com/KelownaCeliac
Chief Officer(s):
Irene Thompson, President
rithomp@telus.net
Marie Ablett, Help-line Contact
dougmarieablett1@shaw.ca

Kingston Chapter
Kingston ON
e-mail: info@kingstonceliac.ca
www.kingstonceliac.ca
Chief Officer(s):
Sue Jennett, President

Kitchener/Waterloo Chapter
PO Box 118, 153 Frederick St., Kitchener ON N2H 2M3
e-mail: kwceliac@sympatico.ca
www.kwceliac.org
Chief Officer(s):
Connie McNeil, President, 519-662-3696

London Chapter
PO Box 27051, London ON N5X 3X5
e-mail: info@londonceliac.org
www.londonceliac.org
Chief Officer(s):
Helen Olmstead, President

Manitoba - West Chapter
#11, 83 Silverbirch Dr., Brandon MB R7B 1A8
Tel: 204-727-8445
e-mail: chapter.mb.westernmanitoba.ca@celiac.ca
Chief Officer(s):
Debbie Barrett, Contact
deborahb22012@yahoo.ca

Manitoba Chapter
#204, 825 Sherbrook St., Winnipeg MB R3A 1M5
Tel: 204-772-6979
e-mail: office@manitobaceliac.com
www.manitobaceliac.com
www.facebook.com/176000709214214
twitter.com/manitobaceliac
Chief Officer(s):
Dorothy Macintyre, President
• Celi-Yak
Type: Newsletter; *Frequency:* Quarterly; *Price:* Free for Manitoba Chapter members
Profile: Food & product information, recipes & restaurants, health news, & upcoming events

Moncton Chapter

PO Box 1576, Moncton NB E1C 9X4
>monctonceliacchapter.org
>www.facebook.com/249496635102956

Chief Officer(s):
Jo-Anne Wilson, President
Aline Farrell, Vice-President
Dave Saunders, Treasurer
• Canadian Celiac Association Moncton Chapter Newsletter
Type: Newsletter; *Editor:* Mike Murphy

Newfoundland & Labrador Chapter
38 East Meadows Ave., St. John's NL A1A 3M5
>celiacnl.ca
>www.facebook.com/199683166751767

Chief Officer(s):
Lisa Dooley, President, 709-693-4213
>glutenfreenuggets@outlook.com

Nova Scotia Chapter
Tacoma Plaza, #14, 50 Tacoma Dr., Dartmouth NS B2W 3E6
Tel: 902-464-9222; *Fax:* 902-435-6747
e-mail: info@celiacns.ca
>www.celiacns.ca
>www.facebook.com/celiacns
>twitter.com/ccaceliac

Chief Officer(s):
Marg Gorveatt, Coordinator, Office Operations
• Canadian Celiac Association Halifax Chapter
Type: Newsletter; *Frequency:* Quarterly
Profile: Recent issues dealing with Celiac Disease & Dermatitis Herpetiformis, chapter updates, & recipes

Ottawa Chapter
PO Box 39035, Stn. Billings Bridge, Ottawa ON K1H 1A1
Tel: 613-786-1335
>www.ottawaceliac.ca

Chief Officer(s):
Samantha Maloney, President
• Ottawa Chapter Newsletter
Type: Newsletter; *Editor:* Quintin Wight; *Price:* Free for Ottawa Chapter members
Profile: Upcoming events, issues, gluten-free product information, & recipes

Peterborough & Area Chapter
Peterborough ON
Tel: 905-372-2361
>www.celiacpeterborough.ca

Chief Officer(s):
Shirley Stewart, Contact
>shirleystewart26@gmail.ca
• Peterborough & Area Chapter Newsletter
Type: Newsletter; *Frequency:* 3 pa; *Accepts Advertising*; *Editor:* Leslee Horton; *Price:* Free with Peterborough & Area Chapter membership

Prince Edward Island Chapter
PO Box 1921, Charlottetown PE C1A 7N5
Tel: 902-724-2189
e-mail: info@celiacpei.ca
>www.celiacpei.ca

Chief Officer(s):
JoAnn Doughart, President
• Canadian Celiac Association Charlottetown Chapter
Type: Newsletter; *Editor:* Jim Hancock; Gay Hancock

Québec Chapter
Montréal QC
Tél: 514-893-9856
Courriel: info@celiacquebec.ca
>celiacquebec.ca

Regina Chapter
PO Box 1773, Regina SK S4P 3C6
e-mail: chapter.sk.regina@celiac.ca

Chief Officer(s):
Audrey Webb, President

Saint John Chapter
NB
e-mail: chapter.nb.saintjohn@celiac.ca

St Catharines Chapter
PO Box 29003, 125 Carlton St., St Catharines ON L2R 7P9
Tel: 905-988-9475
e-mail: chapter.on.st.catharines@celiac.ca

Chief Officer(s):
Lynne Turcotte, President
>lturcotte@cogeco.ca

Saskatoon Chapter
PO Box 8935, Saskatoon SK S7K 6S7
e-mail: chapter.sk.saskatoon@celiac.ca
>www.facebook.com/164568043600499

Chief Officer(s):
Penny Fairbrother, President
• Celiac Digest
Type: Newsletter; *Accepts Advertising*; *Editor:* Jennifer Holmes

Thunder Bay Chapter
739 Harold Cr., Thunder Bay ON P7C 5H8
Tel: 807-623-5572
>www.celiactbay.ca

Chief Officer(s):
Deb Paris, President
• Celiac News
Type: Newsletter; *Frequency:* Y; *Editor:* A. Peat, K. Smith, & B. Knott
Profile: Information with a local emphasis to support & educate people with celiac disease

Toronto Chapter
PO Box 23056, 550 Eglinton Ave. West, Toronto ON M5N 3A8
Tel: 416-781-9140
>www.torontoceliac.org

Chief Officer(s):
Joni Brinder, President
• Toronto Chapter Newsletter
Type: Newsletter; *Accepts Advertising*; *Editor:* Danny Weill & Alanna Weill

Vancouver Chapter
#306, 1385 West 8th St., Vancouver BC V6H 3V9
Tel: 604-736-2229
Toll-Free: 877-736-2240
e-mail: info@vancouverceliac.ca
>www.vancouverceliac.ca
>twitter.com/VancouverCCA

Chief Officer(s):
Jason Klatt, Director
• Celiac News
Type: Newsletter; *Frequency:* 3 pa; *Accepts Advertising*; *Editor:* Jane Kamimura & Joy Swaddling
Profile: Vancouver area news, recipes, restaurant reviews, & upcoming events

Victoria Chapter
PO Box 5457, Stn. B, Victoria BC V8R 6S8
Tel: 250-472-0141
e-mail: victoriaceliacs@hotmail.ca
>www.victoriaceliac.org

Chief Officer(s):
Nancy Adrian, President
• Victoria Celiac News
Type: Newsletter; *Frequency:* Bimonthly; *Accepts Advertising*; *Editor:* Christine Rushforth
Profile: Gluten free diet information

Provincial Associations

QUÉBEC

Fondation québécoise de la maladie coeliaque (FQMC) / Québec Celiac Foundation
#230, 4837, rue Boyer, Montréal QC H2J 3E6
Tél: 514-529-8806; *Téléc:* 514-529-2046
Courriel: info@fqmc.org
>www.fqmc.org

Aperçu: *Dimension:* petite; *Envergure:* provinciale; Organisme sans but lucratif; fondée en 1983
Mission: Diffuser de l'information sur la maladie et le régime sans gluten; faciliter l'approvisionnement; encourager les initiatives des

membres; supporter les membres et défendre leurs droits; favoriser la recherche; soliciter des fonds pour réaliser ses mandats
Membre(s) du bureau directeur:
Suzanne Laurencelle, Directrice Générale

Cerebral Palsy

Cerebral palsy (CP) applies to disorders of voluntary movement resulting from damage to areas in the brain. There are three main types of cerebral palsy: spastic, athetoid and ataxic. People with spastic cerebral palsy—the most common type of CP—have weak, stiff or tight muscles. Athetoid cerebral palsy is characterized by involuntary, uncontrolled movements, usually in the muscles of the arms, trunk and face. People with ataxic cerebral palsy have problems with balance and depth perception, often appearing shaky and unsteady.

Cause

The exact cause of cerebral palsy is often difficult to establish. However, most studies suggest that the majority of cases are due to events that affect brain development before birth. These factors may include infections, exposure to toxins such as nicotine and alcohol, damage to the placenta, maternal diabetes or nutritional deficiencies, genetic disorders and developmental disorders. CP can also be caused by birth trauma, insufficient oxygen supply or premature birth. Suffering from a severe systemic disease, such as meningitis, or experiencing a head injury, seizure or asphyxia (lack of oxygen) during early childhood, may also produce CP.

Symptoms

The symptoms of cerebral palsy vary from person to person, and depend on which areas of the brain have been damaged. Increased spastic movements are the most common symptoms, but children may also show weakness, poor sense of balance, involuntary movements and difficulty with fine motor skills like writing, or with gross motor skills like walking. In more severe cases, difficulty in speaking, hearing problems, vision loss, seizures and intellectual disabilities may also be present. Children with cerebral palsy may not be identified until they reach one to two years of age and may show only lagging motor development. Therefore, children known to be at risk should be followed closely.

Prevalence

There are more than 50,000 people living with cerebral palsy in Canada. According to estimates, approximately one out of every 500 newborns and as many as one in three premature babies are affected by cerebral palsy to some extent. Even with recent advances in neonatal and obstetrical care, the incidence of cerebral palsy has not decreased.

Treatment Options

It often takes months, or even years, before a diagnosis of cerebral palsy is confirmed. The first indications that a child might have CP are delays in reaching milestones such as rolling over, sitting or standing. A baby with CP might also seem floppy or feel stiff. A physician will monitor a child's progress over a period of time—and also rule out other conditions—before making a diagnosis of cerebral palsy. Sometimes CAT (computerized axial tomography) scans and MRI (magnetic resonance imaging) are used to identify lesions in the brain. Motor abnormalities are usually tested with the Gross Motor Function Classification System (GMFCS).

Since there is no known cure for cerebral palsy, the goal of treatment is to develop maximal independence. Therapy may include physical and occupational rehabilitation supplemented by splints, orthotics and casts to help keep joints in place and provide stability. In cases where spasticity is severe, nerve-blocking injections can provide temporary relief. A more recent development is reducing cerebral palsy symptoms with Botox injections. Special orthopedic surgery is sometimes performed to fix the problems that tight muscles can cause in the hips and spines of growing children. A wide range of adaptive equipment including mobility devices such as scooters, walkers, crutches and communication devices such as symbol boards and voice synthesizers are also available for people with CP.

Cerebral palsy is not progressive. Although the effects of CP may change over time, the condition will not get worse. With ongoing treatment and support, many people with cerebral palsy are able to live independent, happy and fulfilling lives.

National Associations

Canadian Cerebral Palsy Sports Association (CCPSA) / Association canadienne de sport pour paralytiques cérébraux (ACPSA)
#104, 720 Belfast Rd., Ottawa ON K1G 0Z5
Tel: 613-748-1430
e-mail: info@ccpsa.ca
www.ccpsa.ca
www.facebook.com/112866075626
Overview: A medium-sized national charitable organization founded in 1985
Mission: To act as umbrella group for all provincial cerebral palsy sport organizations; To design programs that are designed for athletes with cerebral palsy & non-progressive head injuries
Affliation(s): Cerebral Palsy International Sports & Recreation Association; International Paralympic Committee
Chief Officer(s):
Jennifer Larson, Interim Executive Director, 613-748-1430 Ext. 2
jlarson@ccpsa.ca

Provincial Associations

ALBERTA

Alberta Cerebral Palsy Sport Association (ACPSA)
Percy Page Centre, 11759 Groat Rd., Edmonton AB T5M 3K6
Tel: 780-422-2904; *Fax:* 780-422-2663
e-mail: contact@acpsa.ca
www.acpsa.ca
www.facebook.com/165504436855126
twitter.com/AlbertaCPSports
instagram.com/powerchair_sports
Also Known As: Sportability Alberta
Overview: A small provincial charitable organization founded in 1984 overseen by Canadian Cerebral Palsy Sports Association
Mission: To promote recreational & competitive sporting opportunities for persons with cerebral palsy, brain injury & related conditions
Member of: Canadian Cerebral Palsy Sports Association

Cerebral Palsy Association in Alberta (CPAA)
12001 - 44 St. SE, Calgary AB T2Z 4G9
Tel: 403-543-1161; *Fax:* 403-543-1168
Toll-Free: 800-363-2807
e-mail: admin@cpalberta.com
www.cpalberta.com
www.linkedin.com/in/cerebral-palsy-association-in-alberta-b9aa6562
www.facebook.com/CerebralPalsyAlberta
twitter.com/CPAlberta
www.instagram.com/cpalberta
Also Known As: CP Alberta
Overview: A medium-sized provincial organization founded in 1976
Mission: To improve the quality of life of persons with cerebral palsy through a broad range of programs, education, support of research, & the delivery of needed services to people with cerebral palsy & their families; To encourage persons with cerebral palsy to develop & pursue meaningful goals & achievements in life; To raise awareness in society of the abilities of individuals with cerebral palsy
Chief Officer(s):
Janice Bushfield, Executive Director

Mezaun Lakha-Evin, Associate Executive Director
  mezaun@cpalberta.com
Joanne Dorn, Director, Development
  jdorn@cpalberta.com
Mariana Nimara, Director, Administration
  mariana@cpalberta.com
Shyam Poudyal, Manager, Finance
  shyam@cpalberta.com

BRITISH COLUMBIA

British Columbia Centre for Ability Association (BCCFA)
2805 Kingsway, Vancouver BC V5R 5H9
Tel: 604-451-5511; *Fax:* 604-451-5651
www.bc-cfa.org
www.linkedin.com/company/bc-centre-for-ability
twitter.com/bccfa
www.youtube.com/channel/UCIjOVwg7zWgpD5WLT6RNzzA
Previous Name: Children's Rehabilitation & Cerebral Palsy
Association; Children's Centre for Ability
Overview: A medium-sized provincial charitable organization founded
in 1970
Mission: To provide community-based services that promote inclusion
& improve the quality of life for children, youth & adults with disabilities
& their families
Member of: United Way
Chief Officer(s):
Jennifer Baumbusch, President

Cerebral Palsy Association of British Columbia (CPABC)
#330, 409 Granville St., Vancouver BC V6C 1T2
Tel: 604-408-9484; *Fax:* 604-408-9489
Toll-Free: 800-663-0004
e-mail: info@bccerebralpalsy.com
www.bccerebralpalsy.com
www.facebook.com/cerebral.palsy.39
Also Known As: CP Association of BC
Overview: A medium-sized provincial organization founded in 1954
Mission: To raise awareness of cerebral palsy in the community; To
assist those living with cerebral palsy to reach to maximum; To work to
see those living with cerebral palsy realize their place as equals within
a diverse society; To provide support & services that facilitate these
needs; To make a Life Without Limits for people with disabilities
Member of: Better Business Bureau
Chief Officer(s):
Andy Yu, President
Feri Dehdar, Executive Director
Ian Bushfield, Coordinator, Events & Development

SportAbility BC
780 Marine Dr. SW, Vancouver BC V6P 5YZ
Tel: 604-324-1411
e-mail: sportinfo@sportabilitybc.ca
www.sportabilitybc.ca
www.facebook.com/sport.ability.3
twitter.com/SportAbilityBC
www.youtube.com/SportAbilityBC
Previous Name: Cerebral Palsy Sports Association of British Columbia
Overview: A medium-sized provincial charitable organization founded
in 1976 overseen by Canadian Cerebral Palsy Sports Association
Mission: To provide sports & recreational opportunities for people with
cerebral palsy, head injury, stroke & similar disabilities at the local,
regional, provincial & national level; To provide access to appropriate
programming for members including segregated & integrated
opportunities
Affilation(s): Sport BC
Chief Officer(s):
Ross MacDonald, Executive Director
  rossm@sportabilitybc.ca

MANITOBA

Cerebral Palsy Association of Manitoba Inc. (CPAM)
#105, 500 Portage Ave., Winnipeg MB R3C 3X1
Tel: 204-982-4842; *Fax:* 204-982-4844
Toll-Free: 800-416-6166
e-mail: office@cerebralpalsy.mb.ca
www.cerebralpalsy.mb.ca
www.facebook.com/CerebralPalsyAssociationOfMb
twitter.com/CerebralPalsyMB
Overview: A medium-sized provincial charitable organization founded
in 1974
Mission: To enrich the lives of individuals affected by cerebral palsy
through services, advocacy, education & peer support
Chief Officer(s):
David Kron, Director, Membership & Programs
  davidk@cerebralpalsy.mb.ca

Manitoba Cerebral Palsy Sports Association (MCPSA)
MB
Overview: A small provincial organization overseen by Canadian
Cerebral Palsy Sports Association
Mission: To assist in the development of sport for the disabled in
Manitoba by providing an opportunity for a wider participation for
persons with cerebral palsy & other neuromuscular disorders
Member of: Canadian Cerebral Palsy Sports Association

NEWFOUNDLAND AND LABRADOR

Cerebral Palsy Association of Newfoundland & Labrador (CPNL)
PO Box 23059, Stn. Churchill Square, St. John's NL A1B 4J9
Tel: 709-753-9922
www.cerebralpalsynl.com
www.facebook.com/cerebralpalsynl
Previous Name: Newfoundland Cerebral Palsy Association Inc.
Overview: A small provincial charitable organization founded in 1961
Mission: To improve the quality of life of persons with cerebral palsy
through programs, education, support of research & the delivery of
needed services to people with cerebral palsy & their families
Member of: Atlantic Cerebral Palsy Association
Chief Officer(s):
Cindy Bishop, Secretary

ONTARIO

Ontario Cerebral Palsy Sports Association (OCPSA)
PO Box 60082, Ottawa ON K1T 0K9
Tel: 613-723-1806; *Fax:* 613-723-6742
Toll-Free: 866-286-2772
ocpsa.com
Overview: A small provincial organization overseen by Canadian
Cerebral Palsy Sports Association
Mission: To provide, promote & coordinate competitive opportunities
for persons with with cerebral palsy & other neuromuscular disorders in
Ontario.
Member of: Canadian Cerebral Palsy Sports Association
Affilation(s): Canadian Sport Institute - Ontario; Coaches Association
of Ontario; ParaSport Ontario
Chief Officer(s):
Don Sinclair, President

Ontario Federation for Cerebral Palsy (OFCP)
#104, 1630 Lawrence Ave. West, Toronto ON M6L 1C5
Tel: 416-244-9686; *Fax:* 416-244-6543
Toll-Free: 877-244-9686; *TTY:* 866-246-9122
e-mail: info@ofcp.ca
www.ofcp.ca
www.facebook.com/OntarioFederationforCerebralPalsy
twitter.com/OntarioFCP
Overview: A medium-sized provincial charitable organization founded
in 1947
Mission: To improve the quality of life of persons with cerebral palsy
through a broad range of programs, education, support of research &
the delivery of needed services to people with cerebral palsy & other
physical disabilities & their families
Affilation(s): Neurological Health Charities Canada; Ontario
Association of Non-Profit Homes & Services for Seniors

Chief Officer(s):
Gordana Skrba, Interim Executive Director
gordana@ofcp.ca

PRINCE EDWARD ISLAND

Prince Edward Island Cerebral Palsy Association Inc.
PO Box 22034, Charlottetown PE C1A 9J2

Tel: 902-892-9694; *Fax:* 902-628-8751
e-mail: info@peicpa.com
www.peicpa.com

Also Known As: Cerebral Palsy Association of PEI
Overview: A small provincial charitable organization founded in 1953
Mission: To promote individuals with cerebral palsy & their abilities; To advocate for individuals with cerebral palsy; To provide resources, activities & services
Member of: United Way of PEI; Atlantic Cerebral Palsy Association

QUÉBEC

Association de paralysie cérébrale du Québec (APCQ) / Québec Cerebral Palsy Association
CP 1781, Sherbrooke QC J1H 5N8

Tél: 819-829-1144; *Téléc:* 819-829-1144
Ligne sans frais: 800-311-3770
Courriel: info@paralysiecerebrale.com
www.paralysiecerebrale.com

Aperçu: *Dimension:* petite; *Envergure:* provinciale; fondée en 1949
Mission: Favoriser l'amélioration de la qualité de vie et l'intégration sociale des personnes vivant avec une paralysie cérébrale ou toutes autres déficiences; défendre leurs droits; sensibiliser et informer la population, les organismes et les gouvernements; encourager la recherche et découverte de nouvelles thérapies
Membre(s) du bureau directeur:
Joseph Khoury, Président
Michel Larochelle, Directeur général
  m.larochelle@paralysiecerebrale.com

Bureau de Granby
170, rue St-Antoine Nord, Granby QC J2G 5G8

Tél: 450-777-2907

Membre(s) du bureau directeur:
Denise Arès, Responsable
  d.ares@paralysiecerebrale.com

Bureau de Montréal
2000, boul St-Joseph Est, Montréal QC H2M 1E4

Tél: 514-253-9444

Membre(s) du bureau directeur:
Katia Heise-Jensen, Responsable
  k.heise-jensen@paralysiecerebrale.com

Bureau de Saint-Jean-sur-Richelieu
870, rue Curé St-Georges, St-Jean-sur-Richelieu QC J2X 2Z8

Tél: 450-357-2740
Ligne sans frais: 866-849-2740

Membre(s) du bureau directeur:
Monique Laberge, Responsable
  m.laberge@paralysiecerebrale.com

Association québécoise de sports pour paralytiques cérébraux (AQSPC)
4545, av Pierre-de Coubertin, Montréal QC H1V 0B2

Tél: 514-252-3143; *Téléc:* 514-254-1069
www.sportpc.qc.ca
www.facebook.com/189413534433667

Aperçu: *Dimension:* petite; *Envergure:* provinciale surveillé par Canadian Cerebral Palsy Sports Association
Membre de: Canadian Cerebral Palsy Sports Association
Membre(s) du bureau directeur:
José Malo, Directrice générale, 514-252-3143 Ext. 3742
  jmalo@sportpc.qc.ca

SASKATCHEWAN

Saskatchewan Cerebral Palsy Association (SCPA)
2310 Louise Ave., Saskatoon SK S7J 2C7

Tel: 306-955-7272; *Fax:* 306-373-2665
e-mail: saskcpa@shaw.ca
www.saskcp.ca

Overview: A medium-sized provincial charitable organization founded in 1985
Mission: To improve the quality of life of persons with cerebral palsy through a broad range of programs, education, support of research & the delivery of needed services to people with cerebral palsy & their families
Chief Officer(s):
Darren Tkach, President

Local Associations

BRITISH COLUMBIA

Child Development Centre Society of Fort St. John & District
10417 - 106th Ave., Fort St John BC V1J 2M8

Tel: 250-785-3200; *Fax:* 250-785-3202
e-mail: info@cdcfsj.ca
www.cdcfsj.ca

Overview: A small local charitable organization founded in 1973
Mission: To promote the treatment & education of children with special needs, to ensure that they & their families are effectively & locally served with dignity & respect.
Member of: BC Association for Child Development & Intervention
Affliation(s): Cerebral Palsy Association of British Columbia
Chief Officer(s):
Andy Ackerman, President
Penny Gagnon, Executive Director

Quesnel & District Child Development Centre Association (QDCDCA)
488 McLean St., Quesnel BC V2J 2P2

Tel: 250-992-2481; *Fax:* 250-992-3439
www.quesnelcdc.com
www.facebook.com/quesnel.childdevelopmentcentre

Overview: A small local charitable organization founded in 1976
Mission: To assist local children by providing intervention programs which facilitate their physical, social, emotional, communicative & intellectual development
Affliation(s): BC Association for Child Development & Intervention
Chief Officer(s):
Corrina Norman, President

NEW BRUNSWICK

Cerebral Palsy Foundation (St. John) Inc.
PO Box 2152, Saint John NB E2L 3V1

Tel: 506-648-0322
e-mail: mail@cpfsj.ca
www.cpfsj.ca

Overview: A small local organization

NOVA SCOTIA

Halifax Regional Cerebral Palsy Association
PO Box 33075, Stn. Quinpool, Halifax NS B3L 4T6

Tel: 902-423-3025
e-mail: hfxrcpa@gmail.com
www.facebook.com/HalifaxRegionalCerebralPalsyAssociation

Overview: A small local organization
Mission: To improve the lives of individuals in Nova Scotia who are affected by cerebral palsy
Chief Officer(s):
Joy Moulton, President

International Associations

American Academy for Cerebral Palsy & Developmental Medicine (AACPDM)
#1100, 555 East Wells St., Milwaukee WI 53202 USA

Tel: 414-918-3014; *Fax:* 414-276-2146
e-mail: info@aacpdm.org
www.aacpdm.org
www.facebook.com/aacpdm
twitter.com/aacpdm

Overview: A medium-sized international organization founded in 1947
Mission: To foster & stimulate education & research in cerebral palsy & developmental medicine for the welfare of patients & their families
Affiliation(s): Canadian Cerebral Palsy Association
Chief Officer(s):
Unni Narayanan, President
Tracy Burr, Executive Director
  tburr@aacpdm.org
Publications:
• AACPDM [American Academy for Cerebral Palsy & Developmental Medicine] Newsletter
Type: Newsletter; *Frequency:* Quarterly
• Developmental Medicine & Child Neurology [a publication of the American Academy for Cerebral Palsy & Developmental Medicine]
Type: Journal
Profile: Peer reviewed journal

Blissymbolics Communication International (BCI)
#425, 1210 Don Mills Rd., Toronto ON M3B 3N9

www.blissymbolics.ca
Overview: A small international charitable organization founded in 1975
Mission: BCI is a non-profit, charitable organization that has the license for the use and publication of Blissymbols designed for persons with communication, language, & learning difficulties, severe speech & physical impairments.
Affiliation(s): Ontario Federation for Cerebral Palsy
Chief Officer(s):
Shirley McNaughton, Co-Chair

SCOPE for People with Cerebral Palsy
6 Market Rd., London N7 9PW United Kingdom

Tel: 0-20-7619-7100
e-mail: response@scope.org.uk
www.scope.org.uk
www.linkedin.com/companies/165883
www.facebook.com/scope
twitter.com/scope
www.youtube.com/user/scopestories

Previous Name: The Spastics Society
Overview: A small international organization founded in 1952
Mission: To enable men, women & children with cerebral palsy & associated disabilities to claim their rights, lead fulfilling & rewarding lives & play a full part in society; to provide activities & services which respond to individuals' needs, choices & rights
Affiliation(s): Canadian Cerebral Palsy Association
Chief Officer(s):
Richard Hawkes, Chief Executive

Provincial Libraries

Cerebral Palsy Association of British Columbia
#330, 409 Granville St., Vancouver, BC V6C 1T2

Tel: 604-408-9484; *Fax:* 604-408-9489
Toll-Free: 800-663-0004
info@bccerebralpalsy.com
www.bccerebralpalsy.com
Social Media: www.youtube.com/bccerebralpalsy;
twitter.com/CerebralPalsyBC; www.facebook.com/BCCerebralPalsy
Feri Dehdar, Executive Director

Cerebral Palsy Association of Manitoba
#903, 213 Notre Dame Ave., Winnipeg, MB R3B 1N3

Tel: 204-982-4842; *Fax:* 204-982-4844
Toll-Free: 800-416-6166
office@cerebralpalsy.mb.ca
www.cerebralpalsy.mb.ca

David Kron, Director, Membership & Programs
  davidk@cerebralpalsy.mb.ca

Chronic Fatigue Syndrome

Chronic Fatigue Syndrome (CFS) is an illness characterized by longstanding fatigue that does not improve with rest, worsens with physical or mental activity and impairs daily functioning. Profound or life-altering fatigue—the disease's hallmark—usually comes on suddenly and persists for at least six months, and often for years.

Cause
The cause of CFS is controversial. One theory is that a chronic viral infection is involved. Allergic reactions have also been proposed, and various immunologic abnormalities have been reported. Another theory involves proposed disturbances in the hormonal (endocrine) system. Psychological factors may be the cause, although CFS is distinct from typical depression or anxiety. A combination of these factors might also be the trigger for onset of chronic fatigue syndrome.

Symptoms
The fatigue of CFS may be accompanied by sore throat, swollen glands, muscle and joint pain, headaches, sleeplessness, and impaired memory or concentration. Chronic fatigue syndrome can also cause depression and social isolation and interfere with work and day-to-day activities.

Prevalence
In Canada, over 340,000 people have been diagnosed with chronic fatigue syndrome. Prevalence rates of CFS increase with age, and are much higher in women than in men.

Treatment Options
Since the cause is unknown, there is no single test or group of tests that can diagnose CFS. Therefore, the goal in evaluating an individual with presumed CFS is to exclude other treatable illnesses.

Given the difficulty in proving a diagnosis or understanding the cause of CFS, it is not surprising that many treatments have been offered for it. Antidepressants appear to be one of the most successful treatments studied so far; as many as 80 percent of patients report benefit. A combination of psychological counselling and gentle exercise also appears to be effective in the treatment of CFS. Alternative therapies such as acupuncture, massage and yoga or tai chi may be of benefit to some people. Patients with CFS need emotional support from physicians and family, due to the debilitating nature of the disease.

See also Fibromyalgia

Provincial Associations

BRITISH COLUMBIA

MEFM Myalgic Encephalomyelitis & Fibromyalgia Society of British Columbia
PO Box 462, 916 West Broadway Ave., Vancouver BC V5Z 1K7

Tel: 604-878-7707
Toll-Free: 888-353-6322
e-mail: info@mefm.bc.ca
www.mefm.bc.ca

Merged from: British Columbia Fibromyalgia Society; Myalgic Encephalomyelitis Society of British Columbia
Overview: A medium-sized provincial organization
Mission: To provide support to people with (ME) Myalgic Encephalomyelitis, (Chronic Fatigue Syndrome) & (FM) Fibromyalgia & their families; to help educate physicians, paramedical professionals, family members & the community at large regarding ME & FM; to

promote research aimed at improving treatment & ultimately finding a cure; to help to encourage early diagnosis & effective treatment

ONTARIO

Myalgic Encephalomyelitis Association of Ontario (MEAO)
#370, 170 Donway West, Toronto ON M3C 2G3

Tel: 416-222-8820
Toll-Free: 877-632-6682
e-mail: info@meao.ca
www.meao.ca

Overview: A small provincial charitable organization founded in 1992
Mission: To support individuals who have Myalgic Encephalomyelitis/Chronic Fatigue Syndrome & their families; to provide medical professionals, government & the general public with information on the illness & its effects & consequences

National ME/FM Action Network / Réseau national d'action EM/FM encéphalomyélite myalgique/fibromyalgie
#512, 33 Banner Rd., Nepean ON K2H 8V7

Tel: 613-829-6667; *Fax:* 613-829-8518
e-mail: mefminfo@mefmaction.com
www.mefmaction.net
www.facebook.com/MEFMActionNetwork
twitter.com/mefmaction

Also Known As: Myalgic Encephalomyelitis/Chronic Fatique Syndrome & Fibromyalgia Action Network
Overview: A small provincial charitable organization founded in 1993
Mission: To offer support, advocacy, education & research into the many, varied, anomalies connected with Myalgic Encephalomyelitis/Chronic Fatigue Syndrome & Fibromyalgia (ME/FM)
Member of: National Voluntary Health Organization; Health Charities Council of Canada
Affliation(s): Volunteer Ottawa; Volunteer Canada
Chief Officer(s):
Lydia E. Neilson, M.S.M., Founder & CEO

QUÉBEC

Association québécoise de la fibromyalgie (AQF)
#225, 2465, rue Honoré-Mercier, Laval QC H7L 2S9

Tél: 450-933-6530
Courriel: fqf@fibromyalgie-fqf.org
www.aqf.ca

Nom précédent: Association de la fibromyalgie du Québec
Aperçu: *Dimension:* moyenne; *Envergure:* provinciale; fondée en 1989
Mission: Sensibiliser la population face à la maladie par la défense des droits des personnes atteintes dans les différentes régions du Québec

SASKATCHEWAN

Fibromyalgia Association of Saskatchewan (FMAS)
PO Box 7525, Saskatoon SK S7K 4L4

Tel: 306-343-3627
Overview: A small provincial charitable organization founded in 1994
Mission: To improve the quality of life for those directly or indirectly affected by fibromyalgia syndrome (FMS) & chronic fatigue syndrome (CFS).
Affiliation(s): FM-CFS Canada

Local Associations

MANITOBA

Fibromyalgia Support Group of Winnipeg, Inc.
c/o SMD Clearinghouse, 825 Sherbrook St., Winnipeg MB R3A 1M5

Tel: 204-975-3037
e-mail: info@fmswinnipeg.com
www.fmswinnipeg.com

Also Known As: Fibromyalgia Syndrome Winnipeg
Overview: A small local charitable organization founded in 1992
Mission: To sponsor & promote educational services to all persons with fibromyalgia, as well as families, friends, health care professionals & the general public; To promote & sponsor scientific & clinical research relating to causes, treatments & cure of fibromyalgia
Member of: SMD Self-Help Clearinghouse

ONTARIO

Myalgic Encephalomyelitis Association of Halton/Hamilton-Wentworth
#5, 2230 Mountainside Dr., Burlington ON L7P 1B5

Tel: 905-319-7966
Overview: A small local charitable organization
Chief Officer(s):
Sally Hansen, President

Chronic Pain

Chronic pain is defined as pain persisting for more than one month after resolution of an acute injury, or pain that persists or recurs for more than three months.

Cause
The pain may begin for unknown reasons, or may begin with some injury or illness but persist long after the triggering event is gone. In some cases, this persistent pain is due to a problem with pain processing. The chemicals in the brain that control pain may not be functioning properly. Human pain has physiological causes but also has psychological components differing for each person.

Symptoms
The symptoms of chronic pain include stiffness, tightness, soreness and discomfort, and burning, aching, shooting or electrical sensations. Chronic pain can be musculoskeletal, meaning that it affects the ligaments, tendons, muscles and bones; this type of pain is often caused by repetitive strain injuries, sports injuries or health conditions such as fibromyalgia and arthritis. Chronic pain can also affect the nerves and nervous system; health conditions like diabetes, sciatica and shingles may cause nerve pain, as can injuries and health problems that damage the nerves or put pressure on them. Other common types of chronic pain include low back pain, headache, cancer pain and psychogenic pain. It is possible to have more than one type of chronic pain at a time. When pain is chronic, it can lead to other health problems such as sleep disturbances, fatigue, depression and anxiety. Chronic pain can also interfere with school, work and social activities, negatively affecting quality of life.

Prevalence
In Canada, it is estimated that 3.9 million people aged 15 and over suffer from some chronic pain or discomfort. The prevalence of chronic pain increases with age for both sexes. However, rates of chronic pain among women are higher at all ages. The annual cost of chronic pain, including medical treatment and lost income and productivity, now hovers around $10 billion in Canada.

Treatment Options
To diagnose chronic pain, doctors take a detailed medical history that includes questions about what activities cause pain, how long the pain has persisted and what, if anything, relieves the pain. Physical and neurological exams are also performed to try to determine the cause of the pain. To rule out other health problems that might be causing chronic pain, diagnostic tests such as blood tests, x-rays (or other imaging tests), nerve function tests and angiograms are often used.

Doctors and patients have tried almost every conceivable type of therapy for chronic pain. Drug treatments include narcotics (codeine and morphine), non-narcotic painkillers such as acetaminophen, and nonsteroidal anti-inflammatory drugs such as ibuprofen. Use of antidepressants, either alone or in conjunction with pain medications, can be beneficial. Doctors may inject drugs to block the nerves that carry the pain signal, or may even cut the nerve. Physical measures include heat or cold application, application of electrical stimuli (TENS), stretching and general conditioning exercises. Psychological treatment includes psycho-therapy, meditation, hypnosis and biofeedback-relaxation. Because of the complexity of chronic pain and its treatment, some doctors have begun to specialize in management of pain, and have organized multidisciplinary pain clinics which offer expertise from anesthesiology, rheumatology, neurosurgery, psychology and physical therapy.

A realistic goal of therapy is to improve one's daily functioning; for instance, being able to return to work or pleasurable activities. Those able to achieve this status will often state that the pain is still there but that it does not bother them like it once did. Whatever the stage of one's condition, peer support is important, and is available from local in-person support groups or from Internet chat rooms and bulletin boards.

National Associations

Canadian Institute for the Relief of Pain & Disability (CIRPD)
National Office, #204, 916 West Broadway, Vancouver BC V5Z 1K7
Tel: 604-684-4148; *Fax:* 604-684-6247
Toll-Free: 800-872-3105
e-mail: admin@cirpd.org
www.cirpd.org
www.linkedin.com/groups/Canadian-Institute-Relief-Pain-Disability-226 2
www.facebook.com/CIRPD
twitter.com/cirpd
www.youtube.com/user/cirpdadmin
Previous Name: Physical Medicine Research Foundation
Overview: A small national charitable organization founded in 1985
Mission: To improve diagnosis & treatment for pain sufferers; To prevent & reduce pain & disability & improve the quality of life for people who suffer from muscle & joint pain
Affliation(s): Canadian Cochrane Centre
Chief Officer(s):
Marc I. White, Executive Director
Adrienne Hook, President
William Dyer, Secretary
Janette Lyons, Treasurer
Publications:
• Canadian Institute for the Relief of Pain & Disability Annual Report
Type: Yearbook; *Frequency:* Annually

Canadian Pain Society / Société canadienne pour le traitement de la douleur
#301, 250 Consumers Rd., Toronto ON M2J 4V6
Tel: 416-642-6379; *Fax:* 416-495-8723
e-mail: office@canadianpainsociety.ca
www.canadianpainsociety.ca
www.facebook.com/CanadianPain
twitter.com/canadianpain
Overview: A medium-sized national organization founded in 1982
Mission: To foster research on pain; To improve the management of patients with acute & chronic pain
Member of: International Association for the Study of Pain
Chief Officer(s):
Brian Cairns, President
Marsha Campbell-Yeo, Secretary
Karim Mukhida, Treasurer
Emma Roberts, Manager
eroberts@canadianpainsociety.ca
Publications:
• The Canadian Journal of Pain [a publication of the Canadian Pain Society]
Type: Journal; *Frequency:* Quarterly
Profile: Featuring articles & information about the latest developments in the field of pain
• Canadian Pain Society Membership Directory
Type: Directory
Profile: Contact information for members
• CPS [Canadian Pain Society] Newsletter
Type: Newsletter; *Frequency:* Quarterly; *Editor:* Brittany Rosenbloom;
Price: Free with membership in theCanadian Pain Society

Profile: Updates from the Canadian Pain Society, including book reviews, a trainee corner, training opportunities, & forthcoming events

Chronic Pain Association of Canada (CPAC)
PO Box 66017, Stn. Heritage, Edmonton AB T6J 6T4
Tel: 780-482-6727; *Fax:* 780-433-3128
e-mail: cpac@chronicpaincanada.com
www.chronicpaincanada.com
Previous Name: North American Chronic Pain Association of Canada
Overview: A medium-sized national charitable organization founded in 1986
Mission: To advance the treatment & management of chronic intractable pain; to develop research projects to promote the discovery of a cure for this disease; to educate both the health care community & the public
Chief Officer(s):
Terry Bremner, President
Barry Ulmer, Executive Director

Promoting Awareness of RSD & CRPS in Canada (PARC)
PO Box 21026, St Catharines ON L2M 7X2
Tel: 905-934-0261
www.rsdcanada.org/parc
Also Known As: PARC
Overview: A small national charitable organization
Mission: To support persons with CRPS, type 1 & 2 (Reflex Sympathetic Dystrophy & Causalgia), their families, & medical professionals who treat CRPS
Publications:
• PARC [Promoting Awareness of RSD & CRPS in Canada] Pearl
Type: Newsletter; *Frequency:* Quarterly
Profile: Articles by professionals, latest research, coping techniques, resources, & upcoming conferences

Provincial Associations

ALBERTA

Edmonton (Alberta) Nerve Pain Association (EANPA)
14016 - 91 A Ave., Edmonton AB T5R 5A7
Tel: 780-217-9306
e-mail: neuropathy_nervepain@hotmail.com
www.edmontonnervepain.ca
Overview: A medium-sized provincial charitable organization
Mission: To support people suffering from neuropathic pain
Chief Officer(s):
Claude M. Roberto, President

Pain Society of Alberta (PSA)
132 Warwick Rd., Edmonton AB T5X 4P8
Tel: 780-457-5225; *Fax:* 780-475-7968
e-mail: info@painsocietyofalberta.org
painsocietyofalberta.org
Overview: A medium-sized provincial organization
Mission: To provide support for patients & health care professionals in Alberta who are concerned with pain management & treatment
Chief Officer(s):
Dawn Petit, President
Glyn Smith, Administrator
glyn@painsocietyofalberta.org

ONTARIO

Help for Headaches (HFH)
PO Box 1568, Stn. B, 515 Richmond St., London ON N6A 5M3
Tel: 519-434-0008
www.helpforheadaches.org
Also Known As: Headache Support Group
Overview: A small provincial charitable organization founded in 1995
Mission: To provide research, education, advocacy & support for headache sufferers & the public at large
Member of: World Headache Alliance; Canadian Pain Society
Chief Officer(s):
G. Brent Lucas, Director
brent@helpforheadaches.org
Publications:
• Chronic Daily Headache
Type: Book; *Price:* $25.95

• Non-Drug Treatments for Headache
Type: Book; *Price:* $25.25
Profile: Educational book discussing various treatment options for headaches & migraines

International Associations

American Society of Regional Anesthesia & Pain Medicine (ASRA)
#401, 4 Penn Center West, Pittsburgh PA 15276 USA
Tel: 412-471-2718
Toll-Free: 855-795-2772
e-mail: asraassistant@asra.com
www.asra.com
www.linkedin.com/groups?gid=4797719
www.facebook.com/228281927234196
twitter.com/asra_society
Overview: A medium-sized international organization founded in 1923
Mission: To assure excellence in patient care utilizing regional anesthesia & pain medicine; To investigate the scientific basis of the specialty
Chief Officer(s):
Oscar De Leon-Casasola, President
Angie Stengel, Executive Director
astengel@asra.com
Publications:
• ASRA [American Society of Regional Anesthesia & Pain Medicine] News
Type: Newsletter; *Frequency:* Quarterly; *Editor:* Colin McCartney, M.B., F.R.C.A.
Profile: Society news, articles, & meeting reviews
• ASRA [American Society of Regional Anesthesia & Pain Medicine] E-News
Type: Newsletter
Profile: Society announcements, including information about meetings, workshops, awards
• Regional Anesthesia & Pain Medicine
Type: Journal; *Frequency:* Bimonthly; *Editor:* Joseph M. Neal, M.D.
Profile: Peer-reviewed scientific & clinical studies

The Facial Pain Association (TNA)
#602, 408 West University Ave., Gainesville FL 32601 USA
Tel: 352-384-3600; *Fax:* 352-384-3606
Toll-Free: 800-923-3608
www.fpa-support.org
www.facebook.com/facialpainassociation
twitter.com/facialpainassoc
Previous Name: Trigeminal Neuralgia Association
Overview: A large international charitable organization founded in 1990
Mission: To bring people with trigeminal neuralgia & related facial pain conditions together to share their experience & reduce their isolation; to serve as resource/pooling centre for information on trigeminal neuralgia; to provide mutual aid, support & encouragement to those afflicted, their families & other caring individuals; to increase public/professional awareness, visibility & better understanding of the disorder
Member of: National Organization for Rare Disorders (NORD)
Affiliation(s): Centre for Non-Profit Corporations
Chief Officer(s):
John Koff, Chief Executive Officer

Institute for the Study & Treatment of Pain (ISTOP)
#280, 5655 Cambie St., Vancouver BC V5Z 3A4
Tel: 604-264-7867; *Fax:* 604-264-7860
e-mail: istop@istop.org
www.istop.org
Overview: A small international charitable organization founded in 1995
Mission: A non-profit organization dedicated to the understanding & treatment of soft tissue pain
Chief Officer(s):
Chan Gunn, President
Allan Lam, Clinic Director

International Association for the Study of Pain (IASP)
IASP Secretariat, #600, 1510 H St. NW, Washington, DC 20005-1020 USA
Tel: 202-524-5300; *Fax:* 202-524-5301
e-mail: iaspdesk@iasp-pain.org
www.iasp-pain.org
www.linkedin.com/company/1022844
www.facebook.com/IASP.pain
twitter.com/IASPPAIN
Overview: A medium-sized international charitable organization founded in 1973
Mission: To provide a professional forum for science, practice, & education in the field of pain
Member of: World Federation of Neurology; World Federation of Ageing
Affiliation(s): Canadian Pain Society; World Health Organization
Chief Officer(s):
Matthew D'Uva, Executive Director
matthew.duva@iasp-pain.org
Rolf-Detlef Treede, President
Srinivasa Raja, Secretary
Michael Rowbotham, Treasurer
Publications:
• IASP Newsletter
Type: Newsletter; *Frequency:* Quarterly
Profile: Activities of IASP, its chapters, & special interest groups for members
• PAIN
Type: Journal; *Frequency:* 18 pa
Profile: Peer-reviewed, original research on the nature, mechanisms, & treatment of pain
• Pain: Clinical Updates
Type: Newsletter
Profile: Details about pain therapy for clinicians, patients & families

World Federation of Chiropractic (WFC) / La Fédération mondiale de chiropratique
#601, 160 Eglinton Ave. East, Toronto ON M4P 3B5
Tel: 416-484-9978; *Fax:* 416-484-9665
e-mail: info@wfc.org
www.wfc.org
www.facebook.com/WorldFederationofChiropractic
Overview: A medium-sized international organization founded in 1988
Mission: To increase awareness of & access to chiropractic
Member of: Council of International Organizations of Medical Sciences (CIOMS)
Affiliation(s): World Health Organization (WHO)
Chief Officer(s):
Richard Brown, Secretary-General

Cognitive Disorders

Cognitive disorders are a group of conditions characterized by impairments in the ability to think, reason, plan and organize. There are three types of cognitive disorders: delirium, dementia (of which Alzheimer's disease is the most common) and amnestic disorder.

Delirium is a relatively short-term condition in which the level of consciousness waxes and wanes. It is common in patients after surgery or during illness, as with high fever. It resolves when the underlying problem resolves. There are three categories of causes of delirium: a general medical condition, substance-induced and multiple causes. An amnestic disorder, in contrast to delirium or dementia, is a condition in which only memory is impaired; for instance the person is unable to recall important facts or events, making it difficult to function normally. Dementia is a chronic impairment of multiple cognitive functions. Persons with dementia may have severe memory loss and also be unable to plan or prepare for events or to care for themselves. Dementia, Alzheimer's type, is a progressive disorder that slowly kills nerve cells in the brain. Here we will describe only Alzheimer's disease, the most prevalent cognitive disorder.

Alzheimer's Disease

Cause

Alzheimer's disease is a degenerative neurological disease that attacks the brain and impairs memory, thinking faculties and behaviour. In spite of diligent research, the cause of Alzheimer's disease is unknown. However, research has identified several risk factors associated with Alzheimer's disease, the most important of which is aging. The older the person is, the greater the risk. There is also a genetic component to the disease. The chance of developing Alzheimer's disease is three times greater for a person who has a parent or sibling with the disease, and there is even more of a risk if both parents have the disease. Although there is an inherited form of the disease—familial autosomal dominant (FAD) Alzheimer's disease—it is rare, and only a very small percentage of people (5 to 7 percent) have it.

Symptoms

The symptoms of Alzheimer's disease vary from person to person, however the disease generally begins gradually, not with deficits in cognition but with a marked change in personality. For instance, a person may suddenly become given to fits of anger for no apparent reason.

Soon, however, family and acquaintances may notice that the individual begins to mix up facts, or gets lost driving to a familiar place. In the early stages the afflicted individual may become aware of slipping cognitive functions, adding to confusion, fright and depression. After a period, lapses in memory grow more obvious; patients with Alzheimer's are apt to repeat themselves, and may forget the names of grandchildren or longtime friends. They may also be increasingly agitated and combative when family members or other caretakers try to correct them or help with accustomed tasks. The memory lapses in patients with Alzheimer's differ markedly from those in normal aging: a patient with Alzheimer's may often forget entire experiences and rarely remembers them later. The patient only grudgingly acknowledges lapses. In contrast, the individual with normal aging or depression is extremely concerned about, and may even exaggerate, the extent of memory loss. In Alzheimer's, skills deteriorate and a patient is increasingly unable to follow directions, or care for him or herself. The progress of Alzheimer's disease is different for each individual, but symptoms will become more severe over time. Most people suffer from the disease for seven to ten years, but for others, the duration is much longer. Eventually the disease leads to death.

Prevalence

As the most common form of dementia, Alzheimer's disease accounts for 64 percent of the cases of dementia in Canada. Nearly 500,000 Canadians suffer from the illness. It is twice as common in women as in men, affecting primarily older people. In Canada, about 1 in 13 people who are 65 years of age or older have Alzheimer's disease, and in those 85 or older, the statistic is closer to 1 in 3. For people over the age of 65, Alzheimer's disease is the fifth leading cause of death in women and the eighth leading cause of death in men. According to projections, there could be more than 750,000 Canadians suffering from Alzheimer's disease by 2031.

Treatment Options

Since other, serious, treatable disorders can resemble Alzheimer's disease, it is very important for individuals who are losing cognitive functions to be evaluated by a physician. Early detection of Alzheimer's disease, with early treatment, may improve the chances for slowing the rate of decline. In Canada, genetic testing for Alzheimer's disease is limited, and is usually only offered to people with a strong family history of the disease who are participating in research studies.

The diagnosis of Alzheimer's disease is largely based on an interview with the patient and family members, an examination of the patient and a mental status test, although brain imaging tests and blood tests may add helpful information. Some physicians may use the following criteria outlined in the Diagnostic and Statistical Manual of Mental Disorders to confirm a diagnosis of Alzheimer's disease: language disorders; impaired ability to carry out motor activities despite intact motor function; failure to recognize or identify objects despite intact sensory perception; disturbance in executive functioning (planning, organizing, sequencing, abstracting); impairment in social or occupational functioning that represents a decline from previous level of functioning; a gradual and continuous decline; patient does not have other central nervous system conditions such as Parkinson disease, or substance abuse; patient does not have delirium, severe depression or schizophrenia.

Treatment for Alzheimer's disease may include drug therapy. There have been drugs released recently which enhance the transmission of acetylcholine (a neurotransmitter) and can cause at least limited improvement in memory during the early stages of Alzheimer's disease. One drug, memantine, has been developed to slow the progression of advanced disease. However, these drugs do not stop the progression of Alzheimer's, nor do they offer a cure. While definitive treatments are lacking, there is a prodigious amount of research on the condition, some of which suggests that a vaccine may be developed to prevent the condition.

Psychiatrists treating patients with Alzheimer's disease, may also be able to prescribe medications that can treat the depression and anxiety that accompanies the condition. And families are strongly encouraged to take advantage of adjunctive services including support groups, counselling and psychotherapy. There is a high incidence of depression among family members caring at home for persons with Alzheimer's disease.

A healthy lifestyle may reduce the risk of developing Alzheimer's disease. Researchers estimate that close to half of the cases of Alzheimer's disease in the world are related to risk factors that are modifiable. These include depression, smoking, physical inactivity, cognitive inactivity, obesity, diabetes, and high blood pressure. Being physically and socially active, maintaining a healthy weight, reducing stress, and keeping the brain active may reduce the risk of developing Alzheimer's disease.

Because Alzheimer's disease severely affects both patient and family, proper planning, as well as medical and social programs tailored to the individual and to family members are essential. There is much that families and patients can do when the condition is recognized and care and support are sought early in the disorder's progression. A safe and well-structured living environment is the best way to preserve the welfare and dignity of the person with Alzheimer's disease.

See also Aging

National Associations

Alzheimer Society Canada (ASC) / Société Alzheimer Canada
#1600, 20 Eglinton Ave. West, Toronto ON M4R 1K8

Tel: 416-488-8772; *Fax:* 416-322-6656
Toll-Free: 800-616-8816
e-mail: info@alzheimer.ca
www.alzheimer.ca
www.facebook.com/AlzheimerSociety
twitter.com/AlzSociety
www.youtube.com/thealzheimersociety

Overview: A large national charitable organization founded in 1978
Mission: Identifies, develops & facilitates national priorities that enable members to alleviate personal & social consequences of Alzheimer's disease & related disorders; promotes research & leads the search for a cure
Member of: Alzheimer Disease International; Canadian Coalition for Genetic Fairness
Affliation(s): HealthPartners
Chief Officer(s):
John O'Keefe, President

Provincial Associations

ALBERTA

Alzheimer Society of Alberta & Northwest Territories
High Park Corner, #308, 14925 - 111 Ave. NW, Edmonton AB T5M 2P6

Tel: 780-761-0030; *Fax:* 780-761-0031
Toll-Free: 866-950-5465
e-mail: reception@alzheimer.ab.ca
www.alzheimer.ca/ab

Overview: A medium-sized provincial charitable organization founded in 1988 overseen by Alzheimer Society of Canada
Mission: To alleviate the personal & social consequences of Alzheimer's disease through the development, support & coordination of local societies & chapters; To promote the search for a cure through education & research; Registered charity, BN: 129690343RR0001
Affliation(s): Canadian Association on Gerontology; Alberta Association on Gerontology; Canadian Centre for Philanthropy
Chief Officer(s):
Michele Mulder, Chief Executive Officer
mmulder@alzheimer.ab.ca
Christene Gordon, Director, Client Services & Programs
cgordon@alzheimer.ab.ca
Monique Trudelle, Director, Communications
mtrudelle@alzheimer.ab.ca

Edmonton & Area Chapter
10531 Kingsway Ave., Edmonton AB T5H 4K1

Tel: 780-488-2266; *Fax:* 780-488-3055

Chief Officer(s):
Arlene Huhn, Manager, Client Services & Programs
ahuhn@alzheimer.ab.ca

Fort McMurray - Wood Buffalo Chapter
#200, 10010 Franklin Ave., Fort McMurray AB T9H 2K6

Tel: 780-743-6175; *Fax:* 780-791-0088

Chief Officer(s):
Jennifer Kennedy, Community Relations Coordinator
jkennedy@alzheimer.ab.ca

Grande Prairie Chapter
#205, 8712 - 116 Ave., Grande Prairie AB T8V 4B4

Tel: 780-882-8870; *Fax:* 780-882-8780

Chief Officer(s):
Cindy McLeod, Coordinator, First Link/Intake
cmcleod@alzheimer.ab.ca

Lethbridge & Area Chapter
#402, 740 - 4th Ave. South, Lethbridge AB T1J 0N9

Tel: 403-329-3766; *Fax:* 403-327-3711

Chief Officer(s):
Brenda Hill, Manager, Client Services & Programs
hill@alzheimer.ab.ca

Medicine Hat & Area - Palliser Chapter
Hammond Bldg., #401D - 3rd St. SE, Medicine Hat AB T1A 0G8

Tel: 403-528-2700; *Fax:* 403-526-4994

Chief Officer(s):
Alariss Schmid, Community Relations Coordinator
aschmid@alzheimer.ab.ca

Northwest Territories - Yellowknife Chapter
Yellowknife NT

Tel: 867-669-9390

Red Deer & Central Alberta Chapter
#1, 5550 - 45 St., Red Deer AB T4N 1L1

Tel: 403-342-0448; *Fax:* 403-986-3693

Chief Officer(s):
Laurie Grande, Manager, Client Services & Programs
firstlinkreddeer@alzheimer.ab.ca

BRITISH COLUMBIA

Alzheimer Society of British Columbia
#300, 828 West 8th Ave., Vancouver BC V5Z 1E1

Tel: 604-681-6530; *Fax:* 604-669-6907
Toll-Free: 800-667-3742
e-mail: info@alzheimerbc.org
www.alzheimerbc.org
www.linkedin.com/company/alzheimer-society-of-b.c.
www.facebook.com/AlzheimerBC
twitter.com/AlzheimerBC
www.youtube.com/AlzheimerBC

Previous Name: Alzheimer Support Association of BC
Overview: A medium-sized provincial charitable organization founded in 1981 overseen by Alzheimer Society of Canada
Mission: To alleviate the personal & social consequences of Alzheimer disease & related dementias; to promote public awareness & to search for the causes & the cures
Chief Officer(s):
Maria Howard, CEO, 604-742-4901
mhoward@alzheimerbc.org

MANITOBA

Alzheimer Manitoba
#10, 120 Donald St., Winnipeg MB R3C 4G2

Tel: 204-943-6622; *Fax:* 204-942-5408
Toll-Free: 800-378-6699
e-mail: alzmb@alzheimer.mb.ca
www.alzheimer.mb.ca
www.facebook.com/AlzheimerSocietyManitoba
twitter.com/AlzheimerMB
www.youtube.com/AlzheimerMB

Also Known As: Alzheimer Society of Manitoba
Overview: A medium-sized provincial charitable organization founded in 1982 overseen by Alzheimer Society of Canada
Mission: To allieviate the individual, family & social consequences of Alzheimer type dementia while supporting the search for a cure
Chief Officer(s):
Wendy Schettler, CEO
wschettler@alzheimer.mb.ca

NEW BRUNSWICK

Alzheimer Society of New Brunswick / Société alzheimer du nouveau brunswick
PO Box 1553, Stn. A, Fredericton NB E3B 5G2

Tel: 506-459-4280; *Fax:* 506-452-0313
Toll-Free: 800-664-8411
e-mail: info@alzheimernb.ca
www.alzheimernb.ca
www.facebook.com/127071537361985
twitter.com/AlzheimerNB

Overview: A medium-sized provincial organization founded in 1987 overseen by Alzheimer Society of Canada
Mission: To alleviate the personal & social consequences of Alzheimer disease; to promote the search for a cause & cure

NEWFOUNDLAND AND LABRADOR

Alzheimer Society of Newfoundland & Labrador
#107, 835 Topsail Rd., Mount Pearl NL A1N 3J6
Tel: 709-576-0608; *Fax:* 709-576-0798
Toll-Free: 877-776-0608
e-mail: alzheimersociety@nf.aibn.com
www.alzheimernl.org
www.facebook.com/ASNL2
twitter.com/asnl2

Overview: A small provincial charitable organization founded in 1988 overseen by Alzheimer Society of Canada
Mission: To support the search for the cause & cure of Alzheimer Disease; To raise public awareness of the personal & social impact of the disease; To promote the provision of support to families & caregivers in Newfoundland
Chief Officer(s):
Shirley Lucas, Executive Director
slucas@alzheimernl.ca

NOVA SCOTIA

Alzheimer Society of Nova Scotia
#112, 2719 Gladstone St., Halifax NS B3K 4W6
Tel: 902-422-7961; *Fax:* 902-422-7971
Toll-Free: 800-611-6345
e-mail: alzheimer@asns.ca
www.alzheimer.ca/ns
www.facebook.com/alzheimersocietyns
twitter.com/alzheimerns
www.youtube.com/user/alzheimerns

Overview: A medium-sized provincial charitable organization founded in 1983 overseen by Alzheimer Society of Canada
Mission: To enhance the quality of life of people with Alzheimer disease through providing & promoting public education & family support; to engage in advocacy on behalf of people with Alzheimer disease & their families; to promote research at the provincial & national levels
Chief Officer(s):
Lloyd O. Brown, Executive Director
Chris Wilson, President

ONTARIO

Alzheimer Society Ontario / Société Alzheimer Ontario
20 Eglinton Ave. West, 16th Fl., Toronto ON M4R 1K8
Tel: 416-967-5900; *Fax:* 416-967-3826
Toll-Free: 800-879-4226
e-mail: staff@alzheimeront.org
www.alzheimer.ca/en/on
www.facebook.com/AlzheimerSocietyofOntario
twitter.com/alzheimeront
www.youtube.com/alzheimersocietyont

Also Known As: Alzheimer Ontario
Overview: A large provincial charitable organization founded in 1983 overseen by Alzheimer Society of Canada
Mission: To improve the quality of life for persons with Alzheimer disease & their families; to inform & educate the public & health care professionals about Alzheimer disease; to coordinate a chapter network & liaison in order to present a united voice to the Government of Ontario & other provincial groups on matters relating to legal concerns, health care, research, & community needs; to raise funds for research
Chief Officer(s):
Gale Carey, CEO
Rosemary Corbett, Chair

PRINCE EDWARD ISLAND

Alzheimer Society of PEI
166 Fitzroy St., Charlottetown PE C1A 1S1
Tel: 902-628-2257; *Fax:* 902-368-2715
Toll-Free: 866-628-2257
e-mail: society@alzpei.ca
www.alzheimer.ca/pei
www.facebook.com/AlzheimerPEI
twitter.com/AlzheimerPEI
www.youtube.com/user/Alzpei

Overview: A small provincial charitable organization founded in 1989 overseen by Alzheimer Society of Canada
Mission: To support & assist Islanders affected by Alzheimer Disease; To raise the level of awareness & educate the public at large about the disease
Chief Officer(s):
Corrine Hendricken-Eldershaw, CEO

QUÉBEC

Fédération québécoise des sociétés Alzheimer (FQSA) / Federation of Québec Alzheimer Societies
#211, 5165, rue Sherbrooke ouest, Montréal QC H4A 1T6
Tél: 514-369-7891; *Téléc:* 514-369-7900
Ligne sans frais: 888-636-6473
Courriel: info@alzheimerquebec.ca
www.alzheimerquebec.ca
www.facebook.com/LaFederationQuebecoiseDesSocietesAlzheimer
twitter.com/FqsaAlzh
www.youtube.com/user/FQSA1

Aperçu: *Dimension:* grande; *Envergure:* provinciale; Organisme sans but lucratif; fondée en 1985 surveillé par Alzheimer Society of Canada
Mission: Alléger les conséquences personnelles et sociales de la maladie d'Alzheimer; diffuser l'information auprès du public sur la maladie d'Alzheimer et sur les services offerts par notre réseau; soutenir les sociétés qui offrent aide et formation; promouvoir et encourager la recherche sur la maladie d'Alzheimer entre autres par la gestion d'un fonds provincial de la recherche; établir des relations et faire des représentations auprès des autorités concernées
Membre(s) du bureau directeur:
Réal Leahey, Président
Diane Roch, Directrice générale

Bas St-Laurent
Légion canadienne, 114, av St-Jérôme, Matane QC G4W 3A2
Tél: 418-562-2144; *Téléc:* 418-562-7449
Ligne sans frais: 877-446-2144
Courriel: info@alzheimer-bsl.com
www.alzheimer-bsl.com
www.facebook.com/societealzheimer.bassaintlaurent
Membre(s) du bureau directeur:
Denis Bond, Président

Centre du Québec
880, rue Côté, Saint-Charles-de-Drummond QC J2C 4Z7
Tél: 819-474-3666; *Téléc:* 819-474-3133
Courriel: myosotis@aide-internet.org
www.alzheimer-centre-du-quebec.org
Membre(s) du bureau directeur:
Nagui Habashi, Directeur général

Chaudière-Appalaches
CP 1, 440, boul Vachon Sud, Sainte-Marie QC G6E 3B4
Tél: 418-387-1230; *Téléc:* 418-387-1360
Ligne sans frais: 888-387-1230
Courriel: sachap@globetrotter.net
www.alzheimerchap.qc.ca
Membre(s) du bureau directeur:
Sonia Nadeau, Directrice générale

Côte-Nord
373, av Jolliet, Sept-Iles QC G4R 2B1
Tél: 418-968-4673; *Téléc:* 418-962-4161
Ligne sans frais: 866-366-4673
Courriel: sacotenord@globetrotter.net

Estrie
#112, 740, rue Galt Ouest, Sherbrooke QC J1H 1Z3
Tél: 819-821-5127; *Téléc:* 819-820-8649
Courriel: info@alzheimerestrie.com
www.alzheimerestrie.com
www.facebook.com/saeestrie
twitter.com/AlzheimerEstrie
Membre(s) du bureau directeur:
Caroline Giguère, Directrice générale
carolinegiguere@alzheimerestrie.com

Gaspésie/Iles-De-La-Madeleine

114C, av Grand-Pré, Bonaventure QC G0C 1E0
Tel: 418-534-1313; Fax: 418-534-1312
www.alzheimer.ca/fr/gim

Membre(s) du bureau directeur:
Bernard Babin, Directeur général
bernard.sagim@navigue.com

Granby et Région
#3, 356, rue Principale, Granby QC J2G 2W6
Tél: 450-777-3363; Téléc: 450-777-8677
Courriel: sagrinfo@videotron.ca
www.alzheimergranby.ca

Haut-Richelieu
#2, 125, Jacques Cartier nord, Saint-Jean-sur-Richelieu QC J3B 8C9
Tél: 450-347-5500; Téléc: 450-347-7370
Courriel: info@sahr.ca
www.sahr.ca

Lanaudière
190, rue Montcalm, Joliette QC J6E 5G4
Tél: 450-759-3057; Téléc: 450-760-2633
Ligne sans frais: 877-759-3077
Courriel: info@sadl.org
www.sadl.org
www.facebook.com/alzheimerlanaudiere

Membre(s) du bureau directeur:
Janie Duval, Directrice générale

Laurentides
CP 276, #100, 31, rue Principale, Sainte-Agathe-des-Monts QC J8C 3A3
Tél: 819-326-7136; Téléc: 819-326-9664
Ligne sans frais: 800-978-7881
Courriel: admin@salaurentides.ca
www.alzheimerlaurentides.com
www.facebook.com/361627480558344

Membre(s) du bureau directeur:
Catherine Vaudry, Directrice générale
direction@salaurentides.ca

Laval
2525, boul. René-Laennec, Laval QC H7K 0B2
Tél: 450-629-0966; Téléc: 450-975-0517
Courriel: info@alzheimerlaval.org
www.alzheimerlaval.ca

Membre(s) du bureau directeur:
Lise Lalande, Directrice générale
llalande@alzheimerlaval.org

Maskoutains-Vallée des Patriotes
650, rue Girouard Est, Saint-Hyacinthe QC J2S 2Y2
Tél: 450-768-6616; Téléc: 450-768-3716
Courriel: info@alzheimermvp.com
www.alzheimermvp.com
www.facebook.com/alzheimer.mvp

Membre(s) du bureau directeur:
Flore Barrière, Directrice générale

Outaouais québécois
380, boul St-Raymond, Gatineau QC J9A 1V9
Tél: 819-777-4232; Téléc: 819-777-0728
Ligne sans frais: 877-777-0888
Courriel: saoq@saoq.org
www.saoq.org
www.linkedin.com/company/1079874
www.facebook.com/saoq.org
twitter.com/AlzOutaouais
www.youtube.com/channel/UC1rMYxu-ZqK6FTGwHRJ4ecQ

Membre(s) du bureau directeur:
Marie-Josée Williams, Directrice
mjwilliams@saoq.org

Québec
#201, 1040, av Belvédère, Québec QC G1S 3G3
Tél: 418-527-4294; Téléc: 418-527-9966
Ligne sans frais: 866-350-4294
Courriel: info@societealzheimerdequebec.com
www.societealzheimerdequebec.com
www.facebook.com/311740120513
twitter.com/AlzheimerQc

Membre(s) du bureau directeur:
Héléne Thibault, Directrice générale
hthibault@societealzheimerdequebec.com

Rive-Sud
1160, boul Nobert, Longueuil QC J4K 2P1
Tél: 450-442-3333; Téléc: 450-442-9271
Courriel: info@alzheimerrivesud.ca
www.alzheimerrivesud.ca

Membre(s) du bureau directeur:
Geneviève Grégoire, Directrice générale
ggregoire@alzheimerrivesud.ca

Rouyn-Noranda
CP 336, 58, Monseigneur Tessier Est, Rouyn-Noranda QC J9X 5C3
Tél: 819-764-3554; Téléc: 819-764-3534
Courriel: sarn@cablevision.qc.ca

Sagamie
1657, av du Pont Nord, Alma QC G8B 5G2
Tél: 418-668-0161; Téléc: 418-668-2639
Courriel: alzheimersag@bellnet.ca
www.alzheimersagamie.com
www.facebook.com/pages/Société-Alzheimer-de-la-Sagamie/595496990477731
twitter.com/FqsaAlzh
www.youtube.com/user/FQSA1

Membre(s) du bureau directeur:
Josée Pearson, Directrice générale

Société Alzheimer Society Montréal
#410, 5165, rue Sherbrooke ouest, Montréal QC H4A 1T6
Tél: 514-369-0800; Téléc: 514-369-4103
Courriel: info@alzheimermontreal.ca
www.alzheimer.ca/montreal
www.facebook.com/Montreal.Alzheimer
twitter.com/AlzMtl
www.youtube.com/user/montrealalzheimer

Membre(s) du bureau directeur:
Gérald Hubert, Directeur général
ghubert@alzheimermontreal.ca

Suroît
#101, 340, boul du Havre, Salaberry-de-Valleyfield QC J6S 1S6
Tél: 450-373-0303; Téléc: 450-373-0388
Ligne sans frais: 877-773-0303
Courriel: info@alzheimersuroit.com
www.alzheimersuroit.com

Membre(s) du bureau directeur:
Ian Worthington, Président

Val d'or
734, 4e Ave., Val-d'Or QC J9P 1J2
Tél: 819-825-7444; Téléc: 819-825-7448
Courriel: sco.alz.valdor@tlb.sympatico.ca

SASKATCHEWAN

Alzheimer Society Of Saskatchewan Inc. (ASOS)
#301, 2550 - 12 Ave., Regina SK S4P 3X1
Tel: 306-949-4141
Toll-Free: 800-263-3367
e-mail: info@alzheimer.sk.ca
www.alzheimer.sk.ca
www.facebook.com/217901721605861
twitter.com/AlzheimerSK
www.youtube.com/thealzheimersociety

Previous Name: Saskatchewan Alzheimer & Related Diseases Association
Overview: A medium-sized provincial charitable organization founded in 1982 overseen by Alzheimer Society of Canada
Mission: To alleviate the personal & social consequences of Alzheimer's disease & related disorders & to promote the search for a cause & a cure
Chief Officer(s):
Joanne Bracken, CEO
ceo@alzheimer.sk.ca
Publications:
• Prairie View [a publication of the Alzheimer Society of Saskatchewan]

Frequency: 3 pa; *Price:* Free with online subscription
Profile: A publication with important updates about the ASC

Local Associations

ALBERTA

Alzheimer Society of Calgary
#201, 222 - 58 Ave. SW, Calgary AB T2H 2S3
Tel: 403-290-0110
Toll-Free: 877-569-4357
e-mail: info@alzheimercalgary.com
www.alzheimercalgary.com
www.facebook.com/116306041728999
twitter.com/alzcalgary
Overview: A medium-sized local charitable organization founded in 1981
Mission: To offer educational & support services to individuals & families in the Calgary region experiencing Alzheimer Disease & related disorders (dementia), as well as to professionals in the field; to support research
Affiliation(s): Alzheimer Society of Canada; Alzheimer Society of Alberta
Chief Officer(s):
Barb Ferguson, Executive Director

BRITISH COLUMBIA

Prince George Alzheimer's Society
#202, 575 Quebec St., Prince George BC V2L 1W6
Tel: 250-564-7533; *Fax:* 250-564-1642
Toll-Free: 866-564-7533
Overview: A small local charitable organization founded in 1985
Mission: To provide information about Alzheimer's Disease in the Prince George, British Columbia area; To help people concerned with or facing dementia
Member of: Alzheimer Society British Columbia
Chief Officer(s):
Leanne Jones, Coordinator, Support & Education
ljones@alzheimerbc.org
Laurie De Croos, Coordinator, First Link
ldecroos@alzheimerbc.org

NEW BRUNSWICK

Alzheimer Society of Miramichi
PO Box 205, Miramichi NB E1N 3A6
Tel: 506-773-7093; *Fax:* 506-773-7093
Toll-Free: 800-664-8411
e-mail: alzmir@nb.aibn.com
www.alzheimernb.ca
Overview: A small local organization
Mission: To alleviate the personal and social consequences of Alzheimer Disease and related disorders and to promote research.

Alzheimer Society of Moncton
960 St. George Blvd., Moncton NB E1E 3Y3
Tel: 506-858-8380; *Fax:* 506-855-7697
Toll-Free: 800-664-8411
e-mail: moncton@alzheimernb.ca
www.alzheimernb.ca
Overview: A small local charitable organization founded in 1986
Mission: To alleviate the personal & social consequencs of Alzheimer's Disease & related diseases in the Moncton New Brunswick region
Member of: Société Alzheimer Society New Brunswick / Nouveau-Brunswick
Chief Officer(s):
Joanne Sonier, Regional Coordinator

Saint John Alzheimer Society
152 Westmorland Rd., Saint John NB E2J 2E7
Tel: 506-634-8722; *Fax:* 506-648-9404
e-mail: saintjohn@alzheimernb.ca
www.alzheimernb.ca
Overview: A small local charitable organization founded in 1983

Mission: To alleviate the personal & social consequences of Alzheimer disease & related dementia; to promote the search for a cause & cure
Member of: Alzheimer Society of New Brunswick

ONTARIO

Alzheimer Society London & Middlesex (ASLM)
435 Windermere Rd., London ON N5X 2T1
Tel: 519-680-2404; *Fax:* 519-680-2864
Toll-Free: 888-495-5855
e-mail: info@alzheimerlondon.ca
www.alzheimerlondon.ca
www.facebook.com/alzheimerlondon
twitter.com/alzheimerldn
www.youtube.com/user/evokemediasolutions
Overview: A small local charitable organization founded in 1979
Mission: To provide support services & education for persons affected by Alzheimer's Disease & related dementias in Ontario's London & Middlesex region
Chief Officer(s):
Betsy Little, CEO
blittle@alzheimerlondon.ca
Rose Brochu, Manager, Accounting & Operations
rbrochu@alzheimerlondon.ca
Leslie Rand, Manager, Fund Development
lrand@alzheimerlondon.ca
Bruce Wray, Manager, Communications
bwray@alzheimerlondon.ca
Publications:
• Connections [a publication of Alzheimer Society London & Middlesex]
Type: Newsletter; *Frequency:* Quarterly
Profile: New developments plus volunteer news, fundraising activities, & upcoming events from the Alzheimer Society of London & Middlesex

Alzheimer Society of Belleville/Hastings/Quinte
Bay View Mall, #63, 470 Dundas St. East, Belleville ON K8N 1G1
Tel: 613-962-0892; *Fax:* 613-962-1225
Toll-Free: 800-361-8036
www.alzheimer.ca/bhq
www.facebook.com/AlzheimerBHQ
twitter.com/AlzBHQ
www.youtube.com/AlzBHQ
Overview: A small local organization founded in 1987
Mission: To alleviate the personal & social consequences of Alzheimer disease & to promote research
Affiliation(s): Alzheimer Society of Ontario
Chief Officer(s):
Jon Leavens, President
Laura Hare, Executive Director
laura.hare@alzheimerhpe.ca

North Hastings
PO Box 1786, 1 Manor Lane, Bancroft ON K0K 1C0
Tel: 613-332-4614; *Fax:* 613-332-0432
www.alzheimer.ca/en/chapters-on/bhq
Chief Officer(s):
Sarah Krieger, Coordinator, Education & Support

Alzheimer Society of Brant
#701, 6 Bell Lane, Brantford ON N3T 0C3
Tel: 519-759-7692; *Fax:* 519-759-8353
www.alzbrant.ca
www.facebook.com/alzhbrant
Overview: A small local organization
Mission: To alleviate the personal & social consequences of Alzheimer Disease and related disorders and to promote research.
Member of: Alzheimer Association of Ontario
Chief Officer(s):
Mary Burnett, CEO

Alzheimer Society of Chatham-Kent
36 Memory Lane, Chatham ON N7L 5M8
Tel: 519-352-1043; *Fax:* 519-352-3680
e-mail: info@alzheimerchathamkent.ca
www.alzheimer.ca/chathamkent
www.facebook.com/321344923495
www.youtube.com/thealzheimersociety
Overview: A small local charitable organization founded in 1983

Mission: To alleviate the personal & social consequences of Alzheimer Disease and related disorders and to promote research.
Member of: Alzheimer Soceity of Canada
Chief Officer(s):
Mary Ellen Parker, CEO

Alzheimer Society of Cornwall & District
106B - 2 St. West, Cornwall ON K6H 6N6
Tel: 613-932-4914; *Fax:* 613-932-6154
Toll-Free: 888-222-1445
e-mail: alzheimer.info@one-mail.on.ca
www.alzheimer.ca/cornwall

Overview: A small local charitable organization
Mission: To alleviate the personal & social consequences of Alzheimer Disease and related disorders and to promote research.

Alzheimer Society of Dufferin County
#1, 25 Centennial Rd., Orangeville ON L9W 1R1
Tel: 519-941-1221; *Fax:* 519-941-1730
e-mail: info@alzheimerdufferin.org
www.alzheimerdufferin.org
www.facebook.com/Alzheimerdufferin

Overview: A small local charitable organization founded in 1999
Mission: To alleviate the personal & social consequences of Alzheimer Disease and related disorders and to promote research.
Member of: Alzheimer Society of Ontario
Chief Officer(s):
Diane Cowen, Interim Executive Director
dianecowen@alzheimerdufferin.org

Alzheimer Society of Durham Region (ASDR)
Oshawa Executive Centre, Oshawa Centre, #207, 419 King St. West, Oshawa ON L1J 2K5
Tel: 905-576-2567; *Fax:* 905-576-2033
Toll-Free: 888-301-1106
e-mail: information@alzheimerdurham.com
www.alzheimerdurham.com
www.facebook.com/alzheimer.durham
twitter.com/AlzheimerDurham
www.youtube.com/thealzheimersociety

Also Known As: Alzheimer Durham
Overview: A small local charitable organization founded in 1979
Mission: To improve the quality of life of persons with Alzheimer's Disease, or related dementias, & their caregivers in Ontario's Durham Region
Member of: Alzheimer Society of Ontario
Chief Officer(s):
Denyse Newton, Executive Director
dnewton@alzheimerdurham.com
Michelle Pepin, Director, Family Support
mpepin@alzheimerdurham.com
Loretta Tanner, Director, Public Education
ltanner@alzheimerdurham.com
Brenda Davie, Coordinator, Family Support & Education
bdavie@alzheimerdurham.com
Karen Morley, Coordinator, Caregiver
kmorley@alzheimerdurham.com
Publications:
• Staying Connected: A Newsletter from Alzheimer Society of Durham Region
Type: Newsletter; *Frequency:* Quarterly; *Price:* Free with membership in the Alzheimer Society of Durham Region
Profile: Notices about forthcoming events, education, & support groups

Alzheimer Society of Grey-Bruce
753 - 2nd Ave. East, Owen Sound ON N4K 2G9
Tel: 519-376-7230; *Fax:* 519-376-2428
Toll-Free: 800-265-9013
e-mail: info@alzheimergreybruce.com
www.alzheimer.ca/greybruce
www.facebook.com/AlzheimerSocietyofGreyBruce
twitter.com/AlzheimerSGB

Overview: A small local charitable organization founded in 1986
Mission: Exists to alleviate the personal and social consequences of Alzheimer's Disease and related disorders and to promote research.
Member of: Alzheimer Association of Ontario
Chief Officer(s):

Deborah Barker, Executive Director
dbarker@alzheimergreybruce.com

Alzheimer Society of Haldimand Norfolk
645 Norfolk St. North, Simcoe ON N3Y 3R2
Tel: 519-428-7771; *Fax:* 519-428-2968
Toll-Free: 800-565-4614
www.alzhn.ca
www.facebook.com/alzhbrant

Overview: A small local charitable organization founded in 1993
Mission: To help people as they deal with the consequences of Alzheimer's Disease & related disorders
Chief Officer(s):
Mary Burnett, Chief Executive Officer
mary.burnett@alzda.ca

Alzheimer Society of Hamilton Halton
#700, 1575 Upper Ottawa St., Hamilton ON L8W 3E2
Tel: 905-529-7030; *Fax:* 905-529-3787
Toll-Free: 888-343-1017
www.alzheimerhamiltonhalton.org
www.facebook.com/alzhbrant

Overview: A small local charitable organization founded in 1982
Mission: To provide programs & services to help caregivers handle the challenges associated with caring for people with Alzheimer's Disease & related disorders in the communities of Ancaster, Dundas, Flamborough, Glanbrook, Hamilton, & Stoney Creek within the City of Hamilton, & the the communities of Burlington, Halton Hills, Milton & Oakville within Halton Region
Chief Officer(s):
Mary Burnett, Chief Executive Officer
mary.burnett@alzda.ca
JoAnne Chalifour, Regional Director, Operations
joanne.chalifour@alzda.ca
Trevor Clark, Regional Director, Development
trevor.clark@alzda.ca

Alzheimer Society of Hastings - Prince Edward
Bay View Mall, #63, 470 Dundas St. East, Belleville ON K8N 1G1
Tel: 613-962-0892; *Fax:* 613-962-1225
Toll-Free: 800-361-8036
www.alzheimer.ca/hpe
www.facebook.com/AlzheimerHPE

Overview: A small local charitable organization founded in 1985
Mission: To help people diagnosed with Alzheimer's Disease or a related dementia in Prince Edward County of southeastern Ontario
Member of: South East Local Health Integration Network (LHIN)
Chief Officer(s):
Maureen Corrigan, Executive Director, 613-962-0892 Ext. 7012
maureen.corrigan@alzheimerhpe.ca

Alzheimer Society of Huron County
PO Box 639, 317 Huron Rd., Clinton ON N0M 1L0
Tel: 519-482-1482; *Fax:* 519-482-8692
Toll-Free: 800-561-5012
e-mail: admin@alzheimerhuron.on.ca
www.alzheimerhuron.on.ca
www.facebook.com/AlzheimerSocietyHuron
twitter.com/AlzSociety
www.youtube.com/user/AlzheimerSouthwest

Overview: A small local organization
Mission: To alleviate the personal and social consequences of Alzheimer Disease and related disorders and to promote research.
Chief Officer(s):
Cathy Ritsema, Executive Director
cathy@alzheimerhuron.on.ca

Alzheimer Society of Kenora/Rainy River Districts
618 - 9th St. North, Kenora ON P9N 2S9
Tel: 807-468-1516; *Fax:* 807-468-9013
Toll-Free: 800-682-0245
e-mail: info@alzheimerkrr.com
www.alzheimer.ca/krr
www.facebook.com/Alzheimerkrr

Overview: A small local charitable organization founded in 1991
Mission: To alleviate the personal and social consequences of Alzheimer Disease and related disorders and to promote research.
Chief Officer(s):

Lynn Moffatt, Executive Director
lynn@alzheimerkrr.com

Alzheimer Society of Kingston, Frontenac, Lennox & Addington
#4, 400 Elliot Ave., Kingston ON K7K 6M9

Tel: 613-544-3078; Fax: 613-544-6320
Toll-Free: 800-266-7516
e-mail: reception@alzking.com
www.alzheimer.ca/kfla
www.facebook.com/AlzheimerKingston
twitter.com/AlzSocKing
www.youtube.com/thealzheimersociety

Overview: A small local charitable organization founded in 1986
Mission: To improve the quality of life of people with Alzheimer disease & other dementias & their caregivers
Member of: Alzheimer Association of Ontario
Chief Officer(s):
Jan White, President
Vicki Poffley, Executive Director

Alzheimer Society of Lanark County
115 Christie Lake Rd., Perth ON K7H 3C6

Tel: 613-264-0307
Toll-Free: 800-511-1911
e-mail: alz@storm.ca
www.alzheimer.ca/lanark
www.facebook.com/pages/Alzheimer-Society-Lanark-County/71569937
1806903
twitter.com/1ASLC

Overview: A small local organization
Mission: To alleviate the personal and social consequences of Alzheimer Disease and related disorders and to promote research.
Member of: Alzheimer Association of Ontario
Chief Officer(s):
Don McDiarmid, President
Louise Noble, Executive Director
alzlnoble@storm.ca

Alzheimer Society of Leeds-Grenville
c/o Garden Street Site, Brockville General Hospital, 42 Garden St., Brockville ON K6V 2C3

Tel: 613-345-7392; Fax: 613-345-3186
Toll-Free: 866-576-8556
e-mail: administrator@alzheimerleedsgrenville.ca
www.alzheimer.ca/en/lg
www.facebook.com/alzheimerleedsgrenville

Overview: A small local charitable organization founded in 1987
Mission: To help persons diagnosed with Alzheimer's Disease or a related dementia in the Leeds-Grenville region of Ontario
Chief Officer(s):
Louise Noble, Interim Executive Director
administrator@alzheimerleedsgrenville.ca
Sean McFadden, Coordinator, Education & Support
education@alzheimerleedsgrenville.ca
Publications:
• Alzheimer Society of Leeds-Grenville Newsletter
Type: Newsletter; Frequency: 3 pa; Price: Free with membership in the Alzheimer Society of Leeds-Grenville
Profile: Updates about the society's activities, plus educational information, caregiver tips, & research reports
• Alzheimer Update
Type: Newsletter
Profile: Medical information & resources for physicians in the Leeds-Grenville region

Alzheimer Society of Muskoka
#205, 230 Manitoba St., Bracebridge ON P1L 2E1

Tel: 705-645-5621; Fax: 705-645-4397
Toll-Free: 800-605-2076
e-mail: alzmusk@muskoka.com
www.alzheimer.ca/en/muskoka
www.facebook.com/alzheimersocietyofmuskoka
twitter.com/alz_muskoka

Overview: A small local charitable organization founded in 1995
Mission: To assist persons living with Alzheimer's Disease & other dementias in the Muskoka region of Ontario; To provide education

programs; To promote research
Member of: Alzheimer Society of Ontario
Chief Officer(s):
Karen Quernby, Executive Director

Alzheimer Society of Niagara Region
#1, 403 Ontario St., St Catharines ON L2N 1L5

Tel: 905-687-3914; Fax: 905-687-9952
Toll-Free: 877-818-3202
e-mail: niagara@alzheimerniagara.ca
www.alzheimer.ca/niagara
www.facebook.com/106624255247
twitter.com/alzheimerniagar
www.youtube.com/user/alzheimerniagara

Overview: A small local charitable organization founded in 1984
Mission: To ensure quality services for individuals with Alzheimer disease & related dementias; to support & advocate for individuals, families, caregivers & community through counselling, education & the promotion of research to compassionately respond to the very special needs of those experiencing dementia
Chief Officer(s):
Judy Willems, President
Teena Kindt, CEO

Alzheimer Society of North Bay & District
1180 Cassells St., North Bay ON P1B 4B6

Tel: 705-495-4342; Fax: 705-495-0329
www.alzheimer.ca/northbay
www.facebook.com/alzheimersmnbd

Overview: A small local charitable organization founded in 1978
Mission: To alleviate the personal & social consequences of Alzheimer Disease & related disorders & to promote research
Member of: Alzheimer Society of Ontario
Chief Officer(s):
Linda Brown, Family Counsellor & Site Supervisor
lbrown@alzheimernorthbay.com

Alzheimer Society of Ottawa & Renfrew County / Société Alzheimer d'Ottawa et Renfrew County
#1742, 1750 Russell Rd., Ottawa ON K1G 5Z6

Tel: 613-523-4004
e-mail: info@asorc.org
www.alzheimerottawa.ca
www.linkedin.com/company/alzheimer-society-of-ottawa-and-renfrew-count
www.facebook.com/alzheimerOttawa
twitter.com/AlzheimerOttawa
www.youtube.com/user/ASOttawa

Previous Name: Alzheimer Society of Ottawa
Overview: A medium-sized local charitable organization founded in 1980
Mission: To increase the understanding of, & to alleviate the personal & social consequences of Alzheimer disease through patient & family support, information & education & promotion of research
Member of: Alzheimer Society of Ontario; Alzheimer Society of Canada
Affliation(s): Perley & Rideau Veterans' Health Centre; Care for Health & Community Services; Champlain Dementia Network
Chief Officer(s):
Kathy Wright, Executive Director, 613-369-5628
Debbie Seto, Manager, 613-369-5634
Publications:
• Société Alzheimer Society Ottawa & Renfrew County Annual Report
Type: Yearbook; Frequency: Annually
Profile: A review of the year's events
• Société Alzheimer Society Ottawa & Renfrew County Newsletter
Type: Newsletter
Profile: Information about programs & services provided by the society, plus research & education updates

Alzheimer Society of Oxford (ASO)
575 Peel St., Woodstock ON N4S 1K6

Tel: 519-421-2466; *Fax:* 519-421-3098
e-mail: info@alzheimer.oxford.on.ca
www.alzheimer.ca/oxford
www.facebook.com/alzoxford
twitter.com/AlzSociety
www.youtube.com/thealzheimersociety

Overview: A small local charitable organization founded in 1989
Mission: To improve the quality of life for people with Alzheimer disease or related dementias & their caregivers
Member of: Alzheimer Society of Ontario
Chief Officer(s):
Andrew Szasz, President

Alzheimer Society of Peel
60 Briarwood Ave., Mississauga ON L5G 3N6

Tel: 905-278-3667; *Fax:* 905-278-3964
www.alzheimerpeel.com
www.facebook.com/112857568321
twitter.com/AlzPeel

Overview: A small local charitable organization founded in 1983
Mission: To alleviate the personal and social consequences of Alzheimer Disease and related disorders and to promote research.
Member of: Alzheimer Association of Ontario
Chief Officer(s):
Mary-Lynn Peters, President

Alzheimer Society of Perth County
#5, 1020 Ontario St., Stratford ON N5A 6Z3

Tel: 519-271-1910; *Fax:* 519-271-1231
Toll-Free: 888-797-1882
e-mail: info@alzheimerperthcounty.com
www.alzheimerperthcounty.com
www.facebook.com/AlzheimerSocietyPerth
twitter.com/Alzperth

Overview: A small local charitable organization founded in 1988
Mission: To assist those affected by Alzheimer's Disease & other types of dementia
Chief Officer(s):
Debbie Deichert, Executive Director
debdeichert@wightman.ca
Publications:
• The Helping Hand
Type: Newsletter; *Price:* Free with Alzheimer Society of Perth County membership
Profile: Articles to help caregivers & upcoming events

Alzheimer Society of Sarnia-Lambton
420 East St. North, Sarnia ON N7T 6Y5

Tel: 519-332-4444; *Fax:* 519-332-6673
e-mail: info@alzheimersarnia.ca
alzheimer.sarnia.com
www.facebook.com/alzheimersarnialambton
twitter.com/AlzheimerSociet

Overview: A small local charitable organization founded in 1986
Mission: To improve the quality of live of people with Alzheimer disease or related dementia, & their caregivers
Member of: Alzheimer Society of Ontario
Affliation(s): Ministry of Health, Long-Term Care; Ontario Trillium Foundation
Chief Officer(s):
Bill Seymour, Chair
Judy Doan, CEO

Alzheimer Society of Sault Ste. Marie & District of Algoma
341 Trunk Rd., Sault Ste Marie ON P6A 3S9

Tel: 705-942-2195; *Fax:* 705-256-6777
Toll-Free: 877-396-7888
e-mail: info@alzheimeralgoma.org
www.alzheimeralgoma.org

Overview: A small local charitable organization founded in 1987
Mission: To improve the quality of life for people with Alzheimer disease & related disorders & to provide support for their caregivers
Member of: Alzheimer Association of Ontario
Chief Officer(s):
Graham Clark, President

Terry Caporossi, Executive Director

Alzheimer Society of Simcoe County
PO Box 1414, Barrie ON L4M 5R4

Tel: 705-722-1066; *Fax:* 705-722-9392
Toll-Free: 800-265-5391
e-mail: simcoecounty@alzheimersociety.ca
www.alzheimersociety.ca
www.facebook.com/AlzheimerSocietySimcoeCounty
twitter.com/AlzheimerSimcoe

Previous Name: Alzheimer Society of Barrie & District, Alzheimer Society of Greater Simcoe County
Merged from: Alzheimer Society of Greater Simcoe County & Alzheimer Society of North East Simcoe County
Overview: A small local charitable organization founded in 1985
Mission: To improve the quality of life of persons who are directly affected by Alzheimer's diseases or related dementias
Chief Officer(s):
Debbie Islam, Executive Director
dislam@alzheimersociety.ca

Alzheimer Society of Thunder Bay (ASTB)
#310, 180 Park Ave., Thunder Bay ON P7B 6J4

Tel: 807-345-9556; *Fax:* 807-345-1518
Toll-Free: 800-879-4226; *TTY:* 888-887-5140
e-mail: info@alzheimerthunderbay.ca
www.alzheimer.ca/thunderbay
www.facebook.com/ASTBAY

Overview: A small local charitable organization founded in 1986
Mission: To improve the quality of life of persons with Alzheimer disease or related dementia & their caregivers; to promote the rights & well-being of persons with the disease & their caregivers; to support the delivery of programmes for individuals affected by the disease; to provide funds for research
Chief Officer(s):
Laraine Tapak, President
Kelly Brunwin-Harding, Coordinator, Family Support
kelly@alzheimerthunderbay.ca

Alzheimer Society of Timmins/Porcupine District
70 Cedar St. South, Timmins ON P4N 2G6

Tel: 705-268-4554; *Fax:* 705-360-4492
ww.alzheimer.ca/en/timmins
www.facebook.com/AlzheimerSocietyTimmins

Overview: A small local charitable organization founded in 1986
Mission: To alleviate the personal & social consequences of Alzheimer disease; To promote the search for the causes & cure of the disease
Member of: Alzheimer Association of Ontario
Chief Officer(s):
Tracy Koskamp-Bergeron, Executive Director
director@alzheimertimmins.com

Alzheimer Society of Toronto
20 Eglinton Ave. West, 16th Fl., Toronto ON M4R 1K8

Tel: 416-322-6560; *Fax:* 416-322-6656
e-mail: write@alzheimertoronto.org
www.alzheimertoronto.org
www.linkedin.com/company/alzheimer-society-of-toronto
www.facebook.com/AlzheimerToronto
twitter.com/alztoronto
www.youtube.com/user/alzheimertoronto

Overview: A medium-sized local charitable organization founded in 1982
Mission: To enhance the lives of persons with Alzheimer Disease & their caregivers by providing family support, raising awareness & advocating for services & research
Member of: Alzheimer Society of Ontario
Chief Officer(s):
Cathy Barrick, Chief Ececutive Officer
cbarrick@alzheimertoronto.org
Neil Jacoby, Chair

Alzheimer Society of Windsor/Essex County
2135 Richmond St., Windsor ON N8Y 0A1
Tel: 519-974-2220; *Fax:* 519-974-9727
e-mail: generalinformation@aswecare.com
www.alzheimerwindsor.com
www.facebook.com/AlzheimerSocietyOfWindsorEssexCounty
twitter.com/ASWE_Care
Overview: A small local charitable organization founded in 1981
Mission: To improve the quality of life of those affected by Alzheimer disease or other dementia
Member of: Alzheimer Association of Ontario
Affliation(s): Windsor & District Chamber of Commerce, Alzheimer Association of Canada
Chief Officer(s):
Gaston Franklyn, Chair
Sally Bennett Olczak, CEO

Alzheimer Society of York Region
#2, 240 Edward St., Aurora ON L4G 3S9
Tel: 905-726-3477; *Fax:* 905-726-1917
Toll-Free: 888-414-5550
e-mail: info@alzheimer-york.com
www.alzheimer-york.com
www.facebook.com/AlzheimerSocietyYork
twitter.com/AlzheimerYork
Overview: A small local charitable organization founded in 1985
Mission: To support individuals & families, in Ontario's York Region, who cope with Alzheimer's Disease & related disorders; To promote research
Chief Officer(s):
Loren Freid, Chief Executive Officer
Janice Clarke, Manager, Finance & Support Services
Publications:
• Alzheimer Society York Region Newsletter
Type: Newsletter
Profile: Articles about Alzheimer's Disease & dementia, plus information about support groups & workshops for caregivers & forthcoming events in the area

Alzheimer Society Peterborough, Kawartha Lakes, Northumberland, & Haliburton (ASPKLNH)
183 Simcoe St., Peterborough ON K9H 2H6
Tel: 705-748-5131; *Fax:* 705-748-6174
Toll-Free: 800-561-2588
e-mail: info@alzheimerjourney.ca
www.alzheimer.ca/pklnha
www.facebook.com/AlzheimerPKLNH
twitter.com/Alzheimerpklnh
www.youtube.com/thealzheimersociety
Overview: A small local charitable organization founded in 1981
Mission: To improve the quality of life of persons affected by Alzheimer's Disease & related dementias in the Peterborough, Kawartha Lakes, Northumberland & Haliburton regions of Ontario
Chief Officer(s):
Carolyn Hemminger, Interim Executive Director
carolyn@alzeimerjourney.ca
Publications:
• Alzheimer Society Peterborough, Kawartha Lakes, Northumberland, & Haliburton eNewsletter
Type: Newsletter
Profile: Reports & forthcoming events in the region

Kawartha Lakes & Haliburton Office
#201, 55 Mary St., Lindsay ON K9V 5Z6
Tel: 705-878-0126; *Fax:* 705-878-0127
Toll-Free: 800-765-0515
e-mail: admin@alzheimerjourney.ca
www.alzheimer.ca/pklnh
Chief Officer(s):
Pat Finkle, Client Support Coordinator
pat@alzheimerjourney.ca

Lindsay Office
#201, 55 Mary St., Lindsay ON K9V 5Z6
Tel: 705-878-0126; *Fax:* 705-878-0127
Toll-Free: 800-765-0515
e-mail: info@alzheimerjourney.ca
Chief Officer(s):

Carolyn Hemminger, Coordinator, Public Education
carolyn@alzheimerjourney.ca

Alzheimer Society Waterloo Wellington
1145 Concession Rd., Cambridge ON N3H 4L6
Tel: 519-650-1628; *Fax:* 519-742-1862
e-mail: asww@alzheimerww.ca
www.alzheimer.ca/ww
www.facebook.com/alzsocww
twitter.com/alzsocww
www.pinterest.com/alzsocietyww
Merged from: Alzheimer Societies of Cambridge, Guelph-Wellington & Kitchener-Waterloo
Overview: A small local charitable organization founded in 2014
Mission: To enhance the lives of persons with Alzheimer disease or related dementias & their care-givers by providing support, information, education, public awareness, advocacy & promotion of research
Member of: Alzheimer Society of Ontario
Affliation(s): Alzheimer Society of Canada
Chief Officer(s):
Nancy Kauffman-Lambert, Chair
Jennifer Gillies, Executive Director
jgillies@alzheimerww.ca

Guelph Office
#207, 255 Woodlawn Rd. West, Guelph ON N1H 8J1
Tel: 519-836-7672; *Fax:* 519-742-1862

Kitchener Office
831 Frederick St., Kitchener ON N2B 2B4
Tel: 519-742-1422; *Fax:* 519-742-1862

Société Alzheimer Society Sudbury-Manitoulin (SASSM)
960B Notre Dame Ave., Sudbury ON P3A 2T4
Tel: 705-560-0603; *Fax:* 705-560-6938
Toll-Free: 800-407-6369
e-mail: info@alzheimersudbury.ca
www.alzheimersudbury.ca
www.facebook.com/alzheimersmnbd
Overview: A small local organization founded in 1983
Member of: Alzheimer Canada
Affliation(s): Alzheimer Society of Ontario
Chief Officer(s):
Lorraine LeBlanc, Executive Director
lleblanc@alzheimersudbury.ca

International Associations

International Society for Vascular Behavioural & Cognitive Disorders
c/o Newcastle University Campus for Ageing & Vitality, NIHR Biomedical Research Building, 1st Fl., Newcastle upon Tyne NE4 5PL United Kingdom
Tel: 44-191-248-1352; *Fax:* 44-191-248-1301
e-mail: vascogsoc@gmail.com
www.vas-cog.org
Also Known As: The Vas-Cog Society
Overview: A medium-sized international organization founded in 2001
Mission: To study the vascular causes of various brain disorders by bringing together diverse basic sciences & clinical research interests
Chief Officer(s):
Christopher Chen, Chair
Raj Kalaria, Secretariat

Conduct Disorder

Conduct disorder is characterized by a repetitive and persistent pattern of behaviour in which societal norms and the basic rights of others are violated. These behaviours are exhibited at school, home or in public and can include physical harm to people or animals, damage to property, deceitfulness or theft, and extreme violations of rules. It is important to note that troublesome behaviour can also result from adverse circumstances; the circumstances need to be fully investigated, and attempts to rectify adversity made, before conduct disorder is diagnosed. The diagnosis can be divided into two types, depending on the age of diagnosis: childhood-onset type and adolescent-onset type.

Cause

Conduct disorder appears to be caused by both genetic and environmental factors. A child is more likely to have conduct disorder if one or both parents experienced childhood or adolescent conduct problems. Peer rejection, family neglect/abuse and poverty might also be factors involved in the development of conduct disorder.

Symptoms

Children and adolescents with conduct disorder can show aggression and physical cruelty to people and animals. Other symptoms can include bullying; picking fights; using weapons; forcing someone into sexual activity; destruction of property; deceitfulness; and theft, including breaking into someone's house, lying to obtain goods or favours, or shoplifting. Violations of rules, including staying out past curfews, running away from home and truancy from school are also common symptoms. Conduct disorder is often associated with early onset of sexual activity, drinking and smoking. The disorder leads to school disruption, problems with the police, sexually transmitted diseases, unplanned pregnancy and injury from accidents and fights. Suicide and suicidal attempts are more common among adolescents with conduct disorder, probably both because they have a history of abuse and neglect and because their behaviour results in adverse consequences. Individuals with conduct disorder appear to have little remorse for their acts, though they may learn that expressing guilt can diminish punishment, and they often show little or no empathy for the feelings, wishes and well-being of others.

Prevalence

Conduct disorder is the third most prevalent childhood mental disorder. In Canada, the estimated prevalence in children under 15 years of age is 4.2 percent. The disorder seems to be more common in boys than girls. Onset can be before the age of 10, or in adolescence.

Treatment Options

There is no specific test used to diagnose conduct disorder. Assessment is generally based upon a thorough medical and family/social history, observation of the child and reports from parents, teachers and peers. To be diagnosed with conduct disorder, a child must be under the age of 18 and have demonstrated conduct problems that significantly interfere with school, home and community life for at least a year.

Both psychotherapy (usually cognitive behavioural therapy with a focus on anger management techniques) and medication can be useful in treating conduct disorder. This condition is stressful for family members of the affected child or adolescent; it is crucial that they are supported and involved in the treatment.

Early diagnosis and intensive, structured, individualized therapy is essential to help children and adolescents with conduct disorder make a successful transition to adulthood.

National Associations

Canadian Families & Corrections Network (CFCN)
PO Box 35040, Kingston ON K7L 5S5

Tel: 613-541-0743
Toll-Free: 888-371-2326
e-mail: national@cfcn-rcafd.org
www.cfcn-rcafd.org

Overview: A small national charitable organization
Mission: To assist families affected by criminal behaviour, incarceration, & community reintegration
Chief Officer(s):

Louise Leonardi, Executive Director
Publications:
• Child-Friendly Practices within the Prison Setting
 Number of Pages: 26; *Author:* Margaret Holland
Profile: Written with Lori Ann Bevins-Yeomans & Joyce Waddell-Townsend of Children Visiting Prisons-Kingston Inc.
• Families & Corrections Journal
Type: Journal; *Price:* Free
Profile: Articles with news & information about Canadian families & corrections
• One Day at a Time: Writings on Facing the Incarceration of a Friend or Family Member
 Number of Pages: 39
• Staying Involved: A Guide for Incarcerated Fathers
Type: Guide
Profile: A joint initiative of Pro Bono Queen's University & Canadian Families & Corrections Network
• Time Together & The Directory of Canadian Services to the Families of Adult Offenders
 Number of Pages: 95; *Author:* Lloyd Withers
Profile: A survival guide for families & friends visiting in Canadian federal prisons
• Time's Up: A Reintegration Toolkit for families
 Number of Pages: 36; *ISBN:* 0-9688923-5-3
• Waiting at the Gate: Families, Corrections, & Restorative Justice
 Number of Pages: 242; *Price:* $25

Provincial Associations

ONTARIO

Association of Parent Support Groups in Ontario Inc. (APSGO)
PO Box 27581, Stn. Yorkdale, Toronto ON M6A 3B8

Toll-Free: 800-488-5666
e-mail: mail@apsgo.ca
www.apsgo.ca
twitter.com/APSGOca

Overview: A small provincial charitable organization founded in 1985
Mission: To enable parents to develop strategies to deal with their children's disruptive behaviour
Chief Officer(s):
Maureen MacNeil, President
Publications:
• Parent to Parent
Type: Newsletter; *Editor:* Sue Kranz

Local Associations

ONTARIO

Counselling Services of Belleville & District (CSBD)
12 Moira St. East, Belleville ON K8P 2R9

Tel: 613-966-7413; *Fax:* 613-966-2357
e-mail: csbd@csbd.on.ca
www.csbd.on.ca

Overview: A small local charitable organization founded in 1978 overseen by Family Service Ontario
Mission: To offer behavioural assessment & counselling, advocacy & support to families & individuals.
Affiliation(s): YMCA, for summer camps

Helping Other Parents Everywhere Inc. (HOPE)
1740 Kingston Rd., Pickering ON L1V 2R2

Tel: 905-239-3577
Toll-Free: 866-492-1299
e-mail: info@hope4parents.ca
www.hope4parents.ca

Overview: A small local organization
Mission: To provide support, resources, & education to parents of disruptive youth; To offer a confidential & non-judgemental environment for parents who want to deal more effectively with the behaviour of their children; To empower concerned parents to handle situations with their children
Chief Officer(s):
Leanne Lewis, President
 president@hope4parents.ca

York Region Family Services (Markham)
#203, 4261 Hwy. 7, Unionville ON L3R 1L5
Tel: 905-415-9719; *Fax:* 905-415-9706
Toll-Free: 888-820-9986
www.fsyr.ca

Also Known As: FSYR Markham
Overview: A medium-sized local organization founded in 1968 overseen by Family Service Ontario
Mission: To assist people experiencing emotional, behavioural, relational &/or financial challenges through counselling, educational & assessment programs & services designed to improve functioning & coping skills in daily life
Member of: Ontario Psychological Association; Ontario Association of Credit Counselling Services
Affliation(s): Canadian Register of Health Service Providers in Psychology; United Way of York Region
Chief Officer(s):
Elisha Laker, Executive Director
elaker@fsyr.ca

Congenital Heart Disease

Congenital Heart Disease (CHD) represents the most common group of congenital (present from birth) anomalies.

Cause

CHD can be thought of as a group of disorders that result from the abnormal formation of the heart in utero. The heart develops between the 2nd and 6th week of gestation, and may be affected by genetic mutation, rubella infection, maternal diabetes, maternal exposure to medications (for example, chemotherapy drugs, antiseizure drugs, thalidomide) or maternal alcohol abuse. However, in most cases, the exact cause of congenital heart disease is not known.

About half of cardiac defects are considered to be minor and can be followed clinically while the other half fall into the categories of major CHD. This latter group often requires surgery early in life to either completely repair the heart defect or in some cases, to redirect blood through the cardiovascular system to palliate the structural abnormality.

CHD can be divided into three major categories: left to right shunting lesions, left heart obstructive lesions and those that lead to marked cyanosis (decreased oxygen delivery to the organs and tissues), the so-called cyanotic heart diseases.

The left to right shunting lesions are the most common of the three groups and include the ventricular septal defect (VSD), the atrial septal defect (ASD), the atrioventricular septal defect (also referred to as the AV canal), and the patent ductus arteriosus. In all of these left to right shunting lesions, there is a progressive increase in the amount of blood sent from the left side of the heart across the given defect (hole) into the right side that delivers blood to the lungs. There is as a result, too much blood entering the pulmonary circuit and this can lead to problems with breathing and feeding for infants in the first few months of life.

The more common left heart obstructive diseases include aortic stenosis, coarctation of the aorta and hypoplastic left heart syndrome. Each of these can lead to a marked reduction in the amount of blood flow that is able to leave the left side of the heart and be delivered to the organs and tissues. This leads to abnormalities in the way the organs and tissues function and can cause serious and emergent problems for infants in the first week or two of life.

Cyanotic heart defects are those cardiac malformations that lead to a bluish discolouration of the baby as there is insufficient oxygenated blood that is delivered to the body with or without inadequate blood delivered to the lungs to pick up oxygen. The more common disorders in this group are tetralogy of Fallot, transposition of the great arteries, tricuspid atresia and truncus arteriosus.

Symptoms

The most common symptoms of congenital heart disease include shortness of breath, fast breathing, heart murmur and fatigue during physical activity (in older children). Infants with congenital heart disease exhibit poor weight gain and poor feeding behaviour and often have a bluish tint to their lips, skin and fingernails.

Prevalence

In Canada, about 1 in every 100 babies is born with some type of heart defect. Around 257,000 Canadians are currently living with congenital heart disease.

Treatment Options

Congenital heart defects can be diagnosed before birth (through prenatal testing), shortly after birth or in adulthood. After a thorough medical history is taken, and a physical examination is performed, diagnosis is confirmed through tests that may include chest X-ray, electrocardiogram (ECG), echocardiogram, magnetic resonance imaging (MRI) and cardiac catheterization.

Medications such as ACE inhibitors, beta-blockers, diuretics and digoxin are prescribed to treat some types of heart defects. In other cases, surgical and non-surgical procedures are needed to fix holes in the heart, replace heart valves and repair blood vessels. With the remarkable advances in neonatal cardiac surgery and interventional cardiac catheterization, almost all of the cardiac malformations can be aggressively addressed with excellent results, even in the youngest and smallest of patients. Overall, survival from all cardiac surgeries in children with CHD is greater than 95%, and even for the most complex of CHD, it is approaching 90%. These children often require long-term follow-up from a pediatric cardiologist, but the vast majority lead healthy, active lives.

See also Birth Defects

National Associations

Canadian Adult Congenital Heart Network (CACH)
c/o BB&C, #100, 2233 Argentia Rd., Mississauga ON L5N 2K7
Tel: 905-826-6665; *Fax:* 905-826-4873
www.cachnet.org
Overview: A small national organization founded in 1991
Mission: To promote the interests of Canadians born with heart defects
Affiliation(s): Toronto Congenital Cardiac Centre for Adults; Adult Congenital Heart Council
Chief Officer(s):
Erwin Oechslin, President
Publications:
• The Beat
Type: Newsletter; *Editor:* Laura-Lee Walter
Profile: Stories, overviews, & clinic updates

Children's Heart Association for Support & Education (CHASE)
Tel: 416-410-2427
e-mail: kidheart@angelfire.com
www.angelfire.com/on/chase
Overview: A small national organization founded in 1984
Mission: Organization committed to promoting awarness about congenital heart disease; to provide encouragement to families affected by CHD; driven to become the leading provider of resoures to education & support those who seek an understanding of the disease.

International Associations

International Society of Hypertension (ISH)
ISH Secretariat, The Conference Collective Ltd., 8 Waldegrave Rd., Teddington TW11 8GT United Kingdom

Tel: +44 (0) 20 8977 7997
e-mail: secretariat@ish-world.com
www.ish-world.com
www.facebook.com/ISHNIN
twitter.com/ISHNIN

Overview: A medium-sized international charitable organization
Mission: To advance scientific knowledge in all aspects of research; To promote application of research to the prevention & management of heart disease & stroke in hypertension & related cardiovascular diseases
Affliation(s): Canadian Hypertension Society; World Hypertension League; American Society of Hypertension; Council for High Blood Pressure Research of the AHA; Cuban National Committee for the Study of Hypertension; Hypertension societies throughout Africa, The Middle East, Asia, Australasia, Europe, & South America
Chief Officer(s):
Neil Poulter, President
Alta Schutte, Vice-President
Maciej Tomaszewski, Secretary
Masatsugu Horiuchi, Treasurer
Publications:
• Hypertension News
Type: Newsletter; *Frequency:* Quarterly; *Price:* Free with International Society of Hypertension membership
• Journal of Hypertension
Type: Journal; *Frequency:* Monthly; *Price:* Free with International Society of Hypertension membership
Profile: Primary papers from experts, authoritative reviews, recent developments, special reports, & time-sensitive information

Cooley's Anemia

Cause
Cooley's anemia, or beta-Thalassemia major, is an inherited disorder characterized by abnormal production of hemoglobin in the red blood cells. There are three forms of beta-Thalassemia: beta-Thalassemia minor, in which the person has no real symptoms; beta-Thalassemia intermedia, in which there are varying symptoms ranging from mild to moderately severe; and beta-Thalassemia major, or Cooley's anemia, which is a severe, debilitating disease.

Symptoms
Beta-Thalassemia minor often goes undiagnosed because the only real symptom is mild anemia. The symptoms of people with beta-Thalassemia intermedia range from mild to moderate anemia to more serious health problems like spleen enlargement and bone deformities. Although a baby who has Cooley's anemia appears normal at birth, growth rates are impaired, and puberty may be significantly delayed or absent. Without therapy, there is a general decline. The skin becomes pale or jaundiced, facial bones become more prominent and pronounced, and the spleen becomes enlarged. In children with untreated Cooley's anemia, heart failure and infection are the leading causes of death.

Prevalence
Beta-Thalassemia is the most common form of thalassemia found in Canada. The disorder is typically found in people of Mediterranean, African or Asian descent. A child of parents who are both carriers of beta-Thalassemia minor has a 25 percent risk of having beta-Thalassemia major.

Treatment Options
Cooley's anemia is typically diagnosed by two blood tests: complete blood count (CBC) to identify anemia, and hemoglobin electrophoresis to show if an abnormal form of hemoglobin is present. Because there is no cure, genetic screening of at-risk populations is very important. Prenatal diagnosis from chorionic villus sampling (CVS) or amniocentesis can also be performed.

Treatments such as blood transfusions can reduce some symptoms of the disease. However, children with Cooley's anemia should receive as few transfusions as possible because of the danger of iron overload from the "heme" portion of hemoglobin. Iron overload can eventually cause diabetes, liver scarring and heart failure. Therefore, chelation, or binding, of the excess iron associated with multiple, repetitive transfusions is important, and is accomplished with deferoxamine (an iron-binding agent). Removal of the spleen may reduce transfusion requirements.

With medical advances, the quality of life and life expectancy for people with beta-Thalassemia major has improved and should continue to improve.

National Associations

Institute for Optimizing Health Outcomes
#600, 151 Bloor St. West, Toronto ON M5S 1S4

Tel: 416-969-7431
www.optimizinghealth.org

Previous Name: Anemia Institute for Research & Education
Overview: A small national organization
Mission: Promotes patient-centred programs, education, research & advocacy to improve care & support for persons at risk for, or living with, health conditions (including, but not limited to, anemia)
Affiliation(s): Ontario Patient Self-Management Network

Thalassemia Foundation of Canada
338 Falstaff Ave., Toronto ON M6L 3E7

Tel: 416-242-8425; *Fax:* 416-242-8425
e-mail: info@thalassemia.ca
www.thalassemia.ca

Overview: A small national charitable organization founded in 1982
Mission: To raise public awareness of Thalassemia; To raise money for Thalassemia research & treatment; To support families of children with Thalassemia
Chief Officer(s):
Helen Ziavras, President

Crohn's Disease

Crohn's disease is a chronic inflammation in the lining of the digestive tract, generally in the lower part of the small bowel or the upper end of the colon.

Cause
The cause of Crohn's disease is unknown, although it is believed that a combination of genetic and environmental factors are involved. The disease is more common in some families and racial groups, and is diagnosed more often in developed countries. Although not a proven cause, periods of emotional stress have been linked with flare-ups of the disease.

Symptoms
Common symptoms include diarrhea, weight loss, fever, abdominal pain, nausea and loss of appetite. People with Crohn's disease go through periods when their symptoms are active (flare-ups), and times when their symptoms are in remission. If the disease is extensive it may cause deficiencies of essential vitamins and other nutrients. Sometimes inflammation occurs outside the gut, attacking the eyes, joints or skin. Children with Crohn's disease may experience delays in growth and sexual development. Local complications include bowel perforation with formation of abscesses or fistulae which drain out to the skin. Established chronic Crohn's disease is characterized by lifelong exacerbations that can affect work, travel, relationships, family life and mental health. These patients carry an increased risk of cancer of the small bowel and colon/rectum.

Prevalence

Canada has one of the highest prevalence rates of Crohn's disease in the world. There are approximately 112,000 Canadians living with Crohn's disease; of that total, 3,300 are under the age of 20. The disease typically occurs before age 30, and more females than males are affected. People with Crohn's disease have a 47 percent greater risk of premature death compared to people without the disease.

Treatment Options

To diagnose Crohn's disease, the physician takes a complete medical history and performs a physical examination. Tests are also undertaken to rule out other conditions that might be causing the symptoms. These may include blood tests, stool samples and X-ray examinations of the upper intestine or bowel. Sometimes an endoscopy is performed; this is a procedure where a long, flexible video camera is used to look inside the rectum and large bowel.

Since there is no cure for Crohn's disease, the main goal of treatment is to bring symptoms under control and into remission, and then to maintain remission. Depending on the severity of the symptoms, drug treatment can range from simple anti-diarrheal medications to anti-inflammatory drugs, such as 5-ASA (5-Aminosalicylates), to corticosteroids, to immune modifiers, to biological therapies such as infliximab and adalimumab. Surgery may be necessary to treat complications such as abscesses, fistulae, or narrowing or scarring of the bowel, and is also considered when medications aren't working. In all cases, careful attention should be paid to the patient's nutritional status and psychological well-being.

People with Crohn's disease must deal with unpredictable symptoms and ongoing medication needs. However, most of the time, they can lead normal, active and productive lives.

See also Gastrointestinal Disorders and Celiac Disease

National Associations

Crohn's & Colitis Canada / Crohn's et Colitis Canada

#600, 60 St. Clair Ave. East, Toronto ON M4T 1N5

Tel: 416-920-5035; *Fax:* 416-929-0364
Toll-Free: 800-387-1479
e-mail: support@crohnsandcolitis.ca
www.crohnsandcolitis.ca
www.linkedin.com/company/crohn's-and-colitis-foundation-of-canada
www.facebook.com/crohnsandcolitis.ca
twitter.com/getgutsyCanada
www.youtube.com/user/getgutsy

Previous Name: Crohn's & Colitis Foundation of Canada; Canadian Foundation for Ileitis & Colitis
Overview: A medium-sized national charitable organization founded in 1974
Mission: To find a cure for Crohn's disease & ulcerative colitis; To raise funds for medical research; To educate individuals with inflammatory bowel disease, their families, health professionals, & the public
Chief Officer(s):
Mina Mawani, President & CEO
Tim Berry, Vice-President, Finance
Angie Specic, Vice-President, Marketing & Communications

Alberta/NWT Region
#3100, 246 Stewart Green SW, Calgary AB T3H 3C8
Toll-Free: 888-884-2232
Chief Officer(s):
Patricia Glenn, Regional Director
pglenn@crohnsandcolitis.ca

Atlantic Canada Region

PO Box 173, Lower Sackville NS B4C 2S9
Tel: 902-297-1649; *Fax:* 902-422-6552
Toll-Free: 800-265-1101
Chief Officer(s):
Edna Mendelson, Regional Director
emendelson@crohnsandcolitis.ca

British Columbia/Yukon Region
PO Box 47147, Stn. City Square, Vancouver BC V5Z 4L6
Toll-Free: 800-513-8202
e-mail: britishcolumbia@crohnsandcolitis.ca
Chief Officer(s):
Colleen Hauck, Regional Director
chauck@crohnsandcolitis.ca

Bureau du Québec
#420, 1980, rue Sherbrooke Ouest, Montréal QC H3H 1E8
Tél: 514-342-0666; *Téléc:* 514-342-1011
Ligne sans frais: 800-461-4683
Chief Officer(s):
Edna Mendelson, Directrice régionale
emendelson@crohnsandcolitis.ca

Manitoba/Saskatchewan/Nunavut Region
PO Box 20009, 3310 Portage Ave., Winnipeg MB R3K 2E5
Tel: 204-231-2115; *Fax:* 204-237-8214
Toll-Free: 866-856-8551
e-mail: centralcanada@ccfc.ca
Chief Officer(s):
Shair Wolsey, Regional Director
swolsey@crohnsandcolitis.ca

Ontario Region
#600, 60 St. Clair Ave. East, Toronto ON M4T 1N5
Tel: 613-806-7956; *Fax:* 416-929-0364
Toll-Free: 800-387-1479
Chief Officer(s):
Jacqueline Alvarez, Regional Director
jalvarez@crohnsandcolitis.ca

The 3C Foundation of Canada / Fondation Canadienne des 3c

#200, 1 Hines Rd., Kanata ON K2K 3C7
Tel: 613-237-6690
e-mail: info@3cfoundation.org
www.3cfoundation.org
www.facebook.com/GutTogether

Overview: A medium-sized national charitable organization founded in 1997
Chief Officer(s):
Michele Hepburn, President

Provincial Associations

BRITISH COLUMBIA

CHILD Foundation (CHILD)

U.B.C. Campus, #201, 2150 Western Parkway, Vancouver BC V6T 1V6
Tel: 604-736-0645; *Fax:* 604-228-0066
e-mail: info@child.ca
www.child.ca
www.facebook.com/pages/The-CHILD-Foundation/1414072748840373

Also Known As: Children with Intestinal & Liver Disorders
Overview: A small provincial charitable organization founded in 1995
Mission: To help an almost forgotten group of youngsters who suffer from incurable digestive disorders such as Crohn's Disease, Ulcerative Colitis & related IBD (intestinal & bowel disorders) & liver disorders; To find a cure through research for these disorders
Member of: Vancouver Board of Trade
Affiliation(s): CHILD Foundation USA
Chief Officer(s):
Grace M. McCarthy, Chair
Mary Parsons, President & CEO

International Associations

American Society of Colon & Rectal Surgeons
#550, 85 West Algonquin Rd., Arlington Heights IL 60005 USA
Tel: 847-290-9184; *Fax:* 847-427-9656
e-mail: ascrs@fascrs.org
www.fascrs.org
www.linkedin.com/company/the-american-society-of-colon-and-rectal-s
urg
www.facebook.com/fascrs
twitter.com/fascrs_updates
Overview: A medium-sized international organization
Mission: To advance the science & practice of the treatment of
patients with diseases & disorders that affect the colon, rectum, & anus
Chief Officer(s):
Patricia L. Roberts, MD, President
David A. Margolin, MD, Vice-President
Tracy L. Hull, MD, Secretary
Neil H. Hyman, MD, Treasurer
Publications:
• ASCRS [American Society of Colon & Rectal Surgeons] News
Type: Newsletter; *Frequency:* Semiannually
Profile: Information from the society of interest to its members

Cystic Fibrosis

Cystic fibrosis (CF) is an inherited disease of the exocrine (mucus-producing) glands, primarily affecting the gastrointestinal and respiratory tracts. The mucus that is secreted by persons with the disease is especially thick, thus blocking, rather than lubricating, passageways in the lungs and digestive tract.

Cause
The disease occurs when a child inherits a defective copy of the gene responsible for cystic fibrosis from both parents. One in 25 people in Canada is a carrier of the CF gene, however most of the time people do not realize that they are carriers until they have a child with cystic fibrosis.

Symptoms
In the newborn with CF, thick fecal material may cause partial obstruction of the intestine, which may then contort and rupture. Later in life, blockage of secretions from the pancreas results in frequent, foul-smelling, fatty stools, distention of the abdomen and slowed growth. Many people with cystic fibrosis have great difficulty digesting food and need a high calorie diet. Approximately 31 percent of women and 19 percent of men with CF are diagnosed as being underweight, and 85 percent of people with CF need to take pancreatic enzymes so that they can digest food. Damage to the lung occurs as thick mucus secretions plug airways. Fifty percent of all patients develop breathing problems marked by a chronic cough, wheezing and repeated lung infections. CF-related diabetes is a common complication of the disease, affecting more than one quarter of people with CF who are 35 years of age or older.

Prevalence
CF is the most common life-shortening genetic disease in the white population, occurring in 1 in 3,600 live births in Canada, but it occurs in people of all ethnic and racial backgrounds. Each week, one person in Canada dies of cystic fibrosis.

Treatment Options
In Canada, all provinces and territories with the exception of Quebec screen newborns for cystic fibrosis by pricking the baby's heel to take a small blood sample. A sweat test that measures the amount of salt in sweat can also be used to diagnose cystic fibrosis. If results of the sweat test are inconclusive, DNA testing can be done to identify mutations in the gene responsible for CF. About 60 percent of people with cystic fibrosis are diagnosed before they are one year old, and approximately 90 percent are di-

agnosed before the age of ten. Prenatal screening for CF can be done by chorionic villi sampling (CVS), a procedure where a small piece of the placenta is removed, or by amniocentesis.

Treatment of cystic fibrosis is individualized, and depends on the severity of the symptoms. A variety of drugs are used including mucolytics (to loosen mucus in the lungs), bronchodilators (to expand airways), steroids (to decrease lung inflammation) and antibiotics (to prevent lung infections). People with cystic fibrosis also use a variety of techniques to keep their airways clear so that it is less likely for thick mucus to build up in their lungs. Adequate nutrition, to maintain health and help fight infection, and psychosocial support, are also important. In some cases, people with CF undergo double lung transplantation. In Canada, this surgical procedure has doubled in the last decade.

The first CF gene therapy research began in 1993, and scientists have identified mutations in a CF regulator gene that cause cells to produce abnormally thick mucus. Gene therapy to replace the defective gene with a functional copy is currently under study. Genetic screening is now available, but it is not infallible.

The course of CF is usually determined by the degree to which the lungs are affected, and varies greatly from patient to patient. Although there is no cure for cystic fibrosis, advances in therapy have helped many survive well into adulthood. In Canada, around 50 percent of people with cystic fibrosis are expected to live into their forties, and even beyond.

National Associations

Cystic Fibrosis Canada / Fibrose Kystique Canada
National Office, #800, 2323 Yonge St., Toronto ON M4P 2C9
Tel: 416-485-9149; *Fax:* 416-485-0960
Toll-Free: 800-378-2233
e-mail: info@cysticfibrosis.ca
www.cysticfibrosis.ca
www.facebook.com/CysticFibrosisCanada
twitter.com/CFCanada
www.youtube.com/CysticFibrosisCanada
Previous Name: Canadian Cystic Fibrosis Foundation
Overview: A large national charitable organization founded in 1960
Mission: To help people with Cystic Fibrosis through funding research towards a cure or control; To support high quality care; To promote public awareness; To raise & allocate funds
Member of: Canadian Centre for Philanthropy; Canadian Coalition for Genetic Fairness
Affiliation(s): Cystic Fibrosis Worldwide
Chief Officer(s):
Norma Beauchamp, President & CEO
Publications:
• Breathe - Final Report [a publication of Cystic Fibrosis Canada]
Type: Report
• Canadian Patient Data Registry Report [a publication of Cystic Fibrosis Canada]
Type: Report
• Candid Facts [a publication of Cystic Fibrosis Canada]
Type: Newsletter; *Frequency:* Quarterly; *ISSN:* 0226-2347
Profile: News about events, research, & treatments for CFC members, donors, partners, & friends
• CFC [Cystic Fibrosis Canada] Annual Report
Type: Yearbook; *Frequency:* Annually
• Circle of Friends [a publication of Cystic Fibrosis Canada]
Frequency: Semiannually; *Editor:* Carole Varin; *Price:* Free for adults with CF & other interested persons
Profile: National newsletter for Canadian adults with cystic fibrosis
• Cystic Fibrosis Canada Grants & Awards Guide [a publication of Cystic Fibrosis Canada]
Type: Guide
• The Guide: Resources for the CF Community [a publication of Cystic Fibrosis Canada]
Type: Guide

• Insights [a publication of Cystic Fibrosis Canada]
Type: Newsletter
Profile: For the CF community, support groups, & other interested persons

Provincial Associations

QUÉBEC

Fibrose kystique Québec (FKQ) / Cystic Fibrosis Québec (CFQ)
#505, 625 av du Président-Kennedy, Montréal QC H3A 1K2
Tél: 514-877-6161; *Téléc:* 514-877-6116
Ligne sans frais: 800-363-7711
www.fibrosekystique.ca/quebec
www.facebook.com/FKQuebec
twitter.com/FKQuebec
plus.google.com/106908476349956061911
Nom précédent: Association québécoise de la fibrose kystique (AQFK)
Aperçu: *Dimension:* moyenne; *Envergure:* provinciale; Organisme sans but lucratif; fondée en 1981
Mission: Sensibiliser la population sur la fibrose kystique; amasser des fonds pour la recherche médicale; améliorer la qualité de vie des personnes atteintes de FK; découvrir un remède ou un moyen de contrôler la fibrose kystique
Membre de: Cystic Fibrosis Canada
Membre(s) du bureau directeur:
Neil Beaudette, Directeur général par intérim
nbeaudette@fkq.ca

Section Charlevoix-ouest
Baie-Saint-Paul QC
Membre(s) du bureau directeur:
Sylvian Lajoie, Président
lajoie300@hotmail.com

Section Côte-Nord
Baie-Comeau QC
Membre(s) du bureau directeur:
Sophie Girard, Présidente
pizzaroyale@globetrotter.net

Section Estrie
Sherbrooke QC
Membre(s) du bureau directeur:
Michael Roy, Président
michel.roy488@gmail.com

Section La Malbaie
La Malbaie QC
Membre(s) du bureau directeur:
Girard Dorothée, Présidente
dorothee.aurele@sympatico.ca

Section Mauricie/Centre-du-Québec
Trois-Rivières QC
Membre(s) du bureau directeur:
Lisette Tremblay, Présidente
sourislisette@hotmail.com

Section Montréal
Montréal QC
Membre(s) du bureau directeur:
Nicole Laberge, Présidente
labergenicole@gmail.com

Section Outaouais
Gatineau QC
Membre(s) du bureau directeur:
Mario Gagnon, Président
1mariogagnon@gmail.com

Section Québec
#227, 2750, ch Sainte-Foy, Québec QC G1V 1V6
Tél: 418-653-2086
Ligne sans frais: 877-653-2086
Courriel: info@fkquebec.com
www.fkquebec.com

Membre(s) du bureau directeur:

Terry Hall, Président
terry.hall@hotmail.com

Section Saguenay
Chicoutimi QC
Membre(s) du bureau directeur:
Andrée-Anne Guay, Présidente
andree-anne.guay@csjonquiere.qc.ca

Diabetes Mellitus

Diabetes mellitus is a condition in which the body lacks enough insulin to control its own blood glucose (sugar) level. Ordinarily, the pancreas releases enough of this hormone to let the body's cells absorb and metabolize glucose. In type 1 diabetes (formerly called juvenile-onset diabetes and affecting 10 percent of diabetic patients), the pancreas simply stops producing insulin. In type 2, commonly affecting overweight individuals older than 40, the pancreas might release normal, reduced or even elevated levels of insulin, but the body's cells are resistant to the insulin's action. In either case, blood glucose levels rise (hyperglycemia) until the kidney starts to dump sugar into the urine.

Cause
Type 1 appears to be caused by both genetic predisposition and exposure to viruses. Genetic factors are important in type 2 diabetes which runs strongly in families. It is much more common in obese people (especially when weight is carried around the middle), as well as among people of African, Hispanic, Asian, South Asian and Aboriginal descent. Other risk factors include having high blood pressure or high cholesterol, having gestational diabetes and having a diagnosis of schizophrenia, polycystic ovary syndrome or acanthosis nigricans (darkened patches of skin).

Symptoms
Symptoms of diabetes can include excessive thirst and urination, hunger, extreme fatigue, weakness, blurred vision, numbness or tingling in the hands or feet, slow-to-heal cuts and bruises, frequent infections and weight change (gain or loss). Some people with type 2 diabetes do not have any symptoms of the disease. In extreme cases, when there is either insufficient insulin or the body undergoes stress, or strenuous exercise, a person with untreated diabetes may lapse into a coma. Other long-term complications of untreated or improperly managed diabetes include an increased risk of coronary heart disease and other vascular diseases, such as stroke, vision loss and kidney failure.

Prevalence
In Canada, there are more than 2,000,000 people aged 12 and over who have been diagnosed with diabetes. However, the number of people with diabetes could actually be much higher since many people do not know that they have the disease. Due to rising obesity rates and an ever more sedentary lifestyle, the prevalence of type 2 diabetes is increasing in Canada, and the disease is now appearing in children. As people age, diabetes also becomes more prevalent, affecting one in six elderly men and one in seven elderly women. It is estimated that the annual cost of diabetes to the Canadian healthcare system will be $16.9 billion by 2020.

Treatment Options
A diagnosis of diabetes is confirmed by a blood test that measures blood sugar. A fasting plasma glucose test measures the blood glucose level after a person fasts for eight hours, whereas an oral glucose tolerance test measures the blood glucose level at intervals after a person fasts for eight hours and then has a very sweet drink.

Some individuals with type 2 diabetes can control their disease through diet, exercise and weight loss alone. Some will have to take oral medication that helps the pancreas make more insulin or makes the body more sensitive to insulin. Some type 2 diabetics, and all type 1 diabetics, need to take insulin. Research has shown that tight control of diabetes through frequent blood testing and proper adjustment of the dosage of insulin is most beneficial. Insulin is generally given in multiple injections throughout the day, with preparations varying by length of effectiveness. Closest control of glucose levels is achieved by giving insulin through a continuously connected insulin pump. Pancreas transplantation is considered only for patients who also need some other organ, generally a kidney.

Prevention of acute and long-term complications of diabetes requires careful management including maintaining the proper diet and exercise, blood glucose monitoring and medications. Thorough education of the patient and relevant family members is absolutely critical. People who commit to careful management of their diabetes can lead full, independent and active lives.

National Associations

Canadian Diabetes Association (CDA) / Association canadienne du diabète
#1400, 522 University Ave., Toronto ON M5G 2R5
Tel: 416-363-3373; *Fax:* 416-363-7465
Toll-Free: 800-226-8464
Other Communication: Donations: donation@diabetes.ca
e-mail: info@diabetes.ca
www.diabetes.ca
www.linkedin.com/company/canadian-diabetes-association
www.facebook.com/CanadianDiabetesAssociation
twitter.com/DiabetesAssoc
www.youtube.com/user/CDA1927
Overview: A large national charitable organization founded in 1953
Mission: To advance the welfare of Canadians with diabetes; to support research into the causes, complications, treatment, & cure of diabetes; To promote & strengthen services for people affected by diabetes & their families; To work with health professionals to improve standards in care & treatment of diabetes; To develop guidelines for diabetes education in Canada; To promote the rights of Canadians affected by diabetes in an effort to bring about positive change in the areas of public awareness, government policy, health policy issues, & employment
Member of: International Diabetes Federation
Affliation(s): Association du diabète du Québec
Chief Officer(s):
Jim Newton, Chair
Rick Blickstead, President & CEO
John Reidy, Chief Financial Officer
Russell Williams, Vice President, Government Relations & Public Policy
Janelle Robertson, Vice President, National Diabetes Trust, 709-747-4598
Jovita Sundaramoorthy, Vice President, Research & Education, 416-408-7090
Publications:
• Canadian Diabetes Clinical & Scientific Section (C&SS) Connect [a publication of the Canadian Diabetes Association]
Type: Newsletter; *Frequency:* q.; *Number of Pages:* 4; *Editor:* Sara J. Meltzer; *Price:* free with C&SS membership to CDA
• Canadian Journal of Diabetes (CJD) [a publication of the Canadian Diabetes Association]
Type: Journal; *Frequency:* bi-m.; *Editor:* David C.W. Lau
Profile: Peer-reviewed, interdisciplinary journal for diabetes healthcare professionals, including articles, news from theClinical & Scientific Section & the Diabetes Educators Section of the Canadian Diabetes Association, & resource reviews
• CDA [Canadian Diabetes Association] Annual Report
Frequency: a.
• The Diabetes Communicator [a publication of the Canadian Diabetes Association]
Type: Newsletter; *Number of Pages:* 16; *Editor:* Colleen Rand; *Price:* free with DES membership to CDA
Profile: Information on the Diabetes Educator Section (DES)

• Diabetes Current [a publication of the Canadian Diabetes Association]
Type: Newsletter; *Frequency:* monthly; *Price:* Free
Profile: Electronic newsletter containing information on association news, research, medical breakthroughs & more
• Diabetes Dialogue [a publication of the Canadian Diabetes Association]
Type: Magazine; *Frequency:* q.
Profile: Information about research, medical updates, nutrition, exercise, lifestyle management, & resources
• Diet & Nutrition: Beyond the Basics [a publication of the Canadian Diabetes Association]
Type: Book; *Price:* $29.95
Profile: Meal planning guidelines based on CDA's clinical practice guidelines & current scientific evidence.
• Pacesetter [a publication of the Canadian Diabetes Association]
Type: Newsletter; *Frequency:* Monthly; *Price:* Free
Profile: E-newsletter for Team Diabetes members, featuring information about upcoming marathon events, news, training & fundraising tips, & human intereststories

Calgary & District Branch
#204, 2323 - 32 Ave. NE, Calgary AB T2E 6Z3
Tel: 403-266-0620; *Fax:* 403-269-8927

Edmonton & District Branch
#104, 12220 Stony Plain Rd., Edmonton AB T5N 3Y4
Tel: 780-423-1232; *Fax:* 780-423-3322

GTA Regional Leadership Centre
#1400, 522 University Ave., Toronto ON M5G 2R5
Tel: 416-363-3373; *Fax:* 416-363-7465
Chief Officer(s):
Kerry Bruder, Regional Director

Manitoba & Nunavut Regional Leadership Centre
#200, 310 Broadway, Winnipeg MB R3C 0S6
Tel: 204-925-3800; *Fax:* 204-949-0266
Chief Officer(s):
Andrea Kwasnicki, Regional Director
andrea.kwasnicki@diabetes.ca

New Brunswick Region
730 McLeod Ave., Fredericton NB E3B 1V5
Tel: 506-452-9009; *Fax:* 506-455-4728
Toll-Free: 800-884-4232
Chief Officer(s):
Lisa Matte, Regional Director, Martimes
lisa.matte@diabetes.ca

Newfoundland & Labrador Regional Leadership Centre
#2007, 29-31 Pippy Pl., St. John's NL A1B 3X2
Tel: 709-754-0953; *Fax:* 709-754-0734
Chief Officer(s):
Felicia Chapman, Contact
felicia.chapman@diabetes.ca

North Saskatchewan Regional Leadership Centre
#104, 2301 Ave. C North, Saskatoon SK S7L 5Z5
Tel: 306-933-1238; *Fax:* 306-244-2012
Toll-Free: 800-996-4446

Nova Scotia Leadership Centre
#101, 137 Chain Lake Dr., Halifax NS B3S 1B3
Tel: 902-453-4232; *Fax:* 902-453-4440
Toll-Free: 800-326-7712
Chief Officer(s):
Lisa Matte, Regional Director, Maritimes
lisa.matte@diabetes.ca

Ottawa & District Branch
45 Montreal Rd., Ottawa ON K1L 6E8
Tel: 613-521-1902; *Fax:* 613-521-3667

Prince Edward Island Region
Sherwood Business Centre, 161 St. Peter's Rd., Charlottetown PE C1A 5P7
Tel: 902-894-3195; *Fax:* 902-368-1928
Chief Officer(s):
Terry Lewis, Manager, Community Engagement
terry.lewis@diabetes.ca

Canadian Pediatric Endocrine Group (CPEG) / Groupe canadien d'endocrinologie pédiatrique (GCEP)

c/o Robert Barnes, M.D., Montreal Children's Hospital, #316E, 2300, rue Tupper, Montréal QC H3H 1P3

Tel: 514-412-4315; *Fax:* 514-412-4264
www.cpeg-gcep.net

Overview: A small national organization
Mission: To promote the study of pediatric endocrinology
Chief Officer(s):
Robert Barnes, Secretary-Treasurer

Canadian Society of Endocrinology & Metabolism (CSEM) / Société canadienne d'endocrinologie et métabolisme (SCEM)

#1403, 222 Queen St., Ottawa ON K1P 5V9

Tel: 613-594-0005; *Fax:* 613-569-6574
e-mail: info@endo-metab.ca
www.endo-metab.ca

Overview: A small national organization founded in 1972
Mission: To advance the endocrinology & metabolism field in Canada
Chief Officer(s):
Connie Chik, President
Alice Cheng, Secretary-Treasurer

Juvenile Diabetes Research Foundation Canada (JDRF)

#800, 2550 Victoria Park Ave., Toronto ON M2J 5A9

Tel: 647-789-2000; *Fax:* 416-491-2111
Toll-Free: 877-287-3533
e-mail: general@jdrf.ca
www.jdrf.ca
www.facebook.com/JDRFCanada
twitter.com/JDRF_Canada
www.youtube.com/JDRFCanada

Previous Name: Diabetes Research Foundation
Overview: A medium-sized national charitable organization founded in 1974
Mission: To support research to find a cure for diabetes & its complications; To increase awareness of diabetes, particularly Juvenile (Type 1) diabetes
Chief Officer(s):
Matt Varey, Chair
Dave Prowten, President/CEO
David Kozloff, Secretary
Alex Davidson, Treasurer

Calgary
#204, 1608 - 17th Ave. SW, Calgary AB T2T 0E3

Tel: 403-255-7100; *Fax:* 403-253-6683
Toll-Free: 877-287-3533
e-mail: calgary@jdrf.ca

Edmonton
17321 - 107 Ave., Edmonton AB T5S 1E9

Tel: 780-428-0343; *Fax:* 780-428-0348
Toll-Free: 855-428-0343
e-mail: edmonton@jdrf.ca

Chief Officer(s):
Cheryl Vickers, Coordinator, Fundraising & Development
cvickers@jdrf.ca

Halifax Region
Bedford Place Mall, #2055, 1658 Bedford Hwy., Bedford NS B4A 2X9

Tel: 902-453-1009; *Fax:* 902-453-2528
Toll-Free: 888-439-5373

Chief Officer(s):
Marilyn Holm, Atlantic Regional Manager
mholm@jdrf.ca

Hamilton
#12, 442 Millen Rd., Stoney Creek ON L8E 6H2

Tel: 905-664-1432; *Fax:* 905-664-2408
Toll-Free: 866-602-6662

London
309 Commissioners Rd. West, #A, London ON N6J 1Y4

Tel: 519-641-7006; *Fax:* 519-641-7837
e-mail: london@jdrf.ca

Québec

#330, 615 Rene-Levesque Blvd. West, Montréal QC H3B 1P5

Tel: 514-744-5537; *Fax:* 514-744-0516
Toll-Free: 877-634-2238
e-mail: montreal@jdrf.ca
www.facebook.com/FRDJQuebec

Chief Officer(s):
Francine Bourdeau, Regional Director, 514-744-0516 Ext. 243
fbourdeau@jdrf.ca

Saskatoon
959 Patrick Way, Saskatoon SK S7M 0G1

Tel: 306-380-1588
e-mail: saskatoon@jdrf.ca

South Saskatchewan
PO Box 3924, Regina SK S4P 3S9

Tel: 306-789-8474
e-mail: regina@jdrf.ca
www.facebook.com/JdrfRegina

Toronto-York
#800, 2550 Victoria Park Ave., Toronto ON M2J 5A9

Tel: 647-789-2000; *Fax:* 416-491-2111
Toll-Free: 877-287-3533
www.facebook.com/jdrftoronto
twitter.com/jdrftoronto

Chief Officer(s):
Shannon Carkner, Regional Director
scarkner@jdrf.ca

Vancouver
Sperling Plaza II, #150, 6450 Roberts St., Burnaby BC V5G 4E1

Tel: 604-320-1937; *Fax:* 604-320-1938
e-mail: vancouver@jdrf.ca
twitter.com/jdrf_bc

Chief Officer(s):
Chris Lowe, Regional Manager
clowe@jdrf.ca

Waterloo
#103, 684 Belmont Ave. West, Kitchener ON N2M 1N6

Tel: 519-745-2426; *Fax:* 519-745-2626
e-mail: waterloo@jdrf.ca

Winnipeg
#1101, 191 Lombard Ave., Winnipeg MB R3B 0X1

Tel: 204-953-4477; *Fax:* 204-953-4470
e-mail: winnipeg@jdrf.ca

National Aboriginal Diabetes Association Inc. (NADA)

#B1, 90 Garry St, Winnipeg MB R3C 4H1

Tel: 204-927-1220; *Fax:* 204-927-1222
Toll-Free: 877-232-6232
e-mail: diabetes@nada.ca
www.nada.ca
www.facebook.com/nadasugarfree
twitter.com/nadasugarfree

Overview: A small national organization founded in 1995
Mission: To be the driving force in addressing diabetes & Aboriginal people as a priority health issue by working together with people, Aboriginal communities & organizations in the culturally respectful manner in promoting healthy lifestyles among Aboriginal people today & for future generations
Chief Officer(s):
Anita Ducharme, Executive Director
Alisher Kabildjanov, Program Assistant

Provincial Associations

ALBERTA

Alberta Diabetes Foundation
#1-020, Li Ka Shing Centre for Health Research Innovation, 8602 112 St., Edmonton AB T6G 2E1
Tel: 780-492-6537; *Fax:* 780-492-0979
Toll-Free: 800-563-2450
e-mail: info@abdiabetes.com
www.albertadiabetesfoundation.com
www.linkedin.com/company/alberta-diabetes-foundation
www.facebook.com/AlbertaDiabetesFoundation
twitter.com/adfdiabetes
Overview: A medium-sized provincial charitable organization founded in 1988
Mission: To support research on the prevention & treatment of diabetes; To search for a cure for diabetes
Affiliation(s): Funds pilot projects; studentships; & post-doctoral fellowships.
Chief Officer(s):
Lynn Hamilton, Chair
Gillian Clarke, Vice-Chair
Carla Woodward, Treasurer
Brad Fournier, Executive Director
Hardik Patel, Manager, Finance & Human Resources
Twyla McGann, Coordinator, Communications & Events
Publications:
• inFocus: Working towards a Cure
Type: Newsletter
Profile: Articles about diabetics, research, & giving options, plus recipes & upcoming events

QUÉBEC

Association des médecins endocrinologues du Québec
CP 216, Succ. Desjardins, #3000, 2, Complexe Desjardins, Montréal QC H5B 1G8
Tél: 514-350-5135; *Téléc:* 514-350-5049
Ligne sans frais: 800-561-0703
Courriel: ameq@fmsq.org
www.ameq.qc.ca
Aperçu: *Dimension:* petite; *Envergure:* provinciale surveillé par Fédération des médecins spécialistes du Québec
Mission: L'Association est un porte-parole des endocrinologues; elle favorise les intérêts scientifiques de ses membres et organise plusieurs réunions afin de permettre une formation médicale continue des endocrinologues

Diabète Québec (ADQ) / Diabetes Quebec
#300, 8550, boul Pie-IX, Montréal QC H1Z 4G2
Tél: 514-259-3422; *Téléc:* 514-259-9286
Ligne sans frais: 800-361-3504
Courriel: info@diabete.qc.ca
www.diabete.qc.ca
www.facebook.com/diabetequebec
twitter.com/DiabeteQuebec
Également appelé: Association Diabète Québec
Nom précédent: Association du Diabète du Québec
Aperçu: *Dimension:* moyenne; *Envergure:* provinciale; fondée en 1954
Mission: Regrouper les diabétiques et favoriser l'entraide; les renseigner sur les façons de faire face à la maladie; informer le grand public et le sensibiliser à la condition de personnes souffrant du diabète; ouvrir de nouvelles voies dans le domaine de la recherche pour en venir à triompher du diabète
Membre de: Fédération Internationale du Diabète
Membre(s) du bureau directeur:
Sylvie Lauzon, Présidente
direction@diabete.qc.ca
Marcelle Paquette, Directeur, Finances et administration
paquette@diabete.qc.ca
Publications:
• Plein Soleil
Type: Magazine; *Editor:* Louise Bouchard
Profile: Traite des sujets en relation avec le diabète : alimentation, traitement, activité physique, recherche, vivre avec le diabète, etc.

Fondation pour enfants diabétiques
#100, 306, rue Saint-Zotique est, Montréal QC H2S 1L6
Tél: 514-731-9683; *Téléc:* 514-731-2683
Ligne sans frais: 800-731-9683
Courriel: info@diabete-children.ca
www.diabete-children.ca
www.linkedin.com/company/la-fondation-pour-enfants-diabétiques
www.facebook.com/DiabeteEnfants
twitter.com/DiabeteEnfants
Aperçu: *Dimension:* moyenne; *Envergure:* provinciale; fondée en 1974
Mission: Subvenir au développement de camp spécialisé pour enfants et adolescents diabétiques; soutenir des projets d'enseignement et d'information sur les soins en diabète pédiatrique; faire la promotion de soins de santé optimaux pour les enfants diabétiques
Membre(s) du bureau directeur:
Danielle Brien, Directrice générale
dbrien@diabete-enfants.ca

International Associations

International Society for Pediatric & Adolescent Diabetes (ISPAD)
c/o KIT Group GmbH, Kurfürstendamm 71, Berlin 10709 Germany
Tel: +49 30 24603210; *Fax:* +49 30 24603200
e-mail: secretariat@ispad.org
www.ispad.org
Overview: A medium-sized international organization
Mission: To promote research, science, education, & advocacy in childhood & adolescent diabetes
Chief Officer(s):
Joseph Wolfsdorf, President
David M. Maahs, Secretary General
Andrea Scaramuzza, Treasurer
Publications:
• International Society for Pediatric & Adolescent Diabetes Membership Directory
Type: Directory
Profile: A listing of society members with contact information
• ISPAD [International Society for Pediatric & Adolescent Diabetes] Newsletter
Type: Newsletter
Profile: Society activities, including meeting reviews, educational opportunities, forthcoming events
• Pediatric Diabetes
Type: Journal; *Price:* Free with International Society for Pediatric & Adolescent Diabetes memberships

National Publications

Diabetes Dialogue
#1400, 522 University Ave., Toronto, ON M5G 2R5
Tel: 416-363-3373 *Toll-Free:* 800-226-8464
Circulation: 45,510 *Frequency:* Quarterly
Official magazine of the Canadian Diabetes Association.
Denise Barnard, Editor

National Libraries

Canadian Agency for Drugs & Technologies in Health (CADTH)/ Agence canadienne des mèdicaments et des technologies de la santé
#600, 865 Carling Ave., Ottawa, ON K1S 5S8
Tel: 613-226-2553; *Fax:* 613-226-5392
Toll-Free: 866-988-1444
www.cadth.ca
Social Media: www.youtube.com/user/CADTHACMTS;
twitter.com/cadth_acmts; www.linkedin.com/company/cadth
Collection: Reports; reviews; implementation tools
Brian O'Rourke, President & CEO

Canadian Diabetes Association
#360, 1385 West 8th Ave., Vancouver, BC V6H 3V9
Tel: 604-732-1331; *Toll-Free:* 800-665-6526
www.diabetes.ca

Collection: Chinese resource centre, with educational books, videotapes, pamphlets related to diabetes & its management; reference collection of diabetes consumer magazines & medical research journals related to diabetes & its management

Provincial Libraries

Information & Support Centre (Winnipeg)
#401, 1 Wesley Ave., Winnipeg, MB R3C 4C6
Tel: 204-925-3800; *Fax:* 204-949-0266
mbinfo@diabetes.ca
www.diabetes.ca

Dissociative Disorders

Dissociative disorders are a cluster of mental disorders, characterized by a profound change in consciousness or a disruption in continuity of consciousness. People with a dissociative disorder may abruptly take on different personalities, or undergo long periods in which they do not remember anything that happened; in some cases, individuals may embark on lengthy international travels, returning home with no recollection of where they have been or why they had gone.

Dissociative disorders are uncommon, mysterious and somewhat controversial; reports of dissociative disorders have grown more frequent in recent years and a degree of debate surrounds the validity of these reports. Some professionals say the disorders are far more rare than is reported, and that these individuals are highly vulnerable to the suggestions of others.

Cause
Dissociative disorders are believed to be related in many cases to severe trauma, although the historical validity of these cases is often difficult to determine. People who suffered from sexual, physical or emotional abuse during childhood are more likely to develop dissociative disorders. There are four main types of dissociative disorders: dissociative amnesia, dissociative fugue, dissociative identity disorder and depersonalization disorder.

Dissociative Amnesia

Dissociative amnesia is characterized by memory loss that is not caused by a health condition, and is more serious than regular forgetfulness. People with this disorder have no memory of traumatic events which have occurred during their lives.

Symptoms
Patients with dissociative amnesia may feel confused, emotionally distressed and depressed. They often experience impairment in work or interpersonal relationships, and they may practise self-mutilation or have aggressive and suicidal impulses. They may also have symptoms typical of a mood or personality disorder. Individuals with dissociative amnesia often report severe physical or sexual abuse in childhood. Controversy surrounds the accuracy of these reports, in part because of the unreliability of some childhood memories.

Prevalence
The incidence of dissociative amnesia in the general population in Canada is unknown. In fact, many Canadian psychiatrists do not think that there is strong evidence for the scientific validity of a diagnosis of dissociative amnesia.

Treatment Options
To diagnose dissociative amnesia, the physician usually takes a medical history, orders blood tests and urine tests and performs a physical exam of the patient to rule out other medical conditions that may be causing memory loss. Some physicians may use the following criteria outlined in the Diagnostic and Statistical Manual of Mental Disorders to confirm a diagnosis of dissociative amne-

sia: one or more episodes of inability to recall important personal information, usually of a traumatic or stressful nature, that is too extensive to be explained by ordinary forgetfulness; the disturbance does not occur exclusively during the course of any other dissociative disorder and is not due to the direct physiological effects of a substance abuse or general medical condition; the symptoms cause clinically significant distress or impairment in social, occupational or other important areas of functioning.

Treatment for dissociative amnesia may first include supportive psychotherapy or hypnosis to help the patient recover memories. A second stage of psychotherapy may then be initiated to help the patient deal with the traumatic memories that have been uncovered.

Dissociative Fugue

A person experiencing an episode of dissociative fugue will suddenly leave home for a new location, often taking on a new identity in the process, and then have no memory of what has happened when the fugue is over.

Symptoms
The symptoms of dissociative fugue usually only last for a few hours, but on rare occasions, they may continue for a number of months. People experiencing dissociative fugue are commonly confused or distressed when they cannot remember recent events or recognize that their sense of identity is missing.

Prevalence
For dissociative fugue, a prevalence rate of 0.2 percent in the general population has been reported.

Treatment Options
The following criteria outlined in the Diagnostic and Statistical Manual of Mental Disorders are usually used to confirm a diagnosis of dissociative fugue: a sudden, unexpected travel away from home or work, with inability to recall one's past; confusion about personal identity or assumption of a new identity; the disturbance does not occur exclusively during the course of any other dissociative disorder and is not due to the direct physiological effects of a substance or a general medical condition; the symptoms cause clinically significant distress or impairment in social, occupational or other important areas of functioning.

The principal treatment for dissociative fugue is often psychotherapy. Patients learn to recognize traumatic events from the past that may have caused the disorder, and are shown strategies that they can use to cope with the disturbing emotions that they are experiencing.

Dissociative Identity Disorder

Dissociative identity disorder (formerly known as multiple personality disorder) is a condition which causes people to switch to a different identity during periods of stress. People with this disorder may sense that they live with one or more personalities in their heads, each with his or her own unique qualities.

Symptoms
The main symptoms of dissociative identity disorder are amnesia, depersonalization (a feeling of being detached from one's body), derealization (a perception that one's external environment and feelings are not real) and identity disturbances. Individuals with dissociative identity disorder often report severe physical or sexual abuse in childhood and may also have symptoms typical of post-traumatic stress disorder, as well as mood, substance abuse, sexual, eating or sleep disorders.

Prevalence

Dissociative identity disorder is diagnosed three to nine times more frequently in females than in males. It should be noted that many Canadian psychiatrists do not think that there is strong evidence for the scientific validity of a diagnosis of dissociative identity disorder.

Treatment Options

Because many of the symptoms of dissociative identity disorder are similar to those of other conditions such as schizophrenia, borderline personality disorder, psychosomatic disorder and panic disorder, misdiagnosis is common. These mental health problems, along with other medical conditions that may cause overlapping symptoms must first be ruled out. To confirm a diagnosis of dissociative identity disorder, some physicians may refer to the following criteria outlined in the Diagnostic and Statistical Manual of Mental Disorders: the presence of two or more distinct identities or personality states that take control of the person's behaviour, inability to recall important personal information, and the disturbance is not due to the direct physiological effects of a substance or a general medical condition.

Treatment for dissociative identity disorder is often lengthy (five to seven years, in some cases) and may include hypnosis, psychotherapy, family therapy and group therapy. Medications such as antidepressants and anti-anxiety agents may also be prescribed.

Depersonalization Disorder

Depersonalization disorder is characterized by a feeling of being outside one's own body. Symptoms of depersonalization caused by sleep deprivation, stressful situations and certain anesthetics are a common occurrence in the general population. However, if symptoms interfere with everyday life and result in emotional distress, depersonalization disorder may be diagnosed.

Symptoms

People with depersonalization disorder may feel as if they are watching themselves from afar, or as if they are on automatic pilot. Commonly, they experience a sense of emotional detachment. Symptoms of depersonalization disorder may be short-term, or may wax and wane over a period of many years.

Prevalence

Women are twice as likely as men to suffer from depersonalization disorder.

Treatment Options

To rule out other medical conditions that might be causing the symptoms, a physician usually takes a medical history, performs a physical examination of the patient and orders blood and urine tests. To confirm a diagnosis of depersonalization disorder, the following criteria outlined in the Diagnostic and Statistical Manual of Mental Disorders must be met: persistent or recurrent experiences of feeling detached from one's body and mental processes; during the depersonalization experience, reality testing remains intact; the depersonalization causes clinically significant distress or impairment in social, occupational or other important areas of functioning; the depersonalization does not occur during the course of another dissociative disorder or as a direct physiological effect of a substance or general medical condition.

Sometimes, depersonalization disorder resolves on its own without therapy. In other cases, hypnosis, psychodynamic psychotherapy (in which the focus is on unconscious thoughts and how they are revealed in a patient's behaviour) or cognitive behavioural therapy (in which the patient learns to replace negative beliefs and behaviours with positive ones) may be used to treat the symptoms. Medications including benzodiazepine tranquilizers, tricyclic antidepressants and selective serotonin reuptake inhibitors (SSRIs) may also be prescribed.

With early diagnosis and appropriate therapy, the prognosis for recovery is good for most people with dissociative disorders.

National Associations

Canadian Mental Health Association (CMHA) / Association canadienne pour la santé mentale (ACSM)
#1110, 151 Slater St., Ottawa ON K1P 5H3

Tel: 613-745-7750
e-mail: info@cmha.ca
www.cmha.ca
www.facebook.com/CANMentalHealth
twitter.com/CMHA_NTL
www.youtube.com/user/cmhanational

Overview: A large national charitable organization founded in 1918
Mission: To promote mental health as well as support the resilience & recovery of people experiencing mental illness, through advocacy, education, research & service
Affliation(s): Canadian Alliance on Mental Illness & Mental Health; Canadian Health Network
Chief Officer(s):
Patrick Smith, National Chief Executive Officer
Cal Crocker, Chair
Sarika Gundu, National Director, Workplace Mental Health Program
Fardous Hosseiny, National Director, Policy
Publications:
• CMHA [Canadian Mental Health Association] Annual Report
Type: Report; *Frequency:* a.
Profile: Details of CMHA initiatives & achievements

Alberta Division
Capital Place, #320, 9707 - 110 St. NW, Edmonton AB T5K 2L9
Tel: 780-482-6576; Fax: 780-482-6348
e-mail: alberta@cmha.ab.ca
alberta.cmha.ca

William (Bill) Bone, Chair

British Columbia Division
#1200, 1111 Melville St., Vancouver BC V6E 3V6
Tel: 604-688-3234; Fax: 604-688-3236
Toll-Free: 800-555-8222
e-mail: info@cmha.bc.ca
www.cmha.bc.ca
www.facebook.com/CMHABCDIVISION
twitter.com/cmhabc
www.youtube.com/cmhabc

Chief Officer(s):
Beverly Gutray, Chief Executive Officer
bev.gutray@cmha.bc.ca

Division du Québec
#326, 911, rue Jean-Talon Est, Montréal QC H2R 1V5
Tél: 514-849-3291; Téléc: 514-849-8372
Courriel: info@acsm.qc.ca
www.acsm.qc.ca
www.facebook.com/189002251132456
twitter.com/ACSMDivisionQc
www.youtube.com/user/ACSMQC

Chief Officer(s):
Renée Ouimet, Directrice
reneeouimet@acsm.qc.ca

Manitoba Division
930 Portage Ave., Winnipeg MB R3G 0P8
Tel: 204-982-6100; Fax: 204-982-6128
e-mail: office@cmhawpg.mb.ca
winnipeg.cmha.ca
www.facebook.com/cmha.manitoba
twitter.com/MbDivisionCMHA
www.youtube.com/user/CMHAWpg

Chief Officer(s):
Stephanie Skakun, Acting Executive Director

New Brunswick Division

#202, 403 Regent St., Fredericton NB E3B 3X6
Tel: 506-455-5231; *Fax:* 506-459-3878
cmhanb.ca
www.facebook.com/CMHANB

Chief Officer(s):
Christa Baldwin, Executive Director
christa.baldwin@cmhanb.ca

Newfoundland & Labrador Division
70 The Boulevard, 1st Fl., St. John's NL A1A 1K2
Tel: 709-753-8550; *Fax:* 709-753-8537
Toll-Free: 877-753-8550
e-mail: office@cmhanl.ca
www.cmhanl.ca
www.facebook.com/247087668665555
twitter.com/CMHANL
www.youtube.com/user/cmhanational

Chief Officer(s):
George Skinner, Executive Director

Nova Scotia Division
63 King St., Dartmouth NS B2Y 2R7
Tel: 902-466-6600; *Fax:* 902-466-3300
Toll-Free: 877-466-6606
e-mail: cmhans@bellaliant.com
novascotia.cmha.ca
www.facebook.com/cmhansdivision
twitter.com/cmhansdivision
pinterest.com/cmhanovascotia

Chief Officer(s):
Gail Gardiner, Executive Director

Ontario Division
#2301, 180 Dundas St. West, Toronto ON M5G 1Z8
Tel: 416-977-5580; *Fax:* 416-977-2813
Toll-Free: 800-875-6213
e-mail: info@ontario.cmha.ca
ontario.cmha.ca
www.facebook.com/cmha.ontario
twitter.com/CMHAOntario
www.youtube.com/cmhaontario

Chief Officer(s):
Camille Quenneville, CEO
cquenneville@ontario.cmha.ca

Prince Edward Island Division
PO Box 785, 178 Fitzroy St., Charlottetown PE C1A 7L9
Tel: 902-566-3034; *Fax:* 902-566-4643
e-mail: division@cmha.pe.ca
pei.cmha.ca
www.facebook.com/CMHAPEIDivision

Chief Officer(s):
Reid Burke, Executive Director

Saskatchewan Division
2702 - 12th Ave., Regina SK S4T 1J2
Tel: 306-525-5601; *Fax:* 306-569-3788
Toll-Free: 800-461-5483
e-mail: contactus@cmhask.com
www.cmhask.com
www.facebook.com/255440253328

Chief Officer(s):
Dave Nelson, Executive Director
daven@cmhask.com

Yukon Division
6 Bates Cres., Whitehorse YT Y1A 4T8
Tel: 867-668-7144
e-mail: cmha.ca@gmail.com
twitter.com/CMHAYukon

Chief Officer(s):
Dudley Morgan, Executive Director

Centre for Addiction & Mental Health (CAMH) / Centre de toxicomanie et de santé mentale
250 College St., Toronto ON M5T 1R8
Tel: 416-535-8501
Toll-Free: 800-463-6273
e-mail: info@camh.net
www.camh.net
www.linkedin.com/company/camh
www.facebook.com/CentreforAddictionandMentalHealth
twitter.com/CAMHnews
www.youtube.com/camhtv

Previous Name: Addiction Research Foundation
Overview: A large provincial charitable organization founded in 1998
Mission: To provide treatment for & research into substance abuse & mental health issues. Clinical & research sites in Toronto & across Ontario
Affliation(s): University of Toronto; University of Western Ontario; WHO
Chief Officer(s):
Catherine Zahn, President/CEO

Down Syndrome

Cause
Down syndrome is a genetic condition caused by an extra chromosome. Instead of having the usual 46 chromosomes, people with Down syndrome have 47. In most cases, people with Down syndrome have three copies of chromosome 21 instead of two (trisomy 21). This extra genetic material can result in delays in physical growth and intellectual development.

Symptoms
Down syndrome is associated with a wide variety of clinical signs, although most individuals do not possess all of them. Common findings include decreased muscle tone, slanting eyes with folds of skin in the inside corners, white spots appearing in the irises of the eyes, and single creases across the palms of one or both hands. Physically, children with Down syndrome can have broad feet with short toes, short ears and necks, small heads and small oral cavities. Mild to moderate intellectual disabilities are seen in most children with Down syndrome. Hearing and speech abilities may also be hampered, however, many children with Down syndrome can reach high levels of achievement. Congenital heart disease is found in nearly half of children with Down syndrome, and vision problems, hypothyroidism and respiratory problems are also fairly common. There is an increased susceptibility to acute leukemia, and problems such as dementia may increase with age.

Prevalence
There are approximately 45,000 Canadians with Down syndrome. The overall incidence is about 1 in every 800 births in Canada, but there is a marked variability depending on maternal age. In mothers under the age of 30, the incidence is less than 1 in 1000 live births; for mothers over 40, it rises to at least 1 in 100 and increases even further with advancing age.

Treatment Options
Prenatal diagnosis of Down syndrome is available to pregnant women. Screening tests that assess the risk of having a baby with Down syndrome include ultrasound and the triple screen blood test. Diagnostic tests that can tell whether a baby has Down syndrome include amniocentesis, chorionic villus sampling (CVS) and percutaneous umbilical blood sampling.

At birth, a diagnosis of Down syndrome is usually based on physical characteristics that are common in babies with Down syndrome. A karyotype (chromosome study) is used to confirm the diagnosis.

It is essential that parents enroll a child with Down syndrome in an infant development program. These early intervention programs advise parents on how to help a child with Down syndrome develop language, cognitive, social and motor skills. Speech, physical and developmental therapies are often advised. Inclusive education is believed to be the best learning environment for students with Down syndrome.

Today, people with Down syndrome have improved opportunities for inclusion in their schools, workplaces and communities. With proper health care, they can lead healthy lives, and many live into their fifties and sixties.

National Associations

Canadian Down Syndrome Society (CDSS) / Société canadienne du syndrome de Down
#103, 2003 - 14 St. NW, Calgary AB T2M 3N4
Tel: 403-270-8500; *Fax:* 403-270-8291
Toll-Free: 800-883-5608
www.cdss.ca
www.facebook.com/cdndownsyndrome
twitter.com/CdnDownSyndrome
www.youtube.com/user/CdnDownSyndrome
Overview: A medium-sized national charitable organization founded in 1987
Mission: To ensure equitable opportunities for all Canadians with Down Syndrome
Chief Officer(s):
Laura LaChance, Chair
Kirk Crowther, Executive Director
Lynette Gowie, Office Manager
Kaitlyn Pecson, Manager, Communications
Jenny Morrow, Manager, Development
Corrine Grieve, Manager, Resource
Shannon Thomas, Coordinator, Communications & Membership
Publications:
• Canadian Down Syndrome Society Newsletter
Type: Newsletter; *Frequency:* Quarterly
• CDSS [Canadian Down Syndrome Society] Calendar
Frequency: Annually
• CDSS [Canadian Down Syndrome Society] Information Series
Profile: Topics include Teaching Children with Down Syndrome, Toilet Training Your Child with Down Syndrome, Stubborn Behaviour, Registered Educational Savings Plan, Taxation,Wills & Trusts, Obstructive Sleep Apnea Syndrome, & Stop Running by Building Skills: Behavioural Approach

Down Syndrome Research Foundation (DSRF)
1409 Sperling Ave., Burnaby BC V5B 4J8
Tel: 604-444-3773; *Fax:* 604-431-9248
e-mail: info@dsrf.org
www.dsrf.org
www.linkedin.com/company/down-syndrome-research-foundation
www.facebook.com/DSRFCanada
twitter.com/DSRFcanada
www.instagram.com/dsrfcanada
Overview: A small national charitable organization founded in 1995
Mission: To maximize the ability of people with Down Syndrome to lead independent lives & to participate in the community in which they live; To provide educational programs & services that are guided by foundational research; To collaborate with researchers, professionals & families to empower people with Down Syndrome
Member of: Down Syndrome International
Chief Officer(s):
Geoff Griffiths, Chair
Dawn McKenna, Executive Director
 dawn@dsrf.org
Publications:
• Hand in Hand [a publication of the Down Syndrome Research Foundation]
Type: Newsletter; *Frequency:* Quarterly; *Editor:* Glen Hoos

Provincial Associations

MANITOBA

Manitoba Down Syndrome Society (MDSS)
#204, 825 Sherbrook St., Winnipeg MB R3A 1M5
Tel: 204-992-2731; *Fax:* 204-975-3027
www.manitobadownsyndromesociety.com
www.facebook.com/ManitobaDownSyndromeSociety
twitter.com/manitobadss
Overview: A small provincial charitable organization founded in 1991
Mission: To provide support, information & opportunities for individuals with Down Syndrome, parents, professionals and other interested persons; To seek resolutions to issues of concern
Affliation(s): Canadian Down Syndrome Society
Chief Officer(s):
Lorraine Baydack, President
Val Surbey, Vice-President

ONTARIO

Down Syndrome Association of Ontario (DSAO)
300 Sunset Blvd., Peterborough ON K9H 5L3
Tel: 905-439-6644
Toll-Free: 855-921-3726
www.dsao.ca
www.facebook.com/DSAOntario
twitter.com/DSAOntario
Overview: A small provincial charitable organization
Mission: To ensure equality for people with Down Syndrome

Local Associations

ONTARIO

Down Syndrome Association of Toronto (DSAT)
PO Box 40039, Stn. Liberty Village, Toronto ON M5V 0K7
Tel: 416-966-0990
e-mail: info@dsat.ca
www.dsat.ca
www.facebook.com/dsatoronto
twitter.com/DSAToronto
www.youtube.com/user/DSAToronto
Overview: A small local charitable organization founded in 1987
Mission: To pursue civil & human rights, equality of opportunity & the full integration of persons with Down syndrome; To ensure that all students with Down syndrome are welcomed in regular classes in neighbourhood schools with appropriate support services
Chief Officer(s):
Bhaskar Thiagarajan, President
Publications:
• Down Syndrome Association of Toronto Newsletter
Type: Newsletter

Windsor-Essex Down Syndrome Parent Association
#206, 5060 Tecumseh Rd. East, Windsor ON N8T 1C1
Tel: 519-973-6486
www.upaboutdown.org
www.facebook.com/upaboutdown
Also Known As: Up About Down
Overview: A small local charitable organization founded in 1990
Mission: To enhance the lives of individuals with Down syndrome & their families; To provide positive & accurate information through advocacy & education thereby raising awareness throughout the community
Chief Officer(s):
Suzanne Cyr, President

Local Schools

ALBERTA

Calgary: **Calgary Quest School**
3405 Spruce Dr. SW, Calgary, AB T3C 0A5
Tel: 403-253-0003; *Fax:* 403-253-0025
info@calgaryquestschool.com
www.calgaryquestschool.com

Grades: Pre.-12 *Enrollment:* 160 *Note:* Calgary Quest School offers a program for children with special challenges.
Angela Rooke, Executive Director

Calgary: Third Academy
North Campus
510 - 77th Ave. SE, Calgary, AB T2H 1C3
Tel: 403-288-5335; *Fax:* 403-288-5804
info@thirdacademy.com
www.thirdacademy.com
Grades: 1-12 *Note:* The Third Academy offers an Individualized Program Plan that addresses the needs of students with learning disorders.
Sunil Mattu, LLB (Hons) Law, BEd, Executive Director
S. Lal Mattu, Founder & Ambassador at Large
Rehana Mattu, Principal
Bruce Freeman, Communications Officer & Manager, Transportation
Sabu Alexander, Chief Accountant

Campuses
South Campus
P.O. Box 4
Site 22, RR#8, Calgary, AB T2J 2T9
Tel: 403-201-6335; *Fax:* 403-201-2036
Joe Smith, Principal

Edmonton: Elves Child Development Centre
Elves Special Needs Society
10825 - 142 St., Edmonton, AB T5N 3Y7
Tel: 780-454-5310; *Fax:* 780-454-5889
inquiries@elves-society.com
www.elves-society.com
Grades: Pre.-12 *Note:* The Elves Special Needs Society offers programs for pre-school & older children, youth & adults with disabilities & special needs, as well as outreach to students unable to attend school for extended periods of time.
Barb Tymchak Olafson, Executive Director

MANITOBA

Winnipeg: St. Amant School
440 River Rd., Winnipeg, MB R2M 3Z9, Canada
Tel: 204-256-4301; *Fax:* 204-257-4349
inquiries@stamant.ca
www.stamant.mb.ca
www.facebook.com/pages/St-Amant/123434846345
twitter.com/StAmantMB
www.linkedin.com/company/st-amant
www.youtube.com/user/StAmantMB
Grades: K.-12
John Leggat, President & CEO

ONTARIO

Toronto: Bloorview School Authority
150 Kilgour Rd., Toronto, ON M4G 1R8, Canada
Tel: 416-424-3831; *Fax:* 416-425-2981
school@hollandbloorview.ca
www.bloorviewschool.ca
www.facebook.com/HBKRH
twitter.com/#!/bloorviewpr
www.linkedin.com/company/holland-bloorview
www.youtube.com/user/PRBloorview
Note: Bloorview School Authority provides school programs to children & youth with special needs.
Rachee Allen, Chair

Waterloo: KidsAbility School Authority Board
500 Hallmark Dr., Waterloo, ON N2K 3P5, Canada
Tel: 519-886-8886; *Fax:* 519-886-7291
Toll-Free: 1-888-372-2259
info@kidsability.ca
www.kidsability.ca/en/school
www.facebook.com/184568644892738
twitter.com/kidsability
www.youtube.com/user/KidsAbility1957#p/a
Number of Schools: 5 *Note:* KidsAbility School Authority Board serves children with a wide range of special needs. Programs & services

include a kindergarten program, individual education plans, composite classes, communication classes, & language classes.
Deirdre Large, Chair - Advisory Council
Linda Rogers, Principal & Secretary to the Board, 519-886-8886, ext. 1225
lrogers@kidsability.ca
Joanne Cotter, Executive Assistant, 519-886-8886, ext. 1227
jcotter@kidsability.ca
Cynthia Davis, Chair - Authority Board
schoolauthoritychair@kidsability.ca

Windsor: John McGivney Children's Centre School Authority
John McGivney Children's Centre
3945 Matchette Rd., Windsor, ON N9C 4C2, Canada
Tel: 519-282-7281; *Fax:* 519-252-5873
school@jmccentre.ca
www.jmccentre.ca
www.facebook.com/243715438993933
Number of Schools: 1 *Note:* The John McGivney Children's Centre School Authority governs the John McGivney Children's Centre School, formerly known as the Children's Rehabilitation Centre School. The school provides a post trauma / post operative rehabilitation program for students from ages four to twenty-one, who live in Windsor / Essex County.
Grant Gagnon, Chair
Elaine Whitmore, CEO, 519-252-7281, ext. 221
Dr. Brenda Roberts-Santarossa, Secretary & Principal
Adelina Irvine, Treasurer

National Libraries

Canadian Down Syndrome Society
#103, 2003 - 14 St. NW, Calgary, AB T2M 3N4
Tel: 403-270-8500; *Fax:* 403-270-8291
Toll-Free: 800-883-5608
www.cdss.ca
Social Media: www.youtube.com/cdndownsyndrome;
twitter.com/cdndownsyndrome; www.facebook.com/cdndownsyndrome
Collection: Articles & publications relating to Down syndrome & disabilities for parents & professionals
Corrine Grieve, Resource Manager
Kirk Crowther, Executive Director

Provincial Libraries

Down Syndrome Research Foundation
1409 Sperling Ave., Burnaby, BC V5B 4J8
Tel: 604-444-3773; *Fax:* 604-431-9248
Toll-Free: 888-464-3773
Other Numbers: www.youtube.com/user/DSRFCANADA
info@dsrf.org
www.dsrf.org
Social Media: twitter.com/DSRFcanada;
www.facebook.com/DSRFCanada
Dawn McKenna, Executive Director
Pat Hanbury, Director, Programs & Services

Eating Disorders

Eating is integral to human health, and for many people food is a pleasure that can be enjoyed without too much thought. But an increasing number of people (mostly, but not exclusively, women) have eating disorders, which cause them to use food and dieting in ways that are extremely unhealthy, even life-threatening. In Canada, approximately 1.5 percent of women aged 15 to 24 have an eating disorder. The two principal eating disorders are anorexia nervosa and bulimia nervosa; though different in the symptoms they manifest, the two disorders are quite similar in their underlying pathology: an obsessive concern with food, body image and body weight.

Many people believe that eating disorders are, in part, culturally determined: in the Western world a pervasive cultural preference for slimness causes many people to spend extraordinary amounts of time, money and energy dieting and exercising to stay slim. At the same time, people are flooded with media; celebrations of anorexia, and suggested strategies for remaining thin, can be easily found on the internet, on television and in magazines. Cultural preference is likely to exert pressure on people, especially young women, who may be genetically or psychologically predisposed to the illness. It is important to be wary of media, including the internet, which can expose young people to counterproductive influences. Overeating is another type of eating disorder, one that reflects the paradox that, as society values thinness more and more, more and more people are obese.

Anorexia Nervosa

Anorexia is a psychiatric disorder in which dieting and a desire for thinness lead to excessive weight loss.

Cause
The cause of anorexia is unknown, although social factors appear to play an important role, including advertisements that equate thinness with desirability. People who have suffered a traumatic event or have self-image problems are at risk of developing anorexia. Familial factors, such as how someone has been raised or taught to behave, can also be involved. Many people with anorexia are also struggling with emotional difficulties that they cannot face or resolve. Finally, there appears to be a genetic predisposition to anorexia.

Symptoms
Anorexia nervosa is characterized by self-starvation, food preoccupation and rituals, compulsive exercising, and often a resulting absence of menstrual cycles. People with anorexia usually have a distorted body image which makes them think that they are fat, no matter how thin they really are. Over 50 percent of patients develop bulimic symptoms, usually within the first five years of developing the disorder.

Other physical complications of anorexia may include abdominal pain, cold intolerance, fatigue, cardiac arrhythmias, kidney problems and osteoporosis. Patients with anorexia nervosa may be severely depressed, and may experience insomnia, irritability and diminished interest in sex. These features may be exacerbated if the patient is severely underweight. People with anorexia also share many of the features of obsessive compulsive disorder. For instance, they may have an excessive interest in food; they may hoard food, or spend unusual amounts of time reading and researching about foods, recipes and nutrition. People with anorexia nervosa may also exhibit a strong need to control their environment, and may be socially and emotionally withdrawn. Approximately 20 to 30 percent of patients attempt suicide.

Prevalence
A large majority of the people with this disorder are female, although males can be affected. The onset usually occurs during adolescence, but some sufferers are in their 60s. Prevalence studies in females have found rates of 0.5 to 1 percent for anorexia nervosa. The prevalence of the disorder in males is approximately 0.3 percent.

Treatment Options
A diagnosis of anorexia nervosa is based on the following criteria outlined in the Diagnostic and Statistical Manual of Mental Disorders: refusal to maintain body weight at or above eighty-five percent of a minimally normal weight for age and height; intense fear of gaining weight or becoming fat, even though underweight; disturbance in the way one's body weight or shape is experienced, undue influence of body weight or shape on self-evaluation, or denial of the seriousness of the current low body weight; in menstruating females, the absence of at least three consecutive menstrual cycles; physical damage such as imbalances in body

chemicals often occurs, which, if severe, can cause cardiac arrest; purging often erodes tooth enamel, in which case a dentist might make the diagnosis. Anorexia is associated with amenorrhea and infertility, which may lead patients to seek help from a gynecologist, who must then make the diagnosis.

Denial is a prominent feature of anorexia, and sufferers usually resist treatment.

Anorexia may do lasting physical damage; because of this, treatment must first aim to restore a patient to a safe and healthy body weight. Initial treatment may require hospitalization for physical stabilization. Longer-term nutritional counselling and monitoring is often vital to maintain proper body weight.

It is critical to recognize that anorexia, in addition to being life-threatening, is extremely complex; simply restoring the patient to an acceptable body weight is not enough. Many patients have complex and conflicting psychological issues that trigger the morbid fear of gaining weight. These issues need to be addressed by psychotherapy. Forms of psychotherapy that may be useful in treating eating disorders include family therapy, psychodynamic psychotherapy (in which longstanding and sometimes unconscious emotional issues related to the eating disorder are explored) and cognitive behavioural therapy (which aims to identify the thought patterns that trigger the eating disorder and to establish healthy eating habits).

Recent literature suggests that psychotherapeutic approaches are often more effective than medications in the treatment of anorexia. However, SSRIs (Selective Serotonin Reuptake Inhibitors, which were originally developed as antidepressants), are sometimes prescribed to help restore and build self-esteem, and thereby help the patient maintain a positive attitude as well as a safe and healthy body image and body weight.

In Canada, clinical trials are currently underway to investigate the effectiveness of deep-brain electrical stimulation as a therapy for people with severe anorexia. The hope is that by sending a current of electricity to a specific part of the brain (the subcallosal cingulate) that is associated with anxiety, depression and mood, doctors will be able to reduce a patient's obsessive thoughts about food, and improve her or his mood. Initial results are promising.

Anorexia is serious—untreated it can kill a patient. In fact, the disorder is associated with a 10 percent death rate, generally from a sudden disturbance of heart rhythm. This is the highest mortality rate of any mental illness. Treatment may be required over a course of many years, but fortunately, around half of sufferers recover within five years. Eventually, many others return to a normal or near-normal body weight, as well. However, they may continue to struggle with body image and unhealthy eating patterns.

Bulimia Nervosa

Bulimia nervosa is characterized by recurring episodes of binge eating followed by efforts to avoid weight gain, such as purging through self-induced vomiting or abuse of laxatives or diuretics (water pills). Unlike patients with anorexia, those with bulimia usually have normal weight. Binges are often triggered by psychological stress and are carried out in secret.

Cause
The exact cause of bulimia is not known, however social and cultural factors appear to be involved. Obesity during adolescence, a history of sexual abuse, peer pressure, low self-esteem and perfectionism may contribute to development of the disorder.

Symptoms

Warning signs of bulimia include eating uncontrollably, frequent use of the bathroom, erosion of dental enamel of the front teeth (from vomiting), swollen salivary glands, fatigue and amenorrhea. Bulimia may coexist with anorexia.

Individuals with bulimia nervosa are often within the normal weight range, but prior to the development of the disorder they may be overweight. Depression and other mood disorders are common among people with bulimia, and patients often ascribe their bulimia to the mood disorders. Substance abuse occurs in about one-third of individuals with bulimia. Anxiety disorders are common, and fear of social situations can be a precipitating factor in binging episodes.

Prevalence

The prevalence of bulimia among adolescent females is approximately 1 to 3 percent. The rate of the disorder among males is approximately 0.5 percent.

Treatment Options

Diagnosis of bulimia nervosa is based on the following criteria outlined in the Diagnostic and Statistical Manual of Mental Disorders: recurrent episodes of binge eating characterized by eating more food than most people would eat during a similar period of time and under similar circumstances; a sense of loss of control over eating; recurrent inappropriate behaviour in order to prevent weight gain, such as self-induced vomiting or misuse of laxatives, and excessive fasting or exercise; the binge-eating and inappropriate behaviours both occur, on average, at least twice a week for three months; self-evaluation is unduly influenced by body shape and weight; the disturbance does not occur exclusively during episodes of anorexia nervosa.

Treatment for bulimia is similar to that for anorexia. For a complete description, please see Treatment Options in the anorexia nervosa entry above.

Poor prognosis in bulimia patients is usually related to a history of substance abuse, or the presence of a personality disorder. Fortunately, most people with bulimia who are appropriately treated can and do recover.

See also Obesity

National Associations

Eating Disorder Association of Canada (EDAC) / Association des Troubles Alimentaires du Canada (ATAC)
ON

e-mail: edacatac@gmail.com
www.edac-atac.ca
twitter.com/EDACATAC

Overview: A small national organization
Mission: EDAC-ATAC aims to serve the needs of those whose lives are impacted by eating disorders.
Chief Officer(s):
Jadine Cairns, President

Jessie's Hope Society
#400, 601 West Broadway St., Vancouver BC V5Z 4C2
Tel: 604-466-4877; *Fax:* 604-466-4897
Toll-Free: 877-288-0877
www.jessieshope.org
Previous Name: Association for Awareness & Networking around Disordered Eating
Overview: A small national organization founded in 1985
Chief Officer(s):
Heather Quick Rajala

National Eating Disorder Information Centre (NEDIC)
200 Elizabeth St., #ES7-421, Toronto ON M5G 2C4
Tel: 416-340-4156; *Fax:* 416-340-4736
Toll-Free: 866-633-4220
e-mail: nedic@uhn.ca
www.nedic.ca
www.facebook.com/thenedic
Overview: A small national charitable organization founded in 1985
Mission: To provide information & resources on eating disorders, food & weight preoccupation; To raise public awareness about eating disorders & related issues
Member of: Toronto General Hospital
Chief Officer(s):
Elizabeth Pottinger, Officer, Development
  elizabeth.pottinger@uhn.ca
Suzanne Phillips, Manager, Program
  suzanne.phillips@uhn.ca
Marbella Carlos, Coordinator, Education & Outreach
  marbella.carlos@uhn.ca

Provincial Associations

ALBERTA

College of Dietitians of Alberta
#740, 10707 - 100 Ave., Edmonton AB T5J 3M1
Tel: 780-448-0059; *Fax:* 780-489-7759
Toll-Free: 866-493-4348
e-mail: office@collegeofdietitians.ab.ca
www.collegeofdietitians.ab.ca
Overview: A small provincial licensing organization overseen by Dietitians of Canada
Mission: The College is the regulatory body of registered dieticians/nutritionists in Alberta, setting entry requirements, standards of practice. It is accountable to both the government & the public.
Chief Officer(s):
Doug Cook, Executive Director & Registrar

BRITISH COLUMBIA

College of Dietitians of British Columbia (CDBC)
#409, 1367 West Broadway, Vancouver BC V6H 4A7
Tel: 604-736-2016; *Fax:* 604-736-2018
Toll-Free: 877-736-2016
e-mail: info@collegeofdietitiansbc.org
www.collegeofdietitiansofbc.org
Overview: A medium-sized provincial licensing organization founded in 2004 overseen by Dietitians of Canada
Mission: To serve & protect the nutritional health of the public through quality dietetic practice
Chief Officer(s):
Fern Hubbard, Registrar
Mélanie Journoud, Deputy Registrar, Quality Assurance
Chi Cejalvo, Deputy Registrar, Registration & Communication

MANITOBA

College of Dietitians of Manitoba
#36, 1313 Border St., Winnipeg MB R3H 0X4
Tel: 204-694-0532; *Fax:* 204-889-1755
Toll-Free: 866-283-2823
e-mail: office.cdm@mts.net
www.manitobadietitians.ca
Overview: A small provincial organization overseen by Dietitians of Canada
Mission: To act as the regulating body within the province for dietitians & the profession of dietetics; To set education standards; To ensure competency of members
Member of: Alliance of Dietetic Regulatory Bodies
Chief Officer(s):
Michelle Hagglund, Registrar

NEW BRUNSWICK

New Brunswick Association of Dietitians (NBAD) / Association des diététistes du Nouveau-Brunswick (ADNB)
PO Box 27002, 471 Smythe St., Fredericton NB E3B 9M1
Tel: 506-457-9396; *Fax:* 506-450-9375
e-mail: registrar@adnb-nbad.com
www.adnb-nbad.com
Overview: A medium-sized provincial licensing organization overseen by Dietitians of Canada
Mission: To regulate the practice of dietitians within New Brunswick
Chief Officer(s):
Catherine MacDonald, President

NEWFOUNDLAND AND LABRADOR

Newfoundland & Labrador College of Dietitians (NLCD)
PO Box 1756, Stn. C, St. John's NL A1C 5P5
Tel: 709-753-4040; *Fax:* 709-781-1044
Toll-Free: 877-753-4040
e-mail: registrar@nlcd.ca
www.nlcd.ca
Overview: A medium-sized provincial licensing organization overseen by Dietitians of Canada
Mission: To regulate Registered Dietitians & to ensure competency in the dietetic profession, in the interest of the people in Newfoundland
Member of: Alliance of Canadian Regulatory Boards
Chief Officer(s):
Cynthia Whalen, Registrar

NOVA SCOTIA

Nova Scotia Dietetic Association (NSDA)
#301, 380 Bedford Hwy., Halifax NS B3M 2L4
Tel: 902-493-3034
e-mail: info@nsdassoc.ca
www.nsdassoc.ca
Overview: A medium-sized provincial licensing organization founded in 1953 overseen by Dietitians of Canada
Mission: To regulate dietitians & nutritionists in the province, & register & discipline (when necessary) practitioners to ensure safe, ethical & competent dietetic practice
Chief Officer(s):
Melissa Campbell, President
Jennifer Garus, Executive Manager (ex-officio)

ONTARIO

College of Dietitians of Ontario (CDO) / L'Ordre des diététistes de l'Ontario
PO Box 30, #1810, 5775 Yonge St., Toronto ON M2M 4J1
Tel: 416-598-1725; *Fax:* 416-598-0274
Toll-Free: 800-668-4990
e-mail: information@collegeofdietitians.org
www.collegeofdietitians.org
www.facebook.com/CollegeDietitiansOntario
twitter.com/CDOntario
Also Known As: CDO
Overview: A medium-sized provincial licensing charitable organization founded in 1993 overseen by Dietitians of Canada
Mission: To promote awareness of & access to competent, high quality nutritional care for Ontarians
Member of: The Federation of Health Regulatory Bodies of Ontario; Alliance of Canadian Dietetic Regulatory Bodies; Council of Licensure, Enforcement and Regulation
Chief Officer(s):
Melisse L. Willems, Registrar & Executive Director, 416-598-1725 Ext. 228
melisse.willems@collegeofdietitians.org

PRINCE EDWARD ISLAND

Prince Edward Island Dietetic Association (PEIDA)
c/o Prince Edward Island Dietitians Registration Board, PO Box 362, Charlottetown PE C1A 7K7
e-mail: peidietitians@gmail.com
www.peidietitians.ca
www.facebook.com/peidieteticassociation

Overview: A small provincial organization founded in 1965 overseen by Dietitians of Canada
Mission: To promote, encourage & improve the status of dietitians & nutritionists in the province of PEI; To promote & increase the knowledge & proficiency of its members in all matters relating to nutrition & dietetics; To promote public awareness
Chief Officer(s):
Doreen Pippy, President

QUÉBEC

Ordre professionnel des diététistes du Québec (OPDQ)
#1855, 550, rue Sherbrooke ouest, Montréal QC H3A 1B9
Tél: 514-393-3733; *Téléc:* 514-393-3582
Ligne sans frais: 888-393-8528
Courriel: opdq@opdq.org
www.opdq.org
Aperçu: *Dimension:* moyenne; *Envergure:* provinciale; Organisme de réglementation; fondée en 1956 surveillé par Dietitians of Canada
Mission: Assurer la protection du public en contrôlant notamment l'exercice de la profession par ses membres
Membre(s) du bureau directeur:
Annie Chapados, Directrice générale et secrétaire
achapados@opdq.org

SASKATCHEWAN

Saskatchewan Dietitians Association (SDA)
#17, 2010 - 7th Ave., Regina SK S4R 1C2
Tel: 306-359-3040; *Fax:* 306-359-3046
e-mail: registrar@saskdietitians.org
www.saskdietitians.org
Overview: A small provincial licensing organization founded in 1958 overseen by Dietitians of Canada
Mission: To protect the public by registering competent dietitians; To set standards of practice; To uphold codes of conduct; To provide a framework for continuing competence, consisting of a self-assessment tool, a learning plan, & a quality assurance audit
Affliation(s): Network of Interprofessional Regulatory Organizations; Alliance of Dietetic Regulatory Bodies
Chief Officer(s):
Laurel Leushen, President
Lana Moore, Registrar

Local Associations

ONTARIO

Bulimia Anorexia Nervosa Association (BANA) / Association de la boulimie et d'anorexie mentale
#100, 1500 Ouellette Ave., Windsor ON N8X 1K7
Tel: 519-969-2112; *Fax:* 519-969-0227
e-mail: info@bana.ca
www.bana.ca
www.linkedin.com/groups/Bulimia-Anorexia-Nervosa-Association-2223288
www.facebook.com/277063735753721
twitter.com/BANAWindsor
banawindsor.tumblr.com
Overview: A medium-sized local charitable organization founded in 1982
Mission: To reduce the incidence of bulimia & anorexia nervosa with preventative programs; To offer services in the form of group, family & individual counselling; To provide a hotline for the community; To maintain a library for community use; To provide an educational, preventative curriculum
Chief Officer(s):
Luciana Rosu-Sieza, Executive Director
luciana@bana.ca

Sheena's Place
87 Spadina Rd., Toronto ON M5R 2T1
Tel: 416-927-8900; *Fax:* 416-927-8844
e-mail: info@sheenasplace.org
www.sheenasplace.org
www.facebook.com/pages/Sheenas-Place/118354831586196
twitter.com/sheenasplace
www.youtube.com/user/SheenasPlace

Overview: A small local organization
Mission: To offer hope & support for people with eating disorders
Chief Officer(s):
Deborah Berlin-Romalis, Executive Director
  dberlin-romalis@sheenasplace.org

National Publications

Canadian Journal of Dietetic Practice & Research / Revue canadienne de la pratique et de la recherche en diété
c/o Dietitians of Canada, #604, 480 University Ave., Toronto, ON M5G 1V2

Tel: 416-596-0857; *Fax:* 416-596-0603
editor@dietitians.ca

Frequency: Quarterly
Dawna Royall, Editor

National Libraries

National Eating Disorder Information Centre
200 Elizabeth St., #ES 7-421, Toronto, ON M5G 2C4

Tel: 416-340-4156; *Fax:* 416-340-4736
Toll-Free: 866-633-4220
nedic@uhn.ca
www.nedic.ca
Social Media: www.youtube.com/user/NEDIC85; twitter.com/thenedic
www.facebook.com/thenedic

Suzanne Phillips, Program Manager
  suzanne.phillips@uhn.ca
Marbella Carlos, Education & Outreach Coordinator
  marbella.carlos@uhn.ca

Provincial Libraries

Homewood Health Centre
150 Delhi St., Guelph, ON N1E 6K9

Tel: 519-824-1010; *Fax:* 519-824-8751
www.homewoodhealth.com

Collection: Collection includes pamphlets, consumer health information, fiction, magazines, newspaper, reference material, large-print books; talking books; music. The staff library includes clinical text books; professional journals; e-journals; college/university catalogues; hospital archives; quick reference; EbscoHost full text databases.
Jagoda Pike, President & CEO

Endometriosis

Endometriosis is a hormonal condition in which the tissue that normally lines the inside of the uterus (endometrium) is also found outside the uterus, generally on the outer surface of pelvic organs, and also on the bowel and bladder. These cells respond to the woman's hormonal cycles, and swell and bleed at the time of menses. This causes pain, generally worse with each period; pelvic masses; and alterations of the menstrual cycle.

Cause
The exact cause of endometriosis is not known, but some theories suggest that the condition could be the result of an autoimmune disorder, or the inability of the body to break down retrograde menstruation. Some studies claim that it could have a genetic origin. The chance of having endometriosis is three to ten times greater for a woman who has a mother or sister(s) with the condition. If a woman is having trouble conceiving, or has blocked reproductive tracts, she may also have an increased risk for endometriosis.

Symptoms
The symptoms of endometriosis vary. Some women have no symptoms and are not even aware that they have the condition, while others experience severe pain that is sometimes debilitating. Pelvic pain before and during menstruation is most common. However, pain can also be experienced at other times, and in other places such as the abdomen and back. The pain may be aggravated by intercourse or defecation. Nausea, constipation and diarrhea are also common symptoms. In very rare cases, shortness of breath, leg pain or rectal bleeding might be experienced. For some women, the pain associated with endometriosis can affect work, relationships, family life and mental health.

Prevalence
Although the reported incidence varies, endometriosis is commonly found in 10 to 15 percent of women between the ages of 25 and 44 years. It is estimated that 25 to 50 percent of infertile women have this disorder. Close to 40 percent of women with endometriosis experience symptoms before they are 15 years of age.

Treatment Options
Since the symptoms of endometriosis are similar to those of many other conditions, it can be difficult to diagnose. A physician can do a physical and internal examination, but to make a definitive diagnosis, laparoscopy is performed. In this procedure, a laparoscope—a fiber-optic tube with a lens at one end—is inserted through a small cut in the abdomen to check for endometrial implants on the abdominal walls.

Treatment depends on the severity of the symptoms and the age and reproductive wishes of the patient. The pain associated with mild cases may be treated with non-steroidal anti-inflammatory drugs. More severe cases may respond to suppression of ovarian function. Alternative therapies (such as acupuncture), stress management techniques, exercise and nutritional supplements might also help relieve the symptoms of endometriosis in some women. Laparoscopic surgery may destroy some of the collection of tissue, and is often used in hopes of improving fertility. Hysterectomy (removal of the uterus) is used for intractable cases, especially in women who do not desire future pregnancy.

With early diagnosis and proper medical treatment, most women with endometriosis will find relief from their symptoms.

National Associations

The Endometriosis Network
790 Bay St., 8th Fl., Toronto ON M5G 1N8

Tel: 416-591-3963
e-mail: support@endometriosisnetwork.ca
www.endometriosisnetwork.ca
www.facebook.com/TheEndoNetwork
twitter.com/theendonetwork

Previous Name: Toronto Endometriosis Network
Overview: A small national organization founded in 1987
Mission: To increase public & professional awareness of endometriosis; To encourage professional medical research toward early diagnosis & cure of endometriosis; To provide support & education to sufferers & their families
Affiliation(s): Endometriosis Sisterhood
Chief Officer(s):
Katie McLeod, Director, Support
  katie@endometriosisnetwork.ca

International Associations

Endometriosis Association, Inc. (EA) / Association de l'endometriose inc.
International Headquarters, 8585 North 76th Pl., Milwaukee WI 53223 USA

Tel: 414-355-2200; *Fax:* 414-355-6065
e-mail: endo@endometriosisassn.org
www.endometriosisassn.org
www.facebook.com/EndoAssn

Overview: A large international charitable organization founded in 1980

Mission: To establish network for women with endometriosis to share information & mutual support; to educate women, families, friends, & community about endometriosis & about living with this chronic disease; to promote & conduct research on endometriosis; to provide advocacy for women with endometriosis, when necessary, either on an individual or on a group level; to support groups & chapters in Canadian centers
Member of: Society of Obstetricians & Gynacologists of Canada; Canadian Fertility/Andrology Society
Chief Officer(s):
Mary Lou Ballweg, President/Executive Director
   support@EndometriosisAssn.org
Publications:
• The Endometriosis Sourcebook
Type: Book; *Author:* Mary Lou Ballweg; *Price:* $12.95
• Endometriosis: The Complete Reference for Taking Charge of Your Health
Type: Book; *Author:* Mary Lou Ballweg; *Price:* $15.95
• Overcoming Endometriosis
Type: Book

Epilepsy

Epilepsy is characterized by recurrent, sudden, rapid changes in brain function caused by abnormalities in the electrical activity of the brain. A person may have an isolated, nonrecurring seizure due to a high fever in childhood, head trauma, lack of oxygen or some other disease (metabolic abnormality or brain tumour). However, if a person has two or more unprovoked seizures, the disorder is referred to as epilepsy.

Cause
If there is a known cause for the seizures, such as fever, lack of sleep, heat, skipping meals, medication changes, stress, hormonal changes or flashing lights (strobe lights), it is called symptomatic epilepsy. If the seizures seem to be related to a brain structure abnormality, it is referred to as cryptogenic epilepsy. In 50 to 60 percent of cases, there is no apparent cause for the disorder, and it is therefore called idiopathic epilepsy.

Symptoms
Seizures can be classified as generalized, affecting the whole brain at once, or partial, affecting a part of the brain. Generalized absence (petit mal) attacks are seizures in which there is only a brief (10 to 30 second) loss of consciousness, with eye and muscle fluttering but no loss of muscle tone. A generalized tonic-clonic seizure (grand mal) usually lasts 1 to 2 minutes, and includes loss of consciousness, falling and involuntary contractions of the arms and legs. Some patients report that they see flashing lights, feel anxious, hear a sound, or experience a heightened sense of taste and smell (known as an aura) that indicates they are about to have a seizure. During a simple partial (focal) seizure, a person usually experiences strange sensations such as an unusual odour or visual distortion. Other symptoms may include hearing disturbances, stomach discomfort, sudden movements and feelings of fear. Simple partial seizures are categorized as sensory, motor, psychic or autonomous, according to the brain region affected. A complex partial (psychomotor) seizure is characterized by confusion and is often preceded by an aura. The person may engage in repeated motions (automatisms) such as mumbling, head turning or random wandering. A change in memory or consciousness is also possible. Around two-thirds of people with epilepsy experience complex partial seizures. Myoclonic seizures, which are often characterized by jerking muscle movements, and atonic seizures, which are associated with a sudden loss of muscle tone, are more common in children than adults.

Prevalence
Roughly 300,000 Canadians suffer from epilepsy, with half of the cases found in children and adolescents.

Treatment Options
To diagnose epilepsy, a physician usually takes a medical history that includes a complete description of any seizures that have occurred. A physical exam is performed, and various tests are commonly ordered. These may include an electroencephalographic recording (EEG) to identify any changes in the electrical activity of the brain, a computerized tomography (CT) or a magnetic resonance imaging (MRI) scan of the brain to detect any abnormalities such as a tumour or infection, and blood tests to rule out any other medical conditions that might be causing the seizures.

Treatment aims primarily to control seizures. Causative or precipitating factors should be eliminated. Drug treatment is the mainstay of therapy for most types of seizures. In order to limit toxic effects, an attempt is made to use only a single drug though some patients may need to take more than one. In most cases, acceptable control can be achieved with medications alone. Rarely, seizures will not respond to drugs, and surgery on the brain will be recommended. In this procedure, the surgeon tries to identify and remove the part of the brain that is triggering the seizures.

Advancements in the drug treatment of epilepsy have greatly improved the quality of life of people with this disorder. With appropriate therapy, many people can control their seizures, and even eliminate them completely.

National Associations

Canadian Association of Electroneurophysiology Technologists Inc. (CAET) / Association canadienne des technologues en electroneurophysiologie inc. (ACTE)
c/o St. Boniface Hospital, 409 Taché Ave., Winnipeg MB R2H 2A6
Tel: 204-233-8563
www.caet.org
Overview: A small national organization founded in 1951
Mission: To advance the knowledge, science, & technology of electroneurophysiology in Canada
Affliation(s): Canadian Board of Registration of Electroencephalograph Technologists Inc. (CBRET)
Chief Officer(s):
Joanne Nikkel, President
   joanne.nikkel@caet.org
Bruce Goddard, Vice-President
   bruce.goddard@caet.org
Jodi Kent, Secretary & Registrar
   jodi.kent@caet.org
Publications:
• Canadian Association of Electroneurophysiology Technologists Inc. Membership Directory
Type: Directory

Canadian Epilepsy Alliance (CAE) / L'Alliance canadienne de l'épilepsie (ACE)
c/o President, 351 Kenmount Rd., St. John's NL A1B 3P9
Tel: 709-722-0502; *Fax:* 709-722-0999
www.epilepsymatters.com
Overview: A medium-sized national charitable organization founded in 1998
Mission: To promote independence & quality of life for people with epilepsy & their families, through support services, information, advocacy, & public awareness
Chief Officer(s):
Gail Dempsey, President
   executivedirector@epilepsynl.com
Publications:
• Epilepsy Matters: The Newsletter of the Canadian Epilepsy Alliance
Type: Newsletter; *Frequency:* 3 pa

Profile: National thematic journal about epilepsy issues for persons with epilepsy & their caregivers

Canadian League Against Epilepsy (CLAE)
c/o Secretariat Central, #6, 20 Crown Steel Dr., Markham ON L3R 9X9
Tel: 905-415-3917
e-mail: clae@secretariatcentral.com
www.claegroup.org
Overview: A small national organization
Mission: To help Canadians affected by epilepsy; To develop therapeutic & preventative strategies to prevent the effects of epilepsy
Affiliation(s): Canadian Epilepsy Alliance; American Epilepsy Society; North American Commission for Epilepsy
Chief Officer(s):
Jorge Burneo, President
Mary Lou Smith, Secretary
David Steven, Treasurer

Canadian Neurological Sciences Federation (CNSF) / Fédération des sciences neurologiques du Canada
143N - 8500 Macleod Trail SE, Calgary AB T2H 2N1
Tel: 403-229-9544; *Fax:* 403-229-1661
www.cnsfederation.org
Previous Name: Canadian Congress of Neurological Sciences
Overview: A medium-sized national organization
Mission: To support the neuroscience professions in Canada, particularly those members of the CNSF Societies, through education, advocacy, membership services & research promotion
Chief Officer(s):
Dan Morin, Chief Executive Officer
dan-morin@cnsfederation.org
Marika Fitzgerald, Manager, Finance & Administration
marika-fitzgerald@cnsfederation.org
Donna Irvin, Administrator, Membership Services
donna-irvin@cnsfederation.org
Publications:
• Canadian Journal of Neurological Sciences
Type: Journal; *Frequency:* 6 pa; *Editor:* Dr. Robert Chen
Profile: Published through Cambridge Journals Online, a peer-reviewed clinical & basic neuroscience research articles, covering neurology, neurosurgery, clinicalneurophysiology, & pediatric neurology

Canadian Neurological Society (CNS) / Société canadienne de neurologie
#709, 7015 Macleod Trail SW, Calgary AB T2H 2K1
Tel: 403-229-9544; *Fax:* 403-229-1661
www.cnsfederation.org
Overview: A medium-sized national organization overseen by Canadian Neurological Sciences Federation
Mission: To promote & encourage all aspects of neurology, including research, education, assessment & accreditation; provide for annual scientific sessions to promote the knowledge & practice of neurology
Chief Officer(s):
Dan Morin, CNSF CEO
dan-morin@cnsfederation.org
Marika Fitzgerald, CNSF Controller
marika-fitzgerald@cnsfederation.org
Publications:
• The Canadian Journal of Neurological Sciences
Type: Journal; *Frequency:* Bimonthly; *Accepts Advertising; Editor:* G. Bryan Young; *Price:* Free with CNS membership
Profile: Peer-reviewed original articles

Epilepsy Canada (EC) / Épilepsie Canada
#2B, 2900 John St., Markham ON L3R 5G3
Fax: 905-764-1231
Toll-Free: 877-734-0873
e-mail: epilepsy@epilepsy.ca
www.epilepsy.ca
Overview: A medium-sized national charitable organization founded in 1966
Mission: To enhance the quality of life for persons affected by epilepsy; To promote & support research into all aspects of epilepsy; To facilitate educational initiatives; To increase public & professional awareness of epilepsy; To fund research; To encourage governments to address the needs of people with epilepsy

Member of: International Bureau for Epilepsy (IBE); Canadian League Against Epilepsy
Chief Officer(s):
Jacques Brunelle, National President
jbrunelle@tennistremblant.com
Gary N. Collins, Executive Director
garycollins@4growth.ca

Epilepsy Foundation of America (EFA)
8301 Professional Place, Landover MD 20785-7223 USA
Tel: 301-459-3700; *Fax:* 301-577-4941
Toll-Free: 800-332-1000
e-mail: ContactUs@efa.org
www.epilepsyfoundation.org
www.facebook.com/EpilepsyFoundationofAmerica
twitter.com/epilepsyfdn
www.youtube.com/epilepsyfoundation
Overview: A small national charitable organization founded in 1967
Mission: To work for people affected by seizures through research, education, advocacy & service
Affiliation(s): Epilepsy Canada
Chief Officer(s):
Eric R. Hargis, President & CEO

Provincial Associations

BRITISH COLUMBIA

British Columbia Epilepsy Society (BCES)
#2500, 900 West 8 Ave., Vancouver BC V7E 6L3
Tel: 604-875-6704; *Fax:* 604-875-0617
e-mail: info@bcepilepsy.com
www.bcepilepsy.com
www.facebook.com/265298573586670
twitter.com/BCEpilepsy
www.youtube.com/BCEpilepsySociety
Also Known As: BC Epilepsy
Overview: A medium-sized provincial charitable organization founded in 1959
Mission: To serve the well-being of people living with epilepsy; To provide & promote services & education to those with epilepsy; To improve the lives of British Columbians with epilepsy & their families through education, support & research; To advance awareness, understanding & acceptance of epilepsy in British Columbia
Member of: Canadian Epilepsy Alliance
Chief Officer(s):
Lisa Westermark, Executive Director
lisa@bcepilepsy.com
Marlyn Chow, Coordinator, Support Services
marlyn@bcepilepsy.com

British Columbia Society of Electroneurophysiology Technologists (BCSET)
c/o EEG Department, Penticton Regional Hospital, 550 Carmi Ave., Penticton BC V2A 3G6
Tel: 250-492-1000; *Fax:* 250-492-9037
e-mail: webmaster@bcset.org
www.bcset.org
Overview: A small provincial organization
Mission: A professional non-profit association dedicated to fostering excellence in diagnostic electroneurophysiology, furthering education and providing a forum for discussion and interaction.
Affiliation(s): Canadian Association of Electroneurophysiology Technologists
Chief Officer(s):
Tara Cassidy, President

MANITOBA

Epilepsy & Seizure Association of Manitoba
#4, 1805 Main St., Winnipeg MB R2V 2A2
Tel: 204-783-0466; *Fax:* 204-784-9689
e-mail: esam@manitobaepilepsy.org
www.manitobaepilepsy.org
Also Known As: Manitoba Epilepsy Association
Overview: A small provincial charitable organization founded in 1975

Mission: To improve the quality of life of persons with epilepsy by providing programs & education, & supporting research & services
Member of: Canadian Epilepsy Alliance
Chief Officer(s):
Diane Wall, President
Chris Kullman, Vice-President
Krys Kirton, Secretary

NOVA SCOTIA

Epilepsy Association of Nova Scotia (EANS)
#306, 5880 Spring Garden Rd., Halifax NS B3H 1Y1
Tel: 902-429-2633; *Fax:* 902-425-0821
Toll-Free: 866-374-5377
www.epilepsyns.com
www.facebook.com/epilepsyns.org
twitter.com/epilepsy_ns
www.instagram.com/epilepsy_ns
Overview: A small provincial charitable organization founded in 1980
Mission: To provide support for people with epilepsy; To promote awareness & public understanding of epilepsy; To encourage research into the causes, treatment & prevention of epilepsy
Member of: Epilepsy Foundation of America; Canadian Epilepsy Alliance
Chief Officer(s):
Debbi Tobin, Executive Director
Publications:
• Epicure [a publication of the Epilepsy Association of Nova Scotia]
Type: Newsletter; *Frequency:* 3 pa

ONTARIO

Epilepsy Ontario / Épilepsie Ontario
#803, 3100 Steeles Ave. East, Toronto ON L3R 8T3
Tel: 905-474-9696; *Fax:* 905-474-3663
Toll-Free: 800-463-1119
e-mail: info@epilepsyontario.org
www.epilepsyontario.org
www.facebook.com/epilepsy.ontario
twitter.com/EpilepsyOntario
Overview: A medium-sized provincial charitable organization founded in 1956
Mission: To promote optimal quality of life for people living with seizure disorders; To advocate for awareness, support services & research into these disorders & maintains a network of local agencies, contacts & associates to provide services, counselling & referrals
Affiliation(s): Canadian Epilepsy Alliance; Epilepsy Canada
Chief Officer(s):
Paul Raymond, Executive Director
paul@epilepsyontario.org

Durham Region
#3, 310 Byron St. South, Whitby ON L1N 4P8
Tel: 905-430-3090; *Fax:* 905-430-3080
e-mail: support@epilepsydurham.com
www.epilepsydurham.com
www.facebook.com/EpilepsyDurham
twitter.com/Epilepsy_Durham
www.youtube.com/user/DurhamEpilepsy
Chief Officer(s):
Dianne McKenzie, Executive Director
dianne.mckenzie@epilepsydurham.com

Halton Peel Hamilton Region
#4, 2160 Dunwin Dr., Mississauga ON L5L 5M8
Tel: 905-450-1900
Toll-Free: 855-734-2111
e-mail: info@epilepsysco.org
ehph.org
www.youtube.com/channel/UCMs-90lDVPBUXoUi4tUv0Zw
Chief Officer(s):
Cynthia Milburn, Executive Director
cynthia@epilepsysco.org

London & Area

690 Hale St., London ON N5W 1H4
Tel: 519-433-4073; *Fax:* 519-433-4079
Toll-Free: 866-374-5377
e-mail: support@epilepsysupport.ca
www.epilepsysupportcentre.com
www.facebook.com/epilepsysupport
twitter.com/EpilepsySWO
www.youtube.com/user/EpilepsyLondon
Chief Officer(s):
Michelle Franklin, Executive Director
michelle@epilepsysupport.ca

Ottawa-Carleton
#207, 211 Bronson Ave., Ottawa ON K1R 6H5
Tel: 613-594-9255; *Fax:* 613-594-5189
Toll-Free: 866-374-5377
e-mail: info@epilepsyottawa.ca
www.epilepsyottawa.ca
www.facebook.com/EpilepsyOttawa
twitter.com/Epilepsy_Ottawa
www.youtube.com/channel/UCkeb41QGDCVAVSIyUAIVNKA
Chief Officer(s):
Peter Andrews, President

Peterborough & Area
Unit 6, Charlotte Mews, PO Box 2453, 203 Simcoe St., Peterborough ON K9J 7Y8
Tel: 705-874-1897
Toll-Free: 800-463-1119
e-mail: epilepsyptbo@yahoo.ca
epilepsyontario.org/agency/epilepsy-peterborough-and-area
Chief Officer(s):
Tom Appleby, Executive Director

Simcoe County
Victoria Village, #7, 72 Ross St., Barrie ON L4N 1G3
Tel: 705-737-3132; *Fax:* 705-737-5045
Toll-Free: 866-374-5377
e-mail: epilepsysimcoecounty@rogers.com
www.epilepsysimcoecounty.ca
www.facebook.com/epilepsysimcoecountybarrie
twitter.com/simcoeepilepsy
Chief Officer(s):
Sue Donovan, Executive Director

Southeastern Ontario
#205, 920 Princess St., Kingston ON K7L 1H1
Tel: 613-542-6222; *Fax:* 613-548-4162
Toll-Free: 866-374-5377
e-mail: admin@epilepsyresource.org
www.epilepsyresource.org
www.facebook.com/EpilepsyResourceCentre
twitter.com/EpilepsyResourc
Chief Officer(s):
Tom Coke, Executive Director
tcoke@epilepsyresource.org

Timmins
733 Ross Ave. East, Timmins ON P4N 8S8
Tel: 705-264-2933; *Fax:* 705-264-0350
Toll-Free: 866-374-5377
e-mail: info@seizurebraininjurycentre.com
www.seizurebraininjurycentre.com
www.facebook.com/seizurebraininjurycentre
twitter.com/letstalkbrain
Chief Officer(s):
Rhonda Latendresse, Executive Director
rhondal@seizurebraininjurycentre.com
Jacques Arbic, President

Toronto
#210, 468 Queen St. East, Toronto ON M5A 1T7
Tel: 416-964-9095; *Fax:* 416-964-2492
e-mail: info@epilepsytoronto.org
www.epilepsytoronto.org
www.facebook.com/epilepsytoronto
twitter.com/epilepsytoronto
www.youtube.com/channel/UCTZiK0J7kSc1LR4blViMcyA
Chief Officer(s):

Geoff Bobb, Executive Director, 416-964-9095 Ext. 214
gbobb@epilepsytoronto.org

Waterloo/Wellington
#5, 165 Hollinger Cres., Kitchener ON N2K 2Z2
Tel: 519-745-2112; *Fax:* 519-745-2435
e-mail: epilepsy@epilww.com
www.epilww.com
www.facebook.com/epilww

Chief Officer(s):
Jennifer Lyon, Executive Director

Windsor/Essex County
Epilepsy Support Centre, 690 Hale St., London ON N5W 1H4
Tel: 519-890-6614
e-mail: communications@epilepsysupport.ca
epilepsysupport.ca
www.facebook.com/epilepsysupport
twitter.com/EpilepsySC
www.youtube.com/user/EpilepsyLondon

Chief Officer(s):
Mary Secco, Director, Strategic Initiatives
mary@epilepsysupport.ca

York Region
11181 Yonge St., Richmond Hill ON L4S 1L2
Tel: 905-508-5404; *Fax:* 905-508-0920
e-mail: info@epilepsyyork.org
www.epilepsyyork.org
www.facebook.com/epilepsyyorkregion
twitter.com/epilepsyyork

Chief Officer(s):
Claudia Cozza, Executive Director
ccozza@epilepsyyork.org

QUÉBEC

Association québécoise de l'épilepsie
#204, 1650, boul de Maisonneuve ouest, Montréal QC H3H 2P3
Tél: 514-875-5595; *Téléc:* 514-875-6734
Courriel: aqe@cooptel.qc.ca
www.associationquebecoiseepilepsie.com
Aperçu: *Dimension:* moyenne; *Envergure:* provinciale; Organisme sans but lucratif; fondée en 1960
Mission: Veiller au mieux-être des personnes épileptiques et à leurs familles; promouvoir les droits des personnes épileptiques; sensibiliser le public à l'épilepsie; promouvoir l'intégration scolaire et au travail

Épilepsie - Section de Québec
1411, boulevard Père-Lelièvre, Québec QC G1M 1N7
Tél: 418-524-8752; *Téléc:* 418-524-5882
Courriel: epilepsiequebec@megaquebec.net
www.epilepsiequebec.com

Membre(s) du bureau directeur:
Nicole Bélanger, Directrice générale

Épilepsie Abitibi-Témiscamingue
115, rue du Terminus ouest, Rouyn-Noranda QC J9X 2P7
Tél: 819-279-7992
Courriel: epilepsieat@yahoo.fr
www.ae-at.qc.ca

Membre(s) du bureau directeur:
Jacques Bouffard, Président

Épilepsie Côte-Nord
652, av Dequen, Sept-Iles QC G4R 2R5
Tél: 418-968-2507
Ligne sans frais: 866-968-2507
Courriel: epilepsiecn@globetrotter.net

Épilepsie Gaspésie-sud
176, boul. Gérard D. Lévesque Ouest, Paspébiac QC G0C 2K0
Tél: 418-752-6819; *Téléc:* 418-752-5959
Courriel: info@epilepsiegaspesiesud.com
www.epilepsiegaspesiesud.com

Membre(s) du bureau directeur:
Gilles Aspirot, Président

Épilepsie Granby et régions

17, boul. Mountain nord, 2e étage, Granby QC J2G 9M5
Tél: 450-378-8876
Ligne sans frais: 866-374-5377
Courriel: info@epilepsiegranby.com
www.epilepsiegranby.com

Membre(s) du bureau directeur:
Anne Roy, Coordonnatrice, Membres
anie@epilepsiegranby.com

Épilepsie Outaouais
#111, 115, boul Sacré-Coeur, Gatineau QC J8X 1C5
Tél: 819-595-3331; *Téléc:* 819-771-3286
Courriel: EpilepsieOutaouais@videotron.ca
www.epilepsieoutaouais.org

Membre(s) du bureau directeur:
Roger Hébert, Directeur général

Épilepsie régionale pour personnes épileptiques de la région 02
CP 1633, 371, rue Racine est, Chicoutimi QC G7H 6Z5
Tél: 418-549-9888; *Téléc:* 418-549-3547
Courriel: arpe@bellnet.ca

Membre(s) du bureau directeur:
Nicole Bouchard, Coordonnatrice

Local Associations

ALBERTA

Edmonton Epilepsy Association (EEA)
11215 Groat Rd. NW, Edmonton AB T5M 3K2
Tel: 780-488-9600; *Fax:* 780-447-5486
Toll-Free: 866-374-5377
e-mail: info@edmontonepilepsy.org
www.edmontonepilepsy.org
Overview: A small local charitable organization founded in 1961
Mission: To ensure the well-being of persons with epilepsy through increased public awareness & education to further to address specific concerns both personal & social that these individuals experience
Member of: United Way
Affliation(s): Canadian Epilepsy Alliance; Epilepsy Canada
Chief Officer(s):
Gary Sampley, Executive Director/COO
gary@edmontonepilepsy.org
Publications:
• Focus on Epilepsy [a publication of the Edmonton Epilepsy Association]
Type: Newsletter; *Frequency:* s-a.
Profile: Association news, stories from members

Epilepsy Association of Calgary / Association d'épilepsie de Calgary
4112 - 4th St. NW, Calgary AB T2K 1A2
Tel: 403-230-2764; *Fax:* 403-230-5766
Toll-Free: 866-374-5377
e-mail: info@epilepsycalgary.com
www.epilepsycalgary.com
www.facebook.com/EpilepgyCalgary
twitter.com/epilepsycalgary
Overview: A small local charitable organization founded in 1955
Mission: To address community needs related to epilepsy; to improve the quality of life of persons with epilepsy through a broad range of programs, education, advocacy, support
Affliation(s): Canadian Epilepsy Alliance/Alliance Canadienne d'Epilepsié
Chief Officer(s):
Kathy Fyfe, Executive Director
kathyf@epilepsycalgary.com
Publications:
• Epigram [a publication of Epilepsy Association of Calgary]
Type: Newsletter; *Frequency:* Irregular
Profile: News, updates, & important dates

Central Alberta Office
4811 - 48th St., Red Deer AB T4N 1S6
Tel: 403-358-3358; *Fax:* 403-358-3595

Chief Officer(s):
Norma Jaskela, Program Coordinator
centralabinfo@epilepsycalgary.com

BRITISH COLUMBIA

Victoria Epilepsy & Parkinson's Centre Society
#202, 1640 Oak Bay Ave., Victoria BC V8R 1B2
Tel: 250-475-6677; *Fax:* 250-475-6619
e-mail: help@vepc.bc.ca
www.vepc.bc.ca
twitter.com/VEPC
Overview: A small local charitable organization founded in 1983
Mission: To provide education & support services to those affected by epilepsy or Parkinson's Disease, individuals & family members; To promote excellence in care through collaboration with the health care community; To increase public understanding of these conditions & expand awareness & support of the services provided
Affiliation(s): Canadian Epilepsy Alliance
Chief Officer(s):
Mira Laurence, Executive Director
 mlaurence@vepc.bc.ca
Della Cronkrite, Office Manager
Shannon Oatway, Coordinator, Community Education & Awareness

SASKATCHEWAN

Epilepsy Saskatoon
PO Box 1792, Saskatoon SK S7K 4J1
Tel: 306-665-1939
www.facebook.com/EpilepsySaskatoon
Overview: A small local charitable organization founded in 1978
Mission: To improve the quality of life of persons with epilepsy through a broad range of programs, education, support of research & the delivery of needed services to people with epilepsy & their families
Member of: Canadian Epilepsy Alliance

Provincial Libraries

Epilepsy & Seizure Association of Manitoba
#4, 1805 Main St., Winnipeg, MB R2V 2A2
Tel: 204-783-0466; *Fax:* 204-784-9689
esam@manitobaepilepsy.org
www.manitobaepilepsy.org

Diane Wall, President

Epilepsy Association of Calgary
4112 - 4th St. NW, Calgary, AB T2K 1A2
Tel: 403-230-2764; *Fax:* 403-230-5766
Toll-Free: 866-374-5379
info@epilepsycalgary.com
www.epilepsycalgary.com
Social Media: twitter.com/epilepsycalgary
Kathy Fyfe, Executive Director
 kathyf@epilepsycalgary.com

Headway Victoria Epilepsy & Parkinson's Centre Society
#202, 1640 Oak Bay Ave., Victoria, BC V8R 1B2
Tel: 250-475-6677; *Fax:* 250-475-6619
help@vepc.bc.ca
www.vepc.bc.ca
Mira Laurence, Executive Director
 mlaurence@vepc.bc.ca

Montréal Neurological Institute & Hospital
#285, 3801, rue University, Montréal, QC H3A 2B4
Tel: 514-398-1980; *Fax:* 514-398-5077
library.neuro@mcgill.ca
Social Media: www.facebook.com/MNIHLIB
Collection: Neurosciences collection
Alex Amar, Librarian
 alex.amar@muhc.mcgill.ca

Local Hospitals & Health Centres

QUÉBEC

MONTRÉAL: Centre universitaire de santé McGill - Hôpital neurologique de Montréal
Affiliée à: CIUSSS du Centre-Ouest-de-l'Île-de-Montréal
3801, rue University, Montréal, QC H3A 2B4
Tél: 514-398-6644
www.mni.mcgill.ca

Nombre de lits: 65 lits de soins de courte durée; 14 lits de soins neurologiques intensifs
Guy Rouleau, Directeur général

Fabry Disease

Cause
Fabry disease is a rare, inherited fat storage disorder caused by deficiency of alpha-galactosidase A, an enzyme involved in the biodegradation of lipids (fats). As abnormal storage of the fatty compound increases with time, blood vessels become narrowed, leading to decreased blood flow. The problem occurs in all blood vessels in the body, but affects in particular the skin, kidneys, heart, brain, inner ear and nervous system.

Fabry is a faulty gene in the X chromosome. A mother with the faulty gene has a 50 percent chance of passing the faulty gene to her children. A father with the faulty gene will pass it to all his daughters, but to none of his sons.

Symptoms
In children, Fabry disease begins with pain and burning sensations in the hands and feet that is worse with exercise and hot weather. Other symptoms include a dark red rash (known as angiokeratomas) that can appear anywhere on the body, but is usually found between the knees and belly button, decreased ability to perspire, tinnitus (ringing in the ears) and cloudiness of the cornea, which usually does not affect vision.

As those with Fabry disease grow older, they may have impaired circulation, leading to early heart attacks and strokes. As kidneys become more involved, many patients require kidney transplants or dialysis. Gastrointestinal symptoms include frequent bowel movements shortly after eating.

Prevalence
Fabry disease is called an orphan disease because its rate of occurrence is less than 1 in 200,000. It is estimated that there are between 200 and 400 Canadians with Fabry disease, most of whom live in Nova Scotia, since that is where a "carrier" of the disease first moved 16 generations ago.

Treatment Options
Since some of the symptoms of Fabry disease are common to other disorders, the disease is sometimes mistakenly diagnosed as multiple sclerosis, arthritis, Crohn's disease or rheumatic fever. To diagnose Fabry disease, a thorough medical history is taken and a physical exam is performed. A blood test is usually done to measure the level of alpha-galactosidase A in the blood. Since women sometimes show low to normal levels of alpha-galactosidase A, mutation analysis is the definitive method of diagnosis for females.

There is no cure for Fabry disease and treatment typically deals with controlling its symptoms. Pain in hands and feet responds to several medications. Gastrointestinal hyperactivity may be controlled by taking a nutritional supplement.

In Canada, enzyme replacement therapy (ERT) was approved in 2004. ERT is given intravenously once every two weeks either at home or in hospital, and reduces lipid (fat) accumulation in many types of cells. However, the cost of ERT is high, and research shows that its usefulness may be limited.

In January 2013, researchers in Canada launched the first gene therapy trial in the world for Fabry disease. In this trial, stem cells will be removed from the blood of a person with Fabry disease. Then, a working copy of the gene that makes the enzyme Fabry disease patients are missing will be inserted into the stem cells using a modified virus (lentivirus). The goal is that the new working copy of the gene will make the missing enzyme when the stem cells are transplanted back into the patient. Researchers hope that one day this therapy will provide a cure for Fabry disease.

Currently, patients with Fabry disease usually survive into adulthood but have a reduced life expectancy.

National Associations

Canadian Association of Centres for the Management of Hereditary Metabolic Diseases
c/o Pierre Allard, Secretary-Treasurer, Hôpital Ste-Justine, Service de génétique médicale, pièce 6711, 3175 Côte Ste-Catherine, Montréal, QC H3T 1C5

www.garrod.ca

Also Known As: GARROD Association
Overview: A small national organization
Mission: To coordinate of the management of inherited metabolic disorders; to provide a forum for the exchange of information & develops guidelines for the investigation & treatment of the diseases.
Affliation(s): Western Group of Investigators of Inborn Errors of Metabolism; Canadian Paediatric Society; Canadian Dietetic Association; Canadian Society for Metabolic Diseases; CORD (Canadian Organization of Rare Disorders); Canadian College of Medical Geneticists (CCMG); SIMD; National Food Distribution Centre for the Treatment of Hereditary Metabolic Diseases
Chief Officer(s):
Sylvia Stockler, Chair/President
 sstockler@cw.bc.ca
Pierre Allard, Secretary-Treasurer, 514-345-4931
 pierre.allard.hsj@ssss.gouv.qc.ca

Canadian Fabry Association / L'association canadienne de fabry
52 Glen Forest Dr., Hamilton ON L8K 5V8

www.fabrycanada.com

Overview: A medium-sized national organization
Mission: To educate the public & offer information on treatments; To encourage & support research; To increase facilities for those suffering from the disease
Chief Officer(s):
Gina Costantino, President

Fibromyalgia

Fibromyalgia (FM) is a condition of widespread muscular pain and fatigue. The pain ranges from mild discomfort to complete disability and may vary from day to day.

Cause
The exact cause of fibromyalgia is unknown, but it is likely that a number of factors are involved. Since fibromyalgia tends to run in families, it is possible that there is a genetic link to the disorder. Other triggers for fibromyalgia may include infections, physical or emotional trauma, an increased sensitivity in the brain to pain signals and sleep disturbances. Physical over-exertion, changes in weather, drafty environments, stress, depression and hormonal changes can all contribute to flare-ups in FM symptoms.

Symptoms
Widespread pain is the main symptom of fibromyalgia. Most people with FM wake up in pain. Some find that their pain improves as the day progresses, and then gets worse at night, while others experience pain all the time. FM also causes a decreased sense of energy, disturbances of sleep and varying degrees of anxiety and depression. Other medical conditions sometimes associated with fibromyalgia include tension headaches, migraine, irritable bowel syndrome, temporomandibular joint (TMJ) disorders, premenstrual tension syndrome, chronic fatigue syndrome, cold intolerance and restless leg syndrome.

Prevalence
It is estimated that close to 400,000 Canadians have been diagnosed with fibromyalgia, more than half of whom are between the ages of 45 and 64. Over 80 percent of people who are affected by fibromyalgia are women.

Treatment Options
A physician's diagnosis of FM is usually based on the following criteria: widespread musculoskeletal pain for at least three months and tenderness at 11 or more of 18 specific tender points which include the thighs, shoulders, rib cage, neck, lower back, knees, chest, buttocks and elbows. Other tests may also be done to rule out conditions with similar symptoms.

There is currently no commonly accepted cure for this condition, therefore treatment for FM is aimed at relieving pain and helping the individual cope with the symptoms. Aspirin and other drugs used to treat musculoskeletal pain partially improve symptoms. Antidepressant drugs, taken in low doses, have been shown to provide restorative sleep and to ease pain. Anti-convulsants are also sometimes helpful in reducing pain. Patients may also benefit from regular aerobic exercises, local applications of heat, gentle massage and reduced stress in their lives.

Fibromyalgia may remit spontaneously with decreased stress, but can recur at frequent intervals or become chronic.

See also Chronic Fatigue Syndrome

Provincial Associations

BRITISH COLUMBIA

MEFM Myalgic Encephalomyelitis & Fibromyalgia Society of British Columbia
PO Box 462, 916 West Broadway Ave., Vancouver BC V5Z 1K7

Tel: 604-878-7707
Toll-Free: 888-353-6322
e-mail: info@mefm.bc.ca
www.mefm.bc.ca

Merged from: British Columbia Fibromyalgia Society; Myalgic Encephalomyelitis Society of British Columbia
Overview: A medium-sized provincial organization
Mission: To provide support to people with (ME) Myalgic Encephalomyelitis, (Chronic Fatique Syndrome) & (FM) Fibromyalgia & their families; to help educate physicians, paramedical professionals, family members & the community at large regarding ME & FM; to promote research aimed at improving treatment & ultimately finding a cure; to help to encourage early diagnosis & effective treatment

ONTARIO

Myalgic Encephalomyelitis Association of Ontario (MEAO)
#370, 170 Donway West, Toronto ON M3C 2G3

Tel: 416-222-8820
Toll-Free: 877-632-6682
e-mail: info@meao.ca
www.meao.ca

Overview: A small provincial charitable organization founded in 1992
Mission: To support individuals who have Myalgic Encephalomyelitis/Chronic Fatigue Syndrome & their families; to provide medical professionals, government & the general public with information on the illness & its effects & consequences

National ME/FM Action Network / Réseau national d'action EM/FM encéphalomyélite myalgique/fibromyalgie
#512, 33 Banner Rd., Nepean ON K2H 8V7

Tel: 613-829-6667; *Fax:* 613-829-8518
e-mail: mefminfo@mefmaction.com
www.mefmaction.net
www.facebook.com/MEFMActionNetwork
twitter.com/mefmaction

Also Known As: Myalgic Encephalomyelitis/Chronic Fatigue Syndrome & Fibromyalgia Action Network

Overview: A small provincial charitable organization founded in 1993
Mission: To offer support, advocacy, education & research into the many, varied, anomalies connected with Myalgic Encephalomyelitis/Chronic Fatigue Syndrome & Fibromyalgia (ME/FM)
Member of: National Voluntary Health Organization; Health Charities Council of Canada
Affliation(s): Volunteer Ottawa; Volunteer Canada
Chief Officer(s):
Lydia E. Neilson, M.S.M., Founder & CEO

QUÉBEC

Association québécoise de la fibromyalgie (AQF)
#225, 2465, rue Honoré-Mercier, Laval QC H7L 2S9
Tél: 450-933-6530
Courriel: fqf@fibromyalgie-fqf.org
www.aqf.ca

Nom précédent: Association de la fibromyalgie du Québec
Aperçu: *Dimension:* moyenne; *Envergure:* provinciale; fondée en 1989
Mission: Sensibiliser la population face à la maladie par la défense des droits des personnes atteintes dans les différentes régions du Québec

SASKATCHEWAN

Fibromyalgia Association of Saskatchewan (FMAS)
PO Box 7525, Saskatoon SK S7K 4L4
Tel: 306-343-3627
Overview: A small provincial charitable organization founded in 1994
Mission: To improve the quality of life for those directly or indirectly affected by fibromyalgia syndrome (FMS) & chronic fatigue syndrome (CFS).
Affliation(s): FM-CFS Canada

Local Associations

MANITOBA

Fibromyalgia Support Group of Winnipeg, Inc.
c/o SMD Clearinghouse, 825 Sherbrook St., Winnipeg MB R3A 1M5
Tel: 204-975-3037
e-mail: info@fmswinnipeg.com
www.fmswinnipeg.com

Also Known As: Fibromyalgia Syndrome Winnipeg
Overview: A small local charitable organization founded in 1992
Mission: To sponsor & promote educational services to all persons with fibromyalgia, as well as families, friends, health care professionals & the general public; To promote & sponsor scientific & clinical research relating to causes, treatments & cure of fibromyalgia
Member of: SMD Self-Help Clearinghouse

QUÉBEC

Association de la fibromyalgie de la Montérégie
#205, 570 boul Roland-Therrien, Longueuil QC J4H 3V7
Tél: 450-928-1261
Ligne sans frais: 888-928-1261
Courriel: info@fibromyalgiemonteregie.ca
www.fibromyalgiemonteregie.ca

Aperçu: *Dimension:* petite; *Envergure:* locale
Mission: Fournir des informations et des soutien pour des personnes atteintes de fibromyalgie
Membre(s) du bureau directeur:
Zina Manoka, Coordonnatrice, Services aux membres

Association de la Fibromyalgie des Laurentides
366, rue Laviolette, Saint-Jérôme QC J7Y 2S9
Tél: 450-569-7766; *Téléc:* 450-569-7769
Ligne sans frais: 877-705-7766
Courriel: afl@videotron.ca
www.fibromyalgie-des-laurentides.ca
www.facebook.com/376578422426237
twitter.com/FibromyaLaurent

Aperçu: *Dimension:* moyenne; *Envergure:* locale; Organisme sans but lucratif; fondée en 1995
Membre de: Fédération québécoise de la fibromyalgie; Regroupement des Organismes communautaires des Laurentides; Réseau de concertation pour les personnes handicapées des Laurentides

Membre(s) du bureau directeur:
Lise Cloutier, Directrice générale

Association de la fibromyalgie région Ile-De-Montréal
CP 48681, Succ. Outremont, Montréal QC H2V 4T9
Tél: 438-496-7448
Courriel: info@afim.qc.ca
www.afim.qc.ca
www.facebook.com/fibromyalgie.montreal
www.youtube.com/channel/UCCJ__R9NjtU_1-XBrYEOuCA

Aperçu: *Dimension:* petite; *Envergure:* locale; fondée en 1995
Mission: Défendre les intérêts des personnes atteintes de fibromyalgie dans la région de l'Ile-de-Montréal
Membre de: Société québécoise de la fibromyalgie
Membre(s) du bureau directeur:
Alain Larivière, Président

Gastrointestinal Disorders

The digestive tract is responsible for taking food into the body, processing it into simple chemicals that can be absorbed to nourish the body, and expelling the remainder.

Motility disorders of the gastrointestinal (GI) tract are conditions in which there is a failure of normal top-to-bottom movement of gastric contents. In Canada, it is estimated that more than 20 million people are affected by digestive disorders. The incidence of gastrointestinal ulcers in this country is the highest in the world. Every year, close to 30,000 Canadians die of digestive system diseases.

Gastro-Esophageal Reflux Disease (GERD)

In reflux (also known as GERD, or gastro-esophageal reflux disease), the food content moves from the stomach back into the esophagus, causing irritation, inflammation, and sometimes even ulceration of the esophagus. It is a problem in infants but also occurs in adults, especially with advancing age. Occasionally, an ulcer may develop in a segment of the GI tract, typically in the stomach or duodenum.

Symptoms
People suffering from GERD may experience heartburn, indigestion, problems swallowing, hoarseness or coughing, regurgitation, weight loss and tarry, black stools. Children with GERD may fail to grow.

Treatment Options
Diagnosis of gastrointestinal disorders is usually made on the basis of symptoms presented. However, depending on the disorder, there are tests that can be done to confirm the diagnosis. For GERD, tests such as an esophagram and upper GI series (X-rays of the esophagus and upper gastrointestinal tract), a gastroscopy (a camera investigation of the upper gastrointestinal tract), an esophageal motility study (a measurement of esophageal contractions) and a 24-hour pH test (a measurement of acidity) can be used to evaluate the esophagus.

For GERD, medical therapy is the preferred treatment and may include antacids, proton pump inhibitors, prokinetics and histamine receptor antagonists. For people with particularly troubling symptoms, surgery may be an option.

Peptic Ulcer Disease

Cause
An infectious agent, H. pylori, plays a central role in peptic ulcer disease.

Symptoms
Peptic ulcers are often characterized by indigestion, burning pain in the upper abdomen, nausea, weight loss and vomiting.

Prevalence

Approximately 8 to 10 million are infected with H. pylori.

Treatment Options

Tests for peptic ulcers may also include a gastroscopy and an upper GI series, as well as a blood test and a breath test. The recommended treatment for peptic ulcers is a combination of two antibiotics (to get rid of the H. pylori infection), along with an acid-suppressing drug such as a proton pump inhibitor.

Achalasia

In achalasia, a rare disorder, the normal movement of food down the GI tract by peristalsis is disrupted, and contents of the esophagus are unable to move into the stomach. As a result, the person chokes on food or liquid. Although achalasia can occur at any age, it mostly affects middle-aged and older adults.

Symptoms

People affected by achalasia may experience coughing, difficulty swallowing, heartburn, regurgitation, chest pain and weight loss.

Treatment Options

A diagnosis of achalasia is often confirmed using tests such as a gastroscopy, an esophageal motility study and upper GI series.

The main goal of achalasia therapy is to reduce the pressure in the lower esophageal sphincter. This can be achieved with medication (long-acting nitrates or calcium channel blockers) or surgery.

Hirschsprung's disease

Cause

Other motility disorders reflect the bowel's inability to move its contents forward properly. Children may be born with Hirschsprung's disease in which peristalsis is absent or abnormal in the large bowel, resulting in partial or complete obstruction. This disease occurs more frequently in males than females, and is the cause of 25 percent of intestinal blockages in newborns.

Symptoms

Symptoms of Hirschsprung's disease in infants may include difficulty with bowel movements, explosive but infrequent stools, jaundice, trouble feeding, poor weight gain and vomiting. In older children with Hirschsprung's disease symptoms may include worsening constipation, swollen belly, malnutrition and slow growth.

Treatment Options

To help diagnose Hirschsprung's disease, tests including abdominal X-ray, rectal biopsy and anal manometry (a procedure where a balloon is inflated in the rectum to measure pressure) may be used. The treatment for Hirschsprung's disease is surgery to remove the abnormal section of the colon.

Irritable bowel syndrome

The most common motility disorder in adults is called irritable bowel syndrome; also known as functional bowel or spastic colitis, it causes variable degrees of abdominal pain and bloating, diarrhea and constipation, and affects significantly more women than men.

Symptoms

Irritable bowel syndrome symptoms may include abdominal pain, gas, bloating, cramps, irregular bowel patterns, diarrhea or constipation, mucus within the stool, heartburn and nausea.

Prevalence

Around five million Canadians suffer from irritable bowel syndrome.

Treatment Options

A blood test, stool sample and a colonoscopy (a procedure where a flexible tube with a video camera at the end is used to look at the colon) may also be used to help rule out other diseases in the diagnosis of irritable bowel syndrome.

People with irritable bowel syndrome may be able to reduce their symptoms by eating a low-fat, high-fiber diet, reducing stress and exercising. Medication may also be used to prevent diarrhea and reduce pain.

Diverticular disease

Cause

In diverticular disease, outpouchings in the walls of the lower GI tract, called diverticula, sometimes trap nutrient waste, and may become infected, bleed and rupture. The major risk factor for diverticular disease is advanced age.

Symptoms

People suffering from diverticular disease may experience abdominal pain (usually on the lower left side) and constipation or diarrhea.

Prevalence

More than 130,000 Canadians have diverticular disease.

Treatment Options

A CT scan is the most common method used to diagnose diverticular disease. Antibiotics are usually used to treat mild cases of diverticular disease. In more serious cases, surgery may be required.

Hemochromatosis

Cause

The digestive tract may fail in its primary task of absorbing nutrients, known as malabsorption syndromes. Rarely, it will absorb too much of something. In hemochromatosis, for instance, the bowel takes in too much iron from the diet, and the excess is stored in and damages the liver, pancreas, heart and gonads. More commonly, the body absorbs too little nutrient rather than too much.

Symptoms

Hemochromatosis symptoms may include fatigue, joint pain, abdominal pain, darkening of the skin, loss of sexual desire, loss of body hair and weight loss.

Treatment Options

Blood tests that measure iron levels and liver function tests may be used to help diagnose hemochromatosis. The goal of therapy for hemochromatosis is to remove excess iron from the body. A procedure called phlebotomy where a certain amount of blood is removed from the body each week is used to achieve and maintain normal iron levels.

Lactose intolerance

Lactose intolerance is an inability to digest a carbohydrate in dairy products.

Symptoms

People affected by lactose intolerance may experience nausea, diarrhea, bloating, gas and cramps.

Prevalence

Over seven million Canadians are affected by lactose intolerance.

Treatment Options

The simplest way of diagnosing lactose intolerance is to remove all lactose products from the diet for one to two weeks and see if symptoms disappear. People who are lactose intolerant should avoid dairy products. Taking lactase enzymes can help reduce the effects of lactose intolerance.

Gastrointestinal disorders can interfere with an individual's personal and professional life. However, with proper diagnosis and appropriate treatment, most people with gastrointestinal disorders can find relief for their symptoms.

National Associations

Canadian Association for Enterostomal Therapy (CAET) / Association canadienne des stomathérapeutes
66 Leopolds Dr., Ottawa ON K1V 7E3

Fax: 613-834-6351
Toll-Free: 888-739-5072
e-mail: office@caet.ca
www.caet.ca

Overview: A small national charitable organization founded in 1981
Mission: To promote high standards for nursing practice in the area of enterostomal therapy
Chief Officer(s):
Paulo DaRosa, President
  paulo_darosa@rogers.com
Elise Rodd-Nielsen, Treasurer
  eliserodd@hotmail.com
Catherine Harley, Executive Director
  catherine.harley@sympatico.ca
Publications:
• CAET [Canadian Association for Enterostomal Therapy] Membership Directory
Type: Directory
• The Link: The Official Publication of the CAET [Canadian Association for Enterostomal Therapy]
Type: Newsletter; *Frequency:* 3 pa; *Accepts Advertising*; *Price:* Free to CAET members
Profile: Reports, research projects, clinical papers, review articles, & industry news

Canadian Association of Gastroenterology / Association canadienne de gastroentérologie
#224, 1540 Cornwall Rd., Oakville ON L6J 7W5

Tel: 905-829-2504; *Fax:* 905-829-0242
Toll-Free: 888-780-0007
e-mail: general@cag-acg.org
www.cag-acg.org
www.linkedin.com/company/canadian-association-of-gastroenterology
www.facebook.com/canadianassociationofgastroenterology
twitter.com/CanGastroAssn

Overview: A small national organization founded in 1962
Mission: To support & engage in the study of gastroenterology; To promote patient care, research, teaching & professional development in the field; To promote & maintain the highest ethical standards of practice
Affliation(s): Canadian Medical Association; World Organization of Gastroenterology
Chief Officer(s):
Paul Sinclair, Executive Director
Sandra Daniels, Senior Manager
Cathy Mancini, Office Administrator

Canadian Digestive Health Foundation (CDHF) / Fondation canadienne for la promotion de la santé digestive
#455, 2525 Old Bronte Rd., Oakville ON L6M 4J2

Tel: 905-847-2002
www.cdhf.ca
www.linkedin.com/company/649009
www.facebook.com/CDHFdn
twitter.com/TheCDHF
www.youtube.com/user/CDHFtube

Overview: A medium-sized national charitable organization founded in 1994 overseen by Canadian Association of Gastroenterology

Mission: To raise funds for the protection, promotion, & improvement of digestive health
Chief Officer(s):
Richard Fedorak, President
Catherine Mulvale, Executive Director
Publications:
• Canadian Digestive Health Foundation Newsletter
Type: Newsletter
Profile: Current information from digestive health experts across Canada

GI (Gastrointestinal) Society
#231, 3665 Kingsway, Vancouver BC V5R 5W2

Tel: 604-873-4876; *Fax:* 604-875-4429
Toll-Free: 866-600-4875
www.badgut.org
www.facebook.com/CISociety
twitter.com/GISociety
www.youtube.com/user/badgutcanada

Overview: A medium-sized national organization
Mission: To improve the lives of people with GI and liver conditions, support research, advocate for appropriate patient access to healthcare & promote gastrointestinal & liver health
Chief Officer(s):
Lynda Cranston, Chairperson
Gail Attara, Co-Founder & President/CEO

Ostomy Canada Society
#210, 5800 Ambler Dr., Mississauga ON L4W 4J4

Tel: 905-212-7111; *Fax:* 905-212-9002
Toll-Free: 888-969-9698
e-mail: info1@ostomycanada.ca
www.ostomycanada.ca
www.linkedin.com/company/united-ostomy-association-of-canada-inc-
www.facebook.com/OstomyCanada
twitter.com/OstomyCanada
www.youtube.com/user/ostomycanada

Previous Name: United Ostomy Association of Canada
Overview: A medium-sized national charitable organization founded in 1997
Mission: To assist all persons with gastrointestinal or urinary diversions, as well as their families & caregivers, by providing emotional & practical support & help, information & instruction
Affiliation(s): United Ostomy Association - USA
Chief Officer(s):
Ann Ivol, President
Carol Wells, Secretary

Provincial Associations

ONTARIO

Ontario Association of Gastroenterology (OAG)
#210, 2800 - 14 Ave., Markham ON L3R 0E4

Tel: 416-494-7233; *Fax:* 416-491-1670
Toll-Free: 866-560-7585
e-mail: info@gastro.on.ca
www.gastro.on.ca
twitter.com/ontario_gastros

Overview: A small provincial organization
Mission: Serves the practice of gastroenterology in Ontario, promoting, maintaining & improving its knowledge & standards; Represents Ontario gastroenterologists in discussions, meetings & communications with other organizations
Chief Officer(s):
Melonie Hart, Director, Operations

QUÉBEC

Association des gastro-entérologues du Québec (AGEQ)
CP 216, Succ. Desjardins, 2, Complexe Desjardins, Montréal QC H5B 1G8

Tél: 514-350-5112; *Téléc:* 514-350-5146
www.ageq.net

Aperçu: *Dimension:* petite; *Envergure:* !E!; fondée en 1965 surveillé par Fédération des médecins spécialistes du Québec

Mission: D'informer et de formations aux médecins de première ligne, aux patients souffrant de pathologies gastro-intestinales et aux autres médecins intéressés par la gastro-entérologie; de créer des liens avec la communauté médicale internationale

Membre(s) du bureau directeur:
Josée Parent, Présidente
Sylvie Bergeron, Directrice, Administration
sbergeron@fmsq.org

Local Associations

ONTARIO

Zane Cohen Centre for Digestive Diseases Familial Gastrointestinal Cancer Registry (FGICR)
Mount Sinai Hospital, Zane Cohen Centre, PO Box 24, 60 Murray St., Toronto ON M5T 3L9

Tel: 416-586-4800; *Fax:* 416-586-5924
Toll-Free: 877-586-5112
e-mail: zcc@mtsinai.on.ca
www.zanecohencentre.ca

Previous Name: Familial GI Cancer Registry
Overview: A small local organization founded in 1980
Mission: The Registry is an interdisciplinary program dedicated to the specialty care of families affected with rare forms of inherited colorectal cancer.
Publications:
• Network [a publication of the Familial Gastrointestinal Cancer Registry]
Type: Newsletter; *Editor:* Terri Berk

International Associations

Irritable Bowel Syndrome Self Help & Support Group
PO Box 94074, Toronto ON M4N 3R1

Tel: 416-932-3311; *Fax:* 416-932-8909
www.ibsgroup.org
www.facebook.com/ibsgroup
twitter.com/ibsgroup

Also Known As: IBS Self Help Group
Overview: A medium-sized international organization founded in 1987
Mission: To educate & provide support for people who have IBS; To use membership to encourage both medical & pharmaceutical research to make the lives of those with IBS easier
Member of: Self Help Resource Centre; American Self-Help Clearinghouse
Affliation(s): IBS Association
Chief Officer(s):
Jeffrey Roberts, Founder

National Publications

Canadian Journal of Gastroenterology & Hepatology (CJGH) / Journal Canadien de Gastroenterologie
Owned By: Hindawi Publishing Corp.
#3070, 315 Madison Ave., New York, NY

cjgh@hindawi.com

Frequency: Monthly
Official journal of the Canadian Association of Gastroenterology and the Canadian Association for the Study of the Liver.
John Marshall, Editor-in-chief
Eric Yoshida, Editor-in-chief

Canadian Journal of General Internal Medicine
Owned By: Dougmar Publishing Group
Canadian Society of Internal Medicine, #200, 421 Gilmour St., Ottawa, ON K2P 0R5

Tel: 613-422-5977; *Fax:* 613-249-3326
Toll-Free: 855-893-2746

Frequency: 4 times a year
Official publication of the Canadian Society of Internal Medicine.
Scott Bryant, Managing Editor, sbryant@dougmargroup.com

Gaucher Disease

Gaucher disease is an inherited disorder of metabolism of fats. These metabolic products can not be broken down properly because of a deficiency of an enzyme called glucocerebrosidase. The fatty substance accumulates in cells that then build up in the spleen, liver, bone marrow and, sometimes, the lungs.

There are three types of Gaucher disease. Type 1 (the most common type) affects the organs and tissues but not the brain. Type 2 is very rare. It progresses rapidly, affecting the brain and organs, and is usually fatal. Type 3 (also rare) affects the brain and organs, but progresses more slowly, and is less severe than Type 2.

Cause
Gaucher disease is an autosomal recessive genetic disorder. This means that to have the disease a person must have two abnormal genes—one inherited from each parent. If both parents are carriers of the abnormal gene, there is a one in four chance that they will have a child with Gaucher disease.

Symptoms
The symptoms of Gaucher disease, which vary from person to person and can develop in childhood or in adulthood, may include fatigue, anemia, bleeding problems (such as nosebleeds and easy bruising), enlargement of the spleen or liver, bone pain, easily fractured bones and brown pigmentation of the skin. Gaucher disease is progressive, and if left untreated, can worsen over time.

Prevalence
Gaucher disease is one of the most common lipid storage disorders. Type 1 affects approximately 1 in 40,000 to 50,000 people, while types 2 and 3 each affect fewer than 1 in 100,000.

Treatment Options
Diagnosis of Gaucher disease is confirmed by a blood test that measures glucocerebrosidase enzyme activity. DNA testing can also be done to identify gene mutations.

The treatment for Gaucher disease is enzyme replacement therapy, administered intravenously every two weeks. In more severe cases, removal of the spleen, blood transfusions or bone marrow transplantation may be necessary. Current research is aimed at genetic therapy.

Children with type 2 Gaucher disease usually do not live beyond their second year. However, life expectancy is close to normal for people with mild cases of Gaucher disease.

National Associations

Canadian Association of Centres for the Management of Hereditary Metabolic Diseases
c/o Pierre Allard, Secretary-Treasurer, Hôpital Ste-Justine, Service de génétique médicale, pièce 6711, 3175 Côte Ste-Catherine, Montréal, QC H3T 1C5

www.garrod.ca

Also Known As: GARROD Association
Overview: A small national organization
Mission: To coordinate of the management of inherited metabolic disorders; to provide a forum for the exchange of information & develops guidelines for the investigation & treatment of the diseases.
Affliation(s): Western Group of Investigators of Inborn Errors of Metabolism; Canadian Paediatric Society; Canadian Dietetic Association; Canadian Society for Metabolic Diseases; CORD (Canadian Organization of Rare Disorders); Canadian College of Medical Geneticists (CCMG); SIMD; National Food Distribution Centre for the Treatment of Hereditary Metabolic Diseases
Chief Officer(s):
Sylvia Stockler, Chair/President
sstockler@cw.bc.ca

Pierre Allard, Secretary-Treasurer, 514-345-4931
  pierre.allard.hsj@ssss.gouv.qc.ca

**Canadian Society of Endocrinology & Metabolism (CSEM) /
Société canadienne d'endocrinologie et métabolisme (SCEM)**
#1403, 222 Queen St., Ottawa ON K1P 5V9
Tel: 613-594-0005; *Fax:* 613-569-6574
e-mail: info@endo-metab.ca
www.endo-metab.ca
Overview: A small national organization founded in 1972
Mission: To advance the endocrinology & metabolism field in Canada
Chief Officer(s):
Connie Chik, President
Alice Cheng, Secretary-Treasurer

Provincial Associations

QUÉBEC

**Québec Society of Lipidology, Nutrition & Metabolism Inc.
(QSLNM) / Société québécoise de lipidologie, de nutrition et de
métabolisme (SQLNM)**
2705, boul Laurier, Sainte-Foy QC G1V 4G2
Tel: 418-656-4141; *Fax:* 418-654-2145
e-mail: sqlnm@crchul.ulaval.ca
www.lipidologie.qc.ca
Overview: A small provincial charitable organization founded in 2000
Mission: To promote training, education & research in lipidology,
nutrition, metabolism & cardiovascular health
Chief Officer(s):
Pierre Julien, PhD, President
  pierre.julien@crchul.ulaval.ca

Gender Dysphoria

With a wide scope of questions and confusion surrounding human sexuality and gender-explicit roles in the modern era, many children, adolescents and adults have been perplexed by the concepts of homosexuality and cross-gender identification. Homosexuality is a matter of sexual orientation: whether one is sexually attracted to men or women. Gender identity, in contrast, is a matter of what gender one feels oneself to be; people with gender dysphoria feel that their psychological experience conflicts with the physical body with which they were born. Gender dysphoria, formerly referred to as gender identity disorder, can have serious social and occupational repercussions.

Symptoms

Typically, boys with gender dysphoria prefer to dress as girls, fantasize and role play as females, prefer to sit while urinating, are often stressed by their penises and interact primarily with girls. Girls who exhibit gender dysphoria are often mistaken for boys due to attire and hair style, and may assert that they will develop into men. For adolescents and adults, ostracism in school and the workplace is likely to occur.

Those who have gender dysphoria are at risk of mental and physical harm resulting, not from the condition itself, but from the reactions of other people to the condition. In children, a manifestation of separation anxiety disorder, generalized anxiety disorder and symptoms of depression may result. For adolescents, depression and suicidal thoughts or ideas, as well as actual suicide attempts can result from prolonged feelings of ostracism by peers. Relationships with either one or both parents may weaken from resentment, lack of communication and misunderstanding; many with this condition may drop out of or avoid school due to peer teasing. For many, lives are built around attempts to decrease gender distress. They are often preoccupied with appearance. In extreme cases, males with the condition perform their own castration. Prostitution has been linked with the disorder because young people who are rejected by their families and ostracized by others may resort to prostitution as the only way to support themselves, a practice which increases the risk of acquiring sexually transmitted diseases. Some people with the disorder resort to substance abuse and other forms of self-abuse in an attempt to deal with the associated stress.

Prevalence

In most cases, the age of onset for gender dysphoria is in the preschool years. It should be noted, however, that gender dysphoria in childhood does not always continue into adulthood. Canadian studies show that between 2.9 percent and 20 percent of boys who exhibited gender dysphoria as children continued to experience gender incongruence in adulthood. In contrast, in adolescents who experience gender dysphoria, the persistence of the condition into adulthood is between 43.2 percent and 66 percent.

Treatment Options

There is some controversy about the diagnosis; some groups protest that their condition, like homosexuality, should not be classified as a mental illness, nor referred to as a disorder. For this reason, in the fifth edition of the Diagnostic and Statistical Manual of Mental Disorders, which was published in May 2013, the condition is no longer referred to as gender identity disorder, but as gender dysphoria. The wording of the criteria for diagnosis has also been changed. The condition is now described as "a marked incongruence between one's experienced/expressed gender and assigned gender."

Psychological assistance can help individuals to gain acceptance of themselves, and can teach methods of dealing with discrimination, prejudice and violence. Supportive counselling may also help families accept the gender identity of their family member with gender dysphoria.

Treatment for youth with gender dysphoria may include hormone blockers (medications that suppress the physical changes of puberty) and cross-sex hormone therapy (which usually begins at the age of 16). Treatment for adults may include supportive counselling and hormone replacement therapy. Some people with gender dysphoria may decide to live as members of the opposite sex; some choose to undergo sex change surgery.

To reduce the risk of depression and emotional distress and increase the chance of a happy, productive life outcome, it is crucial that people with gender dysphoria receive the support and therapy that they need.

National Associations

PFLAG Canada Inc.
251 Bank St., 2nd Fl., Ottawa ON K2P 1X3
Fax: 888-959-4128
Toll-Free: 888-530-6777
e-mail: inquiries@pflagcanada.ca
www.pflagcanada.ca
www.facebook.com/PFLAGCA
twitter.com/pflagcanada
Also Known As: Parents, Families & Friends of Lesbians & Gays
Previous Name: Parents & Friends of Lesbians & Gays (Parents
FLAG)
Overview: A medium-sized national charitable organization founded in 2003
Mission: To support individuals with questions & concerns about sexual orientation or gender identity; To make Canada a more accepting place for persons of all gender identities & sexual orientations
Chief Officer(s):
Bev Belanger, President
  president@pflagcanada.ca
Donny Potts, Vice-President
  donnypotts@pflagcanada.ca

Daniel Snoek, Treasurer
  treasurer@pflagcanada.ca
Tanya Dawson, Secretary
  secretary@pflagcanada.ca
Louis Duncan-He, Director, Marketing
  louishe@pflagcanada.ca
Steven Keddy, Director, Communications
  stevenkeddy@pflagcanada.ca
Ross Wicks, Director, Governance
  rwicks@pflagcanada.ca

Rainbow Association of Canadian Artists (Spectra Talent Contest)
Toronto ON

www.spectrashowcase.com

Overview: A small national organization founded in 2012
Mission: A community encouraging amateur artistic expression regardless of cultural background, sexual orientation &/or gender identity
Chief Officer(s):
Paul Bellini, Chair
Ralph Hamelmann, Director
  producer@spectrashowcase.com

Local Associations
MANITOBA

Rainbow Resource Centre
170 Scott St., Winnipeg MB R3L 0L3
Tel: 204-474-0212; *Fax:* 204-478-1160
Toll-Free: 855-437-8523
www.rainbowresourcecentre.org
www.facebook.com/RainbowResourceCentre
twitter.com/RainbowResCtr
www.instagram.com/rainbowresourcecentre
Also Known As: Gays for Equality
Previous Name: Campus Gay Club (University of Manitoba)
Overview: A small local charitable organization founded in 1972
Mission: To work toward an equal & diverse society, free of homophobia & discrimination, by encouraging visibility & fostering health & self-acceptance through education, support, resources & outreach
Chief Officer(s):
Mike Tutthill, Executive Director

QUÉBEC

Centre d'orientation sexuelle de l'université McGill (COSUM) / McGill University Sexual Identity Centre (MUSIC)
Dép. de psychiatrie, Hôpital général de Montréal, #A2-160, 1650, av Cedar, Montréal QC H3G 1A4
Tél: 514-934-1934; *Téléc:* 514-934-8471
Courriel: music-cosum@mcgill.ca
www.mcgill.ca/cosum
Aperçu: *Dimension:* petite; *Envergure:* locale
Mission: Offre des psychothérapies individuelles à court terme, psychothérapies de groupe & de couple ou familiales
Membre(s) du bureau directeur:
Karine J. Igartua, Psychiatre

National Libraries

Sex Information & Education Council of Canada (SIECCAN)
#400, 235 Danforth Ave., Toronto, ON M4K 1N2
Tel: 416-466-5304; *Fax:* 416-778-0785
www.sieccan.org
Alex McKay, Executive Director
Jocelyn Wentland, Project Manager & Research Associate

Provincial Libraries

Calgary Sexual Health Centre
#304, 301 - 14 St. NW, Calgary, AB T2N 2A1
Tel: 403-283-5580; *Fax:* 403-270-3209
generalmail@calgarysexualhealth.ca
www.calgarysexualhealth.ca
Social Media: www.youtube.com/user/CalgarySexualHealth;
twitter.com/yycsexualhealth;
www.facebook.com/CalgarySexualHealthCentre
Profile: CBCA offers non-judgmental support and information to help you make confident, well-informed decisions. Pregnancy options - abortion, adoption, parenting, birth control, sexually transmitted diseases (STD), sexual orientation. **Collection:** Canadian Government Publications; Parenting & Sex Education of Children; Contraception; Sexuality; Social Work; Women's Issues; Fiction; Poetry

Sexuality Education Resource Centre
#200, 226 Osborne St. North, Winnipeg, MB R3C 1V4
Tel: 204-982-7800; *Fax:* 204-982-7819
www.serc.mb.ca
Social Media: www.youtube.com/user/sercmbca;
www.facebook.com/sercmb

Genetic Disorders

Genetic disorders are a broad classification for an extensive group of diseases caused by mutations of the DNA. These abnormalities can involve a single-base mutation or the addition or subtraction of an entire chromosome.

Cause
Some gene mutations or chromosome abnormalities are heritable while others are linked to environmental factors. Most are caused by a combination of the two.

There are three categories of genetic disorders: monogenetic, multifactorial inheritance, and chromosome.

Monogenetic disorders are caused by the mutation of a single gene. They can be either dominant (one gene required from one parent) or recessive (one gene required by both parents). Examples of monogenic disorders are sickle-cell disease, cystic fibrosis, and Tay-Sachs disease.

Multifactorial inheritance disorders are caused by a combination of small inherited variations in genes and environmental factors. Heart disease, diabetes, most cancers, and spina bifida are some examples.

Chromosome disorders are caused by an excess or deficiency in the number of chromosomes, or by chromosome structural changes. They are rarely inherited. Down syndrome, the most common type of chromosome abnormality, is caused by an extra copy of chromosome 21 (trisomy 21) and results in physical and mental delays.

Symptoms
Symptoms vary greatly depending on the specific mutation (see Tay-Sachs, Spina Bifida and Down Syndrome for more details.)

Prevalence
Tay-Sachs disease is most prevalent in Ashkenazi Jews and French Canadians who live near the St. Lawrence River. In these groups, the carrier rate is about 1 in 27 in comparison to the rate of 1 in 250 in the general population.

It is estimated that 1 in 2,500 babies born in Canada have some form of spina bifida.

Approximately 45,000 Canadians have Down syndrome. The overall incidence is about 1 in every 800 births in Canada, but occurrence varies greatly with maternal age. For mothers under the age of 30, the incidence is less than 1 in 1000 live births. At age 40, it rises to 1 in 100 and increases with advancing age.

Treatment Options

Prenatal testing is possible for numerous genetic disorders including Tay-Sachs, spina bifida and Down syndrome. Methods can include in vitro blood samples, ultrasounds and amniocentesis.

There is no cure for Tay-Sachs disease, so therapy is aimed at symptom management. Treatment for children with Tay-Sachs may include anti-seizure medication, chest physiotherapy, assistive feeding devices and physical therapy.

Spina bifida requires surgery to put the spinal cord and exposed tissue back into the body. Post-surgery treatments require a united effort by a team of specialists and depend on the severity of the defect.

Down syndrome infants require early intervention programs to help develop language and cognitive, social and motor skills.

Gene therapy may offer hope in treating many genetic disorders, although scientists caution not all will be cured. It is an experimental approach to treating genetic disease where the faulty gene is fixed, replaced or supplemented with a healthy gene so that it can function normally.

National Associations

Alström Syndrome Canada
PO Box 204, RR#2, Finch ON K0C 1K0
Overview: A small national organization
Mission: To raise awareness within the medical community about the existence of Alström Syndrome & its symptoms; To raise money for research; To support the children & families living with Alström Syndrome
Affiliation(s): Alström Syndrome International
Chief Officer(s):
Randy Douglas, Director
  randydouglas@sympatico.ca

Batten Disease Support & Research Association - Canadian Chapter (BDSRA)
www.bdsra.org
www.facebook.com/bdsra
twitter.com/bdsra
Overview: A small national charitable organization founded in 1994
Chief Officer(s):
Margie Frazier, Executive Director, BDSRA
  mfrazier@bdsra.org
Bev Maxim, Canada President
  bevmaxim@yahoo.ca

Canadian Association for Williams Syndrome (CAWS)
19 Pereverzoff Pl., Prince Albert SK S6X 1A8
Tel: 306-922-3230; *Fax:* 306-922-3457
caws.sasktelwebhosting.com
Overview: A small national charitable organization founded in 1984
Mission: To support William syndrome individuals & their families; To advance education, research, & knowledge of the genetic disorder known as Williams Syndrome
Chief Officer(s):
Gloria Manhussier, Editor/Secretary
  mahussier.m@sasktel.net
Publications:
• Canadian Association for Williams Syndrome Newsletter
Type: Newsletter; *Frequency:* Quarterly
Profile: News, resources, & medical & educational information from across Canada

CAWS - Alberta
c/o Mary Kueller, 10733 St. Gabriel Rd., Edmonton AB T6A 3S7
Chief Officer(s):

Misty Kuefler, Chairperson
  MKuefler@vsm.ab.ca

CAWS - British Columbia
c/o Cindy Sanford, PO Box 26206, Richmond BC V6Y 3V3
Chief Officer(s):
Cindy Sanford, Provincial Contact, 604-564-7779
  cawsbc@yahoo.com

CAWS - Manitoba
c/o Coralee Crowe, 27 Regis Dr., Winnipeg MB R2N 1J9
Chief Officer(s):
Coralee Crowe, Vice Chair, 204-479-7734
  dcrowe@mymts.net

CAWS - New Brunswick
c/o Michelle Dobbin, 28 West Ave., Sackville NB E4L 4P1
Chief Officer(s):
Michelle Dobbin, Provincial Contact, 506-536-0821
  dobbinwm@gmail.com

CAWS - Newfoundland
c/o April Williams, 1680 A. Torbay Rd., Torbay NL A1K 1H2
Chief Officer(s):
April Williams, Provincial Contact
  aprildswilliams@hotmail.com

CAWS - Nova Scotia
c/o Christena Cote, NS
Tel: 902-422-8670

CAWS - Ontario
c/o Monique & John Plessas, 163 Wolverleigh Blvd., Toronto ON M4C 1S1
Tel: 416-269-7030
Chief Officer(s):
Monique Plessas, Toronto Contact
John Plessas, Toronto Contact
  momslilangel@rogers.com

CAWS - Québec
c/o Jocelyne Z'Graggen, 108, av 59ème, Saint-Hippolyte QC J8A 1N9
Chief Officer(s):
Jocelyne Z'Graggen, Provincial Contact, 450-563-3574
  coeurachanter@bellnet.ca

CAWS - Saskatchewan
c/o Gloria Mahussier, 19 Pereverzoff Pl., Prince Albert SK S6X 1A8
Chief Officer(s):
Kelly Fraser, Provincial Contact
  schmister@hotmail.com

Canadian Association of Genetic Counsellors (CAGC) / Association Canadienne des conseillers en génétique (ACCG)
PO Box 52083, Oakville ON L6J 7N5
Tel: 905-847-1363; *Fax:* 905-847-3855
Other Communication: president@cagc-accg.ca
e-mail: CAGCOffice@cagc-accg.ca
www.cagc-accg.ca
Overview: A small national organization
Mission: To promote high standards of practice; To encourage professional growth; To increase public awareness of the profession; To offer certification in genetic counselling

Canadian Coalition for Genetic Fairness (CCGF) / Coalition Canadienne pour L'Equité Génétique (CCEG)
#400, 151 Frederick St., Kitchener ON N2H 2M2
Tel: 519-749-7063; *Fax:* 519-749-8965
Toll-Free: 800-998-7398
e-mail: info@ccgf-cceg.ca
www.ccgf-cceg.ca
www.facebook.com/pages/Fighting-Genetic-Discrimination/218530198
176435
twitter.com/GeneticFairness
Overview: A medium-sized national organization
Mission: The CCGF/CCEG is a coalition of organizations dedicated to preventing genetic discrimination for all Canadians.

Canadian College of Medical Geneticists (CCMG) / Collège canadien de généticiens médicaux
#310, 4 Cataraqui St., Kingston ON K7K 1Z7

Tel: 613-507-8345; *Fax:* 866-303-0626
e-mail: info@ccmg-ccgm.org
www.ccmg-ccgm.org

Overview: A small national licensing charitable organization founded in 1975
Mission: To establish & maintain professional & ethical standards for medical genetics services in Canada; To certify individuals who provide medical genetics services; to encourage research activities
Affliation(s): Canadian Association of Genetic Counsellors (CAGC)
Chief Officer(s):
Gail Graham, President
Sean Young, Treasurer
Publications:
• CCMG [Canadian College of Medical Geneticists] Newsletter
Type: Newsletter
• CCMG [Canadian College of Medical Geneticists] Membership Directory
Type: Directory

Canadian Genetic Diseases Network (CGDN) / Réseau canadien sur les maladies génétiques (RCMG)
#201, 2150 Western Pkwy., Vancouver BC V6T 1Z4

Tel: 604-221-7300

Overview: A medium-sized national organization founded in 1990
Mission: A nation-wide consortium of Canada's top investigators & core-technology facilities in human genetics, partnered with colleagues from industry to conduct leading-edge research within an "Institute without Walls"; to achieve international competitiveness in scientific research with social & economic benefits
Publications:
• CGDN [Canadian Genetic Diseases Network] Annual Report
Type: Yearbook; *Frequency:* Annually

CHARGE Syndrome Canada
PO Box 61509, Stn. Fennell, Hamilton ON L8T 5A1

Tel: 519-752-4685; *Fax:* 519-758-9919
e-mail: admin@chargesyndrome.ca
www.chargesyndrome.ca

Overview: A small national charitable organization founded in 2003
Mission: To raise money for the sufferers of CHARGE Syndrome, as well as CHARGE Syndrome research

Kabuki Syndrome Network Inc. (KSN)
8060 Struthers Cres., Regina SK S4Y 1J3

Tel: 306-543-8715
e-mail: margot@kabukisyndrome.com
kabukisyndrome.com

Overview: A small national charitable organization founded in 1997
Mission: To provide information on Kabuki syndrome
Chief Officer(s):
Dean Schmiedge, Contact
Margot Schmiedge, Contact

Shwachman-Diamond Syndrome Canada
2152 Gatley Rd., Mississauga ON L5H 3L9

Toll-Free: 866-462-8907
e-mail: info@shwachman.org
www.shwachman.org
www.facebook.com/shwachmandiamondcanada

Also Known As: SDS-Canada
Overview: A small national charitable organization
Mission: To raise funds to support research; to disseminate current medical information; to heighten awareness of SDS in the medical community to allow earlier diagnosis & treatment; to develop network of contacts & resources for people & families with SDS
Chief Officer(s):
Zoé Nakata, President

Ontario Rett Syndrome Association (ORSA)
PO Box 50030, London ON N6A 6H8

Tel: 519-474-6877; *Fax:* 519-850-1272
www.rett.ca
www.facebook.com/OntarioRettSyndromeAssociation
twitter.com/OntarioRettSA

Overview: A small provincial charitable organization founded in 1991
Mission: To ensure that girls & women with Rett Syndrome are enabled to achieve their full potential & enjoy the highest quality of life within their community
Chief Officer(s):
Terry Boyd, President
Darcy Balak, Secretary
Scott Campbell, Coordinator, Membership

International Genetics Federation (IGF)
Dept. of Evolution & Ecology, University of California - Davis, 1 Shields Ave., Davis CA 95616-8554 USA

Tel: 530-752-4085; *Fax:* 530-752-1449
e-mail: info@meiosis.org
www.internationalgeneticsfederation.org

Overview: A small international organization founded in 1968
Mission: To promote the advancement of the science of genetics
Member of: International Union of Biological Sciences
Affliation(s): Genetics Society of Canada
Chief Officer(s):
Alfred Nordheim, President
 alred.nordheim@uni-tuebingen.de
Charles H. Langley, Secretary-General
 chlangley@ucdavis.edu

Growth Disorders

Cause
Malnutrition is the main cause of growth disorders in Canada, but there are a number of conditions that make a child grow more slowly than average. Any sort of severe chronic illness, especially one involving the digestive system, may cause this. Certain genetic conditions such as Turner's syndrome and Klinefelter's syndrome (sex chromosome abnormalities) or Prader-Willi syndrome (caused by a genetic abnormality on chromosome 15) will predictably limit growth and eventual adult height. Endocrine, or hormonal, causes of short stature include underactivity of the thyroid gland (hypothyroidism) or pituitary gland, where growth hormone (GH) is normally formed. Finally, there are many cases where the child's height is significantly below that of peers, yet none of these conditions is present. This may reflect two parents who are themselves quite short, or may be completely unexplained.

Symptoms
Symptoms of growth disorders can include the inability to grow strong bones, failure to gain weight or grow taller, and delayed sexual development.

Prevalence
Most growth disorders other than malnutrition are rare. For example, the prevalence of Turner's syndrome is one in 2,500 female births.

Treatment Options
Genetic tests, diagnostic assays and karyotyping can be used to diagnose many growth disorders before, or shortly after birth. Growth disorders such as Turner's syndrome and Prader-Willi syndrome are often diagnosed through genetic tests that examine DNA. Diagnostic assays—procedures that identify and measure substances like DNA, enzymes and proteins—are often

used to diagnose growth disorders caused by hypothyroidism or hormone deficiencies. Karyotypes—genetic tests that examine a person's chromosomal map for additional, deleted or abnormal chromosomes—can be used to diagnose growth disorders such as Klinefelter's syndrome and Turner's syndrome.

After birth, a doctor usually measures a baby within one to two weeks; at one, two, four, six, nine, 12, 18 and 24 months; and then on an annual basis. A child who has stopped growing, or is not growing as quickly as the rest of his or her peers, should receive a complete evaluation by a pediatric endocrinologist or other growth specialist. Tests such as blood tests, bone age X-rays or magnetic resonance imaging (MRI) scans of the brain or other parts of the body are often ordered to determine the cause of the growth failure. Sometimes, a growth hormone stimulation test is also done to check the pituitary gland's ability to produce growth hormone (GH).

If slow growth is related to low levels of GH, therapy with GH can be effective. Regular injections will be necessary for a prolonged period until an acceptable height is reached. If an endocrine disorder like hypothyroidism is diagnosed, the child may be treated with thyroid replacement pills. Children with Turner's syndrome and Klinefelter's syndrome can be treated with genetically engineered versions of sex hormones (estrogen or testosterone).

Children diagnosed with growth disorders require parental support to build self-esteem and a sense of self-worth. Children who are extremely self-conscious about their height may benefit from treatment by a mental health professional.

National Associations

Canadian Angelman Syndrome Society (CASS) / Societé canadienne du syndrome d'Angelman (SCSA)
PO Box 37, Priddis AB T0L 1W0
Tel: 403-931-2415
www.angelmancanada.org
Overview: A small national organization
Mission: To educate concerned families, medical & educational communities & the general public about Angelman Syndrome; To establish & maintain support systems; To promote research activities on the diagnosis, treatment, management & prevention of Angelman Syndrome; To fundraise
Chief Officer(s):
John Carscallen, Secretary-Treasurer
cass@davincibb.net

Foundation for Prader-Willi Research in Canada (FPWR Canada)
#370, 19 - 13085 Yonge St., Richmond Hill ON L4E 0K2
Toll-Free: 866-993-7972
www.fpwr.ca
www.facebook.com/fpwr.org
www.youtube.com/user/fpwrcanada
Previous Name: Canadian Prader-Willi Syndrome Association
Overview: A small national charitable organization founded in 2006
Mission: To educate families & inform community services on behalf of individuals with Prader-Willi Syndrome, about the special needs of persons with this condition in Canada
Member of: International Prader-Willi Syndrome Organization
Affliation(s): Ontario Prader-Willi Syndrome Association; British Columbia Prader-Willi Syndrome Association; Alberta Prader-Willi Association; Foundation for Prader Willi Research
Chief Officer(s):
Keegan Johnson, President & Chair
Carole Barron, Executive Director
carole.barron@fpwr.ca
Michelle Cordeiro, Director, Operations
michelle.cordeiro@fpwr.ca
Carole Elkhal, Director, Community
carole.elkhal@fpwr.ca

Turner's Syndrome Society (TSS) / Société du syndrome de Turner
#9, 30 Clearly Ave., Ottawa ON K2A 4A1
Tel: 613-321-2267; *Fax:* 613-321-2268
Toll-Free: 800-465-6744
e-mail: info@turnersyndrome.ca
www.turnersyndrome.ca
www.facebook.com/TurnerSyndromeSocietyOfCanada
Overview: A small national charitable organization founded in 1981
Mission: To improve the quality of life for individuals & families affected by Turner's Syndrome; to strive to accomplish this through providing public & professional awareness about the needs & concerns of individuals with Turner's Syndrome & their families through the development of communication networks to provide mutual support
Chief Officer(s):
Krista Kamstra-Cooper, President

Provincial Associations

ALBERTA

Prader-Willi Syndrome Association of Alberta
9006 - 120 St. NW, Edmonton AB T6G 1X7
Tel: 780-459-1959
Other Communication: 403-217-8587 (Calgary); 403-340-1057 (Red Deer)
www.pwsaa.ca
Also Known As: PWSA of AB
Overview: A small provincial charitable organization founded in 1986
Mission: To advocate for individuals affected by Prader-Willi Syndrome; To improve the quality of life for affected individuals
Affliation(s): Canadian Prader-Willi Syndrome Association
Chief Officer(s):
Lise Dunn, Contact, Edmonton
lisedunn@shaw.ca
Brooke Gibson, Contact, Calgary
brookergibson@gmail.com
Jill Hockin, Contact, Red Deer
reddeerbean@shaw.ca
Publications:
• Prader-Willi Syndrome Association of Alberta Newsletter
Type: Newsletter
Profile: Association reports, stories, & events

BRITISH COLUMBIA

British Columbia Prader-Willi Syndrome Association (BCPWSA)
2133 Chilcotin Cres., Kelowna BC V1V 2N9
www.bcpwsa.com
www.facebook.com/bcpwsa
Overview: A small provincial charitable organization founded in 1982
Mission: To provide an understanding & awareness of PWS by supporting those who have the syndrome, their families & all who come in contact with PWS
Chief Officer(s):
Heather Beach, President
president@bcpwsa.com
Cheryl Gagne, Treasurer
treasurer@bcpwsa.com
Frances Robinson, Secretary
secretary@bcpwsa.com

ONTARIO

Ontario Prader-Willi Syndrome Association (OPWSA)
PO Box 73514, Toronto ON M6C 4A7
Tel: 416-481-8657; *Fax:* 416-981-7788
e-mail: opwsa@rogers.com
www.opwsa.com
www.facebook.com/106828009519275
Overview: A small provincial charitable organization founded in 1982
Mission: To enhance the quality of life for individuals with Prader-Willi Syndrome
Affliation(s): International Prader-Willi Syndrome Association
Chief Officer(s):

Jessie Phillips, Family Services Coordinator
  jessie.opwsa@gmail.com
Dan Yashinsky, Co-chair
  dan_yashinsky@hotmail.com
Cathy Mallove, Co-chair
  cmallove@sympatico.ca

QUÉBEC

Association du Syndrome de Turner du Québec
1484, Montée Gagnon, Val-David QC J0T 2N0

Tél: 819-320-0409
Courriel: turnerquebec@gmail.com
www.syndrometurnerquebec.com

Aperçu: *Dimension:* petite; *Envergure:* provinciale; Organisme sans but lucratif; fondée en 1984
Mission: Faire connaître les personnes atteintes du S.T.; faire circuler l'information médicale; créer des nouveaux contacts
Membre(s) du bureau directeur:
Marie-Claude Doire, Présidente
Jocelyne Jeanneau, Coordonnatrice

Guillain-Barré Syndrome

Guillain-Barré Syndrome is a condition in which a person's immune system attacks the peripheral nerves—those located outside the brain and spinal cord—resulting in muscle weakness, loss of sensation in the extremities and paralysis in the worst cases. It is most common in adults, particularly males, but can affect people of all ages.

Cause
GBS is often preceded by an infection, either bacterial or viral. Recently, the Zika virus in particular has been linked to the syndrome. Surgery and vaccinations have also been known to trigger the condition, although only in rare cases.

Symptoms
The symptoms of GBS usually last for a few weeks, depending on the severity of the case. Most individuals recover without any long-term effects, although some continue to experience a degree of weakness for weeks, months or even years after the original attack. Initial symptoms include weakness or tingling in the legs, which spreads to the arms and face. In some cases, the weakness and tingling can begin in the upper body instead. Paralysis can also occur, including in the chest muscles, resulting in breathing difficulty. Bladder and bowel control, speech and the ability to swallow can also be impaired. Around 3 to 5 percent of patients die from severe complications including breathing difficulty, blood infections, blood clots and cardiac arrest.

Prevalence
GBS is considered a rare disorder, affecting around 2 to 3 people per 100,000, per year.

Treatment Options
There is no known cure for GBS, but because of the potentially life-threatening nature of the syndrome, patients are usually hospitalized and monitored for complications, often in intensive care. Complications can include abnormal heart beat, high or low blood pressure, blood clots and infections. Patients who experience difficulty breathing are often put on a ventilator. Manual movement of the patient's limbs may be necessary to aid in blood flow, and to keep the muscles flexible. Treatment may also be required for additional complications such as pneumonia and bed sores, common among paralyzed patients. Immunotherapy is common during the condition's acute phase, within 7 to 14 days of the initial symptoms, while physiotherapy may be required for patients who experience weakness after the acute phase has passed. Recovery can be 3 to 6 months or longer.

See also Muscular Dystrophy

Guillain-Barré Support Group of Canada
c/o Muscular Dystrophy Canada, #901, 2345 Yonge St., Toronto ON M4P 2E5

Tel: 416-488-2699; *Fax:* 416-488-7523
Toll-Free: 800-567-2873
e-mail: info@muscle.ca
www.muscle.ca

Also Known As: GBS Support Group of Canada
Overview: A small national organization overseen by Muscular Dystrophy Canada
Mission: To offer support to persons who have Guillain-Barré Syndrome.
Chief Officer(s):
Lynn Potvin, Coordinator, Client Services

Guillain-Barré Syndrome Foundation of Canada (GBSFCI)
PO Box 80060, Stn. Rossland Garden, 3100 Garden St., Whitby ON L1R 0H1

Tel: 647-560-6842
Toll-Free: 866-224-3301
www.gbs-cidp.org/canada
www.facebook.com/gbscidp

Overview: A medium-sized national charitable organization founded in 1985
Mission: To provide information about GBS & CIDP; To provide education, research, & support to individuals, families & friends affected by GBS, CIDP & related disorders
Affliation(s): Guillain-Barré Syndrome Foundation International
Chief Officer(s):
Donna Hartlen, Executive Director

Gulf War Syndrome

War syndromes have plagued soldiers for centuries. Though symptoms may vary, soldiers may become affected by various postulated physiological diseases as well as psychological illnesses. Gulf War Syndrome (GWS) or Persian Gulf War Syndrome is a constellation of illnesses experienced by veterans after returning from the Persian Gulf Wars in the 1990s and 2000s.

Cause
The cause of GWS is unknown. Many causes have been suggested, but none have been definitely identified or eliminated. These include effects of chemical or biological weapons, exposure to pesticides, smoke from oil well fires, airborne contamination from munitions plants destroyed in Iraq, exposure to depleted uranium used as a material in some munitions, and exposure to volatile solvents used in the normal course of equipment maintenance. None of these exposures have been convincingly linked to a cause of the illness.

Symptoms
Symptoms are predominately neurological and consist of impaired cognition, with problems of attention, memory, reasoning, insomnia, depression and headaches. Complaints of muscle and joint pain, gastrointestinal difficulties, vertigo and weakness are also common. As veterans resumed family life, various birth defects became more common than usual in their children.

A 2005 study by Statistics Canada shows that Gulf War personnel are more likely than others to report depression, symptoms similar to post-traumatic stress disorder, chronic fatigue, cognitive difficulties, bronchitis, asthma, fibromyalgia, alcohol abuse, anxiety and sexual dysfunction. However, it also concluded that neither the mortality rate nor the prevalence of cancer was higher in Gulf War veterans than in the general population.

Prevalence

Approximately 4,600 members of the Canadian Forces served in the Gulf War. It is estimated that around one-third of veterans are affected by chronic symptoms of illness related to their service in the Gulf War.

Treatment Options

Given the range of reported GWS effects, treatment is highly individualized and symptomatic. Some patients may benefit from drug therapy (for example, selective serotonin reuptake inhibitors and serotonin norepinephrine reuptake inhibitors). Cognitive behavioural therapy may also help reduce symptoms. In addition, alternative therapies such as acupuncture and biofeedback may be useful. Research into the effectiveness of anti-oxidant supplements in relieving the symptoms of GWS is currently underway.

Some Gulf War veterans do not believe that Veterans Affairs Canada is doing enough to help them with illnesses from which they have been suffering for over 20 years. They would like Canada to acknowledge their symptoms as characteristic of a true illness. A 2013 report from the Institute of Medicine in the United States names the illness experienced by Gulf War veterans as chronic multisymptom illness (CMI), and suggests ways to improve treatment for people who suffer from this ailment.

National Associations

Army, Navy & Air Force Veterans in Canada (ANAVETS) / Les Anciens combattants de l'armée, de la marine et des forces aériennes au Canada
#2, 6 Beechwood Ave., Ottawa ON K1L 8B4
Tel: 613-744-0222; *Fax:* 613-744-0208
e-mail: anavets@storm.ca
www.anavets.ca

Overview: A medium-sized national organization founded in 1917
Mission: To unite veterans & their supporters to maintain entitlements & benefits; To provide a fraternal milieu for members by acquiring & operating clubs & homes; To strive to promote patriotism in Canada, & nurture cooperation & unity within the British Commonwealth
Chief Officer(s):
Deanna Fimrite, Secretary-Treasurer
Laila Saikaley, Administrative Assistant
Publications:
• ANAVETS [Army, Navy & Air Force Veterans in Canada] Shoulder to Shoulder
Type: Magazine; *Frequency:* Quarterly; *Accepts Advertising*; *Editor:* Derek Walter

Alberta Provincial Command
c/o Command Secretary, 8106 - 168 St., Edmonton AB T5R 2V4

British Columbia Provincial Command
#200, 951 - 8th Ave. East, Vancouver BC V5T 4L2
Tel: 604-874-8105; *Fax:* 604-874-0633
e-mail: bcanavets@telus.net

Manitoba & Northwestern Ontario Provincial Command
3584 Portage Ave., Winnipeg MB R2Y 0V5
Tel: 204-896-9897; *Fax:* 204-896-8837
e-mail: anavets@mts.net

Nova Scotia Provincial Command
422 Heelen St., New Waterford NS B1H 3C7
e-mail: anavetsnscommand@gmail.com

Ontario Provincial Command
1655 Weston Rd., Toronto ON M9N 1V2
Tel: 416-259-4145; *Fax:* 416-259-1677
e-mail: anaf_opc@bellnet.ca

Québec Provincial Command
18, rue Massawippi, Sherbrooke QC J1M 1L2

Saskatchewan Provincial Command
c/o Stephanie Minion, 254 Langevin Cres., Saskatoon SK S7L 5R3
Tel: 306-384-0106; *Fax:* 306-653-4760
e-mail: aands2@shaw.ca

Canadian Aboriginal Veterans & Serving Members Association (CAV)
34 Kingham Pl., Victoria BC V9B 1L8
Tel: 250-900-5768
e-mail: national-president@nationalalliance.ca
canadianaboriginalveterans.ca
Overview: A small national organization

Canadian Association of Veterans in United Nations Peacekeeping (CAVUNP) / Association Canadienne des Vétérans des Forces de la Paix pour les Nations Unies
PO Box PO Box 46026, RPO Beacon Hill, 2339 Ogilvie Rd., Gloucester ON K1J 9M7
Tel: 613-746-3302
e-mail: cavunp@rogers.com
www.cavunp.org
Overview: A small national organization founded in 1986
Mission: To perpetuate the memories of fallen comrades; to provide assistance to serving & retired Canadian peacekeepers & their families; to provide education about peacekeeping & peacekeepers
Member of: Veterans Affairs Canada Advisory Committee on the New Veterans Charter; Veterans Affairs Canada Veterans Week Advisory Committee; Veterans Affairs Canada Pacific Region Advisory Council; The Joint Veterans Affairs & National Defence Centre for the Care of Injured and Retired Members of the CF
Chief Officer(s):
Ronald R. Griffis, National President, 902-538-3399
J. Robert O'Brien, Chair
gunkeob@yahoo.com
Paul Greensides, National Secretary-Treasurer
cavunp@rogers.com
Publications:
• The Thin Blue Line / Sur la corde raide en bleu
Type: Newsletter; *Editor:* John Stuart
Profile: Association news & activities from chapters across the country

Buffalo 461 Chapter (Hamilton)
c/o Chapter President, 28 Goldwin St., Hamilton ON L9G 6V9
Tel: 905-385-8045

Chief Officer(s):
Douglas Furchner, President
retiredppcli@yahoo.ca
Paul A. Hale, Contact, Chapter Membership, 905-794-2109
cavunpbuffalo461@hotmail.com

Calgary Chapter
c/o Chapter President, 39 Cedardale Hill SW, Calgary AB T2W 5A6
Tel: 403-251-0056
www.cavunp.ab.ca

Chief Officer(s):
Robert F.M. Titus, President
rfmtitus@shaw.ca
Barry T. Wood, Contact, Chapter Membership, 403-254-2882
bwood.un@shaw.ca

Camp Maple Leaf Chapter
c/o Chapter President, 412 Court St. North, Thunder Bay ON P7A 4X1
Tel: 807-475-0803

Chief Officer(s):
Robert L. Manns, President, 807-475-0803
Sydney Bouchard, Contact, Chapter Membership, 807-475-4475

Central Ontario Chapter
c/o Chapter President, 69 Brown Wood Drive, Barrie ON L4M 6M6
Tel: 705-727-1746

Chief Officer(s):
Fernand O. Taillefer, President
taillefer1746@rogers.com
Laurette G. Bedard, Contact, Chapter Membership, 705-429-1547
mlbedard@sympatico.ca

Colonel John Gardam Chapter
c/o Chapter President, 1815 Chopin Place, Orléans ON K1C 5G1
Tel: 613-834-9274

Chief Officer(s):
Wayne R. MacCullough, President
wrmac50@rogers.com

Trevor E. Luten, Contact, Chapter Membership, 613-830-7437
trevor.luten@sympatico.ca

Dartmouth - Halifax Chapter
NS

cavunp-dartmouth.tripod.com

Chief Officer(s):
Shawn E. Kennedy, President
shawn.kennedy450@gmail.com
Al J. Simpson, Contact, Chapter Membership, 902-465-6761
jackdusty51@gmail.com

Edmonton Chapter
c/o Chapter President, #4PH, 8340 Jasper Ave., Edmonton AB T5H
4C6

Tel: 780-429-7232

Chief Officer(s):
Arthur Adamson, President
artadamson@shaw.ca

Kingston Limestone Chapter
c/o Chapter President, 69 Chesterfield Drive, Amherstview ON K7N
1M5

Tel: 613-384-8527

Chief Officer(s):
Jim (Harold) James, President
hethjim@cogeco.ca

LCpl David W. Young Chapter
c/o Chapter President, 11 Goshen St., Tillsonburg ON N4G 2T7

Tel: 519-688-9212

Chief Officer(s):
Edward J. Weil, President
e-mweil@kwic.com

LGen. R.R. Crabbe Chapter
c/o Chapter President, 212 Moorgate St., Winnipeg MB R3J 2L2

Tel: 204-888-0156
www.cavunp-winnipeg.com

Chief Officer(s):
Murdoch (Doc) T.M. Jardine, President
piperdoc@shaw.ca
Gordon A. Criggar, Contact, Chapter Membership, 204-837-1844
gcriggar@mb.sympatico.ca

MCpl Mark Isfeld Memorial Chapter
c/o Chapter President, 909 Foreshaw Road, Victoria BC V9A 6M1

Tel: 250-383-8227

Chief Officer(s):
James P. MacMillan-Murphy, President, 250-889-0944
macmurph2@shaw.ca
Scott Laird, Contact, Chapter Membership, 250-383-2808
slaird2@telus.net

MGen. Lewis W. Mackenzie Chapter
c/o Chapter President, 37 Highland Drive, George's River NS B1Y
3G3

Tel: 902-794-8908
cavunplewis.tripod.com

Chief Officer(s):
Ronald V. Clarke, President, 902-794-8908
babetootie@eastlink.ca
John R. Horvath, Contact, Chapter Membership, 902-539-9953
jhorvath@syd.eastlink.ca

Niagara Chapter
c/o Chapter President, 4525 Garden Gate Terrace, Beamsville ON
L0R 1B9

Tel: 905-563-9911

Chief Officer(s):
Kevin Wadden, President
kwadden@cogeco.ca
Earle Topley, Contact, Chapter Membership, 905-574-4164

North Saskatchewan Chapter
c/o Chapter President, 307 Cowley Rd., Saskatoon SK S7N 3Z3

Tel: 306-933-9847
members.shaw.ca/nschapter

Chief Officer(s):
Michael W. Titus, President
mjtitus@shaw.ca

Kenneth W. Lowther, Contact, Chapter Membership, 306-384-8208
kwl1@shaw.ca

Peterborough Chapter
c/o Bill Steedman, #205, 811 Sherbrooke St., Peterborough ON K9J
2R2

Tel: 705-743-0115

Chief Officer(s):
Bob Ware, President

Prince Edward Island Chapter
c/o Chapter President, #11, 319 Shakespeare Dr., Stratford PE C1B
2Y4

Tel: 902-892-4403

Chief Officer(s):
Peter R. Van Iderstine, President, 902-892-4403
vanider@pei.sympatico.ca

Prince George & Northern British Columbia Chapter
c/o Branch 43, Royal Canadian Legion, 6076 Trent Drive, Prince
George BC V2N 2G3

Tel: 250-964-1822

Chief Officer(s):
Bruce R. Gabriel, President
brgabriel@shaw.ca
Peter M. Engensperger, Contact, Chapter Membership,
250-981-0140
pdt@canada.com

Pte Alexander LeRue Chapter
c/o Chapter President, RR#1, Lower L'Ardoise NS B0E 1W0

Tel: 902-587-2729

Chief Officer(s):
Raymond L. Gracie, President
rlgracie@ns.sympatico.ca
Harris C. MacLean, Contact, Chapter Membership, 902-625-1366
hcmaclean@ns.sympatico.ca

South Saskatchewan Chapter
c/o Chapter President, 37 Lake St., Regina SK S4S 4A7

Tel: 306-584-7308

Chief Officer(s):
Kenneth C. Garbutt, President
kgarbutt@accesscomm.ca
Wesley D. Kopp, Contact, Chapter Membership, 306-584-0678

Spr Christopher Holopina Chapter
c/o Chapter President, 533 - 16th Street, Brandon MB R7A 4Y2

Tel: 204-728-7951

Chief Officer(s):
Yves Lacerte, President, 204-728-7951
good2sea_u@yahoo.com
Martin Haller, Contact, Chapter Membership, 204-727-5009
bdfc@mts.net

Stony Plain Chapter
c/o Chapter President, Box 17, Site 12, RR#2, Carvel AB T0E 0H0

Tel: 780-963-7768

Chief Officer(s):
Norman A. Westwell, President
njwest@telus.net
Herbert Ross Reid, Contact, Chapter Membership, 780-963-8636
hrreid@telus.net

Succursale MGén Alain R. Forand
23 rue Létourneau, Saint-Jean-sur-Richelieu QC J3W 1B3

Tél: 450-359-4776
onuforand.org

Chief Officer(s):
Robert Chouinard, Président, 450-359-4776
choufam@videotron.ca
France Gagné, Secrétaire de Succursale, 514-772-8519
gafrance@hotmail.com

Wainwright Chapter
c/o Chapter President, 1833 - 1A Street Crescent, Wainwright AB
T9W 1N4

Tel: 780-842-6495

Chief Officer(s):
Ronald F. McBride, President, 780-842-6495
mcbride3@telus.net

Western Newfoundland Chapter
c/o Chapter President, 18 Hillside Road, Corner Brook NL A2H 1A6
Tel: 709-639-1163
Chief Officer(s):
Michael S. Martin, President
michaelmartin@nf.sympatico.ca
Winston Childs, Chapter Secretary, 709-634-6428
wdchilds@nl.rogers.com

William C. Hall VC, Greenwood Chapter
c/o Chapter President, PO Box 1152, 883 Carol St., Greenwood NS
B0P 1N0
Tel: 902-765-6755
Chief Officer(s):
Nelson G. Mullen, President
nelbel@eastlink.ca

Canadian Merchant Navy Veterans Association Inc. (CMNVA) / L'Association des Anciens Combattants de la marine marchande canadienne Inc.
2108 Melrick Pl., Sooke BC V9Z 0M9
Tel: 250-642-2638; *Fax:* 250-642-3332
Overview: A medium-sized national organization founded in 1990
Mission: To renew old friendships & bring together ex-Canadian merchant seamen; to promote increased recognition of the role of the merchant navy during wartime; to liaise with government to obtain full benefits & pension as recognized veterans
Chief Officer(s):
Bruce Ferguson, President

Canadian Peacekeeping Veterans Association (CPVA)
PO Box 905, Kingston ON K7L 4X8
Tel: 506-627-6437
e-mail: info@cpva.ca
www.cpva.ca
Overview: A small national organization founded in 1991
Mission: To assist Canadians who have served on peacekeeping missions
Member of: National Council of Veterans
Chief Officer(s):
Ray Kokkonen, President
kokkonen@nbnet.nb.ca

National Council of Veteran Associations (NCVA) / Conseil national des associations d'anciens combattants au Canada (CNAAC)
2827 Riverside Dr., Ottawa ON K1V 0C4
Tel: 613-731-3821; *Fax:* 613-731-3234
Toll-Free: 800-465-2677
e-mail: ncva@waramps.ca
www.ncva-cnaac.ca
twitter.com/NCVACanada
Overview: A medium-sized national organization
Mission: To provide a voice on issues which are of significant interest to the Veterans' community
Chief Officer(s):
Brian N. Forbes, Chair

Trauma Association of Canada (TAC) / Association canadienne de traumatologie
PO Box 8862, Halifax NS B3K 5M5
Fax: 902-850-2289
Toll-Free: 855-403-5463
e-mail: info@traumacanada.org
www.traumacanada.org
twitter.com/TraumaCanada
Overview: A small national organization founded in 1984
Mission: To promote the highest standards of care for the injured patient; To encourage research & education related to trauma
Member of: Royal College of Physicians & Surgeons of Canada
Chief Officer(s):
Paula Poirier, President
president@traumacanada.org
Tracey Taulu, Secretary
director2.secretary@traumacanada.org
Morad Hameed, Treasurer
director1.treasurer@traumacanada.org

Kate Mahon, Executive Director
exec.director@traumacanada.org
Publications:
• Trauma Association of Canada Newsletter
Type: Newsletter; *Frequency:* Semiannually

Union of Veterans' Affairs Employees (UVAE) / Syndicat des employé(e)s des affaires des anciens combattants (SEAC)
#703, 233 Gilmour St., Ottawa ON K2P 0P2
Tel: 613-560-5460; *Fax:* 613-237-8282
uvae-seac.ca
Overview: A small national organization overseen by Public Service Alliance of Canada (CLC)
Mission: To represent the interests of employees of Veterans' Affairs Canada
Chief Officer(s):
Carl Gannon, National President
gannonc@psac.com

The War Amputations of Canada / Les Amputés de guerre du Canada
2827 Riverside Dr., Ottawa ON K1V 0C4
Tel: 613-731-3821; *Fax:* 613-731-3234
Toll-Free: 800-465-2677
e-mail: communications@waramps.ca
www.waramps.ca
www.facebook.com/TheWarAmps
twitter.com/thewaramps
www.youtube.com/warampsofcanada
Also Known As: The War Amps
Overview: A medium-sized national charitable organization founded in 1919
Mission: To provide a wide range of assistance to all Canadian war amputees & child amputees; To promote the advancement of prosthetics through grants to facilities undertaking research in field of prosthetics
Member of: National Council of Veteran Associations
Chief Officer(s):
David Saunders, Chief Operating Officer
Danita Chisholm, Executive Director, Communications

National Hospitals
ONTARIO

OTTAWA: Canadian Forces Health Care Centre Ottawa
Affiliated with: Champlain Local Health Integration Network
713 Montreal Rd., Ottawa, ON K1K 0T2
Tel: 613-945-1111
www.forces.gc.ca/en/caf-community-bases-wings-cfsu-ottawa/dental-medical.page

Note: Hospital Specialties: Primary health care services to the military community in the National Capital Region (613-945-1502); Laboratory services; Surgery; Cardio Pulmonary Unit; Operational Trauma & Stress Support Centre (613-945-1060); Mental health (613-945-1060); Addiction counselling (613-945-1060); Ophthalmology (613-945-1550); & Physiotherapy (613-945-1585).
BGen H.C. MacKay, Commander, Canadian Forces Health Services Group

Local Hospitals & Health Centres
ALBERTA

CALGARY: Carewest Colonel Belcher
Affiliated with: Alberta Health Services
1939 Veterans Way NW, Calgary, AB T3B 5Y8
Tel: 403-944-7800 *Fax:* 403-944-7870
www.carewest.ca
Year Founded: 2003
Number of Beds: 175 residents in seniors' residence, most of whom are veterans
Note: Services include: adult day support; continuing care; & respite care.

CALGARY: Carewest Operational Stress Injury Clinic
Affiliated with: Alberta Health Services
Also Known As: Carewest OSI Clinic
Market Mall, 3625 Shaganappi Trail NW, Calgary, AB T3A 0E2
Tel: 403-216-9860 *Fax:* 403-216-9861
www.carewest.ca

Note: Provides programs & services to help deal with mental health problems caused by shock or stress for veterans, Canadian Forces members, RCMP members, & their families.

ONTARIO

OTTAWA: Perley & Rideau Veterans' Health Centre
1750 Russell Rd., Ottawa, ON K1G 5Z6
Tel: 613-526-7170 *Fax:* 613-526-7172
www.perleyrideau.ca
Social Media: www.facebook.com/perleyrideau
Year Founded: 1995
Number of Beds: 250 beds
Note: Specialties: Geriatric care; Recreation services; Dementia programming; Respite care for people in the mid-stages of dementia; Convalescent care
Akos Hoffer, Chief Executive Officer
Mary Boutette, Chief Operating Officer
Ross Quane, Chief Financial Officer
Dr. Benoit Robert, Medical Director
Carolyn Vollicks, Director, Community Outreach & Programming
Jay Innes, Director, Communications
Russ Tattersall, Director, Human Resources
Jennifer Plant, Director, Clinical Practice
Lorie Stuckless, Director, Support Services
Doris Jenkins, Director, Nursing Operations

YUKON TERRITORY

WHITEHORSE: Front Street Senion's Residence
1190 Front St., Whitehorse, YT Y1A 0P4

Year Founded: 2016
Number of Beds: 48 unites

Head Injuries

Cause
Head injuries cover a range of severity, from a minor bump on the head to a traumatic brain injury. The most common injury is concussion, a mild brain injury which occurs after a blow to the head, or a violent shaking of the head. Damage can also result from penetration of the skull or from acceleration/deceleration of the brain that occurs in severe automobile accidents. Injuries can include brain bruising and bleeding into the brain, resulting in swelling that can be life threatening because the skull, as a rigid structure, cannot expand. The major causes of head injuries are falls, motor vehicle accidents, sports and recreational activities, and assault and homicide.

Symptoms
Symptoms of a head injury can range from mild to severe, and can appear right away, or come on more slowly over a period of several hours or days. Concussion symptoms can include clumsiness, temporary loss of consciousness, amnesia, forgetfulness, behaviour or personality changes, and a dazed or stunned appearance. Post-concussion syndrome sometimes follows a concussion and can include more chronic symptoms such as headaches, dizziness, sensitivity to noise or light, mild mental slowing and fatigue.

Symptoms of moderate head or brain injuries can include loss of consciousness, confusion, seizures, headaches, memory loss, drowsiness, nausea and vomiting and bleeding from the nose, mouth or ears. Loss of consciousness for greater than two minutes implies a worse outcome, such as cognitive and psychologi-

cal impairments lasting many months or even permanently. A severe injury almost always results in prolonged unconsciousness or coma lasting days to weeks or longer. People who sustain a severe head or brain injury often have brain contusions, hematomas (a collection of blood) or damage to the nerve fibers or axons.

Prevalence
Each year, approximately 50,000 Canadians suffer a brain injury. Young men are about twice as likely to suffer a brain injury as young women. In youth aged 12 to 19, around 30,000 concussions (66 percent of which are sports-related) are reported each year in Canada.

Treatment Options
To diagnose a concussion, a physician often performs a neurological exam to check the patient's balance, reflexes, coordination, vision, hearing and strength. In some cases, a computerized tomography (CT) scan of the brain is done.

The severity of a traumatic brain injury is usually assessed using the Glasgow Coma Scale, a 15-point test that scores the patient's speech coherence, body movements and ability to follow directions. Other tests such as an intracranial pressure monitor (to measure pressure in the skull) and a CT scan or magnetic resonance imaging (MRI) of the brain are also often used to diagnose traumatic brain injuries.

In order to allow the brain to recover, the recommended treatment for concussion is rest (physical and mental). Acetaminophen can be used to reduce headache pain. Normal activity can be resumed when concussion symptoms are gone.

Emergency treatment for traumatic brain injuries is initially focused on maintaining the patient's blood pressure and ensuring adequate blood and oxygen supply. Medications to reduce brain pressure and prevent seizures, and surgery to repair skull fractures, and reduce brain pressure and bleeding may also be required. Depending on the severity of the brain injury, and the area of the brain that was injured, a patient may need some form of rehabilitation that could include speech therapy, physical therapy, occupational therapy and vocational and mental health counselling.

Most people with a mild head injury will recover fully. Many people who sustain a severe brain injury make significant improvements in the first year or two. After that, improvement tends to slow down, but may continue for years. Some physical and cognitive impairments can be permanent.

See also Brain Tumours

National Associations

Brain Injury Association of Canada (BIAC) / Association canadienne des lésés cérébraux
#200, 440 Laurier Ave. West, Ottawa ON K1R 7X6
Tel: 613-762-1012; *Fax:* 613-782-2228
Toll-Free: 866-977-2492
e-mail: info@braininjurycanada.ca
www.braininjurycanada.ca
www.facebook.com/braininjurycanada
twitter.com/BIACACLC
www.youtube.com/user/BrainInjuryCanada
Overview: A medium-sized national organization founded in 2003
Mission: To improve the quality of life for persons affected by acquired brain injury; To promote the prevention of brain injuries, through legislation & education in Canada
Chief Officer(s):
Barb Butler, Co-President
RJ Riopelle, Co-President

Harry Zarins, Executive Director
Publications:
• Brain Injury Association of Canada Annual Report
Type: Yearbook
• Impact: Pathways Ahead [a publication of Brain Injury Canada]
Type: Newsletter; *Editor:* Barb Butler
Profile: Happenings at the Brain Injury Association of Canada, plus news from across Canada

Canadian Society of Clinical Neurophysiologists (CSCN) / Société canadienne de neurophysiologistes cliniques
#709, 7015 Macleod Trail SW, Calgary AB T2H 2K6
Tel: 403-229-9544; *Fax:* 403-229-1661
www.cnsfederation.org
Overview: A small national organization founded in 1990 overseen by Canadian Neurological Sciences Federation
Mission: To promote & encourage all aspects of neurophysiology, including research & education, in addition to assessment & accreditation in the field
Member of: Canadian Neurological Sciences Federation
Affliation(s): Cdn. Brain Tumour Consortium; Cdn. Epilepsy Consortium; Cdn. Stroke Consortium; Cdn. League Against Epilepsy; Cdn. Headache Society; Cdn. Movement Disorders Group; Cdn. Network of MS Clinics; Cdn. Neurocritical Care Group; Amyotrophic Lateral Sclerosis Research Foundation; Consortium of Canadian Centres for Clinical Cognitive Research; Associate Societies: Assn. of Electromyography Technologists of Canada; Canadian Assn. of Electroneurophysiology Technologists; Canadian Assn. of Neuroscience; Canadian Assn. of Neuroscience Nurses; Canadian Assn. of Physical Medicine & Rehabilitation
Chief Officer(s):
Dan Morin, CNSF CEO
dan-morin@cnsfederation.org
Publications:
• Canadian Journal of Neurological Sciences
Type: Journal; *Frequency:* Bimonthly; *Accepts Advertising;* *Editor:* G. Bryan Young
Profile: Peer-reviewed original articles

Canadian Society of Otolaryngology - Head & Neck Surgery (CSO-HNS) / Société canadienne d'otolaryngologie et de chirurgie cervico-faciale
Administrative Office, 68 Gilkison Rd., Elora ON N0B 1S0
Tel: 519-846-0630; *Fax:* 519-846-9529
Toll-Free: 800-655-9533
www.entcanada.org
Overview: A medium-sized national charitable organization founded in 1947
Mission: To improve patient care in otolaryngology - head & neck surgery; To maintain high professional & ethical standards
Chief Officer(s):
S. Mark Taylor, President
Trina Uwiera, Secretary
John Yoo, Treasurer
Donna Humphrey, General Manager
cso.hns@sympatico.ca
Publications:
• Journal of Otolaryngology - Head & Neck Surgery
Type: Journal; *Editor:* Dr. Erin Wright; Dr. Hadi Seikaly
Profile: Available for Society members

Provincial Associations

ALBERTA

Association for the Rehabilitation of the Brain Injured (ARBI)
3412 Spruce Dr. SW, Calgary AB T3C 3A4
Tel: 403-242-7116; *Fax:* 403-242-7478
e-mail: info@arbi.ca
arbi.ca
twitter.com/arbi_ca
Overview: A medium-sized provincial charitable organization founded in 1972
Mission: To improve the quality of life of individuals with severe acquired brain injury through long-term personalized rehabilitation
Chief Officer(s):
Mary Ellen Neilson, Executive Director

Bruce Murray, President

Brain Injury Association of Alberta (BIAA)
4916 - 50th St., Red Deer AB T4N 1X7
Tel: 403-309-0866; *Fax:* 403-342-3880
Toll-Free: 888-533-5355
biac-aclc.ca/alberta
Overview: A small provincial organization founded in 1986 overseen by Brain Injury Association of Canada
Mission: To support acquired brain injury survivors, their families, caregivers, & professionals in Alberta; To provide information for individuals & organizations working with brain injury communities
Chief Officer(s):
Meloni Lyon, President
Shelly Wieser, Secretary

BRITISH COLUMBIA

British Columbia Brain Injury Association (BCBIA)
c/o Sea to Sky Meeting Management Inc., #206, 201 Bewicke Ave., North Vancouver BC V7M 3M7
Tel: 604-984-1212; *Fax:* 604-984-6434
Toll-Free: 877-858-1788
e-mail: info@brainstreams.ca
www.brainstreams.ca
www.facebook.com/brainstreams
twitter.com/brainstreams
www.youtube.com/user/brainstreams
Overview: A small provincial organization founded in 1982 overseen by Brain Injury Association of Canada
Mission: To promote a better quality of life for those living with acquired brain injury in British Columbia
Chief Officer(s):
Patti Flaherty, President
Publications:
• The Synaptic Post
Type: Newsletter; *Frequency:* Quarterly

MANITOBA

Manitoba Brain Injury Association Inc.
#204, 825 Sherbrook St., Winnipeg MB R3A 1M5
Tel: 204-975-3280; *Fax:* 204-975-3027
Toll-Free: 866-327-1998
e-mail: info@mbia.ca
www.mbia.ca
www.facebook.com/449153225157899
Also Known As: MBIA
Overview: A small provincial charitable organization founded in 1987 overseen by Brain Injury Association of Canada
Mission: To improve the quality of life & give hope to those affected by acquired brain injury; To support persons affected by acquired brain injury in Manitoba
Chief Officer(s):
Kristyn Cain, President
David Sullivan, Executive Director
david@mbia.ca
Satoshi Yamashita, Office Administrator
Publications:
• MBIA [Manitoba Brain Injury Association] News
Type: Newsletter; *Frequency:* Quarterly
Profile: Association activities, provincial news, meetings, events, & programs, plus member information

NEWFOUNDLAND AND LABRADOR

Newfoundland & Labrador Brain Injury Association (NLBIA)
PO Box 21063, St. John's NL A1A 5B8
Tel: 709-579-3070
e-mail: nlbia2011@gmail.com
www.nlbia.ca
www.facebook.com/119669344782709
Overview: A small provincial organization founded in 1987 overseen by Brain Injury Association of Canada
Mission: To meet the needs of acquired brain injury survivors & their families in Newfoundland & Labrador; To improve access to care & services
Chief Officer(s):

Chava Finkler, Coordinator, Programs & Services
Michelle Ploughman, President
Marina White, Vice-President
Glen Russell, Treasurer

NOVA SCOTIA

Brain Injury Association of Nova Scotia (BIANS)
PO Box 8804, Halifax NS B3K 5M4

Tel: 902-473-7301; *Fax:* 902-473-7302
e-mail: info@braininjuryns.com
braininjuryns.com
www.facebook.com/357100817645932

Previous Name: Nova Scotia Head Injury Association
Overview: A small provincial organization founded in 1988 overseen by Brain Injury Association of Canada
Mission: To promote an environment throughout Nova Scotia that is responsive to the lifelong needs of persons affected by acquired brain injury
Chief Officer(s):
Leona Burkey, Executive Director
Ryan Blood, President
Shelley Pick, Vice-President
Patrick MacConnell, Secretary
Publications:
• BIANS News
Type: Newsletter; *Accepts Advertising; Editor:* Mary Bourgeois
Profile: Association happenings, such as upcoming events & chapter news, plus articles & profiles

ONTARIO

Ontario Brain Injury Association (OBIA)
3550 Schmon Parkway, 2nd Fl., Thorold ON L2V 4Y6

Tel: 905-641-8877; *Fax:* 905-641-0323
Toll-Free: 800-263-5404
e-mail: obia@obia.on.ca
www.obia.ca
www.linkedin.com/company/ontario-brain-injury-association
www.facebook.com/OntarioBIA
twitter.com/OntarioBIA

Overview: A medium-sized provincial organization founded in 1987 overseen by Brain Injury Association of Canada
Mission: To provide on-going support to persons in Ontario whose lives have been affected by acquired brain injury
Chief Officer(s):
Barbara Claiman, President
Brad Borkwood, Treasurer
Ruth Wilcock, Executive Director
  rwilcock@obia.on.ca
Publications:
• Directory of ABI Services [a publication of the Ontario Brain Injury Association]
Type: Directory
Profile: Company listings with program descriptions
• OBIA [Ontario Brain Injury Association] Review
Type: Newsletter; *Frequency:* Quarterly; *Accepts Advertising; Editor:* Jennifer Norquay
Profile: Feature articles, survivor stories, upcoming events, & training information

Belleville
Core Centre, 223 Pinnacle St., Belleville ON K8N 3A7

Tel: 613-967-2756
Toll-Free: 866-894-8884
e-mail: biaqd@bellnet.ca
www.biaqd.ca
www.facebook.com/154337841305196

Chief Officer(s):
Mary-Ellen Thompson, President
Kris Bonn, Vice-President
Monique Chartrand, Office Administrator
• On the Sunnier Side
Type: Newsletter; *Frequency:* Monthly; *Accepts Advertising*
Profile: Notices of upcoming events, information about programs & services, plus prevention updates

Chatham

9 Maple Leaf Dr., Chatham ON N7M 6H2

Tel: 519-351-0297; *Fax:* 519-351-7600
e-mail: lgall@newbeginnings-cksl.com
newbeginnings-cksl.com
www.facebook.com/370648369630107

Chief Officer(s):
Lori Gall, Executive Director
Sean St.Amand, Community Integration Director
  sean@newbeginnings-cksl.com
Greg Davenport, Vice-President
Cathy Weir, Vice-President
Kevin Deacon, Treasurer

Fort Erie
649 Niagara Blvd., Fort Erie ON L2A 3H7

Tel: 905-871-7789; *Fax:* 905-871-7832
e-mail: hiafeadmin@bellnet.ca

Chief Officer(s):
Donna Summerville, Coordinator, Programs
Julie Anthony, President
  hiafepresident@bellnet.ca
Shirley Athoe, Treasurer
  hiafetreasure@bellnet.ca

Hamilton-Wentworth
822 Main St. East, Hamilton ON L8M 1L6

Tel: 905-521-2100; *Fax:* 905-521-7927
e-mail: info@hbia.ca
www.hbia.ca

Chief Officer(s):
Jane Grech, President
Ted Newbigging, Vice-President
Diana Velikonja, Secretary
Shannon Moffat, Treasurer
• Headstrong
Type: Newsletter; *Frequency:* Quarterly; *Accepts Advertising; Editor:* Sandra Best; Celeste Gallant
Profile: Updates on association events & groups, plus new developments related to acquired brain injuries

Kingston
c/o Epilepsy Kingston, 100 Stuart St., Kingston ON K7L 2V6

Tel: 613-547-6969; *Fax:* 613-548-4162
e-mail: BIASEO@epilepsykingston.org
braininjuryhelp.ca
www.facebook.com/407323819294054
twitter.com/abi_help

Chief Officer(s):
Kim Smith, Contact, 613-536-1555

London
201 King St., London ON N6A 1C9

Tel: 519-642-4539; *Fax:* 519-642-4124
e-mail: info@braininjurylondon.on.ca
www.braininjurylondon.on.ca
ca.linkedin.com/company/brain-injury-association-of-london-&-region
www.facebook.com/braininjuryassociationoflondonandregion
twitter.com/braininjuryon
www.youtube.com/user/braininjurylondonon

Chief Officer(s):
Donna Thomson, Executive Director
Alysia Chrisiaen, President
Colin Fitchett, Vice-President
Julie Willsie, Vice-President
Carla Robertson, Treasurer
Stephanie McGill, Coordinator, Communications & Services
• The Monarch [a publication of the Brain Injury Association of London & Region]
Type: Newsletter; *Frequency:* Quarterly; *Accepts Advertising*

Mississauga
#204, 2155 Leanne Blvd., Mississauga ON L5K 2K8

Tel: 905-823-2221; *Fax:* 905-823-9960
Toll-Free: 800-565-8594
e-mail: biaph@biaph.com
www.biaph.com
facebook.com/biaph
twitter.com/BrainAwareBIAPH

Chief Officer(s):

Alexis Moskal, Contact

North Bay
280 Oakwood Ave., North Bay ON P1B 9G2
Tel: 705-840-8882
e-mail: contact@bianba.ca
www.bianba.ca

Chief Officer(s):
Katy Snoddon, Chair
Robert McKay, Secretary
Michael Cairns, Treasurer

Oshawa
#24, 850 King St. West, Oshawa ON L1J 8N5
Tel: 905-723-2732; Fax: 905-723-4936
Toll-Free: 866-354-4464
e-mail: headinjassoc@rogers.com

Chief Officer(s):
Frank Murphy, Executive Director
fmurphy@biad.ca
Frank Welling, President
• The Front Page
Type: Newsletter; Frequency: Monthly
Profile: Association activities & forthcoming events

Ottawa
#300A, 211 Bronson Ave., Ottawa ON K1R 6H5
Tel: 613-233-8303; Fax: 613-233-8422
e-mail: braininjuryottawavalley@bellnet.ca
www.biaov.org

Chief Officer(s):
Wendy Charbonneau, President
Lise Marcoux, Vice-President
Robert Allen, Secretary-Treasurer

Peterborough
#100, 160 Charlotte St., Peterborough ON K9J 2T8
Tel: 705-741-1172; Fax: 705-741-5129
Toll-Free: 800-854-9738
e-mail: biapr@nexicom.net
biapr.ca
twitter.com/biapeterboro

Chief Officer(s):
Cheryl-Ann Hassan, Executive Director
Jeff Lanctot, President
• Heads & Tales
Type: Newsletter; Frequency: Monthly; Accepts Advertising
Profile: Information about the association & acquired brain injuries for members

Richmond Hill
11181 Yonge St., 3rd Fl., Richmond Hill ON L4S 1L2
Tel: 905-780-1236; Fax: 905-780-1524
Toll-Free: 800-263-5404
e-mail: daveblakemore@rogers.com

Chief Officer(s):
Dave Blakemore, President
• The Headway
Type: Newsletter
Profile: Current information related to acquired brain injury in York Region

St. Catharines
c/o Stokes Community Village, PO Box 2338, 4-36 Page Street, St Catharines ON L2R 4A7
Tel: 905-984-5058; Fax: 905-984-5354

Chief Officer(s):
Pat Dracup, Program Director
• Brain Injury Association of Niagara Newsletter
Type: Newsletter; Frequency: Quarterly
Profile: Association activities for members

Sarnia-Lambton
#1032, 1705 London Line, Sarnia ON N7S 1B2
Tel: 519-337-5657; Fax: 519-337-1024
e-mail: info@sarniabiasl.ca
www.sarniabiasl.ca

Chief Officer(s):
Roy Marshall, Contact, 519-542-2151

Sault Ste Marie

#127, 31 Old Garden River Rd., Sault Ste Marie ON P6B 5Y7
Tel: 705-946-0172; Fax: 705-946-0594
e-mail: biassmd@shaw.ca
www.braininjuryssm.ca/bia.htm

Chief Officer(s):
Frank Halford, President
Jennifer Trepasso, Secretary
Karen McKinley, Treasurer
Dawn Kuhlenbaumer, Coordinator, Peer Support
• Brain Injury Association of Sault Ste Marie & District Newsletter
Type: Newsletter

Sudbury & District
2750 Bancroft Dr., Sudbury ON P3B 1T9
Tel: 705-670-0200; Fax: 705-670-1462
e-mail: info@biasd.com
www.biasd.com

Chief Officer(s):
Sean Parsons, President, Chair-Executive

Thunder Bay
#217, 1100 Memorial Ave., Thunder Bay ON P7B 4A3
Tel: 807-621-4164
e-mail: info@biatba.org
www.biatba.org

Timmins
733 Ross Ave. E., Timmins ON P4N 8S8
Tel: 705-264-2933; Fax: 705-264-0350
www.seizurebraininjurycentre.com
www.facebook.com/seizurebraininjurycentre
twitter.com/letstalkbrain

Chief Officer(s):
Rhonda Latendresse, Executive Director
rhondal@seizurebraininjurycentre.com
Stacey DeLaurier, Communications Officer
staceyd@seizurebraininjurycentre.com
Samantha Saley, Client Services Coodinator
sams@seizurebraininjurycentre.com

Toronto
#205, 40 St. Clair Ave. East, Toronto ON M4T 1M9
Tel: 416-830-1485
e-mail: info@bist.ca
www.bist.ca

Chief Officer(s):
Judy Moir, Chair
Paul McCormack, Vice-Chair & Treasurer
Gary Gerber, Secretary
Todd Gotlieb, Treasurer
• BIST Beacon
Type: Newsletter; Frequency: Irregular
Profile: Information about the Brain Injury Society of Toronto, available to members & donors to the society

Waterloo-Wellington
#1, 871 Victoria St. North, Kitchener ON N2B 3S4
Tel: 519-579-5300; Fax: 519-579-0118
e-mail: biaww@bellnet.ca
www.biaww.com
www.linkedin.com/groups/Brain-Injury-Association-WaterlooWellington-38
www.facebook.com/biaww

Chief Officer(s):
Patti Lehman, Executive Director

Windsor-Essex
#201, 200 West Grand Blvd., Windsor ON N9E 3W7
Tel: 519-981-1329
e-mail: info@biawe.com
www.biawe.com
www.facebook.com/BIAWE
www.youtube.com/channel/UC-VWaZbdUVoC4zw-_9jrKFA

Chief Officer(s):
Melanie Gardin, President
Lois Caldwell, Vice-President
Cheryl Henshaw, Secretary
Nancy Nicholson, Treasurer

• Step Ahead!
Type: Newsletter; *Accepts Advertising*
Profile: Review of association activites & announcements of future events

Ontario Neurotrauma Foundation (ONF)
#601, 90 Eglinton Ave. East, Toronto ON M4P 2Y3
Tel: 416-422-2228; *Fax:* 416-422-1240
e-mail: info@onf.org
www.onf.org
twitter.com/OntNeurotrauma
Overview: A medium-sized provincial organization founded in 1998
Mission: To reduce the impact, incidence & prevalence of neurotrauma injuries, through knowledge creation, Research Capacity Building, & knowledge mobilization
Chief Officer(s):
Mimi Lowi-Young, Chair
Kent Bassett-Spiers, Chief Executive Officer
    kent@onf.org

PRINCE EDWARD ISLAND

Brain Injury Coalition of Prince Edward Island (BICPEI)
#5, 81 Prince St., Charlottetown PE C1A 4R3
Tel: 902-314-4228
e-mail: info@biapei.com
www.bicpei.com
www.facebook.com/243812565693892
Overview: A small provincial organization overseen by Brain Injury Association of Canada
Mission: To contribute to an environment that is responsive to the needs of peoples affected with a brain injury in Prince Edward Island; To promote brain injury prevention

QUÉBEC

Association québécoise des traumatisés craniens (AQTC)
#106, 911, rue Jean-Talon est, Montréal QC H2R 1V5
Tél: 514-274-7447; *Téléc:* 514-274-1717
www.aqtc.ca
www.facebook.com/AQTC.montreal.laval
Aperçu: *Dimension:* moyenne; *Envergure:* provinciale; Organisme sans but lucratif; fondée en 1986
Mission: De défendre et promouvoir les droits et les intérêts des personnes traumatisés cranio-cérébrales et de leurs familles et de favoriser le maintien ou l'amélioration de la qualité de vie; AQTC Laval: 220, av du Parc, (514) 274-7447
Membre(s) du bureau directeur:
Pierre Mitchell, Directeur général
Pascal Brodeur, Adjoint à la direction, 514-274-7447 Ext. 233

Association québécoise des traumatisés crâniens (AQTC)
#106, 911, rue Jean-Talon Est, Montréal QC H2R 1V5
Tél: 514-274-7447; *Téléc:* 514-274-1717
www.aqtc.ca
www.facebook.com/AQTC.montreal.laval
Aperçu: *Dimension:* petite; *Envergure:* provinciale; fondée en 1989
Mission: Accompagner les victimes de lésions cérébrales traumatiques en fournissant des loisirs activites, ateliers de groupe, et des informations
Membre de: Regroupement des associations de personnes traumatisées craniocérébrals du Québec / Coalition of Associations of Craniocerebral Trauma in Quebec
Membre(s) du bureau directeur:
Pierre Mitchell, Executive Director, 514-274-7447 Ext. 224
Manon Beaudoin, Présidente
Céline Martel, Vice-présidente
Denyse Rousselet, Secrétaire
Nathalie Boucher, Intervenante psychosociale, 514-274-7447 Ext. 222
Publications:
• Association québécoise des traumatisés crâniens rapport annuel
Type: Yearbook; *Frequency:* Annually
• Phoenix
Type: Newspaper; *Frequency:* Quarterly
Profile: Reports & photographs of association happenings

Regroupement des associations de personnes traumatisées craniocérébrales du Québec (RAPTCCQ) / Coalition of Associations of Craniocerebral Trauma in Quebec
220, av du Parc, Laval QC H7N 3X4
Tél: 514-274-7447; *Téléc:* 514-274-1717
Courriel: info@raptccq.com
www.raptccq.com
www.facebook.com/RAPTCCQ
Aperçu: *Dimension:* petite; *Envergure:* provinciale; fondée en 1999 surveillé par Brain Injury Association of Canada
Mission: Pour soutenir les personnes vivant avec une lésion cérébrale au Québec
Membre(s) du bureau directeur:
Nicole Tremblay, Présidente
Denis Veilleux, Vice-Président
Pascal Brodeur, Secrétaire et trésorier
Guy Lemieux, Directeur

SASKATCHEWAN

Saskatchewan Brain Injury Association (SBIA)
PO Box 3843, Saskatoon SK S4P 3Y3
Tel: 306-373-1555
Toll-Free: 888-373-1555
www.sbia.ca
www.facebook.com/SaskBrainInjury
twitter.com/SKBrainInjury
www.youtube.com/user/sbiaPrograms?feature=mhee
Previous Name: Saskatchewan Head Injury Association
Overview: A small provincial charitable organization founded in 1985 overseen by Brain Injury Association of Canada
Mission: To improve the quality of life for person living with an acquired brain injury, their families, & service providers throughout Saskatchewan; To provide support, information, & services to persons living with the effects of acquired brain injury
Chief Officer(s):
Gordon MacFadden, President
Glenda James, Executive Director
Publications:
• Connections [a publication of the Saskatchewan Brain Injury Association]
Type: Newsletter
Profile: Association activities & event reviews & announcements

Local Associations

ALBERTA

Brain Care Centre (BCC)
Royal Alex Place, #229, 10106 - 111th Ave., Edmonton AB T5G 0B4
Tel: 780-477-7575; *Fax:* 780-474-4415
Toll-Free: 800-425-5552
www.braincarecentre.com
www.facebook.com/pages/Brain-Care-Centre/291605290917593
twitter.com/BrainCareCentre
www.youtube.com/user/braincarecentreyeg
Previous Name: Northern Alberta Brain Injury Society
Overview: A small local charitable organization founded in 1983
Mission: To support people affected by acquired brain injury in northern Alberta
Chief Officer(s):
Garnet Cummings, Executive Director
Stephanie Boldt, President
Publications:
• NABIS News
Type: Newsletter; *Frequency:* Quarterly; *Price:* Free with membership in the Northern Alberta Brain Injury Society

Southern Alberta Brain Injury Society (SABIS)
#102, 2116 - 27th Ave. NE, Calgary AB T2E 7A6
Tel: 403-521-5212; *Fax:* 403-283-5867
e-mail: sabis@sabis.ab.ca
www.sabis.ab.ca
www.facebook.com/226816920793215
twitter.com/SABISCalgary
Overview: A medium-sized local charitable organization founded in 1985

Mission: To promote lifelong support for persons with acquired brain injury, their families & support networks; To raise community awareness of brain injury; To assist persons with acquired brain injury to live as independently as possible

Chief Officer(s):
Natasha Bodei, Executive Director
  natasha@sabis.ab.ca
Cheryl Sayward, Program Manager
  cheryl@sabis.ab.ca

Publications:
• Southern Alberta Brain Injury Society Newsletter
Type: Newsletter; *Frequency:* Quarterly; *Price:* Free with membership in the Southern Alberta Brain Injury Society
• Southern Alberta Brain Injury Society Annual Report
Type: Yearbook; *Frequency:* Annually; *Price:* Free with membership in the Southern Alberta Brain Injury Society

---

Westward Goals Support Services Inc.
PO Box 2292, Rocky Mountain House AB T4T 1B7
Tel: 403-845-2922; *Fax:* 403-845-2277
e-mail: wwgoals@telusplanet.net
www.westwardgoals.ca

Overview: A small local organization founded in 1991
Mission: To assist mentally handicapped/brain injured persons in maximizing independence through supported programs; to offer residential support, community networking & outreach support for adults; to provide children with outreach & family support, including in-home support, rehabilitation aides & host family services

Chief Officer(s):
Marla Hills, Executive Director

BRITISH COLUMBIA

Prince George Brain Injured Group (PGBIG)
1237 - 4 Ave., Prince George BC V2L 3J7
Tel: 250-564-2447; *Fax:* 250-564-6928
Toll-Free: 866-564-2447
e-mail: info@pgbig.ca
pgbig.ca

Overview: A small local organization founded in 1987
Mission: To provide assistance to adults whose lives have changed as a result of an acquired brain injury
Member of: Prince George United Way
Chief Officer(s):
Alison Hagreen, Executive Director

South Okanagan Similkameen Brain Injury Society (SOSBIS)
#2, 996 Main St., Penticton BC V2A 5E4
Tel: 250-490-0613; *Fax:* 250-490-3912
e-mail: info@sosbis.com
www.sosbis.com
www.facebook.com/SOSBIS

Overview: A small local charitable organization
Mission: To assist survivors of acquired brain injuries & their families in acheiving independence & quality of life; To prevent brain injuries
Chief Officer(s):
Linda Sankey, Executive Director

Publications:
• Brain Waves [a publication of the South Okanagan Similkameen Brain Injury Society]
Type: Newsletter; *Frequency:* Quarterly
Profile: Organization news; upcoming events; stories; strategies to cope with acquired brain injury

---

QUÉBEC

Association des neurotraumatisés de l'Outaouais (ANO)
#1, 115 boul Sacré-Coeur, Gatineau QC J8X 1C5
Tél: 819-770-8804; *Télec:* 819-770-5863
Courriel: ano@ano.ca
www.ano.ca
www.facebook.com/ano.ca

Aperçu: *Dimension:* petite; *Envergure:* locale; fondée en 1990
Mission: Pour aider les personnes dans la région québécoise de l'Outaouais qui ont subi un traumatisme crânien ou un AVC
Membre de: Regroupement des associations de personnes traumatisées craniocérébrals du Québec; Regroupement des associations de personnes handicapées de l'Outaouais; CDC Rond Point

Membre(s) du bureau directeur:
Julie Larochelle, Présidente
Georgette Lachance, Vice-présidente
Servane Chesnais, Secrétaire
Raphaëlle Robidoux, Trésorière

Publications:
• Le Mieux Etre [publication d'Association des neurotraumatisés de l'Outaouais]
Type: Newsletter; *Frequency:* 3 pa
Profile: Information sur les services de santé et services sociaux et loisirs pour les membres de l'Association des neurotraumatisés de l'Outaouais

---

Association des personnes accidentées cérébro-vasculaires, aphasiques et traumatisées crânio-cérébrales du Bas-Saint-Laurent (ACVA-TCC du BSL)
391, boul Jessop, Rimouski QC G5L 1M9
Tél: 418-723-2345
Ligne sans frais: 888-302-2282
Courriel: acvatcc@globetrotter.net
www.acvatcc.com
www.facebook.com/pages/ACVA-TCC-du-Bas-Saint-Laurent/61441702
8571908

Aperçu: *Dimension:* petite; *Envergure:* locale; fondée en 1991
Mission: Pour soutenir les personnes dans la région du Bas-Saint-Laurent qui ont été touchés par une lésion cérébrale, accident vasculaire cérébral, ou d'aphasie.
Membre de: Regroupement des associations de personnes traumatisées craniocérébrales du Québec / Coalition of Associations of Craniocerebral Trauma in Quebec
Membre(s) du bureau directeur:
Mathieu Lajoie, Directeur

Association des TCC (le traumatisme cranio-cérébral) et ACV (un accident vasculaire cérébral) de la Gaspésie et des Iles-de-la-Madeleine Inc.
CP 308, Maria QC G0C 1Y0
Tél: 418-759-5120; *Télec:* 418-759-8188
Ligne sans frais: 888-278-2280
Courriel: tccacv@globetrotter.net
www.tccacvgim.org

Nom précédent: Association des personnes traumatisées cranio-cérébrales de la Gaspésie et des Iles-de-la-Madeleine inc.
Aperçu: *Dimension:* petite; *Envergure:* locale; fondée en 1993
Mission: Pour informer et aider les personnes cranio-cérébral, traumatisme et leurs familles, en Gaspésie et les Iles de la Madeleine
Membre de: Regroupement des associations de personnes traumatisées craniocérébrales du Québec / Coalition of Associations of Craniocerebral Trauma in Quebec
Publications:
• La Bulle
Type: Newsletter; *Frequency:* Quarterly
Profile: Association activities

Association des traumatisés crâniens de l'Abitibi-Témiscamingue (Le Pilier)
3. 9e rue, Rouyn-Noranda QC J9X 2A9
Tél: 819-762-7478; *Télec:* 819-797-8313
Courriel: pilieratcat@cablevision.qc.ca
www.pilieratcat.qc.ca

Aperçu: *Dimension:* petite; *Envergure:* locale
Mission: Pour fournir des services de soutien aux personnes qui ont subi une lésion cérébrale acquise, et leurs familles, dans la région de l'Abitibi-Témiscamingue du Québec
Membre de: Regroupement des associations de personnes traumatisées craniocérébrales du Québec / Coalition of Associations of Craniocerebral Trauma in Quebec
Membre(s) du bureau directeur:
Francine Chalifoux, Directrice générale et responsable clinique, 819-762-7478 Ext. 47421

Association des Traumatisés cranio-cérébraux de la Montérégie (ATCCM)

#D-131, 308, rue Montsabré, Beloeil QC J3G 2H5
Tél: 450-446-1111; *Téléc:* 450-446-6405
Ligne sans frais: 877-661-2822
Courriel: atcc@atccmonteregie.qc.ca
www.atccmonteregie.qc.ca

Aperçu: *Dimension:* petite; *Envergure:* locale; fondée en 1994
Mission: Pour fournir des services de soutien aux personnes de la région de la Montérégie du Québec qui ont subi une lésion cérébrale traumatique ou un accident vasculaire cérébral; Pour favoriser la réinsertion et les expériences d'apprentissage
Membre de: Regroupement des associations de personnes traumatisées craniocérébrales du Québec / Coalition of Associations of Craniocerebral Trauma in Quebec
Membre(s) du bureau directeur:
Chantal Bourguignon, Directrice générale
c.bourguignon@atccmonteregie.qc.ca

Association des traumatisés cranio-cérébraux des deux rives (Québec-Chaudière-Appalaches)

Territoire de Québec et de Chaudiere-Appalaches, 14, rue Saint-Amand, Loretteville QC G2A 2K9
Tél: 418-842-8421; *Téléc:* 418-842-9616
Ligne sans frais: 866-844-8421
Courriel: tcc2rives@oricom.ca
www.tcc2rives.qc.ca

Aperçu: *Dimension:* petite; *Envergure:* locale; fondée en 1989
Mission: Pour aider les victimes, les parents, les amis, et les professionnels touchés par une lésion cérébrale traumatique dans la région Chaudière-Appalaches du Québec.
Membre de: Regroupement des associations de personnes traumatisées craniocérébrales du Québec / Coalition of Associations of Craniocerebral Trauma in Quebec
Publications:
• L'En Tête
Type: Newspaper; *Frequency:* Quarterly
Profile: Information about the association's services

Association des traumatisés cranio-cérébraux Mauricie-Centre-du-Québec (ATCC)

39, rue Bellerive, Trois-Rivières QC G8T 6J4
Tél: 819-372-4993
Courriel: atcc@assotcc.org
www.associationtcc.org
www.facebook.com/381058281920939

Aperçu: *Dimension:* petite; *Envergure:* locale
Mission: Pour soutenir les personnes touchées par une lésion cérébrale traumatique en Mauricie-Centre-du-Québec
Membre de: Regroupement des associations de personnes traumatisées craniocérébrales du Québec / Coalition of Associations of Craniocerebral Trauma in Quebec

Association renaissance des personnes traumatisées crâniennes du Saguenay-Lac-Saint-Jean (ARPTC)

2223, boul du Saguenay, Jonquière QC G7S 4H5
Tél: 418-548-9366; *Téléc:* 418-548-9369
Ligne sans frais: 855-548-9366
Courriel: arptc@arptc.org
www.arptc.org

Aperçu: *Dimension:* petite; *Envergure:* locale; fondée en 1995
Mission: Pour aider les personnes dans la région du Saguenay-Lac-Saint-Jean du Québec qui ont été touchés par les conséquences de lésions cérébrales; Pour aider les membres de la famille des personnes qui ont subi une lésion cérébrale
Membre de: Regroupement des associations de personnes traumatisées craniocérébrales du Québec / Coalition of Associations of Craniocerebral Trauma in Quebec
Membre(s) du bureau directeur:
Jonathan Jean-Vézina, Directeur général
direction@arptc.org

Centre d'aide personnes traumatisées crâniennes et handicapées physiques Laurentides (CAPTCHPL)

CP 11, Saint-Jérôme QC J7Z 5T7
Tél: 450-431-2860; *Téléc:* 450-431-7955
Ligne sans frais: 888-431-3437
Courriel: lecaptchpl@sympatico.ca
www.captchpl.org
twitter.com/Captchpl

Aperçu: *Dimension:* petite; *Envergure:* locale
Mission: Pour aider les personnes souffrant de lésions cérébrales et physiquement handicapées dans la région des Laurentides du Québec; Pour favoriser l'intégration sociale des personnes handicapées physiques et de lésions cérébrales
Membre de: Regroupement des associations de personnes traumatisées craniocérébrales du Québec / Coalition of Associations of Craniocerebral Trauma in Quebec
Membre(s) du bureau directeur:
Michel Lajeunesse, Directeur général

International Associations

American Academy of Neurology (AAN)

201 Chicago Ave., Minneapolis MN 55415 USA
Tel: 612-928-6000; *Fax:* 612-454-2746
Toll-Free: 800-879-1960
e-mail: memberservices@aan.com
www.aan.com
www.linkedin.com/groups/2386034
www.facebook.com/AmericanAcademyofNeurology
twitter.com/AANMember
www.youtube.com/AANChannel

Overview: A large international organization
Mission: To advance the art & science of neurology; To promote the best possible care for patients with neurological disorders
Chief Officer(s):
Catherine M. Rydell, Executive Director & CEO
crydell@aan.com
Jason Kopinski, Deputy Executive Director
jkopinski@aan.com
Timothy Engel, Chief Financial Officer
tengel@aan.com
Angela Babb, Chief Communications Officer
ababb@aan.com
Chris Becker, Chief Business Development Officer
cbecker@aan.com
Lynee Koester, Project Manager, Health Policy
lkoester@aan.com
Publications:
• AANnews [a publication of the American Academy of Neurology]
Type: Newsletter; *Frequency:* Monthly; *Price:* Free with American Academy of Neurology membership
Profile: American Academy of Neurology & practice information
• American Academy of Neurology Patient Education Series
Type: Books
Profile: Information & treatment options for patients & caregivers
• Continuum: Lifelong Learning in Neurology
Frequency: Bimonthly; *Editor:* Steven L. Lewis, MD
Profile: A self-study continuing medical education publication
• Neurology
Type: Journal; *Editor:* Robert A. Gross, MD, PhD, FAAN
Profile: The official scientific journal of the American Academy of Neurology, directed to physicians concerned with diseases & conditions of the nervous system
• Neurology Now
Type: Magazine; *Frequency:* Bimonthly
Profile: Updated & important information for neurology patients, families, & caregivers
• Neurology Today
Type: Newspaper; *Frequency:* Biweekly
Profile: Clinical, policy, research, & practice news, for neurologists

National Publications

Canadian Journal of Neurological Sciences
c/o Canadian Neurological Sciences Federation, 143N Heritage Square, #8500 Macleod Trail SE, Calgary, AB T2H 2N1
Tel: 403-229-9544; *Fax:* 403-229-1661
Circulation: 1,200 *Frequency:* Bi-monthly
The journal is the official publication of the four member societies of the Canadian Neurological Sciences Federation: Canadian Neurological Society (CNS), Canadian Neurosurgical Society (CNSS), Canadian Association of Child Neurology (CACN), & the Canadian Society of Clinical Neurophysiologists (CSCN). Peer reviewed articles about the neurosciences are published in the Canadian Journal of Neurological Sciences. The journal is circulated to society members, non-members, & institutions in Canada & around the world.
Lisa Arrington, Managing Editor, larrington@cambridge.org

Journal of Psychiatry & Neuroscience (JPN) / Revue de psychiatrie & de neuroscience
Owned By: Canadian Medical Association
1867 Alta Vista Dr., Ottawa, ON K1G 5W8
Toll-Free: 888-855-2555
jpn@cma.ca
Frequency: 6 times a year
Wendy Carroll, Managing Editor

Provincial Libraries

Alberta Hospital - Ponoka
PO Box 1000, Ponoka, AB T4J 1R8
Tel: 403-783-7691; *Fax:* 403-783-7695
krs@albertahealthservices.ca
www.albertahealthservices.ca
Profile: At the Centennial Centre for Mental Health and Brain Injury, people suffering from brain injury or psychiatric disorders receive care and treatment. **Collection:** Archive for AHP history
Lori Maisey, Library Technician
lori.maisey@albertahealthservices.ca

Centennial Centre for Mental Health & Brain Injury Site
Dave Russell Education Complex, 46 St. South, Ponoka, AB T4J 1R8
Tel: 403-783-7691; *Fax:* 403-783-7695

Ontario Brain Injury Association
3550 Schmon Pkwy., 2nd Fl., Thorold, ON L2V 4Y6
Tel: 905-641-8877; *Fax:* 905-641-0323
obia@obia.on.ca
www.obia.ca
Social Media: twitter.com/OntarioBIA; www.facebook.com/OntarioBIA
Collection: Books & materials on brain injury; articles, journals, & research available on the website
Ruth Wilcock, Executive Director
rwilcock@obia.on.ca

Saskatchewan Brain Injury Association
#422, 230 Ave. R South, Saskatoon, SK S7M 2Z1
Tel: 306-373-1555; *Toll-Free:* 888-373-1555
www.sbia.ca
Social Media: www.youtube.com/user/sbiaPrograms; twitter.com/SKBrainInjury; www.facebook.com/SaskBrainInjury
Glenda James, Executive Director

Local Hospitals & Health Centres

BRITISH COLUMBIA

KELOWNA: Central Okanagan Brain Injury Society
Affiliated with: Interior Health Authority
#11, 368 Industrial Ave., Kelowna, BC V1Y 4N7
Tel: 250-762-3233
www.interiorhealth.ca

Note: Services for people affected by brain injury, as well as their families.

ONTARIO

TORONTO: Community Head Injury Resource Services (CHIRS)
Former Name: Ashby House
62 Finch Ave. West, Toronto, ON M2N 7G1
Tel: 416-240-8000 *Fax:* 416-240-1149
Chirs@chirs.com
www.chirs.com
Social Media: www.facebook.com/chirstoronto
Year Founded: 1974
Number of Employees: 160
Note: A range of residential services are offered for persons living with the effects of acquired brain injury. Community Head Injury Resource Services serves the Greater Toronto Area.
Hedy Chandler, Contact
hedyc@rogers.com

Hearing Loss

Hearing loss is a common problem that affects people of all ages and backgrounds. The degree of loss can range from slight (trouble hearing in a noisy environment) to profound (deafness). There are four types of hearing loss: conductive, sensorineural, mixed and central. Conductive hearing loss is caused by a defect in the external ear canal or middle ear, and can often be corrected by hearing aids, medical treatment or surgery.

Cause
Sensorineural hearing loss, the most common type of permanent hearing loss, results from damage to the inner ear and to the primary nerve that transmits sound waves to the brain. Usually, it cannot be corrected surgically or medically. Mixed hearing loss is a combination of conductive and sensorineural defects. Central hearing loss results from impairment of brain function, and is rare.

Hearing loss may be present at birth due to an inherited condition, premature birth, birth injury, infection (such as rubella) or maternal alcohol or drug use. Causes of hearing loss after birth include infections (such as meningitis), injury, prolonged noise exposure, aging, tumours, hereditary diseases and side effects of certain drugs.

Symptoms
Children with a hearing loss may have slow or inaccurate speech development, or problems with concentration. They may also have difficulty understanding what people are saying, fail to respond when called, complain of earaches, watch TV at a loud volume and have academic or behavioural problems. Adults may suspect a hearing loss if they find it difficult to hear voices on the telephone, are always asking people to repeat themselves, need to watch TV at a loud volume or have trouble hearing conversations in noisy situations. Hearing loss in adults, if moderate or severe, is usually obvious. In young children, however, the problem is easily overlooked and the opportunity for early intervention can be lost.

Prevalence
In Canada, over one million adults report that they have a hearing-related disability. However, since there are probably many more Canadians suffering from a hearing loss who fail to report their condition, the actual number could be closer to three million.

Treatment Options
Most newborns are screened for hearing loss shortly after birth. In older children and adults, hearing loss is usually diagnosed by an audiologist who takes a medical history, performs a physical exam and conducts hearing evaluation tests. These tests may include pure tone testing (to determine the faintest tones that can be heard at certain frequencies), speech testing (to determine the

faintest speech that can be heard) and tests of middle ear function.

Amplification of sound with hearing aids helps almost all persons with mild-to-severe conductive or sensorineural hearing loss. Profoundly deaf persons who cannot be helped by hearing aids may benefit from a cochlear implant, a specialized device inserted into the inner ear.

If hearing loss is not managed properly, it can interfere with a person's work, education and personal life. However, early diagnosis and treatment usually helps children improve their auditory ability, through the use of hearing aids, educational programs and speech therapy. Other recent advancements in technology such as personal communication devices, captioning, assistive devices and text telephones have also greatly improved quality of life for people with a hearing loss.

National Associations

Accessible Media Inc. (AMI)
#200, 1090 Don Mills Rd., Toronto ON M3C 3R6
Tel: 416-422-4222; Fax: 416-422-1633
Toll-Free: 800-567-6755
e-mail: info@ami.ca
www.ami.ca
www.linkedin.com/company/accessible-media-inc-
www.facebook.com/AccessibleMediaInc
twitter.com/AccessibleMedia
www.youtube.com/user/accessiblemedia
Overview: A medium-sized national charitable organization
Mission: To bring media in an alternate form to those not able to follow in traditional ways
Affliation(s): Achilles Canada; Canadian Council of the Blind; CNIB; Courage Canada; Sight Night; Foundation Fighting Blindness
Chief Officer(s):
David Errington, President & CEO
John Melville, Vice-President, Programming & Production
Line Gendreau, Vice-President, Finance
Terry Reid, Vice-President, Human Resources
Peter Burke, Vice-President, Marketing & Communications
Darrel Sauerlender, Vice-President, Technology Services
Chris O'Brien, Accessibility Officer

Canadian Academy of Audiology (CAA) / Académie canadienne d'audiologie (ACA)
PO Box 22531, 300 Coxwell Ave., Toronto ON M4L 3B6
Tel: 647-794-7305
Toll-Free: 800-264-5106
e-mail: contact@canadianaudiology.ca
www.canadianaudiology.ca
www.linkedin.com/groups/4068951
www.facebook.com/CanadianAcademyofAudiology
twitter.com/caaudiology
Overview: A medium-sized national organization founded in 1996
Mission: To represent the audiological community in Canada; To provide quality hearing health care & education to persons with, or at risk for, hearing or vestibular disorders; To maintain & advance ethical standards of practice
Chief Officer(s):
Marlene Bagatto, President
Salima Jiwani, President-Elect

Canadian Association of the Deaf (CAD) / Association des sourds du Canada (ASC)
#606, 251 Bank St., Ottawa ON K2P 1X3
Tel: 613-565-2882; Fax: 613-565-1207; TTY: 613-565-8882
e-mail: info@cad.ca
www.cad.ca
www.facebook.com/1940CADASC
twitter.com/CADASC
Overview: A medium-sized national charitable organization founded in 1940
Mission: To protect & promote the rights, needs, & concerns of deaf Canadians

Affliation(s): World Federation of the Deaf; Council of Canadians with Disabilities
Chief Officer(s):
Frank Folino, President
ffolino@cad.ca
James Roots, Executive Director
Pavel Chernousov, Project Coordinator

Canadian Cultural Society of The Deaf, Inc. (CCSD)
The Distillery Historic District, 34 Distillery Lane, Toronto ON M5A 3C4
e-mail: info@deafculturecentre.ca
www.deafculturecentre.ca
www.facebook.com/pages/Deaf-Culture-Centre/93708438725
twitter.com/DeafCulture
Also Known As: Deaf Culture Centre
Overview: A medium-sized national charitable organization founded in 1973
Mission: To ensure that the cultural needs of deaf & hard-of-hearing people are being met; To concentrate efforts in the areas of the performing arts, sign language, deaf literature, the visual arts, & heritage resources
Chief Officer(s):
Joanne Cripps, Executive Director
jcripps@deafculturecentre.ca

Canadian Deaf Curling Association (CDCA) / Association de Curling des Sourdes du Canada
Vancouver BC
Tel: 604-734-2250; Fax: 604-734-2254; TTY: 250-539-3264
www.deafcurlcanada.org
Also Known As: Deaf Curl Canada
Overview: A small national organization overseen by Canadian Deaf Sports Association
Mission: To provide deaf & hard of hearing curlers with opportunities across Canada
Member of: Canadian Deaf Sports Association; Canadian Curling Association
Affliation(s): British Columbia Deaf Sports Federation; Alberta Deaf Curling Association; Saskatchewan Deaf Sports Association; Manitoba Deaf Curling Association; Ontario Deaf Curling Assocation; Association de Curling des Sourds du Quebec; Nova Scotia Deaf Curling Association
Chief Officer(s):
Bradford Bentley, President
president@deafcurlcanada.org
Allard Thomas, Vice-President
Susanne Beriault, Secretary
cdca-secretary@gmail.com
David Pickard, Treasurer
dpickard@telus.net
Dean Sutton, Chief Technical Director
curlingtd@shaw.ca

Canadian Deaf Golf Association (CDGA) / Association Canadienne de Golf des Sourds
#20, 51 Sholto Drive, London ON N6G 2E9
cdga1993.wixsite.com/cdga
Overview: A small national organization overseen by Canadian Deaf Sports Association
Mission: To aid in the development of leadership & golfing skills among deaf golfers across Canada
Member of: Canadian Deaf Sports Association
Chief Officer(s):
Dana McCarthy, President
cdgapresident@gmail.com
Peter Mitchell, Vice-President
pmitchell25@rogers.com
Paul Landry, Secretary
pauljlandry@shaw.ca
Adam Redmond, Treasurer
cdgatreasurer@gmail.com
Aurele Bourgeois, Director
abourgeois10@cogeco.ca

Canadian Deaf Ice Hockey Federation (CDIHF)

ON

www.cdihf.deafhockey.com
www.facebook.com/canada.deafhockey?fref=ts&ref=br_tf
twitter.com/CDNdeafhockey

Previous Name: Canadian Hearing Impaired Hockey Association
Overview: A small national charitable organization founded in 1983 overseen by Canadian Deaf Sports Association
Mission: To offer ice hockey programs for deaf & hard of hearing participants; To administer a hockey team to represent Canada internationally
Member of: Canadian Deaf Sports Association
Affiliation(s): Canadian Hockey Association; Ontario Deaf Sports Association, Inc.
Chief Officer(s):
Mark Dunn, President
mark.dunn@deafhockey.com

Canadian Deaf Sports Association (CDSA) / Association des sports des sourds du Canada (ASSC)

#202, 10217 boul Pie IX, Montréal QC H1H 3Z5
Tel: 514-321-8686; *Fax:* 514-321-8349; *TTY:* 514-321-2937
e-mail: info@assc-cdsa.com
www.assc-cdsa.com
www.facebook.com/assc.cdsa
twitter.com/ASSC_CDSA

Overview: A medium-sized national licensing charitable organization founded in 1964
Mission: To promote & facilitate the practice of fitness, amateur sports & recreation among deaf people of all ages in Canada from the local recreational level to Olympics calibre
Member of: Canadian Deaf & Hard of Hearing Forum; Canadian Paralympic Committee; Canadian Sports Coalition.
Affiliation(s): International Committee of Sports for the Deaf
Chief Officer(s):
Alain Turpin, Chief Executive Officer
alain.turpin@assc-cdsa.com
Gigi Fiset, Manager, Operational Services & Events
gigi.fiset@assc-cdsa.com

Canadian Deafblind Association (National) (CDBA) / Association canadienne de la surdicécité (Bureau National)

PO Box 421, #14, 1860 Appleby Line, Burlington ON L7L 7H7
Fax: 905-319-2027
Toll-Free: 866-229-5832
e-mail: info@cdbanational.com
www.cdbanational.com
www.facebook.com/cdbanational
twitter.com/CDBANational

Overview: A medium-sized national charitable organization
Mission: To promote awareness, education & support for people who are deafblind, in order to enhance their well-being
Chief Officer(s):
Carolyn Monaco, President
carolyn.monaco@sympatico.ca
Tom McFadden, National Executive Director

Alberta Chapter
AB

Tel: 780-554-6083
www.deafblindalberta.ca

Chief Officer(s):
Nicole Sander, Vice-President
nicsander@me.com

British Columbia Chapter
227 - 6th St., New Westminster BC V3L 3A5
Tel: 604-528-6170; *Fax:* 604-528-6174
www.cdbabc.ca

Chief Officer(s):
Theresa Tancock, Coordinator, Family Services
theresa@cdbabc.ca

Canadian Deafblind Association - New Brunswick Inc.
#495 B Prospect St., #H, Fredericton NB E3B 9M4
Tel: 506-452-1544; *Fax:* 506-451-8309; *TTY:* 506-452-1544
www.cdba-nb.ca
www.facebook.com/CDBANB

Chief Officer(s):
Kevin Symes, Executive Director
k.symes@cdba-nb.ca

Ontario Chapter
50 Main St., Paris ON N3L 2E2
Tel: 519-442-0463; *Fax:* 519-442-1871
Toll-Free: 877-760-7439; *TTY:* 519-442-6641
e-mail: info@cdbaontario.com
www.cdbaontario.com
www.facebook.com/cdbaontario
twitter.com/CDBAOntario

Chief Officer(s):
Cathy Proll, Executive Director

Saskatchewan Chapter
83 Tucker Cres., Saskatoon SK S7H 3H7
Tel: 306-374-0022; *Fax:* 306-374-0004
e-mail: cdba.sk@shaw.ca

Chief Officer(s):
Dana Heinrichs, Executive Director

Canadian Hard of Hearing Association (CHHA) / Association des malentendants canadiens (AMEC)

#205, 2415 Holly Lane, Ottawa ON K1V 7P2
Tel: 613-526-1584; *Fax:* 613-526-4718
Toll-Free: 800-263-8068; *TTY:* 613-526-2692
e-mail: chhanational@chha.ca
www.chha.ca
www.facebook.com/CHHANational
twitter.com/CHHA_AMEC

Overview: A medium-sized national charitable organization founded in 1982
Mission: To act as the voice of all hard of hearing Canadians; To promote the integration of hard of hearing people into society
Chief Officer(s):
Lorin MacDonald, President
Glenn Martin, Executive Director
gmartin@chha.ca
Publications:
• Listen / Écoute [a publication of the Canadian Hard of Hearing Association]
Type: Magazine; *Frequency:* 3 pa; *Accepts Advertising;* *Price:* $5
Profile: Hearing health issues, technology, & the concerns of hard of hearing individuals

Alberta - Calgary Branch
c/o 63 Cornell Rd. NW, Calgary AB T2L 0L4
Tel: 403-284-6224; *Fax:* 403-824-6224
e-mail: info@chha-calgary.ca
www.chha-calgary.ca

Chief Officer(s):
Terry Webb, President

Alberta - Edmonton Branch
#10, 9912 - 106 St., Edmonton AB T5K 1C5
Tel: 780-428-6622; *Fax:* 780-420-6661; *TTY:* 780-628-6622
e-mail: chha-ed@shaw.ca
www.chha-ed.com

Chief Officer(s):
Marilyn Kingdon, President

Alberta - Lethbridge Branch
1010 - 18A St. North, Lethbridge AB T1H 3J3
Tel: 403-328-2929

Chief Officer(s):
Doreen Gyorkos, President
dgyorkos@telusplanet.net

British Columbia - BC Main Chapter
#101, 9300 Nowell St., Chilliwack BC V2P 4V7
Tel: 604-795-9238; *Fax:* 604-795-9628
Toll-Free: 866-888-2442
e-mail: info@chha-bc.org
www.chha-bc.org
www.facebook.com/127952830548757

Chief Officer(s):
Marilyn Dahl, President

British Columbia - BC Parents' Branch

c/o 10150 Gillanders Rd., Chilliwack BC V2P 6H4
Tel: 604-819-5312; Fax: 604-794-3960
e-mail: info@chhaparents.bc.ca
www.chhaparents.bc.ca

Chief Officer(s):
Willetta Les, Administrator

British Columbia - Chilliwack Branch
c/o BC Chapter, #101, 9300 Nowell St., Chilliwack BC V2P4V71
Tel: 604-795-9238
e-mail: info@chha-bc.org

Chief Officer(s):
Scott Secord, President

British Columbia - Comox Valley
PO Box 433, Lazo BC V0R 2K0
Tel: 250-339-5770

Chief Officer(s):
Sarah Trotter, President
fstrotter@shaw.ca

British Columbia - HEAR Branch
#60, 5221 Oakmount Cres., Burnaby BC V5H 4R4
Tel: 604-438-2500

Chief Officer(s):
Betty MacGillivray, Acting President
bettymac@telus.net

British Columbia - North Shore Branch
600 West Queens Rd., North Vancouver BC V7N 2L3
Tel: 604-926-5222; Fax: 604-925-2286
e-mail: chha_nsb@telus.net
www.chha-nsb.com

Chief Officer(s):
Mike Hocevar, President
mikehocevar@gmail.com

British Columbia - Vancouver Branch
c/o 2125 West 7th Ave., Vancouver BC V6K 1X9
Tel: 778-358-9955
e-mail: chhavancouver@gmail.com
www.chhavancouver.ca

Chief Officer(s):
Ruth Warick, President

Manitoba Chapter
c/o SMD Self-Help Clearinghouse, 825 Sherbrook St., Winnipeg MB R3A 1M5
Tel: 204-975-3037; Fax: 204-975-3027
e-mail: mbchha@mts.net
www.chha-mb.ca

Chief Officer(s):
Gladys Nielsen, Contact

New Brunswick - Moncton Branch
809 Bernard St., Dieppe NB E1A 5Y2
Tel: 506-855-3799

Chief Officer(s):
Rhéal Léger, President
legerrh@rogers.com

New Brunswick Chapter
74 Alvic Pl., Saint John NB E2M 5G1
Tel: 506-657-7643; Fax: 506-657-7643
e-mail: winslow@nbnet.nb.ca

Chief Officer(s):
Ian Hamilton, President

Newfoundland - Exploits Valley Branch
576 Main St., Bishops Falls NL A0H 1C0
e-mail: chha-evb@nl.rogers.com

Chief Officer(s):
Lillian Menchenton, President

Newfoundland - Gander Branch
77 Fraser Rd., Gander NL A1V 1L1
Tel: 709-256-7935

Chief Officer(s):
Cal Carter, President
c-carter@nl.rogers.com

Newfoundland - Happy Valley Goose Bay Branch

Happy Valley-Goose Bay NL A0P 1C0
Chief Officer(s):
Cyril Peach, President
cgpeach@hotmail.com

Newfoundland - Labrador West Branch
813 Carol Dr., Labrador City NL A2V 1S9
Tel: 709-944-5253

Chief Officer(s):
Jerome Gover, President
rgover@nf.sympatico.ca

Newfoundland - Western NL Branch
4 Ingrid Ave., Corner Brook NL A2H 6P2
Tel: 709-639-9547

Chief Officer(s):
Virginia Brake, President
vbrake@nf.sympatico.ca

Newfoundland & Labrador Chapter
1081 Topsail Rd., Mount Pearl NL A1N 5G1
Tel: 709-753-3224; Fax: 709-753-5640
e-mail: info@chha-nl.ca
www.chha-nl.nl.ca

Chief Officer(s):
Robert Young, President

Northwest Territories - Yellowknife Branch
Aven Court, #5A, 5710 - 50th Ave., Yellowknife NT X1A 1E9
Tel: 867-873-4735

Chief Officer(s):
Esther Braden, President
ebraden@theedge.ca

Ontario - Hamilton Branch
c/o #122, 762 Upper James St., Hamilton ON L9C 3A2
Tel: 905-575-4964
e-mail: info@chha-hamilton.ca
www.chha-hamilton.ca

Chief Officer(s):
Rob Diehl, President

Ontario - Kingston Hard of Hearing Club
#517, 829 Norwest Rd., Kingston ON K7P 2N3
Tel: 613-378-2457

Chief Officer(s):
Margaret Shenton, President
mshenton@sympatico.ca

Ontario - National Capital Region
c/o #205, 2415 Holly Lane, Ottawa ON K1V 7P2
Tel: 613-526-1584; Fax: 613-526-4718
e-mail: alena@chhancr.com
chhancr.com

Chief Officer(s):
Louise Normand, President
alena@chhancr.com

Ontario - Sudbury Branch
#101, 435 Notre Dame Ave., Sudbury ON P3C 5K6
Tel: 705-523-5695; Fax: 705-523-8621
Toll-Free: 866-300-2442; TTY: 705-523-5695
e-mail: chha@vianet.ca
www.chhasudbury.com

Chief Officer(s):
Lorraine O'Brien, President

Ontario - York Branch
147 Primeau Dr., Aurora ON L4G 6Z6
www.chha-york.com

Chief Officer(s):
Dan McDonnell, President
dmac773@gmail.com

Prince Edward Island Chapter
RR#1 Augustine Cove, Borden-Carleton PE C0B 1X0
Tel: 902-855-2382; Fax: 902-885-3282

Chief Officer(s):
Annie Lee MacDonald, President
annmerdon@pei.sympatico.ca

Québec - Outaouais Branch

25, rue des Rapides, Gatineau QC J8T 5K2
Chief Officer(s):
Carole Willans, Interim President
cwillans@chha.ca

Québec Chapter
25, rue des Rapides, Gatineau QC J8T 5K2
Chief Officer(s):
Carole Willans, President
cwillans@chha.ca

Saskatchewan - Regina Branch
c/o 2341 Broad St., Regina SK S4P 1Y9
Tel: 306-457-3259; *Fax:* 306-757-3252
Toll-Free: 800-565-3323
Chief Officer(s):
Gloria Knous, President
glochha@sasktel.net

Canadian Hearing Instrument Practitioners Society (CHIPS)
#259, 185-9040 Blundell Rd., Richmond BC V6Y 1K3
www.chipscanada.com
Overview: A small national organization founded in 1998
Mission: The national professional organization for Hearing Instrument Practitioners who provide hearing healthcare services for hard of hearing people in Canada.
Member of: International Hearing Society
Chief Officer(s):
Allen Kirkham, Chair

Canadian Hearing Society (CHS) / Société canadienne de l'ouïe
271 Spadina Rd., Toronto ON M5R 2V3
Tel: 416-928-2535; *Fax:* 416-928-2506
Toll-Free: 877-347-3427; *TTY:* 877-216-7310
e-mail: info@chs.ca
www.chs.ca
www.facebook.com/pages/The-Canadian-Hearing-Society/164604840229034
twitter.com/wwwCHSca
www.youtube.com/user/CHSCanadaTV
Overview: A large national charitable organization founded in 1940
Mission: To provide services that enhance the independence of deaf, deafened, & hard of hearing people, & that encourage prevention of hearing loss
Chief Officer(s):
Julia Dumanian, President/CEO
Stephanus Greeff, Vice-President, Finance & Corporate Services
Gary Malkowski, Vice-President, Stakeholder & Employer Relations

Barrie Office
#1412, 64 Cedar Pointe Dr., Barrie ON L4N 5R7
Tel: 705-737-3190; *Fax:* 705-722-0381; *TTY:* 877-872-0585

Belleville Office
Bayview Mall, #51, 470 Dundas St. East, Belleville ON K8N 1G1
Tel: 613-966-8995; *Fax:* 613-966-8365; *TTY:* 877-872-0586
Chief Officer(s):
Jen Vander Heyden, Program Assistant
jvanderheyden@chs.ca

Brantford Office
#139, 225 Colborne St., Brantford ON N3T 2H2
Tel: 519-753-3162; *Fax:* 519-753-7447; *TTY:* 877-843-0370
Chief Officer(s):
Victoria Baby, Regional Director

Brockville Sub-Office
#205, 68 William St., Brockville ON K6V 4V5
Tel: 613-498-3933; *Fax:* 613-498-0363
Toll-Free: 877-817-8209; *TTY:* 877-817-8209
e-mail: info@chs.ca
Chief Officer(s):
Brian McKenzie, Regional Director

Chatham-Kent Office
75 Thames St., 2nd Fl., Chatham ON N7L 1S4
Tel: 519-354-9347; *Fax:* 519-354-2083; *TTY:* 877-872-0589
Chief Officer(s):
Brian McKenzie, Regional Director

Cornwall Office
#203, 4 Montreal Rd., Cornwall ON K6H 1B1
Fax: 613-521-0838
Toll-Free: 877-866-4445; *TTY:* 888-697-3650
Chief Officer(s):
Michel David, Regional Director

Durham Regional Office
Braemor Center Plaza, #7, 575 Thornton Rd. North, Oshawa ON L1J 8L5
Tel: 905-404-8490; *Fax:* 905-404-2012
Toll-Free: 888-697-3617; *TTY:* 888-697-3617
e-mail: webmaster@chs.ca
Chief Officer(s):
Maggie Doherty-Gilbert, Regional Director

Elliot Lake Office
c/o St. Joseph's General Hospital, 70 Spine Rd., Elliot Lake ON P5A 1X2
Tel: 705-848-5306; *Fax:* 705-848-3937
Toll-Free: 877-634-0179
Chief Officer(s):
Silvy Coutu, Regional Director

Guelph Office
#200, 2 Quebec St., Guelph ON N1H 2T3
Tel: 519-821-4242; *Fax:* 519-821-8846
Toll-Free: 888-697-3611
e-mail: webmaster@chs.ca
Chief Officer(s):
Victoria Baby, Regional Director

Hamilton Office
21 Hunter St. East, 2nd Fl., Hamilton ON L8N 1M2
Tel: 905-522-0755; *Fax:* 905-522-1336
Toll-Free: 888-224-7247; *TTY:* 877-817-8208

Kingston Regional Office
Frontenac Mall, 1300 Bath Rd., #D4, Kingston ON K7M 4X4
Tel: 613-544-1927; *Fax:* 613-544-1975
Toll-Free: 877-544-1927; *TTY:* 877-817-8209
Chief Officer(s):
Deborah Martin, Manager, Administration & Support Services
dmartin@chs.ca

London Regional Office
181 Wellington St., London ON N6B 2K9
Tel: 519-667-3325; *Fax:* 519-667-9668; *TTY:* 888-697-3613

Mississauga
#300, 2227 South Millway, Mississauga ON L5L 3R6
Tel: 905-608-0271; *Fax:* 905-608-8241
Toll-Free: 866-603-7161; *TTY:* 877-634-0176
Chief Officer(s):
Victoria Baby, Regional Director

Muskoka Office
#103, 175 Manitoba Street, Bracebridge ON P1L 1S3
Tel: 705-645-8882; *Fax:* 705-645-0182
Toll-Free: 877-840-8882; *TTY:* 877-872-0585
e-mail: webmaster@chs.ca
Chief Officer(s):
Maggie Doherty-Gilbert, Regional Director

North Bay Office
#7, 140 King St. West, North Bay ON P1B 5Z7
Tel: 705-474-8090; *Fax:* 705-474-6075; *TTY:* 877-634-0174
Chief Officer(s):
Silvy Coutu, Regional Director

Ottawa Regional Office
#600, 2197 Riverside Dr., Ottawa ON K1H 7X3
Tel: 613-521-0509; *Fax:* 613-521-0838; *TTY:* 888-697-3650
Chief Officer(s):
Michel David, Regional Director
mdavid@chs.ca

Peterborough Office
315 Reid St., Peterborough ON K9J 3R2
Tel: 705-743-1573; *Fax:* 705-741-0708
Toll-Free: 800-213-3848; *TTY:* 888-697-3623

Sarnia Office

420 East St. North, Sarnia ON N7T 6Y5
Tel: 519-337-8307; *Fax:* 519-337-6886
Toll-Free: 877-634-0178; *TTY:* 877-634-0178
Chief Officer(s):
Marilyn Reid, Regional Director

Sault Ste. Marie Regional Office
130 Queen St. East, Sault Ste Marie ON P6A 1Y5
Tel: 705-946-4320; *Fax:* 705-256-7231
Toll-Free: 855-819-9169; *TTY:* 877-634-0179
Chief Officer(s):
Wayne King, Regional Program Manager

Simcoe York Regional Office
#105, 713 Davis Dr., Newmarket ON L3Y 2R3
Tel: 905-715-7511; *Fax:* 905-715-7109
Toll-Free: 877-715-7511; *TTY:* 877-817-8213
e-mail: webmaster@chs.ca
Chief Officer(s):
Maggie Doherty-Gilbert, Regional Director

Sudbury Regional Office
1233 Paris St., Sudbury ON P3E 3B6
Tel: 705-522-1020; *Fax:* 705-522-1060
Toll-Free: 800-479-4562; *TTY:* 877-817-8205
Chief Officer(s):
Maureen Beaudry, Counsellor

Thunder Bay Regional Office
Victoriaville Centre, #35, 125 Syndicate Ave. South, Thunder Bay ON P7E 6H8
Tel: 807-623-1646; *Fax:* 807-623-4815
Toll-Free: 866-646-0514; *TTY:* 877-634-0183

Timmins Office
20 Wilcox St., Timmins ON P4N 3K6
Tel: 705-268-0771; *Fax:* 705-268-4598
Toll-Free: 877-872-0580; *TTY:* 877-872-0580
e-mail: webmaster@chs.ca
Chief Officer(s):
Silvy Coutu, Regional Director

Toronto (Central) Region
271 Spadina Rd., Toronto ON M5R 2V3
Tel: 416-928-2504; *Fax:* 416-928-2523
Toll-Free: 877-215-9530
e-mail: tr.frontdesk@chs.ca
Chief Officer(s):
Stephanie Ozorio, Regional Director

Waterloo Regional Office
#200, 120 Ottawa St. North, Kitchener ON N2H 3K5
Tel: 519-744-6811; *Fax:* 519-744-2390
Toll-Free: 800-668-5815; *TTY:* 888-697-3611

Windsor Regional Office
300 Giles Blvd. East, #A3, Windsor ON N9A 4C4
Tel: 519-253-7241; *Fax:* 519-253-6630; *TTY:* 877-216-7302

Canadian Tinnitus Foundation
#404, 1688 - 152 St., Surrey BC V4A 4N2
Tel: 604-317-2952
e-mail: info@findthecurenow.org
www.findthecurenow.org
www.facebook.com/CanadianTinnitusFoundation
Overview: A medium-sized national organization
Mission: A not-for-profit organization working to expand awareness & generate funding for tinnitus research
Chief Officer(s):
Nathan Nowak, President
John Jabat, Vice-President
Brian Cassidy, Treasurer
Elizabeth Eayrs, Secretary

Communicative Disorders Assistant Association of Canada (CDAAC)
PO Box 55009, 1800 Sheppard Ave. East, Toronto ON M2J 3Z6
e-mail: info@cdaac.ca
www.cdaac.ca
www.linkedin.com/groups/Communicative-Disorders-Assistant-Association-
www.facebook.com/106123889530114
twitter.com/CDAAC
Overview: A small national organization
Mission: To unite members of the profession & protect the character & status of the profession; To maintain & improve the qualifications & standards of the profession; to represent the members in their relationships with other associations, government, colleges, & other national & international organizations; To promote & achieve statutory regulations for members; To provide the public with information regarding our profession & membership; To provide support & share information for the mutual benefit of members

Dog Guides Canada
152 Wilson St., Oakville ON L6K 0G6
Tel: 905-842-2891; *Fax:* 905-842-3373
Toll-Free: 800-768-3030; *TTY:* 905-842-1585
e-mail: info@dogguides.com
www.dogguides.com
www.facebook.com/LFCDogGuides
twitter.com/LFCDogGuides
Also Known As: Lions Foundation of Canada Dog Guides and Sibtech Creations
Previous Name: Canine Vision Canada
Overview: A medium-sized national organization founded in 1985
Mission: To provide Dog Guides to Canadians through various programs, including Canine Vision Canada, Hearing Ear Dogs of Canada, & Service Dog Guides
Member of: Lions Foundation of Canada
Chief Officer(s):
Sandy Turney, Executive Director
sandyturney@dogguides.com
Julie Jelinek, Director, Development
jjelinek@dogguides.com
Alex Ivic, Director, Programs
aivic@dogguides.com
Sarah Miller, Manager, Communications
smiller@dogguides.com

Hands on Summer Camp Society
1309 Hillside Ave., Victoria BC V8T 2B3
Tel: 250-995-6425; *Fax:* 250-995-6428
e-mail: info@handsonsummercamp.com
www.handsonsummercamp.com
Also Known As: Elizabeth Buckley School
Overview: A small national charitable organization
Mission: To foster & promote recreational & educational opportuniities for all children; To meet their individual communication needs, with an emphasis on Sign Language
Chief Officer(s):
Choloe Elias, Camp Director

Hearing Foundation of Canada / La Fondation canadienne de l'ouïe
#1801, 1 Yonge St., Toronto ON M5J 2N8
Tel: 416-364-4060; *Fax:* 416-369-0515
Toll-Free: 866-432-7968
e-mail: info@hearingfoundation.ca
www.hearingfoundation.ca
www.linkedin.com/company/the-hearing-foundation-of-canada
www.facebook.com/TheHearingFoundationofCanada
twitter.com/HearFdnCan
Previous Name: Canadian Hearing Society Foundation
Overview: A medium-sized national charitable organization founded in 1979
Mission: To eliminate the devastating effects of hearing loss on the quality of life of Canadians by promoting prevention, early diagnosis, leading edge medical research & successful intervention
Member of: Association of Development Professionals; Canadian Society of Association Executives
Chief Officer(s):

John Pepperell, Chair Ext. 2
Andrea Swinton, Executive Director Ext. 2

Lions Foundation of Canada
152 Wilson St., Oakville ON L6J 5E8

Tel: 905-842-2891; *Fax:* 905-842-3373
Toll-Free: 800-768-3030; *TTY:* 905-842-1585
e-mail: info@dogguides.com
www.dogguides.com
www.facebook.com/LFCDogGuides
twitter.com/LFCDogGuides

Overview: A small national charitable organization founded in 1983
Mission: To provide service to physically challenged Canadians in the areas of mobility, safety & independence
Affiliation(s): Lions Clubs of Canada
Chief Officer(s):
Sandy Turney, Executive Director, 905-842-2891 Ext. 224
  sandyturney@dogguides.com
Julie Jelinek, Director of Development, 905-842-2891 Ext. 223
  jjelinek@dogguides.com

Silent Voice Canada Inc.
#300, 50 St. Clair Ave. East, Toronto ON M4T 1M9

Tel: 416-463-1104; *Fax:* 416-778-1876; *TTY:* 416-463-3928
e-mail: silent.voice@silentvoice.ca
www.silentvoice.ca
www.facebook.com/silentvoice.canada
twitter.com/silentvoiceca

Also Known As: Silent Voice
Overview: A small national charitable organization founded in 1975
Mission: To serve deaf children, deaf youth & adults & their families in the GTA; to improve communication & relationships between the deaf & hearing in families & in our community; to provide services in a sign language environment
Member of: Catholic Charities of the Archdiocese of Toronto
Chief Officer(s):
Kelly MacKenzie, Executive Director
  k.mackenzie@silentvoice.ca
Mike Cyr, Director, Child & Family Services
  mikecyr@silentvoice.ca

Speech-Language & Audiology Canada (SAC) / Orthophonie et Audiologie Canada (OAC)
#1000, 1 Nicholas St., Ottawa ON K1N 7B7

Tel: 613-567-9968; *Fax:* 613-567-2859
Toll-Free: 800-259-8519
e-mail: info@sac-oac.ca
www.sac-oac.ca
www.linkedin.com/groups/4226965/profile
www.facebook.com/sac.oac
twitter.com/sac_oac
www.youtube.com/channel/UCmg6LP26_eRR72hBEFfnRug

Previous Name: Canadian Association of Speech-Language Pathologists & Audiologists
Overview: A medium-sized national charitable organization founded in 1964
Mission: To support & represent the professional needs & development of speech-language pathologists & audiologists; To champion the needs of people with communication disorders
Affiliation(s): International Association of Logopedics & Phoniatrics; International Society of Audiology; International Communication Project
Chief Officer(s):
Joanne Charlebois, Chief Executive Officer, 613-567-9968 Ext. 262
  joanne@sac-oac.ca
Phil Bolger, Chief Financial Officer
  phil@sac-oac.ca
Jessica Bedford, Director, Communications & Marketing, 800-259-8519 Ext. 241
  jessica@sac-oac.ca
Michelle Jackson, Manager, Professional Development, 800-259-8519 Ext. 244
  michelle@sac-oac.ca
Publications:
• Canadian Association of Speech-Language Pathologists & Audiologists Communiqué
Type: Newsletter; *Frequency:* Quarterly; *ISSN:* 0842-1196

• The Canadian Journal of Speech-Language Pathology & Audiology (CJSLPA)
Type: Journal; *Frequency:* Quarterly; *Accepts Advertising; ISSN:* 1913-200X
• SAC [Speech-Language & Audiology Canada] Membership Directory
Type: Directory

Provincial Associations

ALBERTA

Alberta Association of the Deaf (AAD)
#204, 11404 - 142 St., Edmonton AB T5M 1V1

www.aadnews.ca
www.facebook.com/deaf.alberta
twitter.com/deafalberta
www.youtube.com/deafalberta

Overview: A small provincial charitable organization
Mission: To promote equal rights for deaf people in Alberta; to improve the quality of life for deaf people in general
Affiliation(s): Calgary Association of the Deaf; Edmonton Association for the Deaf; Edmonton Fellowship of the Deaf Blind; Alberta Cultural Society of the Deaf; Alberta Deaf Sports Association; Association of Sign Language Interpreters of Alberta
Chief Officer(s):
Donald McCarthy, President
  donmcthy@shaw.ca

Alberta College of Speech-Language Pathologists & Audiologists (ACSLPA)
#209, 3132 Parsons Rd., Edmonton AB T6N 1L6

Tel: 780-944-1609; *Fax:* 780-408-3925
Toll-Free: 800-537-0589
e-mail: admin@acslpa.ab.ca
www.acslpa.ab.ca

Previous Name: Speech Language Hearing Association of Alberta
Overview: A small provincial licensing charitable organization founded in 1965
Mission: To provide leadership & coordination among speech-language pathologists & audiologists & the public in order to promote speech, language, & hearing health for Albertans
Affiliation(s): Canadian Association of Speech-Language Pathologists & Audiologists
Chief Officer(s):
Harpreet Chaggar, President
  president@acslpa.ab.ca
Michael Neth, CEO & Registrar
  registrar@acslpa.ab.ca
Leanne Kisilevich, Coordinator, Communications & Office

Alberta Cultural Society of the Deaf (ACSD)
#206, 11404 - 142 St., Edmonton AB T5M 1V1

Tel: 780-453-5053; *Fax:* 780-453-5053; *TTY:* 780-453-5033
e-mail: info@acsd.ca
www.acsd.ca
www.facebook.com/AlbertaCulturalSocietyOfTheDeaf

Overview: A small provincial charitable organization
Mission: To provide educational programs for deaf & hard of hearing people; to raise awareness of deaf education; to foster & preserve deaf culture
Affiliation(s): Canadian Cultural Society of the Deaf
Chief Officer(s):
Sandra Reid, President
  sreid04@telus.net

Alberta Deaf Sports Association (ADSA)
#205, 11404 - 142 St., Edmonton AB T5M 1V1

e-mail: info@albertadeafsports.ca
www.albertadeafsports.ca
www.facebook.com/AlbertaDeafSports

Also Known As: Federation of Silent Sports of Alberta
Overview: A medium-sized provincial charitable organization founded in 1974 overseen by Canadian Deaf Sports Association
Mission: To coordinate sport & recreation activities for deaf people in Alberta; To promote competition at the local, provincial, regional, & national levels; To select Alberta athletes to compete in national

championships for the World Games of the Deaf
Member of: Canadian Deaf Sports Association
Chief Officer(s):
Grant Underschultz, President
Brenda Hillcox, Secretary
Publications:
• Alberta Deaf Sports Newsletter
Type: Newsletter
Profile: Highlights of past events & notice of future events

College of Hearing Aid Practitioners of Alberta (CHAPA)
4017 - 63 St., Camrose AB T4V 2X2
Tel: 403-510-1863; *Fax:* 780-678-3282
Toll-Free: 866-990-4327
e-mail: registrar@chapa.ca
www.chapa.ca
Overview: A medium-sized provincial organization founded in 2002
Mission: To regulate the hearing aid practitioner profession; To ensure clients receive the best possible treatment & equipment so that they are able to hear to the best of their ability
Chief Officer(s):
Allen Kirkham, Executive Director
Holly Barry, Registrar

BRITISH COLUMBIA

BC Hands & Voices
1965 Rodger Ave., Port Coquitlam BC V3C 1B8
e-mail: info@bchandsandvoices.com
www.bchandsandvoices.com
Overview: A small provincial charitable organization
Mission: BC Hands & Voices supports families with children who are deaf or hard of hearing.

British Columbia Association of Speech-Language Pathologists & Audiologists (BCASLPA)
#402, 1755 Broadway West, Vancouver BC V6J 4S5
Tel: 604-420-2222; *Fax:* 604-736-5606
Toll-Free: 877-222-7572
e-mail: contact@bcaslpa.ca
www.bcaslpa.ca
www.linkedin.com/groups/4281068/profile
www.facebook.com/bcaslpa
twitter.com/bcaslpa
Overview: A small provincial charitable organization founded in 1957
Mission: To connect people with language, swallowing & hearing disorders with professionals in BC; To represent speech & hearing professionals; To provide information about disorders & treatments
Member of: Pan-Canadian Alliance of Speech-Language Pathology and Audiology Associations
Affiliation(s): Canadian Association of Speech Language Pathologists & Audiologists
Chief Officer(s):
Kate Chase, President
kate.chase@yahoo.ca
Publications:
• Vibrations [a publication of the British Columbia Association of Speech-Language Pathologists & Audiologists]
Editor: Marianne Bullied

British Columbia Deaf Sports Federation (BCDSF)
#4, 320 Columbia St., New Westminster BC V3L 1A6
Fax: 604-526-5010; *TTY:* 604-526-5010
e-mail: info@bcdeafsports.bc.ca
www.bcdeafsports.bc.ca
www.facebook.com/139556792849947
twitter.com/bcdeafsports
Overview: A medium-sized provincial charitable organization founded in 1975 overseen by Canadian Deaf Sports Association
Mission: To provide & support the development of competitive sporting events in BC among deaf & hard of hearing athletes; to encourage training for deaf coaches; to provide financial assistance to deaf athletes to participate in local, provincial & national competitions
Member of: Canadian Deaf Sports Association
Affiliation(s): BC Sport & Fitness Council for the Disabled
Chief Officer(s):

Marilyn Loehr, Director, Membership
mloehr@bcdeafsports.bc.ca

Deaf Children's Society of B.C. (DCS)
#200, 7355 Canada Way, Burnaby BC V3N 4Z6
Tel: 604-525-6056; *Fax:* 604-525-7307; *TTY:* 604-525-9390
www.deafchildren.bc.ca
www.facebook.com/pages/Deaf-Childrens-Society-of-BC/14657619874
5766
Previous Name: Deaf Children's Society of British Columbia
Overview: A small provincial charitable organization founded in 1975
Mission: To help deaf children and their families in the province
Chief Officer(s):
Janice Springfield, Executive Director

Western Institute for the Deaf & Hard of Hearing (WIDHH)
2125 West 7th Ave., Vancouver BC V6K 1X9
Tel: 604-736-7391; *Fax:* 604-736-4381; *TTY:* 604-736-2527
e-mail: info@widhh.com
www.widhh.com
www.facebook.com/92914429597
twitter.com/widhh
Also Known As: Western Institute
Overview: A small provincial charitable organization founded in 1956
Mission: To address the needs of the deaf, deafened & hard of hearing individuals by providing products, services & programs that work towards ensuring accessibility to their environment which is equal to that of the hearing public
Member of: United Way; Better Business Bureau
Chief Officer(s):
Ruth Warick, President
Susan Masters, Executive Director
masters@widhh.com

MANITOBA

College of Audiologists and Speech-Language Pathologists of Manitoba (CASLPM) / Association des orthophonistes et des audiologistes du Manitoba
#1, 333 Vaughan St., Winnipeg MB R3B 3J9
Tel: 204-453-4539; *Fax:* 204-477-1881
e-mail: office@caslpm.ca
www.caslpm.ca
Previous Name: Manitoba Speech & Hearing Association
Overview: A small provincial licensing organization founded in 1958
Mission: To ensure that members of the association provide high quality speech-language pathology & audiology services to persons with commmunication disorders & their families
Chief Officer(s):
Caroline Wilson, Director, Professional Practice
carolinewilson@caslpm.ca
Lori McKietiuk, Registrar
lorimckietiuk@caslpm.ca
Leitta Taylor, Administrator

Manitoba Cultural Society of the Deaf (MCSD)
101-285 Pembina Hwy., Winnipeg MB R3L 2E1
Tel: 204-284-0802; *Fax:* 204-284-0802; *TTY:* 204-284-0802
www.deafmanitoba.org
Overview: A small provincial organization
Affiliation(s): Winnipeg Community Centre of the Deaf; Canadian Cultural Society of the Deaf
Chief Officer(s):
Sheila Montney, Executive Director

Manitoba Deaf Sports Association Inc. (MDSA)
c/o Sport Manitoba, 145 Pacific Ave., Winnipeg MB R3B 2Z6
www.mdsaassoc.com
Overview: A small provincial organization overseen by Canadian Deaf Sports Association
Mission: To provide sporting opportunities for deaf people in Manitoba
Member of: Canadian Deaf Sports Association
Chief Officer(s):
Brenda Comte, President
mdsapresident72@gmail.com
Shawna Joynt, Vice-President
Kenneth Anderson, Treasurer
Joseph Comte, Technical Director

NEW BRUNSWICK

New Brunswick Association of Speech-Language Pathologists & Audiologists (NBASLPA) / Association des orthophonistes et des audiologistes du Nouveau-Brunswick
147 Ellerdale Ave., Moncton NB E1A 3M8

Tel: 506-858-1788; *Fax:* 506-854-0343
Toll-Free: 877-751-5511
e-mail: nbaslpa@nb.aibn.com
www.nbaslpa.ca

Previous Name: New Brunswick Speech & Hearing Association
Overview: A small provincial licensing organization founded in 1976
Mission: To represent the professions of speech language pathology & audiology including registration of members which outlines requirements for working in New Brunswick
Member of: Canadian Association of Speech-Language Pathologists & Audiologists
Chief Officer(s):
Darin Quinn, President
  president.nbaslpa@gmail.com

NEWFOUNDLAND AND LABRADOR

Newfoundland & Labrador Association of Speech-Language Pathologists & Audiologists (NLASLPA)
PO Box 21212, St. John's NL A1A 5B2

e-mail: info@nlaslpa.ca
www.nlaslpa.ca
www.facebook.com/nlaslpa
twitter.com/nlaslpa

Previous Name: Newfoundland Speech & Hearing Association
Overview: A medium-sized provincial organization founded in 1979
Mission: To foster highest quality of service to the communicatively handicapped; to advance knowledge of speech-language pathology & audiology in the region
Member of: Canadian Association of Speech-Language Pathologists & Audiologists
Chief Officer(s):
Ashley Rossiter, President

Newfoundland & Labrador Association of the Deaf (NLAD)
21 Merrymeeting Rd., 3rd Fl., St. John's NL A1C 2V6

Tel: 709-726-6672; *Fax:* 709-726-6650; *TTY:* 709-726-6672
e-mail: nlad@nlad.org
www.nlad.org

Overview: A small provincial organization founded in 1947
Mission: To protect & promote the rights, needs & concerns of people who have severe hearing disabilities & are profoundly deaf within the Province of Newfoundland & Labrador
Affliation(s): Canadian Association of the Deaf
Chief Officer(s):
Jodie Burke, Chair
  jodie.burke@bellaliant.net

Newfoundland & Labrador Deaf Sports Association (NLDSA)
58 First St., Mount Pearl NL A1N 1Y3
Overview: A small provincial organization overseen by Canadian Deaf Sports Association
Mission: To govern fitness, amateur sports & recreation for deaf people in Newfoundland & Labrador
Member of: Canadian Deaf Sports Association
Chief Officer(s):
Bryan Johnson, Acting President
  bryan.johnson@nf.sympatico.ca

NORTHWEST TERRITORIES

Association of Northwest Territories Speech Language Pathologists & Audiologists (ANTSLPA)
PO Box 982, Yellowknife NT X1A 2N7
Overview: A small provincial organization
Mission: Supports and represents the professional needs of speech-language pathologists, audiologists and supportive personnel inclusively within one organization.

NOVA SCOTIA

Atlantic Provinces Special Education Authority / Commission d'enseignement spécial des provinces de l'Atlantique
5940 South St., Halifax NS B3H 1S6

Tel: 902-424-8500; *Fax:* 902-423-8700; *TTY:* 902-424-8500
e-mail: apsea@apsea.ca
www.apsea.ca

Overview: A small provincial organization founded in 1975
Mission: To provide educational services to children & youth who are visually impaired & hard of hearing
Chief Officer(s):
Bertram Tulk, Superintendent
  tulkb@apsea.ca
Publications:
• Seen and Heard [a publication of the Atlantic Provinces Special Education Authority]
Type: Newsletter
Profile: News & updates for members

Deafness Advocacy Association Nova Scotia (DAANS)
Halifax NS

Tel: 902-425-0240; *TTY:* 902-425-0119
e-mail: daans@ns.sympatico.ca
www.facebook.com/109727935783155

Overview: A small provincial charitable organization founded in 1979
Mission: The Association promotes the rights & needs of the deaf, hard-of-hearing, late-deafened & deafblind in the province.
Member of: Canadian Association of the Deaf

Nova Scotia Deaf Sports Association (NSDSA)
5516 Spring Garden Rd., 4th Fl., Halifax NS B3J 1G6
Overview: A small provincial organization overseen by Canadian Deaf Sports Association
Mission: To govern fitness, amateur sports & recreation for deaf people in Nova Scotia.
Member of: Canadian Deaf Sports Association
Chief Officer(s):
Matt Ayyash, President

Nova Scotia Hearing & Speech Foundation
PO Box 120, #401, 5657 Spring Garden Rd., Halifax NS B3S 3R4

Tel: 902-492-8201
e-mail: contact@hearingandspeech.ca
www.hearingandspeech.ca
twitter.com/NSHSF

Overview: A medium-sized provincial organization founded in 1999
Mission: To provide hearing services to all Nova Scotians & speech-language services to preschool children & adults; To work with community volunteer leaders, the families & friends of those who are hearing or speech impaired, our partners in government, & the medical & academic communities; To raise funds to support critical Centres' needs
Chief Officer(s):
Gordon Moore, Chair

Society of Deaf & Hard of Hearing Nova Scotians (SDHHNS)
#805, 1888 Brunswick St., Halifax NS B3J 3J8

Tel: 902-422-7130; *Fax:* 902-492-8110; *TTY:* 902-422-7130
e-mail: sdhhns@ns.sympatico.ca
www.sdhhns.org
www.facebook.com/SDHHNSCB

Overview: A small provincial organization founded in 1980
Mission: To provide services that meet the needs of Deaf, hard of hearing and late deafened people with dignity, integrity and respect.
Chief Officer(s):
Frank O'Sullivan, Executive Director
  fosullivan@ns.sympatico.ca
Rosalind Wright, Regional Manager, Cape Breton-Sydney Office, 902-564-0003
  rwright@ns.aliantzinc.ca

Speech & Hearing Association of Nova Scotia

PO Box 775, Stn. Halifax Central CRO, Halifax NS B3J 2V2

Tel: 902-423-9331
e-mail: webmaster@shans.ca
www.shans.ca
www.facebook.com/SpeechAndHearing
twitter.com/SpeechHearingNS

Overview: A medium-sized provincial charitable organization
Mission: To allow audiology & speech language pathology professionals to pursue professional development in order to benefit the public
Affiliation(s): Canadian Association of Speech-Language Pathologists & Audiologists (CASLPA)
Chief Officer(s):
Patricia Cleave, President
president@shans.ca

ONTARIO

Association of Hearing Instrument Practitioners of Ontario (AHIP)

#211, 55 Mary St. West, Lindsay ON K9V 5Z6

Tel: 705-328-0907; *Fax:* 705-878-4110
Toll-Free: 888-745-2447
e-mail: office@ahip.ca
www.helpmehear.ca

Overview: A small provincial organization
Mission: AHIP is a non-profit organization that serves as a regulatory & lobbying body for it membership of hearing healthcare professoinals. It ensures education requirements, a code of ethics, & ultimately an improvement of services by its members to the public.
Chief Officer(s):
B. Maggie Arzani, President
Joanne Sproule, Executive Director

Association ontarienne des Sourd(e)s francophones (AOSF)

3349, ch Navan, Orléans ON K4B 1H9

www.aosf-ontario.ca
www.facebook.com/aosfontario
vimeo.com/aosfontario

Aperçu: *Dimension:* petite; *Envergure:* provinciale; fondée en 1995
Mission: L'AOSF est un organisme sans but lucratif qui favorise le regroupement des personnes franco-ontariennes vivant avec une surdité afin de répondre à leurs besoins et à leurs aspirations. Son but est de permettre à la communauté sourde de s'épanouir et de se développer.
Membre(s) du bureau directeur:
Michael McGuire, Président
mmcguire.aosf@hotmail.com

College of Audiologists & Speech-Language Pathologists of Ontario (CASLPO) / Ordre des audiologistes et des orthophonistes de l'Ontario (OAOO)

PO Box 71, #5060, 3080 Yonge St., Toronto ON M4N 3N1

Tel: 416-975-5347; *Fax:* 416-975-8394
Toll-Free: 800-993-9459
e-mail: caslpo@caslpo.com
www.caslpo.com

Overview: A medium-sized provincial licensing organization
Mission: To regulate the practice of the professions & govern the members; To develop, establish & maintain standards of qualification; To assure the quality of the practice of the professions; Develop & maintain a code of ethics & standards
Chief Officer(s):
Scott Whyte, President
Brian O'Riordan, Registrar, 416-975-5347 Ext. 215
boriordan@caslpo.com

Ontario Association of Speech-Language Pathologists & Audiologists (OSLA)

410 Jarvis St., Toronto ON M4Y 2G6

Tel: 416-920-3676; *Fax:* 416-920-6214
Toll-Free: 800-718-6752
e-mail: mail@osla.on.ca
www.osla.on.ca
www.linkedin.com/groups?home=&gid=4453106
www.facebook.com/162240417157549
twitter.com/osla_ontario

Overview: A medium-sized provincial organization founded in 1958
Mission: Represents & promotes the professional interests of its members; provides a comprehensive range of services that support its professional members in their work on behalf of people with communication disorders
Chief Officer(s):
Mary Cook, Executive Director
mcook@osla.on.ca

Ontario Deaf Sports Association (ODSA)

ON

Overview: A small provincial organization founded in 1964 overseen by Canadian Deaf Sports Association
Member of: Canadian Deaf Sports Association

VOICE for Hearing Impaired Children

#302, 177 Danforth Ave., Toronto ON M4K 1N2

Tel: 416-487-7719; *Fax:* 416-487-7423
Toll-Free: 866-779-5144; *TTY:* 416-487-7719
e-mail: info@voicefordeafkids.com
www.voicefordeafkids.com
www.facebook.com/VOICEforHearingImpairedChildren
twitter.com/VOICE4DEAFKIDS
www.youtube.com/channel/UCtqS6zWzpmW9Tq6DRRbZubw

Overview: A small provincial charitable organization founded in 1972
Mission: To ensure that all hearing impaired children have the right to develop their ability to listen & speak & have access to services which will enable them to listen & speak
Member of: Canadian Society of Association Executives
Affiliation(s): Alexander Graham Bell Association

PRINCE EDWARD ISLAND

Prince Edward Island Speech & Hearing Association (PEISHA)

PO Box 20076, Charlottetown PE C1A 9E3

www.peispeechhearing.ca

Overview: A small provincial organization
Mission: To promote the study, research, discussion & dissemination of information concerning the process of human communication in speech & hearing; To encourage the development & improvement of skills in the diagnosis & treatment of human communication disorders
Member of: Canadian Association of Speech-Language Pathologists & Audiologists
Chief Officer(s):
Jennifer Bartlett-Bitar, President

QUÉBEC

Association des implantés cochléaires du Québec (AICQ)

#130, 5100 rue des Tournelles, Québec QC G2J 1E4

Tél: 418-623-7417; *Téléc:* 418-623-7462
Courriel: aicq@bellnet.ca
www.aicq-implant.org

Aperçu: *Dimension:* petite; *Envergure:* provinciale; Organisme sans but lucratif; fondée en 1995
Mission: Promouvoir l'implant cochléaire; supporter le patient et sa famille; offrir des activités
Membre(s) du bureau directeur:
Cécile Viel, Présidente

Association des Sourds de Québec inc.

4100, 3e Av Ouest, Québec QC G1H 6E1

Tél: 418-614-0652; *Téléc:* 418-614-0672
Courriel: asq1964@hotmail.com
sourdsquebec.com

Aperçu: *Dimension:* petite; *Envergure:* provinciale; Organisme sans but lucratif; fondée en 1964
Membre(s) du bureau directeur:

Richard Dagenault, Président

Association du Québec pour enfants avec problèmes auditifs (AQEPA)
3700, rue Berri, #A-446, Montréal QC H2L 4G9

Tél: 514-842-8706; *Téléc:* 514-842-4006
Ligne sans frais: 877-842-4006
Courriel: info@aqepa.org
www.aqepa.org
www.facebook.com/AQEPA
twitter.com/AQEPA

Aperçu: *Dimension:* moyenne; *Envergure:* provinciale; Organisme sans but lucratif; fondée en 1969
Mission: Regrouper les parents d'enfants sourds et malentendants; informer et sensibiliser les parents et le public
Publications:
• Entendre [publication de l'Association du Québec pour enfants avec problèmes auditifs]
Type: Journal

Association québécoise des orthophonistes et des audiologistes (AQOA)
#102, 7229 rue St-Denis, Montréal QC H2R Ee3

Tél: 514-369-8929
Courriel: admin@aqoa.qc.ca
www.aqoa.qc.ca

Aperçu: *Dimension:* petite; *Envergure:* provinciale; Organisme sans but lucratif; fondée en 1996
Mission: Défendre les droits et les intérêts des orthophonistes et audiologistes du Québec auprès de diverses instances, gouvernementales, syndicales, etc.
Affliation(s): Ordre des orthophonistes et audiologistes du Québec, Mouvement pour l'adhésion aux traitements, Orthophonie et audiologie Canada, Association des jeunes bègues du Québec
Membre(s) du bureau directeur:
Philippe Fournier, Président

Association sportive des sourds du Québec inc. (ASSQ)
4545, av Pierre-de Coubertin, Montréal QC H1V 0B2

Tél: 514-252-3049
www.assq.org
www.facebook.com/ASSQ1
twitter.com/@ASSQ_Nouvelles
www.youtube.com/user/1ASSQ

Nom précédent: Association amateur des sports des sourds du Québec; Fédération sportive des sourds du Québec inc.
Aperçu: *Dimension:* moyenne; *Envergure:* provinciale; fondée en 1968 surveillé par Canadian Deaf Sports Association
Mission: Promouvoir le sport, les loisirs et l'activité physique chez les personnes sourdes et malentendantes du Québec
Membre de: Canadian Deaf Sports Association
Membre(s) du bureau directeur:
Suzanne Laforest, Directrice générale
    slaforest@assq.org
Audrey Beauchamp, Coordinatrice, Projets et des communications
    abeauchamp@assq.org
Caroline Hould, Chargée des programmes
    chould@assq.org

Audition Québec
#001, 1951, boul de Maisonneuve est, Montréal QC H2K 2C9

Tél: 514-278-9633; *Téléc:* 514-278-9075
www.auditionquebec.org
www.facebook.com/auditionquebec
twitter.com/auditionquebec

Nom précédent: Association des devenus sourds et des malentendants du Québec
Aperçu: *Dimension:* petite; *Envergure:* provinciale; fondée en 1982
Mission: Défense des droits; intégration des personnes avec problèmes auditifs; assistance à la recherche sur la surdité; assistance pour l'obtention des aides techniques aux personnes ayant un handicap auditif
Membre(s) du bureau directeur:
Daniel Morel, Président
Ronald Choquette, Secrétaire

Centre québécois de la déficience auditive (CQDA) / Québec Centre of Hearing Impaired
#202, 2494, boul Henri-Bourassa est, Montréal QC H2B 1T9

Tél: 514-278-8703; *Téléc:* 514-278-8238; *TTY:* 514-278-8704
Courriel: info@cqda.org
www.cqda.org

Aperçu: *Dimension:* petite; *Envergure:* provinciale; Organisme sans but lucratif; fondée en 1975
Mission: Regrouper les organismes dans le domaine de la surdité au Québec; aider les personnes déficientes auditives; identifier leurs besoins; sensibiliser le public à leur problématique; surveiller et défendre leurs droits et leurs intérêts; créer plus de services répondant à leurs besoins
Membre de: Confédération des organismes de personnes handicapées du Québec
Affliation(s): Confédération des organismes de personnes handicapées du Québec; Conseil des canadiens avec déficiences; KEROUL; Association des sourds du Canada; Association des Malentendants canadiens

Coalition sida des sourds du Québec (CSSQ)
Edifice Plessis, #320, 2075, rue Plessis, Montréal QC H2L 2Y4

Ligne sans frais: 877-535-5556
Courriel: info@cssq.org
www.cssq.org

Aperçu: *Dimension:* petite; *Envergure:* provinciale; Organisme sans but lucratif; fondée en 1992 surveillé par Canadian AIDS Society
Mission: Informer et mettre en garde la communauté sourde du Québec contre les risques de contracter le Sida et les ITSS (Infections transmissibles sexuellement par le sang); dispenser des services et activités aux personnes sourdes et malentendantes atteintes du VIH/Sida et de l'ITSS
Affliation(s): Coalition des organismes communautaires québécois de lutte contre le sida
Membre(s) du bureau directeur:
Darren Saunders, Président
Michel Turgeon, Directeur général
    direction@cssq.org

Fondation des sourds du Québec inc.
3348, boul Mgr-Gauthier, Beauport QC G1E 2W2

Tél: 418-660-6800; *Téléc:* 418-666-0123
Ligne sans frais: 800-463-5617
www.fondationdessourds.net

Aperçu: *Dimension:* petite; *Envergure:* provinciale; Organisme sans but lucratif; fondée en 1986
Mission: Aider les sourds dans leurs activités quotidiennes afin de contribuer à l'amélioration de la qualité de vie, dans une société d'entendants
Membre(s) du bureau directeur:
Daniel Forgues, Président

Ordre des audioprothésistes du Québec (OAQ)
#202-A, 11370, rue Notre-Dame est, Montréal QC H1B 2W6

Tél: 514-640-5117; *Téléc:* 514-640-5291
Ligne sans frais: 866-676-5117
Courriel: oaq@ordreaudio.qc.ca
www.ordreaudio.qc.ca

Nom précédent: Corporation professionnelle des audioprothésistes du Québec
Aperçu: *Dimension:* petite; *Envergure:* provinciale
Mission: Protéger le public qui fait appel aux services professionnels d'un audioprothésiste
Membre(s) du bureau directeur:
Sophie Gagnon, Présidente
    sgagnon@ordreaudio.qc.ca

Ordre des orthophonistes et audiologistes du Québec (OOAQ)
#601, 235, boul René-Levesque Est, Montréal QC H2X 1N8

Tél: 514-282-9123; *Téléc:* 514-282-9541
Ligne sans frais: 888-232-9123
Courriel: info@ooaq.qc.ca
www.ooaq.qc.ca

Aperçu: *Dimension:* moyenne; *Envergure:* provinciale; Organisme de réglementation; fondée en 1973
Mission: D'assurer la protection du public en regard du domaine d'exercice de ses membres, soit les troubles de la communication

humaine; surveiller l'exercice professionnel des orthophonistes et des audiologistes et voir à favoriser l'accessibilité du public à des services de qualité; contribuer à l'intégration sociale des individus et à l'amélioration de la qualité de vie de la population québécoise
Membre(s) du bureau directeur:
Louise Chamberland, Directrice générale
  directiongenerale@ooaq.qc.ca

Saskatchewan Association of Speech-Language Pathologists & Audiologists (SASLPA)
#11, 2010 - 7th Ave., Regina SK S4R 1C2
Tel: 306-757-3990; *Fax:* 306-757-3986
Toll-Free: 800-757-3990
e-mail: saslpa@sasktel.net
www.saslpa.ca
twitter.com/SASLPA
Overview: A small provincial licensing organization founded in 1957
Mission: To encourage public awareness, professional development & quality service in the fields of speech-language pathology & audiology in the province
Member of: Canadian Association of Speech-Language Pathologists & Audiologists
Chief Officer(s):
Kathy Carroll, Executive Director
  ed.saslpa@sasktel.net
Publications:
• Private Practice Directory [a publication of the Saskatchewan Association of Speech-Language Pathologists & Audiologists]
Type: Directory

Saskatchewan Cultural Society of the Deaf
511 Main St. East, Saskatoon SK S7N 0C2
Overview: A small provincial organization
Chief Officer(s):
Laurie Eva-Miller, Acting President
  le-miller1@shaw.ca

Saskatchewan Deaf & Hard of Hearing Services Inc. (SDHHS)
2341 Broad St., Regina SK S4P 1Y9
Tel: 306-352-3323; *Fax:* 306-757-3252
Toll-Free: 800-565-3323
Other Communication: Video Phone: 306-352-3322
e-mail: regina@sdhhs.com
www.sdhhs.com
www.facebook.com/SDHHSinc
twitter.com/SDHHSinc
Overview: A small provincial charitable organization founded in 1981
Mission: To promote independence of deaf, late deafened, & hard of hearing persons; To provide services for persons with a hearing loss in order to enhance their quality of life
Affiliation(s): Canadian Hard of Hearing Association; Canadian Association of the Deaf; Regina Association of the Deaf; Saskatchewan Institute of Applied Science & Technology; United Way; United Way of Regina; United Way of Saskatoon
Chief Officer(s):
Nairn Gillies, Executive Director
Dale Birley, President

Saskatoon Office
#3, 511 - 1st Ave. North, Saskatoon SK S7K 1X5
Tel: 306-665-6575; *Fax:* 306-665-7746
Toll-Free: 800-667-6575
e-mail: saskatoon@sdhhs.com

Saskatchewan Deaf Sports Association (SDSA)
PO Box 932, Fort Qu'Appelle SK S0G 1S0
Overview: A small provincial charitable organization overseen by Canadian Deaf Sports Association
Mission: To foster sporting opportunities to members of the deaf & hard-of-hearing communities; To select & train deaf & hard-of-hearing athletes for international competitions
Member of: Canadian Deaf Sports Association
Affiliation(s): Regina Deaf Athletic Club; Saskatoon Deaf Athletic Club; Saskatchewan Sport Inc.
Chief Officer(s):

Kevin Goodfeather, President
  nivek26@hotmail.com

Yukon Speech-Language Pathology & Audiology Association (YSLPAA)
c/o 80 Falcon Dr., Whitehorse YT Y1A 6C7
e-mail: yslpaa@gmail.com
Overview: A small provincial organization
Mission: Supports and represents the professional needs of speech-language pathologists, audiologists and supportive personnel in the Yukon.
Chief Officer(s):
Karen Rach, President

Calgary Association of the Deaf (CgyAD)
63 Cornell Rd. NW, Calgary AB T2L 0L4
e-mail: info@cad1935.ca
www.facebook.com/CgyAD
Overview: A small local organization
Affiliation(s): Alberta Association of the Deaf
Chief Officer(s):
Robyn Mackie, President

Connect Society - D.E.A.F. Services
6240 - 113 St., Edmonton AB T6H 3L2
Tel: 780-454-9581; *Fax:* 780-447-5820; *TTY:* 780-454-9581
e-mail: info@connectsociety.org
www.connectsociety.org
www.facebook.com/connectsocietyedmonton
www.youtube.com/user/ConnectSociety50
Previous Name: Association for the Hearing Handicapped
Overview: A small local charitable organization founded in 1963
Mission: To bring about the full participation in society of deaf & hard of hearing individuals & their families
Chief Officer(s):
Cheryl Rehead, CEO
  redhead@connectsociety.org

Edmonton Association of the Deaf (EAD)
#203, 11404 - 142 St., Edmonton AB T5M 1V1
Overview: A small local charitable organization
Affiliation(s): Alberta Association of the Deaf; Alberta Cultural Society Deaf; Alberta Deaf Sports Association
Chief Officer(s):
Matthew Kuntz, President
  02mathewkuntz@gmail.com

Pax Natura Society for Rehabilitation of the Deaf
11460 - 60th Ave. NW, Edmonton AB T6H 1J5
Tel: 780-434-1671; *Fax:* 780-435-7788; *TTY:* 780-434-1671
Overview: A small local charitable organization founded in 1975
Mission: To administer & employ its property, assets & rights for the purpose of promoting or aiding in the promotion of programs to benefit the deaf community
Chief Officer(s):
R.A. Bauer, Executive Director

Greater Vancouver Association of the Deaf (GVAD)
2125 West 7th Ave., Vancouver BC V6K 1X9
Fax: 604-738-4645; *TTY:* 604-738-4644
e-mail: gvadoffice@gmail.com
www.gvad.com
www.facebook.com/gvad.vancouver
twitter.com/GVAD2
Overview: A small local charitable organization founded in 1926
Mission: To promote all matters of the welfare of the deaf; to foster the social, cultural, educational & recreational activities of the deaf; To affiliate & serve with provincial, regional & national organizations of the deaf & hard of hearing; To ensure that the activities of the society always be intended to contribute positively to the Greater Vancouver

area or to any other district within the society's areas of operation
Affiliation(s): BC Deaf Sports Federation
Chief Officer(s):
Leanor Vlug, President

Island Deaf & Hard of Hearing Centre (IDHHC)
#201-754 Broughton St., Victoria BC V8W 1E1
Tel: 250-592-8144; *Fax:* 250-592-8199
Toll-Free: 800-667-5448; *TTY:* 250-592-8147
e-mail: victoria@idhhc.ca
www.idhhc.ca
www.facebook.com/145668377075
twitter.com/IDHHC

Overview: A small local charitable organization founded in 1991
Mission: To enable individuals who are deaf, hard of hearing or deafened, their supporters & the communities they represent, to have full & active access, recognition & involvement in society
Chief Officer(s):
Denise Robertson, Executive Director

Nanaimo Branch Office
#101, 75 Front St., Nanaimo BC V9R 5G9
Tel: 250-753-0999; *Fax:* 250-753-9601
Toll-Free: 877-424-3323; *TTY:* 250-753-0977
e-mail: nanaimo@idhhc.ca
www.idhhc.ca

Chief Officer(s):
Alexandra Walker, Office Manager
alex@idhhc.ca

NEW BRUNSWICK

Saint John Deaf & Hard of Hearing Services, Inc (SJDHHS)
324 Duke St. West, Saint John NB E2M 1V2
Tel: 506-633-0599; *Fax:* 506-652-3382; *TTY:* 506-634-8037
e-mail: sjdhhs@nb.sympatico.ca
www.sjdhhs.ca
www.facebook.com/sj.dhhs

Overview: A small local charitable organization founded in 1979
Mission: To empower deaf, hard of hearing & late deafened people to live independent, productive lives with the same full access to services & opportunites as the hearing population
Member of: United Way
Chief Officer(s):
Lynn LeBlanc, Executive Director

ONTARIO

The Bob Rumball Centre for the Deaf (BRCD)
2395 Bayview Ave., Toronto ON M2L 1A2
Tel: 416-449-9651; *Fax:* 416-449-8881; *TTY:* 416-449-2728
e-mail: info@bobrumball.org
www.bobrumball.org
www.facebook.com/86097284911

Overview: A large local organization founded in 1979
Mission: To provide opportunities for a higher quality of life for deaf people while preserving & promoting their language & culture; To foster & develop good relations with the community at large & actively promote the Centre; To work closely with the various ministries of the provincial government & related agencies
Member of: Ontario Mission of the Deaf
Chief Officer(s):
Jane Hooey, Chair

Bob Rumball Foundation for the Deaf
2395 Bayview Ave., Toronto ON M2L 1A2
Tel: 416-449-9651; *TTY:* 416-449-2728
Other Communication: 416-640-0723
e-mail: fundraising@bobrumball.org
www.bobrumball.org
www.facebook.com/86097284911
twitter.com/BobRumball
www.instagram.com/bobrumball

Previous Name: Ontario Mission of the Deaf
Overview: A small local organization founded in 1872
Mission: To meet the social, recreational, educational & spiritual needs of the deaf community & raise funds for The Bob Rumball Centre for the Deaf in Toronto, The Bob Rumball Associations for the Deaf in

Milton, The Bob Rumball Long Term Care Home for the Deaf in Barrie & The Bob Rumball Camp for the Deaf in Parry Sound.
Chief Officer(s):
Derek Rumball, Executive Director

Durham Deaf Services (DDS)
750 King St. East, Oshawa ON L1H 1G9
Tel: 905-579-3328; *Fax:* 905-728-1183; *TTY:* 905-579-6495
e-mail: info@durhamdeaf.org
www.durhamdeaf.org
www.facebook.com/durhamdeafservices
www.youtube.com/user/DurhamDeafServices

Overview: A small local charitable organization founded in 1982
Mission: To offer services & educational programs to promote self-reliance within the deaf, deafened & hard-of-hearing community; to increase awareness of deaf culture.
Affliation(s): Ontario Association of the Deaf, Canadian Association of the Deaf
Chief Officer(s):
Yvonne Brown, Executive Director

Windsor Association for the Deaf (WAD)
c/o Shoppers Drug Mart, PO Box 28036, 500 Tecumseh Rd. East, Windsor ON N8X 2S2
e-mail: deafwad@gmail.com
deafwad.weebly.com
www.facebook.com/deafwad
twitter.com/deafwad
pinterest.com/deafwad

Overview: A small local organization founded in 1959
Mission: Social & recreational activities for persons deafened or hard of hearing; provides social gatherings; offers special events & traveling sports tournaments; promotes the welfare of deaf members, preserves Deaf Culture & ASL, offers social interaction between cultures, encourage the promotion of Deaf Awareness; offer workshops for deaf, hearing, & parents of deaf children & deaf parents of hearing children
Chief Officer(s):
Gary Vassallo, President
wadpresident1@gmail.com
Michelle Walls-Carr, Vice-President
wasvicepresident2@gmail.com
Ken Brockway, Treasurer
wadtreasurer3@gmail.com

QUÉBEC

Association des Sourds de l'Estrie Inc. (ASE)
#100, 359, rue King est, Sherbrooke QC J1G 1B3
Tél: 819-563-1186; *Téléc:* 819-563-3476; *TTY:* 819-563-1186
Courriel: sourdestrie@videotron.ca
www.sourdestrie.com
www.facebook.com/sourdestrie

Aperçu: *Dimension:* petite; *Envergure:* locale; Organisme sans but lucratif; fondée en 1968
Mission: Briser l'isolement des sourds; sensibilisation des intervenants et de la population en général sur la surdité
Membre de: Centre québécois de la déficience auditive; Regroupement québécois pour le sous-titrage inc.
Affliation(s): Coalition Sida des sourds de Québec; Regroupement Canadien des Enseignants et Enseignantes Sourds en Langue des Signes Québécois
Membre(s) du bureau directeur:
Céline Martineau, Directrice
Alain Ouellette, Adjoint administratif
Publications:
• Nouvellestrie [a publication of Association des Sourds de l'Estrie inc.]
Type: Journal; *Frequency:* Trimestriel

Association des Sourds de Lanaudière
200, rue de Salaberry, local 312, Joliette QC J6E 4G1
Tel: 450-752-1426; *TTY:* 450-752-1426
e-mail: asl@cepap.ca
www.asljoliette.org
www.facebook.com/ASLanaudiere

Overview: A small local organization
Chief Officer(s):
Richard Geoffroy, Président

Centre de la Communauté sourde du Montréal métropolitain (CCSMM)

#203, 2200, boul Crémazie est, Montréal QC H2E 2Z8
Tél: 514-903-2200; *Téléc:* 514-279-5373; *TTY:* 514-279-7609
Courriel: ccsmm@videotron.ca
www.ccsmm.net
www.facebook.com/ccsmm.centrecommunautesourde

Aperçu: *Dimension:* petite; *Envergure:* locale; Organisme sans but lucratif; fondée en 1978
Mission: Promouvoir les droits et intérêts des personnes sourdes; offrir des activitiés d'information afin de renseigner notre clientèle; offrir de l'assistance pour la résolution de conflits d'ordre juridique ou autre
Affliation(s): Regroupement de l'Organisme de Sourds du Québec, ROPMM, COPHAN, CDEC, RIOCm, RUTA
Membre(s) du bureau directeur:
Gilles Read, Directeur général
Jeanne d'Arc Paradis, Adjointe
  ccsmm.membres@videotron.ca
Marc-André Saucier, Agent des services communautaires et sociaux
  ccsmm.service@videotron.ca
Yann Lacroix, Service de développement de l'employabilité
  ccsmm.acces@videotron.ca

Regroupement des Sourds de Chaudière-Appalaches (RSCA)

1294, chemin Filteau, Saint-Nicolas QC G7A 2L7
Tél: 418-831-3723; *Téléc:* 418-831-3723; *TTY:* 418-831-3723
Courriel: rsca@globetrotter.net
www.facebook.com/834524883229339

Nom précédent: Association des Sourds de Beauce
Aperçu: *Dimension:* petite; *Envergure:* locale; Organisme sans but lucratif; fondée en 1982
Mission: Travailler à l'amélioration des conditions de vie des personnes sourdes et malentendantes; les regrouper; les représenter et les supporter afin qu'elles aient accès et reçoivent tous les services auxquels elles ont droit et ce, dans leur langue respective; défense de droits
Membre de: Centre québécois de la déficience auditive; Regroupement des associations de personnes handicapées région Chaudière-Appalaches; Coallitions Sida des sourds du Québec
Membre(s) du bureau directeur:
Michel Laurent, Directeur

International Associations

International Association of Physicians in Audiology

c/o Dept. Audiovestibular Medicine, University College London Hospital, London United Kingdom
www.iapa-audiovestibularmedicine.com
Overview: A small international organization founded in 1980
Mission: To promote & improve clinical, ethical & scientific standards in the field of audiological medicine
Chief Officer(s):
Quiju Wang, President
Chrysa Spyridakou, Honorary Secretary

International Catholic Deaf Association (ICDA)

e-mail: mhysell@op.dspt.edu
www.icdacanadasection.wordpress.com
www.facebook.com/ICDACanadianSection
Also Known As: ICDA-Canada
Overview: A small international organization founded in 1949
Mission: To promote religion, religious education, fellowship & leadership among deaf people of all ages; to promote in Canada & the ICDA various programs in foreign countries with a view to enhancing the life of deaf people
Chief Officer(s):
Wanda Berrette, President
  wberrette@rogers.com
Giuliana Grobelski, Vice-President
  julianamusso3@hotmail.com
John Shores, Treasurer
  jshores@shaw.ca

International Committee of Sports for the Deaf (ICSD) / Comité international des Sports des Sourds (CISS)

Maison du Sport International, Av. de Rhondanie 54, Lausanne CH-1007 Switzerland
Tel: 41 78 733 35 67; *Fax:* 7 (499) 255 04 36
e-mail: office@ciss.org
www.ciss.org
Also Known As: International Deaflympics
Overview: A medium-sized international charitable organization founded in 1924
Mission: To organize sporting events for deaf & hard of hearing athletes
Member of: International Olympic Committee; General Assembly of International Sports Federations
Affliation(s): Canadian Deaf Sports Association
Chief Officer(s):
Valery Rukhledev, President
  president@ciss.org

World Federation of the Deaf (WFD) / Fédération mondiale des sourds

PO Box 65, Helsinki FIN-00401 Finland
Tel: 358-9-580-3573; *Fax:* 358-9-580-3572
e-mail: info@wfd.fi
www.wfdeaf.org
www.facebook.com/Wfdeaf.org
Overview: A medium-sized international organization founded in 1951
Mission: To promote the unification of national associations, federations & other organizations of & for deaf people at both regional & international levels; To ensure that the government in each country observe all international declarations & recommendations on human rights & the rights of deaf persons & other persons with disabilities; To promote the creation & development of national organizations of deaf people & organizations providing services to deaf people where such organizations do not exist; to disseminate scientific & legal materials about deafness & the current needs of deaf people; To promote the coordination & conduct of research & studies in all fields of deafness, including other categories of hearing loss; To facilitate the efforts of deaf people to make contributions to cultural enrichment in every country
Affliation(s): Disabled Persons International; International Sign Language Association; International Federation of the Hard of Hearing; Rehabilitation International; International Committee of Sport for the Deaf; World Blind Union; Inclusion International; World Federation of Deaf Blind; United Nations; World Health Organization; International Labor Organization; UN Educational, Scientific & Cultural Organization (UNESCO); World Association of Sign Language Interpreters
Chief Officer(s):
Colin Allen, President
Joseph Murray, Vice-President
Nafisah Rantasalmi, Development Officer

National Publications

The Chronicle of Neurology & Psychiatry

Owned By: Chronicle Companies
#306, 555 Burnhamthorpe Rd., Toronto, ON M9C 2Y3
Tel: 416-916-2476; *Fax:* 416-352-6199
Toll-Free: 866-632-4766
health@chronicle.org

Circulation: 6,189 *Frequency:* 6 times a year
Mitchell Shannon, Publisher
R. Allan Ryan, Editorial Director

Local Schools

ALBERTA

Edmonton: Alberta School for the Deaf (ASD)
6240 - 113 St., Edmonton, AB T6H 3L2
Tel: 780-439-3323; *Fax:* 780-436-0385
abschdeaf@epsb.ca
asd.epsb.ca
TTY: 780-439-3323
Grades: 1-12 *Note:* Provides educational services for Deaf & Hard of Hearing students in Alberta & beyond.
Joanne Aldridge, Principal

Sandra Mason, Supervisor
Melanie St. Martin, Manager, Business

BRITISH COLUMBIA

Burnaby: BC Provincial School for the Deaf
c/o Burnaby South Secondary School
5455 Rumble St., Burnaby, BC V5J 2B7
Tel: 604-296-6880; *Fax:* 604-296-6883
TTY: 604-664-8563

Grades: K-12 *Enrollment:* 75
Lisa Meneian-Cecile, Principal

MANITOBA

Winnipeg: Manitoba School for the Deaf (MSD)
242 Stradford St., Winnipeg, MB R2Y 2C9
Tel: 204-945-8934; *Fax:* 204-945-1767
principal@msd.ca
www.msd.ca
TTY: 204-945-8934

Grades: JK-12 *Enrollment:* 100
Ricki Hall, Principal
rhall@msd.ca

NOVA SCOTIA

Halifax: Atlantic Provinces Special Education Authority (APSEA)
5940 South St., Halifax, NS B3H 1S6, Canada
Tel: 902-424-8500; *Fax:* 902-424-0543
apsea@apsea.ca
www.apsea.ca
TTY: 902-424-8500
Note: The Atlantic Provinces Special Education Authority (APSEA) is an interprovincial cooperative agency established in 1975 by joint agreement among the Ministers of Education of New Brunswick, Newfoundland, Nova Scotia, and Prince Edward Island.
Bertram R. Tulk, Supt.

ONTARIO

Belleville: The Sir James Whitney School for the Deaf
350 Dundas St. West, Belleville, ON K8P 1B2
Tel: 613-967-2823; *Toll-Free:* 800-501-6240
www.psbnet.ca/eng/schools/sjw
TTY: 613-967-2823

Enrollment: 110
Janice Drake, Principal

Brantford: The W. Ross Macdonald School for the Blind
350 Brant Ave., Brantford, ON N3T 3J9
Tel: 519-759-0730; *Toll-Free:* 866-618-9092
www.psbnet.ca/eng/schools/wross
Enrollment: 217
Donald Neale, Principal, Blind/Low Vision Program
Martha Martino, Principal, Deaf/Blind Program

London: The Robarts School for the Deaf
1515 Cheapside St., London, ON N5V 3N9
Tel: 519-453-4400
www.psbnet.ca/eng/schools/robarts
TTY: 519-453-4400
Linda Wall, Vice Principal

Milton: Ernest C. Drury School for the Deaf
255 Ontario St. South, Milton, ON L9T 2M5
Tel: 905-878-2851
www.psbnet.ca/eng/schools/ecd
TTY: 905-878-7195
Jeanne Leonard, Principal

Ottawa: Centre Jules-Léger
281, av Lanark, Ottawa, ON K1Z 6R8
Tél: 613-761-9300; *Téléc:* 613-761-9301
Other Information: ATS: 613-761-9302
Note: Services aux enfants (et leurs familles) en difficultés d'apprentissage, avec ou sans déficit d'attention/hyperactivité, qui sont sourds ou malentendant, qui sont aveugles ou en basse vision, ou qui sont sourds et aveugles.

Ginette Faubert, Surintendante

QUÉBEC

Montréal: Mackay Centre School
3500, boul Decarie, Montréal, QC H4A 3J5
Tel: 514-482-0001; *Fax:* 514-485-7254
www.emsb.qc.ca/mackay

Grades: Pre.-6 *Enrollment:* 170
Number of Employees: 29 teachers (3 for the deaf, 26 for the physically disabled) *Note:* School for the deaf/hearing impaired & children with disabilities.
Patrizia Ciccarelli, Principal, 514-482-0001, ext. 1600
pciccarelli@emsb.qc.ca
Denise Maroun, Vice-Principal, 514-482-0001, ext. 1602
dmaroun@emsb.qc.ca
Sharon Wood, Secretary, 514-482-0001, ext. 1606
swood@emsb.qc.ca

Westmount: École orale de Montréal pour le sourds
Montreal Oral School for the Deaf
4670, Ste. Catherine St. ouest, Westmount, QC H3Z 1S5
Tel: 514-488-4946; *Fax:* 514-488-0802
info@montrealoralschool.com
www.montrealoralschool.com
TTY: 514-488-4946
Note: School for the deaf with programs in both French and English.

National Libraries

Canadian Association of the Deaf
#606, 251 Bank St., Ottawa, ON K2P 1X3
Tel: 613-565-2882; *Fax:* 613-565-1207
TTY: 613-565-288
info@cad.ca
www.cad.ca
Social Media: www.youtube.com/user/1940CADASC;
twitter.com/CADASC; www.facebook.com/1940CADASC
Collection: Documents on & by deaf organizations
James Roots, Executive Director

Canadian Cultural Society of the Deaf Inc.
The Distillery Historic District, 15 Mill St., Toronto, ON M5A 346

info@deafculturecentre.ca
www.deafculturecentre.ca
Social Media: twitter.com/DeafCulture;
www.facebook.com/deafculturecentre

Collection: Archives
Joanne Cripps, Executive Director
jcripps@deafculturecentre.ca

Canadian Hard of Hearing Association
#205, 2415 Holly Lane, Ottawa, ON K1V 7P2
Tel: 613-526-1584; *Fax:* 613-526-4718
Toll-Free: 800-263-8068
TTY: 613-526-269
chhanational@chha.ca
www.chha.ca
Glenn Martin, National Executive Director

Provincial Libraries

Association du Québec pour enfants avec problèmes auditifs
3700, rue Berri, #A-446, Montréal, QC H2L 4G9
Tél: 514-842-8706; *Téléc:* 514-842-4006
Ligne sans frais: 877-842-4006
info@aqepa.org
www.aqepa.org
Collection: Surdité chez les enfants et familles handicapées

Deaf Children's Society of BC
#200, 7355 Canada Way, Burnaby, BC V3N 4Z6
Tel: 604-525-6056; *Fax:* 604-525-7307
TTY: 604-525-939
deafchildren.bc.ca/resources/library
Social Media: www.facebook.com/146576198745766

Collection: Sign language; deaf culture; professional resources; parenting/children's books
Karen Harvey, Office Manager

Institut Raymond-Dewar
3600, rue Berri, Montréal, QC H2L 4G9
Tél: 514-284-2214; *Téléc:* 514-284-5086
TTY: 514-284-374
biblio@raymond-dewar.gouv.qc.ca
www.raymond-dewar.qc.ca
Collection: Vidéocassettes, dictionnaires de langues des signes du monde

Manitoba School for the Deaf
242 Stradford St., Winnipeg, MB R2Y 2C9
Tel: 204-945-8934; *Fax:* 204-945-1767
TTY: 204-945-893
principal@msd.ca
www.msd.ca

Collection: American Sign Language, Deaf Culture, Deaf Education, Technology for the Deaf, Sign Language Dictionaries, Bilingualism/Biculturalism, Deaf Studies, English as a Second Language
Diane Bilyj, Assistant, Multimedia Centre

Local Hospitals & Health Centres

MANITOBA

WINNIPEG: 285 Pembina Inc.
Bethania Group
Affiliated with: Winnipeg Regional Health Authority
Also Known As: Deaf Centre
285 Pembina Hwy., Winnipeg, MB R3L 2E1
Tel: 204-284-0802 *Fax:* 204-474-0073
www.bethania.ca
Number of Beds: 57 beds
Note: Independent living residence for adults who are deaf or hard of hearing, & students enrolled in the Deaf Studies Program.

NOVA SCOTIA

HALIFAX: Nova Scotia Hearing & Speech Centres
Provincial Centre, Park Lane Terraces, PO Box 120, #401, 5657 Spring Garden Rd., Halifax, NS B3J 3R4
Tel: 902-492-8289 *Fax:* 902-423-0532
Toll-Free: 888-780-3330
info@nshsc.nshealth.ca
www.nshsc.nshealth.ca

Note: Specialties: Speech-language pathology services; Audiology services; Augmentative communication program; Cochlear implant program; Industrial & community audiology; Newborn hearing screening program
Anne Mason-Browne, President & CEO

ONTARIO

TORONTO: Bob Rumball Centre for the Deaf
2395 Bayview Ave., Toronto, ON M2L 1A2
Tel: 416-449-9651 *Fax:* 416-449-8881
TTY: 416-449-2728
info@bobrumball.org
www.bobrumball.org
Number of Beds: 56 beds
Note: Long-term care facility for the deaf
Jane Hooey, Chair

QUÉBEC

MONTRÉAL: Institut Raymond-Dewar
Affiliée à: CIUSSS du Centre-Sud-de-l'Ile-de-Montréal
3600, rue Berri, Montréal, QC H2L 4G9
Tél: 514-284-2581 *Téléc:* 514-284-5086
www.ciusss-centresudmtl.gouv.qc.ca

Note: Centre de réadaptation (déficience auditive et de la parole et du langage)

Heart Disease

In Canada, heart disease is one of the three leading causes of death, accounting for about 29 percent of all deaths. Approximately 1.6 million Canadians suffer from heart disease.

There is a wide range of heart (cardiac) diseases that can be divided into four major categories: heart failure, problems in electrical conduction (heart rate and rhythm), malfunction of the heart valves and coronary disease. Coronary disease relates to the arteries that supply oxygen to the heart muscle itself.

Heart Failure

Heart failure is the general inability of the heart to function effectively as the pumping mechanism to distribute oxygenated blood and nutrients to the cells and tissues. As the heart's pumping action declines, blood does not get distributed properly and normal circulation gets disrupted. As a result, the fluid accumulates, or piles up.

Cause
The most common causes of heart failure are damage to the heart muscle from a heart attack, and high blood pressure. Other causes may include diabetes, obesity, thyroid disease or anemia, high blood cholesterol, substance abuse, heart valve disease and heart infections (endocarditis and myocarditis).

Symptoms
Heart failure may cause swelling (edema) in the body, often noticeable in the ankles, as well as within the lungs (pulmonary edema) causing difficulty in breathing. Extreme fatigue, increased urination, loss of appetite and an ongoing cough or cold symptoms are other possible symptoms of heart failure.

Treatment Options
To diagnose heart failure, a physician takes a medical history, does a physical exam and orders tests including an electrocardiogram (a procedure which measures the electrical activity of the heart), a chest X-ray, an echocardiogram (a test which uses sound waves to create an image of the heart), a stress test (where the heart's response to the stress of exercise is measured on an electrocardiogram) and a coronary angiogram (an X-ray that shows whether the coronary arteries are blocked or narrowed).

Numerous mechanisms are responsible for heart failure so treatment is aimed at the underlying causes, improving heart contractibility (and thus pump efficiency), and removal of excess fluid through the kidneys. Drug therapy may include angiotensin converting enzyme (ACE) inhibitors, beta-blockers, diuretics, digoxin and aldosterone receptor antagonists. Surgery for blocked coronary arteries may include coronary angioplasty (a procedure used to open narrowed arteries) and bypass surgery (a procedure used to improve blood flow to the heart muscle). Other surgical procedures used to treat coronary artery disease may include cardiac resynchronization therapy or bi-ventricular pacing (a pacemaker for both the left and right-sided heart chambers), implantable cardioverter defibrilator (a device that shocks the heart to restore it to a normal rhythm), left ventricular assist device (to help the heart pump blood from one chamber of the heart to the rest of the body) and heart transplantation.

Electrical Conduction Problems

Cause
Problems in the electrical conduction that makes the heart contract result in irregular heart rate and rhythm, either slower, faster or, in life-threatening situations, absence of heartbeat or ineffective heart contractions. The most common type of irregular heart

rhythm (arrhythmia) is atrial fibrillation. Causes of atrial fibrillation may include high blood pressure, heart infection (pericarditis or myocarditis), hyperthyroidism, congenital heart disease, substance abuse, blood clots in the lung (pulmonary embolism) and structural abnormalities. Other heart rhythm disturbances are inherited. Inherited rhythm disorders include arrhythmogenic right ventricular cardiomyopathy, hypertrophic cardiomyopathy, long QT syndrome, Wolff-Parkinson-White syndrome, Brugada syndrome, catecholaminergic polymorphic ventricular tachycardia and short QT intervals.

Symptoms

Symptoms of arrhythmia may include heart palpitations, breathlessness, dizziness, lightheadedness, fatigue, chest pain or discomfort, and an irregular or slow or fast heartbeat. Sometimes inherited rhythm disorders cause no symptoms. Common warning signs may include fainting during physical activity or when excited, distressed or startled.

Prevalence

Atrial fibrillation is estimated to affect 350,000 people in Canada.

Treatment Options

To diagnose arrhythmia, a physician usually takes a medical history, family history and orders tests that may include an electrocardiogram (a procedure which measures the electrical activity of the heart), echocardiogram (a test which uses sound waves to create an image of the heart), a stress test (where the heart's response to the stress of exercise is measured on an electrocardiogram), electrophysiology studies (to determine the type of arrhythmia) and holter and event monitoring (to determine the cause of palpitations or dizziness).

Blood thinners and other drugs such as beta-blockers, calcium channel blockers and digitalis/digoxin may be prescribed to treat arrhythmia. Sometimes, electrical cardioversion (a controlled electrical shock) is used to return the heart to a normal rhythm. On rare occasions, catheter ablation (a procedure where small burns are made in the heart tissue to stabilize irregular electrical impulses) is performed.

Heart Valve Disorders

Cause

There are three different types of valve disorders: stenosis (a narrowing of the valve that restricts the amount of blood flow), prolapse (when the valve doesn't close securely) and regurgitation (a backward flow of blood through a valve that doesn't close securely).

Symptoms

Symptoms of a heart valve disorder may include chest pain, palpitations (irregular heartbeat), breathlessness, dizzy spells, faintness and swelling in the hands, wrists, feet and ankles.

Treatment Options

To diagnose a heart valve disorder, a physician usually performs a physical examination. A stethoscope can often easily pick up the murmuring sound that is characteristic of a valve disorder. Other tests such as an electrocardiogram (a procedure which measures the electrical activity of the heart), and an echocardiogram (which uses sound waves to make an image of the heart) may also be ordered.

Mild heart valve disorders are usually treated with medications such as diuretics. Surgical advances enable successful repair and replacement of defective or diseased valves.

Coronary Disease

Cause

The arteries that directly supply the heart (known as coronary arteries) can also be affected by disease processes. Deposits or fatty plaques may cause narrowing of the arteries, or the arteries can become blocked by a clot that originated somewhere else in the body. Either way, the heart may be deprived of oxygenated blood and the particular muscle that is fed by the artery is injured or dies. Angina is chest pain produced when the heart is not receiving enough oxygen but no direct damage occurs. A heart attack (or myocardial infarction) occurs when the heart is deprived of its blood for a significant amount of time.

Symptoms

Symptoms of coronary artery disease may include pain, fatigue and dizziness. Angina symptoms may also include a squeezing, burning feeling in the centre of the chest that moves to the throat, jaw, neck and back, feelings of indigestion, discomfort in the back between the shoulder blades and numbness in the shoulders, arms or wrists. In addition to chest pain and discomfort in the upper body, heart attack symptoms may include nausea, lightheadedness, breathlessness and sweating.

Prevalence

Coronary artery disease is the most common form of heart disease. Each year, there are approximately 70,000 heart attacks in Canada, and close to 16,000 people die of a heart attack.

Treatment Options

To diagnose coronary artery disease, a physician usually does a physical exam, takes a medical history and orders chest X-rays. Other tests including an electrocardiogram (a procedure which measures the electrical activity of the heart), an echocardiogram (which uses sound waves to make an image of the heart) and angiography (an X-ray that shows whether the coronary arteries are blocked or narrowed) may also be used to confirm a diagnosis of coronary artery disease.

Although there is no cure for coronary artery disease, medications and surgical procedures can be used to treat symptoms and slow the progress of the disease. Drug therapy for coronary artery disease may include anti-platelets, angiotensin converting enzyme (ACE) inhibitors, beta-blockers, calcium channel blockers and nitrates. Percutaneous coronary intervention (PCI) (a procedure where a catheter is used to put in a stent to open up narrowed blood vessels in the heart) and coronary bypass surgery (a surgical procedure used to improve blood flow to the heart muscle) are sometimes performed.

The outcome of a heart attack depends on the amount of damage sustained by the affected heart muscle and the speed with which treatment is started. Immediate medical intervention has a marked effect on long-term prognosis. Administration of agents that dissolve the clot (blood thinners, antithrombotics) significantly reduces heart attack deaths when given within six hours of the onset of chest pain.

Due to improved drug treatments and surgical procedures, as well as enhanced prevention strategies, the death rate from heart disease in Canada has decreased by close to 40 percent in the last decade.

See also Congenital Heart Disease

National Associations

Advanced Coronary Treatment (ACT) Foundation of Canada / La fondation des soins avancés en urgence coronarienne du Canada
379 Holland Ave., Ottawa ON K1Y 0Y9

Tel: 613-729-3455
Toll-Free: 800-465-9111
Other Communication: www.flickr.com/photos/actfoundation
e-mail: act@actfoundation.ca
www.actfoundation.ca
www.facebook.com/theactfoundation
twitter.com/actfoundation
www.youtube.com/theactfoundation

Also Known As: ACT Foundation
Overview: A small national charitable organization founded in 1985
Mission: To work with health professionals, governments, & the community in educating the public about the prevention, management, & treatment of illnesses that can lead to prehospital health emergencies
Chief Officer(s):
Sandra Clarke, Executive Director

Canadian Adult Congenital Heart Network (CACH)
c/o BB&C, #100, 2233 Argentia Rd., Mississauga ON L5N 2K7
Tel: 905-826-6665; *Fax:* 905-826-4873
www.cachnet.org

Overview: A small national organization founded in 1991
Mission: To promote the interests of Canadians born with heart defects
Affiliation(s): Toronto Congenital Cardiac Centre for Adults; Adult Congenital Heart Council
Chief Officer(s):
Erwin Oechslin, President
Publications:
• The Beat
Type: Newsletter; *Editor:* Laura-Lee Walter
Profile: Stories, overviews, & clinic updates

Canadian Association of Cardio-Pulmonary Technologists (CACPT)
PO Box 848, Stn. A, Toronto ON M5W 1G3
e-mail: contactus@cacpt.ca
www.cacpt.ca

Overview: A small national organization founded in 1970
Mission: To establish maintain high standards for Registered Cardio-Pulmonary Technologists
Affliation(s): Canadian Cardiovascular Society; Canadian Cardiovascular Congress
Chief Officer(s):
Glenda Ryan, President
  president@cacpt.ca

Canadian Association of Cardiovascular Prevention & Rehabilitation (CACPR)
1390 Taylor Ave., Winnipeg MB R3M 3V8
Tel: 204-928-7870
e-mail: admin@cacpr.ca
www.cacpr.ca
www.facebook.com/1CACPR
twitter.com/CACPR_1

Overview: A small national organization founded in 1991
Mission: To provide research & advocacy in cardiovascular disease prevention & rehabilitation
Chief Officer(s):
Linda Smith, Executive Director
  lsmith@cacpr.ca
Katelin Gresty, Special Projects
  kgresty@cacpr.ca
Publications:
• Current Issues in Cardiac Rehabilitation & Prevention (CICRP)
Type: Newsletter; *Frequency:* Semiannually; *Editor:* Scott Lear; *Price:* Free to members
Profile: Articles, research, reviews, national news, & events
• Journal of Cardiopulmonary Rehabilitation & Prevention (JCRP)
Type: Journal; *Price:* Free for members; $263 non-members

Canadian Association of Interventional Cardiology (CAIC) / Association canadienne de cardiologie d'intervention
3, boul Lakeview, Beaconsfield QC H9W 4P8
Toll-Free: 877-990-9044
e-mail: info@caic-acci.org
www.caic-acci.org

Overview: A small national organization
Mission: To advance the discipline, development, & implementation of interventional cardiology
Member of: Canadian Cardiology Society
Chief Officer(s):
Eric Cohen, President
Kevin McKenzie, Executive Director
Warren J. Cantor, Treasurer

Canadian Cardiovascular Society (CCS) / Société canadienne de cardiologie
#1403, 222 Queen St., Ottawa ON K1P 5V9
Tel: 613-569-3407; *Fax:* 613-569-6574
Toll-Free: 877-569-3407
e-mail: info@ccs.ca
www.ccs.ca
www.facebook.com/141084722576966
twitter.com/SCC_CCS

Previous Name: Canadian Heart Association
Overview: A medium-sized national organization founded in 1947
Mission: To promote cardiovascular health & care through knowledge translation, dissemination of research & encouragement of best practices, professional development & leadership in health policy
Member of: World Heart Federation; Inter-American Society of Cardiology; Canadian Coalition for High Blood Pressure Prevention & Control; American Society of Cardiology
Affiliation(s): Canadian Society of Clinical Perfusionists; Canadian Society of Cardiology Technologists; Canadian Association of Cardiopulmonary Technologists; Canadian Medical Association; Royal College of Physicians & Surgeons of Canada; Canadian Council of Cardiovascular Nursing
Chief Officer(s):
Heather Ross, President
Anne Ferguson, Chief Executive Officer
Publications:
• The Canadian Journal of Cardiology
Type: Journal; *Editor:* Dr. E.R. Smith; *Price:* Free with CCS membership
Profile: Research reports, health outcomes, ethics, review articles, policy, political issues, & case reports concerning cardiovascular medicine

Canadian Council of Cardiovascular Nurses (CCCN) / Conseil canadien des infirmières et infirmiers en nursing cardiovasculaire (CCINC)
#202, 300 March Rd., Ottawa ON K2K 2E2
Tel: 613-599-9210; *Fax:* 613-595-1155
e-mail: info@cccn.ca
www.cccn.ca
www.facebook.com/124535634406687

Overview: A medium-sized national organization founded in 1973
Mission: To promote & maintain high standards of cardiovascular nursing through education, research, health promotion, strategic alliances, & advocacy
Member of: Canadian Nursing Association; Canadian Society of Association Executives
Affliation(s): Heart & Stroke Foundation of Canada; Canadian Coalition for High Blood Pressure Prevention & Control; Canadian Cardiovascular Society
Chief Officer(s):
David Miriguay, Executive Director, 613-599-9210 Ext. 1
  david@cccn.ca
Publications:
• Canadian Council of Cardiovascular Nurses Annual Report
Type: Yearbook; *Frequency:* Annually
Profile: A review of the council's year
• Canadian Council of Cardiovascular Nurses Newsletter
Type: Newsletter; *Frequency:* Monthly
Profile: Current events of the council, including conferences, award presentations, & members in the news

• **Canadian Journal of Cardiovascular Nursing (CJCN)**
Type: Journal; *Frequency:* Quarterly; *Accepts Advertising*; *Editor:* Suzanne Fredericks; *Price:* Free for members of the Canadian Council of Cardiovascular Nurses; $75 non-members
Profile: The peer reviewed official publication of the Canadian Journal of Cardiovascular Nursing, featuring original articles about healthcare issues related to cardiovascular health & illness & research information

Canadian Society of Atherosclerosis, Thrombosis & Vascular Biology (CSATVB) / Société canadienne d'Athérosclérose, de Thrombose et de Biologie Vasculaire (SCATBV)
c/o Laurence Boudreault, Centre de recherche du CHU de Quebec, 2705, boul Laurier, #TR-93, Québec QC G1V 4G2
Tel: 418-656-4141; *Fax:* 418-654-2145
www.csatvb.ca
Previous Name: Canadian Atherosclerosis Society
Overview: A medium-sized national charitable organization founded in 1983
Mission: To provide a means of communication between Canadian professionals interested in atherosclerosis & cardiovascular disease; To promote research & education
Affiliation(s): International Atherosclerosis Society
Chief Officer(s):
Peter Julien, Treasurer
Laurence Boudreault, Contact
laurence.boudreault@crchuq.ulaval.ca

Canadian Society of Cardiac Surgeons / Société des chirurgiens cardiaques
#1403, 222 Queen St., Ottawa ON K1P 5V9
Tel: 613-569-3407; *Fax:* 613-569-6574
Toll-Free: 877-569-3407
www.ccs.ca
www.facebook.com/SCC.CCS.ca
twitter.com/SCC_CCS
Previous Name: Canadian Society of Cardiovascular & Thoracic Surgeons
Overview: A small national organization
Mission: To represent cardiovascular clinicians & scientists in Canada
Chief Officer(s):
Catherine Kells, President
Anne Ferguson, Chief Executive Officer
ferguson@ccs.ca
Linda Palmer, Director, Membership & CCS Affiliate Services
palmer@ccs.ca
Susan Oliver, Director, Strategic Initiatives
oliver@ccs.ca
Melissa Keown, Director, Professional Development
keown@ccs.ca
Erin McGeachie, Manager, Health Policy
mcgeachie@ccs.ca
Julie Graves, Coordinator, Marketing & Communications
graves@ccs.ca
Carol DeHaros, Coordinator, Finance & Administration
deharos@ccs.ca

Canadian Society of Cardiology Technologists Inc. (CSCT) / Société canadienne des technologues en cardiologie inc.
PO Box 3121, Winnipeg MB R3C 4E6
Other Communication: education@csct.ca
e-mail: info@csct.ca
www.csct.ca
Overview: A medium-sized national organization
Mission: To ensure a standard of excellence in the practice of cardiology technology in Canada
Affiliation(s): Canadian Cardiovascular Society (CCS)
Chief Officer(s):
Shauna Ryall, President

Cardiac Health Foundation of Canada
#306, 901 Lawrence Ave. West, Toronto ON M6A 1C3
Tel: 416-730-8299; *Fax:* 416-730-0421
e-mail: info@cardiachealth.ca
www.cardiachealth.ca
www.facebook.com/CardiacHealth
twitter.com/CardiacHealth
Previous Name: Canadian Cardiac Rehabilitation Foundation

Overview: A medium-sized national charitable organization
Mission: To lower instances of, & support recovery from, cardiovascular disease; To aid in the development of cardiovascular rehabilitation & education services & initiatives in Canada
Chief Officer(s):
Barbara Kennedy, Executive Director
bkennedy@cardiachealth.ca
Christina Mellos, Manager, Operations
cmellos@cardiachealth.ca

Heart & Stroke Foundation of Canada (HSFC) / Fondation des maladies du coeur du Canada
#1402, 222 Queen St., Ottawa ON K1P 5V9
Tel: 613-569-4361; *Fax:* 613-569-3278
www.heartandstroke.ca
www.facebook.com/heartandstroke
twitter.com/TheHSF
www.youtube.com/heartandstrokefdn
Overview: A medium-sized national charitable organization founded in 1983
Mission: To further the study, prevention & reduction of disability & death from heart disease & stroke through research, education & the promotion of healthy lifestyles
Member of: Imagine Canada
Affiliation(s): International Society & Federation of Cardiology; Canadian Coalition for High Blood Pressure Prevention & Control
Chief Officer(s):
David Sculthorpe, Chief Executive Officer

Provincial Associations

ALBERTA

Heart & Stroke Foundation of Alberta, NWT & Nunavut (HSFA)
#100, 119 - 14 St. NW, Calgary AB T2N 1Z6
Tel: 403-351-7030; *Fax:* 403-237-0803
Toll-Free: 888-473-4636
www.hsf.ab.ca
Previous Name: Heart & Stroke Foundation of Alberta
Overview: A medium-sized provincial charitable organization founded in 1956 overseen by Heart & Stroke Foundation of Canada
Mission: To disseminate information about heart disease & stroke; to promote research into new drugs, therapies, treatments in disorders leading to heart disease & stroke; to conduct several events to campaign for funds.
Chief Officer(s):
Michael Hill, Chair
Donna Hastings, CEO

Edmonton Office
10985 - 124 St., Edmonton AB T5M 0H9
Tel: 780-451-4545; *Fax:* 780-454-1593

Lethbridge Office
PO Box 2211, Lethbridge AB T1J 4K7
Tel: 403-327-3239; *Fax:* 403-327-9928

Medicine Hat Office
#124, 430 - 6 Ave. SE, Medicine Hat AB T1A 2S8
Tel: 403-527-0028; *Fax:* 403-526-9655

Red Deer Office
#202, 5913 - 50 Ave., Red Deer AB T4N 4C4
Tel: 403-342-4435; *Fax:* 403-342-7088

BRITISH COLUMBIA

Cardiology Technologists' Association of British Columbia (CTABC)
PO Box 2575, 349 West Georgia St., Vancouver BC V6B 3W8
Toll-Free: 866-280-6535
e-mail: info@ctabc.ca
www.ctabc.ca
Overview: A small provincial organization founded in 1975
Mission: To raise standards of practice & of patient care provided by cardiology technologists in British Columbia
Member of: Canadian Society of Cardiology Technologists (CSCT)
Affiliation(s): Canadian Cardiovascular Society (CCS)
Chief Officer(s):

Shauna Ryall, CTABC President
  president@ctabc.ca
Cheryl West, CTABC / CSCT Registrar
  registrar@ctabc.ca
Jiannan Yu, Treasurer
  treasurer@ctabc.ca
Publications:
• Heart Copy: Cardiology Technologists' Association of BC Newsletter
Type: Newsletter
Profile: Association reports

Heart & Stroke Foundation of British Columbia & Yukon (HSFBCY)
#200, 1212 West Broadway, Vancouver BC V6H 3V2
Tel: 778-372-8000
www.heartandstroke.bc.ca
www.facebook.com/heartandstrokebcyukon
Previous Name: BC & Yukon Heart Foundation
Overview: A large provincial charitable organization founded in 1955 overseen by Heart & Stroke Foundation of Canada
Mission: To further the study, prevention & relief of cardiovascular disease
Chief Officer(s):
Adrienne Bakker, CEO

  Coastal Vancouver Area Office - Vancouver/North Shore
  1216 West Broadway, Vancouver BC V6H 1G6
  Tel: 778-372-8052; *Fax:* 604-736-4087

  Fraser North & East Area Office - Tri-Cities/Fraser
    Valley/Burnaby/New Westminster
  2239C McAllister Ave., Port Coquitlam BC V3C 2A5
  Tel: 604-342-8070; *Fax:* 604-472-0055
  Toll-Free: 877-472-0045

  Kamloops Area Office - Kamloops/Cariboo
  729 Victoria St., Kamloops BC V2C 2B5
  Tel: 250-372-3938; *Fax:* 250-372-3940

  Kelowna Area Office - Okanagan/Kootenays
  #4, 1551 Sutherland Ave., Kelowna BC V1Y 9M9
  Tel: 778-313-8090; *Fax:* 250-860-8790
  Toll-Free: 866-432-7833

  Prince George Area Office Northern BC/Yukon
  1480 - 7th Ave., Prince George BC V2L 3P2
  Tel: 250-562-8611; *Fax:* 250-562-8614
  Toll-Free: 866-226-6784

  Richmond Office - Richmond/South Delta
  #260, 7000 Minoru Blvd., Richmond BC V6Y 3Z5
  Tel: 778-234-8080; *Fax:* 604-279-7134

  Surrey Area Office -
    Surrey/Langley/Whiterock/Cloverdale/Aldergrove/North Delta
  #101, 13569 - 76th Ave., Surrey BC V3W 2W3
  Tel: 778-612-8063; *Fax:* 604-591-2624

  Vancouver Island Area Office - Nanaimo
  #401, 495 Dunsmuir St., Nanaimo BC V9R 6B9
  Tel: 250-754-5274; *Fax:* 250-754-2575

  Victoria Office
  #106, 1001 Cloverdale Ave., Victoria BC V8X 4C9
  Tel: 250-410-8091; *Fax:* 250-382-0231

MANITOBA

Heart & Stroke Foundation of Manitoba (HSFM)
The Heart & Stroke Bldg., #200, 6 Donald St., Winnipeg MB R3L 0K6
Tel: 204-949-2000; *Fax:* 204-957-1365
www.heartandstroke.mb.ca
Previous Name: Manitoba Heart Foundation
Overview: A medium-sized provincial charitable organization founded in 1957 overseen by Heart & Stroke Foundation of Canada
Mission: To eliminate heart disease & stroke through education, advocacy, & research
Chief Officer(s):
Debbie Brown, CEO

Manitoba Cardiac Institute (Reh-Fit) Inc.
1390 Taylor Ave., Winnipeg MB R3M 3V8
Tel: 204-488-8023; *Fax:* 204-488-4819
e-mail: reh-fit@reh-fit.com
www.reh-fit.com
Also Known As: Kinsmen Reh-Fit Centre
Overview: A small provincial organization
Mission: To enhance the health and well-being of its members and the community by providing innovative health and fitness services through assessment, education, and exercise in a suportive environment.
Chief Officer(s):
Rosanna Buonpensiere, Director

NEW BRUNSWICK

Heart & Stroke Foundation of New Brunswick / Fondation des maladies du coeur du Nouveau-Brunswick
133 Prince William St., 5th Fl, Saint John NB E2L 2B5
Tel: 506-634-1620; *Fax:* 506-648-0098
Toll-Free: 800-663-3600
www.heartandstroke.nb.ca
Previous Name: New Brunswick Heart Foundation
Overview: A medium-sized provincial organization founded in 1967 overseen by Heart & Stroke Foundation of Canada
Mission: To improve the health of residents of New Brunswick by preventing & reducing disability & death from heart disease & stroke, through research, health promotion & advocacy
Chief Officer(s):
Kurtis Sisk, CEO

New Brunswick Society of Cardiology Techologists (NBSCT)
NB
www.nbsct.ca
Overview: A small provincial organization founded in 1968
Mission: To operate in accordance with An Act Respecting the New Brunswick Society of Cardiology Technologists; To maintain high standards for the practice of cardiology technology in New Brunswick
Member of: Canadian Society of Cardiology Technologists
Affliation(s): Canadian Medical Association
Chief Officer(s):
Kathy Walker, Registrar
  nbsct.registrar@hotmail.com
Kelsey McEachern, Secretary
  nbsct.secretary@hotmail.com
Nadine Hebert, Treasurer
  treasurer_nbsct@hotmail.com
Kristine McLaughlin, Coordinator, Provincial Education
  nbsct.education@hotmail.com

NEWFOUNDLAND AND LABRADOR

Heart & Stroke Foundation of Newfoundland & Labrador
1037 Topsail Rd., Mount Pearl NL A1N 5E9
Tel: 709-753-8521; *Fax:* 709-753-3117
www.heartandstroke.nf.ca
Overview: A medium-sized provincial organization founded in 1964 overseen by Heart & Stroke Foundation of Canada
Mission: To work in Newfoundland & Labrador to advance research, advocate, & promote healthy lifestyles so that heart disease & stroke will be eliminated & their impact reduced
Chief Officer(s):
Mary Ann Butt, CEO

NOVA SCOTIA

Heart & Stroke Foundation of Nova Scotia (HSFNS)
Park Lane - Mall Level 3, PO Box 245, 5657 Spring Garden Rd., Halifax NS B3J 3R4
Tel: 902-423-7530; *Fax:* 902-492-1464
Toll-Free: 800-423-4432
www.heartandstroke.ns.ca
Previous Name: Nova Scotia Heart Foundation
Overview: A medium-sized provincial charitable organization founded in 1958 overseen by Heart & Stroke Foundation of Canada
Mission: To eliminate heart disease & stroke; To advance research; To promote healthy living; To engage in advocacy activities
Member of: The Heart and Stroke Foundation of Canada
Chief Officer(s):

Menna MacIsaac, CEO

ONTARIO

Cardiac Care Network of Ontario
#502, 4100 Yonge St., Toronto ON M2P 2B5
Tel: 416-512-7472; *Fax:* 416-512-6425
e-mail: mail@ccn.on.ca
www.ccn.on.ca

Overview: A small provincial organization
Mission: To work as an advisory body to the Ministry of Health &
Long-Term Care; To improve the quality of cardiovascular care in
Ontario
Chief Officer(s):
Kori Kingsbury, Chief Executive Officer

Cardiac Rehabilitation Network of Ontario (CRNO)
347 Rumsey Rd., Toronto ON M4G 1R7
Tel: 416-597-3422; *Fax:* 416-597-7027
www.crno.ca

Overview: A small provincial organization founded in 2002 overseen
by Canadian Association of Cardiovascular Prevention & Rehabilitation
Mission: Dedicated to the rehabilitation of individuals with cardiac
disease, as well as the prevention of cardiac disease; advocacy on
behalf of the patient through the advancement of health care services
in Ontario
Chief Officer(s):
Terry Fair, Chair, 905-895-4521 Ext. 2805
TFair@southlakeregional.org
Andrew Lotto, Treasurer/Registrar, 905-895-4521 Ext. 6896
alotto@southlakeregional.org

Heart & Stroke Foundation of Ontario (HSFO)
PO Box 2414, #1300, 2300 Yonge St., Toronto ON M4P 1E4
Tel: 416-489-7111; *Fax:* 416-489-6885
Previous Name: Ontario Heart Foundation
Overview: A medium-sized provincial charitable organization founded
in 1952 overseen by Heart & Stroke Foundation of Canada
Mission: To eliminate heart disease & stroke by advancing research &
promoting healthy living; To advocate in areas such as a smoke-free
world, equal access to quality stroke care, obesity targeting, elimination
of trans-fat, & resuscitation/CPR
Member of: Heart & Stroke Foundation of Canada
Chief Officer(s):
Darrell Reid, Chief Executive Officer

Barrie Office
#1, 112 Commerce Park Dr., Barrie ON L4N 8W8
Tel: 705-737-1020; *Fax:* 705-737-0902
www.heartandstroke.on.ca

Belleville Office
#106A, 121 Dundas St. East, Belleville ON K8N 1C3
Tel: 613-962-2502; *Fax:* 613-962-6080
www.heartandstroke.on.ca

Brantford Office
442 Grey St., #A, Brantford ON N3S 7N3
Tel: 519-752-1301; *Fax:* 519-752-5554
www.heartandstroke.on.ca

Brockville Office
Brockville General Hospital, 75 Charles St., Brockville ON K6V 1S8
Tel: 613-345-5645; *Fax:* 613-345-8348
www.heartandstroke.on.ca
Chief Officer(s):
Jay Bhatt, Director

Chatham-Kent Office
214 Queen St., Chatham ON N7M 2H1
Tel: 519-354-6232; *Fax:* 519-354-6351
www.heartandstroke.on.ca

Chinese Canadian Council
PO Box 2414, #1300, 2300 Yonge St., Toronto ON M4P 1E4
Tel: 416-489-7111; *Fax:* 416-489-9179
www.heartandstroke.on.ca

Cornwall Office

36 - 2nd St. East, Cornwall ON K6H 1Y3
Tel: 613-938-8933; *Fax:* 613-938-0655
www.heartandstroke.on.ca

Durham Regional Office
#2, 105 Consumers Dr., Whitby ON L1N 1C4
Tel: 905-666-3777; *Fax:* 905-666-9956
www.heartandstroke.on.ca

Guelph Office
#204, 21 Surrey St. West, Guelph ON N1H 3R3
Tel: 519-837-4858; *Fax:* 519-837-9209
www.heartandstroke.on.ca

Halton Region Office
#7, 4391 Harvester Rd., Burlington ON L7L 4X1
Tel: 905-634-7732; *Fax:* 905-634-1353
www.heartandstroke.on.ca

Hamilton Office
#7, 1439 Upper Ottawa St., Hamilton ON L8W 3J6
Tel: 905-574-4105; *Fax:* 905-574-4380
www.heartandstroke.on.ca

Kingston Office
720 Progress Ave., Kingston ON K7M 4W9
Tel: 613-384-2871; *Fax:* 613-384-2899
www.heartandstroke.on.ca

Kitchener Office
#2A, 1373 Victoria St. North, Kitchener ON N2B 3R6
Tel: 519-571-9600; *Fax:* 519-571-9832
www.heartandstroke.on.ca

London Office
#180, 633 Colborne St., London ON N6B 2V3
Tel: 519-679-0641; *Fax:* 519-679-6898
www.heartandstroke.on.ca

Niagara District Office
#3, 300 Bunting Rd., St Catharines ON L2M 7X3
Tel: 905-938-8800; *Fax:* 905-938-8811
www.heartandstroke.on.ca

Ottawa Office
#100, 1101 Prince of Wales Dr., Ottawa ON K2C 3W7
Tel: 613-727-5060; *Fax:* 613-727-1895
www.heartandstroke.on.ca

Owen Sound Office
795 - 1st Ave. East, Owen Sound ON N4K 2C6
Tel: 519-371-0083; *Fax:* 519-371-8164
www.heartandstroke.on.ca

Peel Office
#306, 201 County Court Blvd., Brampton ON L6W 4L2
Tel: 905-451-0021; *Fax:* 905-452-0503
www.heartandstroke.on.ca

Peterborough Office
#3, 824 Clonsilla Ave., Peterborough ON K9J 5Y3
Tel: 705-749-1044; *Fax:* 705-749-1470
www.heartandstroke.on.ca

Sarnia Office
774 London Rd., Sarnia ON N7T 4Y1
Tel: 519-332-1415; *Fax:* 519-332-3139
www.heartandstroke.on.ca

Sault Ste. Marie Office
59 Great Northern Rd., Sault Ste Marie ON P6B 4Y7
Tel: 705-253-3775; *Fax:* 705-946-5760
www.heartandstroke.on.ca

Stratford Office
556 Huron St., Stratford ON N5A 5T9
Tel: 519-273-5212; *Fax:* 519-273-7024
www.heartandstroke.on.ca

Sudbury Office
#130, 43 Elm St., Sudbury ON P3C 1S4
Tel: 705-673-2228; *Fax:* 705-673-7406
www.heartandstroke.on.ca

Thunder Bay Office

#104, 979 Alloy Dr., Thunder Bay ON P7B 5Z8
Tel: 807-623-1118; Fax: 807-622-9914
www.heartandstroke.on.ca

Timmins Office
#301, 60 Wilson Ave., Timmins ON P4N 2S7
Tel: 705-267-4645; Fax: 705-268-6721
www.heartandstroke.on.ca

Toronto Office
#1300, 2300 Yonge St., Toronto ON M4P 1E4
Tel: 416-489-7111; Fax: 416-489-6885
www.heartandstroke.on.ca

Windsor Office
#350, 4570 Rhodes Dr., Windsor ON N8W 5C2
Tel: 519-254-4345; Fax: 519-254-4215
www.heartandstroke.on.ca

York Region North Office
#29, 17665 Leslie St., Newmarket ON L3Y 3E3
Tel: 905-853-6355; Fax: 905-853-7961
www.heartandstroke.on.ca

York South Office
#204, 9251 Yonge St., Richmond Hill ON L4C 9T3
Tel: 905-709-4899; Fax: 905-709-0883
www.heartandstroke.on.ca

PRINCE EDWARD ISLAND

Heart & Stroke Foundation of Prince Edward Island Inc.
PO Box 279, 180 Kent St., Charlottetown PE C1A 7K4
Tel: 902-892-7441
Overview: A medium-sized provincial charitable organization overseen by Heart & Stroke Foundation of Canada
Mission: To improve the health of Islanders through the funding of heart disease & stroke research & the provision of heart & stroke education & programs
Chief Officer(s):
Charlotte Comrie, Chief Executive Officer
  charlotte.comrie@heartandstroke.ca
Sarah Crozier, Manager, Health Promotion

QUÉBEC

Association des cardiologues du Québec (ACQ)
CP 216, Succ. Desjardins, #3000, 2, Complexe Desjardins, Montréal QC H5B 1G8
Tél: 514-350-5106; Téléc: 514-350-5156
Courriel: acq@fmsq.org
Aperçu: *Dimension:* petite; *Envergure:* provinciale surveillé par Fédération des médecins spécialistes du Québec
Membre(s) du bureau directeur:
Gilles O'Hara, Président
Louise Girard, Directrice

Association des Perfusionnistes du Québec Inc. (APQI)
CP 32172, Succ. Saint-André, Montréal QC H2L 4Y5
www.apqi.com
Aperçu: *Dimension:* petite; *Envergure:* provinciale
Membre(s) du bureau directeur:
Alina Parapuf, Présidente, 514-415-7622
Audrey Chapman, Vice-Présidente, 514-406-2186
Catherine André-Guimont, Trésorière
Thierry Lamarre-Renaud, Secrétaire, 514-406-4676

Fondation des maladies du coeur du Québec (FMCQ) / Heart & Stroke Foundation of Québec
#500, 1434, rue Sainte-Catherine ouest, Montréal QC H3G 1R4
Tél: 514-871-1551; Téléc: 514-871-9385
Ligne sans frais: 800-567-8563
www.fmcoeur.qc.ca
www.facebook.com/fmcoeur
twitter.com/FMCoeur
www.youtube.com/heartandstrokefdn
Nom précédent: Fondation du Québec des maladies du coeur
Aperçu: *Dimension:* grande; *Envergure:* provinciale; Organisme sans but lucratif; fondée en 1955 surveillé par Heart & Stroke Foundation of Canada

Mission: Forte de l'engagement de ses donateurs, de ses bénévoles et de ses employés, a pour mission de contribuer à l'avancement de la recherche et de promouvoir la santé du coeur, afin de réduire les invalidités et les décès dus aux maladies cardiovasculaires et aux accidents vasculaires cérébraux
Membre(s) du bureau directeur:
Edmée Métivier, Chef de la direction
Éric Champagne, Président du conseil

Bas St-Laurent et Gaspésie
33, boul René-Lepage est, Rimouski QC G5L 1N8
Tél: 418-869-1022; Téléc: 418-869-2748
Ligne sans frais: 888-473-4636
Membre(s) du bureau directeur:
Louiselle Bérubé, Directrice régionale

Côte-Nord
1, rue Arnaud, Les Escoumins QC G0T 1K0
Tél: 418-233-2119; Téléc: 418-233-3771
Membre(s) du bureau directeur:
Liliane Larouche, Personne responsable

Estrie
#100, 2630, rue King ouest, Sherbrooke QC J1J 2H1
Tél: 819-562-7942; Téléc: 819-564-0690
Membre(s) du bureau directeur:
Manon Thibodeau, Directrice régionale

La Capitale
#261, 4715, av des Replats, Québec QC G2J 1B8
Tél: 418-682-6387; Téléc: 418-682-8214
Membre(s) du bureau directeur:
Jocelyn Thémens, Directeur régional

Laval/Laurentides/Lanaudière
Tour A, #410, 1600, boul Saint-Martin est, Laval QC H7G 4R8
Tél: 450-669-6909; Téléc: 450-669-8987
Membre(s) du bureau directeur:
Carol Pincox, Directrice régionale

Mauricie/Centre du Québec
137, rue Radisson, Trois-Rivières QC G9A 2C5
Tél: 819-375-9565; Téléc: 819-375-0233

Ouest de Montréal
#18, 795, av Carson, Dorval QC H9S 1L7
Tél: 514-636-4599; Téléc: 514-636-8576
Membre(s) du bureau directeur:
Dalia Solo, Directrice régionale

Outaouais
#007, 109, rue Wright, Gatineau QC J8X 2G7
Tél: 819-771-8595; Téléc: 819-771-7070
Membre(s) du bureau directeur:
Gabrielle Ouzilleau, Directrice régionale

Rive-Sud/Montérégie
#200, 1194, ch de Chambly, Longueuil QC J4J 2W6
Tél: 450-442-6387; Téléc: 450-442-3329
Membre(s) du bureau directeur:
Hélène Gagné, Directrice régionale

Saguenay/Lac Saint-Jean
#251, 152, rue Racine est, Chicoutimi QC G7H 1R8
Tél: 418-543-8959; Téléc: 418-543-5872
Membre(s) du bureau directeur:
Martine Paradis, Directrice régionale

SASKATCHEWAN

Heart & Stroke Foundation of Saskatchewan (HSFS) / Fondation des maladies du coeur de la Saskatchewan
#26, 1738 Quebec Ave., Saskatoon SK S7K 1V9
Fax: 306-664-4016
Toll-Free: 888-473-4636
www.linkedin.com/company/heart-and-stroke-foundation-saskatchewan
www.youtube.com/saskheart
Overview: A medium-sized provincial charitable organization founded in 1956 overseen by Heart & Stroke Foundation of Canada
Mission: To eliminate & reduce the impact of heart disease & stroke; To advance research, promote healthy living, & advocates a healthy public policy

Chief Officer(s):
Dale Oughton, Director, Development

Local Associations

ALBERTA

Children's Heart Society
#128, 9920 63 Ave., Edmonton AB T6E 0G9

Tel: 780-454-7665
e-mail: childrensheart@shaw.ca
www.childrensheart.ca
www.facebook.com/childrenshearts
twitter.com/childrenshearts

Overview: A small local organization
Mission: To support children with heart disease & their families
Chief Officer(s):
Andrea Luft, President
chsgalaedmonton@gmail.com
Danielle Tailleur, Director, Membership
dtailleur@ellisdon.com

QUÉBEC

Fondation Cardio-Montérégienne (FOCAM)
#230, 1750, boul Marie-Victorin, Longueuil QC J4G 1A5

Tél: 450-468-3333; *Téléc:* 450-468-3334
www.fondationcardio-monteregienne.ca

Aperçu: *Dimension:* petite; *Envergure:* locale
Mission: Encourager et soutenir l'avancement de la science médicale au moyen de dons permettant l'acquisition d'équipements reliés à la médecine cardiaque.

Institut de cardiologie de Montréal (ICM) / Montréal Heart Institute (MHI)
5000, rue Bélanger, Montréal QC H1T 1C8

Tél: 514-376-3330
Ligne sans frais: 855-922-6387
www.icm-mhi.org
www.facebook.com/institutcardiologiemontreal
twitter.com/ICMtl
www.youtube.com/user/InstitutdeCardioMtl

Aperçu: *Dimension:* petite; *Envergure:* locale; fondée en 1954
Mission: Un centre uniquement consacré au développement des traitements des maladies cardiovasculaires
Membre(s) du bureau directeur:
Pierre Anctil, Président
Denis Roy, Directeur général

International Associations

American Society of Echocardiography (ASE)
#310, 2100 Gateway Centre Blvd., Morrisville NC 27560 USA

Tel: 919-861-5574; *Fax:* 919-882-9900
e-mail: ase@asecho.org
www.asecho.org
www.linkedin.com/groups/55219
www.facebook.com/asecho
twitter.com/ase360
www.youtube.com/user/AmericanSocietyofEch

Overview: A medium-sized international organization founded in 1975
Mission: To promote excellence in cardiovascular ultrasound & its application to patient care
Chief Officer(s):
Allan Klein, President
president@asecho.org
Robin Wiegerink, Chief Executive Officer
rwiegerink@asecho.org

Society of Cardiovascular Anesthesiologists (SCA)
#300, 8735 West Higgins Rd., Chicago IL 60631 USA

Fax: 847-375-6323
Toll-Free: 855-658-2828
e-mail: info@scahq.org
www.scahq.org
www.facebook.com/210665095719456

Overview: A large international organization

Mission: To promote excellence in clinical care & research in perioperative care for patients undergoing cardiothoracic & vascular procedures
Chief Officer(s):
Colleen Lawler, Executive Director
clawler@scahq.org
Andrea King, Manager, Operations
aking@scahq.org
Publications:
• Annual Update of Cardiopulmonary Bypass
Type: Yearbook; *Frequency:* Annually
• SCA [Society of Cardiovascular Anesthesiologists] Bulletin
Type: Newsletter; *Frequency:* Bimonthly
• Society of Cardiovascular Anesthesiologists Annual Meeting Syllabi
Type: Yearbook; *Frequency:* Annually
• TEE Review Courses [a publication of the Society of Cardiovascular Anesthesiologists]

World Hypertension League (WHL)
168 South Hills Rd., Clancy MT 59634 USA

Tel: 406-861-6844
www.worldhypertensionleague.org

Overview: A large international organization founded in 1984
Mission: To promote the detection, control & prevention of arterial hypertension in populations; To assist national bodies by providing internationally applicable programs
Member of: International Society of Hypertension
Affliation(s): Canadian Coalition for High Blood Pressure Prevention & Control; WHO
Chief Officer(s):
Norman Campbell, M.D., President
ncampbel@ucalgary.ca
Mark Niebylski, CEO
CEO@whleague.org
Publications:
• WHL [World Hypertension League] Newsletter
Type: Newsletter; *Frequency:* q.; *Editor:* Dr. Daniel T. Lackland

National Publications

Canadian Journal of Cardiology
Owned By: Elsevier Inc.
Canadian Cardiovascular Society, #1403, 222 Queen St., Toronto, ON K1P 5V9

Tel: 613-569-3407; *Fax:* 613-569-6574
Toll-Free: 877-569-3407

Circulation: 15,500 *Frequency:* 14 times a year
The official journal of the Canadian Cardiovascular Society (CCS).
Dr. Stanley Nattel, Editor-in-Chief, stanley.nattel@icm-mhi.org
Jennifer Bacchi, Managing Editor, jenniferanne.bacchi@icm-mhi.org
Jane Grochowski, Publisher, j.grochowski@elsevier.com

Provincial/Local Publications

HeartBeat
Owned By: Newman Publishing
PO Box 1, Site 100, RR#1, Carvel, AB T0E 0H0

Tel: 780-892-2910; *Fax:* 780-893-3401

Circulation: 4,600 *Frequency:* Annually
Pauline Newman, Managing Editor

Provincial Libraries

Heart & Stroke Foundation of Alberta, NWT & Nunavut
#100, 119 - 14th St. NW, Calgary, AB T2N 1Z6

Tel: 403-264-5549; *Fax:* 403-237-0803
Toll-Free: 888-473-4636
www.heartandstroke.ca
Social Media: www.youtube.com/heartandstrokefdn;
twitter.com/TheHSF; www.facebook.com/heartandstroke

Collection: Research; Statistics; Videos; Printed literature
Donna Hastings, CEO

Heart & Stroke Foundation of BC & Yukon
#200, 1212 West Broadway, Vancouver, BC V6H 3V2

Tel: 778-372-8000; *Fax:* 604-736-8732
www.heartandstroke.ca

Heart & Stroke Foundation of Nova Scotia
Park Lane, Mall Level 3, 5657 Spring Garden Rd., Halifax, NS B3J 3R4
Tel: 902-423-7530; *Fax:* 902-492-1464
Toll-Free: 800-423-4432
www.heartandstroke.ca
Social Media: twitter.com/TheHSF

Heart & Stroke Foundation of Prince Edward Island
180 Kent St., Charlottetown, PE C1A 7K4
Tel: 902-892-7441; *Fax:* 902-368-7068
www.heartandstroke.ca

Institut de cardiologie de Montréal
5000, rue Bélanger, Montréal, QC H1T 1C8
Tél: 514-376-3330; *Téléc:* 514-593-2565
Ligne sans frais: 855-922-6387
www.icm-mhi.org
Média social: www.facebook.com/institutcardiologiemontreal

Institut universitaire de cariologie et de pneumologie de Québec
#Y2244, 2725, ch Sainte-Foy, Québec, QC G1V 4G5
Tél: 418-656-4563; *Téléc:* 418-656-4720
biblio@criucpq.ulaval.ca
iucpq.qc.ca/fr/enseignement/bibliotheque/heures-d-ouverture
Francine Aumont, Bibliothécaire
francine.aumont@criucpq.ulaval.ca
Julie Émond, Technicienne
Diane St-Pierre, Technicienne

Rumsey Centre - Cardiac
#224, 347 Rumsey Rd., Toronto, ON M4G 1R7
Tel: 416-597-3422
Maureen Pakosh, Information Specialist

University of Ottawa Heart Institute
40 Ruskin St., #H2353, Ottawa, ON K1Y 4W7
Tel: 613-761-4753; *Fax:* 613-761-5309
Toll-Free: 866-399-4432
pwc@ottawaheart.ca
www.ottawaheart.ca
Profile: Specializes in cardiovascular health & healthy lifestyle information

Local Hospitals & Health Centres

ALBERTA

EDMONTON: Mazankowski Alberta Heart Institute
University of Alberta Hospital
Affiliated with: Alberta Health Services
11220 - 83 Ave., Edmonton, AB T6G 2B7
Tel: 780-407-8407
maz@ahs.ca
www.albertahealthservices.ca/maz/maz.aspx
Year Founded: 2001
Note: Programs & services include: cardiac surgery, cardiology services, & patient education.
Mishaela Houle, Executive Director, Cardiac Sciences, Edmonton Zone

BRITISH COLUMBIA

CRANBROOK: East Kootenay Area Heart Function Clinic
Affiliated with: Interior Health Authority
20 - 23rd Ave. South, Cranbrook, BC V1C 5V1
Tel: 250-489-6414
www.interiorhealth.ca
Note: Support for patients diagnosed with heart failure

KAMLOOPS: Kamloops Pacemaker Clinic
Affiliated with: Interior Health Authority
311 Columbia St., 2nd Fl., Kamloops, BC V2C 2T1
Tel: 250-314-2100
www.interiorhealth.ca
Note: Provides support & services for patients with pacemakers, defibrillators, loop recorders, & other implanted devices

KAMLOOPS: TCS Heart Function Clinic
Affiliated with: Interior Health Authority
311 Columbia St., Kamloops, BC V2C 2T1
Tel: 250-314-2727
www.interiorhealth.ca
Note: Support for patients with chronic heart failure. Also includes the Vascular Improvement Clinic.

KELOWNA: Central Okanagan Heart Function Clinic
Affiliated with: Interior Health Authority
505 Doyle Ave., Kelowna, BC V1Y 0C5
Tel: 250-469-7070
www.interiorhealth.ca
Note: Support for patients diagnosed with heart failure

KELOWNA: Kelowna Pacemaker Clinic
Affiliated with: Interior Health Authority
2268 Pandosy St., Kelowna, BC V2Y 1T2
Tel: 250-862-4450
www.interiorhealth.ca
Note: Provides support & services for patients with pacemakers, defibrillators, loop recorders, & other implanted devices

NELSON: Chronic Disease Management Clinic
Affiliated with: Interior Health Authority
#443, 3 View St., Nelson, BC V1L 2V1
Tel: 250-354-2397
www.interiorhealth.ca
Note: Heart function clinic with cardiac rehab

OLIVER: Oliver Cardiac Rehab Clinic
Affiliated with: Interior Health Authority
36003 - 79th St., Oliver, BC V0H 1T0
Tel: 250-770-5507
www.interiorhealth.ca
Note: Offers a 5-week supervised exercise program to improve lung & heart health

OSOYOOS: Osoyoos Cardiac Rehab Clinic
Affiliated with: Interior Health Authority
8505 - 68th Ave., Osoyoos, BC V0H 1V0
Tel: 250-770-5507
www.interiorhealth.ca
Note: Offers a 5-week supervised exercise program to improve lung & heart health

PENTICTON: IHC Heart Function Clinic (HFC)
Affiliated with: Interior Health Authority
Also Known As: Cardiopulmonary Wellness Clinic
740 Carmi Ave., Penticton, BC V2A 8P9
Tel: 250-770-3530
www.interiorhealth.ca
Note: For patients with a diagnosis of heart failure

PENTICTON: Penticton Pacemaker Clinic
Affiliated with: Interior Health Authority
550 Carmi Ave., Penticton, BC V2A 3G6
Tel: 250-492-4000
www.interiorhealth.ca
Note: Offers support & services to patients with implanted cardiac devices

SALMON ARM: Salmon Arm Pacemaker Clinic
Affiliated with: Interior Health Authority
601 - 10th St. NE, Salmon Arm, BC V1E 4N6
Tel: 250-833-3636
www.interiorhealth.ca

TRAIL: Trail Heart Function Clinic
Affiliated with: Interior Health Authority
1500 Columbia Ave., Trail, BC V1R 1J9

Tel: 250-364-6297
www.interiorhealth.ca

Note: Offers treatment & services to patients with congestive heart failure

TRAIL: Trail Pacemaker Clinic
Affiliated with: Interior Health Authority
1200 Hospital Bench, Trail, BC V1R 4M1

Tel: 250-368-3311
www.interiorhealth.ca

Note: Provides support & services for patients with pacemakers, defibrillators, loop recorders, & other implanted devices

VERNON: North Okanagan Heart Function Clinic
Affiliated with: Interior Health Authority
2101 - 32nd St., Vernon, BC V1T 5L2

Tel: 250-558-1200
www.interiorhealth.ca

Note: Support for patients with chronic heart failure. Secondary phones: 250-306-9700 & 250-503-8805.

VERNON: Vernon Cardiac Rehab Clinic
Affiliated with: Interior Health Authority
2101 - 32nd St., Vernon, BC V1T 5L2

Tel: 250-503-3712
www.interiorhealth.ca

Note: Also includes the Vernon Pacemaker Clinic (250-558-1200)

QUÉBEC

MONTRÉAL: Institut de cardiologie de Montréal
Affiliée à: CIUSSS de l'Est-de-l'Ile-de-Montréal
5000, rue Bélanger, Montréal, QC H1T 1C8

Tél: 514-376-3330 *Ligne sans frais:* 855-922-6387
www.icm-mhi.org
Média social: www.facebook.com/institutcardiologiemontreal;
twitter.com/ICMtl; www.youtube.com/user/InstitutdeCardioMtl
Nombre de lits: 153 lits
Personnel: 1900
Dr. Denis Roy, Président-directeur général

QUÉBEC: Institut universitaire de cardiologie et de
pneumologie de Québec (IUCPQ)
Affiliée à: CIUSSS de la Capitale-Nationale
Ancien nom: Hôpital Laval
2725, ch Sainte-Foy, Québec, QC G1V 4G5

Tél: 418-656-8711 *Téléc:* 418-656-4829
iucpq.qc.ca
Média social: twitter.com/IUCPQ; www.youtube.com/IUCPQ;
www.linkedin.com/company/iucpq
Fondée en: 1918
Personnel: 3000
Note: Spécialisé dans la santé des personnes souffrant de maladies cardio-pulmonaires et dans le traitement des troubles liés à l'obésité. Affilié à l'Université Laval.

Hemophilia

Cause
Hemophilia is a genetic disorder that disrupts the body's normal blood clotting function because there is a deficiency of specific proteins known as clotting factors—specifically, factor VIII in hemophilia A and factor IX in hemophilia B. Depending on the amount of clotting factor in the blood, hemophilia can be classified as mild (5 to 30 percent of normal clotting factor), moderate (1 to 5 percent of normal clotting factor), or severe (less than 1 percent of normal clotting factor).

Hemophilia is linked to the X-chromosome because that is where both factor genes are located. As a result, hemophilia affects males almost exclusively, with females being carriers, whose sons have a 50 percent chance of having the disorder.

Symptoms
Hemophiliacs, like anyone else, will bleed if injured, but they will bleed for a longer time if untreated. The extent of the bleeding (also called hemorrhages) varies depending on the severity of the hemophilia. A person with hemophilia may also bleed in response to injuries that are inconsequential in other people. For instance, normal daily activities may cause bleeding within a joint, leading to severe pain and swelling, and over time destroying the joint. A serious complication of untreated hemophilia is internal bleeding in the brain which may be characterized by headaches, vomiting, sleepiness, vision problems and seizures.

Prevalence
Hemophilia is a rare disorder that affects approximately 3,100 Canadians: about 2,500 people in Canada have hemophilia A, and around 600 have hemophilia B.

Treatment Options
Prenatal diagnostic testing can be done as early as the tenth week of pregnancy in women who are known to be carriers of hemophilia. After birth, severe cases of hemophilia are usually diagnosed during the first year of life. However, milder forms of the disease may not be identified until a person reaches adulthood. To confirm a diagnosis of hemophilia, a physician often takes a medical history, does a physical exam and orders blood tests to check for missing or low levels of clotting factors.

Currently, there is no cure for hemophilia. The main treatment for the disease is clotting factor therapy, a procedure in which a person receives an infusion (injection into the vein) of the missing or low clotting factor. This therapy can either be given as needed to stop bleeding when it happens (demand therapy) or on a regular basis to prevent bleeding (prophylactic therapy).

Since the 1970s, most hemophiliacs in Canada have been treated at hemophilia treatment centres (HTC), which offer not just factor replacement but multi-specialty expertise, sophisticated laboratory testing, physical therapy and psychological support.

Gene therapy research that aims to find a way to correct the faulty gene that causes hemophilia is currently underway in Canada and other parts of the world. Due to advances in the treatment of hemophilia, people born with this disease can now lead normal, healthy lives.

National Associations

Association of Hemophilia Clinic Directors of Canada (AHCDC)
70 Bond St., Toronto ON M5B 1X3

Tel: 416-864-5042; *Fax:* 416-864-5251
e-mail: ahcdc@smh.ca
www.ahcdc.ca
Overview: A small national organization founded in 1994
Mission: To improve the treatment of people with hemophilia
Affiliation(s): Canadian Hemophilia Society
Chief Officer(s):
Annie Kaplan, Contact

Canadian Hematology Society (CHS) / Société canadienne
d'hématologie
#199, 435 St. Laurent Blvd., Ottawa ON K1K 2Z8

Tel: 613-748-9613; *Fax:* 613-748-6392
e-mail: chs@uniserve.ca
www.canadianhematologysociety.org
Overview: A small national organization founded in 1971

Mission: To represent members of the Society & provide information about hematology
Chief Officer(s):
Aaron Schimmer, President
Publications:
• Canadian Hematology Society Membership Directory
Type: Directory
• Canadian Hematology Society Newsletter
Type: Newsletter; *Frequency:* 3 pa

Canadian Hemophilia Society (CHS) / Société canadienne de l'hémophilie (SCHQ)
#301, 666 Sherbrooke St. West, Montréal QC H3A 1E7
Tel: 514-848-0503; *Fax:* 514-848-9661
Toll-Free: 800-668-2686
e-mail: chs@hemophilia.ca
www.hemophilia.ca
www.facebook.com/CanadianHemophiliaSociety
twitter.com/CHShemophilia
www.youtube.com/user/CanadianHemophilia

Overview: A medium-sized national charitable organization founded in 1953
Mission: To find a cure & to provide services to people with hemophilia or other inherited bleeding disorders; To serve persons infected with HIV or hepatitis through blood & blood products; To enhance the health & quality of life of individuals affected by inherited bleeding disorders
Affliation(s): World Federation of Hemophilia
Chief Officer(s):
David Page, National Executive Director
  dpage@hemophilia.ca
Hélène Bourgaize, National Director, Chapter Relations & Human Resources
  hbourgaize@hemophilia.ca
Deborah Franz Currie, National Director, Resource Development
  dcurrie@hemophilia.ca
Publications:
• All About Carriers
Number of Pages: 133
Profile: Comprehensive guide, for carriers of hemophilia A or B
• All About von Willebrand Disease
Number of Pages: 86
Profile: A comprehensive guide, for persons with the disease
• Canadian Hemophilia Society Annual Report & Financial Statement
Frequency: Annually
• Factor Deficiencies
Profile: A series of publications, with topics such as Factor XI Deficiency, An Inherited Bleeding Disorder, for patients, families, & healthcare providers
• Hemophilia Today
Type: Magazine; *Frequency:* 3 pa; *Editor:* François Laroche
Profile: Current news & relevant issues to inform the hemophilia & bleeding disorders community

Alberta Chapter
PO Box 44171, Edmonton AB T5V 1N6
Toll-Free: 800-668-2686
e-mail: albertachapter@hemophilia.ca
www.hemophilia.ca/en/provincial-chapters/alberta
Chief Officer(s):
Hillary Nemeth, Co-President
Sheri Spady, Co-President

British Columbia Chapter
PO Box 21161, Stn. Maple Ridge Sq., Maple Ridge BC V2X 1P7
Tel: 778-230-9661
e-mail: chsbc@shaw.ca
www.hemophiliabc.ca
Chief Officer(s):
Curtis Brandell, President

Hemophilia Manitoba

944 Portage Ave., Winnipeg MB R3G 0R1
Tel: 204-775-8625; *Fax:* 204-774-9403
Toll-Free: 866-775-8625
e-mail: info@hemophiliamb.ca
www.hemophiliamb.ca
www.facebook.com/186587534783298
twitter.com/HemophiliaMB
www.youtube.com/user/hemophiliamb
Chief Officer(s):
Christine Keilback, Executive Director

Hemophilia Ontario
#10100, 4711 Yonge St., Toronto ON M2N 6K8
Tel: 416-972-0641; *Fax:* 888-958-0307
Toll-Free: 888-838-8846
www.hemophilia.ca/en/provincial-chapters/ontario
Chief Officer(s):
Matthew Maynard, Interim Executive Director
  mmaynard@hemophilia.on.ca

Hemophilia Saskatchewan
2366 Ave. C North, Saskatoon SK S7L 5X5
Tel: 306-653-4366
Toll-Free: 866-953-4366
e-mail: hemosask@hemophilia.ca
www.hemophiliask.ca/hemophilia-saskatchewan.html
www.facebook.com/HemophiliaSaskatchewan
twitter.com/HemophiliaSask
Chief Officer(s):
Wendy Quinn, President

New Brunswick Chapter
#173, 337 Rothesay Ave., Saint John NB E2J 2C3
Tel: 506-608-0031
www.hemophilia.ca/en/provincial-chapters/new-brunswick
Chief Officer(s):
Victoria Watts, President
  president@chsnb.com

Newfoundland & Labrador Chapter
25 Main Rd., Cavendish NL A0B 1J0
e-mail: chsnlcc@nf.sympatico.ca
hemophilia.ca/en/provincial-chapters/newfoundland-and-labrador
Chief Officer(s):
Jenny Jacobs, President

Nova Scotia Chapter
17 Malcolm Lucas Dr., Enfield NS B2T 1A8
Tel: 902-883-7111
e-mail: nshemophiliasociety@hotmail.com
www.hemophilia.ca/en/provincial-chapters/nova-scotia
Chief Officer(s):
Betty-Anne Hines, President

Prince Edward Island Chapter
PO Box 2951, Charlottetown PE C1A 8C5
www.hemophilia.ca/en/provincial-chapters/prince-edward-island
Chief Officer(s):
Shelley Mountain, President

Section Québec
#514, 2120, rue Sherbrooke Est, Montréal QC H2K 1C3
Tél: 514-848-0666; *Téléc:* 514-904-2253
Ligne sans frais: 877-870-0666
Courriel: info@schq.org
www.hemophilia.ca/fr/sections-provinciales/quebec
www.facebook.com/27424888399
Chief Officer(s):
François Laroche, Président

Provincial Associations

QUÉBEC

Association des médecins hématologistes-oncologistes du Québec (AMHOQ)
CP 216, Succ. Desjardins, 2, Complexe Desjardins, Montréal QC H5B 1G8

Tél: 514-350-5121; *Téléc:* 514-350-5126
Courriel: info@amhoq.org
amhoq.org
www.facebook.com/311775155609901

Aperçu: *Dimension:* petite; *Envergure:* provinciale; Organisme sans but lucratif; fondée en 1976 surveillé par Fédération des médecins spécialistes du Québec
Membre(s) du bureau directeur:
Daniel Bélanger, Président
Nathalie Latendresse, Directrice administrative

International Associations

World Federation of Hemophilia (WFH) / Fédération mondiale de l'hémophilie (FMH)
#1010, 1425, boul René-Lévesque ouest, Montréal QC H3G 1T7
Tel: 514-875-7944; *Fax:* 514-875-8916
e-mail: wfh@wfh.org
www.wfh.org
www.facebook.com/wfhemophilia
twitter.com/wfhemophilia
www.youtube.com/user/WFHcommunications

Overview: A medium-sized international licensing organization founded in 1963
Mission: To introduce, improve & maintain care for people with hemophilia & related blood disorders around the world
Affliation(s): World Health Organization; International Society of Blood Transfusion; International Committee on Thrombosis & Haemostasis; International Society of Haematology; Société internationale de chirurgie orthopédique (SICOT)
Chief Officer(s):
Alain Baumann, Chief Executive Officer
Sarah Ford, Director, Strategy & Communications
  sford@wfh.org

Hepatitis

Cause
Hepatitis, or inflammation of the liver, has multiple causes and several stages. Hepatitis is usually caused by viruses or by excess alcohol consumption. Less common causes include prescription medications, accidental poisoning and auto-immune diseases in which the body attacks its own liver.

There are a number of different forms of viral hepatitis. The four most common types are A, B, C and D. Type A is spread by contaminated food and water, and generally causes a mild to moderately severe illness that runs its course over several weeks and disappears without further damage. Type B is spread by bodily fluids, generally through blood transfusion, sexual intercourse, or sharing needles or other contaminated items like razors. The disease may resolve without further consequences, but frequently becomes chronic and may lead to cirrhosis as well as chronic infections. Hepatitis C is spread through contact with contaminated blood, injection drug use and body piercing and tattooing. Although it is not usually severe at onset, it can lead to the same serious consequences as type B. Finally, there is type D, which is spread by contaminated blood products, and only infects people who already have Type B. Type D is more severe.

Symptoms
The severity of hepatitis is highly variable. At an early stage, hepatitis may cause no symptoms, mild symptoms or overwhelming disease. Early symptoms include vague abdominal pain, jaundice, fever, loss of appetite and nausea. If the disease becomes chronic, it may lead to irreversible scarring, or cirrhosis, which causes weakness, fatigue and weight loss. Late stage disease includes fluid accumulation in the abdominal cavity, gastrointestinal bleeding and mental changes. Abdominal pain and liver enlargement are generally present. Advanced cirrhosis is a risk factor for cancer of the liver.

Prevalence
In Canada, hepatitis A, B and C are the most common types of viral hepatitis, causing 90 percent of infections. The incidence rate of hepatitis A in Canada is about 2.9 cases per 100,000 people, while the estimated rate of hepatitis B is 0.74 cases per 100,000 people. The number of Canadians currently infected with hepatitis C is estimated to be between 700 and 900 per 100,000 people. Only about 30 percent of these people are aware that they have hepatitis C.

Treatment Options
Viral hepatitis is usually diagnosed through a blood test. Since hepatitis B and C can cause damage to the liver before any symptoms of infection are exhibited, people who are at a high risk for coming into contact with the virus are often screened for hepatitis B and C, even if they seem healthy.

Prevention of any of the forms of viral hepatitis depends on avoiding the usual routes of transmission (by washing hands, practising safe sex, not sharing needles or syringes). In addition, there are effective vaccines available to protect against the hepatitis A and B viruses.

Treatment of acute (short-lived) hepatitis A and B is largely supportive, but antiviral drugs are often used to treat chronic hepatitis B and hepatitis C infections. End-stage or overwhelming infection may necessitate liver transplantation.

Although many people recover completely from viral hepatitis, early diagnosis and treatment are crucial in order to prevent serious liver damage and avoid spreading the infection to others.

See also Liver Disease

National Associations

Canadian Association of Hepatology Nurses (CAHN) / Association canadienne des infirmières et infirmiers en hépatologie
c/o Lori Lee Walston, 506 Fader St., New Westminster BC V3L 3T5
www.livernurses.org

Overview: A small national organization
Mission: To represent & support hepatology nurses throughout Canada; To encourage liver health & prevent illness; To improve the standards of practice in hepatology nursing; To promote the excellent care of persons with liver related health problems & disorders
Affliation(s): Canadian Nurses Association (CNA); Canadian Association for the Study of Liver Disease (CASL); Canadian Liver Foundation (CLF)
Chief Officer(s):
Denise Thomas, President
  president@cahn.ca
Lesley Gallagher, Vice-President
  lesley.gallagher@vch.ca
Lori Lee Walston, Treasurer
  treasurer@cahn.ca
Donna Zukowski, Director, Education
  dzukow@shaw.ca
Sharon Bojarski, Co-Director, Conference
  sharonbojarski@hotmail.com
Kathy Poldre, Co-Director, Conference
  kathy.poldre@uhn.on.ca
Publications:
• Canadian Association of Hepatology Nurses Newsletter
Type: Newsletter; *Frequency:* Quarterly

Profile: Updates on issues affecting hepatology nurses, forthcoming educational opportunities, award information, & association membership news

Provincial Associations

NOVA SCOTIA

Hepatitis Outreach Society of Nova Scotia (HepNS)
PO Box 29120, RPO Halifax Shopping Centre, Dartmouth NS B2Y 1C3
Tel: 902-420-1767; *Fax:* 902-463-6725
Toll-Free: 800-521-0572
e-mail: info@hepns.ca
www.hepns.ca
www.facebook.com/114379611934070
twitter.com/HepNSca
www.youtube.com/user/HepNSca
Overview: A medium-sized provincial organization
Mission: To educate Nova Scotians about Hepatitis & its prevention; To reduce social stigmatization & isolation; To prevent the spread of Hepatitis
Chief Officer(s):
Carla Densmore, Executive Director
   director@hepns.ca

Local Associations

BRITISH COLUMBIA

Living Positive Resource Centre, Okanagan (LPRC)
168 Asher Rd., Kelowna BC V1X 3H6
Tel: 778-753-5830; *Fax:* 778-753-5832
e-mail: info@lprc.ca
www.livingpositive.ca
www.facebook.com/lprcokanagen
Previous Name: ARC, AIDS Resource Centre, Okanagan & Region
Overview: A small local charitable organization founded in 1992
Mission: To educate & inform the public about HIV/AIDS & hepatitis, its transmission, prevention, treatment & care, providing the most accurate & up-to-date information available; to develop & promote community based partnerships for the delivery of education & support; to dispel the myths & misunderstandings & to promote awareness of the discrimination & marginalization of persons infected & affected by HIV/AIDS & hepatitis & to advocate for change; to advocate & lobby for programs & services, necessary to promote wellness & quality of life of persons infected & affected by HIV/AIDS & hepatitis; to facilitate access to emotional, spiritual, social & practical support for persons infected & affected by HIV/AIDS & hepatitis, respectful of their right to determine the direction of their lives; to provide accessible services in non-judgmental, safe, confidential environments; to identify & seek solutions to existing gaps in services
Member of: Canadian AIDS Society; Pacific AIDS Network
Affiliation(s): Central Okanagan Hospice Society; Vernon Hospice; Salmon Arm Hospice; North Okanagan Youth & Family Services; Columbia-Shuswap HIV/AIDS Project; Outreach Health Services
Chief Officer(s):
Clare Overton, Executive Director

Huntington Disease

Huntington disease is an inherited and debilitating brain disorder that causes the breakdown of the brain's nerve cells. It affects a person's ability to control their muscles, leading to cognitive and psychiatric disorders, and eventually death.

Cause

Huntington disease is caused by mutations in the Huntington gene, found on chromosome 4, that disrupt the production of a protein, also called Huntington. This disruption results in a malformed protein to be produced which progressively damages brain cells (through mechanisms not completely understood).

Huntington disease is an autosomal dominant disorder, meaning only one copy of the defective gene inherited from one parent is necessary to produce the disease.

Symptoms

Symptoms of Huntington disease usually begin in middle age but can also appear in children (juvenile HD). Generally, the first signs of the disease include subtle cognition problems, such as appearing forgetful or a difficulty coping with new activities or making decisions.

Increased irritability and slight changes in moods and behaviour may also occur. Minor physical changes may be present, including fidgeting, twitching of extremities and excessive restlessness.

As the disease progresses, symptoms become more pronounced and debilitating. Further loss of muscle control results in involuntary movements such as jerking and twitching of the head, neck, arms and legs. At the advanced stage, people with Huntington disease typically exhibit fewer involuntary movements but experience more rigidity. Difficulties with swallowing, communication and weight loss are common. It is a progressive disease that gradually leads to physical incapacitation. Mental capabilities usually diminish to the point of dementia.

Prevalence

It is estimated that one in every 7,000 Canadians has Huntington disease and approximately one in every 5,500 is at risk of developing the disease. People with Huntington disease have a 50 percent chance of passing on the disease to their children, with male and female children having an equal chance of inheriting the disease.

Treatment Options

Diagnosis for Huntington disease often begins with neurological and psychological tests, along with a review of family history. A genetic test, developed in 1993, can confirm a diagnosis. This test is also used to identify carriers of the defective gene who are not yet ill.

Genetic counselling is strongly recommended to help weigh the risks and benefits of taking the test for individuals who have yet to exhibit symptoms. Persons with Huntington disease can greatly benefit from the services of numerous healthcare professionals, including a psychiatrist to deal with depression, a clinical social worker to provide coping skills, and a physiotherapist and speech therapist.

Death usually occurs as a result of complications, including pneumonia, heart disease, physical injuries from falls, and occasionally suicide. The life expectancy of person with this disease is typically 20 years from onset, although juvenile HD usually progresses faster.

National Associations

Huntington Society of Canada (HSC) / Société Huntington du Canada
#400, 151 Frederick St., Kitchener ON N2H 2M2
Tel: 519-749-7063; *Fax:* 519-749-8965
Toll-Free: 800-998-7398
e-mail: info@huntingtonsociety.ca
www.huntingtonsociety.ca
www.linkedin.com/company/huntington-society-of-canada
www.facebook.com/HuntingtonSC
twitter.com/HuntingtonSC
www.youtube.com/user/HuntSocCanada
Also Known As: Huntington Society
Overview: A medium-sized national charitable organization founded in 1973
Mission: To aspire for a world free of Huntington disease; To maximize the quality of life of people living with HD
Member of: Canadian Coalition for Genetic Fairness; Health Charities Coalition of Canada; HealthPartners; Neurological Health Charities Coalition of Canada; International Huntington Association

Chief Officer(s):
Bev Heim-Myers, CEO
bheimmyers@huntingtonsociety.ca

East Central Ontario Resource Centre
PO Box 103, 71 Old Kingston Rd., Ajax ON L1T 3A6
Tel: 905-426-4333
Toll-Free: 855-426-4333

Chief Officer(s):
Marilyn Mitchell, Director
mmitchell@huntingtonsociety.ca

Individual & Family Services
PO Box 31355, Richmond Hill ON L4C 0V7
Tel: 905-787-8359
Toll-Free: 877-573-7011

Chief Officer(s):
Rozi Andrejas, Director
randrejas@huntingtonsociety.ca

Manitoba Resource Centre
200 Woodlawn St., Winnipeg MB R3J 2H7
Tel: 204-772-4617; *Fax:* 204-940-8414
www.hdmanitoba.ca

Chief Officer(s):
Sandra Funk, Director
sfunk@huntingtonsociety.ca

Newfoundland/Labrador Resource Centre
NL
Tel: 709-745-1155
Toll-Free: 877-745-1155

Chief Officer(s):
Elaine Smith, Director
esmith@huntingtonsociety.ca

Northern Alberta Resource Centre
#102, 11747 Kingsway NW, Edmonton AB T5G 0X5
Tel: 780-434-3229

Chief Officer(s):
Bernadette Modrovsky, Director
bmodrovsky@huntingtonsociety.ca

Nova Scotia & PEI Resource Centre
#101, 3845 Joseph Howe Dr., Halifax NS B3L 4H9
Tel: 902-446-4803

Chief Officer(s):
Barbara Horner, Director
bhorner@huntingtonsociety.ca

Saskatoon & Area
PO Box 26012, Saskatoon SK S7K 8C1
Tel: 306-979-9111
e-mail: hdsaskatoon@gmail.com
www.facebook.com/HuntingtonSocietyOfCanadaSaskatoon

Chief Officer(s):
June Nichol, President

Southern Alberta Resource Centre
Westech Bldg., #102, 5636 Burbank Cres. SE, Calgary AB T2H 1Z6
Tel: 403-532-0609; *Fax:* 403-532-3952

Chief Officer(s):
Shannon MacKinnon, Director
smackinnon@huntingtonsociety.ca

Provincial Associations

QUÉBEC

Société Huntington du Québec (SHQ) / Huntington Society of Québec (HSQ)
2300, boul René-Lévesque ouest, Montréal QC H3R 3R5
Tél: 514-282-4272
Ligne sans frais: 800-220-0226
Courriel: shq@huntingtonqc.org
www.huntingtonqc.org
www.facebook.com/138147292892093

Aperçu: *Dimension:* petite; *Envergure:* provinciale; Organisme sans but lucratif; Organisme de réglementation; fondée en 1986 surveillé par Huntington Society Of Canada

Mission: Pour aider les personnes atteintes de la maladie de Huntington à faire face
Membre de: Huntington Society of Canada
Membre(s) du bureau directeur:
Francine Lacroix, Directrice générale

Hydrocephalus

The normal brain and spinal cord are surrounded with a watery substance called cerebro-spinal fluid, or CSF, which collects within the brain in several larger pools called ventricles, connected to one another through tiny channels. CSF is formed in some of these ventricles, circulates widely and is eventually re-absorbed. If CSF production exceeds re-absorption, or if the fluid is blocked from circulating, it may build up pressure that expands the ventricles and presses on the normal brain tissue, causing hydrocephalus, or water on the brain.

Cause
The exact cause of hydrocephalus is often unknown. It may be congenital, that is, present from birth, and due to bleeding within the ventricles (as a complication of premature birth), an infection such as rubella or syphilis that causes inflammation in the developing baby's brain, or an abnormal development of the baby's central nervous system. At any age, excess CSF may be in response to an infection such as meningitis or mumps, blockage of CSF movement by a tumour, or bleeding in the brain after a head injury or stroke.

Symptoms
The symptoms of hydrocephalus vary from person to person, and are dependent on the age of the patient. If hydrocephalus occurs in a child whose skull bones have not yet fused together, it may cause the head to enlarge. In older children and adults, hydrocephalus can cause headache, visual loss, vomiting, lethargy, coordination and balance problems, memory loss, weakness and changes in behaviour.

Prevalence
It is estimated that one in 300 babies is born with hydrocephalus in Canada. Each year, around 10,000 Canadians require surgery to treat hydrocephalus. The condition is more common in babies—about 60 percent of cases occur in infancy.

Treatment Options
Diagnosis of hydrocephalus is usually based on a physical exam, a neurological exam and brain imaging tests such as ultrasound, MRI (magnetic resonance imaging) and CT (computerized tomography).

Treatment and outlook depend on the underlying cause. Medical therapy with diuretics may cause limited temporary improvement. However, in about 75 percent of cases, surgical treatment is needed to correct the underlying cause. Most often, hydrocephalus is treated by placement of a shunt which allows extra CSF to drain from the ventricles to some other part of the body. The shunt is usually kept in place for life, and is monitored regularly. In a smaller number of patients, ventriculostomy may be performed. In this procedure, a hole is made in one of the ventricles to allow CSF to drain from the brain. After both types of surgery, diuretics are often prescribed to remove excess fluid from the body. Because hydrocephalus can affect physical and cognitive development, additional treatment such as occupational and developmental therapy may be required for some patients.

Progressive hydrocephalus can be fatal if left untreated. However, with early diagnosis, successful treatment and rehabilitative and educational therapy when required, many children with hydrocephalus can lead normal lives.

National Associations

Spina Bifida & Hydrocephalus Association of Canada (SBHAC) / Association de spina-bifida et d'hydrocephalie du Canada
#647, 167 Lombard Ave., Winnipeg MB R3B 0V3

Tel: 204-925-3650; *Fax:* 204-925-3654
Toll-Free: 800-565-9488
e-mail: info@sbhac.ca
www.sbhac.ca
www.facebook.com/167743789940812

Overview: A medium-sized national charitable organization founded in 1981
Mission: To improve the quality of life of all individuals with spina bifida &/or hydrocephalus & their families through awareness, education, advocacy & research; to reduce the incidence of neural tube defects
Member of: Canadian Coalition for Genetic Fairness
Affiliation(s): International Federation for Hydrocephalus & Spina Bifida
Chief Officer(s):
Colleen Talbot, President

Provincial Associations

ALBERTA

Spina Bifida & Hydrocephalus Association of Southern Alberta (SBHASA)
PO Box 6837, Stn. D, Calgary AB T2P 2E9

www.sbhasa.ca
Previous Name: Spina Bifida Association of Southern Alberta
Overview: A small provincial charitable organization founded in 1981 overseen by Spina Bifida & Hydrocephalus Association of Canada
Mission: To raise awareness about spina bifida & hydrocephalus & to provide help to people & families who suffer from these conditions
Chief Officer(s):
Minh Ho, President
minh.ho@plainsmidstream.com

BRITISH COLUMBIA

Spina Bifida & Hydrocephalus Association of British Columbia (SBHABC)
4480 Oak St., Vancouver BC V6H 3V4

Tel: 604-878-7000; *Fax:* 604-677-6608
www.sbhabc.org
Previous Name: Lower Mainland Spina Bifida Association
Overview: A medium-sized provincial licensing charitable organization founded in 1977
Mission: To improve the quality of life of all individuals with spina bifida &/or hydrocephalus & their families, through awareness, education & research
Chief Officer(s):
Colleen Talbot, President

MANITOBA

Spina Bifida Association of Manitoba (SBAM)
#647, 167 Lombard Ave., Winnipeg MB R3B 0V3

Tel: 204-925-3653; *Fax:* 204-925-3654
manitoba.sbhac.ca
Overview: A small provincial charitable organization founded in 1965 overseen by Spina Bifida & Hydrocephalus Association of Canada
Mission: To provide resources & support to people & families suffering from spina bifida & hydrocephalus

NEW BRUNSWICK

Spina Bifida & Hydrocephalus Association of New Brunswick
1325 Mountain Rd., Moncton NB E1C 2T9

Tel: 506-857-9947
e-mail: spinabifidanb@hotmail.com
Overview: A small provincial organization overseen by Spina Bifida & Hydrocephalus Association of Canada
Mission: To improve the quality of life of those persons who have spina bifida &/or hydrocephalus; to gather information on spina bifida & hydrocephalus & to disseminate it to all interested persons & organizations; to encourage research into the causes & to advance more effective treatment & care

NOVA SCOTIA

Spina Bifida & Hydrocephalus Association of Nova Scotia (SBHANS)
PO Box 341, Coldbrook NS B4R 1B6

Tel: 902-679-1124
Toll-Free: 800-304-0450
e-mail: info@sbhans.ca
www.sbhans.ca
Overview: A small provincial charitable organization founded in 1984 overseen by Spina Bifida & Hydrocephalus Association of Canada
Mission: To eliminate spina bifida & hydrocephalus in newborns by promoting preventative measures; to help individuals with spina bifida &/or hydrocephalus to reach their full potential by promoting independence & improved quality of life

Cape Breton Chapter
20 Deanna Dr., Glace Bay NS B1A 6Y1

Tel: 902-849-4401

ONTARIO

Spina Bifida & Hydrocephalus Association of Ontario (SB&H)
PO Box 103, #1006, 555 Richmond St. West, Toronto ON M5V 3B1

Tel: 416-214-1056; *Fax:* 416-214-1446
Toll-Free: 800-387-1575
e-mail: provincial@sbhao.on.ca
www.sbhao.on.ca
www.facebook.com/SpinaBifidaHydrocephalusOntario
twitter.com/SBH_Ontario
www.youtube.com/channel/UC3psi9zf8KapVlgJ9p0f1EQ?
Overview: A medium-sized provincial charitable organization founded in 1973
Mission: To build awareness & drive education, research, support, care & advocacy to help find a cure while working to improve the quality of life of all individuals with spina bifida &/or hydrocephalus
Affiliation(s): Spina Bifida & Hydrocephalus Association of Canada
Chief Officer(s):
Elaine Wilson, Executive Director
ewilson@sbhao.on.ca

PRINCE EDWARD ISLAND

Spina Bifida & Hydrocephalus Association of Prince Edward Island
PO Box 3332, Charlottetown PE C0A 1R0

Tel: 902-628-8875
Overview: A small provincial charitable organization overseen by Spina Bifida & Hydrocephalus Association of Canada
Chief Officer(s):
Lurlean Palmer, Contact
lurleanpalmer@eastlink.ca

QUÉBEC

L'Association de spina-bifida et d'hydrocéphalie du Québec (ASBHQ)
#303, 55, av Mont-Royal Ouest, Montréal QC H2T 2S6

Tél: 514-340-9019
Ligne sans frais: 800-567-1788
Courriel: info@spina.qc.ca
www.spina.qc.ca
www.facebook.com/asbhq
twitter.com/ASBHQ
Aperçu: *Dimension:* moyenne; *Envergure:* provinciale; Organisme sans but lucratif; fondée en 1975 surveillé par Spina Bifida & Hydrocephalus Association of Canada
Mission: Promouvoir et défendre les droits, les intérêts et le bien-être des personnes ayant le spina-bifida et l'hydrocéphalie; sensibiliser le public à la nature du spina-bifida et de l'hydrocéphalie ainsi qu'aux besoins des personnes ayant ces malformations; favoriser et soutenir la recherche sur les causes, les nouveaux traitements et les techniques de prévention du spina-bifida et de l'hydrocéphalie
Membre de: Confédération des organismes provinciaux de personnes handicappées du Québec
Affliation(s): Institut de réadaptation en déficience physique de Québec; Hôpital Shriners, Centre de réadaptation Constance-Lethbridge, Centre de réadaptation en déficience physique Chaudière-Appalaches

Membre(s) du bureau directeur:
Marc Picard, Président

A.S.B.H. Région Estrie
928, rue Fédéral, Sherbrooke QC J1H 5A7
Tél: 819-822-3772; *Téléc:* 819-822-4529
Courriel: asbhestrie@hotmail.com
www.spina.qc.ca/estrie

Membre(s) du bureau directeur:
René Labonté, Président
Aline Nault, Coordonnatrice

A.S.B.H. Région Montréal
#448, 14115, Prince-Arthur, Montréal QC H1A 1A8
Tél: 514-739-5515; *Téléc:* 514-739-5505
Courriel: asbhrm@mainbourg.org
www.spina.qc.ca
www.facebook.com/asbhq.quebec
twitter.com/ASBHQ

Membre(s) du bureau directeur:
André Bougie, Président

SASKATCHEWAN

Spina Bifida & Hydrocephalus Association of South Saskatchewan
PO Box 37115, Stn. Landmark, Regina SK S4S 7K3
Tel: 306-586-2222
e-mail: regina@sbhac.ca
Overview: A small provincial organization
Mission: To improve the quality of life for those afflicted with spina bifida &/or hydrocephalus
Member of: Spina Bifida & Hydrocephalus Association of Canada

North Chapter
351 Kenderdine Rd., Saskatoon SK S7N 3S9
Tel: 306-249-1362
www.sbhasn.ca

Chief Officer(s):
Laurel Scherr, President

South Chapter
PO Box 37115, Regina SK S4S 7K3
Tel: 306-359-6049
e-mail: regina@sbhac.ca

Local Associations

ALBERTA

Spina Bifida & Hydrocephalus Association of Northern Alberta (SBHANA)
PO Box 35025, 10818 Jasper Ave., Edmonton AB T5J 0B7
Tel: 780-451-6921; *Fax:* 888-881-7172
e-mail: info@sbhana.org
www.sbhana.org
www.facebook.com/sbhana01
twitter.com/SBHANA1
www.youtube.com/user/TheSBHANA
Previous Name: Spina Bifida Association of Northern Alberta
Overview: A small local charitable organization founded in 1981
Mission: To enhance the lives of individuals & families affected by spina bifida &/or hydrocephalus through public awareness, education & research
Member of: Spina Bifida & Hydrocephalus Association of Canada; Alberta Disablility Forum; Albera Committee for Citizens with Disabilities
Chief Officer(s):
Cindy Smith, President
Megan Gergatz, Program Manager

Provincial Libraries

Spina Bifida & Hydrocephalus Association of Ontario
#1006, 555 Richmond St. West, Toronto, ON M5V 3B1
Tel: 416-214-1056; *Fax:* 416-214-1446
Toll-Free: 800-387-1575
provincial@sbhao.on.ca
www.sbhao.on.ca
Social Media: twitter.com/SBH_Ontario;
www.facebook.com/SpinaBifidaHydrocephalusOntario
Collection: Vertical file of articles related to Spina Bifida & Hydrocephalus
Elaine Wilson, Executive Director
ewilson@sbhao.on.ca
Shauna Beaudoin, Information & Services Coordinator
sbeaudoin@sbhao.on.ca

Hypertension

Hypertension is an abnormal elevation of blood pressure. Blood pressure is noted as a top number (systolic) over a bottom number (diastolic) with a reading of 120/80 being recognized as normal. Hypertension is defined as a systolic pressure at or greater than 140 or a diastolic pressure at or greater than 90. For people with diabetes or chronic kidney disease, a reading of 130/80 is considered high.

Cause

Primary, or essential, hypertension is the most common form, and it has no known cause. It is more prevalent in males and those with a family history of high blood pressure. Other risk factors include obesity, diabetes, high levels of fat and cholesterol, excess dietary sodium, smoking, sedentary lifestyle and psychological stress. Hypertension is a significant risk factor for coronary heart disease, heart failure, stroke and kidney failure, and may also be associated with sexual problems and dementia.

Symptoms

Patients with hypertension generally have no symptoms. For this reason, high blood pressure is often called "a silent killer."

Prevalence

High blood pressure is a common disorder that affects about six million Canadians, or 22 percent of the population aged 20 and over. Hypertension becomes more common with advanced age. Approximately 53.2 percent of Canadians aged 60 to 70 years have high blood pressure, whereas about 18.4 percent of Canadians aged 40 to 59 have the condition. It is estimated that 17 percent of people are not aware that they have high blood pressure.

Treatment Options

Diagnosis of hypertension is made by simple measurement with a blood pressure cuff. It is advised that adults have their blood pressure checked once a year so that hypertension can be diagnosed before it causes health problems.

Treatment of hypertension is done in a step-wise fashion beginning with lifestyle modifications (weight reduction, regular exercise, smoking cessation, a low salt, fat and cholesterol diet, limiting alcohol and reducing stress). If medications are necessary, doctors can choose from a wide variety of effective and usually well-tolerated drugs including diuretics, beta blockers, ACE (angiotensin converting enzyme) inhibitors, ARBs (angiotensin receptor blockers), calcium channel blockers and direct renin inhibitors (aliskiren). Most people with high blood pressure require two or more medications, and therapy generally must be continued for life.

Occasionally the blood pressure may be refractory, or difficult to control with medicines. In this instance, screening is needed for unusual causes of hypertension, such as renovascular disease (narrowing of the arteries feeding the kidneys), hyperaldosteronism (a tumour or overgrowth of the adrenal gland which secretes hormones that raise the blood pressure), or aortic coarctation (a congenital malformation of the major blood vessels near the heart.) If no specifically treatable cause is identified, the patient will require combination therapy with high doses of drugs.

When high blood pressure is diagnosed early and treated successfully with medication or lifestyle modifications, there is a significant positive effect on general health, and a decreased risk of premature death or disability.

National Associations

Hypertension Canada
#211, 3780 - 14th Ave., Markham ON L3R 9Y5
Tel: 905-943-9400; *Fax:* 905-943-9401
www.hypertension.ca
twitter.com/HTNCANADA
www.youtube.com/user/hypertensioncanada
Merged from: Blood Pressure Canada; Canadian Hypertension Society; & Canadian Hypertension Education Program
Overview: A medium-sized national organization
Mission: To advance health by preventing & controlling high blood pressure
Chief Officer(s):
Nadia Khan, President
Angelique Berg, Chief Executive Officer
Glen Doucet, Vice-President
Trevor Hudson, Treasurer
Publications:
• Hypertension Therapeutic Guide
Type: Textbook
Profile: A reference tool to help physicians, nurses, & pharmacists in the management of hypertension

International Associations

International Society of Hypertension (ISH)
ISH Secretariat, The Conference Collective Ltd., 8 Waldegrave Rd., Teddington TW11 8GT United Kingdom
Tel: +44 (0) 20 8977 7997
e-mail: secretariat@ish-world.com
www.ish-world.com
www.facebook.com/ISHNIN
twitter.com/ISHNIN
Overview: A medium-sized international charitable organization
Mission: To advance scientific knowledge in all aspects of research; To promote application of research to the prevention & management of heart disease & stroke in hypertension & related cardiovascular diseases
Affliation(s): Canadian Hypertension Society; World Hypertension League; American Society of Hypertension; Council for High Blood Pressure Research of the AHA; Cuban National Committee for the Study of Hypertension; Hypertension societies throughout Africa, The Middle East, Asia, Australasia, Europe, & South America
Chief Officer(s):
Neil Poulter, President
Alta Schutte, Vice-President
Maciej Tomaszewski, Secretary
Masatsugu Horiuchi, Treasurer
Publications:
• Hypertension News
Type: Newsletter; *Frequency:* Quarterly; *Price:* Free with International Society of Hypertension membership
• Journal of Hypertension
Type: Journal; *Frequency:* Monthly; *Price:* Free with International Society of Hypertension membership
Profile: Primary papers from experts, authoritative reviews, recent developments, special reports, & time-sensitive information

World Hypertension League (WHL)
168 South Hills Rd., Clancy MT 59634 USA
Tel: 406-861-6844
www.worldhypertensionleague.org

Overview: A large international organization founded in 1984
Mission: To promote the detection, control & prevention of arterial hypertension in populations; To assist national bodies by providing internationally applicable programs
Member of: International Society of Hypertension
Affliation(s): Canadian Coalition for High Blood Pressure Prevention & Control; WHO
Chief Officer(s):
Norman Campbell, M.D., President
ncampbel@ucalgary.ca
Mark Niebylski, CEO
CEO@whleague.org
Publications:
• WHL [World Hypertension League] Newsletter
Type: Newsletter; *Frequency:* q.; *Editor:* Dr. Daniel T. Lackland

Impulse Control Disorder

Everyone has experienced a situation in which they are tempted to do something that is harmful to themselves or others. This kind of behaviour only becomes a disorder when a person is repeatedly and persistently unable to resist a temptation which is always harmful to them or to others. Usually the person feels a rising tension before acting on the need, feels pleasure and relief when giving in to the impulse and, sometimes, feels remorse and guilt afterwards. Five different disorders are included in this category: intermittent explosive disorder, kleptomania, pathological gambling, pyromania and trichotillomania.

Intermittent Explosive Disorder

Intermittent explosive disorder is characterized by impulsive, aggressive behaviour that provides immediate relief from tension, but is usually followed by feelings of guilt and remorse.

Symptoms
The behaviour of a person with this disorder can have very serious consequences, including job loss, loss of relationships and divorce. Injuries as a result of fighting and accidents are common. People with paranoid or obsessive characteristics may be especially likely to have explosive outbursts. Intermittent explosive disorder is also associated with substance abuse disorders and certain neurological disorders but should not be confused with the aggression seen in other forms of psychiatric and organic brain disorders, such as antisocial personality disorder, borderline personality disorder, head trauma and substance withdrawal.

Prevalence
Intermittent explosive disorder is more common in men than women. Symptoms usually begin to emerge in the period between late childhood and the early 20s. It is a rare disorder.

Treatment Options
Diagnosis of intermittent explosive disorder is usually based on the following criteria outlined in the Diagnostic and Statistical Manual of Mental Disorders: several clear episodes of inability to resist aggressive impulses resulting in serious assault or destruction of property; the extent of aggression is out of proportion to any precipitating stressful event.

Treatment for intermittent explosive disorder usually includes cognitive behaviour therapy (in which the patient learns to replace negative beliefs and behaviours with positive ones) and medications such as carbamazepine, propranolol and lithium.

In some cases, the symptoms of intermittent explosive disorder may become less severe with increased age, but in others, the condition is chronic.

Kleptomania

People with kleptomania repeatedly fail in their attempts to resist the urge to steal.

Symptoms

Kleptomania should not be confused with thefts which are deliberate and for personal gain, or those that are sometimes done by adolescents on a dare or as a rite of passage. Kleptomania is strongly associated with depression, anxiety disorders and eating disorders.

Prevalence

Kleptomania appears to be very rare; fewer than 5 percent of shoplifters have the disorder. However, kleptomania is usually kept secret by the person, so this estimate may be low. It is much more common among females than males and may continue in spite of convictions for shoplifting.

Treatment Options

Diagnosis of kleptomania is usually based on the following criteria outlined in the Diagnostic and Statistical Manual of Mental Disorders: recurrent failure to resist the impulse to steal objects; often they are objects the individual could have paid for or doesn't particularly want; increased sense of tension immediately before the theft; pleasure and relief during the stealing; the theft is not due to anger, delusions or hallucinations; awareness that stealing is senseless and wrong; feelings of depression and guilt after stealing.

Treatment for kleptomania may include cognitive behaviour therapy (in which the patient learns to replace negative beliefs and behaviours with positive ones) and prescription of antidepressants. A combination of therapy and medication is most likely to help the person curb the impulse to steal while treating some of the underlying problems.

Pathological Gambling

Pathological gambling is characterized as compulsive gambling that creates problems for the person, his or her family and the community.

Symptoms

Compulsive gamblers are distorted in their thinking. They are superstitious, deny they have a problem and may be overconfident. They believe that money is the cause of, and solution to, all their problems. They are often competitive and easily bored. They may be extravagantly generous and very concerned with other people's approval. Compulsive gamblers are prone to medical problems such as hypertension and migraine. They also have a higher rate of attention-deficit/hyperactivity disorder. In Canada, up to 24 percent of problem gamblers suffer from depression, 42 percent report high levels of stress, 15 percent abuse alcohol and 18 percent are reported to have contemplated suicide.

Prevalence

Both males and females can be compulsive gamblers. Men usually begin gambling in adolescence, women somewhat later. Women are more likely to use gambling as an escape from depression. The prevalence of problem gambling is high and rising. According to the Canadian Problem Gambling Index, around 76 percent of Canadians aged 15 and over spent money gambling in 2002. Approximately 1.2 million Canadians are problem gamblers or have the potential to become problem gamblers.

Treatment Options

Diagnosis of pathological gambling is usually based on the following criteria outlined in the Diagnostic and Statistical Manual of Mental Disorders: gambles recurrently; gambling disrupts family, personal and work activities; shows preoccupation with gambling, thinking about past plays, planning future gambling and how to get money for more gambling; seeks excitement more than money; increases bets and risks to produce the needed excitement; continues gambling despite repeated efforts to stop, with accompanying restless and irritability; may gamble to escape depression, anxiety, guilt; chasing losses may become a pattern; may lie to family, therapists and others to conceal gambling; may turn to criminal behaviour—forgery, fraud, theft—to get money for gambling; may lose job, relationships, career opportunities; shows bailout behaviour, that is turning to family and others when in desperate financial straits.

Pathological gambling is a difficult disorder to treat, but psychotherapy that concretely targets the behaviour can be successful. Gamblers Anonymous, a 12-step program, may enable some to stop gambling. Treatment of any other underlying mental health disorders and involving family members may also be helpful.

It is important to note that, as specified in the American Psychiatric Association's Diagnostic and Statistical Manual of Mental Disorders, a psychiatric diagnosis, including this one, does not and is not meant to exonerate an individual from responsibility for criminal behaviour.

Pyromania

People affected by pyromania deliberately set fires to gain pleasure and tension relief.

Symptoms

Many people with this disorder make complicated preparations for setting a fire, and seem not to care about the serious consequences. Instead, they may get satisfaction from the destruction. Most juveniles who set fires also have symptoms of attention—deficit/hyperactivity disorder or adjustment disorder. Adults with this disorder may also experience depression, suicidal thoughts and interpersonal conflict.

Prevalence

Among children, the disorder is rare. Fire setting occurs mostly among adult males, and is more common in those with alcohol problems, learning problems and poor social skills.

Treatment Options

Diagnosis of pyromania is usually based on the following criteria outlined in the Diagnostic and Statistical Manual of Mental Disorders: purposefully setting fires more than once; increased tension before the deed; fascination with and curiosity about fire and its paraphernalia; pleasure or relief when setting or watching fires; the fire is not set for financial gain, revenge or political reasons.

A variety of treatment approaches are usually used with children and adolescents and may include training in anger management, problem-solving and aggression replacement, as well as cognitive behaviour therapy (in which the patient learns to replace negative beliefs and behaviours with positive ones). Pyromania is difficult to treat in adults because the person usually does not take responsibility for the fire setting, and is in denial. A combination of psychotherapy and antidepressants is considered the most effective treatment.

In most cases, the prognosis for recovery from pyromania is better in children who receive therapy than in adults.

Trichotillomania

Trichotillomania is characterized by persistent, uncontrollable urges to pull out one's hair. In many cases, the condition interferes with family and social life, school and job performance and everyday functioning.

Symptoms

Symptoms of trichotillomania may include examining the hair root, pulling the hair between the teeth, or eating hairs (trichophagia). Rarely, if enough hair is swallowed, a hairball may form in the digestive system. This can lead to pain, bloating, weight loss and constipation or diarrhea, and requires prompt medical attention.

Hair pulling is usually done in private or in the presence of close family members. Pain is not usually reported. The hair pulling is mostly denied and concealed by wigs, hairstyling and cosmetics. People with this disorder may also be affected by depression, general anxiety disorder or an eating disorder.

Prevalence

Among children, both males and females can have the disorder, but among adults, it is far more frequent in females. Symptoms usually emerge around the age of 13, but the condition may also affect children as young as five.

Treatment Options

Diagnosis of trichotillomania is usually based on the following criteria outlined in the Diagnostic and Statistical Manual of Mental Disorders: repeated hair pulling so that hair loss is noticeable; increasing tension just before the behaviour or when trying to resist it; pleasure or relief when pulling; causes clear distress and problems in personal work, or social functioning.

There is no agreement about the cause of this disorder, making treatment more difficult. Professionals are often not consulted. Treatments that have been proposed include hypnosis and stress reduction. However, cognitive behaviour therapy (in which the patient learns to replace negative beliefs and behaviours with positive ones) is considered the most effective treatment for trichotillomania. Studies suggest a success rate of at least 90 percent for cognitive behaviour therapy in the treatment of trichotillomania. Medications such as serotonin reuptake inhibitors (SSRIs) are sometimes prescribed if cognitive behaviour therapy is not successful.

Early diagnosis and appropriate treatment is crucial for people affected by this condition.

Provincial Associations

ALBERTA

Lieutenant Governor's Circle on Mental Health & Addiction
#208, 14925 - 111th Ave., Edmonton AB T5M 2P6
Tel: 780-453-2201
e-mail: execdir@lgcirclealberta.ca
www.lgcircle.ca
www.facebook.com/LGCircle
Overview: A small provincial organization
Chief Officer(s):
Sol Rolingher, Chair

ONTARIO

Centre for Addiction & Mental Health (CAMH) / Centre de toxicomanie et de santé mentale
250 College St., Toronto ON M5T 1R8
Tel: 416-535-8501
Toll-Free: 800-463-6273
e-mail: info@camh.net
www.camh.net
www.linkedin.com/company/camh
www.facebook.com/CentreforAddictionandMentalHealth
twitter.com/CAMHnews
www.youtube.com/camhtv

Previous Name: Addiction Research Foundation
Overview: A large provincial charitable organization founded in 1998
Mission: To provide treatment for & research into substance abuse & mental health issues. Clinical & research sites in Toronto & across Ontario
Affiliation(s): University of Toronto; University of Western Ontario; WHO
Chief Officer(s):
Catherine Zahn, President/CEO

Responsible Gambling Council (Ontario) (RGC(O)) / Le Conseil ontarien pour le jeu responsable
#205, 411 Richmond St. East, Toronto ON M5A 3S5
Tel: 416-499-9800; *Fax:* 416-499-8260
www.responsiblegambling.org
www.linkedin.com/company/responsible-gambling-council
twitter.com/RGCouncil
www.youtube.com/user/RGCouncilCanada
Previous Name: Canadian Foundation on Compulsive Gambling (Ontario)
Overview: A small provincial charitable organization founded in 1983
Mission: To increase awareness of compulsive gambling among families, community & service club leaders; To support research into the causes & treatment
Affiliation(s): Responsible Gambling Council of Canada
Chief Officer(s):
Robin Boychuk, Chair
Jon E. Kelly, Chief Executive Officer, 416-490-2060
jonk@rgco.org

Incontinence

Urinary incontinence is the involuntary leakage of urine, whether during waking or sleeping hours.

Cause

One common type is urge incontinence, resulting from involuntary bladder contractions. The person feels a sudden urge to urinate, so intense that it may not be controlled long enough to reach the toilet. Common causes of urge incontinence are urinary tract infections, spinal cord injury and kidney stones. Stress incontinence is the instantaneous leakage of urine without bladder contractions. It manifests as loss of urine during coughing, sneezing, laughing, exercise or lifting. This may occur in women due to weak bladder tone from multiple pregnancies. In men, stress incontinence can occur after prostate removal or trauma to the bladder. Overflow incontinence, in which the bladder cannot control urine output, can be caused by nerve injury, alcoholism and some diseases. Other types of incontinence include mixed incontinence, a combination of urge and stress incontinence; functional incontinence, a problem in getting to the toilet due to physical or psychological barriers; and nocturnal enuresis, or bedwetting.

Symptoms

Symptoms include urgency, frequency (having to urinate more often) and nocturia (having to urinate at night).

Prevalence

It is estimated that over 3.3 million people in Canada experience incontinence. Incontinence affects males and females of all ages (10 percent of six-year-olds, 25 percent of women who are middle-aged or older, and 15 percent of men who are 60 years or over). Only about 26 percent of people affected by incontinence seek help for their condition.

Treatment Options

Blood tests and urinalysis are often used to diagnose incontinence. Sometimes people affected by urinary incontinence are also asked to keep a bladder diary. Specialized testing may be required to diagnose incontinence. Such tests include pelvic ultrasound, cystogram (an X-ray of the bladder), cystoscopy (a procedure in which a thin tube with a small lens is inserted into the urethra to check for abnormalities), urodynamic testing (a procedure in which the pressure in the bladder is measured at rest and when filling) and postvoid residual measurement (a procedure in which urine output and residual urine in the bladder are measured).

Treatment of incontinence focuses on therapy for the underlying causes. Behaviour therapy is sometimes recommended as the first treatment for urinary incontinence. This includes education on healthy bladder behaviours and pelvic muscle exercises. Medical treatments such as estrogen therapy and injections of bulking agents such as collagen are sometimes used, as well. Drug therapies for overactive bladder include anticholinergic medications, tricyclic antidepressants and combined anticholinergics and smooth muscle relaxants. Other therapies include biofeedback and electrical stimulation. Severe cases may require surgical repair. Research is currently being undertaken to see if stem cells can be used in the treatment of urinary incontinence.

Because people are often embarrassed to discuss this condition with a health practitioner, urinary incontinence remains a largely neglected problem, despite the fact that it can often be successfully treated.

National Associations

The Canadian Continence Foundation / Fondation d'aide aux personnes incontinentes (Canada)
PO Box 417, Peterborough ON K9J 6Z3
Tel: 705-750-4600; *Fax:* 705-750-1770
Toll-Free: 800-265-9575
www.canadiancontinence.ca
www.linkedin.com/groups/Canadian-Continence-Foundation-3694602
www.facebook.com/canadian.continence
twitter.com/cdncontinence
www.youtube.com/user/canadiancontinence
Previous Name: The Simon Foundation for Continence Canada
Overview: A large national charitable organization founded in 1986
Mission: To act as a source of information, education & support for incontinent individuals; to increase public awareness & influence government policy
Affiliation(s): Simon Foundation-USA
Chief Officer(s):
Jacqueline Cahill, Executive Director
Adrian Wagg, President
Publications:
• The Informer: Your Canadian Continence Resource
Type: Newsletter
Profile: Research, issues & foundation news

Canadian Urologic Oncology Group (CUOG)
c/o Dr. Fred Saad, CUOG Chairman, 1560 Sherbrooke est, Montréal QC H2L 4M1
Tel: 514-890-8000
e-mail: fred.saad.chum@ssss.gouv.qc.ca
www.cuog.org
Overview: A small national organization
Mission: Clinical research investigator network committed to furthering urology research in Canada
Affiliation(s): Canadian Urological Association
Chief Officer(s):
Neil Fleshner, Chair

Canadian Urological Association (CUA) / Association des urologues du Canada
#401, 185 av Dorval, Dorval QC H9S 5J9
Tel: 514-395-0376; *Fax:* 514-395-1664
e-mail: cua@cua.org
www.cua.org
www.linkedin.com/company/canadian-urological-association-journal-cuaj-
www.facebook.com/CanadianUrologyAssociation
twitter.com/CanUrolAssoc

Overview: A medium-sized national organization founded in 1945
Mission: To advance the urology field; To promote high standards of urologic care in Canada
Affiliation(s): Canadian Medical Association
Chief Officer(s):
Tiffany Pizioli, Executive Director
  tiffany.pizioli@cua.org
Nadia Pace, Director, Communications
  nadia.pace@cua.org
Denise Toner, Manager, Advertising & Membership
  denise.toner@cua.org
Publications:
• Canadian Urological Association Journal (CUAJ) / Journal de l'Association des urologues du Canada (JAUC)
Type: Journal; *Frequency:* Bimonthly; *Editor:* Adriana Modica
Profile: Peer-reviewd original scientific research, reviews, resident studies, & casereports
• CUA News: Newsletter of the Canadian Urological Association
Type: Newsletter; *Frequency:* Semiannually
Profile: CUA activities, programs, events, awards, professional development, & committee reports

Urology Nurses of Canada
c/o 62 Barrie St., Kingston ON K7L 3J7
e-mail: membership@unc.org
www.unc.org

Overview: A small national organization
Mission: To promote the specialty of urologic nursing in Canada by promoting education, research & clinical practice.
Affiliation(s): Canadian Urological Association; Canadian Nurses' Association
Chief Officer(s):
Gina Porter, President
  president@unc.org
LuAnn Pickard, Secretary
  secretary@unc.org
Nancy Carson, Treasurer
  treasurer@unc.org
Publications:
• Pipeline
Type: Newsletter; *Frequency:* Semiannually; *Editor:* Brenda Bonde

Calgary
Calgary AB

Edmonton
Chief Officer(s):
Elizabeth Smits, Contact
  lizsmits@shaw.ca

Halifax
Halifax NS
Chief Officer(s):
Liette Connor, Contact
  liette.connor@cdha.nshealth.ca

Kingston
Chief Officer(s):
Sylvia Robb, Contact
  sylviamrobb@gmail.com

Montréal
Montréal QC
Chief Officer(s):
Raquel DeLeon, Contact
  raquel.deleon@muhc.mcgill.ca

New Brunswick
Chief Officer(s):
Gina Porter, Contact
  gina.porter@rogers.com

Newfoundland & Labrador
Chief Officer(s):
Sue Hammond, Contact
  hammond_so@yahoo.ca

Ottawa
Chief Officer(s):
Susan Freed, Contact
  freeds@teksavvy.com

Nancy Bauer, Secretary
Judy St. Germain, Treasurer

Toronto
Chief Officer(s):
Frances Stewart, Contact
  bladderqueen@hotmail.com

Victoria
Chief Officer(s):
Jill Jeffery, Contact
jpjeffery@shaw.ca

Provincial Associations

ONTARIO

Society of Urologic Surgeons of Ontario (SUSO)
#510, 3030 Lawrence Ave. East, Toronto ON M1P 2T7
Tel: 416-438-9948; *Fax:* 416-438-9590
e-mail: executive@suso.ca
www.suso.ca

Overview: A small provincial organization
Mission: Dedicated to ensuring patient access to urological care with a commitment to excellence, education, research & sharing of information
Chief Officer(s):
Allan Toguri, Executive Director

QUÉBEC

Association des urologues du Québec (AUQ) / Quebec Urological Association (QUA)
Tour de l'est, 2, Complexe Desjardins, 32e étage, Montréal QC H5B 1G8
Tél: 514-350-5131; *Téléc:* 514-350-5181
Courriel: info@auq.org
www.auq.org

Aperçu: *Dimension:* petite; *Envergure:* provinciale surveillé par Fédération des médecins spécialistes du Québec
Membre(s) du bureau directeur:
Serge Carrier, Président
Steven Lapointe, Secrétaire

International Associations

International Continence Society (ICS)
19 Portland Sq., Bristol BS2 8SJ United Kingdom
Tel: +44 117 9444881; *Fax:* +44 117 9444882
e-mail: info@icsoffice.org
www.icsoffice.org

Overview: A medium-sized international charitable organization
Mission: To further education, clinical practice, & scientific research; To remove the stigma of incontinence
Chief Officer(s):
Daniel Snowdon, Director, Administration
Dominic Turner, Director, Information Technology
Avicia Burchill, Manager, Project & Events
Publications:
• ICS [International Continence Society] Newsletter
Type: Newsletter; *Price:* Free with International Continence Society membership
• International Continence Society Membership Directory
Type: Directory
Profile: Continence professionals throughout the world
• Neurourology & Urodynamics
Type: Journal; *Frequency:* Bimonthly; *Price:* Free with International Continence Society membership

Infertility

Infertility is defined as the failure to achieve conception by couples who have not used contraception for at least one year.

Cause
Female causes of infertility may include age, sexually transmitted diseases, dysfunction of the ovaries, blockage of the tubes con-necting the ovaries to the uterus, endometriosis, hypothyroidism and hormone imbalances. Infertility in males is mostly related to sperm disorders, either insufficient production of sperm, ineffective sperm, or defective delivery of sperm, but may also be due to sexually transmitted diseases, hormone imbalances and genital injuries or abnormalities. Sometimes the cause of infertility is unknown (idiopathic infertility).

Symptoms
Medical consultation for infertility is usually suggested after one year of trying to get pregnant for women under the age of 35, or after six months for women over the age of 35. It is often recommended that a woman seek medical assistance sooner if she has endometriosis, irregular periods or a family history of infertility, or if she has previously had miscarriages, sexually transmitted diseases or abdominal/uterine surgery.

Prevalence
It is estimated that infertility affects between 12 and 16 percent of heterosexual couples in Canada. When trying to get pregnant, close to one in seven Canadian couples seek medical assistance. Since infertility increases as a woman ages, couples in which the woman is between the ages of 35 and 44 are two to three times more likely to seek help to get pregnant than couples in which the woman is between the ages of 25 and 29. About one in five couples who seek medical help to conceive use assisted reproductive technologies, while two in five use fertility-enhancing drugs.

Treatment Options
To diagnose infertility, a physician usually performs a physical exam and takes a detailed medical history to identify factors that could be affecting fertility. A variety of tests can also be used to determine the exact cause of infertility. For women, these tests may include urinalysis, blood hormone level tests, pelvic ultrasound and an X-ray dye test to check for blockage in the Fallopian tubes. Tests for men commonly include urinalysis, blood hormone level tests and semen analysis.

Once the cause of infertility has been determined, appropriate treatment options are identified. Infertility treatments for women can include surgery (for fibroids, uterine scarring or Fallopian tube blockages), fertility drugs (hormone treatments to induce or regulate ovulation), intrauterine insemination and assisted reproductive technology (for example, in vitro fertilization [IVF] and embryo transfer). Infertility treatment for men may include surgery to correct ejaculation problems and to repair varicose veins in the testes. Failure to conceive can be an emotional burden on couples, so counselling and psychological support are also important parts of treatment.

Infertility treatments can significantly increase the chances of becoming pregnant. However, it is important to note that age does influence the success rates of these therapies.

National Associations

Canadian Fertility & Andrology Society (CFAS) / Société canadienne de fertilité et d'andrologie
#301, 1719 rue Grand Trunk, Montréal QC H3K 1M1
Tel: 514-524-9009; *Fax:* 514-524-2163
e-mail: info@cfas.ca
www.cfas.ca

Previous Name: Canadian Society for the Study of Fertility
Merged from: Canadian Andrology Society
Overview: A medium-sized national charitable organization founded in 1954
Mission: To speak on behalf of interested parties in the field of assisted reproductive technologies & research in reproductive sciences
Chief Officer(s):

Jeff Roberts, President
Jason Min, Vice-President
Jason Hitkari, Director, Continuing Professional Development
Jay Baltz, Treasurer
Publications:
• CFAS [Canadian Fertility & Andrology Society] Communiqué
Type: Newsletter
Profile: CFAS information & events, plus articles
• Presidents' Annual Report [a publication of the Canadian Fertility & Andrology Society]
Type: Yearbook; *Frequency:* Annually

Infertility Awareness Association of Canada (IAAC) / Association canadienne de sensibilisation à l'infertilité (ACSI)
#201, 475 av Dumont, Dorval QC H9S 5W2

Tel: 514-633-4494
Toll-Free: 800-263-2929
e-mail: info@iaac.ca
www.iaac.ca
www.facebook.com/57435550753
twitter.com/iaac_acsi
www.pinterest.com/iaac1

Overview: A medium-sized national charitable organization founded in 1990
Mission: To offer assistance, support & education to individuals with infertility concerns; to increase the awareness & understanding of the causes, treatments & the emotional impact of infertility through the development of educational programs.
Member of: International Federation of Infertility Patient Associations (IFIPA)
Affliation(s): Canadian Fertility & Andrology Society; Society of Obstetricians & Gynaecologists of Canada
Chief Officer(s):
Janet Fraser, President

Infertility Network
160 Pickering St., Toronto ON M4E 3J7

Tel: 416-691-3611; *Fax:* 416-690-8015
e-mail: info@infertilitynetwork.org
www.infertilitynetwork.org

Overview: A small national charitable organization founded in 1990
Mission: To provide information, support & referral on infertility & related issues; To help people make informed choices for family-building options; To advocate for reform of gamete donation practices
Chief Officer(s):
Patricia Silver, President
Diane Allen, Executive Director

Marguerite Bourgeoys Family Centre Fertility Care Programme (MBFC)
Coxwell Medical Bldg., #100, 688 Coxwell Ave., Toronto ON M4C 3B7

Tel: 416-465-2868; *Fax:* 416-465-3538
www.fertilitycare.ca
www.facebook.com/FertilityCareToronto
twitter.com/FertilityCareTO

Overview: A small national charitable organization
Mission: To help families manage & care for their reproductive health, by providing health care & resources; To educate women, couples, & youth about sexuality, fertility, & family relationships, in the framework of Catholic values; To respect the dignity & differences of people
Member of: ShareLife Catholic Charities
Affliation(s): Archdiocese of Toronto
Chief Officer(s):
Krystyna Zasowski, President
Hemingway Karen, CFCS, Executive Director

Natural Family Planning Association
c/o #205, 3050 Yonge St., Toronto ON M4N 2K4

Tel: 416-481-5465
www.naturalfamilyplanning.ca

Also Known As: The Billings Group
Overview: A small national charitable organization
Mission: To promote the Billings Ovulation Method of natural family planning which is based on an awareness of a woman's physical systems to gauge optimum fertility state.
Member of: WOOMB International

Chief Officer(s):
Christian Elia, Executive Director

International Associations

World Organization Ovulation Method Billings Inc.
1506 Dansey Ave., Coquitlam BC V3K 3J1

Tel: 604-936-4472; *Fax:* 604-936-5690
www.woomb.ca

Also Known As: WOOMB Canada Inc.
Overview: A small international organization founded in 1982
Mission: To teach fertility awareness & natural family planning
Affliation(s): WOOMB International - Australia

Kidney Disease

Cause
The diseases that affect the kidney can be divided into diseases of the kidney itself, such as nephritis, polycystic kidney disease, kidney infections and stones, and diseases of other body systems that cause damage to the kidneys, such as diabetes, high blood pressure and lupus. In all of the above, disruption of kidney function results in failure to remove excess fluids and wastes from the blood. This may lead to end stage kidney, or renal, failure.

Chronic kidney disease is defined as damage to the kidney, or a reduced level of kidney function that has been present for three or more months. There are five stages of chronic kidney disease, and in many cases, the disease progresses slowly and silently through the early stages, presenting no symptoms until the advanced stages. At stage 5, or end-stage renal disease, kidney function is less than 15 percent of normal. Rapid onset of kidney failure, called acute kidney failure, is most often caused by kidney infection and injury.

Symptoms
Symptoms of kidney disease and their severity depend on the underlying cause. If there is damage or disease in the urinary tract, there can be pain when urinating, blood in the urine or changes in frequency and urgency of urination. If excess fluid cannot be removed, there may be swelling around the eyes and ankles. When the kidney is damaged directly, back or flank tenderness may be present.

Prevalence
It is estimated that two million people in Canada have some form of kidney disease, and that as many as 600,000 Canadians could be at risk for kidney disease and not even know it. Of the more than 4,300 Canadians on the organ transplantation wait list, close to 80 percent are in need of a kidney.

Treatment Options
Since people in the early stages of kidney disease often have no symptoms, the disease can be difficult to detect. Usually, tests such as urinalysis (to identify protein and blood in the urine) and blood tests (to check the level of serum creatine) are used to diagnose early-stage kidney disease.

Treatment is directed to the cause, and may include antibiotics for infections; removal of kidney stones by surgery or ultrasound waves; management of the systemic disease such as diabetes; dietary modification, especially of salt and protein intake; medication; and close monitoring and correction of fluids and electrolytes. Treatment may also include control of high blood pressure, which can be caused by kidney disease and further damage the kidney. The most severe cases of kidney failure require either dialysis, in which the blood's toxins are mechanically filtered and removed, or a kidney transplant.

Due to advances in transplant techniques and increases in transplant success rates, a kidney transplant is now often considered the best form of treatment for end-stage renal disease in many people.

National Associations

Canadian Association of Nephrology Nurses & Technologists (CANNT) / Association canadienne des infirmières et infirmiers et technologues de néphrologie (ACITN)

PO Box 10, 59 Millmanor Place, Delaware ON N0L 1E0

Tel: 519-652-6767; *Fax:* 519-652-5015
Toll-Free: 877-720-2819
e-mail: cannt@cannt.ca
www.cannt.ca
www.facebook.com/160999717295820
twitter.com/CANNT1

Overview: A small national organization founded in 1968
Mission: To improve the care of renal patients through support of educational opportunities for association members; To evaluate the performance & competence of nephrology nurses & technologists against the CANNT Standards of Practice
Affliation(s): Kidney Foundation of Canada; Canadian Nurses Association
Chief Officer(s):
Anne Moulton, RN, CNeph(C), President, 905-522-1155 Ext. 33916
    CANNT.president@gmail.com
Melanie Wiggins, Treasurer & Coordinator, Website
    CANNT.webtreasurer@gmail.com
Publications:
• CANNT [Canadian Association of Nephrology Nurses & Technologists] Journal / Journal ACITN
Type: Journal; *Frequency:* Quarterly; *Editor:* Gillian Brunier; *Price:* Free with CANNT membership

Canadian Society of Nephrology (CSN) / Société canadienne de néphrologie (SCN)

PO Box 25255, Stn. RDP, Montréal QC H1E 7P9

Tel: 514-643-4985
e-mail: info@csnscn.ca
www.csnscn.ca
www.facebook.com/1498868453774190
twitter.com/CSNSCN

Overview: A small national organization founded in 1966
Mission: To advance the practice of Nephrology; To promote the highest quality of care for patients with renal diseases, by setting high standards for medical training & education; To encourage research in biomedical sciences related to the kidney, kidney disorders & renal replacement therapies
Member of: International Society of Nephrology
Affliation(s): Royal College of Physicians & Surgeons of Canada
Chief Officer(s):
Braden Manns, President
Filomena Picciano, Director, Operations
Publications:
• CSN [Canadian Society of Nephrology] Newsletter
Type: Newsletter; *Frequency:* Quarterly

Canadian Urological Association (CUA) / Association des urologues du Canada

#401, 185 av Dorval, Dorval QC H9S 5J9

Tel: 514-395-0376; *Fax:* 514-395-1664
e-mail: cua@cua.org
www.cua.org
www.linkedin.com/company/canadian-urological-association-journal-cuaj-
www.facebook.com/CanadianUrologyAssociation
twitter.com/CanUrolAssoc

Overview: A medium-sized national organization founded in 1945
Mission: To advance the urology field; To promote high standards of urologic care in Canada
Affliation(s): Canadian Medical Association
Chief Officer(s):
Tiffany Pizioli, Executive Director
    tiffany.pizioli@cua.org

Nadia Pace, Director, Communications
    nadia.pace@cua.org
Denise Toner, Manager, Advertising & Membership
    denise.toner@cua.org
Publications:
• Canadian Urological Association Journal (CUAJ) / Journal de l'Association des urologues du Canada (JAUC)
Type: Journal; *Frequency:* Bimonthly; *Editor:* Adriana Modica
Profile: Peer-reviewd original scientific research, reviews, resident studies, & casereports
• CUA News: Newsletter of the Canadian Urological Association
Type: Newsletter; *Frequency:* Semiannually
Profile: CUA activities, programs, events, awards, professional development, & committee reports

Kidney Cancer Canada Association

#226, 4936 Yonge St., Toronto ON M2N 6S3

Tel: 416-603-0277; *Fax:* 416-603-0277
Toll-Free: 866-598-7166
e-mail: info@kidneycancercanada.ca
www.kidneycancercanada.ca
www.linkedin.com/company/kidney-cancer-canada
www.facebook.com/KidneyCancerCanada
twitter.com/KidneyCancer_Ca
www.youtube.com/KidneyCancerCanada

Also Known As: Kidney Cancer Canada
Overview: A medium-sized national charitable organization founded in 2007
Mission: To support & improve the lives of patients & families living with kidney cancer; To raise awareness of kidney cancer treatment options; To promote quality care across Canada; To increase funding for kidney cancer research
Chief Officer(s):
Andrew Weller, Chair
    aweller@kidneycancercanada.ca
Heather Chappell, Executive Director
    hchappell@kidneycancercanada.ca
Jan Coleman, Coordinator, Administration & Program Development
Publications:
• KCC [Kidney Cancer Canada] Newsletter
Type: Newsletter
• Kidney Cancer Canada Brochure
Type: Brochure

Kidney Foundation of Canada (KFOC) / Fondation canadienne du rein

#310, 5160, boul Decarie, Montréal QC H3X 2H9

Tel: 514-369-4806; *Fax:* 514-369-2472
Toll-Free: 800-361-7494
Other Communication: Website Management: webmaster@kidney.ca
e-mail: info@kidney.ca
www.kidney.ca
www.facebook.com/kidneyfoundation
twitter.com/kidneycanada
www.youtube.com/kidneycanada

Overview: A large national charitable organization founded in 1964
Mission: To improve the health & quality of life of people living with kidney disease; To fund research & related clinical education; To provide services for the special needs of individuals living with kidney disease; To advocate for access to high quality health care; To actively promote awareness of & commitment to organ donation
Member of: National Voluntary Organization; Healthpartners; Canadian Centre for Philanthrophy; Health Charities Coalition; Canadian Coalition for Genetic Fairness
Chief Officer(s):
Paul Kidston, National President
Silvana Anania, Interim National Executive Director
Elisabeth Fowler, National Director, Research
Teresa Havill, National Director, Human Resources
Carole Larouche, National Director, Finance
Publications:
• Living with Kidney Disease
Type: Manual
Profile: Published in English, French, Italian, Chinese, & Punjabi

Atlantic Canada Branch

#204, 56 Avonlea Ct., Fredericton NB E3C 1N8
Tel: 506-453-0533; Fax: 506-454-3639
Toll-Free: 877-453-0533
e-mail: kidneyatlantic@kidney.ca
www.kidney.ca/atlantic

Chief Officer(s):
Trina Ralph, Executive Director
trina.ralph@kidney.ca

British Columbia & Yukon Branch
#200, 4940 Canada Way, Burnaby BC V5G 4K6
Tel: 604-736-9775; Fax: 604-736-9703
Toll-Free: 800-567-8112
e-mail: info@kidney.bc.ca
www.kidney.ca/BC

Chief Officer(s):
Pia Schindler, Executive Director, 604-558-6875
pias@kidney.bc.ca

Division du Québec
2300, boul René-Lévesque ouest, Montréal QC H3H 2R5
Tél: 514-938-4515; Téléc: 514-938-4757
Ligne sans frais: 800-565-4515
Courriel: infoquebec@kidney.ca
www.kidney.ca/quebec

Chief Officer(s):
Martin Munger, Directeur général
martin.munger@kidney.ca

Eastern Ontario Chapter
#401, 1376 Bank St., Ottawa ON K1H 7Y3
Tel: 613-724-9953; Fax: 613-722-5907
Toll-Free: 800-724-9953

Chief Officer(s):
Sarah Hart, Program Coordinator
shart@kidney.on.ca

Hamilton & District Chapter
#201, 1599 Hurontario St., Mississauga ON L5G 4S1
Fax: 905-271-4990
Toll-Free: 800-387-4474

Chief Officer(s):
Tony Tirone, Contact
ttirone@kidney.on.ca

Kingston Chapter
PO Box 24003, Stn. Barriefield, Kingston ON K7L 0B4
Tel: 613-542-2121
Toll-Free: 800-387-4474

Chief Officer(s):
Kerry McCloy, Fund Development Officer
kmccloy@kidney.on.ca

Manitoba Branch
#1, 452 Dovercourt Dr., Winnipeg MB R3Y 1G4
Tel: 204-989-0800
Toll-Free: 800-729-7176
e-mail: info@kidney.mb.ca
www.kidney.ca/manitoba
twitter.com/KidneyFdnMB

Chief Officer(s):
Valerie Dunphy, Executive Director
vdunphy@kidney.mb.ca

Niagara & District Chapter
#201, 1599 Hurontario St., Mississauga ON L5G 4S1
Fax: 905-271-4990
Toll-Free: 800-387-4474

Chief Officer(s):
Jennifer Fraser, Chapter Manager
jfraser@kidney.on.ca

Northern Alberta & The Territories Branch
#202, 11227 Jasper Ave. NW, Edmonton AB T5K 0L5
Tel: 780-451-6900; Fax: 780-451-7592
Toll-Free: 800-461-9063
e-mail: info@kidney.ab.ca
www.kidney.ca/Page.aspx?pid=266

Chief Officer(s):
Flavia Robles, Executive Director

Northern Superior Chapter - Thunder Bay
PO Box 22043, Stn. Northwood, Thunder Bay ON P7E 6P2
Tel: 807-624-2680

Chief Officer(s):
Marion Harms, Fundraising Coordinator
mharms@tbaytel.net

Ontario Branch
#201, 1599 Hurontario St., Mississauga ON L5G 4S1
Tel: 905-278-3003; Fax: 905-271-4990
Toll-Free: 800-387-4474
e-mail: kidney@kidney.on.ca
www.kidney.ca/ontario
twitter.com/kidneyontario

Chief Officer(s):
Jim O'Brien, Executive Director, 905-278-3003 Ext. 4950
jobrien@kidney.on.ca

Outaouais-Québécois Chapter
CP 89027, Succ. Cité des jeunes, 207, boul Mont-Bleu, Gatineau QC J8Z 3G3
Tél: 819-661-5079

Chief Officer(s):
Bruno Tousignant, Responsable
bruno.tousignant@kidney.ca

Prince Edward Island Chapter
565 North River Rd., Charlottetown PE C1E 1J7
Tel: 902-892-9009
Toll-Free: 877-892-9009
e-mail: kidneypei@kidney.ca

Chief Officer(s):
Harry McLellan, Fundraising Coordinator
harry.mclellan@kidney.ca

Québec Chapter
#101, 1675, ch Ste-Foy, Québec QC G1S 2P7
Tél: 418-683-1449; Téléc: 418-683-7079

Chief Officer(s):
Maryse Neron, Coordonnatrice
maryse.neron@kidney.ca

Regina & District Chapter
1545C McAra St., Regina SK S4N 6H4
Tel: 306-347-0711; Fax: 306-586-8287
e-mail: regina@kidney.sk.ca

Chief Officer(s):
Iris Lord, Fund Development Manager
ilord@kidney.sk.ca

Saguenay/Lac Saint-Jean Chapter
#301, 23, rue Racine est, Chicoutimi QC G7H 1P4
Tél: 418-543-9644

Chief Officer(s):
Nathalie Sauliner, Coordinatrice
nathalie.saulnier@kidney.ca

Sarnia-Lambton Chapter
#405B, 546 Christina St. North, Sarnia ON N7T 5W6
Tel: 519-344-3462; Fax: 519-344-4038

Chief Officer(s):
Elaine Hayter, Senior Development Manager
ehayter@kidney.on.ca

Saskatchewan Branch
#1, 2217 Hanselman Ct., Saskatoon SK S7L 6A8
Tel: 306-664-8588; Fax: 306-653-4883
Toll-Free: 888-664-8588
e-mail: info@kidney.sk.ca
www.kidney.ca/sk

Chief Officer(s):
Joyce VanDeurzen, Executive Director
executivedirector@kidney.sk.ca

Sault Ste Marie Chapter
PO Box 20057, RPO Churchill Place, Sault Ste Marie ON P6A 6W3
Tel: 705-949-0400

Chief Officer(s):
Tannis McMillan, Fund Development Officer
tmcmillan@kidney.on.ca

Southern Alberta Branch

6007 - 1A St. SW, Calgary AB T2H 0G5
Tel: 403-255-6108; *Fax:* 403-255-9590
Toll-Free: 800-268-1177
e-mail: info@kidneyfoundation.ab.ca
www.kidney.ca/sab
Chief Officer(s):
Joyce Van Deurzen, Executive Director
joyce.vandeurzen@kidneyfoundation.ab.ca
Karen Thomas, Director, Community Relations
karen.thomas@kidneyfoundation.ab.ca

Southwestern Ontario Chapter
#203, 785 Wonderland Rd. South, London ON N6K 1M6
Fax: 519-850-5360
Toll-Free: 800-667-3597
Chief Officer(s):
Rizwana Ramzanali, Fund Development Officer
rramzanali@kidney.on.ca

Timmins-Porcupine Chapter
11357 Hwy. 101 East, Connaught ON P0N 1A0
Tel: 705-235-3233; *Fax:* 705-235-3237
Marlene Smith, President

Western Ontario Chapter
#201, 1599 Hurontario St., Mississauga ON L5G 4S1
Fax: 905-271-4990
Toll-Free: 800-387-4474
Chief Officer(s):
Evelina Turney, Fund Development Officer
eturney@kidney.on.ca

Windsor & District Chapter
PO Box 22033, 11500 Tecumseh Rd. East, Windsor ON N8N 5G6
Tel: 519-977-9211
Toll-Free: 800-387-4474
Chief Officer(s):
Anne Brinkman, Ontario Program Manager
peersupport@kidney.ca

Urology Nurses of Canada
c/o 62 Barrie St., Kingston ON K7L 3J7
e-mail: membership@unc.org
www.unc.org

Overview: A small national organization
Mission: To promote the specialty of urologic nursing in Canada by promoting education, research & clinical practice.
Affliation(s): Canadian Urological Association; Canadian Nurses' Association
Chief Officer(s):
Gina Porter, President
president@unc.org
LuAnn Pickard, Secretary
secretary@unc.org
Nancy Carson, Treasurer
treasurer@unc.org
Publications:
• Pipeline
Type: Newsletter; *Frequency:* Semiannually; *Editor:* Brenda Bonde

Calgary
Calgary AB

Edmonton
Chief Officer(s):
Elizabeth Smits, Contact
lizsmits@shaw.ca

Halifax
Halifax NS
Chief Officer(s):
Liette Connor, Contact
liette.connor@cdha.nshealth.ca

Kingston
Chief Officer(s):
Sylvia Robb, Contact
sylviamrobb@gmail.com

Montréal

Montréal QC
Chief Officer(s):
Raquel DeLeon, Contact
raquel.deleon@muhc.mcgill.ca

New Brunswick
Chief Officer(s):
Gina Porter, Contact
gina.porter@rogers.com

Newfoundland & Labrador
Chief Officer(s):
Sue Hammond, Contact
hammond_so@yahoo.ca

Ottawa
Chief Officer(s):
Susan Freed, Contact
freeds@teksavvy.com
Nancy Bauer, Secretary
Judy St. Germain, Treasurer

Toronto
Chief Officer(s):
Frances Stewart, Contact
bladderqueen@hotmail.com

Victoria
Chief Officer(s):
Jill Jeffery, Contact
jpjeffery@shaw.ca

Provincial Associations

BRITISH COLUMBIA

British Columbia Provincial Renal Agency (BCPRA)
#700, 1380 Burrard St., Vancouver BC V6Z 2H3
Tel: 604-875-7340
e-mail: bcpra@bcpra.ca
www.bcrenalagency.ca
www.facebook.com/BCRenalAgency
twitter.com/BCRenalAgency
www.youtube.com/user/BCRenalAgency

Overview: A large provincial organization founded in 1997
Mission: To make BC a leader in kidney care delivery in Canada, through enhancing the network of kidney care, providing a coordinated patient-focused information system & monitoring & maintaining quality & standards of care
Publications:
• PROMIS UpDate
Type: Newsletter
Profile: Up-to-date information about projects & system features, distributed every eight to ten weeks
• Renal News [a publication of the British Columbia Provincial Renal Agency]
Type: Newsletter; *Frequency:* Quarterly
Profile: Information about projects & practices across British Columbia's renal network

ONTARIO

Society of Urologic Surgeons of Ontario (SUSO)
#510, 3030 Lawrence Ave. East, Toronto ON M1P 2T7
Tel: 416-438-9948; *Fax:* 416-438-9590
e-mail: executive@suso.ca
www.suso.ca

Overview: A small provincial organization
Mission: Dedicated to ensuring patient access to urological care with a commitment to excellence, education, research & sharing of information
Chief Officer(s):
Allan Toguri, Executive Director

QUÉBEC

Association des néphrologues du Québec
CP 216, Succ. Desjardins, #3000, 2, Complexe Desjardins, Montréal
QC H5B 1G8

Tél: 514-350-5134; *Téléc:* 514-350-5151
Courriel: nephrologie@fmsq.org
Aperçu: *Dimension:* petite; *Envergure:* provinciale surveillé par
Fédération des médecins spécialistes du Québec
Membre(s) du bureau directeur:
Robert Charbonneau, Président
Lillian Plasse, Directrice, Administration

**Association des urologues du Québec (AUQ) / Quebec
Urological Association (QUA)**
Tour de l'est, 2, Complexe Desjardins, 32e étage, Montréal QC H5B
1G8

Tél: 514-350-5131; *Téléc:* 514-350-5181
Courriel: info@auq.org
www.auq.org
Aperçu: *Dimension:* petite; *Envergure:* provinciale surveillé par
Fédération des médecins spécialistes du Québec
Membre(s) du bureau directeur:
Serge Carrier, Président
Steven Lapointe, Secrétaire

Association générale des insuffisants rénaux (AGIR)
4865, boul. Gouin est, Montréal QC H1G 1A1

Tél: 514-852-9297; *Téléc:* 514-323-1231
Ligne sans frais: 888-852-9297
Courriel: reins@agir.ca
www.agir.ca
www.facebook.com/groups/assoagir
Aperçu: *Dimension:* moyenne; *Envergure:* provinciale; fondée en 1979
Mission: Pour soutenir les personnes atteintes de maladies rénales et
qui ont eu des greffes de rein et pour aider à améliorer leur vie
Membre de: Office des personnes handicapées du Québec
Membre(s) du bureau directeur:
Berthe Martin, Directrice générale

Local Associations

QUÉBEC

La Fondation canadienne du rein, section Chibougamau
CP 462, Chibougamau QC G8P 2Y8
Aperçu: *Dimension:* petite; *Envergure:* locale surveillé par The Kidney
Foundation of Canada
Membre(s) du bureau directeur:
Hélène Ross-Arseneault

National Publications

Canadian Journal of General Internal Medicine
Owned By: Dougmar Publishing Group
Canadian Society of Internal Medicine, #200, 421 Gilmour St., Ottawa,
ON K2P 0R5

Tel: 613-422-5977; *Fax:* 613-249-3326
Toll-Free: 855-893-2746
Frequency: 4 times a year
Official publication of the Canadian Society of Internal Medicine.
Scott Bryant, Managing Editor, sbryant@dougmargroup.com

Local Hospitals & Health Centres

BRITISH COLUMBIA

CRANBROOK: Cranbrook Community Dialysis Clinic
Affiliated with: Interior Health Authority
13 - 24th Ave. North, Cranbrook, BC V1C 3H9
Tel: 250-417-3588   *Toll-Free:* 866-288-8082
www.interiorhealth.ca

Note: Provides renal programs & hemodialysis services

CRANBROOK: East Kootenay CKD Clinic
Affiliated with: Interior Health Authority
20 - 23rd Ave. South, Cranbrook, BC V1C 5V1

Tel: 250-489-6414
www.interiorhealth.ca

Note: Hemodialysis clinic

CRESTON: Creston Community Dialysis Clinic
Affiliated with: Interior Health Authority
312 - 15th Ave. North, Creston, BC V0B 1G5

Tel: 250-428-3830
www.interiorhealth.ca

Note: Offers renal programs & hemodialysis services

GRAND FORKS: Grand Forks Community Dialysis Clinic
Affiliated with: Interior Health Authority
7649 - 22nd St., Grand Forks, BC V0H 1H0

Tel: 250-443-2119
www.interiorhealth.ca

Note: Offers hemodialysis services

KAMLOOPS: Kamloops Community Dialysis Clinic
Affiliated with: Interior Health Authority
795 Tranquille Rd., Kamloops, BC V2B 3J3

Tel: 250-314-2100
www.interiorhealth.ca

Note: Offers hemodialysis services

**KAMLOOPS: Thompson Cariboo Shuswap Chronic Kidney
Disease Clinic**
Affiliated with: Interior Health Authority
Royal Inland Hospital, 311 Columbia St., Kamloops, BC V2C 2T1

Tel: 250-314-2849
www.interiorhealth.ca

Note: Also the Thompson Cariboo Shuswap Peritoneal Hemodialysis
Clinic (250-314-2100, ext. 3259), Thompson Cariboo Shuswap Home
Hemodialysis Clinic, Thompson Cariboo Shuswap In-Center
Hemodialysis Clinic & Thompson Cariboo Shuswap Transplant Clinic
(250-314-2260).

KELOWNA: Kelowna Chronic Kidney Disease Clinic
Affiliated with: Interior Health Authority
2268 Pandosy St., Kelowna, BC V1Y 1T2

Tel: 250-862-4156
www.interiorhealth.ca

Note: Also the Kelowna Peritoneal Dialysis Clinic, Kelowna Home
Hemodialysis Clinic & the Kelowna In-Centre Hemodialysis Clinic
(250-862-4345).

KELOWNA: Kelowna Transplant Clinic
Affiliated with: Interior Health Authority
2268 Pandosy St., Kelowna, BC V1Y 1T2

Tel: 250-862-4156
www.interiorhealth.ca

Note: Follow-up care for organ transplant recipients, primarily renal
transplant.

KELOWNA: Rutland Community Dialysis
Affiliated with: Interior Health Authority
125 Park Rd., Kelowna, BC V1X 3E3

Tel: 250-491-7613
www.interiorhealth.ca

Note: Offers hemodialysis services

KIMBERLEY: Kidney Care Clinic
Affiliated with: Interior Health Authority
260 - 4th Ave., Kimberley, BC V1A 2R6

www.interiorhealth.ca

Note: Offers services for individuals & families affected by chronic kidney disease

PENTICTON: Penticton Chronic Kidney Disease Clinic
Affiliated with: Interior Health Authority
Penticton Health Centre, 740 Carmi Ave., Penticton, BC V2A 8P9
Tel: 250-770-3530
www.interiorhealth.ca

Note: Offers hemodialysis services

PENTICTON: Penticton Home Hemodialysis Clinic
Affiliated with: Interior Health Authority
550 Carmi Ave., Penticton, BC V2A 3G6
Tel: 250-492-4000
www.interiorhealth.ca

Note: Also the Penticton In-Centre Hemodialysis Clinic (250-492-9059), Penticton Peritoneal Dialysis Clinic (250-492-4000, ext. 2650) & Penticton Transplant Clinic (250-492-4000, ext. 2603).

SPARWOOD: Sparwood Community Dialysis Clinic
Affiliated with: Interior Health Authority
570 Pine Ave., Sparwood, BC V0B 2G0
Tel: 250-425-4527
www.interiorhealth.ca

Note: Offers hemodialysis services

TRAIL: Kootenay Boundary Chronic Kidney Disease Clinic
Affiliated with: Interior Health Authority
1200 Hospital Bench, Trail, BC V1R 4M1
Tel: 250-364-6270
www.interiorhealth.ca

Note: Also the Kootenay Boundary Home Hemodialysis Clinic, Kootenay Boundary In-Center Hemodialysis Clinic, & Kootenay Boundary Peritoneal Dialysis Clinic (250-364-3450).

TRAIL: Kootenay Boundary Transplant Clinic
Affiliated with: Interior Health Authority
1200 Hospital Bench, Trail, BC V1R 4M1
Tel: 250-364-3494
www.interiorhealth.ca

Note: Follow-up care for organ transplant recipients, primarily renal transplant.

VERNON: Vernon Renal Clinic
Affiliated with: Interior Health Authority
#700, 3115 - 48th Ave., Vernon, BC V1T 3R5
Tel: 250-503-3320
www.interiorhealth.ca

Note: Offers services to patients with chronic kidney disease

WILLIAMS LAKE: Williams Lake Community Dialysis
Affiliated with: Interior Health Authority
517 - 6th Ave. North, Williams Lake, BC V2G 2G8
Tel: 250-302-3209
www.interiorhealth.ca

Note: Offers hemodialysis services

Leprosy

Leprosy, or Hansen's disease, is a chronic bacterial infection that causes skin sores, nerve damage and muscle weakness. Severe cases can result in disfiguration, crippling and blindness. Leprosy has two main types, tuberculoid and lepromatous.

Cause

Leprosy is caused by the bacterium Mycobacterium leprae, which multiplies slowly and has an average incubation period of five years. The bacteria attacks and damages the sensory nerves. Leprosy is believed to be spread by an infected person through coughing and sneezing. These droplets from the nose or mouth can be transmitted when in close and prolonged contact with an infected person.

Symptoms

Leprosy symptoms can take as long as twenty years to manifest and can vary depending on a person's resistance to the disease. Early symptoms typically include skin lesions that have decreased sensation and are slightly red, lighter or darker than a person's normal skin colour, and do not heal. Lepromatous, the most severe type of leprosy, can also produce large, disfiguring lumps (nodules). Damage to the sensory nerves can cause loss of sensation in the hands and feet, leaving them vulnerable to burns and injuries. Numbness can cause small muscles to become paralyzed, which leads to deformities such as a dropped foot or a clawed hand. Facial nerve damage can prevent the eyes from blinking, leaving them susceptible to infection and can lead to blindness. Contrary to popular belief, leprosy does not cause fingers and toes to fall off. Rather, recurring injuries and infections of numb areas can cause the bones and tissues around fingers and toes to shrink, making them appear shorter.

Prevalence

An estimated 211,973 new cases of leprosy were reported in 2015, compared to 407,791 in 2004. Leprosy, however, remains endemic in poorer parts of the world, namely Southeast Asia, with India recording the highest number of cases worldwide. In Canada, two to ten cases are typically diagnosed annually, with most infected individuals having immigrated to Canada from India, Indonesia, the Philippines or Myanmar. Children are more likely than adults to get the disease. It is estimated that 3 million people are living with some permanent disability due to leprosy.

Treatment Options

Leprosy is usually diagnosed during a physical examination, although a skin lesion biopsy or a skin smear can be used to confirm the disease. The lepromin skin test, which involves the injection of a sample of inactivated leprosy-causing bacteria, can distinguish the type of leprosy a person has contracted.

Leprosy can now be cured. Treatment typically consists of a combination of three drugs: rifampicin, clofazimine and dapsone. Since 1995, WHO (World Health Organization) has supplied this multi-drug treatment free for all leprosy patients worldwide. Fear of social consequences, as well as ignorance of the availability of effective and free treatment, remain obstacles that infected people face while trying to obtain treatment.

With early treatment, the damage caused by leprosy can be limited and the spreading of the disease can be stopped and a person with leprosy can live a normal life.

International Associations

effect:hope
#200, 90 Allstate Pkwy., Markham ON L3R 6H3
Tel: 905-886-2885; *Fax:* 905-886-2887
Toll-Free: 888-537-7679
e-mail: info@effecthope.org
effecthope.org
www.linkedin.com/company/3068053
www.facebook.com/effecthope
twitter.com/effecthope
www.youtube.com/user/effecthope

Also Known As: The Leprosy Mission Canada
Previous Name: The Mission to Lepers
Overview: A medium-sized international organization founded in 1892
Mission: To provide care & support to leprosy patients in many parts of the world including India, Bangladesh, & Nigeria
Member of: Canadian Council of Christian Charities
Affliation(s): The Leprosy Mission International

Chief Officer(s):
Peter Derrick, Executive Director

Heiser Program for Research in Leprosy & Tuberculosis
c/o The New York Community Trust, 909 - 3rd Ave., New York NY 10022 USA

Tel: 212-686-0010; *Fax:* 212-532-8528

Overview: A small international charitable organization
Mission: To award grants to fund research into leoprosy, tuberculosis & their bacterial agents to find measures for prevention & cure.
Chief Officer(s):
Gilla Kaplan, Chair, Scientific Advisory Committee
Len McNally, Director
 lm@nyct-cfi.org

Liver Disease

Liver disease covers a wide range of disorders that can result in chronic liver damage, such as scarring (fibrosis) or the development of cirrhosis.

Cause
There are more than 100 different forms of liver disease that may be caused by factors including infection (such as viral hepatitis), chronic alcoholism or drug abuse, obesity, genetics, medications and autoimmune disorders. Severe disease can permanently damage the liver, causing it to fail totally.

Symptoms
Common signs of liver damage are fatigue, loss of appetite, nausea and tea-colored urine. Yellowing of the skin and the whites of the eye (jaundice) is seen in 50 percent of cases. Other symptoms include liver enlargement and tenderness, and fluid collection in the abdominal cavity. A shrivelling liver indicates more chronic and severe damage.

Prevalence
An estimated 2,788 Canadians die each year from liver disease. Over 145 babies are born with liver disease every year in Canada.

Treatment Options
Because the symptoms of liver disease are often similar to those of other health problems, diagnosis can be difficult. To confirm a diagnosis of liver disease, a physician usually performs a physical exam and takes a medical history to identify factors that may be putting a person at risk for liver disease. Other tests may also be ordered including liver tests (blood tests to determine the presence of liver inflammation) and liver biopsy (a procedure where a small piece of liver tissue is obtained and examined).

Treatment for liver disease depends on the underlying cause and may include dietary modifications, medications or surgery. Liver transplantation is accepted as appropriate treatment for end-stage liver dysfunction.

The prognosis for a person with liver disease varies. In less serious cases (such as viral hepatitis), the liver can completely recover due to its remarkable capacity to heal itself. Other liver diseases are managed rather than cured.

See also Hepatitis

National Associations

Canadian Association for the Study of the Liver (CASL) / Association canadienne pour l'étude du foie
c/o BUKSA Strategic Conference Services, #307, 10328 - 81st Ave., Edmonton AB T6C 3T5

Tel: 780-436-0983
e-mail: casl@hepatology.ca
www.hepatology.ca

Overview: A small national organization
Mission: To eliminate liver disease
Affliation(s): International Association for the Study of the Liver (IASL)
Chief Officer(s):
Rick Schreiber, President
Kelly Burak, Secretary-Treasurer
Marc Bilodeau, President-Elect
Publications:
• Canadian Journal of Gastroenterology & Hepatology [a publication of the Canadian Association for the Study of the Liver]
Type: Journal; *Price:* Free with membership in the Canadian Association for the Study of the Liver

Canadian Liver Foundation (CLF) / Fondation canadienne du foie (FCF)
#801, 3100 Steeles Ave. East, Toronto ON L3R 8T3

Tel: 416-491-3353; *Fax:* 905-752-1540
Toll-Free: 800-563-5483
e-mail: clf@liver.ca
www.liver.ca
www.facebook.com/6584473365
twitter.com/CdnLiverFdtn
www.youtube.com/user/clfwebmaster

Overview: A large national charitable organization founded in 1969
Mission: To reduce the incidence & impact of all liver disease by funding liver research & education; promote liver health through programs & publications
Chief Officer(s):
Morris Sherman, Chairman
Elliot M. Jacobson, Sec.-Treas.
Publications:
• Canadian Liver Foundation Annual Report
Type: Yearbook; *Frequency:* Annually

Atlantic Canada Regional Office/Halifax Chapter
#103-406, 287 Lacewood Dr., Halifax NS B3M 3Y7
Tel: 902-423-8538; *Fax:* 902-423-8811
Toll-Free: 866-423-8538
e-mail: atlantic@liver.ca
Chief Officer(s):
Shayla Steeves, Regional Director

British Columbia/Yukon Regional Office
#109, 828 West 8th Ave., Vancouver BC V5Z 1E2
Tel: 604-707-6430; *Fax:* 604-681-6067
Toll-Free: 800-856-7266
Chief Officer(s):
Mark Mansfield, Regional Manager
 mmansfield@liver.ca

Chatham/Kent Chapter
PO Box 23, Chatham ON N7M 5K1
Tel: 519-682-9805; *Fax:* 519-682-2184
e-mail: clfchatham@liver.ca
Chief Officer(s):
Sheila Hughes, Development Manager

Eastern Ontario Regional Office
#641, 1500 Bank St., Ottawa ON K1H 1B8
Toll-Free: 844-316-6990
Chief Officer(s):
Gary O'Byrne, Regional Manager
 GOByrne@liver.ca

London Chapter
Royal Bank Bldg., #1206, 383 Richmond St., London ON N6A 3C4
Fax: 905-752-1540
Toll-Free: 800-563-5483
e-mail: clf@liver.ca

Manitoba Chapter
#210, 375 York Ave., Winnipeg MB R3C 3J3
Tel: 204-831-6231
Chief Officer(s):
Bianca Pengelly, Reginal Coordinator
 bpengelly@liver.ca

Moncton Chapter
#110, 1127B Main St., Moncton NB E1C 1H1
e-mail: atlantic@liver.ca

Chief Officer(s):
Shayla Steeves, Regional Director

Montréal Chapter
#1430, 1000, rue de la Gauchetière Ouest, Montréal QC H3B 4W5
Tél: 514-876-4170; *Téléc:* 514-876-4172
Courriel: montrealevents@liver.ca

Chief Officer(s):
Betty Esperanza, Regional Director
besperanza@liver.ca

Southern Alberta/Calgary Regional Office
#309, 1010 - 1st Ave. NE, Calgary AB T2E 7W7
Tel: 403-276-3390; *Fax:* 403-276-3423
Toll-Free: 888-557-5516

Debralee Fernets, Regional Manager
debralee@liver.ca

Toronto/GTA Chapter
#801, 3100 Steeles Ave. East, Markham ON L3R 8T3
Tel: 416-491-3353; *Fax:* 905-752-1540
Toll-Free: 800-563-5483
e-mail: clf@liver.ca

Chief Officer(s):
Steven Foster, Regional Manager
sfoster@liver.ca

Lung Disease

In Canada, more than three million people suffer from one of the five most serious lung diseases: asthma, lung cancer, cystic fibrosis, tuberculosis and chronic obstructive pulmonary disease (COPD). The cost to Canada's economy for just three of these chronic lung diseases—lung cancer, asthma and COPD—was approximately $12 billion in 2010. These diseases, along with influenza, pneumonia and other lung disorders that are secondary to clots originating from other sites in the body, systemic illness and skeletal abnormalities that interfere with chest expansion during breathing affect people of all ages and backgrounds. Because asthma, lung cancer, cystic fibrosis and tuberculosis are discussed in detail in other chapters of this book, the focus of this description will be COPD.

Chronic Obstructive Pulmonary Disease

Cause
Chronic obstructive pulmonary disease is characterized by progressive damage to the airways that makes breathing difficult. In about 80 percent of cases, COPD is caused by smoking. Other possible causes include air pollution, secondhand smoke and frequent lung infections in childhood. High-risk occupations for COPD include mining, farming, building construction and certain types of manufacturing.

Symptoms
Symptoms of COPD may include an ongoing cough, sputum production, breathlessness, wheezing and chest tightness. Possible complications associated with COPD include heart problems, osteoporosis, eye problems (such as glaucoma), malnutrition, pulmonary hypertension and frequent chest infections. Lung cancer is often seen in people with COPD, because the two conditions have similar causes.

Prevalence
Approximately 804,043 people in Canada have chronic obstructive pulmonary disease. Due to an increase in smoking among women, COPD is now more common in women under the age of 75 than in men.

Treatment Options
Diagnosis of COPD depends on a very careful history, physical examination, chest X-ray, aerial blood gas testing (to check the levels of oxygen and carbon dioxide in the blood) and lung function testing. Spirometry is the test most commonly used to diagnose COPD. Patients are asked to blow as hard as possible into a tube that is hooked up to a machine (spirometer) that monitors the rate at which air is breathed out, as well as the amount of air that is breathed out. These measures are also important in following disease progression and response to treatment.

Management of COPD includes avoiding tobacco or exposure to other irritants such as dust and fumes. Drug therapy may include antibiotics to control heavy sputum production, bronchodilators to open up the narrowed airways and inhaled steroids to reduce lung inflammation. Pulmonary rehabilitation may also be recommended. The goal of this therapy is to give people with COPD exercise and diet advice, counselling and disease management training. In advanced cases, breathing oxygen directly by nasal prongs improves quality of life and survival.

Lung disease has a significant impact on the lives of many Canadians. Studies suggest that more direct strategies to reduce smoking, improve air quality and lessen exposure to secondhand smoke would help reduce the prevalence of chronic lung disease in Canada.

National Associations

Action on Smoking & Health (ASH)
PO Box 4500, Stn. South, Edmonton AB T6E 6K2
Tel: 780-426-7867; *Fax:* 780-488-7195
e-mail: info@ash.ca
www.ash.ca
twitter.com/actiononsmoking
Overview: A small national charitable organization founded in 1979
Mission: To act as a tobacco control agency in western Canada
Publications:
• Action on Smoking & Health Newsletter
Type: Newsletter; *Price:* Free, with membership in Action on Smoking & Health
Profile: News & events from Action on Smoking & Health

Canadian Association of Cardio-Pulmonary Technologists (CACPT)
PO Box 848, Stn. A, Toronto ON M5W 1G3
e-mail: contactus@cacpt.ca
www.cacpt.ca
Overview: A small national organization founded in 1970
Mission: To establish maintain high standards for Registered Cardio-Pulmonary Technologists
Affliation(s): Canadian Cardiovascular Society; Canadian Cardiovascular Congress
Chief Officer(s):
Glenda Ryan, President
president@cacpt.ca

Canadian Association of Thoracic Surgeons (CATS) / Association canadienne des chirurgiens thoraciques
#300, 421 Gilmour St., Ottawa ON K2P 0R5
e-mail: cats@canadianthoracicsurgeons.ca
www.canadianthoracicsurgeons.ca
Overview: A medium-sized national organization
Mission: To represent thoracic surgeons across Canada
Chief Officer(s):
Drew Bethune, President
Andrew Seely, Secretary-Treasurer & Chair, Programs

Canadian Board for Respiratory Care Inc. (CBRC) / Le Conseil canadien des soins respiratoires inc. (CCSR)
#103, 1083 Queen St., Halifax NS B3H 0B2
Tel: 902-492-4387; *Fax:* 902-492-0045
e-mail: cbrc@cbrc.ca
www.cbrc.ca
Overview: A small national organization founded in 1989
Mission: To produce examinations used to test respiratory therapists prior to entering active practice
Chief Officer(s):

Julie Brown, Secretary/Treasurer

Canadian Council for Tobacco Control (CCTC) / Conseil canadien pour le contrôle du tabac

#508, 75 Albert St., Ottawa ON K1P 5E7

Tel: 613-567-3050; *Fax:* 613-567-2730
Toll-Free: 800-267-5234
www.facebook.com/158829997464616
twitter.com/CdnCouncilTC

Previous Name: Canadian Council on Smoking & Health
Overview: A medium-sized national charitable organization founded in 1974
Mission: To envision a strong & effective tobacco control movement; To diminish the adverse impact to the health of Canadians caused by tobacco industry products; To increase the effectiveness & capacity of individuals & organizations involved in tobacco control, to achieve a smoke free society in Canada; To prevent tobaccco use; To persuade & help smokers to stop using tobacco products; To educate Canadians about the marketing strategies & tactics of the tobacco industry & the adverse effects tobacco products have on the health of Canadians

Canadian Lung Association (CLA) / Association pulmonaire du Canada

National Office, #300, 1750 Courtwood Cres., Ottawa ON K2C 2B5

Tel: 613-569-6411
Toll-Free: 888-566-5864
e-mail: info@lung.ca
www.lung.ca
www.facebook.com/canadianlungassociation
twitter.com/canlung
www.youtube.com/user/TheLungAssociation

Previous Name: The Canadian Association for the Prevention of Consumption & Other Forms of Tuberculosis; The Canadian Tuberculosis & Respiratory Disease Association
Overview: A large national charitable organization founded in 1900
Mission: To improve & promote lung health across Canada
Chief Officer(s):
Debra Lynkowski, President & Chief Executive Officer
Terry Dean, Senior Vice President, Federation Development & Partnerships
Debbie Smith, Vice President, Finance & Operations
Janet Sutherland, Director, Canadian Thoracic Society/Canadian Respiratory Health Professiona
Marketa Stastna, Manager, Marketing & Communications
Amy Henderson, Manager, Public Policy & Health Communications
Kristen Curren, Manager, Education & Knowledge Translation
Publications:
• Canadian Lung Association Annual Report
Type: Yearbook; *Frequency:* Annually

Canadian Network for Respiratory Care (CNRC) / Réseau Canadien pour les soins respiratoires (RCSR)

16851 Mount Wolfe Rd., Caledon ON L7E 3P6

Tel: 905-880-1092; *Fax:* 905-880-9733
Toll-Free: 855-355-4672
e-mail: info@cnrchome.net
www.cnrchome.net

Previous Name: Canadian Network for Asthma Care
Overview: A small national charitable organization founded in 1994
Mission: To certify healthcare professionals as asthma & rspiratory educators (CAEs & CREs)
Chief Officer(s):
Cheryl Connors, Executive Director

Canadian Respiratory Health Professionals (CRHP)

c/o Canadian Thoracic Society, #300, 1750 Courtwood Cres., Ottawa ON K2C 2B5

Tel: 613-569-6411; *Fax:* 613-569-8860
e-mail: crhpinfo@lung.ca
crhp.lung.ca
www.facebook.com/334691136607567

Merged from: Cdn Nurses Respiratory, Cdn Physiotherapy Cardio-Respiratory, & Respiratory Therapy Societies
Overview: A small national organization founded in 2004 overseen by Canadian Lung Association
Mission: To promote lung health & the prevention of lung disease
Affiliation(s): Canadian Thoracic Society

Chief Officer(s):
Janet Sutherland, Executive Director
Publications:
• Airwaves - The Newsletter of the Canadian Respiratory Health Professionals
Type: Newsletter; *Price:* Free with CRHP membership
Profile: Information for Canadian Respiratory Health Professionals members

Canadian Society of Respiratory Therapists (CSRT) / La Société canadienne des thérapeutes respiratoires (SCTR)

#201, 2460 Lancaster Rd., Ottawa ON K1B 4S5

Tel: 613-731-3164; *Fax:* 613-521-4314
Toll-Free: 800-267-3422
www.csrt.com
www.facebook.com/csrt.sctr
twitter.com/@CSRT_tweets

Overview: A medium-sized national organization founded in 1964
Mission: To provide leadership toward the advancement of cardiorespiratory care; To achieve excellence through the definition of roles, standards, & scope of clinical practice
Chief Officer(s):
Jeff Dionne, President
Adam Buettner, Treasurer
Christiane Ménard, Executive Director, 800-267-3422 Ext. 222
cmenard@csrt.com

Centre for Immunization & Respiratory Infectious Diseases (CIRID)

c/o Public Health Agency of Canada, 130 Colonnade Rd., Ottawa ON K1A 0K9

www.phac-aspc.gc.ca/irid-diir

Overview: A small national organization
Mission: To decrease & eradicate instances of vaccine-preventable & infectious respiratory diseases; To lessen the negative impact of respiratory infections
Chief Officer(s):
Rhonda Kropp, Director General, 613-960-2893

Non-Smokers' Rights Association (NSRA) / Association pour les droits des non-fumeurs

#221, 720 Spadina Ave., Toronto ON M5S 2T9

Tel: 416-928-2900; *Fax:* 416-928-1860
e-mail: toronto@nsra-adnf.ca
www.nsra-adnf.ca
twitter.com/nsra_adnf

Overview: A medium-sized national organization founded in 1974
Mission: To promote public health by stopping illness & death due to tobacco, including second-hand smoke
Affliation(s): Smoking & Health Action Foundation (SHAF)
Chief Officer(s):
Lorraine Fry, Executive Director

Physicians for a Smoke-Free Canada / Médecins pour un Canada sans fumée

134 Caroline Ave., Ottawa ON K1Y 0S9

Tel: 613-297-3590; *Fax:* 613-728-9049
e-mail: psc@nospamsmoke-free.ca
www.smoke-free.ca

Overview: A medium-sized national organization founded in 1985
Mission: To address tobacco issues; To promote reduced smoking & prevent tobacco-caused illness
Chief Officer(s):
Atul Kapur, President
James Walker, Secretary-Treasurer

Provincial Associations

ALBERTA

Alberta & Northwest Territories Lung Association
PO Box 4500, Stn. South, #208, 17420 Stony Plain Rd., Edmonton AB
T6E 6K2

Tel: 780-488-6819; *Fax:* 780-488-7195
Toll-Free: 888-566-5864
e-mail: info@ab.lung.ca
www.ab.lung.ca
www.facebook.com/lungassociationabnwt
twitter.com/lungabnwt
Overview: A medium-sized provincial charitable organization founded
in 1939 overseen by Canadian Lung Association
Mission: To educate the public & medical professionals about lung
health
Chief Officer(s):
Paul Borrett, Chair
Evangeline Berube, Vice-Chair & Treasurer
Kate Hurlburt, Secretary
Publications:
• Alberta & Northwest Territories Lung Association Annual Report
Type: Yearbook; *Frequency:* Annually
Profile: Highlights of fundraising activities, advocacy activities, & patient
support programs

**College & Association of Respiratory Therapists of Alberta
(CARTA)**
#218, 6715 - 8 St. NE, Calgary AB T2E 7H7
Tel: 403-274-1828; *Fax:* 403-274-9703
Toll-Free: 800-205-2778
www.carta.ca
Previous Name: Alberta College & Association of Respiratory Therapy
Overview: A medium-sized provincial licensing organization founded in
1971
Mission: To serve & protect the public interest by regulating the
respiratory therapy profession; To provide professional services to
members
Member of: Federation of Regulated Health Professions of Alberta
Affiliation(s): Respiratory Therapy Labour Mobility Consortium
Chief Officer(s):
Irina Charania, President
Bryan Buell, Executive Director
  bryan.buell@carta.ca

BRITISH COLUMBIA

Airspace Action on Smoking & Health
PO Box 18004, 1215C - 56th St., Delta BC V4L 2M4
Tel: 778-899-4832
airspace.bc.ca
www.facebook.com/234024210003649
twitter.com/airspace_bc
Previous Name: AIRSPACE Non-Smokers' Rights Society
Overview: A medium-sized provincial organization founded in 1981
Mission: To educate non-smokers on the effects that smoking has on
them & of their legal right to smoke-free air; to help establish laws to
protect the comfort, safety & health of non-smokers; to help reduce the
number of future smokers
Affiliation(s): Non-Smokers' Rights Association; Canadian Council on
Smoking & Health

British Columbia Lung Association (BCLA)
2675 Oak St., Vancouver BC V6H 2K2
Tel: 604-731-5864; *Fax:* 604-731-5810
Toll-Free: 800-665-5864
e-mail: info@bc.lung.ca
www.bc.lung.ca
www.facebook.com/BCLungAssociation
twitter.com/BCLungAssoc
Previous Name: Anti-Tuberculosis Society
Overview: A medium-sized provincial charitable organization founded
in 1906 overseen by Canadian Lung Association
Mission: To support lung health research, education, prevention, &
advocacy; To help people manage respiratory diseases, including

asthma, COPD (chronic bronchitis & emphysema), lung cancer, sleep
apnea, & tuberculosis
Chief Officer(s):
Scott McDonald, President & CEO
Kelly Ablog-Morrant, Director, Health Education & Program Services
Chris Lam, Manager, Development
Katrina van Bylandt, Manager, Communications
Debora Wong, Manager, Finance & Administration
Marissa McFadyen, Coordinator, Special Events
Publications:
• British Columbia Lung Association Annual Report
Type: Yearbook; *Frequency:* Annually
• Your Health [a publication of the British Columbia Lung Association]
Type: Magazine; *Frequency:* Semiannually; *Editor:* Katrina van Bylandt
Profile: Health information for medical & health promoters, educators,
donors to the Lung Association, & persons interested in
respiratoryhealth

British Columbia Society of Respiratory Therapists (BCSRT)
PO Box 4760, Vancouver BC V6B 4A4
Tel: 604-623-2227
www.bcsrt.ca
Overview: A medium-sized provincial organization founded in 1977
Mission: To represent the interests of the respiratory therapy
profession in British Columbia; To promote best practices within the
occupation; To uphold the British Columbia Society of Respiratory
Therapists Standards for Professional Conduct, Code of Ethics, &
Standards of Practice
Chief Officer(s):
Mike Giesbrecht, President
  preselect.bcsrt@gmail.com

TB Vets
1410 Kootenay St., Vancouver BC V5K 4R1
Tel: 604-874-5626
Toll-Free: 888-874-5626
e-mail: information@tbvets.org
www.tbvets.org
www.facebook.com/tbvets
twitter.com/tbvets
plus.google.com/115497261163706842951
Overview: A medium-sized provincial charitable organization founded
in 1945
Mission: Operates a key return service, with proceeds & donations
going to respiratory disease research, treatments & education; annually
sends out over 350,000 keytags to BC residents
Chief Officer(s):
Eric Beddis, Chair
Kanys Merola, Executive Director
Publications:
• TB Vets e-newsletter
Type: Newsletter; *Frequency:* Quarterly

MANITOBA

**Manitoba Association of Registered Respiratory Therapists,
Inc. (MARRT) / L'Association des thérapeutes respiratoires du
Manitoba, inc.**
#206, 629 McDermot Ave., Winnipeg MB R3A 1P6
Tel: 204-944-8081
www.marrt.org
Overview: A medium-sized provincial licensing organization founded in
1981
Affliation(s): Canadian Society of Respiratory Therapists
Chief Officer(s):
Cory Campbell, President
Shane McDonald, Registrar

Manitoba Lung Association
#301, 1 Wesley Ave., Winnipeg MB R3C 4C6
Tel: 204-774-5501
e-mail: info@mb.lung.ca
www.mb.lung.ca
www.facebook.com/manitobalungassociation
twitter.com/ManitobaLung
www.youtube.com/channel/UC3OyzjhurY-5KBPZvsG1G4Q

Overview: A small provincial charitable organization founded in 1904 overseen by Canadian Lung Association
Mission: To improve lung health
Member of: Sanatorium Board of Manitoba
Chief Officer(s):
Deborah Harri, Chair
Bill Pratt, President & CEO
Kathi Neal, Director, Fund Development
Malcolm Harwood, Coordinator, Finance
Tracy Fehr, Coordinator, Tobacco Reduction
Publications:
• Manitoba Lung Association Annual Report
Type: Yearbook; *Frequency:* Annually

Manitoba Tobacco Reduction Alliance
192 Goulet St., Winnipeg MB R2H 0R8
Tel: 204-784-7030; *Fax:* 204-784-7039
e-mail: info@mantrainc.ca
www.mantrainc.ca
Also Known As: ManTRA
Previous Name: Council for a Tobacco-Free Manitoba
Overview: A small provincial organization founded in 1977
Mission: To strive for a tobacco-free society for Manitobans; to encourage & support legislation to restrict smoking in public places & workplaces; to maintain awareness of the hazards of tobacco consumption to identified high-risk target groups
Member of: Canadian Council on Smoking & Health
Chief Officer(s):
Rick Lambert, Chair
Murray Gibson, Executive Director

NEW BRUNSWICK

The New Brunswick Association of Respiratory Therapists Inc. (NBART) / L'Association des thérapeutes respiratoires du Nouveau-Brunswick inc. (ATRNB)
500 St. George St., Moncton NB E1C 1Y3
Tel: 506-389-7813; *Fax:* 506-389-7814
Toll-Free: 877-334-1851
e-mail: info@nbart.ca
www.nbart.ca
www.facebook.com/nbartinfo
twitter.com/nbart_info
Overview: A medium-sized provincial organization founded in 1984 overseen by Canadian Society of Respiratory Therapists
Mission: To protect the public by ensuring that the respiratory therapists practicing in the province of New Brunswick deliver safe & ethical care
Chief Officer(s):
Pam Taylor, President
president@nbart.ca
Troy Denton, Registrar
registrar@nbart.ca
Publications:
• New Brunswick Association of Respiratory Therapists Membership Registry
Type: Directory
Profile: A listing of active, associate, & student members

New Brunswick Lung Association / Association pulmonaire du Nouveau-Brunswick
65 Brunswick St., Fredericton NB E3B 1G5
Tel: 506-455-8961; *Fax:* 506-462-0939
Toll-Free: 888-566-5864
e-mail: info@nb.lung.ca
www.nb.lung.ca
www.facebook.com/nblung
twitter.com/NBlung
Overview: A small provincial charitable organization overseen by Canadian Lung Association
Mission: To promote wellness throughout New Brunswick & prevent lung disease
Chief Officer(s):
Barbara MacKinnon, President & CEO
Ted Allingham, Director, Finance & Administration
Monica Brewer, Director, Fundraising & Donor Relations
Barbara Walls, Director, Health Initiatives

Liz Smith, Director, Public Education
Roshini Kassie, Director, Community Outreach Programs
Maggie Estey, Manager, Marketing & Development

NEWFOUNDLAND AND LABRADOR

Newfoundland & Labrador Association of Respiratory Therapists (NLART)
#133, Bldg. 50, Hamlyn Rd. Plaza, St. John's NL A1A 5X7
e-mail: nlarrt@gmail.com
www.nlart.ca
Overview: A medium-sized provincial organization overseen by Canadian Society of Respiratory Therapists
Mission: To improve & maintain the standards of respiratory care in Newfoundland & Labrador
Affliation(s): Canadian Society of Respiratory Therapists (CSRT)

Newfoundland & Labrador Lung Association (NLLA)
PO Box 13457, Stn. A, St. John's NL A1B 4B8
Tel: 709-726-4664; *Fax:* 709-726-2550
Toll-Free: 888-566-5864
e-mail: info@nf.lung.ca
www.nf.lung.ca
www.facebook.com/NLLung
twitter.com/nllung
Overview: A small provincial charitable organization founded in 1944 overseen by Canadian Lung Association
Mission: To achieve healthy breathing for the people of Newfoundland & Labrador
Chief Officer(s):
Greg Noel, President & CEO
greg.noel@nf.lung.ca
Publications:
• Newfoundland & Labrador Lung Association Newsletter
Type: Newsletter

NOVA SCOTIA

The Lung Association of Nova Scotia (LANS)
#200, 6331 Lady Hammond Rd., Halifax NS B3K 2S2
Tel: 902-443-8141; *Fax:* 902-445-2573
Toll-Free: 888-566-5864
e-mail: info@ns.lung.ca
www.ns.lung.ca
www.linkedin.com/company/the-lung-association-of-nova-scotia
www.facebook.com/LungNS
twitter.com/NSLung
www.youtube.com/LungNovaScotia
Overview: A small provincial charitable organization founded in 1909 overseen by Canadian Lung Association
Mission: To control & prevent lung disease in Nova Scotia; To help people who live with lung disease
Chief Officer(s):
Louis Brill, President & Chief Executive Officer, 902-443-8141 Ext. 22
louisbrill@ns.lung.ca
Robert MacDonald, Manager, Health Initiatives
robertmacdonald@ns.lung.ca
Maria Caines, Senior Manager, Finance
mariacaines@ns.lung.ca
Caitlin Gray, Manager, Communications & Special Events
caitlingray@ns.lung.ca
Lynette Hollett, Manager, Donor Relations
lynettehollett@ns.lung.ca
Sam Warshick, Senior Manager, Fund Development
samanthawarshick@ns.lung.ca

Nova Scotia College of Respiratory Therapists (NSCRT)
#1301, 1959 Upper Water St., Halifax NS B3J 3N2
Tel: 902-423-3229; *Fax:* 902-422-2388
e-mail: registrar@nscrt.com
www.nscrt.com
Overview: A small provincial organization founded in 2007
Mission: To serve as the regulatory body of respiratory therapy in Nova Scotia; To establish professional & ethical standards for respiratory therapy practice; To promote excellence & leadership in cardio-respiratory care practice
Chief Officer(s):

Shannon McDonald, Registrar
registrar@nscrt.com
Tara Planetta, Deputy Registrar
deputyregistrar@nscrt.com

ONTARIO

College of Respiratory Therapists of Ontario (CRTO)
#2103, 180 Dundas St. West, Toronto ON M5G 1Z8
Tel: 416-591-7800; *Fax:* 416-591-7890
Toll-Free: 800-261-0528
e-mail: questions@crto.on.ca
www.crto.on.ca
twitter.com/theCRTO
www.youtube.com/user/TheCRTO
Overview: A medium-sized provincial licensing organization
Mission: To regulate the profession of respiratory care in Ontario
Chief Officer(s):
David Jones, President

The Ontario Campaign for Action on Tobacco
c/o Ontario Medical Association, #900, 150 Bloor St. West, Toronto ON M5S 3C1
Tel: 416-340-2992; *Fax:* 416-340-2995
e-mail: ocat@oma.org
www.ocat.org
Overview: A small provincial organization founded in 1992
Mission: To secure the passage of Ontario's Tobacco Control Act (TCA)
Chief Officer(s):
Michael Perley, Director

Ontario Home Respiratory Services Association (OHRSA)
#600, 55 University Ave., Toronto ON M5J 2H7
Tel: 416-961-8001
www.ohrsa.ca
twitter.com/OHRSAOntario
Overview: A small provincial organization founded in 1985
Mission: To foster & promote an innovative & viable home respiratory services industry; To provide opportunities for future growth; To offer quality products & services through members
Member of: Ontario Health Providers Alliance
Chief Officer(s):
Shane Walsh, Chair
Al Benton, Secretary-Treasurer

Ontario Lung Association (OLA)
#401, 18 Wynford Dr., Toronto ON M3C 0K8
Tel: 416-864-9911; *Fax:* 416-864-9916
Toll-Free: 888-344-5864
e-mail: olalung@on.lung.ca
www.on.lung.ca
www.facebook.com/OntarioLungAssociation?ref=ts
twitter.com/OntarioLung
www.youtube.com/user/ONLungAssociation
Overview: A large provincial charitable organization founded in 1945 overseen by Canadian Lung Association
Mission: To provide lung health information & support to people affected by lung disease; To prevent & control chronic lung disease
Chief Officer(s):
John Granton, Chair
George Habib, President & Chief Executive Officer
John Martin, Treasurer
Publications:
• Asthma Action
Type: Newsletter
• Breathworks
Type: Newsletter
• Oxygen
Type: Newsletter
Profile: Lung health information, donor & research profiles, & forthcoming events

Belleville Office (Hastings & Prince Edward Counties)
#339, 110 North Front St. A3, Belleville ON K8P 0A6
Tel: 613-969-0323
www.on.lung.ca
Chief Officer(s):

Lola McMurter, Coordinator, Special Events
lmcmurter@on.lung.ca

Brantford Office (Brant County)
410 Colborne St., Lower Level, Brantford ON N3S 3N6
Tel: 519-753-4682; *Fax:* 519-753-4667
e-mail: brant@on.lung.ca
www.on.lung.ca

Hamilton Office (Hamilton, Brant County, Niagara, Haldimand & Norfolk Counties, & Waterloo & Wellington Regions)
#255, 245 King George St., Brantford ON N3R 7N7
Tel: 905-383-1616
Toll-Free: 800-790-5527
e-mail: hamilton@on.lung.ca
www.on.lung.ca

Kingston Office (Kingston & the Thousand Islands)
#339, 110 North Front St. A3, Belleville ON K8P 0A6
Tel: 613-545-3462
www.on.lung.ca
Chief Officer(s):
Lola McMurter, Coordinator, Volunteer & Fund Development
lmcmurter@on.lung.ca

London Office (Bluewater-Thames Valley)
#2, 639 Southdale Rd. East, London ON N6E 3M2
Tel: 519-453-9086; *Fax:* 519-453-9184
Chief Officer(s):
Lori Pallen, Regional Manager
lpallen@on.lung.ca

Ottawa Office (Ottawa, Renfrew County, & Cornwall Area)
#500, 2319 St. Laurent Blvd., Ottawa ON K1G 4J8
Tel: 613-230-4200; *Fax:* 613-230-5210
Chief Officer(s):
Melanie Estable-Porter, Officer, Corporate & Community Development
melanie@on.lung.ca

Sault Ste Marie Office (Algoma Area)
514 Queen St. East, 1st Fl., Sault Ste Marie ON P6A 2A1
Tel: 705-256-2335; *Fax:* 705-256-1210
Chief Officer(s):
Grace Briglio, Coordinator, Volunteer & Fund Development
gbriglio@on.lung.ca

Stratford Office (Huron-Perth)
#105, 356 Ontario St., Stratford ON N5A 7X6
Tel: 519-271-7500; *Fax:* 519-271-7503
Chief Officer(s):
Deedee Herman, Area Manager
dherman@on.lung.ca

Toronto Office (Greater Toronto Area West)
#401, 18 Wynford Dr., Toronto ON M3C 0K8
Fax: 416-864-9916
Toll-Free: 888-344-5864
e-mail: olalung@on.lung.ca

Windsor Office (Windsor-Essex & Chatham-Kent Area)
#210, 3041 Dougall Ave., Windsor ON N9E 1S3
Tel: 519-256-3433
Chief Officer(s):
Julie Bortolotti, Coordinator, Volunteer & Fund Development
jbortolotti@on.lung.ca
• Windsor-Essex & Chatham-Kent Area Breathworks Support Group Newsletter
Type: Newsletter; *Frequency:* Monthly
Profile: Support & advice for patients with COPD & their caregivers

Ontario Respiratory Care Society (ORCS)
#401, 18 Wynford Dr., Toronto ON M3C 0K8
Tel: 416-864-9911; *Fax:* 416-864-9916
e-mail: info@on.lung.ca
www.on.lung.ca
Overview: A medium-sized provincial charitable organization
Mission: To improve lung health through the provision of excellent interdisciplinary respiratory care
Chief Officer(s):
Bruce Cooke, Chair

George Habib, President & CEO
Publications:
• ORCS [Ontario Respiratory Care Society] Update
Type: Newsletter; *Frequency:* 3 pa; *Price:* Free with membership in the Ontario Respiratory Care Society
Profile: ORCS activities & respiratory articles
• Research Review [a joint publication of the Ontario Respiratory Care Society & the Ontario Thoracic Society]
 Frequency: Annually; *Price:* Free with membership in the Ontario Respiratory Care Society
Profile: Highlights of researchers & their studies
• RHEIG [Respiratory Health Educators Interest Group] Connections
 Frequency: 3 pa; *Price:* Free with membership in the Ontario Respiratory Care Society
Profile: Published by the Respiratory Health Educators Interest Group for members of the group

Ontario Thoracic Society (OTS)
c/o Ontario Lung Association, #401, 18 Wynford Dr., Toronto ON M3C 0K8

Tel: 416-864-9911
e-mail: olalung@on.lung.ca
www.on.lung.ca

Overview: A medium-sized provincial charitable organization founded in 1961
Mission: To promote respiratory health through medical research & education
Member of: Ontario Lung Association
Affiliation(s): Canadian Thoracic Society
Chief Officer(s):
Thomas Kovesi, Chair

Respiratory Therapy Society of Ontario (RTSO) / Société de la thérapie respiratoire de l'Ontario
#440, 160-2 Country Court Blvd., Brampton ON L6W 4V1

Tel: 647-729-2717; *Fax:* 647-729-2715
Toll-Free: 855-297-3089
e-mail: office@rtso.ca
www.rtso.ca

Overview: A medium-sized provincial organization founded in 1972 overseen by Canadian Society of Respiratory Therapists
Mission: To represent & advance the professional interests of Ontario's respiratory therapists; To develop & maintain standards of practice for respiratory therapy
Chief Officer(s):
Kyle Davies, President
Mike Keim, Treasurer
Publications:
• Airwaves
Type: Newsletter; *Price:* Free with RTSO membership
Profile: Society reports, events, & information plus articles

PRINCE EDWARD ISLAND

Prince Edward Island Lung Association
81 Prince St., Charlottetown PE C1A 4R3

Tel: 902-892-5957
Toll-Free: 888-566-5864
e-mail: info@pei.lung.ca
www.pei.lung.ca
www.facebook.com/196098560534899
twitter.com/PEI_Lung

Previous Name: PEI Tuberculosis League
Overview: A small provincial charitable organization founded in 1936 overseen by Canadian Lung Association
Mission: To improve the respiratory health of Islanders through education, advocacy & research; To raise funds to support medical research
Chief Officer(s):
Joanne Ings, Executive Director
jings@pei.lung.ca

QUÉBEC

Association des handicapés respiratoires de Québec
#204, 1001 rte de l'Église, Québec QC G1V 3V7

Tél: 418-657-2477; *Téléc:* 418-657-4823
Courriel: ahrq@videotron.ca
pages.videotron.com/ahrq1984

Aperçu: *Dimension:* petite; *Envergure:* provinciale
Mission: D'améliorer la qualité de vie des personnes aux prises avec une maladie respiratoire

Association des pneumologues de la province de Québec (APPQ)
CP 216, #3000, 2, Complexe Desjardins, Montréal QC H5B 1G8

Tél: 514-350-5117; *Téléc:* 514-350-5153
Courriel: appq@fmsq.org
www.fmsq.org

Aperçu: *Dimension:* petite; *Envergure:* provinciale surveillé par Fédération des médecins spécialistes du Québec
Mission: Promouvoir les intérêts professionnels et économiques de ses membres; se préoccuper du maintien de leur compétence; se prononcer sur les problématiques de la pneumologie dans les meilleurs intérêts de la population
Membre de: Fédération des médecins spécialistes du Québec
Membre(s) du bureau directeur:
Pierre Mayer, Président
Elsa Fournier, Directrice, Administration

Conseil québécois sur le tabac et la santé / Québec Council on Tobacco & Health
#302, 4126, rue St-Denis, Montréal QC H2W 2M5

Tél: 514-948-5317; *Téléc:* 514-948-4582
Courriel: info@cqts.qc.ca
www.cqts.qc.ca
twitter.com/cqts

Aperçu: *Dimension:* moyenne; *Envergure:* provinciale; Organisme sans but lucratif; fondée en 1976
Mission: Promouvoir la santé du fumeur et du non-fumeur; faire le lien entre les associations, groupes bénévoles et autres intéressés à la santé publique; trouver des approches et des moyens pour améliorer l'éducation face à l'usage du tabac
Membre de: Conseil canadien pour le contrôle du tabac
Membre(s) du bureau directeur:
Mario Bujold, Directeur général
Claire Harvey, Agente, Communications et relations médias

Ordre professionnel des inhalothérapeutes du Québec (OPIQ)
#721, 1440, rue Sainte-Catherine Ouest, Montréal QC H3G 1R8

Tél: 514-931-2900; *Téléc:* 514-931-3621
Ligne sans frais: 800-561-0029
Courriel: info@opiq.qc.ca
www.opiq.qc.ca
www.facebook.com/opiq.qc.ca
twitter.com/OPIQMEDSOC

Aperçu: *Dimension:* moyenne; *Envergure:* provinciale; Organisme sans but lucratif; fondée en 1969
Mission: Protection du public; surveillance de l'exercice professionnel de l'inhalothérapie
Affliation(s): Alliance nationale des organismes de réglementation de la thérapie respiratoire
Membre(s) du bureau directeur:
Jocelyn Vachon, Présidente
Josée Prud'Homme, Directrice générale et secrétaire

Québec Lung Association (QLA) / Association pulmonaire du Québec (APQ)
#104, 6070, rue Sherbrooke Est, Montréal QC H1N 1C1

Tel: 514-287-7400; *Fax:* 514-287-1978
Toll-Free: 888-768-6669
e-mail: info@pq.poumon.ca
www.pq.poumon.ca
www.facebook.com/poumon.qc
twitter.com/AssoPulmonaireQ
www.youtube.com/user/PoumonAPQ

Overview: A medium-sized provincial charitable organization founded in 1938 overseen by Canadian Lung Association
Mission: To provide resources in Québec about lung cancer, chronic obstructive pulmonary disease, sarcoidosis, tuberculosis, asthma,

chronic bronchitis, sleep apnea, pneumonia, & emphysema
Member of: World Health Organization; International Union against Tuberculosis & Lung Disease; American Lung Association; European Lung Association
Chief Officer(s):
Dominique Massie, Executive Director, 514-975-5382 Ext. 224
  dominique.massie@pq.poumon.ca
Raymond Jabbour, Chief Financial Officer & Director, Direct Marketing & Information Technology, 514-975-5382 Ext. 226
Mathieu Leroux, Admisor, Development & Communications,
  514-975-5382 Ext. 235
  mathieu.leroux@pq.poumon.ca
Publications:
• Le Bulletin de l'association pulmonaire du Québec
Type: Newsletter; *Editor:* Louis P. Brisson; *ISSN:* 0843-381X
Profile: Respiratory health information, plus donation news
• Le Rapport annuel de l'association pulmonaire du Québec
Type: Yearbook; *Frequency:* Annually

SASKATCHEWAN

Saskatchewan Coalition for Tobacco Reduction (SCTR)
1080 Winnipeg St., Regina SK S4R 8P8
Tel: 306-766-6327; *Fax:* 306-766-6945
Previous Name: Saskatchewan Interagency Council on Smoking & Health
Overview: A small provincial organization founded in 1975
Mission: To advocate, coordinate & educate to ensure a tobacco-free Saskatchewan for all its residents
Member of: Canadian Centre for Tobacco Control
Chief Officer(s):
Lynn Greaves, Contact
  sctr@rqhealth.ca

Saskatchewan Lung Association
Saskatoon Office, 1231 - 8 St. East, Saskatoon SK S7H 0S5
Tel: 306-343-9511; *Fax:* 306-343-7007
Toll-Free: 888-566-5864
e-mail: info@sk.lung.ca
www.sk.lung.ca
www.facebook.com/LungSask
twitter.com/lungsk
www.youtube.com/user/LungAssociation1
Previous Name: Saskatchewan Anti-Tuberculosis League
Overview: A medium-sized provincial charitable organization founded in 1911 overseen by Canadian Lung Association
Mission: To improve respiratory health & overall quality of life; To advocate for support of education & research
Chief Officer(s):
Pat Smith, Chair
Karen Davis, Vice-Chair
Brian Graham, President & CEO
Jennifer Miller, Vice-President, Health Promotion
Sharon Kremeniuk, Vice-President, Development
Melissa Leib, Vice-President, Finance & Operations
Donna Crooks, Treasurer
Publications:
• Breathworks: COPD Newsletter
Type: Newsletter
Profile: Educational articles plus notices of forthcoming support group meetings
• Lung Association of Saskatchewan Annual Report
Type: Yearbook; *Frequency:* Annually
• Nightly Nezzz Newsletter
Type: Newsletter; *Frequency:* Quarterly
Profile: Information for persons with sleep apnea & their families

Local Associations

ONTARIO

Smoking & Health Action Foundation
#221, 720 Spadina Ave., Toronto ON M5S 2T9
Tel: 416-928-2900; *Fax:* 416-928-1860
e-mail: toronto@nsra-adnf.ca
www.nsra-adnf.ca
twitter.com/nsra_adnf

Overview: A small local organization founded in 1974
Mission: To conduct public policy research & education designed to reduce tobacco-related disease & death
Chief Officer(s):
Lorraine Fry, Executive Director

International Associations

American Association for Thoracic Surgery (AARS)
#4550, 500 Cummings Center, Beverly MA 01915 USA
Tel: 978-927-8330; *Fax:* 978-524-0498
www.aats.org
www.facebook.com/AATS1917
twitter.com/AATSHQ
Overview: A medium-sized international organization founded in 1917
Mission: To promote scholarship & scientific research in thoracic & cardiovascular surgery
Chief Officer(s):
Thoralf M. Sundt, President
Publications:
• Journal of Thoracic & Cardiovascular Surgery
Type: Journal; *Editor:* Richard Weisel
Profile: Original articles about the chest, heart, lungs, & great vessels where surgical intervention is indicated
• Operative Techniques in Thoracic & Cardiovascular Surgery: A Comparative Atlas
 Editor: J. William Gaynor
Profile: Technique-based articles in cardiovascular & thoracic surgery by renowned surgeons in the field
• Pediatric Cardiac Surgery Annual
Type: Journal; *Frequency:* Annually; *Editor:* Robert D.B. Jaquiss
Profile: Developments in pediatric cardiac surgery
• Seminars in Thoracic & Cardiovascular Surgery
Type: Journal; *Editor:* Harvey Pass; Todd Rosengart
Profile: Topics & issues faced by practising surgeons in clinical practice
• Thoracic Surgery News
Type: Newspaper; *Frequency:* 10 pa; *Editor:* Michael Liptay
Profile: News of general thoracic surgery, adult cardiac surgery, transplantation, & congenital heart disease

American College of Chest Physicians (ACCP)
2595 Patriot Blvd., Glenview IL 60062-2348 USA
Tel: 224-521-9800; *Fax:* 224-521-9801
Toll-Free: 800-343-2227
www.chestnet.org
Overview: A medium-sized international organization founded in 1935
Mission: To improve cardiopulmonary health & critical care worldwide; To promote the prevention & treatment of diseases of the chest
Chief Officer(s):
Stephen J. Welch, Interim Chief Executive Officer
P. Stratton Davies, Chief Financial Officer & Sr. Vice-President
Jennifer Nemkovich, Chief Strategy Officer
Robert Musacchio, Senior Vice-President, Business Development
Nicole Augustyn, Senior Vice-President, Education
Sue Reimbold, Senior Vice-President, Marketing & Communications
Publications:
• ACCP [American College of Chest Physicians] Critical Care Medicine Board Review
 ISBN: 978-0-916609-76-4
Profile: Review chapters developed to complement the American College of Chest Physicians Critical Care Medicine Board Review course,directed toward an audience of physicians in critical care & pulmonary medicine, emergency departments, anesthesiology, & surgery, as well as nurses & respiratory therapists
• ACCP [American College of Chest Physicians] Pulmonary Medicine Board Review
 ISBN: 978-0-916609-77-1
Profile: A text covering current pulmonary literature & management strategies for critically ill patients, written for physicians & fellows incritical care pulmonary medicine, as well as advanced critical care nurse practitioners & respiratory therapy practitioners
• ACCP [American College of Chest Physicians] Sleep Medicine Board Review
 ISBN: 978-0-916609-75-7
Profile: Review chapters of major topics from the American College of Chest Physicians Sleep Medicine Board Review course, intended for

physiciansin sleep medicine, physicians in pulmonary medicine, neurologists, respiratory therapists, & nurses
• ACCP [American College of Chest Physicians] / AAP Pediatric Pulmonary Board Review
ISBN: 978-0-916609-85-6
Profile: Review chapters of major topics from the American College of Chest Physicians / American Academy of Pediatrics PediatricPulmonary Medicine Board Review course, of interest to pediatric pulmonologists, family physicians, pediatric intensivists, allergists, & general pediatricians
• CHEST [a publication of the American College of Chest Physicians]
Type: Journal; *Frequency:* Monthly; *Accepts Advertising*; *Editor:* Richard S. Irwin, MD, FCCP; *ISSN:* 0012-3692
Profile: Original research in the multidisciplinary specialties of chest medicine, of interest to specialists in pulmonology,critical care medicine, sleep medicine, thoracic surgery, cardiorespiratory interactions, & related specialists
• Chest Physician
Type: Newspaper; *Frequency:* Monthly; *Accepts Advertising*; *Editor:* Vera A. De Palo, MD, MBA, FCCP
Profile: News from chest medicine specialties, clinical information, American College of Chest Physicians activities, & updoming events

American Lung Association (ALA)
#1150, 55 West Wacker Dr., Chicago IL 60601 USA
Fax: 202-452-1805
Toll-Free: 800-586-4872
www.lungusa.org
www.facebook.com/lungusa
twitter.com/lungassociation
www.youtube.com/user/americanlung
Overview: A large international charitable organization founded in 1904
Mission: To prevent lung disease & promote lung health
Affliation(s): American Thoracic Society
Chief Officer(s):
Kathryn A. Forbes, Chair
Harold Wimmer, President & CEO

Canadian Thoracic Society (CTS) / Société canadienne de thoracologie (SCT)
c/o National Office, The Lung Association, #300, 1750 Courtwood Cres., Ottawa ON K2C 2B5
Tel: 613-569-6411; *Fax:* 613-569-8860
e-mail: ctsinfo@lung.ca
cts.lung.ca
Overview: A medium-sized international charitable organization founded in 1958 overseen by Canadian Lung Association
Mission: To enhance the prevention & treatment of respiratory diseases
Affliation(s): AllerGen; American College of Chest Physicians; American Thoracic Society; Canadian COPD Alliance; Canadian Respiratory Health Professionals; Canadian Society of Allergy & Clinical Immunology; European Respiratory Society; Guidelines International Network
Chief Officer(s):
Andrew Halayko, President
John Granton, Secretary
Catherine Lemière, Treasurer
Janet Sutherland, Executive Director
Publications:
• Canadian Thoracic Society Annual Report
Type: Yearbook; *Frequency:* Annually
• Canadian Thoracic Society E-Bulletin
Type: Newsletter
Profile: Updates for all members of the Society

International Primary Care Respiratory Group (IPCRG)
c/o Samantha Louw, PO Box 11961, Westhill AB32 9AE Scotland
Tel: 44-1224-743-753; *Fax:* 44-1224-743-753
e-mail: businessmanager@theipcrg.org
www.theipcrg.org
Overview: A medium-sized international organization
Mission: To represent international primary care perspectives in respiratory medicine; To raise standards of care worldwide
Chief Officer(s):

Siân Williams, Executive Officer
execofficer@theipcrg.org
Publications:
• Primary Care Respiratory Journal
Type: Journal
Profile: Original research papers, review, & discussion papers on respiratory conditions commonly found in primary & community settings in countries around the world

Society for Research on Nicotine & Tobacco (SNRT)
2424 American Lane, Madison WI 53704 USA
Tel: 608-443-2462; *Fax:* 608-443-2474
e-mail: info@srnt.org
www.srnt.org
Overview: A small international organization
Mission: To generate new knowledge about nicotine
Chief Officer(s):
Bruce Wheeler, Executive Director, 608-443-2462 Ext. 143
Dianne Benson, Financial Contact, 608-443-2462 Ext. 147
Publications:
• Nicotine & Tobacco Research: The Journal of SRNT [Society for Research on Nicotine & Tobacco]
Type: Journal; *Frequency:* Monthly; *ISSN:* 1462-2203
Profile: Peer reviewed articles about the study of nicotine & tobacco
• Society for Research on Nicotine & Tobacco Annual Meeting Abstracts
Type: Yearbook; *Frequency:* Annually
• SRNT [Society for Research on Nicotine & Tobacco] Newsletter
Type: Newsletter; *Editor:* Karen Cropsey
Profile: Current society information for members, featuring reviews, meetings, publications, position openings, & funding news
• SRNT [Society for Research on Nicotine & Tobacco] Membership Directory
Type: Directory

National Publications

Canadian Respiratory Journal
Owned By: Hindawi Publishing Corp.
#3070, 315 Madison Ave., New York, NY

crj@hindawi.com
Frequency: 8 times a year

Provincial Libraries

BC Lung Association
2675 Oak St., Vancouver, BC V6H 2K2
Tel: 604-731-5864; *Fax:* 604-731-5810
Toll-Free: 800-665-5864
info@bc.lung.ca
www.bc.lung.ca
Social Media: www.youtube.com/user/TheBCLungAssociation;
twitter.com/bclungassoc; www.facebook.com/BCLungAssociation
Profile: Material is provided free of charge to residents of British Columbia; materials can be mailed or picked up at the association's Vancouver office **Collection:** Material on lung health & air quality issues
Kelly Ablog-Morrant, Director, Health Education & Program Services

Institut universitaire de cariologie et de pneumologie de Québec
#Y2244, 2725, ch Sainte-Foy, Québec, QC G1V 4G5
Tél: 418-656-4563; *Téléc:* 418-656-4720
biblio@criucpq.ulaval.ca
iucpq.qc.ca/fr/enseignement/bibliotheque/heures-d-ouverture
Francine Aumont, Bibliothécaire
francine.aumont@criucpq.ulaval.ca
Julie Émond, Technicienne
Diane St-Pierre, Technicienne

New Brunswick Lung Association/ Association Pulmonaire du Nouveau-Brunswick
65 Brunswick St., Fredericton, NB E3B 1G5
Tel: 506-455-8961; *Fax:* 506-462-0939
Toll-Free: 888-566-5864
info@nb.lung.ca
www.nb.lung.ca
Barbara MacKinnon, President & CEO

Ontario Lung Association
#401, 18 Wynford Dr., Toronto, ON M3C 0K8
Tel: 416-864-9911; *Fax:* 416-864-9916
info@on.lung.ca
www.on.lung.ca
George Habib, President & CEO

Local Hospitals & Health Centres

BRITISH COLUMBIA

OLIVER: Oliver Cardiac Rehab Clinic
Affiliated with: Interior Health Authority
36003 - 79th St., Oliver, BC V0H 1T0
Tel: 250-770-5507
www.interiorhealth.ca

Note: Offers a 5-week supervised exercise program to improve lung & heart health

OSOYOOS: Osoyoos Cardiac Rehab Clinic
Affiliated with: Interior Health Authority
8505 - 68th Ave., Osoyoos, BC V0H 1V0
Tel: 250-770-5507
www.interiorhealth.ca

Note: Offers a 5-week supervised exercise program to improve lung & heart health

Lupus Erythematosus

Lupus erythematosus refers to two distinct but overlapping conditions. Systemic lupus erythematosus (SLE) is a chronic multi-organ inflammatory illness that may involve the brain, skin, kidneys, joints, bowel and eyes. It is the most common form of lupus. Discoid lupus erythematosus (DLE) is a much less serious disease that is limited to the skin. In DLE, patches of skin may turn red and develop white scales, followed by thinning and scarring. About 10 percent of patients with DLE will go on to develop SLE; roughly 25 percent of patients with SLE also have the manifestations of DLE.

Cause
Although the cause of lupus is unclear, research suggests that there could be genetic and hormonal factors involved. Environmental factors such as infection, stress, ultraviolet light and antibiotics may also act as triggers. In any case, SLE causes its damage through auto-immune mechanisms. The body's own immune system, designed to fight off invasion from micro-organisms, produces antibodies (called autoantibodies) that attack its own tissues and organs.

Symptoms
Symptoms of SLE include fatigue, fever, loss of appetite, nausea, weight loss, hair loss, skin rash, sensitivity to light (photophobia), joint pain, headaches, personality changes, eye irritation and mouth ulcers. In more severe cases, there may be kidney, lung, heart or neurological damage.

Prevalence
In Canada, around 15,000 people have SLE. Of SLE cases, 90 percent are women, and the disease usually develops between the ages of 15 and 44.

Treatment Options
Lupus is sometimes hard to diagnose because it can affect so many of the body's tissues and organs. For this reason, lupus is often called "the disease with a thousand faces." After taking a medical history and performing a physical exam, a physician will usually order a blood test to check for elevated levels of antinuclear antibodies. To confirm a diagnosis of SLE, four of the following criteria must also be present: butterfly rash on the face, skin rash, mouth ulcers, sensitivity to light, arthritis in two or more joints, kidney disorder, neurological disorder, immunological disorder, blood count abnormalities and serositis (inflammation of the lining around the heart, lungs or abdomen).

Since there is currently no cure for SLE, the aim of treatment is inflammation reduction and organ protection. Mild SLE symptoms are usually treated with anti-malarial agents and NSAIDs (non-steroidal anti-inflammatories). If there is more serious organ involvement, immunosuppressants are often prescribed. Corticosteroids may also be used when there is organ involvement, and to manage flare-ups of SLE. Some of these therapies may be associated with long-term complications.

In general, the course of SLE is chronic and relapsing, often with long periods (years) of remission. It may only be mild but can also progress toward more serious illness. Due to improved methods of diagnosis and treatment, most people with SLE now lead full lives and have a normal life expectancy.

National Associations

Canadian Network for Improved Outcomes in Systemic Lupus Erythematosus (CaNIOS)
Health Sciences Centre, #RR149, 800 Sherbrook St., Winnipeg MB R3A 1M4
Tel: 204-787-4734; *Fax:* 204-787-2475
www.canios.ca
www.facebook.com/CaniosRacple
twitter.com/Canios1
Overview: A medium-sized national organization founded in 1995
Mission: To allow Canadian researchers to address questions important to patients with lupus & their families
Chief Officer(s):
Christine Peschken, Chair
Publications:
• CaNIOSIn Touch: CaNIOS Research Participants Newsletter
Type: Newsletter; *Frequency:* Semiannually

Lupus Canada
#306, 615 Davis Dr., Newmarket ON L3Y 2R2
Tel: 905-235-1714
Toll-Free: 800-661-1468
e-mail: info@lupuscanada.org
www.lupuscanada.org
www.facebook.com/LupusCanada
twitter.com/lupuscanada
Overview: A medium-sized national charitable organization founded in 1987
Mission: To improve the lives of people living with lupus; To encourage cooperation among the lupus organizations in Canada
Chief Officer(s):
Tanya Carlton, President
Malcolm Gilroy, Vice-President
Patricia Morzenti, Treasurer
Leanne Mielczarek, Executive Director
leanne.mielczarek@lupuscanada.org

Provincial Associations

ALBERTA

Lupus Society of Alberta (LESA)
#202, 1055 - 20 Ave. NW, Calgary AB T2M 1E7
Tel: 403-228-7956; *Fax:* 403-228-7853
Toll-Free: 888-242-9182
e-mail: lupuslsa@shaw.ca
www.lupus.ab.ca
www.youtube.com/channel/UCAvO7nEVN3TdOzMo_pJif4Q
Overview: A small provincial charitable organization founded in 1973 overseen by Lupus Canada
Mission: To provide education & support on lupus issues & enable research to find a cure
Member of: Imagine Canada; Leave a Legacy Calgary; Volunteer Calgary
Chief Officer(s):
Mike Sewell, President
Rosemary E. Church, Executive Director

BRITISH COLUMBIA

British Columbia Lupus Society (BCLS)
#210, 888 West 8th Ave., Vancouver BC V5Z 3Y1
Tel: 604-714-5564
Toll-Free: 866-585-8787
e-mail: info@bclupus.org
www.bclupus.org
Also Known As: BC Lupus Society
Overview: A medium-sized provincial charitable organization founded in 1977 overseen by Lupus Canada
Mission: To provide education & support to Lupus patients & their friends & families; to increase public awareness of lupus
Chief Officer(s):
Josie Bradley, President

MANITOBA

Lupus Society of Manitoba
#105, 386 Broadway Ave., Winnipeg MB R3X 1G2
Tel: 204-942-6825; *Fax:* 204-942-4894
e-mail: lupus@mymts.net
www.lupusmanitoba.com
www.facebook.com/lupus.manitoba
Overview: A small provincial charitable organization founded in 1988 overseen by Lupus Canada
Mission: To provide support, encouragement & education to lupus patients & their families
Chief Officer(s):
Debbie Dohan, President

NEW BRUNSWICK

Lupus New Brunswick
#17, 55 Grant St., Moncton NB E1A 3R3
Tel: 506-384-6227
Toll-Free: 877-303-8080
e-mail: lupins@rogers.com
www.lupusnb.ca
Overview: A small provincial organization founded in 1986 overseen by Lupus Canada
Mission: To promote eduction & public awareness of lupus; To bring together lupus patients, friends, family, & other interested persons for a network of support
Member of: Lupus Canada
Chief Officer(s):
Nancy Votour, President

NEWFOUNDLAND AND LABRADOR

Lupus Newfoundland & Labrador
PO Box 8121, Stn. A, St. John's NL A1B 3M9
Tel: 709-368-8130
e-mail: lupus.nl.ca@gmail.com
www.envision.ca/webs/lupusnfldlab
Previous Name: Lupus Society of Newfoundland

Overview: A small provincial charitable organization overseen by Lupus Canada
Mission: To support individuals with lupus; to promote education & awareness of lupus; to support research & treatment of the disease

ONTARIO

Lupus Foundation of Ontario (LFO)
PO Box 687, 294 Ridge Rd. North, Ridgeway ON L0S 1N0
Tel: 905-894-4611; *Fax:* 905-894-4616
Toll-Free: 800-368-8377
e-mail: lupusont@vaxxine.com
www.vaxxine.com/lupus
Overview: A medium-sized provincial charitable organization founded in 1977 overseen by Lupus Canada
Mission: To serve the lupus patient community as a charitable organization
Chief Officer(s):
Laurie Kroeker, President

Lupus Ontario
#10, 25 Valleywood Dr., Toronto ON L3R 5L9
Tel: 905-415-1099; *Fax:* 905-415-9874
Toll-Free: 877-240-1099
e-mail: info@lupusontario.org
www.lupusontario.org
twitter.com/LupusON
Merged from: Ontario Lupus Association; Lupus Society of Hamilton
Overview: A medium-sized provincial charitable organization founded in 2004 overseen by Lupus Canada
Mission: To serve the needs of Lupus sufferers in Ontario
Member of: Lupus Canada
Chief Officer(s):
Linda Keill, President
Karen Furlotte, Office Manager & Coordinator
   kfurlotte@lupusontario.org

Kingston Branch
Kingston ON
Chief Officer(s):
Sherrill Ritchie, Contact

Kitchener Branch
Zehrs Laurentian, 750 Ottawa St. South, Kitchener ON N2E 1B6
Toll-Free: 877-240-1099

London Branch
London ON
e-mail: lupuslondononario@gmail.com

Mississauga/Oakville/Brampton/West Toronto Branch
Toronto ON
Toll-Free: 877-240-1099
Chief Officer(s):
Juanita Butler, Contact, Support Group
   jbutler@lupusontario.org

Ottawa Branch
Ottawa ON
Toll-Free: 877-240-1099
Chief Officer(s):
David Boal, Contact
   david.boal@sympatico.ca

Sudbury Branch
Sudbury ON
Tel: 705-280-0900
Chief Officer(s):
Ruth Tarvudd, Contact
   rtarvudd@gmail.com

Thunder Bay Branch
Thunder Bay ON
e-mail: info@lupusontario.org

Timmins Branch
Timmins ON
Tel: 705-268-5299; *Fax:* 877-240-1099
Chief Officer(s):

Juanita Butler, Contact, Support Group
jbutler@lupusontario.org

Windsor Branch
1395 Albert Rd., Windsor ON N8Y 3R1

Tel: 519-919-6717

Chief Officer(s):
Kevin Stannard, President
kevin.stannard@sympatico.ca

PRINCE EDWARD ISLAND

Lupus PEI
PO Box 23002, Charlottetown PE C1E 1Z6

Tel: 902-892-3875; Fax: 902-626-3585
Toll-Free: 800-661-1468
e-mail: info@lupuscanada.org
www.lupuscanada.org/pei

Overview: A small provincial organization founded in 1993 overseen by Lupus Canada
Mission: To promote public awareness of lupus on PEI, while offering support & educational materials to lupus patients, their families & friends.

SASKATCHEWAN

Lupus SK Society
c/o Royal University Hospital, PO Box 88, 103 Hospital Dr., Saskatoon SK S7N 0W8

Toll-Free: 877-566-6123
e-mail: lupus@lupussk.com
www.lupussk.com
www.facebook.com/Lupus-SK-254959414545218
twitter.com/Lupus_SK
www.youtube.com/user/sasklupus?

Overview: A small provincial charitable organization founded in 1981 overseen by Lupus Canada
Mission: To assist individuals affected by lupus by providing education, raising awareness, & supporting research
Chief Officer(s):
Tammy Hinds, First Vice-President
Katie Thompson, Secretary

Lymphatic Disorders

Lymphatic disorders are a classification of diseases that affect the lymphatic system's ability to function and protect the body from infection. Lymphatic diseases can be inherited or are a result of other diseases present in the body.

Cause
The lymphatic system plays a major role in the body as it clears away infection and keeps the body's fluids in balance. Three common lymphatic disorders are: lymphedema, lymphadenitis, and lymphoma. Lymphedema is caused by an accumulation of lymphatic fluid within the body, causing swelling of the arms and legs. Lymphedema can occur on its own or as a result of the surgical removal of lymph nodes, mainly due to cancer. Lymphadenitis, or lymphadenopathy, is caused by bacterial infection. The glands become enlarged due to swelling, often in response to bacteria, viruses, or fungi. Lymphoma is a type of blood cancer that begins in the lymph nodes and is caused by the body producing too many abnormal white blood cells (see Lymphoma for more details.)

Symptoms
Lymphedema symptoms include swelling of part or the entire arm or leg, including fingers or toes. Other signs include a feeling of heaviness or tightness, a restricted range of motion, aching or discomfort, recurring infections, and hardening and thickening of the skin.

Lymphadenitis is typically noticed when red, tender skin over a lymph node is discovered, along with swollen, tender, or hard lymph nodes. Lymph nodes may feel rubbery if an abscess has formed or they have become inflamed. Tender, swollen lymph nodes typically occur in the area where the infection originated, such as tonsillitis that causes the infection to move to the lymph nodes in the neck.

The most common symptom of lymphoma cancer is a painless swelling of a lymph node (see Lymphoma for more details.)

Prevalence
In Ontario, it is estimated that over 63,000 children and adults live with lymphedema. Up to one in four breast cancer survivors will develop lymphedema as a result of surgical lymph node removal.

In 2016, about 9,000 Canadians were estimated to be diagnosed with lymphoma, with 8,000 of these cases involving non-Hodgkin's lymphoma. Among cancers in Canada, lymphoma is the fifth most common.

Treatment Options
Lymphedema can be diagnosed during a physical examination for high-risk patients who have had their lymph nodes surgically removed. In other cases, imaging tests, such as a MRI, can confirm diagnosis. There is no cure for lymphedema. Treatment focuses on reducing swelling and controlling pain. It can include light exercise of the affected limb to help with lymph fluid drainage, bandage wrapping to encourage fluid to flow back toward the trunk of the body, and manual lymph drainage massages. The wearing of compression garments (long sleeves or stockings) and the use of a compression device (a pump connected to a sleeve on the arm) can aid the flow of the lymph fluid out of the affected limb.

Lymphadenitis is typically diagnosed during a physical examination that includes feeling the lymph nodes and looking for signs of injury or infection around any swollen nodes. A biopsy and culture of the affected area or node may show the cause of the inflammation. Blood cultures may reveal the spread of infection into the bloodstream. Treatment typically includes antibiotics to treat infection, painkillers, anti-inflammatory medications, and cool compresses to reduce inflammation and pain. Prompt antibiotic treatment usually leads to a complete recovery, although swelling may remain for months.

Lymphoma can be diagnosed by conducting a lymph node biopsy, a bone marrow aspiration and other biopsies. Traditional cancer treatments are used to treat lymphoma (see Lymphoma for details.)

National Associations

The Leukemia & Lymphoma Society of Canada (LLSC) / Société de leucémie et lymphome du Canada
#804, 2 Lansing Square, Toronto ON M2J 4P8

Tel: 416-661-9541; Fax: 416-661-7799
Toll-Free: 877-668-8326
e-mail: AdminCanada@lls.org
www.llscanada.org
www.linkedin.com/company/5127044
www.facebook.com/LeukemiaandLymphomaSocietyofCanada
twitter.com/llscanada
www.youtube.com/llscanada

Previous Name: Leukemia Research Fund of Canada
Overview: A medium-sized national charitable organization founded in 1955
Mission: To cure leukemia, lymphoma, Hodgkin's disease & myeloma, & to improve the quality of life of patients & their families
Affliation(s): Canadian Centre for Philanthropy
Chief Officer(s):
Shelagh Tippet-Fagyas, President
Ted Moroz, Chair

Atlantic Canada Branch
#H2, 1660 Hollis St., Halifax NS B3J 1V7
Tel: 902-422-5999
Toll-Free: 855-515-5572
www.llscanada.org/atlantic-region
www.facebook.com/llscatlantic
Chief Officer(s):
Joe DiPenta, Regional Director, 905-422-5999 Ext. 7520, Fax:
  902-422-5968
  joe.dipenta@lls.org

British Columbia/Yukon Branch
#303, 1401 West Broadway, Vancouver BC V6H 1H6
Tel: 604-733-2873
Toll-Free: 866-547-5433
Chief Officer(s):
Donna McLennan, Regional Director
  donna.mclennan@lls.org
Sharon Paulse, Manager, Patient Services
  sharon.paulse@lls.org
Scott Kehoe, Manager, Fund Development
  scott.kehoe@lls.org

Ontario Branch
#804, 2 Lansing Sq., Toronto ON M2J 4P8
Tel: 647-253-5530
Chief Officer(s):
Sandra Harris, Regional Director

Ontario Branch - Ottawa
#701, 116 Albert St., Ottawa ON K1P 5G3
Tel: 613-234-1274

Prairies/Territories Branch - Calgary
#316, 1212 31 Avenue NE, Calgary AB T2E 7S8
Tel: 403-263-5300
www.llscanada.org/prairies-region
Chief Officer(s):
Lauren Atkinson, Regional Director, Fax: 403-263-5303
  lauren.atkinson@lls.org

Prairies/Territories Branch - Edmonton
#208, 10240 - 124th St., Edmonton AB T5N 3W6
Tel: 780-758-4261

Prairies/Territories Branch - Saskatoon
#202, 402 - 21st St. East, Saskatoon SK S7K 0C3
Tel: 306-242-6611

Québec Branch
#602, 740, rue St-Maurice, Montréal QC H3C 1L5
Tel: 514-875-1000
Chief Officer(s):
Andy Fratino, Acting Regional Director
  andy.fratino@lls.org

Provincial Associations

BRITISH COLUMBIA

BC Lymphedema Association (BCLA)
PO Box 42603, Stn. Columbia Square, New Westminster BC V3M 6L7
Toll-Free: 866-991-2252
e-mail: info@bclymph.org
www.bclymph.org
Overview: A medium-sized provincial charitable organization founded
in 2006
Mission: To raise awareness about lymphedema; To represent &
support lymphedema patients
Chief Officer(s):
Lucette Wesley, President

QUÉBEC

**Association Québécoise du Lymphoedème (AQL) /
Lymphedema Association of Québec (LAQ)**
6565 St. Hubert, Montréal QC H2S 2M5
Tél: 514-979-2463
Courriel: aql@infolympho.ca
www.infolympho.ca
www.facebook.com/AQL.LAQ

Aperçu: *Dimension:* moyenne; *Envergure:* provinciale; Organisme
sans but lucratif

Mental Illness

Cause
Mental illness touches Canadians of all ages, backgrounds and
income levels. In fact, over the course of their lives, around 20
percent of people in Canada will be personally affected by a
mental health problem. Mental illness includes disorders of
mood, thinking and behaviour that cause emotional distress and
interfere with everyday living over extended periods of time. Psychiatry is the branch of medicine responsible for their study, diagnosis, treatment and prevention. Mental illness may be
determined by genetic, physical, chemical, psychological and
social factors.

Symptoms
Symptoms of mental illness can range from mild to severe, and
people can experience more than one mental health problem at
the same time. Mental or emotional illness includes such conditions as major depression, schizophrenia, bipolar disorder (also
called manic depression), panic and other anxiety disorders, substance abuse and dependence, and dementia and other cognitive disorders. Mental illness may have a significant impact on
education, employment, relationships and family life. People affected by a mental health problem may also have to deal with the
stigma and discrimination that are too often still attached to
mental illness.

Prevalence
In most cases, symptoms of mental illness first appear in adolescence or young adulthood. Mental illness affects more women
than men. In Canada, the most prevalent mental illness in adults
is anxiety disorders, followed by depression, however nearly 50
percent of those who suffer from these disorders have never consulted a physician about their anxiety or depression. It is estimated that mental illness costs the Canadian health care system
close to $8 billion per year.

Treatment Options
In Canada, psychiatric diagnoses generally are based on criteria
outlined in the Diagnostic and Statistical Manual of Mental Disorders (DSM), published by the American Psychiatric Association.
The fifth edition of DSM was published in May 2013. A number of
Canadian experts were among the 1,500 contributors to the
revised edition of the DSM.

Most mental illnesses can be treated. Depending on the specific
diagnosis, therapy can include medication, counselling, behaviour modification, psychotherapy, occupational therapy and modification of the patient's environment. Education about mental
health services and the support of self-help programs are important for people affected by mental illness, and their families.

At some point, all Canadians will be indirectly affected by mental
illness through a friend, family member or colleague. According to
the Canadian Alliance for Mental Illness and Mental Health
(CAMIMH), a critical first step in enhancing the mental health of
all people in Canada is to fight the stigma of mental illness, and
ensure that people affected by mental illness are protected from
discrimination. Public education will be the cornerstone in promoting improved acceptance and understanding of mental illness
in Canada.

See also Adjustment Disorders, Alcohol/Substance Abuse and
Dependence, Anxiety Disorders, Attention Deficit Hyperactivity
Disorder, Autism Spectrum Disorders, Child and Adolescent
Mental Health Issues, Cognitive Disorders, Conduct Disorder,

Dissociative Disorders, Eating Disorders, Gender Dysphoria, Gulf War Syndrome, Impulse Control Disorder, Mood Disorders, Personality Disorders, Perversions, Psychosomatic Disorders, Schizophrenia, Sexual Disorders, Sleep Disorders, Suicide, Tourette Syndrome

National Associations

Anxiety Disorders Association of Canada (ADAC) / Association Canadienne des Troubles Anxieux (ACTA)
PO Box 117, Stn. Cote-St-Luc, Montréal QC H4V 2Y3

Tel: 514-484-0504
Toll-Free: 888-223-2252
e-mail: contactus@anxietycanada.ca
www.anxietycanada.ca
twitter.com/anxietycanada

Overview: A medium-sized national charitable organization founded in 2002
Mission: To promote the prevention, treatment & management of anxiety disorders, & to improve the lives of people who suffer from them
Chief Officer(s):
Lynn Miller, President

L'Arche Canada
1280 Bernard Ave. West, Outremont QC H1H 1H1

Tel: 514-844-1661; *Fax:* 514-844-1960
e-mail: office@larche.ca
www.larche.ca

Overview: A medium-sized national charitable organization founded in 1969
Mission: To provide care & a sense of belonging for people who have developmental disabilities
Member of: L'Arche International

L'Arche Foundation
#300, 10271 Yonge St., Richmond Hill ON L4C 3B5

Tel: 905-770-7696; *Fax:* 905-884-4819
Toll-Free: 800-571-0212
e-mail: info@larchefoundation.ca
www.larchefoundation.ca
www.facebook.com/larchecanadafoundation
www.twitter.com/LArcheCanadaF1

Overview: A medium-sized national charitable organization overseen by L'Arche Canada
Mission: To raise money to support the activities of L'Arche Canada
Member of: L'Arche International
Chief Officer(s):
Gary Sim, President & CEO

Association des psychothérapeutes pastoraux du Canada (APPC) / Association of Pastoral Psychotherapists of Canada
892, rue Bernard Pilon, McMasterville QC J3G 5W8

Tél: 450-446-9058; *Téléc:* 450-446-9058
Aperçu: *Dimension:* petite; *Envergure:* nationale; fondée en 1985
Mission: Regrouper tous les psychothérapeutes pastoraux qui s'intéressent à la dimension pastorale en relation d'aide; assurer la spécificité de la psychothérapie pastorale afin d'empêcher tout empiètement dans les domaines connexes, et de sauvegarder ainsi l'autonomie de chaque profession concernée par la relation d'aide; veiller de manière efficace à la compétence vérifiée des psychothérapeutes pastoraux membres de l'Association pour éviter les dangers du charlatanisme; promouvoir la psychothérapie pastorale étant donnée son importance pour assurer le respect réel de la personne totale dans la relation d'aide

Canadian Academy of Child & Adolescent Psychiatry (CACAP) / Académie canadienne de psychiatrie de l'enfant et de l'adolescent
#701, 141 Laurier Ave. West, Ottawa ON KIP 5J3

Tel: 613-288-0408; *Fax:* 613-234-9857
e-mail: info@cacap-acpea.org
www.cacap-acpea.org

Previous Name: Canadian Academy of Child Psychiatry
Overview: A small national charitable organization founded in 1980

Mission: To advance the mental health of children, youth, & families; To promote the highest standards of patient care & service to children, youth, & families, incorporating a psychological, social, & biological approach
Chief Officer(s):
Wade Junek, President
Elizabeth Waite, Executive Director
Alexa Bagnell, Secretary-Treasurer
Publications:
• Journal of the Canadian Academy of Child & Adolescent Psychiatry
Type: Journal; *Frequency:* Quarterly; *Accepts Advertising*; *Editor:* Normand Carrey; *ISSN:* 1719-8429
Profile: Featuring original articles, clinical perspectives, & book reviews

Canadian Academy of Geriatric Psychiatry (CAGP) / L'Académie canadienne de psychiatrie gériatrique (ACPG)
#6, 20 Crown Steel Dr., Markham ON L3R 9X9

Tel: 905-415-3917; *Fax:* 905-415-0071
Toll-Free: 855-415-3917
e-mail: cagp@secretariatcentral.com
www.cagp.ca
www.facebook.com/CanadianAcademyofGeriatricPsychiatry

Overview: A small national organization
Mission: To promote mental health for elderly people in Canada
Member of: Council of Academies of the Canadian Psychiatric Association
Chief Officer(s):
Mark Rapoport, President
Maria Kardaris, Manager
Nancy Vasil, Co-Chair, Communications
Publications:
• CAGP [Canadian Academy of Geriatric Psychiatry] E-newsletter
Type: Newsletter; *Frequency:* Quarterly
Profile: CAGP reports, meetings, awards, & statistics
• Canadian Journal of Geriatric Medicine & Psychiatry
Type: Journal
Profile: Peer-reviewed original research on the health & care of older adults, co-sponsored by the Canadian Academy of Geriatric Psychiatry & the Canadian Geriatrics Society

Canadian Academy of Psychiatry & the Law (CAPL) / L'Académie canadienne de psychiatrie et droit (ACPD)
c/o Katie Hardy, Canadian Psychiatric Association, #701, 141 Laurier Ave. West, Ottawa ON K1P 5J3

Tel: 613-234-2815; *Fax:* 613-234-9857
e-mail: capl@cpa-apc.org
www.capl-acpd.org

Overview: A small national organization founded in 1995 overseen by Canadian Psychiatric Association
Mission: To advance the science & practice of forensic psychiatry; To promote high standards of patient care & professional practice; To address issues related to forensic psychiatry
Chief Officer(s):
Johann Brink, MB ChB, FCPsych, President
Brad Booth, MD, FRCPC, DABP, Secretary
Publications:
• CAPL [Canadian Academy of Psychiatry & the Law] Newsletter
Type: Newsletter
Profile: Review of meeting presentations for CAPL members

Canadian Alliance on Mental Illness & Mental Health (CAMIMH)
#702, 141 Laurier Ave. West, Ottawa ON K1P 5J3

Tel: 613-237-2144; *Fax:* 613-237-1674
www.facebook.com/FaceMentalIllness
twitter.com/miawcanada
www.flickr.com/photos/45033589@N02

Overview: A medium-sized national organization founded in 1998
Mission: An alliance of mental health organizations comprised of health care providers and organizations representing persons with mental illness and their families and caregivers.

Canadian Assembly of Narcotics Anonymous (CANA)
PO Box 812, Stn. Edmonton Main, Edmonton AB T5J 2L4

www.canaacna.org

Previous Name: Narcotics Anonymous
Overview: A small national organization founded in 1989
Mission: To help addicts who suffer from the disease of addiction

British Columbia Region
PO Box 1695, Stn. A, Vancouver BC V6C 2P7
Tel: 604-873-1018
www.bcrna.ca

Canada Atlantic Region
PO Box 26025, 407 Westmorland Rd., Saint John NB E2J 4M3
Toll-Free: 800-564-0228
e-mail: contact.us@carna.ca
www.carna.ca

Golden Triangle Area
#311, 23-500 Fairway Rd. South, Kitchener ON N2C 1X3
Tel: 519-651-1121
Toll-Free: 866-311-1611
www.gtascna.org

Hamilton Area
PO Box 57067, Stn. Jackson, 2 King St. West, Hamilton ON L8P 4W9
Tel: 905-522-0332; *Crisis Hot-Line:* 888-811-3887
www.nahamilton.org

Narcotiques Anonymes
5496 rue Notre-Dame est, Montréal QC H1N 2C4
Ligne sans frais: 855-544-6362
Courriel: info@naquebec.org
www.naquebec.org

Ontario Region
PO Box 5939, Stn. A, Toronto ON M5W 1P3
www.orscna.org

Canadian Association for Educational Psychology (CAEP) / L'association Canadienne en psychopedagogie (ACP)

C/O Nancy Perry, University Of British Columbia, 2125 Main Mall, Vancouver BC V6T 1Z4
Tel: 604-822-6410
caepacp.wordpress.com
www.facebook.com/CAEP.ACP

Overview: A small national organization founded in 1997
Mission: To research, discuss, & encourage the study of educational psychology
Member of: Canadian Society for Studies in Education
Chief Officer(s):
Sylvie Cartier, Co-President
sylvie.cartier@umontreal.ca
Deborah Butler, Co-President
deborah.butler@ubc.ca
Publications:
• Canadian Association for Educational Psychology Newsletter
Type: Newsletter; *Frequency:* Semiannually

Canadian Association for Sandplay Therapy (CAST)

c/o Dave Rogers, Treasurer, #232, 220 Century Rd., Spruce Grove AB T7X 3X7
www.sandplay.ca

Overview: A small national organization founded in 1993
Mission: To promote the development of sandplay in Canada by providing training, offering opportunities for professional exchange, and maintaining guidelines for professional practice.
Member of: International Society for Sandplay Therapy (ISST)
Chief Officer(s):
Barbara Dalziel, President

Canadian Association for Supported Employment (CASE)

c/o AiMHi, 950 Kerry St., Prince George BC V2M 5A3
Tel: 250-564-6408; *Fax:* 250-564-6801
www.supportedemployment.ca
www.facebook.com/CanadianAssocSupportedEmployment
twitter.com/casecanada

Overview: A medium-sized national organization
Mission: To promote workplace inclusion for Canadians with disabilities through supported employment
Chief Officer(s):
Tracy Williams, President

Canadian Coalition for Seniors Mental Health (CCSMH)

c/o Baycrest, West Wing, Old Hospital, #311, 3560 Bathurst St., Toronto ON M6A 2E1
Tel: 613-233-1619; *Fax:* 613-614-9450
www.ccsmh.ca
twitter.com/CCSMH

Overview: A small national organization founded in 2002
Mission: To promote the mental health of seniors by connecting people, ideas and resources.
Chief Officer(s):
Bonnie Schroeder, Executive Director
director@ccsmh.ca

Canadian Counselling & Psychotherapy Association (CCPA) / L'Association canadienne de counseling et de psychothérapie (ACCP)

#6, 203 Colonnade Rd. South, Ottawa ON K2E 7K3
Tel: 613-237-1099; *Fax:* 613-237-9786
Toll-Free: 877-765-5565
www.ccpa-accp.ca
www.facebook.com/CCPA.ACCP
twitter.com/ccpa_accp

Previous Name: Canadian Counselling Association
Overview: A medium-sized national organization founded in 1965
Mission: To enhance the counselling profession in Canada; To promote policies & practices which support the provision of accessible, competent, & accountable counselling services throughout the human lifespan, & in a manner sensitive to the pluralistic nature of society
Chief Officer(s):
Natasha Caverley, President
president@ccpa-accp.ca
Barbara MacCallum, Chief Executive Officer
bmaccallum@ccpa-accp.ca

Alberta & Northwest Territories Chapter
AB
Chief Officer(s):
Kathy Offet Gartner, President
president@abnwtchapter.ca

British Columbia Chapter
BC
www.ccpa-accp.ca/en/chapters/britishcolumbia
Chief Officer(s):
Paul Yeung, President

Career Development Chapter
www.ccpa-accp.ca/en/chapters/careercounsellors
Chief Officer(s):
Jessica Isenor, President
jisen010@uottawa.ca

Counsellor Educators Chapter
www.ccpa-accp.ca/en/chapters/counselloreducator
Chief Officer(s):
Patrice Keats, President

Creative Arts in Counselling Chapter
www.ccpa-accp.ca/en/chapters/creativeartsincounselling
Chief Officer(s):
Amy Mackenzie, President
amy.mackenzie@gmail.com

Indigenous Circle Chapter
www.ccpa-accp.ca/chapters/indigenous-circle
Chief Officer(s):
Jamie Warren, President
jwarrencounselling@gmail.com

National Capital Region Chapter
Ottawa ON
Chief Officer(s):
Nicholas Renaud, President
nicholas.renaud@gmail.com

Pastoral & Spiritual Care in Counselling Chapter
www.ccpa-accp.ca/en/chapters/pastoralspiritualcare
Chief Officer(s):
Gerard Vardy, President

Private Practitioners Chapter

www.ccpa-accp.ca/en/chapters/privatepractitioners
Chief Officer(s):
Corrine Hendricken-Eldershaw, President
  corrinealz@eastlink.ca

School Counsellors Chapter
www.ccpa-accp.ca/en/chapters/schoolcounsellors
Chief Officer(s):
Belinda Josephson, President
  gjosephson@eastlink.ca

Social Justice Chapter
www.ccpa-accp.ca/en/chapters/socialjustice
Chief Officer(s):
Linda Wheeldon, Chair
  linda.wheeldon@acadiau.ca
Andria Hill-Lehr, Chair
  andrialehr@yahoo.ca

Canadian Depression Research & Intervention Network (CDRIN)
c/o CDRIN Secretariat, Mood Disorders Society of Canada, #736, 304 Stone Rd. West, Guelph ON N1G 4W4
e-mail: info@cdrin.org
www.cdrin.org
www.linkedin.com/company/canadian-depression-research-and-intervention
www.facebook.com/CDRIN.org
twitter.com/CDRINorg
Overview: A medium-sized national organization founded in 2013
Mission: To create & share knowledge that leads to more effective prevention, early diagnosis, & treatment of depression, Post-Traumatic Stress Disorder, & related illnesses
Affiliation(s): Mood Disorders Society of Canada; Mental Health Commission of Canada
Chief Officer(s):
David Pilon, Chair
Zul Merali, Scientific Director
Phil Upshall, Officer

Canadian Federation of Mental Health Nurses (CFMHN) / Fédération canadienne des infirmières et infirmiers en santé mentale
#109, 1 Concorde Gate, Toronto ON M3C 3N6
Tel: 416-426-7029; *Fax:* 416-426-7280
www.cfmhn.ca
twitter.com/CFMHN
Overview: A medium-sized national organization
Mission: To serve as the voice of psychiatric & mental health (PMH) nursing; To develop & implement standards of psychiatric & mental health nursing practice; To address mental health issues; To examine government policy; To work with national or international groups with similar professional interests; To provide educational & networking resources for members
Affiliation(s): Canadian Nurses Association
Chief Officer(s):
Florence Budden, President
Doug Rosser, General Manager
  drosser@firststageinc.com

Canadian Group Psychotherapy Association (CGPA)
c/o First Stage Enterprises, #109, 1 Corcorde Gate, Toronto ON M3C 3N6
Tel: 416-426-7229; *Fax:* 416-726-7280
Toll-Free: 866-433-9695
e-mail: admin@cgpa.ca
www.cgpa.ca
www.linkedin.com/company/5054194
twitter.com/National_CGPA
Overview: A small national organization founded in 1990
Mission: To promote excellence in standards of training, practice, & research; To encourage & provide for the education of mental health professionals in group psychotherapy
Member of: International Association for Group Psychotherapy & Group Processes (IAGP)
Chief Officer(s):
Joan-Dianne Smith, President
Colleen Wilkie, Secretary

Jessica Kerr, Contact
Publications:
• The Chronicle: The Newsletter of the Canadian Group Psychotherapy Association
Type: Newsletter; *Editor:* Colleen Wilkie, PhD
Profile: Articles, committee reports, section news, & Canadian Group Psychotherapy Foundation news

Canadian Institute for Child & Adolescent Psychoanalytic Psychotherapy (CICAPP)
17 Saddletree Trail, Brampton ON L6X 4M5
Tel: 416-690-5464; *Fax:* 416-690-2746
e-mail: info@cicapp.ca
www.cicapp.ca
Previous Name: Toronto Child Psychoanalytic Program
Overview: A small national organization founded in 1981
Mission: To provide training in psychodynamic child therapy; to foster the growth of the profession in Canada; to have input in shaping government policies; to promote ongoing research in child psychotherapy
Chief Officer(s):
Suzanne Pearen, Administrator
  suzanne_pearen@rogers.com

Canadian Institute of Stress (CIS)
Toronto ON
Tel: 416-236-4218
e-mail: info@stresscanada.org
www.stresscanada.org
www.facebook.com/TheCanadianInstituteOfStress
Overview: A small national organization founded in 1979
Mission: To provide programs & tools for individuals & workplaces to handle stress
Chief Officer(s):
Richard Earle, Managing Director
  earle@stresscanada.org

Canadian Positive Psychology Association (CAPPA)
#703, 1 Eglinton Ave. East, Toronto ON M4P 3A1
Tel: 416-481-8930
e-mail: info@positivepsychologycanada.com
www.positivepsychologycanada.com
Overview: A small national organization
Mission: A representative association for scholars and academics who are engaged in rigorous academic research in the field of positive psychology.
Chief Officer(s):
Louisa Jewell, President

Canadian Psychiatric Association (CPA) / Association des psychiatres du Canada
#701, 141 Laurier Ave. West, Ottawa ON K1P 5J3
Tel: 613-234-2815; *Fax:* 613-234-9857
Toll-Free: 800-267-1555
e-mail: cpa@cpa-apc.org
www.cpa-apc.org
Overview: A medium-sized national organization founded in 1951
Mission: To forge a strong, collective voice for Canadian psychiatrists & to promote an environment that fosters excellence in the provision of clinical care, education & research
Affliation(s): Canadian Medical Association; World Psychiatric Association
Chief Officer(s):
Glenn Brimacombe, Chief Executive Officer
  gbrimacombe@cpa-apc.org
Brenda Fudge, Director, Finance & Administration
  bfudge@cpa-apc,org
Katie Hardy, Director, Professional & Membership Services
  khardy@cpa-apc.org
Jadranka Bacic, Associate Director, Communications
  jbacic@cpa-apc.org

Canadian Psychoanalytic Society (CPS) / Société canadienne de psychanalyse (SCP)
7000 Côte-des-Neiges Chemin, Montréal QC H3S 2C1
Tel: 514-738-6105
www.psychoanalysis.ca

Overview: A small national licensing organization founded in 1967
Mission: To promote psychoanalysis treatments & professionals
Affiliation(s): International Psychoanalytic Association
Chief Officer(s):
Andrew Brook, President

CPS Western Canadian Branch
c/o Nancy Briones, 7755 Yukon St., Vancouver BC V5X 2Y4
e-mail: info1@wbcps.org
www.wbcps.org

Chief Officer(s):
David Heilbrunn, President

Ottawa Psychoanalytic Society
c/o Somerset Psychologists, #201, 125 Somerset St. West, Ottawa ON K2P 0H7
Tel: 613-236-5608
e-mail: contact@ottawaps.ca
ottawaps.ca
www.facebook.com/OttawaPsychoanalyticSociety

Chief Officer(s):
Arthur Leonoff, Director

Québec English Branch
7000, ch Côte des Neiges, Montréal QC H3S 2C1
Tel: 514-342-7444; *Fax:* 514-342-1062
e-mail: cpsqeb@qc.aira.com
www.psychoanalysismontreal.com

Chief Officer(s):
Erica Robertson, President

Société psychanalytique de Montréal
7000, ch de la Côte-des-Neiges, Montréal QC H3S 2C1
Tél: 514-342-5208; *Téléc:* 514-342-9990
Courriel: spsymtl@qc.aira.com
www.psychanalysemontreal.org

Chief Officer(s):
Louis Brunet, Président

Société psychanalytique de Québec
1180, rue Charles-Albanel, Sainte-Foy QC G1X 4T9
Tél: 418-877-8445; *Téléc:* 418-877-7056
Courriel: info@spq-scp.ca
www.spq-scp.ca

South Western Ontario Psychoanalytic Society
London ON

Toronto Psychoanalytic Society
#203, 40 St. Clair Ave. East, Toronto ON M4T 1M9
Tel: 416-922-7770; *Fax:* 416-922-9988
torontopsychoanalysis.com
www.facebook.com/TorontoPsychoanalyticSociety

Chief Officer(s):
Rukhsana Bukhari, President

Canadian Psychological Association (CPA) / Société canadienne de psychologie (SCP)

#702, 141 Laurier Ave. West, Ottawa ON K1P 5J3
Tel: 613-237-2144; *Fax:* 613-237-1674
Toll-Free: 888-472-0657
e-mail: cpa@cpa.ca
www.cpa.ca
www.facebook.com/146082642130174
twitter.com/CPA_SCP
www.youtube.com/user/CPAVideoChannel

Overview: A medium-sized national organization founded in 1939
Mission: To improve the health & welfare of Canadians by promoting psychological research, education, & practice
Affiliation(s): Canadian Register of Health Service Providers in Psychology; Council of Provincial Associations of Psychologists; International Union of Psychological Science; Canadian Federation for the Humanities & Social Sciences
Chief Officer(s):
Karen R. Cohen, Chief Executive Officer, 613-237-2144 Ext. 323
executiveoffice@cpa.ca
Lisa Votta-Bleeker, Deputy CEO & Director, Science Directorate, 613-237-2144 Ext. 323
executiveoffice@cpa.ca

Phil Bolger, Chief Financial Officer, 613-237-2144 Ext. 329
pbolger@cpa.ca
Rozen Alex, Director, Practice Directorate, 613-237-2144 Ext. 334
practicedirectorate@cpa.ca
Seán Kelly, Director, Events, Membership & Association Development, 613-237-2144 Ext. 335
skelly@cpa.ca
Publications:
• Canadian Journal of Behavioural Science / La revue canadienne des sciences du comportement
Type: Journal; *Frequency:* Quarterly; *Accepts Advertising*; *Editor:* Todd Morrison; *Price:* $119 + GST/HST individuals in Canada; $289.00 + GST/HSTinstitutions in Canada
Profile: Original, empirical articles in the following areas of psychology:abnormal, behavioural, community, counselling, educational, environmental, developmental, health, industrial-organizational, clinical neuropsychological, personality, psychometrics, & social
• The Canadian Journal of Experimental Psychology
Type: Journal; *Frequency:* Quarterly; *Accepts Advertising*; *Editor:* Doug J. Mewhort; *ISSN:* 0008-4255; *Price:* $119 + GST/HST individuals in Canada; $289.00 + GST/HST institutions in Canada
Profile: A journal of original research papers from the field of experimental psychology, published in partnershipwith the American Psychological Association
• Canadian Psychology
Type: Journal; *Frequency:* Quarterly; *Accepts Advertising*; *Editor:* Martin Drapeau, Ph.D.; *Price:* $119 + GST/HST individuals in Canada; $289.00 + GST/HST institutions inCanada
Profile: Generalist articles in areas of theory, research, & practice
• CPA [Canadian Psychological Association] News
Type: Newsletter; *Price:* Free with membership in the Canadian Psycological Association
Profile: Current information for members
• Psynopsis: Canada's Psychology Magazine
Type: Magazine; *Frequency:* Quarterly; *Accepts Advertising*; *Editor:* Karen R. Cohen; *ISSN:* 1187-11809
Profile: Articles of interest to scientists, educators, & practitioners in psychology

Canadian Society for Brain, Behaviour & Cognitive Science (CSBBCS) / Société Canadienne des Sciences du Cerveau, du Comportement et de la Cognition

c/o Dept. of Psychology, University of British Columbia, Vancouver BC V6T 1Z4
e-mail: secretary@csbbcs.org
www.csbbcs.org

Overview: A small national organization
Mission: To advance Canadian research in experimental psychology & behavioral neuroscience
Member of: National Consortium of Scientific & Educational Societies
Chief Officer(s):
Penny Pexman, President
Peter Graf, Secretary-Treasurer

Child Development Institute (CDI)

197 Euclid Ave., Toronto ON M6J 2J8
Tel: 416-603-1827; *Fax:* 416-603-6655
e-mail: info@childdevelop.ca
www.childdevelop.ca
ca.linkedin.com/company/child-development-institute
www.facebook.com/childdevelop
twitter.com/officialcdi
www.youtube.com/user/CDICanada

Overview: A medium-sized international charitable organization
Mission: An accredited children's mental health agency that develops innovative programming for children ages 0-12 and youth ages 13-18 and their families in the areas of Early Intervention Services, Family Violence Services and Healthy Child Development.
Chief Officer(s):
Tony Diniz, Chief Executive Officer
tdiniz@childdevelop.ca
Shauna Klein, Director, Fund Development, Marketing and Communications
sklein@childdevelop.ca

Children and Youth in Challenging Contexts Network (CYCC)
PO Box 15000, 6420 Coburg Rd., Halifax ON B3H 4R2

Tel: 902-494-4087
cyccnetwork.org
www.facebook.com/CYCCNetwork
twitter.com/CYCCNetwork
www.youtube.com/user/cyccnetwork

Overview: A medium-sized national organization
Mission: The CYCC Network is a knowledge mobilization network that was created to improve mental health and well-being for vulnerable and at-risk children and youth in Canada.
Chief Officer(s):
Lisa Lachance, Executive Director
  lisa.lachance@dal.ca

General Practice Psychotherapy Association (GPPA)
312 Oakwood Ct., Newmarket ON L3Y 3C8

Tel: 416-410-6644; *Fax:* 866-328-7974
e-mail: info@gppaonline.ca
www.gppaonline.ca

Overview: A small national organization founded in 1984
Mission: To support & encourage quality psychotherapy by physicians in Canada; To promote professional development through ongoing education & collegial interaction
Chief Officer(s):
Carol Ford, Manager

Goodwill, The Amity Group
225 King William St., Hamilton ON L8R 1B1

Tel: 905-526-8482
www.goodwillonline.ca
www.facebook.com/GoodwillCareerCentre
twitter.com/JobsGoodwill
www.youtube.com/GoodwillIntl

Previous Name: Amity Goodwill Industries
Overview: A medium-sized national organization founded in 1935
Mission: To enrich the community by providing vocational rehabilitation programs & services to assist people challenged by disabilities & special needs to achieve maximum employment, community participation & self-fulfillment
Affliation(s): Canadian Association of Goodwill Industries; Goodwill Industries International
Chief Officer(s):
Tim Dobbie, Chair
Paul Chapin, President & CEO, 905-526-8482 Ext. 2222
Albert Deveau, Vice-President, Retail & Donated Goods Operations,
  905-875-3533
Publications:
• Goodwill, The Amity Group Newsletter
Type: Newsletter

Healthy Minds Canada
#300, 1920 Yonge St., Toronto ON M4S 3E2

Tel: 416-351-7757
Toll-Free: 800-915-2773
e-mail: admin@healthymindscanada.ca
www.healthymindscanada.ca
www.linkedin.com/company/healthy-minds-canada
www.facebook.com/healthymindscanada
twitter.com/Healthy_Minds
www.instagram.com/healthymindscanada

Overview: A medium-sized national charitable organization founded in 1980
Mission: To support & enhance the well-being of individuals with mental health issues & addictions; To emphasize the value of mental health to society
Chief Officer(s):
Katie Robinette, Executive Director
  krobinette@healthymindscanada.ca
Chelsea Ricchio, Manager, Communications
  chelsea@healthymindscanada.ca
Publications:
• Healthy Minds Canada Annual Report
Type: Yearbook; *Frequency:* Annually
• HMC [Healthy Minds Canada] Newsletter
Type: Newsletter; *Editor:* Chelsea Ricchio

• When Something's Wrong: Ideas for Families
Type: Handbook
Profile: For parents & caregivers to help children
• When Something's Wrong: Strategies for the Workplace
Type: Handbook
Profile: For employers, human resource personnel, managers, disability management providers, occupational health & safety personnel, union representatives, & employees
• When Something's Wrong: Strategies for Teachers
Type: Handbook
Profile: For elementary & secondary school teachers & administrators

Jack.org
#505, 192 Spadina Ave., Toronto ON MST 2C2

Tel: 416-425-2494
www.jack.org
www.facebook.com/jackdotorg
twitter.com/jackdotorg
www.instagram.com/jackdotorg

Overview: A medium-sized national charitable organization
Mission: To eliminate the stigmatization of mental illness; To enhance the lives of young people through programs, initiatives & outreach
Chief Officer(s):
Eric Windeler, Executive Director

KickStart Disability Arts & Culture
PO Box 2749, Stn. Terminal, Vancouver BC V6B 3X2

Tel: 604-559-6626
e-mail: info@kickstart-arts.ca
www.kickstart-arts.ca
www.facebook.com/318968627521

Previous Name: Society for Disability Arts & Culture
Overview: A small national organization founded in 1998
Mission: Kickstart's mission is to produce and present works by artists with disabilities and to promote artistic excellence among artists with disabilities working in a variety of disciplines.
Chief Officer(s):
Nisse Gustafson, Operations Director
Emma Kivisild, Artistic Director

National Network for Mental Health (NNMH)
#604, 55 King St., St Catharines ON L2R 3H5

Tel: 905-682-2423; *Fax:* 905-682-7469
Toll-Free: 888-406-4663
e-mail: info@nnmh.ca
www.nnmh.ca
www.facebook.com/pages/National-Network-for-Mental-Health/525630
59509
twitter.com/NNMH_RNSM

Overview: A small national organization founded in 1992
Mission: To advocate, educate & provide expertise & resources for the increased health & well-being of the Canadian mental health consumer/survivor community
Chief Officer(s):
Julie L. Flatt, Executive Director
Jean Beckett, President

The Organization for Bipolar Affective Disorder (OBAD)
1019 - 7th Ave. SW, Calgary AB T2P 1A8

Tel: 403-263-7408
Toll-Free: 866-263-7408
e-mail: obad@obad.ca
www.obad.ca

Overview: A medium-sized national charitable organization
Mission: To assist people affected directly or indirectly by bipolar disorder, depression, & anxiety
Chief Officer(s):
Kaj Korvela, Executive Director

Partners For Mental Health
#1100, 151 Slater St., Ottawa ON K1P 5H3

Tel: 613-798-5862; *Fax:* 613-683-3760
e-mail: info@partnersformh.ca
www.partnersformh.ca
www.facebook.com/partnersformh
twitter.com/partnersformh
www.youtube.com/partnersformh

Overview: A small national charitable organization founded in 2007

Mission: Partners for Mental Health is a national charity that aims to improve mental health in Canada by mobilizing and engaging Canadians to drive fundamental changes.
Chief Officer(s):
Jeff Moat, President, 613-683-3743
  jmoat@partnersformh.ca

Psychosocial Rehabilitation Canada / Réadaptation Psychosociale Canada (RPS)
PO Box 13060, 140 Holland St. West, Bradford ON L3Z 2Y5
Fax: 705-456-9786
Toll-Free: 866-655-8548
e-mail: registrar@psrrpscanada.ca
www.psrrpscanada.ca

Also Known As: PSR Canada/RPS Canada
Overview: A small national organization founded in 2002
Mission: To achieve full community participation of persons with mental health issues; To promote the principles & practice of psychosocial rehabilitation through practice standards, education, quality, outcome measures, advocacy & public policy
Affiliation(s): International Association of Psychosocial Rehabilitation Services; Ontario Federation of Community Mental Health & Addictions Programs; Association québécoise pour la readaptation psychosociale; Psychosocial Rehabilitation Manitoba, BC, Atlantic Region, Ont.
Chief Officer(s):
John Higenbottam, President
Sue Carr, Vice-President
Dorothy Edem, Secretary

Rehtaeh Parsons Society
NS
rehtaehparsons.ca
www.facebook.com/angelrehtaehofficial
twitter.com/angelrehtaeh

Overview: A small national organization founded in 2014
Mission: To prevent sexual assault & cyber-harassment; to raise awareness of suicide & mental health; to support victims & engage in public education of healthy relationships
Chief Officer(s):
Glen Canning, Co-founder
Leah Parsons, Co-founder

Vocational Rehabilitation Association of Canada (VRA Canada)
PO Box 370, #3, 247 Barr St., Renfrew ON K7V 1J6
Fax: 613-432-6840
Toll-Free: 888-876-9992
www.vracanada.com
www.facebook.com/VRACanada
twitter.com/VRACanada

Previous Name: Canadian Association of Rehabilitation Professionals Inc.
Overview: A small national organization founded in 1970
Mission: To support members in promoting & providing vocational & pre-vocational rehabilitation services
Member of: Commission on Rehabilitation Counselor Certification
Affiliation(s): Canadian Association for Vocational Evaluation & Work Adjustment
Chief Officer(s):
Tricia Gueulette, President

Alberta Society
Calgary AB
e-mail: vrac.ab@gmail.com

Chief Officer(s):
Shelley Langstaff, President

Atlantic Society
PO Box 757, 14 Weymouth Street, Charlottetown PE C1A 7L7
Tel: 902-569-7730; *Fax:* 902-368-6359
e-mail: amaxwell@wcb.pe.ca
www.vraatlantic.com

Chief Officer(s):
Ann Maxwell, BBA, RRP, President

Manitoba Society

VRAC Manitoba, c/o 299 Truro Street, Winnipeg MB R3J 2A2
Tel: 204-799-8842
e-mail: kerrihiebert@mts.net
vracanada.com/manitoba.php

Chief Officer(s):
Kerri Hiebert, Contact

Ontario Society
#200, 411 Richmond St. East, Toronto ON M5A 3S5
Tel: 647-875-8046
e-mail: office@vracanadaon.com
www.vracanadaon.com

Chief Officer(s):
Ravi Persaud, President

Saskatchewan Society
1440 Broadway Ave., Regina SK S4P 1E2
Tel: 306-522-8571

Chief Officer(s):
Rhonda Teichreb, Contact

Provincial Associations

ALBERTA

Ability Society of Alberta (ASA)
#302, 327 - 41 Ave. NE, Calgary AB T2E 2N4
Tel: 403-262-9445; *Fax:* 403-262-4539
www.abilitysociety.org
www.linkedin.com/in/abilitysociety
www.facebook.com/AbilitySociety
twitter.com/AbilitySociety
plus.google.com/114873957698483644364

Previous Name: Society for Technology & Rehabilitation
Overview: A medium-sized provincial charitable organization founded in 1984
Mission: To build a caring community; to provide innovative, appropriate, & needed technical aids to individuals with any type of disability, seniors, their families, & support systems; to provide access to technology that is used as a tool by a person with a disability to live with dignity
Chief Officer(s):
Adrian Bohach, President/CEO
  adrian@abilitysociety.org

Alberta Alliance on Mental Illness & Mental Health
Capital Place, #320, 9707 - 110 St., Edmonton AB T5K 2L9
Tel: 780-482-4993; *Fax:* 780-482-6348
www.aamimh.ca

Overview: A small provincial organization
Mission: To act as a voice for the mental health & mental illness community; To ensure mental health & mental illness issues are prominent on health & social policy agendas in Alberta
Chief Officer(s):
Orrin Lyseng, Executive Director
  executivedirector@aamimh.ca

Alberta Association of Rehabilitation Centres (AARC)
#19, 3220 - 5 Ave. NE, Calgary AB T2A 5N1
Tel: 403-250-9495; *Fax:* 403-291-9864
e-mail: acds@acds.ca
www.acds.ca

Overview: A medium-sized provincial organization founded in 1972
Mission: To support organizations that provide services & supports to people with disabilities; To act as a voice for the field of community rehabilitation to the political & administrative arms of government; To focus on human resource initiatives for the services sector; To provide in-service training opportunities for people employed in the field; To accredit & certify service in Alberta
Chief Officer(s):
Ann Nicol, CEO, 403-250-9495 Ext. 238
Helen Ficocelli, President
Bob Diewold, Vice-President

Alberta Psychiatric Association (APA)
#400, 1040 - 7 Ave. SW, Calgary AB T2P 3G9
Tel: 403-244-4487; *Fax:* 403-244-2340
e-mail: info@albertapsych.org
www.albertapsych.org

Overview: A small provincial organization
Affiliation(s): Canadian Psychiatric Association
Chief Officer(s):
Thomas Raedler, President

L'Arche Western Region
307 - 57 Ave. SW, Calgary AB T2H 2T6
Tél: 403-571-0155; *Téléc:* 403-255-1354
Aperçu: *Dimension:* moyenne; *Envergure:* provinciale; Organisme sans but lucratif surveillé par L'Arche Canada
Mission: Regional office contact information for the communities of L'Arche in Western Canada
Membre de: L'Arche International
Membre(s) du bureau directeur:
Pat Favaro, Regional Coordinator
pfavaro@larchecalgary.org

L'Arche Calgary
307 - 57th Ave. SW, Calgary AB T2H 2T6
Tel: 403-571-0155; *Fax:* 403-255-1354
e-mail: office@larchecalgary.org
www.larchecalgary.org
www.facebook.com/pages/LArche-Calgary/117157234970135
twitter.com/larchecalgary
www.pinterest.com/larchecalgary
Membre(s) du bureau directeur:
Garth Reesor, Community Leader
GReesor@larchecalgary.org

L'Arche Comox Valley
1225C England Ave., Courtenay BC V9N 2P1
Tel: 250-334-8320; *Fax:* 250-334-8321
e-mail: office@larchecomoxvalley.org
www.larchecomoxvalley.org
www.facebook.com/pages/LArche-Comox-Valley
Membre(s) du bureau directeur:
Christine Monier, Community Leader

L'Arche Edmonton
Fulton Place, 10310 - 56 St. NW, Edmonton AB T6A 2J2
Tel: 780-465-0618; *Fax:* 780-465-8091
e-mail: edmoffice@larcheedmonton.org
www.larcheedmonton.org
www.facebook.com/pages/LArche-Edmonton/174434082672376
twitter.com/larcheedmonton
Membre(s) du bureau directeur:
Pat Desnoyers, Executive Director & Community Leader Ext. 205
pdesnoyers@larcheedmonton.org

L'Arche Greater Vancouver
7401 Sussex Ave., Burnaby BC V5J 3V6
Tel: 604-435-9544
e-mail: office@larchevancouver.org
www.larchevancouver.org
www.facebook.com/LArcheV
Membre(s) du bureau directeur:
Denise Haskett, Executive Diretor & Community Leader,
604-435-9544 Ext. 27
dhaskett@larchevancouver.org

L'Arche Lethbridge
240 - 12C St. North, Lethbridge AB T1H 2M7
Tel: 403-328-3735; *Fax:* 403-320-6737
e-mail: office@larchelethbridge.org
www.larchelethbridge.org
Membre(s) du bureau directeur:
Tim Wiebe, Community Leader

L'Arche Saskatoon
PO Box 23006, Saskatoon SK S7J 5H3
Tel: 306-262-7243; *Fax:* 306-373-5746
www.larchesaskatoon.org
www.facebook.com/larchesaskatoon
Membre(s) du bureau directeur:

Wyndham Thiessen, Community Leader
wthiessen@larchesaskatoon.org

L'Arche Winnipeg
118 Regent Ave. East, Winnipeg MB R2C 0C1
Tel: 204-237-0300; *Fax:* 204-237-0316
e-mail: office@larchewinnipeg.org
www.larchewinnipeg.org
Membre(s) du bureau directeur:
Jim Lapp, Community Leader Ext. 6
jimlapp@larchewinnipeg.org

Caregivers Alberta
c/o Fulton Place School, 10310 - 56th St. NW, Edmonton AB T6A 2J2
Tel: 780-453-5088; *Fax:* 780-465-5089
Toll-Free: 877-453-5088
e-mail: office@caregiversalberta.ca
www.caregiversalberta.ca
www.linkedin.com/company/alberta-caregivers-association
www.facebook.com/AlbertaCaregivers
twitter.com/ABcaregivers
www.youtube.com/user/ABcaregivers

Also Known As: Alberta Caregivers Association
Overview: A small provincial charitable organization founded in 2001
Mission: To support family caregivers in Alberta, in order to ensure their well-being
Chief Officer(s):
Arlene Baron, Office Manager
abaron@caregiversalberta.ca
Debbie Cameron-Laninga, Coordinator, Program
dcameron-laninga@caregiversalberta.ca
Andy King, Advisor, Communications
aking@caregiversalberta.ca
Publications:
• Caregivers Alberta Newsletter
Type: Newsletter
Profile: Information for family caregivers in Alberta, including articles, caregiver stories, training programs, & forthcoming activities

College of Alberta Psychologists
Sun Life Place, #2100, 10123 - 99th St. NW, Edmonton AB T5J 3H1
Tel: 780-424-5070
Toll-Free: 800-659-0857
e-mail: psych@cap.ab.ca
www.cap.ab.ca

Overview: A small provincial organization
Mission: To develop ethical & practice standards for the profession of psychology in Alberta
Chief Officer(s):
Lorraine Stewart, President
Richard Spelliscy, Registrar

College of Registered Psychiatric Nurses of Alberta
#201, 9711 - 45 Ave., Edmonton AB T6E 5V8
Tel: 780-434-7666; *Fax:* 780-436-4165
Toll-Free: 877-234-7666
e-mail: crpna@crpna.ab.ca
www.crpna.ab.ca
Previous Name: Registered Psychiatric Nurses Association of Alberta
Overview: A medium-sized provincial organization
Mission: To protect & serve the public interest by ensuring members provide safe, competent & ethical practice; To address the needs of members & the public through education, regulation, & advocacy
Chief Officer(s):
Mary Haase, President
Barbara Lowe, Executive Director
barbara.lowe@crpna.ab.ca

Goodwill Industries of Alberta
8761 - 51 Ave., Edmonton AB T6E 5H1
Tel: 780-944-1414
Toll-Free: 866-927-1414
e-mail: media@goodwill.ab.ca
www.goodwill.ab.ca
www.facebook.com/GoodwillAB
twitter.com/goodwilab
instagram.com/goodwill_ab

Overview: A medium-sized provincial charitable organization founded in 1951
Mission: To help persons with disabilities & disadvantages; To build a strong future through rehabilitation & training
Member of: Goodwill Industries International
Affliation(s): United Way of the Capital Region
Chief Officer(s):
Larry Brownoff, Chair
Dale Monaghan, President & CEO

Psychologists Association of Alberta (PAA)
#103, 1207 - 91 St. SW, Edmonton AB T6X 1E9
Tel: 780-424-0294; *Fax:* 780-423-4048
Toll-Free: 888-424-0297
www.psychologistsassociation.ab.ca
www.facebook.com/169589246436220
Overview: A medium-sized provincial licensing organization founded in 1960
Mission: To enhance & promote the profession of psychology
Chief Officer(s):
Bonnie Rude-Weisman, President
Judi Malone, Acting Executive Director
judim@paa-ab.ca

REHOBOTH Christian Ministries
3920 - 49th Ave., Stony Plain AB T7Z 2J7
Tel: 780-963-4044; *Fax:* 780-963-3075
e-mail: provincial_admin@rehoboth.ab.ca
rehoboth.ab.ca
Also Known As: Christian Association for the Mentally Handicapped of Alberta
Overview: A medium-sized provincial charitable organization founded in 1976
Mission: To convey God's love to persons with disabilities through support, advocacy & public education, & by providing opportunities for personal growth & meaningful participation in society
Member of: Alberta Council of Disability Services; Canadian Centre for Philanthropy
Affliation(s): Christian Stewardship Services
Chief Officer(s):
Ron Bos, Executive Director
ron.bos@rehoboth.ab.ca

BRITISH COLUMBIA

Adlerian Psychology Association of British Columbia (APABC)
#440, 2184 West Broadway, Vancouver BC V6K 2E1
Tel: 604-742-1818; *Fax:* 604-742-1811
e-mail: apabc@adler.bc.ca
www.adlercentre.ca
www.facebook.com/Adler-Centre-1401879176699468
twitter.com/AdlerCentre
Also Known As: Adler School of Professional Psychology
Previous Name: Adlerian Psychological Association of British Columbia
Overview: A small provincial charitable organization founded in 1973 overseen by North American Society of Adlerian Psychology
Member of: North American Society of Adlerian Psychologists; Canadian Guidance & Counselling Association
Chief Officer(s):
James Skinner, Executive Director, 204-742-1818
Publications:
• Canadian Journal of Adlerian Psychology [a publication of the Adlerian Psychology Association of British Columbia]

Anxiety Disorders Association of British Columbia
#103, 237 Columbia St. East, New Westminster BC V3L 3W4
Tel: 604-525-7566; *Fax:* 604-525-7586
e-mail: info@anxietybc.com
www.anxietybc.com
www.facebook.com/AnxietyBC
twitter.com/AnxietyBC
www.youtube.com/user/AnxietyBC/
Also Known As: AnxietyBC
Overview: A small provincial organization founded in 1999 overseen by Anxiety Disorders Association of Canada

Mission: To increase awareness of anxiety disorders, including panic disorder, phobias, obsessive-compulsive disorder, and post-traumatic stress disorder; To provide information and resources for individuals wanting to manage their own anxiety
Member of: BC Partners for Mental Health and Addictions Information
Affliation(s): Anxiety BC
Chief Officer(s):
Amir Rasheed, President
Judith Law, Executive Director

British Columbia Art Therapy Association (BCATA)
#101, 1001 West Broadway, Dept. 123, Vancouver BC V6H 4E4
Tel: 604-878-6393
Other Communication: admin@bcarttherapy.com
e-mail: info@bcarttherapy.com
www.bcarttherapy.com
Overview: A small provincial organization founded in 1978
Mission: To foster the professional development of art therapy in British Columbia; To govern the standards & practice of the profession of art therapy & its practitioners; To uphold the British Columbia Art Therapy Association Code of Ethics
Chief Officer(s):
Michelle Oucharek-Deo, President
president@bcarttherapy.com
Debora Broadhurst, Vice-President
vp@bcarttherapy.com
Carolyn Simpson, Corresponding Secretary
corresponding@bcarttherapy.com
Charlotte Spafford, Treasurer
treasurer@bcarttherapy.com
Morgan Reinsbakken, Chair, Membership
membership@bcarttherapy.com
Publications:
• BCATA [British Columbia Art Therapy Association] Newsletter
Type: Newsletter; *Frequency:* Quarterly; *Editor:* Geri Nolan Hilfiker
Profile: Information about professional development workshops, book reviews, updates about the association, & regionalnews for art therapists in British Columbia & western Canada

British Columbia Association for Behaviour Analysis (BC-ABA)
PO Box 64743, Stn. Sunwood Square, Coquitlam BC V3B 6S0
e-mail: info@bc-aba.org
bc-aba.org
Overview: A small provincial organization

British Columbia Association of School Psychologists (BCASP)
c/o Barbara Nichols, 7715 Loedel Cres., Prince George BC V2N 0A5
e-mail: executives@bcasp.ca
www.bcasp.ca
Overview: A small provincial organization
Mission: To represent the interests of school psychologists and to further the standards of school psychology practice in order to promote effective service to all students and their families.
Chief Officer(s):
Douglas Agar, President
president@bcasp.ca

British Columbia Psychogeriatric Association (BCPGA)
PO Box 47028, 1030 Denman St., Vancouver BC V6G 3E1
Fax: 888-835-2451
www.bcpga.com
www.facebook.com/pages/BC-Psychogeriatric-Association/138869817
8027128
twitter.com/BCPGA1
Overview: A small provincial organization founded in 1997
Mission: A professional association of clinicians working in the field of mental health and older adults.
Chief Officer(s):
Nancy Jokinen, Co-President, 250-960-5111
jokinenn@unbc.ca
Dawn Hemingway, Co-President, 250-960-5694
Dawn.Hemingway@unbc.ca

British Columbia Psychological Association (BCPA)
#402, 1177 West Broadway, Vancouver BC V6H 1G3
Tel: 604-730-0501; *Fax:* 604-730-0502
Toll-Free: 800-730-0522
www.psychologists.bc.ca
www.linkedin.com/groups/3997897
www.facebook.com/bcpsychologists
twitter.com/bcpsychologists
www.youtube.com/user/bcpsychologists

Overview: A medium-sized provincial organization
Mission: To promote & advance the profession of psychology in British Columbia
Chief Officer(s):
Rick Gambrel, Executive Director
  rick.gambrel@psychologists.bc.ca
Inky Kang, Coordinator, Marketing & Advertising
  inkyung.kang@psychologists.bc.ca
Priya Bangar, Coordinator, Education
  priya.bangar@psychologists.bc.ca

Coast Foundation Society (CFS)
293 East 11 Ave., Vancouver BC V5T 2C4
Tel: 604-872-3502; *Fax:* 604-879-2363
Toll-Free: 877-602-6278
e-mail: info@coastmentalhealth.com
www.coastmentalhealth.com
www.facebook.com/coastmentalhealth
twitter.com/CoastMH

Overview: A medium-sized provincial charitable organization founded in 1974
Mission: To promote recovery of persons with mental illness
Member of: Canadian Council of Health Services Association
Chief Officer(s):
Isabela Zabava, Executive Director
  isabelaz@coastmentalhealth.com

College of Psychologists of British Columbia (CPBC)
#404, 1755 West Broadway, Vancouver BC V6J 4S5
Tel: 604-736-6164; *Fax:* 604-736-6133
Toll-Free: 800-665-0979
www.collegeofpsychologists.bc.ca

Overview: A medium-sized provincial organization
Mission: To regulate the profession of psychology in British Columbia by establishing practice standards & taking action when standards are not met
Chief Officer(s):
Andrea Kowaz, Registrar & CEO
Amy Janeck, Deputy Registrar
Susan Turnbull, Director, Practice Support
David Perry, Director, Policy & External Relations
Publications:
• The Chronicle [a publication of the College of Psychologists of British Columbia]
Type: Newsletter

College of Registered Psychiatric Nurses of B.C. (CRPNBC)
#307, 2502 St. Johns St., Port Moody BC V3H 2B4
Tel: 604-931-5200; *Fax:* 604-931-5277
Toll-Free: 800-565-2505
e-mail: crpnbc@crpnbc.ca
www.crpnbc.ca

Overview: A small provincial organization
Mission: To serve & protect the public through self-regulation, assuring a safe, accountable, & ethical level of psychiatric nursing practice
Chief Officer(s):
Kyong-ae Kim, CEO
  kkim@crpnbc.ca
Fiona Ramsay, Registrar & Director, Operations
  framsay@crpnbc.ca
Publications:
• College of Registered Psychiatric Nurses of BC Annual Report
Type: Yearbook; *Frequency:* Annually

College of Registered Psychiatric Nurses of British Columbia
#307, 2502 St. Johns St., Port Moody BC V3H 2B4
Tel: 604-931-5200; *Fax:* 604-931-5277
Toll-Free: 800-565-2505
www.crpnbc.ca

Previous Name: Registered Psychiatric Nurses Association of British Columbia
Overview: A medium-sized provincial organization founded in 1974
Mission: To serve & protect the public; to assure a safe, accountable & ethical level of psychiatric nursing practice
Chief Officer(s):
Dorothy Jennings, Chair
Kyong-ae Kim, Executive Director & Registrar
Publications:
• The Communicator
Type: Magazine; *Frequency:* Quarterly; *Accepts Advertising*; *Editor:* Dr. Jacqollyne Keath

Greater Vancouver Community Services Society (GVCSS)
#500, 1212 West Broadway, Vancouver BC V6H 3V1
Tel: 604-737-4900; *Fax:* 604-737-2922
e-mail: info@gvcss.bc.ca
www.gvcss.bc.ca

Overview: A small provincial organization
Mission: Non-profit provider of in-home health care services to the elderly and individuals with physical and/or developmental disabilities
Chief Officer(s):
Ron McLeod, CEO

MANITOBA

Anxiety Disorders Association of Manitoba (ADAM)
#100, 4 Fort St., Winnipeg MB R3C 1C4
Tel: 204-925-0600; *Fax:* 204-925-0609
Toll-Free: 800-805-8885
e-mail: adam@adam.mb.ca
www.adam.mb.ca
www.facebook.com/anxietydisordersassociationofmanitoba

Overview: A small provincial charitable organization founded in 1986 overseen by Anxiety Disorders Association of Canada
Mission: A peer-led organization for the support of people with anxiety, and to share knowledge and hope with others.
Chief Officer(s):
Richard Shore, Chair

College of Registered Psychiatric Nurses of Manitoba (CRPNM)
1854 Portage Ave., Winnipeg MB R3J 0G9
Tel: 204-888-4841; *Fax:* 204-888-8638
www.crpnm.mb.ca

Previous Name: Registered Psychiatric Nurses Association of Manitoba
Overview: A medium-sized provincial licensing organization founded in 1960
Mission: To ensure that members of the profession provide safe & effective psychiatric nursing services to the public of Manitoba, in accordance with the Registered Psychiatric Nurses Act
Chief Officer(s):
Laura Panteluk, Executive Director
Publications:
• Annual Report of The College of Registered Psychiatric Nurses of Manitoba
Type: Yearbook; *Frequency:* Annually
• CRPNM [College of Registered Psychiatric Nurses of Manitoba] Advisor

Manitoba Association for Behaviour Analysis (MABA)
PO Box 53017, Stn. South St. Vital, Winnipeg MB R2N 3X2
e-mail: president@maba.ca
www.maba.ca

Overview: A small provincial organization
Chief Officer(s):
Genevieve Roy-Wsiaki, President
  president@maba.ca

Manitoba Association of School Psychologists Inc.
#562, 162 - 2025 Corydon Ave., Winnipeg MB R3P 0N5
www.masp.mb.ca

Overview: A small provincial organization founded in 1981
Mission: To promote & support school psychology in Manitoba; to develop a network of communication among practitioners of school psychology in Manitoba; to encourage & provide information to educators & the public regarding the practice of school psychology & other related educational issues
Chief Officer(s):
Barry Mallin, President

Manitoba League of Persons with Disabilities (MLPD)
#909, 294 Portage Ave., Winnipeg MB R3C 0B9
Tel: 204-943-6099; *Fax:* 204-943-6654
Toll-Free: 888-330-1932; *TTY:* 204-943-6099
e-mail: contact@mlpd.mb.ca
www.mlpd.mb.ca

Overview: A medium-sized provincial charitable organization founded in 1974
Mission: To remove systemic barriers to community participation for people with disabilities
Member of: Council of Canadians with Disabilities
Affliation(s): Disabled Peoples' International
Chief Officer(s):
Jennifer Sande, Provincial Coordinator

Psychological Association of Manitoba (PAM) / Association des psychologues du Manitoba
#253, 162-2025 Corydon Ave., Winnipeg MB R3P 0N5
Tel: 204-487-0784; *Fax:* 204-489-8688
e-mail: pam@mymts.net
www.cpmb.ca

Overview: A small provincial licensing organization founded in 1966
Mission: To provide screening & examination of candidates &, if eligible, registration as a psychologist; to protect the public from fraudulent services & provide referral to & liaison with psychologists
Chief Officer(s):
John Arnett, President
Alan Slusky, Registrar

NEW BRUNSWICK

College of Psychologists of New Brunswick (CPNB) / Collège des psychologues du Nouveau-Brunswick
PO Box 201, Stn. A, Fredericton NB E3B 4Y9
Tel: 506-382-1994; *Fax:* 506-857-9813
e-mail: cpnb@nbnet.nb.ca
www.cpnb.ca

Overview: A small provincial licensing organization founded in 1965
Mission: To regulate the practice of psychology; to represent the interests of its members
Chief Officer(s):
Jeffrey Landine, President
Carole Cormier-Rioux, Registrar
carole.c.rioux@nb.aibn.com

NEWFOUNDLAND AND LABRADOR

Association of Psychology Newfoundland & Labrador (APNL)
PO Box 26061, Stn. LeMarchant Rd., St. John's NL A1E 0A5
Tel: 709-739-5405
e-mail: info@apnl.ca
www.apnl.ca
www.facebook.com/479381738747827
twitter.com/apnladvocacy

Previous Name: Association of Psychology in Newfoundland & Labrador; Association of Newfoundland Psychologists (ANP)
Overview: A small provincial organization founded in 1976
Mission: To promote all areas of professional psychology in Newfoundland & Labrador
Member of: Canadian Psychological Association
Chief Officer(s):
Janine Hubbard, President
janine@janinehubbard.com

NORTHWEST TERRITORIES

Association of Psychologists of the Northwest Territories
PO Box 1320, Yellowknife NT X1A 2L9
Tel: 867-920-8058
e-mail: psych@theedge.ca

Overview: A small provincial organization
Affliation(s): Canadian Provincial Association of Psychologists (CPAP)
Chief Officer(s):
Robert O'Rourke, President

NOVA SCOTIA

L'Arche Atlantic Region
1381 Orangedale Rd., Orangedale NS B0E 2K0
Tel: 902-295-0050; *Fax:* 902-895-6349
e-mail: office@larcheatlantic.ca
www.larcheatlantic.ca
www.facebook.com/pages/LArche-Atlantic-Region-Canada/382786644
28

Overview: A medium-sized provincial charitable organization founded in 1983 overseen by L'Arche Canada
Mission: Regional office contact information for the Atlantic Canada communities of L'Arche
Member of: L'Arche International
Chief Officer(s):
Jenn Power, Regional Leader

L'Arche Antigonish
4 West St., Antigonish NS B2G 1R8
Tel: 902-863-5000; *Fax:* 902-863-8224
www.larcheantigonish.ca
www.facebook.com/larcheantigonish

Chief Officer(s):
Beth Wolters, Community Leader

L'Arche Cape Breton
3 L'Arche Lane, Whycocomagh NS B0E 3M0
Tel: 902-756-3162; *Fax:* 902-756-3381
e-mail: office@larchecapebreton.org
www.larchecapebreton.org
www.facebook.com/pages/LArche-Cape-Breton-Community/12898192
3841453
www.youtube.com/user/larchecapebreton

Chief Officer(s):
Lisa Poirier-Sinclair, Community Leader

L'Arche Halifax
5512 Sullivan St., Halifax NS B3K 1X7
Tel: 902-407-5512; *Fax:* 902-405-9755
e-mail: office@larchehalifax.org
www.larchehalifax.org

Chief Officer(s):
Rosaire Geddes-Pfaff, Community Leader

L'Arche Homefires
10 Gaspereau Ave., Wolfville NS B4P 2C2
Tel: 902-542-3520; *Fax:* 902-542-7686
e-mail: office@larchehomefires.org
www.larchehomefires.org

Chief Officer(s):
Ingrid Blais, Director
director@larchehomefires.org

L'Arche Saint-John
623 Lancaster Ave., Saint John NB E2M 2M3
Tel: 506-672-6504
e-mail: larchesaintjohn@nb.aibn.com
www.larchesaintjohn.org

Chief Officer(s):
Jocelyn Worster, Community Leader

Association of Psychologists of Nova Scotia (APNS)
#435, 5991 Spring Garden Rd., Halifax NS B3H 1Y6
Tel: 902-422-9183; *Fax:* 902-462-9801
e-mail: apns@apns.ca
www.apns.ca
www.facebook.com/AssociationofPsychologistsofNovaScotia
twitter.com/apnsPsych

Overview: A small provincial organization founded in 1965
Mission: To represent psychology in Nova Scotia; to establish professional guidelines; to promote psychology as a science & a profession for human welfare
Affiliation(s): Council of Provincial Associations of Psychology; Canadian Psychological Association (CPAP); Canadian Register of Health Service Providers in Psychology (CRHSPP); American Psychological Association (APA).
Chief Officer(s):
Shelley Goodwin, President
Publications:
• The APNS Private Practice Directory
Type: Directory

Caregivers Nova Scotia (CNS)
#2, 3433 Dutch Village Rd., Halifax NS B3N 2S7
Tel: 902-421-7390; *Fax:* 902-421-7338
Toll-Free: 877-488-7390
e-mail: info@caregiversns.org
www.caregiversns.org
www.facebook.com/CaregiversNS
twitter.com/CaregiversNS

Also Known As: CaregiversNS
Previous Name: Family Caregivers Association of Nova Scotia
Overview: A small provincial organization founded in 1998
Mission: To support caregivers throughout Nova Scotia
Affliation(s): Canadian Caregiver Coalition
Chief Officer(s):
Kathleen Rothwell, President
Angus Campbell, Executive Director
director@caregiversns.org
Jennifer Briand, Coordinator, Western Region Caregiver Support
western@caregiversns.org
Maggie Roach-Ganaway, Coordinator, Cape Breton Region Support
capebreton@caregiversns.org
Cindie Smith, Coordinator, Northern & Eastern Mainland Region Support
northern@Caregiversns.org
Publications:
• The Caregiver's Handbook [a publication of Caregivers Nova Scotia]
Type: Handbook; *Editor:* Angus Campbell
Profile: Information for unpaid family & friend caregivers in Nova Scotia
• Caregivers Nova Scotia News [a publication of Caregivers Nova Scotia]
Type: Newsletter; *Frequency:* Quarterly
Profile: Information about caregiving issues, forthcoming workshops, plus the experiences & concerns of caregivers

NUNAVUT

Pamiqsaiji Association for Community Living
PO Box 708, Rankin Inlet NU X0C 0G0
Tel: 867-645-2542; *Fax:* 867-645-2543
e-mail: pamiqad@qiniq.com
Overview: A small provincial charitable organization overseen by Nunavummi Disabilities Makinnasuaqtiit Society
Mission: To provide support for adults with intellectual disabilities
Member of: Canadian Association for Community Living

ONTARIO

Anxiety Disorders Association of Ontario (ADAO)
Heartwood House, 404 McArthur Ave., Ottawa ON K1K 1G5
Tel: 613-729-6761
Toll-Free: 877-308-3843
e-mail: info@anxietydisordersontario.ca
www.anxietydisordersontario.ca
www.facebook.com/anxietyottawa
twitter.com/AnxietyOttawa
www.youtube.com/user/anxietyottawa
Overview: A small provincial charitable organization founded in 1997 overseen by Anxiety Disorders Association of Canada
Mission: ADAO's mission is to empower, in an holistic way, the lives of those affected by anxiety through advocacy, education, research support and community programming.
Chief Officer(s):
Joan Riggs, BA, B.S.W., M.S, President

L'Arche Ontario
186 Floyd Ave., Toronto ON M4J 2J1
Tel: 416-406-2869
larcheontario.org
www.facebook.com/larcheontario
Overview: A medium-sized provincial charitable organization overseen by L'Arche Canada
Mission: Regional office contact information for the Ontario communities of L'Arche
Member of: L'Arche International
Chief Officer(s):
John Guido, Regional Coordinator
johnguido@larche.ca

L'Arche Arnprior
#103, 16 Edward St., Arnprior ON K7S 3W4
Tel: 613-623-7323
e-mail: office@larchearnprior.org
www.larche.ca/en/communities/arnprior
Chief Officer(s):
Jeanette Fraser, Community Leader

L'Arche Daybreak
11339 Yonge St., Richmond Hill ON L4S 1L1
Tel: 905-884-3454; *Fax:* 905-884-0584
e-mail: office@larchedaybreak.com
www.larchedaybreak.com
www.facebook.com/larchedaybreak

L'Arche Hamilton
664 Main St. East, Hamilton ON L8M 1K2
Tel: 905-312-0162; *Fax:* 905-312-0165
e-mail: office@larcheham.com
www.larche.ca/en/communities/hamilton
Chief Officer(s):
Lynn Godfrey, Community Leader

L'Arche London
#121, 4056 Meadowbrook Dr., London ON N6L 1E3
e-mail: office@larchelondon.org
larchelondon.org
www.facebook.com/larchelondon
Chief Officer(s):
Marietta Drost, Community Leader

L'Arche North Bay
102 - 1st Ave. East, North Bay ON P1B 1J6
Tel: 705-474-0081; *Fax:* 705-497-3447
e-mail: office_larchenorthbay@bellnet.ca
www.larchenorthbay.ca
www.facebook.com/pages/Friends-of-LArche-North-Bay/224163822118
Chief Officer(s):
Martina Getz, Community Leader

L'Arche Ottawa
11 Rossland Ave., Ottawa ON K2G 2K2
Tel: 613-228-7136; *Fax:* 613-228-8829
e-mail: office@larcheottawa.org
www.larche.ca/en/communities/ottawa
Chief Officer(s):
Raphael Amato, Community Leader

L'Arche Stratford
PO Box 522, Stn. Main, Stratford ON N5A 6T7
Tel: 519-271-9751; *Fax:* 519-271-1861
e-mail: info@larche.stratford.on.ca
www.larchestratford.on.ca
www.facebook.com/pages/LArche-Stratford/115312341812477
Chief Officer(s):
Stephanie Calma, Community Leader
commleader@larche.stratford.on.ca

L'Arche Sudbury
1173 Rideau St., Sudbury ON P3A 3A5
Tel: 705-525-1015; *Fax:* 705-525-4448
e-mail: larchesudbury@larchesudbury.org
www.larchesudbury.org
Chief Officer(s):

Jennifer McCauley, Community Leader
jennifer.mccauley@larchesudbury.org

L'Arche Toronto
186 Floyd Ave., Toronto ON M4J 2J1

Tel: 416-406-2869
e-mail: office@larchetoronto.org
www.larchetoronto.org
www.facebook.com/larchetoronto
twitter.com/larchetoronto
www.youtube.com/larchetoronto

Chief Officer(s):
Raphael Arens, Community Leader
raphael@larchetoronto.org

Children's Mental Health Ontario (CMHO) / Santé Mentale pour Enfants Ontario (SMEO)
#309, 40 St. Clair Ave. East, Toronto ON M4T 1M9

Tel: 416-921-2109; *Fax:* 416-921-7600
e-mail: info@cmho.org
www.cmho.org
www.linkedin.com/company/747188
www.facebook.com/kidsmentalhealth
twitter.com/kidsmentalhlth
www.youtube.com/user/ChangeTheView2016

Also Known As: Ontario Association of Children's Mental Health Centres
Overview: A medium-sized provincial charitable organization founded in 1972
Mission: To promote, support & strengthen a sustainable system of mental health services for children, youth & their families
Member of: Child Welfare League of Canada
Chief Officer(s):
Kimberly Moran, Chief Executive Officer
kmoran@cmho.org

The College of Psychologists of Ontario (CPO)
#500, 110 Eglinton Ave. West, Toronto ON M4R 1A3

Tel: 416-961-8817; *Fax:* 416-961-2635
Toll-Free: 800-489-8388
e-mail: cpo@cpo.on.ca
www.cpo.on.ca

Overview: A large provincial licensing organization
Mission: To monitor & regulate the practice of psychology in Ontario
Chief Officer(s):
Robert Gauthier, College Council President
Catherine Yarrow, Registrar & Executive Director
Publications:
• The College of Psychologists of Ontario Standards of Professional Conduct
Type: Manual; *Number of Pages:* 22
Profile: Members of the College of Psychologists must adhere to the standards while practicing the profession
• e-Bulletin [a publication of the College of Psychologists of Ontario]
Type: Newsletter
Profile: Articles, discipline proceedings, by-law amendments, & committee & council news

College of Registered Psychotherapists of Ontario (CRPO)
163 Queen St. East, 4th Fl., Toronto ON M5A 1S21

Tel: 416-862-4801; *Fax:* 416-974-4079
Toll-Free: 888-661-4801
e-mail: info@crpo.ca
www.crpo.ca

Overview: A small provincial licensing organization
Mission: To regulate the profession of psychotherapy & to maintain professional, ethical standards.
Chief Officer(s):
Joyce Rowlands, Registrar

Distress Centres Ontario (DCO)
#1016, 30 Duke St. West, Kitchener ON N2H 3W5

Tel: 416-486-2242; *Fax:* 519-342-0970
e-mail: info@dcontario.org
www.dcontario.org

Previous Name: Ontario Association of Distress Centres
Overview: A medium-sized provincial charitable organization founded in 1971

Mission: To transfer best practices between member centres; To promote, support & sustain member agencies
Chief Officer(s):
Karen Letofsky, Chair
Elizabeth Fisk, Executive Director

Ontario Association for Behaviour Analysis (ONTABA)
#413, 283 Danforth Ave., Toronto ON M4K 1N2

e-mail: contact@ontaba.org
www.ontaba.org
twitter.com/ONTABA1

Overview: A small provincial organization
Affiliation(s): Association for Behaviour Analysis International
Chief Officer(s):
Albert Malkin, President

Ontario Association of Consultants, Counsellors, Psychometrists & Psychotherapists (OACCPP) / Association des consultants et conseillers en santé mentale, psychométriciens, et psychothérapeutes de l'Ontario
#410, 586 Eglinton Ave. East, Toronto ON M4P 1P2

Tel: 416-298-7333; *Fax:* 416-298-9593
Toll-Free: 888-622-2779
e-mail: oaccpp@oaccpp.ca
www.oaccpp.ca
www.linkedin.com/company/2202979?trk=tyah
twitter.com/OACCPP

Overview: A small provincial organization founded in 1978
Mission: The OACCPP is a provincial body of mental health service providers that provides for the professional needs of its members, and meets the needs of the community in identifying and certifying practitioners.
Chief Officer(s):
James Whetstone, President
Carol Cox, Administrative Director
admin-director@oaccpp.ca
Publications:
• Psychologica Magazine
Type: Magazine; *Frequency:* 2 pa

Ontario Association on Developmental Disabilities (OADD)
2 Surrey Pl., Toronto ON M5S 2C2

Tel: 416-429-3720; *Fax:* 647-260-2016
e-mail: oadd@oadd.org
www.oadd.org

Overview: A medium-sized provincial organization
Mission: To support professionals & students in the field of developmental disabilities through the promotion of the highest standards of research, education, & practice
Affiliation(s): Great Lakes Society for Developmental Services of Ontario (GLS); Research Special Interest Group (RSIG)
Chief Officer(s):
Tony Vipond, Chair
Publications:
• BrOADDcast [a publication of the Ontario Association on Developmental Disabilities]
Type: Newsletter
Profile: Brief articles submitted by families, service providers, students, & researchers
• Journal on Developmental Disabilities
Editor: Maire Percy et. al.; *Price:* oadd@oadd.org
Profile: A peer-reviewed journal, featuring research on issues relevant to developmental disabilities for both a Canadian & international audience

Ontario Community Support Association (OCSA) / Association ontarienne de soutien communautaire
#104, 970 Lawrence Ave. West, Toronto ON M6A 3B6

Tel: 416-256-3010; *Fax:* 416-256-3021
Toll-Free: 800-267-6272
e-mail: reception@ocsa.on.ca
www.ocsa.on.ca
twitter.com/OCSAtweets

Previous Name: Meals on Wheels Ontario Inc.
Overview: A medium-sized provincial charitable organization founded in 1992

Mission: To support & represent the common goals of community-based, not-for-profit health & social service organizations which assist individuals to live at home in their own community
Member of: Canadian Centre for Philanthropy
Chief Officer(s):
Deborah Simon, Chief Executive Officer
  deborah.simon@ocsa.on.ca

Ontario Council of Alternative Businesses (OCAB)
#203, 1499 Queen St. West, Toronto ON M6R 1A3
Tel: 416-504-1693; Fax: 416-504-8063
Toll-Free: 866-504-1693
e-mail: ocab@on.aibn.com
www.ocab.ca
Overview: A small provincial organization founded in 1994
Mission: To increase economic opportunities for psychiatric survivors by developing community businesses; To reduce discrimination & ignorance of general public in regards to psychiatric survivors
Chief Officer(s):
Joyce Brown, Co-Director
  jmbrown@on.aibn.com
Becky McFarlane, Co-Director
  becky@on.aibn.com

Ontario Mental Health Foundation
180 Bloor St. West, #UC101, Toronto ON M5S 2V6
Tel: 416-920-7721; Fax: 416-920-0026
www.omhf.on.ca
www.linkedin.com/company/ontario-mental-health-foundation
www.facebook.com/TheOMHF
twitter.com/the_omhf
Overview: A small provincial charitable organization
Mission: To promote the mental health of people in Ontario; To improve the diagnosis & treatment of mental illness
Chief Officer(s):
Andrea Swinton, Executive Director
  andreas@omhf.on.ca
Lauren Edding-Lee, Acting Officer, Program
  laurene@omhf.on.ca
Publications:
• Ontario Mental Health Foundation Annual Report
Type: Yearbook; *Frequency:* Annually

Ontario Psychiatric Association (OPA)
#100, 2233 Argentia Rd., Mississauga ON L5N 2X7
Tel: 905-813-0105; Fax: 905-826-4873
e-mail: opa@eopa.ca
www.eopa.ca
www.linkedin.com/groups/4618836
www.facebook.com/146883128706932
twitter.com/OntPsychAssoc
Overview: A medium-sized provincial organization founded in 1956
Mission: To represent Ontario psychiatrists to government, universities & other associations; To promote high standards of professional development & practice; To promote the exchange of information; To advocate for people with mental disorders
Chief Officer(s):
Diana Kljenak, President

Ontario Psychological Association (OPA)
#403, 21 St. Clair Ave. East, Toronto ON M4T 1L8
Tel: 416-961-5552; Fax: 416-961-5516
e-mail: opa@psych.on.ca
www.psych.on.ca
www.facebook.com/ONPsych
twitter.com/onpsych
Overview: A medium-sized provincial organization founded in 1947
Mission: To advance the practice & science of psychology in Ontario communities; To promote the highest ethical standards in the profession
Chief Officer(s):
Sylvain Roy, President
Janet Kasperski, Chief Executive Officer
Publications:
• Psychology Ontario
Type: Magazine

Ontario Society of Psychotherapists (OSP)
#1, 189 Queen St. East, Toronto ON M5A 1S2
Tel: 416-923-4050; Fax: 416-968-6818
e-mail: mail@psychotherapyontario.org
psychotherapyontario.com
twitter.com/psychotherapyon
Overview: A small provincial organization
Mission: The Ontario Society of Psychotherapists is committed to the continuing development of ethically responsible and self-reflective psychotherapists
Chief Officer(s):
Christina Becker, President

Parents for Children's Mental Health (PCMH)
PO Box 20004, St Catharines ON L2N 7W7
Tel: 416-220-0742
Toll-Free: 855-254-7264
e-mail: admin@pcmh.ca
www.pcmh.ca
www.facebook.com/PCMHOntario
twitter.com/PCMHontario
Overview: A small provincial organization founded in 1994
Mission: To provide a voice for children & families in Ontario who are affected by mental health problems
Chief Officer(s):
Michele Sparling, Chair
Sarah Cannon, Executive Director

Post Traumatic Stress Disorder Association
93 Dufferin Ave., Toronto ON N6A 1K3
Tel: 604-525-7566; Fax: 604-525-7586
e-mail: info@ptsdassociation.com
ptsdassociation.com
Overview: A small provincial charitable organization
Mission: To empower individuals suffering from Post Traumatic Stress Disorder through education, linkages with appropriate services, facilitation of research and discovery into the causation.
Chief Officer(s):
Roméo A. Dallaire, O.C., C.M.M., G, Honorary Chair
Ute Lawrence-Fisher, President & Founder

Saint Elizabeth Health Care (SEHC) / Les soins de santé Sainte-Elizabeth
#300, 90 Allstate Pkwy., Markham ON L3R 6H3
Tel: 905-940-9655; Fax: 905-940-9934
Toll-Free: 800-463-1763; TTY: 800-855-0511
e-mail: communications@saintelizabeth.com
www.saintelizabeth.com
www.linkedin.com/company/saint-elizabeth-health-care
www.facebook.com/SaintElizabethSEHC
twitter.com/stelizabethSEHC
www.youtube.com/user/SaintElizabethSEHC
Previous Name: Saint Elizabeth Visiting Nurses' Association of Ontario
Overview: A medium-sized provincial charitable organization founded in 1908
Mission: To serve the physical, emotional, & spiritual needs of people in their homes & communities
Member of: Nursing Best Practice Research Unit, through the RNAO & the University of Ottawa
Affliation(s): Canadian Council on Health Services Accreditation
Chief Officer(s):
Noreen Taylor, Chair
Shirlee Sharkey, President & CEO
Heather McClure, Treasurer
Don McCutchan, Secretary
Publications:
• Saint Elizabeth Health Care e-Newsletter
Type: Newsletter
• Saint Elizabeth Health Care Foundation Newsletter
Type: Newsletter
• SEHC [Saint Elizabeth Health Care] Research Activity Report
Type: Report
Profile: Highlights of research achievements

Barrie - North Simcoe Muskoka Service Delivery Centre

#104, 85 Ferris Lane, Barrie ON L4M 6B9
Fax: 877-619-4033
Toll-Free: 888-737-5055
e-mail: info@saintelizabeth.com

Cornwall - Eastern Counties Service Delivery Centre
#5, 1916 Pitt St., Cornwall ON K6H 5H3
Tel: 613-936-8668; *Fax:* 866-619-4059
e-mail: info@saintelizabeth.com

Hamilton - Hamilton, Niagara, Haldimand & Brant Service Delivery Centre
1525 Stone Church Rd. East, Hamilton ON L8W 3P8
Fax: 866-619-4062
Toll-Free: 888-275-2299
e-mail: info@saintelizabeth.com

Kingston - South East Service Delivery Centre
#410, 1471 John Counter Blvd., Kingston ON K7M 8S8
Tel: 613-530-3400; *Fax:* 866-619-4063
e-mail: info@saintelizabeth.com

London - South West Service Delivery Centre
#15, 1100 Dearness Dr., London ON N6E 1N9
Tel: 519-668-2997; *Fax:* 866-619-4065
e-mail: info@saintelizabeth.com

Markham - Central Service Delivery Centre
#201, 90 Allstate Pkwy., Markham ON L3R GH3
Tel: 905-944-1743; *Fax:* 866-619-4074
e-mail: info@saintelizabeth.com

Mississauga - Peel Service Delivery Centre
#5, 6745 Century Ave., Mississauga ON L5N 1V9
Tel: 905-826-0854; *Fax:* 905-826-0854
e-mail: info@saintelizabeth.com

Ottawa - Champlain Service Delivery Centre
#225, 30 Colonnade Rd., Ottawa ON K2E 7J6
Tel: 613-738-9661; *Fax:* 877-619-4038
e-mail: info@saintelizabeth.com

Seaforth - Huron Service Delivery Centre
87 Main St. South, Seaforth ON N0K 1W0
Fax: 519-600-0105
Toll-Free: 888-823-1626
e-mail: info@saintelizabeth.com

Thunder Bay - North West Service Delivery Centre
#103, 920 Tungsten St., Thunder Bay ON P7B 5Z6
Tel: 807-344-2002; *Fax:* 807-344-1999
e-mail: info@saintelizabeth.com

Toronto - Toronto Central Service Delivery Centre
#600, 2 Lansing Sq., Toronto ON M2J 4P8
Tel: 416-498-8600; *Fax:* 416-498-0213
e-mail: info@saintelizabeth.com

Whitby - Central East Service Delivery Centre
1549 Victoria St. East, Whitby ON L1N 8R1
Fax: 416-398-3206
Toll-Free: 877-397-1035

Windsor - Erie St. Clair Service Delivery Centre
2473 Ouellette Ave., Windsor ON N8X 1L5
Tel: 519-972-3895; *Fax:* 866-619-4073
e-mail: info@saintelizabeth.com

Woodstock - Oxford County Service Delivery Centre
#5, 695 Canterbury Ave., Woodstock ON N4S 8W7
Tel: 519-539-9807; *Fax:* 866-619-4070
e-mail: info@saintelizabeth.com

PRINCE EDWARD ISLAND

Prince Edward Island Council of People with Disabilities (PEICOD)
Landmark Plaza, #2, 5 Lower Malpeque Rd., Charlottetown PE C1E 1R4
Tel: 902-892-9149; *Fax:* 902-566-1919
Toll-Free: 888-473-4263
e-mail: peicod@peicod.pe.ca
www.peicod.pe.ca
www.facebook.com/PEICOD

Overview: A small provincial charitable organization founded in 1974
Mission: To improve the quality of life of people with disabilities on PEI
Member of: Prince Edward Island Literacy Alliance Inc.
Chief Officer(s):
Marcia Carroll, Executive Director

Psychological Association of Prince Edward Island (PAPEI)
PE
www.peipsychology.org/papei

Overview: A small provincial organization
Chief Officer(s):
Nadine DeWolfe, Ph.D., President

QUÉBEC

L'Arche Québec
1280, rue Bernard Ouest, Outremont QC H2V 1V9
Tél: 514-849-0110
Courriel: aaq@larche.ca
archequebec.ca
www.facebook.com/arche.quebec
twitter.com/archequebec
plus.google.com/+ArchequebecCa

Aperçu: *Dimension:* moyenne; *Envergure:* provinciale; Organisme sans but lucratif surveillé par L'Arche Canada
Mission: Régional d'information contacter le bureau pour les collectivités du Québec de L'Arche
Membre de: L'Arche International
Membre(s) du bureau directeur:
Sylvie Morin, Directrice régionale
smorin-aaq@larche.ca

L'Arche Abitibi-Témiscamingue
42, rue Principale Sud, Amos QC J9T 3A5
Tél: 819-732-1265
Courriel: courrier@larcheamos.org
www.larcheamos.org

Membre(s) du bureau directeur:
Perrine Forgeot D'Arc, Responsable de communauté

L'Arche Agapè
19, rue Hanson, Gatineau QC J8Y 3M4
Tél: 819-770-2000; *Téléc:* 819-770-3907
Courriel: arche.agape@bellnet.ca
www.larcheagape.org
www.facebook.com/larche.agape

Membre(s) du bureau directeur:
Nancy Lamothe, Responsable de communauté

L'Arche Beloeil
221, rue Bernard-Pilon, Beloeil QC J3G 1V2
Tél: 450-446-1061; *Téléc:* 450-446-2396
Courriel: archebelo@qc.aira.com
www.larche.ca/en/communities/beloeil
www.facebook.com/larchebeloeil

Membre(s) du bureau directeur:
Marie Fréchette, Responsable de communauté

L'Arche Joliette
#3-21, 144, rue St-Joseph, Beloeil QC J6E 5C4
Tél: 450-759-0408; *Téléc:* 450-759-8266
Courriel: larchejoliette@bellnet.ca
www.larche.ca/en/communities/joliette

Membre(s) du bureau directeur:
Elisabeth Richard, Responsable de communauté

L'Arche l'Étoile
218, rue St-Sauveur, Québec QC G1N 4S1
Tél: 418-527-8839; *Téléc:* 418-527-8738
Courriel: larcheletoile@videotron.ca
arche-quebec.ca
www.facebook.com/cdjetoile

Membre(s) du bureau directeur:
Lynda St-Pierre, Responsable de communauté

L'Arche Le Printemps

1375, rue Principale, Saint-Malachie QC G0R 3N0

Tél: 418-642-5785
Courriel: archeleprintemps@globetrotter.net
www.larche.ca/en/communities/le_printemps

Membre(s) du bureau directeur:
Geneviève Moutquin, Responsable de communauté

L'Arche Mauricie
570, rue St-Paul, Trois-Rivières QC G9A 1H8

Tél: 819-373-8781
Courriel: archemauricie@qc.aira.com
www.larchemauricie.org
www.facebook.com/LARCHEMAURICIE

Membre(s) du bureau directeur:
Patrice Paradis, Responsable de communauté

L'Arche Montréal
6105, rue Jogues, Montréal QC H4E 2W2

Tél: 514-761-7307
Courriel: info@larche-montreal.org
www.larche-montreal.org

Membre(s) du bureau directeur:
Alain Ouedraogo, Directeur
  direction@larche-montreal.org

Association des groupes d'intervention en défense de droits en santé mentale du Québec (AGIDD-SMQ)
#210, 4837, rue Boyer, Montréal QC H2J 3E6

Tél: 514-523-3443; *Téléc:* 514-523-0797
Ligne sans frais: 866-523-3443
Courriel: info@agidd.org
www.agidd.org

Aperçu: *Dimension:* moyenne; *Envergure:* provinciale; fondée en 1990
Mission: Au service des personnes qui ont des problèmes et qui ont besoin d'aide et de soutien pour exercer et faire valoir leurs droits
Membre(s) du bureau directeur:
Doris Provencher, Directrice générale

Association des médecins-psychiatres du Québec (AMPQ) / Québec Psychiatrists' Association
CP 216, Succ. Desjardins, Montréal QC H5B 1G8

Tél: 514-350-5128; *Téléc:* 514-350-5198
www.ampq.org

Aperçu: *Dimension:* moyenne; *Envergure:* provinciale; fondée en 1953
Mission: Promouvoir les intérêts professionnels et économiques de ses membres
Membre(s) du bureau directeur:
Karine J. Igartua, Présidente
Guillaume Dumont, Secrétaire

Association des psychothérapeutes psychanalytiques du Québec
#310, 911, rue Jean-Talon Est, Montréal QC H2R 1V5

Tél: 514-383-1240
e-mail: info@appq.com
www.appq.com

Overview: A small provincial organization founded in 1985
Mission: Développer chez ses membres un sentiment d'appartenance à un groupe partageant des vues théoriques et thérapeutiques communes basées sur la pensée psychanalytique
Chief Officer(s):
Thérèse Nadeau, Présidente
Marie Gauthier, Trésorière

Association Québécoise pour la Santé Mentale des Nourrisson (AQSMN)
CP 10009, Saint-Jean-sur-Richelieu QC J2W 0G6

Tél: 514-598-8413
Courriel: info@aqsmn.org
www.aqsmn.org

Aperçu: *Dimension:* petite; *Envergure:* provinciale
Mission: De promouvoir la recherche dans les domaines de la santé et le développement mental du nourrisson; pour étudier la santé mentale des parents.
Membre(s) du bureau directeur:
Alain Lebel, Président

Association/Troubles de l'Humeur et d'Anxiété au Québec (ATHAQ)
QC

Courriel: info@athaq.com
www.athaq.com

Nom précédent: Association/Troubles Anxieux du Québec
Aperçu: *Dimension:* petite; *Envergure:* provinciale; Organisme sans but lucratif; fondée en 1991 surveillé par Anxiety Disorders Association of Cnada
Mission: Formée par un groupe de professionnels oeuvrant dans le domaine des troubles anxieux et de ses comorbidités avec pour but de collaborer au niveau des soins, de l'enseignement, de la recherche, de la formation médicale et de l'information du public
Membre(s) du bureau directeur:
Cédric Aubé, Consultant

Centre Psycho-Pédagogique de Québec Inc.
École Saint-François, 1000, rue du Joli-Bois, Québec QC G1V 3Z6

Tél: 418-650-1171; *Téléc:* 418-650-1145
www.cppq.qc.ca

Aperçu: *Dimension:* petite; *Envergure:* provinciale
Membre(s) du bureau directeur:
Donald Gilbert, Président

Confédération des Organismes de Personnes Handicapées du Québec (COPHAN)
#300, 2030, boul Pie-IX, Montréal QC H1V 2C8

Tél: 514-284-0155; *Téléc:* 514-284-0775
Courriel: info@cophan.org
www.cophan.org

Nom précédent: Confédération des organismes provinciaux de personnes handicapées du Québec
Aperçu: *Dimension:* moyenne; *Envergure:* provinciale; Organisme sans but lucratif; fondée en 1985
Mission: Milite pour la défense des droits et la promotion des intérêts des personnes ayant des limitations fonctionnelles, de tous âges
Membre de: Conseil de canadiens avec déficiences
Membre(s) du bureau directeur:
Richard Lavigne, Directeur général
  direction@cophan.org
Véronique Vézina, Présidente

Entre-amis Lavallois inc
4490, 10e rue, Laval QC H7R 6A9

Tél: 450-962-4058

Aperçu: *Dimension:* petite; *Envergure:* provinciale
Mission: Offrir une activité culturelle et de rencontre aux personnes atteintes de déficience intellectuelle

Fédération des familles et amis de la personne atteinte de maladie mentale (FFAPAMM) / Federation of Families & Friends of Persons with a Mental Illness
#203, 1990, rue Cyrille-Duquet, Québec QC G1N 4K8

Tél: 418-687-0474; *Téléc:* 418-687-0123
Ligne sans frais: 800-323-0474
Courriel: info@ffapamm.com
www.ffapamm.com

Aperçu: *Dimension:* moyenne; *Envergure:* provinciale; Organisme sans but lucratif; fondée en 1986
Mission: Défendre et promouvoir les intérêts de ses membres; de les soutenir dans leur développement; de sensibiliser l'opinion publique aux problèmes reliés à la maladie mentale; de créer des programmes de communication et d'éducation
Membre(s) du bureau directeur:
Hélène Fradet, Directrice générale

Fondation des maladies mentales / Mental Illness Foundation
#804, 55, av du Mont-Royal West, Montréal QC H2T 2S6

Tél: 514-529-5354; *Téléc:* 514-529-9877
Ligne sans frais: 888-529-5354
Courriel: info@fondationdesmaladiesmentales.org
www.fondationdesmaladiesmentales.org

Nom précédent: Fondation québécoise des maladies mentales
Aperçu: *Dimension:* petite; *Envergure:* provinciale; fondée en 1980
Mission: Pour mettre des services cliniques en place et les maintenir; prévenir les maladies mentales
Membre(s) du bureau directeur:

Isabelle Limoges, Directrice générale
ilimoges@fondationdesmaladiesmentales.org

Fondation québécoise de la déficience intellectuelle (FQDI)
6275, boul des Grandes-Prairies, Montréal QC H1P 1A5
Tél: 514-725-9797; *Téléc:* 514-725-3530
www.fqdi.ca
www.facebook.com/pages/FQDI/473133932730673

Aperçu: *Dimension:* petite; *Envergure:* provinciale; Organisme sans but lucratif; fondée en 1988
Mission: Amasse des fonds pour venir en aide aux organismes oeuvrant à l'intégration et à l'amélioration de la qualité de vie des personnes présentant une déficience intellectuelle
Affliation(s): Association du Québec pour l'intégration sociale
Membre(s) du bureau directeur:
Philippe Siebes, Directeur général

Institut de réadaptation en déficience physique de Québec (IRDPQ)
525, boul Wilfrid-Hamel, Québec QC G1M 2S8
Tél: 418-529-9141; *TTY:* 418-649-3733
Courriel: communications@irdpq.qc.ca
www.irdpq.qc.ca
www.facebook.com/IRDPQ
www.youtube.com/user/VideosIRDPQ

Nom précédent: Institut de réadaptation physique de Québec
Aperçu: *Dimension:* petite; *Envergure:* provinciale; fondée en 1996
Mission: Offrir des services de réadaptation, d'adaptation et de soutien à l'intégration sociale aux enfants, adultes et ainés qui ont des incapacités et vivent des situations de handicap en raison de leur déficience auditive, motrice, neurologique, visuelle, de la parole ou du langage, de même que des services d'accompagnement et de soutien à l'entourage
Membre de: Association des établissements de réadaptation en déficience physique du Québec
Membre(s) du bureau directeur:
Marc Prenevost, Directeur général

L'Ordre des psychologues du Québec (OPQ)
#510, 1100, av Beaumont, Montréal QC H3P 3H5
Tél: 514-738-1881; *Téléc:* 514-738-8838
Ligne sans frais: 800-363-2644
Courriel: info@ordrepsy.qc.ca
www.ordrepsy.qc.ca

Aperçu: *Dimension:* moyenne; *Envergure:* provinciale; fondée en 1962
Mission: Assurer la protection du public; contrôler l'exercice de la profession par ses membres; veiller à la qualité des services dispensés par ses membres; favoriser le développement de la compétence professionnelle, le respect des normes déontologiques et l'accessibilité aux services psychologiques
Affliation(s): American Psychological Association
Membre(s) du bureau directeur:
Rose-Marie Charest, Présidente
presidence@ordrepsy.qc.ca

Société québécoise des psychothérapeutes professionnels (SQPP)
CP 34, Succ. Ahuntsic, Montréal QC H3L 3N5
Tél: 514-990-3403
Courriel: info@sqpp.org
www.sqpp.org

Aperçu: *Dimension:* petite; *Envergure:* provinciale; fondée en 1991
Mission: Un regroupement multidisciplinaire de psychothérapeutes qui sont des professionnels de la psychothérapie régis par un code de déontologie; possèdent une formation académique universitaire ou son équivalent et une solide formation à la psychothérapie; ont accompli une démarche psychothérapeutique approfondie
Membre(s) du bureau directeur:
Andrée Thauvette-Poupart, Présidente

SASKATCHEWAN

Psychology Association of Saskatchewan
PO Box 4528, Regina SK S4P 3W7
e-mail: info@psychsask.ca
psychsask.ca
twitter.com/PsychSask

Overview: A small provincial organization

Mission: To represent the interests of its members & to further & promote interest in psychology
Member of: Council of Provincial Associations of Psychologists
Chief Officer(s):
Kristi Wright, President

Registered Psychiatric Nurses Association of Saskatchewan (RPNAS)
2055 Lorne St., Regina SK S4P 2M4
Tel: 306-586-4617; *Fax:* 306-586-6000
www.rpnas.com

Overview: A large provincial licensing organization founded in 1948
Mission: To regulate psychiatric nursing as a distinct profession
Chief Officer(s):
Marion Palidwor, President
Robert Allen, Executive Director

Saskatchewan Abilities Council
2310 Louise Ave., Saskatoon SK S7J 2C7
Tel: 306-374-4448; *Fax:* 306-373-2665
e-mail: provincialservices@abilitiescouncil.sk.ca
www.abilitiescouncil.sk.ca
www.linkedin.com/company/saskatchewan-abilities-council
www.facebook.com/saskatchewanabilitiescouncil
twitter.com/skabilitiesyqr

Also Known As: Easter Seals Saskatchewan
Previous Name: Saskatchewan Council for Crippled Children & Adults
Overview: A medium-sized provincial charitable organization founded in 1950 overseen by Easter Seals Canada
Mission: To enhance the independence & community participation of people of varying abilities in Saskatchewan
Chief Officer(s):
Ian Wilkinson, Executive Director

Saskatchewan College of Psychologists (SCP)
1026 Winnipeg St., Regina SK S4R 8P8
Tel: 306-352-1699; *Fax:* 306-352-1697
e-mail: skcp@sasktel.net
www.skcp.ca

Previous Name: Saskatchewan Psychological Association
Overview: A small provincial licensing organization
Mission: To protect the public by guiding & regulating the professional conduct of Saskatchewan psychologists
Chief Officer(s):
Karen Litke, President
Karen Messer-Engel, M.A., R.Psych., Executive Director & Registrar

Saskatchewan Psychiatric Association
Saskatoon SK
sask-psychiatrists.tripod.com

Overview: A small provincial organization
Mission: To increase psychiatric knowledge in Saskatchewan
Affliation(s): Canadian Psychiatric Association

Local Associations

Emotions Anonymous
PO Box 4245, St. Paul MN 55104-0245 USA
Tel: 651-647-9712; *Fax:* 651-647-1593
e-mail: info2gh99jsd@emotionsanonymous.org
www.emotionsanonymous.org

Overview: A small local organization
Mission: To help people overcome emotional difficulties

ALBERTA

Calgary Association of Self Help
1019 - 7th Ave. SW, Calgary AB T2P 1A8
Tel: 403-266-8711; *Fax:* 403-266-2478
e-mail: info@calgaryselfhelp.com
calgaryselfhelp.com
www.facebook.com/CalgaryAssociationofSelfHelp
twitter.com/yycselfhelp

Overview: A medium-sized local charitable organization founded in 1973
Mission: To provide client-centred, flexible services promoting the abilities of adults with mental illness through rehabilitation, counselling & social/leisure programs

Chief Officer(s):
Anneisa Lauchlan, Chief Executive Officer, 403-266-8711 Ext. 222

BRITISH COLUMBIA

Communitas Supportive Care Society
#103, 2776 Bourquin Cres. West, Abbotsford BC V2S 6A4
Tel: 604-850-6608; *Fax:* 604-850-2634
Toll-Free: 800-622-5455
e-mail: office@communitascare.com
www.communitascare.com
www.linkedin.com/company/communitas-supportive-care-society
www.facebook.com/CommunitasCare
twitter.com/CommunitasCare
Previous Name: Mennonite Central Committee Supportive Care Services Society
Overview: A small local organization
Mission: Provide various resources to persons living & dealing with mental, physical &/or emotional disabilities.
Member of: Association for Community Living; Community Social Services Employers Association; Psychosocial Rehabilitation Canada; BC Association for Child Development & Intervention; Denominational Health Association; Fraser Valley Brain Injury Association
Affiliation(s): Jean Vanier; Henri Nouwen; Copeland Centre for Wellness & Recovery; International Initiative for Mental Health; Living Room; Mental Health Commission of Canada; STEP Enterprises; Mennonite Central Committee (British Columbia & Canada); Mennonite Disaster Service; Ten Thousand Villages
Chief Officer(s):
Karyn Santiago, Chief Executive Officer
Gary Falk, Chair
Jacquie Lepp, CPA, Treasurer

Helping Spirit Lodge Society (HSLS)
3965 Dumfries St., Vancouver BC V5N 5R3
Tel: 604-874-6629; *Fax:* 604-873-4402
e-mail: reception@hsls.ca
www.hsls.ca
Overview: A small local organization founded in 1991
Mission: To provide support & a safe place for aboriginal women & children affected by family violence; to provide holistic education programs
Chief Officer(s):
Doris Peters, President

North Okanagan Neurological Association (NONA)
2802 - 34th St., Vernon BC V1T 5X1
Tel: 250-549-1281; *Fax:* 250-549-3771
e-mail: administration@nona-cdc.com
www.nona-cdc.com
www.facebook.com/NONAChildDevelopmentCentre
Overview: A small local organization founded in 1975
Mission: To provide services for the treatment, education & support of special needs children & their families
Member of: B.C. Association of Child Development & Rehabilitation
Affiliation(s): Cerebral Palsy Association of British Columbia
Chief Officer(s):
Janice Foster, Executive Director

Open Door Group
#300, 30 East 6 Ave., Vancouver BC V5T 1J4
Tel: 604-876-0770; *Fax:* 604-873-1758
Toll-Free: 866-377-3670
e-mail: info@opendoorgroup.org
www.opendoorgroup.org
www.facebook.com/OpenDoorGroup
Previous Name: Arbutus Vocational Society; THEO BC
Overview: A medium-sized local charitable organization founded in 1976
Mission: To assist psychiatrically, emotionally, & socially disadvantaged people to develop the necessary skills to lead more satisfying lives
Chief Officer(s):
Tom Burnell, Chief Executive Officer
tom.burnell@opendoorgroup.org

Naomi Bullock, Executive Director, Program Management & Development
naomi.bullock@opendoorgroup.org
Alona Puehse, Executive Director, Corporate Development
alona.puehse@opendoorgroup.org
Christine Buchanan, Director, Diversity & Disability Services
christine.buchanan@opendoorgroup.org
Katrina Welsh, Director, Human Resources
katrina.welsh@opendoorgroup.org
Joey Alain, Director, Information Technology
joey.alain@opendoorgroup.org

NOVA SCOTIA

Golden Opportunities Vocational Rehabilitation Centre Workshop
PO Box 887, 32 Industrial Park, Springhill NS B0M 1X0
Tel: 902-597-3158
www.nsnet.org/govrc
Also Known As: GOVRC Workshop
Overview: A small local organization
Mission: To offer vocational training for mentally challenged adults
Member of: DIRECTIONS Council for Vocational Services Society
Chief Officer(s):
Paul Williams, Executive Director

Inverness Cottage Workshop (ICW)
PO Box 485, 46 Lower Railway St., Inverness NS B0E 1N0
Tel: 902-258-3316; *Fax:* 902-258-3351
www.invernesscottageworkshop.ca
www.facebook.com/ICottageWorkshop
twitter.com/InvernessCW
Overview: A small local organization founded in 1981
Member of: DIRECTIONS Council for Vocational Services Society
Chief Officer(s):
Donna MacLean, President
Cindy O'Neill, Executive Director/Manager

Regional Occupation Centre Society
3 MacQuarrie Dr., Port Hawkesbury NS B9A 3A3
Tel: 902-625-0132; *Fax:* 902-625-5344
www.rocsociety.ca
Also Known As: ROC Society
Overview: A small local organization founded in 1975
Mission: To support individuals with disabilities through vocational & community programs
Member of: DIRECTIONS Council for Vocational Services Society
Chief Officer(s):
Tom Gunn, President

Self-Help Connection Clearinghouse Association
#800, 11 Akerley Blvd., Dartmouth NS B2Y 2R7
Tel: 902-466-2011; *Fax:* 902-404-3205
Toll-Free: 866-765-6639
www.selfhelpconnection.ca
Overview: A small local charitable organization founded in 1987
Mission: To enable Nova Scotians to improve control over their health by increasing their knowledge, skills & resources for individual & collective action
Member of: Canadian Network of Self-Help Centres; International Network of Mutual Help Centres
Affiliation(s): National Network for Mental Health; Canadian Coalition of Mental Health Resources

ONTARIO

Catholic Family Services of Toronto (CFS Toronto) / Services familiaux catholiques de Toronto
Catholic Pastoral Centre, #200, 1155 Yonge St., Toronto ON M4T 1W2
Tel: 416-921-1163; *Fax:* 416-921-1579
e-mail: info@cfstoronto.com
www.cfstoronto.com
Previous Name: Catholic Welfare Bureau
Overview: A medium-sized local charitable organization founded in 1922
Mission: To help individuals & families develop their potential by providing wellness programs & treatment services

Member of: Catholic Charities of the Archdiocese of Toronto
Affiliation(s): Family Service Canada; Family Service Ontario
Chief Officer(s):
Ivana Zanardo, President
Denis Costello, Executive Director & Secretary

North Toronto Office
#300, 5799 Yonge St., Toronto ON M2M 3V3
Tel: 416-222-0048; *Fax:* 416-222-3321

C.G. Jung Foundation of Ontario
14 Elm St., Toronto ON M5G 157
Tel: 416-961-9767; *Fax:* 416-961-6659
e-mail: info@cgjungontario.com
www.cgjungontario.com

Also Known As: Ontario Association of Jungian Analysts
Overview: A small local charitable organization founded in 1971
Mission: To disseminate information about the psychological teachings of Carl Gustav Jung through lectures, seminars, workshops, a library & a bookstore; a list of Jungian analysts is available for referral
Member of: International Association of Jungian Analysts
Chief Officer(s):
Catherine Johnson, Administrator
Publications:
• Chiron [a publication of the C.G. Jung Foundation of Ontario]
Type: Newsletter; *Editor:* Robert Black; *ISSN:* 1918-6142

Chai-Tikvah The Life & Hope Foundation
#313, 4600 Bathurst St., Toronto ON M2R 3V2
Tel: 416-634-3050
e-mail: info@lifeandhope.ca
www.lifeandhope.ca

Overview: A small local charitable organization
Mission: To support individuals with mental illness by providing secure housing options & services, & promoting their inclusion in society
Chief Officer(s):
David Drutz, Chair
Rochelle Goldman-Brown, Executive Director

Community Counselling Centre of Nipissing / Centre communautaire de counselling du Nipissing
361 McIntyre St. East, North Bay ON P1B 1C9
Tel: 705-472-6515; *Fax:* 705-472-4582; *Crisis Hot-Line:* 866-887-0015
e-mail: info@cccnip.com
www.cccnip.com

Previous Name: Family Life Centre
Overview: A small local charitable organization founded in 1972 overseen by Ontario Association of Credit Counselling Services
Mission: To provide professional community & credit counselling services, plus developmental, addiction, & sexual assault services, to individuals, couples, & families in North Bay & the surrounding community
Member of: Ontario Association of Credit Counselling Services
Chief Officer(s):
Alan McQuarrie, Executive Director
amcquarrie@cccnip.com

Community Torchlight Guelph/Wellington/Dufferin
PO Box 1027, Guelph ON N1H 6N1
Tel: 519-821-3761; *Fax:* 519-821-8190; *Crisis Hot-Line:* 888-821-3760
e-mail: info@communitytorchlight.com
www.communitytorchlight.com
www.linkedin.com/pub/community-torchlight/23/2a2/236
twitter.com/CommunityTorch

Previous Name: Distress Centre Wellington/Dufferin; Guelph Distress Centre
Overview: A small local charitable organization founded in 1969 overseen by Distress Centres Ontario
Mission: To provide a free, 24-hour listening, referral & crisis assistance telephone service to Guelph & rural Wellington & Dufferin counties
Chief Officer(s):
Katherine Johnson, Manager, Services
kjohnson@communitytorchlight.com
Judith Rosenberg, Coordinator, Community Development & Recruitment
jrosenberg@communitytorchlight.com

Crisis Centre North Bay
PO Box 1407, North Bay ON P1B 8K6
Tel: 705-472-6204; *Fax:* 705-472-6236
e-mail: info@crisiscentre-nb.on.ca
www.crisiscentre-nb.on.ca

Overview: A small local charitable organization founded in 1972 overseen by Distress Centres Ontario
Mission: To help people in crises by providing temporary room & board as well as rehabilitation services

Distress Centre Niagara Inc.
PO Box 25014, Stn. Pen Centre-Glendale Ave., St Catharines ON L2T 2C4
Fax: 905-682-7959; *Crisis Hot-Line:* 905-688-3711
e-mail: dcniagara@distresscentreniagara.com
distresscentreniagara.com

Overview: A small local organization founded in 1970 overseen by Distress Centres Ontario
Mission: To provide a no-cost confidential telephone support service by trained volunteers to assist anyone in need in the Niagara area

Distress Centre North Halton
PO Box 85, Georgetown ON L7G 4T1
Tel: 905-877-0655; *Fax:* 905-877-0655; *Crisis Hot-Line:* 905-877-1211
e-mail: dcnhalton@bellnet.ca
www.dchalton.ca

Overview: A small local organization founded in 1973 overseen by Distress Centres Ontario
Mission: To provide confidential listening, emotional support, referrals & information, & crisis intervention

Distress Centre of Durham Region (DCD)
306 Brock St. North, Whitby ON L1N 4H7
Tel: 905-430-3511; *Crisis Hot-Line:* 800-452-0688
e-mail: dcd@distresscentredurham.com
www.distresscentredurham.com
www.facebook.com/DurhamDistress
twitter.com/DurhamDistress

Overview: A small local charitable organization founded in 1970
Mission: To help people in distress to cope, by providing emotional support, crisis/suicide management & community education
Member of: Distress Centres Ontario; Canadian Association of Suicide Prevention
Chief Officer(s):
Victoria Kehoe, Executive Director
victoria@distresscentredurham.com

Distress Centre of Ottawa & Region (DCOR) / Centre de détresse d'Ottawa et la région
PO Box 3457, Stn. C, Ottawa ON K1Y 4J6
Tel: 613-238-1089; *Fax:* 613-722-5217
www.dcottawa.on.ca
www.facebook.com/DistressCentreOR
twitter.com/DistressCentreO

Also Known As: Distress Centre Ottawa
Previous Name: Distress Centre Ottawa/Carleton
Overview: A small local charitable organization founded in 1969 overseen by Distress Centres Ontario
Mission: The Distress Centre is a non-profit organization that provides 24/7 confidential telephone services for emotional support, suicide prevention/intervention, postvention, crisis intervention, information referral & education services. It is a registered charity, BN: 108079815RR0001
Affiliation(s): American Association of Suicidology; Canadian Association for Suicide Prevention; International Association for Suicide Prevention

Distress Centres of Toronto
PO Box 243, Stn. Adelaide, Toronto ON M5C 2J4
Tel: 416-598-0166; *TTY:* 416-408-0007; *Crisis Hot-Line:* 416-408-4357
e-mail: info@torontodistresscentre.com
www.torontodistresscentre.com
www.facebook.com/1536691786591642
twitter.com/DC_TO

Overview: A small local organization founded in 1967

Mission: To assist emotionally distressed individuals deal with those issues they are currently unable to manage
Affliation(s): Ontario Association of Distress Centres
Chief Officer(s):
Karen Letofsky, Executive Director, 416-598-0168
  karen@torontodistresscentre.com

Distress Line Sarnia
Bldg. 1030, 1086 Modeland Rd., Sarnia ON N7S 6L2
  Tel: 519-336-0120; *Fax:* 519-336-8517
  Toll-Free: 800-831-3031; *Crisis Hot-Line:* 888-347-8737
  www.familycounsellingctr.com
Also Known As: Family Counselling Centre
Overview: A small local charitable organization founded in 1973 overseen by Distress Centres Ontario
Mission: To help strengthen people & their relationships with others
Member of: Distress Centres Ontario
Chief Officer(s):
Don Pitt, Executive Director
  don.pitt@familycounsellingctr.com

Eli Bay Relaxation Response Institute
226 Wychwood Ave., Toronto ON M6C 2T3
  Tel: 416-932-2784
  Other Communication: Presentation & Workshop e-mail:
  info@kmprod.com
  www.elibay.com
Also Known As: The Relaxation Response Ltd.
Overview: A small local organization founded in 1978
Mission: To empower individuals & organizations with mind-body skills proven to effectively release stress anywhere & anytime
Chief Officer(s):
Eli Bay, Founder

Family Service Centre of Ottawa-Carleton / Centre de service familial d'Ottawa-Carleton
312 Parkdale Ave., Ottawa ON K1Y 4X5
  Tel: 613-725-3601; *Fax:* 613-725-5651; *TTY:* 613-725-6175
  e-mail: fsfo@familyservicesottawa.org
  www.familyservicesottawa.org
  www.facebook.com/familyservicesottawa
Overview: A medium-sized local organization founded in 1914 overseen by Family Service Ontario
Mission: To strengthen all aspects of family & community living through the provision of family focused, professional social services in the areas of counselling, family life education, social planning & advocacy
Affliation(s): Family Service Canada
Chief Officer(s):
Kathryn Ann Hill, Executive Director

Good Shepherd Refuge Social Ministries
412 Queen St. East, Toronto ON M5A 1T3
  Tel: 416-869-3619
  www.goodshepherd.ca
  www.linkedin.com/company/good-shepherd-ministries
  www.facebook.com/goodshepherdTO
  twitter.com/goodshepherd_to
  www.youtube.com/user/GoodShepherdToronto
Also Known As: Good Shepherd Ministries
Previous Name: Good Shepherd Refuge
Overview: A small local charitable organization founded in 1963
Mission: To provide services to homeless, disadvantaged & marginalized people; To provide the basic necessities of food, shelter & ancillary services, ensuring each client justice, equality, dignity & acceptance; To provide human services that will assist clients in regaining freedom from homelessness
Member of: Ontario Hostels Association
Chief Officer(s):
Werner Zapfe, Chair
David Lynch, Executive Director
Aklilu Wendaferew, Assistant Executive Director
Publications:
• Good Shepherd Journal
Type: Newsletter; *Frequency:* Bi-annually; *Editor:* Adrienne Urquhart;
Price: Free to supporters
Profile: Provides client, service & donor updates.

Goodwill Industries
255 Horton St., London ON N6B 1L1
  Tel: 519-850-9000
  www.goodwillindustries.ca
  twitter.com/Goodwill_OGL
  www.youtube.com/user/GoodwillOGLakes
Previous Name: London Goodwill Industries Association
Overview: A medium-sized local charitable organization founded in 1943
Mission: To provide programs & services that enhance the employability of people with barriers or diminished opportunities; To provide & recycle goods
Member of: Goodwill Industries International Inc.
Chief Officer(s):
Michelle Quintyn, President & CEO
  mquintyn@goodwillindustries.ca
Terry Off, Chief Financial Officer
Scott Louch, Chief Operations Officer

Goodwill Industries Essex Kent Lambton
1121 Wellington St., Sarnia ON N7S 6J7
  Tel: 519-332-0440
  www.goodwillekl.com
  www.facebook.com/GoodwillEKL
  twitter.com/goodwillekl
  www.youtube.com/user/GoodwillIntl
Overview: A small local charitable organization founded in 1933
Mission: To promote dignity & independence; To provide employment & training programs to assist people with employment barriers; To help people develop life skills
Chief Officer(s):
Kevin Smith, Chief Executive Officer
  ksmith@goodwillekl.com
Maryam Foroughian, Chief Financial Officer
  mforoughian@goodwillekl.com
Michelle Repuski, Director, Workforce Development
  mrepuski@goodwillccc.com
Heather Allen, Manager, Marketing & Communication
  hallen@goodwillekl.com
Mary Lynn Bouman, Manager, Human Resources
  mbouman@goodwillekl.com
Craig Watters, Manager, Operations
  cwatters@goodwillekl.com

Hincks-Dellcrest Treatment Centre & Foundation
440 Jarvis St., Toronto ON M4Y 2H4
  Tel: 416-924-1164; *Fax:* 416-924-8208
  Toll-Free: 855-944-4673
  e-mail: info@hincksdellcrest.org
  www.hincksdellcrest.org
  www.facebook.com/hincksdellcrest
  twitter.com/hincksdellcrest
  www.youtube.com/thehincksdellcrest
Overview: A small local organization founded in 1998
Mission: To offer a comprehensive range of mental health services to infants, children, youth, & their families; to provide a variety of programs, including prevention & early intervention, outpatient & residential treatment.
Affliation(s): University of Toronto
Chief Officer(s):
Ian Smith, Chair
Donna Duncan, President & CEO

Homestead Christian Care
249 Caroline St. South, #A, Hamilton ON L8P 3L6
  Tel: 905-529-0454; *Fax:* 905-529-0355
  Toll-Free: 866-529-0454
  e-mail: info@hscc.ca
  homesteadchristiancare.ca
  www.facebook.com/homesteadchristiancare
Overview: A small local charitable organization founded in 1974
Mission: To assist those with mental illness, through affordable housing & rehabilitation services, in order to help them reach personal recovery goals
Chief Officer(s):
Jeffrey Neven, Executive Director

Hong Fook Mental Health Association (HFMHA)
#201, 3320 Midland Ave., Toronto ON M1V 5E6
Tel: 416-493-4242; *Fax:* 416-493-2214
www.hongfook.ca
Overview: A small local charitable organization founded in 1982 overseen by Ontario Council of Agencies Serving Immigrants
Mission: To empower Canadians, including those of Cambodian, Chinese, Korean & Vietnamese, & other Asian communities, who reside within the Greater Toronto Area; to obtain ethno-racial equity in the mental health system & to achieve optimal mental health status through activities of direct services, promotion & prevention & system advocacy.
Affliation(s): Ontario Federation of Community Mental Health & Addiction Programs; Canadian Mental Health Association
Chief Officer(s):
Bonnie Wong, Executive Director

Downton Branch
130 Dundas St. West, 3rd Fl., Toronto ON M5G 1C3
Tel: 416-493-4242; *Fax:* 416-595-6332

Mid-Toronto Community Services (MTCS)
192 Carlton St., 2nd Fl., Toronto ON M5A 2K8
Tel: 416-962-9449; *Fax:* 416-962-5541
e-mail: admin@midtoronto.com
www.midtoronto.com
Overview: A small local charitable organization founded in 1965
Mission: Provides programs & services to support the independence of seniors & adults with disabilities to continue living in their own homes
Member of: Ontario Community Support Association
Chief Officer(s):
Kaarina Luoma, Executive Director
kluoma@midtoronto.com
Susan Burns, Chair

Oakville Distress Centre
PO Box 776, Oakville ON L6K 0A9
Tel: 905-849-4559; *Crisis Hot-Line:* 905-849-4541
e-mail: info@dchalton.ca
www.dchalton.ca
www.linkedin.com/company/distress-centre-oakville
twitter.com/DCOakville
Overview: A small local charitable organization founded in 1974 overseen by Distress Centres Ontario
Mission: To provide telephone, crisis intervention, & support services for the community of Oakville, Milton, & surrounding areas; To develop & provide outreach & suicide prevention programs to meet the needs of the community

A Post Psychiatric Leisure Experience (APPLE)
Bronson Center, 211 Bronson Ave., Ottawa ON K1R 6H5
Tel: 613-238-1209; *Fax:* 613-238-5806
e-mail: contact_apple@hotmail.com
www.appledropin.com
www.facebook.com/appledropin
Overview: A small local organization founded in 1981
Mission: To enhance the quality of life for their members by offering support & activities; to prevent hospitalization of their members

Self-Help Resource Centre (SHRC)
#307, 40 St. Clair Ave. East, Toronto ON M4T 1M9
Tel: 416-487-4355; *Fax:* 416-487-0344
Toll-Free: 888-283-8806
e-mail: shrc@selfhelp.on.ca
www.selfhelp.on.ca
twitter.com/selfhelprc
Overview: A small local charitable organization founded in 1987
Mission: To promote self-help/mutual aid; to increase awareness about self-help/mutual aid in the community & among helping professionals; to facilitate the growth & development of self-help groups, networks & resources
Affliation(s): Centre of Health Promotion; Canadian Health Network
Chief Officer(s):
Jennifer Poole, President
Mark Freeman, Executive Director

Spectra Helpline
#402, 7700 Hurontario St., Brampton ON L6Y 4M3
Tel: 289-569-1200; *Fax:* 888-658-8577; *Crisis Hot-Line:* 905-459-7777
e-mail: info@spectrahelpline.org
www.spectrahelpline.org
www.linkedin.com/company/spectra-community-support-services
www.facebook.com/SpectraHelpline
twitter.com/spectrasupport
Previous Name: Telecare Distress Centre Brampton
Overview: A small local charitable organization founded in 1973 overseen by Distress Centres Ontario
Mission: To provide a 24-hour-a-day telephone service to people in need; To aim to be a listening ministry, not a problem-solving, advice-giving institution
Affliation(s): Telecare Teleministries of Canada Inc.; Life Line International
Chief Officer(s):
Alison Caird, Executive Director

STRIDE
#26, 55 Ontario St. South, Milton ON L9T 2M3
Tel: 905-693-4252; *Fax:* 905-875-9262
e-mail: stride@stride.on.ca
www.stride.on.ca
Also Known As: Supported Training & Rehabilitation in Diverse Environments
Overview: A small local organization
Chief Officer(s):
Anita Lloyd, Executive Director, 905-693-4252 Ext. 224
alloyd@stride.on.ca

Tel-Aide Outaouais (TAO)
CP 7218, Succ. Vanier, Ottawa ON K1L 8E3
Tél: 819-776-2649; *Téléc:* 888-765-7040
Courriel: administration@telaideoutaouais.ca
www.telaideoutaouais.ca
Aperçu: *Dimension:* petite; *Envergure:* locale; Organisme sans but lucratif; fondée en 1974
Mission: Offrir un service d'écoute téléphonique en français pour toute personne ayant besoin d'aide, de soutien et de référence; développer et offrir des services d'écoute en français pour la population de l'Outaouais et de l'Ontario; favoriser l'implication sociale de la communauté par le biais du bénévolat; sensibiliser et éduquer le public à la nécessité d'être à l'écoute des gens vivant dans la détresse; susciter et entretenir des partenariats avec des organismes du milieu de la santé et des services sociaux; promouvoir les services de Tel-Aide Outaouais auprès de la population
Membre de: Ontario Association of Distress Centres; Association québécois de suicidologie
Affliation(s): Regroupement des organismes communautaires en santé mentale de l'Outaouais
Membre(s) du bureau directeur:
Jean-François Parent, Executive Director
direction@telaideoutaouais.ca

Telephone Aid Line Kingston (TALK)
PO Box 1325, Kingston ON K7L 5C6
Tel: 613-531-8529; *Fax:* 613-531-3312; *Crisis Hot-Line:* 613-544-1771
e-mail: director@telephoneaidlinekingston.com
www.telephoneaidlinekingston.com
www.facebook.com/telephoneaidlinekingston
Overview: A small local organization founded in 1973 overseen by Distress Centres Ontario
Mission: To provide telephone & support services, as well as community outreach & education, to meet the needs of the community

Thunder Bay Counselling Centre
544 Winnipeg Ave., Thunder Bay ON P7B 3S7
Tel: 807-684-1880; *Fax:* 807-344-3782
Toll-Free: 888-204-2221
e-mail: community@tbaycounselling.com
www.tbaycounselling.com
www.facebook.com/thunderbaycounsellingcentre
twitter.com/tbcounselling
Previous Name: Family Services Thunder Bay
Overview: A medium-sized local charitable organization founded in 1967 overseen by Ontario Association of Credit Counselling Services

Mission: To provide community based support services to individuals, couples, & families in the Thunder Bay area; To offer confidential counselling
Member of: Ontario Association of Credit Counselling Services; United Way of Thunder Bay
Chief Officer(s):
Nancy Chamberlain, Executive Director
Publications:
• The Solution Source [a publication of the Thunder Bay Counselling Centre]
Type: Newsletter; *Frequency:* Quarterly; *ISSN:* 1481-2568
Profile: Issue topics include benefits of counselling, living with uncertainty, compassion fatigue, single parent families, & understanding teens& substance abuse

Toronto Art Therapy Institute (TATI)
8 Prince Arthur Ave., 2nd Fl., Toronto ON M5R 1A9
Tel: 416-924-6221
e-mail: torontoarttherapyassistant@gmail.com
www.tati.on.ca
Overview: A small local charitable organization founded in 1968
Mission: To train individuals who want to become art therapists; To use art therapy to promote growth & healing within communities
Affiliation(s): Lesley College, Cambridge, MA
Chief Officer(s):
Debbie Anderson, Chair
Helene Burt, Executive Director

Waypoint Centre for Mental Health Care / Waypoint centre de soins de santé mentale
500 Church St., Penetanguishene ON L9M 1G3
Tel: 705-549-3181
e-mail: info@waypointcentre.ca
www.waypointcentre.ca
Overview: A small local organization founded in 2008
Mission: To provide psychiatric inpatient & outpatient services & mental health programs to individuals in Simcoe County, Dufferin County & Muskoka/Parry Sound
Chief Officer(s):
Betty Valentine, Chair
Carol Lambie, President & CEO

QUÉBEC

Action Autonomie
3958, rue Dandurand, Montréal QC H1X 1P7
Tél: 514-525-5060; Télec: 514-525-5580
Courriel: lecollectif@actionautonomie.qc.ca
www.actionautonomie.qc.ca
Aperçu: *Dimension:* petite; *Envergure:* locale
Mission: Protéger les droits des personnes vivant des problèmes de santé mentale par une approche d'éducation

Association de loisirs pour personnes handicapées psychiques de Laval (ALPHPL)
6600, av 29e, Laval QC H7R 3M3
Tél: 450-627-4525; Télec: 450-627-4370
Courriel: alphpl@videotron.ca
www.alphpl.org
Aperçu: *Dimension:* petite; *Envergure:* locale; Organisme sans but lucratif; fondée en 1983
Mission: Promouvoir l'évolution sociale des personnes handicapées psychiques en stimulant leurs intérêts pour des activités physiques, socio-culturelles et des loisirs; les soutenir dans leur apprentissage, l'entraînement et l'utilisation des ressources et équipments socio-communautaires; créer un sentiment d'appartenance du participant dans son milieu
Membre de: Association régionale pour personnes handicapées des Laurentides; Association québécoise pour la réadaptation psychosociale; Regroupement des ressources alternatives en santé mentale du Québec; l'Association canadienne pour la santé mentale
Membre(s) du bureau directeur:
François Bullock, Directeur général

Association des alternatives en santé mentale de la Montérégie (AASMM)
#309, 170 rue Saint-Antoine nord, Granby QC J2G 5G8
Tél: 450-375-5868; Télec: 450-375-5319
Courriel: info@aasmm.com
www.aasmm.com
Aperçu: *Dimension:* petite; *Envergure:* locale; Organisme sans but lucratif; fondée en 1986
Mission: Promouvoir la vie associative par des action concrètes; promouvoir les expertises de ses ressources membres; soutenir et défendre les intérêts de ses ressources membres; promouvoir l'idéologie alternative en santé mentale auprès de ses ressources membres et auprès des communautés
Membre(s) du bureau directeur:
André Leduc, Président
Joseph-Anne St-Hilaire, Vice-Présidente

Association des parents et amis de la personne atteinte de maladie mentale Rive-Sud (APAMM-RS)
#206, 10, boul Churchill, Greenfield Park QC J4V 2L7
Tél: 450-766-0524; Crisis Hot-Line: 450-679-8689
www.apammrs.org
www.facebook.com/apammrs
Aperçu: *Dimension:* petite; *Envergure:* locale; Organisme sans but lucratif
Mission: Aide des familles qui sont touchées par la maladie mentale et soutient des recherches sur les maladies mentales
Membre(s) du bureau directeur:
Guy Savoie, Président
Patricia Arnaud, Directrice générale

Association des personnes handicapées physiques et sensorielles du secteur Joliette (APHPSSJ)
200 rue de Salaberry, Joliette QC J6E 4G1
Tel: 450-759-3322; Fax: 450-759-8749
Toll-Free: 888-756-3322
e-mail: aphpssj@cepap.ca
www.aphpssj.com
Previous Name: Association of Physically Disabled Joliette - L'Assomption; Association of People with Physical Disabilities Joliette
Overview: A small local organization founded in 1977
Mission: To promote the rights of people with physical & sensory disabilities in the Joliette region; To encourage social integration of disabled people
Member of: Regroupement des associations de personnes traumatisées craniocérébrales du Québec / Coalition of Associations of Craniocerebral Trauma in Quebec
Chief Officer(s):
Jocelyn Picard, Président
Jacynthe Arseneau, 1ère Vice-président
Michel Lacourse, 2e Vice-président
François Gagnon, Secretaire
Murielle Desrosiers, Trésorière
Publications:
• Dynamic Player
Type: Newsletter
Profile: Association updates, announcements, & forthcoming activities

Centre d'aide personnes traumatisées crâniennes et handicapées physiques Laurentides (CAPTCHPL)
CP 11, Saint-Jérôme QC J7Z 5T7
Tél: 450-431-2860; Télec: 450-431-7955
Ligne sans frais: 888-431-3437
Courriel: lecaptchpl@sympatico.ca
www.captchpl.org
twitter.com/Captchpl
Aperçu: *Dimension:* petite; *Envergure:* locale
Mission: Pour aider les personnes souffrant de lésions cérébrales et physiquement handicapées dans la région des Laurentides du Québec; Pour favoriser l'intégration sociale des personnes handicapées physiques et de lésions cérébrales
Membre de: Regroupement des associations de personnes traumatisées craniocérébrales du Québec / Coalition of Associations of Craniocerebral Trauma in Quebec
Membre(s) du bureau directeur:
Michel Lajeunesse, Directeur général

L'Écluse des Laurentides

22A, rue Goyer, Saint-Sauveur QC J0R 1R0

Tel: 450-744-1393; *Fax:* 450-744-1335
e-mail: ecluse@cgocable.ca
www.ecluse.org

Overview: A small local organization founded in 1991
Chief Officer(s):
Émilie Rouleau, Directrice

The EJLB Foundation

#1050, 1350, rue Sherbrooke Ouest, Montréal QC H3G 1J1
Fax: 514-843-4080
e-mail: general@fondationecho.ca
www.ejlb.qc.ca

Overview: A small local organization founded in 1983
Mission: Provides grants to organizations with areas of interest in mental health and the environment
Chief Officer(s):
Kevin Leonard, Executive Director

International Associations

American Association on Intellectual & Developmental Disabilities (AAIDD)

#200, 501 - 3rd St. NW, Washington DC 20001 USA
Tel: 202-387-1968; *Fax:* 202-387-2193
e-mail: admin@aaidd.org
aaidd.org
www.linkedin.com/groups/American-Association-on-Intellectual-Develo
pme
www.facebook.com/350322627779
twitter.com/_aaidd
www.youtube.com/user/aaiddvideos

Previous Name: American Association on Mental Retardation
Overview: A large international organization founded in 1876
Mission: To provide leadership in the field of intellectual & developmental disabilities throughout the world
Chief Officer(s):
William Gaventa, MDiv, President
Margaret A. Nygren, EdD, Executive Director & CEO
  mnygren@aaidd.org
Paul D. Aitken, CPA, Director, Finance & Administration
  pdaitken@aaidd.org
Corinne Carpenter, Coordinator, Communications & Membership
  ccarpenter@aaidd.org
Publications:
• American Journal on Intellectual & Developmental Disabilities
Type: Journal; *Frequency:* Bimonthly; *Editor:* Deborah Fidler; *ISSN:* 1944-7558
Profile: Scientific, scholarly & archival journal for original contributions of knowledge of intellectual disability, including its causes,treatment & prevention.
• Inclusion [a publication of the American Association on Intellectual & Developmental Disabilities]
Type: Journal; *Frequency:* Bimonthly; *Editor:* Michael Wehmeyer; Karrie Shogren; *ISSN:* 2326-6988
Profile: Peer-reviewed journal that discusses strategies that promote the inclusion ofpeople with intellectual & developmental disabilities in society.
• Intellectual & Developmental Disabilities
Type: Journal; *Frequency:* Bimonthly; *Editor:* James R. Thompson; *ISSN:* 1934-9556
Profile: Peer-reviewed journal of policy, practices & perspectives.

American Psychological Association (APA)

750 - 1st St. NE, Washington DC 20002-4242 USA
Tel: 202-336-5500; *Fax:* 202-335-5997
Toll-Free: 800-374-2721; *TTY:* 202-336-6123
e-mail: executiveoffice@apa.org
www.apa.org
www.linkedin.com/groups?gid=58284
www.facebook.com/AmericanPsychologicalAssociation
twitter.com/apa
plus.google.com/109392714004041510585
Overview: A large international organization founded in 1892

Mission: To advance psychology as a science, profession & as a means of promoting human welfare
Member of: American Council of Learned Societies
Chief Officer(s):
Barry S. Anton, President
Norman Anderson, CEO

International Academy of Law & Mental Health (IALMH) / Académie internationale de droit et de santé mentale (AIDSM)

c/o Philippe Pinel, Faculty of Medicine, University of Montreal, PO Box 6128, Stn. Centre-Ville, Montréal QC H3C 3J7
Tel: 514-343-5938; *Fax:* 514-343-2452
e-mail: admin@ialmh.org
www.ialmh.org

Overview: A small international organization founded in 1981
Chief Officer(s):
George Woods, President
Publications:
• International Journal of Law and Psychiatry [a publication of the International Academy of Law & Mental Health]
Type: Journal; *Frequency:* q.; *ISSN:* 0160-2527
Profile: Multidisciplinary forum for the exchange of information and ideas among professionals that relate tothe intersection of law and psychiatry

International Association for Cross-Cultural Psychology (IACCP)

Institute for Psychology, Hungarian Academy of Sciences, Victor Hugo utca 18-22, Budapest 1132 Hungary
Tel: 36-70-313-87
www.iaccp.org
twitter.com/iaccp

Overview: A small international organization founded in 1972
Mission: To facilitate communication among persons interested in cross-cultural psychology issues
Affliation(s): International Union of Psychological Science
Chief Officer(s):
Fons van de Vijver, President
Márta Fülöp, Secretary General
  martafulop@yahoo.com
Sharon Glazer, Treasurer
  sharon.glazer@usa.net
Publications:
• Cross-Cultural Psychology Bulletin
Type: Journal; *Editor:* William K. Gabrenya Jr.; *Price:* Free to IACCP members
• Journal of Cross-Cultural Psychology
Type: Journal; *Frequency:* Bimonthly; *Editor:* Deborah Best; *ISSN:* 0022-0221
Profile: Papers focussing on the interrelationships between culture & psychological processes

International PhotoTherapy Association

Photo Therapy Centre, 890 The Grove Rd., Gambier Island BC V0N 1V0
Tel: 604-202-3431
www.phototherapy-centre.com
www.facebook.com/groups/PhotoTherapy.and.Therapeutic.Photograph
y

Overview: A small international organization
Mission: To educate about therapeutic uses of still & video photography
Chief Officer(s):
Judy Weiser, Contact
  jweiser@phototherapy-centre.com

International Society for Affective Disorders (ISAD)

c/o Caroline Holebrook, Institute of Psychiatry, King's College London, PO72 De Crespigny Park, Denmark Hill, London SE5 8AF UK
Tel: +44 (0) 20 7848 0295; *Fax:* +44 (0) 20 7848 0298
Other Communication: help@isad.org.uk
e-mail: enquiry@isad.org.uk
www.isad.org.uk
twitter.com/ISADTweet

Overview: A large international charitable organization founded in 2001

Mission: To advance research into affective disorders through all relevant scientific disciplines
Chief Officer(s):
Allan Young, President
Anthony Cleare, Treasurer
John Rush, Regional Representative, North America (Canada & the United States)
Caroline Holebrook, Administrator
  caroline.loveland@kcl.ac.uk
Publications:
• Journal of Affective Disorders
Type: Journal; *Editor:* Jair Soares; Paolo Brambilla

North American Society of Adlerian Psychology (NASAP)
#276, 429 East Dupont Rd., Fort Wayne IN 46825 USA
Tel: 260-267-8807; *Fax:* 260-818-2098
e-mail: info@alfredadler.org
www.alfredadler.org
www.linkedin.com/company/nasap-north-american-society-of-adlerian-psyc

Overview: A medium-sized international organization
Mission: To promote the teaching, understanding, & application of the core concepts of Adlerian (Individual) Psychology; To maintain the principles of Adlerian Psychology; To foster research, knowledge, & training; To operate according to the Codes of Ethics of the American Psychological Association, the International Coach Federation, & the National Board of Certified Counselors
Affiliation(s): Adler Graduate School of Minesota; Adler International Learning Inc.; Adler School of Professional Psychology; Aderian Psychology Association of British Columbia; Adlerian Society of Arizona; Adlerian Student Affiliate; Alfred Adler Institute of New York; ALFREDS - Adler Learning Federation for Research, Education & Delivery of Services; Central PA Society of Adlerian Psychology; Georgia Society of Adlerian Psychology; McAbee Adlerian Psychology Society (MAPS); Parent Encouragement Program (PEP); South Carolina Society of Adlerian Psychology; The Individual Psychology Society - Chicago (TIPS)
Chief Officer(s):
Susan Belangee, Vice-President
Michele Frey, Secretary
Susan Brokaw, Treasurer
Publications:
• Journal of Individual Psychology
Type: Journal; *Frequency:* Quarterly; *Editor:* Bill Curlette; Roy Kern
• NASAP [North American Society of Adlerian Psychology] Newsletter
Type: Newsletter; *Frequency:* Bimonthly

World Federation for Mental Health (WFMH) / Fédération mondiale pour la santé mentale
PO Box 807, Occoquan VA 22125 USA
Fax: 703-490-6926
e-mail: info@wfmh.com
www.wfmh.org
www.facebook.com/WFMH1
twitter.com/WFMHDC
Overview: A large international charitable organization founded in 1948
Mission: To promote mental health through advocacy, transfer of knowledge & consultation; to prevent or reduce the incidence & disabling consequences of mental illness throughout the world
Affliation(s): World Health Organization
Chief Officer(s):
George Christodoulou, President
Ellen R. Mercer, Vice-President, Program Development
Juan Mezzich, Vice-President, Government
Larry Cimino, Corporate Secretary

National Publications

Canadian Journal of Community Mental Health
c/o Department of Psychiatry, University of British Columbia, 2255 Wesbrook Mall, Vancouver, BC V6T 2A1

Frequency: 4 times a year
Covers mental health issues in community settings.
John Higenbottam, Editor-in-Chief, john_a@dccnet.com

Canadian Journal of Psychiatry
#701, 141 Laurier Ave. West, Ottawa, ON K1P 5J3
Tel: 613-234-2815; *Fax:* 613-234-9857
Toll-Free: 800-267-1555
Frequency: 12 times a year
Dr. Scott Patten, Editor-in-chief

Canadian Journal of Psychoanalysis / Revue canadienne de psychanalyse
Becker Associates, #202, 10 Morrow Ave., Toronto, ON M6R 2J1
Tel: 416-538-1650; *Fax:* 416-489-1713
journals@beckerassociates.ca
Circulation: 650 *Frequency:* Bi-annually
Charles Levin, Editor

The Chronicle of Neurology & Psychiatry
Owned By: Chronicle Companies
#306, 555 Burnhamthorpe Rd., Toronto, ON M9C 2Y3
Tel: 416-916-2476; *Fax:* 416-352-6199
Toll-Free: 866-632-4766
health@chronicle.org
Circulation: 6,189 *Frequency:* 6 times a year
Mitchell Shannon, Publisher
R. Allan Ryan, Editorial Director

Journal of Psychiatry & Neuroscience (JPN) / Revue de psychiatrie & de neuroscience
Owned By: Canadian Medical Association
1867 Alta Vista Dr., Ottawa, ON K1G 5W8
Toll-Free: 888-855-2555
jpn@cma.ca
Frequency: 6 times a year
Wendy Carroll, Managing Editor

Transcultural Psychiatry
Previous Name: Transcultural Psychiatric Research Review
Dept. of Psychiatry, McGill University, 1033, av des Pins ouest, Montréal, QC H3A 1A1
Tel: 514-398-7302; *Fax:* 514-375-1459
transcultural.psychiatry@mcgill.ca
Circulation: 500 *Frequency:* 5 times a year
Laurence J. Kirmayer, Editor M.D.

Local Schools

ALBERTA

Edmonton: Phoenix Academy
#145, 10403 - 172 St., Edmonton, AB T5S 1K9
Tel: 780-440-0708; *Fax:* 780-440-0760
www.upcs.org
Grades: K-12 *Note:* School for students who struggle with behavioural disorders and learning disabilities
Kathy King, Contact
  kking@upcs.org

Red Deer: Parkland School
6016 - 45 Ave., Red Deer, AB T4N 3M4
Tel: 403-347-3911; *Fax:* 403-342-2677
prkland@shaw.ca
www.parklandschool.org
Grades: 4-19 yrs old; Special Ed.
Number of Employees: 45
Trudy Lewis, Chief of Educational Services

MANITOBA

Brandon: Child & Adolescent Treatment Centre (CATC)
1240 - 10th St., Brandon, MB R7A 7L6
Tel: 204-727-3445; *Fax:* 204-727-3451
Toll-Free: 866-403-5459
www.brandonrha.mb.ca/en/Mental_Health/CATC
Other Information: After Hours Phone: 204-571-7278
Grades: 4-12 *Note:* The CATC provides mental health services to children, including a day program, Crisis Stabilization Unit, Early Intervention Services, & educational services
Brian Schoonbaert, CEO, Brandon Regional Health Authority, 204-578-2301
  schoonbaertb@brandonrha.mb.ca

Jayne Troop, VP, Community Services & Long-Term Care,
204-578-2304
troopj@brandonrha.mb.ca
Elizabeth McLeod, Program Manager, 204-571-7255

St Norbert: Behavioural Health Foundation
P.O. Box 250
35 av de la Digue, St Norbert, MB R3V 1L6, Canada
Tel: 204-269-3430; *Fax:* 204-269-8049
info@bhf.ca
www.bhf.ca

Note: The Behavioural Health Foundation provides long term
residential addictions treatment programming for men, women, teens
and family units experiencing a variety of addiction problems and
co-occurring mental health concerns.
Maureena Downing, Contact, 204-269-3430
maureenad@bhf.ca

NOVA SCOTIA

Wolfville: Landmark East School
708 Main St., Wolfville, NS B4P 1G4
Tel: 902-542-2237; *Fax:* 902-542-4147
Toll-Free: 800-565-5887
admissions@landmarkeast.org
www.landmarkeast.org
twitter.com/landmarkeast
www.youtube.com/lmeschoolcanada

Grades: 3-12 *Enrollment:* 60 *Note:* The international school serves
students with learning disabilities. Landmark East has an overall
student-teacher ratio of 3:1.
Jim Sotvedt, Chair
Peter Coll, Headmaster
pcoll@landmarkeast.org
Glen Currie, Director, Students
gcurrie@landmarkeast.org

QUÉBEC

Saint-Laurent: Summit School
École le Sommet
1750, rue Deguire, Saint-Laurent, QC H4L 1M7
Tel: 514-744-2867; *Fax:* 514-744-6410
admin@summit-school.com
www.summit-school.com

Grades: Pre./Elem./Sec.; Spec. Ed.; Eng. *Enrollment:* 600 *Note:*
Educational services for special needs students, from ages 4 to 21,
with developmental disabilities such as autism, behavioural
disturbances & other associated problems.
Herman Erdogmus, Director General
Bena Finkelberg, Vice-Principal
Ron Bergamin, Director, Finance

National Libraries

Canadian Mental Health Association
#1110, 151 Slater St., Ottawa, ON K1P 5H3
Tel: 613-745-7750; *Fax:* 613-745-5522
www.cmha.ca

Collection: Research reports; Discussion papers; Backgrounders;
Publications; Guides; Pamphlets

Provincial Libraries

Alberta Hospital - Ponoka
PO Box 1000, Ponoka, AB T4J 1R8
Tel: 403-783-7691; *Fax:* 403-783-7695
krs@albertahealthservices.ca
www.albertahealthservices.ca

Profile: At the Centennial Centre for Mental Health and Brain Injury,
people suffering from brain injury or psychiatric disorders receive care
and treatment. **Collection:** Archive for AHP history
Lori Maisey, Library Technician
lori.maisey@albertahealthservices.ca

Allan Memorial Institute of Psychiatry/ Institut psychiatrie Allan Memorial
#P2.033, 1025, av des Pins ouest, Montréal, QC H3A 1A1
Tel: 514-934-1934; *Fax:* 514-843-1731
ami.library@muhc.mcgill.ca

Association de Montréal pour la déficience intellectuelle/ Montréal Association for the Intellectually Handicapped
#100, 633, boul Crémazie est, Montréal, QC H2M 1L9
Tel: 514-381-2300; *Fax:* 514-381-0454
info@amdi.info
www.amdi.info

BC Mental Health & Substance Use Services
4500 Oak St., Vancouver, BC V6H 3N1
Tel: 604-524-7734
feedback@bcmhsus.bc.ca
bcmhsus.ca

Collection: Rating Scales; Practice Guidelines

Bibliothèque Albert-Prévost
#298, Pavillon Albert-Prévost, 6555, boul Gouin ouest, Montréal, QC
H4K 1B3
Tél: 514-338-2222
www.hscm.ca/enseignement/bibliotheques

Canadian Mental Health Association - Peterborough Branch
466 George St. North, Peterborough, ON K9H 3R7
Tel: 705-748-6711; *Fax:* 705-748-2577
Toll-Free: 866-990-9956
info@cmhahkpr.ca
www.cmhahkpr.ca
Social Media: twitter.com/cmhahkpr;
www.facebook.com/148148298570293

Collection: Books; periodicals; videos; audio cassettes
Jack Veitch, Health Promotion & Education Contact
jveitch@cmhahkpr.ca

Centennial Centre for Mental Health & Brain Injury Site
Dave Russell Education Complex, 46 St. South, Ponoka, AB T4J 1R8
Tel: 403-783-7691; *Fax:* 403-783-7695

Centre for Addiction & Mental Health
33 Russell St., Toronto, ON M5S 2S1
Tel: 416-535-8501; *Fax:* 416-595-6601
library@camh.ca
www.camh.ca
Social Media: www.youtube.com/camhtv; twitter.com/CAMHnews;
www.facebook.com/CentreforAddictionandMentalHealth
Collection: Temperance Collection, Social & Cultural History of
Drinking, Addiction Research Foundation Publications, Drug Education
Materials, C.K. Clarke Archives, Clarke Institute of Psychiatry
Publications
Tim Tripp, Director, Library
tim.tripp@camh.ca
416-535-8501 ext. 36999

Centre for Addiction & Mental Health Archives
1001 Queen St. West, Toronto, ON M6J 1H4
Tel: 416-535-8501; *Fax:* 416-583-1355
Collection: Institutional & manuscript records
John Court, Archivist
john.court@camh.ca

Centre intégré universitaire de santé et de services sociaux du Saguenay-Lac-Saint-Jean
305, rue St-Vallier, Chicoutimi, QC G7H 5H6
Tél: 418-541-1234; *Téléc:* 418-541-1145
www.santesaglac.com

Douglas Institute/ Institut Douglas
Pavillon Perry, 6875 LaSalle Blvd., #E-4501, Montréal, QC H4H 1R3
Tél: 514-762-3029; *Fax:* 514-762-3039
biblio@douglas.mcgill.ca
www.douglas.qc.ca/page/charles-cahn-library

Benoît Cameron, Librarian
benoit.cameron@douglas.mcgill.ca
514-762-3029 ext. 2486

Marie-Line Rioux, Library Technician
514-762-3029 ext. 2485

Le GIFRIC (Groupe interdisciplinaire freudien de recherches et d'interventions cliniques)
342, boul René-Lévesque ouest, Québec, QC G1S 1R9
Tél: 418-687-4350; *Téléc:* 418-683-1935
gifric@gifric.com
www.gifric.com

Hincks-Dellcrest Centre
114 Maitland St., Toronto, ON M4Y 1E1
Tel: 416-972-1935; *Fax:* 416-924-9808
jackman.library@hincksdellcrest.org
www.hincksdellcrest.org

Collection: Fellows' research papers & theses
Wylie Burke, Interim Director
wburke@hincksdellcrest.org

Hôpital Maisonneuve-Rosemont
Rez-de-chaussée, Pavillon J.A.-DeSève, 5415, boul de l'Assomption, Montréal, QC H1T 2M4
Tél: 514-252-3463
biblio.hmr.qc.ca

Richard Coveney, Bibliothécaire
rcoveney.hmr@ssss.gouv.qc.ca
514-252-3400 ext. 3686
Odette Hinse, Technicienne en documentation
ohinse.hmr@ssss.gouv.qc.ca
514-252-3400 ext. 3685
Lucie Grisé, Technicienne en documentation
lgrise.hmr@ssss.gouv.qc.ca
514-252-3462
Olivier Lafortune, Technicien en documentation
olafortune.hmr@ssss.gouv.qc.ca
514-252-3463

Hôpital Rivière-des-Prairies
7070, boul Perras, Montréal, QC H1E 1A4
Tél: 514-323-7260
bibliotheque.hrdp@ssss.gouv.qc.ca
www.hrdp.qc.ca

Isabelle Barrette, Responsable
isabelle.barrette.hrdp@ssss.gouv.qc.ca

Institut universitaire en santé mentale de Montréal
Pavillon Bédard, 7401, rue Hochelaga, 3e étage, #BE-316-34, Montréal, QC H1N 3M5
Tél: 514-251-4000; *Téléc:* 514-251-0270
centrededocumentation.iusmm@ssss.gouv.qc.ca
www.iusmm.ca/centre-de-documentation.html
Collection: Les monographies; Les périodiques; Les documents audiovisuels (VHS ou DVD)

Institut universitaire en santé mentale de Québec
#1639J, 2601, ch de la Canardière, Québec, QC G1J 2G3
Tél: 418-663-5300; *Téléc:* 418-666-9416
biblio@crulrg.ulaval.ca
www.institutsmq.qc.ca/en/enseignement/centre-de-documentation

Institute of Community & Family Psychiatry/ L'Institut de psychiatrie communautaire et familiale
4333, ch de la Côte Ste-Catherine, 2è étage, Montréal, QC H3T 1E4
Tél: 514-340-8222; *Fax:* 514-340-8104
icfplib.jgh@mail.mcgill.ca
www.jgh.ca
Profile: The library provides lending & specialized services to the staff & students of the Jewish General Hospital's Department of Psychiatry & its affiliated programs. **Collection:** Books, journals, & audiovisual material on the subject of general psychiatry, clinical psychiatry, & psychotherapies
Teodora Constantinescu, Librarian

North Bay Regional Health Centre
50 College Dr., North Bay, ON P1B 0A4
Tel: 705-474-8600
www.nbrhc.on.ca
Collection: Audio Digest Tapes on Psychiatry, Medical Videos
Bonnie Brownstein, Librarian

Ontario Shores Centre for Mental Health Sciences
700 Gordon St., Whitby, ON L1N 5S9
Tel: 905-430-4015; *Fax:* 905-430-4014
Toll-Free: 800-341-6323
www.ontarioshores.ca
Collection: Audio Digest series on Psychiatry

Pacific Region
33344 King Rd., Abbotsford, BC V2S 6J5
Tel: 604-870-7700; *Fax:* 604-870-7746

Parkwood Institute - Mental Health Care Building
550 Wellington Rd., #F2-191, London, ON N6C 0A7
Tel: 519-646-6100
www.sjhc.london.on.ca

Laurel Lamarre, Contact
519-646-6100 ext. 47440

PhotoTherapy Centre
890 The Grove Rd., Gambier Island, BC V0N 1V0
Tel: 604-202-3431
www.phototherapy-centre.com
Collection: PhotoTherapy techniques, using therapy clients' personal snapshots & family photographs as catalysts for therapeutic communication & personal healing
Judy Weiser, Director
jweiser@phototherapy-centre.com

Prairie Region
2520 Central Ave. North, Saskatoon, SK S7K 3X5
Tel: 306-975-5442; *Fax:* 306-975-6024

Providence Care - Mental Health Services
752 King St. West, Kingston, ON K7L 4X3
Tel: 613-548-5567
www.providencecare.ca
Collection: Staff Publications
Karen Gagnon, Director, Library Services
gagnonk@providencecare.ca

St. Joseph's Care Group
580 Algoma St. North, Thunder Bay, ON P7B 5G4
Tel: 807-343-4351
Other Numbers: 807-343-4356
sjcglibs@tbh.net
www.sjcg.net/departments/library

Selkirk Mental Health Centre Archives Collection Inc.
825 Manitoba Ave., Selkirk, MB R1A 2B5
Tel: 204-482-3810
smhc-archives.com
Profile: Collects & preserves records documenting the development of mental health services & psychiatric nursing in Manitoba, with a focus on Selkirk Mental Health Centre **Collection:** Letters; publications; photographs; artefacts; oral histories
Brian Kaltenberger, Archival Request Contact

Society for Manitobans with Disabilities
825 Sherbrook St., Winnipeg, MB R3A 1M5
Tel: 204-975-3010; *Fax:* 204-975-3073
Toll-Free: 866-282-8041
TTY: 204-975-308
www.smd.mb.ca
Collection: Online resources

Southwest Centre for Forensic Mental Health Care - St. Thomas
401 Sunset Dr., #C2-550, St. Thomas, ON N5R 3C6
Tel: 519-631-8510
www.sjhc.london.on.ca

Waterford Hospital
306 Waterford Bridge Rd., St. John's, NL A1E 4J8
Tel: 709-777-3300

Waypoint Centre for Mental Health Care
500 Church St., Penetanguishene, ON L9M 1G3
Tel: 705-549-3181
info@waypointcentre.ca
www.waypointcentre.ca

Collection: Staff Publications, Forensic Psychiatry
Carol Lambie, President & CEO

Provincial Government

Addiction & Mental Health Services / Services de traitement des dépendances et de santé mentale

Tel: 506-444-4442
Fax: 506-453-8711

Executive Director, Gisèle Maillet
Tel: 506-381-0854
gisele.maillet@gnb.ca
Director, Child & Youth Services, Yvette Doiron
Tel: 506-869-6118
yvette.doiron-brun@gnb.ca
Director, Adult Services, Sylvie Martin
Tel: 506-473-7588
sylvie.martin@gnb.ca

National Hospitals

BRITISH COLUMBIA

ABBOTSFORD: Pacific Institution / Regional Treatment Centre
Correctional Services Canada, Dept. of the Solicitor General
Former Name: Regional Health Centre (Pacific)
Also Known As: Pacific Institution
PO Box 3000, 33344 King Rd., Abbotsford, BC V2S 4P4
Tel: 604-870-7700 Fax: 604-870-7746
www.csc-scc.gc.ca/institutions/001002-5008-eng.shtml
Year Founded: 1972
Number of Beds: 122 beds
Note: Psychiatric care unit, health centre, rehabilitation unit, regional reception/assessment centre, & intensive program unit

SASKATCHEWAN

SASKATOON: Regional Psychiatric Centre (Prairies)
PO Box 9243, 2520 Central Ave. North, Saskatoon, SK S7K 3X5
Tel: 306-975-5400 Fax: 306-975-6024
www.csc-scc.gc.ca/institutions/001002-4009-eng.shtml
Year Founded: 1978
Number of Beds: 204 beds
Tim Krause, Assistant Warden, Management Services

Local Hospitals & Health Centres

ALBERTA

AIRDRIE: Airdrie - 209 Centre Avenue West
Affiliated with: Alberta Health Services
209 Centre Ave. West, Airdrie, AB T4B 3L8
Tel: 403-948-8553 Fax: 403-912-3307
Toll-Free: 866-332-2322
www.albertahealthservices.ca

AIRDRIE: Airdrie Provincial Building
Affiliated with: Alberta Health Services
Former Name: Airdrie Mental Health Clinic
104 - 1 Ave. NW, Airdrie, AB T4B 0R2
Tel: 403-948-3878 Fax: 403-948-7926
Toll-Free: 877-652-4700
www.albertahealthservices.ca

ATHABASCA: Athabasca Community Health Services
Affiliated with: Alberta Health Services
3401 - 48 Ave., Athabasca, AB T9S 1M7
Tel: 780-675-5404 Fax: 780-675-3111
www.albertahealthservices.ca

BANFF: Banff - Mineral Springs Hospital
Banff Community Health Centre
Affiliated with: Alberta Health Services
303 Lynx St., Banff, AB T1L 1B3
Tel: 403-762-4451 Fax: 403-762-5570
www.albertahealthservices.ca

Note: Provides assessment, treatment, counselling, & referral services for people experiencing mental health issues

BARRHEAD: Barrhead Healthcare Centre
Affiliated with: Alberta Health Services
PO Box 4504, 4815 - 51 Ave., Barrhead, AB T7N 1M1
Tel: 780-674-8243 Fax: 780-674-8352
www.albertahealthservices.ca

BLACK DIAMOND: Black Diamond Mental Health Centre at Oilfields General Hospital
Affiliated with: Alberta Health Services
717 Government Rd., Black Diamond, AB T0L 0H0
Tel: 403-933-3800 Fax: 403-933-4353
Toll-Free: 877-652-4700
www.albertahealthservices.ca

Note: Services include: assessment; treatment; group therapy; & geriatric services.

BLAIRMORE: Crowsnest Pass Provincial Building
Affiliated with: Alberta Health Services
PO Box 206, 12501 - 20 Ave., Blairmore, AB T0K 0E0
Tel: 403-562-3222
www.albertahealthservices.ca

BON ACCORD: Oak Hill Boys Ranch
PO Box 97, 56119 - Range Rd. 240, Bon Accord, AB T0A 0K0
Tel: 780-921-2121
www.oakhillboysranch.ca
Number of Beds: 32 beds
Note: Residential treatment facility for young males (11-16) suffering from issues such as mental health & substance abuse.
Anton Smith, Executive Director

BONNYVILLE: Bonnyville New Park Place
Affiliated with: Alberta Health Services
Bonnyville Remax Bldg., 5201 - 44 St., Bonnyville, AB T9N 2G5
Tel: 780-826-2404 Fax: 780-826-6114
www.albertahealthservices.ca

BOW ISLAND: Bow Island Provincial Building
Affiliated with: Alberta Health Services
Former Name: Bow Island Mental Health Clinic
802 - 6 St. East, Bow Island, AB T0K 0G0
Tel: 403-529-3500 Fax: 403-529-3562
www.albertahealthservices.ca

BROOKS: Brooks Community Mental Health Clinic
Affiliated with: Alberta Health Services
440 - 3rd St. East, Brooks, AB T1R 1C5
Tel: 403-793-6655 Fax: 403-793-6656
www.albertahealthservices.ca

CALGARY: Arnika Centre
Affiliated with: Alberta Health Services
3465 - 26 Ave. NE, Calgary, AB T1Y 6L4
Tel: 403-943-8301 Fax: 403-943-8367
www.albertahealthservices.ca

Note: Psychiatric assessment for people 16 years & older

CALGARY: Bridgeland Seniors Health Centre
Affiliated with: Alberta Health Services
1070 Mcdougall Rd. NE, Calgary, AB T2E 7Z2
Tel: 403-955-1555 Fax: 403-955-1564
www.albertahealthservices.ca

CALGARY: Calgary - 316-7 Avenue SE
Affiliated with: Alberta Health Services
316 - 7 Ave. SE, Calgary, AB T2G 0J2
Tel: 403-428-3308
www.albertahealthservices.ca

CALGARY: Carewest Operational Stress Injury Clinic
Affiliated with: Alberta Health Services
Also Known As: Carewest OSI Clinic
Market Mall, 3625 Shaganappi Trail NW, Calgary, AB T3A 0E2
Tel: 403-216-9860 *Fax:* 403-216-9861
www.carewest.ca

Note: Provides programs & services to help deal with mental health problems caused by shock or stress for veterans, Canadian Forces members, RCMP members, & their families.

CALGARY: Distress Centre Calgary (DCC)
Affiliated with: Alberta Health Services
#300, 1010 - 8th Ave. SW, Calgary, AB T2P 1J2
Tel: 403-266-1601
info@distresscentre.com
www.distresscentre.com
Info Line: 403-266-4357
Social Media: www.facebook.com/distresscentre;
twitter.com/Distress_Centre;
www.youtube.com/user/DistressCentreYYC

Note: Offers crisis support, professional counselling, & referrals to people in distress
Joan Roy, Executive Director
Bing Hu, Chief Financial Officer
Jerilyn Dressler, Director, Operations
Diane Jones Konihowski, Director, Fund Development & Communications

CALGARY: East Calgary Health Centre
Affiliated with: Alberta Health Services
4715 - 8 Ave. SE, Calgary, AB T2A 3N4
Tel: 403-955-1010 *Fax:* 403-955-1013
www.albertahealthservices.ca

Note: Perinatal mental health; child & adolescent addiction & mental health

CALGARY: Northeast Calgary Mental Health Clinic
Affiliated with: Alberta Health Services
Sunridge Mall, #200, 2580 - 32 St. NE, Calgary, AB T1Y 7M8
Tel: 403-944-9700
www.albertahealthservices.ca

Note: Provides mental health assessment, treatment, & therapy services.

CALGARY: Northwest Community Mental Health Centre
Affiliated with: Alberta Health Services
Former Name: Foothills Professional Building
#280, 1620 - 29th St. NW, Calgary, AB T2N 4L7
Tel: 403-943-1500 *Toll-Free:* 866-943-1500
www.albertahealthservices.ca

CALGARY: Society for Treatment of Autism (STA)
404 - 94 Ave. SE, Calgary, AB T2J 0E8
Tel: 403-253-2291 *Fax:* 403-253-6974
Toll-Free: 888-301-2872
consultation@sta-ab.com
www.sta-ab.com
Number of Beds: 20 beds
Note: Programs & services for people with autism & other pervasive developmental disorders
Dave Mikkelsen, Executive Director

CALGARY: South Calgary Health Centre
Affiliated with: Alberta Health Services
31 Sunpark Plaza SE, 2nd Fl., Calgary, AB T2X 3W5
Tel: 403-943-9374
www.albertahealthservices.ca

Note: Mental health urgent care & walk-in services
Sue Ramsden, Site Manager

CALGARY: Sunridge Professional Building
Affiliated with: Alberta Health Services
#201, 2675 - 36 St. NE, Calgary, AB T1Y 6H6
Tel: 403-943-4596 *Fax:* 403-219-3521
www.albertahealthservices.ca

Note: Mental health forensic assessment services

CALGARY: Wood's Homes - Bowness Campus
Affiliated with: Alberta Health Services
9400 - 48 Ave. NW, Calgary, AB T3B 2B2
Tel: 403-247-6751 *Fax:* 403-286-0878
askus@woodshomes.ca
www.woodshomes.ca
Social Media: www.facebook.com/woodshomesnfp;
twitter.com/ChildMntlHealth; www.youtube.com/user/WoodsHomes1;
www.linkedin.com/company/wood%27s-homes
Number of Beds: 110 beds

CALGARY: Wood's Homes - Parkdale Campus
805 - 37 St. NW, Calgary, AB T2N 4N8
Tel: 403-270-4102 *Fax:* 403-283-9735
askus@woodshomes.ca
www.woodshomes.ca
Info Line: 800-563-6106
Social Media: www.facebook.com/woodshomesnfp;
twitter.com/ChildMntlHealth; www.youtube.com/user/WoodsHomes1;
www.linkedin.com/company/wood%27s-homes
Year Founded: 1914
Number of Beds: 150 beds
Area Served: Alberta; Northwest Territories
Population Served: 20000
Number of Employees: 500
Specialties: Crisis counselling & outreach services; residential treatment
Note: Foster care; homeless youth shelters; specialized learning; day treatment; residential treatment; outreach services; & child welfare services.
Sylvia MacIver, Communications Manager
403-270-1768, sylvia.maciver@woodshomes.ca

CAMROSE: Camrose Addiction & Mental Health Clinic
Affiliated with: Alberta Health Services
4911 - 47 St., Camrose, AB T4V 1J9
Tel: 780-679-1181 *Fax:* 780-679-1740
www.albertahealthservices.ca

CANMORE: Canmore Provincial Building
Affiliated with: Alberta Health Services
800 Railway Ave., Canmore, AB T1W 1P1
Tel: 403-678-4696 *Fax:* 403-678-1951
www.albertahealthservices.ca

CARDSTON: Cardston Community Mental Health Clinic
Affiliated with: Alberta Health Services
576 Main St., Cardston, AB T0K 0K0
Tel: 403-653-5240 *Fax:* 403-653-2926
www.albertahealthservices.ca

CHESTERMERE: Chestermere Community Health Centre
Affiliated with: Alberta Health Services
288 Kinniburgh Blvd., Chestermere, AB T1X 0V8
Tel: 403-365-5400 *Toll-Free:* 877-652-4700
www.albertahealthservices.ca

Note: Provides mental health assessment & treatment as well as addiction prevention services

CLARESHOLM: Claresholm Centre for Mental Health & Addictions
Affiliated with: Alberta Health Services
PO Box 490, 139 - 43 Ave. West, Claresholm, AB T0L 0T0
Tel: 403-682-3563 *Fax:* 403-625-4318
claresholmcentre@albertahealthservices.ca
www.claresholmcentre.com
Year Founded: 1933
Number of Beds: 108 beds

Note: Programs & services include: active rehabilitation; concurrent disorders; extended treatment; & transitions

CLARESHOLM: Claresholm Mental Health Clinic
Affiliated with: Alberta Health Services
4901 - 2nd St. West, Claresholm, AB T0L 0T0

Tel: 403-625-4068

Note: Services include: assessment; treatment; information; & referral.

COCHRANE: Cochrane Addiction & Mental Health Clinic
Affiliated with: Alberta Health Services
60 Grande Blvd., Cochrane, AB T4C 0S4

Tel: 403-851-6100 *Fax:* 403-851-6101
www.albertahealthservices.ca

COLD LAKE: Cold Lake Healthcare Centre
Affiliated with: Alberta Health Services
#208, 314 - 25 St., Cold Lake, AB T9M 1G6

Tel: 780-639-4922 *Fax:* 780-639-4990
www.albertahealthservices.ca

CONSORT: Consort Community Health Centre
Affiliated with: Alberta Health Services
5410 - 52 Ave., Consort, AB T0C 1B0

Tel: 403-577-3770 *Fax:* 403-577-2235
www.albertahealthservices.ca

DIDSBURY: Didsbury District Health Services
Affiliated with: Alberta Health Services
1210 - 20 Ave., Didsbury, AB T0M 0W0

Tel: 403-335-7285 *Fax:* 403-335-7227
www.albertahealthservices.ca

DRAYTON VALLEY: Drayton Valley Mental Health Clinic
Affiliated with: Alberta Health Services
4110 - 50 Ave., Drayton Valley, AB T7A 0B3

Tel: 780-542-3140 *Fax:* 780-542-4461
www.albertahealthservices.ca

DRUMHELLER: Drumheller Health Centre
Affiliated with: Alberta Health Services
351 - 9 St. NW, Drumheller, AB T0J 0Y1

Tel: 403-820-7863 *Fax:* 403-820-7865
www.albertahealthservices.ca

EDMONTON: Addiction Services Edmonton
Affiliated with: Alberta Health Services
10010 - 102A Ave. NW, Edmonton, AB T5J 0G5

Tel: 780-427-2736 *Fax:* 780-427-4180
Toll-Free: 866-332-2322
www.albertahealthservices.ca

Note: Addiction prevention & mental health promotion

EDMONTON: Alberta Hospital Edmonton
Affiliated with: Alberta Health Services
17480 Fort Rd., Edmonton, AB T5J 2J7

Tel: 780-342-5555
www.albertahealthservices.ca

Year Founded: 1923
Number of Beds: 410 beds
Note: Provides assessment, diagnosis, treatment, education, & consultation. Conducts research. Programs & services include: acute inpatient services; early psychosis intervention; group home support; inpatient intensive care; inpatient rehabilitation; & wellness recovery. Donna Tchida, Site Director

EDMONTON: Edmonton 108 Street Building
Affiliated with: Alberta Health Services
9942 - 108th St. NW, Edmonton, AB T5K 2J5

Tel: 780-342-7700 *Fax:* 780-342-7621
www.albertahealthservices.ca

EDMONTON: Forensic & Community Services
Affiliated with: Alberta Health Services
10225 - 106 St., Edmonton, AB T5J 1H5

Tel: 780-342-6400
www.albertahealthservices.ca

Note: Offers counselling as well as addiction &/or mental health treatment

EDMONTON: Hys Medical Centre
Affiliated with: Alberta Health Services
11010 - 101 St., Edmonton, AB T5H 4B9

Tel: 780-342-9100 *Fax:* 780-424-4964
www.albertahealthservices.ca

Note: Geriatric psychiatry & laboratory services

EDMONTON: Northeast Community Health Centre
Affiliated with: Alberta Health Services
14007 - 50 St., Edmonton, AB T5A 5E4

Tel: 780-342-4027
www.albertahealthservices.ca

Note: Addictions & mental health services

EDMONTON: Villa Caritas
Covenant Health
Affiliated with: Alberta Health Services
16515 - 88 Ave. NW, Edmonton, AB T5R 0A4

Tel: 780-342-6500
www.covenanthealth.ca/hospitals-care-centres/villa-caritas
Number of Beds: 120 acute geriatric psychiatry beds; 30 geriatric psychiatry transitional beds
Note: Acute mental health facility for seniors, located on the Misericordia Community Hospital campus.

EDSON: Edson Provincial Building
Affiliated with: Alberta Health Services
Former Name: Edson Mental Health Centre
#100, 111 - 54 St., Edson, AB T7E 1T2

Tel: 780-723-8294 *Fax:* 780-723-8297
www.albertahealthservices.ca

FAIRVIEW: Fairview Health Complex
Affiliated with: Alberta Health Services
PO Box 2201, 10628 - 110 St., Fairview, AB T0H 1L0

Tel: 780-835-6149 *Fax:* 780-835-6185
www.albertahealthservices.ca
Info Line: 877-303-2642

FORT MACLEOD: Fort Macleod Community Health
Affiliated with: Alberta Health Services
744 - 26 St., Fort MacLeod, AB T0L 0Z0

Tel: 403-553-5340 *Fax:* 403-553-4940
www.albertahealthservices.ca

FORT MCMURRAY: Northern Lights Regional Health Centre
Affiliated with: Alberta Health Services
7 Hospital St., Fort McMurray, AB T9H 1P2

Tel: 780-791-6194 *Fax:* 780-791-6219
www.albertahealthservices.ca

FORT SASKATCHEWAN: Fort Saskatchewan Community Hospital
Affiliated with: Alberta Health Services
Former Name: Fort Saskatchewan Health Centre
9401 - 86 Ave., Fort Saskatchewan, AB T8L 0C6

Tel: 780-342-2388 *Fax:* 780-342-3348
www.albertahealthservices.ca

Note: Provides addiction & mental health assessment & treatment services

FORT VERMILION: St. Theresa General Hospital
Affiliated with: Alberta Health Services
4506 - 46 Ave., Fort Vermilion, AB T0H 1N0

Tel: 780-841-3229 *Fax:* 780-926-3738
Toll-Free: 877-823-6433
www.albertahealthservices.ca

Note: Provides mental health treatment & information services.

FOX CREEK: Fox Creek Healthcare Centre
Affiliated with: Alberta Health Services
600 - 3rd St., Fox Creek, AB T0H 1P0
Tel: 780-622-5106 *Fax:* 780-622-3474
www.albertahealthservices.ca

GRANDE CACHE: Pine Plaza Building
Affiliated with: Alberta Health Services
PO Box 120, 702 Pine Plaza NW, Grande Cache, AB T0E 0Y0
Tel: 780-827-4998 *Fax:* 780-827-7207
www.albertahealthservices.ca
Info Line: 877-303-2642

Note: Addictions & mental health services

GRANDE PRAIRIE: Grande Prairie Nordic Court
Affiliated with: Alberta Health Services
Former Name: Nordic Court Mental Health Clinic
#600, 10014 - 99th St., Grande Prairie, AB T8V 3N4
Tel: 780-538-5160 *Fax:* 780-538-6279
www.albertahealthservices.ca

HANNA: Hanna Health Centre
Affiliated with: Alberta Health Services
904 Centre St. North, Hanna, AB T0J 1P0
Tel: 403-854-5276 *Fax:* 403-854-5280
www.albertahealthservices.ca

HIGH LEVEL: Northwest Health Centre
Affiliated with: Alberta Health Services
11202 - 100 Ave., High Level, AB T0H 1Z0
Tel: 780-841-3229 *Fax:* 780-926-3738
Toll-Free: 877-823-6433
www.albertahealthservices.ca

HIGH PRAIRIE: High Prairie Health Complex
Affiliated with: Alberta Health Services
4620 - 53 Ave., High Prairie, AB T0G 1E0
Tel: 780-523-6490 *Fax:* 780-523-6491
Toll-Free: 877-823-6433
www.albertahealthservices.ca

HIGH RIVER: High River Addiction & Mental Health Clinic
Affiliated with: Alberta Health Services
#200, 617 - 1 St. West, High River, AB T1V 1M5
Tel: 403-652-8340 *Fax:* 403-601-8016
Toll-Free: 877-652-4700
www.albertahealthservices.ca

Jill McEwen, Manager, Administration

HINTON: Hinton Community Health Services
Affiliated with: Alberta Health Services
Former Name: Hinton Mental Health Centre
1280A Switzer Dr., Hinton, AB T7V 1T5
Tel: 780-865-8247 *Fax:* 780-865-8327
www.albertahealthservices.ca

INNISFAIL: Innisfail Health Centre
Affiliated with: Alberta Health Services
5023 - 42 St., Innisfail, AB T4G 1A9
Tel: 403-227-4601 *Fax:* 403-227-5683
www.albertahealthservices.ca

JASPER: Seton - Jasper Healthcare Centre
Affiliated with: Alberta Health Services
PO Box 310, 518 Robson St., Jasper, AB T0E 1E0
Tel: 780-852-6640 *Fax:* 780-852-3413
Toll-Free: 877-303-2642
www.albertahealthservices.ca

KILLAM: Killam 4811 - 49 Avenue
Affiliated with: Alberta Health Services
4811 - 49 Ave., Killam, AB T0B 2L0
Tel: 780-385-7161 *Fax:* 780-385-3329
www.albertahealthservices.ca

Note: Provides assessment, treatment, & rehabilitation services for individuals experiencing mental health issues

LA CRETE: La Crete Continuing Care Centre
Affiliated with: Alberta Health Services
10601 - 100 Ave., La Crete, AB T0H 2H0
Tel: 780-928-2410 *Fax:* 877-853-5380
Toll-Free: 877-823-6433
www.albertahealthservices.ca

LAC LA BICHE: Lac La Biche Provincial Building
Affiliated with: Alberta Health Services
Former Name: Lac La Biche Community Health Services
PO Box 297, 9503 Beaver Hill Rd., Lac La Biche, AB T0A 2C0
Tel: 780-623-5230 *Fax:* 780-623-5232
www.albertahealthservices.ca

LACOMBE: Lacombe Mental Health Centre
Affiliated with: Alberta Health Services
5033 - 52 St., Lacombe, AB T4L 2A6
Tel: 403-782-3413 *Fax:* 403-782-3878
www.albertahealthservices.ca

LAMONT: Lamont Health Care Centre
Affiliated with: Alberta Health Services
PO Box 479, 5216 - 53 St., Lamont, AB T0B 2R0
Tel: 780-895-5817 *Fax:* 780-895-7305
www.lamonthealthcarecentre.com

Note: Affiliated with the United Church of Canada.
Harold James, Executive Director
 harold.james@ahs.ca

LEDUC: Leduc Addiction & Mental Health Clinic
Affiliated with: Alberta Health Services
Centre Hope Bldg., 4906 - 49 Ave., Leduc, AB T9E 6W6
Tel: 780-986-2660 *Fax:* 780-986-9292
www.albertahealthservices.ca

LEDUC: Leduc Neighbourhood Centre
Affiliated with: Alberta Health Services
4901 - 50 Ave., Leduc, AB T9E 6W7
Tel: 780-980-7580 *Fax:* 780-980-7581
Toll-Free: 866-332-2322
www.albertahealthservices.ca

Note: Addiction & mental health services

LETHBRIDGE: Chinook Regional Hospital
Affiliated with: Alberta Health Services
Former Name: Lethbridge Regional Hospital
960 - 19 St. South, Lethbridge, AB T1J 1W5
Tel: 403-388-6244 *Fax:* 403-388-6250
www.albertahealthservices.ca

Note: Child & adolescent mental health; day treatment centre

LETHBRIDGE: Lethbridge Provincial Building
Affiliated with: Alberta Health Services
#103, 200 - 5th Ave. South, Lethbridge, AB T1J 4L1
Tel: 403-381-5260 *Fax:* 403-382-4518
www.albertahealthservices.ca

Note: Addictions & mental health services

MAYERTHORPE: Mayerthorpe Healthcare Centre
Affiliated with: Alberta Health Services
PO Box 30, 4417 - 45 St., Mayerthorpe, AB T0E 1N0
Tel: 780-786-2279 *Fax:* 780-786-2023
www.albertahealthservices.ca

Note: Provides mental health assessment, diagnosis, treatment, therapy, support, & referral services

MEDICINE HAT: Medicine Hat Provincial Building
Affiliated with: Alberta Health Services
Former Name: Medicine Hat Community Mental Health
346 - 3 St. SE, Medicine Hat, AB T1A 0G7
Tel: 403-529-3500 *Fax:* 403-529-3562
www.albertahealthservices.ca

MEDICINE HAT: Regional Resource Centre
Affiliated with: Alberta Health Services
631 Prospect Dr. SW, Medicine Hat, AB T1A 4C2
Tel: 403-529-8030 *Fax:* 403-502-8618
www.albertahealthservices.ca

Note: Programs & services include: child & adolescent mental health program; mental health diversion services for adults with low risk minor criminal offences; & mental health outreach

MORINVILLE: Morinville Provincial Building
Affiliated with: Alberta Health Services
10008 - 107 St., Morinville, AB T8R 1L3
Tel: 780-342-2620 *Fax:* 780-939-1216
www.albertahealthservices.ca

Note: Addiction & mental health community clinics

OKOTOKS: Okotoks Mental Health Centre
Affiliated with: Alberta Health Services
11 Cimarron Common, Okotoks, AB T1S 2E9
Tel: 403-995-2712 *Toll-Free:* 877-652-4700
www.albertahealthservices.ca

Note: Addiction prevention & mental health assessment & treatment services

OLDS: Olds Provincial Building
Affiliated with: Alberta Health Services
#212, 5025 - 50th St., Olds, AB T4H 1R9
Tel: 403-507-8174 *Fax:* 403-556-1584
www.albertahealthservices.ca

Note: Addictions & mental health services

ONOWAY: Onoway Community Health Services
Affiliated with: Alberta Health Services
PO Box 1047, 5115 Lac St. Anne Trail, Onoway, AB T0E 1V0
Tel: 780-967-9117 *Fax:* 780-967-2547
www.albertahealthservices.ca

PEACE RIVER: Peace River Mental Health Clinic
Affiliated with: Alberta Health Services
10015 - 98 St., Peace River, AB T8S 1T4
Tel: 780-624-6151 *Fax:* 780-624-6565
www.albertahealthservices.ca

PINCHER CREEK: Pincher Creek Community Mental Health Clinic
Affiliated with: Alberta Health Services
#212, 782 Main St., Pincher Creek, AB T0K 1W0
Tel: 403-627-1121 *Fax:* 403-627-1145
www.albertahealthservices.ca

PONOKA: Centennial Centre for Mental Health & Brain Injury
Affiliated with: Alberta Health Services
PO Box 1000, 46 St. South, Ponoka, AB T4J 1R8
Tel: 403-783-7600
www.albertahealthservices.ca

Note: Specialized mental health & brain injury treatment & care

PONOKA: Ponoka Provincial Building
Affiliated with: Alberta Health Services
#223, 5110 - 49th Ave., Ponoka, AB T4J 1R6
Tel: 403-783-7903 *Fax:* 403-785-7926
www.albertahealthservices.ca

Note: Addictions & mental health services

PROVOST: Provost Provincial Building
Affiliated with: Alberta Health Services
5419 - 44 St., Provost, AB T0B 3S0
Tel: 780-753-2575 *Fax:* 780-753-8096
www.albertahealthservices.ca

RAYMOND: Prairie Ridge
Good Samaritan Society
Affiliated with: Alberta Health Services
Former Name: Prairie Ridge Hospital
PO Box 630, 328 Broadway South, Raymond, AB T0K 2S0
Tel: 403-752-3441 *Fax:* 403-752-3250
goodsaminfo@gss.org
www.gss.org
Number of Beds: 50 supportive living suites; 30 geriatric mental health care beds; 5 community support beds
Note: Services include assisted living & dementia care.
Shawn Terlson, President & CEO, Good Samaritan Society
sterlson@gss.org

RAYMOND: Raymond Health Centre
Affiliated with: Alberta Health Services
150 North - 4 St. East, Raymond, AB T0K 2S0
Tel: 403-752-5440 *Fax:* 403-752-4147
www.albertahealthservices.ca

RED DEER: Red Deer - 49th Street Community Health Centre
Affiliated with: Alberta Health Services
4733 - 49 St., Red Deer, AB T4N 1T6
Tel: 403-340-5466 *Fax:* 403-340-4874
www.albertahealthservices.ca

ROCKY MOUNTAIN HOUSE: Rocky Mountain House Health Centre
Affiliated with: Alberta Health Services
5016 - 52 Ave., Rocky Mountain House, AB T4T 1T2
Tel: 403-844-5235 *Fax:* 403-844-5236
www.albertahealthservices.ca

Note: Provides assessment, treatment, & rehabilitation services for people with mental health issues

SHERWOOD PARK: Strathcona County Health Centre
Affiliated with: Alberta Health Services
2 Brower Dr., Sherwood Park, AB T8H 1V4
Tel: 780-342-4600
www.albertahealthservices.ca
Info Line: 877-303-2642

SLAVE LAKE: Slave Lake Mental Health Services
Affiliated with: Alberta Health Services
101 Main St. SE, Slave Lake, AB T0G 2A3
Tel: 780-805-3502 *Fax:* 780-805-3550
www.albertahealthservices.ca

SMOKY LAKE: George McDougall - Smoky Lake Healthcare Centre
Affiliated with: Alberta Health Services
Smoky Lake Health Unit, 4212 - 55 Ave., Smoky Lake, AB T0A 3C0
Tel: 780-656-3595 *Fax:* 780-656-2242
www.albertahealthservices.ca

SPIRIT RIVER: Spirit River Community Health Services
Affiliated with: Alberta Health Services
Former Name: Mistahia Health Unit - Spirit River
5003 - 45 Ave., Spirit River, AB T0H 3G0
Tel: 780-538-5160 *Fax:* 780-538-6279
Toll-Free: 877-823-6433
www.albertahealthservices.ca

Note: Provides assessment, diagnosis, treatment, therapy, support, & referral services for individuals experiencing mental health issues.

SPRUCE GROVE: Stan Woloshyn Building
Affiliated with: Alberta Health Services
205 Diamond Ave., Spruce Grove, AB T7X 3A8
Tel: 780-342-1344
www.albertahealthservices.ca

Note: Addiction & mental health services for children, youth, & adults

ST ALBERT: St. Albert Provincial Building
Affiliated with: Alberta Health Services
30 Sir Winston Churchill Ave., St Albert, AB T8N 3A3
Tel: 780-342-1410 *Fax:* 780-460-7152
www.albertahealthservices.ca

ST. PAUL: St. Therese - St. Paul Healthcare Centre
Affiliated with: Alberta Health Services
4713 - 48 Ave., St. Paul, AB T0A 3A3
Tel: 780-645-1850 *Fax:* 780-645-2788
www.albertahealthservices.ca

STANDOFF: Kainai Wellness Centre
Blood Tribe Department of Health Inc.
PO Box 229, Standoff, AB T0L 1Y0
Tel: 403-737-3883 *Fax:* 403-737-2036
btdh.ca/staff/kainai-wellness-centre
Year Founded: 1985
Note: Provides programs & services for the Blood Tribe Community, including criss intervention & prevention, mental health, alcohol & drug abuse programs, counselling, stress management, relaxation therapy, mental illness education, grief & loss recovery, & wellness.
Sandy Many Chief, Director
sandi.mc@btdh.ca

STETTLER: Stettler Hospital & Care Centre
Affiliated with: Alberta Health Services
5912 - 47 Ave., Stettler, AB T0C 2L0
Tel: 403-743-2000 *Fax:* 403-740-8880
www.albertahealthservices.ca

STONY PLAIN: WestView Health Centre
Affiliated with: Alberta Health Services
4405 South Park Dr., Stony Plain, AB T7Z 2M7
Tel: 780-963-6151 *Fax:* 780-963-7186
Toll-Free: 866-332-2322
www.albertahealthservices.ca

Note: Addiction prevention & mental health promotion services

SWAN HILLS: Swan Hills Healthcare Centre
Affiliated with: Alberta Health Services
PO Box 261, 29 Freeman Dr., Swan Hills, AB T0G 2C0
Tel: 780-333-4241 *Fax:* 780-333-7009
www.albertahealthservices.ca

SYLVAN LAKE: Sylvan Lake Community Health Centre
Affiliated with: Alberta Health Services
4602 - 49 Ave., Sylvan Lake, AB T4S 1M7
Tel: 403-887-6777 *Fax:* 403-887-6721
www.albertahealthservices.ca

Note: Provides mental health assessment, treatment, & rehabilitation programs & services

TABER: Taber Health Centre
Affiliated with: Alberta Health Services
4326 - 50 Ave., Taber, AB T1G 1N9
Tel: 403-223-7244 *Fax:* 403-223-7236
www.albertahealthservices.ca

Note: Offers assessment, treatment, counselling, & other addiction & mental health services.

THREE HILLS: Three Hills Provincial Building
Affiliated with: Alberta Health Services
Former Name: Three Hills Mental Health Centre
128 - 3 Ave. SE, Three Hills, AB T0M 2A0
Tel: 403-443-8532 *Fax:* 403-443-8541
www.albertahealthservices.ca

Note: Addictions (403-820-7863) & mental health services

TOFIELD: Tofield - 5024-51 Avenue
Affiliated with: Alberta Health Services
5024 - 51 Ave., Tofield, AB T0B 4J0
Tel: 780-672-1181 *Fax:* 780-679-1737
www.albertahealthservices.ca

Note: Child & adolescent addiction & mental health services.

VEGREVILLE: Vegreville Community Health Centre
Affiliated with: Alberta Health Services
5318 - 50 St., Vegreville, AB T9C 1R1
Tel: 780-632-2714 *Fax:* 780-632-4954
www.albertahealthservices.ca

VERMILION: Vermilion Provincial Building
Affiliated with: Alberta Health Services
4701 - 52 St., Vermilion, AB T9X 1J9
Tel: 780-581-8000 *Fax:* 780-851-8001
www.albertahealthservices.ca

VULCAN: Vulcan Community Health Centre
Affiliated with: Alberta Health Services
610 Elizabeth St. South, Vulcan, AB T0L 2B0
Tel: 403-485-3356
www.albertahealthservices.ca

Note: Offers mental health assessment, treatment, counselling, & referral services

WAINWRIGHT: Wainwright Provincial Building
Affiliated with: Alberta Health Services
810 - 14 Ave., Wainwright, AB T9W 1R2
Tel: 780-842-7522 *Fax:* 780-842-3151
www.albertahealthservices.ca

WESTLOCK: Westlock Community Health Services
Affiliated with: Alberta Health Services
10024 - 107 Ave., Westlock, AB T7P 2E3
Tel: 780-349-5246 *Fax:* 780-349-5846
www.albertahealthservices.ca

Note: Mental health assessment, diagnosis, treatment, therapy, support, & referral services

WETASKIWIN: Wetaskiwin Provincial Building
Affiliated with: Alberta Health Services
#101, 5201 - 50 Ave., Wetaskiwin, AB T9A 0S7
Tel: 780-361-1245 *Fax:* 780-361-1387
www.albertahealthservices.ca

WHITECOURT: Whitecourt Healthcare Centre
Affiliated with: Alberta Health Services
20 Sunset Blvd., Whitecourt, AB T7S 1M8
Tel: 780-706-3281 *Fax:* 780-706-7154
www.albertahealthservices.ca

BRITISH COLUMBIA

100 MILE HOUSE: 100 Mile Mental Health
Affiliated with: Interior Health Authority
555 Cedar Ave. South, 100 Mile House, BC V0K 2E0
Tel: 250-395-7676
www.interiorhealth.ca

Note: Services include: assessment; treatment; crisis intervention; counselling; & mental health support.

ABBOTSFORD: Abbotsford Mental Health Office
Affiliated with: Fraser Health Authority
32700 George Ferguson Way, Abbotsford, BC V2T 4V6
Tel: 604-870-7800 *Fax:* 604-870-7801

ASHCROFT: Ashcroft Mental Health
Affiliated with: Interior Health Authority
700 Ash-Cache Creek Hwy., Ashcroft, BC V0K 1A0
Tel: 250-453-2211 *Toll-Free:* 877-499-6599
www.interiorhealth.ca

Note: Services include: assessment; treatment; crisis intervention; counselling; & mental health support.

BARRIERE: Barriere Mental Health
Affiliated with: Interior Health Authority
4936 Barriere Town Rd., Barriere, BC V0E 1A0
Tel: 250-672-9773
www.interiorhealth.ca

Note: Services include: assessment; treatment; crisis intervention; counselling; & mental health support.

BURNABY: The Burnaby Centre for Mental Health & Addiction (BCMHA)
Affiliated with: Interior Health Authority
3405 Willingdon Ave., Burnaby, BC V5G 3H4
Tel: 604-675-3950 Fax: 604-675-3955
burnabycentreinfo@interiorhealth.ca
www.interiorhealth.ca
Number of Beds: 100 beds
Note: Six to nine-month residential treatment program for BC residents with concurrent disorders

BURNABY: Burnaby Mental Health Office
Affiliated with: Fraser Health Authority
3935 Kincaid St., Burnaby, BC V5G 2X6
Tel: 604-453-1930 Fax: 604-453-1929

BURNABY: Craigend Rest Home
5488 Patterson Ave., Burnaby, BC V5H 2M5
Tel: 604-433-8600
Number of Beds: 10 beds

CASTLEGAR: Castlegar Mental Health
Affiliated with: Interior Health Authority
707 - 10th St., Castlegar, BC V1N 2H7
Tel: 250-304-1846
www.interiorhealth.ca

Note: Services include: adult community support; counselling; early psychosis intervention; eating disorders; intake, urgent response, & emergency; & seniors mental health.

CHASE: Chase Mental Health
Affiliated with: Interior Health Authority
825 Thompson Ave., Chase, BC V0E 1M0
Tel: 250-679-3312
www.interiorhealth.ca

Note: Services include: assessment; treatment; crisis intervention; counselling; & mental health support.

CLEARWATER: Clearwater Mental Health
Affiliated with: Interior Health Authority
612 Park Dr., Clearwater, BC V0E 1N1
Tel: 250-674-2600
www.interiorhealth.ca

Note: Services include: adult community support; counselling; early psychosis intervention; eating disorders; intake, urgent response, & emergency services; & seniors mental health.

COQUITLAM: BC Mental Health & Substance Use Services Forensic Psychiatric Hospital
70 Colony Farm Rd., Coquitlam, BC V3C 5X9
Tel: 604-524-7700 Fax: 604-524-7905
feedback@bcmhs.bc.ca
www.bcmhsus.ca
Number of Beds: 190 beds
Note: Facility providing specialized clinical services & rehabilitative & vocational programs.
Angela Draude, Provincial Executive Director, Forensic Psychiatric Services
angela.draude@forensic.bc.ca

CRANBROOK: Clover Club House
Affiliated with: Interior Health Authority
400 Victoria Ave. North, Cranbrook, BC V1C 3Y3
Tel: 250-426-0102
www.interiorhealth.ca

Note: Services include: adult community support; assessment; treatment; crisis intervention; counselling; & mental health support.

CRANBROOK: Cranbrook Development Disability Mental Health Services
Affiliated with: Interior Health Authority
1212 - 2nd St. North, Cranbrook, BC V1C 4T6
Tel: 250-417-2534
www.interiorhealth.ca

Note: Provides developmental disability mental health services.

CRANBROOK: Cranbrook Mental Health
Affiliated with: Interior Health Authority
20 - 23rd Ave. South, Cranbrook, BC V1C 5V1
Tel: 250-420-2210
www.interiorhealth.ca

Note: Services include: adult community support; assessment; treatment; crisis intervention; counselling; & mental health support.

CRANBROOK: Tamarack Cottage
Affiliated with: Interior Health Authority
2005 - 5th St. North, Cranbrook, BC V1C 4Y2
Tel: 250-417-0103
www.interiorhealth.ca
Number of Beds: 5 tertiary specialized residential beds; 2 tertiary rehabilitative beds
Note: Offers tertiary psychiatric services & a tertiary rehabilitation & recovery program.

CRESTON: Creston Mental Health Centre
Affiliated with: Interior Health Authority
243 - 16th Ave. North, Creston, BC V0B 1G0
Tel: 250-428-8734
www.interiorhealth.ca

Note: Services include: adult community support; counselling; early psychosis intervention; eating disorders; intake, urgent response, & emergency; & seniors mental health.

DELTA: Delta-North Mental Health Office
Affiliated with: Fraser Health Authority
6345 - 120th St., Delta, BC V4E 2A6
Tel: 604-592-3700 Fax: 604-591-2302

DELTA: Delta-South Mental Health Office
Affiliated with: Fraser Health Authority
1835 - 56 St., Delta, BC V4L 2L8
Tel: 604-948-7010 Fax: 604-943-0872

GOLDEN: Golden Mental Health
Affiliated with: Interior Health Authority
835 - 9th Ave. South, Golden, BC V0A 1H0
Tel: 250-344-3015
www.interiorhealth.ca

Note: Services include: adult community support; assessment; treatment; crisis intervention; counselling; & mental health support.

GRAND FORKS: Boundary Mental Health & Substance Use Services
Affiliated with: Interior Health Authority
7441 2nd St., Grand Forks, BC V0H 1H0
Tel: 250-442-0330
www.interiorhealth.ca

Note: Services include: adult community support; counselling; early psychosis intervention; eating disorders; intake, urgent response, & emergency; & seniors mental health.

GRAND FORKS: Granby Clubhouse
Affiliated with: Interior Health Authority
8443 Riverside Dr., Grand Forks, BC V0H 1H0
Tel: 250-442-2465
www.interiorhealth.ca

Note: Services include: adult community support; assessment; treatment; crisis intervention; & mental health support.

HAZELTON: Hazelton Mental Health & Addictions
Affiliated with: Northern Health Authority
2506 Hwy. 62, Hazelton, BC V0J 1Y0
Tel: 250-842-5144 *Fax:* 250-842-2179
www.northernhealth.ca
Info Line: 888-562-1214

Note: Programs & services include: assessment & treatment; life skills training; recreational therapy; observation unit; perinatal depression; supportive recovery; & community response unit.

INVERMERE: Invermere Mental Health
Affiliated with: Interior Health Authority
850 - 10th Ave., Invermere, BC V0A 1K0
Tel: 250-342-2363
www.interiorhealth.ca

Note: Services include: adult community support; assessment; treatment; crisis intervention; counselling; & mental health support.

KAMLOOPS: Apple Lane Tertiary Mental Health Geriatric Unit
Affiliated with: Interior Health Authority
#200, 945 Southill St., Kamloops, BC V2B 7Z9
Tel: 250-554-5590
www.interiorhealth.ca
Number of Beds: 6 beds
Note: Provides care for elderly patients who have been diagnosed with a serious mental illness. Offers tertiary psychiatric services & a tertiary rehabilitation & recovery program.

KAMLOOPS: Development Disability Mental Health Child, Youth & Children's Assessment Network
Affiliated with: Interior Health Authority
624 Tranquille Rd., Kamloops, BC V2B 3H6
Tel: 250-554-0085
www.interiorhealth.ca

Note: Offers developmental disability mental health services.

KAMLOOPS: Forensic Psychiatric Services Commission (B.C.) Kamloops Clinic
#5, 1315 Summit Dr., Kamloops, BC V2C 5R9
Tel: 250-377-2660 *Fax:* 250-377-2688
www.bcmhsus.ca/regional-clinics

KAMLOOPS: Hillside Centre
Affiliated with: Interior Health Authority
311 Columbia St., Kamloops, BC V2C 2T1
Tel: 250-314-2700
www.interiorhealth.ca
Year Founded: 2006
Number of Beds: 44 beds
Note: Offers services to individuals with acute illness &/or severely dysfunctional behaviours.

KAMLOOPS: Kamloops Developmental Disability Mental Health Services
Affiliated with: Interior Health Authority
#202, 300 Columbia St., Kamloops, BC V2C 6L1
Tel: 250-377-6500
www.interiorhealth.ca

Note: Provides mental health services for people with developmental disabilities.

KAMLOOPS: Kamloops Mental Health & Substance Use
Affiliated with: Interior Health Authority
200 - 235 Lansdowne St., Kamloops, BC V2C 1X8
Tel: 250-377-6500
www.interiorhealth.ca

Note: Services include: adult community support; counselling; early psychosis intervention; eating disorders; intake, urgent response, & emergency; & seniors mental health.

KAMLOOPS: South Hills Tertiary Psychiatric Rehabilitation Centre
Affiliated with: Interior Health Authority
#200, 945 Southill St., Kamloops, BC V2B 7Z9
Tel: 250-554-5590
www.interiorhealth.ca
Number of Beds: 40 beds
Note: Provides a rehabilitation & recovery program for adults with a serious mental illness.

KAMLOOPS: Youth Forensic Psychiatric Services Kamloops Outpatient Clinic
#8 Tudor Village, 1315 Summit Dr., Kamloops, BC V2C 5R9
Tel: 250-828-4940 *Fax:* 250-828-4946

Note: For young offenders directed by court/probation to assessment/treatment

KASLO: Kaslo Mental Health
Affiliated with: Interior Health Authority
673 A Ave., Kaslo, BC V0G 1M0
Tel: 250-353-2291
www.interiorhealth.ca

Note: Services include: adult community support; assessment; treatment; crisis intervention; counselling; & mental health support.

KELOWNA: Cara Centre
Affiliated with: Interior Health Authority
160 Nickel Rd., Kelowna, BC V1X 4E6
Tel: 250-763-4144
www.interiorhealth.ca
Year Founded: 2011
Number of Beds: 11 beds
Note: Provides tertiary psychiatric services & a tertiary rehabilitation & recovery program for individuals who have a mental illness or psychiatric concerns. Admission is by referral only.

KELOWNA: Central Okanagan Brain Injury Society
Affiliated with: Interior Health Authority
#11, 368 Industrial Ave., Kelowna, BC V1Y 4N7
Tel: 250-762-3233
www.interiorhealth.ca

Note: Services for people affected by brain injury, as well as their families.

KELOWNA: Kelowna Developmental Disability Mental Health Services
Affiliated with: Interior Health Authority
505 Doyle Ave., Kelowna, BC V1Y 0C5
Tel: 250-469-7070
www.interiorhealth.ca

Note: Provides mental health services for people with developmental disabilities.

KELOWNA: Kelowna Mental Health & Substance Use
Affiliated with: Interior Health Authority
505 Doyle Ave., Kelowna, BC V1Y 0C5
Tel: 250-469-7070
www.interiorhealth.ca

Note: Services include: adult community support; assessment; treatment; crisis intervention; counselling; & mental health support.

KELOWNA: Seniors Mental Health & Eating Disorders Program
Affiliated with: Interior Health Authority
#100, 540 Groves Ave., Kelowna, BC V1Y 4Y7
Tel: 250-870-5777
www.interiorhealth.ca

Note: Services include: adult community support; assessment; treatment; crisis intervention; counselling; & mental health support.

KELOWNA: White Heather Manor
3728 Casorso Rd., Kelowna, BC V1W 4M8
Tel: 250-763-6554 *Fax:* 250-763-6754
Number of Beds: 44 beds

KEREMEOS: Princeton/Keremeos Mental Health Centre
Affiliated with: Interior Health Authority
700 - 3rd St., Keremeos, BC V0X 1N3
Tel: 250-499-3029 *Toll-Free:* 800-663-7867
www.interiorhealth.ca

Note: Services include: adult community support; assessment; treatment; crisis intervention; counselling; & mental health support.

KIMBERLEY: Kimberley Mental Health
Affiliated with: Interior Health Authority
260 - 4th Ave., Kimberley, BC V1A 2R6
Tel: 250-427-2215
www.interiorhealth.ca

Note: Services include: adult community support; assessment; treatment; crisis intervention; counselling; & mental health support.

LILLOOET: Lillooet Mental Health
Affiliated with: Interior Health Authority
951 Murray St., Lillooet, BC V0K 1V0
Tel: 250-256-1343
www.interiorhealth.ca

Note: Services include: adult community support; counselling; early psychosis intervention; eating disorders; intake, urgent response, & emergency; & seniors mental health.

LOGAN LAKE: Logan Lake Mental Health
Affiliated with: Interior Health Authority
5 Beryl Dr., Logan Lake, BC V0K 1W0
Tel: 250-523-9414
www.interiorhealth.ca

Note: Services include: adult community support; assessment; treatment; crisis intervention; counselling; & mental health support.

LYTTON: Lytton Mental Health
Affiliated with: Interior Health Authority
533 Main St., Lytton, BC V0K 1Z0
Tel: 250-455-2216
www.interiorhealth.ca

Note: Services include: adult community support; counselling; early psychosis intervention; eating disorders; intake, urgent response, & emergency; & seniors mental health.

MAPLE RIDGE: Trejan Lodge Ltd.
25402 Hilland Ave., Maple Ridge, BC V4R 1G3
Tel: 604-467-3377 *Fax:* 604-467-0705
Annabelle Cariaso, Manager

MERRITT: Merritt Mental Health
Affiliated with: Interior Health Authority
3451 Voght St., Merritt, BC V1K 1C6
Tel: 250-378-3401
www.interiorhealth.ca

Note: Services include: adult community support; assessment; treatment; crisis intervention; counselling; & mental health support.

MIDWAY: Boundary Access Centre
Affiliated with: Interior Health Authority
7th Ave., Midway, BC V0H 1M0
Tel: 250-449-2887
www.interiorhealth.ca

Note: Services include: assessment; treatment; crisis intervention; counselling; & mental health support.

NAKUSP: Nakusp Mental Health
Affiliated with: Interior Health Authority
97 - 1st Ave. NE, Nakusp, BC V0G 1R0
Tel: 250-265-5253
www.interiorhealth.ca

Note: Services include: adult community support; assessment; treatment; crisis intervention; counselling; & mental health support.

NAKUSP: Terra Pondera Clubhouse
Affiliated with: Interior Health Authority
97 - 2nd Ave. NW, Nakusp, BC V0G 1R0
Tel: 250-265-0064
www.interiorhealth.ca

Note: Services include: adult community support; assessment; treatment; crisis intervention; counselling; & mental health support.

NANAIMO: Forensic Psychiatric Services Commission (B.C.) Nanaimo Clinic
Former Name: Nanaimo Adult Forensic Psychiatric Community Services
#101, 190 Wallace St., Nanaimo, BC V9R 5B1
Tel: 250-739-5000 *Fax:* 250-739-5001
www.bcmhsus.ca/regional-clinics

NANAIMO: Youth Forensic Psychiatric Services Nanaimo Outpatient Clinic
1 - 1925 Bowen Rd., Nanaimo, BC V9S 1H1
Tel: 250-760-0409
www.mcf.gov.bc.ca/yfps/index.htm

Note: Mental health assessment & treatment services for youth involved in the criminal justice system
André Picard, Provincial Director
778-452-2202

NELSON: McKim Cottage
Affiliated with: Interior Health Authority
916 - 11th St., Nelson, BC V1L 7A6
Tel: 250-352-2022
www.interiorhealth.ca

Note: Services include: adult community support; assessment; treatment; crisis intervention; counselling; & mental health support.

NELSON: Nelson Friendship Outreach Clubhouse
Affiliated with: Interior Health Authority
818 Vernon Rd., Nelson, BC V1L 4G4
Tel: 250-352-7730
www.interiorhealth.ca

Note: Services include: adult community support; assessment; treatment; crisis intervention; counselling; & mental health support.

NELSON: Nelson Mental Health
Affiliated with: Interior Health Authority
333 Victoria St., Nelson, BC V1L 4K3
Tel: 250-505-7248
www.interiorhealth.ca

Note: Services include: adult community support; assessment; treatment; crisis intervention; counselling; & mental health support.

OLD MASSET: Old Masset Adult Day Program
Affiliated with: Northern Health Authority
510 Naanii Rd., Old Masset, BC V0T 1M0
Tel: 250-565-2649 *Fax:* 250-565-2640
Toll-Free: 866-565-2999
www.northernhealth.ca

Note: Offers programs & services designed to help seniors & adults with disabilities to continue to live in their own homes.

OLIVER: Desert Sun Counselling & Resource Centre
Affiliated with: Interior Health Authority
PO Box 1890, 762 Fairview Rd., Oliver, BC V0X 1C0
Tel: 250-498-2538   Toll-Free: 877-723-3911
www.desertsuncounselling.ca
Social Media: www.facebook.com/desertsuncounselling
Year Founded: 1998
Note: Services include: counselling; crisis help; parenting resources; seniors' resources; & community outreach.
Patricia Batchelor, Chair

OLIVER: Robert Bateman House
Affiliated with: Interior Health Authority
538 Fairview Rd., Oliver, BC V0H 1T0
Tel: 250-485-0043
www.interiorhealth.ca
Note: Services include: adult community support; assessment; treatment; crisis intervention; counselling; & mental health support.

OSOYOOS: Country Squire Retirement Villa
Affiliated with: Interior Health Authority
9707 North 87 St., Osoyoos, BC V0H 1V0
Tel: 250-495-6568   Fax: 250-495-7466
www.interiorhealth.ca
Note: Provides tertiary psychiatric services
Deb McCartney, Contact
deb.mccartney@thecountrysquire.ca

OSOYOOS: Osoyoos Mental Health
Affiliated with: Interior Health Authority
4816 - 89 St., Osoyoos, BC V0H 1V1
Tel: 250-495-6433
www.interiorhealth.ca
Note: Services include: adult community support; assessment; treatment; crisis intervention; counselling; & mental health support.

PENTICTON: Braemore Lodge
Affiliated with: Interior Health Authority
2402 South Main St., Penticton, BC V2A 5H9
Tel: 250-492-2969
www.interiorhealth.ca
Number of Beds: 16 beds (4 tertiary specialized residential beds)
Note: Offers tertiary psychiatric & psychosocial rehabilitation services to individuals with a serious mental illness.

PENTICTON: Penticton Mental Health
Affiliated with: Interior Health Authority
#117 - 437 Martin St., Penticton, BC V1L 5L1
Tel: 250-770-3555
www.interiorhealth.ca
Note: Services include: adult community support; assessment; treatment; crisis intervention; counselling; & mental health support.

PRINCE GEORGE: AiMHi - Prince George Association for Community Living
950 Kerry St., Prince George, BC V2M 5A3
Tel: 250-564-6408 Fax: 250-564-6801
aimhi@aimhi.ca
www.aimhi.ca
Social Media: www.facebook.com/AiMHibc; twitter.com/AiMHiBC
Note: Non-profit, supports individuals with developmental disabilities & children with special needs
Melinda Heidsma, Executive Director

PRINCE GEORGE: Forensic Psychiatric Services Commission (B.C.)
Prince George Clinic
1584 - 7 Ave., 2nd Fl., Prince George, BC V2L 3P4
Tel: 250-561-8060 Fax: 250-561-8075
www.bcmhsus.ca/regional-clinics
Note: Outpatient mental health services

PRINCE GEORGE: Hazelton Street Residence
Affiliated with: Northern Health Authority
2554 Hazelton St., Prince George, BC V2L 1H1
Tel: 250-960-1499
www.northernhealth.ca
Number of Beds: 6 long-term beds
Note: Programs & services include: assistance with daily activities; medication management; & support & education for clients, families & caregivers. Managed by Western Human Resource Corporation.

PRINCE GEORGE: Iris House
Affiliated with: Northern Health Authority
1111 Lethbridge St., Prince George, BC V2M 7E9
Tel: 250-649-7245 Fax: 250-563-2706
www.northernhealth.ca
Year Founded: 2002
Number of Beds: 20 beds
Note: Tertiary rehabilitation & residential facility for adults with long-term mental illness. Affiliated with Seven Sisters in Terrace, BC.

PRINCE GEORGE: Urquhart House
Affiliated with: Northern Health Authority
4418 Urquhart Cres., Prince George, BC V2M 5H1
Tel: 250-564-0987 Fax: 250-564-2847
www.northernhealth.ca
Note: Community residential services for adults.

PRINCETON: Anchorage Drop-In Centre
Affiliated with: Interior Health Authority
136 Vermillion Ave., Princeton, BC V0X 1W0
Tel: 250-295-6936
www.interiorhealth.ca
Note: Services include: assessment; treatment; crisis intervention; counselling; & mental health support.

QUEEN CHARLOTTE: Queen Charlotte City Health Centre
Affiliated with: Northern Health Authority
302 - 2nd Ave., Queen Charlotte, BC V0T 1S0
Tel: 250-559-8765 Fax: 250-559-8765
www.northernhealth.ca
Note: Programs & services include: mental health & addictions; home care nursing; & home support.

QUESNEL: Quesnel Mental Health Team & QUESST Unit
Affiliated with: Northern Health Authority
543 Front St., Quesnel, BC V2J 2K7
Tel: 250-985-5608
www.northernhealth.ca
Number of Beds: 5 beds
Note: Short-term intensive services including assessment, stabilization, consultation, brief treatment, & discharge planning. QUESST stands for Quesnel Unit for Emergency Short Stay Treatment.

REVELSTOKE: Revelstoke Mental Health
Affiliated with: Interior Health Authority
1200 Newlands Rd., Revelstoke, BC V0E 2S0
Tel: 250-814-2241
www.interiorhealth.ca
Note: Services include: adult community support; assessment; treatment; crisis intervention; counselling; & mental health support.

SALMO: Salmo Mental Health
Affiliated with: Interior Health Authority
311 Railway Ave., Salmo, BC V0G 1Z0
Tel: 250-357-2277
www.interiorhealth.ca
Note: Services include: adult community support; counselling; early psychosis intervention; eating disorders; intake, urgent response, & emergency; & seniors mental health.

SALMON ARM: Mental Health/Addictions & Public Health
Affiliated with: Interior Health Authority
433 Hudson Rd., Salmon Arm, BC V1E 4S1

www.interiorhealth.ca

SALMON ARM: Salmon Arm Mental Health
Affiliated with: Interior Health Authority
851 - 16th St. NE, Salmon Arm, BC V1E 4N7

Tel: 250-833-4100
www.interiorhealth.ca

Note: Services include: adult community support; assessment; treatment; crisis intervention; counselling; & mental health support.

TERRACE: Birchwood Place
Affiliated with: Northern Health Authority
3183 Kofoed Dr., Terrace, BC V8G 3P8

Tel: 250-635-2171 *Fax:* 250-635-7057
www.northernhealth.ca

Number of Beds: 8 beds
Note: Supported living residential care

TERRACE: Seven Sisters Residence
Affiliated with: Northern Health Authority
2815 Tetrault St., Terrace, BC V8G 2W6

Tel: 250-631-4121 *Fax:* 250-631-4129
www.northernhealth.ca

Note: Tertiary rehabilitation & residential facility for adults with long-term mental illness. Affiliated with Iris House in Prince George, BC.

TERRACE: Terrace Community Mental Health Services
Affiliated with: Northern Health Authority
#34, 3412 Kalum St., Terrace, BC V8G 0G5

Tel: 250-631-4202 *Fax:* 250-631-4282
www.northernhealth.ca
Info Line: 250-638-4082

Note: Programs & services include: intake; crisis response; counselling; case management; life skills support; medication management; education; & psychiatric consultation.

TRAIL: Friend of Friends Clubhouse
Affiliated with: Interior Health Authority
1454 - 2nd Ave., Trail, BC V1R 1M2

Tel: 250-368-6343
www.interiorhealth.ca

Note: Services include: adult community support; assessment; treatment; crisis intervention; counselling; & mental health support.

TRAIL: Harbour House
Affiliated with: Interior Health Authority
1100 Hospital Bench, Trail, BC V1R 4M1

Tel: 250-364-9995
www.interiorhealth.ca
Number of Beds: 6 tertiary specialized residential beds; 3 tertiary rehabilitative beds
Note: Provides services for clients in need of longer-term residential psychosocial rehabilitation.

TRAIL: Trail Mental Health
Affiliated with: Interior Health Authority
#3, 1500 Columbia Ave., Trail, BC V1R 1J9

Tel: 250-364-6262
www.interiorhealth.ca

Note: Services include: adult community support; assessment; treatment; crisis intervention; counselling; & mental health support.

TUMBLER RIDGE: Tumbler Ridge Mental Health & Addictions
Affiliated with: Northern Health Authority
PO Box 1205, 220 Front St., Tumbler Ridge, BC V0C 2W0

Tel: 250-242-5505 *Fax:* 250-242-3595
www.northernhealth.ca

Note: Services include: case management; counselling; crisis

response; education; intake; life skills support; medication management; & psychiatric consultation.

VANDERHOOF: Vanderhoof Health Unit
Affiliated with: Northern Health Authority
3299 Hospital Rd., Vanderhoof, BC V0J 3A2

Tel: 250-567-5994 *Fax:* 250-567-6171
www.northernhealth.ca

VERNON: Aberdeen House
Affiliated with: Interior Health Authority
9604 Shamanski Dr., Vernon, BC V1B 2L7

Tel: 250-542-9350
aberdeenhouse@shawbiz.ca
www.interiorhealth.ca
Number of Beds: 14 beds (7 tertiary specialized residential)
Note: Provides specialized mental health services

VERNON: Okanagan House
Affiliated with: Interior Health Authority
4007 - 24th Ave., Vernon, BC V1T 4N7

Tel: 250-549-5737
www.interiorhealth.ca

Note: Services include: adult community support; assessment; treatment; crisis intervention; counselling; & mental health support.

VERNON: Vernon Mental Health
Affiliated with: Interior Health Authority
1440 - 14th Ave., Vernon, BC V1B 2T1

Tel: 250-549-5737
www.interiorhealth.ca

Note: Services include: adult community support; assessment; treatment; group therapy; crisis intervention; counselling; & mental health support.

VERNON: Willowview
Affiliated with: Interior Health Authority
1808 - 30th St., Vernon, BC V1T 5C5

Tel: 250-542-4890
www.interiorhealth.ca

Note: Services include: adult community support; assessment; treatment; crisis intervention; counselling; community residential programs; geriatric programs; group therapy; & mental health support.

VICTORIA: Pacific Operational Trauma & Stress Support Centre (OTSSC)
Canadian Forces Health Services
1200 Colville Rd., Victoria, BC V9A 7N2

Tel: 250-363-4411
Year Founded: 1999
Note: Specialties: Assistance to serving members of the Canadian Forces & their families, who are dealing with psychological, emotional, spiritual, & social problems stemming from military operations, especially deployments abroad; Psychiatry; Psychology; Social work; Community health nursing; Educational programs; Chaplain services

VICTORIA: Youth Forensic Psychiatric Services
Victoria Outpatient Clinic
1515 Quadra St., Victoria, BC V8V 3P4

Tel: 250-387-2830
www.mcf.gov.bc.ca/yfps/index.htm

WILLIAMS LAKE: Gateway Crisis Stabilization Unit
Affiliated with: Interior Health Authority
517 North 6th Ave., 3rd Fl., Williams Lake, BC V2G 2P3

Tel: 250-392-8261
www.interiorhealth.ca

Note: Services include: adult community support; assessment; treatment; crisis intervention; counselling; & mental health support.

WILLIAMS LAKE: Williams Lake Mental Health Centre
Affiliated with: Interior Health Authority
487 Borland St., Williams Lake, BC V2G 1R9

Tel: 250-392-1483
www.interiorhealth.ca

Note: Services include: adult community support; counselling; early psychosis intervention; eating disorders; intake, urgent response, & emergency; & seniors mental health.

MANITOBA

ALTONA: Blue Sky Opportunities Inc.
PO Box 330, 122 - 10th Ave. NW, Altona, MB R0G 0B0
Tel: 204-324-5401 *Fax:* 204-324-5094
bsoinc@mymts.net
www.blueskyop.com

Note: Employment & training opportunities as well as non-vocational services for adults with intellectual disabilities.
Richard Neufeld, General Manager
204-324-5401, bsogm@mymts.net

ARBORG: Riverdale Place Homes Inc.
PO Box 968, 332 Ingolfs St., Arborg, MB R0C 0A0
Tel: 204-376-2940 *Fax:* 204-376-5051
riverdale@mts.net
Year Founded: 1977
Number of Beds: 19 beds
Note: Provides residential services to adults with intellectual disabilities.

BOISSEVAIN: Prairie Partners Inc.
298 South Railway St., Boissevain, MB R0K 0E0
Tel: 204-534-2956
residential@prairiepartners.ca
www.prairiepartners.ca

Note: Residential & employment services for adults with intellectual disabilities.
Jason L. Dyck, Executive Director & CEO
Helen Nantais, CFO
Misheyla Iwasiuk, Program Manager

BRANDON: Brandon Community Options Inc.
136 - 11th St., Brandon, MB R7A 4J4
Tel: 204-571-5770 *Fax:* 204-571-5780
bdnco@mts.net
www.brandoncommunityoptionsinc.com

Note: Residential & day programs for adults with mental disabilities.
Juliette Popplestone, Chair

BRANDON: Brandon Support Services
1540 Rosser Ave., Brandon, MB R7A 0M6
Tel: 204-728-2025 *Fax:* 204-728-2052
admin@bssmb.ca
www.bssmb.ca
Area Served: Brandon, Portage La Prairie, MacGregor & Carberry
Note: Community-based agency providing supportive services to individuals with intellectual &/or physical disabilities
Barry Foster, Director, Community Development

BRANDON: Centre for Adult Psychiatry (CAP)
Affiliated with: Prairie Mountain Health
Brandon Regional Health Centre, 150 McTavish Ave. East, Brandon, MB R7A 2B3
Tel: 204-578-4555
www.prairiemountainhealth.ca
Number of Beds: 25 beds
Note: Acute services for adults 18-64 experiencing a psychiatric illness (DSM IV diagnosis) &/or severe psychosocial crisis.

BRANDON: Centre for Geriatric Psychiatry
Affiliated with: Prairie Mountain Health
150 McTavish Ave. East, Brandon, MB R7A 2B3
Tel: 204-578-4000
www.prairiemountainhealth.ca
Number of Beds: 22 beds
Area Served: Parkland, Assiniboine, Brandon
Note: Provides assessment & short-term treatment for adults 65 years & over experiencing difficulties with day to day functioning due to mental health issues.
Pamela Gulay, Manager

BRANDON: Child & Adolescent Treatment Centre (CATC)
Affiliated with: Prairie Mountain Health
1240 - 10 St., Brandon, MB R7A 7L6
Tel: 204-578-2700 *Fax:* 204-578-2850
Toll-Free: 866-403-5459
www.prairiemountainhealth.ca

Note: Programs & services include: mental health assessments & treatment; crisis stabilization; individualized treatment plans; individual, group, & family therapy; & mental health education/promotion.

BRANDON: Community Mental Health Services
Affiliated with: Prairie Mountain Health
800 Rosser Ave., #B13, Brandon, MB R7A 6N5
Tel: 204-578-2400 *Fax:* 204-578-2822
www.prairiemountainhealth.ca

Note: Services include counselling, resource coordination, & group programming.
Jayne Troop, Vice-President, Community & Long Term Care

BRANDON: Family Visions Inc.
2705 Victoria Ave., Brandon, MB R7B 0N1
Tel: 204-726-5602 *Fax:* 204-571-0907
reception@familyvisions.ca
www.familyvisions.ca
Year Founded: 2000
Note: Residential & day services for adults with intellectual disabilities.
Kim Longstreet, Executive Director
executive.director@familyvisions.ca

BRANDON: Westman Crisis Services
Affiliated with: Prairie Mountain Health
Brandon, MB
Tel: 204-725-4411 *Toll-Free:* 888-379-7699
www.prairiemountainhealth.ca
Area Served: Brandon & Assiniboine regions
Note: Services include Mobile Crisis Unit (assessment, screening, & intervention) & Crisis Stabilization Unit (residential unit providing short-term intensive care for individuals experiencing a mental health crisis).

NINETTE: Southwest Community Options Inc. (SWCO)
PO Box 46, 210 Queen St. North, Ninette, MB R0K 1R0
Tel: 204-528-5060 *Fax:* 877-919-8681
www.swco.ca
Year Founded: 2000
Note: Residential & day services for adults with intellectual disabilities.
Linda Stephenson, Executive Director
Susie Prankie, Financial Officer

NOTRE DAME DE LOURDES: Mountain Industries
Also Known As: Atelier la Montagne
65 Notre-Dame Ave., Notre Dame de Lourdes, MB R0G 1M0
Tel: 204-248-2154
www.mountainindustries.ca
Year Founded: 1978
Note: Provides a day program for over 25 individuals with special needs

PINE FALLS: Wings of Power Inc.
PO Box 66, 39 Pine St., Pine Falls, MB R0E 1M0
Tel: 204-367-9641 *Fax:* 204-367-9784
www.wingsofpower.org

Note: Community & family resource centre. Programs & services include: prenatal/postnatal; children's; summer; school; & programs for adults with disabilities.
Guy Borlase, Executive Director
gbwingsdirector@mymts.net

PORTAGE LA PRAIRIE: Manitoba Developmental Centre
#840, 3rd St. NE, Portage la Prairie, MB R1N 3C6
Tel: 204-856-4200 *Fax:* 204-856-4258
csd@gov.mb.ca
www.gov.mb.ca/fs/mdc/index.html
Number of Beds: 180 resident capacity
Note: Developmental centre for residents with an intellectual disability.

Programs & services include: Extended Care Program & Habilitation/Specialty Program.

PORTAGE LA PRAIRIE: Portage ARC Industries Inc.
1675 Saskatchewan Ave. West, Portage la Prairie, MB R1N 0R4
Tel: 204-857-7752 *Fax:* 204-239-0968
portagearc@mymts.net

Note: Activities for individuals with special needs
Tara Ryzner, Executive Director

SELKIRK: Hearthstone Community Group
209 Superior Ave., Selkirk, MB R1A 0Z7
Tel: 204-817-1996 *Fax:* 204-817-1997
www.hearthstone-community-group.ca

Note: Community living homes & day programs for people with developmental disabilities
Lori Zdebiak, General Manager
Karen Fraser, Office Manager

SELKIRK: Selkirk Mental Health Centre
Affiliated with: Interlake-Eastern Regional Health Authority
PO Box 9600, 825 Manitoba Ave., Selkirk, MB R1A 2B5
Tel: 204-482-3810 *Fax:* 204-785-8936
Toll-Free: 800-881-3073
smhc@gov.mb.ca
www.gov.mb.ca/health/smhc
Number of Beds: 252 beds
Note: Long-term mental health inpatient care & rehabilitation; also provides mental health services to people from the Territory of Nunavut.
D. Bellehumeur, Chief Executive Officer
Dr. M. Teillet, Medical Director
R. Cromarty, Chief Nursing Officer & Director, Programs
B. Wynnobel, Director, Operations

ST MALO: Smile of St. Malo Inc.
112 St. Malo Ave., St Malo, MB R0A 1T0
Tel: 204-347-5418
www.epicsmile.ca

Note: Provides residential & day programs for adults with intellectual disabilities.
Helene Lariviere, Executive Director
helene@epicsmile.ca

ST NORBERT: The Behavioural Health Foundation, Inc. (BHF)
Affiliated with: Winnipeg Regional Health Authority
PO Box 250, 35, av de la Digue, St Norbert, MB R3V 1L6
info@bhf.ca
www.bhf.ca

Note: Long-term residential addictions treatment for men, women, teens & families
Jean Doucha, Executive Director
jeand@bhf.ca

STEINBACH: enVision Community Living
84 Brandt St., Steinbach, MB R5G 0E1
Tel: 204-326-7539 *Fax:* 204-346-3639
info@envisioncl.com
www.envisioncl.com
Social Media: www.facebook.com/envisioncl; twitter.com/enVisioncl

Note: Offers residential & daytime support services to adults with intellectual disabilities.
Jeannette Delong, Executive Director
jdelong@envisioncl.com

WINKLER: Gateway Resources Inc.
PO Box 1448, 1582 Pembina Ave. West, Winkler, MB R6W 4B4
Tel: 204-325-7304 *Fax:* 204-325-1958
gradmin@gatewayresourcesinc.com
www.gatewayresourcesinc.com
Social Media: www.facebook.com/575874922554789; twitter.com/gateway1582

Area Served: Winkler/Morden area of South Central Manitoba
Note: Operates 13 group homes that provide services & programs for individuals with an intellectual disability.
Kimberly Nelson, Chief Executive Officer
kim@gatewayresourcesinc.com
Bonnie Dobson, Director, Human Resources
bonnie@gatewayresourcesinc.com
Ron Gerbrandt, Director, Operations
ron@gatewayresourcesinc.com
Dianne Hildebrand, Director, Housing
dianne@gatewayresourcesinc.com
Brenda Pohl, Director, Programs
brenda@gatewayresourcesinc.com

WINNIPEG: Arcane Horizon Inc. (AHI)
#62, 1313 Border St., Winnipeg, MB R3H 0X4
Tel: 204-897-5482
www.arcanehorizon.org
Social Media: www.facebook.com/arcanehorizon

Note: Support services for adults living with developmental disabilities.

WINNIPEG: L'Avenir Cooperative Inc.
80 Sherbrook St., Winnipeg, MB R3C 2B3
Tel: 204-789-9777 *Fax:* 204-837-8614
www.lavenircoop.ca
Year Founded: 1983
Note: Provides support services to people with intellectual &/or physical disabilities.
Marc Piché, Executive Director
mpiche@lavenircoop.ca
Mariano Bautista, Finance & Administration Head
mbautista@lavenircoop.ca
Tess De Jesus, Manager, Finance
tdjesus@lavenircoop.ca

WINNIPEG: Changes
200 - 395 Stafford St., Winnipeg, MB R3M 2X4
Tel: 204-953-5300 *Fax:* 204-953-5305
info@changeswinnipeg.ca
changeswinnipeg.ca

Note: Services for adults who need support in their homes & communities.

WINNIPEG: Clubhouse of Winnipeg, Inc.
Affiliated with: Winnipeg Regional Health Authority
172 Sherbrook St., Winnipeg, MB R3C 2B6
Tel: 204-783-9400 *Fax:* 204-783-9890

Note: Employment & educational opportunities to people coping with mental illness.
Mark Elie, Director

WINNIPEG: Community Respite Service Inc.
1155 Notre Dame Ave., Winnipeg, MB R3E 3G1
Tel: 204-953-2400 *Fax:* 204-775-6214
www.communityrespiteservice.ca
Year Founded: 1984
Note: Respite care for families & individuals with intellectual & physical disabilities.
Nancy Morgan, Chair

WINNIPEG: Crisis Response Centre (CRC)
Affiliated with: Winnipeg Regional Health Authority
Also Known As: Adult Mental Health Crisis Response Centre
817 Bannatyne Ave., Winnipeg, MB R3E 0Y1
Tel: 204-940-1781
TTY: 204-779-8902
www.wrha.mb.ca/facilities/crisis-response-centre.php
Year Founded: 2013
Note: Provides 24/7 walk-in & schedules urgent care services; acts as a base for a Mobile Crisis Team.
James Bolton, Medical Director

WINNIPEG: DASCH Inc.
Also Known As: Direct Action in Support of Community Homes
#1, 117 Victor Lewis Dr., Winnipeg, MB R3P 1J6
Tel: 204-987-1550 *Fax:* 204-987-1552
www.dasch.mb.ca
Social Media: twitter.com/dasch_inc

Year Founded: 1974
Note: Provides residential, day program, respite & foster care programs & services for people with developmental disabilities
Karen Fonseth, Chief Executive Officer
Brenda Martinussen, Chief Operating Officer
Angela Bakker, Administrative Officer
Nadeen Haverstock, Director, Operations
Scott Smith, Director, Operations

WINNIPEG: Friends Housing Inc.
Affiliated with: Winnipeg Regional Health Authority
#100, 890 Sturgeon Rd., Winnipeg, MB R2Y 0L2
Tel: 204-953-1160 *Fax:* 204-953-1162
fhousing@mymts.net
www.friendshousinginc.ca

Note: Provides housing & daily living support for people with mental illnesses, or people in need of subsidized housing.
Edward Harting, Director, Operations

WINNIPEG: Innovative LIFE Options Inc. (LIFE)
Also Known As: Living in Friendship Everyday
#4, 120 Maryland St., Winnipeg, MB R3G 1L1
Tel: 204-772-3557 *Fax:* 204-784-4816
Toll-Free: 866-516-5445
info@icof-life.ca
www.icof-life.ca
Social Media:
www.facebook.com/LifeIsGoodInTheCompanyOfFriendsicof;
twitter.com/lifeisgoodicof

Year Founded: 2000
Note: Provides guidance, resources, training, & information to individuals receiving funding through Manitoba Family Service's program In the Company of Friends (ICOF).
Patti Chiappetta, Executive Director
204-784-4814, patti@icof-life.ca
Laureen Spitzke, Office Manager
204-784-4810
Liz Allen, Financial Coordinator
204-414-6398, liz@icof-life.ca

WINNIPEG: Manitoba Adolescent Treatment Centre Inc. (MATC)
Affiliated with: Winnipeg Regional Health Authority
120 Tecumseh St., Winnipeg, MB R3E 2A9
Tel: 204-477-6391
info@matc.ca
www.matc.ca

Number of Beds: 14 beds
Note: Mental health services for children, youth, & families

WINNIPEG: Norshel Inc.
Also Known As: Norshel Centre
890 Nairn Ave., Winnipeg, MB R2L 0X8
Tel: 204-654-6117
www.norshel.mb.ca
Social Media: www.facebook.com/309500839098006

Note: Provides support for adults with physical & developmental disabilities.
Colin Rivers, Executive Director
colinrivers@norshel.mb.ca

WINNIPEG: Opportunities For Independence, Inc.
1070 Portage Ave., Winnipeg, MB R3G 0S3
Tel: 204-786-0100 *Fax:* 204-786-0109
www.ofii.ca

Year Founded: 1983
Number of Employees: 100
Note: Programs & services for adults with intellectual disabilities who engage in high-risk behaviour, including: residential; alternative vocational programming; living skills training; & therapeutic programs.
Donald Welch, Staff Representative

WINNIPEG: Pulford Community Living Services Inc. (PCLS)
#5, 1146 Waverley St., Winnipeg, MB R3T 0P4
Tel: 204-284-2255 *Fax:* 204-453-5657
www.pulford.ca
Year Founded: 1986
Note: Provides housing & support services for people with developmental disabilities.
John Pollard, President & Treasurer

WINNIPEG: The Salvation Army Community Venture
1350 Church Ave., Winnipeg, MB R2X 1G4
Tel: 204-946-9418 *Fax:* 204-946-5347
www.communityventure.mb.ca

Note: Programs & services for adults living with developmental disabilities include: day programs; residential services; transportation; outreach; & respite.
Kim Park, Executive Director
director@communityventure.mb.ca
Regina Caligagan, Coordinator, Administration & Support Services
office@communityventure.mb.ca

WINNIPEG: Sara Riel Inc.
Affiliated with: Winnipeg Regional Health Authority
#101, 66 Moore Ave., Winnipeg, MB R2M 2C4
Tel: 204-237-9263 *Fax:* 204-233-2564
info@sararielinc.com
www.sararielinc.com
Year Founded: 1977
Note: Provides housing support, rehabilitation, & employment counselling to individuals with mental health issues.
Diane Lau, Executive Director

WINNIPEG: Shalom Residences Inc.
1033 McGregor St., Winnipeg, MB R2V 3H4
Tel: 204-582-7064 *Fax:* 204-582-7162
shalom@mts.net
www.shalomresidences.com

Note: Community-based care homes for adults with intellectual disabilities; Judaic-oriented programs.
Nancy Hughes, Executive Director
Maureen Baskin, Coordinator
Shelley Nagle, Coordinator
Meaghan Spenchuk, Office Manager

WINNIPEG: Special People in Kildonan East Inc. (SPIKE)
Also Known As: SPIKE House
1303 Dugald Rd., #B, Winnipeg, MB R2J 0H3
Tel: 204-338-0773 *Fax:* 204-338-1129
www.spikeinc.org
Year Founded: 1978
Note: Permanent & respite care for mentally &/or physically disabled individuals.
Peter Court, Executive Director
204-339-2990, pcourt@spikeinc.org

WINNIPEG: Turning Leaf Community Support Services Inc.
Also Known As: Turning Leaf Inc.
2585 Portage Ave., 2nd Fl., Winnipeg, MB R3J 0P5
Tel: 204-221-5594 *Fax:* 204-219-1821
Toll-Free: 855-221-5594
info@turningleafservices.com
www.turningleafservices.com
Social Media: www.facebook.com/TurningLeafWpg;
twitter.com/turningleafwpg; instagram.com/turningleafwpg;
www.linkedin.com/company-beta/3634827

Note: Provides treatment & support for youth & adults with intellectual challenges & mental illnesses.
Barkley Engel, Founder & CEO
204-221-5594, bjengel@turningleafservices.com
Jennifer Biggs, Director, Supported Independent Living
jbiggs@turningleafservices.com

Renee Voss, Director, Residential Services
  reneevoss@turningleafservices.com
Samneek Sandhu, Director, Finance
  samneeksandhu@turningleafservices.co
Leanne Peters, Director, Community Relations
  leannepeters@turningleafservices.com
Carol Rusnak, Office Manager
  carolrusnak@turningleafservices.com

WINNIPEG: Visions of Independence Inc.
#211, 530 Century St., Winnipeg, MB R3H 0Y4
Tel: 204-453-5982 *Fax:* 204-452-0714
www.visionsofindependence.org
Social Media: www.facebook.com/visionsofindependenceMB;
twitter.com/VofIndependence

Note: Provides housing & programs to people with intellectual disabilities. Programs & services include: residential; day programs; & supported independent living/respite.
Jennifer Hagedorn, Executive Director
  jhagedorn@visionsofindependence.org
Ven Block, Director, Finance
  vblock@visionsofindependence.org
Shannon Harley, Director, Services
  sharley@visionsofindependence.org
Kevin Young, Manager, Human Resources
  careers@visionsofindependence.org
Melissa Van Soelen, Coordinator, Program Development
  mvansoelen@visionsofindependence.org

NEW BRUNSWICK

CAMPBELLTON: Centre Hospitalier Restigouche
Affiliée à: Vitalité Health Network
CP 10, 63, ch Gallant, Campbellton, NB E3N 3G2
Tél: 506-789-7000 *Téléc:* 506-789-7065
info@vitalitenb.ca
www.vitalitenb.ca

Nombre de lits: 172 lits

CAMPBELLTON: Duguay's Special Care Home
20 Dover St., Campbellton, NB E3N 1P3
Tel: 506-789-1208

Note: Duguay's is a licensed special care home in New Brunswick.
Susan Duguay, Administrator

MONCTON: Ritchie V Manor II
Affiliated with: Horizon Health Network
2031 Mountain Rd., Moncton, NB E1G 1B1
Tel: 506-384-7658 *Fax:* 506-855-8994
Number of Beds: 20 beds
Debbie Teakles, Proprietor

MONCTON: Smith Special Care Home Ltd.
Affiliated with: Horizon Health Network
56 Dorchester St., Moncton, NB E1E 3A7
Tel: 506-874-0757
Number of Beds: 10 beds
Connie Whitman, Contact

RATTERS CORNER: Wilson Special Care Home
510 Drury's Cove Rd., Ratters Corner, NB E4E 3L4
Tel: 506-433-5532
Number of Beds: 2 beds
Sharon Wilson, Proprietor

SAINT JOHN: Centracare Saint John Inc.
Affiliated with: Horizon Health Network
PO Box 3220 Stn. B, 414 Bay St., Saint John, NB E2M 4H7
Tel: 506-649-2550 *Fax:* 506-649-2520
horizonnb.ca
Number of Beds: 50 beds

SAINT JOHN: Forest Hills Special Care Home
Affiliated with: Horizon Health Network
Former Name: Burnside Special Care Home
30 Mountain Rd., Saint John, NB E2J 2W8
Tel: 506-633-0743

Number of Beds: 10 beds
Janet Hebert, Proprietor

SHIPPAGAN: Pavillon St-Jérôme Inc.
150, 17e rue, Shippagan, NB E8S 1G4
Tel: 506-336-8609 *Fax:* 506-336-8652
pavillon.stj@nb.aibn.com

Number of Beds: 12 lits
Note: Résidence pour adultes handicapés intellectuels
Marie-Reine Hébert, Directrice

TITUSVILLE: Yvonne's Special Care Home
1773 Rte. 860, Titusville, NB E5N 3W2
Tel: 506-832-7186

Number of Beds: 18 units
Note: Yvonne's is a special care home for the elderly.
Yvonne Clark, Proprietor

NEWFOUNDLAND & LABRADOR

ST. JOHN'S: Waterford Hospital
Affiliated with: Eastern Regional Health Authority
306 Waterford Bridge Rd., St. John's, NL A1E 4J8
Tel: 709-777-3300 *Fax:* 709-777-3993
www.easternhealth.ca

Note: Programs & services include: mental health program; acute & outpatient care; dialysis services; blood collection; & x-ray.

NORTHWEST TERRITORIES

FORT LIARD: Fort Liard Mental Health & Addictions Program
Affiliated with: Northwest Territories Health & Social Services Authority
General Delivery, Fort Liard, NT X0G 0A0
Tel: 867-770-4770 *Fax:* 867-770-4813

FORT SIMPSON: Fort Simpson Mental Health & Addictions Program
Affiliated with: Northwest Territories Health & Social Services Authority
PO Box 246, Fort Simpson, NT X0E 0N0
Tel: 867-695-2293 *Fax:* 867-695-2920

YELLOWKNIFE: Yellowknife Mental Health Clinic
Affiliated with: Northwest Territories Health & Social Services Authority
PO Box 608, Yellowknife, NT X1A 2N5
Tel: 867-873-7042 *Fax:* 867-873-0487

NOVA SCOTIA

CANNING: Tibbetts Home Wilmot
PO Box 70, 9711 Main St., Canning, NS B0P 1H0
Tel: 902-582-7157 *Fax:* 902-582-7157
tibbco2001@yahoo.com
annapolisvalleychamber.ca
Number of Beds: 25 beds
Wanda Tibbetts, Administrator

DARTMOUTH: East Coast Forensic Psychiatric Hospital
Affiliated with: Nova Scotia Health Authority
88 Gloria McCluskey Ave., Dartmouth, NS B3B 2B8
Tel: 902-460-7300
www.nshealth.ca
Number of Beds: 30 rehabilitation beds; 24 inpatient beds

DARTMOUTH: The Nova Scotia Hospital
Affiliated with: Nova Scotia Health Authority
PO Box 1004, 300 Pleasant St., Dartmouth, NS B2Y 3S3
Tel: 902-464-3111 *Fax:* 902-464-6032
www.cdha.nshealth.ca

Note: Specialties: Mental health programs
John McCarthy, Board Development Officer
  john.mccarthy@cdha.nshealth.ca

GLACE BAY: Jones Manor
Affiliated with: Nova Scotia Health Authority
1 Minto St., Glace Bay, NS B1Z 5B2

Tel: 902-849-1605

Number of Beds: 7 beds
Calvin Jones, Administrator

HALIFAX: IWK Health Centre
Halifax Community Mental Health & Central Referral Service
Former Name: Atlantic Child Guidance Center
#1001, 6080 Young St., Halifax, NS B3K 5L2

Tel: 902-464-4110 *Fax:* 902-464-3008
Toll-Free: 855-635-4110
www.iwk.nshealth.ca

Tracy Kitch, President & CEO

HALIFAX: Metro Community Housing Association
#280, 7071 Bayers Rd., Halifax, NS B3L 2C2

Tel: 902-453-6444 *Fax:* 902-453-1188
info@mcha.ns.ca
www.mcha.ns.ca

Social Media: www.facebook.com/metrocommunityhousingassociation
Number of Beds: 86 residential capacity & 79 supported apartments
Note: Specialties: Support & residential services to persons who have experienced mental health difficulties
Cathy Crouse, Executive Director

NUNAVUT

IQALUIT: Akausisarvik Mental Health Facility
PO Box 1000, Iqaluit, NU X0A 0H0

Tel: 867-979-7631

Number of Beds: 13 beds

ONTARIO

BELLEVILLE: Cheshire Homes (Hastings - Prince Edward) Inc.
41 Pinnacle St. South, Belleville, ON K8N 3A1

Tel: 613-966-2941 *Fax:* 613-966-2461
receptionist@cheshirehpe.ca
www.cheshirehpe.ca

Year Founded: 1973
Note: Cheshire Homes offers support housing & an outreach program to physically disabled adults.

BELLEVILLE: Welcome to Community Living Belleville & Area
Former Name: Plainfield Community Homes; Plainfield Children's Home
91 Millennium Pkwy., Belleville, ON K8N 4Z5

Tel: 613-969-7407 *Fax:* 613-969-7775
www.communitylivingbelleville.org
Social Media: www.facebook.com/communitylivingbellevilleandarea;
twitter.com/CLBelleville

Year Founded: 1951
Note: Community Living Belleville & Area works toward the full inclusion in community life of persons with intellectual disabilities.
John B. Klassen, Executive Director
Stephen Ollerenshaw, Director, Finance
Katherine Potts, Director, Human Resources
Christine Semark, Director, Services
Jim Burgess, Manager, Buildings & Property
Sharon Wright, Manager, Community Development & Volunteer
 Services

BRANTFORD: Participation House Brantford
10 Bell Lane, Brantford, ON N3T 5W5

Tel: 519-756-1430
dhunt@participationhousebrantford.org
www.participationhousebrantford.org

Number of Beds: 30 beds
Note: Non-for-profit organization serving the needs of adults with physical disabilities
Steve Leighfield, Executive Director

BROCKVILLE: Brockville Mental Health Centre
Royal Ottawa Health Care Group
Former Name: Brockville Psychiatric Hospital
PO Box 1050, 1804 Hwy. 2 East, Brockville, ON K6V 5W7

Tel: 613-345-1461 *Fax:* 613-342-6194
mharc@theroyal.ca
www.theroyal.ca

Number of Beds: 161 inpatient beds
George Weber, President & CEO
 613-722-6521

COCHRANE: Cochrane Community Living
PO Box 2330, 18 2nd Ave., Cochrane, ON P0L 1C0

Tel: 705-272-2999
iccl@puc.net
www.communitylivingontario.ca

Number of Beds: 12 beds in 3 facilities
Mac Hiltz, Interim Executive Director

COLLINGWOOD: Canford House
695 St. Marie St., Collingwood, ON L9Y 3L4

Tel: 705-445-5203 *Fax:* 705-445-7357

Number of Beds: 32 beds
Wayne Canning, Administrator

CORNWALL: Open Hands Residential Services
17383 South Branch Rd., Cornwall, ON K6K 1T3

Tel: 613-933-0012 *Fax:* 613-932-5134
www.ocapdd.on.ca

Note: The non-profit agency offers both residential & daytime community support services to persons with development disabilities. Open Hands is operated by the Ottawa Carleton Association for Persons with Developmental Disabilities (OCAPDD).
David A. Ferguson, Executive Director
 dferguson@ocapdd.on.ca

DRYDEN: Patricia Gardens Care Home
35 Van Horne Ave., Dryden, ON P8N 3B4

Tel: 807-223-5278 *Fax:* 807-223-5273
info@drydenseniorservices.ca
www.drydenseniorservices.ca

Penney Bradley, Program Coordinator
 penney.bradley@drytel.net

EAST GARAFRAXA: Dufferin Association for Community Living
065371 County Rd. 3, East Garafraxa, ON L9W 7J8

Tel: 519-941-8971 *Fax:* 519-941-9121
info@communitylivingdufferin.ca
www.communitylivingdufferin.ca
Social Media: www.facebook.com/communitylivingdufferin;
twitter.com/cldufferin; www.youtube.com/user/CLDufferin/videos

Note: Dufferin Association for Community Living assists children & adults with developmental disabilities.
Residential services include supported independent living, the operation of group homes & a home for adults with Prader Willi Syndrome, a family home program, a transitional living co-operative, & respite care. The association's group homes provide accommodations for 56 adults with developmental disabilties.
Sheryl Chandler, Executive Director
 sheryl@communitylivingdufferin.ca
Diane Slater, Director, Adult Services
 diane@communitylivingdufferin.ca
Ann Somerville, Director, Business & Finance
 ann@communitylivingdufferin.ca
Karen Bowen, Manager, Preschool Resource Program
 karen@communitylivingdufferin.ca
Nadene Buck, Manager, Residential
 nadene@communitylivingdufferin.ca
Joyce Cook, Manager, Options
 joyce@communitylivingdufferin.ca
Teresa Donaldson, Manager, Systems
 teresa@communitylivingdufferin.ca
Darlene Morrow, Manager, Residential
 darlene@communitylivingdufferin.ca

Lindsay Pendleton, Manager, Residential
  lindsay@communitylivingdufferin.ca
Catherine Ryan, Manager, Residential
  cryan@communitylivingdufferin.ca
Denyse Small, Manager, Employment Services
  denyse@communitylivingdufferin.ca

FERGUS: Canadian Mental Health Association - Waterloo Wellington
Fergus
Former Name: Trellis Mental Health & Developmental Services
234 St. Patrick St. East, Fergus, ON N1M 1M6
Fax: 519-843-7608
Toll-Free: 844-264-2993
www.cmhaww.ca

Note: Services include counselling & treatment, psychiatry assessment, developmental services, support groups, education & training, family support, crisis support, geriatric services, respite services, & mental health & justice services.
Janet Kaufman, President

GRAVENHURST: Doe Lake Residence
1750 Gravenhurst Pkwy., Gravenhurst, ON P1P 1R3
Tel: 705-687-6285 *Fax:* 705-687-0100
doelakeresidence@hotmail.com

Angie Joseph, Manager

GUELPH: Homewood Health Centre
150 Delhi St., Guelph, ON N1E 6K9
Tel: 519-824-1010 *Fax:* 519-824-8751
healthcentre@homewoodhealth.com
www.homewoodhealth.com
Social Media: www.facebook.com/HomewoodHealth;
twitter.com/homewoodhc;
www.linkedin.com/company/homewood-health-centre
Year Founded: 1883
Number of Beds: 300 beds
Number of Employees: 650
Specialties: Mental Health
Note: Specialty: Behavioural, addiction & psychiatric services
Jagoda Pike, President & CEO
Marg Bellman, Executive Vice-President, Return to Work Services
Francine Bolduc, Executive Vice-President, Human Resources
Jared Landry, Executive Vice-President, Growth & Strategy
Al Van Leeuwen, Executive Vice-President, Operations
Dr. Ann Malain, Executive Vice-President, Stay at Work Services
Kimberly Mirotta, Executive Vice-President, Finance & Administration
Sean Slater, Executive Vice-President, Sales & Marketing

HAMILTON: Good Shepherd Centre
PO Box 1003, 10 Delaware Ave., Hamilton, ON L8N 3R1
Tel: 905-528-9109 *Fax:* 905-528-6967
info@goodshepherdcentres.ca
www.goodshepherdcentres.ca
Year Founded: 1961
Richard MacPhee, Executive Director

HAMILTON: Lynwood Hall Child & Family Centre
526 Upper Paradise Rd., Hamilton, ON L9C 5E3
Tel: 905-389-1361
info@lynwoodhall.com
www.lynwoodhall.com

Note: Specialties: Mental health services, including day treatment, home-based services, & residential services
Alex Thomson, Executive Director

HAMILTON: McMaster Children's Hospital
Hamilton Health Sciences
Affiliated with: Hamilton Niagara Haldimand Brant Local Health Integration Network
1200 Main St. West, Hamilton, ON L8N 3Z5
Tel: 905-521-2100
www.mcmasterchildrenshospital.ca
Social Media: www.facebook.com/140084176009847;
twitter.com/hamhealthsc; www.vimeo.com/hamiltonhealthsciences

Year Founded: 1988
Number of Beds: 165 acute care beds; 6 mental health day beds; 4 eating disorder day beds
Specialties: Acute pediatrics
Note: Provides tertiary health care services for children in Hamilton & the surrounding region. Programs & services include: 2G, 2Q & 3E child & youth clinic; audiology; Child Advocacy & Assessment Program (CAAP); child & youth mental health program; children's exercise & nutrition centre; emergency; outpatient clinical services for children with diabetes; pediatric eating disorders program; pharmacy; & sexual assault & domestic violence care centre.
Rob MacIsaac, President & CEO, Hamilton Health Sciences
Dr. Peter Fitzgerald, President, McMaster Children's Hospital

HAMILTON: McMaster Children's Hospital - Chedoke Site
Hamilton Health Sciences
Affiliated with: Hamilton Niagara Haldimand Brant Local Health Integration Network
PO Box 2000 Stn. A, Sanitorium Road, MPO, Hamilton, ON LC9 1C4
Tel: 905-521-2100
www.hamiltonhealthsciences.ca
Social Media: www.facebook.com/140084176009847;
twitter.com/hamhealthsc; www.vimeo.com/hamiltonhealthsciences
Year Founded: 1906
Note: Programs & services include: autism spectrum disorder service (Hamilton Autism Intervention Program); child & youth mental health programs; cleft lip & palate program; developmental pediatrics & rehabilitation; family resource centre; pediatric lipid clinic; specialized developmental & behavioural services; & technology access clinic.
Rob MacIsaac, President & CEO, Hamilton Health Sciences
president@hhsc.ca
Dr. Peter Fitzgerald, President & CEO, McMaster Children's Hospital

HAMILTON: St. Joseph's Healthcare Hamilton - Mental Health & Addiction Services
St. Joseph's Health System
PO Box 585, 100 - 5 St. West, Hamilton, ON L8N 3K7
Tel: 905-522-1155
www.stjoes.ca
Social Media: www.facebook.com/stjosephshealthcarefoundation;
twitter.com/STJOESHAMILTON; www.youtube.com/Stjoesfoundation

Specialties: Mental Health
Dr. David Higgins, President
905-522-1155, president@stjoes.ca

HAMILTON: St. Joseph's Healthcare Hamilton - West 5th Campus
St. Joseph's Health System
Affiliated with: Hamilton Niagara Haldimand Brant Local Health Integration Network
100 West 5th St., Hamilton, ON L9C 0E3
Tel: 905-522-1155
www.stjosham.on.ca
Info Line: 905-522-4941
Social Media: www.facebook.com/stjosehshealthcarefoundation;
twitter.com/STJOESHAMILTON; www.youtube.com/Stjoesfoundation;
www.linkedin.com/company/st-joseph's-healthcare-hamilton

Note: Offers mental health & medical services, as well as teaching & research facilities. Affiliated with the Faculty of Health Sciences at McMaster University & Mohawk College.
Dr. David Higgins, President
Romeo Cercone, Vice-President, Quality & Strategic Planning, & Mental Health & Addiction Programs

HANMER: Kingsley Residential Home
PO Box 118, 36 Oscar St., Hanmer, ON P3P 1X6
Tel: 705-969-5538
Number of Beds: 6 beds
Jeannine Kingsley, Proprietor

HANOVER: Community Living Hanover
521 - 11th Ave., Hanover, ON N4N 2J3
Tel: 519-364-6100 *Fax:* 519-364-7488
www.clhanover.com
Number of Beds: 15 beds
Charlie Caudle, Executive Director

HOLLAND LANDING: Cedar Lane Residential Home
19704 Holland Landing Rd., Holland Landing, ON L9N 1M8
Tel: 905-836-4272 *Fax:* 905-836-8277
Cathy Dowling, Contact

HOLLAND LANDING: Porter Place, Men's Shelter
18838 Hwy. 11, Holland Landing, ON L9N 0C5
Tel: 905-898-1015 *Fax:* 905-898-6414
Toll-Free: 888-554-5525
www.bluedoorshelters.ca
Number of Beds: 19 beds
Monica Auerbach, Executive Director

HOLLAND LANDING: Southdown Institute
18798 Old Yonge St., Holland Landing, ON L9N 0L1
Tel: 905-727-4214 *Fax:* 905-895-6296
www.southdown.on.ca
Number of Beds: 44 beds
Note: Specialties: Residential & outpatient psychological treatment to clergy & religious; Psychodynamic group therapy; Individual & group addiction counselling; 12-step groups; Specialized group treatment for persons who have violated sexual boundaries; Art therapy; Health education
Dorothy Heiderscheit, CEO
Brenda Allison, Office Manager

KESWICK: Pipe & Slipper Home
2926 Old Homestead Rd., Keswick, ON L4P 3E9
Tel: 905-989-0907
Note: Residential care is provided for adults. Referral is necessary.

KINGSTON: Ongwanada Hospital
191 Portsmouth Ave., Kingston, ON K7M 8A6
Tel: 613-548-4417 *Fax:* 613-548-8135
www.ongwanada.com
Social Media: www.facebook.com/Ongwanada1;
twitter.com/ongwanada
Year Founded: 1948
Number of Beds: 227 beds
Note: Specialties: Support for persons with developmental disabilities; Day support; Vocational & life skills training; Occupational therapy; Physiotherapy; Hydrotherapy; Snoezelen Room; Community behavioural services; Research. Number of employees: 494
Dr. Robert W. Seaby, Executive Director

KINGSTON: Providence Care - Mental Health Services
Affiliated with: Providence Care
Former Name: Kingston Psychiatric Hospital
752 King St. West, Kingston, ON K7L 4X3
Tel: 613-546-1101 *Fax:* 613-548-5588
www.providencecare.ca
Number of Beds: 198 beds
Note: Adult Treatment & Rehabilitation, Geriatric Psychiatry, Forensic Psychiatry. Affilated with Queen's University.
Maurio Ruffolo, Vice-President, Patient & Client Care
ruffolom@providencecare.ca

KITCHENER: Sunbeam Lodge
389 Pinnacle Dr., Kitchener, ON N2G 3W5
Tel: 519-886-4222 *Fax:* 519-885-1580
teena@sunbeamlodge.com
www.sunbeamlodge.com
Info Line: 519-886-4700
Number of Beds: 22 beds
Note: Specialties: Lont-term residential care & treatment for children with special needs; Day program; Physiotherapy treatment; Kinesiology; Communications programs; Independent living skills program. Number of Employees: 9 Registered Nurses & Registered Practical Nurses + 2 Kinessiologists + 1 Program Coordinator + 21 Child Care Attendants + 1 Dietician + 2 Housekeepers + 1 Executive Secretary
John Vos, Administrator
Shabnam Vos, Administrator

KITCHENER: Sunbeam Residential Development Centre
2749 Kingsway Dr., Kitchener, ON N2C 1A7
Tel: 519-893-6200 *Fax:* 519-893-9034
www.sunbeamcentre.com

Year Founded: 1956
Note: Specialties: Care for individuals with diverse & complex developmental challenges; Long-term & short-term support; Activation; Sensory stimulation
Dr. Shaune Lawton, Executive Director

LINDSAY: Chimo Youth & Family Services
227 Kent St. West, Lindsay, ON K9V 2Z1
Tel: 705-324-3300 *Fax:* 705-324-3304
Toll-Free: 888-454-6275
info@chimoyouth.ca
www.chimoyouth.ca
Note: Chimo Youth & Family Services is accredited under Children's Mental Health Ontario. Programs include clinical & crisis care, group meetings, day treatment, & residential & respite care.

LONDON: Child & Parent Resource Institute (CPRI)
600 Sanatorium Rd., London, ON N6H 3W7
Tel: 519-858-2774 *Fax:* 519-858-3913
Toll-Free: 877-494-2774
www.cpri.ca
Number of Beds: 75 beds
Note: Provides outpatient, intensive/residential, support, & referral services for children & youth with developmental disabilities or mental health needs
Dr. Shannon Stewart, Program Manager

LONDON: Parkwood Institute
Affiliated with: St. Joseph's Health Care, London
Former Name: Parkwood Hospital; Regional Mental Healthcare London
550 Wellington Rd. South, London, ON N6C 0A7
Tel: 519-646-6100
www.sjhc.london.on.ca
Number of Beds: 403 beds
Note: Programs & services include: geriatric services; Veterans Care program; mental health care programs; & rehabilitation programs & assessments.
Roy Butler, Vice-President, Patient Care & Risk Management

LUCAN: Crest Support Services
13570 Elginfield Rd., RR#1, Lucan, ON N0M 2J0
Tel: 519-227-6766 *Fax:* 519-227-6768
www.crestsupportservices.ca
Note: Specialties: Services for adults with mental health or developmental disabilities; Accommodation services; Operation of three small businesses to provide training & employment opportunities
David Ragobar, Executive Director
david@thecrestcentre.com

MARKHAM: Kinark Child & Family Services
Corporate Office, #200, 500 Hood Rd., Markham, ON L3R 9Z3
Tel: 905-474-9595 *Fax:* 905-474-1448
Toll-Free: 800-230-8533
info@kinark.on.ca
www.kinark.on.ca
Social Media: www.facebook.com/kinark; twitter.com/mykinark;
www.youtube.com/user/mykinark
Year Founded: 1916
Number of Employees: 800
Note: Services include crisis services, therapeutic family programs, child care, day treatment, residential treatment, adventure-based programming, autism services, & youth justice services.
Cathy Paul, President & CEO

MARKHAM: Participation House
204 - 4261 Hwy. 7, Markham, ON L3R 9W6
Tel: 905-294-0944 *Fax:* 905-294-7834
postmaster@participationhouse.net
www.participationhouse.net
Number of Beds: 52 beds
Note: Provides services designed to enhance the qualify of life of people with disabilities
Sharon M. Lawlor, Executive Director

NEPEAN: Total Communication Environment (TCE)
#5, 203 Colonnade Rd. South, Nepean, ON K2E 7K3
Tel: 613-228-0999 Fax: 613-228-1402
TTY: 613-228-8669
tceadmin@tceottawa.org
www.tceottawa.org

Year Founded: 1979
Note: Specialties: Services for adults with multiple disabilities & special communication needs; Respite care; Day services; Outreach to long-term care homes
Karen Anderson, Executive Director

NEWMARKET: Brigitta's Residential Home Inc.
128 Arden Ave., Newmarket, ON L3Y 4H6
Tel: 905-895-5890

Number of Beds: 22 beds
Brigitta Miller, Administrator

NEWMARKET: Brown's Residential Home
399 Queen St., Newmarket, ON L3Y 2G9
Tel: 905-898-1955 Fax: 905-898-1955

Note: Supportive residential care is provided for adults.

NEWMARKET: Heritage Lodge
508 College St., Newmarket, ON L3Y 1C6
Tel: 905-853-1587 Fax: 905-853-1587

Note: Heritage Lodge is a home for special care to assist persons with a mental health disability.

NORTH BAY: Community Living North Bay
161 Main St. East, North Bay, ON P1B 1A9
Tel: 705-476-3288 Fax: 705-476-4788
info@communitylivingnorthbay.org
www.communitylivingnorthbay.org

Year Founded: 1954
Jennifer Valenti, Executive Director

NORTH BAY: North Bay Regional Health Centre - Mental Health Clinic
Former Name: North Bay Psychiatric Hospital
120 King St. West, North Bay, ON P1B 5Z7
Tel: 705-494-3050 Fax: 705-494-3092
www.nbrhc.on.ca

OAKVILLE: Central West Specialized Developmental Services
Former Name: Oaklands Regional Centre
53 Bond St., Oakville, ON L6K 1L8
Tel: 905-844-7864 Fax: 905-844-3545
www.cwsds.ca
Year Founded: 1975
Note: Specialties: Care & support to persons with multiple developmental disabilities; Basic life skill development; Psychiatry; Behaviour therapy; Occupational therapy; Speech therapy; Respite care
James Duncan, Executive Director

OTTAWA: Roberts/Smart Centre
1199 Carling Ave., Ottawa, ON K1Z 8N8
Tel: 613-728-1946 Fax: 613-728-4986
Toll-Free: 800-279-9941
info@rsc-crs.com
www.robertssmartcentre.com
Number of Beds: 47 beds
Cameron Macleod, Executive Director

OTTAWA: Royal Ottawa Mental Health Centre
1145 Carling Ave., Ottawa, ON K1Z 7K4
Tel: 613-722-6521 Toll-Free: 800-987-6424
www.theroyal.ca
Social Media: www.facebook.com/TheRoyalMHC;
twitter.com/TheRoyalMHC

Year Founded: 1910
Number of Beds: 190
George Weber, President & CEO
Dr. Raj Bhatla, Psychiatrist-in-Chief & Chief of Staff
Dr. A.G. Ahmed, Associate Chief, Integrated Forensic Program
Cal Crocker, Chief Financial Officer

Joanne Bezzubetz, Vice-President, Patient Care Services
Nicole Loreto, Vice-President, Communications & Partnerships
Susan Engels, Chief Nursing Executive & Vice-President, Quality & Professional Practice

OWEN SOUND: Kent Residential Home
Former Name: Tucker's Residential Home
1065 - 9th Ave. West, Owen Sound, ON N4K 2G5
Tel: 519-371-5029 Fax: 519-371-3237
Number of Beds: 18 beds
Note: residential home for people with mental illness
Yvonne Kent

OXFORD MILLS: Old Mill Guest Home
12 Bridge St., Oxford Mills, ON K0G 1S0
Tel: 613-258-3366
Number of Beds: 22 beds
Note: Specialties: Residential services for post-psychiatric patients; Social programs

PENETANGUISHENE: Waypoint Centre for Mental Health Care
Former Name: Penetanguishene Mental Health Centre
500 Church St., Penetanguishene, ON L9M 1G3
Tel: 705-549-3181 Fax: 705-549-3778
Toll-Free: 877-341-4729
info@waypointcentre.ca
www.waypointcentre.ca

Year Founded: 1859
Number of Beds: 301
Number of Employees: 1200
Specialties: Mental Health
Note: Offers psychiatric services to Simcoe County, Muskoka, & parts of Dufferin County & Parry Sound
Carol Lambie, President & CEO
Linda Adams, Chief Nursing Executive & Vice-President, Quality & Professional Practice
Rob Desroches, Vice-President, Clinical Services
Lorraine Smith, Vice-President, Corporate Services
Terry McMahon, Vice-President, Human Resources & Organizational Development
Bob Savage, Vice-President, Redevelopment
Deborah Duncan, Vice-President, Clinical Support Services
Dr. Jeff Van Impe, Psychiatrist-in-Chief

PETERBOROUGH: Community Living Peterborough
223 Aylmer St., Peterborough, ON K9J 3K3
Tel: 705-743-2411 Fax: 705-743-3722
www.communitylivingpeterborough.ca
Social Media: www.facebook.com/CommunityLivingPtbo;
twitter.com/CLPeterborough;
www.youtube.com/user/CommunityLivingPtbo

Year Founded: 1953
Note: The following services are provided: supported housing for adults over the age of 21; family support; community access; & employment options.
Jack Gillan, Chief Executive Officer
Barb Hiland, Director, Operations
Cindy Hobbins, Manager, Community Development, Communications, & Quality Enhancement
Pat McNamara, Manager
Edna O'Toole, General Manager, Supportive Housing

PETROLIA: Lambton County Developmental Services
Former Name: Lambton County Association for Mentally Handicapped
PO Box 1210, 339 Centre St., Petrolia, ON N0N 1R0
Tel: 519-882-0933 Fax: 519-882-3386
administration@lcds.on.ca
www.lcds.on.ca
Number of Beds: 68 beds
Note: Provides services to persons with intellectual disabilities
Don Seymour, Executive Director

POWASSAN: Eide's Residential Home
532 Main St., Powassan, ON P0H 1Z0
Tel: 705-724-2748

SAINT-PASCAL-BAYLON: St. Pascal Residential Home
2454 du Lac Rd., RR#1, Saint-Pascal-Baylon, ON K0A 3N0
Tel: 613-488-2626 *Fax:* 613-488-2626
admin@stpascalresidence.com
www.stpascalresidence.com

SEVERN BRIDGE: Trentview House
1647 Kilworthy Rd., RR#1, Severn Bridge, ON L0K 2B0
Tel: 705-689-5685
Year Founded: 1979
Number of Beds: 25 beds
Note: Specialties: Services for adults with mental health disabilities

ST AGATHA: Carizon Family & Community Services
Former Name: kidsLINK
PO Box 190, 1855 Notre Dame Dr., St Agatha, ON N0B 2L0
Tel: 519-746-5437
Social Media: www.facebook.com/carizonupdates; twitter.com/carizon;
www.linkedin.com/company/carizon-family-and-community-services

Note: Mental health & counselling services for children, youth, &
families
Tracy Elop, CEO
Jennifer Berry, Director, Communications

ST CATHARINES: Montebello Place
Former Name: Horvath Residence
1 Montebello St., St Catharines, ON L2R 6B5
Tel: 905-984-6506
caringplaces.ca/montebello-place.html
Year Founded: 1973
Number of Beds: 15 beds
Sharon Okum, Co-Owner
David Okum, Co-Owner

ST THOMAS: Tara Hall Residential Care Home
38 Chester St., St Thomas, ON N5R 1V2
Tel: 519-631-4937 *Fax:* 519-631-1526
tarahall@rogers.com
Year Founded: 1988
Number of Beds: 36 beds
Note: Specialties: Assisted living for adults with an intellectual disability,
brain injury, or mental illness
James Akey, Manager

**ST. THOMAS: Southwest Centre for Forensic Mental Health
Care**
Affiliated with: St. Joseph's Health Care, London
401 Sunset Dr., St. Thomas, ON N5R 3C6
Tel: 519-646-6100
www.sjhc.london.on.ca
Dr. Gillian Kernaghan, President & CEO
askgillian@sjhc.london.on.ca

**SUDBURY: North Bay Regional Health Centre (NBRHC)/Centre
régional de santé de North Bay**
Kirkwood Place
**Former Name: Northeast Mental Health Centre, Sudbury
Campus**
680 Kirkwood Dr., Sudbury, ON P3E 1X3
Tel: 705-675-9193 *Fax:* 705-675-6817
pr@nbrhc.on.ca
www.nbrhc.on.ca
Social Media: www.facebook.com/nbrhc; twitter.com/nbrhc;
www.youtube.com/thenbrhc

Tanya Nixon, Vice-President, Mental Health

SUDBURY: Sudbury Mental Health and Addictions Centre
Kirkwood Place
Affiliated with: Health Sciences North
680 Kirkwood Dr., Sudbury, ON P3E 1X3
Tel: 705-675-5900
www.hsnsudbury.ca

Note: Acute inpatient psychiatry services
Dr. Denis-Richard Roy, President & CEO, Health Sciences North
Dr. Chris Bourdon, Chief of Staff, Health Sciences North

THUNDER BAY: Lakehead Psychiatric Hospital
St. Joseph's Care Group
580 Algoma St. North, Thunder Bay, ON P7B 5G4
Tel: 807-343-4300 *Fax:* 807-343-4373

Specialties: Mental Health
Tracy Buckler, President & CEO

THUNDER BAY: Marcinowsky Residential Home
601 Alice Ave., RR#14, Thunder Bay, ON P7G 1X1
Tel: 807-767-6199

TORONTO: Bellwood Health Services
Edgewood Health Network Inc.
**Affiliated with: Toronto Central Local Health Integration
Network**
175 Brentcliffe Rd., Toronto, ON M4G 0C5
Tel: 416-495-0926 *Fax:* 416-495-7943
Toll-Free: 800-387-6198
info@bellwood.ca
www.bellwood.ca
Social Media: www.facebook.com/bellwoodhealthservices;
twitter.com/BellwoodHealth; www.youtube.com/user/BellwoodHealth
Year Founded: 1984
Number of Beds: 88
Specialties: Addiction & eating disorders
Note: Serves men & women aged 19 years & over. Programs &
services include: treatment & education for individuals & families
struggling with addictions, including alcohol & drugs, gambling, sex,
eating disorders, workplace trauma with or without concurrent
addiction; assessments; detox services; funded residential treatment
program for alcohol addiction of Ontario residents with valid OHIP card;
continuing care programs; family services; & outpatient individual &
group counselling services.
Cara Vaccarino, Chief Operating Officer
cvaccarino@bellwood.ca
Kristen Cleary, Clinical Director
kcleary@bellwood.ca
Joshua Montgomery, Operations Director
jmontgomery@bellwood.ca

TORONTO: Centre for Addiction & Mental Health
ARF Site
Former Name: Addiction Research Foundation
33 Russell St., Toronto, ON M5S 2S1
Tel: 416-595-6000 *Fax:* 416-595-9997
Toll-Free: 800-463-2338
info@camh.ca
www.camh.ca
Social Media: www.facebook.com/CentreforAddictionandMentalHealth;
twitter.com/CAMHnews; www.youtube.com/camhtv;
www.linkedin.com/company/camh

Note: Drug rehabilitation centre
David Cunic, Vice-President, Redevelopment & Support Services

**TORONTO: Centre for Addiction & Mental Health (Corporate
Office)**
1001 Queen St. West, Toronto, ON M6J 1H4
Tel: 416-535-8501 Toll-Free: 800-463-2338
info@camh.ca
www.camh.ca
Social Media: www.facebook.com/CentreforAddictionandMentalHealth;
twitter.com/CAMHnews; www.youtube.com/user/CAMHTV;
www.linkedin.com/company/camh
Number of Beds: 530 inpatient beds
Note: Addiction treatment
Dr. Catherine Zahn, President & CEO

TORONTO: Child Development Institute
Former Name: West End Creche Child & Family Clinic
197 Euclid Ave., Toronto, ON M6J 2J8
Tel: 416-603-1827 *Fax:* 416-603-6655
info@childdevelop.ca
www.childdevelop.ca
Social Media: www.facebook.com/childdevelop; twitter.com/officialcdi;
www.youtube.com/user/CDICanada;
www.linkedin.com/company/child-development-institute

Year Founded: 1909
Note: Provides mental health programs & services for children & youth
Tony Diniz, CEO
  tdiniz@childdevelop.ca
Steve Blake, COO
  sblake@childdevelop.ca
Dr. Leena Augimeri, Director, Scientific & Program Development
  laugimeri@childdevelop.ca
Shauna Klein, Director, Fund Development, Marketing &
  Communications
  sklein@childdevelop.ca
Linda Levely, Director, Finance & Administration
  llevely@childdevelop.ca

TORONTO: Community Outreach Services (COS)
Michael Garron Hospital
671 Danforth Ave., 2nd Fl., Toronto, ON M4J 1L3
Tel: 416-461-2000
ptrep@tegh.on.ca (Patients); community@tegh.on.ca (Community)
www.tegh.on.ca

Note: Specialties: Community based mental health services;
Counselling to adults; Supported housing; Psychiatric treatment;
Psycho-social rehabilitation; Family support program; Community &
school outreach program

TORONTO: Griffin Centre
24 Silverview Dr., Toronto, ON M2M 2B3
Tel: 416-222-1153 *Fax:* 416-222-1321
contact@griffin-centre.org
www.griffin-centre.org

Number of Beds: 10 beds
Laurie Dart, Executive Director

TORONTO: Hincks-Dellcrest Treatment Centre
440 Jarvis St., Toronto, ON M4Y 2H4
Tel: 416-924-1164 *Fax:* 416-924-8208
info@hincksdellcrest.org
www.hincksdellcrest.org
Social Media: www.facebook.com/255128254500066;
twitter.com/hincksdellcrest; www.youtube.com/thehincksdellcrest

Note: Children's mental health
John Spekkens, Executive Director

TORONTO: Salvation Army Broadview Village
1132 Broadview Ave., Toronto, ON M4K 2S5
Tel: 416-425-1052 *Toll-Free:* 888-333-1229
www.salvationarmy.ca

Number of Beds: 61 beds
Note: Facility for adults with developmental disabilities
Capt. Glenda Davis, Director

TORONTO: The Scarborough Hospital - Birchmount Campus
Scarborough & Rouge Hospital
Affiliated with: Central East Local Health Integration Network
Former Name: The Scarborough Hospital - Grace Campus
3030 Birchmount Rd., Toronto, ON M1W 3W3
Tel: 416-495-2400
www.tsh.to
Social Media: www.facebook.com/ScarboroughHospital;
twitter.com/ScarboroughHosp;
www.youtube.com/user/TSHCommunications;
www.linkedin.com/company/the-scarborough-hospital
Number of Beds: 215 beds
Number of Employees: 3105
Note: A health facility with emphasis on emergency outpatient
psychiatric concerns, notably its Regional Crisis Program, an
emergency response team to acute psychiatric crises. Affiliated with the
University of Toronto.
Robert Biron, President & CEO
Dr. Tom Chan, Chief of Medical Staff
Linda Calhoun, Chief Nursing Executive & Vice-President, Integrated
  Care & Patient Experience

TORONTO: Youthdale Treatment Centres
227 Victoria St., Toronto, ON M5B 1T8
Tel: 416-368-4896
www.youthdale.ca

Year Founded: 1969
Note: Youthdale provides mental health services to approximately
5,000 children & their families each year. A crisis service line is
available (416-363-9990). The non-profit, charitable community
agency also offers clinical services, including psychiatric crisis
response, residential treatment, & outpatient consultation.

VARS: Pine Rest Residence
PO Box 109, 5876 Bearbrook Rd., Vars, ON K0A 3H0
Tel: 613-835-2849 *Fax:* 613-835-9335
Number of Beds: 33 residential capacity
Note: Specialties: Residential care for persons with developmental
disabilities, psychiatric disabilities, or those who suffer from alcoholism;
Medication supervision; Respite care
Raymond Meloche, Administrator

VARS: Résidence Ste-Marie
5855, rue Buckland RR#2, Vars, ON K0H 3H0
Tel: 613-835-2525
Number of Beds: 40 lits
Note: Spécialisée à la prestation des soins aux personnes atteintes de
maladie mentale grave; soins infirmiers, activités hebdomadaires
Gaétan Brisson, Propriétaire
Suzanne Brisson, Propriétaire

VINELAND: Amber Lodge
4024 Martin Rd., Vineland, ON L0R 2E0
Tel: 905-562-7272 *Fax:* 905-892-9700
William Ram, Administrator/Owner

VINELAND: Bethesda Home for the Mentally Handicapped Inc.
3950 Fly Rd., Vineland, ON L0R 2C0
Tel: 905-684-6918 *Fax:* 905-684-6918
info@bethesdaservices.com
www.bethesdaservices.com
Number of Beds: 42 beds
Donald Boese, Executive Director

WATERLOO: Children's Mental Health Services
Lutherwood
285 Benjamin Rd., Waterloo, ON N2J 3Z4
Tel: 519-884-1470 *Fax:* 519-886-8479
www.lutherwood.ca
Number of Beds: 6 beds (Bridgelands program); 10 beds (Woodlands
program)
Note: Specialties: Day treatment program; Residential treatment
program; Group & individual skills training; Individual & family
counselling; Home support; Community integration; Crisis support

WATERLOO: Lutherwood
285 Benjamin Rd., Waterloo, ON N2J 3Z4
Tel: 519-884-7755 *Fax:* 519-884-9071
www.lutherwood.ca
Social Media: www.facebook.com/lutherwoodjobs;
twitter.com/lutherwood; www.youtube.com/user/LutherwoodCanada;
www.linkedin.com/company/lutherwood
Year Founded: 1970
Number of Employees: 500
Note: Specialties: Mental health services for children & families,
including assessment, a youth shelter, housing support services,
residential treatment, family crisis & prevention counselling, a
community services program, & school-based interventions; Senior
services, including independent & supported living resources
John Colangeli, CEO

WATERLOO: Underhill Residential Home
127 Erb St. West, Waterloo, ON N2L 1T7
Tel: 519-884-7160 *Fax:* 519-884-5936

Note: Specialties: Residential & personal care services for seniors &
persons with mental health concerns

WHITBY: Ontario Shores Centre for Mental Health Sciences
Former Name: Whitby Mental Health Centre
700 Gordon St., Whitby, ON L1N 5S9
Tel: 905-430-4055 *Toll-Free:* 800-341-6323
centralizedreferral@ontarioshores.ca
www.ontarioshores.ca
Year Founded: 1919
Number of Employees: 1200
Specialties: Mental Health
Note: Specialized, tertiary mental health care on an inpatient/outpatient basis. Community service sites in Newmarket, Lindsay, Peterborough, & Whitby
Karim Mamdani, President & CEO

PRINCE EDWARD ISLAND

CHARLOTTETOWN: Hillsborough Hospital & Special Care Centre
Affiliated with: Health PEI
PO Box 1929, 115 Murchison Lane, Charlottetown, PE C1A 7N5
Tel: 902-368-5400 *Fax:* 902-368-5467
Number of Beds: 75 beds
Note: Specialties: Psychiatry; Medical services for persons with acute or long-term mental illnesses or mental handicaps, & psychogeriatric patients; Day services for former patients; Assessment; Behavioural management

CHARLOTTETOWN: Sherwood Home
Affiliated with: Health PEI
75 Murchison Lane, Charlottetown, PE C1N 7N5
Tel: 902-368-4141 *Fax:* 902-368-4931

Note: Sherwood Home is a provincial residential service for persons with physical and/or developmental disabilities. The home offers residential, respite and day program services.

QUÉBEC

LACHINE: Centre de réadaptation de l'Ouest de Montréal (CROM/WMR)/West Montreal Readaptation Centre
Affiliée à: CIUSSS de l'Ouest-de-l'Ile-de-Montréal
8000, rue Notre-Dame, Lachine, QC H8R 1H2
Tél: 514-363-3025 *Téléc:* 514-364-0608
infocrom@ssss.gouv.qc.ca
www.crom.ca
Média social: www.facebook.com/CROM.WMRC
Région desservi: CSSS de l'Ouest de l'Ile; CSSS Cavendish; CSSS de la Montagne
Spécialités: Services spécialisés pour des adultes et enfants présentant une déficience intellectuelle ou un trouble du spectre autistique
Dre. Katherine Moxness, Directrice générale

MALARTIC: Hôpital psychiatrique de Malartic
Affiliée à: CISSS de l'Abitibi-Témiscamingue
1141, rue Royale, Malartic, QC J0Y 1Z0
Tél: 819-825-5858 *Téléc:* 819 825-7739
Nombre de lits: 34 lits
Note: Services de santé mentale et psychiatrie; soins aigus; soins de longue durée.

MONTRÉAL: Hôpital Rivière-des-Prairies
Affiliée à: CIUSSS du Nord-de-l'Ile-de-Montréal
7070, boul Perras, Montréal, QC H1E 1A4
Tél: 514-323-7260 *Téléc:* 514-323-8622
www.hrdp.qc.ca
Nombre de lits: 125 lits

MONTRÉAL: L'Institut universitaire en santé mentale de Montréal
Affiliée à: CIUSSS de l'Est-de-l'Ile-de-Montréal
Ancien nom: Hôpital Louis-H. Lafontaine
7401, rue Hochelaga, Montréal, QC H1N 3M5
Tél: 514-251-4000 *Téléc:* 514-251-0856
www.iusmm.ca
Nombre de lits: 389 lits
Denise Fortin, Directrice générale
Frédéric Doutrelepont, Directeur, Services multidisciplinaire

QUÉBEC: Centre de réadaptation en santé mentale
Également connu sous le nom de: La Maisonnée
855, boul Louis XIV, Québec, QC G1H 1A6
Tél: 418-628-2572 *Téléc:* 418-628-5440
www.csssqn.qc.ca
Région desservi: Région de la Capitale-Nationale

QUÉBEC: L'Institut universitaire en santé mentale de Québec
Ancien nom: Centre hospitalier Robert Giffard
2601, ch. de la Canardière, Quebec, QC G1J 2G3
Tél: 418-663-5000 *Téléc:* 418-663-9774
www.institutsmq.qc.ca
Fondée en: 1976
Nombre de lits: 513 lits
Note: Affilié à l'Université Laval.
Dr. Simon Racine, Directeur général
Sylvie Laverdière, Directrice générale adjointe
Dr. Pierre Laliberté, Directeur des services professionnels et hospitaliers
Sylvain Pouliot, Directeur des Programmes-clientèles
Carl Parent, Directeur des ressources humaines
Dr. Philip Baruch, Directeur de l'enseignement
Dr. Evens Villeneuve, Chef du Département régional de psychiatrie
Dr. Yves de Koninck, Directeur de la recherche
Gilles Grondin, Directeur des ressources informationnelles

RIMOUSKI: L'hôpital de jour santé mentale et psychiatrie
Affiliée à: CISSS du Bas-St-Laurent
95, rue de l'Évêché Ouest, Rimouski, QC G5L 4H4
Tél: 418-725-0544

Population desservi: 21000
Jocelyne Morissette, Responsable

SHERBROOKE: Centre de réadaptation Estrie (CRE)
Affiliée à: CIUSSS de l'Estrie
#200, 300, rue King est, Sherbrooke, QC J1G 1B1
Tél: 819-346-8411 *Téléc:* 819-346-4580
www.santeestrie.qc.ca
Média social: www.youtube.com/user/readaptationestrie

Spécialités: Réadaptation fonctionnelle intensive; Ressources résidentielles et d'hébergement

SASKATCHEWAN

ARBORFIELD: Arborfield Special Care Lodge
Affiliated with: Kelsey Trail Regional Health Authority
PO Box 160, 509 - 5th Ave., Arborfield, SK S0E 0A0
Tel: 306-769-8757 *Fax:* 306-769-8759
ww.kelseytrailhealth.ca
Number of Beds: 36 beds
Sharon Frisky, Community Coordinator

ARCOLA: Arcola Mental Health Clinic
Affiliated with: Sun Country Health Region
PO Box 419, Arcola, SK S0C 0G0
Tel: 306-455-2159

Note: Programs & services include: children's mental health.

BATTLEFORD: Battlefords District Care Centre
Affiliated with: Prairie North Health Region
PO Box 69, Battleford, SK S0M 0E0
Tel: 306-446-6900 *Fax:* 306-937-2258

CANORA: Canora Gateway Lodge
Affiliated with: Sunrise Regional Health Authority
PO Box 1387, 212 Centre Ave. East, Canora, SK S0A 0L0
Tel: 306-563-5685 *Fax:* 306-563-5711
Number of Beds: 63 long-term beds; 1 respite

CARROT RIVER: Pasquia Special Care Home
Affiliated with: Kelsey Trail Regional Health Authority
PO Box 250, 4101 - 1st Ave West, Carrot River, SK S0E 0L0
Tel: 306-768-2725 *Fax:* 306-768-3233
Number of Beds: 35 long-term care beds

CUMBERLAND HOUSE: Cumberland House Addiction Services
Affiliated with: Kelsey Trail Regional Health Authority
PO Box 218, Cumberland House, SK S0E 0S0
Tel: 306-888-2155 *Fax:* 306-888-4633

DALMENY: Spruce Manor Special Care Home
Affiliated with: Saskatoon Health Region
PO Box 190, 701 - 1st St., Dalmeny, SK S0K 1E0
Tel: 306-254-2101 *Fax:* 306-254-2178
sprucemanor.mennonite.net
Year Founded: 1950
Number of Beds: 36 beds

ESTERHAZY: Centennial Special Care Home
Affiliated with: Sunrise Regional Health Authority
PO Box 310, 300 James St., Esterhazy, SK S0A 0X0
Tel: 306-745-6444 *Fax:* 306-745-2741
Number of Beds: 52 long term care beds; 1 respite bed

ESTEVAN: Estevan Mental Health Clinic
Affiliated with: Sun Country Health Region
1174 Nicholson Rd., Estevan, SK S4A 2V3
Tel: 306-637-3610
Note: Programs & services include: children's mental health.

FORT QU'APPELLE: Echo Lodge Special Care Home
Affiliated with: Regina Qu'Appelle Health Region
PO Box 1790, 560 Broadway St. West, Fort Qu'appelle, SK S0G 1S0
Tel: 306-332-4300 *Fax:* 306-332-5708
Number of Beds: 50 beds
Note: Adult day care & respite care are available.

HERBERT: Herbert Nursing Home Inc.
Affiliated with: Cypress Regional Health Authority
PO Box 520, 405 Herbert Ave., Herbert, SK S0H 2A0
Tel: 306-784-2466
Year Founded: 1951
Number of Beds: 48 beds

HUMBOLDT: St. Mary's Villa
Affiliated with: Saskatoon Health Region
PO Box 1360, 1109 - 13 St. North, Humboldt, SK S0K 2A0
Tel: 306-682-2628 *Fax:* 306-682-3211
Number of Beds: 85 beds

KIPLING: Kipling Mental Health Clinic
Affiliated with: Sun Country Health Region
PO Box 420, Kipling, SK S0G 2S0
Tel: 306-736-2638
Note: Programs & services include: children's mental health.

LANGENBURG: Centennial Special Care Home
Affiliated with: Sunrise Regional Health Authority
PO Box 370, 407 - 2 St. South, Langenburg, SK S0A 2A0
Tel: 306-743-2232 *Fax:* 306-743-5025
Number of Beds: 44 long-term care beds; 2 respite beds; 1 palliative care bed

LLOYDMINSTER: Lloydminster Mental Health & Addictions Services
Affiliated with: Prairie North Health Region
3830 - 43 Ave., Lloydminster, SK S9V 1Y3
Tel: 306-820-6250 *Fax:* 306-820-6256

MANKOTA: Prairie View Health Centre
Affiliated with: Cypress Regional Health Authority
PO Box 390, 241 - 1 Ave., Mankota, SK S0H 2W0
Tel: 306-478-2200
Number of Beds: 20 beds

MEADOW LAKE: Northland Pioneers Lodge Inc.
Affiliated with: Prairie North Health Region
515 - 3 St. West, Meadow Lake, SK S9X 1L1
Tel: 306-236-5812

MELFORT: Sakwatamo Lodge
Affiliated with: Prince Albert Parkland Health Region
PO Box 3917, Melfort, SK S0E 1A0
Tel: 306-864-3631 *Fax:* 306-864-2204
Note: Programs & services include: addiction services; family support; suicide prevention.

NORTH BATTLEFORD: Villa Pascal
Affiliated with: Prairie North Health Region
Also Known As: Société Joseph Breton Inc.
1301 - 113 St., North Battleford, SK S9A 3K1
Tel: 306-445-8465 *Fax:* 306-445-5117

PRINCE ALBERT: Addiction Services Prince Albert
Affiliated with: Prince Albert Parkland Health Region
101 - 15th St. East, Prince Albert, SK S6V 1G1
Tel: 306-765-6550 *Fax:* 306-765-6567

PRINCE ALBERT: Mont St. Joseph Home Inc.
Affiliated with: Prince Albert Parkland Regional Health Authority
777 - 28 St. East, Prince Albert, SK S6V 8C2
Tel: 306-953-4500 *Fax:* 306-953-4550
montstjoseph.org
Social Media:
www.facebook.com/pages/Mont-St-Joseph-Home/176717885855784
Year Founded: 1956
Number of Beds: 120 beds
Note: Special care home
Brian Martin, Executive Director

PRINCE ALBERT: White Buffalo Youth Inhalant Treatment Centre
Affiliated with: Prince Albert Parkland Health Region
PO Box 2350, Prince Albert, SK S6V 6Z1
Tel: 306-764-5250 *Fax:* 306-764-5255
Note: Programs & services include: family support; suicide prevention; addiction services.

RAYMORE: Silver Heights Special Care Home
Affiliated with: Regina Qu'Appelle Health Region
PO Box 549, 402 McLean St., Raymore, SK S0A 3J0
Tel: 306-746-5744 *Fax:* 306-746-5747
Number of Beds: 29 beds
Population Served: 600

REGINA: Salvation Army William Booth Special Care Home
Affiliated with: Regina Qu'Appelle Health Region
50 Angus Rd., Regina, SK S4R 8P6
Tel: 306-543-0655 *Fax:* 306-543-1292
www.williamboothregina.ca
Number of Beds: 53 beds
Ivy Scobie, Executive Director

SASKATOON: Circle Drive Special Care Home Inc.
Affiliated with: Saskatoon Health Region
3055 Preston Ave. South, Saskatoon, SK S7T 1C3
Tel: 306-955-4800 *Fax:* 306-955-2376
circlecare@saskatoonhealthregion.ca
circledrivespecialcarehome.ca
Number of Beds: 53 beds
Diane Martin, Director of Care
Clint Kinchen, Administrator
Brad Traill, Board Chair

SASKATOON: Extendicare - Preston
Extendicare Canada
Affiliated with: Saskatoon Health Region
2225 Preston Ave., Saskatoon, SK S7J 2E7
Tel: 306-374-2242 *Fax:* 306-373-2203
cnh_preston@extendicare.com
www.extendicarecanada.com/saskatoon/index.aspx
Number of Beds: 82 beds

WARMAN: Warman Mennonite Special Care Home
Affiliated with: Saskatoon Health Region
PO Box 100, 201 Centennial Blvd., Warman, SK S0K 4S0
Tel: 306-933-2011 *Fax:* 306-933-2782
Number of Beds: 31 beds

WEYBURN: Weyburn Mental Health Clinic
Affiliated with: Sun Country Health Region
PO Box 2003, Weyburn, SK S4H 2Z9
Tel: 306-842-8660

Note: Programs & services include: children's mental health.

WEYBURN: Weyburn Special Care Home
Affiliated with: Sun Country Health Region
PO Box 2003, 704 - 5th St. NE, Weyburn, SK S4H 2Z9
Tel: 306-842-4455

Note: Programs & services include: dietician; home care; palliative care; respite care.
Debbie Obst, Contact

YORKTON: Sunrise Regional Health Authority Mental Health & Addiction Services
Affiliated with: Sunrise Regional Health Authority
270 Bradbrooke Dr., Yorkton, SK S3N 2K6
Tel: 306-786-0558 *Fax:* 306-786-0556
Number of Beds: 18 inpatient and assessment beds
Note: Programs & services include: adult community services; rehabilitation services; child & youth services.

Metabolic Disorders

Metabolic disorders are illnesses that occur when the body is unable to process fats (lipids), proteins, sugars (carbohydrates) or nucleic acids properly.

Cause
Most metabolic disorders are inherited and are caused by genetic mutations that result in missing or dysfunctional enzymes that are needed for the cell to perform metabolic processes. Hunter syndrome, also called Mucopolysaccharidosis type II, is an example of an inherited metabolic disorder. The condition is caused by a lack of the enzyme iduronate sulfatase. Without this enzyme, mucopolysaccharides build up in various body tissues, eventually causing permanent damage. This affects appearance, mental development, organ function and physical abilities. The affected gene for Hunter syndrome is on the X chromosome, which means boys are most often affected.

Metabolic disorders can also be caused when organs, such as the liver or pancreas, become diseased or do not function normally. Diabetes mellitus is an example of when the pancreas fails to work properly. Diabetes is a disorder of carbohydrate metabolism, characterized by inadequate production or utilization of insulin and results in excessive amounts of glucose in the blood and urine (see Diabetes Mellitus for details.)

Symptoms
Hunter syndrome symptoms usually occur between two and four years of age. Early onset of the disease, which is the severe form, begins shortly after two. Late-onset causes less severe symptoms to appear later in life. Symptoms can include a large head and brow, broad nose and thick lips, recurrent respiratory infections, chronic runny nose, respiratory problems, including noisy breathing and snoring, recurrent ear infections, hearing loss, heart murmur, enlarged belly due to an enlarged liver and spleen, hernias, recurrent watery diarrhea, joint stiffness leading to clumsiness, developmental delay, and speech delay. As the disease progresses, numerous complications can arise, including airway obstruction, carpal tunnel syndrome and progressive hearing loss. Mental functions can decline over time and a person can lose the ability to complete daily living tasks.

Symptoms of diabetes can include excessive thirst and urination, hunger, extreme fatigue, weakness, blurred vision, numbness or tingling in the hands or feet, slow-to-heal cuts and bruises, frequent infections and weight change (see Diabetes Mellitus for details.)

Prevalence
Hunter Syndrome affects at least 1 in 162,000 male live births. It is inherited as an X-linked recessive disease. It is a rare disease that affects an estimated 30 to 40 people in Canada.

In Canada, there are more than 2,000,000 people aged 12 and over who have been diagnosed with diabetes.

Treatment Options
Tests for the diagnosis of Hunter syndrome can include an enzyme study, genetic testing for a change (mutation) in the iduronate sulfatase gene and a urine test for heparan sulfate and dermatan sulfate. Prenatal testing is available by measuring I2S enzymatic activity in amniotic fluid (a sample of the fluid that surrounds the baby in utero) or in chorionic villus (placental) tissue. Prenatal diagnosis is also available via mutation analysis. Genetic counselling is recommended for couples who want to have children and who have a family history of Hunter syndrome.

There is no cure for Hunter syndrome. Treatment of Hunter syndrome involves management of symptoms and complications. Enzyme therapy, a treatment that uses genetically engineered enzymes, can be given weekly through intravenous. The drug idursulfase (Elaprase) can also be used in treatment and, if given early enough, may delay or prevent some of the symptoms of Hunter syndrome. In milder forms of Hunter syndrome, bone marrow transplants can be used to ease the problems of breathing, mobility, and heart, liver and spleen function. It can also help prevent a child's mental regression, although results can vary.

People with the early-onset (severe) form of Hunter syndrome usually live to 10 - 20 years of age. People with the late-onset (mild) form typically live 20 - 60 years.

A diagnosis of diabetes is confirmed by a blood test that measures blood sugar. Type 1 is controlled by administering insulin; Type 2 diabetes can sometimes be controlled without medication (see Diabetes Mellitus for details.)

National Associations

Canadian Fabry Association / L'association canadienne de fabry
52 Glen Forest Dr., Hamilton ON L8K 5V8
www.fabrycanada.com
Overview: A medium-sized national organization
Mission: To educate the public & offer information on treatments; To encourage & support research; To increase facilities for those suffering from the disease
Chief Officer(s):
Gina Costantino, President

Canadian PKU and Allied Disorders Inc.
#180, 260 Adelaide St. East, Toronto ON M5A 1N1
Tel: 416-207-0064
Toll-Free: 877-226-7581
e-mail: info@canpku.org
www.canpku.org
twitter.com/canpku
Overview: A small national charitable organization founded in 2008
Mission: To provide news, information & support to families and professionals dealing with phenylketonuria and similar, rare, inherited

metabolic disorders
Member of: Canadian Coalition for Genetic Fairness
Chief Officer(s):
John Adams, President & CEO
 john.adams@canpku.org
Publications:
• CanPKU News
Type: Newsletter

Canadian Society for Mucopolysaccharide & Related Diseases Inc.

PO Box 30034, RPO Parkgate, North Vancouver BC V7H 2Y8
Tel: 604-924-5130; *Fax:* 604-924-5131
Toll-Free: 800-667-1846
e-mail: info@mpssociety.ca
www.mpssociety.ca
www.facebook.com/208787789156391
twitter.com/canmpssociety

Also Known As: The Canadian MPS Society
Overview: A small national charitable organization founded in 1984
Mission: To support families affected with MPS & related diseases
Member of: Canadian Organization for Rare Disorders
Chief Officer(s):
Bernie Geiss, Chair
Jamie Myrah, Executive Director
Publications:
• The Canadian MPS Society Annual Report
Type: Yearbook; *Frequency:* Annually; *Price:* Free with Canadian MPS Society membership
• The Canadian MPS Society Family Referral Directory
Type: Directory; *Frequency:* Annually; *Price:* Free with Canadian MPS Society membership
• The Connection
Type: Newsletter; *Frequency:* Quarterly; *Price:* Free with Canadian MPS Society membership
Profile: A resource for families affected with MPS & related diseases, featuring MPS news, care options, new treatment updates, clinical trials, medical updates, current research, events, fundraising, & familynews

Migraine

Classified as a vascular headache, migraine headaches are usually understood to be caused by intracranial vasospasm, that is, alternating swelling and constricting of blood vessels on the surface of the brain. The swelling phase brings on intense pain and nausea, while the constricting phase may cause neurological symptoms such as focal loss of vision or numbness involving one side of the body. Another theory is that migraines are due to a different dysfunction of the neurovascular system that results in the release of a substance that leads to migraine.

Cause

Although the exact cause of migraine is unknown, there may be genetic factors involved. More than 50 percent of patients have a family history of migraine. Migraines also appear to have a hormonal component, being more common in women and often affected by menstrual cycles or pregnancy. There are also a number of other common triggers that bring on migraine attacks in many people including stress, sleep disturbances, weather changes, physical exertion, hunger, perfume, bright light, loud noise, heat, alcohol, smoke and certain foods (such as aspartame, chocolate, aged cheeses and monosodium glutamate).

Symptoms

Migraines are usually characterized by moderate to severe throbbing pain that often occurs on one side of the head. Nausea, vomiting and sensitivity to light and sound may accompany these headaches. The duration of a migraine ranges from several hours to several days, and the frequency varies from two to three per year to two or more per week.

Four stages of migraines have been identified, although a person may not experience all of them. During the first stage (prodrome) which occurs one to two days before a migraine, a person may experience food cravings, diarrhea, constipation, depression, irritability, neck stiffness or hyperactivity. A second stage (aura) may occur 20 minutes to one hour before the headache with symptoms such as vision loss, numbness and tingling, sensory disturbances and visual phenomena like bright spots or flashing lights. In most cases, aura symptoms last for 10 to 30 minutes and are then followed by a headache, the third stage of migraine. After the migraine attack, a person may feel drained out or euphoric. This is the final phase of migraine called postdrome.

Prevalence

It is estimated that more than two million Canadians aged 12 or over have received a diagnosis of migraine. Migraines affect people between the ages of 25 and 54 most frequently, and women are three times more likely than men to suffer from migraines. Each year in Canada, around seven million working days are lost due to migraines.

Treatment Options

Migraines are often diagnosed on the basis of a medical history and physical exam. In some cases, however, various tests may be used to rule out other possible health problems that might be causing pain. These tests may include a computerized tomography (CT) scan or magnetic resonance imaging (MRI) of the brain and a spinal tap (a procedure where a thin needle is used to extract a sample of cerebrospinal fluid for analysis).

Management of migraine begins with careful observation for triggering agents like foods, alcohol or irregular sleep patterns. Acute treatment to stop a migraine involves drugs which are designed to stop symptoms and abort migraines. Pain-relieving therapy for mild migraines includes over-the-counter medications such as ibuprofen and acetaminophen, and migraine-specific drugs that combine aspirin, caffeine and acetaminophen. For more severe migraine pain, triptans such as sumatriptan are usually the drug of choice. Ergot drugs work by helping the swollen blood vessels constrict down to normal size. Although less expensive than triptans, they are often considered less effective. If headaches become very frequent, doctors may recommend preventive therapy, which requires daily drug administration. Drugs used in this way include beta-blockers and calcium-channel blockers, which were originally developed for hypertension and heart disease, and certain medicines ordinarily used for depression or seizures. Pain medication should be used sparingly. Narcotic medications should be avoided except under special circumstances and with strict guidelines.

Most migraine sufferers can be satisfactorily managed by their primary care physician or a neurologist, but for people whose migraines do not respond to standard treatment, a multi-disciplinary headache centre may be of help.

National Associations

Canadian Association for Neuroscience (CAN)

c/o DeArmond Management, 2661 Queenswood Dr., Victoria BC V8N 1X6
Tel: 250-472-7644
e-mail: info@can-acn.org
can-acn.org
www.facebook.com/can.acn
twitter.com/CAN_ACN

Overview: A large national organization
Mission: To promote communication among Canadian neuroscientists & encourage research related to the nervous system; To educate about current neuroscience research
Chief Officer(s):

Julie Poupart, Director, Communications

Headache Network Canada (HNC)
210 Georgian Dr., Oakville ON L6H 6T8
Tel: 905-330-9657
headachenetwork.ca
twitter.com/HeadacheNetwork
Overview: A large national charitable organization
Mission: To raise awareness about headache disorders in Canada; To encourage government assistance to the field; To educate the public about headache disorders
Affiliation(s): Neurological Health Charities Canada
Chief Officer(s):
Valerie South, Executive Director
Publications:
• Canadian Headache Society Guideline for Migraine Prophylaxis
Profile: To assist the doctor in recommending the appropriate medication for a migraine sufferer

Neurological Health Charities Canada (NHCC)
c/o Parkinson Canada, #316, 4211 Yonge St., Toronto ON M2P 2A9
Tel: 416-227-9700; *Fax:* 416-227-9600
Toll-Free: 800-565-3000
e-mail: info@mybrainmatters.ca
www.mybrainmatters.ca
www.facebook.com/MyBrainMatters
twitter.com/MyBrainMatters
www.youtube.com/MyBrainMatters
Overview: A large national charitable organization
Mission: To improve quality of life for persons with chronic brain conditions & their caregivers; To increase awareness in the government about neurological issues; To support research
Chief Officer(s):
Joyce Gordon, Chair
Publications:
• Brain Matters [a publication of Neurological Health Charities Canada]
Type: Newsletter; *Frequency:* s-a.

Provincial Associations

ONTARIO

Help for Headaches (HFH)
PO Box 1568, Stn. B, 515 Richmond St., London ON N6A 5M3
Tel: 519-434-0008
www.helpforheadaches.org
Also Known As: Headache Support Group
Overview: A small provincial charitable organization founded in 1995
Mission: To provide research, education, advocacy & support for headache sufferers & the public at large
Member of: World Headache Alliance; Canadian Pain Society
Chief Officer(s):
G. Brent Lucas, Director
 brent@helpforheadaches.org
Publications:
• Chronic Daily Headache
Type: Book; *Price:* $25.95
• Non-Drug Treatments for Headache
Type: Book; *Price:* $25.25
Profile: Educational book discussing various treatment options for headaches & migraines

Mood Disorders

Life is full of highs and lows, but for people with mood disorders, these periods last longer and are felt more intensely. Mood disorders can also have a significant impact on family life, job performance and everyday functioning. Approximately 7.8 percent of Canadians have been diagnosed with a mood disorder. Some of the more common mood disorders—depression, postpartum depression and bipolar disorder—are discussed in detail below.

Depression

Feelings of sadness are common to everyone, and quite natural in reaction to unfortunate circumstances. The death of a loved one, the end of a relationship and other traumatic life experiences are bound to bring on the blues. But when feelings of sadness and despair persist beyond a reasonable period, arise for no particular reason or begin to affect a person's ability to function, help is needed. Depression is a diagnosis made by a psychiatrist or other mental health professional to describe serious and prolonged symptoms of sadness or despair. While it is quite common, it is also a disease that no one should take lightly; depression can be deadly. Many people who are deeply depressed think about or actually try to commit suicide; some commit suicide. Even a relatively mild depression, if untreated, can disrupt marriages and relationships or impede careers.

Cause
Depression is more common in people with a family history of depression. Research is currently being gathered on the relationship between depression and chemical imbalances in the brain. Clinical depression can also be associated with childhood abuse and trauma, the loss of a loved one, job loss, certain medications and other physical illnesses and chronic disabilities.

Symptoms
Because depression can range from mild to severe, people who are depressed may exhibit a variety of behaviours. Often, people who are depressed are tearful, irritable or brooding; experience changes in appetite or gastrointestinal problems; and lose interest in previously enjoyed activities. Problems sleeping (either insomnia or sleeping too much) are common, as are feelings of inadequacy; difficulty thinking, concentrating and making decisions; and a sense of impending doom. People with depression may also worry unnecessarily about being sick or having a disease, or they may report physical symptoms such as headaches or other pains. Depression can seriously affect people's friendships and intimate relationships.

Depression can make people worry about having a disease, but this is not a central symptom. Depression very frequently coexists with anxiety disorder.

Abuse of alcohol, prescription drugs or illegal drugs is also common among people who are depressed. The most serious risk associated with depression is the risk of suicide. Suicide is the cause of death in approximately 15 percent of untreated patients. People who have tried to commit suicide in the past, or who have family members who have committed suicide are especially at risk. Individuals who have another mental disorder, such as schizophrenia, in addition to depression are also more likely to commit suicide.

Prevalence
Every year close to three million Canadians suffer some type of depressive illness, but less than one-third seek treatment. Depression does not discriminate; anyone can have it. Children, adults and the elderly are susceptible. Nevertheless, studies do indicate that women are twice as likely to have depression as men. Depression has significant adverse effects on children's functioning and development; among adolescents, suicide is believed to be the second leading cause of death. Depression is also common among the elderly, affecting about 5 to 10 percent of those living in the community, and 30 to 40 percent of those living in institutions, and can be treated as an illness distinct from the loneliness or sadness that may accompany old age.

Treatment Options
Depression is a medical disease and does not respond to the usual ways we have of cheering up ourselves or others. In fact, attempts to cheer depressed individuals may have the opposite and unfortunate consequence of making them feel worse, often

because they are frustrated and feel guilty that others' well-meaning efforts do not help. If a person experiences the symptoms of depression, he or she should seek treatment from a qualified professional.

A psychiatrist or other mental health professional should conduct a thorough evaluation, including an interview; a physical examination should be done by a primary care provider. Depression is diagnosed when an individual experiences persistent feelings of sadness or loss of interest or pleasure in usual activities, in addition to five of the following symptoms for at least two weeks: significant weight gain or loss unrelated to dieting; inability to sleep or, conversely, sleeping too much; restlessness and agitation; fatigue or loss of energy; feelings of worthlessness or guilt; diminished ability to think or concentrate; recurrent thoughts of death or suicide; distress is not caused by a medication or the symptoms of a medical illness.

On the basis of a complete evaluation, the appropriate treatment will be prescribed. Treatment must be tailored to the individual and most likely, will include medication or psychotherapy, or both. Drug therapy for depression may include tricyclic antidepressants and monoamine oxidase inhibitors (MAOIs). Newer medications such as selective serotonin reuptake inhibitors (SSRIs), serotonin norepinephrine reuptake inhibitors (SNRIs) and norepinephrine dopamine reuptake inhibitors (NNRIs) are often preferred because they have fewer side effects. Some people may also be prescribed antipsychotics in addition to antidepressants. Antidepressants usually take effect within two to six weeks after treatment has begun. It is important to give medications long enough to work, and to increase dosages or change or add medications if depression does not resolve completely.

The natural (untreated) course of a depressive episode is about nine months. Therefore treatment should be continued for at least that length of time even though the individual feels better. If treatment is discontinued prematurely, the depression is very likely to return. Depression is also a recurring disease; the risk of an episode after a first episode is 50 percent; after two episodes, 67 percent; and after three, over 90 percent. Therefore, some patients prefer to continue taking antidepressant medication indefinitely.

Psychotherapy, or talk therapy, may be used to help the patient improve the way he or she thinks about things and deals with specific life problems. Individual, family or couples therapy may be recommended, depending on the patient's life experiences. If the depression is not severe, treatment can take a few weeks; if the depression has been a longstanding problem, it may take much longer, but in many cases, a patient will experience improvement in 10 to 15 sessions. Self-help groups may also be of benefit to people with depression. Patient and family education can play a crucial role, as well.

The vast majority of people with depression get better when they are treated properly, and virtually everyone gets some relief from their symptoms.

Postpartum Depression

Within days to a year after giving birth, women may experience a spectrum of psychological symptoms related to both the abrupt hormonal changes and the psychological and social demands of motherhood. The mildest of these symptoms, baby blues, is not a psychiatric condition. It consists of a few days of heightened emotionality starting within days after birth that usually resolves spontaneously with reassurance, extra support and adequate sleep.

Cause
A previous history of depression is a risk factor for developing postpartum depression. Studies suggest that the rapid changes in hormone levels that women experience after giving birth may also be involved. The symptoms, which are listed below, are much the same as those of depression that occur at any other time of life.

Symptoms
Symptoms of postpartum depression often develop around four weeks after giving birth. Women with postpartum depression become preoccupied with concerns about their ability to be good mothers. Unlike an average, tired new mother, the depressed woman cannot enjoy her baby. She is often guilty and reluctant to tell her family about it because she knows she is supposed to appreciate her good fortune and be happy. Severe postpartum depression, or postpartum psychosis, which causes confusion, disorientation, delusions and hallucinations, and can cause suicide or infanticide, is a serious medical condition demanding immediate professional attention. Fortunately, there is increasing awareness and understanding of postpartum depression among the general population.

Prevalence
Very mild depression after delivery affects between 50 and 80 percent of postpartum women. Postpartum depression affects between 3 and 20 percent of new mothers in Canada. Postpartum psychosis is estimated to affect 1 in 1,000 women after they give birth.

Treatment Options
The fact that the postpartum period is almost always associated with problems with sleep, appetite, libido, energy and concentration makes those symptoms less useful for diagnosis at this time. Two cardinal questions are: "Are you feeling sad most of the time?" and "Are you unable to enjoy things that you usually enjoy?"

The Diagnostic and Statistical Manual identifies a woman suffering from postpartum depression as demonstrating (in addition to the symptoms above) preoccupation with concerns of being a good mother, inability to rest while the baby is sleeping and inability to enjoy her baby, accompanied with feelings of guilt.

Treatment for postpartum depression is similar to treatment for depression in general. Possible risks of medications taken during pregnancy and breastfeeding have to be weighed against the risks of leaving the depression untreated. Women who discontinue antidepressant medication because they wish to become or they have become pregnant are at a very high risk of relapse.

Bipolar Disorder

Bipolar disorder (formerly referred to as manic depression) is the name for a group of serious mental illnesses characterized by alterations between depression and manic euphoria or irritability. The two states are not independent of each other, but part of the same illness. There are three main forms of bipolar disorder: bipolar I disorder, bipolar II disorder and cyclothymic disorder. A person with bipolar I disorder has manic episodes and usually experiences depression at some point. Bipolar II disorder consists of repeated depressive episodes interspersed with hypomanic (not full blown mania) episodes. The individual with cyclothymic disorder has a history of at least two years of repeated episodes of elevated and depressed mood which don't meet all the criteria for mania or depression but which cause distress or decreased ability to function.

Cause

A number of researchers are closing in on genetic links to the illness. As with all mental disorders, however, the relationship between genetic, physiologic, psychological and environmental causes is complex.

Symptoms

Individuals in the manic phase of bipolar disorder may feel exuberant, invincible or even immortal. They may be awake for days at a time, and be able to work tirelessly; they may rush from one idea to the next carried by a nearly uncontrollable burst of energy that leaves others bewildered and unable to keep up. (Some extraordinarily creative people have had bipolar disorder. Whether or not the disorder makes a positive contribution to creativity is a controversial question.) In the depressed phase which follows a manic high, the patient may be suicidal. The depressed phase of the illness mirrors a major depressive episode.

Bipolar disorder can cause extreme disruption to individual lives and careers, and to whole families. While manic, patients may spend all of a family's money, borrow great sums, engage in indiscriminate sexual activity and behave in other ways that leave lasting negative effects. Suicide is a risk factor in the illness, and an estimated 10 to 15 percent of individuals with bipolar I disorder commit suicide. Abuse of children, spouses or other family members, or other types of violence, may occur during the manic phase of the illness. Untreated mania, during which the individual gets no sleep, little or no nutrition and expends great quantities of energy, can result in death as well.

The cycles of mood changes tend to become more frequent, shorter and more intense as the patient gets older. Disturbances in work, school or social functioning are common, resulting in frequent school truancy or failure, occupational failure, divorce or episodic antisocial behaviour. A variety of other mental disorders may accompany bipolar disorder; these include anorexia nervosa, bulimia nervosa, attention deficit/hyperactivity disorder, panic disorder, social phobia and substance-abuse related disorder.

Prevalence

The average age of onset for bipolar disorder is usually between 18 and 24 years, but it can develop in childhood, or as late as the forties or fifties. It is estimated that bipolar disorder will affect 1 percent of Canadians in their lifetime.

Treatment Options

To diagnose bipolar disorder a physician takes a detailed medical history and does a physical exam to rule out other medical conditions that might be causing the symptoms. To confirm diagnosis reference is made to the following criteria for bipolar disorder outlined in the Diagnostic and Statistical Manual. A manic episode consists of the following: a distinct period of abnormally and persistently elevated, expansive, or irritable mood, lasting at least one week; inflated self-esteem or grandiosity; decreased need for sleep; more talkative than usual; flight of ideas (a succession of topics with little relationship to one another) or a subjective experience that thoughts are racing; distractibility; increase in goal-directed activity; excessive involvement in activities that have a high potential for painful consequences; the mood disturbances are severe enough to cause impairment in social or occupational functioning; the symptoms are not due to the direct physiological effects of a substance. The depressive phase of bipolar disorder consists of the following: depressed mood most of the day, nearly every day, as indicated by either subjective report or observation; markedly diminished interest or pleasure in almost all activities most of the day; significant weight loss when not dieting, weight gain, or decrease or increase in appetite nearly every day; insom-

nia or hypersomnia nearly every night; psychomotor agitation or retardation nearly every day; fatigue or loss of energy nearly every day; feelings of worthlessness or excessive or inappropriate guilt nearly every day.

It is important for patients with depression to be carefully screened for any manic or hypomanic symptoms so that bipolar disorder can be diagnosed and the appropriate treatment prescribed. Most people with bipolar disorder present, or are referred, for care while in the depressive state.

Lithium is the most commonly prescribed drug for bipolar disorder and is effective for stabilizing patients in the manic phase of the illness and preventing mood swings. However, compliance is a problem among patients both because of the nature of the condition (some patients may actually miss the high of their mood swings and other people often envy their enthusiasm, energy and confidence) and because of the side effects associated with the drug. These include weight gain, excessive thirst, tremors and muscle weakness. Lithium is also very toxic in overdose. Blood levels of lithium must be measured daily or weekly to begin with, and in at least six-month intervals thereafter. Several other medications are now available and effective. Anticonvulsants/mood stabilizers, such as valproate, carbamazepine, lamotrigine, gabapentin, and topiramate have also become first-line treatments, as have several antipsychotic medications. Many patients with bipolar disorder need a combination of medications to address both the manic and depressive aspects. It is essential that any individual diagnosed with depression be carefully evaluated to rule out bipolar disorder before antidepressant medication is prescribed. Antidepressant medication alone can precipitate a manic episode in an individual with bipolar disorder.

While medication is quite effective, the disruptive nature of the condition also necessitates the use of psychotherapy and family therapy to help patients rebuild relationships, to maintain compliance with treatment and a positive attitude toward living with chronic illness, and to restore confidence and self-esteem.

Early diagnosis, education about the disorder and appropriate treatment are crucial in preventing future relapses and providing a successful outcome for people with bipolar disorder.

See also Mental Illness and Schizophrenia

National Associations

Canadian Association for Suicide Prevention (CASP) / L'Association canadienne pour la prévention du suicide (ACPS)
285 Benjamin Rd., Waterloo ON N2J 3Z4

Tel: 519-884-1470
e-mail: casp@suicideprevention.ca
www.suicideprevention.ca
www.facebook.com/CanadianAssociationforSuicidePrevention
twitter.com/casp_ca

Overview: A small national charitable organization founded in 1985
Mission: To reduce the suicide rate; To minimize the harmful consequences of suicide
Chief Officer(s):
Karen Letofsky, President
Tana Nash, Executive Director

Mood Disorders Society of Canada (MDSC) / La Société pour les troubles de l'humeur du Canada

#736, 3-304 Stone Rd. West, Guelph ON N1G 4W4
Tel: 519-824-5565; *Fax:* 519-824-9569
e-mail: info@mooddisorderscanada.ca
www.linkedin.com/company/3204824
www.facebook.com/MoodDisordersSocietyCanada
twitter.com/MoodDisordersCa
www.youtube.com/user/MDSofC?

Overview: A large national organization founded in 2001
Mission: The MDSC works nationally to ensure that issues related to mood disorders are understood and considered in the setting of research priorities, the development of treatment strategies, and the creation of government programs and policies. The Mood Disorders Society of Canada is one of the leading national, voluntary health organizations in the fields of depression, bipolar illness, and associated mood disorders
Chief Officer(s):
Phil Upshall, National Executive Director
John Starzynski, President

Your Life Counts (YLC)

Seaway Mall, #GG5B, 800 Niagara St. North, Welland ON L3C 5Z4
Tel: 289-820-5777
e-mail: info@yourlifecounts.org
www.yourlifecounts.org
www.facebook.com/YourLifeCounts
twitter.com/yourlifecounts
www.youtube.com/user/YOURLIFECOUNTSTV

Overview: A small national charitable organization founded in 2000
Mission: Works with youth, families, veterans and emergency services in the battle against trauma, addictions and overwhelming life situations that may lead to thoughts of suicide.
Chief Officer(s):
Kevin Bolibruck, Chair

Provincial Associations

ALBERTA

Centre for Suicide Prevention (CSP)

#320, 105 - 12 Ave. SE, Calgary AB T2G 1A1
Tel: 403-245-3900; *Fax:* 403-245-0299; *Crisis Hot-Line:* 403-266-4357
www.suicideinfo.ca
www.linkedin.com/company/centre-for-suicide-prevention
www.facebook.com/centreforsuicideprevention
twitter.com/cspyyc
suicideinfo.tumblr.com

Previous Name: Suicide Information & Education Centre
Overview: A medium-sized provincial charitable organization founded in 1982
Mission: To educate people about the risk of suicide & suicide prevention
Member of: Canadian Association for Suicide Prevention
Affiliation(s): Canadian Mental Health Association - Alberta Division
Chief Officer(s):
Mara Grunau, Executive Director
  mara@suicideinfo.ca
Hilary Sirman, Director, Impact & Engagement
  hilary@suicideinfo.ca
Crystal Walker, Coordinator, Communications
  crystal@suicideinfo.ca

BRITISH COLUMBIA

Mood Disorders Association of British Columbia (MDA)

#1450, 605 Robson St., Vancouver BC V6B 5J3
Tel: 604-873-0103; *Fax:* 604-873-3095
e-mail: info@mdabc.net
www.mdabc.net
www.facebook.com/mdasupport
twitter.com/MDA_BC

Overview: A small provincial charitable organization founded in 1982
Mission: To provide support & education for people with a mood disorder, & those around them, in order to help them live a healthy & active life

Chief Officer(s):
Martin Addison, Executive Director

MANITOBA

Artists in Healthcare Manitoba (AHM)

#2, 1325 Markham Rd., Winnipeg MB R3T 4J6
Tel: 204-999-0057
e-mail: info@artistsinhealthcare.com
www.artistsinhealthcare.com

Overview: A small provincial charitable organization
Mission: To integrate the creative arts into health care as a way of introducing the healing effects of creative expression to help relieve depression

Mood Disorders Association of Manitoba (MDAM)

#100, 4 Fort St., Winnipeg MB R3C 1C4
Tel: 204-786-0987; *Fax:* 201-786-1906
Toll-Free: 800-263-1460
e-mail: info@mooddisordersmanitoba.ca
www.mooddisordersmanitoba.ca
www.facebook.com/MoodDisordersMB
twitter.com/MoodDisordersMB

Overview: A small provincial charitable organization
Mission: To help others through peer support, education & advocacy; to increase public awareness about mood disorders & empower people to develop & manage mental wellness
Chief Officer(s):
Tara Brousseau, Executive Director
  TaraS@mooddisordersmanitoba.ca

Postpartum Depression Association of Manitoba (PPDAM)

MB
e-mail: info@ppdmanitoba.ca
www.ppdmanitoba.ca

Overview: A small provincial organization
Mission: PPDAM is committed to helping Manitoba families get connected with the help dealing with postpartum depression or related illnesses through education, awareness and resources.

ONTARIO

Mood Disorders Association of Ontario (MDAO)

#602, 36 Eglinton Ave. West, Toronto ON M4R 1A1
Tel: 416-486-8046; *Fax:* 416-486-8127
Toll-Free: 888-486-8236
www.mooddisorders.ca
www.facebook.com/MoodDisordersAssociationON
twitter.com/mooddisorderson
instagram.com/mooddisordersassociation

Overview: A small provincial charitable organization founded in 1985
Mission: To provide information, education & support to those affected by depression & manic depression, their families & friends; to develop & maintain a network of supportive self-help groups; to improve the quality of life of people who experience mood disorders, their families & friends; to advocate for a flexible & responsive system of care
Member of: Federation of Community Mental Health & Addictions; Consumer Survivor Development Initiative
Chief Officer(s):
Ann Marie MacDonald, Executive Director, 416-486-8046 Ext. 226
  annmariem@mooddisorders.ca
Publications:
• Mood Disorders Association of Ontario Fact Sheets
Type: Reports
Profile: A series of fact sheets about various mood disorders

QUÉBEC

Revivre - Association Québécoise de soutien aux personnes souffrant de troubles anxieux, dépressifs ou bipolaires /

Québec Anxiety, Depressive & Bipolar Disorder Support Association

5140, rue Saint-Hubert, Montréal QC H2J 2Y3
Tél: 514-529-3081; *Téléc:* 514-529-3083
Ligne sans frais: 866-738-4873
Courriel: revivre@revivre.org
www.revivre.org
www.linkedin.com/company/revivre
www.facebook.com/revivre.org
twitter.com/revivre_org

Également appelé: Association des dépressifs et maniaco-dépressifs
Nom précédent: Association québécoise des cyclothymiques
Aperçu: *Dimension:* petite; *Envergure:* provinciale; Organisme sans but lucratif; fondée en 1983
Mission: Diffuser de l'information sur les troubles anxieux, dépressifs et bipolaires; favoriser le diagnostic et la prise en charge des personnes atteintes de ces maladies; supporter les personnes atteintes et leurs proches; briser l'isolement de ces personnes; partager notre expertise avec les professionnels et autres intervenants du milieu de la santé
Membre de: Association des professionnels en gestion philantropique
Affliation(s): Réseau alternatif et communautaire des organismes en santé mentale
Membre(s) du bureau directeur:
Martin Enault, Président
Jean-Rémy Provost, Directeur général

Local Associations

BRITISH COLUMBIA

Pacific Post Partum Support Society (PPPSS)

#200, 7342 Winston St., Burnaby BC V5A 2H1
Tel: 604-255-7955; *Fax:* 604-255-7588
Other Communication: Volunteer e-mail: volunteer@postpartum.org
e-mail: admin@postpartum.org
www.postpartum.org
www.facebook.com/120735171295360
twitter.com/postpartumbc

Overview: A small local charitable organization founded in 1984
Mission: To provide support for women affected by postpartum/perinatal distress, depression, & anxiety
Affliation(s): United Way of the Lower Mainland
Chief Officer(s):
Sheila Duffy, Director
Stace Dayment, Manager, Administration

QUÉBEC

Suicide Action Montréal (SAM)

2345, rue Bélanger, Montréal QC H2G 1C9
Tel: 514-723-3594; *Fax:* 514-723-3605
Toll-Free: 866-277-3553; *Crisis Hot-Line:* 514-723-4000
e-mail: info@suicideactionmontreal.qc.ca
www.suicideactionmontreal.org

Overview: A small local charitable organization founded in 1984
Affliation(s): Canadian Association for Suicide Prevention
Chief Officer(s):
Suzanne Carrière, President

Multiple Sclerosis

Multiple sclerosis (MS) is a chronic disease that affects the central nervous system and impairs many of its functions. MS destroys the protective myelin sheath that surrounds nerve fibers. When this special sheath is damaged, it causes interference in the passage of electrical signals between the brain, spinal cord and other parts of the body.

Cause

Although the cause of MS is unknown, an immunologic abnormality is suspected. There also appear to be both genetic and environmental factors involved.

Symptoms

Four different types of MS have been identified: relapsing remitting, primary progressive, secondary progressive and progressive relapsing. The most common type, presented by about 85 percent of people at the time of diagnosis, is relapsing remitting MS. In this form of MS, flare-ups of symptoms lasting from 48 hours to a few months are followed by symptom-free periods (remissions) that can last for months or even years. About 50 percent of people with this form of MS will develop secondary progressive MS (where remissions occur less frequently and disability accumulates) within 10 years of diagnosis. In about 10 percent of cases, the course of MS is primary progressive, meaning that disability progresses slowly without periods of remission. About 5 percent of people diagnosed have progressive relapsing MS. In these individuals, the disease worsens steadily right from the beginning, and they also experience attacks of symptoms from which they may or may not recover.

The symptoms of MS vary from person to person and depend on what area or areas of the myelin are damaged. Symptoms can include: generalized or focal weakness; difficulty walking; clumsiness; slurred speech; easy fatigability; numbness and tingling; pain; dizziness; visual loss; incontinence (loss of bladder and bowel control); loss of sexual function; depression; and problems with short-term memory, judgment, or reason.

Prevalence

It is estimated that 100,000 Canadians have MS. The disease appears to be more common in certain geographic areas; Canada has one of the highest prevalence rates of MS in the world. With age of onset typically between 15 and 40 years, multiple sclerosis is the most common neurological disease affecting young Canadian adults. Women are three times more likely to be affected than men.

Treatment Options

There is no single test used to diagnose MS. Usually, a medical history is taken, and physical and neurological exams are performed. To detect lesions in the central nervous system that might not be causing symptoms, tests such as magnetic resonance imaging (MRI) and evoked potentials are often used. In an evoked potentials test, very small electric shocks are applied to electrodes that have been placed on the head and body. Then, the speed at which these stimuli are registered in the pathways of the central nervous system is measured.

Currently there is no curative treatment for MS, but medications such as corticosteroids, beta interferons, glatiramer acetate and natalizumab can be used to help shorten or prevent relapses. Supportive treatment includes medications to control muscle spasticity (baclofen, tizanidine), fatigue (amantadine) and pain. Maintaining a healthy lifestyle is recommended, as are avoiding fatigue and exposure to excessive heat. Physical therapy may also be helpful. Because of the debilitating nature of MS, counselling, psychiatric support and antidepressant medication may be warranted. Other procedures for treating MS, such as stem cell therapy, and angioplasty to open blocked veins in the head and neck ("liberation procedure" for chronic cerebrospinal venous insufficiency [CCSVI]) are currently under investigation.

Significant strides are being made in both treating and understanding MS. Although the disease can be disabling, MS patients now have a number of options available to manage their symptoms and slow the progress of their disease.

National Associations

Multiple Sclerosis Society of Canada (MS) / Société canadienne de la sclérose en plaques
North Tower, #500, 250 Dundas St. West, Toronto ON M5T 2Z5
Tel: 416-922-6065; *Fax:* 416-922-7538
Toll-Free: 800-268-7582
e-mail: info@mssociety.ca
www.mssociety.ca
www.linkedin.com/company/ms-society-of-canada
www.facebook.com/MSSocietyCanada
twitter.com/mssocietycanada
www.youtube.com/MSSocietyCanada

Also Known As: MS Society
Overview: A medium-sized national charitable organization founded in 1948
Mission: To be a leader in finding a cure for multiple sclerosis & enabling people affected by MS to enhance their quality of life
Member of: Multiple Sclerosis International Federation
Affiliation(s): Canadian Medical Association
Chief Officer(s):
Yves Savoie, President & CEO
Karen Lee, Vice-President, Research
Lori Radke, Vice-President, Marketing & Development
Publications:
• MS Canada [a publication of the Multiple Sclerosis Society of Canada]
Type: Magazine; *Frequency:* Semiannually; *Editor:* Tiffany Regaudie; Meaghan Kelly; *ISSN:* 0315-1131; *Price:* Free with membership inthe Multiple Sclerosis Society of Canada
Profile: MS Society programs & services, plus the latest advance in MS research & treatments

Alberta & Northwest Territories Division
#150, 9405 - 50 St., Edmonton AB T6B 2T4
Tel: 403-463-1190; *Fax:* 403-479-1001
Toll-Free: 800-268-7582
e-mail: info.alberta@mssociety.ca
mssociety.ca/division/alberta-and-northwest-territories-division
Chief Officer(s):
Garry Wheeler, President
garry.wheeler@mssociety.ca

Atlantic Division
#1, 109 Ilsley Ave., Dartmouth NS B3B 1S8
Tel: 902-468-8230; *Fax:* 902-468-5328
Toll-Free: 800-268-7582
e-mail: info.atlantic@mssociety.ca
mssociety.ca/division/atlantic-division
www.facebook.com/170182879748684
twitter.com/MSAtlantic
Chief Officer(s):
Benjamin Davis, President, 800-268-7582 Ext. 1003

British Columbia & Yukon Division
Metrotower II, #1103, 4720 Kingsway, Burnaby BC V5H 4N2
Tel: 604-689-3144; *Fax:* 604-689-0377
e-mail: info.bc@mssociety.ca
www.mssociety.ca/division/bc-and-yukon-division
www.facebook.com/mssocietybcy
twitter.com/mssocietybc
www.flickr.com/photos/mssociety_bcyukon
Chief Officer(s):
Chelsea Seaby, Chair
Tania Vrionis, President, 604-602-3217 Ext. 7241
tania.vrionis@mssociety.ca

Calgary & Area Chapter
Emerson Bldg., #150, 110 Quarry Park Blvd. SE, Calgary AB T2C 3G3
Tel: 403-250-7090; *Fax:* 403-250-8937
e-mail: info.calgary@mssociety.ca
www.mssociety.ca/calgary
www.facebook.com/MSSocietyCalgary
twitter.com/MS_Calgary
www.youtube.com/user/calgaryms
Chief Officer(s):
Darrel Gregory, Southern Regional Director
darrel.gregory@mssociety.ca

Division du Québec
Tour Est, #1010, 550, rue Sherbrooke ouest, Montréal QC H3A 1B9
Tél: 514-849-7591; *Téléc:* 514-849-8914
Ligne sans frais: 800-268-7582
Courriel: info.qc@mssociety.ca
www.mssociety.ca/division/quebec-division
www.linkedin.com/company/soci-t-canadienne-de-la-scl-rose-en-plaqu
es-d
www.facebook.com/SocieteSPCanada
twitter.com/SocCanDeLaSP
www.flickr.com/photos/societesp-quebec
Louis Adam, Executive Director
louis.adam@mssociety.ca

Manitoba Division
#100, 1465 Buffalo Pl., Winnipeg MB R3T 1L8
Tel: 204-943-9595; *Fax:* 204-988-0915
Toll-Free: 800-268-7582
e-mail: info.manitoba@mssociety.ca
mssociety.ca/division/manitoba-division
www.facebook.com/mssocietymanitoba
twitter.com/mssocietyMB
www.instagram.com/mssocietymb
Chief Officer(s):
Erin Kuan, President
erin.kuan@mssociety.ca
Ilona Niemczyk, Director, Development
ilona.niemczyk@mssociety.ca
Darell Hominuk, Director, Programs & Services
darell.hominuk@mssociety.ca

Ontario & Nunavut Division
#500, 250 Dundas St. West, Toronto ON M5T 2Z5
Tel: 416-922-6065; *Fax:* 416-922-7538
Toll-Free: 800-268-7582
e-mail: info.ontario@mssociety.ca
www.mssociety.ca/ontario
twitter.com/MSSocietyON
Chief Officer(s):
Marie Vaillant, Chair

Saskatchewan Division
150 Albert St., Regina SK S4R 2N2
Tel: 306-522-5600; *Fax:* 306-565-0477
Toll-Free: 800-268-7582
e-mail: info.sask@mssociety.ca
mssociety.ca/division/saskatchewan-division
twitter.com/MSSocietySK
www.flickr.com/photos/mssocietysask/
Chief Officer(s):
Lisa Smith, Director, Development
lisa.smith@mssociety.ca
Laurie Murphy, Director, Client Services
laurie.murphy@mssociety.ca

Provincial Associations

QUÉBEC

Société canadienne de la sclérose en plaques (Division du Québec) (SCSP) / Multiple Sclerosis Society of Canada (Québec Division)
Tour Est, #1010, 550, rue Sherbrooke Ouest, Montréal QC H3A 1B9
Tél: 514-849-7591; *Téléc:* 514-849-8914
Ligne sans frais: 800-268-7582
Courriel: info.qc@mssociety.ca
www.mssociety.ca/qc
www.facebook.com/SocieteSPCanada
twitter.com/SocCanDeLaSP
www.youtube.com/SocieteSPCanada

Également appelé: SP - Québec
Aperçu: *Dimension:* moyenne; *Envergure:* provinciale; Organisme sans but lucratif; fondée en 1948
Mission: Soutenir la recherche sur la SP; offrir des services aux personnes atteintes de la maladie et à leurs familles; sensibiliser le public à la sclérose en plaques et maintenir les relations avec les gouvernements.

Membre de: Multiple Sclerosis Society of Canada
Affliation(s): Fédération internationale de la sclérose en plaques
Membre(s) du bureau directeur:
Louis Adam, Directeur général

Local Associations

QUÉBEC

Association Sclérose en Plaques Rive-Sud (ASPRS)
3825, rue Windsor, Saint-Hubert QC J4T 2Z6
Tél: 450-926-5210; *Téléc:* 450-926-5215
Courriel: info@asprs.qc.ca
www.asprs.qc.ca
www.linkedin.com/company/association-sclérose-en-plaques-rive-sud
twitter.com/asprs2
Aperçu: *Dimension:* petite; *Envergure:* locale; fondée en 1976
Mission: Aider des gens qui a sclérose en plaques de surmonter avec leur maladie en s'engageant dans des activités sociales
Membre(s) du bureau directeur:
Nancy Caron, Directrice générale
nancy.caron@asprs.qc.ca

International Associations

Consortium of Multiple Sclerosis Centers (CMSC)
359 Main St., #A, Hackensack NJ 07601 USA
Tel: 201-487-1050; *Fax:* 201-678-2290
www.mscare.org
www.linkedin.com/company/cmsc
www.facebook.com/CMSCmscare
twitter.com/mscare
Also Known As: Consortium of MS Centers
Overview: A medium-sized international organization founded in 1986
Mission: To maximize the ability of multiple sclerosis healthcare professionals to improve the quality of life for people affected by multiple sclerosis; To provide information about the most current research results, clinical trials, treatments, & patient education programs
Chief Officer(s):
Robert Lisak, President
June Halper, Chief Executive Officer
Publications:
• Consortium of Multiple Sclerosis Centers Membership Directory
Type: Directory; *Price:* Free with Consortium of Multiple Sclerosis Centers membership
• International Journal of Multiple Sclerosis Care
Type: Journal; *Frequency:* Quarterly; *Accepts Advertising*; *Editor:* Lael A. Stone, MD
Profile: Peer-reviewed clinical & original research articles on topics of interest to multiple sclerosis healthcare providers

Multiple Sclerosis International Federation (MSIF)
Skyline House, 200 Union St., London SE1 0LX UK
Tel: 44-20-7620-1911
www.msif.org
www.facebook.com/110033075774139
twitter.com/MSIntFederation
www.youtube.com/user/MSIFmedia
Previous Name: International Federation of Multiple Sclerosis Societies
Overview: A medium-sized international charitable organization founded in 1967
Mission: To link the work of national MS societies worldwide; to eliminate MS & its devastating effects; to promote global research, exchange of information, advocacy & development of new & existing MS societies
Affliation(s): Multiple Sclerosis Society of Canada
Chief Officer(s):
Weyman Johnson, President & Chair

National Libraries

Multiple Sclerosis Society of Canada
#500, 250 Dundas St. West, Toronto, ON M5T 2Z5
Tel: 416-922-6065; *Fax:* 416-922-7538
Toll-Free: 800-268-7582
info@mssociety.ca
www.mssociety.ca
Social Media: www.youtube.com/mssocietycanada;
twitter.com/mssocietycanada; www.facebook.com/mssocietycanada
Collection: Multiple Sclerosis genetics, symptoms, diagnosis, treatments, complimentary therapies, psychological issues & current research
Yves Savoie, President & Chief Executive Officer

Provincial Libraries

Atlantic Division Library
#1, 109 Ilsley Ave., Dartmouth, NS B3B 1S8
Tel: 902-468-8230; *Fax:* 902-468-5328
Toll-Free: 800-268-7582
info.atlantic@mssociety.ca
www.mssociety.ca/division/atlantic-division
Social Media: twitter.com/MSAtlantic; www.facebook.com/MSAtlantic
Monica Jordan, Director, Community Programs
monica.jordan@mssociety.ca

Muscular Dystrophy

Muscular dystrophy is a group of genetic disorders marked by progressive weakness and degeneration of the skeletal, or voluntary, muscles that control movement. The muscles of the heart and other involuntary muscles may also be affected, and there may be organ involvement as well. There are a number of different types of muscular dystrophy, the most common of which is Duchenne. Other forms of muscular dystrophy include myotonic, Becker's, limb-girdle, Emery-Dreifuss, distal, mitochondrial, oculopharyngeal and facioscapulohumeral. The different forms are distinguished from each other by factors such as age of onset, rate of disease progression, severity of symptoms, involvement of tissues other than muscle, and pattern of inheritance.

Cause
A particular gene defect is responsible for each form of muscular dystrophy. Most of the time, the genetic mutations are inherited, but sometimes they occur spontaneously.

Symptoms
The symptoms of muscular dystrophy vary according to the form of the disorder. In some types of muscular dystrophy all the muscles are affected, while in others, only certain muscle groups become weak. Those with Duchenne experience progressive weakness and difficulty in climbing, jumping and hopping by age five. Between the ages of eight and ten, leg braces are often required, and eventually walking is impossible. Duchenne is also associated with heart problems and intellectual impairment that affects verbal ability more than performance. Death usually occurs in the third decade of life, often as a result of pneumonia.

Prevalence
Muscular dystrophy is a rare disorder that affects people of both sexes and all ages. Duchenne muscular dystrophy appears in childhood and affects males almost exclusively, but other forms may not appear until middle age or later. In Canada, it is estimated that more than 50,000 people are affected by muscular dystrophy of one form or another.

Treatment Options
Genetic testing is available to detect female carriers of the defective gene that causes muscular dystrophy, enabling genetic counselling for families and couples considering conception. Prenatal testing for muscular dystrophy can also be performed. In children

and adults, muscular dystrophy is usually diagnosed after a physical exam is performed and a detailed medical history is taken. Information about when and where muscle weakness first occurred, and its severity, is very helpful in classifying the type of muscular dystrophy. Blood tests are often used to measure levels of creatine kinase, an enzyme released by damaged muscles. If the level is high, and there has been no injury to the muscles, a muscle disorder such as muscular dystrophy may be suspected. Electromyography is another test commonly used to help diagnose muscular dystrophy. In this procedure, electrodes are inserted into the muscle to check for the electrical activity patterns that characterize the disorder. Studying a small piece of muscle tissue can also indicate whether the disorder is muscular dystrophy, and which form of the disease it is.

No specific treatment exists for muscular dystrophy. Corticosteroids, such as prednisone, may be of significant benefit in improving muscle strength, but owing to their numerous side effects, they should be reserved for patients with major functional decline. Other treatment includes physical therapy, which can help minimize the shortening of the muscles that occurs around the joints; assistive devices such as wheelchairs and braces; and avoidance of prolonged immobility. Research into gene therapy for muscular dystrophy is currently underway, and scientists are also investigating muscular injections of a human protein called Wnt7A as a possible therapy for Duchenne muscular dystrophy.

Although muscular dystrophy is progressive in all cases, the severity of disability varies. Some types (such as Duchenne) are fatal, but people with other forms of muscular dystrophy have a normal life expectancy.

See also Guillain-Barré Syndrome

National Associations

Association of Electromyography Technologists of Canada (AETC)

e-mail: info@aetc.ca
www.aetc.ca

Overview: A small national organization founded in 1976
Mission: To enhance the standards & education of individuals involved in the electromyography (EMG) technology field
Chief Officer(s):
Jodi Beswick, President
  jodi.beswick@aetc.ca
Angela Scott, Vice-President
  angela.scott@aetc.ca
Nancy Verreault, Secretary-Treasurer
  nancy.verreault@aetc.ca

Muscular Dystrophy Canada (MDC) / Dystrophie musculaire Canada (DMC)

#900, 2345 Yonge St., Toronto ON M4P 2E5
Fax: 416-488-7523
Toll-Free: 866-687-2538
e-mail: info@muscle.ca
www.muscle.ca
www.linkedin.com/company/466761
www.facebook.com/muscle.ca
twitter.com/md_canada
www.youtube.com/user/musculardystrophycan

Overview: A large national charitable organization founded in 1954
Mission: To improve the quality of life of persons who have muscular dystrophy through a broad range of programs, education, support of research & the delivery of needed services to people with muscular dystrophy & their families
Member of: Canadian Coalition for Genetic Fairness
Chief Officer(s):
Buzz Green, Chair
Barbara Stead-Coyle, Chief Executive Officer

Melanie Towell, Chief Financial Officer
  melanie.towell@muscle.ca

Atlantic Regional Office
100 Ilsley Ave., #N, Dartmouth NS B3B 1L3
Tel: 902-429-6322; *Fax:* 902-425-4226
Toll-Free: 800-884-6322
e-mail: infoatlantic@muscle.ca

Ontario & Nunavut Regional Office
#901, 2345 Yonge St., Toronto ON M4P 2E5
Tel: 416-488-2699; *Fax:* 416-488-0107
Toll-Free: 800-567-2873
e-mail: infoontario@muscle.ca

Québec Regional Office
#506, 1425, René-Lévesque ouest, Montréal QC H3G 1T7
Tel: 514-393-3522; *Fax:* 514-393-8113
Toll-Free: 800-567-2236
e-mail: infoquebec@muscle.ca

Western Canada Regional Office
#302, 601 West Broadway, Vancouver BC V5Z 4C2
Tel: 604-732-8799; *Fax:* 604-731-6127
Toll-Free: 800-336-8166
e-mail: infowest@muscle.ca
www.facebook.com/MDCBCYUKON

International Associations

American Association of Neuromuscular & Electrodiagnostic Medicine (AANEM)

2621 Superior Dr. NW, Rochester MN 55901 USA
Tel: 507-288-0100; *Fax:* 507-288-1225
e-mail: aanem@aanem.org
www.aanem.org
www.facebook.com/AANEMorg
twitter.com/aanemorg

Overview: A medium-sized international organization founded in 1953
Mission: To advance neuromuscular, musculoskeletal, & electrodiagnostic medicine; To increase members' knowledge of neurophysiology, pathophysiology, instrumentation, & electrodiagnostic medicine; To improve the quality of patient care
Chief Officer(s):
Shirlyn A. Adkins, Executive Director
  sadkins@aanem.org
Patrick Aldrich, Director, Finance
  paldrich@aanem.org
Millie Suk, Director, Health Policy
  msuk@aanem.org
Laurie Mona, Manager, Communications
  lmona@aanem.org
Publications:
• AANEM [American Association of Neuromuscular & Electrodiagnostic Medicine] News
Type: Newsletter; *Frequency:* Quarterly
Profile: Association activities, science in brief, legislative issues, & information about coding
• Muscle & Nerve
Type: Journal; *Accepts Advertising; ISSN:* 0148-639X
Profile: Readership includes neurologists, physiatrists, & physical & rehabilitative medical specialists

Society for Muscular Dystrophy Information International (SMDI)

PO Box 7490, Bridgewater NS B4V 2X6
Tel: 902-685-3961; *Fax:* 902-685-3962
e-mail: smdi@auracom.com
www.nsnet.org/smdi

Overview: A medium-sized international charitable organization founded in 1983
Mission: To facilitate international contact by producing website, & publications (newsletters, books) & by the sharing of neuromuscular & disability information between those concerned with muscular dystrophy &/or allied disorders

Myasthenia Gravis

Myasthenia gravis is an autoimmune disease of the neuromuscular junction—the structure which carries the nerve's chemical signal that tells the muscle to contract.

Cause
In acquired myasthenia gravis, circulating antibodies attack this junction, leading to weakness of voluntary muscles. In inherited myasthenia gravis, a genetic mutation causes a flaw in the neuromuscular junction that affects nerve impulse transmission.

Symptoms
Although myasthenia gravis may have a sudden onset, it is more common for early symptoms of the disease to develop slowly and subtly. The disease is characterized by weakness and fatigue that increases after exercise, and as the day progresses. Any muscle may be involved, but muscles in the face and throat are especially susceptible. The disease therefore especially affects chewing, swallowing, coughing and facial expressions. Double vision is also a common symptom. These manifestations fluctuate in intensity over a period lasting from a few hours to a few days, and usually improve with rest.

Prevalence
Myasthenia gravis affects approximately one in 5,000 to 10,000 people, and is almost twice as common in women as it is in men. Although the disease can affect anyone at any age, it is more common in women between the ages of 20 and 40 and in men over the age of 40.

Treatment Options
To diagnose myasthenia gravis, a physician usually takes a medical history, performs a physical exam and orders blood tests to detect acetylcholine receptor antibodies. Two other tests are also commonly used to confirm diagnosis: electromyography (to check the function of the muscles and the nerves that control the muscles) and a Tensilon test (to determine if muscle strength is improved by an injection of edrophonium).

Because myasthenia gravis is caused by an overactive immune system, most treatments target this system. These include corticosteroids; immunosuppressive drugs, such as azathioprine; plasmapheresis (filtration of the blood with retention of the cells and removal of the plasma); intravenous immunoglobulins; and surgical removal of the thymus gland. In addition, anticholinesterase drugs like pyridostigmine increase the level of the messenger chemical at the neuromuscular junction, thereby increasing muscle strength. Because progressive weakness is often associated with this disease, physical therapy and assistive devices are sometimes required, as well.

Although myasthenia gravis can be serious and cause life-threatening respiratory problems in certain cases, most people affected by this disease have a normal life expectancy.

Provincial Associations
BRITISH COLUMBIA

Myasthenia Gravis Association of British Columbia (MGABC)
2805 Kingsway, Vancouver BC V5R 5H9
Tel: 604-451-5511; *Fax:* 604-451-5651
e-mail: mgabc@centreforability.bc.ca
www.myastheniagravis.ca
Overview: A small provincial charitable organization founded in 1955
Mission: To provide information & support to British Columbians who suffer from Myasthenia Gravis (Grave Muscular Disease) & to their caregivers; to increase public awareness of the disease; to gather & disseminate specific information on Myasthenia Gravis to healthcare providers in British Columbia; to foster & support research into the causes & treatment of Myasthenia Gravis
Chief Officer(s):
Brenda Kelsey, President
North Island MG Association
BC
Chief Officer(s):
John Skalos, Contact
lisaandjohn@shaw.ca
Victoria
Victoria BC

Neurofibromatosis

Neurofibromatosis (NF) or von Recklinghausen disease, named after a German pathologist, is a genetic disorder. The term neurofibromatosis covers three separate disorders—neurofibromatosis type 1 (NF1), neurofibromatosis type 2 (NF2) and Schwannomatosis—all of which are characterized by the growth of benign tumours. The skin and the nervous system are the primary target organs.

Cause
In many instances, NF is inherited. Each child of a parent with the disease has a 50 percent chance of inheriting the gene. However, between 30 percent and 50 percent of new cases are due to a spontaneous change in a person's genes.

Symptoms
NF1 (the most common form of neurofibromatosis) is characterized by skin lesions (large, flat brown freckles, called caf_ au lait spots, owing to their light coffee color). They are apparent at birth or in infancy in more than 90 percent of patients. Tumours that grow on a nerve or nerves under the skin (neurofibromas) usually appear in late childhood between the ages of 10 and 15 years. Other symptoms include tumours on the iris of the eye or on the optic nerve, scoliosis (curvature of the spine) and bone deformities. NF1 symptoms are usually mild, but can be debilitating in some cases. NF2 is characterized by tumours on the eighth cranial nerve that occur on both sides of the body. These tumours, called vestibular schwannomas, may cause symptoms such as hearing loss, tinnitus, poor balance, facial pain or numbness and headaches. The symptoms of NF2 vary from person to person, but in some cases, the tumours can cause damage to nearby cranial nerves and the brainstem that can be life-threatening. Schwannomatosis is characterized by multiple tumours that may develop anywhere in the body except for on the eighth cranial nerve. The main symptom is pain.

Prevalence
Estimates put the number of Canadians currently living with neurofibromatosis at approximately 11,000. NF1 occurs about once in every 4,000 births. NF2 and Schwannomatosis are rarer, each affecting about one in 40,000 people.

Treatment Options
Before birth, inherited NF1 and NF2 can be identified through prenatal diagnostic tests such as amniocentesis and chorionic villus sampling. In children, a diagnosis of neurofibromatosis is usually made after a physical exam. For familial NF1 and NF2, genetic analysis can also be used to confirm the diagnosis. Magnetic resonance imaging (MRI) now allows for the detection and early treatment of very small tumours.

There is no cure for this condition, so the aim of treatment is symptom control. Tumours that produce severe symptoms or become cancerous can be surgically removed or irradiated.

Although neurofibromatosis can be severely debilitating, symptom management allows most people with this disorder to lead normal, full lives.

National Associations

Children's Tumor Foundation (CTF)
120 Wall St., 16th Fl., New York NY 10005-3904 USA
Tel: 212-344-6633; *Fax:* 212-747-0004
Toll-Free: 800-323-7938
e-mail: info@ctf.org
www.ctf.org
www.linkedin.com/company/children's-tumor-foundation
www.facebook.com/childrenstumor
twitter.com/childrenstumor
Previous Name: National NF Foundation
Overview: A medium-sized national charitable organization founded in 1978
Mission: To sponsor research to find the cause of & cure for both types of neurofibromatosis - NF1 & NF2; To promote clinical activities which assure individuals with NF ready access to the highest calibre of medical care; To develop programs to increase public awareness of NF; To provide support services for patients & families, with referrals to qualified healthcare professionals
Member of: International NF Association
Affliation(s): NF Associations worldwide
Chief Officer(s):
Annette Bakker, President & Chief Scientific Officer
Simon Vukelj, Vice-President, Marketing & Communications
Salvo La Rosa, Vice-President, Research & Development

Provincial Associations

BRITISH COLUMBIA

British Columbia Neurofibromatosis Foundation (BCNF)
PO Box 5339, Victoria BC V8R 6S4
Toll-Free: 800-385-2263
e-mail: info@bcnf.bc.ca
www.bcnf.bc.ca
www.facebook.com/10150157765325565
twitter.com/BC_NF
Overview: A small provincial charitable organization founded in 1984
Mission: To empower individuals with NF & their families to reach their full potential by providing support, education & research funding to find a cure
Member of: INFA - International NF Association
Affliation(s): National NF Foundation
Chief Officer(s):
Desirée Sher, Executive Director

ONTARIO

Neurofibromatosis Society of Ontario (NFSO)
2004 Underhill Ct., Pickering ON L1X 2M6
Tel: 905-683-0811
Toll-Free: 866-843-6376
e-mail: info@nfon.ca
www.nfon.ca
www.facebook.com/NFOntario
Also Known As: NF Society of Ontario
Overview: A small provincial charitable organization founded in 1985
Mission: To be a source of information; develop a participating membership; increase public awareness
Affliation(s): National NF Foundation
Chief Officer(s):
Angela Bobbett, President
a.bobbett@nfon.ca

QUÉBEC

L'Association de la Neurofibromatose du Québec (ANFQ)
CP 150, Succ. St-Michel, Montréal QC H2A 3B0
Tél: 514-385-6702; *Téléc:* 514-385-1420
Ligne sans frais: 888-385-6702
www.anfq.org

Aperçu: *Dimension:* petite; *Envergure:* provinciale; Organisme sans but lucratif; fondée en 1989
Mission: Regrouper les membres et leurs familles; diffuser l'information sur la NF auprès des membres et des professionnels de la santé et de l'éducation; favoriser la recherche
Membre de: Confédération des organismes de personnes handicapées; National Neurofibromatosis Foundation; Association québécoise pour les troubles d'apprentissage; NF Canada
Membre(s) du bureau directeur:
Louise L'Africain, Chair

SASKATCHEWAN

Neurofibromatosis Association of Saskatchewan
450 Kirkpatrick Ct., Saskatoon SK S7L 6Z3
Tel: 306-384-3540
Also Known As: NF Association of Saskatchewan
Overview: A small provincial charitable organization founded in 1985
Affliation(s): National NF Foundation

International Associations

AboutFace
PO Box 702, 1057 Steeles Ave. West, Toronto ON M2R 3X1
Tel: 416-597-2229; *Fax:* 416-597-8494
Toll-Free: 800-665-3223
e-mail: info@aboutface.ca
www.aboutface.ca
www.facebook.com/AboutFaceInternational
twitter.com/AboutFace
www.youtube.com/user/AboutFaceEvents
Overview: A small international charitable organization founded in 1985
Mission: To provide emotional support & information to, & on behalf of, individuals who have a facial difference & their families
Chief Officer(s):
Anna Pileggi, Executive Director
 anna@aboutface.ca
Emily Rivers, Manager, Communications & Database
 emily@aboutface.ca
Amanda Lizon, Manager, Client Programs & Outreach
 amanda@aboutface.ca

Local Hospitals & Health Centres

QUÉBEC

MONTRÉAL: Centre universitaire de santé McGill - Hôpital neurologique de Montréal
Affiliée à: CIUSSS du Centre-Ouest-de-l'Île-de-Montréal
3801, rue University, Montréal, QC H3A 2B4
Tél: 514-398-6644
www.mni.mcgill.ca
Nombre de lits: 65 lits de soins de courte durée; 14 lits de soins neurologiques intensifs
Guy Rouleau, Directeur général

Obesity

Obesity refers to a condition in which there is an excessive accumulation of fat in subcutaneous and other tissues of the body. Being obese and being overweight are not necessarily synonymous, as people who are overweight may have increased body size as a result of increased muscle or skeletal tissue mass.

Obesity may develop at any age, but peak development periods are the first 12 months of life, between the ages of five and six years, and the adolescent years in children. In adults, obesity may develop at any time, but many people may find that weight gain progresses most significantly between the third and sixth decades.

Cause
Obesity may result from an increase in the actual number of fat cells or from an increase in the size of the individual fat cells. Re-

searchers believe that fat cells increase in number in proportion to caloric intake increase and that this increase is particularly evident in the first 12 months of life. As children grow, increases in fat cell populations continue at a slower rate. Because the number of fat cells cannot be decreased—except surgically—later weight loss must result from the reduction of fat in individual cells.

Obesity usually results when caloric intake exceeds the energy demands of the body, thus increasing the storage of body fat. Fat accumulation is usually a progressive process, resulting from repeated episodes of food intake exceeding the body's demand for energy (calories). Patterns of behaviour that may lead to obesity are often established as early as infancy. For example, if parents or caregivers persistently use a bottle to pacify a crying baby, the baby may learn that food is equivalent to relief of stress. Many other factors may influence appetite or obesity, including environmental influences; psychosocial disturbances that may be induced by emotional upset or trauma; brain lesions that may involve a certain area of the brain such as the hypothalamus or the pituitary gland (both essential to hormone production); an overabundance of insulin in the body (hyperinsulinism); and genetic influences. In addition, in rare instances, obesity may be a feature of certain genetic disorders (see Prader-Willi syndrome). The most common cause in North America however, is the excessive intake of calories, particularly those from fats and sugars, and the concomitant lack of physical exercise and activity that uses calories.

Symptoms

Complications of obesity in the child and the adult may include respiratory difficulties, such as shortness of breath; increased cardiovascular risk factors, such as high blood pressure; elevated total cholesterol levels as well as increased bad, or LDL, cholesterol and decreased good, or HDL, cholesterol; and increased levels of fatty acid and glycerol compounds (triglycerides). These are risk factors for the development of coronary artery disease, one of the leading causes of mortality in North America. In addition, obesity may be associated with a resistance to the hormone insulin that aids in the metabolism of glucose, fats, carbohydrates and proteins. This resistance may lead to excessive levels of circulating insulin in the body (hyperinsulinism); however, the body is not able to appropriately use this insulin and high blood sugar (hyperglycemia) may occur. This condition is known as type II diabetes mellitus and its incidence in the population is also increasing dramatically in both children and adults. Finally, being obese puts a person at risk for other illnesses such as osteoarthritis; gall bladder disease; sleep apnea; and breast, colon and endometrial cancer.

Prevalence

It is clear from numerous public health studies that there has been a dramatic increase recently in obesity rates in adults and youth in Canada. For example, over the past 25 years, the number of obese children in Canada has tripled. Approximately 20 percent of Canadian adults are obese, and 28.5 percent of boys and 17 percent of girls are overweight or obese. The highest prevalence of obesity is in adults aged 45 to 64, particularly men.

Treatment Options

The diagnosis of obesity in children, adolescents and adults is usually determined through a physical exam and medical history that includes questions about a person's eating and exercise habits. In adults, certain screening methods such as measurement of the body mass index (BMI) as well as waist circumference (WC) are also used to diagnose obesity.

Treatment for obesity should include the cooperation and support of the entire family and may be directed toward behaviour modification, as well as individual and family counselling. Weight management programs that promote a combination of balanced diet, regular exercise and healthy eating habits are a mainstay in treating obesity. Sometimes a weight-loss medication such as orlistat is prescribed. In cases where lifestyle changes are not successful, gastric bypass surgery may be performed. In this procedure, the size of the stomach is reduced making it uncomfortable to eat anything more than a small amount of food.

Obesity is a significant public health issue in Canada. However, by diligently following a weight management program, most people can achieve and maintain a healthy body weight, decrease the medical risks associated with obesity and improve their quality of life.

See also Eating Disorders

National Associations

Active Healthy Kids Canada / Jeunes en forme Canada
#1205, 77 Bloor St. West, Toronto ON M5S 1M2
Tel: 416-913-0238; *Fax:* 416-913-1541
e-mail: info@activehealthykids.ca
www.activehealthykids.ca
www.facebook.com/ActiveHealthyKidsCanada
twitter.com/ActiveHealthyKi
www.youtube.com/user/ActiveHealthyKids
Previous Name: The Foundation for Active Healthy Kids
Overview: A small national charitable organization founded in 1994
Mission: To advocate the importance of quality, accessible & enjoyable physical activity participation experiences for children & youth; To provide expertise & direction to decision makers at all levels, from policy-makers to parents, in order to increase the attention given to, investment in, & effective implementation of physical activity opportunities for all Canadian children & youth
Chief Officer(s):
Jennifer Cowie Bonne, Chief Executive Officer

Canadian Association of Bariatric Physicians & Surgeons (CABPS) / L'Association canadienne des medecins et chirurgiens bariatrique (ACMCB)
#210, 2800 - 14th Ave., Markham ON L3R 0E4
Tel: 416-491-2886; *Fax:* 416-491-1670
e-mail: cabps@associationconcepts.ca
cabps.ca
www.linkedin.com/company/cabps
www.facebook.com/pages/CABPS/215143185313177#
twitter.com/Cabps_Obesity
Overview: A small national organization
Mission: Represents Canadian specialists interested in the treatment of obesity and severe obesity for the purposes of professional development and coordination and promotion of common goals.
Affliation(s): International Federation for the Surgery of Obesity and Metabolic Disorders
Chief Officer(s):
Mehran Anvari, President, 905-522-2951
anvari@mcmaster.ca

Canadian Obesity Network (CON) / Réseau Canadien en Obésité (RCO)
Li Ka Shing Centre for Health Research & Innovation, Univ. of Alberta, #1-116, 8602 - 112 St., Edmonton AB T6G 2E1
Tel: 780-492-8361; *Fax:* 780-492-9414
e-mail: info@obesitynetwork.ca
www.obesitynetwork.ca
twitter.com/CanObesityNet
Overview: A small national organization founded in 2006
Mission: To foster knowledge translation, capacity building, & partnerships in the area of obesity in Canada; To find innovative & effective ways to treat & prevent obesity; To reduce the mental, physical, & economic burden of obesity
Chief Officer(s):
Anton Hart, Chair
Arya M. Sharma, Scientific Director

Publications:
• Best Weight: A Practical Guide to Office-Based Obesity Management
Number of Pages: 100; *Author:* Dr. Y. Freedhoff; Dr. A.M. Sharma
Profile: A practical guide to managing obesity in a clinical setting
• Conduit
Type: Magazine; *Frequency:* Quarterly; *Accepts Advertising; Editor:* Brad Hussey
Profile: Articles about obesity research & networking activities throughout Canada
• Obesity + (Online Best Evidence Service In Tackling Obesity Plus)
Profile: Latest evidence for clinical practice on obesity

Childhood Obesity Foundation (COF)
Robert H.N. Ho Research Centre, VGH Hospital Campus, 771A - 2635 Laurel St., Vancouver BC V5Z 1M9

Tel: 604-251-2229
e-mail: info@childhoodobesityfoundation.ca
www.childhoodobesityfoundation.ca
www.facebook.com/pages/Childhood-Obesity-Foundation/4970958836 47517
twitter.com/COF_5210

Overview: A small national charitable organization founded in 2004
Mission: Aims to reduce the prevalence of childhood obesity in Canada.
Chief Officer(s):
Tom Warshawski, Chair

Fondation Lucie et André Chagnon / Lucie & André Chagnon Foundation
#1000, 2001, av McGill College, Montréal QC H3A 1G1

Tél: 514-380-2001; *Téléc:* 514-340-8434
Courriel: info@fondationchagnon.org
www.fondationchagnon.org
twitter.com/FondChagnon
www.youtube.com/user/FondationChagnon

Aperçu: *Dimension:* moyenne; *Envergure:* nationale
Mission: Contribuer au développement et à l'amélioration de la santé par la prévention de la pauvreté et de la maladie en agissant principalement auprès des enfants et de leurs parents
Membre(s) du bureau directeur:
André Chagnon, Président du conseil

Provincial Associations

TOPS Club, Inc.
PO Box 070360, 4575 South Fifth St., Milwaukee WI 53207-0360
United States

Tel: 414-482-4620
e-mail: wondering@tops.org
www.tops.org

Also Known As: Take Off Pounds Sensibly
Overview: A small provincial organization
Mission: To help overweight persons attain & maintain their goal weight
Chief Officer(s):
Sandra Seidlitz, Area Coordinator, AB, BC, MB, NT, NU, ON, SK, YT
Debra-Ann MacLean, Area Coordinator, NB, NL, NS, PE, QC

ALBERTA

College of Dietitians of Alberta
#740, 10707 - 100 Ave., Edmonton AB T5J 3M1

Tel: 780-448-0059; *Fax:* 780-489-7759
Toll-Free: 866-493-4348
e-mail: office@collegeofdietitians.ab.ca
www.collegeofdietitians.ab.ca

Overview: A small provincial licensing organization overseen by Dietitians of Canada
Mission: The College is the regulatory body of registered dieticians/nutritionists in Alberta, setting entry requirements, standards of practice. It is accountable to both the government & the public.
Chief Officer(s):
Doug Cook, Executive Director & Registrar

BRITISH COLUMBIA

College of Dietitians of British Columbia (CDBC)
#409, 1367 West Broadway, Vancouver BC V6H 4A7

Tel: 604-736-2016; *Fax:* 604-736-2018
Toll-Free: 877-736-2016
e-mail: info@collegeofdietitiansbc.org
www.collegeofdietitiansofbc.org

Overview: A medium-sized provincial licensing organization founded in 2004 overseen by Dietitians of Canada
Mission: To serve & protect the nutritional health of the public through quality dietetic practice
Chief Officer(s):
Fern Hubbard, Registrar
Mélanie Journoud, Deputy Registrar, Quality Assurance
Chi Cejalvo, Deputy Registrar, Registration & Communication

MANITOBA

College of Dietitians of Manitoba
#36, 1313 Border St., Winnipeg MB R3H 0X4

Tel: 204-694-0532; *Fax:* 204-889-1755
Toll-Free: 866-283-2823
e-mail: office.cdm@mts.net
www.manitobadietitians.ca

Overview: A small provincial organization overseen by Dietitians of Canada
Mission: To act as the regulating body within the province for dietitians & the profession of dietetics; To set education standards; To ensure competency of members
Member of: Alliance of Dietetic Regulatory Bodies
Chief Officer(s):
Michelle Hagglund, Registrar

NEW BRUNSWICK

New Brunswick Association of Dietitians (NBAD) / Association des diététistes du Nouveau-Brunswick (ADNB)
PO Box 27002, 471 Smythe St., Fredericton NB E3B 9M1

Tel: 506-457-9396; *Fax:* 506-450-9375
e-mail: registrar@adnb-nbad.com
www.adnb-nbad.com

Overview: A medium-sized provincial licensing organization overseen by Dietitians of Canada
Mission: To regulate the practice of dietitians within New Brunswick
Chief Officer(s):
Catherine MacDonald, President

NEWFOUNDLAND AND LABRADOR

Newfoundland & Labrador College of Dietitians (NLCD)
PO Box 1756, Stn. C, St. John's NL A1C 5P5

Tel: 709-753-4040; *Fax:* 709-781-1044
Toll-Free: 877-753-4040
e-mail: registrar@nlcd.ca
www.nlcd.ca

Overview: A medium-sized provincial licensing organization overseen by Dietitians of Canada
Mission: To regulate Registered Dietitians & to ensure competency in the dietetic profession, in the interest of the people in Newfoundland
Member of: Alliance of Canadian Regulatory Boards
Chief Officer(s):
Cynthia Whalen, Registrar

NOVA SCOTIA

Nova Scotia Dietetic Association (NSDA)
#301, 380 Bedford Hwy., Halifax NS B3M 2L4

Tel: 902-493-3034
e-mail: info@nsdassoc.ca
www.nsdassoc.ca

Overview: A medium-sized provincial licensing organization founded in 1953 overseen by Dietitians of Canada
Mission: To regulate dietitians & nutritionists in the province, & register & discipline (when necessary) practitioners to ensure safe, ethical & competent dietetic practice
Chief Officer(s):
Melissa Campbell, President

Jennifer Garus, Executive Manager (ex-officio)

ONTARIO

College of Dietitians of Ontario (CDO) / L'Ordre des diététistes de l'Ontario

PO Box 30, #1810, 5775 Yonge St., Toronto ON M2M 4J1

Tel: 416-598-1725; *Fax:* 416-598-0274
Toll-Free: 800-668-4990
e-mail: information@collegeofdietitians.org
www.collegeofdietitians.org
www.facebook.com/CollegeDietitiansOntario
twitter.com/CDOntario

Also Known As: CDO
Overview: A medium-sized provincial licensing charitable organization founded in 1993 overseen by Dietitians of Canada
Mission: To promote awareness of & access to competent, high quality nutritional care for Ontarians
Member of: The Federation of Health Regulatory Bodies of Ontario; Alliance of Canadian Dietetic Regulatory Bodies; Council of Licensure, Enforcement and Regulation
Chief Officer(s):
Melisse L. Willems, Registrar & Executive Director, 416-598-1725 Ext. 228
  melisse.willems@collegeofdietitians.org

PRINCE EDWARD ISLAND

Prince Edward Island Dietetic Association (PEIDA)

c/o Prince Edward Island Dietitians Registration Board, PO Box 362, Charlottetown PE C1A 7K7

e-mail: peidietitians@gmail.com
www.peidietitians.ca
www.facebook.com/peidieteticassociation

Overview: A small provincial organization founded in 1965 overseen by Dietitians of Canada
Mission: To promote, encourage & improve the status of dietitians & nutritionists in the province of PEI; To promote & increase the knowledge & proficiency of its members in all matters relating to nutrition & dietetics; To promote public awareness
Chief Officer(s):
Doreen Pippy, President

QUÉBEC

Ordre professionnel des diététistes du Québec (OPDQ)

#1855, 550, rue Sherbrooke ouest, Montréal QC H3A 1B9

Tél: 514-393-3733; *Téléc:* 514-393-3582
Ligne sans frais: 888-393-8528
Courriel: opdq@opdq.org
www.opdq.org

Aperçu: *Dimension:* moyenne; *Envergure:* provinciale; Organisme de réglementation; fondée en 1956 surveillé par Dietitians of Canada
Mission: Assurer la protection du public en contrôlant notamment l'exercice de la profession par ses membres
Membre(s) du bureau directeur:
Annie Chapados, Directrice générale et secrétaire
  achapados@opdq.org

SASKATCHEWAN

Saskatchewan Dietitians Association (SDA)

#17, 2010 - 7th Ave., Regina SK S4R 1C2

Tel: 306-359-3040; *Fax:* 306-359-3046
e-mail: registrar@saskdietitians.org
www.saskdietitians.org

Overview: A small provincial licensing organization founded in 1958 overseen by Dietitians of Canada
Mission: To protect the public by registering competent dietitians; To set standards of practice; To uphold codes of conduct; To provide a framework for continuing competence, consisting of a self-assessment tool, a learning plan, & a quality assurance audit
Affliation(s): Network of Interprofessional Regulatory Organizations; Alliance of Dietetic Regulatory Bodies
Chief Officer(s):
Laurel Leushen, President
Lana Moore, Registrar

Local Associations

ONTARIO

Canadian Association for Size Acceptance (CASA)

#511, 99 Dalhousie St., Toronto ON M5B 2N2

Tel: 416-861-0217; *Fax:* 416-861-1668

Overview: A small local organization founded in 1997
Mission: To lobby against & raises awareness of discrimination towards people of size.
Member of: International Size Acceptance Association; National Association to Advance Fat Acceptance

QUÉBEC

ÉquiLibre - Groupe d'action sur le poids

#304, 7200, rue Hutchison, Montréal QC H3N 1Z2

Tél: 514-270-3779; *Téléc:* 514-270-1974
Ligne sans frais: 877-270-3779
Courriel: info@equilibre.ca
www.equilibre.ca
www.facebook.com/GroupeEquiLibre
twitter.com/groupeequilibre
www.youtube.com/user/groupeequilibre

Nom précédent: Collectif action alternative en obésité
Aperçu: *Dimension:* petite; *Envergure:* locale; Organisme sans but lucratif
Mission: Favoriser la prévention et la diminution des problèmes reliés au poids et à l'image corporelle par l'élaboration d'actions de sensibilisation, et la conception de programmes et d'outils éducatifs à l'intention de la population et des professionnels de la santé
Membre(s) du bureau directeur:
Roxanne Léonard, Directrice générale
  roxanne.leonard@equilibre.ca

International Associations

Outremangeurs Anonymes

312, rue Beaubien est, Montréal QC H2S 1R8

Tél: 514-490-1939
Ligne sans frais: 877-509-1939
Courriel: reunions@outremangeurs.org
outremangeurs.org

Aperçu: *Dimension:* grande; *Envergure:* internationale; fondée en 1960
Mission: Aide les hommes et les femmes de maîtriser les problèmes ils ont avec la suralimentation

National Publications

Obesity Surgery
Owned By: Springer

Social Media: twitter.com/clinmedjournals
Circulation: 2,300 Frequency: 12 times a year
Scott Shikora, Editor-in-Chief

Osteogenesis Imperfecta

Osteogenesis imperfecta (OI), often called "brittle bone" disease, is actually a group of genetic disorders that are characterized by abnormally fragile bones that break or fracture easily. There are at least eight distinct forms of the disorder, with type I being the most common and mildest, and type II being the most severe. A person with OI has either less collagen (the major protein of the connective tissue around which bone is formed), or a poorer quality collagen.

Cause

Most types of OI (85 to 90 percent) are inherited in an autosomal dominant pattern. This means that for a child to have OI, only one copy of the gene mutation (inherited from a parent or as a spontaneous mutation) is necessary. In the other 10 to 15 percent of cases, OI is inherited in an autosomal recessive pattern. This means that the child receives a copy of the gene mutation from both parents (parents do not have OI, but are carriers of the gene mutation).

Symptoms

The symptoms of OI vary in severity. Children with the mildest type of OI may have bones that fracture easily; loose joints and muscle weakness; a blue tint to the whites of the eyes; brittle teeth; and possible hearing loss. Infants born with more severe forms of OI may have multiple bone fractures, and routine vaginal delivery may lead to significant bone fracture, hemorrhage into the brain and other major problems. Survivors develop shortened extremities and other bony abnormalities.

Prevalence

Approximately one in 20,000 babies is born with some form of OI.

Treatment Options

Prenatal testing for OI can be performed through chorionic villus sampling (CVS) or amniocentesis. After birth, diagnosis of OI can often be based on clinical (characteristic) features. A collagen biopsy test or DNA test may also be used to confirm a diagnosis of OI.

At present, there is no cure for this disorder, so the aim of treatment is to control symptoms and reduce pain and complications. Bisphosphonates are sometimes prescribed to increase bone density and strength, and to reduce fractures and bone pain. Gentle exercise and physical therapy are directed at preventing fractures and increasing function. Rodding surgery (a procedure where metal rods are placed in the long bones of the legs) is sometimes used to increase bone strength and prevent deformities.

The prognosis for people with OI varies depending on the severity of their symptoms. Although they must deal with multiple fractures and limited physical activity, most people with OI still lead full and productive lives.

National Associations

Osteoporosis Canada / Ostéoporose Canada
#301, 1090 Don Mills Rd., Toronto ON M3C 3R6
Tel: 416-696-2663; *Fax:* 416-696-2673
Toll-Free: 800-463-6842
www.osteoporosis.ca
www.linkedin.com/company/2610844
www.facebook.com/osteoporosiscanada
twitter.com/OsteoporosisCA
www.youtube.com/osteoporosisca

Previous Name: Osteoporosis Society of Canada
Overview: A large national charitable organization founded in 1982
Mission: To encourage research into the prevention, diagnosis, & treatment of osteoporosis; To improve access to osteoporosis care & support
Member of: Canadian Coalition for Genetic Fairness
Chief Officer(s):
Famida Jiwa, President & CEO
Emily Bartens, Chair
Publications:
• Osteoblast
Type: Newsletter; *Frequency:* 3 pa; *Price:* Free for members
Profile: Scientifically based information on osteoporosis & Osteoporosis Canada activities, for members & donors

Calgary - Alberta Chapter
Bldg. B8, Currie Barracks, #104, 2526 Battleford Ave. SW, Calgary AB T3E 7J4
Tel: 403-237-7022; *Fax:* 403-220-1727
e-mail: alberta@osteoporosis.ca
Chief Officer(s):
Chloe Kilkenny, Contact

Dartmouth - Nova Scotia Chapter

#206, 44 - 46 Portland St., Dartmouth NS B2Y 1H4
Tel: 902-407-4053
e-mail: novascotia@osteoporosis.ca
Chief Officer(s):
Charmaine Hollett, Chair

Hamilton - Hamilton-Burlington Chapter
75 MacNab St. South, Hamilton ON L8P 3C1
Tel: 905-525-5398; *Fax:* 905-577-0396
e-mail: hamilton@osteoporosis.ca
Chief Officer(s):
Juanita Gledhill, Chair
• Osteoporosis Canada, Hamilton-Burlington Chapter Newsletter
Type: Newsletter; *Frequency:* Semiannually

Kelowna Chapter
PO Box 21072, Stn. Orchard Park, Kelowna BC V1Y 9N8
Tel: 250-861-6880
e-mail: kelowna@osteoporosis.ca
Chief Officer(s):
Trish Gunning, Chair

Laval - Greater Montreal Chapter
274, rue Antoine Forestier, Laval QC H7M 6B9
Tel: 514-212-5549
Toll-Free: 800-977-1778
e-mail: montreal@osteoporosis.ca

London - London & Thames Valley Chapter
PO Box 32017, London ON N5V 5K4
Tel: 519-457-0624; *Fax:* 519-457-0624
e-mail: london-thamesvalley@osteoporosis.ca
Chief Officer(s):
Joanne Legros-Kelly, Chair

Mid-Island Chapter
110 Moss Ave., #B, Parksville BC V9P 1L5
Tel: 250-951-0243; *Fax:* 250-951-0343
e-mail: mid-island@osteoporosis.ca
Chief Officer(s):
Lisa Leger, Chair

Mississauga Chapter
c/o/ #76, 6797 Formentera Ave., Mississauga ON L5N 2L6
Tel: 416-696-2663
e-mail: mississauga@osteoporosis.ca
Chief Officer(s):
Bev Nickle, Chair
Elizabeth St. Onge, Chair

Moncton - Greater Moncton Chapter
Moncton NB
e-mail: greatermoncton@osteoporosis.ca
Chief Officer(s):
Linda Hopper, Chair

Peterborough Chapter
PO Box 373, Stn. Main, Peterborough ON K9J 6Z3
Tel: 705-740-2776
e-mail: peterborough@osteoporosis.ca
Chief Officer(s):
Heather Drysdale, Chair

Québec - Québec City Chapter
#100, 1200, av Germain-des-Prés, Québec QC G1V 3M7
Tél: 418-651-8661; *Téléc:* 418-650-3916
Ligne sans frais: 800-977-1778
Courriel: sectiondequebec@osteoporosecanada.ca

Regina Chapter
90C Cavendish St., Regina SK S4N 5G7
Tel: 306-757-2663; *Fax:* 306-789-2663
e-mail: regina@osteoporosis.ca
Chief Officer(s):
Sylvia Fiske, Chair

St. Catharines - Niagara Chapter
264 Welland Ave., St Catharines ON L2R SP8
Tel: 905-685-1225
e-mail: niagara@osteoporosis.ca
Chief Officer(s):
Phyllis Kerkhoven, Chair

Saskatoon Chapter
PO Box 25179, Stn. River Heights, Saskatoon SK S7K 8B7
Tel: 306-931-2663; *Fax:* 306-249-9065
e-mail: saskatoon@osteoporosis.ca

Chief Officer(s):
Carole Young, Chair

Surrey / White Rock Chapter
#207, 1558 - 1st St., White Rock BC V4B 4B7
Tel: 604-538-2500
e-mail: surrey-whiterock@osteoporosis.ca

Chief Officer(s):
Margaret Willson, Chair

Winnipeg - Manitoba Chapter
123 St. Anne's Rd., Winnipeg MB R2M 2Z1
Tel: 204-772-3498; *Fax:* 204-772-4200
e-mail: manitoba@osteoporosis.ca

Chief Officer(s):
Cherylle Unryn, Chair

Provincial Associations

ALBERTA

Prairie Osteopathic Association
1603 - 20 Ave NW, Calgary AB T2M 1G9
Tel: 403-282-7165; *Fax:* 403-289-8269
Overview: A small provincial organization
Affiliation(s): Canadian Osteopathic Association
Chief Officer(s):
C.E. (Ted) Findlay, President

Osteoporosis

Osteoporosis is a general term for many conditions which result in a reduction in bone mass and deterioration of bone tissue and lead to fracture risk.

Cause

Most cases occur in post-menopausal women because estrogen loss is associated with decreased bone mass. Risk factors for osteoporosis include age, cigarette smoking, thin body build and early menopause and it is more common amongst white women. Men can develop a similar condition, but decline is generally more gradual. Excessive activity of the adrenal glands (Cushing's syndrome), the thyroid gland (thyrotoxicosis), the parathyroid glands (hyperparathyroidism), and the pituitary gland (hyperprolactinemia) causes bones to thin, as does under-activity of the testes or ovaries. Anorexia nervosa and prolonged administration of cortisone or heparin will also thin the bones.

Symptoms

Because bone loss can occur over the course of many years without any symptoms, osteoporosis is often called "the silent thief." The wrist, spine, shoulder and hip are the most common fracture sites in people with osteoporosis. Post-menopausal osteoporosis may also cause marked reduction in a woman's height, as multiple vertebral bodies in the spine compress downwards over the years. Osteoporosis can interfere with quality of life since it often reduces mobility, decreases independence and lowers self-esteem.

Prevalence

In Canada, at least two million people are affected by osteoporosis. As many as one in three women and one in five men will experience a fracture due to osteoporosis during their lifetime. It is estimated that treating osteoporosis costs the healthcare system more than two billion dollars every year in Canada.

Treatment Options

Bone mineral density (BMD) tests are often used to diagnose osteoporosis. The most common of these tests is dual energy X-ray absorptiometry (DXA). In this procedure, an X-ray detector is used to scan the bones to indicate how dense they are. Two other fracture risk assessment tools—CAROC (launched by the Canadian Association of Radiologists and Osteoporosis Canada) and FRAX (a Fracture Risk Assessment tool launched by the World Health Organization)—are now available in Canada. These tools calculate a person's 10-year absolute risk of fracture.

Treatment of osteoporosis is in part nonspecific, and can include surgery or other immobilization to treat fractures of the hip or wrist, control of pain with medications and physical therapy to encourage return to pre-fracture function. Specific therapy includes calcium and Vitamin D supplementation and weight-bearing exercises. Drug therapy for osteoporosis may include bisphosphonates, such as alendronate, SERMs (selective estrogen receptor modulators), such as raloxifene, hormone therapy (estrogen/progesterone), calcitonin (Miacalcin), denosumab (Prolia) and parathyroid hormone (teriparatide injection).

Osteoporosis can be a debilitating disease. Early diagnosis of bone loss and proper medical therapy are crucial in preventing future fractures.

National Associations

Osteoporosis Canada / Ostéoporose Canada
#301, 1090 Don Mills Rd., Toronto ON M3C 3R6
Tel: 416-696-2663; *Fax:* 416-696-2673
Toll-Free: 800-463-6842
www.osteoporosis.ca
www.linkedin.com/company/2610844
www.facebook.com/osteoporosiscanada
twitter.com/OsteoporosisCA
www.youtube.com/osteoporosisca
Previous Name: Osteoporosis Society of Canada
Overview: A large national charitable organization founded in 1982
Mission: To encourage research into the prevention, diagnosis, & treatment of osteoporosis; To improve access to osteoporosis care & support
Member of: Canadian Coalition for Genetic Fairness
Chief Officer(s):
Famida Jiwa, President & CEO
Emily Bartens, Chair
Publications:
• Osteoblast
Type: Newsletter; *Frequency:* 3 pa; *Price:* Free for members
Profile: Scientifically based information on osteoporosis & Osteoporosis Canada activities, for members & donors

Calgary - Alberta Chapter
Bldg. B8, Currie Barracks, #104, 2526 Battleford Ave. SW, Calgary AB T3E 7J4
Tel: 403-237-7022; *Fax:* 403-220-1727
e-mail: alberta@osteoporosis.ca

Chief Officer(s):
Chloe Kilkenny, Contact

Dartmouth - Nova Scotia Chapter
#206, 44 - 46 Portland St., Dartmouth NS B2Y 1H4
Tel: 902-407-4053
e-mail: novascotia@osteoporosis.ca

Chief Officer(s):
Charmaine Hollett, Chair

Hamilton - Hamilton-Burlington Chapter
75 MacNab St. South, Hamilton ON L8P 3C1
Tel: 905-525-5398; *Fax:* 905-577-0396
e-mail: hamilton@osteoporosis.ca

Chief Officer(s):
Juanita Gledhill, Chair
• Osteoporosis Canada, Hamilton-Burlington Chapter Newsletter
Type: Newsletter; *Frequency:* Semiannually

Kelowna Chapter

PO Box 21072, Stn. Orchard Park, Kelowna BC V1Y 9N8
Tel: 250-861-6880
e-mail: kelowna@osteoporosis.ca

Chief Officer(s):
Trish Gunning, Chair

Laval - Greater Montreal Chapter
274, rue Antoine Forestier, Laval QC H7M 6B9
Tel: 514-212-5549
Toll-Free: 800-977-1778
e-mail: montreal@osteoporosis.ca

London - London & Thames Valley Chapter
PO Box 32017, London ON N5V 5K4
Tel: 519-457-0624; *Fax:* 519-457-0624
e-mail: london-thamesvalley@osteoporosis.ca

Chief Officer(s):
Joanne Legros-Kelly, Chair

Mid-Island Chapter
110 Moss Ave., #B, Parksville BC V9P 1L5
Tel: 250-951-0243; *Fax:* 250-951-0343
e-mail: mid-island@osteoporosis.ca

Chief Officer(s):
Lisa Leger, Chair

Mississauga Chapter
c/o/ #76, 6797 Formentera Ave., Mississauga ON L5N 2L6
Tel: 416-696-2663
e-mail: mississauga@osteoporosis.ca

Chief Officer(s):
Bev Nickle, Chair
Elizabeth St. Onge, Chair

Moncton - Greater Moncton Chapter
Moncton NB
e-mail: greatermoncton@osteoporosis.ca

Chief Officer(s):
Linda Hopper, Chair

Peterborough Chapter
PO Box 373, Stn. Main, Peterborough ON K9J 6Z3
Tel: 705-740-2776
e-mail: peterborough@osteoporosis.ca

Chief Officer(s):
Heather Drysdale, Chair

Québec - Québec City Chapter
#100, 1200, av Germain-des-Prés, Québec QC G1V 3M7
Tél: 418-651-8661; *Téléc:* 418-650-3916
Ligne sans frais: 800-977-1778
Courriel: sectiondequebec@osteoporosecanada.ca

Regina Chapter
90C Cavendish St., Regina SK S4N 5G7
Tel: 306-757-2663; *Fax:* 306-789-2663
e-mail: regina@osteoporosis.ca

Chief Officer(s):
Sylvia Fiske, Chair

St. Catharines - Niagara Chapter
264 Welland Ave., St Catharines ON L2R SP8
Tel: 905-685-1225
e-mail: niagara@osteoporosis.ca

Chief Officer(s):
Phyllis Kerkhoven, Chair

Saskatoon Chapter
PO Box 25179, Stn. River Heights, Saskatoon SK S7K 8B7
Tel: 306-931-2663; *Fax:* 306-249-9065
e-mail: saskatoon@osteoporosis.ca

Chief Officer(s):
Carole Young, Chair

Surrey / White Rock Chapter
#207, 1558 - 1st St., White Rock BC V4B 4B7
Tel: 604-538-2500
e-mail: surrey-whiterock@osteoporosis.ca

Chief Officer(s):
Margaret Willson, Chair

Winnipeg - Manitoba Chapter
123 St. Anne's Rd., Winnipeg MB R2M 2Z1
Tel: 204-772-3498; *Fax:* 204-772-4200
e-mail: manitoba@osteoporosis.ca

Chief Officer(s):
Cherylle Unryn, Chair

Provincial Associations

ALBERTA

Prairie Osteopathic Association
1603 - 20 Ave NW, Calgary AB T2M 1G9
Tel: 403-282-7165; *Fax:* 403-289-8269
Overview: A small provincial organization
Affliation(s): Canadian Osteopathic Association
Chief Officer(s):
C.E. (Ted) Findlay, President

International Associations

American Society for Bone & Mineral Research (ASBMR)
#800, 2025 M St. NW, Washington DC 20036-3309 USA
Tel: 202-367-1161; *Fax:* 202-367-2161
Other Communication: Publications email: jbmroffice@wiley.com
e-mail: asbmr@asbmr.org
www.asbmr.org
www.facebook.com/ASBMR
twitter.com/ASBMR

Overview: A medium-sized international organization
Mission: To promote study in the field of bone & mineral metabolism
Chief Officer(s):
Jane Cauley, President
Ann L. Elderkin, Executive Director
Douglas Fesler, Associate Executive Director
Deborah Kroll, Director, Development
Brenda Malottke, Director, Finance
Amanda Darvill, Director, Marketing & Communications
Katie Duffy, Director, Publications
Lauren Taggart, Manager, Operations
Angela Cangemi, Manager, Programs
Publications:
• ASBMR [American Society for Bone & Mineral Research] e-news
Type: Newsletter; *Frequency:* Monthly
Profile: Information from the American Society for Bone & Mineral Research, including upcoming events, grant announcements, membership benefits, committee & task forcehighlights, & program updates
• Journal of Bone & Mineral Research
Type: Journal; *Accepts Advertising; Editor:* Juliet E. Compston
Profile: Up-to-date basic & clinical research in the pathophysiology & treatment of bone & mineral disorders
• Primer on the Metabolic Bone Diseases & Disorders of Mineral Metabolism
Type: Primer; *Editor:* Clifford Rosen, M.D.; *Price:* A free copy & on-line access for American Society for Bone & Mineral Research members
Profile: A resource for scientists & students seeking an overview of the bone & mineral field, as well as for clinicians who care forpatients with disorders of bone & mineral metabolism

National Libraries

Osteoporosis Canada
#500, 1200 Eglinton Ave. East, Toronto, ON M3C 1H9
Tel: 416-696-2663; *Fax:* 416-696-2673
Toll-Free: 800-463-6842
Other Numbers: French Toll-Free: 1-800-977-1778
www.osteoporosis.ca
Tanya Long, National Education Manager
416-696-2663 ext. 2229

Paget's Disease

Paget's disease is a chronic disorder of the bone which typically results in enlarged and deformed bones in one or more regions of the skeleton. Excessive bone breakdown and formation cause new bone to be dense but fragile. Paget's disease most frequently affects the spine, skull, pelvis, collarbone and legs.

Cause

The cause of Paget's disease is unknown. It is sometimes familial—between 10 and 40 percent of people with Paget's disease have a family member who is also affected. Researchers have discovered several genes associated with the disease, and have even identified one gene (the sequestosome 1 gene) that predisposes people to develop Paget's. Studies suggest that there may also be an environmental factor, such as a virus, involved.

Symptoms

Many people with Paget's disease have no symptoms, and only become aware that they have the disease when they start to experience complications. Early symptoms of Paget's disease include bone and joint pain and fatigue, as well as headaches and hearing loss when the skull is affected. Deformities of bone such as enlargement of the forehead, bowing of a limb, and curvature of the spine may occur as the disease progresses.

The course of the disease varies greatly and may range from complete stability to rapid progression. Generally, symptoms progress slowly in affected bones, and usually do not spread to unaffected ones.

Complications of Paget's disease may include osteoarthritis, heart disease, kidney stones and, in rare cases, bone cancer.

Prevalence

Paget's disease affects both men and women, and is most often diagnosed in people over the age of 40. In older adults, the prevalence of Paget's disease is estimated to be about three percent.

Treatment Options

Paget's disease is often detected through X-rays, bone scans or blood tests. An elevated level of serum alkaline phosphatase (a bone-forming enzyme) in a blood test, or some areas of bone which are thick and porous and others that are thinner, are all signs that may indicate Paget's disease. Bone scans can help to determine the extent of the disease.

There is currently no cure for Paget's disease, so treatment is aimed at pain relief and prevention of disease progression. Drugs that suppress disease activity include bisphosphonates (such as Aclasta, Actonel or Fosamax) and calcitonins (such as Caltine or Calcimar). Analgesics and anti-inflammatory drugs may also be used to reduce pain. Orthopedic surgery for joint replacement or stabilization may be recommended.

Paget's disease usually progresses slowly, and is rarely fatal. Serious complications of the disease can be prevented with early and appropriate medical treatment.

National Associations

Canadian Orthopaedic Association (COA) / Association canadienne d'orthopédie
#620, 4060 rue Ste-Catherine ouest, Westmount QC H3Z 2Z3
Tel: 514-874-9003; *Fax:* 514-874-0464
www.coa-aco.org
twitter.com/CdnOrthoAssoc
Overview: A medium-sized national organization founded in 1948
Mission: To provide continuing medical education & training for orthopaedic surgeons
Chief Officer(s):
Douglas C. Thomson, Chief Executive Officer
Publications:
• COA [Canadian Orthopaedic Association] Newsletter
Type: Newsletter; *Frequency:* Quarterly; *Accepts Advertising*; *Editor:*

Dr. Alastair Younger; *Price:* Free with COA membership
Profile: Current events & ideas in orthopaedics

Canadian Orthopaedic Foundation (COF) / Fondation orthopédique du Canada (FOC)
PO Box 1036, Toronto ON M5K 1P2
Tel: 416-410-2341; *Fax:* 416-352-5078
Toll-Free: 800-461-3639
e-mail: mailbox@canorth.org
www.canorth.org
www.facebook.com/pages/Canadian-Orthopaedic-Foundation/1751633
19218018
twitter.com/CanOrthoFound
Overview: A medium-sized national charitable organization founded in 1965
Mission: To foster excellence in the provision of health care to patients with musculoskeletal disease or injury, in a cost effective manner, based on significant outcome studies, by supporting research, educating its members & securing funding from government & other health care funding agencies
Affliation(s): World Orthopaedic Concern; Canadian Medical Association
Chief Officer(s):
Geoffrey Johnston, Chair & President
James Hall, Vice Chair
Publications:
• OrthoLink
Type: Newsletter; *Frequency:* Quarterly
Profile: Information & practical tips for people interested in building & maintaining bone & joint health

Canadian Orthopaedic Nurses Association (CONA) / Association canadienne des infirmières et infirmiers en orthopédie
7714 - 80 Ave., Edmonton AB T6C 0S4
www.cona-nurse.org
Overview: A medium-sized national organization founded in 1978
Mission: To foster professional growth of the membership in the assessment, treatment & rehabilitation of individuals with neuromuscular & skeletal alterations; To promote nursing research related to orthopaedics
Affliation(s): Canadian Nurses Association
Chief Officer(s):
Candace Kenyon, President
Publications:
• Orthroscope [a publication of the Canadian Orthopaedic Nurses Association]
Type: Newsletter; *Frequency:* Quarterly; *Price:* Free with CONA membership
Profile: National newsletter with current events in orthopaedic nursing

Canadian Orthopaedic Residents Association (CORA) / L'Association Canadienne des Residents en Orthopédie (ACRO)
#450, 4150, rue Sainte-Catherine ouest, Montréal QC H3Z 2Y5
Tel: 514-874-9003; *Fax:* 514-874-0464
e-mail: coraweb@canorth.org
www.coraweb.org
Overview: A small national organization
Mission: To foster & promote research & education in the field of Orthopaedic Surgery
Chief Officer(s):
Nadia Murphy, President
nlmurphy@dal.ca

Canadian Society of Orthopaedic Technologists (CSOT) / Société canadienne des technologistes en orthopedie
#715A, 18 Wynford Dr., Toronto ON M3C 3S2
Tel: 416-445-4516; *Fax:* 416-489-7356
e-mail: csot@look.ca
www.pappin.com/csot
Overview: A small national licensing organization founded in 1972
Mission: To promote & develop training programs & professional standards; To encourage uniform training programs & examinations; To promote & facilitate cooperation between Orthopaedic Technologists & the medical profession
Chief Officer(s):

Alba Greco, President
    agreco3@cogeco.ca
Pamela Smith, Office Manager & Registrar
Publications:
• BodyCast [a publication of the Canadian Society of Orthopaedic Technologists]
Type: Journal; *Frequency:* s-a.; *Editor:* Tony Romeo
• NewsCast [a publication of the Canadian Society of Orthopaedic Technologists]
Type: Newsletter; *Frequency:* s-a.

Alberta Chapter
303 Chaparral Dr. SE, Calgary AB T2X 3L9

Tel: 403-201-2423

Chief Officer(s):
Pam Nadon, President

Graham Bell Chapter
26 Geneva Crt., Brantford ON L6S 1B8

Tel: 905-791-7970

Chief Officer(s):
Adam Bradley, President

Manitoba Chapter
c/o Pan Am Clinic, 75 Poseidon Bay, Winnipeg MB R3M 3E4

Tel: 204-925-1522

Chief Officer(s):
Mary Kate Turner, President

Niagara Chapter
22 Lyndon St. West, Thorold ON L2V 3J7

Tel: 906-321-6201

Chief Officer(s):
Stephanie Koch, President

Northtechs Chapter
6211-149 Ave., Edmonton AB T5A 1W1

Tel: 780-342-4056

Chief Officer(s):
Ellanore Gallagher, President

Wascana Chapter
200 Angus St., Regina SK S4R 3K4

Tel: 306-775-2100

Chief Officer(s):
Dustin Livingstone, President

Provincial Associations

QUÉBEC

Association d'orthopédie du Québec
Tour de L'Est, CP 216, Succ. Desjardins, 2, Complexe Desjardins, 30e étage, Montréal QC H5B 1G8

Tél: 514-844-0803; *Téléc:* 514-844-6786
Courriel: aoq@fmsq.org
www.orthoquebec.ca

Aperçu: *Dimension:* moyenne; *Envergure:* provinciale surveillé par Fédération des médecins spécialistes du Québec
Mission: Valoriser le statut professionnel de ses membres; promouvoir leurs intérêts économiques; contribuer au développement de la chirurgie orthopédique et de la traumatologie par le biais d'activités de formation médicale continue
Membre(s) du bureau directeur:
Robert Turcotte, Président
Jean-François Joncas, Secrétaire-trésorier

Paraphilias

Paraphilias are sexual disorders or perversions in which sexual intercourse is not the desired goal. Instead, the desire is to use non-human objects or non-sexual body parts for sexual activities sometimes involving the suffering of, or inflicting pain onto, non-consenting partners. According to the Diagnostic and Statistical Manual of Mental Disorders the criteria for paraphilias include recurrent, intense, sexually arousing fantasies, urges or behaviour involving the particular perversion for at least six months; the fantasies, urges or behaviour cause distress or disruption in the person's functioning in social, work and interpersonal areas.

Paraphiliacs are almost exclusively male. Very few volunteer to disclose their activities or to seek treatment. It is estimated that most have deficits in interpersonal or sexual relationships. In one study, two thirds were diagnosed with mood disorders and 50 percent had alcohol or drug abuse problems.

Recent studies provide evidence that the great majority of paraphiliacs are active in more than one form of sexually perverse behaviour; less than 10 percent have only one form; and 38 percent engage in five or more sexually deviant behaviours. At the same time, the incidence and prevalence of some sexual perversions are hard to estimate, or unknown, because they are rarely reported or the people involved do not come into contact with authorities.

There are eight paraphilias: exhibitionism, fetishism, frotteurism, pedophilia, sexual masochism, sexual sadism, transvestic fetishism and voyeurism.

Exhibitionism

Symptoms
Exhibitionism is characterized by the compulsion to expose the genitals to a stranger or group of strangers. The person with this problem often has an urge to shock or sexually arouse his victims. The "flasher" does not usually engage in sexual contact with the victim, but sometimes masturbates during exposure.

Prevalence
The onset of this disorder usually occurs before age 18 and becomes less severe after age 40. In almost all cases, exhibitionists are male.

Treatment Options
A diagnosis of exhibitionism is made after a psychiatric evaluation, neurological examination (to rule out other medical conditions that might be causing the symptoms) and assessment of responses to a sexual behaviour questionnaire.

Therapy for exhibitionism may include psychotherapy and medications such as selective serotonin reuptake inhibitors (SSRIs), female hormones such as medroxyprogesterone acetate (MPA) and anti-androgens (agents that reduce the level of testosterone in the blood).

Fetishism

Symptoms
Fetishism is characterized by the use of non-living objects, known as fetishes, for sexual gratification. Objects commonly used by men with the disorder include women's underwear, shoes or other articles of women's clothing. The person with this problem often masturbates while holding, rubbing or smelling the fetish object.

Prevalence
This chronic disorder usually begins in adolescence; it is rarely diagnosed in women.

Treatment Options
A diagnosis of fetishism is usually made by direct observation, or after taking a detailed history. It is rare for people with a fetish to seek professional treatment.

Frotteurism

Symptoms

Frotteurism is characterized by sexual arousal, and sometimes masturbation to orgasm, while rubbing against a non-consenting, unfamiliar person. The behaviour is usually planned to occur in a crowded place, such as on a bus, subway or in a swimming pool, where detection is less likely.

Prevalence

Frotteurism usually begins in adolescence, is most frequent between the ages of 15 and 25, then gradually declines. Most acts of frotteurism are performed by males.

Treatment Options

It is rare for people with this problem to seek professional treatment. If referred to a mental health professional, diagnosis is usually confirmed by means of an interview with the patient, and possibly the victim or other people who observed the act of frotteurism.

Treatment may include behaviour therapy and medication such as medroxyprogesterone acetate (MPA).

Pedophilia

Symptoms

Pedophilia is characterized by sexual activity with a child, generally 13 years or younger. The pedophiliac must be at least 16 and at least five years older than his victim when the behaviour occurs. Pedophiliacs are usually attracted to children in one particular age range. The frequency of the behaviour may be associated with the degree of stress in the person's life.

Prevalence

Pedophilia usually begins in adolescence and is chronic. Pedophiles may be married, but have a higher than average incidence of marital discord. Men are more likely than women to engage in pedophilia.

Treatment Options

It is rare for pedophiles to voluntarily seek professional treatment. If referred to a mental health professional, a pedophile would be treated with long-term psychotherapy. However, the success rate for this form of therapy is not high. Pedophilia may also be treated with medication including female hormones such as medroxyprogesterone acetate (MPA), luteinizing hormone-releasing hormone (LHRH) agonists and anti-androgens (agents that reduce the level of testosterone in the blood). In some cases, surgical castration is offered as a therapy option for pedophiles.

Sexual Masochism

Symptoms

Sexual masochists engage in acts of bondage, beating, humiliation, or some other sort of suffering in order to become sexually aroused. The behaviours can be self-inflicted or performed with a partner, and include physical bondage, blindfolding and humiliation.

Prevalence

Masochistic sexual fantasies are likely to have been present since childhood. The activities themselves begin at different times but are common by early adulthood; they are usually chronic. The severity of the behaviours may increase over time.

Treatment Options

It is not uncommon for consenting adults to engage in masochism, but most of the time, these activities are acted out and do not cause real pain. Sexual masochism is diagnosed when acts that cause suffering and humiliation make a person sexually aroused.

The behaviour must also cause significant distress and interfere with work, social and everyday life.

Many people with this disorder do not seek treatment. If therapy is sought out, behavioural therapy and medication to reduce fantasies are often used. Medications prescribed to treat sexual masochism may include female hormones such as medroxyprogesterone acetate (MPA), anti-androgen medications (which reduce the level of testosterone in the blood) and selective serotonin reuptake inhibitors (SSRIs).

Sexual Sadism

Symptoms

Sexual sadism is characterized by acts in which the person becomes sexually excited through the physical or psychological suffering of someone else. Some sexual sadists may conjure up the sadistic fantasies during sexual activity without acting on them. Others act on their sadistic urges with a consenting partner (who may be a sexual masochist), or act on their urges with a non-consenting partner. The behaviour may involve forcing the other person to crawl, be caged or tortured. When the disorder is severe or coupled with antisocial personality disorder, the person is likely to seriously injure or kill his victim.

Prevalence

Sadistic sexual fantasies are likely to have been present in childhood. The onset of the behaviour varies but most commonly occurs by early adulthood. The disorder is usually chronic, and severity tends to increase over time.

Treatment Options

As with masochism, it is not uncommon for consenting adults to engage in sadism, but most of the time, these activities are acted out and do not cause real pain. Sexual sadism is diagnosed when real acts that cause suffering and humiliation make a person sexually aroused. The behaviour must also cause significant distress and interfere with work, social and everyday life.

Many people with this disorder do not seek treatment. If therapy is sought out, behavioural therapy and medication to reduce fantasies are often used. Medications prescribed to treat sexual sadism may include female hormones such as medroxyprogesterone acetate (MPA), anti-androgen medications (which reduce the level of testosterone in the blood) and selective serotonin reuptake inhibitors (SSRIs).

Transvestic Fetishism

Symptoms

Transvestic fetishism consists of heterosexual males dressing in women's clothes and makeup to become sexually aroused. When not cross-dressed, the man looks like an ordinary man. It is important to note that there is considerable controversy over this diagnosis; some people who cross-dress seem to have little distress and function normally.

Prevalence

This condition typically begins in childhood or adolescence. Often the cross-dressing is not done publicly until adulthood.

Treatment Options

Transvestic fetishism is only diagnosed as a mental health disorder if it causes a person significant distress and interferes with his work, social or family life. Most people do not seek treatment for cross-dressing.

Voyeurism

Symptoms

Voyeurism, sometimes called Peeping Tom disorder, involves the act of observing one or more unsuspecting persons (usually strangers) who are naked, in the process of undressing, or engaged in sexual activity, in order for the voyeur to become sexually excited. Sexual activity with the people being observed is not usually sought. The voyeur may masturbate during the observation or later.

Prevalence

The onset of this disorder is usually before age 15. It tends to be chronic and is more common in men.

Treatment Options

Voyeurism is only diagnosed as a mental health disorder if it causes a person significant distress and interferes with his or her work, social or family life. Most people do not seek treatment for voyeurism, but when they do, behavioural therapy is most commonly used.

All the paraphilias are difficult to treat. In some cases (for example, exhibitionism, frotteurism, pedophilia, sexual sadism), treatment is associated with the risk of reporting and punishment; so many individuals do not have any real interest in being treated. They may deliberately deceive the professional, or deny the problem. Sex offenders are also more likely to exaggerate treatment gains, resist treatment or end treatment prematurely.

The fact that these conditions are classified as mental disorders does not relieve individuals who violate laws of criminal responsibility.

National Associations

Canadian Counselling & Psychotherapy Association (CCPA) / L'Association canadienne de counseling et de psychothérapie (ACCP)
#6, 203 Colonnade Rd. South, Ottawa ON K2E 7K3
Tel: 613-237-1099; *Fax:* 613-237-9786
Toll-Free: 877-765-5565
www.ccpa-accp.ca
www.facebook.com/CCPA.ACCP
twitter.com/ccpa_accp
Previous Name: Canadian Counselling Association
Overview: A medium-sized national organization founded in 1965
Mission: To enhance the counselling profession in Canada; To promote policies & practices which support the provision of accessible, competent, & accountable counselling services throughout the human lifespan, & in a manner sensitive to the pluralistic nature of society
Chief Officer(s):
Natasha Caverley, President
president@ccpa-accp.ca
Barbara MacCallum, Chief Executive Officer
bmaccallum@ccpa-accp.ca

Alberta & Northwest Territories Chapter
AB
Chief Officer(s):
Kathy Offet Gartner, President
president@abnwtchapter.ca
British Columbia Chapter
BC
www.ccpa-accp.ca/en/chapters/britishcolumbia
Chief Officer(s):
Paul Yeung, President
Career Development Chapter
www.ccpa-accp.ca/en/chapters/careercounsellors
Chief Officer(s):
Jessica Isenor, President
jisen010@uottawa.ca

Counsellor Educators Chapter
www.ccpa-accp.ca/en/chapters/counselloreducator
Chief Officer(s):
Patrice Keats, President
Creative Arts in Counselling Chapter
www.ccpa-accp.ca/en/chapters/creativeartsincounselling
Chief Officer(s):
Amy Mackenzie, President
amy.mackenzie@gmail.com
Indigenous Circle Chapter
www.ccpa-accp.ca/chapters/indigenous-circle
Chief Officer(s):
Jamie Warren, President
jwarrencounselling@gmail.com
National Capital Region Chapter
Ottawa ON
Chief Officer(s):
Nicholas Renaud, President
nicholas.renaud@gmail.com
Pastoral & Spiritual Care in Counselling Chapter
www.ccpa-accp.ca/en/chapters/pastoralspiritualcare
Chief Officer(s):
Gerard Vardy, President
Private Practitioners Chapter
www.ccpa-accp.ca/en/chapters/privatepractitioners
Chief Officer(s):
Corrine Hendricken-Eldershaw, President
corrinealz@eastlink.ca
School Counsellors Chapter
www.ccpa-accp.ca/en/chapters/schoolcounsellors
Chief Officer(s):
Belinda Josephson, President
gjosephson@eastlink.ca
Social Justice Chapter
www.ccpa-accp.ca/en/chapters/socialjustice
Chief Officer(s):
Linda Wheeldon, Chair
linda.wheeldon@acadiau.ca
Andria Hill-Lehr, Chair
andrialehr@yahoo.ca

General Practice Psychotherapy Association (GPPA)
312 Oakwood Ct., Newmarket ON L3Y 3C8
Tel: 416-410-6644; *Fax:* 866-328-7974
e-mail: info@gppaonline.ca
www.gppaonline.ca
Overview: A small national organization founded in 1984
Mission: To support & encourage quality psychotherapy by physicians in Canada; To promote professional development through ongoing education & collegial interaction
Chief Officer(s):
Carol Ford, Manager

Provincial Associations

QUÉBEC

Association des sexologues du Québec (ASQ)
CP 22147, Succ. Iberville, Montréal QC H1Y 3K8
Tél: 514-270-9289
www.associationdessexologues.com
www.facebook.com/144131012376823
twitter.com/Asso_Sexologues
Aperçu: *Dimension:* petite; *Envergure:* provinciale; fondée en 1978
Mission: Susciter auprès du public une meilleure connaissance de la sexologie et du rôle du sexologue, en favorisant et en maintenant les normes scientifiques et professionnelles les plus élevées dans l'exercice de la sexologie et dans la formation des sexologues
Membre de: Sex Information & Education Council of Canada; World Association of Sexology

ONTARIO

Waypoint Centre for Mental Health Care / Waypoint centre de soins de santé mentale
500 Church St., Penetanguishene ON L9M 1G3

Tel: 705-549-3181
e-mail: info@waypointcentre.ca
www.waypointcentre.ca

Overview: A small local organization founded in 2008
Mission: To provide psychiatric inpatient & outpatient services & mental health programs to individuals in Simcoe County, Dufferin County & Muskoka/Parry Sound
Chief Officer(s):
Betty Valentine, Chair
Carol Lambie, President & CEO

Parkinson's Disease

Parkinson's disease is a chronic, degenerative neurological condition characterized by slow and decreased movement. In people with Parkinson's, the cells that produce dopamine (a chemical in the brain that controls movement) die, or are damaged.

Cause
The cause of Parkinson's is unknown, but both genetic and environmental factors may play a role. In a minority of cases, Parkinson's develops after repeated head trauma, carbon monoxide poisoning, drug use or viral infections that affect the brain.

Symptoms
The progression of Parkinson's varies from person to person. The most common symptoms of Parkinson's include tremor (shaking), muscle stiffness, slow movement and balance problems. Other symptoms may include fatigue, soft speech, reduced facial expression, sleep disturbances, depression and memory problems. As the disease progresses, voluntary movements, such as walking and eating, become more and more difficult. Rigidity and postural instability (difficulty standing up) develop and there is an increased risk of dementia.

Prevalence
Parkinson's affects about 100,000 people in Canada—1 percent of the population over the age of 60, and 2 percent of the population over the age of 70. Twenty percent of people diagnosed with Parkinson's are under the age of 50.

Treatment Options
There are no specific tests used to diagnose Parkinson's disease. Diagnosis is usually based on a medical history and physical and neurological exam. Sometimes other tests (such as blood tests) are used to rule out other health problems that could be causing the symptoms.

Because Parkinson's disease is characterized by reduced levels of dopamine in the brain, drug therapy focuses on increasing dopamine levels, or imitating the action of dopamine. Levodopa, a drug which is converted to dopamine in the brain, is the mainstay of treatment and is associated with improvement of all Parkinson's symptoms. Other medications for Parkinson's disease include dopamine agonists, amantadine, monoamine oxidase type B inhibitors and anticholinergic medications. In cases where drug therapy is no longer effective, surgical treatment of Parkinson's is sometimes considered. In deep brain stimulation an electric charge is sent to areas of the brain that control movement to help block the abnormal signals that Parkinson's produces.

General supportive care should not be neglected, and includes physical therapy and an exercise program to help optimize mobility.

With ongoing monitoring and effective symptom management, many people with Parkinson's disease can remain active and maintain their quality of life.

Parkinson Society Canada (PSC) / Société Parkinson Canada
#316, 4211 Yonge St., Toronto ON M2P 2A9

Tel: 416-227-9700; *Fax:* 416-227-9600
Toll-Free: 800-565-3000
e-mail: general.info@parkinson.ca
www.parkinson.ca

Previous Name: Parkinson Foundation of Canada
Overview: A small national organization founded in 1965
Mission: To raise funds for research into the causes & treatment of Parkinsons; to provide services which support Parkinsonians & their families; to disseminate information about the condition to individuals & organizations across Canada
Member of: Neurological Health Charities Canada; Health Partners; Canadian Coalition for Genetic Fairness
Chief Officer(s):
Joyce Gordon, President & CEO
Marina Joseph, Director, Marketing & Communication
communications@parkinson.ca
Publications:
• ParkinsonPost
Type: Newsletter; *Frequency:* 5 pa; *Editor:* Marina Joseph
Profile: An online subscription for Canada's Parkinson's community, distributed 5 times per year.

ALBERTA

Parkinson Alberta Society (PAS)
Westech Building, #102, 5636 Burbank Cres. SE, Calgary AB T2H 1Z6

Tel: 403-243-9901; *Fax:* 403-243-8283
Toll-Free: 800-561-1911
e-mail: info@parkinsonalberta.ca
www.parkinsonalberta.ca
www.facebook.com/281448621909497
twitter.com/ParkinsonAB
www.youtube.com/user/ParkinsonAlberta

Overview: A small provincial charitable organization founded in 1981 overseen by Parkinson Society Canada
Mission: PAS is dedicated to helping people and families of Southern Alberta who live with Parkinson's and related disorders
Chief Officer(s):
John Petryshen, CEO
jpetryshen@parkinsonalberta.ca
Publications:
• Parkinson Pulse
Type: Newsletter

Edmonton Office
#102, 11748 Kingsway Ave., Edmonton AB T2G 0X5
Tel: 780-425-6400; *Fax:* 780-425-6425

Grande Prairie Office
#103, 10901 - 100 St., Grande Prairie AB T8V 2M9
Tel: 780-882-6640

Chief Officer(s):
Krlsteva Dowling, Coordinator, Client Services
KDowling@parkinsonalberta.ca

Lethbridge Office
St. John's Ambulance Building, 1254 - 3 Ave. South, Lethbridge AB T1J 0J9
Tel: 403-317-7710; *Fax:* 403-327-2820

Chief Officer(s):
Brian Treadwell, Coordinator, Client Services
btreadwell@parkinsonalberta.ca

Medicine Hat Office
United Way of South Eastern Alberta, #101, 928 Allowance Ave. SE, Medicine Hat AB T1A 3G7
Tel: 403-526-5521; *Fax:* 403-526-5244

Chief Officer(s):

Beth Metcalf, Coordinator, Client Services
bmetcalf@parkinsonalberta.ca

Red Deer Office
The Lending Cupboard Society, 5406D - 43 St., Red Deer AB T4P 1C9

Tel: 403-346-4463

Chief Officer(s):
Marilynne Herron, Coordinator, Client Services
mherron@parkinsonalberta.ca

BRITISH COLUMBIA

Parkinson Society British Columbia (PSBC)
#600, 890 West Pender St., Vancouver BC V6C 1J9
Tel: 604-662-3240; *Fax:* 604-687-1327
Toll-Free: 800-668-3330
e-mail: info@parkinson.bc.ca
www.parkinson.bc.ca
www.facebook.com/191326604220827
twitter.com/ParkinsonsBC
www.youtube.com/user/ParkinsonSocietyBC

Overview: A medium-sized provincial organization founded in 1969 overseen by Parkinson Society Canada
Chief Officer(s):
Jean Blake, CEO
jblake@parkinson.bc.ca

MANITOBA

Parkinson Society Manitoba
#7, 414 Westmount Dr., Winnipeg MB R2J 1P2
Tel: 204-786-2637
Toll-Free: 866-999-5558
e-mail: parkinson@mymts.net
www.parkinsonmanitoba.ca
www.facebook.com/ParkinsonSocietyManitobaSuperwalk2013

Previous Name: Parkinson Society Canada - Manitoba Region
Overview: A medium-sized provincial organization overseen by Parkinson Society Canada
Chief Officer(s):
Howard Koks, CEO
howard.koks@parkinson.ca

Brandon/Westman Office
Scotia Towers, #228, 1011 Rosser Ave., Brandon MB R7A 0L5
Tel: 204-726-1702

NEWFOUNDLAND AND LABRADOR

Parkinson Society Newfoundland & Labrador
The Viking Bldg., #305, 136 Crosbie Rd., St. John's NL A1B 3K3
Tel: 709-574-4428; *Fax:* 709-754-5868
Toll-Free: 800-567-7020
e-mail: parkinson@nf.aibn.com
www.parkinsonnl.ca
www.facebook.com/ParkinsonSocietyNewfoundlandAndLabrador
twitter.com/Parkinsons_NL

Overview: A medium-sized provincial organization overseen by Parkinson Society Canada
Chief Officer(s):
Derek Staubitzer, Executive Director

NOVA SCOTIA

Parkinson Society Maritime Region (PSMR) / Société Parkinson - Region Maritime (SPRM)
#150, 7071 Bayers Rd., Halifax NS B3L 2C2
Tel: 902-422-3656; *Fax:* 902-422-3797
Toll-Free: 800-663-2468
e-mail: psmr@parkinsonmaritimes.ca
www.parkinsonmaritimes.ca
www.facebook.com/parkinsonmaritimes
twitter.com/psmr
www.youtube.com/channel/UCo1IYTO_WaeylOiUhkrnjXg

Overview: A small provincial charitable organization overseen by Parkinson Society Canada
Mission: To give information to people with Parkinson & their family, children & caregivers

Chief Officer(s):
Jim Horwich, Chair
Robert Shaw, Regional CEO

QUÉBEC

Société Parkinson du Québec / Parkinson Society Québec
#1080, 550 rue Sherbrooke Ouest, Montréal QC H3A 1B9
Tél: 514-861-4422
Ligne sans frais: 800-720-1307
Courriel: info@parkinsonquebec.ca
www.parkinsonquebec.ca
www.facebook.com/pages/Societe-Parkinson-du-Quebec/4420047026 08772
twitter.com/parkinsonquebec
www.youtube.com/channel/UCMo6s0d7FXkc46ThRFScExQ

Aperçu: *Dimension:* moyenne; *Envergure:* provinciale; Organisme sans but lucratif surveillé par Parkinson Society Canada
Membre(s) du bureau directeur:
Nicole Charpentier, Directrice générale
ncharpentier@parkinsonquebec.ca

SASKATCHEWAN

Parkinson Society Saskatchewan (PSS)
610 Duchess St., Saskatoon SK S7K 0R1
Tel: 306-933-4481; *Fax:* 888-775-1402
Toll-Free: 888-685-0059
e-mail: saskatchewan@parkinson.ca
www.parkinsonsaskatchewan.ca

Overview: A medium-sized provincial charitable organization founded in 1972 overseen by Parkinson Society Canada
Mission: To provide education & support services in Saskatchewan to ease the burdens of people living with Parkinson's disease & their families; To support research to find a cure for Parkinson's disease
Member of: Parkinson Society Canada / Société Parkinson Canada
Chief Officer(s):
Travis Low, Executive Director
traivs.low@parkinson.ca

Local Associations

BRITISH COLUMBIA

Victoria Epilepsy & Parkinson's Centre Society
#202, 1640 Oak Bay Ave., Victoria BC V8R 1B2
Tel: 250-475-6677; *Fax:* 250-475-6619
e-mail: help@vepc.bc.ca
www.vepc.bc.ca
twitter.com/VEPC

Overview: A small local charitable organization founded in 1983
Mission: To provide education & support services to those affected by epilepsy or Parkinson's Disease, individuals & family members; To promote excellence in care through collaboration with the health care community; To increase public understanding of these conditions & expand awareness & support of the services provided
Affliation(s): Canadian Epilepsy Alliance
Chief Officer(s):
Mira Laurence, Executive Director
mlaurence@vepc.bc.ca
Della Cronkrite, Office Manager
Shannon Oatway, Coordinator, Community Education & Awareness

ONTARIO

Parkinson Society Central & Northern Ontario
#321, 4211 Yonge St., Toronto ON M2P 2A9
Tel: 416-227-1200; *Fax:* 416-227-1520
Toll-Free: 800-565-3000
e-mail: info.cno@parkinson.ca
www.cno.parkinson.ca
www.facebook.com/101248525517
twitter.com/ParkinsonCNO

Previous Name: Parkinson Society Canada - Central & Northern Ontario Region
Overview: A small local organization overseen by Parkinson Society Canada
Chief Officer(s):

Debbie Davis, CEO
   debbie.davis@parkinson.ca

Parkinson Society of Eastern Ontario / Société Parkinson de l'est de l'Ontario

#1, 200 Colonnade Rd., Ottawa ON K2E 7M1
Tel: 613-722-9238; *Fax:* 613-722-3241
e-mail: psoc@toh.on.ca
www.parkinsons.ca
twitter.com/ParkinsonEastOn

Previous Name: Parkinson Society Ottawa
Overview: A small local organization founded in 1978 overseen by Parkinson Society Canada
Mission: To improve the lives of individuals & families affected by Parkinson's disease
Affliation(s): Parkinson Society of Canada
Chief Officer(s):
Alan Muir, Manager, Resource Development
   alan.muir@parkinson.ca
Ginette Trottier, Coordinator, Community Development
Publications:
• The Parkinson Paper
Type: Newsletter; *Frequency:* Quarterly

Parkinson Society Southwestern Ontario

Meadowbrook Business Park, #117, 4500 Blakie Rd., London ON N6L 1G5
Tel: 519-652-9437; *Fax:* 519-652-9267
Toll-Free: 888-851-7376
e-mail: info@parkinsonsociety.ca
www.parkinsonsociety.ca
www.facebook.com/parkinsonsociety
twitter.com/ParkinsonSWO

Previous Name: Parkinson Society Canada - Southwestern Ontario Region
Overview: A small local organization overseen by Parkinson Society Canada
Chief Officer(s):
Chris Maciejowski, President
Joanne Bernard, Manager, Administration

QUÉBEC

Association des personnes handicapées physiques et sensorielles du secteur Joliette (APHPSSJ)

200 rue de Salaberry, Joliette QC J6E 4G1
Tel: 450-759-3322; *Fax:* 450-759-8749
Toll-Free: 888-756-3322
e-mail: aphpssj@cepap.ca
www.aphpssj.com

Previous Name: Association of Physically Disabled Joliette - L'Assomption; Association of People with Physical Disabilities Joliette
Overview: A small local organization founded in 1977
Mission: To promote the rights of people with physical & sensory disabilities in the Joliette region; To encourage social integration of disabled people
Member of: Regroupement des associations de personnes traumatisées craniocérébrales du Québec / Coalition of Associations of Craniocerebral Trauma in Quebec
Chief Officer(s):
Jocelyn Picard, Président
Jacynthe Arseneau, 1ère Vice-président
Michel Lacourse, 2e Vice-président
François Gagnon, Secretaire
Murielle Desrosiers, Trésorière
Publications:
• Dynamic Player
Type: Newsletter
Profile: Association updates, announcements, & forthcoming activities

Provincial Libraries

Headway Victoria Epilepsy & Parkinson's Centre Society

#202, 1640 Oak Bay Ave., Victoria, BC V8R 1B2
Tel: 250-475-6677; *Fax:* 250-475-6619
help@vepc.bc.ca
www.vepc.bc.ca

Mira Laurence, Executive Director
   mlaurence@vepc.bc.ca

Pediatric Mental Health Issues

Mental illness is a significant health issue for Canadian children—as many as 13 to 22 percent are affected by mental health problems. Although the media is full of reports about increasing use of psychiatric medications in children, and, tragically, from time to time, stories of children who commit suicide or murder, many young people with mental health problems suffer in silence. Parents, other relatives, guardians and teachers are understandably concerned about not missing the signs of a treatable disorder while, at the same time, not subjecting the child to unnecessary and potentially stigmatizing diagnosis and treatment. Studies suggest that as many as 57 percent of Canadian parents are worried about their children's mental health.

Symptoms

It is often difficult to know whether a child's behaviour is normal for his or her age, if a child is being adversely influenced by circumstances, what the warning signs for a mental disorder are and what constitutes a mental disorder. Canadian studies also show that close to one third of teen girls and nearly half of teen boys do not discuss their concerns about mental health, and only 10 percent of youth share their worries with a family member.

Warning signs of mental illness in children and youth may include self-harm, substance abuse, sudden and unexplained weight loss, difficulty focusing, drastic behaviour changes, dangerous or out-of-control behaviour, unexplained and overwhelming feelings of fear, drastic mood swings and feelings of sadness that last for at least two weeks.

In general, a child or adolescent is evaluated not only on the basis of particular behaviours that cause concern, but also with respect to meeting the milestones expected at his or her age. A child should be increasingly able to relate to other people, both children and adults, and to learn. An untreated mental disorder can deprive a child of essential years of social and educational growth.

It is common for parents to wait and see how a child's mental health symptom (for example, constant moodiness or persistent anxiety about school) will play out before they seek therapy for their child. However, this may cause untreated mental health problems to become more severe.

Prevalence

It is estimated that over 1.25 million Canadian children and youth have mental health problems. The most common mental illness affecting children and youth in Canada is anxiety, followed by conduct disorder and attention deficit disorder. Amongst 12- to 19-year-olds, approximately 5 percent of males and 12 percent of females have been affected by major depression.

Treatment Options

Anyone concerned about a child should start with the child's pediatrician. A child should not be given a diagnosis or prescribed medication without a complete physical health evaluation; specialized observation; and interviews with parents, teachers and others familiar with him or her. There should be no hesitation to obtain a second opinion. Health professionals should be able to explain why a child was or wasn't given a specific diagnosis, and the pros and cons of the treatment choices.

There is a shortage of fully qualified experts in child and adolescent mental health; it may require considerable persistence to ensure that a child receives the attention necessary. Wait times for psychologists and psychiatrists are often as long as six months in Canada, and studies suggest that as many as one in five Canadian children who need therapy for mental health problems do not get it. There are recent initiatives underway in Canada that intend to improve the situation. The Child and Youth Mental Health Practice Support Program in British Columbia is one example. The aim of this program is to train family doctors in the province to diagnose and treat mental health problems in children and teens. Making better use of the school setting to promote child and youth mental health is also under investigation. The Canadian Academy of Child and Adolescent Psychiatry is in the process of developing a page on their website (www.cacap-acpea.org) which will provide families with improved access to child and adolescent mental health information.

Experts suggest that early identification of mental illness in children and youth will improve life outcomes, and reduce the incidence of adult mental health problems. More than 70 percent of adults with a mental illness first experienced symptoms of their condition in childhood or early adolescence. Successful early intervention with children and teens could also go a long way toward changing perceptions about mental illness.

National Associations

Ability Online Support Network / En ligne directe
PO Box 18515, 250 Wincott Dr., Toronto ON M9R 4C8
Tel: 416-650-6207; *Fax:* 866-829-6780
Toll-Free: 866-650-6207
e-mail: information@abilityonline.org
www.abilityonline.org
www.facebook.com/AbilityOnline
twitter.com/Ability_Online
Also Known As: Ability Online
Overview: A small national charitable organization founded in 1992
Mission: To enhance the lives of children with disabilities or illness by providing an online community for friendship, support & skill development
Chief Officer(s):
Michelle McClure, Executive Director
Michael Teixeira, Chair
  miket@abilityonline.org
George Kyriakis, Vice-Chair

Association for Vaccine Damaged Children
67 Shier Dr., Winnipeg MB R3R 2H2
Overview: A small national organization founded in 1986
Mission: To inform parents of the risks of immunization; To support parents in any challenging situation with public health authorities
Chief Officer(s):
Mary James, Co-Founder
  tjames4@shaw.ca

Canadian Academy of Child & Adolescent Psychiatry (CACAP) / Académie canadienne de psychiatrie de l'enfant et de l'adolescent
#701, 141 Laurier Ave. West, Ottawa ON KIP 5J3
Tel: 613-288-0408; *Fax:* 613-234-9857
e-mail: info@cacap-acpea.org
www.cacap-acpea.org
Previous Name: Canadian Academy of Child Psychiatry
Overview: A small national charitable organization founded in 1980
Mission: To advance the mental health of children, youth, & families; To promote the highest standards of patient care & service to children, youth, & families, incorporating a psychological, social, & biological approach
Chief Officer(s):
Wade Junek, President
Elizabeth Waite, Executive Director
Alexa Bagnell, Secretary-Treasurer
Publications:
• Journal of the Canadian Academy of Child & Adolescent Psychiatry
Type: Journal; *Frequency:* Quarterly; *Accepts Advertising*; *Editor:*

Normand Carrey; *ISSN:* 1719-8429
Profile: Featuring original articles, clinical perspectives, & book reviews

Canadian Association for Child & Play Therapy
PO Box 24010, Guelph ON N1E 6V8
Tel: 519-827-1506; *Fax:* 519-827-1825
e-mail: membership@cacpt.com
www.cacpt.com
Overview: A small national organization
Mission: To advance & promote play therapy; To set high professional & ethical play therapy practice standards; To support research & professional training in the play therapy field
Chief Officer(s):
Elizabeth A. Sharpe, Executive Director
  elizabeth@cacpt.com
Publications:
• Playground Magazine [a publication of the Canadian Association for Child & Play Therapy]
Type: Magazine; *Frequency:* Quarterly; *Accepts Advertising*; *Editor:* Lorie Walton
Profile: Information on Play Therapy; Association information & upcoming events

Canadian Association of Paediatric Health Centres (CAPHC) / Association canadienne des centres de santé pédiatriques
c/o Canadian Association of Paediatric Health Centres, #104, 2141 Thurston Dr., Ottawa ON K1G 6C9
Tel: 613-738-4164; *Fax:* 613-738-3247
e-mail: info@caphc.org
www.caphc.org
www.facebook.com/ACCSP.CAPHC
twitter.com/CAPHCTweets
Previous Name: Canadian Association of Paediatric Hospitals
Overview: A medium-sized national organization founded in 1968
Mission: To improve the health of children within Canada through research activities & through advocacy with governments & health care organizations; To provide information exchange amongst members
Chief Officer(s):
Elaine Orrbine, President & Chief Executive Officer
  eorrdine@caphc.org
Doug Maynard, Associate Director
  dmaynard@caphc.org

Canadian Association of Paediatric Surgeons (CAPS) / Association de la chirurgie infantile canadienne
c/o Children's Hospital Of Winnipeg, 840 Sherbrook St., #AE401, Winnipeg MB R3A 1S1
Tel: 204-787-1246; *Fax:* 204-787-4618
e-mail: admin@caps.ca
www.caps.ca
www.facebook.com/CAPSsurgeons
twitter.com/CAPSsurgeons
Overview: A medium-sized national organization
Mission: To improve the surgical care of infants & children in Canada
Chief Officer(s):
B.J. Hancock, Secretary-Treasurer

Canadian Association of Pregnancy Support Services
#304 - 4820 Gaetz Ave., Red Deer AB T4N 4A4
Tel: 403-347-2827; *Fax:* 403-343-2847
Toll-Free: 866-845-2151
www.capss.com
www.facebook.com/CanadianAssociationOfPregnancySupportServices?ref=str
twitter.com/CAPSS_RD
Overview: A small national organization
Mission: A Christian national ministry dedicated to providing support for life and sexual health by partnering with Pregnancy Centres across Canada.
Affiliation(s): Evangelical Fellowship of Canada; Canadian Council of Christian Charities
Chief Officer(s):
Lola French, Executive Director, 403-347-2827
  lola@capss.com

Canadian Institute for Child & Adolescent Psychoanalytic Psychotherapy (CICAPP)
17 Saddletree Trail, Brampton ON L6X 4M5
Tel: 416-690-5464; *Fax:* 416-690-2746
e-mail: info@cicapp.ca
www.cicapp.ca

Previous Name: Toronto Child Psychoanalytic Program
Overview: A small national organization founded in 1981
Mission: To provide training in psychodynamic child therapy; to foster the growth of the profession in Canada; to have input in shaping government policies; to promote ongoing research in child psychotherapy
Chief Officer(s):
Suzanne Pearen, Administrator
suzanne_pearen@rogers.com

Canadian Institute of Child Health (CICH) / Institut canadien de la santé infantile
#300, 384 Bank St., Ottawa ON K2P 1Y4
Tel: 613-230-8838; *Fax:* 613-230-6654
e-mail: cich@cich.ca
profile.cich.ca
www.facebook.com/313427342097626
twitter.com/CICH_ICSI

Overview: A medium-sized national charitable organization founded in 1977
Mission: To promote the health & well-being of Canadian children through consultation, collaboration, research & advocacy by building alliances & coalitions & by creating resources on health promotion, disease & injury prevention relevant to child & family health in Canada; To identify issues of concern by monitoring the health & well-being of children in Canada; To promote & improve the health & well-being of mothers & infants in all settings; To promote the healthy physical development of children in a safe environment & reduce childhood injuries; To promote the healthy psycho-social development of children in supportive & nurturing environments; To facilitate empowerment of individuals & communities to achieve the above goals for Canadian children & their families; To facilitate collaborative work between consumers, professional, non-professional & government agencies that results in appropriate actions for identified needs
Member of: Canadian Coalition for the Prevention of Developmental Disabilities; Coalition of National Voluntary Organizations; Canadian Coalition on the Rights of the Child; Children's Alliance; Breastfeeding Committee for Canada; National Literacy & Health Program
Affliation(s): Canadian Children's Environmental Health Network; Key Institution of Childwatch International; International Network for Child Health, Environment & Safety; WHO/European Environment Agency Working Group on the Environment & Children's Health
Chief Officer(s):
Janice Sonmen, Executive Director
Publications:
• Child Health [a publication of the Canadian Institute of Child Health]
Type: Newsletter; *Frequency:* Quarterly; *ISSN:* 0838-9683; *Price:* Free with CICH membership
Profile: National news about child health & well-being issues

Canadian Lactation Consultant Association (CLCA) / Association canadienne des consultantes en lactation
4 Innovation Dr., Dundas ON L9H 793
Tel: 905-689-3980; *Fax:* 905-689-1465
e-mail: clca-accl@gmail.com
www.clca-accl.ca
www.linkedin.com/groups/Canadian-Lactation-Consultant-Association-CLCA
www.facebook.com/welcomeback/requests/#!/CLCA.ACCL
twitter.com/cdnlactation

Overview: A small national organization founded in 1986
Affliation(s): International Lactation Consultant Association
Chief Officer(s):
Lauretta Williams, Administrator

Canadian Paediatric Society (CPS) / Société canadienne de pédiatrie
#100, 2305 St. Laurent Blvd., Ottawa ON K1G 4J8
Tel: 613-526-9397; *Fax:* 613-526-3332
www.cps.ca
www.linkedin.com/company/canadian-paediatric-society
www.facebook.com/CanadianPaediatricSociety
twitter.com/canpaedsociety
www.youtube.com/canpaedsociety

Overview: A medium-sized national organization founded in 1922
Mission: To advocate for the health needs of children & youth; To provide continuing education to paediatricians; To establish national guidelines for paediatric care & practice
Member of: International Paediatric Association
Chief Officer(s):
Jonathan Kronick, President
Marie Adèle Davis, Executive Director
madavis@cps.ca
Elizabeth Moreau, Director, Communications & Knowledge Translation
elizabethm@cps.ca
Publications:
• CPS [Canadian Paediatric Society] News
Type: Newsletter; *Frequency:* 5 pa; *Accepts Advertising*; *Price:* Free with CPS membership
Profile: Current society activities for CPS members
• Paediatrics & Child Health [a publication of the Canadian Paediatric Society]
Type: Journal; *Accepts Advertising*; *Price:* Free with CPS membership
Profile: Educational information & research reports for clinicians, parents, & caregivers

Canadian Pediatric Endocrine Group (CPEG) / Groupe canadien d'endocrinologie pédiatrique (GCEP)
c/o Robert Barnes, M.D., Montreal Children's Hospital, #316E, 2300, rue Tupper, Montréal QC H3H 1P3
Tel: 514-412-4315; *Fax:* 514-412-4264
www.cpeg-gcep.net

Overview: A small national organization
Mission: To promote the study of pediatric endocrinology
Chief Officer(s):
Robert Barnes, Secretary-Treasurer

Canadian Pediatric Foundation (CPF) / La fondation canadienne de pédiatrie
#100, 2305 St. Laurent Blvd., Ottawa ON K1G 4J8
Tel: 613-526-9397; *Fax:* 613-526-3332
www.cps.ca
www.linkedin.com/company/canadian-paediatric-society
www.facebook.com/CanadianPaediatricSociety
twitter.com/canpaedsociety
www.youtube.com/canpaedsociety

Overview: A medium-sized national organization founded in 1985
Mission: To promote improved health care & social well-being for the children of Canada, particularly for disadvantaged groups; To promote better standards of health care for children throughout the world, particularly where Canadian aid is active
Chief Officer(s):
Marie Adèle Davis, Executive Director, 613-526-9397 Ext. 226
madavis@cps.ca
Elizabeth Moreau, Director, Communications & Knowledge Translation
elizabethm@cps.ca
Jackie Millette, Director, Education, Committees & Sections
jackiem@cps.ca
Jane Cheesman, Director, Finance & Administration
janec@cps.ca

Childhood Cancer Canada Foundation
#801, 21 St. Clair Ave. East, Toronto ON M4T 1L9
Tel: 416-489-6440; *Fax:* 416-489-9812
Toll-Free: 800-363-1062
e-mail: info@childhoodcancer.ca
www.childhoodcancer.ca
www.facebook.com/ChildhoodCancerCanada
twitter.com/chldhdcancercan

Overview: A large national organization founded in 1987
Mission: To help improve the lives of children suffering from cancer through family support programs; to fund cancer research

Chief Officer(s):
Glenn Fraser, Chair

British Columbia Childhood Cancer Parent's Association
British Columbia Children's Hospital, #A127A, 4480 Oak St.,
   Vancouver BC V6H 3B8
Tel: 604-875-2345

Candlelighters Newfoundland & Labrador
PO Box 5846, St. John's NL A1C 5X3
Tel: 709-745-4448
Toll-Free: 866-745-4448
e-mail: info@Candlelightersnl.ca
www.candlelightersnl.ca
www.facebook.com/CandlelightersNL
twitter.com/CandlelighterNL

Chief Officer(s):
Amanada Kinsman, Coordinator, Provincial Family Program
   coordinator@candlelightersnl.ca

Manitoba - Candlelighters Childhood Cancer Support Group
PO Box 350, RR#1, Winkler MB R6W 4A1
e-mail: support@manitobacandlelighters.ca
www.manitobacandlelighters.ca

Chief Officer(s):
Denis Foidart, Chair, 204-737-2684
   denlis@wiband.ca

ON - Candlelighters Simcoe
6 Emily Ct., Barrie ON L4N 6B4
Tel: 705-737-4296; *Fax:* 705-737-4836

Chief Officer(s):
Barbara Johnson, Coordinator
   albarbjohnson@sympatico.ca

SK - Candlelighters - Prince Albert
350 - 30th St. East, Prince Albert SK S6V 1Z4
Tel: 306-763-7356

SK - Regina Candlelighters
100 cardinal Cres., Regina SK S4S 4Y7
Tel: 306-529-3292
e-mail: sask.candlelighters@sasktel.net

Chief Officer(s):
David Achter, Contact
Tangy Achter, Contact

Children's Heart Association for Support & Education (CHASE)
Tel: 416-410-2427
e-mail: kidheart@angelfire.com
www.angelfire.com/on/chase
Overview: A small national organization founded in 1984
Mission: Organization committed to promoting awarness about congenital heart disease; to provide encouragement to families affected by CHD; driven to become the leading provider of resoures to education & support those who seek an understanding of the disease.

Provincial Associations
BRITISH COLUMBIA

British Columbia Play Therapy Association (BCPTA)
#335, 2818 Main St., Vancouver BC V5T 0C1
Tel: 778-710-7529
bcplaytherapy.ca
www.facebook.com/196439843813637
Overview: A small provincial organization founded in 1993
Mission: To promote the status of play therapy in British Columbia, encourage sound play therapy principles; promote high standards of professional and ethical conduct; and nurture the professional development of play therapists within a supportive association.

ONTARIO

Association of Parent Support Groups in Ontario Inc. (APSGO)
PO Box 27581, Stn. Yorkdale, Toronto ON M6A 3B8
Toll-Free: 800-488-5666
e-mail: mail@apsgo.ca
www.apsgo.ca
twitter.com/APSGOca

Overview: A small provincial charitable organization founded in 1985
Mission: To enable parents to develop strategies to deal with their children's disruptive behaviour
Chief Officer(s):
Maureen MacNeil, President
Publications:
• Parent to Parent
Type: Newsletter; *Editor:* Sue Kranz

Children's Mental Health Ontario (CMHO) / Santé Mentale pour Enfants Ontario (SMEO)
#309, 40 St. Clair Ave. East, Toronto ON M4T 1M9
Tel: 416-921-2109; *Fax:* 416-921-7600
e-mail: info@cmho.org
www.cmho.org
www.linkedin.com/company/747188
www.facebook.com/kidsmentalhealth
twitter.com/kidsmentalhlth
www.youtube.com/user/ChangeTheView2016
Also Known As: Ontario Association of Children's Mental Health Centres
Overview: A medium-sized provincial charitable organization founded in 1972
Mission: To promote, support & strengthen a sustainable system of mental health services for children, youth & their families
Member of: Child Welfare League of Canada
Chief Officer(s):
Kimberly Moran, Chief Executive Officer
   kmoran@cmho.org

Kinark Child & Family Services
#200, 500 Hood Rd., Markham ON L3R 9Z3
Tel: 905-944-7086; *Fax:* 905-474-1448
Toll-Free: 800-230-8533
e-mail: info@kinarkfoundation.org
www.kinarkfoundation.org
www.facebook.com/kinark
twitter.com/mykinark
Overview: A small provincial organization founded in 1972
Mission: To strengthen the well-being of children & their families, thereby contributing to safe & healthy communities; seek to achieve this goal by being a provider of choice in the delivery of the highest quality services to our clients in partnership with community resources
Affiliation(s): Children's Mental Health Ontario
Chief Officer(s):
Cheri Smith, Director, Development
   cheri.smith@kinarkfoundation.org

Ontario Association of Children's Aid Societies (OACAS) / Association ontarienne des sociétés de l'aide à l'enfance
#308, 75 Front St. East, Toronto ON M5E 1V9
Tel: 416-987-7725; *Fax:* 416-366-8317
Toll-Free: 800-718-7725
e-mail: public_editor@oacas.org
www.oacas.org
www.linkedin.com/company/ontario-association-of-children-s-aid-societi
twitter.com/our_children
Overview: A medium-sized provincial organization founded in 1912
Mission: To provide leadership for the achievement of excellence in the protection of children & in the promotion of their well-being within their families & communities
Chief Officer(s):
Nancy MacGillivray, Executive Director
Publications:
• Ontario Association of Children's Aid Societies Child Welfare Report
Type: Report; *Frequency:* Annually
Profile: Outlines recommendations & areas of priority for the child welfare sector
• Ontario Association of Children's Aid Societies Journal
Type: Journal; *Frequency:* s-a.; *Number of Pages:* Y; *Editor:* Bernadette Gallagher; *ISSN:* 0381-985X; *Price:* $16
Profile: Features articles & news on child welfare practice & research in Ontario
• Ontario Association of Children's Aid Societies Annual Report
Type: Report; *Frequency:* Annually
• The Voice [a publication of the Ontario Association of Children's Aid Societies]

Type: Newsletter; *Frequency:* Monthly
Profile: Contains association initiatives & advocacy effort, public engagement opprtunities, & other child welfare sector news

Ontario Association of Children's Rehabilitation Services (OACRS) / Association ontarienne des services de réhabilitation pour enfants (AOSRE)
150 Kilgour Rd., Toronto ON M4G 1R8

Tel: 416-424-3864
e-mail: info@oacrs.com
www.oacrs.com
www.facebook.com/OACRS
twitter.com/OACRS
www.youtube.com/OACRS

Previous Name: Association of Treatment Centres of Ontario
Overview: A medium-sized provincial charitable organization founded in 1973
Mission: To promote a province-wide, coordinated, community-based service system for children & youth with multiple disabilities & their families; To support members centres to achieve responsive, family-centred care
Affliation(s): Kid's Coalition
Chief Officer(s):
Jennifer Churchill, Chief Executive Officer
   jchurchill@oacrs.com

Parents for Children's Mental Health (PCMH)
PO Box 20004, St Catharines ON L2N 7W7

Tel: 416-220-0742
Toll-Free: 855-254-7264
e-mail: admin@pcmh.ca
www.pcmh.ca
www.facebook.com/PCMHOntario
twitter.com/PCMHontario

Overview: A small provincial organization founded in 1994
Mission: To provide a voice for children & families in Ontario who are affected by mental health problems
Chief Officer(s):
Michele Sparling, Chair
Sarah Cannon, Executive Director

QUÉBEC

Association des pédiatres du Québec
CP 216, Succ. Desjardins, #3000, 2, Complexe Desjardins, Montréal QC H5B 1G8

Tél: 514-350-5127; *Téléc:* 514-350-5177
Courriel: pediatrie@fmsq.org
www.pediatres.ca

Aperçu: *Dimension:* moyenne; *Envergure:* provinciale surveillé par Fédération des médecins spécialistes du Québec
Membre de: Fédération des Médcins Spécialistes du Québec (FMSQ)
Affliation(s): Association des allergologues et immunologues du Québec; Association des anesthésiologistes du Québec; Association des médecins biochimistes du Québec; Association des cardiologues du Québec; Association des chirurgiens cardio-vasculaires et thoraciques du Québec; Association québécoise de chirurgie; Association des chirurgiens vasculaires du Québec; Association des spécialistes en chirurgie plastique et esthétique du Québec; Association des dermatologistes du Québec; Association des médecins endocrinologues du Québec; Association des gastro-entérologues du Québec
Membre(s) du bureau directeur:
May Dagher, Directrice, Administration

SASKATCHEWAN

Ranch Ehrlo Society
Pilot Butte Campus, PO Box 570, Pilot Butte SK S0G 3Z0

Tel: 306-781-1800; *Fax:* 306-757-0599
e-mail: inquiries@ranchehrlo.ca
www.ehrlo.ca
www.facebook.com/RanchEhrlo
twitter.com/RanchEhrlo
www.youtube.com/user/ranchehrlo1

Previous Name: Saskatchewan Council on Children & Youth
Overview: A medium-sized provincial charitable organization

Mission: To provide a range of quality assessment, treatment, education & support services that improve the social & emotional functioning of children & youth
Chief Officer(s):
Andrea Brittin, President & CEO

Local Associations

ALBERTA

Big Brothers Big Sisters Edmonton & Area
10135 - 89 St., Edmonton AB T5H 1P6

Tel: 780-424-8181; *Fax:* 780-426-6689
Toll-Free: 855-424-8181
bgcbigs.ca
www.facebook.com/BGCBigs
twitter.com/BGCBigs

Overview: A small local charitable organization
Mission: To ensure the healthy development of children & their families through wellness programs & professionally supported volunteer mentoring relationships
Affliation(s): Big Brothers Big Sisters of Canada; United Way, Alberta Capital Region; Boys & Girls Clubs of Edmonton & Area
Chief Officer(s):
Liz O'Neill, Executive Director
Kerry Woodland, Director, Service Delivery
Dawna Morgan, Manager, Finance
Danisha Bhaloo, Manager, Development
Lana Tordoff, Manager, Marketing & Communications

Calgary Children's Foundation
c/o CHQR FM, #170, 200 Barclay Parade SW, Calgary AB T2P 4R5

Tel: 403-444-4337

Overview: A small local organization
Mission: To promote the mental & physical health & welfare of children & certain adults who are disadvantaged & reside within Alberta
Chief Officer(s):
Betty Jo Kaiser, Administrator
   bettyjo.kaiser@corusent.com

Children's Heart Society
#128, 9920 63 Ave., Edmonton AB T6E 0G9

Tel: 780-454-7665
e-mail: childrensheart@shaw.ca
www.childrensheart.ca
www.facebook.com/childrenshearts
twitter.com/childrenshearts

Overview: A small local organization
Mission: To support children with heart disease & their families
Chief Officer(s):
Andrea Luft, President
   chsgalaedmonton@gmail.com
Danielle Tailleur, Director, Membership
   dtailleur@ellisdon.com

Churchill Park Family Care Society
3311 Centre St. NW, Calgary AB T2E 2X7

Tel: 403-266-4656; *Fax:* 403-264-5657
e-mail: cpfirst@churchillpark.ca
www.churchillpark.ca
www.facebook.com/133191603370805

Overview: A small local organization founded in 1970
Mission: To offer quality child care; To help families & caregivers access support & emergency assistance
Chief Officer(s):
Sharon Reib, Executive Director
Dionne Maier, Senior Director, Human Resources
Don Ballance, Director, Finance
Christie Scarlett, Director, Operations

Kids Kottage Foundation
10107 - 134 Ave., Edmonton AB T5E 1J2

Tel: 780-448-1752; *Crisis Hot-Line:* 780-944-2888
e-mail: info@kidskottage.org
www.kidskottage.org
www.facebook.com/kidskottageYEG
twitter.com/KidsKottageEDM

Previous Name: Canadian Foundation for the Love of Children

Overview: A medium-sized local charitable organization founded in 1987
Mission: To promote the health & well-being of children & their families; To prevent child abuse & neglect by supporting families in crisis
Chief Officer(s):
Lori Reiter, Executive Director
Dianne Petersen, Program Manager

Variety Club of Southern Alberta
Calgary AB

Tel: 403-228-6168
e-mail: info@varietyalberta.ca
www.varietyalberta.ca
www.facebook.com/VarietyAlberta

Overview: A small local charitable organization founded in 1982
Mission: To provide disabled & disadvantaged children with the means to enjoy quality life experiences; to support research for below the knee amputee children; to provide assistance & bursaries to children in special situations
Affiliation(s): Variety Children's Lifeline

BRITISH COLUMBIA

Cariboo Chilcotin Child Development Centre Association (CDC)
690 - 2nd Ave. North, Williams Lake BC V2G 4C4
Tel: 250-392-4481; Fax: 250-392-4432
www.cccdca.org

Overview: A medium-sized local organization founded in 1975
Mission: To work in partnership with families & the community; To provide a comprehensive continuum of quality developmental support services for children & their families
Member of: BC Association for Child Development & Rehabilitation
Chief Officer(s):
Jerry Tickner, President

Centre for Child Development
9460 - 140th St., Surrey BC V3V 5Z4
Tel: 604-584-1361; Fax: 604-583-5113
e-mail: info@centreforchilddevelopment.ca
www.the-centre.org
www.facebook.com/thecentreforchilddevelopment
twitter.com/Centreforchild
www.youtube.com/user/Centreforchild

Previous Name: South Fraser Child Development Centre; Lower Fraser Valley Cerebral Palsy Association
Overview: A medium-sized local charitable organization founded in 1953
Mission: To provide services for children with special needs & their families
Affiliation(s): BC Association of Child Development & Rehabilitation; Cerebral Palsy Association of BC; Commission on the Accreditation of Rehabilitation Facilities Canada (CARF)
Chief Officer(s):
Joe Hall, Chair
Gerard Bremault, Chief Executive Officer
  gerard@the-centre.org
Amber Robinson, Vice-President, Marketing Communications
  amber@the-centre.org

Kitimat Child Development Centre
1515 Kingfisher Ave., Kitimat BC V8C 1S5
Tel: 250-632-3144; Fax: 250-632-3120
e-mail: info@kitimatcdc.ca
www.kitimatcdc.ca

Overview: A small local organization founded in 1974
Mission: To ensure that special needs children have equal opportunities to be the best that they can be
Member of: BC Association for Community Living; Canadian Council for Exceptional Children; Spina Bifida Association of BC; Child Development & Rehabilitation Network; Association for the Care of Children's Health
Chief Officer(s):
Margaret Warcup, Executive Director
  mwarcup@kitimatcdc.ca

McCreary Centre Society (MCS)
3552 Hastings St. East, Vancouver BC V5K 2A7
Tel: 604-291-1996; Fax: 604-291-7308
e-mail: mccreary@mcs.bc.ca
www.mcs.bc.ca

Previous Name: Friends of the McCreary Centre Society
Overview: A small local charitable organization founded in 1977
Mission: To raise awareness & understanding of youth health & related issues; To address the health needs of young people through the development of projects & initiatives
Member of: Canadian Health Network
Chief Officer(s):
Annie Smith, Executive Director

Quesnel & District Child Development Centre Association (QDCDCA)
488 McLean St., Quesnel BC V2J 2P2
Tel: 250-992-2481; Fax: 250-992-3439
www.quesnelcdc.com
www.facebook.com/quesnel.childdevelopmentcentre

Overview: A small local charitable organization founded in 1976
Mission: To assist local children by providing intervention programs which facilitate their physical, social, emotional, communicative & intellectual development
Affiliation(s): BC Association for Child Development & Intervention
Chief Officer(s):
Corrina Norman, President

Starbright Children's Development Centre
1546 Bernard Ave., Kelowna BC V1Y 6R9
Tel: 250-763-5100; Fax: 250-862-8433
Toll-Free: 877-763-5100
e-mail: info@starbrightokanagan.ca
iwishimight.ca
www.facebook.com/iwishimight
www.pinterest.com/starbrightchild

Previous Name: Central Okanagan Child Development Association; Okanagan Neurological Association
Overview: A medium-sized local charitable organization founded in 1966
Mission: To support families in promoting the optimum development of children with challenges
Affiliation(s): British Colombia Association of Child Development Centres
Chief Officer(s):
Rhonda Nelson, Executive Director

Step-By-Step Child Development Society
PO Box 47601, Stn. Blue Mountain, Coquitlam BC V3K 6T3
Tel: 604-931-1977
www.step-by-step.ca

Overview: A small local charitable organization founded in 1979
Mission: To provide preschool education to children requiring extra supports; To operate an equipment loans cupboard for children requiring specialized equipment; To provide physiotherapy & occupational therapy services to children; To provide outreach support services to neighbourhood child care centres; To promote inclusion of children needing extra supports
Member of: British Columbia Association Child Development & Rehabilitation
Chief Officer(s):
Carla Arrano, Manager

Victoria Youth Empowerment Society
533 Yates St., Victoria BC V8W 1K7
Tel: 250-383-3514; Fax: 250-383-3812
e-mail: office_manager@vyes.ca
www.vyes.ca

Merged from: Alliance Club; Association for Street Kids
Overview: A small local charitable organization founded in 1992
Mission: To assist youth to remove themselves from the high risk environment of the street & make the transition to healthier & more constructive life situations; To help youth make positive choices which will prevent involvement in at risk behaviour or connection with the street scene
Member of: Federation of Child & Family Services of BC; United Way

MANITOBA

Child & Family Services of Western Manitoba (C&FS Western)
800 McTavish Ave., Brandon MB R7A 7L4

Tel: 204-726-6030; *Fax:* 204-726-6775
Toll-Free: 800-483-8980
e-mail: info@cfswestern.mb.ca
www.cfswestern.mb.ca

Previous Name: Children's Aid Society of Western Manitoba
Overview: A medium-sized local charitable organization founded in 1899
Mission: To ensure children are safe in strong loving families within caring communities
Member of: Child Welfare League of Canada
Chief Officer(s):
Phil Shaman, President
Candace Kowalchuk, Specialist, Human Resources
  hr@cfswestern.mb.ca
Susan Cable, Coordinator, Community Education
  commed@cfswestern.mb.ca

Jewish Child & Family Services (JCFS)
123 Doncaster St., #C200, Winnipeg MB R3N 2B2

Tel: 204-477-7430; *Fax:* 204-477-7450
Other Communication: After Hours Emergency Phone: 204-946-9510
e-mail: info@jcfswinnipeg.org
www.jcfswinnipeg.org
www.linkedin.com/company/jewish-child-and-family-service

Overview: A small local charitable organization founded in 1952
Mission: To provide social services that focus on 3 areas: care of children, family problems, & concern for the needs of recent immigrants
Chief Officer(s):
Al Benarroch, Executive Director

NOVA SCOTIA

Adsum for Women & Children
2421 Brunswick St., Halifax NS B3K 2Z4

Tel: 902-423-5049; *Fax:* 902-423-9336; *Crisis Hot-Line:* 902-423-4443
e-mail: adsum@adsumforwomen.org
www.adsumforwomen.org
www.facebook.com/pages/Adsum-for-Women-Children/111571128907431
twitter.com/AdsumForWomen
www.youtube.com/user/adsumforwomen

Previous Name: Association for Women's Residential Facilities
Overview: A medium-sized local charitable organization founded in 1983
Mission: To administer Adsum House; To provide emergency shelter for homeless women & children
Chief Officer(s):
Sheri Lecker, Executive Director
  sheri.lecker@adsumforwomen.org

Chisholm Services for Children
5724 South St., Halifax NS B3H 1S4

Tel: 902-423-9871; *Fax:* 902-422-3725
e-mail: info@chisholm4children.ca
www.chisholm4children.ca
twitter.com/chisholm4c

Overview: A medium-sized local charitable organization founded in 2004
Mission: To offer residential care, support, & early intervention programs for children in need; To provide resources, education, & advocacy to meet the needs of children
Chief Officer(s):
Wade Johnston, Executive Director
  wjohnston@chisholm4children.ca
Daniel Abar, Director, Clinical Services
  dabar@chisholm4children.ca
Geoff Hurst, Director, Business Development
  ghurst@chisholm4children.ca

ONTARIO

Alva Foundation
c/o Graham Hallward, 199 Albertus Ave., Toronto ON M4R 1J6

e-mail: info@alva.ca
www.alva.ca

Previous Name: Southam Foundation
Overview: A medium-sized local charitable organization founded in 1965
Mission: To fund research into risk factors in early childhood development (pre-natal to 3 years of age); To fund pilot programs on demonstrations of new therapies serving the constituency described above
Chief Officer(s):
Christopher Kerrigan, President
Graham F. Hallward, Chair, Donations Committee

Brant Family & Children's Services
PO Box 774, 70 Chatham St., Brantford ON N3T 5R7

Tel: 519-753-8681; *Fax:* 519-753-6090
Toll-Free: 888-753-8681; *TTY:* 519-753-8323
www.brantfacs.ca

Previous Name: Children's Aid Society of Brant
Overview: A small local organization founded in 1894
Mission: To provide child welfare & family services in Brantford, Brant, Six Nations, & New Credit; To foster & build healthy families & family relationships through guidance & education
Member of: Ontario Association of Children's Aid Societies
Affliation(s): Contact Brant; Lansdowne Children's Centre; St. Leonard's Community Services; Brant County Health Unit; Nova Vita Domestic Violence Prevention Services
Chief Officer(s):
Andrew Koster, Executive Director

Bruce Grey Child & Family Services (BGCFS)
1290 - 3rd Ave. East, Owen Sound ON N4K 2L5

Tel: 519-371-4453; *Fax:* 519-376-8934
Toll-Free: 855-322-4453
www.bgcfs.ca

Previous Name: Bruce Children's Aid Society
Merged from: The Children's Aid Societies of Bruce & Grey Counties
Overview: A small local organization founded in 2012
Mission: To protect children by providing supportive services to children & families through partnerships
Chief Officer(s):
David F. Wyles, President
Phyllis Lovell, Executive Director

Catholic Children's Aid Society of Hamilton (CCAS)
735 King St. East, Hamilton ON L8M 1A1

Tel: 905-525-2012; *Fax:* 905-525-5606
Other Communication: Emergency After Hours Phone: 905-525-5606
www.hamiltonccas.on.ca
www.facebook.com/hamiltonccas
twitter.com/HamiltonCCAS
www.youtube.com/channel/UCfI8rgJy4r8oMcepjfErppw/feed

Overview: A small local charitable organization founded in 1954
Mission: To provide child welfare & family services to the Hamilton community; To ensure that services are guided by Catholic values
Member of: Ontario Association of Children's Aid Societies
Affliation(s): Council of Catholic Service Organziations
Chief Officer(s):
Ersilia DiNardo, Executive Director

Catholic Children's Aid Society of Toronto (CCAS)
26 Maitland St., Toronto ON M4Y 1C6

Tel: 416-395-1500; *Fax:* 416-395-1581
e-mail: communications@torontoccas.org
www.ccas.toronto.on.ca

Previous Name: Catholic Children's Aid Society of Metropolitan Toronto
Overview: A medium-sized local charitable organization founded in 1894
Mission: To provide social services that protect children, strengthen family life & are reflective of Catholic values
Member of: Catholic Charities of the Archdiocese of Toronto
Affliation(s): Ministry of Children and Youth Services

Chief Officer(s):
Janice Robinson, Executive Director
Publications:
• Catholic Children's Aid Society of Toronto Annual Report
Type: Report; *Frequency:* a.
• Connections [a publication of the Catholic Children's Aid Society of Toronto]
Type: Newsletter; *Frequency:* 3 pa

East Toronto Branch
1880 Birchmount Rd., Toronto ON M1P 2J7
Chief Officer(s):
Nancy DiNatale, Branch Manager

North West Toronto Branch
30 Drewry Ave., Toronto ON M2M 4C4
Chief Officer(s):
Nyron Sookraj, Branch Manager

Scarborough Branch
843 Kennedy Rd., Toronto ON M1K 2E3
Chief Officer(s):
Domenic Gratta, Branch Manager

South Toronto Branch
Dufferin Mall, #219, 900 Dufferin St., Toronto ON M6H 4B1
Chief Officer(s):
Renée Walsh, Branch Manager

Child & Parent Resource Institute (CPRI)
600 Sanatorium Rd., London ON N6H 3W7
Tel: 519-858-2774; *Fax:* 519-858-3913
Toll-Free: 877-494-2774; *TTY:* 519-858-0257
www.cpri.ca

Previous Name: Children's Psychiatric Research Institute
Overview: A medium-sized local organization founded in 1960
Mission: To enhance the quality of life of children & youth with complex mental health or developmental challenges; to assist their families so these children & youth can reach their full potential
Member of: Ontario Association of Children's Mental Health Centres

Children's Aid Society of Algoma / Société de l'aide à l'enfance d'Algoma
191 Northern Ave. East, Sault Ste Marie ON P6B 4H8
Tel: 705-949-0162; *Fax:* 705-949-4747
Toll-Free: 888-414-3571
www.algomacas.org

Overview: A small local organization founded in 1902
Mission: To protect the children of Algoma; to promote their well-being in a manner that reflects community standards & the spirit or legislation, while making efficient use of community & society resources
Member of: Ontario Association of Children's Aid Societies
Chief Officer(s):
Kim Streich-Poser, Executive Director

Blind River Office
9 Lawton St., Blind River ON P0R 1B0
Tel: 705-356-1464; *Fax:* 705-356-0773

Elliot Lake Office
29 Manitoba Rd., Elliot Lake ON P5A 2A7
Tel: 705-848-8000; *Fax:* 705-848-5145

Hornepayne Office
#7, 8 - 2nd St., Hornepayne ON P0M 1Z0
Tel: 807-868-2624

Wawa Office
31 Algoma St., Wawa ON P0S 1K0
Tel: 705-856-2960; *Fax:* 705-856-7379

Children's Aid Society of Ottawa (CASO) / La Société de l'aide à l'enfance d'Ottawa
1602 Telesat Ct., Gloucester ON K1B 1B1
Tel: 613-747-7800; *Fax:* 613-747-4456; *TTY:* 613-742-1617
e-mail: yourcasquestion@casott.on.ca
www.casott.on.ca
www.facebook.com/ottawacas
twitter.com/OttawaCas
www.youtube.com/user/casott123
Previous Name: Ottawa-Carleton Children's Aid Society

Overview: A small local charitable organization founded in 1893
Mission: To protect the children & youth of the Ottawa area from abuse & neglect, as regulated by Ontario's Ministry of Children & Youth Services & as governed by the Child & Family Services Act
Chief Officer(s):
Tess Porter, Executive Director
Publications:
• Children's Aid Society of Ottawa Annual Report
Type: Report; *Frequency:* a.

Children's Aid Society of Oxford County
712 Peel St., Woodstock ON N4S 0B4
Tel: 519-539-6176; *Fax:* 519-421-0123
Toll-Free: 800-250-7010
e-mail: info@casoxford.on.ca
www.casoxford.on.ca

Also Known As: CAS Oxford
Previous Name: Oxford Family & Child Services
Overview: A small local organization founded in 1895
Mission: To serve & promote the best interests, protection & well-being of children, while supporting the autonomy, integrity & cultural diversity of families and communities
Member of: Ontario Association of Children's Aid Societies
Chief Officer(s):
Bruce Burbank, Executive Director

Children's Aid Society of the District of Nipissing & Parry Sound / La Société d'aide à l'enfance Nipissing & Parry Sound
433 McIntyre St. West, North Bay ON P1B 2Z3
Tel: 705-472-0910; *Fax:* 705-472-9743
Toll-Free: 877-303-0910
www.parnipcas.org

Previous Name: Nipissing Children's Aid Society for the District of Nipissing & Parry Sound
Overview: A small local licensing charitable organization founded in 1907
Mission: To promote the well-being & protection of children & youth, and advocates for their fundamental rights
Member of: Ontario Association of Children's Aid Societies
Chief Officer(s):
Joe Rogers, President

Children's Aid Society of the Districts of Sudbury & Manitoulin (CAS) / La Société d'aide à l'enfance des districts de Sudbury et de Manitoulin
#3, 319 Lasalle Blvd., Sudbury ON P3A 1W7
Tel: 705-566-3113; *Fax:* 705-521-7372
Toll-Free: 800-272-4334
www.casdsm.on.ca

Merged from: Sudbury Children's Aid Society; Manitoulin Children's Aid Society
Overview: A medium-sized local charitable organization founded in 1971
Mission: To protect the well-being of children in the community
Member of: Ontario Association of Children's Aid Societies
Chief Officer(s):
Elaina Groves, Executive Director

Chapleau Office
34 Birch St. East, Chapleau ON P0M 1K0
Tel: 705-864-0329; *Fax:* 705-864-2133

Children's Aid Society of the Region of Peel
West Tower, 6860 Century Ave., Mississauga ON L5N 2W5
Tel: 905-363-6131; *Fax:* 905-363-6133
Toll-Free: 888-700-0996
e-mail: mail@peelcas.org
www.peelcas.org
www.youtube.com/user/PeelChildrensAid

Also Known As: Peel Children's Aid
Overview: A medium-sized local charitable organization founded in 1944
Mission: To protect children & strengthen families & communities through partnership
Chief Officer(s):
Rav Bains, Executive Director

Children's Hospital of Eastern Ontario Foundation
415 Smyth Rd., Ottawa ON K1H 8M8

Tel: 613-737-2780; *Fax:* 613-738-4818
Toll-Free: 800-561-5638
www.cheofoundation.com
www.facebook.com/CHEOkids
twitter.com/cheohospital
www.youtube.com/user/CHEOvideos

Also Known As: Children's Hospital Foundation
Overview: A medium-sized local charitable organization founded in 1974
Mission: To advance the physical, mental, & social well-being of children & their families in Eastern Ontario & Western Quebec by raising, managing, & disbursing funds; To support the Children's Hospital of Eastern Ontario
Member of: Children's Miracle Network Telethon
Chief Officer(s):
Mahesh Mani, Chair
Len Hanes, Director, Communications
lhanes@cheofoundation.com

Family & Children's Services Niagara (FACS)
PO Box 24028, St Catharines ON L2R 7P7

Tel: 905-937-7731; *Fax:* 905-646-7085
Toll-Free: 888-937-7731
e-mail: info@facsniagara.on.ca
www.facsniagara.on.ca
www.facebook.com/familyandchildrensservicesniagara
twitter.com/FACSNiagara

Also Known As: FACS Niagara
Overview: A large local charitable organization founded in 1898
Mission: To protect children & support those in need of safe homes; To provide guidance & counselling services to families; To investigate all reports of possible child abuse or neglect
Member of: Ontario Association of Children's Aid Societies
Chief Officer(s):
Chris Steven, Executive Director

Family & Children's Services of Frontenac, Lennox & Addington
817 Division St., Kingston ON K7K 4C2

Tel: 613-545-3227; *Fax:* 613-542-4428
Toll-Free: 855-445-3227
e-mail: info@facsfla.ca
www.facsfla.ca
www.facebook.com/facsfla
twitter.com/FACSFLA
www.youtube.com/user/FACSFLA

Merged from: Children's Aid Society of the City of Kingston and County of Frontenac; Lennox & Addington CAS
Overview: A small local charitable organization founded in 1994
Mission: To provide professional child protection services which safeguard children, support nurturing environments & strengthen families
Member of: Ontario Association of Children's Aid Societies
Affliation(s): Community Living Kingston; Kingston Interval House; Northern Frontenac Community Services; Frontenac Community Mental Health Services; Pathways for Children & Youth; Youth Diversion Program
Chief Officer(s):
Steve Woodman, Executive Director

Family & Children's Services of Guelph & Wellington County (F&CS)
PO Box 1088, 275 Eramosa Rd., Guelph ON N1H 6N3

Tel: 519-824-2410; *Fax:* 519-763-9628
Toll-Free: 800-265-8300
e-mail: info@fcsgw.org
www.fcsgw.org
www.facebook.com/371460589598793
twitter.com/fcsgw

Also Known As: Children's Aid Society of Guelph & Wellington County
Overview: A small local charitable organization founded in 1934
Mission: To provide help & support services for families to ensure that children are protected from physical & emotional abuse or neglect.
Member of: Ontario Association of Children's Aid Societies
Chief Officer(s):

Daniel Moore, Executive Director

Family & Children's Services of Renfrew County
#100, 77 Mary St., Pembroke ON K8A 5V4

Tel: 613-735-6866; *Fax:* 613-735-6641
Toll-Free: 800-267-5878
e-mail: inquiries@fcsrenfrew.on.ca
www.fcsrenfrew.on.ca

Previous Name: Renfrew Family & Child Services
Overview: A medium-sized local charitable organization founded in 1935
Mission: To support & enhance the lives of children, youth, & families in Ontario's County of Renfrew by providing essential, mandated, & volutary services; To improve the quality of life for children, youth, & adults with developmental disabilities
Member of: Ontario Association of Children's Aid Societies
Chief Officer(s):
Arijana Tomicic, Executive Director

Family & Children's Services of the District of Rainy River (FACS)
820 Lakeview Dr., Kenora ON P9N 3P7

Tel: 807-467-5437; *Fax:* 807-467-5539; *Crisis Hot-Line:* 800-465-1100
www.krrcfs.ca

Also Known As: Kenora-Patricia Child & Family Services
Overview: A small local charitable organization founded in 1935
Mission: To ensure the safety of children & youth; to provide a variety of services to protect them; to investigate any concerns of their abuse or neglect.
Member of: Ontario Association of Children's Aid Societies; Children's Mental Health Associations of Ontario
Chief Officer(s):
Bill Leonard, Executive Director
Publications:
• Developmental Services Newsletter [a publication of the Family & Children's Services of the District of Rainy River]
Type: Newsletter; *Frequency:* Bimonthly
• Family & Children's Services of the District of Rainy River Newsletter
Type: Newsletter; *Frequency:* 7 pa

Halton Children's Aid Society
1445 Norjohn Ct., Burlington ON L7L 0E6

Tel: 905-333-4441; *Fax:* 905-333-1844
Toll-Free: 866-607-5437
www.haltoncas.ca

Overview: A large local charitable organization founded in 1914
Mission: To protect children & youth while respecting their diverse needs; To strengthen families
Member of: Ontario Association of Children's Aid Societies
Chief Officer(s):
Nancy MacGillivray, Executive Director

Hamilton District Society for Disabled Children (HDSDC)
325 Wellington St., Hamilton ON L8L 0A4

Tel: 905-385-5391

Overview: A small local organization founded in 1951
Mission: To assist in addressing the needs of children (under 21 years of age) who have physical disabilities that affect gross or fine motor control & that limit their ability to function in activities of daily living, by providing financial assistance to projects not funded by other agencies or government
Chief Officer(s):
Mark Matson, President

Helping Other Parents Everywhere Inc. (HOPE)
1740 Kingston Rd., Pickering ON L1V 2R2

Tel: 905-239-3577
Toll-Free: 866-492-1299
e-mail: info@hope4parents.ca
www.hope4parents.ca

Overview: A small local organization
Mission: To provide support, resources, & education to parents of disruptive youth; To offer a confidential & non-judgemental environment for parents who want to deal more effectively with the behaviour of their children; To empower concerned parents to handle situations with their children
Chief Officer(s):

Leanne Lewis, President
president@hope4parents.ca

Highland Shores Children's Aid
363 Dundas St. West, Belleville ON K8P 1B3
Tel: 613-962-9291; *Fax:* 613-966-3868
Toll-Free: 800-267-0570; *TTY:* 613-962-1019
e-mail: info@highlandshorescas.com
www.highlandshorescas.com
Previous Name: Hastings Children's Aid Society
Overview: A small local charitable organization founded in 1907
Member of: Ontario Association of Children's Aid Societies
Chief Officer(s):
Michael McLeod, President

Cobourg
1005 Burnham St., Cobourg ON K9A 5J6
Tel: 905-372-1821; *Fax:* 905-372-5284
Toll-Free: 800-267-0570

North Hastings
PO Box 837, #104, 16 Billa St., Bancroft ON K0L 1C0
Tel: 613-332-2425; *Fax:* 613-332-5686
Toll-Free: 866-532-2269

Picton
16 MacSteven Dr., Picton ON K0K 2T0
Tel: 613-476-7957; *Fax:* 613-476-2316
Toll-Free: 800-267-0570; *TTY:* 613-962-1019

Quinte West
469 Dundas St. West, Trenton ON K8V 3S4
Tel: 613-965-6261; *Fax:* 613-965-0930
Toll-Free: 800-267-0570

Hincks-Dellcrest Treatment Centre & Foundation
440 Jarvis St., Toronto ON M4Y 2H4
Tel: 416-924-1164; *Fax:* 416-924-8208
Toll-Free: 855-944-4673
e-mail: info@hincksdellcrest.org
www.hincksdellcrest.org
www.facebook.com/hincksdellcrest
twitter.com/hincksdellcrest
www.youtube.com/thehincksdellcrest
Overview: A small local organization founded in 1998
Mission: To offer a comprehensive range of mental health services to infants, children, youth, & their families; to provide a variety of programs, including prevention & early intervention, outpatient & residential treatment.
Affliation(s): University of Toronto
Chief Officer(s):
Ian Smith, Chair
Donna Duncan, President & CEO

Infant Feeding Action Coalition
533 Colborne St., London ON N6B 2T5
Tel: 416-595-9819
e-mail: info@infactcanada.ca
www.infactcanada.ca
Also Known As: INFACT Canada
Previous Name: Infant/Maternal Nutrition Education Association
Overview: A small local organization
Mission: To protect, promote & support breastfeeding in Canada & globally; to promote better infant & maternal health; to foster appropriate mother & infant nutrition
Member of: Canadian Council for International Cooperation
Chief Officer(s):
Elisabeth Sterken, National Director
esterken@infactcanada.ca

Jewish Family & Child (JFCS)
4600 Bathurst St., 1st Fl., Toronto ON M2R 3V3
Tel: 416-638-7800; *Fax:* 416-638-7943
e-mail: info@jfandcs.com
www.jfandcs.com
www.linkedin.com/company/jewish-family-&-child
www.facebook.com/JFandCS
www.youtube.com/user/jewishfamilyandchild
Overview: A small local charitable organization founded in 1868

Mission: To support the healthy development of individuals, families & communities in the Greater Toronto Area through prevention, protection, counselling, education & advocacy services, within the context of Jewish values
Affliation(s): Family Service Ontario; Association of Jewish Family & Children's Agencies; Canadian Family Services Accreditation Program; Children's Mental Health Ontario; Council on Accreditation; Ontario Association of Children's Aid Societies; Ontario Association of Social Workers; Ontario College of Social Workers and Social Service Workers
Chief Officer(s):
Brian Prousky, Executive Director
Publications:
• Family Matters [a publication of Jewish Family & Child]
Type: Newsletter; *Frequency:* monthly
Profile: Contains agency updates & important news
• Jewish Family & Child Annual Report
Type: Report; *Frequency:* a.

Kawartha-Haliburton Children's Aid Society
1100 Chemong Rd., Peterborough ON K9H 7S2
Tel: 705-743-9751; *Fax:* 757-437-858
Toll-Free: 800-661-2843
www.khcas.on.ca
Overview: A small local organization
Mission: To protect children, youth, & young adults by engaging & cooperating with families & the wider community
Member of: Ontario Association of Children's Aid Societies
Chief Officer(s):
Deirdre Thomas, President

Haliburton
HALCO Plaza, PO Box 958, 83 Maple Ave., Haliburton ON K0M 1S0
Tel: 705-457-1661
Toll-Free: 800-661-1979

Lindsay
42 Victoria Ave. North, Lindsay ON K9V 4G2
Tel: 705-324-3594
Toll-Free: 800-567-9136

London-Middlesex Children's Aid Society
PO Box 7010, 1680 Oxford St. East, London ON N5Y 5R8
Tel: 519-455-9000; *Fax:* 519-455-4355
Toll-Free: 888-661-6167; *TTY:* 519-455-6498
e-mail: info@caslondon.on.ca
www.caslondon.on.ca
www.linkedin.com/company/children's-aid-society-of-london-&-middlesex
Overview: A small local organization
Mission: To protect & care for at-risk children & families
Member of: Ontario Association of Childrens' Aid Societies
Chief Officer(s):
Regina Bell, Interim Executive Director

Multiple Birth Families Association (MBFA)
PO Box 5532, Stn. F, Ottawa ON K2C 3M1
Tel: 613-860-6565
www.mbfa.ca
Previous Name: Ottawa Twins' Parents Association
Overview: A small local charitable organization founded in 1961
Mission: Giving parents an opportunity to get together & share ideas on raising multiples - the joys & the pitfalls
Chief Officer(s):
Olga Kutikov, President
president@mbfa.ca

North Eastern Ontario Family & Children's Services / Services à la famille et à l'enfance du Nord Est de l'Ontario
707 Ross Ave. East, Timmins ON P4N 8R1
Tel: 705-360-7100; *Fax:* 705-360-7200
www.neofacs.org
Previous Name: Child & Family Services of Timmins & District
Overview: A medium-sized local organization
Mission: To ensure the well-being of children & families
Chief Officer(s):
Don Anderson, President

Our Place (Peel)
3579 Dixie Rd., Mississauga ON L4Y 2B3

Tel: 905-238-6916
e-mail: info@ourplacepeel.org
www.ourplacepeel.org

Overview: A small local charitable organization founded in 1985
Mission: To provide emergency shelter & residential services for disadvantaged & homeless youth, from ages 16 to 21, in Peel Region
Chief Officer(s):
Christy Upshall, Executive Director
 cupshall@ourplacepeel.org

Ronald McDonald House Toronto
240 McCaul St., Toronto ON M5T 1W5

Tel: 416-977-0458; *Fax:* 416-977-8807
e-mail: info@rmhtoronto.ca
www.rmhtoronto.ca
www.linkedin.com/company/ronald-mcdonald-house-toronto
www.facebook.com/RMHCToronto
twitter.com/RMHToronto

Also Known As: Toronto Children's Care Inc.
Previous Name: Children's Oncology Care of Ontario Inc.
Overview: A small local charitable organization founded in 1981
Mission: To provide a home & support services for out-of-town families whose children are receiving treatment in Toronto hospitals for serious illness
Chief Officer(s):
Sally Ginter, Chief Executive Officer
 sginter@rmhctoronto.ca
Anita Price, Office Manager
 aprice@rmhctoronto.ca

Toronto Parents of Multiple Births Association (TPOMBA)
#356, 1920 Ellesmere Rd., Toronto ON M1H 3G1

Tel: 416-760-3944
e-mail: info@tpomba.org
www.tpomba.org
www.facebook.com/TorontoParentsOfMultipleBirthsAssociation
twitter.com/TPOMBA
plus.google.com/u/0/b/116137137302949869664

Previous Name: Toronto Parents of Twins Club
Overview: A small local organization founded in 1976
Mission: To provide guidance & help to adjust to multiple birth situations through educational meetings, support groups, social events for families & adults, & member services; to enable families to cope with their unique situation & therefore lead a full life
Chief Officer(s):
Camille Kloppenburg, President

Windsor-Essex Children's Aid Society (WECAS)
1671 Riverside Dr. East, Windsor ON N8Y 5B5

Tel: 519-256-1171; *Fax:* 519-256-2739
e-mail: foundation@wecas.on.ca
www.wecaf.on.ca

Overview: A small local organization founded in 1899
Mission: Dedicated to the well being & safety of every child by advocating for & partnering with our children, families & communities
Member of: Ontario Association of Children's Aid Societies
Chief Officer(s):
Cheryl Sprague, Interim President

York Region Children's Aid Society
Kennedy Place, 16915 Leslie St., Newmarket ON L3Y 9A1

Tel: 905-895-2318; *Fax:* 905-895-2113
Toll-Free: 800-718-3850
www.yorkcas.org

Also Known As: York Region CAS
Previous Name: Children & Family Services for York Region
Overview: A small local charitable organization
Mission: To protect children & promote a safe, healthy & caring environment for them in partnership with a diverse community
Member of: Ontario Association of Children's Aid Societies
Chief Officer(s):
Colette Prévost, Executive Director

QUÉBEC

Association de balle des jeunes handicapés de Laval-Laurentides-Lanaudière (ABJHLLL)
2020, av Laplante, Laval QC H7S 1E7

Tél: 450-689-4668

Également appelé: Association de balle des jeunes handicapés de Laval/ABJHL
Aperçu: *Dimension:* petite; *Envergure:* locale; Organisme sans but lucratif; fondée en 1995
Mission: Etablir et opérer des équipes de balle pour la détente de l'esprit et du corps de jeunes handicapés physiques et/ou intellectuels, garçons et filles, principalement des régions de Laval, Laurentides et Lanaudière. Organiser et maintenir toute autre activités social, sportive et culturelle connexe pour promouvoir les buts de la corporations
Membre de: La petite ligue de baseball du Québec (Division Challenger)
Membre(s) du bureau directeur:
Tony Condello, Responsable
 tcondello@videotron.ca

Association de parents d'enfant trisomique-21 de Lanaudière
245, ch des Anglais, Mascouche QC J7L 3P3

Tél: 450-477-4116; *Téléc:* 560-477-3534
www.apetl.org
www.facebook.com/199268050113168

Aperçu: *Dimension:* petite; *Envergure:* locale; fondée en 1990
Affliation(s): Association du Québec pour l'intégration sociale
Membre(s) du bureau directeur:
Chantal Lamarre, Directrice générale

Association des parents d'enfants handicapés du Témiscamingue inc.
#1, 3, rue Industrielle, Ville-Marie QC JV9 1S3

Tél: 819-622-1126; *Téléc:* 819-622-0021
Courriel: apeht@cablevision.qc.ca

Aperçu: *Dimension:* petite; *Envergure:* locale
Mission: Offrir des services d'aide aux personnes vivant avec un handicap physique et intellectuel ainsi qu'à leurs familles.
Affliation(s): Association du Québec pour l'intégration sociale

Batshaw Youth & Family Centres
5 Weredale Pk., Westmount QC H3Z 1Y5

Tel: 514-989-1885
www.batshaw.ca

Overview: A small local organization founded in 1992
Mission: To intervene with children and families in situations of abuse, neglect, abandonment & when youth have serious behaviour problems, providing psychosocial, rehabilitation & social integration services.
Chief Officer(s):
Judy Martin, President
Lesley Hill, Executive Director

Les Centres jeunesse de l'Outaouais (CJO)
105, boul Sacré-Coeur, Gatineau QC J8X 1C5

Tél: 819-771-6631
www.cjoutaouais.qc.ca

Merged from: Centre de services sociaux de l'Outaouais; Centre de réadaptation les jeunes de l'Outaouais
Aperçu: *Dimension:* petite; *Envergure:* locale; Organisme sans but lucratif; fondée en 1942
Mission: Nous assurons la protection des jeunes; nous amenons les jeunes à assumer leurs responsabilités et à se réadapter à la société en les aidant à retrouver un équilibre personnel et social; nous aidons enfants et adultes à se préparer à une adoption; nous aidons les enfants adoptés et parents naturels à reprendre contact; nous offrons notre expertise dans certaines causes de divorce; nous assurons aux jeunes un éventail de ressources d'hébergement
Membre de: Association des Centres jeunesse du Québec
Membre(s) du bureau directeur:
Luc Cadieux, Directeur général
 Luc_Cadieux@ssss.gouv.qc.ca

Head & Hands / A deux mains
5833, rue Sherbrooke ouest, Montréal QC H4A 1X4

Tel: 514-481-0277; *Fax:* 514-481-2336
e-mail: info@headandhands.ca
www.headandhands.ca
www.facebook.com/headandhands
twitter.com/headandhands
www.youtube.com/user/HeadandHands

Overview: A small local charitable organization founded in 1970
Mission: Medical, social, and legal services with an approach that is harm-reductive, holistic, and non-judgmental.
Chief Officer(s):
Jon McPhedran Waitzer, Director
  admin@headandhands.ca
Juniper Belshaw, Contact, Fundraising and Development
  membres@headandhands.ca

Mouvement contre le viol et l'inceste (MCVI)
CP 50009, Succ. Jarry, Montréal QC H2P 0A1

Tél: 514-278-9383; *Téléc:* 514-278-9385
Courriel: mcvi@contreleviol.org
www.mcvicontreleviol.org
www.facebook.com/mcvicontreleviol

Aperçu: *Dimension:* petite; *Envergure:* locale; Organisme sans but lucratif; fondée en 1976
Mission: Contrer la violence sexuelle dont sont victimes les femmes et les enfants
Affliation(s): Regroupement québécois des Centre d'aide et de lutte contre les agressions à caractère sexuel

SASKATCHEWAN

Early Childhood Intervention Program (ECIP) Sask. Inc.
2220 College Ave., 2nd Fl., Regina SK S4P 4V9

Fax: 306-787-0277
www.saskatchewan.ca/residents/family-and-social-support

Overview: A small local charitable organization founded in 1981
Mission: To provide a link between families & other professionals, working collaboratively with child care providers, speech & language pathologists, phyiotherapists, occupational therapists, nurses, physicians, teachers & school administrators to build trust & achieve mutually identified goals for the children & families

Kindersley - West Central ECIP Inc.
PO Box 775, 125 - 1st Ave. East, Kindersley SK S0L 1S0
Tel: 306-463-6822; *Fax:* 306-463-6898
e-mail: westcentralecip@sasktel.net

La Ronge - Children North ECIP Inc.
#106, 708 La Ronge Ave., La Ronge SK S0J 1L0
Tel: 306-425-6600; *Fax:* 306-425-6667
e-mail: ChildrenNorthECIP@mcrrha.sk.ca
Chief Officer(s):
Daina Lapworth, Contact
  daina.lapworth@mcrrha.sk.ca

Lloydminster - Midwest Family Connections
Co-op Plaza, #103, 4910 - 50th St., Lower Level, Lloydminster SK S9V 0Y5
Tel: 306-825-5911; *Fax:* 306-825-5912
Toll-Free: 866-651-5911
e-mail: info@midwestfamilyconnections.ca
www.midwestfamilyconnections.ca
Chief Officer(s):
Sherri Husch Foote, Executive Director
  sherri@midwestfamilyconnections.ca

Moose Jaw - South Central ECIP Inc.
#37, 1322 - 11th Ave. NW, Moose Jaw SK S9H 4L9
Tel: 306-692-2616; *Fax:* 306-692-2377
e-mail: southcentral.ecip@sasktel.net

North Battleford - Battlefords ECIP Inc.
PO Box 1297, North Battleford SK S9A 3L8
Tel: 306-446-4545; *Fax:* 306-446-0575
e-mail: becip@sasktel.net
www.becip.org
www.facebook.com/saskatchewan.ecip
Chief Officer(s):
Colleen Sabraw, Executive Director

Prince Albert - Prince Albert ECIP Inc.
3041 Sheman Dr., Prince Albert SK S6V 7B7
Tel: 306-922-3247; *Fax:* 306-763-5244
e-mail: paecip@sasktel.net

Regina - Regina Region ECIP
#305, 1102 - 8th Ave., Regina SK S4R 1C9
Tel: 306-374-5021
e-mail: ecip.rr@sasktel.net

Saskatoon - Prairie Hills ECIP Inc.
Kinsmen Children's Centre, 1319 Colony St., Saskatoon SK S7N 2Z1
Tel: 306-655-1083; *Fax:* 306-655-1449
Chief Officer(s):
Arlene Trask, Contact

Swift Current - Swift Current ECIP Inc.
El Wood Bldg., PO Box 486, 350 Cheadle St. West, 3rd Fl., Swift Current SK S9H 3W3
Tel: 306-773-3600; *Fax:* 306-778-6633
e-mail: swiftcurrentecip@sasktel.net
Chief Officer(s):
Wayne Cormier, Executive Director

Tisdale - North East ECIP Inc.
PO Box 1675, 610 - 100A St., Tisdale SK S0E 1T0
Tel: 306-873-3411; *Fax:* 306-873-3452
e-mail: neecip@sasktel.net

Weyburn - Holy Family RCSSD 140
110 Souris Ave., Weyburn SK S4H 2Z8
Tel: 306-842-7025; *Fax:* 306-842-7033
e-mail: wec.ecip@sasktel.net
Chief Officer(s):
Lynn Colquhoun, Contact
  lynn.colquhoun@holyfamilyrcssd.ca

Weyburn - Weyburn & Area ECIP Inc.
405 Coteau Ave., Weyburn SK S4H 1H2
Tel: 306-842-2686; *Fax:* 306-842-0723
e-mail: wecip@sasktel.net

Yorkton - Parkland ECIP Inc.
83 North St., Yorkton SK S3N 0G9
Tel: 306-786-6988; *Fax:* 306-786-7116
e-mail: parklandecip@sasktel.net
Chief Officer(s):
Michelle Yaschuk, Executive Director

International Associations

Academic Pediatric Association (APA)
6728 Old McLean Village Dr., McLean VA 22101 USA
Tel: 703-556-9222; *Fax:* 703-556-8729
e-mail: info@academicpeds.org
www.ambpeds.org
www.facebook.com/AcademicPeds
twitter.com/academicpeds

Overview: A large international organization
Mission: To improve the health of children & adolescents; To provide leadership in education of child health professionals; To engage in research & disseminate knowledge
Chief Officer(s):
Jessica O'Hara, Executive Director
  jessica@academicpeds.org
Stephanie Blyskal, Manager
  stephanie@academicpeds.org
Jennifer Padilla, Manager
  jennifer@academicpeds.org
Publications:
• Academic Pediatrics [a publication of the Academic Pediatric Association]
Type: Journal; *Frequency:* Bimonthly; *Editor:* Peter Szilagyi, MD, MPH; *Price:* Free with Academic Pediatric Association membership
Profile: The peer-reviewed publication is the official journal of the Academic Pediatric Association, featuring research &educational information for health professionals who care for children

• APA [Academic Pediatric Association] Focus
Type: Newsletter; *Frequency:* Bimonthly; *Price:* Free with Academic Pediatric Association membership

American Society of Pediatric Hematology / Oncology (ASPHO)

#300, 8735 West Higgins Rd., Chicago IL 60631 USA
Tel: 847-375-4716; *Fax:* 847-375-6483
e-mail: info@aspho.org
www.aspho.org
www.facebook.com/aspho.org

Overview: A medium-sized international organization founded in 1974
Mission: To promote optimal care of children & adolescents with blood disorders & cancer; To advance research, education, treatment, & professional practice
Chief Officer(s):
Amy Billett, President
Sally Weir, Executive Director
Bruce Hammond, Director, Governance & Operations
Judith Greifer, Manager, Marketing & Membership
Publications:
• Pediatric Blood & Cancer
Type: Journal; *Frequency:* Monthly; *Editor:* Peter E. Newburger, MD
Profile: Official journal of the American Society of Pediatric Hematology / Oncology & the International Society of Pediatric Oncology

Association of Children's Prosthetic-Orthotic Clinics (ACPOC)

#727, 6300, North River Rd., Rosemont IL 60018-4226 USA
Tel: 847-698-1637; *Fax:* 847-823-0536
e-mail: acpoc@aaos.org
www.acpoc.org

Overview: A small international organization founded in 1978
Mission: To provide prosthetic-orthotic care for children with limb loss or orthopaedic disabilities.
Chief Officer(s):
David B. Rotter, President

Casa - Pueblito

#107A, 2238 Dundas St. West, Toronto ON M6R 3A9
Tel: 416-642-5781
e-mail: info@casapueblito.org
www.casapueblito.org
www.facebook.com/CasaPueblito
twitter.com/CasaPueblito
instagram.com/casapueblito

Merged from: Pueblito Canada Incorporated; Casa Canadiense
Overview: A small international charitable organization founded in 1974
Mission: To work in partnership with Latin American organizations; To support the development of local programs for children in health care, childcare & education
Chief Officer(s):
Maria Paola Wong, Interim Executive Director
Publications:
• Casa - Pueblito Newsletter
Type: Newsletter; *Frequency:* Monthly
Profile: News & updates for members

Christian Children's Fund of Canada (CCFC)

1200 Denison St., Markham ON L3R 8G6
Tel: 905-754-1001; *Fax:* 905-754-1002
Toll-Free: 800-263-5437
Other Communication: media@ccfcanada.ca
e-mail: donor-relations@ccfcanada.ca
www.ccfcanada.ca
www.facebook.com/CCFC
twitter.com/CCFCanada
www.youtube.com/c/ccfcanada

Overview: A large international charitable organization founded in 1960
Mission: To focus upon community development ministry, starting with basic assistance & leading to programs stressing self-help & eventual independence; To work with colleagues & partners in developing countries; To reach out to children & families of all faiths
Member of: Canadian Council of Christian Charities; Better Business Bureau; ChildFund Alliance; Imagine Canada

Affliation(s): Canadian Marketing Association; Association of Fundraising Professionals
Chief Officer(s):
Douglas Ellenor, Chair
Terrance M Slobodian, Vice-President, Fund Development & Communications
Jim Carrie, Vice-President, Global Operations
Jeff Hogan, CPA; CA; CSR-P, Vice-President, Finance & Corporate Services
Publications:
• Child Essentials Newsletter
Type: Newsletter; *Frequency:* monthly
• ChildVoice
Type: Magazine; *Frequency:* s-a.; *Editor:* Vicki Quigley
Profile: Magazine for donors featuring stories of sponsored children

Compassion Canada

PO Box 5591, London ON N6A 5G8
Tel: 519-668-0224; *Fax:* 866-685-1107
Toll-Free: 800-563-5437
e-mail: info@compassion.ca
www.compassion.ca

Overview: A medium-sized international charitable organization founded in 1963
Mission: To provide sponsors for children in Third World countries; To aid community development projects in cooperation with Canadian International Development Agency; To be an advocate for children, to release them from their spiritual, economic, social & physical poverty & to enable them to become responsible & fulfilled Christian adults
Member of: Better Business Bureau; Canadian Council of Christian Charities; Association of Evangelical Relief & Development Organizations; Evangelical Fellowship of Canada
Chief Officer(s):
Barry Slauenwhite, President & CEO
Jim Bartholomew, Vice-President, Strategy & Marketing
Tim DeWeerd, Vice-President, Business Services
Deb Wilkins, Vice-President, Engagement

International Pediatric Association (IPA) / Association internationale de pédiatrie

418 Webster Forest Dr., Webster Groves MO 63119 USA
Tel: 847-434-7507
e-mail: adminoffice@ipa-world.org
www.ipa-world.org
www.facebook.com/InternationalPediatricAssociation
twitter.com/ipaworldorg

Overview: A large international organization founded in 1910
Mission: To promote the physical, mental, & social health of all children; To realize high standards of health for newborns, children, & adolescents in all countries of the world
Chief Officer(s):
Zulfiqar Bhutta, President
William J. Keenan, Executive Director
Publications:
• IPA [International Pediatric Association] Quarterly Newsletter
Type: Newsletter; *Frequency:* Quarterly

International Society for Pediatric & Adolescent Diabetes (ISPAD)

c/o KIT Group GmbH, Kurfürstendamm 71, Berlin 10709 Germany
Tel: +49 30 24603210; *Fax:* +49 30 24603200
e-mail: secretariat@ispad.org
www.ispad.org

Overview: A medium-sized international organization
Mission: To promote research, science, education, & advocacy in childhood & adolescent diabetes
Chief Officer(s):
Joseph Wolfsdorf, President
David M. Maahs, Secretary General
Andrea Scaramuzza, Treasurer
Publications:
• International Society for Pediatric & Adolescent Diabetes Membership Directory
Type: Directory
Profile: A listing of society members with contact information
• ISPAD [International Society for Pediatric & Adolescent Diabetes] Newsletter

Type: Newsletter
Profile: Society activities, including meeting reviews, educational opportunities, forthcoming events
• Pediatric Diabetes
Type: Journal; *Price:* Free with International Society for Pediatric & Adolescent Diabetes memberships

Pediatric Endocrine Society (PES)
6728 Old McLean Village Dr., McLean VA 22101 USA
Tel: 703-556-9222; *Fax:* 703-556-8729
e-mail: info@pedsendo.org
www.pedsendo.org
www.facebook.com/410788862293625
twitter.com/PedsEndoSociety
Previous Name: Lawson Wilkins Pediatric Endocrine Society
Overview: A medium-sized international organization
Mission: To promote the acquisition of knowledge about endocrine & metabolic disorders, from conception through adolescence
Chief Officer(s):
Stephen M. Rosenthal, President
Maureen Thompson, Executive Director
Janice Wilkins, Association Manager
John Fuqua, Secretary
Peter A. Lee, Treasurer
Publications:
• Pediatric Endocrine Society Membership Directory
Type: Directory
• PES [Pediatric Endocrine Society] Newsletter
Type: Newsletter
Profile: Pediatric Endocrine Society news, including award winners, meeting reviews, forthcoming meetings, & workshops

Society for Adolescent Health & Medicine (SAHM)
#800, 1 Parkview Plaza, Oakbrook Terrace IL 60181 USA
Tel: 847-686-2246; *Fax:* 847-686-2251
e-mail: info@adolescenthealth.org
www.adolescenthealth.org
www.facebook.com/adolescenthealth.medicine
twitter.com/SAHMtweets
www.youtube.com/SAHMAdolescentHealth
Overview: A medium-sized international organization founded in 1968
Mission: To advance the physical & psychosocial health & well-being of adolescents & young adults; To improve the delivery of health services for adolescents; To promote the field of adolescent medicine & health
Chief Officer(s):
Ryan Norton, Executive Director
Caitlyn Gibson, Director, Administration
Justin Dreyfuss, Manager, Marketing Communications
Publications:
• Journal of Adolescent Health
Type: Journal; *Frequency:* Monthly; *Editor:* Charles E. Irwin, Jr., M.D., FSAM; *Price:* Free with Society forAdolescent Medicine membership dues
Profile: Peer-reviewed articles on clinical medicine, public health policy, youth development, international health, & behavioral science
• SAHM [Society for Adolescent Health & Medicine] Newsletter
Type: Newsletter; *Frequency:* Quarterly
Profile: News from programs & members, presidential messages, announcements, committee reports, special interest group reports, professional development opportunities,& chapter activities

Teamwork Children's Services International
5983 Ladyburn Cres., Mississauga ON L5M 4V9
Tel: 905-542-1047
www.teamworkchildrenservices.com
Overview: A small international charitable organization
Mission: To provide a safe environment for disadvantaged children in rural areas of Africa; To help children become productive citizens through the provision of physical & mental care, education, & vocational training
Chief Officer(s):
Joel Chacha, Executive Director
jchacha@teamworkchildrenservices.com

National Publications

Baby & Child Care Encyclopedia
Owned By: Parents Canada Group
65 The East Mall, Toronto, ON M8Z 5W3
Tel: 416-537-2604; *Fax:* 416-538-1794
admin@parentscanada.com
Circulation: 100,000 *Frequency:* 2 times a year (May & Nov.)
A child care guide for parents of newborns & children through age five.
Amy Bielby, Editor, amyb@parentscanada.com

Canadian Family Physician
College of Family Physicians of Canada, 2630 Skymark Ave., Mississauga, ON L4W 5A4
Tel: 905-629-0900; *Fax:* 905-629-0893
Toll-Free: 800-387-6197
CFPmedia@cfpc.ca
Social Media: twitter.com/CanFamPhysician
Frequency: Monthly
Kathryn Taylor, Managing Editor

The Compleat Mother - The Magazine of Pregnancy, Birth & Breastfeeding
PO Box 38033, Calgary, AB T3K 5G9
Tel: 403-255-0246
thecompleatmother@shaw.ca
Frequency: 4 times a year
Angela van Son, Distributor

The Hospital Activity Book for Children
Owned By: Suggitt Publishing Ltd.
10177 105 St. NW, Edmonton, AB T5J 1E2
Fax: 877-463-6185
Toll-Free: 877-413-6163
reception@habfc.com
Activity books for children ages 4-12 who are undergoing medical treatment.
Robert Suggitt, President, rob@habfc.com
Melanie Smith, General Manager, St. John's Office,
melanie@habfc.com

Journal of Obstetrics & Gynaecology Canada
c/o Society of Obstetricians & Gynaecologists of Canada, #200, 2781 Lancaster Rd., Ottawa, ON K1B 1A7
Tel: 613-730-4192; *Fax:* 613-730-4314
Toll-Free: 800-561-2416
info@sogc.com
Social Media: twitter.com/JOGC_Social
www.facebook.com/JOGCsocial
Frequency: Monthly
Togas Tulandi, Editor-in-Chief MD, MHCM, FRCSC

Paediatrics & Child Health
Canadian Paediatric Society, #100, 2305 St. Laurent Blvd., Ottawa, ON K1G 4J8
Tel: 613-526-9397; *Fax:* 613-526-3332
journal@cps.ca
Circulation: 14,500 *Frequency:* 10 times a year
Official journal of the Canadian Paediatric Society.
Lindsay Conboy, Editorial Coordinator, lindsayc@cps.ca

Parents Canada
Owned By: Parents Canada Group
65 The East Mall, Toronto, ON M8Z 5W3
Tel: 416-537-2604; *Fax:* 416-538-1794
admin@parentscanada.com
Social Media: twitter.com/ParentsCanada
www.facebook.com/ParentsCanada
Janice Biehn, Editor, 416-537-2604,ext.349,
janiceb@parentscanada.com

Parents Canada Best Wishes
Owned By: Parents Canada Group
65 The East Mall, Toronto, ON M8Z 5W3
Tel: 416-537-2604; *Fax:* 416-538-1794
admin@parentscanada.com
Circulation: 135,000 *Frequency:* 2 times a year (May & Nov.)
Provides information & advice on parenthood.

Parents Canada Expecting
Owned By: Parents Canada Group
65 The East Mall, Toronto, ON M8Z 5W3
Tel: 416-537-2604; *Fax:* 416-538-1794
Toll-Free: 866-457-3320
admin@parentscanada.com

Parents Canada Group
Owned By: Family Communications Inc.
65 The East Mall, Toronto, ON M8Z 5W3
Tel: 416-537-2604; *Fax:* 416-538-1794
Social Media: twitter.com/ParentsCanada
www.facebook.com/ParentsCanada

Publishes 9 parenting magazines.
Donald G. Swinburne, President
Amy Bielby, Contact, 416-537-2604 ext.238,
  amyb@parentscanada.com

Parents Canada Labour & Birth Guide
Owned By: Parents Canada Group
65 The East Mall, Toronto, ON M8Z 5W3
Tel: 416-537-2604; *Fax:* 416-538-1794
Toll-Free: 866-457-3320
admin@parentscanada.com

Parents Canada Naissance
Détenteur: Parents Canada Group
65 The East Mall, Toronto, ON M8Z 5W3
Tél: 416-537-2604; *Téléc:* 416-538-1794
Ligne sans frais: 866-457-3320
admin@parentscanada.com

Today's Parent Pregnancy
Previous Name: Great Expectations
Owned By: Rogers Media Inc.
1 Mount Pleasant Rd., 7th Fl., Toronto, ON M4Y 2Y5
Tel: 416-764-2000; *Fax:* 416-764-3934
Circulation: 150,000 (English), 35,000 (French) *Frequency:* 2 times a year

Provincial/Local Publications

Enfants Québec
Détenteur: Les Éditions Rogers limitée
1101, av Victoria, Saint-Lambert, QC J4R 1P8
Tél: 514-875-9612
serviceclient@enfantsquebec.com
Médias sociaux:
www.facebook.com/enfantsquebec
Tirage: 60,506 *Fréquence:* 8 fois par an
Mathilde Singer, Rédactrice

Poupon
Anciennement: Mère Nouvelle
Détenteur: Les Éditions Rogers limitée
#800, 1200, av McGill College, Montréal, QC H3B 4G7
Tél: 514-845-5141
Tirage: 34,500 *Fréquence:* 2 fois par an
French magazine for new parents.

Local Schools

ALBERTA

Edmonton: **Columbus Academy**
#145, 10403 - 172 St., Edmonton, AB T5S 1K9
Tel: 780-440-0708; *Fax:* 780-440-0760
www.upcs.org
Grades: 7-12 *Note:* The school is a special education, private school in Alberta. Students are referred from social service agencies, surrounding school jurisdictions, & parents.
Kathy King, Contact
  kking@upcs.org

BRITISH COLUMBIA

Kelowna: **Venture Academy**
#338, 101 - 1865 Dilworth Dr., Kelowna, BC V1Y 9T1
Tel: 250-491-4593; *Fax:* 250-491-0251
Toll-Free: 866-762-2211
info@ventureacademy.ca
www.ventureacademy.ca
Grades: 7-12 *Note:* A therapeutic program & boarding school for troubled teens; also has locations in Alberta & Ontario
Gordon Hay, B.G.S., Founder & Executive Director
Leanne Stanley, B.Sc., Kin, B.Ed., Executive Director
Jeff Brain, MA, CTS, CEP, Director, Admissions & Program
  Development

Langley: **Whytecliff Agile Learning Centres**
Langley School
20561 Logan Ave., Langley, BC V3A 7R3
Tel: 604-532-1268; *Fax:* 604-532-1269
focus@focusfoundation.ca
www.focusfoundation.ca
www.facebook.com/focusfoundationBC
Grades: 8-12 *Enrollment:* 41 *Note:* Whytecliff Agile Learning Centres are provincially accredited, independent schools for boys & girls, aged 13-19, who face personal or behavioural challenges. Many of the students have dropped out of school, or have been excluded or expelled.
Laura Quarin, Principal

Campuses
Whytecliff Agile Learning Centre - Burnaby
3450 Boundary Rd., Burnaby, BC V5M 4A5
Tel: 604-438-4451; *Fax:* 604-438-5572
Grades: 8-12

SASKATCHEWAN

Pilot Butte: **Ranch Ehrlo Society**
P.O. Box 570
Pilot Butte, SK S0G 3Z0
Tel: 306-781-1800; *Fax:* 306-757-0599
inquiries@ranchehrlo.ca
www.ehrlo.com
www.facebook.com/RanchEhrlo
twitter.com/RanchEhrlo
www.youtube.com/user/ranchehrlo1
Enrollment: 192 *Note:* Ranch Ehrlo Society is a residential school for children, youth, & young adults who are experiencing social, psychological, mental, psychiatric, &/or physical difficulties. The Ranch offers holistic, psycho-social therapies, as well as community & family programming.
Andrea Brittin, President

Campuses
Buckland Campus
P.O. Box 1892
Prince Albert, SK S6V 6J9
Tel: 306-764-4511; *Fax:* 306-764-0042
buckland@ranchehrlo.ca

Corman Park Campus
P.O. Box 580
Martensville, SK S0K 2T0
Tel: 306-659-3100; *Fax:* 306-956-2570

National Libraries

Baby's Breath
PO Box 21053, St Catharines, ON L2M 7X2
Tel: 905-688-8884; *Fax:* 905-688-3300
Toll-Free: 800-363-7437
www.babysbreathcanada.ca
Social Media: twitter.com/babysbreathca;
www.facebook.com/babysbreathca

Provincial Libraries

Alberta Children's Hospital Knowledge Centre
2888 Shaganappi Trail NW, Calgary, AB T3B 6A8
Tel: 403-955-7077
krs@albertahealthservices.ca
krs.albertahealthservices.ca

Association du Québec pour enfants avec problèmes auditifs
3700, rue Berri, #A-446, Montréal, QC H2L 4G9
Tél: 514-842-8706; *Téléc:* 514-842-4006
Ligne sans frais: 877-842-4006
info@aqepa.org
www.aqepa.org

Collection: Surdité chez les enfants et familles handicapées

Bristol Circle Site
#100, 2381 Bristol Circle, Oakville, ON L6H 5S9
Tel: 905-855-2690

Children's Hospital London Health Sciences Centre
800 Commissioners Rd. East, #C3-300, London, ON N6A 4G5
Tel: 519-685-8484; *Fax:* 519-685-8103
rathbunlibrary@lhsc.on.ca
www.lhsc.on.ca

Children's Hospital of Eastern Ontario/ Hôpital pour enfants de l'est de l'Ontario
401 Smyth Rd., Ottawa, ON K1H 8L1
Tel: 613-738-3942; *Fax:* 613-738-4806
library@cheo.on.ca
www.cheo.on.ca/en/kaitlinatkinsonfrl
Social Media: www.youtube.com/user/CHEOvideos;
twitter.com/cheohospital; www.facebook.com/CHEOkids

CHU Sainte-Justine/Centre de réadaptation Marie-Enfant
5200, rue Bélanger est, #SS-036, Montréal, QC H1T 1C9
Tél: 514-374-1710
biblio.crme@ssss.gouv.qc.ca
readaptation.chusj.org

Collection: Réadaptation pédiatrique, éducation specialisée

ErinoakKids Centre for Treatment & Development
Burloak Site, Westbury Business Park, 1122 International Blvd., 5th Fl., Burlington, ON L7L 6Z8
Tel: 905-855-2690; *Toll-Free:* 877-374-6625
www.erinoakkids.ca/Resources/Resource-Centre.aspx
Social Media: www.youtube.com/ErinoakKidsCentre;
twitter.com/ErinoakKids; www.facebook.com/ErinoakKids

Collection: Information & resources on skill development; toys; books
Bridget Fewtrell, President & CEO
Sandra Black, Assistant, Family Resource Centres
905-855-2690 ext. 2480

Family Resource Library
#5850, 5980 University Ave., Halifax, NS B3K 6R8
Tel: 902-470-8351
www.iwk.nshealth.ca

Collection: Books; health videos; video games; multicultural children's books in Arabic, Simplified Chinese & Mi'kmaq
Andrea Kuttner, Librarian & Coordinator
andrea.kuttner@iwk.nshealth.ca
902-470-8982

Glenrose Rehabilitation Hospital
10230 - 111th Ave., #GE0613, Edmonton, AB T5G 0B7
Tel: 780-735-8823; *Fax:* 780-735-8863
glenroselibrary@albertahealthservices.ca
Donna Gordon, Library Technician
donna.gordon@albertahealthservices.ca

Hincks-Dellcrest Centre
114 Maitland St., Toronto, ON M4Y 1E1
Tel: 416-972-1935; *Fax:* 416-924-9808
jackman.library@hincksdellcrest.org
www.hincksdellcrest.org

Collection: Fellows' research papers & theses
Wylie Burke, Interim Director
wburke@hincksdellcrest.org

Holland Bloorview Kids Rehabilitation Hospital
Grocery Foundation Resource Centre, 150 Kilgour Rd., 1st Fl., Toronto, ON M4G 1R8
Tel: 416-425-6220; *Toll-Free:* 800-363-2440
library@hollandbloorview.ca
www.hollandbloorview.ca

Pui-Ying Wong, Librarian
416-425-6220 ext. 3517
Winky Yeung, Library & Archives Technician
416-425-6220 ext. 3291

Hôpital Rivière-des-Prairies
7070, boul Perras, Montréal, QC H1E 1A4
Tél: 514-323-7260
bibliotheque.hrdp@ssss.gouv.qc.ca
www.hrdp.qc.ca

Isabelle Barrette, Responsable
isabelle.barrette.hrdp@sssss.gouv.qc.ca

Hospital for Sick Children
#1301, 555 University Ave., Black Wing, Toronto, ON M5G 1X8
Tel: 416-813-6693; *Fax:* 416-813-7523
hsclink@sickkids.ca
www.sickkids.ca/Learning/HospitalLibrary

IWK Health Centre
5850/5980 University Ave., Halifax, NS B3K 6R8
Tel: 902-470-7058; *Fax:* 902-470-7122
www.iwk.nshealth.ca/page/health-sciences-library
Social Media: www.youtube.com/iwkhealthcentre;
twitter.com/iwkhealthcentre; www.facebook.com/iwkhealthcentre

Collection: Over 3,000 journals (electronic & print); books; audiovisual materials; reference materials
Darlene Chapman, Manager, Library Services
darlene.chapman@iwk.nshealth.ca
902-470-6729

J.P. Das Centre on Developmental & Learning Disabilities
#6-123C, Education Bldg. North, University of Alberta, Edmonton, AB T6G 2G5
Tel: 780-492-3696
dascentre.educ.ualberta.ca

Rauno Parrila, Director
rauno.parrila@ualberta.ca

Montréal Children's Hospital of the McGill University Health Centre/ Hôpital de Montréal pour enfants du centre universitaire de santé McGill
#RC-1107, 1001, boul Décarie, Montréal, QC H4A 3J1
Tel: 514-412-4400
bibliofam@muhc.mcgill.ca
www.mchfamilylibrary.ca

Collection: Pain Management resources

Ottawa Children's Treatment Centre
395 Smyth Rd., Ottawa, ON K1H 8L2
Tel: 613-737-0871; *Fax:* 613-523-5167
www.octc.ca/lending-library.php

Collection: Switch adapted & non-switch adapted toys, fine motor & gross motor toys, software & peripherals, communication aids, books & videos, games, puzzles
Anne Huot, Executive Director

Paediatric Family Resource Centre
Zone B, 1st Fl., #006 (B1-006), 800 Commissioners Rd. East, London, ON N6A 5W9
Tel: 519-685-8500
pfrc@lhsc.on.ca
www.lhsc.on.ca/pfrc

Collection: Medical Reference Books; Parent Guides; Bereavement Books and Resources; Pamphlets
Darren Connolly, Family Advisor

Quinte Health Care - Trenton Memorial
100 Station St., Belleville, ON K8N 2S5
Tel: 613-966-9427; *Fax:* 613-966-8819
www.familyspace.ca

Kelly Allan, Executive Director

Quinte Health Care - Trenton Memorial
Charlotte Sills Wing, 265 Dundas St. East, Belleville, ON K8N 5A9
Tel: 613-969-7400; *Fax:* 613-968-9154
www.quintectc.com
Collection: Medical texts, journals & electronic resource

South Millway Site
2277 South Millway, Mississauga, ON L5L 2M5
Tel: 905-855-2690

Torbram Site
8177 Torbram Rd., 1st Fl., Brampton, ON L6T 5C5
Tel: 905-855-2690

Provincial Government

Alberta Office of the Child & Youth Advocate (OCYA)
#600, 9925 - 109 St. NW, Edmonton, AB T5K 2J8
Tel: 780-422-6056
Fax: 780-422-3675
Toll-Free: 800-661-3446
ca.information@ocya.alberta.ca
www.ocya.alberta.ca
Other Communication: Southern Alberta Advocacy Services, Phone:
403-297-8435, Fax: 403-297-4456
Secondary Address: #2420, 801 - 6 Ave. SW
South Office
Calgary, AB T2P 3W3
twitter.com/AlbertaCYA
As of April 1, 2012, the Child & Youth Advocate is an independent officer reporting to the Legislature under the Child & Youth Advocate Act.

Child & Youth Advocate, Del Graff
Tel: 780-422-6056
Fax: 780-422-3675
del.graff@ocya.alberta.ca

Executive Director, Child & Youth Advocacy, Jackie Stewart
Tel: 780-644-2363
jackie.stewart@ocya.alberta.ca

Director, Engagement & Education, Randy Baker
Tel: 780-644-2632
Fax: 780-644-8833
randy.baker@ocya.alberta.ca

Director, Investigations & Legal Representation, Terri Pelton
Tel: 780-415-8936
Fax: 780-644-7227
terri.pelton@ocya.alberta.ca

Director, Strategic Support, Bonnie Russell
Tel: 780-422-2966
Fax: 780-638-3718
bonnie.russell@ocya.alberta.ca

British Columbia Ministry of Children & Family Development (MCFD)
Customer Service Centre, PO Box 9770 Stn. Prov Govt, Victoria, BC V8W 9S5
Tel: 250-387-7027
Fax: 250-356-5720
Toll-Free: 877-387-7027
TTY: 800-667-4770
MCF.CorrespondenceManagement@gov.bc.ca
www.gov.bc.ca/mcf
Other Communication: Helpline for Children: 310-1234; Emergencies outside office hours: 1-800-663-9122
The Ministry of Children & Family Development works to support healthy child development, to maximize the potential of children & youth, & to achieve meaningful outcomes for children, youth, & families. A client-centered approach is used to deliver services. The following services are available to families throughout British Columbia: adoption services; early childhood development & child care services; child safety, family support, & children in care services;

services for children & youth with special needs; mental health services for children & youth; & youth justice services.

Minister, Children & Family Development, Hon. Stephanie Cadieux
Tel: 250-387-9699
Fax: 250-387-9722
MCF.Minister@gov.bc.ca
PO Box 9057 Prov Govt Sta.
Victoria, BC V8W 9E2

Deputy Minister, Lori Wanamaker
Tel: 250-387-1541
Fax: 250-356-2920
mcf.deputyminister@gov.bc.ca
PO Box 9721 Prov Govt Sta.
Victoria, BC V8W 9S2

Aboriginal Services
PO Box 9777 Stn. Prov Govt, Victoria, BC V8W 9S5
Tel: 250-356-9791
Fax: 250-387-1732
Executive Director, Divisional Operations, Shane DeMeyer
Tel: 250-387-7081
Director, Practice, Cindy Ghostkeeper
Tel: 250-565-6645

Provincial Services
PO Box 9717 Stn. Prov Govt, Victoria, BC V8W 9S1
Tel: 250-387-0978
Fax: 250-356-2079
Executive Director, Youth Custody Services, Lenora Angel
Tel: 604-356-1970
Fax: 604-356-2079
PO Box 9719 Prov Govt Sta.
Victoria, BC V8W 9S5
Provincial Director, Youth Forensic Psychiatric Services, Andre Picard
Tel: 778-452-2202
Fax: 778-452-2201
Provincial Clinical Director, Youth Forensic Psychiatric Services, Dr. Kulwant Riar
Tel: 778-452-2205
Fax: 778-452-2201
Office Manager, Provincial Services for Deaf & Hard of Hearing, Elaine Bains
Tel: 604-660-1800
Fax: 604-660-1859
psdhh@gov.bc.ca
Other Communications: TTY: 604-660-1807
TTY: 800-667-4770

Policy & Provincial Services
PO Box 9738 Stn. Prov Govt, Victoria, BC V8W 9S2
Tel: 250-387-5954
Fax: 250-387-2481
Assistant Deputy Minister, Christine Massey
Tel: 250-387-7090
Fax: 250-387-2481
Executive Director, Child Care Programs & Services Branch, Jonathan Barry
Tel: 250-387-7762
Toll-free: 888-338-6622
Fax: 250-387-2997
Executive Director, CW, Permanency, QA & Aboriginal Policy, Cheryl May
Tel: 250-356-5581
Executive Director, Children & Youth with Special Needs Policy, Aleksandra Stevanovic
Tel: 250-387-1828
Aleksandra.Stevanovic@gov.bc.ca
Executive Director, Child & Youth Mental Health Policy, Sandy Wiens
Tel: 250-216-3657
Fax: 250-356-0580
MCF.ChildYouthMentalHealth@gov.bc.ca
Director, Child & Youth Mental Health Policy, Robert Lampard
Tel: 250-356-5201
Director, Aboriginal Policy, Lise LeLievre
Tel: 250-356-2777

Director, Vancouver After Hours, Lesley Renshaw
Tel: 604-660-4927
Toll-free: 800-663-9122
Director, Child Welfare Policy, James Wale
Tel: 250-387-7075
James.Wale@gov.bc.ca
Director, Policy Initiatives & Coordination, Sonja Yli-Kahila
Tel: 250-953-4360
Sonja.YliKahila@gov.bc.ca

Provincial Office for the Early Years
PO Box 9721 Stn. Prov Govt, Victoria, BC V8W 9S2

Tel: 250-387-5942
Fax: 250-356-0311

Acting Executive Director, Emily Horton
Tel: 250-413-7608
Director, Danielle Smith
Tel: 250-387-9714
Director, Stakeholder Engagement & Coordination, Jan White
Tel: 778-679-9646

Provincial Office of Domestic Violence & Strategic Priorities
PO Box 9768 Stn. Prov Govt, Victoria, BC V8W 9S5

Tel: 250-356-9808
Fax: 250-387-8000

Acting Assistant Deputy Minister, Tami Currie
Tel: 250-356-5332
Executive Director, Strategic Priorities Branch, Linda Bradford
Tel: 250-387-7423
Executive Director, Provincial Office of Domestic Violence, Catherine Talbott
Tel: 250-387-7044
Director, System & Service Coordination, Provincial Office of Domestic Violence, Clark Russell
Tel: 250-952-0893

Office of the Provincial Director of Child Welfare
PO Box 9721 Stn. Prov Govt, Victoria, BC V8W 9S2

Tel: 250-356-9791
Fax: 250-356-6534

Assistant Deputy Minister & Provincial Director, Child Welfare, Cory Heavener
Tel: 250-356-9791
Deputy Director, Child Welfare, Alex Scheiber
Tel: 250-387-7418
Executive Director, Guardianship, Adoption & Permanency Planning, Anne Clayton
Tel: 250-387-2281
MCF.AdoptionsBranch@gov.bc.ca
Director, Adoption Services, Renaa Bacy
Tel: 250-387-7069
MCF.AdoptionsBranch@gov.bc.ca

Families & Children / Familles et des enfants

Tel: 506-453-2181
Fax: 506-453-2164

Assistant Deputy Minister, Lisa Doucette
Tel: 506-453-2181
Lisa.Doucette@gnb.ca
Director, Community & Individual Development, Amélie Deschênes
Tel: 506-444-4213
Amélie.Deschenes@gnb.ca
Director, Child & Youth Services, William Innes
Tel: 506-453-3622
bill.innes@gnb.ca
Director, Wellness, Marlien McKay
Tel: 506-444-4633
marlien.mckay@gnb.ca

Newfoundland & Labrador Department of Children, Seniors & Social Development
PO Box 8700 St. John's, NL A1B 4J6

Tel: 709-729-0862
Fax: 709-729-0870
TTY: 855-229-2044
CSSDInfo@gov.nl.ca
www.cssd.gov.nl.ca

In August 2016, the Department of Child, Youth & Family Services & the Department of Seniors, Wellness and Social Development

combined to create the Department of Children, Seniors and Social Development. The Department focuses on child protection, youth services, aging, seniors, health promotion, sport & general wellness. The Department is also responsible for the Poverty Reduction Strategy & the Disability Policy Office.

Minister, Hon. Sherry Gambin-Walsh
Tel: 709-729-0659
Fax: 709-729-0662
sherrygambinwalsh@gov.nl.ca

Deputy Minister, Bruce Cooper
Tel: 709-729-0958
brucecooper@gov.nl.ca

Assistant Deputy Minister, Policies & Programs, Rick Healey
Tel: 709-729-0088
rhealey@gov.nl.ca

Assistant Deputy Minister, Corporate Services, Jean Tilley
Tel: 709-729-0656
jeantilley@gov.nl.ca

Assistant Deputy Minister, Services Delivery & Regional Operations, Susan Walsh
Tel: 709-729-3473
swalsh@gov.nl.ca

Director of Communications, Children & Youth, Melony O'Neill
Tel: 709-729-5148
melonyoneill@gov.nl.ca

Director of Communications, Seniors & Wellness, Roger Scaplen
Tel: 709-729-0928
rogerscaplen@gov.nl.ca

Child Protection & In Care Division

Tel: 709-729-2668

Director, Michelle Shallow
Tel: 709-729-6078
mshallow@gov.nl.ca
Director, Youth Corrections, Paul Ludlow
pludlow@gov.nl.ca

Healthy Living Division

Tel: 709-729-6243

Acting Director, Linda Carter
Tel: 709-729-3117
lindacarter@gov.nl.ca
Coordinator, Eat Great & Participate, Stephanie O'Brien
Tel: 709-729-4432
StephanieOBrien@psnl.ca

Poverty Reduction Strategy

Fax: 709-729-5139
Toll-Free: 866-883-6600
povertyreduction@gov.nl.ca

Director, Aisling Gogan
Tel: 709-729-1287
aislinggogan@gov.nl.ca

Recreation & Sport

Tel: 709-729-2829
Fax: 709-729-5293

Director, Michelle Healey
Tel: 709-729-5241
MichelleHealey@gov.nl.ca
Manager, Programs & Strategic Initiatives, Jaime Collins
Tel: 709-729-0855
Jaimecollins@gov.nl.ca

Children, Youth & Families
www.novascotia.ca/coms/families
Executive Director, Children & Family Services, Leonard Doiron
Tel: 902-424-3867
Director, Child Protection Services, Wendy Marie Leiper
Tel: 902-424-7433

Ontario Ministry of Children & Youth Services

Macdonald Block, #M-1B114, 900 Bay St., Toronto, ON M7A 1N3

Tel: 416-212-7432
Fax: 416-212-1977
Toll-Free: 866-821-7770
TTY: 800-387-5559
mcsinfo@mcys.gov.on.ca
www.children.gov.on.ca
twitter.com/OntYouth

Working collaboratively with community partners, as well as the Ministries of Education, Health & Long-Term Care, Community & Social Services, Citizenship, Immigration & International Trade, & Tourism, Culture & Sport, to integrate a number of Ontario's children & youth programs & services. By bringing these programs under one roof, the government seeks to make children a top priority & to make it easier for families to access services at all stages of a child's development.

Minister, Hon. Michael Coteau
Tel: 416-212-7432
Fax: 416-212-7431
michael.coteau@ontario.ca

Deputy Minister, Nancy Matthews
Tel: 416-212-2280
nancy.matthews@ontario.ca

Director, Communications & Marketing, Melissa Hogg
Tel: 416-326-3512
Fax: 416-212-1977
melissa.hogg@ontario.ca

Business Planning & Corporate Services

Hepburn Block, 80 Grosvenor St., 6th Fl., Toronto, ON M7A 1E9

Tel: 416-325-5595
Fax: 416-325-5615

Assistant Deputy Minister & Chief Administrative Officer, Nadia Cornacchia
Tel: 416-325-5588
nadia.cornacchia@ontario.ca
Senior Manager, Emergency Management Program, Mark Bett
Tel: 416-327-4813
mark.bett@ontario.ca
Manager, Organizational Health & Effectiveness, Andrew Bizzarro
Tel: 416-326-0803
andrew.bizzarro@ontario.ca

Children, Youth & Social Services Cluster, I & IT

Hepburn Block, 80 Grosvenor St., 6th Fl., Toronto, ON M7A 1E9

Tel: 416-314-9694

Chief Information Officer, Dafna Carr
Tel: 416-326-0770
Dafna.Carr@ontario.ca
Director, Child Protection Information Network (CPIN), Shelley Edworthy
Tel: 613-548-6688
shelley.edworthy@ontario.ca
Coordinator, Issues & Special Projects, Bryan Marks
Tel: 416-218-4034
Bryan.Marks@ontario.ca

Policy Development & Program Design Division

56 Wellesley St. West, 14th Fl., Toronto, ON M5S 2S3

Tel: 416-212-1961
Fax: 416-314-1862

Acting Assistant Deputy Minister, Jennifer Morris
Tel: 416-212-1961
jennifer.morris@ontario.ca
Director, Ontario Autism Program Project Team, Sarah Hardy
Tel: 416-325-8409
sarah.hardy@ontario.ca
Director, Child Welfare Reform Project Team, Esther Levy
Tel: 416-314-0175
esther.levy@ontario.ca
Director, Children & Youth at Risk, Marian Mlakar
Tel: 416-212-5205
Fax: 416-212-2021
marian.mlakar@ontario.ca

Acting Director, Child Welfare Secretariat, Peter Kiatipis
Tel: 416-325-3560
Fax: 416-326-8098
peter.kiatipis@ontario.ca

Service Delivery Division

56 Wellesley St. West, 14th Fl., Toronto, ON M5S 2S3

Tel: 416-212-5663
Fax: 416-314-1862

Assistant Deputy Minister, Rachel Kampus
Tel: 416-212-3141
rachel.kampus@ontario.ca
Director, Resource Management, Harrison Moon
Tel: 416-212-8480
harrison.moon@ontario.ca
Director, Client Services, Judy Switson
Tel: 416-326-3170
Fax: 416-325-9631
judy.switson@ontario.ca
Director, Child & Parent Resource Institute, Children's Facilities, Anne Stark
Tel: 519-858-2774 ext: 2010
anne.stark@ontario.ca
Administrator, Thistletown Regional Centre, Vacant
Tel: 416-326-0741
Fax: 416-326-9078

Strategic Policy & Planning Division

56 Wellesley St., 14th Fl., Toronto, ON M5S 2S3

Tel: 416-327-9460
Fax: 416-314-1862

Assistant Deputy Minister, Darryl Sturtevant
Tel: 416-327-9481
Fax: 416-314-1862
darryl.sturtevant@ontario.ca
Director, Strategic Policy & Aboriginal Relationships, Sarah Caldwell
Tel: 416-326-1051
Fax: 416-327-0570
sarah.caldwell@ontario.ca
Director, Youth Strategies, Sean Twyford
Tel: 416-325-4699
Fax: 416-327-0570
sean.twyford@ontario.ca
Manager, Early Intervention Policy & Programs Unit, Lisa M. Butler
Tel: 416-212-9887
lisa.m.butler@ontario.ca
Acting Manager, Child Development Policy & Programs Unit, Rachael Manson-Smith
Tel: 416-325-4483
rachael.manson-smith3@ontario.ca
Manager, Aboriginal Strategy Unit, Martin Rukavina
Tel: 416-327-9135
martin.rukavina@ontario.ca

Youth Justice Services

56 Wellesley St. West, 14th fl., Toronto, ON M5S 2S3

Tel: 416-314-3502
Fax: 416-327-0478

Assistant Deputy Minister, JoAnn Miller-Reid
Tel: 416-327-9910
david.mitchell3@ontario.ca
Director, Direct Operated Facilities, John Scarfo
Tel: 905-826-1505
Toll-free: 844-805-3805
Fax: 905-826-1707
john.scarfo@ontario.ca
Manager, Mental Health & Specialized Client Services, Brian Smegal
Tel: 416-212-6286
Fax: 416-327-0944
brian.smegal@ontario.ca

Office of the Provincial Advocate for Children & Youth
#2200, 401 Bay St., Toronto, ON M7A 0A6

Tel: 416-325-5669
Fax: 416-325-5681
Toll-Free: 800-263-2841
TTY: 416-325-2648
advocacy@provincialadvocate.on.ca
www.provincialadvocate.on.ca
Secondary Address: #3, 905 Victoria Ave. East
Thunder Bay, ON P7C 1B3
Other Communication: Toll-Free Phone: 1-888-342-1380
twitter.com/OntarioAdvocate
www.facebook.com/OPACY1
www.youtube.com/user/ProvincialAdvocate

The Office's mandate is to provide an independent voice for children & youth (including those with special needs & First Nations children) by reporting directly to the Legislature.

Provincial Advocate, Irwin Elman

Director, Strategic Development, Laura Arndt

Director, Investigation, Diana Cooke

Director, Advocacy, Trevor McAlmont

Project Lead, Research & Quality Assurance, Dr. Fred Matthews

Prince Edward Island Department of Family & Human Services
Jones Bldg., 11 Kent St., 2nd Fl., PO Box 2000Charlottetown, PE C1A 7N8

Tel: 902-620-3777
Fax: 902-894-0242
Toll-Free: 866-594-3777
www.gov.pe.ca/sss

The Department of Family & Human Services strives to develop healthy & self-reliant individuals & to support vulnerable members of the province. Programs & services are offered to promote social & economic prosperity & the creation of work environments that contribute to a safe, healthy & engaged workforce.

Minister, Hon. Tina M. Mundy
Tel: 902-368-6520
Fax: 902-368-4740
tmmundy@gov.pe.ca

Deputy Minister, Teresa Hennebery
Tel: 902-368-6520
tahennebery@gov.pe.ca

Senior Communications Officer, Darlene Gillis
Tel: 902-620-3409
ddgillis@gov.pe.ca

Child & Family Services
The Child & Family Services Division offers a wide range of programs & services to care for Prince Edward Island's children & families.
Examples of programs include child protection, foster care, & adoption services.
Director, Child & Family Services, Rona Smith
Tel: 902-368-5396
Fax: 902-368-4258
ronasmith@gov.pe.ca
Director, Child Protection, Wendy L. McCourt
Tel: 902-368-6515
Fax: 902-620-3776
wlmccourt@gov.pe.ca
Provincial Coordinator, Residential Services, Barry L. Chandler
Tel: 902-368-6180
Fax: 902-368-3362
blchandler@ihis.org
Provincial Coordinator, Child Protection, Maureen G. MacEwen
Tel: 902-368-6161
Fax: 902-620-3362
mgmacewen@gov.pe.ca
Family Violence Coordinator, Dr. Wendy Verhoek-Oftedahl
Tel: 902-368-6712

Fax: 902-620-3362
wverhoekoftedahl@gov.pe.ca

Yukon Child & Youth Advocate Office
#19, 2070 Second Ave., Whitehorse, YT Y1A 1B1

Tel: 867-456-5575
Fax: 867-456-5574
Toll-Free: 800-661-0408
www.ycao.ca
www.facebook.com/116941835050317
www.youtube.com/user/YukonChildAdvocate

Yukon Child & Youth Advocate, Annette King
annette.king@ycao.ca

Deputy Child & Youth Advocate, Bengie Clethero
bengie.clethero@ycao.ca

Local Hospitals & Health Centres

ALBERTA

BON ACCORD: Oak Hill Boys Ranch
PO Box 97, 56119 - Range Rd. 240, Bon Accord, AB T0A 0K0
Tel: 780-921-2121
www.oakhillboysranch.ca
Number of Beds: 32 beds
Note: Residential treatment facility for young males (11-16) suffering from issues such as mental health & substance abuse.
Anton Smith, Executive Director

CALGARY: Alberta Children's Hospital
Affiliated with: Alberta Health Services
Former Name: Alberta Crippled Children's Hospital; Junior Red Cross Hospital
West Campus, University of Calgary, 2888 Shaganappi Trail NW, Calgary, AB T3B 6A8
Tel: 403-955-7211
www.albertahealthservices.ca/Facilities/ACH/
Social Media: www.facebook.com/179579998746821;
twitter.com/AHS_media; www.youtube.com/AHSChannel
Year Founded: 2006
Note: Programs & services include: Aboriginal services; angiography; pediatrics (birth to age 18); emergency services; surgery; complex pain service; diagnostic imaging; burn treatment; eating disorder program - day treatment; sexual assault response team; child abuse service; child & adolescent mental health inpatient services; community education service; & Infant Headshape Program.
Margaret Fullerton, Senior Operating Officer

CALGARY: Wood's Homes - Bowness Campus
Affiliated with: Alberta Health Services
9400 - 48 Ave. NW, Calgary, AB T3B 2B2
Tel: 403-247-6751 *Fax:* 403-286-0878
askus@woodshomes.ca
www.woodshomes.ca
Social Media: www.facebook.com/woodshomesnfp;
twitter.com/ChildMntlHealth; www.youtube.com/user/WoodsHomes1;
www.linkedin.com/company/wood%27s-homes
Number of Beds: 110 beds

CALGARY: Wood's Homes - Parkdale Campus
805 - 37 St. NW, Calgary, AB T2N 4N8
Tel: 403-270-4102 *Fax:* 403-283-9735
askus@woodshomes.ca
www.woodshomes.ca
Info Line: 800-563-6106
Social Media: www.facebook.com/woodshomesnfp;
twitter.com/ChildMntlHealth; www.youtube.com/user/WoodsHomes1;
www.linkedin.com/company/wood%27s-homes
Year Founded: 1914
Number of Beds: 150 beds
Area Served: Alberta; Northwest Territories
Population Served: 20000
Number of Employees: 500
Specialties: Crisis counselling & outreach services; residential treatment
Note: Foster care; homeless youth shelters; specialized learning; day

treatment; residential treatment; outreach services; & child welfare services.
Sylvia MacIver, Communications Manager
  403-270-1768, sylvia.maciver@woodshomes.ca

EDMONTON: Edmonton Addiction Youth Services
Affiliated with: Alberta Health Services
12325 - 140 St. NW, Edmonton, AB T5L 2C9
Tel: 780-422-7383
www.albertahealthservices.ca

EDMONTON: Santa Rosa
Affiliated with: Alberta Health Services
6705 - 120 Ave., Edmonton, AB T5B 0C7
Tel: 780-644-3627
www.albertahealthservices.ca

Note: Youth detoxification & stabilization

EDMONTON: Stollery Children's Hospital
University of Alberta Hospital
Affiliated with: Alberta Health Services
8440 - 112 St., Edmonton, AB T6G 2B7
Tel: 780-407-8822
www.albertahealthservices.ca
Area Served: Northern & Central Alberta; parts of Manitoba
Specialties: Organ transplantation
Note: Western Canada's referral centre for pediatric cardiac surgery. Programs & services include: clinics; audiology; Child & Adolescent Protection Centre; chronic pain service; Diabetes Education Centre; diagnostic imaging; endocrinology; gastroenterology & nutrition; hematology; home nutrition support/dietician; infectious diseases; medicine; Neonatal Intensive Care Unit; Northern Alberta Children's Cancer Program; Northern Alberta Pediatric Sleep Program; occupational & physical therapy; otolaryngology; palliative care; Pediatric Comprehensive Epilepsy Program; feeding & swallowing service; hemophilia; intensive care; Medicine/Surgical Ambulatory Unit; neurology; social work; speech language pathology; & surgery.

EDMONTON: University of Alberta Hospital
Affiliated with: Alberta Health Services
8440 - 112 St. NW, Edmonton, AB T6G 2B7
Tel: 780-407-8822
www.albertahealthservices.ca
Social Media: www.facebook.com/179579998746821;
twitter.com/AHS_media; www.youtube.com/ahschannel
Number of Beds: 687 beds
Specialties: Organ & Tissue Transplant Program
Note: A clinical, research & teaching facility, its specialized services include cardiac sciences, neurosciences, surgery, medicine, renal, critical & trauma care, & a burn unit. Other areas of focus include: anaesthesiology; angiography; audiology; bronchoscopy; cardiology; CT scans; dental clinic; ENT; ears nose & throat surgery; eating disorders; endoscopy; fluoroscopy; gastroenterology & hepatology; general surgery; general systems intensive care unit; geriatric assessment; hemodialysis; laboratory; MRI; nuclear medicine; nutrition counselling; occupational therapy; palliative care; physical therapy; plastic surgery; psychiatry; pulmonary medicine; respiratory therapy; rheumatology; sexual assault response; social work; speech language pathology; spiritual care; stroke; surgery; transplantation; tuberculosis; ultrasound; & vascular interventional neuro radiology. Also located within the facility are the Mazankowski Alberta Heart Institute & the Stollery Children's Hospital, specializing in pediatric cardiac surgery & organ transplantation.
Dr. Verna Yiu, President/CEO, AHS
Dr. Francois Belanger, Interim CMO & Vice-President, Quality

GRANDE PRAIRIE: Grande Prairie Aberdeen Centre
Affiliated with: Alberta Health Services
#300, 9728 Montrose Ave., Grande Prairie, AB T8V 5B6
Tel: 780-538-6330 *Fax:* 780-538-5256
Toll-Free: 866-332-2322
www.albertahealthservices.ca

LETHBRIDGE: Lethbridge Community Health Centre
Affiliated with: Alberta Health Services
801 - 1 Ave. South, Lethbridge, AB T1J 4L5
Tel: 403-388-6666 *Fax:* 403-328-5934
www.albertahealthservices.ca

Note: Includes prenatal education

LETHBRIDGE: Lethbridge Youth Treatment Centre
Affiliated with: Alberta Health Services
402 - 6th Ave. North, Lethbridge, AB T1H 6J9
Tel: 403-388-7600 *Fax:* 403-388-7619
www.albertahealthservices.ca

Note: Addictions counselling & treatment

LETHBRIDGE: Sifton Family & Youth Services
528 Stafford Dr. North, Lethbridge, AB T1H 2B2
Tel: 403-381-5411 *Fax:* 403-382-4565

Note: Provides a treatment program for young people with behavioural &/or emotional challenges

MEDICINE HAT: Regional Resource Centre
Affiliated with: Alberta Health Services
631 Prospect Dr. SW, Medicine Hat, AB T1A 4C2
Tel: 403-529-8030 *Fax:* 403-502-8618
www.albertahealthservices.ca

Note: Programs & services include: child & adolescent mental health program; mental health diversion services for adults with low risk minor criminal offences; & mental health outreach

SPRUCE GROVE: Stan Woloshyn Building
Affiliated with: Alberta Health Services
205 Diamond Ave., Spruce Grove, AB T7X 3A8
Tel: 780-342-1344
www.albertahealthservices.ca

Note: Addiction & mental health services for children, youth, & adults

TOFIELD: Tofield - 5024-51 Avenue
Affiliated with: Alberta Health Services
5024 - 51 Ave., Tofield, AB T0B 4J0
Tel: 780-672-1181 *Fax:* 780-679-1737
www.albertahealthservices.ca

Note: Child & adolescent addiction & mental health services.

BRITISH COLUMBIA

CRANBROOK: Cranbrook Family Connections
Affiliated with: Interior Health Authority
209A - 16th Ave. North, Cranbrook, BC V1V 5S8
Tel: 250-489-5011
www.interiorhealth.ca

GRAND FORKS: Glanville Family Centre
Boundary Family & Individual Services Society
Affiliated with: Interior Health Authority
PO Box 2498, 1200 Central Ave., Grand Forks, BC V0H 1H0
Tel: 250-442-2267 *Toll-Free:* 877-442-5355
info@bfiss.org
www.boundaryfamily.org

Note: Programs for children, youth, women & families

KAMLOOPS: Development Disability Mental Health Child,
Youth & Children's Assessment Network
Affiliated with: Interior Health Authority
624 Tranquille Rd., Kamloops, BC V2B 3H6
Tel: 250-554-0085
www.interiorhealth.ca

Note: Offers developmental disability mental health services.

PRINCE GEORGE: AiMHi - Prince George Association for Community Living
950 Kerry St., Prince George, BC V2M 5A3
Tel: 250-564-6408 *Fax:* 250-564-6801
aimhi@aimhi.ca
www.aimhi.ca
Social Media: www.facebook.com/AiMHibc; twitter.com/AiMHiBC

Note: Non-profit, supports individuals with developmental disabilities & children with special needs
Melinda Heidsma, Executive Director

PRINCE GEORGE: Prince George Family Resource Centre
Affiliated with: Northern Health Authority
1200 Lasalle Ave., Prince George, BC V2L 4J8
Tel: 250-614-9449 *Fax:* 250-614-9448
www.northernhealth.ca

VANCOUVER: BC Children's Hospital
Affiliated with: Provincial Health Services Authority
Former Name: Crippled Children's Hospital; Children's Hospital
4480 Oak St., Vancouver, BC V6H 3N1
Tel: 604-875-2345 *Toll-Free:* 888-300-3088
comm@cw.bc.ca
www.bcchildrens.ca

Year Founded: 1928
Note: Programs & services include: Children's Heart Centre; child & youth mental health; clinical, diagnostic, & family services; critical care; endocrinology & diabetes; emergency; family support; pain service; medical genetics; neurosciences; oncology, hematology, & BMT; specialized pediatrics; Sunny Hill Health Centre; surgery; & trauma service.
Sarah Bell, Interim Chief Operating Officer

VANCOUVER: Sunny Hill Health Centre for Children
Affiliated with: Provincial Health Services Authority
3644 Slocan St., Vancouver, BC V5M 3E8
Tel: 604-453-8300 *Fax:* 604-453-8301
Toll-Free: 888-300-3088
TTY: 604-453-8315
www.bcchildrens.ca
Number of Beds: 18 beds
Note: Provincial rehabilitation & assessment centre for children with disabilities

VICTORIA: Queen Alexandra Centre for Children's Health
Affiliated with: Vancouver Island Health Authority
2400 Arbutus Rd., Victoria, BC V8N 1V7
Tel: 250-519-5390
www.viha.ca
Social Media: www.facebook.com/135150073228437; twitter.com/vanislandhealth

Note: Acute & extended care
Dr. Brendan Carr, President & CEO, VIHA

MANITOBA

BRANDON: Child & Adolescent Treatment Centre (CATC)
Affiliated with: Prairie Mountain Health
1240 - 10 St., Brandon, MB R7A 7L6
Tel: 204-578-2700 *Fax:* 204-578-2850
Toll-Free: 866-403-5459
www.prairiemountainhealth.ca

Note: Programs & services include: mental health assessments & treatment; crisis stabilization; individualized treatment plans; individual, group, & family therapy; & mental health education/promotion.

WINNIPEG: Manitoba Adolescent Treatment Centre Inc. (MATC)
Affiliated with: Winnipeg Regional Health Authority
120 Tecumseh St., Winnipeg, MB R3E 2A9
Tel: 204-477-6391
info@matc.ca
www.matc.ca

Number of Beds: 14 beds
Note: Mental health services for children, youth, & families

WINNIPEG: New Directions for Children, Youth, Adults & Families
Former Name: Children's Home of Winnipeg
#500, 717 Portage Ave., Winnipeg, MB R3G 0M8
Tel: 204-786-7051 *Fax:* 204-774-6468
TTY: 204-774-8541
www.newdirections.mb.ca

Year Founded: 1885
Note: Programs & services in the following categories: Counselling, Assessment, Support & Prevention Programs; Training & Education Programs; & Residential & Support Programs.
Dr. Jennifer Frain, Chief Executive Officer

WINNIPEG: Rehabilitation Centre for Children (RCC)
Affiliated with: Winnipeg Regional Health Authority
1155 Notre Dame Ave., Winnipeg, MB R3E 3G1
Tel: 204-452-4311 *Fax:* 204-477-5547
www.rccinc.ca

Note: Offers services to children with physical & developmental challenges.

NEWFOUNDLAND & LABRADOR

ST. JOHN'S: Janeway Children's Health & Rehabilitation Centre
Affiliated with: Eastern Regional Health Authority
300 Prince Philip Dr., St. John's, NL A1B 3V6
Tel: 709-777-6300
client.relations@easternhealth.ca
www.easternhealth.ca
Social Media: www.facebook.com/EasternHealthNL; twitter.com/EasternHealthNL

Number of Beds: 83 beds
Note: Teaching hospital for the Memorial University of Newfoundland Faculty of Medicine. Programs & services include: children & women's health; diagnostic services; dialysis; emergency services; inpatient services; laboratory; outpatient services; radiography; & surgery.

NOVA SCOTIA

KENTVILLE: Evergreen Home for Special Care
655 Park St., Kentville, NS B4N 3V7
Tel: 902-678-7355 *Fax:* 902-678-5996
evergreen@evergreenhome.ns.ca
www.evergreenhome.ns.ca
Number of Beds: 97 beds; 19 children's beds; 2 respite beds
Note: Seniors' Centre; Childrens' Centre
Fred Houghton, Administrator
Dr. Jim Seaman, Medical Director

ONTARIO

AJAX: Carea Community Health Centre - Ajax Office
Former Name: The Youth Centre; Barbara Black Centre for Youth Resources
#5, 360 Bayly St., Ajax, ON L1S 1P1
Tel: 905-428-1212 *Fax:* 905-428-9151
info@careachc.ca
www.careachc.ca
Social Media: www.facebook.com/CareaCHC; twitter.com/careachc

Note: Offers community health & wellness programs, as well as primary care, counselling, & chronic disease management services
Andrea Peckham, Chair

BELLEVILLE: Welcome to Community Living Belleville & Area
Former Name: Plainfield Community Homes; Plainfield Children's Home
91 Millennium Pkwy., Belleville, ON K8N 4Z5
Tel: 613-969-7407 *Fax:* 613-969-7775
www.communitylivingbelleville.org
Social Media: www.facebook.com/communitylivingbellevilleandarea; twitter.com/CLBelleville

Year Founded: 1951
Note: Community Living Belleville & Area works toward the full inclusion in community life of persons with intellectual disabilities.
John B. Klassen, Executive Director
Stephen Ollerenshaw, Director, Finance
Katherine Potts, Director, Human Resources
Christine Semark, Director, Services
Jim Burgess, Manager, Buildings & Property
Sharon Wright, Manager, Community Development & Volunteer
   Services

BRANTFORD: Lansdowne Children's Centre
39 Mount Pleasant St., Brantford, ON N3T 1S7
Tel: 519-753-3153 *Fax:* 519-753-5927
info@lansdownecc.com
www.lansdownecentre.ca
Social Media: www.facebook.com/127644350608842;
twitter.com/LansdowneBrant; www.youtube.com/user/LansdowneCC

Note: The centre provides services for children & youth with physical, communication & developmental challenges.
Rita-Marie Hadley, Executive Director

CAMBRIDGE: KidsAbility Centre for Child Development
Cambridge
Former Name: Rotary Children's Centre
c/o Chaplin Family YMCA, 250 Hespeler Rd., Cambridge, ON N1R 3H3
Fax: 519-886-7292
Toll-Free: 888-372-2259
www.kidsability.ca
Year Founded: 1957
Note: Specialty: Services for children & young adults with physical, developmental, & communication disabilities
Paola Zimmer, Client Services Manager, Cambridge
   pzimmer@kidsability.ca

CHATHAM: Children's Treatment Centre of Chatham-Kent
Former Name: Prism Centre for Audiology & Children's
Rehabilitation
355 Lark St., Chatham, ON N7L 5B2
Tel: 519-354-0520 *Fax:* 519-354-7355
Toll-Free: 877-352-0089
TTY: 226-996-9967
info@ctc-ck.com
www.ctc-ck.com
Social Media: www.facebook.com/CTCCK; twitter.com/CTC_CK
Year Founded: 1948
Note: Services include: music therapy; occupational therapy; physiotherapy; respite services; & speech therapy.
Donna Litwin-Makey, Executive Director
   519-354-0520, dlitwinmakey@childrenstreatment-ck.c
James Lively, Manager, Finance
   jlively@ctc-ck.com

FERGUS: KidsAbility Centre for Child Development
Fergus
Former Name: Rotary Children's Centre
c/o Community Resource Centre, 160 St. David St. South, Fergus, ON N1M 2L3
Fax: 519-886-7292
Toll-Free: 888-372-2259
www.kidsability.ca
Year Founded: 1957
Note: Specialty: Services for children & young adults with physical, developmental, & communication disabilities
Mary Ellen McIlroy, Client Services Manager, Guelph & Fergus
   memcilroy@kidsability.ca

GUELPH: KidsAbility Centre for Child Development
Guelph
Former Name: Rotary Children's Centre
c/o West End Community Centre, 21 Imperial Rd. South, Guelph, ON N1K 1X3
Fax: 519-780-0470
Toll-Free: 888-372-2259
info@kidsability.ca
www.kidsability.ca

Year Founded: 1957
Note: Specialty: Services for children & young adults with physical, developmental, & communication disabilities
Mary Ellen McIlroy, Client Services Manager, Guelph & Fergus
   memcilroy@kidsability.ca

HAMILTON: McMaster Children's Hospital
Hamilton Health Sciences
Affiliated with: Hamilton Niagara Haldimand Brant Local
Health Integration Network
1200 Main St. West, Hamilton, ON L8N 3Z5
Tel: 905-521-2100
www.mcmasterchildrenshospital.ca
Social Media: www.facebook.com/140084176009847;
twitter.com/hamhealthsc; www.vimeo.com/hamiltonhealthsciences
Year Founded: 1988
Number of Beds: 165 acute care beds; 6 mental health day beds; 4 eating disorder day beds
Specialties: Acute pediatrics
Note: Provides tertiary health care services for children in Hamilton & the surrounding region. Programs & services include: 2G, 2Q & 3E child & youth clinic; audiology; Child Advocacy & Assessment Program (CAAP); child & youth mental health program; children's exercise & nutrition centre; emergency; outpatient clinical services for children with diabetes; pediatric eating disorders program; pharmacy; & sexual assault & domestic violence care centre.
Rob MacIsaac, President & CEO, Hamilton Health Sciences
Dr. Peter Fitzgerald, President, McMaster Children's Hospital

HAMILTON: McMaster Children's Hospital - Chedoke Site
Hamilton Health Sciences
Affiliated with: Hamilton Niagara Haldimand Brant Local
Health Integration Network
PO Box 2000 Stn. A, Sanitorium Road, MPO, Hamilton, ON LC9 1C4
Tel: 905-521-2100
www.hamiltonhealthsciences.ca
Social Media: www.facebook.com/140084176009847;
twitter.com/hamhealthsc; www.vimeo.com/hamiltonhealthsciences
Year Founded: 1906
Note: Programs & services include: autism spectrum disorder service (Hamilton Autism Intervention Program); child & youth mental health programs; cleft lip & palate program; developmental pediatrics & rehabilitation; family resource centre; pediatric lipid clinic; specialized developmental & behavioural services; & technology access clinic.
Rob MacIsaac, President & CEO, Hamilton Health Sciences
   president@hhsc.ca
Dr. Peter Fitzgerald, President & CEO, McMaster Children's Hospital

KINGSTON: Child Development Centre (CDC)/Le Centre de
développement de l'enfant
Hotel Dieu Hospital
c/o Hotel Dieu Hospital, 166 Brock St., Kingston, ON K7L 5G2
Tel: 613-544-3400 *Fax:* 613-545-3557
www.kingstoncdc.ca
Area Served: Kingston & the surrounding area
Note: Most services at the Child Development Centre require physician referral. The Infant Develpment Program accepts children directly from parents.

LONDON: Child & Parent Resource Institute (CPRI)
600 Sanatorium Rd., London, ON N6H 3W7
Tel: 519-858-2774 *Fax:* 519-858-3913
Toll-Free: 877-494-2774
www.cpri.ca
Number of Beds: 75 beds
Note: Provides outpatient, intensive/residential, support, & referral services for children & youth with developmental disabilities or mental health needs
Dr. Shannon Stewart, Program Manager

LONDON: London Health Sciences Centre - Children's Hospital
Affiliated with: South West Local Health Integration Network
PO Box 5010, 800 Commissioners Rd. East, London, ON N6A 5W9
Tel: 519-685-8500
www.lhsc.on.ca
Info Line: 519-685-8380
Social Media: www.facebook.com/LHSCCanada;
twitter.com/LHSCCanada; www.youtube.com/LHSCCanada
Year Founded: 1917
Note: Provides specialized paediatric inpatient & outpatient services, including liver & bowel transplants; oncology; infectious disease programs; trauma; & intensive care.
Murray Glendining, President & CEO
Jackie Schleifer Taylor, Vice-President, Children's Hospital & Women's Care

LONDON: Thames Valley Children's Centre
779 Baseline Rd. East, London, ON N6C 5Y6
Tel: 519-685-8700 *Toll-Free:* 866-590-8822
innovations@tvcc.on.ca
www.tvcc.on.ca
Year Founded: 1949
Note: Specialties: Rehabilitation services for children with physical disabilities, developmental delays, & communication disorders; Assessment & diagnosis services; Autism intervention program; Intensive behavioural intervention; Physiotherapy; Occupational therapy; Research; School support program. Number of Employees: 350+ + 500 volunteers + 55 students
John A. LaPorta, CEO

MISSISSAUGA: Erinoak Kids
2277 South Millway, Mississauga, ON L5L 2M5
Tel: 905-855-2690 *Toll-Free:* 877-374-6625
www.erinoakkids.ca
Social Media: www.facebook.com/ErinoakKids;
twitter.com/ErinoakKids; www.youtube.com/ErinoakKidsCentre
Year Founded: 1978
Number of Employees: 650
Note: Offers autism, communication, hearing, medical, occupational therapy, physiotherapy, & vision services to children & families.
Bridget Fewtrell, President & CEO
Pauline Eaton, Vice-President, Autism Services
Chris Hartley, Vice-President, Clinical Services
Kathy Swaile, Vice-President, Human Resources & Facilities
Christina Djokoto, Vice-President, Quality, Improvement & Operational Readiness

OSHAWA: Grandview Children's Centre
Former Name: Grandview Rehabilitation & Treatment Centre of Durham Region
600 Townline Rd. South, Oshawa, ON L1H 7K6
Tel: 905-728-1673 *Fax:* 905-728-2961
Toll-Free: 800-304-6180
www.grandviewkids.ca
Social Media: www.facebook.com/GrandviewKids;
twitter.com/grandviewkids
Note: A treatment centre for children with physical, developmental & communication disabilities.
Lorraine Sunstrum-Mann, Chief Executive Officer
905-728-1673, lorraine.sunstrum-mann@grandviewkids

OTTAWA: Children's Hospital of Eastern Ontario (CHEO)
Affiliated with: Champlain Local Health Integration Network
401 Smyth Rd., Ottawa, ON K1H 8L1
Tel: 613-737-7600 *Toll-Free:* 866-736-2436
webmaster@cheo.on.ca
www.cheo.on.ca
Social Media: www.facebook.com/CHEOkids; twitter.com/cheohospital;
www.youtube.com/user/CHEOvideos
Year Founded: 1974
Number of Beds: 112 pediatric, oncology, adolescent medicine, & surgery beds; 25 psychiatry beds; 20 neonatal intensive care unit beds; 10 intensive care unit beds
Number of Employees: 1796
Note: Programs & services include: Autism Program of Eastern

Ontario; Centre for Healthy Active Living; child & youth protection service; cleft lip & palate craniofacial clinic; diabetes clinic; Eastern Ontario Regional Genetics Program; inpatient psychiatric units; Kaitlin Atkinson Family Resource Library; mental health outpatient' regional eating disorders program; regional psychiatric emergency service for children & youth; sexually assaulted youth counselling; social work; teen health centre; & Youth Net / Réseau Ado. Has 271 physicians on staff.
Alex Munter, President & CEO
Dr. Lindy Samson, Chief of Staff
Susan Richardson, Vice-President, Patient Care

OTTAWA: The Ottawa Children's Treatment Centre (OCTC)/Le Centre de traitement pour enfants d'Ottawa
395 Smyth Rd., Ottawa, ON K1H 8L2
Tel: 613-737-0871 *Fax:* 613-523-5167
Toll-Free: 800-565-4839
www.octc.ca
Year Founded: 1951
Note: From several locations in Ottawa & area, The Centre provides specialized care for children with multiple physical, developmental & behavioural needs. Services in English & French. Amalgamated with the Children's Hospital of Eastern Ontario in October 2016.
Anne Huot, Executive Director
Lori Raycroft, Chief Financial Officer
Shirley Rogers, Director, Human Resource Services
Dr. Elizabeth Macklin, Medical Director, Medical Services

PETERBOROUGH: Five Counties Children's Centre
872 Dutton Rd., Peterborough, ON K9H 7G1
Tel: 705-748-2221 *Fax:* 705-748-3526
Toll-Free: 888-779-9916
www.fivecounties.on.ca
Social Media: www.facebook.com/FiveCountiesChildrensCentre;
twitter.com/5CountiesKids;
www.youtube.com/user/FiveCountiesChildren
Note: Helps children with special needs 0-19 years of age. Services include speech & language therapy, occupational therapy, physiotherapy, therapautic recreation, & augmentative communication.
Diane Pick, Chief Executive Officer
dpick@fivecounties.on.ca
Darlene Callan, Director, Clinical Services
dcallan@fivecounties.on.ca
Kerri Wellstood, Manager, Finance & Administration
kwellstood@fivecounties.on.ca
Elizabeth Martinell, Manager, Quality & Performance
emartinell@fivecounties.on.ca

SARNIA: Pathways Health Centre for Children
1240 Murphy Rd., Sarnia, ON N7S 2Y6
Tel: 519-542-3471 *Fax:* 519-542-4115
Toll-Free: 855-542-3471
info@pathwayscentre.org
www.pathwayscentre.org
Social Media: www.facebook.com/PathwaysHealthCentreforChildren
Year Founded: 1975
Note: Children's treatment centre
Jenny Greensmith, Executive Director

SAULT STE MARIE: THRIVE Child Development Centre
Former Name: Children's Rehabilitation Centre Algoma
74 Johnson Ave., Sault Ste Marie, ON P6C 2V5
Tel: 705-759-1131 *Fax:* 705-759-0783
Toll-Free: 855-759-1131
info@kidsthrive.ca
www.kidsthrive.ca
Year Founded: 1952
Note: Programs & services include therapy, respite care, & resource support.
Susan Vanagas-Cote, Executive Director
Mirja Keranen, Business Director
Kate Lawrence, Professional Services Manager, Early Childhood Education
Maxine Orr, Professional Services Manager, Occupational Therapy
Scott Nieson, Professional Services Manager, Physiotherapy
Tina Nelson, Professional Services Manager, Speech-Language Pathology

ST AGATHA: Carizon Family & Community Services
Former Name: kidsLINK
PO Box 190, 1855 Notre Dame Dr., St Agatha, ON N0B 2L0
Tel: 519-746-5437
Social Media: www.facebook.com/carizonupdates; twitter.com/carizon;
www.linkedin.com/company/carizon-family-and-community-services

Note: Mental health & counselling services for children, youth, & families
Tracy Elop, CEO
Jennifer Berry, Director, Communications

ST CATHARINES: Niagara Peninsula Children's Centre
567 Glenridge Ave., St Catharines, ON L2T 4C2
Tel: 905-688-3550 Fax: 905-688-1055
Toll-Free: 800-896-5496
info@niagarachildrenscentre.com
www.niagarachildrenscentre.com

Note: Children's rehabilitation centre
Oksana Fisher, CEO
905-688-1890, oksana.fisher@niagarachildrenscentre
Marla Smith, Director, Development
marla.smith@niagarachildrenscentre.c
Dorothy Harvey, Manager, Rehabilitation Services
dorothy.harvey@niagarachildrenscentr
Jackie VanLankveld, Manager, Speech Services
jackie.vanlankveld@niagarachildrensc
Jean Byrnes, Manager, Corporate Services & Finance
jean.byrnes@niagarachildrenscentre.c

SUDBURY: Children's Treatment Centre
Affiliated with: Health Sciences North
41 Ramsey Lake Rd., Sudbury, ON P3E 5J1
Tel: 705-523-7337 Fax: 705-523-7157
www.hsnsudbury.ca
Social Media: www.facebook.com/HSNSudbury;
twitter.com/HSN_Sudbury;
www.youtube.com/user/healthsciencesnorth;
www.linkedin.com/company/health-sciences-north

Note: Outpatient, community-based rehabilitation centre for children & young adults with motor & communication challenges.
Dr. Sean Murray, Medical Director
Joanne Tramontini, Clinical Manager

THUNDER BAY: George Jeffrey Children's Centre (GJCC)
Former Name: George Jeffrey Children's Treatment Centre
200 Brock St. East, Thunder Bay, ON P7E 0A2
Tel: 807-623-4381 Fax: 807-623-7161
Toll-Free: 888-818-7330
www.georgejeffrey.com
Social Media: www.facebook.com/132052553534644
Year Founded: 1948
Note: Services include occupational therapy, physiotherapy, speech & language therapy & social work.
Tom Walters, Chief Executive Officer

TIMMINS: Cochrane Temiskaming Children's Treatment Centre
#1, 733 Ross Ave. East, Timmins, ON P4N 8S8
Tel: 705-264-4700 Fax: 705-268-3585
Toll-Free: 800-575-3210
Year Founded: 1980
Area Served: Districts of Cochrane and Temiskaming
Note: Services include consultation, assessment, treatment and education.
Mary MacKay, Executive Director

TORONTO: Central Toronto Community Health Centres
Shout Clinic
168 Bathurst St., Toronto, ON M5V 2R4
Tel: 416-703-8482
info@ctchc.com
www.ctchc.com
Year Founded: 1992
Note: Walk-in medical clinic providing comprehensive health care services to homeless & street involved youth, 16-24 years of age.

Anne Marie DiCenso, Director, Community Health & Development
adicenso@ctchc.com

TORONTO: Child Development Institute
Former Name: West End Creche Child & Family Clinic
197 Euclid Ave., Toronto, ON M6J 2J8
Tel: 416-603-1827 Fax: 416-603-6655
info@childdevelop.ca
www.childdevelop.ca
Social Media: www.facebook.com/childdevelop; twitter.com/officialcdi;
www.youtube.com/user/CDICanada;
www.linkedin.com/company/child-development-institute
Year Founded: 1909
Note: Provides mental health programs & services for children & youth
Tony Diniz, CEO
tdiniz@childdevelop.ca
Steve Blake, COO
sblake@childdevelop.ca
Dr. Leena Augimeri, Director, Scientific & Program Development
laugimeri@childdevelop.ca
Shauna Klein, Director, Fund Development, Marketing & Communications
sklein@childdevelop.ca
Linda Levely, Director, Finance & Administration
llevely@childdevelop.ca

TORONTO: Holland Bloorview Kids Rehabilitation Hospital
Affiliated with: Toronto Central Local Health Integration Network
Former Name: Bloorview Children's Hospital
150 Kilgour Road, Toronto, ON M4G 1R8
Tel: 416-425-6220 Fax: 416-425-6591
Toll-Free: 800-363-2440
www.hollandbloorview.ca
Social Media: www.facebook.com/HBKRH; twitter.com/HBKidsHospital;
www.youtube.com/user/PRBloorview
Year Founded: 1899
Number of Beds: 75 beds
Note: Pediatric rehabilitation & continuing care complex
Julia Hanigsberg, President & CEO
Marilyn Ballantyne, Chief Nursing Executive
Golda Milo-Manson, Vice-President, Medicine & Academic Affairs
Stewart Wong, Vice-President, Communications, Marketing & Advocacy

TORONTO: The Hospital for Sick Children
Affiliated with: Toronto Central Local Health Integration Network
Also Known As: SickKids
555 University Ave., Toronto, ON M5G 1X8
Tel: 416-813-1500
www.sickkids.ca
Info Line: 416-813-6621
Social Media: www.facebook.com/sickkidsfoundation;
twitter.com/SickKidsNews; www.youtube.com/SickKidsInteractive;
www.linkedin.com/company/the-hospital-for-sick-children
Year Founded: 1875
Number of Beds: 370 beds
Note: Paediatric acute care hospital, with programs & services including: adolescent medicine; allergy; anxiety disorders; audiology; blood & marrow transplant; burns; cancer detection & treatment; cardiology; cleft lip & palate; dental clinic; diabetes clinic; dialysis; eating disorders; emergency; genetic counselling; gynecology; hand clinic; hematology; infectious diseases (including HIV); International Patient Office; Motherisk program; ophthalmology; otolaryngology; pain clinic; psychiatry; psychiatric emergency crisis service; respiratory illnesses; SCAN (Suspected Child Abuse & Neglect) program; sleep disorders; social work; speech language clinic; substance abuse outreach & day treatment; Tay Sachs testing; trauma unit; & Young Families Program (Tots of Teens).
Dr. Michael Apkon, President & CEO
Jeff Mainland, Executive Vice-President, Strategy, Quality, Performance & Communications
Marilyn Monk, Executive Vice-President, Clinical
Dr. Denis Daneman, Chief, Paediatrics

TORONTO: Oakdale Child & Family Service Ltd.

291 Chisholm Ave., Toronto, ON M4C 4W5

Tel: 416-699-5600 *Fax:* 416-699-6547
tor-oakdale@bellnet.ca
www.oakdaleservices.com

Note: Specialties: Long & short term care for children with special needs; Teaching independence in life skills, social & community awareness, & appropriate communication methods

WATERLOO: KidsAbility - Centre for Child Development
Former Name: Rotary Children's Centre

500 Hallmark Dr., Waterloo, ON N2K 3P5

Tel: 519-886-8886 *Fax:* 519-886-7292
Toll-Free: 888-372-2259
info@kidsability.ca
www.kidsability.ca

Social Media: www.facebook.com/KidsAbility; twitter.com/KidsAbility
Year Founded: 1957
Note: Specialties: Services for children & young adults with physical, developmental, & communication disabilities; Autism intervention; Occupational therapy; Physiotherapy; Speech-language therapy; Augmentative communication; Therapeutic recreation; Social work.
Number of Employees: 200 + 300 volunteers
Linda Kenny, CEO
 lkenny@kidsability.ca
Nancy Buchanan, CFO
 nbuchanan@kidsability.ca

WINDSOR: The John McGivney Children's Centre
Former Name: Children's Rehabilitation Centre of Essex County

3945 Matchette Rd., Windsor, ON N9C 4C2

Tel: 519-252-7281 *Fax:* 519-252-5873
info@jmccentre.ca
www.jmccentre.ca
Social Media: www.facebook.com/243715438993933;
twitter.com/JMCCentre

Note: Services include augmentative communication, autism services, & speech, occupational, & physiotherapy.
Elaine Whitmore, Chief Executive Officer

WINDSOR: Teen Health Centre
Affiliated with: Windsor Essex Community Health Centre

#101, 1361 Ouellette Ave., Windsor, ON N8X 1J6

Tel: 519-253-8481 *Fax:* 519-253-4362
www.wechc.org

Note: Specialties: Counselling; Primary care; Special Additions, a prenatal program; Diabetes In Action, a community based diabetes program; Street Health Homeless Initiative Program, a program to serve homeless or at-risk persons in Windsor & Essex County

---

PRINCE EDWARD ISLAND

TRACADIE CROSS: Provincial Adolescent Group Home

171 Station Rd., Tracadie Cross, PE C1A 7N8

Tel: 902-676-3242 *Fax:* 902-676-3241
Number of Beds: 9 beds; 1 emergency 72-hour bed
Note: Adolescent residential treatment

QUÉBEC

BONAVENTURE: Centre de réadaptation pour les jeunes en difficulté d'adaptation de Bonaventure
Affiliée à: CISSS de la Gaspésie
Ancien nom: Centre jeunesse Gaspésie/Les Iles - Unité La Balise

193, av de Port Royal, Bonaventure, QC G0C 1E0

Tél: 418-534-3283
www.cisss-gaspesie.gouv.qc.ca

Nombre de lits: 12 lits

BONAVENTURE: Point de service - Réadaptation et jeunesse de Bonaventure
Affiliée à: CISSS de la Gaspésie

238, av Port-Royal, Bonaventure, QC G0C 1E0

Tél: 418-534-4243 *Téléc:* 418-534-2411

CHANDLER: Centre de protection et de réadaptation pour les jeunes en difficulté d'adaptation du Rocher-Percé
Affiliée à: CISSS de la Gaspésie
Ancien nom: Centre jeunesse Gaspésie/Les Iles - Succursale Rocher-Percé

#102, 105, rue Commerciale Ouest, Chandler, QC G0C 1K0

Tél: 418-689-2286

CHICOUTIMI: Le Centre jeunesse du Saguenay — Lac-Saint-Jean
Affiliée à: CIUSSS du Saguenay-Lac-Saint-Jean

1109, av Bégin, Chicoutimi, QC G7H 4P1

Tél: 418-549-4853 *Téléc:* 418 693-0765
www.cjsaglac.ca
Média social: www.facebook.com/cjsaglac

Laval Dionne, Président, Conseil d'administration
Marc Thibeault, Directeur général
Sylvie Mailhot, Commissaire aux plaintes et à la qualité des services
 plaintes@cjsaglac.ca
Danielle Tremblay, Directrice de la protection de la jeunesse
Brigitte Savaria, Agente d'information

CÔTE SAINT-LUC: CLSC René-Cassin
Affiliée à: CIUSSS du Centre-Ouest-de-l'Ile-de-Montréal

5800, boul Cavendish, Côte Saint-Luc, QC H4W 2T5

Tél: 514-484-7878 *Téléc:* 514-485-2978
www.cssscavendish.qc.ca

Spécialités: Services médicaux; Services psychosociaux; Centre d'éducation pour la santé; Clinique enfance - jeunesse; Services de nutrition; Vaccination

GASPÉ: Centre de réadaptation pour les jeunes en difficulté d'adaptation de Gaspé
Affiliée à: CISSS de la Gaspésie
Ancien nom: Centre jeunesse Gaspésie/Les Iles - Unité La Vigie

418, montée de Wakeham, Gaspé, QC G4X 2P4

Tél: 418-368-5344
www.cisss-gaspesie.gouv.qc.ca

Note: Centre de réadaptation.

GASPÉ: Centre jeunesse Gaspésie/Les Iles - Unité La Rade
Affiliée à: CISSS de la Gaspésie

#100, 205, boul de York Ouest, Gaspé, QC G4X 2V7

Tél: 418-368-1803

GASPÉ: Programme Jeunesse
Affiliée à: CISSS de la Gaspésie
Ancien nom: Centre jeunesse Gaspésie/Les Iles

#100, 205, boul de York ouest, Gaspé, QC G4X 2V7

Tél: 418-368-1803

Nombre de lits: 55 lits

GATINEAU: Les Centres jeunesse de l'Outaouais
Affiliée à: CISSS de l'Outaouais

105, boul Sacré-Coeur, Gatineau, QC J8X 1C5

Tél: 819-771-6631
www.cjoutaouais.qc.ca

Nombre de lits: 149 lits
Note: Centre jeunesse, protection

JOLIETTE: Les Centres jeunesse de Lanaudière (CJL)
Affiliée à: CISSS de Lanaudière

260, rue Lavaltrie Sud, Joliette, QC J6E 5X7

Tél: 450-756-4555 *Téléc:* 450-756-0814
Ligne sans frais: 800-229-1152
www.centresjeunessedelanaudiere.qc.ca

Jacques Perreault, Président, Conseil d'administration
Richard Provost, Vice-président

Christian Gagné, Directeur général & Secrétaire

LAVAL: Centre Jeunesse de Laval
Affiliée à: CISSS de Laval
308, boul Cartier Ouest, Laval, QC H7N 2J2
Tél: 450-975-4150
www.centrejeunessedelaval.ca
Guy Villeneuve, Président, Conseil d'administration
Jean-Guy Blanchet, Premier vice-président, Conseil d'administration
Danièle Dulude, Secrétaire, Conseil d'administration
Yvon Shedleur, Trésorier, Conseil d'administration
Mathieu Vachon, Responsable, services des communications

LES ILES-DE-LA-MADELEINE: Centre de protection et de réadaptation pour les jeunes des les-de-la-Madeleine
Affiliée à: CISSS de la Gaspésie
Ancien nom: Centre jeunesse Gaspésie/Les Iles - Succursale des Iles
539-2, ch Principal, Les Iles-de-la-Madeleine, QC G4T 1E7
Tél: 418-986-2230

LÉVIS: Les Centres jeunesse Chaudière-Appalaches
Affiliée à: CISSS de Chaudière-Appalaches
100, rue Mgr Ignace-Bourget, Lévis, QC G6V 2Y9
Tél: 418-837-1930 *Téléc:* 418-838-8860
Ligne sans frais: 800-461-9331
Nombre de lits: 146 lits
Note: Services de la protection de la jeunesse; service aux jeunes contrevenants; service d'adoption; services de réadaptation.
Installations: Lévis, Saint-Romuald, Montmagny, Sainte-Marie, Saint-Joseph, Saint-Georges & Thetford Mines.

LISTUGUJ: Centre de réadaptation pour les jeunes en difficulté d'adaptation de Listuguj
Affiliée à: CISSS de la Gaspésie
Ancien nom: Centre jeunesse Gaspésie/Les Iles - Unité Gignu
CP 193, 4, Pacific Dr., Listuguj, QC G0C 2R0
Tél: 418-788-5605

LONGUEUIL: Centre jeunesse de la Montérégie (CJM)
Affiliée à: CISSS de la Montérégie-Est
575, rue Adoncour, Longueuil, QC J4G 2M6
Tél: 450-928-5125 *Téléc:* 450-679-3731
Ligne sans frais: 800-641-1315
www.centrejeunessemonteregie.qc.ca
Fondée en: 1992
Personnel: 1 906
Marc Rodier, Président
Catherine Lemay, Directrice générale & Secrétaire
Pierre Henrichon, Trésorier

MONTRÉAL: Centre de protection de l'enfance et de la jeunesse
Affiliée à: CIUSSS du Centre-Sud-de-l'Ile-de-Montréal
Ancien nom: Centre jeunesse de Montréal - Institut universitaire
Fondation du Centre Jeunesse de Montréal, 9335, rue Saint-Hubert, Montréal, QC H2M 1Y7
Tél: 514-593-2676
www.ciusss-centresudmtl.gouv.qc.ca
Média social: www.youtube.com/user/centrejeunessemtl

Jean-Marc Potvin, Directeur général, CIUSSS du Centre-Sud-de-l'Ile-de-Montréal

MONTRÉAL: Hôpital Shriners pour enfants (Québec) inc.
1003 boul Décarie, Montréal, QC H4A 0A9
Tél: 514-842-4464 *Téléc:* 514-842-7553
Ligne sans frais: 800-361-7256
www.shrinershospitalsforchildren.org
Nombre de lits: 40 lits
Christine Boyle, Administrator
Reggie Hamdy, Directeur, Personnel
Emmanuelle Rondeau, Directrice, Communications et marketing

MONTRÉAL: Hôpital Shriners pour enfants (Quebec) inc.
1003, boul Decarie, Montréal, QC H4A 0A9
Tél: 514-842-4464 *Téléc:* 514-842-7553
Ligne sans frais: 800-361-7256
fr.shrinershospitalsforchildren.org/%C3%A9tablissements/lrf/canada
Céline Doray, Directrice générale

RIMOUSKI: Centre jeunesse du Bas-St-Laurent
Affiliée à: CISSS du Bas-St-Laurent
CP 3500, 287, rue Pierre-Saindon, 3e étage, Rimouski, QC G5L 8V5
Tél: 418-723-1255 *Téléc:* 418-722-0620
www.centrejeunessebsl.com
Nombre de lits: 73 lits

SAINT-JÉRÔME: Centre jeunesse des Laurentides
Affiliée à: CISSS des Laurentides
500, boul des Laurentides, Saint-Jérôme, QC J7Z 5M2
Tél: 450-436-7607 *Téléc:* 450-436-4811
Ligne sans frais: 866-492-3263
www.cjlaurentides.qc.ca
Nombre de lits: 160 lits

SHERBROOKE: Centre jeunesse de l'Estrie (CJE)
Affiliée à: CIUSSS de l'Estrie
594, boul Queen Victoria, Sherbrooke, QC J1H 3R7
Tél: 819-564-7100 *Téléc:* 819-564-7109
Ligne sans frais: 800-567-3495
intranet.cje@ssss.gouv.qc.ca
www.cjestrie.ca
Média social: www.facebook.com/CJEstrie; twitter.com/CjEstrie

Personnel: 620
Marie Caron, Directrice générale

SHERBROOKE: Centre Notre-Dame de l'Enfant (Sherbrooke) inc. (CNDE)
CRDITED Estrie
1621, rue Prospect, Sherbrooke, QC J1J 1K4
Tél: 819-346-8471 *Téléc:* 819-346-8473
info.crditedestrie@ssss.gouv.qc.ca
www.crditedestrie.qc.ca
Fondée en: 1965
Note: Le centre de réadaptation en déficience intellectuelle et troubles envahissants du développement Estre (CRDITED Estrie) est composé de deux établissements du réseau de la santé et des services sociaux du Québec, soit le Centre Notre-Dame de l'Enfant (Sherbrooke) inc. et le Centre d'accueil Dixville inc.
Danielle Lareau, Directrice générale

STE-ANNE-DES-MONTS: Programme Jeunesse - Succursale Haute-Gaspésie
Affiliée à: CISSS de la Gaspésie
230, rte du Parc, #EB-132, Ste-Anne-des-Monts, QC G4V 2C4
Tél: 418-763-2251

TROIS-RIVIÈRES: Centre jeunesse de la Mauricie et Centre-du-Québec
Affiliée à: CIUSSS de la Mauricie-et-du-Centre-du-Québec
Centre administratif, 1455, boul du Carmel, Trois-Rivières, QC G8Z 3R7
Ligne sans frais: 855-378-5481
communications_cjmcq@ssss.gouv.qc.ca
www.cjmcq.qc.ca

Robert Nolin, Président, Conseil d'administration
Nathalie Garon, Directrice générale intérimaire
Gérald Milot, Vice-président, Conseil d'administration
Dorothée Leblanc, Secrétaire, Conseil d'administration

VAL-D'OR: Centre jeunesse de l'Abitibi-Témiscamingue
Affiliée à: CISSS de l'Abitibi-Témiscamingue
700, boul Forest, Val-d'Or, QC J9P 2L3
Tél: 819-825-0002 *Téléc:* 819-825-5132
www.cisss-at.gouv.qc.ca
Fondée en: 1996
Nombre de lits: 57 lits
Personnel: 450

VERDUN: Teen Haven
4360, boul Lasalle, Verdun, QC H4G 2A8
Tel: 514-769-5050
teenhaven@b2b2c.ca
www.teenhaven.ca

Number of Beds: 15 lits
Marie Louise Dionne, Administrative Secretary

**WESTMOUNT: Les centres de la jeunesse et de la famille
Batshaw**
Affiliée à: CIUSSS de l'Ouest-de-l'Ile-de-Montréal
**Ancien nom: Les centres de la jeunesse et de la famille
Saint-Georges**
5, rue Weredale Park, Westmount, QC H3Z 1Y5
Tél: 514-989-1885
www.batshaw.qc.ca

Nombre de lits: 243 lits
Note: Centre de réadaptation (déficience motrice) + déficience
sensorielle

Personality Disorders

Personality is deeply rooted in our sense of ourselves and how
others see us; it is formed from a complex intermingling of genetic
factors and life experience. Everyone has personality characteristics that are likable and unlikable, attractive and unattractive, to
others. By adulthood, most of us have personality traits that are
difficult to change. Sometimes, these deeply rooted personality
traits can get in the way of our happiness, hinder relationships
and even cause harm to ourselves or others. For example, a person may have a tendency to be deeply suspicious of other people
with no good reason. Another person may assume a haughty,
arrogant manner that is difficult to be around.

A diagnosis of a personality disorder should be distinguished
from labelling someone as a bad or disagreeable person and not
be used to stigmatize people who are simply unpopular, rebel-
lious or otherwise unorthodox. A personality disorder is not simply
a personality style, but a condition that interferes with successful
living. A personality disorder refers to an enduring pattern or experience and behaviour that is inflexible, long-lasting (often beginning in adolescence or early childhood) and which leads to
distress and impairment. Personality disorders frequently co-exist with substance abuse, sexual problems, eating disorders, suicidal thinking and behaviour, depression and other mental
disorders, and are estimated to affect between 6 and 15 percent
of the general population.

Personality disorders, by definition, do not cause symptoms,
which are experiences that are troublesome to the individual.
They consist of whole sets of distorted experiences of the outside
world that pervade every or nearly every aspect of a person's life,
causing traits and behaviours leading to interpersonal problems
which only secondarily cause distress to the individual. The
problem is blamed on other people.

Cause
The exact cause of personality disorders is not known. Research
suggests that a traumatic event (for example, the loss of a parent), particularly in early childhood, may act as a trigger for the
development of a personality disorder. Social factors (such as
abuse, parental neglect or overprotection), and genetic factors
may also be involved. It also appears that in people with personality disorders, there may be some dysfunction in the regulation of
the brain circuits that control emotion.

Ten distinct personality disorders have been identified: antisocial,
avoidant, borderline, dependent, histrionic, narcissistic, obsessive-compulsive, paranoid, schizoid and schizotypal.

Antisocial Personality Disorder
Antisocial personality disorder is usually characterized by irresponsible behaviour and a disregard for the law, the rights of others and societal norms.

Symptoms
Antisocial personality traits may begin to appear in early childhood or adolescence in the form of lying, stealing, property destruction, trouble-making, disrespect for authority, rule violation
and violent behaviour. Adults with antisocial personality disorder
may exhibit aggression, frustration and reckless behaviour (such
as unsafe sex or excessive speeding); abuse drugs or alcohol;
make irresponsible decisions about money; lead a tumultuous
life (for example, change jobs or relationships in an unpredictable manner) and engage in criminal activities (such as theft or
drug dealing). People with antisocial personality disorder often
use their charm to deceive, trick or manipulate others. They seem
to feel little remorse for the suffering of those affected by their
behaviour.

Prevalence
Antisocial personality disorder is estimated to affect between 1
and 3 percent of the general population. It is much more common
in men than women.

Treatment Options
A clinical diagnosis of antisocial personality disorder is based
upon identification of the following criteria outlined in the Diagnostic and Statistical Manual of Mental Disorders (DSM): the person has demonstrated a pattern of getting into trouble at school,
at home or with the law as a child or teen; the person continues to
show persistent disregard for the rights of others and rules of society. This pattern is manifested in at least three of the following
ways: behaviour that repeatedly results in arrest; repeated de-
ception of others for profit or fun; impulsive behaviour; physical
fights that occur on a regular basis; reckless disregard for personal safety and that of others; lack of concern about holding a
job or meeting financial obligations; lack of remorse about the
consequences of his or her actions; feelings of justification or
indifference about having caused harm or suffering to other
people.

Most people who suffer from antisocial personality disorder do
not see themselves as having psychological problems, and therefore do not seek treatment. Antisocial personality disorder is notably difficult to treat, especially in extreme cases, when the
affected individual lacks all concern for others. For those who do
seek treatment, long-term psychotherapy is the most effective.
This may include cognitive behavioural therapy (in which a patient learns to replace negative beliefs and behaviours with positive ones), psychodynamic therapy (which helps patients
understand unconscious thoughts and behaviours so that they
can change their negative impact) and psychoeducation (which
teaches patients ways to cope with their condition).

Psychotherapeutic treatment should include attention to family
members, stressing the importance of emotional support, reassurance, explanation of the disorder and advice on how to manage and respond to the patient. Group therapy is helpful in many
situations.

There is no specific medication used to treat antisocial personality disorder, however antidepressants, mood stabilizers, anti-anxiety agents and antipsychotic drugs may be prescribed to treat
conditions associated with the disorder.

Antisocial personality disorder is a chronic, lifelong condition. The
impulsive behaviour associated with this disorder commonly re-

sults in imprisonment or premature death due to an accident or suicide. However, it appears that the more serious symptoms of antisocial personality disorder often diminish as people age.

Avoidant Personality Disorder

People with avoidant personality disorder often feel extremely shy and self-conscious in social settings. In fact, they may try to avoid these situations at all costs because they are so terrified that they will say or do something humiliating that will be criticized by others.

Symptoms

The signs of avoidant personality disorder may include self-criticism, hypersensitivity, social inhibition, social awkwardness and social anxiety. Because they are so terrified of rejection, people with avoidant personality disorder may miss school and work and feel unable to participate in social events, even though they do want to have friends and a social life.

Prevalence

Avoidant personality disorder is one of the most common personality disorders with a prevalence of about 6.6 percent in the general population.

Treatment Options

clinical diagnosis of avoidant personality disorder is based upon the following criteria outlined in the Diagnostic and Statistical Manual of Mental Disorders (DSM): in social settings, they have a pattern of feeling hypersensitive, inhibited and inadequate. This pattern is manifested in at least four of the following ways: avoidance of jobs that require a good deal of interpersonal contact due to fear of criticism or rejection; an unwillingness to get to know people without advance assurance that they will be liked; resistance of intimacy for fear of shame or ridicule; worries about being criticized or rejected in social settings; inhibition when meeting new people due to feelings of inadequacy; feelings of inferiority, social ineptitude and unattractiveness; reluctance to take risks or try new things for fear that they might prove embarrassing. The avoidance must also have started early in life, be well beyond normal shyness and interfere significantly with school, work and social life.

The most effective treatment for avoidant personality disorder is psychotherapy. Psychotherapy encourages patients to talk about the personality traits that have a negative impact on their lives, and therefore helps to improve social interactions. It is important for a patient to find a mental health professional with expert knowledge and experience in treating personality disorders.

Psychotherapeutic treatment should include attention to family members, stressing the importance of emotional support, reassurance, explanation of the disorder and advice on how to manage and respond to the patient. Group therapy is helpful in many situations.

Medication can be useful in treating the anxiety and depression that sometimes co-exist with avoidant personality disorder. Therapy can often help people with avoidant personality disorder improve their social skills.

Borderline Personality Disorder

People with borderline personality disorder often engage in impulsive behaviour, have unstable relationships, and are subject to intense mood changes, a high level of anxiety and an ever-changing self-image.

Symptoms

Borderline personality disorder is characterized by unstable behaviour (self-harm, risk-taking, suicidal thoughts or attempts), unstable emotions (extreme anger, intense boredom, severe anxiety or depression), unstable relationships (fear of abandonment, unstable sense of others), unstable sense of identity (lack of self-knowledge, feelings of emptiness) and awareness problems (delusions, hallucinations, feeling separated from mind and body). The symptoms of borderline personality disorder vary from person to person because there are many different combinations of symptoms. Often, symptoms are easier to manage as people grow older, and in many cases, people recover from the disorder by the time they are 50. Other disorders associated with borderline personality disorder include eating disorders, attention-deficit/hyperactivity disorder, anxiety disorders, mood disorders and dissociative disorders.

Prevalence

Borderline is one of the most common personality disorders. About 1 percent of Canadians will be affected by this disorder over the course of their lives. It is usually diagnosed when people are in their twenties.

Treatment Options

A clinical diagnosis of borderline personality disorder is based upon confirming at least five of the following criteria outlined in the Diagnostic and Statistical Manual of Mental Disorders (DSM): extreme fear of abandonment, repeated unstable relationships, unstable sense of self, behaviour that is self-destructive and impulsive, suicidal thinking/behaviour or self-harm, extreme mood swings, feelings of emptiness, anger management problems, episodes of paranoia and loss of contact with reality.

The most effective treatment for borderline personality disorder is psychotherapy. Dialectical behaviour therapy, which combines cognitive behavioural therapy with mindfulness, is commonly used to treat borderline personality disorder. Newer therapies include mentalization-based therapy (which helps patients understand behaviour and the thoughts and feelings associated with it), transference-focused therapy (which helps patients understand relationships) and schema-focused therapy (which focuses on problematic ways of thinking, feeling and behaving).

Psychotherapeutic treatment should include attention to family members, stressing the importance of emotional support, reassurance, explanation of the disorder and advice on how to manage and respond to the patient. Group therapy is helpful in many situations.

Medications can be useful in treating some of the symptoms of borderline personality disorder, and may include mood stabilizers, certain antidepressants and atypical antipsychotics.

Early diagnosis and appropriate therapy is crucial for people with borderline personality disorder. Although the condition tends to stabilize after the age of 30, around 75 to 80 percent of people with borderline personality disorder attempt or threaten suicide, and 8 to 10 percent die of suicide.

Dependent Personality Disorder

People with dependent personality disorder exhibit an excessive need to be taken care of, and to be led in decision-making. They can also be very clingy.

Symptoms

Dependent personality disorder is characterized by feelings of inadequacy, helplessness and incompetence. Because they rely on others so much, people with this disorder may never learn decision-making or self-motivation skills. They may also be under-achievers since they are often afraid to seek employment that requires decision-making or responsibility. Women with dependent personality disorder are often submissive, while men with the disorder tend to be more demanding and pushy, even though they are still dependent on others.

Prevalence
Dependent personality disorder affects close to 1 percent of the general population.

Treatment Options
A clinical diagnosis of dependent personality disorder is based upon confirming at least five of the following criteria outlined in the Diagnostic and Statistical Manual of Mental Disorders (DSM): requires advice and reassurance for normal decision-making, places major life responsibilities on others, hastens to find another relationship to stand in for one that has ended, worries excessively about life without someone to care for him or her, feels uncomfortable when alone, agrees to do unpleasant things in exchange for care, is unmotivated to take action without the help of others and is afraid to disagree with someone if that might mean losing that person's support. These behaviours are exhibited over a long period of time and affect everyday activities, relationships and quality of life.

Treatment of dependent personality disorder may include cognitive behavioural therapy (in which the patient learns to replace negative beliefs and behaviours with positive ones), interpersonal therapy (which helps the patient understand patterns of interaction in relation to dependency issues), group therapy and family/marital therapy. Medication such as antidepressants or anti-anxiety agents may be prescribed.

Many people who receive therapy for dependent personality disorder can learn to become more independent and enjoy an improved quality of life.

Histrionic Personality Disorder
People with histrionic personality disorder are often extremely emotional in social settings. Their behaviour may appear theatrical, even when that is not the intent.

Symptoms
Although it is usually not intended, the seductive behaviour of someone with histrionic personality disorder may seem like a "come on" to other people. Individuals with this disorder may also be obsessively focused on their personal appearance, and have a tendency to be overly sensitive to any perceived criticism about the way they look. A fear of commitment and becoming emotionally intimate often makes interpersonal relationships difficult for people with this disorder.

Prevalence
It is estimated that close to 1 percent of the general population is affected by histrionic personality disorder.

Treatment Options
A clinical diagnosis of histrionic personality disorder is based upon confirming at least five of the following criteria outlined in the Diagnostic and Statistical Manual of Mental Disorders (DSM): discomfort when not the centre of attention; inappropriate provocative behaviour; ever-changing, superficial emotions; focus on physical appearance as attention-seeking measure; overly dramatic social behaviour; misinterpretation of actual intimacy of relationships; and being easily influenced by others.

Treatment for histrionic personality disorder may include group and family therapy. Medication is usually only prescribed if there is a co-existing condition such as depression.

Although people with histrionic personality disorder often have difficulty staying in therapy long enough to benefit from it, many

individuals with the disorder seem to exhibit fewer symptoms as they grow older.

Narcissistic Personality Disorder
People with narcissistic personality disorder tend to seek the admiration of others, feel overly important and lack empathy.

Symptoms
Individuals affected by narcissistic personality disorder may think that they are extremely special and should only associate with people of a similar status. A sense of entitlement may make them feel that it is acceptable to resort to illegal means to get what they want, or to use other people to get ahead. Individuals with this disorder often have problematic interpersonal relationships.

Prevalence
Approximately 2 percent of the population is affected by narcissistic personality disorder.

Treatment Options
A clinical diagnosis of narcissistic personality disorder is based upon confirmation of at least five of the following criteria outlined in the Diagnostic and Statistical Manual of Mental Disorders (DSM): over-inflated sense of self; obsessive fantasies about success, beauty and intelligence; sense of special status; sense of entitlement; lack of empathy; constant jealousy of achievements of others; arrogance; need for admiration of others; and facility in using others for personal gain.

Treatment of narcissistic personality disorder may include psychotherapy, although the benefits may be limited due to the fact that many people with this disorder tend to criticize their therapists. If anxiety or depression co-exists with narcissistic personality disorder, medication may be prescribed to relieve the symptoms of these conditions.

Although some people with narcissistic personality disorder find that they have fewer symptoms in middle age, others may find it extremely painful to lose their looks and relinquish their positions in the labour force as they age.

Obsessive Compulsive Disorder
People with obsessive compulsive disorder (OCD) often have a constant need to be in control and keep things orderly.

Symptoms
OCD is usually characterized by obsession with details and scheduling, a need to constantly recheck things to avoid making a mistake, black-and-white thinking, being overly critical of self and others, workaholic tendencies, inflexibility, hoarding and miserly behaviour.

Prevalence
OCD is one of the most common personality disorders, with an estimated prevalence rate of 7 percent in the general population.

Treatment Options
A clinical diagnosis of OCD is based upon confirmation of at least four of the following criteria outlined in the Diagnostic and Statistical Manual of Mental Disorders (DSM): preoccupation with lists, schedules, details and organization; perfectionism that interferes with everyday living; preoccupation with work to the exclusion of other activities; inflexibility in relation to ethics; inability to throw things out; rigidity; obstinacy; and miserly behaviour.

Treatment for OCD is usually focused on cognitive behavioural therapy (in which the patient learns to replace negative beliefs and behaviours with positive ones). Medication, primarily selective serotonin reuptake inhibitors (SSRIs), may be prescribed.

OCD is a chronic condition, and it is rare to completely resolve all symptoms associated with the disorder. However, most people with OCD can benefit from a combination of drug therapy and psychotherapy.

Paranoid Personality Disorder

Paranoid personality disorder is characterized by a tendency to mistrust others and suspect that they have ulterior motives.

Symptoms

To be diagnosed with paranoid personality disorder, one must show feelings of distrust and suspicion of others, social isolation, aggressiveness, hostility, lack of a sense of humour, and the sense—without any justification—that others intend to harm or exploit the person.

Prevalence

More men than women appear to be affected by paranoid personality disorder; it affects between 0.5 and 2 percent of the general population.

Treatment Options

A clinical diagnosis of paranoid personality disorder is based upon, from at least early adulthood, confirmation of a minimum of four of the following criteria outlined in the Diagnostic and Statistical Manual of Mental Disorders (DSM): the belief that others are not worthy of trust; an unfounded suspicion that people intend to harm, deceive or exploit him or her; the misinterpretation of innocent remarks or neutral events; a tendency to hold grudges; angry and aggressive responses to perceived insults; and jealousy and unfounded suspicions about a partner's sexual faithfulness.

Individual supportive psychotherapy is considered the most effective treatment for paranoid personality disorder. However, since many people with this disorder are suspicious of therapists, gaining the trust of the patient can be difficult. Paranoid personality disorder is not usually treated with medication. If a person is very anxious, anti-anxiety agents are sometimes prescribed. Low doses of antipsychotic medications may be used during times of extreme stress or agitation.

People with paranoid personality disorder often have the condition for life. However, their feelings of paranoia may be at least partially controlled through appropriate therapy.

Schizoid Personality Disorder

People with schizoid personality disorder are often unable to relate to other people, and have a limited range of emotions.

Symptoms

Signs of schizoid personality disorder may include lack of emotion, mechanical behaviour, social isolation, social awkwardness and lack of desire for personal interaction. Because they do not usually enjoy dealing with other people, those with schizoid personality disorder tend to gravitate toward jobs where they can interact with machines or computers rather than people.

Prevalence

Schizoid personality disorder affects slightly more men than women. It has a prevalence of approximately 1 percent in the general population.

Treatment Options

A clinical diagnosis of schizoid personality disorder is based upon, since childhood, confirmation of at least four of the following criteria outlined in the Diagnostic and Statistical Manual of

Mental Disorders (DSM): an avoidance of close relationships; a preference for solitary activities; a lack of interest in sexual relationships; a lack of pleasure in normal activities; a lack of close friends; an indifference to praise or criticism of other people; and emotional detachment.

Treatment for schizoid personality disorder usually includes psychodynamic therapy (in which the therapist builds a relationship with the patient that can be used as a model for other relationships), cognitive behavioural therapy (in which the patient learns to replace negative beliefs and behaviours with positive ones) and group therapy. Medication may be prescribed if anxiety and depression co-exist with the disorder.

Many people with schizoid personality disorder do not seek treatment due to their desire for social isolation. However, if therapy is maintained, it is often of benefit.

Schizotypal Personality Disorder

People with schizotypal personality disorder tend to find close relationships very uncomfortable. They may also have distorted or strange thoughts and feelings.

Symptoms

Signs of schizotypal personality disorder may include passivity, indifference, inappropriate or awkward social behaviour, peculiarities in appearance (such as ill-fitting clothes or poor personal hygiene), lack of emotion and odd mannerisms.

Prevalence

The prevalence of schizotypal personality disorder is between 2 and 4 percent in the general population.

Treatment Options

A clinical diagnosis of schizotypal personality disorder is based upon confirmation of at least five of the following criteria outlined in the Diagnostic and Statistical Manual of Mental Disorders (DSM): strange beliefs that are outside of cultural norms; odd perceptions, thinking and speech patterns; suspicious and paranoid thinking; lack of emotion; odd appearance; lack of friends; and social anxiety.

Schizotypal personality disorder is often difficult to distinguish from schizophrenia. The main difference is that, unlike people with schizotypal personality disorder, people with schizophrenia experience hallucinations and delusions.

Treatment for schizotypal personality disorder may include psychodynamic therapy (in which the therapist builds a relationship with the patient that can be used as a model for other relationships), cognitive behavioural therapy (in which the patient learns to replace negative beliefs and behaviours with positive ones) and family therapy. Medications to treat schizotypal personality disorder may include antipsychotics, tricyclic antidepressants and other antidepressants such as Prozac.

Many people with schizotypal personality disorder are unlikely to seek treatment. When therapy is pursued, it may be of some benefit in milder cases.

National Associations

Canadian Mental Health Association (CMHA) / Association canadienne pour la santé mentale (ACSM)
#1110, 151 Slater St,, Ottawa ON K1P 5H3

Tel: 613-745-7750
e-mail: info@cmha.ca
www.cmha.ca
www.facebook.com/CANMentalHealth
twitter.com/CMHA_NTL
www.youtube.com/user/cmhanational

Overview: A large national charitable organization founded in 1918
Mission: To promote mental health as well as support the resilience & recovery of people experiencing mental illness, through advocacy, education, research & service
Affiliation(s): Canadian Alliance on Mental Illness & Mental Health; Canadian Health Network
Chief Officer(s):
Patrick Smith, National Chief Executive Officer
Cal Crocker, Chair
Sarika Gundu, National Director, Workplace Mental Health Program
Fardous Hosseiny, National Director, Policy
Publications:
• CMHA [Canadian Mental Health Association] Annual Report
Type: Report; *Frequency:* a.
Profile: Details of CMHA initiatives & achievements

Alberta Division
Capital Place, #320, 9707 - 110 St. NW, Edmonton AB T5K 2L9
Tel: 780-482-6576; *Fax:* 780-482-6348
e-mail: alberta@cmha.ab.ca
alberta.cmha.ca

William (Bill) Bone, Chair

British Columbia Division
#1200, 1111 Melville St., Vancouver BC V6E 3V6
Tel: 604-688-3234; *Fax:* 604-688-3236
Toll-Free: 800-555-8222
e-mail: info@cmha.bc.ca
www.cmha.bc.ca
www.facebook.com/CMHABCDIVISION
twitter.com/cmhabc
www.youtube.com/cmhabc

Chief Officer(s):
Beverly Gutray, Chief Executive Officer
bev.gutray@cmha.bc.ca

Division du Québec
#326, 911, rue Jean-Talon Est, Montréal QC H2R 1V5
Tél: 514-849-3291; *Téléc:* 514-849-8372
Courriel: info@acsm.qc.ca
www.acsm.qc.ca
www.facebook.com/189002251132456
twitter.com/ACSMDivisionQc
www.youtube.com/user/ACSMQC

Chief Officer(s):
Renée Ouimet, Directrice
reneeouimet@acsm.qc.ca

Manitoba Division
930 Portage Ave., Winnipeg MB R3G 0P8
Tel: 204-982-6100; *Fax:* 204-982-6128
e-mail: office@cmhawpg.mb.ca
winnipeg.cmha.ca
www.facebook.com/cmha.manitoba
twitter.com/MbDivisionCMHA
www.youtube.com/user/CMHAWpg

Chief Officer(s):
Stephanie Skakun, Acting Executive Director

New Brunswick Division
#202, 403 Regent St., Fredericton NB E3B 3X6
Tel: 506-455-5231; *Fax:* 506-459-3878
cmhanb.ca
www.facebook.com/CMHANB

Chief Officer(s):
Christa Baldwin, Executive Director
christa.baldwin@cmhanb.ca

Newfoundland & Labrador Division

70 The Boulevard, 1st Fl., St. John's NL A1A 1K2
Tel: 709-753-8550; *Fax:* 709-753-8537
Toll-Free: 877-753-8550
e-mail: office@cmhanl.ca
www.cmhanl.ca
www.facebook.com/247087668665555
twitter.com/CMHANL
www.youtube.com/user/cmhanational

Chief Officer(s):
George Skinner, Executive Director

Nova Scotia Division
63 King St., Dartmouth NS B2Y 2R7
Tel: 902-466-6600; *Fax:* 902-466-3300
Toll-Free: 877-466-6606
e-mail: cmhans@bellaliant.com
novascotia.cmha.ca
www.facebook.com/cmhansdivision
twitter.com/cmhansdivision
pinterest.com/cmhanovascotia

Chief Officer(s):
Gail Gardiner, Executive Director

Ontario Division
#2301, 180 Dundas St. West, Toronto ON M5G 1Z8
Tel: 416-977-5580; *Fax:* 416-977-2813
Toll-Free: 800-875-6213
e-mail: info@ontario.cmha.ca
ontario.cmha.ca
www.facebook.com/cmha.ontario
twitter.com/CMHAOntario
www.youtube.com/cmhaontario

Chief Officer(s):
Camille Quenneville, CEO
cquenneville@ontario.cmha.ca

Prince Edward Island Division
PO Box 785, 178 Fitzroy St., Charlottetown PE C1A 7L9
Tel: 902-566-3034; *Fax:* 902-566-4643
e-mail: division@cmha.pe.ca
pei.cmha.ca
www.facebook.com/CMHAPEIDivision

Chief Officer(s):
Reid Burke, Executive Director

Saskatchewan Division
2702 - 12th Ave., Regina SK S4T 1J2
Tel: 306-525-5601; *Fax:* 306-569-3788
Toll-Free: 800-461-5483
e-mail: contactus@cmhask.com
www.cmhask.com
www.facebook.com/255440253328

Chief Officer(s):
Dave Nelson, Executive Director
daven@cmhask.com

Yukon Division
6 Bates Cres., Whitehorse YT Y1A 4T8

Tel: 867-668-7144
e-mail: cmha.ca@gmail.com
twitter.com/CMHAYukon

Chief Officer(s):
Dudley Morgan, Executive Director

Provincial Associations

Ontario Association for the Application of Personality Type (OAAPT)

Toll-Free: 888-424-5455
e-mail: oaaptmail@gmail.com
www.oaapt.ca
www.linkedin.com/groups/OAAPT-2241270
www.facebook.com/pages/Oaapt/484894888194146
twitter.com/oaapt

Overview: A small provincial organization founded in 1985
Mission: To promote direction, mechanisms & resources to a broad-based community, an understanding of psychological type & the most effective applications of the MBTI & other related instruments in

Ontario
Affliation(s): Association of Psychological Type
Chief Officer(s):
Irene Anderson, President

Post-Polio Syndrome

Post-polio syndrome (PPS), also known as the late effects of polio or post polio sequelae, occurs only in people who have previously been infected with poliovirus. It is characterized by new symptoms that occur in people with a history of polio after a long period of stability during which whatever strength they had recovered remained unchanged.

Cause
While the cause of PPS is not clearly understood, two theories exist. One suggests that it is caused by normal muscle loss that accompanies aging. The other is that PPS is caused by the repeated over-use of muscle groups. In both cases, muscle groups not previously known to have been affected by polio are weakened, and it is this weakness that is the major indicator of PPS. A polio survivor with an affected leg may find that his or her arms are newly affected. Whether the arm problems are a result of undetected muscle damage that occurred at the time of the original polio or newer damage resulting from the overuse of the remaining good muscles, or a combination of the two, is not clearly understood.

Prevalence
PPS affects up to 60 percent of polio survivors, 20 to 40 years after the initial episode.

Symptoms
The hallmark of PPS is new weakness. Other symptoms include fatigue, new pain, difficulty breathing and swallowing, intolerance to cold and new muscle atrophy.

Treatment Options
Post-polio syndrome, like most diseases classified as syndromes, does not have a specific diagnostic test, but a diagnosis of exclusion. This means that other medical conditions that may present with symptoms similar to those found in PPS should be considered and excluded, if possible. PPS is frequently emotionally difficult for polio survivors. Many feel they have triumphed over their initial polio, or have come to terms with their resulting disabilities. To think that the polio is coming back is often terrifying. These emotional issues are frequently made more difficult by the fact that PPS is often misdiagnosed as other conditions or normal aging.

Once diagnosis of PPS is determined, treatment is individualized by primary symptoms and may include medications, supervised therapy, physiotherapy and exercise, injections, pacing of activities of daily living, and, in some cases, surgery.

PPS usually responds well to strengthening exercises and many people with the disease can continue to live normal lives and return to employment.

Provincial Associations

BRITISH COLUMBIA

Post-Polio Awareness & Support Society of BC (PPASS/BC)
#222, 2453 Beacon Ave., Sidney BC V8L 1X7
Tel: 250-655-8849; *Fax:* 250-655-8859
e-mail: ppass@ppassbc.com
www.ppassbc.com
Overview: A medium-sized provincial charitable organization founded in 1986

Mission: To develop awareness, communication & education between society & community; To disseminate information concerning research & treatment about Post-Polio Syndrome; To support polio survivors other than through direct financial aid
Chief Officer(s):
Joan Toone, President

MANITOBA

Post-Polio Network Manitoba Inc. (PPN-MB)
c/o SMD Self-Help Clearinghouse, 825 Sherbrook St., Winnipeg MB R3A 1M5
Tel: 204-975-3037; *Fax:* 204-975-3027
e-mail: postpolionetwork@gmail.com
www.postpolionetwork.ca
Overview: A small provincial charitable organization founded in 1986
Mission: To serve as a support group & information centre for polio survivors throughout Manitoba, especially those suffering from post-polio syndrome; To acquaint the medical community & those responsible for government services as to the nature & extent of the problems associated with the late effects of polio
Member of: Society of Manitobans with Disabilities
Affliation(s): Polio Canada; SMD - Fostering Growth & Clearinghouse of Self-Help Organizations
Chief Officer(s):
Cheryl Currie, President
Donna Remillard, Treasurer
Estelle Boissonneault, Secretary

QUÉBEC

Polio Québec
#219A, 3500 boul. Décarie, Montréal QC H4A 3J5
Tél: 514-489-1143
Ligne sans frais: 877-765-4672
Courriel: association@polioquebec.org
www.polioquebec.org
Également appelé: Polio Quebec Association
Aperçu: *Dimension:* moyenne; *Envergure:* provinciale; fondée en 1985
Mission: D'aider toutes les personnes atteintes par la polio et de sensibiliser la population en général sur tous les aspects de la polio, incluant la prévention
Affliation(s): L'Institut et Hôpital Neurologiques de Montréal; Le centre de réadaptation MAB-Mackay; Confédération des organismes de personnes handicapées du Québec (COPHAN); L'Association multi-ethnique pour l'intégration des personnes handicapées (AMEIPH); Le Carrefour familial des personnes handicapées (Québec)
Membre(s) du bureau directeur:
Daniel Montmarquette, Président
Stewart Valin, Vice-président

Local Associations

ALBERTA

Southern Alberta Post Polio Support Society (SAPPSS)
7 - 11 St. NE, Calgary AB T2E 4Z2
Tel: 403-265-5041; *Fax:* 403-265-0162
Toll-Free: 866-265-5049
e-mail: sappss@shaw.ca
www.polioalberta.ca/sappss
Overview: A small local organization founded in 1988
Mission: To bring awareness about Post Polio Syndrome to the Southern Alberta community; to provide support for polio survivors

Wildrose Polio Support Society
132 Warwick Rd. NW, Edmonton AB T5X 4P8
Tel: 780-428-8842; *Fax:* 780-475-7968
e-mail: wpss@polioalberta.ca
www.polioalberta.ca/wildrose
Overview: A small local organization founded in 1999
Mission: To bring awareness about Post Polio Syndrome to the Southern Alberta community; to provide support for polio survivors
Chief Officer(s):
Marleen Henley, President

ONTARIO

Barrie Post Polio Association
57 Henry St., Barrie ON L4N 1C6
Overview: A small local charitable organization
Mission: A self help group working with Ontario March of Dimes for those suffering from the late effects of poliomyelitis & for any other interested persons
Chief Officer(s):
Pauline Berry, Contact
  pberry@marchofdimes.ca

SASKATCHEWAN

Polio Regina
825 McDonald St., Regina SK S4N 2X5

e-mail: polio@accesscomm.ca
nonprofits.accesscomm.ca/polio

Overview: A small local organization
Mission: To provide support & information to those who suffer & have suffered from polio.
Chief Officer(s):
Wilf Tiefenbach, President

Prader-Willi Syndrome

Prader-Willi syndrome (PWS) is a genetic disorder. It was first described by Drs. Prader, Labhart and Willi in 1956 after they examined a group of children who shared common characteristics including small stature, obesity, insatiable hunger and intellectual disability. Dysfunction of the hypothalamus (a part of the brain involved in hunger regulation, puberty, emotions and other body functions) is believed to be responsible for these symptoms.

Cause

In about 70 percent of patients, PWS is caused by a missing piece (deletion) of part of chromosome 15. In close to 30 percent of cases, the child inherits two chromosome 15s from his or her mother and none from his or her father (uniparental disomy). A tiny genetic mutation that makes the genetic material inactive in the Prader-Willi region of chromosome 15 (imprinting mutation) is responsible for the rest of cases. How this genetic abnormality causes hypothalamic dysfunction is unknown.

Symptoms

There are two stages of PWS symptoms. In stage 1, infants show decreased muscle tone and usually have trouble breastfeeding. In general, muscle tone improves with growth, but there are usually delays in reaching motor milestones. In stage 2, which usually begins when a child is between the ages of two and six, many children have insatiable hunger and begin to overeat. Other symptoms include obesity, short stature, hypogonadism (diminished function of the testes or ovaries), small hands and feet, intellectual disability, scoliosis, sleep disturbances and infertility. Some persons with PWS may show signs of obsessive-compulsive disorder, apart from their obsessions with food. Other behavioural symptoms include emotional highs and lows, poor motor skills and cognitive impairment.

Prevalence

Prader-Willi syndrome affects both boys and girls and occurs in about one in every 15,000 births. It is one of the common causes of obesity in children.

Treatment Options

Genetic research has improved diagnosis of PWS. A blood test (DNA methylation test) can now identify cases of PWS at birth.

Human growth hormone (HGH) is now recognized for use in treating PWS. The benefits of this therapy include decreased body fat, increased height, strength and agility and improved weight distribution. Obesity remains the most serious health complication of PWS. There are currently no effective drugs for appetite regulation, so emphasis is placed on nutrition education, specialized diets, food exposure limitations and customized exercise programs and support.

Due to a greater awareness of PWS and improved diagnosis and treatment, the outlook for children with this disorder is more promising. Some patients are now living into their fifties and sixties.

National Associations

Canadian Angelman Syndrome Society (CASS) / Societé canadienne du syndrome d'Angelman (SCSA)
PO Box 37, Priddis AB T0L 1W0

Tel: 403-931-2415
www.angelmancanada.org

Overview: A small national organization
Mission: To educate concerned families, medical & educational communities & the general public about Angelman Syndrome; To establish & maintain support systems; To promote research activities on the diagnosis, treatment, management & prevention of Angelman Syndrome; To fundraise
Chief Officer(s):
John Carscallen, Secretary-Treasurer
  cass@davincibb.net

Foundation for Prader-Willi Research in Canada (FPWR Canada)
#370, 19 - 13085 Yonge St., Richmond Hill ON L4E 0K2

Toll-Free: 866-993-7972
www.fpwr.ca
www.facebook.com/fpwr.org
www.youtube.com/user/fpwrcanada

Previous Name: Canadian Prader-Willi Syndrome Association
Overview: A small national charitable organization founded in 2006
Mission: To educate families & inform community services on behalf of individuals with Prader-Willi Syndrome, about the special needs of persons with this condition in Canada
Member of: International Prader-Willi Syndrome Organization
Affliation(s): Ontario Prader-Willi Syndrome Association; British Columbia Prader-Willi Syndrome Association; Alberta Prader-Willi Association; Foundation for Prader Willi Research
Chief Officer(s):
Keegan Johnson, President & Chair
Carole Barron, Executive Director
  carole.barron@fpwr.ca
Michelle Cordeiro, Director, Operations
  michelle.cordeiro@fpwr.ca
Carole Elkhal, Director, Community
  carole.elkhal@fpwr.ca

Provincial Associations

ALBERTA

Prader-Willi Syndrome Association of Alberta
9006 - 120 St. NW, Edmonton AB T6G 1X7

Tel: 780-459-1959
Other Communication: 403-217-8587 (Calgary); 403-340-1057 (Red Deer)
www.pwsaa.ca

Also Known As: PWSA of AB
Overview: A small provincial charitable organization founded in 1986
Mission: To advocate for individuals affected by Prader-Willi Syndrome; To improve the quality of life for affected individuals
Affliation(s): Canadian Prader-Willi Syndrome Association
Chief Officer(s):
Lise Dunn, Contact, Edmonton
  lisedunn@shaw.ca
Brooke Gibson, Contact, Calgary
  brookergibson@gmail.com
Jill Hockin, Contact, Red Deer
  reddeerbean@shaw.ca

Publications:
• Prader-Willi Syndrome Association of Alberta Newsletter
Type: Newsletter
Profile: Association reports, stories, & events

BRITISH COLUMBIA

British Columbia Prader-Willi Syndrome Association (BCPWSA)
2133 Chilcotin Cres., Kelowna BC V1V 2N9

www.bcpwsa.com
www.facebook.com/bcpwsa

Overview: A small provincial charitable organization founded in 1982
Mission: To provide an understanding & awareness of PWS by supporting those who have the syndrome, their families & all who come in contact with PWS
Chief Officer(s):
Heather Beach, President
    president@bcpwsa.com
Cheryl Gagne, Treasurer
    treasurer@bcpwsa.com
Frances Robinson, Secretary
    secretary@bcpwsa.com

ONTARIO

Ontario Prader-Willi Syndrome Association (OPWSA)
PO Box 73514, Toronto ON M6C 4A7

Tel: 416-481-8657; *Fax:* 416-981-7788
e-mail: opwsa@rogers.com
www.opwsa.com
www.facebook.com/106828009519275

Overview: A small provincial charitable organization founded in 1982
Mission: To enhance the quality of life for individuals with Prader-Willi Syndrome
Affliation(s): International Prader-Willi Syndrome Association
Chief Officer(s):
Jessie Phillips, Family Services Coordinator
    jessie.opwsa@gmail.com
Dan Yashinsky, Co-chair
    dan_yashinsky@hotmail.com
Cathy Mallove, Co-chair
    cmallove@sympatico.ca

Psychosomatic Disorders

Psychosomatic disorders are characterized by multiple physical symptoms with no diagnosed illness, or the conviction that one is ill despite negative medical examinations and laboratory tests. Those who have a psychosomatic disorder persist in believing they are ill, or experience physical symptoms over long periods, and their beliefs negatively affect all areas of their functioning. The two main types of psychosomatic disorders are hypochondria (also referred to as hypochondriasis) and somatization disorder.

Hypochondria

Hypochondria is characterized by the conviction that one is seriously ill despite evidence to the contrary. Physical symptoms become a preoccupation, and are often misinterpreted as signs of disease. For instance, a person with hypochondria may be convinced that a headache is a sign of brain cancer, or that an occasional increase in heart rate signals heart disease. The person with this disorder visits many doctors, but physical examinations and negative lab results neither reassure them nor resolve their symptoms. They often believe they are not getting proper respect or attention, and, indeed, they may be viewed in medical settings as troublesome, since they do not have a physical condition. Fear of developing a specific illness may be magnified by reading about a disease in a newspaper, or hearing about a friend or family member who is suffering from a certain medical condition. Symptoms may also become more intense after a stressful event such as divorce, or the death of a loved one. People with

hypochondriasis do not deliberately produce or falsely complain of physical symptoms; their symptoms are engendered by psychological conflict.

Cause
The exact cause of hypochondria is not known, however one theory suggests that people with this disorder are much more sensitive to normal physical sensations than the general population. Another theory cites catastrophic thinking as a cause for hypochondria. People may also be more likely to develop hypochondria if they have experienced trauma or frequent, serious illnesses as a child. The disorder also appears to run in families.

Symptoms
The symptoms of hypochondria may wax and wane, sometimes lasting for months or years, and then going into long periods of remission. Physical complaints may be non-specific and appear to change over time. People with this disorder may also be preoccupied with illness, have persistent concerns about health, obsessively check for information about feared illnesses in books or on the internet, visit one doctor after another seeking a diagnosis for their symptoms, or avoid anything that has to do with illness and death altogether. People affected by hypochondria often suffer from anxiety and depression, and their preoccupation with feared diseases may interfere with their participation in work or social events.

Prevalence
Hypochondria is equally common in both sexes. The age of onset is usually young adulthood. Its prevalence in the general population is estimated to be 1 to 5 percent. In general medical practice, 2 percent to 7 percent of patients have the disorder. It is usually chronic.

Treatment Options
To rule out other medical conditions that could be causing the symptoms, a number of exams and tests are usually performed including a physical exam, a psychological evaluation and blood tests. The clinical diagnosis of hypochondria is based on the following criteria outlined in the *Diagnostic and Statistic Manual of Mental Disorders (DSM)* : preoccupation with fears of having a serious illness based on a misinterpretation of bodily symptoms or sensations; the preoccupation persists in spite of medical reassurance; the preoccupation is a source of distress and difficulty in social, work and other areas; the duration of the preoccupation is at least six months.

Physical symptoms appearing after a diagnosis of hypochondria is made should not be dismissed completely, however. Sufferers can have general medical disorders at the same time as hypochondria.

Treatment for hypochondria often includes psychological counselling and medication. Cognitive behavioural therapy, which gives people techniques to manage anxiety and modify beliefs about the origin and course of physical symptoms, is usually considered the most effective treatment. Researchers have also found that stress management techniques may be helpful in reducing symptoms. Exposure therapy, a form of treatment in which patients practise confronting their anxieties until they become better able to manage them, is also sometimes used. Medications such as serotonin reuptake inhibitors (SSRIs) and tricyclic antidepressants are sometimes prescribed to treat hypochondria.

Although hypochondria is a chronic condition which can be disabling if left untreated, many people with this disorder find relief from their symptoms with the appropriate psychological counselling and drug therapy.

Somatization Disorder

Somatization disorder is characterized by multiple physical symptoms without a discernible basis. Many of the reported symptoms are similar to those associated with actual diseases, but others are not. Nonetheless, people with somatization disorder suffer pain and discomfort and visit many doctors to try to find a diagnosis. Physical examinations and negative lab results neither reassure them nor resolve their symptoms. They often believe they are not getting proper respect or attention, and, indeed, they may be viewed in medical settings as troublesome, because their problems are "all in their heads."

Cause

The exact cause of somatization disorder is not known. One long-standing theory is that people with this disorder develop physical symptoms in order to avoid psychological distress. Other research cites catastrophic thinking as a cause for somatization disorder.

Symptoms

Symptoms of somatization disorder commonly include nausea, diarrhea, bloating, food sensitivities, menstrual problems, pain during intercourse, erectile dysfunction, headaches, back and joint pain, urinary retention and swallowing and speaking problems. People with somatization disorder may also have neurological problems such as seizures, balance or coordination problems, or paralysis. People with this disorder often suffer from anxiety and depression as well.

Prevalence

It is estimated that between 0.2 percent and 2 percent of the general population suffers from somatization disorder. It is slightly less common among men.

Treatment Options

To rule out other medical conditions that could be causing the symptoms, a number of exams and tests are usually performed including a physical exam, a psychological evaluation and blood tests. The clinical diagnosis of somatization disorder is based on the following criteria outlined in the *Diagnostic and Statistic Manual of Mental Disorders (DSM)* : four pain symptoms related to at least four anatomical areas or functions (such as headaches, back, joint, chest or abdmonial pain); two gastrointestinal problems other than pain (such as nausea or diarrhea); one sexual symptom other than pain (such as irregular menstruation, sexual disinterest or erectile dysfunction); one pseudoneurological symptom other than pain (such as weakness or double vision); symptoms cannot be explained by a medical condition; when a medical condition exists, physical complaints and social difficulties are greater than normal.

Physical symptoms appearing after the diagnosis of somatization disorder is made, however, should not be dismissed completely out of hand. Sufferers can have general medical disorders at the same time as somatization disorder.

Treatment of somatization disorder usually includes cognitive behavioural therapy and medication. Cognitive behavioural therapy gives people techniques to manage anxiety and modify beliefs about the origin and course of physical symptoms. Often, patients are also encouraged to increase their activity level, and are trained in relaxation techniques and communication skills. Antidepressant medications may be used to treat the symptoms of somatization disorder.

Although somatization disorder symptoms can wax and wane and vary in severity over time, it is still a chronic disorder. If left untreated, somatization disorder can seriously interfere with a person's participation in work and social life. However, with the appropriate psychotherapy and drug therapy, many people with somatization disorder can reduce their symptoms, and lead a more active life.

National Associations

Canadian Alliance on Mental Illness & Mental Health (CAMIMH)
#702, 141 Laurier Ave. West, Ottawa ON K1P 5J3
Tel: 613-237-2144; *Fax:* 613-237-1674
www.facebook.com/FaceMentalIllness
twitter.com/miawcanada
www.flickr.com/photos/45033589@N02
Overview: A medium-sized national organization founded in 1998
Mission: An alliance of mental health organizations comprised of health care providers and organizations representing persons with mental illness and their families and caregivers.

Canadian Psychiatric Association (CPA) / Association des psychiatres du Canada
#701, 141 Laurier Ave. West, Ottawa ON K1P 5J3
Tel: 613-234-2815; *Fax:* 613-234-9857
Toll-Free: 800-267-1555
e-mail: cpa@cpa-apc.org
www.cpa-apc.org
Overview: A medium-sized national organization founded in 1951
Mission: To forge a strong, collective voice for Canadian psychiatrists & to promote an environment that fosters excellence in the provision of clinical care, education & research
Affiliation(s): Canadian Medical Association; World Psychiatric Association
Chief Officer(s):
Glenn Brimacombe, Chief Executive Officer
gbrimacombe@cpa-apc.org
Brenda Fudge, Director, Finance & Administration
bfudge@cpa-apc,org
Katie Hardy, Director, Professional & Membership Services
khardy@cpa-apc.org
Jadranka Bacic, Associate Director, Communications
jbacic@cpa-apc.org

Canadian Psychoanalytic Society (CPS) / Société canadienne de psychanalyse (SCP)
7000 Côte-des-Neiges Chemin, Montréal QC H3S 2C1
Tel: 514-738-6105
www.psychoanalysis.ca
Overview: A small national licensing organization founded in 1967
Mission: To promote psychoanalysis treatments & professionals
Affliation(s): International Psychoanalytic Association
Chief Officer(s):
Andrew Brook, President

CPS Western Canadian Branch
c/o Nancy Briones, 7755 Yukon St., Vancouver BC V5X 2Y4
e-mail: info1@wbcps.org
www.wbcps.org
Chief Officer(s):
David Heilbrunn, President

Ottawa Psychoanalytic Society
c/o Somerset Psychologists, #201, 125 Somerset St. West, Ottawa ON K2P 0H7
Tel: 613-236-5608
e-mail: contact@ottawaps.ca
ottawaps.ca
www.facebook.com/OttawaPsychoanalyticSociety
Chief Officer(s):
Arthur Leonoff, Director

Québec English Branch
7000, ch Côte des Neiges, Montréal QC H3S 2C1
Tel: 514-342-7444; *Fax:* 514-342-1062
e-mail: cpsqeb@qc.aira.com
www.psychoanalysismontreal.com
Chief Officer(s):
Erica Robertson, President

Société psychanalytique de Montréal
7000, ch de la Côte-des-Neiges, Montréal QC H3S 2C1
Tél: 514-342-5208; *Téléc:* 514-342-9990
Courriel: spsymtl@qc.aira.com
www.psychanalysemontreal.org

Chief Officer(s):
Louis Brunet, Président

Société psychanalytique de Québec
1180, rue Charles-Albanel, Sainte-Foy QC G1X 4T9
Tél: 418-877-8445; *Téléc:* 418-877-7056
Courriel: info@spq-scp.ca
www.spq-scp.ca

South Western Ontario Psychoanalytic Society
London ON

Toronto Psychoanalytic Society
#203, 40 St. Clair Ave. East, Toronto ON M4T 1M9
Tel: 416-922-7770; *Fax:* 416-922-9988
torontopsychoanalysis.com
www.facebook.com/TorontoPsychoanalyticSociety

Chief Officer(s):
Rukhsana Bukhari, President

Canadian Psychological Association (CPA) / Société canadienne de psychologie (SCP)
#702, 141 Laurier Ave. West, Ottawa ON K1P 5J3
Tel: 613-237-2144; *Fax:* 613-237-1674
Toll-Free: 888-472-0657
e-mail: cpa@cpa.ca
www.cpa.ca
www.facebook.com/146082642130174
twitter.com/CPA_SCP
www.youtube.com/user/CPAVideoChannel
Overview: A medium-sized national organization founded in 1939
Mission: To improve the health & welfare of Canadians by promoting psychological research, education, & practice
Affliation(s): Canadian Register of Health Service Providers in Psychology; Council of Provincial Associations of Psychologists; International Union of Psychological Science; Canadian Federation for the Humanities & Social Sciences
Chief Officer(s):
Karen R. Cohen, Chief Executive Officer, 613-237-2144 Ext. 323
executiveoffice@cpa.ca
Lisa Votta-Bleeker, Deputy CEO & Director, Science Directorate, 613-237-2144 Ext. 323
executiveoffice@cpa.ca
Phil Bolger, Chief Financial Officer, 613-237-2144 Ext. 329
pbolger@cpa.ca
Rozen Alex, Director, Practice Directorate, 613-237-2144 Ext. 334
practicedirectorate@cpa.ca
Seán Kelly, Director, Events, Membership & Association Development, 613-237-2144 Ext. 335
skelly@cpa.ca
Publications:
• Canadian Journal of Behavioural Science / La revue canadienne des sciences du comportement
Type: Journal; *Frequency:* Quarterly; *Accepts Advertising; Editor:* Todd Morrison; *Price:* $119 + GST/HST individuals in Canada; $289.00 + GST/HSTinstitutions in Canada
Profile: Original, empirical articles in the following areas of psychology:abnormal, behavioural, community, counselling, educational, environmental, developmental, health, industrial-organizational, clinical neuropsychological, personality, psychometrics, & social
• The Canadian Journal of Experimental Psychology
Type: Journal; *Frequency:* Quarterly; *Accepts Advertising; Editor:* Doug J. Mewhort; *ISSN:* 0008-4255; *Price:* $119 + GST/HST individuals in Canada; $289.00 + GST/HST institutions in Canada
Profile: A journal of original research papers from the field of experimental psychology, published in partnershipwith the American Psychological Association
• Canadian Psychology
Type: Journal; *Frequency:* Quarterly; *Accepts Advertising; Editor:* Martin Drapeau, Ph.D.; *Price:* $119 + GST/HST individuals in Canada; $289.00 + GST/HST institutions inCanada
Profile: Generalist articles in areas of theory, research, & practice

• CPA [Canadian Psychological Association] News
Type: Newsletter; *Price:* Free with membership in the Canadian Psycological Association
Profile: Current information for members
• Psynopsis: Canada's Psychology Magazine
Type: Magazine; *Frequency:* Quarterly; *Accepts Advertising; Editor:* Karen R. Cohen; *ISSN:* 1187-11809
Profile: Articles of interest to scientists, educators, & practitioners in psychology

Provincial Associations

QUÉBEC

Fondation des maladies mentales / Mental Illness Foundation
#804, 55, av du Mont-Royal West, Montréal QC H2T 2S6
Tél: 514-529-5354; *Téléc:* 514-529-9877
Ligne sans frais: 888-529-5354
Courriel: info@fondationdesmaladiesmentales.org
www.fondationdesmaladiesmentales.org
Nom précédent: Fondation québécoise des maladies mentales
Aperçu: *Dimension:* petite; *Envergure:* provinciale; fondée en 1980
Mission: Pour mettre des services cliniques en place et les maintenir; prévenir les maladies mentales
Membre(s) du bureau directeur:
Isabelle Limoges, Directrice générale
ilimoges@fondationdesmaladiesmentales.org

Raynaud's Disease

Cause
Raynaud's disease is the spasm of blood vessels to fingers, toes, nose and ears resulting in restricted blood supply in response to cold or emotional upset. The condition is referred to as primary Raynaud's when it is not caused by an underlying disease or medical problem. This is the most common form of Raynaud's, and it generally results in no serious consequences. Secondary Raynaud's is the result of other underlying medical conditions, including scleroderma, vascular disease, rheumatoid arthritis and lupus. The secondary form is often a more serious disorder. Certain drugs can also trigger Raynaud's, including ergotamine and a number of beta-blocking drugs that are used in the treatment of heart disease. About 10 percent of Raynaud's cases are related to specific repetitive stress activities such as the operation of pneumatic drills and other hand-held vibrating machinery.

Symptoms
The symptoms of Raynaud's include tingling and numbness. During an episode, which can last from minutes to hours, the arteries contract briefly and the skin, deprived of oxygen, turns pale and then blue. As arteries relax and blood begins to flow, reddening, tingling, or swelling may occur. In most Raynaud's cases, symptoms are discomforting but not serious. In extreme cases, Raynaud's can result in skin ulcerations and infections, tissue atrophy and gangrene.

Prevalence
Raynaud's affects four of every 10,000 Canadians. In approximately 90 percent of all cases, it begins in a woman who is under 40.

Treatment Options
To diagnose Raynaud's, a physician takes a detailed medical history, including symptoms, and performs a physical exam to check for signs of any underlying medical conditions. To rule out other diseases that might be causing the symptoms, blood tests are often ordered. Rheumatologists may perform a nailfold capillaroscopy (a procedure where the tiny blood vessels at the fingernail base are examined under a microscope).

In general, it is recommended that preventative measures including protection from cold (even when taking food out of the refrigerator or freezer), and avoiding smoking and stress are the best way to manage Raynaud's.

Medical treatment of Raynaud's is directed toward improving blood flow to the extremities. In many cases, simple exercises are prescribed, and relaxation techniques, such as biofeedback, teach the body to ignore trivial or transient signals of cold. In other cases, vasodilator drugs which are designed to relax and open blood vessels to improve blood flow are prescribed. In the most extreme cases, surgery may be performed to cut nerves that may be inappropriately triggering the contraction of arteries, although relief may last only one to two years. Herbal remedies have been used in the treatment of Raynaud's and other circulatory conditions, especially the Chinese herb Dong quai. There is also evidence that foods rich in vitamin E, and fish oils, may help to reduce or moderate the vascular spasms that produce Raynaud's symptoms.

Although there is currently no cure for Raynaud's, it can be controlled, and most people find symptom relief.

National Associations

Scleroderma Society of Canada (SSC)
#206, 41 King William St., Hamilton ON L8R 1A2
Toll-Free: 866-279-0632
e-mail: info@scleroderma.ca
www.scleroderma.ca
Overview: A small national organization founded in 2000
Mission: To promote awareness of scleroderma, to support research toward finding a cure and to provide support and information to those affected by the disease.
Chief Officer(s):
Maureen Sauvé, President

Provincial Associations

BRITISH COLUMBIA

Scleroderma Association of British Columbia
PO Box 218, Stn. Delta Main, Delta BC V4K 3N7
Tel: 604-940-9343; Fax: 604-940-9346
Toll-Free: 888-940-9343
www.sclerodermabc.ca
www.facebook.com/scleroderma.bc
Overview: A small provincial charitable organization founded in 1984
Mission: To support, educate & keep informed those diagnosed with scleroderma (in skin form - localized, or in systemic form - systemic sclerosis); To raise research funds
Member of: Scleroderma Society of Canada
Chief Officer(s):
Rosanne Queen, President
rq.sabc@telus.net

ONTARIO

The Scleroderma Society of Ontario (SSO)
Empire Times Bldg., #206, 41 King William St., Hamilton ON L8R 1A2
Tel: 905-544-0343
Toll-Free: 888-776-7776
www.sclerodermaontario.ca
Overview: A small provincial charitable organization
Mission: To promote public awareness; To advance patient wellness; To support research in Scleroderma
Member of: The Arthritis Society
Chief Officer(s):
Anna McCusker, Executive Director
anna@sclerodermaontario.ca

Sarcoidosis

Sarcoidosis is a chronic disease that can affect almost any part of the body. It is characterized by the deposit of small masses of tissue (granulomas) in multiple organs. If the granulomas grow, they may affect organ function.

Cause
The cause of sarcoidosis is unknown, although it is speculated to be related to an immunologic defect or infection.

Symptoms
Sarcoidosis symptoms vary considerably, depending on the site and extent of involvement. Systemic symptoms may include fatigue, weight loss, loss of appetite and fever. Local symptoms may involve any organ, but the most commonly affected are the lungs, skin, eyes and lymph nodes. If the disease becomes severe and life-threatening, it is usually because of lung involvement. Patients may cough or wheeze, develop chest pain and have difficulty breathing.

Prevalence
Sarcoidosis affects about one in 5,000 people worldwide, and is more likely to occur in women than men. In North America, sarcoidosis is more common in African Americans and in adults between the ages of 20 and 40.

Treatment Options
A diagnosis of sarcoidosis is usually based on a medical history, physical exam and biopsy (sampling and analysis) of the affected organ or tissue. If there is lung involvement, lung function tests and a chest X-ray are often used to confirm diagnosis.

In most cases, sarcoidosis runs its course and improves without treatment. If progressive symptoms require therapy, corticosteroids are usually given to suppress inflammation. If these are not effective or tolerated, immunosuppressive drugs such as methotrexate or azathioprine may be tried.

Both the severity and the long-term outlook of sarcoidosis are extremely variable. In most patients, the disease regresses within several months and does not recur. In approximately 25 percent of patients, the disease progresses and causes serious disability due to heart, lung or kidney failure, glaucoma or skin disfigurement. Approximately 5 percent of patients die of respiratory failure.

National Associations

Canadian Lung Association (CLA) / Association pulmonaire du Canada
National Office, #300, 1750 Courtwood Cres., Ottawa ON K2C 2B5
Tel: 613-569-6411
Toll-Free: 888-566-5864
e-mail: info@lung.ca
www.lung.ca
www.facebook.com/canadianlungassociation
twitter.com/canlung
www.youtube.com/user/TheLungAssociation
Previous Name: The Canadian Association for the Prevention of Consumption & Other Forms of Tuberculosis; The Canadian Tuberculosis & Respiratory Disease Association
Overview: A large national charitable organization founded in 1900
Mission: To improve & promote lung health across Canada
Chief Officer(s):
Debra Lynkowski, President & Chief Executive Officer
Terry Dean, Senior Vice President, Federation Development & Partnerships
Debbie Smith, Vice President, Finance & Operations
Janet Sutherland, Director, Canadian Thoracic Society/Canadian Respiratory Health Professiona
Marketa Stastna, Manager, Marketing & Communications
Amy Henderson, Manager, Public Policy & Health Communications
Kristen Curren, Manager, Education & Knowledge Translation

Publications:
• Canadian Lung Association Annual Report
Type: Yearbook; *Frequency:* Annually

Provincial Associations

ALBERTA

Alberta & Northwest Territories Lung Association
PO Box 4500, Stn. South, #208, 17420 Stony Plain Rd., Edmonton AB T6E 6K2

> *Tel:* 780-488-6819; *Fax:* 780-488-7195
> *Toll-Free:* 888-566-5864
> *e-mail:* info@ab.lung.ca
> www.ab.lung.ca
> www.facebook.com/lungassociationabnwt
> twitter.com/lungabnwt

Overview: A medium-sized provincial charitable organization founded in 1939 overseen by Canadian Lung Association
Mission: To educate the public & medical professionals about lung health
Chief Officer(s):
Paul Borrett, Chair
Evangeline Berube, Vice-Chair & Treasurer
Kate Hurlburt, Secretary
Publications:
• Alberta & Northwest Territories Lung Association Annual Report
Type: Yearbook; *Frequency:* Annually
Profile: Highlights of fundraising activities, advocacy activities, & patient support programs

BRITISH COLUMBIA

British Columbia Lung Association (BCLA)
2675 Oak St., Vancouver BC V6H 2K2

> *Tel:* 604-731-5864; *Fax:* 604-731-5810
> *Toll-Free:* 800-665-5864
> *e-mail:* info@bc.lung.ca
> www.bc.lung.ca
> www.facebook.com/BCLungAssociation
> twitter.com/BCLungAssoc

Previous Name: Anti-Tuberculosis Society
Overview: A medium-sized provincial charitable organization founded in 1906 overseen by Canadian Lung Association
Mission: To support lung health research, education, prevention, & advocacy; To help people manage respiratory diseases, including asthma, COPD (chronic bronchitis & emphysema), lung cancer, sleep apnea, & tuberculosis
Chief Officer(s):
Scott McDonald, President & CEO
Kelly Ablog-Morrant, Director, Health Education & Program Services
Chris Lam, Manager, Development
Katrina van Bylandt, Manager, Communications
Debora Wong, Manager, Finance & Administration
Marissa McFadyen, Coordinator, Special Events
Publications:
• British Columbia Lung Association Annual Report
Type: Yearbook; *Frequency:* Annually
• Your Health [a publication of the British Columbia Lung Association]
Type: Magazine; *Frequency:* Semiannually; *Editor:* Katrina van Bylandt
Profile: Health information for medical & health promoters, educators, donors to the Lung Association, & persons interested in respiratoryhealth

MANITOBA

Manitoba Lung Association
#301, 1 Wesley Ave., Winnipeg MB R3C 4C6

> *Tel:* 204-774-5501
> *e-mail:* info@mb.lung.ca
> www.mb.lung.ca
> www.facebook.com/manitobalungassociation
> twitter.com/ManitobaLung
> www.youtube.com/channel/UC3OyzjhurY-5KBPZvsG1G4Q

Overview: A small provincial charitable organization founded in 1904 overseen by Canadian Lung Association

Mission: To improve lung health
Member of: Sanatorium Board of Manitoba
Chief Officer(s):
Deborah Harri, Chair
Bill Pratt, President & CEO
Kathi Neal, Director, Fund Development
Malcolm Harwood, Coordinator, Finance
Tracy Fehr, Coordinator, Tobacco Reduction
Publications:
• Manitoba Lung Association Annual Report
Type: Yearbook; *Frequency:* Annually

NEW BRUNSWICK

New Brunswick Lung Association / Association pulmonaire du Nouveau-Brunswick
65 Brunswick St., Fredericton NB E3B 1G5

> *Tel:* 506-455-8961; *Fax:* 506-462-0939
> *Toll-Free:* 888-566-5864
> *e-mail:* info@nb.lung.ca
> www.nb.lung.ca
> www.facebook.com/nblung
> twitter.com/NBlung

Overview: A small provincial charitable organization overseen by Canadian Lung Association
Mission: To promote wellness throughout New Brunswick & prevent lung disease
Chief Officer(s):
Barbara MacKinnon, President & CEO
Ted Allingham, Director, Finance & Administration
Monica Brewer, Director, Fundraising & Donor Relations
Barbara Walls, Director, Health Initiatives
Liz Smith, Director, Public Education
Roshini Kassie, Director, Community Outreach Programs
Maggie Estey, Manager, Marketing & Development

NEWFOUNDLAND AND LABRADOR

Newfoundland & Labrador Lung Association (NLLA)
PO Box 13457, Stn. A, St. John's NL A1B 4B8

> *Tel:* 709-726-4664; *Fax:* 709-726-2550
> *Toll-Free:* 888-566-5864
> *e-mail:* info@nf.lung.ca
> www.nf.lung.ca
> www.facebook.com/NLLung
> twitter.com/nllung

Overview: A small provincial charitable organization founded in 1944 overseen by Canadian Lung Association
Mission: To achieve healthy breathing for the people of Newfoundland & Labrador
Chief Officer(s):
Greg Noel, President & CEO
greg.noel@nf.lung.ca
Publications:
• Newfoundland & Labrador Lung Association Newsletter
Type: Newsletter

NOVA SCOTIA

The Lung Association of Nova Scotia (LANS)
#200, 6331 Lady Hammond Rd., Halifax NS B3K 2S2

> *Tel:* 902-443-8141; *Fax:* 902-445-2573
> *Toll-Free:* 888-566-5864
> *e-mail:* info@ns.lung.ca
> www.ns.lung.ca
> www.linkedin.com/company/the-lung-association-of-nova-scotia
> www.facebook.com/LungNS
> twitter.com/NSLung
> www.youtube.com/LungNovaScotia

Overview: A small provincial charitable organization founded in 1909 overseen by Canadian Lung Association
Mission: To control & prevent lung disease in Nova Scotia; To help people who live with lung disease
Chief Officer(s):
Louis Brill, President & Chief Executive Officer, 902-443-8141 Ext. 22
louisbrill@ns.lung.ca

SECTION I:
Chronic & Mental Illnesses

Robert MacDonald, Manager, Health Initiatives
robertmacdonald@ns.lung.ca
Maria Caines, Senior Manager, Finance
mariacaines@ns.lung.ca
Caitlin Gray, Manager, Communications & Special Events
caitlingray@ns.lung.ca
Lynette Hollett, Manager, Donor Relations
lynettehollett@ns.lung.ca
Sam Warshick, Senior Manager, Fund Development
samanthawarshick@ns.lung.ca

ONTARIO

Ontario Lung Association (OLA)
#401, 18 Wynford Dr., Toronto ON M3C 0K8
Tel: 416-864-9911; *Fax:* 416-864-9916
Toll-Free: 888-344-5864
e-mail: olalung@on.lung.ca
www.on.lung.ca
www.facebook.com/OntarioLungAssociation?ref=ts
twitter.com/OntarioLung
www.youtube.com/user/ONLungAssociation
Overview: A large provincial charitable organization founded in 1945
overseen by Canadian Lung Association
Mission: To provide lung health information & support to people
affected by lung disease; To prevent & control chronic lung disease
Chief Officer(s):
John Granton, Chair
George Habib, President & Chief Executive Officer
John Martin, Treasurer
Publications:
• Asthma Action
Type: Newsletter
• Breathworks
Type: Newsletter
• Oxygen
Type: Newsletter
Profile: Lung health information, donor & research profiles, &
forthcoming events

Belleville Office (Hastings & Prince Edward Counties)
#339, 110 North Front St. A3, Belleville ON K8P 0A6
Tel: 613-969-0323
www.on.lung.ca
Chief Officer(s):
Lola McMurter, Coordinator, Special Events
lmcmurter@on.lung.ca

Brantford Office (Brant County)
410 Colborne St., Lower Level, Brantford ON N3S 3N6
Tel: 519-753-4682; *Fax:* 519-753-4667
e-mail: brant@on.lung.ca
www.on.lung.ca

Hamilton Office (Hamilton, Brant County, Niagara, Haldimand &
Norfolk Counties, & Waterloo & Wellington Regions)
#255, 245 King George St., Brantford ON N3R 7N7
Tel: 905-383-1616
Toll-Free: 800-790-5527
e-mail: hamilton@on.lung.ca
www.on.lung.ca

Kingston Office (Kingston & the Thousand Islands)
#339, 110 North Front St. A3, Belleville ON K8P 0A6
Tel: 613-545-3462
www.on.lung.ca
Chief Officer(s):
Lola McMurter, Coordinator, Volunteer & Fund Development
lmcmurter@on.lung.ca

London Office (Bluewater-Thames Valley)
#2, 639 Southdale Rd. East, London ON N6E 3M2
Tel: 519-453-9086; *Fax:* 519-453-9184
Chief Officer(s):
Lori Pallen, Regional Manager
lpallen@on.lung.ca

Ottawa Office (Ottawa, Renfrew County, & Cornwall Area)
#500, 2319 St. Laurent Blvd., Ottawa ON K1G 4J8
Tel: 613-230-4200; *Fax:* 613-230-5210

Chief Officer(s):
Melanie Estable-Porter, Officer, Corporate & Community
Development
melanie@on.lung.ca

Sault Ste Marie Office (Algoma Area)
514 Queen St. East, 1st Fl., Sault Ste Marie ON P6A 2A1
Tel: 705-256-2335; *Fax:* 705-256-1210
Chief Officer(s):
Grace Briglio, Coordinator, Volunteer & Fund Development
gbriglio@on.lung.ca

Stratford Office (Huron-Perth)
#105, 356 Ontario St., Stratford ON N5A 7X6
Tel: 519-271-7500; *Fax:* 519-271-7503
Chief Officer(s):
Deedee Herman, Area Manager
dherman@on.lung.ca

Toronto Office (Greater Toronto Area West)
#401, 18 Wynford Dr., Toronto ON M3C 0K8
Fax: 416-864-9916
Toll-Free: 888-344-5864
e-mail: olalung@on.lung.ca

Windsor Office (Windsor-Essex & Chatham-Kent Area)
#210, 3041 Dougall Ave., Windsor ON N9E 1S3
Tel: 519-256-3433
Chief Officer(s):
Julie Bortolotti, Coordinator, Volunteer & Fund Development
jbortolotti@on.lung.ca
• Windsor-Essex & Chatham-Kent Area Breathworks Support Group
Newsletter
Type: Newsletter; *Frequency:* Monthly
Profile: Support & advice for patients with COPD & their caregivers

Ontario Thoracic Society (OTS)
c/o Ontario Lung Association, #401, 18 Wynford Dr., Toronto ON M3C
0K8
Tel: 416-864-9911
e-mail: olalung@on.lung.ca
www.on.lung.ca
Overview: A medium-sized provincial charitable organization founded
in 1961
Mission: To promote respiratory health through medical research &
education
Member of: Ontario Lung Association
Affiliation(s): Canadian Thoracic Society
Chief Officer(s):
Thomas Kovesi, Chair

PRINCE EDWARD ISLAND

Prince Edward Island Lung Association
81 Prince St., Charlottetown PE C1A 4R3
Tel: 902-892-5957
Toll-Free: 888-566-5864
e-mail: info@pei.lung.ca
www.pei.lung.ca
www.facebook.com/196098560534899
twitter.com/PEI_Lung
Previous Name: PEI Tuberculosis League
Overview: A small provincial charitable organization founded in 1936
overseen by Canadian Lung Association
Mission: To improve the respiratory health of Islanders through
education, advocacy & research; To raise funds to support medical
research
Chief Officer(s):
Joanne Ings, Executive Director
jings@pei.lung.ca

QUÉBEC

Association des pneumologues de la province de Québec (APPQ)
CP 216, #3000, 2, Complexe Desjardins, Montréal QC H5B 1G8
Tél: 514-350-5117; *Télec:* 514-350-5153
Courriel: appq@fmsq.org
www.fmsq.org

Aperçu: *Dimension:* petite; *Envergure:* provinciale surveillé par Fédération des médecins spécialistes du Québec
Mission: Promouvoir les intérêts professionnels et économiques de ses membres; se préoccuper du maintien de leur compétence; se prononcer sur les problématiques de la pneumologie dans les meilleurs intérêts de la population
Membre de: Fédération des médecins spécialistes du Québec
Membre(s) du bureau directeur:
Pierre Mayer, Président
Elsa Fournier, Directrice, Administration

Québec Lung Association (QLA) / Association pulmonaire du Québec (APQ)

#104, 6070, rue Sherbrooke Est, Montréal QC H1N 1C1
Tel: 514-287-7400; *Fax:* 514-287-1978
Toll-Free: 888-768-6669
e-mail: info@pq.poumon.ca
www.pq.poumon.ca
www.facebook.com/poumon.qc
twitter.com/AssoPulmonaireQ
www.youtube.com/user/PoumonAPQ
Overview: A medium-sized provincial charitable organization founded in 1938 overseen by Canadian Lung Association
Mission: To provide resources in Québec about lung cancer, chronic obstructive pulmonary disease, sarcoidosis, tuberculosis, asthma, chronic bronchitis, sleep apnea, pneumonia, & emphysema
Member of: World Health Organization; International Union against Tuberculosis & Lung Disease; American Lung Association; European Lung Association
Chief Officer(s):
Dominique Massie, Executive Director, 514-975-5382 Ext. 224
   dominique.massie@pq.poumon.ca
Raymond Jabbour, Chief Financial Officer & Director, Direct Marketing
   & Information Technology, 514-975-5382 Ext. 226
Mathieu Leroux, Admisor, Development & Communications,
   514-975-5382 Ext. 235
   mathieu.leroux@pq.poumon.ca
Publications:
• Le Bulletin de l'association pulmonaire du Québec
Type: Newsletter; *Editor:* Louis P. Brisson; *ISSN:* 0843-381X
Profile: Respiratory health information, plus donation news
• Le Rapport annuel de l'association pulmonaire du Québec
Type: Yearbook; *Frequency:* Annually

SASKATCHEWAN

Saskatchewan Lung Association

Saskatoon Office, 1231 - 8 St. East, Saskatoon SK S7H 0S5
Tel: 306-343-9511; *Fax:* 306-343-7007
Toll-Free: 888-566-5864
e-mail: info@sk.lung.ca
www.sk.lung.ca
www.facebook.com/LungSask
twitter.com/lungsk
www.youtube.com/user/LungAssociation1
Previous Name: Saskatchewan Anti-Tuberculosis League
Overview: A medium-sized provincial charitable organization founded in 1911 overseen by Canadian Lung Association
Mission: To improve respiratory health & overall quality of life; To advocate for support of education & research
Chief Officer(s):
Pat Smith, Chair
Karen Davis, Vice-Chair
Brian Graham, President & CEO
Jennifer Miller, Vice-President, Health Promotion
Sharon Kremeniuk, Vice-President, Development
Melissa Leib, Vice-President, Finance & Operations
Donna Crooks, Treasurer
Publications:
• Breathworks: COPD Newsletter
Type: Newsletter
Profile: Educational articles plus notices of forthcoming support group meetings
• Lung Association of Saskatchewan Annual Report
Type: Yearbook; *Frequency:* Annually

• Nightly Nezzz Newsletter
Type: Newsletter; *Frequency:* Quarterly
Profile: Information for persons with sleep apnea & their families

International Associations

American Lung Association (ALA)

#1150, 55 West Wacker Dr., Chicago IL 60601 USA
Fax: 202-452-1805
Toll-Free: 800-586-4872
www.lungusa.org
www.facebook.com/lungusa
twitter.com/lungassociation
www.youtube.com/user/americanlung
Overview: A large international charitable organization founded in 1904
Mission: To prevent lung disease & promote lung health
Affiliation(s): American Thoracic Society
Chief Officer(s):
Kathryn A. Forbes, Chair
Harold Wimmer, President & CEO

Schizophrenia

Schizophrenia is a chronic mental illness that is characterized by disturbances of thinking, feeling and behaviour. Despite its literal translation of "split mind," schizophrenia is not the same as split personality disorder. Though not a common disorder, it is one of the most destructive, disrupting the lives of sufferers, as well as of family members and loved ones. People with schizophrenia and their families have long borne a burden of stigma because of the lack of understanding of the illness by society.

Cause

Although its specific cause is unknown, schizophrenia is believed to usually result from a complex interaction between biologic, inherited and environmental factors. One theory is that it is a disorder of information processing resulting from a defect in the prefrontal cortex of the brain. Because this system is defective, an individual with schizophrenia is easily overwhelmed by the amount of information and stimuli coming from the environment. People with a family history of schizophrenia are 10 times more likely to develop schizophrenia than the general population. If both parents have schizophrenia, there is a 40 percent chance that their children will also have the disorder. Environmental factors involved in schizophrenia may include viral infections and trauma before birth or during birth.

Symptoms

Schizophrenia is known as a heterogeneous disease, meaning that the illness takes many forms, depending on a variety of individual characteristics and circumstances. Symptoms of schizophrenia vary in type and severity and may include hallucinations, which are sensory experiences in the absence of actual stimuli (hearing voices when no one is speaking), and delusions, which are bizarre beliefs (that the individual is God, that the television is conveying messages specifically aimed at the individual, that some power is removing the individual's thoughts from his or her mind). These are called positive symptoms. Speech may be confused, and the person may have incoherent thought patterns. These are called cognitive symptoms. The individual also loses some normal behaviours and experiences, engaging in little social interaction and displaying catatonic behaviour and a flat or grossly inappropriate emotional state. These are called negative symptoms.

Because their disease causes difficulty in perceiving their environment and responding to it normally, people with schizophrenia often act strange, and have odd beliefs. They sometimes react to stimuli (voices or images originating inside their brains) as though they were originating in their environment. Hallucinations and delusions can make a person's behaviour appear bizarre to others. Anhedonia, the inability to enjoy pleasurable activities, is common in schizophrenia, as are sleep disturbances and abnormalities of psychomotor activity. The latter may take the form of pacing, rocking or immobility. Many people with schizophrenia have limited social relationships, and 60 to 70 percent do not marry. Only between 10 and 40 percent of people with schizophrenia are employed.

Individuals with untreated schizophrenia, under the influence of hallucinations and delusions, have a slightly greater propensity for violence than the general population, but only when there is co-existing alcohol or substance abuse, which is quite common. Up to 80 percent of people with schizophrenia will have a substance abuse problem during their lives. Patients who receive appropriate treatment are not more violent than the general population.

Schizophrenia takes many forms, and there are a number of subtypes of the illness. Paranoid schizophrenia is characterized by frequent and prominent hallucinations and delusions. When the prominent symptoms are mental stupor and muscular rigidity, the subtype is designated as catatonic. In people with disorganized schizophrenia, the prominent symptoms are disorganized behaviour and speech. If the prominent symptoms do not meet the criteria for catatonic, disorganized or paranoid schizophrenia, the diagnosis is undifferentiated schizophrenia, and if there is continuous evidence of schizophrenia without active symptoms, the diagnosis is residual schizophrenia.

It is important to note that psychotic illness does not necessarily affect all aspects of an individual's thinking. People with schizophrenia may have bizarre beliefs or behaviour in one sphere of life, but be perfectly able to make decisions and function in other areas.

Prevalence
The first episode of schizophrenia usually occurs in teenage years, although some cases may occur in the late thirties or forties. Onset prior to puberty is rare. Women have a later average of onset and a better prognosis. It is estimated that about 1 percent of the Canadian population is affected by schizophrenia.

Treatment Options
There is no test to diagnose schizophrenia. A physician must first rule out other disorders that might be causing the symptoms. A diagnosis of schizophrenia is based on the following guidelines developed by the Canadian Psychiatric Association: delusions, hallucinations, withdrawal from social contact, lack of motivation, and thought disorder. The symptoms cause social, educational and occupational dysfunction and have been exhibited most of the time for at least one month, with some signs having persisted for six months. The symptoms must not be related to mood or depressive disorders, substance abuse or general medical conditions.

Drug treatment is the cornerstone of managing schizophrenia. When treated early, patients tend to respond quickly and more fully. Effective drugs have been available for several decades, and have revolutionized treatment of the disease. Older medications, such as Haldol, are effective, but cause more side effects than newer medications, such as Zyprexa and Geodon. Clozapine was the first and is still one of the most effective treatments, but it causes a low incidence of a life-threatening blood disorder; therefore people who take it must have blood tests at regular intervals. The newer medications are more effective in treating the negative, as well as the positive, symptoms.

Often, patients report that antipsychotic medications make them feel foggy, or lethargic. They can have serious side effects, including tardive dyskinesia (a movement disorder). The newer antipsychotic medications are less sedating and have a decreased risk of causing tardive dyskinesia, but are associated with significant weight gain and increased risk of diabetes. There is considerable public controversy as to whether the weight gain and risk of diabetes associated with the newer medications outweigh their advantages.

Having schizophrenia interferes with taking care of oneself and getting proper medical care in several ways. If untreated, schizophrenia can interfere with an individual's ability to understand signs and symptoms of medical disorders. Compliance with medication is often a problem, and failure to continue taking medication is a major cause of relapse.

For this reason, treatment should include supportive therapy, in which a psychiatrist or other mental health professional provides counselling aimed at helping the patient maintain a positive and optimistic attitude focused on staying healthy. Other forms of therapy, such as social skills training, have also found some success and may be useful in helping a person with schizophrenia learn appropriate social and interpersonal behaviour. Cognitive behavioural therapy (CBT) may also be an effective part of the treatment program for people with schizophrenia. In addition, people close to persons with schizophrenia are often very affected by the disease and can be helped by support and advocacy groups.

Schizophrenia is a chronic disease and, once diagnosed, a person often needs treatment for the rest of his or her life. The life expectancy of people with schizophrenia is shorter than the general population for a variety of reasons: suicide is common among people with the disease—about 10 percent die from suicide—and people with schizophrenia often have both poor medical care and poor health. However, great strides have been made in treating the disease and with early diagnosis, appropriate treatment and adherence to therapy many individuals with schizophrenia can hold jobs, marry, parent children and have gratifying and productive lives.

See also Mental Illness/General and Depression

National Associations

Schizophrenia Society of Canada (SSC) / Société canadienne de schizophrénie
#100, 4 Fort St., Winnipeg MB R3C 1C4
Tel: 204-786-1616; *Fax:* 204-783-4898
Toll-Free: 800-263-5545
e-mail: info@schizophrenia.ca
www.schizophrenia.ca
www.facebook.com/pages/Schizophrenia-Society-of-Canada/19708826
3635191
twitter.com/SchizophreniaCa
Previous Name: Canadian Friends of Schizophrenics
Overview: A medium-sized national charitable organization founded in 1979
Mission: To improve the quality of life for those affected by schizophrenia & psychosis; To advocate on behalf of individuals & families affected by schizophrenia for improved treatment & services
Chief Officer(s):
Chris Summerville, D. Min, CPRP, Chief Executive Officer
  chris@schizophrenia.ca
Publications:
• A Future With Hope
Type: Newsletter; *Frequency:* 3 pa; *Price:* Free with membership in the Schizophrenia Society of Canada
Profile: Society activities, executive reports, & current issues

• Psychosis & Substance Use: A Booklet for Youth
Type: Booklet; Number of Pages: 6
• Rays of Hope
Type: Manual; Number of Pages: 268; ISBN: 0-9733913-0-8
Profile: A reference publication for families & caregivers of individuals with schizophrenia
• Reaching Out
Type: Kit
Profile: An awareness & learning resource for students in grades seven to twelve, including a video
• Respite Needs of People Living with Schizophrenia
 Number of Pages: 80; Editor: Michelle Bergin; Heather Stuart
Profile: Results of a national survey of Schizophrenia Society of Canada members
• Schizophrenia & Substance Use: Information for Families
Type: Booklet; Number of Pages: 9
• Schizophrenia & Substance Use: Information for Consumers
Type: Booklet; Number of Pages: 7
• Schizophrenia & Substance Use: Information for Service Providers
Type: Booklet; Number of Pages: 7
• Schizophrenia in Canada: A National Report
Type: Report
Profile: Sections include understanding schizophrenia, stigma & discrination, & solutions
• Schizophrenia Society of Canada Annual Report
Type: Yearbook; Frequency: Annually
• Schizophrenia: The Journey to Recovery, A Consumer & Family Guide to Assessment & Treatment
Type: Booklet; Number of Pages: 48; Author: Mary Metcalfe, M.S.; Editor: Deborah Kelly; Francine Knoops
Profile: A guide produced by the Schizophrenia Society of Canada & the CanadianPsychiatric Association
• Strengthening Families Together: Helping Canadians Live with Mental Illness
Type: Handbook; Number of Pages: 146; Editor: Edna Barker
Profile: A book for facilitators of the Stenghtening Families Together program

Provincial Associations

ALBERTA

Schizophrenia Society of Alberta (SSA)
4809 - 48 Ave., Red Deer AB T4N 3T2
Tel: 403-986-9440; Fax: 403-986-9442
e-mail: info@schizophrenia.ab.ca
www.schizophrenia.ab.ca
www.linkedin.com/groups/Schizophrenia-Society-Alberta-SSA-2604548/abou
www.facebook.com/SchizophreniaSocietyofAlberta
twitter.com/SchizophreniaAB
Previous Name: Alberta Friends of Schizophrenics
Overview: A small provincial charitable organization founded in 1980 overseen by Schizophrenia Society of Canada
Mission: To support individuals with schizophrenia & related illnesses through education, public policy, research, & programs
Affliation(s): Schizophrenia Society of Canada
Chief Officer(s):
Doug Race, Chair
Lesley Vaage, Vice-Chair
Shelley Stigter, Secretary
Publications:
• Opening Minds [a publication of the Schizophrenia Society of Alberta]
Type: Newsletter

Calgary & Area Chapter
#1120 - 53 Ave. NE, Bay 101A, Calgary AB T2E 6N9
Tel: 403-264-5161; Fax: 403-269-1727
Chief Officer(s):
Larry Fedun, Program Coordinator
lfedun@schizophrenia.ab.ca

Camrose & Area Chapter
#206, 5010 - 50 Ave., Camrose AB T4V 3P7
Tel: 780-679-4280
e-mail: aholler@schizophrenia.ab.ca

Edmonton & Area Chapter

5215 - 87 St., Edmonton AB T6E 5L5
Tel: 780-452-4661; Fax: 780-482-3027
e-mail: nnicholson@schizophrenia.ab.ca
• Grey Matters
Type: Newsletter; Frequency: Monthly; Price: Free with membership in the Schizophrenia Society of Alberta, Edmonton & Area Chapter
Profile: Information about local activities & groups involved with mental illness

Lethbridge & Area Chapter
234C - 12th St. B North, Lethbridge AB T1H 2K7
Tel: 403-327-4305; Fax: 403-328-0124
e-mail: jhansen@schizophrenia.ab.ca

Medicine Hat & Area Chapter
526B - 3 St. SE, Medicine Hat AB T1A 0H3
Tel: 403-526-8515
e-mail: wbonertz@schizophrenia.ab.ca

Red Deer & Area Chapter
4811 - 48 St., Red Deer AB T4N 3T2
Tel: 403-342-5760; Fax: 403-342-4866
e-mail: JLund@schizophrenia.ab.ca

Chief Officer(s):
Lyle McKellar, Chair
Don Simpson, Vice-Chair
Gary Lathan, Executive Director
Marion Weidner, Secretary
Roger Goodwin, Treasurer
Lana King Kottman, Coordinator, Education
lana@ssard.com
Chris Thomas, Coordinator, Programs & Services
chris@ssard.com
• Courage
Type: Newsletter; Frequency: Quarterly; Price: Free with Schizophrenia Society of Alberta, Red Deer Chapter, membership
Profile: Information about Red Deer area & provincial events

BRITISH COLUMBIA

British Columbia Schizophrenia Society
#1100, 1200 West 73rd Ave., Vancouver BC V6P 6G5
Tel: 604-270-7841; Fax: 604-270-9861
Toll-Free: 888-888-0029
e-mail: prov@bcss.org
www.bcss.org
www.facebook.com/BCSchizophreniaSociety
twitter.com/BCSchizophrenia
www.youtube.com/user/bcssprov
Previous Name: BC Friends of Schizophrenics
Overview: A small provincial charitable organization founded in 1982 overseen by Schizophrenia Society of Canada
Mission: To alleviate the suffering caused by schizophrenia; To provide support & education; To increase public awareness & understanding of schizophrenia & other persistent mental illnesses; To promote research into the causes, treatment & cure of schizophrenia
Member of: Schizophrenia Society of Canada
Chief Officer(s):
Deborah Conner, Executive Director

MANITOBA

Manitoba Schizophrenia Society, Inc. (MSS)
#100, 4 Fort St., Winnipeg MB R3C 1C4
Tel: 204-786-1616; Fax: 204-783-4898
e-mail: info@mss.mb.ca
www.mss.mb.ca
www.facebook.com/ManitobaSchizophreniaSociety
twitter.com/mbschizophrenia
www.youtube.com/user/recoverytree?
Overview: A medium-sized provincial charitable organization founded in 1979
Mission: To improve the quality of life for individuals affected by schizophrenia / psychosis & co-occurring disorders
Chief Officer(s):
Chris Summerville, Executive Director
chris@mss.mb.ca
Jane Burpee, Coordinator, Public Education
jane@mss.mb.ca

Katrina Tinman, Administrator, Special Events
  katrina@mss.mb.ca
Publications:
• Reasons for Hope [a publication of the Manitoba Schizophrenia Society]
Type: Newsletter; *Frequency:* Quarterly; *Editor:* Chris Summerville; Kim Heidinger
• The Sharing Tree [a publication of the Manitoba Schizophrenia Society]
Type: Newsletter; *Editor:* Jo-Ann Paley

NEW BRUNSWICK

Schizophrenia Society of New Brunswick (SSNB)
PO Box 562, 130 Duke St., Miramichi NB E1V 3T7
Tel: 506-622-1595; *Fax:* 506-622-8927
e-mail: ssnbmiramichi@nb.aibn.com
www.schizophreniasociety.nb.ca
Overview: A small provincial charitable organization founded in 1986 overseen by Schizophrenia Society of Canada
Member of: Schizophrenia Society of Canada
Chief Officer(s):
Barb Johnson, President
  ssbj@rogers.com

Fredericton Chapter
Fredericton NB
Tel: 506-451-7770
www.schizophreniasociety.nb.ca/chapters/fredericton.htm

Moncton Chapter
178 Summer Ave., Moncton NB E1C 8A5
Tel: 506-384-8668; *Fax:* 506-854-7524
e-mail: cormiergc@rogers.com
www.schizophreniasociety.nb.ca/chapters/moncton.htm

Saint John Chapter
55 Union St., Saint John NB E2L 5B7
e-mail: ssbj@rogers.com
schizophreniasocietysj.wordpress.com

NEWFOUNDLAND AND LABRADOR

Schizophrenia Society of Newfoundland & Labrador
UB Waterford Hospital, PO Box 28029, 48 Kenmount Rd., St. John's NL A1B 1X0
Tel: 709-777-3335; *Fax:* 709-777-3224
e-mail: info@ssnl.org
ssnl.org
www.facebook.com/171941232764
twitter.com/schizophreniaNL
Overview: A small provincial charitable organization overseen by Schizophrenia Society of Canada
Mission: To alleviate the suffering caused by schizophrenia
Member of: Schizophrenia Society of Canada

NOVA SCOTIA

Schizophrenia Society of Nova Scotia (SSNS)
#B-23, E.C. Purdy Building, PO Box 1004, Stn. Main, 300 Pleasant St., Dartmouth NS B2Y 3Z9
Tel: 902-465-2601; *Fax:* 902-465-5479
Toll-Free: 800-465-2601
e-mail: ssns@bellaliant.com
www.ssns.ca
www.facebook.com/schizophrenia.society.ns
twitter.com/ssnsc
Previous Name: Nova Scotia Friends of Schizophrenics
Overview: A small provincial charitable organization founded in 1982 overseen by Schizophrenia Society of Canada
Mission: To alleviate the suffering caused by schizophrenia
Member of: Schizophrenia Society of Canada
Chief Officer(s):
Diane MacDougall, Executive Director

ONTARIO

Schizophrenia Society of Ontario (SSO) / Société de schizophrénie de l'Ontario
#302, 130 Spadina Ave., Toronto ON M5V 2L4
Fax: 416-449-8434
Toll-Free: 800-449-6367
www.schizophrenia.on.ca
www.facebook.com/SchizophreniaSocietyON
twitter.com/peace_of_minds
www.youtube.com/user/SSOOntario
Previous Name: Ontario Friends of Schizophrenics
Overview: A medium-sized provincial charitable organization founded in 1979 overseen by Schizophrenia Society of Canada
Mission: To improve the quality of life for families affected by schizophrenia, by offering support to them, & by promoting community awareness of the disease
Chief Officer(s):
Aamir Mian, Chair
Mary Alberti, Chief Executive Officer
  malberti@schizophrenia.on.ca

Halton / Peel Region
136 Cross Ave., Main Fl., Oakville ON L6J 2W6
Tel: 905-338-2112; *Fax:* 905-338-2113
Chief Officer(s):
Marina Sue-Ping, Family & Community Coordinator
  msue-ping@schizophrenia.on.ca

Hamilton/Niagara Region
#405, 20 Hughson St. South, Hamilton ON L8N 2A1
Tel: 905-523-7413; *Fax:* 416-449-8434
Chief Officer(s):
Cassandra Roach, Regional Coordinator

Ottawa Region
c/o ROH, 1145 Carling Ave., Ottawa ON K1Z 7K4
Tel: 613-722-6521; *Fax:* 613-729-8980
Chief Officer(s):
Sheila Deighton, Regional Coordinator Ext. 7775
  sdeighton@schizophrenia.on.ca

Peterborough/Durham Region
#3, 421 Water St., Peterborough ON K9H 3L9
Tel: 705-749-1753; *Fax:* 705-749-6175
Chief Officer(s):
Allyson Susko, Regional Coordinator
  asusko@schizophrenia.on.ca

PRINCE EDWARD ISLAND

Schizophrenia Society of Prince Edward Island (SSPEI)
PO Box 25020, Charlottetown PE C1A 9N4
Tel: 902-368-5850; *Fax:* 902-368-5467
e-mail: schizophreniapei@pei.aibn.com
Overview: A small provincial charitable organization founded in 1984 overseen by Schizophrenia Society of Canada
Mission: To alleviate the suffering caused by schizophrenia
Member of: Schizophrenia Society of Canada

QUÉBEC

Société québécoise de la schizophrénie (SQS)
7401, rue Hochelaga, Montréal QC H1N 3M5
Tél: 514-251-4125; *Téléc:* 514-251-6347
Ligne sans frais: 866-888-2323
Courriel: info@schizophrenie.qc.ca
www.schizophrenie.qc.ca
wwww.facebook.com/SQSchizophrenie
twitter.com/SQSchizophrenie
www.youtube.com/user/SQSchizophrenie1
Nom précédent: Association québécoise de la schizophrénie
Aperçu: *Dimension:* petite; *Envergure:* provinciale; Organisme sans but lucratif; fondée en 1988
Mission: Organisme communautaire dont les services et activités ont pour but d'apporter un soutien essentiel aux familles dont un être cher est atteint de schizophrénie; information, écoute, orientation et accompagnement font entre autres partie de notre mission
Membre de: Société canadienne de schizophrénie; Fédération des familles et amis de la personne atteinte de maladie mentale;

Association canadienne pour la santé mentale; Association québécoise pour la réadaptation psychosociale
Membre(s) du bureau directeur:
Francine Dubé, Directrice générale
fdube@schizophrenie.qc.ca

SASKATCHEWAN

Schizophrenia Society of Saskatchewan (SSS)
PO Box 305, Stn. Main, Regina SK S4P 3A1
Tel: 306-584-2620; *Fax:* 306-584-0525
Toll-Free: 877-584-2620
e-mail: sssprov@sasktel.net
www.schizophrenia.sk.ca
www.facebook.com/201415453215067
twitter.com/SZSask
www.youtube.com/user/SchizophreniaSask
Previous Name: Saskatchewan Friends of Schizophrenics
Overview: A small provincial charitable organization founded in 1982 overseen by Schizophrenia Society of Canada
Mission: The Society provides easily understood information on schizophrenia for concerned families. It works to increase public awareness of the illness with initiatives aimed at all age groups, & speaks on behalf of affected families. It is a registered charity, BN :894249861RR0001.
Member of: Schizophrenia Society of Canada
Chief Officer(s):
Anita Hopfauf, Executive Director
Vonni Widdis, President

Saskatoon Chapter
#219, 230 Ave. R South, Saskatoon SK S7M 2Z1
Tel: 306-374-2224; *Fax:* 306-477-5649
e-mail: ssssaskatoon@sasktel.net
www.schizophrenia-saskatoon.com
www.facebook.com/pages/Sasktoon-Schizophrenia-Society/217889741572764
www.youtube.com/user/SkSchizophrenia

Local Associations

ONTARIO

Hamilton Program for Schizophrenia (HPS)
#102, 350 King St. East, Hamilton ON L8N 3Y3
Tel: 905-525-2832; *Fax:* 905-546-0055
e-mail: info@hpfs.on.ca
www.hpfs.on.ca

Overview: A small local organization founded in 1979
Mission: The organization is a comprehensive, community-based treatment & rehabilitation program for adults with schizophrenia. It promotes an understanding of schizophrenia in the community.
Affiliation(s): McMaster University Clinical Teaching Unit
Chief Officer(s):
Peter E. Cook, Executive Director

QUÉBEC

Le Centre de soutien en santé mentale - Montérégie (CSSM-M)
2510, rue Sainte-Héléne, Longueuil QC J4K 3V2
Tél: 450-677-4347; *Téléc:* 450-748-0503
www.schizophrenie-monteregie.com
schizomonteregie.blogspot.ca
Nom précédent: Société de Schizophrénie de la Montérégie
Aperçu: *Dimension:* petite; *Envergure:* locale
Mission: Aider toute personne atteintes de schizophrénie et leurs familles d'améliorer leur qualité de vie et de sensibilliser aux problèmes de schizophrénie provoque
Membre(s) du bureau directeur:
Lucie Couillard, Dierctrice générale

International Associations

International Schizophrenia Foundation (ISF)
16 Florence Ave., Toronto ON M2N 1E9
Tel: 416-733-2117; *Fax:* 416-733-2352
e-mail: centre@orthomed.org
www.isfmentalhealth.org
www.facebook.com/178337749007188
twitter.com/ISFMentalHealth
Previous Name: Canadian Schizophrenia Foundation
Overview: A medium-sized international charitable organization founded in 1968
Mission: To raise the levels of diagnosis, treatment & prevention of the schizophrenias & related disorders; to reduce the fear & stigma; to provide the best possible treatment & rehabilitation services.
Member of: International Society for Orthomolecular Medicine
Chief Officer(s):
Trevor Roberts, Executive Director

Provincial Libraries

Schizophrenia Society of Nova Scotia
Purdy Bldg., 300 Pleasant St., #B23, Dartmouth, NS B2Y 3Z9
Tel: 902-465-2601; *Fax:* 902-465-5479
Toll-Free: 800-465-2601
contact@ssns.ca
www.ssns.ca
Collection: Educational materials about schizophrenia & psychosis for families & caregivers; Videos
Diane MacDougall, Executive Director
director@ssns.ca
Todd MacMillan, Resource Advisor
todd@ssns.ca

Scleroderma

Scleroderma, literally "hard skin," is a progressive and chronic disorder of the connective and vascular tissue which leads to scarring (sclerosis). Scleroderma can either be localized (affecting the skin and sometimes the bones and muscles beneath), or systemic (affecting the skin, tissues, blood vessels and internal organs).

Cause
The cause of the disease is unknown. One theory suggests that an autoimmune reaction in people with scleroderma causes them to produce too much collagen (the major protein of connective tissue). This excess collagen is deposited in the skin, tissues and organs, causing them to thicken and harden. Other theories suggest that the trigger for the disease may be environmental or viral.

Symptoms
Since almost any organ may be involved, the list of possible scleroderma symptoms is extensive. Important ones include thickening or hardening of the skin, calcium deposits under the skin, muscle weakness, fatigue, joint stiffness, weight loss, shortness of breath, abdominal bloating and pain, diarrhea and irritation of the eyes. Kidney involvement usually causes abrupt acceleration of high blood pressure. A very characteristic symptom, although not unique to this disease, is Raynaud's phenomenon: on exposure to cold, the arteries of the patient's hands and feet contract, causing the skin colour to change from red, to white (blanch), to blue (cyanosis), and resulting in pain and numbness.

Prevalence
It is estimated that approximately 16,000 Canadians are affected by scleroderma. Women are 3 to 5 times as likely as men to get the disease, which typically begins between the ages of 30 and 50. It is comparatively rare in children and the elderly.

Treatment Options
Since the symptoms of scleroderma are similar to those of other autoimmune conditions, it can be difficult to diagnose. Usually a

physician evaluates the history of a patient's symptoms, and performs a physical exam to check for signs that are characteristic of scleroderma, such as thickened and hardened areas of skin, grating sensations in the joints and capillary changes in the fingernails.

At present, there is no cure for scleroderma. Treatment is aimed at symptom reduction and prevention of organ damage. Scleroderma limited to the skin is often treated with corticosteroid creams, while calcium channel blockers (drugs that cause blood vessels to expand, thereby improving blood flow) are often prescribed for Raynaud's. Joint stiffness and pain may be treated with corticosteroids or NSAIDs (non-steroidal anti-inflammatory drugs). Immunosuppressants may also be used to prevent inflammation. Use of ACE inhibitors can prevent high blood pressure caused by kidney damage. When end-stage kidney disease cannot be prevented, dialysis or transplant may be needed.

If scleroderma is limited to the skin the outlook is good, and patients have a normal life expectancy. Involvement of the lungs and kidneys in the systemic form may be fatal, but recent advances in treatment have improved patient survival. Currently, the five-year survival rate for people who have been diagnosed with severe forms of scleroderma is approximately 80 to 85 percent.

National Associations

Scleroderma Society of Canada (SSC)
#206, 41 King William St., Hamilton ON L8R 1A2
Toll-Free: 866-279-0632
e-mail: info@scleroderma.ca
www.scleroderma.ca
Overview: A small national organization founded in 2000
Mission: To promote awareness of scleroderma, to support research toward finding a cure and to provide support and information to those affected by the disease.
Chief Officer(s):
Maureen Sauvé, President

Provincial Associations

BRITISH COLUMBIA

Scleroderma Association of British Columbia
PO Box 218, Stn. Delta Main, Delta BC V4K 3N7
Tel: 604-940-9343; *Fax:* 604-940-9346
Toll-Free: 888-940-9343
www.sclerodermabc.ca
www.facebook.com/scleroderma.bc
Overview: A small provincial charitable organization founded in 1984
Mission: To support, educate & keep informed those diagnosed with scleroderma (in skin form - localized, or in systemic form - systemic sclerosis); To raise research funds
Member of: Scleroderma Society of Canada
Chief Officer(s):
Rosanne Queen, President
rq.sabc@telus.net

ONTARIO

The Scleroderma Society of Ontario (SSO)
Empire Times Bldg., #206, 41 King William St., Hamilton ON L8R 1A2
Tel: 905-544-0343
Toll-Free: 888-776-7776
www.sclerodermaontario.ca
Overview: A small provincial charitable organization
Mission: To promote public awareness; To advance patient wellness; To support research in Scleroderma
Member of: The Arthritis Society
Chief Officer(s):
Anna McCusker, Executive Director
anna@sclerodermaontario.ca

Scoliosis

Scoliosis is a lateral curvature of the spine that usually occurs just before puberty.

Cause
More than 80 percent of scoliosis is idiopathic, that is, there is no known cause. However, it is believed that there is a genetic link since scoliosis tends to run in families. Other possible causes of scoliosis include spine injuries, birth defects and neuromuscular conditions such as cerebral palsy and muscular dystrophy.

Symptoms
Scoliosis may first be suspected when one shoulder appears higher than the other, or clothes don't hang straight. The spinal curve is more pronounced when the person bends forward. Other symptoms include prominent shoulder blades, uneven hip levels and fatigue in the lower back after sitting or standing for prolonged periods of time. In many cases there are no symptoms unless the scoliosis is severe. When a spinal curve is severe, the amount of space in the chest is reduced, which can affect lung function and make breathing difficult. The rib compression in severe scoliosis can also cause back pain and put pressure on other organs.

Prevalence
It is estimated that scoliosis affects up to 12 percent of the general population. Although both boys and girls develop scoliosis, it is more likely for a girl to have a spinal curve that worsens and requires treatment.

Treatment Options
To diagnose scoliosis, a physician usually takes a detailed medical history and performs a physical exam which includes a forward-bending test. During this test, the physician checks the level of the shoulders and examines the ribs to see if they curve differently from one side to the other. X-rays are sometimes used to determine the severity of the spinal curve.

Treatment for scoliosis depends on the site and severity of the curve, and the age of onset of symptoms. The majority of cases require only observation for progression. In cases where scoliosis is progressive, an orthopedic brace is often needed. The brace is usually worn for most of the night and day for a period until a child's bones stop growing. In some cases, spinal fusion surgery is required.

Research suggests that the earlier a diagnosis is made, the better the chance of preventing the progression of scoliosis. In Canada, clinical trials are currently underway to develop genetic tests and blood tests that will identify people with an inherited predisposition to scoliosis.

National Associations

Canadian Orthopaedic Association (COA) / Association canadienne d'orthopédie
#620, 4060 rue Ste-Catherine ouest, Westmount QC H3Z 2Z3
Tel: 514-874-9003; *Fax:* 514-874-0464
www.coa-aco.org
twitter.com/CdnOrthoAssoc
Overview: A medium-sized national organization founded in 1948
Mission: To provide continuing medical education & training for orthopaedic surgeons
Chief Officer(s):
Douglas C. Thomson, Chief Executive Officer
Publications:
• COA [Canadian Orthopaedic Association] Newsletter
Type: Newsletter; *Frequency:* Quarterly; *Accepts Advertising; Editor:* Dr. Alastair Younger; *Price:* Free with COA membership
Profile: Current events & ideas in orthopaedics

Canadian Orthopaedic Foundation (COF) / Fondation orthopédique du Canada (FOC)
PO Box 1036, Toronto ON M5K 1P2

Tel: 416-410-2341; Fax: 416-352-5078
Toll-Free: 800-461-3639
e-mail: mailbox@canorth.org
www.canorth.org
www.facebook.com/pages/Canadian-Orthopaedic-Foundation/175163319218018
twitter.com/CanOrthoFound

Overview: A medium-sized national charitable organization founded in 1965
Mission: To foster excellence in the provision of health care to patients with musculoskeletal disease or injury, in a cost effective manner, based on significant outcome studies, by supporting research, educating its members & securing funding from government & other health care funding agencies
Affiliation(s): World Orthopaedic Concern; Canadian Medical Association
Chief Officer(s):
Geoffrey Johnston, Chair & President
James Hall, Vice Chair
Publications:
• OrthoLink
Type: Newsletter; Frequency: Quarterly
Profile: Information & practical tips for people interested in building & maintaining bone & joint health

Canadian Orthopaedic Nurses Association (CONA) / Association canadienne des infirmières et infirmiers en orthopédie
7714 - 80 Ave., Edmonton AB T6C 0S4

www.cona-nurse.org
Overview: A medium-sized national organization founded in 1978
Mission: To foster professional growth of the membership in the assessment, treatment & rehabilitation of individuals with neuromuscular & skeletal alterations; To promote nursing research related to orthopaedics
Affiliation(s): Canadian Nurses Association
Chief Officer(s):
Candace Kenyon, President
Publications:
• Orthroscope [a publication of the Canadian Orthopaedic Nurses Association]
Type: Newsletter; Frequency: Quarterly; Price: Free with CONA membership
Profile: National newsletter with current events in orthopaedic nursing

Canadian Orthopaedic Residents Association (CORA) / L'Association Canadienne des Residents en Orthopédie (ACRO)
#450, 4150, rue Sainte-Catherine ouest, Montréal QC H3Z 2Y5

Tel: 514-874-9003; Fax: 514-874-0464
e-mail: coraweb@canorth.org
www.coraweb.org
Overview: A small national organization
Mission: To foster & promote research & education in the field of Orthopaedic Surgery
Chief Officer(s):
Nadia Murphy, President
nlmurphy@dal.ca

Canadian Society of Orthopaedic Technologists (CSOT) / Société canadienne des technologistes en orthopedie
#715A, 18 Wynford Dr., Toronto ON M3C 3S2

Tel: 416-445-4516; Fax: 416-489-7356
e-mail: csot@look.ca
www.pappin.com/csot
Overview: A small national licensing organization founded in 1972
Mission: To promote & develop training programs & professional standards; To encourage uniform training programs & examinations; To promote & facilitate cooperation between Orthopaedic Technologists & the medical profession
Chief Officer(s):
Alba Greco, President
agreco3@cogeco.ca
Pamela Smith, Office Manager & Registrar

Publications:
• BodyCast [a publication of the Canadian Society of Orthopaedic Technologists]
Type: Journal; Frequency: s-a.; Editor: Tony Romeo
• NewsCast [a publication of the Canadian Society of Orthopaedic Technologists]
Type: Newsletter; Frequency: s-a.

Alberta Chapter
303 Chaparral Dr. SE, Calgary AB T2X 3L9
Tel: 403-201-2423
Chief Officer(s):
Pam Nadon, President

Graham Bell Chapter
26 Geneva Crt., Brantford ON L6S 1B8
Tel: 905-791-7970
Chief Officer(s):
Adam Bradley, President

Manitoba Chapter
c/o Pan Am Clinic, 75 Poseidon Bay, Winnipeg MB R3M 3E4
Tel: 204-925-1522
Chief Officer(s):
Mary Kate Turner, President

Niagara Chapter
22 Lyndon St. West, Thorold ON L2V 3J7
Tel: 906-321-6201
Chief Officer(s):
Stephanie Koch, President

Northtechs Chapter
6211-149 Ave., Edmonton AB T5A 1W1
Tel: 780-342-4056
Chief Officer(s):
Ellanore Gallagher, President

Wascana Chapter
200 Angus St., Regina SK S4R 3K4
Tel: 306-775-2100
Chief Officer(s):
Dustin Livingstone, President

Provincial Associations

QUÉBEC

Association d'orthopédie du Québec
Tour de L'Est, CP 216, Succ. Desjardins, 2, Complexe Desjardins, 30e étage, Montréal QC H5B 1G8

Tél: 514-844-0803; Téléc: 514-844-6786
Courriel: aoq@fmsq.org
www.orthoquebec.ca
Aperçu: Dimension: moyenne; Envergure: provinciale surveillé par Fédération des médecins spécialistes du Québec
Mission: Valoriser le statut professionnel de ses membres; promouvoir leurs intérêts économiques; contribuer au développement de la chirurgie orthopédique et de la traumatologie par le biais d'activités de formation médicale continue
Membre(s) du bureau directeur:
Robert Turcotte, Président
Jean-François Joncas, Secrétaire-trésorier

International Associations

Association of Children's Prosthetic-Orthotic Clinics (ACPOC)
#727, 6300, North River Rd., Rosemont IL 60018-4226 USA

Tel: 847-698-1637; Fax: 847-823-0536
e-mail: acpoc@aaos.org
www.acpoc.org
Overview: A small international organization founded in 1978
Mission: To provide prosthetic-orthotic care for children with limb loss or orthopaedic disabilities.
Chief Officer(s):
David B. Rotter, President

Sexual Disorders

It is not possible to know what degree of sexual interest, desire or activity is normal; at best, we have averages, not indications of the optimal state. A sexual disorder is diagnosed when lack of desire or activity is repeated, persists over time and causes distress or interferes with the person's functioning in other important areas of life.

It is essential to know whether the problem is lifelong or was precipitated by a recent event, and whether it occurs only with a particular partner or in a particular situation. It is also essential not to make assumptions about sexual activity based on age, socioeconomic status or sexual orientation. The only way to know about an individual's sexual life is to ask.

Sexual disorders are divided into four groups: disorders of sexual desire, disorders of sexual arousal, orgasmic disorders and disorders involving sexual pain.

Sexual Desire Disorders

Symptoms

There are two types of sexual desire disorders. Hypoactive sexual desire disorder (HSDD) is characterized by a persistent or repeated lack of sexual fantasies or desire for sexual activities. The person does not initiate sexual activity, or respond to the partner's initiation attempts. The disorder is often associated with the inability to achieve orgasm in women, and the inability to achieve an erection in men. It can also be associated with other psychiatric and medical problems, including a history of sexual trauma and abuse. Sexual aversion disorder (SAD) is characterized by persistent or repeated extreme aversion to, and avoidance of, all or almost all genital sexual contact with a partner. The most common causes of sexual aversion disorder are interpersonal problems (for example, unhappiness in a relationship) and a previous traumatic experience (for example, rape). The person with a sexual desire disorder commonly has a poor body image and avoids nudity. Both sexual desire disorders cause marked distress or interpersonal problems.

Prevalence

HSDD is common in both men and women but twice as many women as men report it. It is estimated at 20 percent overall. The prevalence of SAD is unknown.

Treatment Options

The diagnosis of sexual desire disorders is usually based on a physical examination (to rule out other medical conditions that might be causing the symptoms) and an interview with the patient and his or her partner.

Treatment of sexual desire disorders usually includes psychotherapy (to treat any underlying psychological problems that might be causing the symptoms) and couples counselling. Testosterone is sometimes prescribed to improve sex drive in post-menopausal women with sexual desire disorders. However, it can have serious side effects.

Sexual Arousal Disorders

Symptoms

There are two types of sexual arousal disorders. Female sexual arousal disorder (FSAD) is characterized by a persistent or repeated inability to attain or maintain adequate lubrication—swelling (sexual excitement) response throughout sexual activity. Male erectile disorder (MED) is characterized by a persistent or repeated inability to maintain an adequate erection throughout sexual activity. Both disorders cause clear distress or interpersonal problems. However, men tend to be more upset by it than

women. Contributing issues include performance anxiety (especially in men), fear of failure, inadequate stimulation and relationship conflicts. Other problems associated with FSAD and MED are childhood sexual trauma, sexual identity concerns, religious orthodoxy, depression, lack of intimacy or trust and power conflicts. MED is frequently associated with diabetes, peripheral nerve disorders and hypertension, and is a side effect of a variety of medications; men with MED must be evaluated for these conditions. In addition, the medications used to treat MED are contraindicated in some medical conditions, such as heart conditions.

Prevalence

Prevalence information varies for FSAD. In one Canadian study, 24 percent of women reported lubrication problems. In a study of happily married couples, about one third of women complained of difficulty in achieving or maintaining sexual excitement.

Erectile difficulties in men are estimated to be very common, affecting close to 50 percent of men aged 40 and over in Canada. The frequency of erectile problems increases steeply with age. The disorder is common among married, single, heterosexual and homosexual men.

Treatment Options

Diagnosis of sexual arousal disorders is usually based on a psychological and medical history, as well as a physical examination to rule out other medical problems that might be causing the symptoms.

In FSAD, cognitive-behavioural psychotherapy is often recommended, including practical help such as the use of water-soluble lubricating products. Hormone treatment, such as testosterone-estrogen compounds, is sometimes helpful. However, the use of testosterone to treat sexual disorders in menopausal women is controversial and can have serious side effects.

An array of treatments is available for male erectile dysfunction, including prosthetic devices for physiological penile problems. In cases of hormonal problems, testosterone treatments have had some results. Viagra has produced success for treating male erectile dysfunction, as have two other medications for MED, vardenafil (Levitra) and tadalafil (Cialis).

When sexual problems are limited to a particular partner or situation, psychotherapy (individual or couple) is necessary to resolve the difficulty.

Orgasmic Disorders

Symptoms

There are three types of orgasmic disorders. Female orgasmic disorder (FOD) and male orgasmic disorder are characterized by a persistent or repeated delay in, or absence of, orgasm, despite a normal sexual excitement phase. When FOD or MOD occurs only in certain situations, difficulty with desire and arousal are often also present. Medical or surgical conditions such as multiple sclerosis, spinal cord injury, surgical prostatectomy (males), and some medications can also play a role in FOD and MOD. Premature ejaculation (PE) is characterized by a persistent or recurring ejaculation with minimal sexual stimulation before, upon or shortly after penetration and earlier than desired. PE is likely to be very disruptive. Some males may have had the disorder all their lives; for others it may be situational. Few illnesses or drugs are associated with PE. All three disorders cause clear distress or interpersonal problems and are associated with poor body image, self-esteem or relationship problems.

Prevalence

FOD is probably the most frequent sexual disorder among females. In general population samples, 15.4 percent of pre-menopausal women report the disorder, and 34.7 percent of postmenopausal women do so. More single than married women report that they have never had an orgasm. There is no association between FOD and race, socioeconomic status, education or religion. MOD is relatively rare; only 3 percent to 8 percent of men seeking treatment report having the disorder, though there is a higher prevalence among homosexual males (10 percent to 15 percent). PE is very common: 16 percent to 24 percent of adult males in Canada report having this problem.

Treatment Options

Diagnosis of orgasmic disorders is usually based on a psychological and medical history and physical examination to rule out other medical problems that might be causing the symptoms.

Psychotherapeutic treatments for orgasmic disorders are similar to those for sexual desire and sexual arousal disorders. In both males and females with orgasmic disorders there may be a lack of desire, performance anxiety, and fear of impregnation or disease. Therapy should take into account contextual and historical information concerning the onset and course of the problem. Cognitive-behavioural methods to help change the assumptions and thinking of the person have sometimes been helpful.

Drug therapy for premature ejaculation may include selective serotonin reuptake inhibitors (SSRIs) such as Zoloft and Prozac. Drug therapy for female orgasmic disorder is under investigation. The second round of clinical trials for a testosterone-based nasal spray called Tefina is currently underway in Canada.

Disorders Involving Pain

There are two sexual disorders involving pain. Dyspareunia is characterized by recurring or persistent pain during sexual intercourse in a male or female. Various physical factors are associated with dyspareunia, such as pelvic inflammatory disease, hymenal scarring and vulvar vestibulitis. Dyspareunia is not a clear symptom of any physical condition. In women it is often combined with depression and interpersonal conflicts. Vaginismus is characterized by a persistent or recurrent involuntary spasm of the vagina that interferes with sexual intercourse. Women with vaginismus tend to avoid gynecological exams, and the disorder is most often associated with psychological and interpersonal issues. Other associated psychosocial factors include religious orthodoxy, low self-esteem, poor body image, poor couple communication and a history of sexual trauma. Both disorders cause clear distress or interpersonal problems, and may be associated with lack of desire or arousal.

Prevalence

Dyspareunia is frequent in females, affecting between 8 and 22 percent over the course of a lifetime, but occurs infrequently in males. Vaginismus is experienced by approximately 2 women of 1,000.

Treatment Options

To diagnose vaginismus and dyspareunia a physician usually performs a physical examination and pelvic examination, and sometimes orders an ultrasound to rule out other possible medical conditions that could be causing the symptoms. A medical history and sex history are also taken in order to identify possible psychological causes for the symptoms.

Probably the most successful treatment for women with these disorders is the reinsertion of a graduated sequence of dilators in the vagina. The woman's sexual partner should be present, and a participant in this treatment. This treatment should be done in conjunction with relaxation training, sensate focusing exercises (which help people focus on the pleasures of sex rather than the performance) and sex therapy.

Many people affected by sexual disorders do not seek treatment. Their lack of desire for sex is often combined with a lack of desire for sex therapy. Even with therapy, relapse is commonly reported. Treatments that have had some success are ones that challenge the cognitive assumptions and distortions of the client(s), such as that without intercourse and without both partners having an orgasm, it isn't real sex or that sex should be perfect.

Provincial Associations

QUÉBEC

Association des sexologues du Québec (ASQ)
CP 22147, Succ. Iberville, Montréal QC H1Y 3K8

Tél: 514-270-9289
www.associationdessexologues.com
www.facebook.com/144131012376823
twitter.com/Asso_Sexologues

Aperçu: *Dimension:* petite; *Envergure:* provinciale; fondée en 1978
Mission: Susciter auprès du public une meilleure connaissance de la sexologie et du rôle du sexologue, en favorisant et en maintenant les normes scientifiques et professionnelles les plus élevées dans l'exercice de la sexologie et dans la formation des sexologues
Membre de: Sex Information & Education Council of Canada; World Association of Sexology

Ordre professionnel des sexologues du Québec (OPSQ)
#300, 4126, rue St-Denis, Montréal QC H2W 2M5

Tél: 438-386-6777
Ligne sans frais: 855-386-6777
Courriel: info@opsq.org
opsq.org

Aperçu: *Dimension:* petite; *Envergure:* provinciale; Organisme de réglementation
Mission: De réglementer la profession des sexologues afin de protéger le public et d'assurer la meilleure qualité de service possible est fournie
Membre(s) du bureau directeur:
Isabelle Beaulieu, Directrice générale et secrétaire de l'Ordre
isabelle.beaulieu@opsq.org

Sexually Transmitted Infections

In Canada, sexually transmitted infections (STIs) are a significant public health issue. The highest rates of STIs occur in young people between the ages of 15 and 24, and there is an upward trend in rates of chlamydia, gonorrhea and syphilis.

More than 20 STIs have been identified, the most common of which include chlamydia, gonorrhea, syphilis, human papillomavirus (HPV) and genital herpes. Two other common STIs—HIV and hepatitis B—are described in detail in separate sections of this book.

Chlamydia

Cause

Chlamydia is caused by the bacteria Chlamydia trachomatis, and is acquired through unprotected vaginal, anal or oral sex with a partner who has the infection. Pregnant women can pass the infection on to their babies when they give birth.

Symptoms

Many people with chlamydia do not have symptoms, and are unaware that they are infected. For this reason, chlamydia is often called "the silent disease." When they are apparent, symptoms usually begin about two to six weeks after infection. In women, symptoms may include vaginal discharge, lower abdominal pain, pain during intercourse, vaginal bleeding after intercourse or between periods and a burning sensation when urinating. Symptoms in men may include testicular pain, discharge from the penis and a burning sensation when urinating. For men, untreated chlamydia can lead to scarring of the urethra and even infertility. For women, untreated chlamydia can cause pelvic inflammatory disease (PID). In this condition, the sensitive pelvic reproductive organs are attacked, leading to fever and lower abdominal pain and occasionally collection of pus in a pelvic abscess. Residual scarring may lead to chronic pelvic pain, pain during intercourse, infertility and ectopic pregnancy, in which the fertilized egg implants in other pelvic structures outside the uterus. Prompt recognition and vigorous antibiotic treatment of the acute attack of PID are important.

Prevalence

In Canada, chlamydia is one of the most common bacterial STIs, affecting close to 83,000 people.

Treatment Options

Diagnosis of chlamydia is usually confirmed through a urine test or swab taken from the cervix or opening of the penis. Chlamydia is commonly treated with antibiotics. To prevent re-infection, any sexual partners of the person with chlamydia need to receive antibiotic treatment, as well.

Gonorrhea

Cause

Gonorrhea is caused by the bacteria Neisseria gonorrhea, and is acquired through unprotected vaginal, oral or anal sex with a partner who has the infection. Pregnant women can pass the infection on to their babies when they give birth.

Symptoms

Early symptoms of gonorrhea are often mild, and some people may not have any symptoms at all. When they do appear, it is usually about two to five days after infection, but sometimes symptoms can take up to a month to develop. Men may experience pain in the testicles, discharge from the penis and a burning sensation when urinating. Women may experience vaginal discharge, abdominal pain, bleeding after intercourse or between periods and a burning sensation when urinating. Gonorrhea can also infect the throat, eyes, rectum, penis or cervix. For women, untreated gonorrhea can cause pelvic inflammatory disease (PID), as in chlamydia (see above).

Prevalence

Gonorrhea is another of the most common STIs in Canada, affecting close to 13,000 people.

Treatment Options

Diagnosis of gonorrhea is usually confirmed through a urine test or swab taken from the cervix or opening of the penis. Gonorrhea is commonly treated with antibiotics. To prevent re-infection, any sexual partners of the person with gonorrhea need to receive antibiotic treatment, as well.

Syphilis

Cause

Syphilis is a bacterial infection acquired through vaginal, oral or anal sex with an infected partner. In some cases, it can be transmitted through injection drug use or broken skin. Pregnant women can pass syphilis on to their unborn babies, possibly causing birth defects, or even death.

Symptoms

Symptoms of syphilis usually appear within a few weeks or months of infection. Because it often causes a variety of symptoms, syphilis is sometimes called "the great imitator." The first sign of syphilis is commonly a sore (chancre) that doesn't heal. A body rash, hair loss and flu-like symptoms may follow. These symptoms often disappear on their own, but if syphilis is left untreated, it can damage the heart, brain and other organs, and may even result in death.

Prevalence

In Canada, about 1,400 people are infected with syphilis. Although it was rare in Canada in the 1990s, the number of cases has been on the rise since 2002.

Treatment Options

Syphilis is usually diagnosed through a blood test. The most common treatment is antibiotics (usually, penicillin injections). To prevent re-infection, any sexual partners of the person with syphilis need to receive antibiotic treatment, as well.

Human Papillomavirus (HPV)

Cause

HPV is a virus acquired through skin-to-skin contact or oral, vaginal or anal sex with an infected partner. There are a number of types of HPV that can affect different parts of the body.

Symptoms

A common symptom of HPV is genital warts. The warts may appear anywhere in the genital and rectal area, making transmission difficult to prevent with a condom. Genital warts in the male, unless quite large, are often just a cosmetic nuisance, although a wart inside the urinary passage may cause discomfort. Women with genital warts not only need to have the warts removed, but to be observed for pre-cancerous changes in the cervix. Although a small percentage of people with HPV develop cancer, most healthy people will be able to get rid of an HPV infection on their own.

Prevalence

HPV is a very common STI in Canada, particularly among teens and young adults. According to estimates, up to 75 percent of people who are sexually active will have at least one HPV infection over the course of their lives. One type of HPV causes about 70 percent of the cases of cervical cancer.

Treatment Options

The genital warts caused by HPV can often be diagnosed through observation. Sometimes a PAP test is used to check for changes in cervical cells that are characteristic of an active HPV infection. Warts are generally destroyed by application of chemicals, but doctors have also used laser beams, freezing and electrical currents to destroy them. Recurrence after treatment is common, even in the absence of re-infection. Fortunately, researchers have developed two vaccines for HPV-Gardasil (for males and females) and Cervarix (for females only)—which are very effective in protecting against certain types of HPV.

Genital Herpes

Cause

Genital herpes is a virus of the herpes family characterized by blisters (vesicles) in the genital area. It is acquired through oral, vaginal or anal sex with an infected person. Rarely, pregnant women can pass the infection to their babies while giving birth.

Symptoms

In many cases, people with genital herpes have no symptoms, and are unaware that they are infected. The appearance of the blisters is often preceded by low-grade fever and by tingling, itching or burning pain in the affected area. The first episode is often the most painful. Herpes infections are self-limited but recurrent because the virus chronically infects nerves that radiate from the spinal column. Under certain conditions, such as febrile illness and physical or emotional stress, the virus reactivates and causes another outbreak.

Prevalence

According to estimates, there are about 50,000 new cases of genital herpes in Canada every year.

Treatment Options

Genital herpes can often be diagnosed through observation of the sores. Sometimes, a swab of the sores is taken, and blood tests are ordered. Specific anti-viral therapy will shorten the duration and intensity of an attack. People with frequent recurrences can lower the risk of repeat attacks by taking a low dose of the anti-viral medication every day.

Fortunately, most STIs are curable with prompt treatment, and do not become chronic. People who suffer from these diseases over long periods almost always do so because of re-infection rather than treatment failure. Fortunately, behavioural changes in sexual practices can drastically reduce the risk of STIs. Abstinence from intercourse or having a long-term, monogamous relationship with an uninfected partner give essentially complete protection. Risk rises with multiple partners, unprotected intercourse, anonymous sex and contact with high-risk individuals, such as prostitutes. Barrier methods, notably condoms, give significant but not complete protection.

See also AIDS and Hepatitis

National Associations

Action Canada for Sexual Health & Rights
251 Bank St., 2nd Fl., Ottawa ON K2P 1X3

Tel: 613-241-4474
Toll-Free: 888-642-2725
Other Communication: Donor inquiries ext 8; Media inquiries ext 7
e-mail: info@sexualhealthandrights.ca
www.sexualhealthandrights.ca
www.facebook.com/actioncanadaSHR
twitter.com/action_canada

Merged from: Canadians for Choice; Canadian Federation for Sexual Health; Action Canada for Population
Overview: A large national charitable organization founded in 2014
Mission: To advance sexual & reproductive health & rights in Canada & abroad through Public education & awareness; Support for the delivery of programs & services in Canada.
Member of: International Planned Parenthood Federation
Chief Officer(s):
Sandeep Prasad, Executive Director
Frédérique Chabot, Health Information Officer
Publications:
• Beyond the Basics: A Sourcebook on Sexual & Reproductive Health Education
Type: Book
Profile: Resource used in schools, public health offices, & community-based health organizations

The AIDS Foundation of Canada
#505, 744 West Hastings St., Vancouver BC V6C 1A5

Tel: 604-688-7294
www.aidsfoundationofcanada.ca
Overview: A medium-sized national organization founded in 1986
Mission: To address the growing problem of HIV disease in Canada; to fund new & innovative ways of assisting infected/affected people with HIV; to support new ways to heighten awareness of HIV disease among the general population

Black Coalition for AIDS Prevention
20 Victoria St., 4th Fl., Toronto ON M5C 2N8

Tel: 416-977-9955; *Fax:* 416-977-7664
e-mail: info@black-cap.com
www.black-cap.com
www.facebook.com/blackcapto

Also Known As: Black CAP
Overview: A medium-sized national organization founded in 1987 overseen by Canadian AIDS Society
Mission: To reduce the spread of HIV infection in Black communities; To enhance the quality of life for Black people living with or affected by HIV/AIDS
Member of: Ontario AIDS Network
Chief Officer(s):
Shannon Thomas Ryan, Executive Director
    s.ryan@black-cap.com

Canadian AIDS Society (CAS) / Société canadienne du sida (SCS)
#100, 190 O'Connor St., Ottawa ON K2P 2R3

Tel: 613-230-3580; *Fax:* 613-563-4998
Toll-Free: 800-499-1986
e-mail: casinfo@cdnaids.ca
www.cdnaids.ca
www.facebook.com/aidsida
twitter.com/CDNAIDS
www.instagram.com/cdnaids

Overview: A medium-sized national charitable organization founded in 1988
Mission: To strengthen the response to HIV/AIDS across Canada; To enrich the lives of people living with HIV/AIDS
Chief Officer(s):
Greg Riehl, Chair
    gregr@cdnaids.ca
Michael Sangster, Vice-Chair
    mikes@cdnaids.ca
Gary Lacasse, Executive Director
    gary.lacasse@cdnaids.ca
Gerry Croteau, Secretary
    gerryc@cdnaids.ca
Janet MacPhee, Treasurer
    janetm@cdnaids.ca
Janne Charbonneau, Officer, Communications
    janne.charbonneau@cdnaids.ca
Lynne Belle-Isle, Manager, National Programs
    lynne.belle-isle@cdnaids.ca
Tobias Keogh, Manager, Fundraising
    tobias.keogh@cdnaids.ca
Publications:
• Canadian AIDS Society Annual Report
Type: Yearbook; *Frequency:* Annually
Profile: Society's achievements, finances, supporters, & volunteers
• InfoCAS
Type: Newsletter; *Frequency:* Quarterly; *Price:* Free
Profile: HIV/AIDS national policy, governmental news, & activities of member groups
• InFocus
Type: Newletter; *Frequency:* Semiannually
Profile: Examination of HIV/AIDS issues, ideas, & information

Canadian AIDS Treatment Information Exchange (CATIE) / Réseau canadien d'info-traitements sida
PO Box 1104, #505, 555 Richmond St. West, Toronto ON M5V 3B1

Tel: 416-203-7122; *Fax:* 416-203-8284
Toll-Free: 800-263-1638
e-mail: info@catie.ca
www.catie.ca
www.linkedin.com/company/canadian-aids-treatment-information-exchange
www.facebook.com/CATIEInfo
twitter.com/CATIEInfo
www.youtube.com/user/catieinfo

Previous Name: Community AIDS Treatment Information Exchange
Overview: A small national charitable organization founded in 1990
Mission: To improve the health & quality of life of all people living with HIV/AIDS (PHAs) in Canada; To provide HIV/AIDS treatment information to PHAs, caregivers & AIDS service organizations who are encouraged to be active partners in achieving informed decision-making & optimal health care; To promote collaboration among affected populations
Member of: Canadian AIDS Society; Ontario AIDS Network; Ontario Hospital Association
Chief Officer(s):

John McCullagh, Chair
   jmccullagh@catie.ca
Laurie Edmiston, Executive Director
   ledmiston@catie.ca
Publications:
• The CATIE [Canadian AIDS Treatment Information Exchange] Exchange
Type: Newsletter; *Editor:* Jim Pollock
Profile: Forum on CATIE & frontline programs
• The Positive Side [a publication of the Canadian AIDS Treatment Information Exchange]
Type: Magazine; *Frequency:* s-a.; *Editor:* Debbie Koenig
Profile: A health & wellness magazine written for people living with HIV

Canadian Foundation for AIDS Research (CANFAR) / Fondation canadienne de recherche sur le SIDA

#602, 200 Wellington St. West, Toronto ON M5V 3C7
   Tel: 416-361-6281; *Fax:* 416-361-5736
   Toll-Free: 800-563-2873
   www.canfar.com
   www.facebook.com/canfar
   twitter.com/canfar
   www.youtube.com/user/CANFAR; www.flickr.com/photos/canfar
Overview: A medium-sized national charitable organization founded in 1987
Mission: To raise awareness in order to fund research into all aspects of HIV infection & AIDS
Chief Officer(s):
Christopher Bunting, President & CEO, 416-361-6281 Ext. 229
   cbunting@canfar.com
Publications:
• CANFAR [Canadian Foundation for AIDS Research] Annual Report
   Frequency: Annually
• Catalyst [a publication of the Canadian Foundation for AIDS Research]
Type: Newsletter
Profile: CANFAR's programs & fundraising events, reports on advances in HIV / AIDS, & updates on research
• Funding Leading-Edge Research: Canada's HIV/AIDS epidemic, the global HIV / AIDS crisis & CANFAR
   Author: S.E. Read, R.S. Remis, J.K. Stewart

Canadian HIV Trials Network (CTN) / Réseau canadien pour les essais VIH

#588, 1081 Burrard St., Vancouver BC V6Z 1Y6
   Tel: 604-806-8327; *Fax:* 604-806-8005
   Toll-Free: 800-661-4664
   e-mail: ctninfo@hivnet.ubc.ca
   www.hivnet.ubc.ca
   www.linkedin.com/company/2287403
   www.facebook.com/CIHR.CTN
   twitter.com/CIHR_CTN
   www.youtube.com/user/CIHRCTN
Overview: A medium-sized national organization founded in 1990
Mission: To develop treatments, vaccines & a cure for HIV disease & AIDS through the conduct of scientifically sound & ethical clinical trials
Chief Officer(s):
Aslam Anis, National Director
Marina Klein, National Co-Director
Sharon Walmsley, National Co-Director

Atlantic Region
QEII Health Sciences Centre - Victoria General Hospital, 5790 University Ave., Halifax NS B3H 1V7
   Tel: 902-473-2700

Ontario Region
University of Ottawa at Ottawa General Hospital, 501 Smyth Rd., Ottawa ON K1H 8L6

Pacific Region
St. Paul's Hospital, John Ruedy Immunodeficiency Clinic, 1081 Burrard St., Vancouver BC V6Z 1Y6

Prairie Region
Southern Alberta HIV Clinic, #3223, 1213 - 4 St. SW, Calgary AB T2R 0X7

Québec Region

Institut thoracique de Montréal, 3650, rue St-Urbain, Montréal QC H2X 2P4

Toronto & Area Office
Sunnybrook Health Science Centre, 2075 Bayview Ave., Toronto ON M4N 3M5
   Tel: 416-480-5900

Canadian HIV/AIDS Legal Network / Réseau juridique canadien VIH/sida

#600, 1240 Bay St., Toronto ON M5R 2A7
   Tel: 416-595-1666; *Fax:* 416-595-0094
   e-mail: info@aidslaw.ca
   www.aidslaw.ca
   www.facebook.com/CanadianHIVAIDSLegalNetwork
   twitter.com/aidslaw
   www.youtube.com/aidslaw
Overview: A medium-sized national charitable organization founded in 1992 overseen by Canadian AIDS Society
Mission: To promote the human rights of people living with & vulnerable to HIV/AIDS, in Canada & internationally; through research, legal & policy analysis, education, advocacy & community mobilization
Chief Officer(s):
Richard Elliot, Executive Director, 416-595-1666 Ext. 229
Janet Butler-McPhee, Director of Communications, 416-595-1666 Ext. 228
Publications:
• HIV / AIDS Policy & Law Review
Type: Journal; *Editor:* David Garmaise; *ISSN:* 1712-624X; *Price:* $75 Canada; $125 international
Profile: Analysis & summaries of current developments in HIV/AIDS-related policy and law from an international perspective
• Legal Network News
ISSN: 1488-0997

Prisoners' HIV/AIDS Support Action Network (PASAN)

526 Richmond St. East, Toronto ON M5A 1R3
   Tel: 416-920-9567; *Fax:* 416-920-4314
   Toll-Free: 866-224-9978
   www.pasan.org
Overview: A small national organization founded in 1991
Mission: Prisoners, ex-prisoners, organizations, activists & individuals working together to provide advocacy, education, & support to prisoners on HIV/AIDS, HCV & related issues
Chief Officer(s):
Glen Brown, Interim Executive Director
   glen@pasan.org

Provincial Associations

ALBERTA

Alberta Reappraising AIDS Society (ARAS)

PO Box 61037, Stn. Kensington, Calgary AB T2N 4S6
   Tel: 403-220-0129
   e-mail: aras@aras.ab.ca
   www.aras.ab.ca
Overview: A small provincial organization founded in 1999
Mission: To provide a science-based alternative information on HIV/AIDS & other infectious diseases; does not provide treatment recommendations
Chief Officer(s):
David Crowe, President, 403-289-6609, Fax: 403-206-7717
   david.crowe@aras.ab.ca
Roger Swan, Treasurer

BRITISH COLUMBIA

Options for Sexual Health (OPT)

3550 East Hastings St., Vancouver BC V5K 2A7
   Tel: 604-731-4252; *Fax:* 604-731-4698
   e-mail: info@optbc.org
   www.optionsforsexualhealth.org
   www.facebook.com/optbc
   twitter.com/optbc
Previous Name: Planned Parenthood Association of British Columbia
Overview: A medium-sized provincial charitable organization founded in 1963 overseen by Canadian Federation for Sexual Health

Mission: To promote optimal sexual health for all British Columbians by supporting reproductive choice, reducing unplanned pregnancy, & providing quality education, information & clinical services
Member of: United Way
Affliation(s): International Planned Parenthood Federation
Chief Officer(s):
Jennifer Breakspear, Executive Director
  jbreakspear@optbc.org

Positive Living BC
803 East Hastings St., Vancouver BC V6A 1R8
Tel: 604-893-2200; *Fax:* 604-893-2251
Toll-Free: 800-994-2437
e-mail: info@positivelivingbc.org
www.positivelivingbc.org
www.facebook.com/positivelivingbc
twitter.com/pozlivingbc

Previous Name: British Columbia Persons with AIDS Society
Overview: A small provincial charitable organization founded in 1986
Mission: To empower persons in British Columbia who live with HIV/AIDS
Member of: CAS; CAAN; Red Road HIV/AIDS Society; BC Health Coalition; Canadian HIV/AIDS Legal Network
Chief Officer(s):
Neil Self, Chair
Tom McAulay, Vice-Chair
Publications:
• British Columbia Persons with AIDS Society Annual Report
Type: Yearbook; *Frequency:* Annually
• British Columbia Persons with AIDS Society HIV/AIDS eNewslist
Type: Newsletter; *Frequency:* Weekly
• eScoop [a publication of Positive Living BC]
Type: Newsletter; *Frequency:* Bimonthly
• Living+ [a publication of Positive Living BC]
Type: Magazine
Profile: Current issues encountered by those infected & affected by HIV/AIDS
• Positive Living Manual
Type: Manual
Profile: Information for BCPWA members, interested individuals, PWAs, AIDS service organizations, & health care workers

MANITOBA

Sexuality Education Resource Centre Manitoba (SERC)
#200, 226 Osborne St. North, Winnipeg MB R3C 1V4
Tel: 204-982-7800; *Fax:* 204-982-7819
www.serc.mb.ca
www.facebook.com/sercmb
www.youtube.com/user/sercmbca

Previous Name: Planned Parenthood Manitoba
Overview: A medium-sized provincial organization founded in 1966 overseen by Canadian Federation for Sexual Health
Mission: To promote universal access to comprehensive, reliable information & services on sexuality & related health issues by fostering awareness, understanding, & support through education
Affliation(s): Canadian Federation for Sexual Health; International Planned Parenthood Federation
Chief Officer(s):
Holly Banner, Acting Executive Director

Brandon Office
1700 Pacific Ave., #C, Brandon MB R7A 7L9
Tel: 204-727-0417; *Fax:* 204-729-8364

NEW BRUNSWICK

AIDS New Brunswick / Sida Nouveau Brunswick
#G17, 65 Brunswick St., Fredericton NB E3B 1G5
Fax: 888-501-6301
Toll-Free: 800-561-4009
e-mail: info@aidsnb.com
www.aidsnb.com
www.linkedin.com/company/aids-nb
www.facebook.com/aidsnb
twitter.com/aidsnb
www.youtube.com/aidsnb
Overview: A small provincial charitable organization founded in 1987

Mission: To facilitate community-based responses to the issue of HIV/AIDS
Member of: Canadian AIDS Society
Affliation(s): Atlantic AIDS Network
Chief Officer(s):
Karen Tanner, President
Stephen Alexander, Executive Director, 800-561-4009 Ext. 105
  stephen@aidsnb.com

NEWFOUNDLAND AND LABRADOR

AIDS Committee of Newfoundland & Labrador (ACNL)
47 Janeway Pl., St. John's NL A1A 1R7
Tel: 709-579-8656; *Fax:* 709-579-0559
Toll-Free: 800-563-1575
www.acnl.net
www.facebook.com/AIDSCommitteeNL
twitter.com/aidscommitteenl

Previous Name: Newfoundland & Labrador AIDS Committee
Overview: A medium-sized provincial charitable organization founded in 1988 overseen by Canadian AIDS Society
Mission: To prevent new HIV infections through education; to provide support to persons living with HIV/AIDS & their families, friends & partners
Member of: Atlantic AIDS Network
Chief Officer(s):
Gerard Yetman, Executive Director

Planned Parenthood - Newfoundland & Labrador Sexual Health Centre (NLSHC)
203 Merrymeeting Rd., St. John's NL A1C 2W6
Tel: 709-579-1009; *Fax:* 709-726-2308
Toll-Free: 877-666-9847
e-mail: info@nlsexualhealthcentre.org
www.nlsexualhealthcentre.org
www.facebook.com/PlannedParenthoodNL
twitter.com/NLSexualHealth

Overview: A medium-sized provincial organization founded in 1972 overseen by Canadian Federation for Sexual Health
Mission: To promote positive sexual health attitudes & practices throughout Newfoundland & Labrador; To support & respect individual choice
Member of: Coalition Against the Sexual Exploitation of Youth
Chief Officer(s):
Angie Brake, Executive Director
Publications:
• The Messenger
Type: Newsletter; *Frequency:* Semiannually; *Price:* Free with NLSHC membership
Profile: Centre reports, informative articles. & upcoming activities

NOVA SCOTIA

AIDS Coalition of Nova Scotia (ACNS)
#200, 5516 Spring Garden Rd., Halifax NS B3J 1G6
Tel: 902-429-7922; *Fax:* 902-422-6200
Toll-Free: 800-566-2437
Other Communication: Alternate Phone: 902-425-4882
acns.ns.ca
www.facebook.com/AIDSNS
twitter.com/AIDS_NS

Previous Name: Nova Scotia PWA Coalition
Overview: A small provincial charitable organization founded in 1995 overseen by Canadian AIDS Society
Mission: To empower persons living with & affected by HIV/AIDS & those at risk through health promotion & mutual support & to reduce the spread of HIV in Nova Scotia
Member of: Canadian AIDS Society; Canadian HIV/AIDS Legal Network
Chief Officer(s):
Michelle Johnson, Coordinator, Programs, 902-425-4882 Ext. 226
  pc@acns.ns.ca

Hepatitis Outreach Society of Nova Scotia (HepNS)
PO Box 29120, RPO Halifax Shopping Centre, Dartmouth NS B2Y 1C3
Tel: 902-420-1767; *Fax:* 902-463-6725
Toll-Free: 800-521-0572
e-mail: info@hepns.ca
www.hepns.ca
www.facebook.com/114379611934070
twitter.com/HepNSca
www.youtube.com/user/HepNSca

Overview: A medium-sized provincial organization
Mission: To educate Nova Scotians about Hepatitis & its prevention;
To reduce social stigmatization & isolation; To prevent the spread of
Hepatitis
Chief Officer(s):
Carla Densmore, Executive Director
director@hepns.ca

ONTARIO

African & Caribbean Council on HIV/AIDS in Ontario (ACCHO)
20 Victoria St., 4th Fl., Toronto ON M5C 2N8
Tel: 416-977-9955; *Fax:* 416-977-7664
e-mail: administration@accho.ca
www.accho.ca
www.facebook.com/ACCHOntario
twitter.com/ACCHOntario
www.youtube.com/ACCHOntario

Overview: A medium-sized provincial organization
Mission: To provide support & resources to members of the African,
Caribbean & Black communities in Ontario who are affected by
HIV/AIDS
Chief Officer(s):
Valérie Pierre-Pierre, Director, 416-977-9955 Ext. 292
v.pierrepierre@accho.ca

Birth Control & Venereal Disease Information Centre
#403, 960 Lawrence Ave. West, Toronto ON M6A 3B5
Tel: 416-789-4541; *Fax:* 416-789-0762
e-mail: info@BirthControlVD.org
www.birthcontrolvd.org

Overview: A small provincial organization founded in 1972
Mission: To help maintain sexual health with an emphasis on
education & prevention. To provide patient-centred service in a caring,
non-judgmental manner.

HALCO
#400, 65 Wellesley St. East, Toronto ON M4Y 1G7
Tel: 416-340-7790; *Fax:* 416-340-7248
Toll-Free: 888-705-8889
e-mail: talklaw@halco.org
www.halco.org

Also Known As: HIV & AIDS Legal Clinic of Ontario
Overview: A small provincial organization founded in 1995
Mission: Community-based legal clinic that provides free legal
services to people living with HIV/AIDS in Ontario
Chief Officer(s):
Ryan Peck, Executive Director

Ontario HIV Treatment Network
#600, 1300 Yonge St., Toronto ON M4T 1X3
Tel: 416-642-6486; *Fax:* 416-640-4245
Toll-Free: 877-743-6486
e-mail: info@ohtn.on.ca
www.ohtn.on.ca
www.facebook.com/theOHTN
twitter.com/theOHTN
www.youtube.com/user/OntarioHIVTreatment

Overview: A small provincial organization
Mission: To optimize the quality of life of people living with HIV in
Ontario & to promote excellence & innovation in treatment, research,
education & prevention through a collaborative network of excellence
representing consumers, providers, researchers & other stakeholders
Chief Officer(s):
Sean Rourke, Scientific & Executive Diretor
srourke@ohtn.on.ca

PRINCE EDWARD ISLAND

AIDS PEI
161 St. Peter's Rd., Charlottetown PE C1A 5P7
Tel: 902-566-2437; *Fax:* 902-626-3400
www.aidspei.com
www.facebook.com/pages/AIDS-PEI/156237431556
twitter.com/aidspei

Overview: A small provincial charitable organization founded in 1990
overseen by Canadian AIDS Society
Mission: To provide education & support to Islanders infected or
affected by HIV/AIDS; To promote the development of greater
understanding & acceptance by the public in relation to persons
affected by HIV/AIDS
Member of: Prince Edward Island Literacy Alliance Inc.
Chief Officer(s):
Alana Leard, Executive Director
director@aidspei.com

QUÉBEC

Coalition des organismes communautaires québécois de lutte contre le sida (COCQ-SIDA)
1, rue Sherbrooke Est, Montréal QC H2X 3V8
Tél: 514-844-2477; *Téléc:* 514-844-2498
Ligne sans frais: 866-535-0481
Courriel: info@cocqsida.com
www.cocqsida.com
www.facebook.com/COCQSIDA
twitter.com/COCQSIDA

Aperçu: *Dimension:* moyenne; *Envergure:* provinciale; Organisme
sans but lucratif; fondée en 1990
Mission: Représenter les membres afin de favoriser l'émergence et le
soutien d'une action concertée dans les dossiers d'intérêt commun;
faire reconnaître l'expertise et l'apport des organismes
communautaires et non-gouvernementaux dans la lutte contre le sida.
Membre(s) du bureau directeur:
Hélène Légaré, Présidente
Ken Monteith, Directeur général
ken.monteith@cocqsida.com

Comité des personnes atteintes du VIH du Québec (CPAVIH)
#310, 2075, rue Plessis, Montréal QC H2L 2Y4
Tél: 514-521-8720; *Téléc:* 514-521-9633
Ligne sans frais: 800-927-2844
Courriel: cpavih@cpavih.qc.ca

Aperçu: *Dimension:* moyenne; *Envergure:* provinciale; Organisme
sans but lucratif; fondée en 1987
Mission: Informer les personnes vivant avec le VIH/SIDA; promouvoir
leurs droits afin d'améliorer leur qualité de vie
Membre de: Canadian AIDS Society

Groupe d'action pour la prévention de la transmission du VIH et l'éradication du Sida (GAP-VIES)
3330, rue Jarry Est, Montréal QC H1Z 2E8
Tél: 514-722-5655; *Téléc:* 514-722-0063
Courriel: gapvies@gapvies.ca
www.gapvies.ca

Nom précédent: Groupe haïtien pour la prévention du sida; Groupe
d'action pour la prévention du sida
Aperçu: *Dimension:* petite; *Envergure:* provinciale; fondée en 1987
surveillé par Canadian AIDS Society
Mission: Prévenir la transmission du VIH/sida et d'aider les personnes
atteintes du virus de l'immunodéficience humaine dans la population en
général et dans la communauté haïtienne en particulier; informer et
d'éduquer sur les implications de la maladie et les moyens de la
prévenir; accompagner les personnes atteintes ainsi que leurs proches
Membre de: Coalition des organismes communautaires québécois de
lutte contre le sida
Membre(s) du bureau directeur:
Joseph Jean-Gilles, Directeur général

Mouvement d'information et d'entraide dans la lutte contre le sida à Québec

625, av Chouinard, Québec QC G1S 3E3

Tél: 418-649-1720; *Téléc:* 418-649-1256
Courriel: miels@miels.org
www.miels.org
www.facebook.com/mielsQC

Également appelé: MIELS-Québec
Aperçu: *Dimension:* petite; *Envergure:* provinciale; fondée en 1986 surveillé par Canadian AIDS Society
Mission: Soutenir les personnes vivant avec le VIH/sida et leurs proches; prévenir la transmission du VIH; accueillir et héberger personnes vivant avec le sida
Affiliation(s): Société canadienne du sida
Membre(s) du bureau directeur:
Martin Masson, Président
Thérèse Richer, Directrice générale
  dgmiels@miels.org

Mouvement d'information, d'éducation et d'entraide dans la lutte contre le sida (MIENS)

CP 723, Chicoutimi QC G7H 5E1

Tél: 418-693-8983; *Téléc:* 418-693-0409
Ligne sans frais: 800-463-3764
Courriel: lemiens@lemiens.com
www.lemiens.com

Aperçu: *Dimension:* petite; *Envergure:* provinciale; Organisme sans but lucratif; fondée en 1988
Mission: Pour fournir des informations sur la prévention du VIH ainsi que de soutenir et d'aider les personnes infectées par le VIH et à leurs proches
Affiliation(s): Coalition des organismes québécois de lutte contre le sida

SIDALYS

3702, rue Ste-Famille, Montréal QC H2X 2L4

Tél: 514-842-4439; *Téléc:* 514-842-2284
Courriel: sidasecours@hotmail.com

Nom précédent: Centre des services sida secours du Québec
Aperçu: *Dimension:* petite; *Envergure:* provinciale surveillé par Canadian AIDS Society
Membre de: Coalition des organismes communautaires québécois de lutte contre le sida (COCQ-SIDA)

SASKATCHEWAN

Persons Living with AIDS Network of Saskatchewan Inc.

PO Box 7123, Saskatoon SK S7K 4J1

Tel: 306-373-7766; *Fax:* 306-374-7746
Toll-Free: 800-226-0944
e-mail: plwa@sasktel.net
www.aidsnetworksaskatoon.ca

Also Known As: PLWA Network of Saskatchewan
Overview: A small provincial charitable organization founded in 1987 overseen by Canadian AIDS Society
Mission: To provide & operate support & social activities for persons diagnosed with HIV disease, as well as their families, friends & partners
Member of: Saskatoon Interagency Council on STD's & AIDS; Canadian Centre for Philanthropy

YUKON TERRITORY

Blood Ties Four Directions Centre

307 Strickland St., Whitehorse YT Y1A 2J9

Tel: 867-633-2437; *Fax:* 867-633-2447
Toll-Free: 877-333-2437
e-mail: bloodties@klondiker.com
www.bloodties.ca

Previous Name: AIDS Yukon Alliance
Overview: A small provincial charitable organization founded in 1988 overseen by Canadian AIDS Society
Mission: To acts as an information & support centre; to promote public awareness of AIDS/AIDS & hepatitis C and aid in their prevention; to assist people living with HIV/AIDS & hep C.
Member of: Pacific AIDS Network
Chief Officer(s):

Patricia Bacon, Executive Director
  executivedirector@bloodties.ca

Local Associations

ALBERTA

Calgary Sexual Health Centre

#304, 301 - 14 St. NW, Calgary AB T2N 2A1

Tel: 403-283-5580; *Fax:* 403-270-3209
e-mail: generalmail@calgarysexualhealth.ca
www.calgarysexualhealth.ca
www.facebook.com/CalgarySexualHealthCentre
twitter.com/yycsexualhealth

Previous Name: Calgary Birth Control Association
Overview: A small local organization founded in 1972
Mission: To offer counselling & education services to help people consider their sexual & reproductive choices in informed & responsible ways.
Member of: Planned Parenthood Alberta; Planned Parenthood Federation of Canada
Chief Officer(s):
Pam Krause, Executive Director
  pkrause@calgarysexualhealth.ca

Central Alberta AIDS Network Society (CAANS)

Turning Point, 4611 - 50th Ave., Red Deer AB T4N 3Z9

Tel: 403-346-8858; *Fax:* 403-346-2352
Toll-Free: 877-346-8858
e-mail: info@caans.org
www.caans.org
www.facebook.com/CentralAlbertaAIDSNetwork
twitter.com@CAANSRedDeer

Overview: A small local charitable organization founded in 1988 overseen by Canadian AIDS Society
Mission: To carry out its charitable mission, which includes responsibility for HIV prevention & support, in the David Thompson Health Region, which extends from Drumheller to Drayton Valley & from Nordegg to the Saskatchewan border
Chief Officer(s):
Jennifer Vanderschaeghe, Executive Director
  jennifer@caans.org

Compass Centre for Sexual Wellness

#50, 9912 - 106 St., Edmonton AB T5K 1C5

Tel: 780-423-3737; *Fax:* 780-425-1782
e-mail: info@compasscentre.ca
www.compasscentre.ca
www.facebook.com/64347076574
twitter.com/CompassCentre

Previous Name: OPTIONS Sexual Health Association; Planned Parenthood Association of Edmonton
Overview: A small local charitable organization founded in 1964
Mission: To promote healthy sexuality for all, through education, counselling, advocacy, in partnership with the community
Member of: Canadian Federation for Sexual Health; International Planned Parenthood
Affiliation(s): Planned Parenthood Alberta

HIV Community Link (ACAA)

#110, 1603 - 10th Ave. SW, Calgary AB T3C 0J7

Tel: 403-508-2500; *Fax:* 403-263-7358
Toll-Free: 877-440-2437
www.hivcl.org
www.linkedin.com/company/aids-calgary-awareness-association
www.facebook.com/AIDSCalgary
twitter.com/hivcommlink

Also Known As: AIDS Calgary
Previous Name: AIDS Calgary Awareness Association
Overview: A small local charitable organization founded in 1983 overseen by Canadian AIDS Society
Mission: To reduce the harm associated with HIV & AIDS for all individuals & communities in the Calgary region; to provide HIV education & support; to enhance the quality of life & advocate on behalf of people living with HIV; to promote awareness & understanding of HIV issues; to work together with partners in the community to create a caring & compassionate society in the face of HIV & AIDS

Member of: Canadian AIDS Society; Alberta Community Council on HIV/AIDS; Canadian HIV/AIDS Legal Network; Calgary Coalition on HIV & AIDS
Chief Officer(s):
Leslie Hill, Executive Director

HIV Network of Edmonton Society
9702 - 111 Ave. NW, Edmonton AB T5G 0B1

Tel: 780-488-5742; *Fax:* 780-488-3735
Toll-Free: 877-388-5742
www.hivedmonton.com
www.facebook.com/home.php#!/hiv.edmonton?fref=ts
twitter.com/HIVEdmonton
www.youtube.com/user/hivedmontonvideo

Also Known As: HIV Edmonton
Previous Name: AIDS Network of Edmonton Society
Overview: A small local charitable organization founded in 1984
Mission: HIV Edmonton is a community-based, not-for-profit organization that works to reduce HIV/AIDS related stigma & discrimination. It works to educate, support & advocate on behalf of those infected & affected by HIV & related conditions.
Member of: Canadian AIDS Society; Canadian Centre for Philanthropy Canadian HIV/AIDS Legal Network; Canadian Palliative Care Association; Chamber of Commerce
Affiliation(s): Alberta Community Council on HIV
Chief Officer(s):
Ken MacDonald, Chair
Shelley Williams, Executive Director
shelley.w@hivedmonton.com

HIV North Society
9607 - 102 St., Grande Prairie AB T8V 2T8

Tel: 780-538-3388; *Fax:* 780-538-3368
www.hivnorth.org
www.facebook.com/106064926090085

Also Known As: HIV North
Previous Name: South Peace AIDS Council of Grande Prairie; Society of the South Peace AIDS Council
Overview: A small local charitable organization founded in 1987 overseen by Canadian AIDS Society
Mission: To provide outreach, education, harm reduction & support programs & services, working collaboratively with other agencies, to fight against HIV/AIDS
Member of: Alberta Community Council on HIV; Canadian AIDS Society; Canadian Society of Association Executives
Chief Officer(s):
Susan Belcourt, Executive Director
director@hivnorth.org

HIV West Yellowhead Society
PO Box 5005, 152 Athabasca Ave., Hinton AB T7V 1X3

Tel: 780-740-0066; *Fax:* 780-740-0060
Toll-Free: 877-291-8811
www.hivwestyellowhead.com

Previous Name: AIDS Jasper Society
Overview: A small local organization founded in 1988 overseen by Canadian AIDS Society
Mission: To promote healthy lifestyles & relationships & prevent the spread of HIV
Member of: Alberta Community Council on HIV
Chief Officer(s):
Lori Phillips, Executive Director
director@hivwestyellowhead.com

Lethbridge HIV Connection (LHC)
1206 - 6th Ave. South, Lethbridge AB T1J 1A4

Tel: 403-328-8186; *Fax:* 403-328-8564
e-mail: info@lethbridgehiv.com
www.lethbridgehiv.com

Previous Name: Lethbridge AIDS Connection Society
Overview: A medium-sized local charitable organization founded in 1986 overseen by Canadian AIDS Society
Mission: To support, educate, advocate & facilitate compassionate & effective community responses to HIV
Member of: Alberta Community Council on HIV; United Way of Southwestern Alberta

Living Positive
#50, 9912 - 106 St., Edmonton AB T5K 1C5

Tel: 780-424-2214
e-mail: living-positive@telus.net
www.facebook.com/LivingPoz

Previous Name: Edmonton Persons Living with HIV Society
Overview: A small local charitable organization founded in 1990 overseen by Canadian AIDS Society
Mission: To provide persons living with HIV infection nurturing, supportive environments in which to develop positive attitudes & self image
Member of: Alberta Community Council on HIV

BRITISH COLUMBIA

AIDS Vancouver (AV)
803 East Hastings St., Vancouver BC V6A 1R8
Tel: 604-893-2201; *Fax:* 604-893-2205; *Crisis Hot-Line:* 604-696-4666
e-mail: contact@aidsvancouver.org
www.aidsvancouver.org
www.facebook.com/aidsvancouver
twitter.com/AIDSVancouver

Also Known As: Vancouver AIDS Society
Overview: A small local charitable organization founded in 1983 overseen by Canadian AIDS Society
Mission: To alleviate individual & collective vulnerability to HIV & AIDS, through care, support, education, advocacy, & research
Member of: Canadian Public Health Association
Chief Officer(s):
Brian Chittock, Executive Director, 604-696-4655
brian@aidsvancouver.org

AIDS Vancouver Island (AVI)
Access Health Centre, 713 Johnson St., 3rd Fl., Victoria BC V8W 1M8
Tel: 250-384-2366; *Fax:* 250-380-9411
Toll-Free: 800-665-2437
e-mail: info@avi.org
www.avi.org
www.facebook.com/aidsvancouverisland?ref=ts
twitter.com/AIDSVanIsle

Overview: A small local charitable organization founded in 1986 overseen by Canadian AIDS Society
Mission: To serve people infected & affected by HIV & Hepatitis C on Vancouver Island & the Gulf Islands, British Columbia; To provide support & combat stigma; To prevent infection
Chief Officer(s):
Katrina Jensen, Executive Director
James Boxshall, Manager, Fund Development & Volunteer Services
Heidi Exner, Manager, Health Promotion & Community Development
George Pine, Manager, Operations
Bryson Hawkins, Director, Finance
Kristen Kvakic, Director, Programs
Publications:
• AVI [AIDS Vancouver Island] Newsletter
Type: Newsletter

Campbell River Office
1371 c. Cedar St., Campbell River BC V9W 2W6
Tel: 250-830-0787; *Fax:* 250-830-0784
Toll-Free: 877-650-8787

Chief Officer(s):
Leanne Cunningham, Contact

Courtenay/Comox Office
355 - 6th St., Courtenay BC V9N 1M2
Tel: 250-338-7400; *Fax:* 250-334-8224
Toll-Free: 877-311-7400

Chief Officer(s):
Sarah Sullivan, Contact

Nanaimo Office
#216, 55 Victoria Rd., Nanaimo BC V9R 5N9
Tel: 250-754-9111; *Fax:* 250-754-9888
e-mail: health.centre@avi.org
avihealthcentre.org

Chief Officer(s):
Dana Becker, Manager

Port Hardy Office

PO Box 52, Port Hardy BC V0N 2P0

Tel: 250-902-2238; *Fax:* 250-949-9953

Chief Officer(s):
Shane Thomas, Manager

ANKORS

West Kootenay Regional Office, 101 Baker St., Nelson BC V1L 4H1

Tel: 250-505-5506; *Fax:* 250-505-5507
e-mail: information@ankors.bc.ca
www.ankors.bc.ca
www.facebook.com/ankors.west
twitter.com/ankorswest

Also Known As: AIDS Network Kootenay Outreach & Support Society
Previous Name: AIDS Network, Outreach & Support Society
Overview: A small local charitable organization founded in 1992
Mission: To provide support, care, outreach & harm reduction services to individuals living with & affected by HIV, AIDS & HepC
Member of: Pacific AIDS Network; Kootenay Pride; Canadian Aids Society; CATIE; Canadian Treatment Action Council; Positive Living BC; Canadian HIV/AIDS Legal Network; HepC BC; Positive Women's Network; Canadian Aboriginial AIDS Network
Affiliation(s): West Kootenay Women's Association; Advocacy Centre; Nelson CARES Society; Nelson Committee on Homelessness
Chief Officer(s):
Cheryl Dowden, Executive Director
    cheryl@ankors.bc.ca

Positive Women's Network (PWN)

#614, 1033 Davie St., Vancouver BC V6E 1M7

Tel: 604-692-3000; *Fax:* 604-684-3126
Toll-Free: 866-692-3001
e-mail: pwn@pwn.bc.ca
www.pwn.bc.ca
www.facebook.com/Positivewomensnetwork
twitter.com/pwn_bc

Overview: A small local charitable organization founded in 1989 overseen by Canadian AIDS Society
Mission: Challenging HIV, Changing Women's Lives
Member of: Pacific AIDS Network; Canadian HIV/AIDS Legal Network
Chief Officer(s):
Marcie Summers, Executive Director
    marcies@pwn.bc.ca

MANITOBA

Kali-Shiva AIDS Services

646 Logan Ave., Winnipeg MB R3A 0S7

Tel: 204-783-8565; *Fax:* 204-772-7237
e-mail: kalishiv@mts.net
www.kalishiva.wix.com/shiva

Overview: A small local charitable organization founded in 1987 overseen by Canadian AIDS Society
Mission: To provide community-based support services for persons with HIV/AIDS

NEW BRUNSWICK

AIDS Moncton / SIDA Moncton

80 Weldon St., Moncton NB E1C 5V8

Tel: 506-859-9616; *Fax:* 506-855-4726
e-mail: sidaidsm@nb.aibn.com
www.sida-aidsmoncton.com
twitter.com/AIDSMoncton

Overview: A small local charitable organization founded in 1989 overseen by Canadian AIDS Society
Mission: To improve the quality of life for persons infected & affected by HIV / AIDS; To reduce HIV & other sexually transmitted infections
Chief Officer(s):
Deborah Warren, Executive Director

AIDS Saint John (ASJ)

62 Waterloo St., Saint John NB E2L 3P3

Tel: 506-652-2437; *Fax:* 506-652-2438
e-mail: info@aidssaintjohn.com
www.aidssaintjohn.com

Overview: A small local charitable organization founded in 1987
Mission: To confront HIV & AIDS through providing education, support, prevention & awareness initiatives; to create supportive social

environments to people living with & affected with HIV/AIDS; to share our resources & build partnerships to promote the collaborative development of a community-based response to AIDS locally, provincially & regionally
Chief Officer(s):
Leslie Jeffrey, President

NOVA SCOTIA

AIDS Coalition of Cape Breton (ACCB)

150 Bentinck St., Sydney NS B1P 4W4

Tel: 902-567-1766
accb.ns.ca
www.facebook.com/CB.4.harmreduction

Overview: A small local organization founded in 1991 overseen by Canadian AIDS Society
Chief Officer(s):
Christine Porter, Executive Director
    christine.porter@bellaliant.com
Frances Macleod, SANE Project Coordinator
    frances.macleod@bellaliant.com

Cape Breton Centre for Sexual Health

PO Box 1598, 150 Bentinck St., Sydney NS B1P 6R8

Tel: 902-539-5158; *Fax:* 902-539-0290
e-mail: pp.cb@eastlink.ca

Previous Name: Planned Parenthood Cape Breton
Overview: A small local organization founded in 1979
Member of: Nova Scotia Association for Sexual Health; Planned Parenthood Federation of Canada

Halifax Sexual Health Centre

#201, 6009 Quinpool Rd., Halifax NS B3K 5J7

Tel: 902-455-9656; *Fax:* 902-429-3853
www.hshc.ca
www.facebook.com/HSHCNS
twitter.com/HfxSexualHealth
www.youtube.com/HSHCTV

Previous Name: Planned Parenthood Metro Clinic
Overview: A small local charitable organization founded in 1970
Mission: To promote sexual & reproductive health within an environment that respects & supports individual choice
Member of: Canadian Federation for Sexual Health
Chief Officer(s):
Kelly Grover, Executive Director

The Northern AIDS Connection Society (NACS)

33 Pleasant St., Truro NS B2N 3R5

Tel: 902-895-0931; *Fax:* 902-895-3353
Toll-Free: 866-940-2437
e-mail: admin@nhcsociety.ca
www.nhcsociety.ca
www.facebook.com/nhcsns

Previous Name: Truro & Area Outreach Project; Pictou County AIDS Coalition
Overview: A small local organization founded in 1996 overseen by Canadian AIDS Society
Mission: To support & promote the health & well-being of individuals living with HIV & those affected by HIV; To provide prevention education within northern region of Nova Scotia
Affiliation(s): Nova Scotia AIDS Coalition
Chief Officer(s):
Albert McNutt, Director
    super@nhcsociety.ca
Dwight Griffiths, Program Coordinator
    programs@nhcsociety.ca
Publications:
• Extreme Reality [a publication of the Northern AIDS Connection Society]
Type: Newsletter; *Frequency:* Quarterly

Sexual Health Centre for Cumberland County

PO Box 661, Amherst NS B4H 4B8

Tel: 902-667-7500; *Fax:* 902-667-0585
e-mail: shccc@ns.aliantzinc.ca
www.amherstsexualhealth.ca
www.facebook.com/25778277501746

Previous Name: Cumberland County Family Planning Association

Overview: A small local organization founded in 1981
Mission: To promote informed, responsible attitudes toward healthy sexuality, & strives to reduce unwanted pregnancy & sexually transmitted diseases; to encourage parents' involvement in their children's sexuality education
Member of: Nova Scotia Association for Sexual Health; Canadian Federation for Sexual Health; United Way of Cumberland County
Affiliation(s): Planned Parenthood Federation of Canada

Sexual Health Centre Lunenburg County
48 Empire St., Bridgewater NS B4V 2L4
Tel: 902-527-2868
e-mail: lunco.ns.sexualhealth@gmail.com
www.sexualhealthlunenburg.com
www.facebook.com/shclc
twitter.com/shclc
Previous Name: Planned Parenthood Bridgewater
Overview: A small local charitable organization founded in 1988
Mission: To ensure that information & services concerning human sexuality & fertility are available; To encourage informed, responsible attitudes toward sexuality from childhood to old age
Chief Officer(s):
Jan Cressman, Co-Chair
Kendra Fevens, Co-Chair
Rhonda Haines, Officer, Finance
Jill Skinner, Secretary

ONTARIO

AIDS Action Now / Le groupe d'action sida
Toronto ON
e-mail: aidsactionnowtoronto@gmail.com
www.aidsactionnow.org
www.facebook.com/AidsActionNow
twitter.com/AIDSActionNow
vimeo.com/channels/152729
Overview: A small local organization founded in 1989 overseen by Canadian AIDS Society
Mission: To fight for improved treatment, care & support for people living with AIDS & HIV infection

AIDS Committee of Cambridge, Kitchener/Waterloo & Area (ACCKWA)
#203, 639 King St. West, Kitchener ON N2G 1C7
Tel: 519-570-3687; *Fax:* 519-570-4034
Toll-Free: 877-770-3687
www.acckwa.com
www.facebook.com/ACCKWA
twitter.com/AIDSCKW
Overview: A small local charitable organization founded in 1987
Mission: To provide support & education services for people affected by & infected with HIV/AIDS; To mobilize community to respond effectively & with compassion to individuals affected by HIV/AIDS; To advocate on behalf of people infected or affected by HIV
Member of: Canadian Public Health Association
Affiliation(s): Ontario AIDS Network; Canadian AIDS Society
Chief Officer(s):
Ruth Cameron, Executive Director
director@acckwa.com

AIDS Committee of Durham Region (ACDR)
#202, 22 King St. West, Oshawa ON L1H 1A3
Tel: 905-576-1445; *Fax:* 905-576-4610
Toll-Free: 877-361-8750
e-mail: info@aidsdurham.com
www.aidsdurham.com
www.facebook.com/AIDSDurham
twitter.com/AIDSDurham
Overview: A small local charitable organization founded in 1992 overseen by Canadian AIDS Society
Mission: To provide HIV/AIDS related services to the infected, affected & general community in the Region of Durham
Member of: Ontario AIDS Network
Affiliation(s): Interagency Coalition on AIDS & Development; Canadian AIDS Treatment Information Exchange; Canadian HIV/AIDS Legal Network; Community Networks; Community Advisory Committee; Local

Planning & Coordinating Group; Feed The Need in Durham; Affrican & Caribbean Council on HIV/AIDS in Ontario
Chief Officer(s):
Margaret McCormack, President
Adrian Betts, Executive Director, 905-576-1445 Ext. 11
director@aidsdurham.com

AIDS Committee of North Bay & Area (ACNBA) / Comité du sida de North Bay et de la région
#201, 269 Main St. West, North Bay ON P1B 2T8
Tel: 705-497-3560; *Fax:* 705-497-7850
Toll-Free: 800-387-3701
e-mail: oaacnba@gmail.com
www.aidsnorthbay.com
www.facebook.com/128216403874712
twitter.com/ACNBA
Overview: A small local organization founded in 1990 overseen by Canadian AIDS Society
Mission: To assist & support all those affected & infected by HIV/AIDS; To limit the spread of the virus through education & awareness strategies
Member of: Ontario AIDS Network
Affiliation(s): Chamber of Commerce Downtown Inprovement Area
Chief Officer(s):
Sal Renshaw, President
Stacey L. Mayhill, Ph.D., Executive Director
acnbaed@gmail.com

AIDS Committee of Ottawa (ACO) / Comité du SIDA d'Ottawa
19 Main St., Ottawa ON K1S 1A9
Tel: 613-238-5014; *Fax:* 613-238-3425
e-mail: info@aco-cso.ca
www.aco-cso.ca
www.linkedin.com/company/1098145
www.facebook.com/acocso
twitter.com/ACOttawa
Overview: A small local charitable organization founded in 1985 overseen by Canadian AIDS Society
Mission: To fight AIDS & HIV infection through advocacy, education & support services
Member of: Ontario AIDS Network
Chief Officer(s):
Khaled Salam, Executive Director, 613-238-5014 Ext. 234
ed@aco-cso.ca

AIDS Committee of Simcoe County (ACSC)
#555, 80 Bradford St., Barrie ON L4N 6S7
Tel: 705-722-6778; *Fax:* 705-722-6560
Toll-Free: 800-372-2272
www.acsc.ca
www.facebook.com/AIDSCommitteeofSimcoeCounty
twitter.com/acsc
Overview: A small local charitable organization overseen by Canadian AIDS Society
Mission: To provide support, education & advocacy to people infected & affected by HIV/AIDS in Simcoe County
Member of: The Canadian AIDS Society; The Ontario AIDS Network; The Greater Barrie Chamber of Commerce
Chief Officer(s):
Gerry L. Croteau, Executive Director
ed@acsc.ca

AIDS Committee of Toronto (ACT)
399 Church St., 4th Fl., Toronto ON M5B 2J6
Tel: 416-340-2437; *Fax:* 416-340-8224
e-mail: ask@actoronto.org
www.actoronto.org
www.facebook.com/ACToronto
twitter.com/ACToronto
www.youtube.com/user/AIDSCommitteeToronto
Overview: A medium-sized local charitable organization founded in 1983 overseen by Canadian AIDS Society
Mission: To provide health promotion, support, education & advocacy for people living with HIV/AIDS & those affected by HIV/AIDS
Member of: Ontario AIDS Network
Chief Officer(s):

John Maxwell, Executive Director, 416-340-2437 Ext. 245
  jmaxwell@actoronto.org
Winston Husbands, Director, Research, 416-340-2437 Ext. 454
Jason Patterson, Director, Development, 416-340-2437 Ext. 268
Don Phaneuf, Director, Employment Services, 416-340-2437 Ext. 262
Publications:
• Being Well: The PWA/ACT Wellness Newsletter

AIDS Committee of Windsor (ACW)
511 Pelissier St., Windsor ON N9A 4L2
Tel: 519-973-0222; *Fax:* 519-973-7389
Toll-Free: 800-265-4858
www.aidswindsor.org
www.facebook.com/aidswindsor
Overview: A small local charitable organization founded in 1985
overseen by Canadian AIDS Society
Mission: To mobilize communities to help people affected by HIV/AIDS
in the Windsor-Essex & Chatham-Kent areas through advocacy,
education & support
Member of: Ontario AIDS Network
Affiliation(s): AIDS Support Chatham Kent; Drouillard Road Clinic
Chief Officer(s):
Michael Brennan, Executive Director
  mbrennan@aidswindsor.org

  AIDS Support Chatham-Kent
  Adelaide Place, 67 Adelaide St. South, Chatham ON N7M 4R1
Tel: 519-352-2121; *Fax:* 519-351-7067
Toll-Free: 800-265-4858
  Chief Officer(s):
  Karyn O'Neil, Associate Director, Development
    koneil@aidswindsor.org

AIDS Committee of York Region
#203, 10909 Yonge St., Richmond Hill ON L4C 3E3
Tel: 905-884-0613; *Fax:* 905-884-7215
Toll-Free: 800-243-7717
e-mail: info@acyr.org
www.acyr.org
www.facebook.com/AIDSCommitteeOfYorkRegion
twitter.com/outreachacyr
Overview: A small local organization
Mission: To provide support & education; To promote access to
dignified care for people living with HIV/AIDS & those affected by
HIV/AIDS
Chief Officer(s):
Vibhuti Mehra, Executive Director

AIDS Niagara
120 Queenston St., St Catharines ON L2R 2Z3
Tel: 905-984-8684; *Fax:* 905-988-1921
Toll-Free: 800-773-9843
e-mail: info@aidsniagara.com
www.aidsniagara.com
www.facebook.com/AIDSNiagara
twitter.com/aidsniagara
Overview: A small local charitable organization founded in 1987
Mission: To improve quality of life for those infected &/or affected by
HIV/AIDS & to reduce the spread of HIV
Member of: United Way
Affiliation(s): Ontario AIDS Network; Canadian AIDS Society
Chief Officer(s):
Francis Gregotski, Chair
Glen Walker, Executive Director, 905-984-8684 Ext. 112
  gwalker@aidsniagara.com

Alliance for South Asian AIDS Prevention (ASAAP)
#315, 120 Carlton st., Toronto ON M5A 4K3
Tel: 416-599-2727; *Fax:* 416-599-6011
e-mail: info@asaap.ca
www.asaap.ca
www.facebook.com/pages/Asaap/262246160480711
twitter.com/ASAAP
www.youtube.com/user/ASAAPTV
Overview: A small local charitable organization founded in 1989
overseen by Canadian AIDS Society
Mission: To prevent the spread of HIV & to promote the health of
South Asians infected with & affected by HIV/AIDS.

Member of: Ontario AIDS Network; Council of Agencies Serving South
Asians; Interagency Coalition on AIDS & Development
Chief Officer(s):
Rupal Shah, Chair
Vihaya Chikermane, Executive Director
  ed@asaap.ca

Asian Community AIDS Services (ACAS)
#410, 260 Spadina Ave., Toronto ON M5T 2E4
Tel: 416-963-4300; *Fax:* 416-963-4371
Toll-Free: 877-630-2227
e-mail: info@acas.org
www.acas.org
www.facebook.com/AsianCommunityAIDSServices
twitter.com/ACAStoronto
www.youtube.com/user/acasorg
**Merged from: Gay Asians Toronto's Gay Asian AIDS Project;
Vietnamese AIDS Project; AIDS Alert Project**
Overview: A small local charitable organization founded in 1994
overseen by Canadian AIDS Society
Mission: To provide education, prevention & support services on
HIV/AIDS to the East & Southeast Asian communities; programs are
based on a proactive & holistic approach to HIV/AIDS & are provided in
a collaborative, empowering & non-discriminatory manner
Member of: Ontario AIDS Network
Chief Officer(s):
Giovanni Temansja, Chair
Noulmook Sutdhibhasilp, Executive Director, 416-963-4300 Ext. 227
  ed@acas.org

Bruce House
#402, 251 Bank St., Ottawa ON K2P 1X3
Tel: 613-729-0911; *Fax:* 613-729-0959
e-mail: admin@brucehouse.org
www.brucehouse.org
www.facebook.com/MoreThanAHouse
twitter.com/MoreThanAHouse
Overview: A small local charitable organization founded in 1988
overseen by Canadian AIDS Society
Mission: To provide housing, compassionate care & support in
Ottawa-Carleton for people living with HIV/AIDS, believing that
everyone has the right to live & die with dignity; to operate a 7-bed
residence staffed 24-hours a day for people who require extensive
support & 34 rent-to-income apartment units for those able to live
independently.
Member of: Ontario AIDS Network; Ontario Non-Profit Housing
Association
Affiliation(s): City of Ottawa, Province of Ontario, government of
Canada, a network of community centers & agencies, local hospitals,
physicians, social service agencies, other local charitable agencies &
organizations

Casey House Hospice Inc.
9 Huntley St., Toronto ON M4Y 2K8
Tel: 416-962-7600; *Fax:* 416-962-5147
e-mail: heart@caseyhouse.on.ca
www.caseyhouse.com
www.linkedin.com/company/casey-house-foundation
www.facebook.com/CaseyHouseTO
twitter.com/caseyhouseTO
www.youtube.com/caseyhousetv
Overview: A small local charitable organization founded in 1988
overseen by Canadian AIDS Society
Mission: To provide treatment, support & health services for people
affected by HIV/AIDS
Member of: Ontario Hospital Association; Canadian Palliative Care
Association
Affiliation(s): St. Michael's Hospital
Chief Officer(s):
Joanne Simons, Chief Executive Officer
Ann Stewart, Medical Director

Elevate NWO (ATB)
574 Memorial Ave., Thunder Bay ON P7B 3Z2

Tel: 807-345-1516; *Fax:* 807-345-2505
Toll-Free: 800-488-5840
e-mail: info@elevatenwo.org
www.elevatenwo.org
www.facebook.com/169997633037453
twitter.com/elevatenwo

Previous Name: AIDS Thunder Bay
Overview: A small local charitable organization founded in 1985
Mission: To confront HIV/AIDS infection through prevention, support, education, & advocacy
Member of: Canadian AIDS Society; Ontario AIDS Network
Chief Officer(s):
Dennis Eeles, President
Holly Gauvin, Executive Director
  hgauvin@elevatenwo.org
Publications:
• Front Line
Type: Newsletter; *Editor:* Selly Pajamaki
Profile: Contains association news & important event dates

Fife House
490 Sherburne St., 2nd Fl., Toronto ON M4X 1K9

Tel: 416-205-9888; *Fax:* 416-205-9919
www.fifehouse.org
www.facebook.com/FifeHouse
twitter.com/FifeHouse

Overview: A medium-sized local charitable organization founded in 1988 overseen by Canadian AIDS Society
Mission: To provide secure, affordable, supportive housing & support services to people living with HIV/AIDS
Member of: Ontario AIDS Network; Ontario Non-Profit Housing Association
Chief Officer(s):
Keith Hambly, Executive Director
  khambly@fifehouse.org

Hamilton AIDS Network (HAN)
#101, 140 King St. East, Hamilton ON L8N 1B2

Tel: 905-528-0854; *Fax:* 905-528-6311
Toll-Free: 866-563-0563
www.aidsnetwork.ca
www.facebook.com/TheAIDSNetwork

Previous Name: Hamilton AIDS Network for Dialogue & Support
Overview: A medium-sized local organization founded in 1986 overseen by Canadian AIDS Society
Mission: To help mobilize community-based responses to the needs created & exacerbated by the HIV epidemic in Hamilton & the surrounding community
Member of: Ontario AIDS Network; Canadian AIDS Society
Chief Officer(s):
Tim McClemont, Executive Director
  tmcclemont@aidsnetwork.ca
James Finlay, Director, Finance & Administration
  jfinlay@aidsnetwork.ca
Leanne Parsons, Director, Support & Volunteer Services
  lparsons@aidsnetwork.ca
Karyn Cooper, Director, Community Engagement
  dcep@aidsnetwork.ca

HIV/AIDS Regional Services (HARS)
844A Princess St., Kingston ON K7L 1G5

Tel: 613-545-3698; *Fax:* 613-545-9809
Toll-Free: 800-565-2209
e-mail: hars@kingston.net
www.hars.ca
www.facebook.com/harskingston

Previous Name: Kingston AIDS Project
Overview: A medium-sized local charitable organization founded in 1986
Mission: To prevent spread of Human Immunodeficiency Virus (HIV); To educate people about AIDS & HIV; To support people affected by AIDS & HIV infection
Affliation(s): Ontario AIDS Network; Canadian AIDS Society; Canadian HIV/AIDS Legal Network
Chief Officer(s):

John MacTavish, Executive Director
Amanda Girling, Coordinator, Education
  amanda@kingston.net

HIV/AIDS Resources and Community Health (ARCH)
#115, 89 Dawson Rd., Guelph ON N1H 1B1

Tel: 519-763-2255; *Fax:* 519-763-8125
Toll-Free: 800-282-4505
e-mail: education@archguelph.ca
www.archguelph.ca
www.facebook.com/archguelph?fref=ts
twitter.com/archguelph

Previous Name: AIDS Committee of Guelph & Wellington County
Overview: A small local charitable organization founded in 1989
Mission: To provide exemplary services, education & support in the area of HIV & AIDS through innovative health promotion strategies & community partnerships
Member of: Ontario AIDS Network; Canadian AIDS Society
Chief Officer(s):
Tom Hammond, Executive Director, 519-763-2255 Ext. 129
  director@archguelph.ca
Tashauna Devonshire, Coordinator, Support Services, 519-763-2255 Ext. 126
  support@archguelph.ca

John Gordon Home
596 Pall Mall St., London ON N5Y 2Z9

Tel: 519-433-3951; *Fax:* 519-433-1314
e-mail: johngordonhome@lrah.ca
www.johngordonhome.ca

Also Known As: London Regional AIDS Hospice
Overview: A small local organization founded in 1991 overseen by Canadian AIDS Society
Mission: To provide compassionate care to people with AIDS & HIV in a comforting, non-discriminatory, homeike environment; to provide medical, psychosocial, spiritual & personal support
Member of: Ontario AIDS Network; Canadian AIDS Society; Ontario Non-Profit Housing Association
Chief Officer(s):
Bruce Rankin, Executive Director
  brucerankin@lrah.ca

Maggie's: The Toronto Sex Workers Action Project
298A Gerrard St. East, 2nd Fl., Toronto ON M5A 2G7

Tel: 416-964-0150
e-mail: maggiescoord@gmail.com
www.maggiestoronto.ca
www.facebook.com/Maggiestoronto

Also Known As: Maggie's
Previous Name: Maggie's: The Toronto Prostitutes' Community Service Project; Prostitute's Safe Sex Project
Overview: A small local charitable organization founded in 1991
Mission: To provide education & support to assist sex workers in our efforts to live & work with safety & dignity
Member of: Ontario AIDS Network

PARN Your Community AIDS Resource Network (PARN)
#302, 159 King St., Peterborough ON K9J 2R8

Tel: 705-749-9110; *Fax:* 705-749-6310
Toll-Free: 800-361-2895; *TTY:* 705-749-9110
e-mail: getinformed@parn.ca
www.parn.ca
www.facebook.com/PARNStaff
twitter.com/PARN4Counties

Previous Name: Peterborough AIDS Resource Network
Overview: A small local charitable organization founded in 1987 overseen by Canadian AIDS Society
Mission: To support people HIV-infected & HIV-affected
Member of: Canadian AIDS Society; Ontario AIDS Network.
Chief Officer(s):
Kim Dolan, Executive Director
John Lyons, Chair
John Curtis, Treasurer
Publications:
• PARN News
Type: Newsletter; *Frequency:* Quarterly; *Accepts Advertising*

Profile: Thematic issues, such as Hepatitis C, testing, harm reduction, & disclosure

Peel HIV/AIDS Network
#1, 160 Traders Blvd., Mississauga ON L4Z 3K7
Tel: 905-361-0523; *Fax:* 905-361-1004
Toll-Free: 866-896-8700
www.phan.ca
www.facebook.com/PeelHIVAIDSNetwork
twitter.com/phanpeel
www.flickr.com/photos/31432883@N05/
Overview: A small local organization
Chief Officer(s):
Phillip Banks, Executive Director
  phillipb@phan.ca

Positive Youth Outreach (PYO)
399 Church St., 4th Fl., Toronto ON M5B 2J6
Tel: 416-340-8484
e-mail: pyo@actoronto.org
www.actoronto.org/home.nsf/pages/positiveyouthoutreach
Overview: A small local organization founded in 1990 overseen by Canadian AIDS Society
Mission: To provide education, support, advocacy & referral to all youth living with HIV/AIDS regardless of the mode of transmission
Member of: AIDS Committee of Toronto; Ontario AIDS Network

Regional HIV/AIDS Connection
#30, 186 King St., London ON N6A 1C7
Tel: 519-434-1601; *Fax:* 519-434-1843
Toll-Free: 866-920-1601
e-mail: info@hivaidsconnection.ca
www.hivaidsconnection.ca
www.facebook.com/189146047805897
twitter.com/_RHAC
www.youtube.com/user/AIDSLondon
Previous Name: AIDS Committee of London
Overview: A small local organization founded in 1985 overseen by Canadian AIDS Society
Mission: To bring people together in partnership to provide leadership in education, support & advocacy to meet the challenge of HIV/AIDS; To create an atmosphere of trust which enables people living with & affected by HIV/AIDS to make informed choices; To serve the counties of Perth, Huron, Lambton, Elgin, Middlesex, & Oxford.
Member of: Ontario AIDS Network
Chief Officer(s):
Brian Lester, Executive Director, 519-434-1601 Ext. 243
  blester@hivaidsconnection.ca
Mana Khami, President

Regroupement des personnes vivant avec le VIH-sida de Québec et la région
#100, 190 O'Connor St., Ottawa ON K2P 2R3
Tél: 613-230-3580; *Téléc:* 613-563-4998
Courriel: casinfo@cdnaids.ca
www.facebook.com/aidsida
twitter.com/CDNAIDS
Aperçu: *Dimension:* petite; *Envergure:* locale; fondée en 1990 surveillé par Canadian AIDS Society
Mission: Regrouper les personnes vivant avec le VIH/sida

Réseau ACCESS Network
#203, 111 Elm St., Sudbury ON P3C 1T3
Tel: 705-688-0500
Toll-Free: 800-465-2437
e-mail: aaninfo@reseauaccessnetwork.com
www.accessaidsnetwork.com
Also Known As: Réseau ACCESS Network HIV/Hepatitis Health & Social Services Services
Previous Name: AIDS Committee of Sudbury; Access AIDS Committee
Overview: A small local organization founded in 1989 overseen by Canadian AIDS Society
Mission: To serve the needs of HIV positive individuals living in Algoma, Sudbury, & Manitoulin.
Affliation(s): Canada Helps; Ontarion Aboriginal HIV/AIDS Strategy; Sudbury Action Centre for Youth; HAVEN Program

The Teresa Group
#104, 124 Merton St., Toronto ON M4S 2Z2
Tel: 416-596-7703; *Fax:* 416-596-7910
e-mail: info@teresagroup.ca
www.teresagroup.ca
www.facebook.com/120076698045376
twitter.com/TheTeresaGroup
Overview: A small local charitable organization founded in 1990 overseen by Canadian AIDS Society
Mission: Serves the needs of children & their families living with or affected by HIV/AIDS
Member of: Ontario AIDS Network; Canadian AIDS Society
Chief Officer(s):
Nicci Stein, Executive Director
Publications:
• Bye-Bye Secrets: A Book About Children Living With HIV or AIDS in their Family
Type: Book; *Number of Pages:* 36; *Price:* $14.95
Profile: The experiences of five girls, aged 8-12 years, who live with HIV/AIDS in their families.
• Early Intervention Programs for Children & Women Living with HIV & AIDS Leaflet
Type: Leaflet
Profile: Descriptions of the following: Pre-Natal, New Moms, Mom & Tots Groups, & The Formula Program
• Hopes, Wishes & Dreams: A Book of Art & Writing by Children Living with HIV/AIDS in their Family
Type: Book; *Number of Pages:* 40; *Price:* $14.95
Profile: Art, poetry & writings by children affected by HIV/AIDS
• How Do I Tell My Kids? A Disclosure Booklet About HIV/AIDS in the Family
Type: Booklet; *Number of Pages:* 48; *Price:* $5.00
Profile: A booklet for adults, designed to help with the process of telling their children that a family member has HIV.
• In Touch [a publication of The Teresa Group]
Type: Newsletter
• Programs & Services Booklet
Type: Brochure
Profile: This brochure outlines what The Teresa Group does.

Toronto PWA Foundation (TPWAF)
200 Gerrard St. East, 2nd Fl., Toronto ON M5A 2E6
Tel: 416-506-1400; *Fax:* 416-506-1404
e-mail: info@pwatoronto.org
www.pwatoronto.org
www.facebook.com/TorontoPWA
twitter.com/TPWA
Also Known As: Toronto People With AIDS Foundation
Previous Name: People with AIDS Foundation
Overview: A small local charitable organization founded in 1987 overseen by Canadian AIDS Society
Mission: To promote the health & well-being of all people living with HIV/AIDS by providing accessible, direct & practical services
Member of: Ontario AIDS Network
Chief Officer(s):
Suzanne Paddock, Interim Executive Director
  spaddock@pwatoronto.org

QUÉBEC

Bureau local d'intervention traitant du SIDA (BLITS)
#116, 59, rue Monfette, Victoriaville QC G6P 1J8
Tél: 819-758-2662; *Téléc:* 819-758-8270
Ligne sans frais: 866-758-2662
Courriel: blits@cdcbf.qc.ca
www.blits.ca
www.facebook.com/BLITSvictoriaville
Aperçu: *Dimension:* petite; *Envergure:* locale; Organisme sans but lucratif; fondée en 1989
Membre(s) du bureau directeur:
Gabrielle Bergeron, Présidente
Maryse Laroche, Directrice
  blitscoordo@cdcbf.qc.ca
Sylvie Bondon, Agente de bureau
Véronique Vanier, Agente d'éducation
  blitsprojet@cdcbf.qc.ca

Bureau régional d'action sida (Outaouais) (BRAS)
#003, 109, rue Wright, Gatineau QC J8X 2G7
Tél: 819-776-2727; *Téléc:* 819-776-2001
Ligne sans frais: 877-376-2727
Courriel: info@lebras.qc.ca
www.lebras.qc.ca
www.facebook.com/bureauregionaldactionsida
Aperçu: *Dimension:* petite; *Envergure:* locale; fondée en 1990
Mission: Développer et promouvoir des actions communautaires vizant l'amelioration de la qualité de vie de la population de l'Outaonais face au VIH/sida
Membre de: Réseau juridique canadien du VIH/Sida; Coalition des organismes communautaires québécois de lutte contre le sida; CATIE, TROCAO, CRIO
Membre(s) du bureau directeur:
Sylvain Laflamme, Directeur général
dg@lebras.qc.ca

Centre d'action sida Montréal (Femmes) (CASMF) / Centre for AIDS Services of Montréal (Women)
1750, rue Saint-André, 3e étage, Montréal QC H2L 3T8
Tél: 514-495-0990; *Téléc:* 514-495-8087
Courriel: casm@netrover.net
www.netrover.com/~casm
Aperçu: *Dimension:* petite; *Envergure:* locale
Mission: Offrir des services aux femmes affectées et infectées par le VIH/SIDA ainsi qu'aux membres de leur famille; ces actions, priorisant les besoins particuliers des femmes, ont pour but d'augmenter leur pouvoir à déterminer la qualité de leur propre vie
Membre de: Canadian AIDS Society; Fédération des femmes du Québec; Conseil des femmes de Montréal; Coalition des organismes communautaires québécois de lutte contre le sida

Centre sida amitié (CSA)
527, rue St-Georges, Saint-Jérôme QC J7Z 5B6
Tél: 450-431-7432; *Téléc:* 450-431-6536
Courriel: csa1@qc.aira.com
twitter.com/Sidaamitie
Aperçu: *Dimension:* petite; *Envergure:* locale; Organisme sans but lucratif; fondée en 1989 surveillé par Canadian AIDS Society

Hébergements de l'envol
6984, rue Fabre, Montréal QC H2E 2B2
Tél: 514-374-1614; *Téléc:* 514-593-9227
Courriel: hebergementlenvol@hotmail.com
pages.infinit.net/lenvol2/
Aperçu: *Dimension:* petite; *Envergure:* locale
Mission: Foyer collectif pour personnes en perte d'autonomie
Affiliation(s): Coalition des organismes communautaires québécois de lutte contre le sida

Intervention régionale et information sur le sida en Estrie
505, rue Wellington Sud, Sherbrooke QC J1H 5E2
Tél: 819-823-6704
www.iris-estrie.com
Également appelé: IRIS/Estrie
Aperçu: *Dimension:* petite; *Envergure:* locale; Organisme sans but lucratif; fondée en 1988
Mission: Stimuler et développer une action communautaire pour faire face à la problématique du Sida dans la région de l'Estrie; pour remplir sa mission, l'organisme a regroupé ses actions dans trois programmes spécifiques: Soutien, Prévention, Intervention
Affiliation(s): Coalition québécoise des organismes communautaires de lutte contre le sida
Membre(s) du bureau directeur:
Yannick Dallaire, Directeur général
ydallaire.irisestrie@hotmail.com

Maison Amaryllis
1462, rue Panet, Montréal QC H2L 2Z3
Tél: 514-526-3635; *Téléc:* 514-521-9209
Courriel: maison.amaryllis@sympatico.ca
Aperçu: *Dimension:* petite; *Envergure:* locale; Organisme sans but lucratif; fondée en 1990 surveillé par Canadian AIDS Society
Affiliation(s): Coalition des organismes communautaires québécois de lutte contre le sida

Maison du Parc
1287, rue Rachel Est, Montréal QC H2J 2J9
Tél: 514-523-6467; *Téléc:* 514-523-6800
Courriel: info@maisonduparc.org
www.maisonduparc.org
Aperçu: *Dimension:* petite; *Envergure:* locale; fondée en 1991 surveillé par Canadian AIDS Society
Membre de: Coalition des Organismes Communautaires Québécois-Sida

Maison Plein Coeur
1611, rue Dorion, Montréal QC H2K 4A5
Tél: 514-597-0554; *Téléc:* 514-597-2788
Courriel: infompc@maisonpleincoeur.org
www.maisonpleincoeur.org
twitter.com/mpleincoeur
Aperçu: *Dimension:* petite; *Envergure:* locale; fondée en 1991
Mission: Contribuer à prévenir le VIH-SIDA, et à promouvoir la santé chez les personnes vivant avec la maladie; offrir des services sans aucune discrimination; favoriser des services communautaires visant à stabiliser la situation des personnes présentant des troubles de santé et d'organisation; améliorer la qualité de vie de la personne en offrant un lieu de partage et d'informations
Membre de: Société canadienne du sida; Coalition des organismes communautaires québécois de lutte contre le sida; Table des Organismes Montréalais de VIH-sida; Centre d'action bénévole de Montréal; Chambre de commerce LGBT du Québec; Conseil canadien de surveillance sur l'accès aux traitements
Membre(s) du bureau directeur:
Elaine Mayrand, Présidente
Chris Lau, Directeur général, 514-597-0554 Ext. 222
chris@maisonpleincoeur.org

Projet d'Intervention auprès des mineurs-res prostitués-ées (PIAMP)
CP 907, Succ. C, 3736, ue St-Hubert, Montréal QC H2L 4V2
Tél: 514-284-1267; *Téléc:* 514-284-6808
Courriel: piamp@piamp.net
piamp.net
Aperçu: *Dimension:* petite; *Envergure:* locale; Organisme sans but lucratif
Mission: Fournit de l'aide et de soutien à la famille et les amis concernés par la prostitution.

RÉZO
CP 246, Succ. C, Montréal QC H2L 4K1
Tél: 514-521-7778; *Téléc:* 514-521-7665
www.rezosante.org
www.facebook.com/REZOsante
twitter.com/rezosante
www.youtube.com/REZOsante
Nom précédent: Action Séro Zéro
Aperçu: *Dimension:* petite; *Envergure:* locale; fondée en 1991
Mission: Développer et coordonner des activités d'éducation et de prévention du VIH-sida et des autres ITSS dans un contexte de promotion de la santé sexuelle auprès des hommes gais, bisexuels et hommes ayant des relations sexuelles avec d'autres hommes de Montréal.
Membre(s) du bureau directeur:
Robert Rousseau, Directeur général, 514-521-7778 Ext. 227
robertrousseau@rezosante.org

Sexual Health Network of Québec Inc. / Réseau de la Santé Sexuelle du Québec inc.
PO Box 22516, 5683 Monkland Ave., Montréal QC H4A 3T4
e-mail: info@shnq.ca
www.shnq.ca
www.facebook.com/shnq.rssq
Previous Name: Planned Parenthood Montréal
Overview: A small local charitable organization founded in 1964
Mission: To advance sexual health
Chief Officer(s):
Laurie Betito, President

Sidaction Mauricie
515, rue Ste-Cécile, Trois-Rivières QC G9A 1K9
Tél: 819-374-5740
Courriel: information@sidactionmauricie.ca
www.sidactionmauricie.ca
Aperçu: *Dimension:* petite; *Envergure:* locale; Organisme sans but lucratif; fondée en 1990 surveillé par Canadian AIDS Society
Mission: Offrir des programmes d'éducation et de prévention au grand public et aux clientèles à risque, en collaboration avec les organismes gouvernementaux et communautaires qui oeuvrent aussi dans le domaine du Sida, et avec les personnes séropositives; l'organisme offre aussi un service de soutien aux personnes atteintes du VIH/Sida et à leurs proches
Membre de: Coalition des organismes communautaires québécois de lutte contre le Sida
Membre(s) du bureau directeur:
Hélène Neault, Adjointe à la coordination

SASKATCHEWAN

AIDS Programs South Saskatchewan (APSS)
2911 - 5th Ave., Regina SK S4T 0L4
Tel: 306-924-8420; *Fax:* 306-525-0904
Toll-Free: 877-210-7623
e-mail: aidsprograms@sasktel.net
www.aidsprogramssouthsask.com
www.facebook.com/aidsprogramssouthsask
twitter.com/aidsprograms
Previous Name: AIDS Regina, Inc.
Overview: A small local charitable organization founded in 1985 overseen by Canadian AIDS Society
Mission: To meet the needs of people living with AIDS & HIV positive persons; To educate society about HIV & AIDS; To address issues in society which may arise as a result of HIV & AIDS
Member of: Canadian AIDS Society
Chief Officer(s):
Stephanie Milla, Executive Director

AIDS Saskatoon
PO Box 4062, Saskatoon SK S7K 4E3
Tel: 306-242-5005; *Fax:* 306-665-9976
Toll-Free: 800-667-6876
e-mail: admin@aidssaskatoon.ca
www.aidssaskatoon.ca
www.facebook.com/aidssaskatoon
Overview: A small local charitable organization founded in 1986 overseen by Canadian AIDS Society
Mission: To provide support to those affected by AIDS & HIV; to educate & inform the community; to have the community embrace the issues addressed by AIDS Saskatoon
Chief Officer(s):
Dave Moors, President
Danielle Genest, Executive Director

International Associations

Africans in Partnership Against AIDS (APAA)
526 Richmond St. East, 2nd Fl, Toronto ON M5A 1R3
Tel: 416-924-5256; *Fax:* 416-924-6575
e-mail: info@apaa.ca
www.apaa.ca
www.facebook.com/162063662030
Overview: A small international charitable organization founded in 1993 overseen by Canadian AIDS Society
Mission: To create a stable organization & community response to the impact of HIV/AIDS through capacity development, partnership, growth, & community development & involvement.
Member of: Ontario AIDS Network; Canadian AIDS Society; African Canadian Social Development Council
Chief Officer(s):
Fanta Ongoiba, Executive Director
Publications:
• Kibaru
Type: Newsletter; *Frequency:* Quarterly

International Council of AIDS Service Organizations (ICASO) / Le Conseil international des organisations de lutte contre le SIDA
#311, 120 Carlton St., Toronto ON M5A 4K2
Tel: 416-921-0018
www.icaso.org
Overview: A small international organization founded in 1990
Mission: To promote & support the work of community-based organizations around the world in the prevention of AIDS, & care & treatment for people living with HIV/AIDS, with particular emphasis on strengthening the response in communities with fewer resources; To accomplish these objectives through information sharing, advocacy & network building
Chief Officer(s):
Mary Ann Torres, Executive Director
maryannt@icaso.org
Margaret Quish, Manager, Finance
margaretq@icaso.org
Zhanna Kasperskaya, Coordinator, Program
zhannak@icaso.org

International Papillomavirus Society (IPVS)
c/o Institut Català d'Oncologia, Av. Gran Via de l'Hospitalet 199-203, L'Hospitalet de Llobregat 08908 Spain
Tel: 34-93-2607812; *Fax:* 34-93-2607787
www.ipvsoc.org
Overview: A medium-sized international organization
Mission: To facilitate research on human & animal papillomaviruses & their associated diseases; To promote the translation of research into applications & policies
Chief Officer(s):
Silvia de Sanjose, President
s.sanjose@iconcologia.net
Margaret Stanley, Vice-President
mas@mole.bio.cam.ac.uk
W. Martin Kast, Treasurer
martin.kast@med.usc.edu
Robert Burk, Secretary
robert.burk@einstein.yu.edu
Publications:
• International Papillomavirus Society Membership Directory
Type: Directory

International Society for Sexually Transmitted Diseases Research (ISSTDR)
c/o Basil Donovan, The Kirby Institute, University of New South Wales, Sidney Australia
www.isstdr.org
Overview: A medium-sized international organization founded in 1977
Mission: To promote research on sexually transmitted diseases
Chief Officer(s):
Michel Alary, Chair & President
michel.alary@uresp.ulaval.ca

International Society for the Study of Trauma & Dissociation (ISSTD)
USA
Tel: 703-610-9037; *Fax:* 703-610-0234
e-mail: info@isst-d.org
www.isst-d.org
www.facebook.com/people/Isstd-Headquarters/100000004676158
twitter.com/isstd
Overview: A medium-sized international organization
Mission: Promotes research and training in the identification and treatment of dissociative disorders and their relationship to developmental, relational, and other traumas.
Chief Officer(s):
Lynette S. Danylchuk, President, 650-773-4476
l.danylchuk@usa.net
Publications:
• Journal of Trauma & Dissociation
Type: Journal; *Editor:* Jennifer J. Freyd

National Libraries

Sex Information & Education Council of Canada (SIECCAN)
#400, 235 Danforth Ave., Toronto, ON M4K 1N2
Tel: 416-466-5304; *Fax:* 416-778-0785
www.sieccan.org

Alex McKay, Executive Director
Jocelyn Wentland, Project Manager & Research Associate

Provincial Libraries

Blood Ties Four Directions Centre
405 Ogilvie St., Whitehorse, YT Y1A 2S5
Tel: 867-633-2437; *Fax:* 867-633-2447
Toll-Free: 877-333-2437
admin@bloodties.ca
www.bloodties.ca

Patricia Bacon, Executive Director
executivedirector@bloodties.ca

Brandon Office
1700 Pacific Ave., #C, Brandon, MB R7A 7L9
Tel: 204-727-0417; *Fax:* 204-729-8364

Calgary Sexual Health Centre
#304, 301 - 14 St. NW, Calgary, AB T2N 2A1
Tel: 403-283-5580; *Fax:* 403-270-3209
generalmail@calgarysexualhealth.ca
www.calgarysexualhealth.ca
Social Media: www.youtube.com/user/CalgarySexualHealth;
twitter.com/yycsexualhealth;
www.facebook.com/CalgarySexualHealthCentre
Profile: CBCA offers non-judgmental support and information to help you make confident, well-informed decisions. Pregnancy options - abortion, adoption, parenting, birth control, sexually transmitted diseases (STD), sexual orientation. **Collection:** Canadian Government Publications; Parenting & Sex Education of Children; Contraception; Sexuality; Social Work; Women's Issues; Fiction; Poetry

Sexuality Education Resource Centre
#200, 226 Osborne St. North, Winnipeg, MB R3C 1V4
Tel: 204-982-7800; *Fax:* 204-982-7819
www.serc.mb.ca
Social Media: www.youtube.com/user/sercmbca;
www.facebook.com/sercmb

Local Hospitals & Health Centres

MANITOBA

WINNIPEG: Nine Circles Community Health Centre
Affiliated with: Winnipeg Regional Health Authority
705 Broadway, Winnipeg, MB R3G 0X2
Tel: 204-940-6000 *Fax:* 204-940-6003
Toll-Free: 888-305-8647
ninecircles@ninecircles.ca
www.ninecircles.ca
Social Media: www.facebook.com/NineCirclesCommunityHealthCentre;
twitter.com/ninecircleschc; instagram.com/ninecircleschc

Note: Non-profit centre specializing in STI/HIV prevention & care services
Michael Payne, Executive Director

QUÉBEC

QUAQTAQ: Dispensaire de Quaqtaq
General Delivery, Quaqtaq, QC J0M 1J0
Tél: 819-492-9090

Région desservi: Nunavik (région sociosanitaire)
Spécialités: Services intégrés de dépistage et de prévention des infections transmissibles sexuellement et par le sang (SIDEP)

Sickle Cell Disease

Sickle cell disease is a group of inherited blood disorders where there is a defect on the gene for hemoglobin, the oxygen-carrying element in the blood. In some circumstances, the normally disc-shaped red blood cell takes on a crescent, or sickle, shape. It then becomes lodged in small capillaries and prevents normal oxygen flow to the tissues. This oxygen deprivation can cause pain, anemia, sickle cell crises and other complications.

Cause
Children with sickle cell trait have received a copy of the sickle cell gene from only one parent. They may have deformed red blood cells, but they usually don't have symptoms. Only if a child receives a copy of the defective gene from both parents will the full-blown disease develop.

Symptoms
Although sickle cell disease affects different people in different ways, pain and anemia are common symptoms. Other symptoms may include headache, paleness, chest pain, cold hands and feet, rapid heartbeat and fatigue. During a sickle cell crisis (an attack of pain that can last from a few hours to several weeks), there may be severe pain in the back, joints, hands and feet. Severe abdominal pain and vomiting, fever and shortness of breath may also occur. Possible triggers for sickle cell crises include sudden weather changes, infections or excessive exercise. Sometimes there is no obvious cause. Possible complications associated with sickle cell disease include gallstones, vision problems, frequent infections, priapism (painful erections), strokes and kidney, liver or lung failure.

Prevalence
Sickle cell disease occurs most frequently in people of African descent, but it also affects people whose ancestors come from India, Spanish-speaking regions, Mediterranean and Middle Eastern countries. It is estimated that about 1 in 400 black babies are born with sickle cell disease in Canada.

Treatment Options
Genetic testing can be conducted to identify carriers of the sickle cell trait. Prenatal testing can also be done to detect sickle cell disease before birth. In children and adults, a physical exam and medical history may reveal symptoms that are characteristic of sickle cell disease. A blood test (hemoglobin electrophoresis) is usually used to confirm the diagnosis, and is also administered as one of the routine screening tests for newborns.

There is no cure for sickle cell disease, so therapy is aimed at preventing and treating infections, maintaining an adequate diet and fluid intake, and managing acute attacks with painkillers, oxygen, antibiotics and blood transfusion. Hydroxyurea has been shown to reduce the number of sickle cell crises, as well as the need for transfusion. In some cases, bone marrow transplantations have been used to treat (and cure) people with sickle cell disease. Research is also currently underway in gene therapy and possible new drug treatments for sickle cell disease.

In the past, death typically occurred because of overwhelming infection or from organ destruction brought about by multiple sickle cell crises. Modern therapy has improved life expectancy dramatically for people with sickle cell disease, but some level of disability is common.

National Associations

Canadian Society of Cytology (CSC) / Société canadienne de cytologie
c/o Canadian Association of Pathologists, #310, 4 Cataraqui St., Kingston ON K7K 1Z7
Tel: 613-507-8528; *Fax:* 866-531-0626
www.cap-acp.org/cytology.php
Previous Name: Canadian Cytology Council
Overview: A small national charitable organization founded in 1961

Mission: To promote & support education in cytology; To maintain a high standard of practice within the discipline of cytopathology; To foster the development of cytopathology in Canada
Member of: Canadian Association of Pathologists / Association canadienne des pathologistes
Chief Officer(s):
Janine Benoit, Chair
    benoitj@shaw.ca
Publications:
• CSC [Canadian Society of Cytology] Bulletin
Type: Newsletter; *Frequency:* 3 pa

Provincial Associations
ALBERTA

Sickle Cell Foundation of Alberta
PO Box 55041, Stn. New Knottwood, 1704 Millwoods Rd. SW, Edmonton AB T6K 3N0
Tel: 780-450-4943
e-mail: scfoa@telus.ca
www.sicklecellfoundationofalberta.org
Overview: A small provincial organization
Mission: To promote awareness about sickle cell disorder in Alberta
Chief Officer(s):
Ekua Yorke, Founder & Coordinator

ONTARIO

Sickle Cell Association of Ontario (SCAO)
#205, 4610 Dufferin St., Toronto ON M3H 5S4
Tel: 416-789-2855; *Fax:* 416-789-1903
www.linkedin.com/company/2437730
www.facebook.com/SickleCellCanada
twitter.com/SCA_O
Overview: A small provincial charitable organization founded in 1981
Mission: To serve the community as a recognized voluntary agency that endeavors to optimize the quality of life for individuals & families with sickle cell disease
Chief Officer(s):
Marie Boyd, Administrative Assistant

Sjogren's Syndrome

Sjogren's syndrome (also called sicca syndrome) is an autoimmune disorder characterized by dryness of the mouth, eyes and mucous membranes. Variable enlargement of the lacrimal (tear) or salivary gland can occur. Sjogren's syndrome is divided into two forms: primary (affecting only the eyes and mouth) and secondary (generalized) and may be associated with connective tissue diseases such as rheumatoid arthritis, systemic lupus erythematosus, polymyositis or scleroderma.

Cause
The disorder has no known cause, but many researchers believe that it has a genetic basis.

Symptoms
Patients who suffer from Sjogren's syndrome often complain initially of a gritty sensation in the eyes or severe dryness of the mouth. Other symptoms include sensitivity to bright light, crusting of the eyelids and eyelashes, teeth deterioration, swollen parotid glands (located on the angles of the jaws) and fatigue. Patients may also develop kidney, skin, neurologic, pulmonary or joint problems. Up to 10 percent of people with Sjogren's may eventually develop a lymph node cancer called non-Hodgkin's B-cell lymphoma.

Prevalence
It is estimated that as many as 430,000 Canadians live with Sjogren's syndrome. Although the disorder most commonly affects women between the ages of 30 and 50, children and the elderly can also have Sjogren's.

Treatment Options
To diagnose Sjogren's, a physician conducts a physical exam and takes a medical history to get detailed information about the symptoms a person is experiencing. To confirm the diagnosis, blood tests, as well as tests to assess the presence of dry eyes or dry mouth may be ordered. Ophthalmologic tests may include the Schirmer test (a procedure where strips of filter paper are attached to the closed lower eyelid to estimate tear flow) and the Rose Bengal/Lissamine green stains and fluorescein test (a staining test where dyes are placed in the eye to see if there are any abnormal cells on the surface of the eye). Salivary gland tests to assess dry mouth may include parotid gland flow (a test to measure unstimulated saliva), salivary scintigraphy (in which the uptake of radio isotope by the salivary gland is measured after exposure to a stimulus) and sialography (an X-ray of the salivary glands). A lip biopsy (where a small piece of lip tissue is removed and analyzed to determine the presence of inflammation) may also be used to diagnose Sjogren's.

Treatment for Sjogren's is mainly symptomatic in the form of artificial tears, sipping fluids throughout the day, chewing gum and using special mouthwash. Pilocarpine may be used to stimulate saliva production. Severe cases, especially if they affect parts of the body outside of the glands, may require corticosteroid therapy. Dental caries (cavities) are a complication of dry mouth, so close dental follow-up is important.

With early diagnosis, appropriate treatment and ongoing monitoring to prevent the development of complications, the prognosis for most people with Sjogren's is an average life expectancy and quality of life.

National Associations

Association du Syndrome de Sjogren, Inc / Sjögren's Syndrome Association
#001, 3155 Hochelaga, Montréal QC H1W 1G4
Tel: 514-934-3666; *Fax:* 514-934-1241
Toll-Free: 877-934-3666
e-mail: sjogren.montreal@qc.aira.com
www.sjogrens.ca
Overview: A small national charitable organization
Mission: To work to draw the attention of medical world to Sjogren's Syndrome & the urgent need to discover a cause & cure; to provide support & education to patients & information to the medical community

International Associations

Sjogren's Syndrome Foundation Inc. (SSF)
#325, 6707 Democracy Blvd., Bethesda MD 20817 USA
Tel: 301-530-4420; *Fax:* 301-530-4415
Toll-Free: 800-475-6473
e-mail: tms@sjogrens.org
www.sjogrens.org
www.facebook.com/SjogrensSyndromeFoundation
twitter.com/MoistureSeekers
Also Known As: The Moisture Seekers
Overview: A medium-sized international charitable organization founded in 1983
Mission: To educate patients & their families about Sjogren's syndrome; to increase public & professional awareness of Sjogren's syndrome; to encourage research into new treatments & a cure; provides patients practical information & coping strategies that minimize the effects of Sjogren's syndrome; Foundation is clearing house for medication information & is the recognized national advocate for Sjogren's syndrome
Chief Officer(s):
Steven Taylor, CEO
    staylor@sjogrens.org

Skin Disorders

The skin is the largest human organ, protecting the muscles, ligaments, bones and internal organs of the body. There are more than 1,200 diseases that involve the skin, the three most common of which are acne, eczema and psoriasis.

Acne

Acne involves the sebaceous glands—glands that produce sebum, a substance that preserves the skin's natural oiliness. In acne, the glands' pores become plugged, trapping the sebum and bacteria. The visible results are pimples, whiteheads, blackheads and cysts.

Cause

There are a number of possible causes for acne flare-ups (breakouts) including cosmetics, sweating, some medications (such as anti-seizure drugs, or certain birth control pills), overwashing with strong cleansers or alcohol-based toners, and hormones (in women before the menstrual cycle).

Symptoms

Acne is seen most commonly on the face, neck, back and shoulders as small, red, tender bumps, with a corresponding blackhead or whitehead. Acne can be mild, consisting of a few lesions that are close to the surface and not inflamed; moderate, characterized by lesions that are deeper and somewhat red; or severe, marked by many red, inflamed lesions that can become pus-filled or even cystic, ranging from 1 mm to 5 mm. In some cases, acne can result in scarring of the skin.

Prevalence

Acne is probably the most common skin disorder, affecting close to 5.6 million Canadians. It can affect all age groups, but typically occurs in adolescents and young adults. In Canada, about 80 percent of people who suffer from acne are between the ages of 12 and 24.

Treatment Options

Treatment for acne starts with keeping affected areas clean. Locally applied creams include retinoic acid, benzoyl peroxide and various antibiotics. Oral antibiotics (tetracycline) are especially effective for large, deep pimples. Oral tretinoin (Accutane) is very effective, but causes birth defects and other side effects and should be used only as a last resort and in consultation with a dermatologist. Oral contraceptives are often helpful in young women. Treatment for acne scarring may include tretinoin creams, chemical or alphahydroxy acid (AHA) peels, microdermabrasion (a procedure in which the uppermost damaged layers of skin are removed), injected fillers (such as collagen injected below the surface of the skin) and laser skin resurfacing.

Eczema

Cause

Eczema is a catchall term for many diseases which involve skin inflammation in response to some irritant. The irritant may be a direct one, such as contact dermatitis from the metal in a belt buckle, or an indirect one, as in atopic dermatitis triggered by various environmental agents (inhalants) and factors (certain foods). Atopic dermatitis is frequently associated with a personal or family history of allergic disorders (hay fever, asthma).

Symptoms

Atopic dermatitis usually begins in infancy or childhood and is most commonly characterized by inflamed, itchy skin patches on the face, neck, hands, the inside of the elbows and behind the knees. Symptoms of other types of eczema may include small, itchy water blisters on the hands and soles of the feet (dyshidrotic); thick, itchy plaques on the neck, wrists, ankles, lower legs and inner thighs (lichen simplex); multiple, round plaques of inflamed, itchy skin on the hands, arms and legs (nummular); and greasy, scaly, yellowish-brown patches on the eyebrows, nose, scalp and chest (seborrheic). In some cases, eczema may result in skin infections characterized by fever and redness and tenderness, or pus-filled bumps on the affected area of skin.

Prevalence

Estimates show that as many as 17 percent of people in Canada are affected by atopic dermatitis at some point in their lives. Most commonly, children suffer from eczema; however, approximately half will grow out of the condition.

Treatment Options

Eczema treatment consists of identifying and eliminating the offending agent (if possible), and applying corticosteroid creams or nonspecific soothing and hydrating substances to the affected area. Topical calcineurin inhibitors are immunosuppressive ointments effective in reducing itch and preventing flare-ups. For severe cases of eczema, phototherapy (a procedure where the skin is exposed to specific rays of ultraviolet light) is sometimes used to relieve symptoms.

Psoriasis

Psoriasis is a chronic inflammatory skin disease characterized by scaly patches, some as small as rain drops, and others a few inches in diameter. There are a variety of forms of psoriasis including guttate, pustular, inverse and erthyrodermic. The most common type is plaque psoriasis which affects about 90 percent of patients. Psoriasis may be chronic or episodic (acting up and then going into remission until the next flare-up). Triggers for flare-ups may include infections, skin injuries, stress, cold, dry weather and certain medications (such as lithium).

Cause

The exact cause of psoriasis is unknown, but research suggests that a malfunction of the immune system, resulting in inflammation, may be involved. Family history is also a risk factor for psoriasis.

Symptoms

Symptoms of psoriasis can range from mild to severe (when 10 percent or more of the body is affected). Typical locations are the scalp, knees and elbows, but any part of the body may be affected. The patches usually develop in the same place on both sides of the body, and are extremely itchy. Compulsive scratching may further damage the skin, and sometimes the lesions may also crack and bleed. In roughly 30 percent of cases there is an associated arthritis.

Prevalence

Psoriasis usually begins in early adult life, and affects approximately one million Canadians.

Treatment Options

Milder cases of psoriasis are treated with steroid creams; tar preparations; or agents such as calcitrol, calcipotriol and tazarotene, which are applied to the skin. Oral drugs such as methotrexate, acitretine and cyclosporine are effective in more severe cases. Injectable biologic response modifiers (biologics) such as alefacept, etanercept, adalimumab, infliximab and ustekinumab are new agents now available to treat psoriasis. Light therapy, both natural and ultraviolet artificial (UV), may also be used to relieve the symptoms of psoriasis.

Although skin disorders such as acne, eczema and psoriasis do not shorten one's life or cause significant disability, they can have a profound effect on one's self-esteem, and may lead to depression, frustration, anger and social withdrawal. Appropriate treatment can greatly improve quality of life for most people with skin disorders.

National Associations

Canadian Dermatology Association (CDA) / Association canadienne de dermatologie (ACD)
#425, 1385 Bank St., Ottawa ON K1H 8N4
Tel: 613-738-1748; *Fax:* 613-738-4695
Toll-Free: 800-267-3376
e-mail: info@dermatology.ca
www.dermatology.ca
www.facebook.com/CdnDermatology
twitter.com/cdndermatology
Overview: A medium-sized national organization founded in 1925
Mission: To advance the science of medicine & surgery related to the health of the skin; To support & advance patient care; To represent dermatologists in Canada
Affliation(s): Canadian Medical Association; American Academy of Dermatology
Chief Officer(s):
Vince Bertucci, President
Chantal Courchesne, Chief Executive Officer
  ccourchesne@dermatology.ca
Robyn Hopkins, Director, Finance
  rhopkins@dermatology.ca
Nimmi Sidhu, Coordinator, Communications
  nsidhu@dermatology.ca
Publications:
• Canadian Dermatology Association eBulletin
Type: Newsletter; *Frequency:* monthly; *Price:* Free with membership in the Canadian DermatologyAssociation
Profile: CDA activities, articles of personal & professional interest, political reports, & news from regional dermatologic associations
• Journal of Cutaneous Medicine & Surgery [a publication of the Canadian Dermatology Association]
Type: Journal; *Accepts Advertising*; *Editor:* Dr. Jason Rivers; *Price:* Free withmembership in the Canadian Dermatology Association
Profile: Reviews, basic & clinical science articles, editorials, case reports, & letters to the editor

Canadian Porphyria Foundation Inc. (CPF) / La Fondation canadienne de la porphyrie
PO Box 1206, Neepawa MB R0J 1H0
Tel: 204-476-2800; *Fax:* 204-476-2800
Toll-Free: 866-476-2801
e-mail: porphyria@cpf-inc.ca
www.cpf-inc.ca
Overview: A small national charitable organization founded in 1988
Mission: Dedicated to improving the quality of life for Canadians affected by the porphyrias through programs of awareness, education, service, advocacy & research; committed to promoting public & medical professional awareness; assembling, printing & distributing up-to-date educational information to physicians, health care personnel, diagnosed patients & others affected by porphyria; offering support programs to affected individuals & their families; promoting the family social welfare of affected individuals; educating & informing physicians & others in health care about the porphyrias so that early diagnosis & proper treatment will be realized; promoting & providing financial assistance for research; committed to encouraging, supporting & serving physicians & researchers in their efforts to find more effective treatments & to increasing physician, patient & community awareness & thereby cultivating support for research
Chief Officer(s):
Lois J. Aitken, President/Executive Director
Publications:
• Canadian Porphyria Foundation National Newsletter
Type: Newsletter; *Frequency:* Semiannually
Profile: General information about porphyria

Canadian Skin Patient Alliance (CSPA)
#383, 136-2446 Bank St., Ottawa ON K1V 1A8
Tel: 613-440-4260; *Fax:* 877-294-1525
Toll-Free: 877-505-2772
e-mail: info@canadianskin.ca
www.canadianskin.ca
www.facebook.com/CanadianSkin
twitter.com/canadianskin
Overview: A large national organization founded in 2007
Mission: To educate the public about skin health & to help patients experience skin health concerns
Affliation(s): AboutFace; Alberta Society of Melanoma; Alliance Québécoise du Psoriasis; BCCNS Life Support Network; British Columbia Lymphedema Association; Canadian Alopecia Areata Foundation; Canadian Burn Survivors Community; Canadian Pemphigus & Pemphigoid Foundation; Canadian Psoriasis Network; Canadian Skin Cancer Foundation; Cutaneous Lymphoma Foundation; DEBRA Canada, Epidermolysis Bullosa; Eczema Society of Canada; Neurofibromatosis Society of Ontario; Save Your Skin; Scieroderma Association of British Columbia; Scleroderma Society of Ontario; Canadian Association of Psoriasis Patients
Chief Officer(s):
Kathryn Andrews-Clay, Executive Director
  kathrynclay@canadianskin.ca
Helen Crawford, Manager, CAPP Programs, Social Media & Governance
  helencrawford@canadianskin.ca
Publications:
• Canadian Skin Magazine
Type: Magazine; *Frequency:* 4 times a year; *Editor:* Sheri Pilon; *ISSN:* 1923-0729
Profile: The magazine publishes articles regarding skin health

Canadian Society of Plastic Surgeons (CSPS) / Société canadienne des chirurgiens plasticiens
PO Box 60192, Stn. Saint-Denis, Montréal QC H2J 4E1
Tel: 514-843-5415; *Fax:* 514-843-7005
e-mail: csps_sccp@bellnet.ca
www.plasticsurgery.ca
Overview: A medium-sized national organization founded in 1947
Mission: To represent, promote & provide leadership for the descipline of plastic surgery across Canada
Affliation(s): Canadian Medical Association
Chief Officer(s):
Peter Lennox, President
Gorman Louie, Vice-President
Bing Gan, Secretary-Treasurer
Karyn Wagner, Executive Director
Publications:
• CSPS News: The Newsletter of the Canadian Society of Plastic Surgeons
Type: Newsletter; *Frequency:* Semiannually; *Editor:* Karyn Wagner
Profile: Message from the president, meeting highlights, upcoming workshops, member news
• Plastic Surgery
Type: Journal; *Editor:* Dr. Edward Buchel

DEBRA Canada
PO Box 76035, #3, 1500 Upper Middle Rd., Oakville ON L6M 3H5
Toll-Free: 800-313-3012
Other Communication: French Phone: 866-433-0676
e-mail: debra@debracanada.org
www.debracanada.org
www.facebook.com/groups/18951212616
twitter.com/DEBRACanada
Overview: A medium-sized national charitable organization
Mission: To support patients of Epidermolysis Bullosa & their families & provide funding for the medical needs of patients
Chief Officer(s):
Tina Boileau, President
  tina@debracanada.org

Eczema Society of Canada / Société d'Eczéma du Canada

PO Box 25009, 417 The Queensway South, Keswick ON L4P 2C7

Toll-Free: 966-329-3621
www.eczemahelp.ca
www.facebook.com/EczemaSocietyofCanada
www.youtube.com/user/EczemaHelp

Previous Name: Canadian Eczema Society for Education & Research
Overview: A small national charitable organization founded in 1997
Mission: To disseminate information about eczema & its treatment to both patients, families & their doctors; To encourage & fund basic research on eczema; To increase public awareness of eczema in society in general
Chief Officer(s):
Amanda Cresswell-Melville, President-Executive Director
director@eczemahelp.ca

Psoriasis Society of Canada / Société psoriasis du Canada

National Office, PO Box 25015, Halifax NS B3M 4H4

Fax: 902-443-2073
Toll-Free: 800-656-4494
www.psoriasissociety.org

Overview: A medium-sized national charitable organization founded in 1983
Mission: To provide programs & services to people who suffer from psoriasis in Canada; to encourage formation of support groups where individual sufferers may share experiences & exchange information; to provide facts about psoriasis to medical community, general public & teaching profession; to promote & encourage research directed towards treatment & cure for psoriasis
Affiliation(s): International Federation of Psoriasis Associations
Chief Officer(s):
Judy Misner, President

Provincial Associations

BRITISH COLUMBIA

Save Your Skin Foundation

#319, 3600 Windcrest Dr., North Vancouver BC V7G 2S5

Toll-Free: 800-460-5832
www.saveyourskin.ca
www.facebook.com/SaveYourSkinFoundation
twitter.com/saveyourskinfdn
www.youtube.com/channel/UCNIKKrfOJ0Gh4SKrEqYpuRw

Overview: A small provincial organization
Mission: To provide help & support to patients with skin cancer; To raise awareness about melanoma; To raise funds for research
Chief Officer(s):
Kathy Barnard, President
kathy@saveyourskin.ca

QUÉBEC

Alliance Québécoise du Psoriasis / Quebec Psoriasis Alliance

#200, 5700 rue J.-B.-Michaud, Lévis QC G6V 0B1

Tel: 418-838-9779
e-mail: info@psoriasisquebec.org
www.facebook.com/211449008933190
twitter.com/psoriasisquebec
www.youtube.com/PsoriasisQuebec

Overview: A small provincial organization founded in 2008
Mission: Pour représenter les patients atteints de psoriasis et de sensibiliser le public sur le psoriasis

Association des dermatologistes du Québec (ADQ) / Association of Dermatologists of Québec

CP 216, Succ. Desjardins, #3000, 2, Complexe Desjardins, Montréal QC H5B 1G8

Tél: 514-350-5111; *Téléc:* 514-350-5161
www.adq.org

Aperçu: *Dimension:* moyenne; *Envergure:* provinciale; Organisme sans but lucratif; fondée en 1950 surveillé par Fédération des médecins spécialistes du Québec
Mission: Syndicat professionnel: assure la défense des intérêts économiques, professionnels et scientifiques de ses membres
Affiliation(s): Fédération des médecins spécialistes du Québec
Membre(s) du bureau directeur:

Dominique Hanna, Présidente

Local Associations

MANITOBA

Mamingwey Burn Survivor Society

#303, 83 Garry St., Winnipeg MB R3C 4J9

Tel: 204-272-0945
e-mail: info@mamingwey.ca
www.mamingwey.ca

Overview: A small local organization
Mission: To offer support to persons with burn injuries
Chief Officer(s):
Barbara-Anne Hodge, Chair

International Associations

International Confederation for Plastic Reconstructive & Aesthetic Surgery (IPRAS)

Zita Congress SA, PO Box 155, 1st km Peanias Markopoulou Ave, Peania Attica 190 02 Greece

Tel: (30) 211 100 1777; *Fax:* (30) 210 664 2216
e-mail: ipras@iprasmanagement.com
www.ipras.org
www.facebook.com/ipras.org

Overview: A large international organization founded in 1955
Mission: To promote plastic surgery both scientifically & clinically; To further education
Chief Officer(s):
Marita Eisenmann-Klein, President
Publications:
• Globalplast
Type: Newsletter; *Frequency:* Annually
• IPRAS [International Confederation for Plastic, Reconstructive & Aesthetic Surgery] Journal
Type: Journal

International League of Dermatological Societies (ILDS)

Wilan House, 4 Fitzroy Sq., London W1T 5HQ United Kingdom

Tel: 44-20-7388-6515; *Fax:* 44-20-7388-3123
e-mail: admin@ilds.org
web.ilds.org

Overview: A medium-sized international organization founded in 1888
Mission: To stimulate the cooperation of societies of dermatology and societies interested in all fields of cutaneous medicine and biology throughout the world; encourage the worldwide advancement of dermatological education, care, and sciences; promote personal and professional relations among the dermatologists of the world; represent dermatology in commisions and international health organizations; and organize a World Congress of Dermatology every five years and to sponsor additional international educational and scientific activities.
Chief Officer(s):
Joanna Groves, Executive Director
Publications:
• International League of Dermatological Societies Newsletter
Type: Newsletter

International Society for Burn Injuries (ISBI)

c/o Administrator, 2172 Hwy. 181 South, Floresville TX 781114 USA

Fax: 830-216-4101
e-mail: lizals@tgti.net
www.worldburn.org

Overview: A small international organization founded in 1965
Mission: To disseminate knowledge; to stimulate burn prevention
Chief Officer(s):
Elisabeth Greenfield McManus, Administrator, Fax: 830-947-3142
lizals@tgti.net
Richard L. Gamelli, President
rgamell@luc.edu
Nicole S. Gibran, Regional Representative, North America
burnadmn@u.washington.edu
Publications:
• Burns
Type: Journal; *Price:* Free with ISBI membership

National Psoriasis Foundation - USA
#300, 6600 SW 92nd Ave., Portland OR 97223-7195 USA
Tel: 503-244-7404; *Fax:* 503-245-0626
Toll-Free: 800-723-9166
e-mail: getinfo@psoriasis.org
www.psoriasis.org
www.facebook.com/National.Psoriasis.Foundation
twitter.com/NPF
www.youtube.com/user/PsoriasisFoundation
Overview: A medium-sized international charitable organization founded in 1968
Mission: To improve the quality of life of people who have psoriasis & psoriatic arthritis; To promote & ensure access to treatment; To support research that will lead to effective management & ultimately a cure
Member of: International Federation of Psoriasis Associations
Affiliation(s): Canadian Psoriasis Foundation
Chief Officer(s):
Randy Beranek, President & CEO

Secours aux lépreux (Canada) inc. (SLC) / Leprosy Relief (Canada) Inc. (LR)
#305, 1805, rue Sauvé ouest, Montréal QC H4N 3H4
Tél: 514-744-3199; *Téléc:* 514-744-9095
Ligne sans frais: 866-744-3199
Courriel: info@slc-lr.ca
www.slc-lr.ca
Aperçu: *Dimension:* petite; *Envergure:* internationale; Organisme sans but lucratif; fondée en 1961
Mission: Venir en aide médicalement et socialement aux personnes affectées par la lèpre.
Membre de: Federation internationale des associations de lutte contre la lèpre
Membre(s) du bureau directeur:
Paul E. Legault, Prèsident
Maryse Legault, Director
maryse.legault@slc-lr.ca
Marie Gilbert, Secretaire
Christiane Beauvois, Trèsorière

National Publications

The Chronicle of Skin & Allergy
Owned By: Chronicle Companies
#306, 555 Burnhamthorpe Rd., Toronto, ON M9C 2Y3
Tel: 416-916-2476; *Fax:* 416-352-6199
Toll-Free: 866-632-4766
health@chronicle.org
Circulation: 7,045 *Frequency:* 8 times a year
R. Allan Ryan, Editorial Director
Mitchell Shannon, Publisher

Sleep Disorders

Sleep disorders are a group of disorders characterized by extreme disruptions in normal sleeping patterns. These include narcolepsy, sleep apnea, circadian rhythm sleep disorder, nightmare disorder, sleep terror disorder and insomnia.

Narcolepsy is characterized by chronic, involuntary and irresistible sleep attacks; a person with the disorder can suddenly fall asleep at any time of the day and during nearly any activity, including driving a car. Fortunately, there is a new drug, Provigil, which helps people with narcolepsy to stay awake.

Sleep apnea is diagnosed when sleep is disrupted by an obstruction of the breathing apparatus.

Circadian rhythm sleep disorder is a disruption of normal sleep patterns leading to a mismatch between the schedule required by a person's environment and his or her sleeping patterns; for example, the individual is irresistibly sleepy when he or she is required to be awake, and awake at those times that he or she should be sleeping.

Nightmare disorder is diagnosed when there is a repeated occurrence of frightening dreams that lead to waking.

Sleep terror disorder is the repeated occurrence of sleep terrors, or abrupt awakenings from sleeping with a shriek or a cry.

Insomnia consists of the inability to sleep, with excessive daytime sleepiness, for at least one month, as evidenced by either prolonged sleep episodes or daytime sleep episodes that occur almost daily. Insomnia is the sleep disorder with the greatest prevalence, and will be the focus of the rest of the discussion.

Insomnia

Insomnia is a common problem that affects people in different ways. Some individuals have trouble falling asleep, while others can't stay asleep or find that they wake up too early. These sleep problems may only last a short time, or they may become chronic. If insomnia affects daytime performance, then it is considered a problem.

Cause

There are many causes of insomnia, the most common of which are stress, anxiety and depression. Other possible causes may include poor sleep hygiene (habits), shift work, chronic pain, other sleep disorders such as sleep apnea (a condition in which a person stops breathing periodically while sleeping) or restless leg syndrome (an uncomfortable sensation in the calf that provokes an urge to move the legs), lack of physical activity, jet lag, caffeine, nicotine and alcohol, certain medications (decongestants and some antidepressants) and medical conditions such as Alzheimer's disease, Parkinson disease and reflux. Individuals with insomnia may also have a history of light sleeping.

Symptoms

Symptoms of insomnia may include inability to fall asleep, inability to stay asleep, inability to get back to sleep after waking too early, not feeling refreshed upon waking, excessive daytime sleepiness, irritability, anxiety, difficulty focusing and headaches. In general, there are few serious complications associated with insomnia, however, interpersonal or work-related problems may arise because of lack of sleep, and accidents and injuries may result from a lack of attentiveness during waking hours. It is also possible that sleep inducing, tranquillizer, or other medications may be misused or abused by people suffering from insomnia.

Prevalence

In Canada, it is estimated that 3.3 million people aged 15 and over suffer from insomnia. Insomnia becomes more prevalent with increased age, and women are more likely than men to suffer from insomnia.

Treatment Options

A diagnosis of insomnia requires an examination by a physician to determine physical condition. Once general medical problems are ruled out, a careful sleep history will often be taken to determine if the individual has poor sleep habits or is reacting to an adverse life situation. A clinical diagnosis of insomnia is made if the following criteria are met: difficulty initiating or maintaining sleep or non-restorative sleep for at least one month; clinically significant distress or impairment in social, occupational or other important areas of functioning; difficulty sleeping that is not due to other sleep-related disorders, another general medical or psychiatric disorder or the direct physiological effects of a substance. Referrals may be made to sleep clinics, where, to determine the cause of sleep disturbances, an individual may undergo interviews, psychological tests and laboratory observation. The patient will sleep in the sleep laboratory while an overnight polysomnography is conducted. In this procedure, the person is wired to electrodes that monitor the various sleep stages. Polysomnography can also determine if the individual is suffering from sleep apnea.

The main treatments for insomnia are behavioural therapy and sleep medications. The behavioural methods used to help people with insomnia include relaxation exercises, planning a transition time for unwinding before bed, going to bed only when sleepy, getting out of bed if unable to sleep, getting up at the same time every morning, reserving the bedroom for sleeping only, avoiding daytime naps and limiting the amount of time in bed to actual sleep time. People with insomnia are also encouraged to practise good sleep habits such as avoiding stimulants and alcohol before bedtime, exercising regularly and keeping the bedroom quiet and dark.

Prescription medications may also be part of the treatment plan for insomnia. Known as hypnotics, or sleeping pills, these drugs include temazepam, Ambien, Sonata and Lunesta. Some medications are more helpful with falling asleep, and others are more helpful with staying asleep; a new formulation of Ambien has been developed in an attempt to address both. Sleep medications can lose effectiveness if taken over extended periods; use should always be supervised by a physician. Melatonin supplementation and over-the-counter medications that contain diphenhydramine may also be of some benefit in treating insomnia.

Studies suggest that 70 to 80 percent of people with insomnia find benefit in behavioural therapy alone. Many cases of insomnia will resolve with improved sleep hygiene, and treatment of pain and other remediable causes.

National Associations

Canadian Sleep Society (CSS) / Société Canadienne du Sommeil (SCS)
c/o Reut Gruber, McGill University, Douglas Institute, 6875 LaSalle Blvd., Montréal QC H4H 1R3
Fax: 877-659-0760
Toll-Free: 866-239-2176
Other Communication: media@canadiansleepsociety.ca
e-mail: info@canadiansleepsociety.ca
www.canadiansleepsociety.ca
Overview: A small national charitable organization founded in 1986
Mission: To further the advancement & understanding of sleep & its disorders through scientific study & public awareness
Chief Officer(s):
Shelly K. Weiss, President
president@canadiansleepsociety.ca

Provincial Associations

QUÉBEC

Fondation Sommeil: Association de personnes atteintes de déficiences reliées au sommeil
#380A, 1600, av de Lorimier, Montréal QC H2K 3W5
Tél: 514-522-3901
Ligne sans frais: 888-622-3901
Courriel: info@fondationsommeil.com
www.fondationsommeil.com
www.linkedin.com/company/5240224
www.facebook.com/FondationSommeilQuebec
twitter.com/FondationSom
Également appelé: Fondation Sommeil
Aperçu: *Dimension:* moyenne; *Envergure:* provinciale; Organisme sans but lucratif; fondée en 1990
Mission: Rejoindre les gens touchés par des troubles du sommeil et les appuyer dans leur démarche
Membre de: Confédération des organismes de personnes handicapées du Québec
Affliation(s): Regroupement des organismes de promotion du Montréal Métropolitain

Membre(s) du bureau directeur:
Jacques Clairoux, Directeur

International Associations

World Association of Sleep Medicine (WASM)
#109, 3270 19th St. NW, Rochester MN 55901 USA
Tel: 507-316-0084; *Fax:* 877-659-0760
e-mail: info@wasmonline.org
www.wasmonline.org
www.facebook.com/wasmf
Overview: A medium-sized international organization
Mission: To advance knowledge about sleep health throughout the world; To improve sleep health; To encourage prevention of sleep disorders; To act as a bridge between different sleep societies & cultures; To encourage standards of practice for sleep medicine
Chief Officer(s):
Luigi Ferini-Strambi, President
Publications:
• Sleep Medicine Worldwide: Sleep Health around the World
Type: Newsletter; *Editor:* Liborio Parrino; Robert Thomas

Speech Impairments

A speech impairment prevents a person from speaking in a clear or understood manner. Speech impairments can be present at birth due to developmental disorders, such as autism, Down syndrome or cerebral palsy. They can also develop as a result of an injury or an illness, such as a stroke.

Cause
There are three common speech disorders: disfluency, articulation disorder, and voice disorders.

Stuttering is considered the most serious disfluency. It is believed that developmental stuttering occurs when a child's speech and language abilities are unable to meet the child's verbal demands. Neurogenic stuttering can be caused by a stroke, head trauma or brain injury. It results in signalling problems between the brain and nerves or muscles.

Articulation disorders can be caused by problems or changes in the structure or shape of the muscles and bones used to make speech sounds. Some speech sound errors can result from a cleft palate or tooth problem. Some cases are due to damage to parts of the brain or the nerves that control how the muscles work together to create speech. Cerebral palsy is an example of this. Articulation disorders, as well as stuttering, can occur in many members of the same family and scientists are discovering the important role genetics play in speech disorders.

Voice disorders are a result of problems that arise when air passes from the lungs, through the vocal cords, and then through the throat, nose, mouth, and lips. A voice disorder may be due to several factors, including: acid from the stomach moving upward; throat cancer; cleft palate or other problems with the palate; conditions that damage the nerves that supply the muscles of the vocal cords; laryngeal webs or clefts (a birth defect in which a thin layer of tissue is between the vocal cords); and non-cancerous growths (such as polyps). It can also occur from overuse of the vocal cords from activities like screaming, constantly clearing the throat, or singing.

Symptoms
Stuttering is the repetition of sounds, words, or part of words or phrases. It can include adding interjections, such as "uh" in a sentence or adding extra letters to words. A person who stutters can become frustrated and embarrassed when trying to communicate. They may also jerk their head and blink their eyes while talking.

Articulation disorders often involve substituting one sound for another, slurring of speech, or indistinct speech. Consonants may be left off, added, changed or even substituted. These substitutes can make it very difficult for the person to be understood.

A person with a voice disorder may speak in a hoarse or raspy manner. Their voice may break in and out and the pitch can change suddenly. They may speak too loudly or too softly and can often run out of air while speaking. Voice quality can be distorted because of hypernasality, a condition in which there is excessive resonance in the nasal cavity when talking; or hyponasality, in which insufficient air comes through the nose.

Prevalence

In Canada, a speech-related disability affects about 67,000 children aged five to 14 (43.3 percent of children with disabilities). Boys are more likely to have this disability than girls (46.6 percent compared with 37.6). Intellectual disability and hearing loss make children more likely to develop speech disorders. Children with speech impairments are four times more likely to have a family history of the disorder than children without an impairment.

Approximately 360,000 or 1.5 percent of Canadians aged 15 and over reported a speech-related disability. At least 30 percent of people suffer loss of language (aphasia) after a stroke.

Treatment Options

Early diagnosis and intervention for a child with a speech impairment disorder is key to the child's success. A referral to a speech-language pathologist is recommended if any of the communication milestones are not being met. A speech-language pathologist can identify a speech impairment by listening to the person and may use a formal articulation test to record sound errors. An oral mechanism examination is also done to determine whether the muscles of the mouth are working correctly. A hearing test may also be performed by an audiologist to rule out a hearing impairment.

Milder forms of speech disorders may disappear on their own. Speech therapy may help with more severe symptoms or speech problems that do not improve. Speech therapy sessions can involve exercises such as sound or word repetitions, rhymes, conversational activities, reading and comprehension activities, puzzles, word or sentence scrambles, and reading aloud.

A physician can diagnosis a voice disorder and the underlying cause by using a laryngoscope, which provides a close look at the voice box. A stroboscopy, a tiny camera attached to a probe, can be used to provide a magnified, high-resolution image to help physicians diagnose small vocal fold scars. Typically, voice disorders are addressed with a combination of treatments, including drugs, voice therapy or surgery. In most cases, voice function can be improved or resolved with appropriate treatment.

National Associations

Canadian Stuttering Association (CSA) / Association canadienne des bègues
PO Box 69001, Stn. St. Clair Centre, Toronto ON M4T 3A1

Tel: 416-840-5169
Toll-Free: 866-840-5169
e-mail: csa-info@stutter.ca
www.stutter.ca
www.facebook.com/111972052148483
twitter.com/CSAStuttering
www.youtube.com/user/canstuttering

Previous Name: Canadian Association for People Who Stutter (CAPS)
Overview: A small national charitable organization founded in 1991
Mission: To support Canadians afflicted with the disorder of stuttering; To increase awareness of stuttering

Chief Officer(s):
Andrew Harding, National Coordinator
Publications:
• CSA [Canadian Stuttering Association] Newsletter
Type: Newsletter; *Frequency:* Quarterly
Profile: Developments in research & therapy, personal stories, news from CSA members, & CSA events

Communicative Disorders Assistant Association of Canada (CDAAC)
PO Box 55009, 1800 Sheppard Ave. East, Toronto ON M2J 3Z6

e-mail: info@cdaac.ca
www.cdaac.ca
www.linkedin.com/groups/Communicative-Disorders-Assistant-Associat ion-
www.facebook.com/106123889530114
twitter.com/CDAAC

Overview: A small national organization
Mission: To unite members of the profession & protect the character & status of the profession; To maintain & improve the qualifications & standards of the profession; to represent the members in their relationships with other associations, government, colleges, & other national & international organizations; To promote & achieve statutory regulations for members; To provide the public with information regarding our profession & membership; To provide support & share information for the mutual benefit of members

Speech-Language & Audiology Canada (SAC) / Orthophonie et Audiologie Canada (OAC)
#1000, 1 Nicholas St., Ottawa ON K1N 7B7

Tel: 613-567-9968; *Fax:* 613-567-2859
Toll-Free: 800-259-8519
e-mail: info@sac-oac.ca
www.sac-oac.ca
www.linkedin.com/groups/4226965/profile
www.facebook.com/sac.oac
twitter.com/sac_oac
www.youtube.com/channel/UCmg6LP26_eRR72hBEFfnRug

Previous Name: Canadian Association of Speech-Language Pathologists & Audiologists
Overview: A medium-sized national charitable organization founded in 1964
Mission: To support & represent the professional needs & development of speech-language pathologists & audiologists; To champion the needs of people with communication disorders
Affiliation(s): International Association of Logopedics & Phoniatrics; International Society of Audiology; International Communication Project
Chief Officer(s):
Joanne Charlebois, Chief Executive Officer, 613-567-9968 Ext. 262
joanne@sac-oac.ca
Phil Bolger, Chief Financial Officer
phil@sac-oac.ca
Jessica Bedford, Director, Communications & Marketing, 800-259-8519 Ext. 241
jessica@sac-oac.ca
Michelle Jackson, Manager, Professional Development, 800-259-8519 Ext. 244
michelle@sac-oac.ca
Publications:
• Canadian Association of Speech-Language Pathologists & Audiologists Communiqué
Type: Newsletter; *Frequency:* Quarterly; *ISSN:* 0842-1196
• The Canadian Journal of Speech-Language Pathology & Audiology (CJSLPA)
Type: Journal; *Frequency:* Quarterly; *Accepts Advertising; ISSN:* 1913-200X
• SAC [Speech-Language & Audiology Canada] Membership Directory
Type: Directory

Provincial Associations

ALBERTA

Alberta College of Speech-Language Pathologists & Audiologists (ACSLPA)
#209, 3132 Parsons Rd., Edmonton AB T6N 1L6
Tel: 780-944-1609; *Fax:* 780-408-3925
Toll-Free: 800-537-0589
e-mail: admin@acslpa.ab.ca
www.acslpa.ab.ca
Previous Name: Speech Language Hearing Association of Alberta
Overview: A small provincial licensing charitable organization founded in 1965
Mission: To provide leadership & coordination among speech-language pathologists & audiologists & the public in order to promote speech, language, & hearing health for Albertans
Affiliation(s): Canadian Association of Speech-Language Pathologists & Audiologists
Chief Officer(s):
Harpreet Chaggar, President
president@acslpa.ab.ca
Michael Neth, CEO & Registrar
registrar@acslpa.ab.ca
Leanne Kisilevich, Coordinator, Communications & Office

BRITISH COLUMBIA

British Columbia Association of People Who Stutter (BCAPS)
8582 Flowering Pl., Burnaby BC V5A 4B4
Fax: 888-301-2227
Toll-Free: 888-301-2227
e-mail: info@bcaps.ca
www.bcaps.ca
www.facebook.com/bcaps123
twitter.com/BCAPS1
Overview: A small provincial organization
Mission: To encourage & assist local support groups for people who stutter
Chief Officer(s):
Kim Block, President
Publications:
• B.C. Blockbuster
Type: Newsletter; *Frequency:* Quarterly

British Columbia Association of Speech-Language Pathologists & Audiologists (BCASLPA)
#402, 1755 Broadway West, Vancouver BC V6J 4S5
Tel: 604-420-2222; *Fax:* 604-736-5606
Toll-Free: 877-222-7572
e-mail: contact@bcaslpa.ca
www.bcaslpa.ca
www.linkedin.com/groups/4281068/profile
www.facebook.com/bcaslpa
twitter.com/bcaslpa
Overview: A small provincial charitable organization founded in 1957
Mission: To connect people with language, swallowing & hearing disorders with professionals in BC; To represent speech & hearing professionals; To provide information about disorders & treatments
Member of: Pan-Canadian Alliance of Speech-Language Pathology and Audiology Associations
Affiliation(s): Canadian Association of Speech Language Pathologists & Audiologists
Chief Officer(s):
Kate Chase, President
kate.chase@yahoo.ca
Publications:
• Vibrations [a publication of the British Columbia Association of Speech-Language Pathologists & Audiologists]
Editor: Marianne Bullied

MANITOBA

College of Audiologists and Speech-Language Pathologists of Manitoba (CASLPM) / Association des orthophonistes et des audiologistes du Manitoba
#1, 333 Vaughan St., Winnipeg MB R3B 3J9
Tel: 204-453-4539; *Fax:* 204-477-1881
e-mail: office@caslpm.ca
www.caslpm.ca
Previous Name: Manitoba Speech & Hearing Association
Overview: A small provincial licensing organization founded in 1958
Mission: To ensure that members of the association provide high quality speech-language pathology & audiology services to persons with commmunication disorders & their families
Chief Officer(s):
Caroline Wilson, Director, Professional Practice
carolinewilson@caslpm.ca
Lori McKietiuk, Registrar
lorimckietiuk@caslpm.ca
Leitta Taylor, Administrator

NEW BRUNSWICK

New Brunswick Association of Speech-Language Pathologists & Audiologists (NBASLPA) / Association des orthophonistes et des audiologistes du Nouveau-Brunswick
147 Ellerdale Ave., Moncton NB E1A 3M8
Tel: 506-858-1788; *Fax:* 506-854-0343
Toll-Free: 877-751-5511
e-mail: nbaslpa@nb.aibn.com
www.nbaslpa.ca
Previous Name: New Brunswick Speech & Hearing Association
Overview: A small provincial licensing organization founded in 1976
Mission: To represent the professions of speech language pathology & audiology including registration of members which outlines requirements for working in New Brunswick
Member of: Canadian Association of Speech-Language Pathologists & Audiologists
Chief Officer(s):
Darin Quinn, President
president.nbaslpa@gmail.com

NEWFOUNDLAND AND LABRADOR

Newfoundland & Labrador Association of Speech-Language Pathologists & Audiologists (NLASLPA)
PO Box 21212, St. John's NL A1A 5B2
e-mail: info@nlaslpa.ca
www.nlaslpa.ca
www.facebook.com/nlaslpa
twitter.com/nlaslpa
Previous Name: Newfoundland Speech & Hearing Association
Overview: A medium-sized provincial organization founded in 1979
Mission: To foster highest quality of service to the communicatively handicapped; to advance knowledge of speech-language pathology & audiology in the region
Member of: Canadian Association of Speech-Language Pathologists & Audiologists
Chief Officer(s):
Ashley Rossiter, President

NORTHWEST TERRITORIES

Association of Northwest Territories Speech Language Pathologists & Audiologists (ANTSLPA)
PO Box 982, Yellowknife NT X1A 2N7
Overview: A small provincial organization
Mission: Supports and represents the professional needs of speech-language pathologists, audiologists and supportive personnel inclusively within one organization.

NOVA SCOTIA

Nova Scotia Hearing & Speech Foundation
PO Box 120, #401, 5657 Spring Garden Rd., Halifax NS B3S 3R4
Tel: 902-492-8201
e-mail: contact@hearingandspeech.ca
www.hearingandspeech.ca
twitter.com/NSHSF
Overview: A medium-sized provincial organization founded in 1999
Mission: To provide hearing services to all Nova Scotians & speech-language services to preschool children & adults; To work with community volunteer leaders, the families & friends of those who are hearing or speech impaired, our partners in government, & the medical & academic communities; To raise funds to support critical Centres' needs
Chief Officer(s):
Gordon Moore, Chair

Speech & Hearing Association of Nova Scotia
PO Box 775, Stn. Halifax Central CRO, Halifax NS B3J 2V2
Tel: 902-423-9331
e-mail: webmaster@shans.ca
www.shans.ca
www.facebook.com/SpeechAndHearing
twitter.com/SpeechHearingNS
Overview: A medium-sized provincial charitable organization
Mission: To allow audiology & speech language pathology professionals to pursue professional development in order to benefit the public
Affiliation(s): Canadian Association of Speech-Language Pathologists & Audiologists (CASLPA)
Chief Officer(s):
Patricia Cleave, President
  president@shans.ca

ONTARIO

College of Audiologists & Speech-Language Pathologists of Ontario (CASLPO) / Ordre des audiologistes et des orthophonistes de l'Ontario (OAOO)
PO Box 71, #5060, 3080 Yonge St., Toronto ON M4N 3N1
Tel: 416-975-5347; *Fax:* 416-975-8394
Toll-Free: 800-993-9459
e-mail: caslpo@caslpo.com
www.caslpo.com
Overview: A medium-sized provincial licensing organization
Mission: To regulate the practice of the professions & govern the members; To develop, establish & maintain standards of qualification; To assure the quality of the practice of the professions; Develop & maintain a code of ethics & standards
Chief Officer(s):
Scott Whyte, President
Brian O'Riordan, Registrar, 416-975-5347 Ext. 215
  boriordan@caslpo.com

Ontario Association of Speech-Language Pathologists & Audiologists (OSLA)
410 Jarvis St., Toronto ON M4Y 2G6
Tel: 416-920-3676; *Fax:* 416-920-6214
Toll-Free: 800-718-6752
e-mail: mail@osla.on.ca
www.osla.on.ca
www.linkedin.com/groups?home=&gid=4453106
www.facebook.com/162240417157549
twitter.com/osla_ontario
Overview: A medium-sized provincial organization founded in 1958
Mission: Represents & promotes the professional interests of its members; provides a comprehensive range of services that support its professional members in their work on behalf of people with communication disorders
Chief Officer(s):
Mary Cook, Executive Director
  mcook@osla.on.ca

The Speech & Stuttering Institute
#2, 150 Duncan Mill Rd., Toronto ON M3B 3M4
Tel: 416-491-7771; *Fax:* 416-491-7215
e-mail: info@speechandstuttering.com
www.speechandstuttering.com
www.facebook.com/pages/The-Speech-Stuttering-Institute/1218324078
56560
twitter.com/SpchStutterInst
Previous Name: Speech Foundation of Ontario
Overview: A medium-sized provincial charitable organization founded in 1977
Mission: To provide treatment of & foster the development of innovative speech/language therapy programs; to support education & research in communication disorders
Chief Officer(s):
Paul L'Heureux, Chair
Robert Kroll, Executive Director

PRINCE EDWARD ISLAND

Prince Edward Island Speech & Hearing Association (PEISHA)
PO Box 20076, Charlottetown PE C1A 9E3
www.peispeechhearing.ca
Overview: A small provincial organization
Mission: To promote the study, research, discussion & dissemination of information concerning the process of human communication in speech & hearing; To encourage the development & improvement of skills in the diagnosis & treatment of human communication disorders
Member of: Canadian Association of Speech-Language Pathologists & Audiologists
Chief Officer(s):
Jennifer Bartlett-Bitar, President

QUÉBEC

Association des jeunes bègues de Québec (AJBQ)
CP 79044, Succ. Bird, Laval QC H7L 5J1
Tél: 514-388-8455
www.ajbq.qc.ca
www.linkedin.com/company/association-des-jeunes-bègues-du-québec
www.facebook.com/assjeunesbeguesquebec
twitter.com/AJBQ_1993
Aperçu: *Dimension:* petite; *Envergure:* provinciale; Organisme sans but lucratif; fondée en 1993
Mission: Contrer la méconnaissance de la société à l'égard du bégaiement; offrir du soutien aux jeunes bègues de 2 à 25 ans; promouvoir les services qui leur sont accessibles ainsi qu'à leurs parents
Membre(s) du bureau directeur:
Julie Tanguy, Présidente
Chantale Baillargeon, Directrice générale

Association des personnes intéressées à l'aphasie et à l'accident vasculaire cérébral (APIA)
#A07, 525, boul Wilfrid-Hamel, Québec QC G1M 2S8
Tél: 418-647-3684; *Téléc:* 418-647-1925
Courriel: apia-avc@bellnet.ca
www.apia-avc.org
Nom précédent: Association des personnes intéressées à l'aphasie
Aperçu: *Dimension:* petite; *Envergure:* provinciale; Organisme sans but lucratif; fondée en 1985
Mission: Répondre à toute demande d'information sur l'aphasie; sensibiliser le public à la problématique de l'aphasie; promouvoir et défendre les droits des personnes aphasiques; améliorer la qualité de vie des personnes aphasiques et de leurs proches
Membre(s) du bureau directeur:
Claude Hébert, Co-Présidente
Claudia-Lynn Pelletier, Co-Présidente

Association québécoise de la dysphasie
3958, rue Dandurand, Montréal QC H1X 1P7
Tél: 514-495-4118; *Téléc:* 514-495-8637
Ligne sans frais: 800-495-4118
Courriel: direction@dysphasie.qc.ca
www.aqea.qc.ca
Nom précédent: Association québécoise pour les enfants atteints d'audimutité

Aperçu: *Dimension:* moyenne; *Envergure:* provinciale; fondée en 1986
Mission: Regrouper les parents d'enfants dysphasiques ou atteints d'audimutité; sensibiliser la communauté à la réalité que vivent ces enfants; informer les parents de leurs droits et des divers services dont ils peuvent bénéficier; identifier leurs besoins; susciter la création de nouveaux services; colliger et encourager les recherches faites sur les dysphasies et l'audimutité
Membre(s) du bureau directeur:
Caroline Ricard, Présidente

SASKATCHEWAN

Saskatchewan Association of Speech-Language Pathologists & Audiologists (SASLPA)
#11, 2010 - 7th Ave., Regina SK S4R 1C2
Tel: 306-757-3990; *Fax:* 306-757-3986
Toll-Free: 800-757-3990
e-mail: saslpa@sasktel.net
www.saslpa.ca
twitter.com/SASLPA
Overview: A small provincial licensing organization founded in 1957
Mission: To encourage public awareness, professional development & quality service in the fields of speech-language pathology & audiology in the province
Member of: Canadian Association of Speech-Language Pathologists & Audiologists
Chief Officer(s):
Kathy Carroll, Executive Director
ed.saslpa@sasktel.net
Publications:
• Private Practice Directory [a publication of the Saskatchewan Association of Speech-Language Pathologists & Audiologists]
Type: Directory

YUKON TERRITORY

Yukon Speech-Language Pathology & Audiology Association (YSLPAA)
c/o 80 Falcon Dr., Whitehorse YT Y1A 6C7
e-mail: yslpaa@gmail.com
Overview: A small provincial organization
Mission: Supports and represents the professional needs of speech-language pathologists, audiologists and supportive personnel in the Yukon.
Chief Officer(s):
Karen Rach, President

Local Associations

ONTARIO

The Hanen Centre
#515, 1075 Bay St., Toronto ON M5S 2B1
Tel: 416-921-1073; *Fax:* 416-921-1225
Toll-Free: 877-426-3655
e-mail: info@hanen.org
www.hanen.org
www.facebook.com/thehanencentre
twitter.com/TheHanenCentre
Overview: A medium-sized local licensing charitable organization founded in 1975
Mission: To provide specialized services & resources to parents, teachers & caregivers of language delayed children; To provide training to speech-language pathologists
Affiliation(s): Canadian Association of Speech-Language Pathologists & Audiologists; American Speech & Hearing Association
Chief Officer(s):
Elaine Weitzman, Executive Director
elaine.weitzman@hanen.org

Ottawa Association of People Who Stutter (OAPWS)
Lakeside Gardens Centre, Britannia Park, 102 Greenview Ave., Ottawa ON K2B 5Z6
Tel: 613-226-7001
e-mail: admin@oapws.ca
oapws.ca
Overview: A small local organization

Mission: A local support groups for people who stutter.

QUÉBEC

Aphasie Rive-Sud
170, De Gaulle, Saint-Hubert QC J4T 1M9
Tél: 450-550-4466
Courriel: info@aphasierivesud.org
www.aphasierivesud.org
Aperçu: *Dimension:* petite; *Envergure:* locale
Mission: Pour amener les gens souffrant d'aphasie ensemble des activités sociales et pour aider à leur réhabilitation
Membre de: Regrouper les associations de personnes aphasiques de Québec
Membre(s) du bureau directeur:
Natalie Taupier, Coordonnatrice

International Associations

International Society for Augmentative & Alternative Communication (ISAAC) / Société internationale de communication non-orale
#216, 312 Dolomite St., Toronto ON M3J 2N2
Tel: 905-850-6848; *Fax:* 905-850-6852
e-mail: isaac@isaac-online.org
www.isaac-online.org
Overview: A small international charitable organization founded in 1983
Mission: To promote the best possible communication for people with complex communication needs
Chief Officer(s):
Gregor Renner, President
gregor.renner@kh-freiburg.de
Franklin Smith, Executive Director
franklin@isaac-online.org
Teraiz El-Deir, Coordinator, Membership
Publications:
• Augmentative and Alternative Communication [pub. of the International Society for Augmentative & Alternative Communication]
Type: Journal; *Frequency:* Quarterly; *Editor:* Martine Smith & Bronwyn Hemsley; *ISSN:* 0743-4618; *Price:* $98 individual; $293 corporate; $59 people who use AAC/Family; $59 retired/student
Profile: Contains scientific articles related to thefield of AAC that report on research, treatment, rehabilitation, education

Spina Bifida

Spina bifida refers to conditions which result in an incomplete closure of the spinal column during fetal development. It is the most serious of a group of disorders called neural tube defects. The severity of spina bifida ranges from mild to severe.

Spina bifida occulta is an opening in one or more vertebrae without damage to the spinal cord. This is the mildest form of spina bifida. In meningocele, the protective covering around the spinal cord (meninges) protrudes into the vertebrae, with little, if any, damage. In myelomeningocele, the most severe form of spina bifida, part of the spinal cord pushes through the back and exposes nerves and tissues.

Cause
The specific cause of spina bifida is unknown. It is most likely that a combination of environmental and genetic factors come into play. For example, women who have a folic acid deficiency or a family history of neural tube defects have a greater risk of having a child with spina bifida. Other risk factors for having a baby with spina bifida include obesity, uncontrolled diabetes, taking anti-seizure medication during pregnancy and a high core body temperature in the early weeks of pregnancy.

Symptoms
Some people with spina bifida occulta have mild symptoms, and are never even diagnosed. However, the effects of spina bifida, in its most extreme state, are serious. They can include paralysis,

loss of bowel and bladder control and hydrocephalus. Other inherited abnormalities, such as deformities of the feet, uneven hips and scoliosis, may also be present.

Prevalence

It is estimated that 120 babies are born with spina bifida every year in Canada.

Treatment Options

It is possible to screen for spina bifida in utero by using a blood test called the maternal serum alpha-fetoprotein test. High levels of a specific protein (alpha-fetoprotein) suggest a neural tube defect. Ultrasound and amniocentesis are other prenatal tests often used to diagnose spina bifida.

Babies with myelomeningocele require surgery to put the spinal cord and exposed tissue back inside the body. This procedure is usually performed within 24 to 48 hours after birth. Prenatal surgery to repair a baby's spine can also be done, but the operation does increase the risk of premature delivery. After initial surgery, treatments for spina bifida require a united effort by a team of specialists, and depend on the severity of the defects.

With proper care, many children with spina bifida live fairly normal lives. Life expectancy has greatly improved in recent years, and many people with spina bifida now live into adulthood.

See also Birth Defects

National Associations

Spina Bifida & Hydrocephalus Association of Canada (SBHAC) / Association de spina-bifida et d'hydrocephalie du Canada
#647, 167 Lombard Ave., Winnipeg MB R3B 0V3
Tel: 204-925-3650; *Fax:* 204-925-3654
Toll-Free: 800-565-9488
e-mail: info@sbhac.ca
www.sbhac.ca
www.facebook.com/167743789940812
Overview: A medium-sized national charitable organization founded in 1981
Mission: To improve the quality of life of all individuals with spina bifida &/or hydrocephalus & their families through awareness, education, advocacy & research; to reduce the incidence of neural tube defects
Member of: Canadian Coalition for Genetic Fairness
Affliation(s): International Federation for Hydrocephalus & Spina Bifida
Chief Officer(s):
Colleen Talbot, President

Provincial Associations

ALBERTA

Spina Bifida & Hydrocephalus Association of Southern Alberta (SBHASA)
PO Box 6837, Stn. D, Calgary AB T2P 2E9
www.sbhasa.ca
Previous Name: Spina Bifida Association of Southern Alberta
Overview: A small provincial charitable organization founded in 1981 overseen by Spina Bifida & Hydrocephalus Association of Canada
Mission: To raise awareness about spina bifida & hydrocephalus & to provide help to people & families who suffer from these conditions
Chief Officer(s):
Minh Ho, President
minh.ho@plainsmidstream.com

BRITISH COLUMBIA

Spina Bifida & Hydrocephalus Association of British Columbia (SBHABC)
4480 Oak St., Vancouver BC V6H 3V4
Tel: 604-878-7000; *Fax:* 604-677-6608
www.sbhabc.org

Previous Name: Lower Mainland Spina Bifida Association
Overview: A medium-sized provincial licensing charitable organization founded in 1977
Mission: To improve the quality of life of all individuals with spina bifida &/or hydrocephalus & their families, through awareness, education & research
Chief Officer(s):
Colleen Talbot, President

MANITOBA

Spina Bifida Association of Manitoba (SBAM)
#647, 167 Lombard Ave., Winnipeg MB R3B 0V3
Tel: 204-925-3653; *Fax:* 204-925-3654
manitoba.sbhac.ca
Overview: A small provincial charitable organization founded in 1965 overseen by Spina Bifida & Hydrocephalus Association of Canada
Mission: To provide resources & support to people & families suffering from spina bifida & hydrocephalus

NEW BRUNSWICK

Spina Bifida & Hydrocephalus Association of New Brunswick
1325 Mountain Rd., Moncton NB E1C 2T9
Tel: 506-857-9947
e-mail: spinabifidanb@hotmail.com
Overview: A small provincial organization overseen by Spina Bifida & Hydrocephalus Association of Canada
Mission: To improve the quality of life of those persons who have spina bifida &/or hydrocephalus; to gather information on spina bifida & hydrocephalus & to disseminate it to all interested persons & organizations; to encourage research into the causes & to advance more effective treatment & care

NOVA SCOTIA

Spina Bifida & Hydrocephalus Association of Nova Scotia (SBHANS)
PO Box 341, Coldbrook NS B4R 1B6
Tel: 902-679-1124
Toll-Free: 800-304-0450
e-mail: info@sbhans.ca
www.sbhans.ca
Overview: A small provincial charitable organization founded in 1984 overseen by Spina Bifida & Hydrocephalus Association of Canada
Mission: To eliminate spina bifida & hydrocephalus in newborns by promoting preventative measures; to help individuals with spina bifida &/or hydrocephalus to reach their full potential by promoting independence & improved quality of life

Cape Breton Chapter
20 Deanna Dr., Glace Bay NS B1A 6Y1
Tel: 902-849-4401

ONTARIO

Spina Bifida & Hydrocephalus Association of Ontario (SB&H)
PO Box 103, #1006, 555 Richmond St. West, Toronto ON M5V 3B1
Tel: 416-214-1056; *Fax:* 416-214-1446
Toll-Free: 800-387-1575
e-mail: provincial@sbhao.on.ca
www.sbhao.on.ca
www.facebook.com/SpinaBifidaHydrocephalusOntario
twitter.com/SBH_Ontario
www.youtube.com/channel/UC3psi9zf8KapVlgJ9p0f1EQ?
Overview: A medium-sized provincial charitable organization founded in 1973
Mission: To build awareness & drive education, research, support, care & advocacy to help find a cure while working to improve the quality of life of all individuals with spina bifida &/or hydrocephalus
Affliation(s): Spina Bifida & Hydrocephalus Association of Canada
Chief Officer(s):
Elaine Wilson, Executive Director
ewilson@sbhao.on.ca

Spina Bifida & Hydrocephalus Association of Prince Edward Island
PO Box 3332, Charlottetown PE C0A 1R0
Tel: 902-628-8875
Overview: A small provincial charitable organization overseen by Spina Bifida & Hydrocephalus Association of Canada
Chief Officer(s):
Lurlean Palmer, Contact
 lurleanpalmer@eastlink.ca

L'Association de spina-bifida et d'hydrocéphalie du Québec (ASBHQ)
#303, 55, av Mont-Royal Ouest, Montréal QC H2T 2S6
Tél: 514-340-9019
Ligne sans frais: 800-567-1788
Courriel: info@spina.qc.ca
www.spina.qc.ca
www.facebook.com/asbhq
twitter.com/ASBHQ
Aperçu: *Dimension:* moyenne; *Envergure:* provinciale; Organisme sans but lucratif; fondée en 1975 surveillé par Spina Bifida & Hydrocephalus Association of Canada
Mission: Promouvoir et défendre les droits, les intérêts et le bien-être des personnes ayant le spina-bifida et l'hydrocéphalie; sensibiliser le public à la nature du spina-bifida et de l'hydrocéphalie ainsi qu'aux besoins des personnes ayant ces malformations; favoriser et soutenir la recherche sur les causes, les nouveaux traitements et les techniques de prévention du spina-bifida et de l'hydrocéphalie
Membre de: Confédération des organismes provinciaux de personnes handicappées du Québec
Affliation(s): Institut de réadaptation en déficience physique de Québec; Hôpital Shriners, Centre de réadaptation Constance-Lethbridge, Centre de réadaptation en déficience physique Chaudière-Appalaches
Membre(s) du bureau directeur:
Marc Picard, Président

A.S.B.H. Région Estrie
928, rue Fédéral, Sherbrooke QC J1H 5A7
Tél: 819-822-3772; *Téléc:* 819-822-4529
Courriel: asbhestrie@hotmail.com
www.spina.qc.ca/estrie
Membre(s) du bureau directeur:
René Labonté, Président
Aline Nault, Coordonnatrice

A.S.B.H. Région Montréal
#448, 14115, Prince-Arthur, Montréal QC H1A 1A8
Tél: 514-739-5515; *Téléc:* 514-739-5505
Courriel: asbhrm@mainbourg.org
www.spina.qc.ca
www.facebook.com/asbhq.quebec
twitter.com/ASBHQ
Membre(s) du bureau directeur:
André Bougie, Président

Spina Bifida & Hydrocephalus Association of South Saskatchewan
PO Box 37115, Stn. Landmark, Regina SK S4S 7K3
Tel: 306-586-2222
e-mail: regina@sbhac.ca
Overview: A small provincial organization
Mission: To improve the quality of life for those afflicted with spina bifida &/or hydrocephalus
Member of: Spina Bifida & Hydrocephalus Association of Canada

North Chapter
351 Kenderdine Rd., Saskatoon SK S7N 3S9
Tel: 306-249-1362
www.sbhasn.ca
Chief Officer(s):
Laurel Scherr, President

South Chapter

PO Box 37115, Regina SK S4S 7K3
Tel: 306-359-6049
e-mail: regina@sbhac.ca

Spina Bifida & Hydrocephalus Association of Northern Alberta (SBHANA)
PO Box 35025, 10818 Jasper Ave., Edmonton AB T5J 0B7
Tel: 780-451-6921; *Fax:* 888-881-7172
e-mail: info@sbhana.org
www.sbhana.org
www.facebook.com/sbhana01
twitter.com/SBHANA1
www.youtube.com/user/TheSBHANA
Previous Name: Spina Bifida Association of Northern Alberta
Overview: A small local charitable organization founded in 1981
Mission: To enhance the lives of individuals & families affected by spina bifida &/or hydrocephalus through public awareness, education & research
Member of: Spina Bifida & Hydrocephalus Association of Canada; Alberta Disablility Forum; Albera Committee for Citizens with Disabilities
Chief Officer(s):
Cindy Smith, President
Megan Gergatz, Program Manager

Spina Bifida & Hydrocephalus Association of Ontario
#1006, 555 Richmond St. West, Toronto, ON M5V 3B1
Tel: 416-214-1056; *Fax:* 416-214-1446
Toll-Free: 800-387-1575
provincial@sbhao.on.ca
www.sbhao.on.ca
Social Media: twitter.com/SBH_Ontario;
www.facebook.com/SpinaBifidaHydrocephalusOntario
Collection: Vertical file of articles related to Spina Bifida & Hydrocephalus
Elaine Wilson, Executive Director
 ewilson@sbhao.on.ca
Shauna Beaudoin, Information & Services Coordinator
 sbeaudoin@sbhao.on.ca

Spinal Cord Injuries

Cause
Spinal cord injuries result from trauma to or disease of the spinal cord. If they are caused by physical trauma due to a sports-related incident, a fall, a violent crime or a motor vehicle accident they are classified as traumatic. When damage is the result of a disease such as cancer, or a congenital disorder like spina bifida, spinal injuries are classified as non-traumatic.

Symptoms
Depending on where the spinal cord was injured, paraplegia (paralysis affecting the legs and lower part of the body) or quadriplegia (paralysis affecting all muscles below the neck and therefore all four limbs), may occur. Other symptoms of spinal cord injuries may include loss of sensation, spasms and difficulty breathing. Bladder and sexual function may also be damaged.

Prevalence
In Canada today, it is estimated that there are about 86,000 people living with a spinal cord injury. About 51 percent of these injuries are the result of physical trauma, and 49 percent have a non-traumatic cause. Traumatic spinal cord injuries occur most frequently in males between the ages of 16 and 34. Each year, there are around 4,300 new cases of spinal cord injury in Canada.

Treatment Options

A physician can sometimes rule out a spinal cord injury resulting from physical trauma after receiving information about the accident, and doing physical and neurological exams to evaluate motor and sensory function. However, further diagnostic testing is often necessary. This may include X-rays, a computerized tomography (CT) scan or magnetic resonance imaging (MRI) of the spine.

Acute (early) treatment of spinal cord injuries focuses on intensive medical care and appropriate surgical stabilization at the time of the injury. In later years, attention is paid to preventing the complications of spinal cord injuries, such as skin breakdown, bladder infection and lung dysfunction. One of the greatest challenges is helping persons with spinal cord injuries to live as productive and independent a life as possible. Rehabilitation should begin as soon as possible after the injury. It usually starts with several weeks at a specialized inpatient facility, then transitions to family-assisted or independent living, depending on the extent of the disability. The multidisciplinary team provides education, emotional support, physical and occupational therapy, assistive devices, braces and beds, and helps arrange special vans or modifications to the patient's home. Many voluntary societies and government agencies can help with the transition to life in the community.

Modern medical and surgical care has dramatically increased both long-term survival and quality of life for victims of spinal cord injuries. Scientists continue to investigate stem cell therapy for spinal cord injuries, and to research new drug therapies to promote nerve cell regeneration and to control inflammation.

National Associations

Canadian Spinal Research Organization (CSRO)

#2, 120 Newkirk Rd., Richmond Hill ON L4C 9S7

Tel: 905-508-4000; *Fax:* 905-508-4002
Toll-Free: 800-361-4004
www.csro.com
www.facebook.com/196341387063476
www.youtube.com/user/CSROVideos

Overview: A medium-sized national organization founded in 1984
Mission: To improve the physical quality of life for people with spinal injuries; to reduce the incidence of spinal cord injuries through awareness programs for the public & prevention programs with targeted groups
Member of: Charities First
Chief Officer(s):
Kent Bassett-Spiers, Executive Director
Barry Munro, President
Publications:
• CSRO [Canadian Spinal Research Organization] Quarterly
Type: Magazine; *Frequency:* Quarterly

Canadian Syringomyelia Network (CSN)

c/o The Forrestall Group, #4, 201 Whitehall Dr., Markham ON L3R 9Y3
Fax: 905-944-4844
www.csn.ca

Overview: A small national charitable organization founded in 1993
Mission: To provide information & support for persons with Syringomyelia & related conditions, plus their caregivers & families
Publications:
• The CSN News
Type: Newsletter; *Frequency:* Quarterly
Profile: Information & updates from the Canadian Syringomyelia Network

Canadian Transverse Myelitis Association (CTMA) / Association Canadienne de myélite transverse

263 Malcolm Circle, Dorval QC H9S 1T6

Tel: 514-636-9337
e-mail: info@mytm.ca
www.mytm.ca
twitter.com/CTMAssociation

Overview: A medium-sized national organization
Mission: To help patients with transverse myelitis & their families build a network of support; To inform patients & families of new research & treatment that has been discovered; To raise awareness about the disorder
Chief Officer(s):
Kimberley Kotar, President & Founder

Rick Hansen Foundation

#300, 3820 Cessna Dr., Richmond BC V7B 0A2

Tel: 604-295-8149; *Fax:* 604-295-8159
Toll-Free: 800-213-2131
e-mail: info@rickhansen.com
www.rickhansen.com
wwww.facebook.com/rickhansenfdn
twitter.com/RickHansenFdn
wwww.youtube.com/user/RickHansenFdn

Overview: A medium-sized national charitable organization founded in 1988
Mission: To improve the quality of life of people with spinal cord injury; To create more accessible & inclusive communities; to advance research
Chief Officer(s):
Lyall Knott, Co-Chair
Rick Hansen, Chief Executive Officer
George Gaffney, Co-Chair
Eric Watt, Treasurer
Publications:
• In Motion: The Rick Hansen Foundation Newsletter
Type: Newsletter; *Frequency:* Quarterly
Profile: Donation information, related news stories, possibilities, & solutions

Spinal Cord Injury Canada / Lésions Médullaires Canada

#104, 720 Belfast Rd., Ottawa ON K1G 6M8

Tel: 416-200-5814
www.sci-can.ca
www.facebook.com/223239864405595

Also Known As: SCI Canada
Previous Name: Canadian Paraplegic Association
Overview: A medium-sized national charitable organization founded in 1945
Mission: To assist persons with spinal cord injuries & other physical disabilitieto to cope with the changes caused by their injury, to become independent & self-reliant, & to lead productive lives
Chief Officer(s):
Bill Adair, Executive Director
bill@sci-can.ca
Publications:
• Canadian Paraplegic Association Annual Report [a publication of Spinal Cord Injury Canada]
Type: Yearbook; *Frequency:* Annually
• The Complete Incomplete Resource [a publication of Spinal Cord Injury Canada]
Price: $6
Profile: Resource dedicated to incomplete SCI
• Fire Safety for People with Disabilities [a publication of Spinal Cord Injury Canada]
Price: $22
Profile: Fire safety training kit for people with disabilities & seniors
• Life After Spinal Cord Injury [a publication of Spinal Cord Injury Canada]
Price: $30 non-members; $15 members
Profile: Information resource for persons with SCI & their family members
• Life Interrupted [a publication of Spinal Cord Injury Canada]
Type: Manual
Profile: Practical information for youth, between the ages of 12 & 21, with SCI

• Opening Doors to Rehabilitation [a publication of Spinal Cord Injury Canada]
Type: Manual
Profile: Information for professional counsellors who work with clients with mobility impairments
• Total Access [a publication of Spinal Cord Injury Canada]
Type: Magazine; *Frequency:* Semiannually; *Price:* $19.99 Canada; $25 International
Profile: Information for people with spinal cord injury & other physical disabilities
• Workforce Participation Survey of Canadians with Spinal Cord Injuries [a publication of Spinal Cord Injury Canada]
Type: Report

Provincial Associations

ALBERTA

Spinal Cord Injury Alberta
#305, 11010 - 101 St., Edmonton AB T5H 4B9
Tel: 780-424-6312; *Fax:* 780-424-6313
Toll-Free: 888-654-5444
e-mail: edmonton@sci-ab.ca
www.sci-ab.ca
www.facebook.com/SpinalCordInjuryAlberta?ref=hl
twitter.com/scialberta
www.youtube.com/cpaalberta
Previous Name: Canadian Paraplegic Association (Alberta)
Overview: A medium-sized provincial organization overseen by Spinal Cord Injury Canada
Chief Officer(s):
Teren Clarke, CEO
Publications:
• Spinal Columns
Type: Magazine; *Frequency:* Quarterly; *Accepts Advertising*; *Price:* $20
Profile: Articles on issues such as advocacy, transportation, employment, & relationships
• Wheel-e
Type: Newsletter; *Frequency:* Monthly
Profile: Association events & announcements

Calgary
5211 - 4th St. NE, Calgary AB T2K 6J5
Tel: 403-228-3001; *Fax:* 403-229-4271
e-mail: calgary@sci-ab.ca

Fort McMurray
Fort McMurray AB
Tel: 587-645-0771
e-mail: fortmcmurray@sci-ab.ca
Chief Officer(s):
Stephanie Myrick, Regional Program Coordinator
stephanie.myrick@sci-ab.ca

Grande Prairie
10 Knowledge Way, Grande Prairie AB T8W 2V9
Tel: 780-532-3305; *Fax:* 780-539-3567
e-mail: grandeprairie@sci-ab.ca

Lethbridge
53 Mount Sundance Rd. West, Lethbridge AB T1J 0B6
Tel: 403-327-7577; *Fax:* 403-320-0269
e-mail: lethbridge@sci-ab.ca

Lloydminster
Lloydminster AB
Tel: 780-871-4542
e-mail: lloydminster@sci-ab.ca

Medicine Hat
#26, 419 - 3rd St. SE, Medicine Hat AB T1A 0G9
Tel: 403-504-4001; *Fax:* 403-504-5172
e-mail: medicinehat@sci-ab.ca

Red Deer
Red Deer AB
Tel: 403-341-5060; *Fax:* 403-343-1630
e-mail: reddeer@sci-ab.ca

St. Paul

PO Box 653, St Paul AB T0A 3A0
Tel: 780-645-5116; *Fax:* 780-645-5141
e-mail: stpaul@sci-ab.ca

BRITISH COLUMBIA

Spinal Cord Injury British Columbia (BCPA)
780 Southwest Marine Dr., Vancouver BC V6P 5Y7
Tel: 604-324-3611; *Fax:* 614-326-1229
e-mail: info@bcpara.org
sci-bc.ca
www.facebook.com/SpinalCordInjuryBC
twitter.com/sci_bc
www.youtube.com/user/BCParaplegic
Previous Name: British Columbia Paraplegic Association; Canadian Paraplegic Association
Overview: A medium-sized provincial organization founded in 1957 overseen by Spinal Cord Injury Canada
Member of: BC SCI Community Services Network
Chief Officer(s):
Edward Milligan, Chair
Chris McBride, Executive Director
cmcbride@sci-bc.ca
Marion Patsis, Manager, Finance & Human Resources
mpastis@sci-bc.ca
Publications:
• Comming into Focus: People Living with Spinal Cord Injury in BC
Type: Report
• Paragraphic
Type: Magazine; *Frequency:* Quarterly; *Accepts Advertising*; *Price:* Free for BCPA supporting members & community partners
Profile: BCPA programs, research information, personal profiles, & updates from the GF Strong Rehabilitation Centre

Prince George
777 Kinsmen Pl., Prince George BC V2M 6Y7
Tel: 250-563-6942; *Fax:* 250-563-6992
e-mail: info@sci-bc.ca
Chief Officer(s):
Brandy Stiles, Coordinator, Peer Program
bstiles@sci-bc.ca

MANITOBA

Canadian Paraplegic Association (Manitoba)
#211, 825 Sherbrook St., Winnipeg MB R3A 1M5
Tel: 204-786-4753; *Fax:* 204-786-1140
Toll-Free: 800-720-4933
e-mail: winnipeg@canparaplegic.org
www.cpamanitoba.ca
Overview: A medium-sized provincial organization overseen by Spinal Cord Injury Canada
Mission: To represent persons with spinal cord injuries in Manitoba
Chief Officer(s):
Ron Burky, Executive Director
rburky@canparaplegic.org
Darlene Cooper, Director, Rehabilitation Services
djcooper@canparaplegic.org

Manitoba Paraplegia Foundation Inc.
825 Sherbrook St., Winnipeg MB R3A 1M5
Tel: 204-786-4753; *Fax:* 204-786-1140
e-mail: winnipeg@canparaplegic.org
www.cpamanitoba.ca/mpf
Overview: A small provincial organization founded in 1980
Mission: To provide support for research & prevention activities; To provide direct aid to paraplegics & quadriplegics for home modifications, vocational aid & other items to assist spinal cord injured Manitobans to lead independent lives within the community; To provide support for special projects undertaken on behalf of spinal cord injured persons in Manitoba
Chief Officer(s):
Doug Finkbeiner, President

Ability New Brunswick / Capacité Nouveau-Brunswick
#102, 440 Wilsey Rd., Fredericton NB E2B 7G5

Tel: 506-462-9555; Fax: 506-458-9134
Toll-Free: 866-462-9555
e-mail: info@abilitynb.ca
www.abilitynb.ca
www.facebook.com/abilitynb
twitter.com/AbilityNB
www.youtube.com/user/abilitynb

Previous Name: Canadian Paraplegic Association (New Brunswick) Inc.
Overview: A medium-sized provincial organization overseen by Spinal Cord Injury Canada
Mission: To respond to the needs of people with spinal cord injuries & their families in New Brunswick
Chief Officer(s):
Bill Leonard, President
Haley Flaro, Executive Director
   haley.flaro@abilitynb.ca
Publications:
• Ability Now! [a publication of Ability New Brunswick]
Type: Newsletter

Moncton
#407, 236 St. George St., Moncton NB E1C 1W1
Tel: 506-858-0311; Fax: 506-858-8290
e-mail: info@abilitynb.ca

Spinal Cord Injury Newfoundland & Labrador (SCI NL)
PO Box 21284, #101, 396 Elizabeth Ave., St. John's NL A1A 5G6
Tel: 709-753-5901; Fax: 709-753-4224
Toll-Free: 877-783-5901
e-mail: info@sci-nl.ca
sci-nl.ca
www.facebook.com/186403331430655
twitter.com/SCI_NL
www.youtube.com/user/CanParaplegicNL

Previous Name: Canadian Paraplegic Association - Newfoundland & Labrador
Overview: A medium-sized provincial organization overseen by Spinal Cord Injury Canada
Mission: To help people with spinal cord injuries and other mobility impairments to become self-reliant and independent
Chief Officer(s):
Michael Burry, Executive Director, 902-753-5901 Ext. 222
   mburry@sci-nl.ca

Bay Roberts
PMC Professional Bldg., PO Box 1309, 25 Bareneed Rd., Bay Roberts NL A0A 1G0
Tel: 709-786-1442; Fax: 709-786-1441

Gander
230 Airport Blvd., Gander NL A1V 1L7
Tel: 709-256-7077; Fax: 709-256-7047

Grand Falls - Windsor
4A Bayley St., Grand Falls-Windsor NL A2A 2T5
Tel: 709-489-8445

Happy Valley - Labrador Office
PO Box 848, Stn. B, 215 Hamilton River Rd., Happy Valley-Goose Bay NL A0P 1E0
Tel: 709-896-7057; Fax: 709-896-3716

Marystown
PO Box 1296, #245, 247 Villa Marie Dr., Marystown NL A0E 2M0
Tel: 709-279-2790; Fax: 709-279-0919
Toll-Free: 877-792-2790

Canadian Paraplegic Association (Nova Scotia)
Mumford Professional Centre, #255, 6960 Mumford Rd., Halifax NS B3L 4P1

Tel: 902-423-1277; Fax: 902-492-1213
Toll-Free: 800-889-1889
e-mail: halifax@canparaplegic.org
www.thespine.ca
www.facebook.com/213554735333572
twitter.com/CPANS
www.youtube.com/user/CPANovaScotia

Overview: A medium-sized provincial organization overseen by Spinal Cord Injury Canada
Chief Officer(s):
Gordon Pye, Chair
Angela Cook, Treasurer
Nancy Beaton, Executive Director
   nbeaton@canparaplegic.org

Spinal Cord Injury Ontario
520 Sutherland Dr., Toronto ON M4G 3V9

Tel: 416-422-5644; Fax: 416-422-5943
Toll-Free: 877-422-1112
www.sciontario.org
www.facebook.com/sciontario.org
twitter.com/SCI_Ontario
www.youtube.com/user/SCIOntarioOrg

Also Known As: SCI Ontario
Previous Name: Canadian Paraplegic Association Ontario
Overview: A medium-sized provincial organization founded in 1979 overseen by Spinal Cord Injury Canada
Mission: To act as the voice of persons with spinal cord injury in Ontario
Publications:
• Outspoken!
Type: Magazine; *Frequency:* Quarterly; *Price:* Free with membership
Profile: CPA Ontario services & activities

Barrie Office
#111, 80 Bradford St., Barrie ON L4N 6S7
Tel: 705-726-4546; Fax: 705-726-5054
Toll-Free: 800-870-5670

Hamilton Office
North Regional Rehabilitation Centre, #B1-3, 300 Wellington St., Hamilton ON L8L 0A4
Tel: 905-383-0216; Fax: 905-383-5021

Kingston Office
PO Box 20105, Kingston ON K7P 2T6
Tel: 613-547-1391; Fax: 613-547-1393
Toll-Free: 866-220-7539

London Office
#3, 1111 Elias St., London ON N5W 5L1
Tel: 519-433-2331; Fax: 519-433-3987
Toll-Free: 866-433-9888

Mississauga/Halton; Peel/Dufferin Office
c/o 520 Sutherland Dr., Toronto ON M4G 3V9
Tel: 905-459-6965; Fax: 905-459-0283
Toll-Free: 866-287-1689

Muskoka Office
PO Box 327, Kearney ON P0A 1M0
Tel: 705-636-5827; Fax: 705-636-7223

Ottawa Office
#104, 720 Belfast Rd., Ottawa ON K1G 0Z5
Tel: 613-723-1033; Fax: 613-688-0373
• Spinal Columns: Ottawa Region Newsletter
Type: Newsletter; *Accepts Advertising*
Profile: Resources, upcoming events, & volunteer opportunities

Peterborough Office
PO Box 131, Warsaw ON K0L 3A0
Tel: 705-652-7496; Fax: 705-652-0786
Toll-Free: 888-643-2507

Sault St. Marie Office
260 Elizabeth St., Sault Ste Marie ON P6A 6J3
Tel: 705-759-0333; *Fax:* 705-759-0335
Toll-Free: 866-531-1513

Thunder Bay Office
1201 Jasper Dr., #B, Thunder Bay ON P7B 6R2
Tel: 807-344-3743; *Fax:* 807-344-9490
Toll-Free: 866-344-4159

Toronto - West Office
#306, 1120 Finch Ave., Toronto ON M3J 3H7
Tel: 416-241-1433; *Fax:* 416-241-2466

Waterloo-Wellington Office
PO Box 1881, 88 Wyndham St. North, Guelph ON N1H 7A1
Tel: 519-893-1267; *Fax:* 519-893-2585
Toll-Free: 888-893-1267

Windsor Office
c/o Tafour Campus, Hotel Dieu Grace Hospital, 1453 Prince Rd.,
Windsor ON N9C 3Z4
Tel: 519-253-7272; *Fax:* 519-253-7279

PRINCE EDWARD ISLAND

Spinal Cord Injury (Prince Edward Island) (SCI-PEI)
40 Enman Cres., Charlottetown PE C1E 1E6
Tel: 902-370-9523
www.sci-pei.ca
www.facebook.com/166802903349902
Previous Name: Canadian Paraplegic Association (Prince Edward
Island)
Overview: A small provincial organization founded in 1990 overseen
by Spinal Cord Injury Canada
Chief Officer(s):
Meagan MacKenzie, Executive Director
mmackenzie@sci-pei.ca

QUÉBEC

Fondation pour la recherche sur la moelle épinière
#400, 6020 rue Jean-Talon Est, Montréal QC H1S 3B1
Tél: 514-341-7272; *Téléc:* 514-341-8884
Ligne sans frais: 877-341-7272
Courriel: info@moelleepiniere.com
www.moelleepiniere.com
www.facebook.com/MEMOQuebec
twitter.com/MEMOQuebec
Nom précédent: Fondation André Sénécal pour la recherche sur la
moelle épinière
Aperçu: *Dimension:* moyenne; *Envergure:* provinciale; fondée en 1994
Mission: A pour but de récolter des fonds pour financer,
principalement, la recherche scientifique et médicale sur les lésions
médullaires
Membre(s) du bureau directeur:
Walter Zelaya, Directeur général
wzelaya@moelleepiniere.com

**Moelle Épinière et Motricité Québec / Quebec Paraplegics
Association**
#400, 6020, rue Jean-Talon Est, Montréal QC H1S 3B1
Tél: 514-341-7272; *Téléc:* 514-341-8884
Ligne sans frais: 877-341-7272
Courriel: info@moelleepiniere.com
www.moelleepiniere.com
www.facebook.com/MEMOQuebec
twitter.com/MEMOQuebec
Aperçu: *Dimension:* moyenne; *Envergure:* provinciale; fondée en 1946
surveillé par Spinal Cord Injury Canada
Mission: Pour aider les personnes souffrant de lésions de la moelle
épinière se réinsérer dans la société
Membre(s) du bureau directeur:
Walter Zelaya, Directeur général
wzelaya@moelleepiniere.com

SASKATCHEWAN

Spinal Cord Injury Saskatchewan
311 - 38th St. East, Saskatoon SK S7K 0T1
Tel: 306-652-9644; *Fax:* 306-652-2957
Toll-Free: 888-282-0186
e-mail: saskatoon@canparaplegic.org
www.spinalcordinjurysask.com
www.facebook.com/CPASaskatchewan
twitter.com/scisask
Previous Name: Canadian Paraplegic Association (Saskatchewan)
Overview: A medium-sized provincial organization overseen by Spinal
Cord Injury Canada
Mission: To provide services to persons with spinal cord injury & other
mobility impairments in Saskatchewan
Chief Officer(s):
Lyn Brown, Executive Director
lbrown@canparaplegic.org

Regina
3928 Gordon Rd., Regina SK S4S 6Y3
Tel: 306-584-0101; *Fax:* 306-584-0008
Toll-Free: 877-582-4483
e-mail: regina@canparaplegic.org
Chief Officer(s):
Blake Lamontagne, Coordinator, Client Service
blamontagne@canparaplegic.org

International Associations

**International Society for the Study of the Lumbar Spine
(ISSLS)**
c/o Institute for Clinical Sciences, Sahlgrenska Academy, PO Box 426,
#MG301, 2075 Bayview Ave., Gothenburg SE-405 30 Sweden
Tel: 46-31-786-44-36
www.issls.org
www.facebook.com/1396088907323562
twitter.com/ISSLS_Society
www.youtube.com/user/ISSLSSociety
Overview: A small international organization founded in 1974
Chief Officer(s):
Keith Luk, President
Katarina Olinder Eriksson, Administrator
katarina.olinder@gu.se

Provincial Libraries

Spinal Cord Injury Ontario
520 Sutherland Dr., Toronto, ON M4G 3V9
Tel: 416-422-5644; *Fax:* 416-422-5943
Toll-Free: 877-422-1112
www.sciontario.org
Social Media: www.youtube.com/user/SCIOntarioOrg;
www.twitter.com/sci_ontario; www.facebook.com/sciontario.org
Collection: Spinal cord injuries; accessible housing; vehicle
modifications; transportation; funding sources for mobility; assistive
devices; sports & recreation

Stroke

Strokes are an interruption of blood flow to the brain. In around 80
percent of cases strokes are ischemic, meaning that they are the
result of a blocked blood vessel. In the other 20 percent, strokes
are hemorrhagic, meaning that they are caused by uncontrolled
bleeding in the brain.

Cause
High blood pressure, atherosclerosis (fatty deposits), heart disease, stress, diabetes, excess weight, smoking and heavy alcohol consumption are the major risk factors predisposing someone
to stroke.

Symptoms
Depending on the severity and location of the damage, symptoms of stroke may include sudden weakness or paralysis (especially on one side of the body), blurred vision, difficulty speaking,

slurred speech, dizziness and falling, extreme headache, stiff neck, altered level of alertness and loss of bladder control.

Prevalence

In Canada, stroke is the fourth leading cause of death. Approximately 16,000 Canadians die of stroke every year. The incidence increases with age, is higher in men and in postmenopausal women, and is higher in First Nations people and those of South Asian and African descent. It is estimated that stroke costs the Canadian economy about $3.6 billion per year.

Treatment Options

A variety of tests can be used to diagnose a stroke. A physician often performs physical and neurological exams to determine what type of stroke has occurred, and how the brain has been affected. A cerebral angiography or carotid ultrasound can be used to examine how blood is flowing through the arteries in the brain and neck. A computerized tomography (CT) scan or magnetic resonance imaging (MRI) of the brain is often conducted to determine the presence and cause of a stroke. An electroencephalogram (EEG) may be performed to see if a stroke has caused any brain damage. Heart tests such as an echocardiogram or transesophageal echocardiogram (TEE) may be used to check heart function.

Preventive therapy of stroke is aimed at treatment of high blood pressure, heart disease and diabetes. If someone has had an ischemic stroke they may be treated with thrombolytic drugs such as tissue plasminogen activator (tPA) that can break up the blood clot causing the stroke. Research has shown that patients who are given one of these agents within three hours of stroke symptoms may have some or total restoration of neurologic function. Surgery is sometimes needed after a stroke to repair broken blood vessels, remove blood that has pooled in the brain or clear plaque from inside the carotid artery. Rehabilitation after the stroke involves physical and occupational therapy. Medications such as blood-thinning agents, antihypertensives (to treat high blood pressure) and cholesterol lowering drugs may also be prescribed.

Many stroke survivors experience depression and difficulty regaining independence, so it is important to provide emotional support for both survivors and their families. With appropriate therapy, most stroke survivors recover some degree of function, and can lead full, productive lives.

National Associations

Canadian Stroke Network (CSN) / Réseau canadien contre les accidents cérébrovasculaires
#301, 600 Peter Morand Cres., Ottawa ON K1G 5Z3
Tel: 613-562-5696; *Fax:* 613-521-9215
e-mail: info@canadianstrokenetwork.ca
www.canadianstrokenetwork.ca
www.linkedin.com/company/canadian-stroke-network
www.facebook.com/canadianstrokenetwork
twitter.com/strokenetwork
www.youtube.com/user/strokenetwork
Overview: A small national organization founded in 1999
Mission: To reduce the physical, social, & economic consequences of stroke on individuals & society through leadership in research; To develop & implement national strategies in stroke research; To maximize health & economic benefits; To build a consensus across Canada on stroke policy
Member of: Canada's Network of Centres of Excellence
Chief Officer(s):
Pierre Boyle, Chair
Antoine Hakim, CEO & Scientific Director
Kevin Willis, Executive Director
Robin Millbank, Manager, Professional Development

Publications:
• Canadian Stroke Network: Reducing the Impact of Stroke
Type: Newsletter
Profile: Information about stroke care

Heart & Stroke Foundation of Canada (HSFC) / Fondation des maladies du coeur du Canada
#1402, 222 Queen St., Ottawa ON K1P 5V9
Tel: 613-569-4361; *Fax:* 613-569-3278
www.heartandstroke.ca
www.facebook.com/heartandstroke
twitter.com/TheHSF
www.youtube.com/heartandstrokefdn
Overview: A medium-sized national charitable organization founded in 1983
Mission: To further the study, prevention & reduction of disability & death from heart disease & stroke through research, education & the promotion of healthy lifestyles
Member of: Imagine Canada
Affiliation(s): International Society & Federation of Cardiology; Canadian Coalition for High Blood Pressure Prevention & Control
Chief Officer(s):
David Sculthorpe, Chief Executive Officer

Provincial Associations

ALBERTA

Heart & Stroke Foundation of Alberta, NWT & Nunavut (HSFA)
#100, 119 - 14 St. NW, Calgary AB T2N 1Z6
Tel: 403-351-7030; *Fax:* 403-237-0803
Toll-Free: 888-473-4636
www.hsf.ab.ca
Previous Name: Heart & Stroke Foundation of Alberta
Overview: A medium-sized provincial charitable organization founded in 1956 overseen by Heart & Stroke Foundation of Canada
Mission: To disseminate information about heart disease & stroke; to promote research into new drugs, therapies, treatments in disorders leading to heart disease & stroke; to conduct several events to campaign for funds.
Chief Officer(s):
Michael Hill, Chair
Donna Hastings, CEO

Edmonton Office
10985 - 124 St., Edmonton AB T5M 0H9
Tel: 780-451-4545; *Fax:* 780-454-1593

Lethbridge Office
PO Box 2211, Lethbridge AB T1J 4K7
Tel: 403-327-3239; *Fax:* 403-327-9928

Medicine Hat Office
#124, 430 - 6 Ave. SE, Medicine Hat AB T1A 2S8
Tel: 403-527-0028; *Fax:* 403-526-9655

Red Deer Office
#202, 5913 - 50 Ave., Red Deer AB T4N 4C4
Tel: 403-342-4435; *Fax:* 403-342-7088

BRITISH COLUMBIA

Heart & Stroke Foundation of British Columbia & Yukon (HSFBCY)
#200, 1212 West Broadway, Vancouver BC V6H 3V2
Tel: 778-372-8000
www.heartandstroke.bc.ca
www.facebook.com/heartandstrokebcyukon
Previous Name: BC & Yukon Heart Foundation
Overview: A large provincial charitable organization founded in 1955 overseen by Heart & Stroke Foundation of Canada
Mission: To further the study, prevention & relief of cardiovascular disease
Chief Officer(s):
Adrienne Bakker, CEO

Coastal Vancouver Area Office - Vancouver/North Shore
1216 West Broadway, Vancouver BC V6H 1G6
Tel: 778-372-8052; *Fax:* 604-736-4087

Fraser North & East Area Office - Tri-Cities/Fraser
Valley/Burnaby/New Westminster
2239C McAllister Ave., Port Coquitlam BC V3C 2A5
Tel: 604-342-8070; *Fax:* 604-472-0055
Toll-Free: 877-472-0045

Kamloops Area Office - Kamloops/Cariboo
729 Victoria St., Kamloops BC V2C 2B5
Tel: 250-372-3938; *Fax:* 250-372-3940

Kelowna Area Office - Okanagan/Kootenays
#4, 1551 Sutherland Ave., Kelowna BC V1Y 9M9
Tel: 778-313-8090; *Fax:* 250-860-8790
Toll-Free: 866-432-7833

Prince George Area Office Northern BC/Yukon
1480 - 7th Ave., Prince George BC V2L 3P2
Tel: 250-562-8611; *Fax:* 250-562-8614
Toll-Free: 866-226-6784

Richmond Office - Richmond/South Delta
#260, 7000 Minoru Blvd., Richmond BC V6Y 3Z5
Tel: 778-234-8080; *Fax:* 604-279-7134

Surrey Area Office -
Surrey/Langley/Whiterock/Cloverdale/Aldergrove/North Delta
#101, 13569 - 76th Ave., Surrey BC V3W 2W3
Tel: 778-612-8063; *Fax:* 604-591-2624

Vancouver Island Area Office - Nanaimo
#401, 495 Dunsmuir St., Nanaimo BC V9R 6B9
Tel: 250-754-5274; *Fax:* 250-754-2575

Victoria Office
#106, 1001 Cloverdale Ave., Victoria BC V8X 4C9
Tel: 250-410-8091; *Fax:* 250-382-0231

Stroke Recovery Association of BC (SRABC)
#301, 1212 West Broadway, Vancouver BC V6H 3V1
Tel: 604-688-3603; *Fax:* 604-688-3660
Toll-Free: 888-313-3377
www.strokerecoverybc.ca
www.facebook.com/StrokeRecoveryBC
twitter.com/StrokeRecovBC
www.youtube.com/user/office814
Overview: A small provincial charitable organization founded in 1979
Mission: To encourage stroke survivors & their families as they adjust themselves to changes in their lives; To foster understanding of strokes within the community; To provide, through local Stoke Recovery branches throughout BC, a resource for stroke survivors living in the community
Chief Officer(s):
Atul Gadhia, President

MANITOBA

Heart & Stroke Foundation of Manitoba (HSFM)
The Heart & Stroke Bldg., #200, 6 Donald St., Winnipeg MB R3L 0K6
Tel: 204-949-2000; *Fax:* 204-957-1365
www.heartandstroke.mb.ca
Previous Name: Manitoba Heart Foundation
Overview: A medium-sized provincial charitable organization founded in 1957 overseen by Heart & Stroke Foundation of Canada
Mission: To eliminate heart disease & stroke through education, advocacy, & research
Chief Officer(s):
Debbie Brown, CEO

Stroke Recovery Association of Manitoba Inc.
247 Provencher Blvd., #B, Winnipeg MB R2H 0G6
Tel: 204-942-2880; *Fax:* 204-944-1982
e-mail: admin@strokerecovery.ca
www.strokerecovery.ca
www.facebook.com/StrokeRecoveryMB
Overview: A small provincial organization overseen by Stroke Recovery Network
Mission: To help improve the lives of stroke victims & their families
Chief Officer(s):
April Takacs, President
Diane O'Neil, Executive Director & Administrator

NEW BRUNSWICK

Heart & Stroke Foundation of New Brunswick / Fondation des maladies du coeur du Nouveau-Brunswick
133 Prince William St., 5th Fl, Saint John NB E2L 2B5
Tel: 506-634-1620; *Fax:* 506-648-0098
Toll-Free: 800-663-3600
www.heartandstroke.nb.ca
Previous Name: New Brunswick Heart Foundation
Overview: A medium-sized provincial organization founded in 1967 overseen by Heart & Stroke Foundation of Canada
Mission: To improve the health of residents of New Brunswick by preventing & reducing disability & death from heart disease & stroke, through research, health promotion & advocacy
Chief Officer(s):
Kurtis Sisk, CEO

NEWFOUNDLAND AND LABRADOR

Heart & Stroke Foundation of Newfoundland & Labrador
1037 Topsail Rd., Mount Pearl NL A1N 5E9
Tel: 709-753-8521; *Fax:* 709-753-3117
www.heartandstroke.nf.ca
Overview: A medium-sized provincial organization founded in 1964 overseen by Heart & Stroke Foundation of Canada
Mission: To work in Newfoundland & Labrador to advance research, advocate, & promote healthy lifestyles so that heart disease & stroke will be eliminated & their impact reduced
Chief Officer(s):
Mary Ann Butt, CEO

NOVA SCOTIA

Heart & Stroke Foundation of Nova Scotia (HSFNS)
Park Lane - Mall Level 3, PO Box 245, 5657 Spring Garden Rd., Halifax NS B3J 3R4
Tel: 902-423-7530; *Fax:* 902-492-1464
Toll-Free: 800-423-4432
www.heartandstroke.ns.ca
Previous Name: Nova Scotia Heart Foundation
Overview: A medium-sized provincial charitable organization founded in 1958 overseen by Heart & Stroke Foundation of Canada
Mission: To eliminate heart disease & stroke; To advance research; To promote healthy living; To engage in advocacy activities
Member of: The Heart and Stroke Foundation of Canada
Chief Officer(s):
Menna MacIsaac, CEO

ONTARIO

Heart & Stroke Foundation of Ontario (HSFO)
PO Box 2414, #1300, 2300 Yonge St., Toronto ON M4P 1E4
Tel: 416-489-7111; *Fax:* 416-489-6885
Previous Name: Ontario Heart Foundation
Overview: A medium-sized provincial charitable organization founded in 1952 overseen by Heart & Stroke Foundation of Canada
Mission: To eliminate heart disease & stroke by advancing research & promoting healthy living; To advocate in areas such as a smoke-free world, equal access to quality stroke care, obesity targeting, elimination of trans-fat, & resuscitation/CPR
Member of: Heart & Stroke Foundation of Canada
Chief Officer(s):
Darrell Reid, Chief Executive Officer

Barrie Office
#1, 112 Commerce Park Dr., Barrie ON L4N 8W8
Tel: 705-737-1020; *Fax:* 705-737-0902
www.heartandstroke.on.ca

Belleville Office
#106A, 121 Dundas St. East, Belleville ON K8N 1C3
Tel: 613-962-2502; *Fax:* 613-962-6080
www.heartandstroke.on.ca

Brantford Office
442 Grey St., #A, Brantford ON N3S 7N3
Tel: 519-752-1301; *Fax:* 519-752-5554
www.heartandstroke.on.ca

Brockville Office

Brockville General Hospital, 75 Charles St., Brockville ON K6V 1S8
Tel: 613-345-5645; *Fax:* 613-345-8348
www.heartandstroke.on.ca

Chief Officer(s):
Jay Bhatt, Director

Chatham-Kent Office
214 Queen St., Chatham ON N7M 2H1
Tel: 519-354-6232; *Fax:* 519-354-6351
www.heartandstroke.on.ca

Chinese Canadian Council
PO Box 2414, #1300, 2300 Yonge St., Toronto ON M4P 1E4
Tel: 416-489-7111; *Fax:* 416-489-9179
www.heartandstroke.on.ca

Cornwall Office
36 - 2nd St. East, Cornwall ON K6H 1Y3
Tel: 613-938-8933; *Fax:* 613-938-0655
www.heartandstroke.on.ca

Durham Regional Office
#2, 105 Consumers Dr., Whitby ON L1N 1C4
Tel: 905-666-3777; *Fax:* 905-666-9956
www.heartandstroke.on.ca

Guelph Office
#204, 21 Surrey St. West, Guelph ON N1H 3R3
Tel: 519-837-4858; *Fax:* 519-837-9209
www.heartandstroke.on.ca

Halton Region Office
#7, 4391 Harvester Rd., Burlington ON L7L 4X1
Tel: 905-634-7732; *Fax:* 905-634-1353
www.heartandstroke.on.ca

Hamilton Office
#7, 1439 Upper Ottawa St., Hamilton ON L8W 3J6
Tel: 905-574-4105; *Fax:* 905-574-4380
www.heartandstroke.on.ca

Kingston Office
720 Progress Ave., Kingston ON K7M 4W9
Tel: 613-384-2871; *Fax:* 613-384-2899
www.heartandstroke.on.ca

Kitchener Office
#2A, 1373 Victoria St. North, Kitchener ON N2B 3R6
Tel: 519-571-9600; *Fax:* 519-571-9832
www.heartandstroke.on.ca

London Office
#180, 633 Colborne St., London ON N6B 2V3
Tel: 519-679-0641; *Fax:* 519-679-6898
www.heartandstroke.on.ca

Niagara District Office
#3, 300 Bunting Rd., St Catharines ON L2M 7X3
Tel: 905-938-8800; *Fax:* 905-938-8811
www.heartandstroke.on.ca

Ottawa Office
#100, 1101 Prince of Wales Dr., Ottawa ON K2C 3W7
Tel: 613-727-5060; *Fax:* 613-727-1895
www.heartandstroke.on.ca

Owen Sound Office
795 - 1st Ave. East, Owen Sound ON N4K 2C6
Tel: 519-371-0083; *Fax:* 519-371-8164
www.heartandstroke.on.ca

Peel Office
#306, 201 County Court Blvd., Brampton ON L6W 4L2
Tel: 905-451-0021; *Fax:* 905-452-0503
www.heartandstroke.on.ca

Peterborough Office
#3, 824 Clonsilla Ave., Peterborough ON K9J 5Y3
Tel: 705-749-1044; *Fax:* 705-749-1470
www.heartandstroke.on.ca

Sarnia Office
774 London Rd., Sarnia ON N7T 4Y1
Tel: 519-332-1415; *Fax:* 519-332-3139
www.heartandstroke.on.ca

Sault Ste. Marie Office
59 Great Northern Rd., Sault Ste Marie ON P6B 4Y7
Tel: 705-253-3775; *Fax:* 705-946-5760
www.heartandstroke.on.ca

Stratford Office
556 Huron St., Stratford ON N5A 5T9
Tel: 519-273-5212; *Fax:* 519-273-7024
www.heartandstroke.on.ca

Sudbury Office
#130, 43 Elm St., Sudbury ON P3C 1S4
Tel: 705-673-2228; *Fax:* 705-673-7406
www.heartandstroke.on.ca

Thunder Bay Office
#104, 979 Alloy Dr., Thunder Bay ON P7B 5Z8
Tel: 807-623-1118; *Fax:* 807-622-9914
www.heartandstroke.on.ca

Timmins Office
#301, 60 Wilson Ave., Timmins ON P4N 2S7
Tel: 705-267-4645; *Fax:* 705-268-6721
www.heartandstroke.on.ca

Toronto Office
#1300, 2300 Yonge St., Toronto ON M4P 1E4
Tel: 416-489-7111; *Fax:* 416-489-6885
www.heartandstroke.on.ca

Windsor Office
#350, 4570 Rhodes Dr., Windsor ON N8W 5C2
Tel: 519-254-4345; *Fax:* 519-254-4215
www.heartandstroke.on.ca

York Region North Office
#29, 17665 Leslie St., Newmarket ON L3Y 3E3
Tel: 905-853-6355; *Fax:* 905-853-7961
www.heartandstroke.on.ca

York South Office
#204, 9251 Yonge St., Richmond Hill ON L4C 9T3
Tel: 905-709-4899; *Fax:* 905-709-0883
www.heartandstroke.on.ca

PRINCE EDWARD ISLAND

Heart & Stroke Foundation of Prince Edward Island Inc.
PO Box 279, 180 Kent St., Charlottetown PE C1A 7K4
Tel: 902-892-7441

Overview: A medium-sized provincial charitable organization overseen by Heart & Stroke Foundation of Canada
Mission: To improve the health of Islanders through the funding of heart disease & stroke research & the provision of heart & stroke education & programs
Chief Officer(s):
Charlotte Comrie, Chief Executive Officer
  charlotte.comrie@heartandstroke.ca
Sarah Crozier, Manager, Health Promotion

QUÉBEC

Fondation des maladies du coeur du Québec (FMCQ) / Heart & Stroke Foundation of Québec
#500, 1434, rue Sainte-Catherine ouest, Montréal QC H3G 1R4
Tél: 514-871-1551; *Téléc:* 514-871-9385
Ligne sans frais: 800-567-8563
www.fmcoeur.qc.ca
www.facebook.com/fmcoeur
twitter.com/FMCoeur
www.youtube.com/heartandstrokefdn

Nom précédent: Fondation du Québec des maladies du coeur
Aperçu: *Dimension:* grande; *Envergure:* provinciale; Organisme sans but lucratif; fondée en 1955 surveillé par Heart & Stroke Foundation of Canada
Mission: Forte de l'engagement de ses donateurs, de ses bénévoles et de ses employés, a pour mission de contribuer à l'avancement de la recherche et de promouvoir la santé du coeur, afin de réduire les invalidités et les décès dus aux maladies cardiovasculaires et aux accidents vasculaires cérébraux
Membre(s) du bureau directeur:
Edmée Métivier, Chef de la direction

Éric Champagne, Président du conseil

Bas St-Laurent et Gaspésie
33, boul René-Lepage est, Rimouski QC G5L 1N8
Tél: 418-869-1022; *Téléc:* 418-869-2748
Ligne sans frais: 888-473-4636
Membre(s) du bureau directeur:
Louiselle Bérubé, Directrice régionale

Côte-Nord
1, rue Arnaud, Les Escoumins QC G0T 1K0
Tél: 418-233-2119; *Téléc:* 418-233-3771
Membre(s) du bureau directeur:
Liliane Larouche, Personne responsable

Estrie
#100, 2630, rue King ouest, Sherbrooke QC J1J 2H1
Tél: 819-562-7942; *Téléc:* 819-564-0690
Membre(s) du bureau directeur:
Manon Thibodeau, Directrice régionale

La Capitale
#261, 4715, av des Replats, Québec QC G2J 1B8
Tél: 418-682-6387; *Téléc:* 418-682-8214
Membre(s) du bureau directeur:
Jocelyn Thémens, Directeur régional

Laval/Laurentides/Lanaudière
Tour A, #410, 1600, boul Saint-Martin est, Laval QC H7G 4R8
Tél: 450-669-6909; *Téléc:* 450-669-8987
Membre(s) du bureau directeur:
Carol Pincox, Directrice régionale

Mauricie/Centre du Québec
137, rue Radisson, Trois-Rivières QC G9A 2C5
Tél: 819-375-9565; *Téléc:* 819-375-0233

Ouest de Montréal
#18, 795, av Carson, Dorval QC H9S 1L7
Tél: 514-636-4599; *Téléc:* 514-636-8576
Membre(s) du bureau directeur:
Dalia Solo, Directrice régionale

Outaouais
#007, 109, rue Wright, Gatineau QC J8X 2G7
Tél: 819-771-8595; *Téléc:* 819-771-7070
Membre(s) du bureau directeur:
Gabrielle Ouzilleau, Directrice régionale

Rive-Sud/Montérégie
#200, 1194, ch de Chambly, Longueuil QC J4J 2W6
Tél: 450-442-6387; *Téléc:* 450-442-3329
Membre(s) du bureau directeur:
Hélène Gagné, Directrice régionale

Saguenay/Lac Saint-Jean
#251, 152, rue Racine est, Chicoutimi QC G7H 1R8
Tél: 418-543-8959; *Téléc:* 418-543-5872
Membre(s) du bureau directeur:
Martine Paradis, Directrice régionale

SASKATCHEWAN

**Heart & Stroke Foundation of Saskatchewan (HSFS) /
Fondation des maladies du coeur de la Saskatchewan**
#26, 1738 Quebec Ave., Saskatoon SK S7K 1V9
Fax: 306-664-4016
Toll-Free: 888-473-4636
www.linkedin.com/company/heart-and-stroke-foundation-saskatchewan
www.youtube.com/saskheart
Overview: A medium-sized provincial charitable organization founded in 1956 overseen by Heart & Stroke Foundation of Canada
Mission: To eliminate & reduce the impact of heart disease & stroke; To advance research, promote healthy living, & advocates a healthy public policy
Chief Officer(s):
Dale Oughton, Director, Development

Local Associations

QUÉBEC

Association des accidentés cérébro-vasculaires et traumatisés crâniens de l'Estrie (ACTE)
68, boul Jacques-Cartier Nord, Sherbrooke QC J1J 2Z8
Tél: 819-821-2799; *Téléc:* 819-821-4599
Courriel: info@acteestrie.com
www.acteestrie.com
www.facebook.com/ACTEEstrie
Aperçu: *Dimension:* petite; *Envergure:* locale; fondée en 1984
Mission: Pour aider les personnes de la région de l'Estrie du Québec qui ont subi un accident vasculaire cérébral ou un traumatisme crânien; regrouper et soutenir les personnes victimes d'AVC et de traumatisme craniocérébral
Membre de: Regroupement des associations de personnes traumatisées craniocérébrales du Québec / Coalition of Associations of Craniocerebral Trauma in Quebec; Regroupement des associations de personnes aphasiques du Québec
Membre(s) du bureau directeur:
Peter Nieman, Directeur général, 819-821-2799
peter.nieman@acteestrie.com
Publications:
• L'Actif [publication de Association des accidentés cérébro-vasculaires et traumatisés crâniens de l'Estrie]
Type: Journal; *ISSN:* 1488-4453
Profile: Journal inspiré par les membres de l'ACTE

Association des neurotraumatisés de l'Outaouais (ANO)
#1, 115 boul Sacré-Coeur, Gatineau QC J8X 1C5
Tél: 819-770-8804; *Téléc:* 819-770-5863
Courriel: ano@ano.ca
www.ano.ca
www.facebook.com/ano.ca
Aperçu: *Dimension:* petite; *Envergure:* locale; fondée en 1990
Mission: Pour aider les personnes dans la région québécoise de l'Outaouais qui ont subi un traumatisme crânien ou un AVC
Membre de: Regroupement des associations de personnes traumatisées craniocérébrals du Québec; Regroupement des associations de personnes handicapées de l'Outaouais; CDC Rond Point
Membre(s) du bureau directeur:
Julie Larochelle, Présidente
Georgette Lachance, Vice-présidente
Servane Chesnais, Secrétaire
Raphaëlle Robidoux, Trésorière
Publications:
• Le Mieux Etre [publication d'Association des neurotraumatisés de l'Outaouais]
Type: Newsletter; *Frequency:* 3 pa
Profile: Information sur les services de santé et services sociaux et loisirs pour les membres de l'Association des neurotraumatisés de l'Outaouais

Association des personnes accidentées cérébro-vasculaires, aphasiques et traumatisées crânio-cérébrales du Bas-Saint-Laurent (ACVA-TCC du BSL)
391, boul Jessop, Rimouski QC G5L 1M9
Tél: 418-723-2345
Ligne sans frais: 888-302-2282
Courriel: acvatcc@globetrotter.net
www.acvatcc.ca
www.facebook.com/pages/ACVA-TCC-du-Bas-Saint-Laurent/61441702
8571908
Aperçu: *Dimension:* petite; *Envergure:* locale; fondée en 1991
Mission: Pour soutenir les personnes dans la région du Bas-Saint-Laurent qui ont été touchés par une lésion cérébrale, accident vasculaire cérébral, ou d'aphasie.
Membre de: Regroupement des associations de personnes traumatisées craniocérébrales du Québec / Coalition of Associations of Craniocerebral Trauma in Quebec
Membre(s) du bureau directeur:
Mathieu Lajoie, Directeur

Association des TCC (le traumatisme cranio-cérébral) et ACV (un accident vasculaire cérébral) de la Gaspésie et des Iles-de-la-Madeleine Inc.

CP 308, Maria QC G0C 1Y0

Tél: 418-759-5120; *Téléc:* 418-759-8188
Ligne sans frais: 888-278-2280
Courriel: tccacv@globetrotter.net
www.tccacvgim.org

Nom précédent: Association des personnes traumatisées cranio-cérébrales de la Gaspésie et des Iles-de-la-Madeleine inc.
Aperçu: *Dimension:* petite; *Envergure:* locale; fondée en 1993
Mission: Pour informer et aider les personnes cranio-cérébral, traumatisme et leurs familles, en Gaspésie et les Iles de la Madeleine
Membre de: Regroupement des associations de personnes traumatisées craniocérébrales du Québec / Coalition of Associations of Craniocerebral Trauma in Quebec
Publications:
• La Bulle
Type: Newsletter; *Frequency:* Quarterly
Profile: Association activities

Association des traumatisés cranio-cérébraux des deux rives (Québec-Chaudière-Appalaches)

Territoire de Québec et de Chaudiere-Appalaches, 14, rue Saint-Amand, Loretteville QC G2A 2K9

Tél: 418-842-8421; *Téléc:* 418-842-9616
Ligne sans frais: 866-844-8421
Courriel: tcc2rives@oricom.ca
www.tcc2rives.qc.ca

Aperçu: *Dimension:* petite; *Envergure:* locale; fondée en 1989
Mission: Pour aider les victimes, les parents, les amis, et les professionnels touchés par une lésion cérébrale traumatique dans la région Chaudière-Appalaches du Québec.
Membre de: Regroupement des associations de personnes traumatisées craniocérébrales du Québec / Coalition of Associations of Craniocerebral Trauma in Quebec
Publications:
• L'En Tête
Type: Newspaper; *Frequency:* Quarterly
Profile: Information about the association's services

Association des traumatisés cranio-cérébraux Mauricie-Centre-du-Québec (ATCC)

39, rue Bellerive, Trois-Rivières QC G8T 6J4

Tél: 819-372-4993
Courriel: atcc@assotcc.org
www.associationtcc.org
www.facebook.com/381058281920939

Aperçu: *Dimension:* petite; *Envergure:* locale
Mission: Pour soutenir les personnes touchées par une lésion cérébrale traumatique en Mauricie-Centre-du-Québec
Membre de: Regroupement des associations de personnes traumatisées craniocérébrales du Québec / Coalition of Associations of Craniocerebral Trauma in Quebec

National Libraries

March of Dimes Canada

10 Overlea Blvd., Toronto, ON M4H 1A4

Tel: 416-425-3463; *Fax:* 416-425-1920
Toll-Free: 800-263-3463
www.marchofdimes.ca
Social Media: www.youtube.com/user/marchofdimescda;
twitter.com/modcanada; www.facebook.com/MarchofDimesCanada
Collection: Downloadable information package; The Phoenix Newsletter; links to other resources
Andria Spindel, President & CEO

Provincial Libraries

Heart & Stroke Foundation of Alberta, NWT & Nunavut

#100, 119 - 14th St. NW, Calgary, AB T2N 1Z6

Tel: 403-264-5549; *Fax:* 403-237-0803
Toll-Free: 888-473-4636
www.heartandstroke.ca
Social Media: www.youtube.com/heartandstrokefdn;
twitter.com/TheHSF; www.facebook.com/heartandstroke
Collection: Research; Statistics; Videos; Printed literature
Donna Hastings, CEO

Heart & Stroke Foundation of BC & Yukon

#200, 1212 West Broadway, Vancouver, BC V6H 3V2

Tel: 778-372-8000; *Fax:* 604-736-8732
www.heartandstroke.ca

Heart & Stroke Foundation of Nova Scotia

Park Lane, Mall Level 3, 5657 Spring Garden Rd., Halifax, NS B3J 3R4

Tel: 902-423-7530; *Fax:* 902-492-1464
Toll-Free: 800-423-4432
www.heartandstroke.ca
Social Media: twitter.com/TheHSF

Heart & Stroke Foundation of Prince Edward Island

180 Kent St., Charlottetown, PE C1A 7K4

Tel: 902-892-7441; *Fax:* 902-368-7068
www.heartandstroke.ca

Stroke Recovery Association of Barrie & District

#111, 80 Bradford St., Barrie, ON L4N 6S7

Tel: 705-737-9202
info@strokerecoverybarrie.com
www.strokerecoverybarrie.com

Local Hospitals & Health Centres

BRITISH COLUMBIA

KELOWNA: Kelowna TIA Clinic
Affiliated with: Interior Health Authority
2251 Pandosy St., Kelowna, BC V1Y 1T1

Tel: 250-980-1392
www.interiorhealth.ca

Note: Services for identifying & treating transient ischemic attack (TIA)

ONTARIO

TORONTO: Apotex Centre, Jewish Home for the Aged & The Louis & Leah Posluns Centre for Stroke & Cognition
3560 Bathurst St., Toronto, ON M6A 2E1

Tel: 416-785-2500
www.baycrest.org

Number of Beds: 472 beds
Note: Care is offered to adults 65 years of age & older within the context of orthodox Jewish traditions.

TORONTO: Sunnybrook Health Sciences Centre - St. John's Rehab
Affiliated with: Toronto Central Local Health Integration Network
285 Cummer Ave., Toronto, ON M2M 2G1

Tel: 416-226-6780 *Fax:* 416-226-6265
www.sunnybrook.ca

Number of Beds: 160 beds
Note: Provides specialized rehabilitation services & care in burn injuries, organ transplant rehabilitation, cancer, cardiovascular surgery, strokes & other neurological conditions, traumatic injuries & complex medical conditions. Teaching site for the University of Toronto & a research facility. A multicultural & multifaith environment dedicated to the values of care of the Sisters of St. John the Divine.
Barry A. McLellan, President & CEO

Substance Abuse and Dependence

Substance abuse is a broad term that refers to any illegal, dangerous or destructive use of some substance. This use may be legal (binge drinking by an adult) or illegal (smoking marijuana). Some abused substances include marijuana, heroin, prescription painkillers and tranquilizers, stimulants such as amphetamines and cocaine and hallucinogens such as LSD. Alcohol, a drug that is widely available and socially approved, is the most abused of all substances, and alcohol addiction is a pervasive mental disorder. Substance dependence refers to a state of strong compulsion to use the substance, in many cases accompanied by physical withdrawal symptoms if the substance is not regularly available.

Substance abuse and addictive disorders are among the most destructive mental disorders in Canada today, contributing to a host of medical and social problems including job loss, arrest, family breakup, automobile and other accidents, birth defects (fetal alcohol syndrome), direct toxic effects (cirrhosis of the liver from alcohol) and infections (HIV or hepatitis B from sharing needles). Substance abuse, unless it occurs in extremely isolated persons, greatly affects family members and loved ones. Family members often deny the reality of the abuse, and may help, or enable, the abuser to cover up the problem and avoid its consequences.

Cause
The cause of substance abuse is very complex, and involves an interplay between the individual's behavioural choices, his or her genetic background and the past and present social environment. Like all addictive disorders, substance abuse is characterized by repeated use despite repeated adverse consequences, and by physical and psychological craving. Scientific understanding of how abused substances work on the body and the brain, and the underlying physiology of addiction, has advanced remarkably in recent years. With the help of brain imaging and other techniques, we can now see that these disorders are associated with structural changes in the brain. Childhood sexual abuse is strongly associated with substance dependence. Some substance abusers also have a definable psychiatric disorder such as depression or schizophrenia; treatment of these dual-disorder patients is especially challenging.

Symptoms
People with a substance abuse problem are physically and psychologically dependent on a certain drug or alcohol. Signs of physical dependence include needing an increased amount of the substance to obtain the same effect and suffering withdrawal symptoms such as headaches, diarrhea, shaking, anxiety and depression when the substance is stopped. Signs of psychological dependence include cravings for the substance and a willingness to go to any length to get the desired substance.

There are many complications associated with substance abuse and dependence. Typically, accidents, injuries and suicide accompany alcohol dependence. Absenteeism, low work productivity and injuries on the job are often caused by alcohol dependence. Alcohol is also the most common cause of preventable birth defects, including fetal alcohol syndrome. Alcohol abuse can severely damage organ systems including the brain, the liver, the heart and the digestive tract.

Many individuals with substance or alcohol-use disorders take more than one substance and suffer from other mental symptoms and disorders as well. Individuals with a wide variety of mental disorders sometimes abuse drugs as an attempt to medicate themselves. Forty-seven percent of people with schizophrenia have drug abuse disorders. People with antisocial personality disorder often abuse substances, including amphetamines such as cocaine. Substance-related disorders can also lead to other mental disorders. Use of the synthetic hallucinogen ecstasy is as-

sociated with acute and paranoid psychoses, and the prolonged use of cocaine (a stimulant) can lead to paranoid psychosis with violent behaviour. Substance use and the effects on an individual's employment and relationships, as well as legal difficulties, can precipitate anxiety and mood disorders. Intravenous substance abuse is associated with a high risk of HIV infections and other medical complications. Chronic drug and alcohol abuse can lead to difficulty in memory and problem solving, and impaired sexual functioning.

Prevalence
Problematic substance abuse affects approximately 11 percent of Canadians. Alcohol dependence and abuse are among the most prevalent mental disorders in the general population. Canadian statistics reveal that about 4 percent of the population over the age of 15 is dependent on alcohol. Substance-related disorders are more common among males than females. About 14 percent of Canadians are estimated to use cannabis (marijuana) and around 279,000 Canadians have reported injection drug use at some point in their life. Those between the ages of 15 and 24 have a high prevalence for abuse of all substances. Early adolescent drug and alcohol use is associated with a slight but significant decline in intellectual abilities. About 4 percent of 15- to 24-year-olds in Canada have used amphetamines; 6 percent have used cocaine/crack; 4 percent have used hallucinogens like LSD and 4 percent have used drugs like ecstasy. Thirty-seven percent of youth in Canada in this age group have reported binge drinking, and of those who do, 12 percent have engaged in this behaviour at least once a week.

Treatment Options
Diagnosis of substance abuse problems is usually based on a detailed medical history and physical exam. Blood and urine tests can indicate substance use, but cannot be used to confirm substance abuse. Criteria for abuse, dependence, tolerance and withdrawal, outlined in the Diagnostic and Statistical Manual of Mental Disorders, follow; they are often used to confirm a diagnosis.

Alcohol and substance abuse symptoms include repeated use resulting in inability to fulfill fundamental obligations at work, school, or home (repeated absences, poor work performance, family neglect); repeated use, resulting in dangerous situation (driving or operating a machine while impaired); repeated alcohol and substance-related legal problems (arrests for disorderly conduct); continued use despite persistent social or interpersonal problems, worsened by the effects of substance abuse.

Alcohol and substance dependence problems include alcohol or substance is often taken in greater amounts or for a longer period than intended; repeated wish or unsuccessful attempts to control use; a great deal of time is taken to get and use alcohol or substance or to recover from its effects; important social, work or recreational activities are missed because of use; use continues in spite of the person knowing about the persistent psychological or physical problems it causes (depression induced by cocaine or continued drinking).

Tolerance symptoms include a need for increased amounts of alcohol or the substance to achieve desired effect; diminished effects with continued use of the same amount of alcohol or substance. Alcohol abuse can occur without tolerance, as in binge drinking, a particular problem for young people on college campuses and elsewhere.

Withdrawal symptoms include characteristic withdrawal syndrome, prolonged taking and then stopping/reducing alcohol or substance causing physical and mental symptoms; same or a related substance is taken to avoid/alleviate the withdrawal symptoms.

There is no quick and universally effective treatment for substance abuse.

Diagnosis and treatment of alcohol dependence has improved as understanding of the physiology of addiction has advanced. But successful treatment still relies on acceptance by the patient that he or she has an illness, as well as support from other people who have gone through the same process. For this reason, medical treatment is most often successful when it is accompanied by involvement in a support group, for both the patient and family members; these may include Alcoholics Anonymous (AA) and Al-Anon, 12-step spiritual programs that have gained popularity over the years. Local groups can be found in almost every community and are listed in the phone book and on the internet. Recently, similar groups have formed that do not emphasize spirituality, as these do, but rely on group support for sobriety.

There is a growing controversy over the need for people who have had an alcohol problem to abstain completely from alcohol for the rest of their lives, one of the central beliefs of AA. Some researchers and clinicians are arguing that it is possible for some former alcoholics to resume controlled social drinking. AA, in the past, has discouraged members from using psychotropic medications; this is often counterproductive. Many alcohol treatment programs have been developed with men's needs and personalities in mind. Successful programs for women are less confrontational than men's programs and include arrangements for child care.

Treatment for alcoholism has been hospital-based in the past, but has increasingly moved to the outpatient setting. Hospital treatment is necessary for withdrawal when alcohol use has been heavy and steady. Delirium tremens, a consequence of very heavy drinking, can be fatal.

Medical treatment of alcohol dependence may include Anabuse, a drug that makes an individual violently ill if alcohol is used. Group or hospital-based treatment may also be useful, and psychotherapy can help the patient more effectively deal with underlying conflicts and interpersonal problems.

Denial of illness and ambivalence about abstinence can make treatment of drug abuse difficult. A patient's cravings can be overwhelmingly intense, and the individual's social circle is often composed of other substance abusers, making it hard for the individual to maintain relationships while becoming or remaining abstinent—the goal in treatment. A wide range of intervention may be needed, including a general assessment of the drug abuse, and evaluation of medical, social and psychological problems. It is best to involve partner, family and friends to help the person gain new understanding of the problem and to make the general assessment complete. An explicit treatment plan should be worked out with the person (and partner/family/friends if appropriate) with concrete goals for which the person takes responsibility, which should include not only stopping substance use, but dealing with associated problems concerning health, personal relationships and work.

Severe withdrawal symptoms may require hospitalization. Another option is maintenance therapy, in which a drug is prescribed that has a slower action and is less addictive than the street drug, for example, methadone vs. heroin. Therapy is added to help with withdrawal and problems associated with drug use. Cognitive-behavioural therapy can help increase the substance abuser's personal skills resulting in less dependency on drugs and the drug

culture. Prescription drugs and relaxation techniques can help with withdrawal symptoms. Rehabilitation in a therapeutic community is another option.

Dropout during treatment and relapse after initial success are common, but many people do achieve life-long cures with abstinence from further substance abuse.

National Associations

Adult Children of Alcoholics (ACA)
#505, 5863 Leslie St., Toronto ON M2H 1J8

Tel: 416-631-3614
e-mail: acatoronto@hotmail.com
www.acatoronto.org

Overview: A small national organization
Mission: To improve members' lives through the 12 step program

Al-Anon Family Groups (Canada), Inc. / Groupe familiaux Al-Anon
#900, 275 Slater St., Ottawa ON K1P 5H9

Tel: 613-723-8484
e-mail: afgwso@al-anon.org
www.al-anon.org
www.facebook.com/AlAnonFamilyGroupsWSO
twitter.com/AlAnon_WSO

Also Known As: AL-ANON/ALATEEN
Overview: A medium-sized national charitable organization founded in 1951
Mission: To provide support for friends & family members of alcoholics

Alcoholics Anonymous (GTA Intergroup) (AA)
#202, 234 Eglinton Ave. East, Toronto ON M4P 1K5
Tel: 416-487-5591; *Fax:* 416-487-5855
Toll-Free: 877-404-5591; *TTY:* 866-831-4657
e-mail: office@aatoronto.org
aatoronto.org

Overview: A large national charitable organization founded in 1947
Mission: Fellowship of men & women who share their experience, strength & hope with each other so that they may solve their common problem & help others recover from alcoholism; the primary purpose is to stay sober & help other alcoholics to achieve sobriety
Publications:
• Better Times [a publication of Alcoholics Anonymous (GTA Intergroup)]
Type: Newsletter; *Frequency:* Monthly

Abbotsford - Intergroup Committee
#17, 1961 Eagle St., Abbotsford BC V2S 3A7
Crisis Hot-Line: 604-850-0811
e-mail: abbotsfordintrgrp@hotmail.com
www.theabbotsfordintergroup-aa.org

Barrie - Barrie & Area Intergroup
#622, 80 Bradford St., Barrie ON L4N 6S7
Tel: 705-725-8682
e-mail: barrieaa@barrieaa.com
www.barrieaa.com

Calgary - Central Service Office
#2, 4015 - 1st St. SE, Calgary AB T2G 4X7
Tel: 403-777-1212; *Fax:* 403-287-6540
e-mail: centraloffice@telus.net
www.calgaryaa.org

Edmonton - AA Central Office
#205, 10544 - 114 St. NW, Edmonton AB T5H 3J7
Tel: 780-424-5900
www.edmontonaa.org

Guelph - Central West District 3
PO Box 210, #17A, 218 Silvercreek Pkwy. North, Guelph ON N1H 8E8
Tel: 519-836-1522
www.centralwest2district3aa.org

Halifax Central Office

PO Box 31338, Halifax NS B3K 5Z1
Tel: 902-461-1119
e-mail: help.aahalifax@gmail.com
www.aahalifax.org

Hamilton - Central Office
#205, 627 Main St. East, Hamilton ON L8M 1J5
Tel: 905-522-8399; *Fax:* 905-522-1946
e-mail: info@aahamilton.org
www.aahamilton.org

London - London Area Intergroup
201 Consortium Crt., London ON
Tel: 519-438-9006
www.aalondon.org

Montréal - Intergroupe de Montréal
3920, rue Rachel est, Montréal QC H1X 1Z3
Tel: 514-374-3688; *Fax:* 514-374-2250
e-mail: region87@aa-quebec.org
aa87.org

Oshawa - Lakeshore Intergroup
200 Thornton Rd. North, Oshawa ON L1J 6T8
Tel: 905-728-1020
e-mail: aa.oshawa@live.com
www.aaoshawa.org

Ottawa - Ottawa Area Intergroup
#108, 211 Bronson Ave., Ottawa ON K1R 6H5
Tel: 613-237-6000
www.ottawaaa.org

Peterborough - Kawartha District Intergroup
625 Cameron St., Peterborough ON K9J 3Z9
Tel: 705-745-6111
e-mail: district86aa@hotmail.com
www.peterboroughaa.org

Prince Edward Island - Green Acres Intergroup
5 Summer St., Summerside PE C1N 3H3
Tel: 902-436-7721

Québec - Northeast Area of Québec Central Office
14, rue St-Amand, Québec QC G2A 2K9
Tel: 418-915-2929; *Fax:* 418-915-4959
e-mail: region89@aa-quebec.org
aa-quebec.org/region89

Québec - Northwest Area of Québec Central Office
PO Box 361, Saint-Jérôme QC J7Z 5V2
Tel: 450-560-3902; *Fax:* 450-560-3903
e-mail: region@aa90.org
www.aa90.org

Regina - Central Office
#107, 845 Broad St., Regina SK S4R 8G9
Tel: 306-545-9300
e-mail: a.a@sasktel.net
www.aaregina.com

St Catharines - Niagara District Intergroup
Tel: 905-682-2140
Toll-Free: 866-311-9042
e-mail: info@aaniagara.org
www.aaniagara.org

St. John's - Central Office
#117, 183 Kenmount Rd., St. John's NL A1B 3P9
Tel: 709-579-6091
Toll-Free: 888-579-5215
e-mail: sjintergroup@nl.rogers.com
www.aastjohns.nf.net

Saskatoon - Saskatoon Central Office
#515, 245 - 3rd Ave. South, Saskatoon SK S7K 1M4
Tel: 306-665-6727; *Fax:* 306-665-6753
e-mail: aasaskatoon@sasktel.net
www.aasaskatoon.org

Trenton - District 30 Quinte West
Toll-Free: 866-951-3711
www.quintewestaa.org

Vancouver - Greater Vancouver Intergroup Society

3457 Kingsway, Vancouver BC V5R 5L5
Tel: 604-434-3933; *Fax:* 604-434-2553
e-mail: staff@vancouveraa.ca
www.vancouveraa.ca

Victoria - AA Central Office
#8, 2020 Douglas St., Victoria BC V8T 4L1
Tel: 250-383-0415; *Fax:* 250-383-0417; *Crisis Hot-Line:* 250-383-7744
e-mail: vicintgpco@shaw.ca
www.aavictoria.ca

Whitehorse - Whitehorse Intergroup
c/o BC/Yukon Area 79, PO Box 42114, Vancouver BC V5S 4R5
Tel: 604-435-2181
e-mail: info@bcyukonaa.org
www.bcyukonaa.org

Winnipeg - Manitoba Central Office
1856 Portage Ave., Winnipeg MB R3J 0G9
Tel: 204-942-0126
Toll-Free: 877-942-0126
e-mail: aambco@mts.net
www.aamanitoba.org

Canadian Addiction Counsellors Certification Federation (CACCF) / Fédération canadienne d'agrément des conseillers en toxicomanie
81 Bruce St., #C, Kitchener ON N2B 1Y7
Tel: 519-772-0533; *Fax:* 519-772-0535
Toll-Free: 866-624-1911
e-mail: info@caccf.ca
canadianaddictioncounsellors.org
www.linkedin.com/company/canadian-addiction-counsellors-certificatio
n-
www.facebook.com/CACCF
twitter.com/CACCF_Canada
Previous Name: Canadian Addiction Counsellors Certification Board
Overview: A medium-sized national organization
Mission: To offer credible certifications to all addiction specific counsellors in Canada; To promote & monitor the competency of addiction specific counsellors in Canada
Member of: International Certification & Reciprocity Consortium / Alcohol & Other Drug Abuse (IC&RC/AODA)
Chief Officer(s):
Jeff Wilbee, Executive Director
  jeff@caccf.ca
Tom Gabriel, President
Publications:
• The Beacon
Type: Newsletter; *Frequency:* Semiannually

Canadian Assembly of Narcotics Anonymous (CANA)
PO Box 812, Stn. Edmonton Main, Edmonton AB T5J 2L4
www.canaacna.org
Previous Name: Narcotics Anonymous
Overview: A small national organization founded in 1989
Mission: To help addicts who suffer from the disease of addiction

British Columbia Region
PO Box 1695, Stn. A, Vancouver BC V6C 2P7
Tel: 604-873-1018
www.bcrna.ca

Canada Atlantic Region
PO Box 26025, 407 Westmorland Rd., Saint John NB E2J 4M3
Toll-Free: 800-564-0228
e-mail: contact.us@carna.ca
www.carna.ca

Golden Triangle Area
#311, 23-500 Fairway Rd. South, Kitchener ON N2C 1X3
Tel: 519-651-1121
Toll-Free: 866-311-1611
www.gtascna.org

Hamilton Area
PO Box 57067, Stn. Jackson, 2 King St. West, Hamilton ON L8P 4W9
Tel: 905-522-0332; *Crisis Hot-Line:* 888-811-3887
www.nahamilton.org

Narcotiques Anonymes
5496 rue Notre-Dame est, Montréal QC H1N 2C4
Ligne sans frais: 855-544-6362
Courriel: info@naquebec.org
www.naquebec.org

Ontario Region
PO Box 5939, Stn. A, Toronto ON M5W 1P3
www.orscna.org

Canadian Centre on Substance Abuse (CCSA) / Centre canadien de lutte contre l'alcoolisme et les toxicomanies (CCLAT)
#300, 75 Albert St., Ottawa ON K1P 5E7
Tel: 613-235-4048; *Fax:* 613-235-8101
e-mail: info@ccsa.ca
www.ccsa.ca
www.linkedin.com/company/canadian-centre-on-substance-abuse-ccsa
twitter.com/CCSAcanada
www.youtube.com/user/CCSACCLAT
Overview: A medium-sized national charitable organization founded in 1988
Mission: To minimize the harm associated with addictions, including substance abuse & problem gambling
Chief Officer(s):
Rita Notarandrea, CEO
Jody Brian, Director, Public Affairs & Communications
Amy Porath-Waller, Interim Director, Research & Policy
Publications:
• Action News [a publication of the Canadian Centre on Substance Abuse]
Type: Newsletter; *Frequency:* Quarterly; *Editor:* Richard Garlick; *ISSN:* 1701-4522
Profile: Current events related to substance abuse
• Canadian Centre on Substance Abuse Annual Report
Type: Yearbook; *Frequency:* Annually
• Directory of Fetal Alcohol Spectrum Disorder (FASD) Information & Support Services in Canada
Type: Directory; *ISSN:* 1715-4197
Profile: Listings of organizations & individuals that provide an FASD related service in Canada

The Canadian Don't Do Drugs Society
PO Box 1053, 7B Pleasant Blvd., Toronto ON M4T 1K2
Tel: 416-923-3779; *Fax:* 416-923-0083
Toll-Free: 800-883-7761
www.skddd.org
www.linkedin.com/company/2802976?trk
www.facebook.com/pages/Smart-Kids-Dont-Do-Drugs/3206626680261
84
twitter.com/SKDDD_SmartKidz
www.youtube.com/user/TheSmartkidz
Also Known As: Smart Kids Don't Do Drugs
Overview: A small national charitable organization founded in 1994
Mission: To aide children & parents in the fight against the ravages of drugs in our society
Chief Officer(s):
Robert O'Reilly, Executive Director

Canadian Harm Reduction Network
#1904, 666 Spadina Ave., Toronto ON M5S 2H8
Tel: 416-928-0279; *Fax:* 416-966-9512
Toll-Free: 800-728-1293
e-mail: noharm@canadianharmreduction.com
www.canadianharmreduction.com
www.facebook.com/noharmcanada
twitter.com/noharmcanada
youtube.com/noharmcanada
Overview: A small national organization
Mission: To reduce the social, health & economic harms associated with drugs & drug policies
Affiliation(s): Drug Policy Alliance

Canadian Society of Addiction Medicine (CSAM) / La Société Medicale Canadienne sur l'Addiction (SMCA)
1444 40th St. NW, Calgary AB T3C 1W7
Tel: 403-246-9393
e-mail: admin@csam-smca.org
www.csam-smca.org
www.linkedin.com/in/csam-smca
www.facebook.com/canadiansocietyofaddictionmedicine
twitter.com/csam_smca
Overview: A small national organization founded in 1989
Mission: To foster & promote medical sciences & clinical practice in the field of substance use disorders in Canada; To establish & promote standards of clinical practice
Affiliation(s): The International Society of Addiction Medicine
Chief Officer(s):
Paul Sobey, President
Publications:
• The Canadian Journal of Addiction [a publication of the Canadian Society of Addiction Medicine]
Type: Journal; *Editor:* Marilyn Dorozio
Profile: Information & scientific materials pertaining to the addiction medicine field
• CSAM [Canadian Society of Addiction Medicine] Bulletin
Type: Newsletter; *Frequency:* 3 pa
Profile: CSAM conferences, reports, membership information, research updates, clinical experiences, & continuing education opportunities related to addiction medicine

Canadian Society of Pharmacology & Therapeutics (CSPT) / Société de pharmacologie du Canada
e-mail: info@pharmacologycanada.org
www.pharmacologycanada.org
Previous Name: Pharmacological Society of Canada; Canadian Society for Clinical Pharmacology
Overview: A medium-sized national organization founded in 1974 overseen by Canadian Federation of Biological Societies
Mission: To promote research & education in the disciplines of pharmacology & experimental therapeutics
Chief Officer(s):
Emanuel Escher, President
Michael Rieder, Vice-President
Gerhard Multhaup, Treasurer
Publications:
• The Canadian Journal of Clinical Pharmacology / Journal canadien de pharmacologie clinique
Type: Journal; *ISSN:* 1710-6222
Profile: Original research papers, case reports, & review articles about clinical pharmacology, drugs, & therapeutics
• Canadian Journal of Physiology & Pharmacology
Type: Journal; *Frequency:* Monthly; *Editor:* Ghassan Bkaily; *ISSN:* 1205-7541
Profile: Current research in pharmacology, physiology, toxicology, & nutrition by scientists & experts, plus award lectures & symposium reviews
• Canadian Society of Pharmacology & Therapeutics Newsletter
Type: Newsletter; *Frequency:* Semiannually; *Price:* Free with membership in the Canadian Society of Pharmacology & Therapeutics
Profile: Societal business plus significant events

Council on Drug Abuse (CODA)
#120, 215 Spadina Ave., Toronto ON M5T 2C7
Tel: 416-763-1491
e-mail: info@drugabuse.ca
www.drugabuse.ca
twitter.com/yacers
Overview: A small national charitable organization founded in 1969
Mission: To prevent & reduce substance abuse, primarily among youth, by sponsoring education programs in schools
Chief Officer(s):
Lorraine Patterson, Chair

National Native Addictions Partnership Foundation (NNAPF) / Fondation autochtone nationale de partenariat pour la lutte contre les dépendances
PO Box 183, Muskoday SK S0J 3H0

Tel: 306-763-4714; Fax: 306-763-5993
Toll-Free: 866-763-4714
e-mail: info@nnapf.org
www.nnapf.org
www.facebook.com/423836911040446
twitter.com/NNAPF

Overview: A small national organization founded in 1998
Mission: To advocate, develop, facilitate, & monitor strategies designed to continuously upgrade & enhance the quality of ideas, information, program methodologies, financial alliociations & skills of service providers comprising the program
Chief Officer(s):
Austin Bear, President
Janice Nicotine, Vice-President

Opération Nez rouge / Operation Red Nose
Maison Couillard, Université Laval, 2539, rue Marie-Fitzbach, Québec QC G1V 0A6

Tél: 418-653-1492; Téléc: 418-653-3315
Ligne sans frais: 800-463-7222
Courriel: info@operationnezrouge.com
www.operationnezrouge.com
www.facebook.com/OperationNezrouge
twitter.com/ORNose
www.youtube.com/user/OperationNezrouge

Aperçu: Dimension: grande; Envergure: nationale; fondée en 1984
Mission: Service de chauffeur privé gratuit & bénévole offert pendant la période des Fêtes à tout automobiliste qui a consommé de l'alcool, our qui ne se sent pas en état de conduire son véhicule
Membre de: Réseau de l'action bénévole du Québec; Chambre de commerce et d'industrie de la ville de Québec
Membre(s) du bureau directeur:
Jean-Philippe Giroux, Directeur général
  jpgiroux@operationnezrouge.com
Monique Mailhot, Directrice, Administration et finances
  mmailhot@operationnezrouge.com

Provincial Associations

ALBERTA

Lieutenant Governor's Circle on Mental Health & Addiction
#208, 14925 - 111th Ave., Edmonton AB T5M 2P6

Tel: 780-453-2201
e-mail: execdir@lgcirclealberta.ca
www.lgcircle.ca
www.facebook.com/LGCircle

Overview: A small provincial organization
Chief Officer(s):
Sol Rolingher, Chair

MANITOBA

Addictions Foundation of Manitoba (AFM) / Fondation manitobaine de lutte contre les dépendances
1031 Portage Ave., Winnipeg MB R3G 0R8

Tel: 204-944-6236; Fax: 204-944-7082
Toll-Free: 866-638-2561
e-mail: execoff@afm.mb.ca
afm.mb.ca

Overview: A medium-sized provincial organization founded in 1956
Mission: To be a sensitive, caring, learning organization dedicated to continuously improving our services related to addiction & to collaborate with community members in providing a holistic approach, resulting in an improved quality of life for Manitobans; provides prevention, education & treatment programs related to addictions to individuals & communities; conducts research into the negative effects of addictions
Chief Officer(s):
Don McCaskill, Chair
Yvonne Block, CEO

Northern Region Office

Polaris Place, 90 Princeton Dr., Thompson MB R8N 0L3
Tel: 204-677-7300; Fax: 204-677-7328
Toll-Free: 866-291-7774
e-mail: northreg@afm.mb.ca

Western Region Office
Parkwood Centre, 510 Frederick St., Brandon MB R7A 6Z4
Tel: 204-729-3838; Fax: 204-729-3844
Toll-Free: 866-767-3838
e-mail: parkwood@afm.mb.ca

Winnipeg Region Office
1031 Portage Ave., Winnipeg MB R3G 0R8
Tel: 204-944-6200; Fax: 204-786-7768
Toll-Free: 866-638-2561
e-mail: wpgreg@afm.mb.ca

Native Addictions Council of Manitoba (NACM)
160 Salter St., Winnipeg MB R2W 4K1

Tel: 204-586-8395; Fax: 204-589-3921
e-mail: info@nacm.ca
www.mts.net/~nacm/

Also Known As: Pritchard House
Overview: A small provincial charitable organization founded in 1972
Mission: To provide traditional holistic healing services to First Peoples through treatment of addictions; each member of First Peoples has the right to wellness.

ONTARIO

Addictions & Mental Health Ontario
#104, 970 Lawrence Ave. West, Toronto ON M6A 2B6

Tel: 416-490-8900; Fax: 866-295-6394
e-mail: info@addictionsandmentalhealthontario.ca
www.addictionsandmentalhealthontario.ca
twitter.com/AMHont

Previous Name: Alcohol and Drug Recovery Association of Ontario
Merged from: Addictions Ontario; Ontario Federation of Community Mental Health & Addiction Programs
Overview: A small provincial charitable organization founded in 1968
Mission: To ensure that the best possible addictions treatment & recovery services are available to people throughout Ontario
Chief Officer(s):
Gail Czukar, Chief Executive Officer
  gail.czukar@addictionsandmentalhealthontario.ca

Jean Tweed Treatment Centre (JTC)
215 Evans Ave., Toronto ON M8Z 1J5

Tel: 416-255-7359; Fax: 416-255-9021
e-mail: info@jeantweed.com
www.jeantweed.com
www.facebook.com/pages/The-Jean-Tweed-Centre/213119005385114
twitter.com/jeantweedcentre

Overview: A small provincial charitable organization founded in 1983
Mission: To provide services for women with substance abuse or gambling problems & their families with a focus on children 0-6
Member of: Federation of Community Mental Health & Addictions Programs; Toronto Area Addictions Services Committee; Residential Addiction Services of Ontario
Chief Officer(s):
Nancy Bradley, Executive Director
Katherine Devlin, Chair
Erin MacRae, Vice Chair/ Treas.

Nar-Anon Family Groups of Ontario
PO Box 20046, 2900 Warden Ave., Toronto ON M1W 3Y9

Tel: 416-239-0096
Toll-Free: 877-239-0096
e-mail: info@naranonontario.com
www.naranonontario.com

Overview: A medium-sized provincial organization
Mission: To support & provide weekly meetings for those who know or have known a feeling of desperation due to the addiction problem of someone close to them

Parent Action on Drugs (PAD)
#121, 7 Hawksdale Rd., Toronto ON M3K 1W3
Tel: 416-395-4970; *Fax:* 866-591-7685
Toll-Free: 877-265-9279
e-mail: pad@parentactionondrugs.org
www.parentactionondrugs.org
www.facebook.com/pages/Parent-Action-on-Drugs-PAD/390301531674
twitter.com/PAD_Ontario
Overview: A small provincial charitable organization founded in 1983
Mission: To address issues of substance use among youth through outreach, prevention, education & parent support; enhances the capacity of parents, youth & communities to promote an environment that encourages youth to make informed choices
Member of: HC Link
Chief Officer(s):
Diane Buhler, Executive Director
pad@sympatico.ca
Publications:
• PAD Parent & COmmunity Handbook
Profile: Facts on tobacco, alcohol, cannabis and other drugs

QUÉBEC

Alcooliques Anonymes du Québec
Bureau des services de la Région 87, 3920, rue Rachel est, Montréal QC H1X 1Z3
Tél: 514-374-3688; *Télec:* 514-374-2250
www.aa-quebec.org
Aperçu: *Dimension:* petite; *Envergure:* provinciale; fondée en 1935
Mission: Demeurer abstinent et aider d'autres alcooliques à le devenir
Membre(s) du bureau directeur:
Marco L., Président
president@aa87.org

Association des intervenants en dépendance du Québec (AIDQ)
#420, 1001 boul de Maisonneuve ouest, Montréal QC H3A 3C8
Tél: 514-287-9625; *Télec:* 514-287-9649
Ligne sans frais: 877-566-9625
Courriel: info@aidq.org
www.aidq.org
Nom précédent: Association des centres de réadaptation en dépendance du Québec
Aperçu: *Dimension:* petite; *Envergure:* provinciale
Mission: Soutenir l'intervention dans le traitement des personnes aux prises avec une dépendance
Membre(s) du bureau directeur:
Lisa Massicotte, Directrice générale
lmassicotte@aidq.org

Éduc'alcool
#1000, 606, rue Cathcart, Montréal QC H3B 1K9
Tél: 514-875-7454; *Télec:* 514-875-5990
Ligne sans frais: 888-252-6651
Courriel: info@educalcool.qc.ca
www.educalcool.qc.ca
www.facebook.com/279669212081870
twitter.com/educalcool
www.youtube.com/user/deuxtroisquatrezero
Aperçu: *Dimension:* moyenne; *Envergure:* provinciale; Organisme sans but lucratif; fondée en 1989
Mission: Promouvoir la consommation équilibrée et responsable de l'alcool par des activités d'éducation, de sensibilisation et de communication; coordonner les actions de différents organismes nationaux oeuvrant dans le même but
Affliation(s): Conseil international sur les problemes de l'alcoolisme et des toxicomanies
Membre(s) du bureau directeur:
Hubert Sacy, Directeur général

Narcotiques Anonymes
Chibougamau QC
Ligne sans frais: 800-463-0162
www.naquebec.org
Aperçu: *Dimension:* petite; *Envergure:* provinciale

Local Associations
ALBERTA

Calgary Alpha House Society
203 - 15 Ave. SE, Calgary AB T2G 1G4
Tel: 403-234-7388; *Fax:* 403-705-0123
e-mail: info@alphahousecalgary.com
www.alphahousecalgary.com
www.facebook.com/AlphaHouseSociety
twitter.com/alphahouseyyc
Also Known As: Alpha House
Overview: A small local organization founded in 1981
Mission: To provide drop-in/overnight shelter & short-term detoxification for males & females with alcohol &/or drug abuse issues
Chief Officer(s):
Kathy Christiansen, Executive Director
kathy@alphahousecalgary.com

BRITISH COLUMBIA

From Grief To Action (FGTA)
c/o St. Mary's Anglican Church, 2490 West 37th Ave., Vancouver BC V6M 1P5
www.fromgrieftoaction.com
Overview: A small local charitable organization founded in 1999
Mission: To serve as a support group for those affected by drug addiction in a family member or friend; To promote the recognition of drug addiction as a health issue; To support a comprehensive continuum of care for drug users, including harm reduction, detoxification, treatment & rehabilitation; To provide educational resources on drug abuse prevention
Chief Officer(s):
Bev Gutray, Director

ONTARIO

Addiction Services of Thames Valley
#260, 200 Queens Ave., London ON N6A 1J3
Tel: 519-673-3242; *Fax:* 519-673-1022
e-mail: intake@adstv.on.ca
www.adstv.on.ca
Overview: A small local organization
Mission: Addiction remedial services in the Thames Valley area of Southwestern Ontario

Caritas Project Community Against Drugs
#1-2, 241 Hanlan Rd., Woodbridge ON L4L 3R7
Tel: 416-748-9988; *Fax:* 416-748-7341
Toll-Free: 800-201-8138
e-mail: info@caritas.ca
www.caritas.ca
www.facebook.com/pages/Caritas-School-of-Life/468788439859031
twitter.com/Caritas4Life
www.youtube.com/user/CaritasFoundation
Also Known As: Caritas
Overview: A small local organization founded in 1980
Mission: To prevent addiction through education & awareness; to provide a therapeutic community in order to rehabilitate those suffering from dependencies; to also aid people with mental health issues, behavioural problems, & family issues
Member of: Therapeutic Communities of America
Affliation(s): Archdiocese of Toronto
Chief Officer(s):
Gianni Carparelli, Founder
Dara Ogus, Executive Director

F.A.S.T.
#7B, 2441 Lakeshore Rd. West, Oakville ON L6L 5V5
Tel: 905-469-6338
Toll-Free: 888-651-5186
www.familytalk.ca
Also Known As: Family Adolescent Straight Talk Inc.
Overview: A small local charitable organization
Mission: F.A.S.T. helps people to recover from substance abuse/addicitons, by providing a safe environment in to receive crisis counselling, reconcile with family, friends and employers, and participate in ongoing individual and group therapy.

Chief Officer(s):
Jim Harkins, Executive Director/Senior Counselor

Greater Toronto Al-Anon Information Services (GTAIS)
PO Box 1304, 145 The West Mall, Toronto ON M9C 1C0
Tel: 416-410-3809
Toll-Free: 888-425-2666
e-mail: gtais.updates@gmail.com
al-anon.alateen.on.ca/gtais

Overview: A small local organization
Mission: The group provides a forum for the Al-Anon & Alateen groups within the Toronto geographic area to exchange information. It also offers a variety of services, such as lists of meeting schedules, post office box, telephone answering.
Affliation(s): Toronto Al-Anon Family Groups Public Outreach

Parkdale Focus Community Project
#103, 1497 Queen St. West, Toronto ON M6R 1A3
Tel: 416-536-1234
www.stchrishouse.org/adults/alcohol-drug-pre-pro
Overview: A small local organization founded in 1991
Member of: St. Christopher House

The Renascent Centres for Alcoholism & Drug Addiction
Lillian & Don Wright Family Health Centre, 38 Isabella St., Toronto ON MR7 1N1
Tel: 416-927-1202; *Fax:* 416-927-0331
Toll-Free: 866-232-1212
e-mail: info@renascent.ca
www.renascent.ca
www.linkedin.com/company/renascent
www.facebook.com/RenascentCanada
twitter.com/renascentcanada

Also Known As: Renascent
Overview: A small local charitable organization founded in 1970
Mission: To facilitate prevention, education & recovery from addiction to alcohol & other drugs through a continuum of programs & services with equitable access
Chief Officer(s):
Patrick Smith, Chief Executive Officer
Publications:
• Renascent Annual Report
Type: Report; *Frequency:* Annually

Southern Ontario Cocaine Anonymous (CA)
c/o Southern Ontario Cocaine Anonymous, PO Box 19032, 360A Bloor St. West, Toronto ON M5S 3C9
Tel: 416-927-7858
Toll-Free: 866-622-4636
www.ca-on.org

Overview: A small local organization founded in 1987
Mission: To help members stay free from cocaine and all other mind-altering substances through the Twelve Step Recovery Program

QUÉBEC

Centre d'intervention et de prévention en toxicomanie de l'Outaouais (CIPTO)
92, rue Saint-Jacques, Gatineau QC J8X 2Z2
Tél: 819-770-7249; *Téléc:* 819-770-9199
Ligne sans frais: 866-778-4372
Courriel: toxico@cipto.qc.ca
www.cipto.qc.ca

Aperçu: *Dimension:* petite; *Envergure:* locale; fondée en 1982
Mission: De développer des actions communautaires et d'offrir des services d'intervention et de prévention en toxicomanie à la population des secteurs Hull/ Grande-Rivière et une partie du Pontiac (Luskville et Quyon).
Membre(s) du bureau directeur:
Yves Séguin, Directeur général
yves.seguin@cipto.org

Centre de réadaptation et dépendance le virage
5110, boul. Cousineau, Saint-Hubert QC J3Y 7G5
Tél: 450-443-2100
Ligne sans frais: 800-363-9434
www.levirage.qc.ca

Nom précédent: Centre de réadaption Montérégie

Aperçu: *Dimension:* petite; *Envergure:* locale; fondée en 1995
Mission: Pour réhabiliter les personnes qui souffrent d'addictions diverses, de sorte qu'ils sont capables de se réinsérer dans la société

L'Écluse des Laurentides
22A, rue Goyer, Saint-Sauveur QC J0R 1R0
Tel: 450-744-1393; *Fax:* 450-744-1335
e-mail: ecluse@cgocable.ca
www.ecluse.org

Overview: A small local organization founded in 1991
Chief Officer(s):
Émilie Rouleau, Directrice

Méta d'âme
2250, rue Florian, Montréal QC H2X 2P5
Tél: 514-528-9000; *Téléc:* 514-527-6999
Courriel: administration@metadame.org
www.metadame.org

Aperçu: *Dimension:* petite; *Envergure:* locale
Mission: Pour prodiguer des soins médicaux aux personnes souffrant de dépendance aux médicaments d'ordonnance et à faciliter leur réinsertion dans la société

International Associations

Alcoholic Beverage Medical Research Foundation (ABMRF)
#310, 1200-C Agora Dr., Bel Air MD 21014 USA
Toll-Free: 800-688-7152
e-mail: info@abmrf.org
www.abmrf.org
www.linkedin.com/company/1137768
www.facebook.com/AlcoholResearch?ref=ts
twitter.com/AlcoholResearch

Also Known As: The Foundation for Alcohol Research
Overview: A small international organization founded in 1982
Chief Officer(s):
Mack C. Mitchell, President
Lisa Hoffberger, Director, Development & Communications
Erin Teigen, Director, Research & Grants Programs

International Council on Alcohol, Drugs & Traffic Safety (ICADTS)
c/o Joris C. Verster, Secretary, Utrecht Institute for Pharmaceutical Sciences, Universiteitsweg 99, Utrecht 3584CG The Netherlands
Tel: +31-30-253-6909
www.icadts.org
twitter.com/ICADTS

Previous Name: International Committee on Alcohol, Drugs & Traffic Safety
Overview: A small international organization founded in 1963
Mission: To reduce traffic related deaths & injuries by designing, promoting & implementing effective programs & policies, based on sound research
Chief Officer(s):
Kathryn Stewart, President
stewart@pire.org
Publications:
• ICADTS [International Council on Alcohol, Drugs & Traffic Safety] Reporter
Type: Newsletter; *Frequency:* Quarterly; *Editor:* Kathryn Stewart; *ISSN:* 1016-0477

National Association of Addiction Treatment Providers
#1303, 1120 Lincoln St., Denver CO 80203 USA
Toll-Free: 888-574-1008
e-mail: info@naatp.org
www.naatp.org

Overview: A small international organization founded in 1978
Mission: To promote, assist & enhance the delivery of ethical, effective, research-based treatment for alcoholism & other drug addictions; To provide its members & the public with accurate, responsible information & other resources related to the treatment of these diseases; To advocate for increased access to & availability of quality treatment for those who suffer from alcoholism & other drug addictions; To work in partnership with other organizations & individuals that share NAATP's mission & goals
Affliation(s): Fifteen treatment centres in Canada

Chief Officer(s):
Carlton Kester, Chair
Marvin Ventrell, Executive Director
Katie Strand, Director, Operations
Jessica Swan, Manager, Outcomes & Surveys
Tiffany Rode, Coordinator, Programs

Nechi Training, Research & Health Promotions Institute
PO Box 2039, Stn. Main, St. Albert AB T8N 2G3

Tel: 780-459-1884; *Fax:* 780-458-1883
Toll-Free: 800-459-1884
www.nechi.com

Also Known As: Nechi Institute
Overview: A small international charitable organization founded in 1974
Mission: To promote holistic healing & healthy, addictions-free lifestyles
Member of: Canadian Society of Association Executives
Affliation(s): First Nations Adult & Higher Education Consortium
Chief Officer(s):
Geraldine Potts, Director, Operations

National Publications

CrossCurrents: The Journal of Addiction & Mental Health
Centre for Addiction & Mental Health, 33 Russell St., Toronto, ON M5S 2S1

Frequency: 4 times a year

Drugs & Addiction Magazine
Owned By: Suggitt Publishing Ltd.
10177 105 St. NW, Edmonton, AB T5J 1E2

Toll-Free: 866-421-5999
reception@dafacts.com
Social Media: twitter.com/dafactscanada
www.facebook.com/534006560033456

A teaching tool given free to young people in order to educate them about the dangers of drug abuse.
Robert Suggitt, Publisher
Melanie Smith, General Manager, melanie@dafacts.com
Elana Sures, Author

Local Schools

ALBERTA

***Stand Off:* Kainai Adolescent Treatment Center**
P.O. Box 120
Stand Off, AB T0L 1Y0

Tel: 403-653-3315; *Fax:* 403-653-3338
www.katcenter.ca

Grades: 12-17 yrs

BRITISH COLUMBIA

***Kelowna:* Venture Academy**
#338, 101 - 1865 Dilworth Dr., Kelowna, BC V1Y 9T1
Tel: 250-491-4593; *Fax:* 250-491-0251
Toll-Free: 866-762-2211
info@ventureacademy.ca
www.ventureacademy.ca
Grades: 7-12 *Note:* A therapeutic program & boarding school for troubled teens; also has locations in Alberta & Ontario
Gordon Hay, B.G.S., Founder & Executive Director
Leanne Stanley, B.Sc., Kin, B.Ed., Executive Director
Jeff Brain, MA, CTS, CEP, Director, Admissions & Program Development

MANITOBA

***St Norbert:* Behavioural Health Foundation**
P.O. Box 250
35 av de la Digue, St Norbert, MB R3V 1L6, Canada
Tel: 204-269-3430; *Fax:* 204-269-8049
info@bhf.ca
www.bhf.ca

Note: The Behavioural Health Foundation provides long term residential addictions treatment programming for men, women, teens and family units experiencing a variety of addiction problems and co-occurring mental health concerns.
Maureena Downing, Contact, 204-269-3430
maureenad@bhf.ca

National Libraries

Canadian Centre on Substance Abuse/ Centre canadien de lutte contre l'alcoolisme et les toxicomanies
#500, 75 Albert St., Ottawa, ON K1P 5E7

Tel: 613-235-4048; *Fax:* 613-235-8101
media@ccsa.ca
www.ccsa.ca
Social Media: www.youtube.com/user/CCSACCLAT;
twitter.com/CCSAcanada;
www.linkedin.com/company/canadian-centre-on-substance-abuse-ccsa

Rita Notarandrea, Chief Executive Officer

Provincial Libraries

BC Mental Health & Substance Use Services
4500 Oak St., Vancouver, BC V6H 3N1

Tel: 604-524-7734
feedback@bcmhsus.bc.ca
bcmhsus.ca

Collection: Rating Scales; Practice Guidelines

Centre for Addiction & Mental Health
33 Russell St., Toronto, ON M5S 2S1

Tel: 416-535-8501; *Fax:* 416-595-6601
library@camh.ca
www.camh.ca
Social Media: www.youtube.com/camhtv; twitter.com/CAMHnews;
www.facebook.com/CentreforAddictionandMentalHealth

Collection: Temperance Collection, Social & Cultural History of Drinking, Addiction Research Foundation Publications, Drug Education Materials, C.K. Clarke Archives, Clarke Institute of Psychiatry Publications
Tim Tripp, Director, Library
tim.tripp@camh.ca
416-535-8501 ext. 36999

Centre for Addiction & Mental Health Archives
1001 Queen St. West, Toronto, ON M6J 1H4

Tel: 416-535-8501; *Fax:* 416-583-1355

Collection: Institutional & manuscript records
John Court, Archivist
john.court@camh.ca

Homewood Health Centre
150 Delhi St., Guelph, ON N1E 6K9

Tel: 519-824-1010; *Fax:* 519-824-8751
www.homewoodhealth.com

Collection: Collection includes pamphlets, consumer health information, fiction, magazines, newspaper, reference material, large-print books; talking books; music. The staff library includes clinical text books; professional journals; e-journals; college/university catalogues; hospital archives; quick reference; EbscoHost full text databases.
Jagoda Pike, President & CEO

National Government

Canadian Centre on Substance Abuse (CCSA) / Centre canadien de lutte contre l'alcoolisme et les toxicomanies (CCLAT)
#500, 75 Albert St., Ottawa, ON K1P 5E7
Tel: 613-235-4048
Fax: 613-235-8101
info@ccsa.ca
www.ccsa.ca
Other Communication: Publications: publications@ccsa.ca; Media: media@ccsa.ca
twitter.com/CCSAcanada
linkedin.com/company/canadian-centre-on-substance-abusse-ccsa-
www.youtube.com/user/CCSACCLAT
CCSA is a non-profit organization working to minimize the harm associated with the use of alcohol, tobacco, & other drugs.

Interim Chair, Paula Tyler
Tel: 613-235-4048 ext: 232

Chief Executive Officer, Rita Notarandrea
Tel: 613-235-4048 ext: 227

Deputy Chief Executive Officer, Rhowena Martin
Tel: 613-235-4048 ext: 239

Interim Director, Public Affairs & Communications, Wendy Cumming
Tel: 613-235-4048 ext: 276

Director, Strategic Partnerships & Knowledge Mobilization, Robert Eves
Tel: 613-235-4048 ext: 260

Interim Director, Finance, Darwin Ewert
Tel: 613-235-4048 ext: 231

Director, Information Systems & Performance Measurement, Rebecca Jesseman
Tel: 613-235-4048 ext: 228

Director, Human Resources, Darlene Pinto
Tel: 613-235-4048 ext: 254

Director, Research & Policy, Amy Porath-Waller
Tel: 613-235-4048 ext: 252

Senior Executive Assistant & Corporate Secretary, Sharon Roy
Tel: 613-235-4048 ext: 232

Provincial Government

Addiction & Mental Health Services / Services de traitement des dépendances et de santé mentale
Tel: 506-444-4442
Fax: 506-453-8711

Executive Director, Gisèle Maillet
Tel: 506-381-0854
gisele.maillet@gnb.ca
Director, Child & Youth Services, Yvette Doiron
Tel: 506-869-6118
yvette.doiron-brun@gnb.ca
Director, Adult Services, Sylvie Martin
Tel: 506-473-7588
sylvie.martin@gnb.ca

Local Hospitals & Health Centres

ALBERTA

BANFF: Cascade Plaza
Affiliated with: Alberta Health Services
#320, 317 Banff Ave., Banff, AB T1L 1B4
Tel: 403-678-3133 *Fax:* 403-678-3138
www.albertahealthservices.ca

Note: Addiction prevention & adult & youth counselling

BARRHEAD: Barrhead - 5143-50 Street
Affiliated with: Alberta Health Services
PO Box 4504, 5143 - 50 St., Barrhead, AB T7N 1A4
Tel: 780-674-8239 *Fax:* 780-674-8294
Toll-Free: 866-332-2322
www.albertahealthservices.ca

Note: Addiction prevention & adult & youth counselling

BLACKFOOT: Thorpe Recovery Centre (TRC)
Affiliated with: Alberta Health Services
Also Known As: Walter A. "Slim" Thorpe Recovery Centre
PO Box 291, Blackfoot, AB T0B 0L0
Tel: 780-875-8890 *Fax:* 780-875-2161
Toll-Free: 877-875-8890
info@thorperecoverycentre.org
www.thorperecoverycentre.org
Social Media: www.facebook.com/thorperecoverycentre
Year Founded: 1975
Note: Detox, residential & transitional services
Teressa Krueckl, Executive Director
Suzie Le Brocq, Clinical Director

BONNYVILLE: Bonnyville Provincial Building
Affiliated with: Alberta Health Services
PO Box 7085, #201, 4904 - 50 Ave., Bonnyville, AB T9N 2J6
Tel: 780-826-8054 *Fax:* 780-826-8057
Toll-Free: 866-332-2322
www.albertahealthservices.ca

Note: Addiction prevention & adult & youth counselling

BROOKS: Brooks - 403-2 Avenue West
Affiliated with: Alberta Health Services
403 - 2nd Ave. West, Brooks, AB T1R 0S3
Tel: 403-362-1265 *Fax:* 403-362-1248
Toll-Free: 866-332-2322
brooks@albertahealthservices.ca
www.albertahealthservices.ca

Note: Addiction prevention & adult & youth counselling

CALGARY: Alcove Addiction Recovery for Women
Affiliated with: Alberta Health Services
Former Name: Youville Women's Residence
1937 - 42 Ave. SW, Calgary, AB T2T 2M6
Tel: 403-242-0722 *Fax:* 403-242-3915
www.alcoverecovery.net
Social Media: twitter.com/AlcoveRecovery;
instagram.com/alcoverecovery
Year Founded: 1977
Note: Provides support & services for women experiencing addiction & mental health issues
Cheryll Nandee, Executive Director
ed@alcoverecovery.net

CALGARY: Alpha House
Affiliated with: Alberta Health Services
203 - 15 Ave. SE, Calgary, AB T2G 1G4
Tel: 403-234-7388 *Fax:* 403-234-7391
info@alphahousecalgary.com
www.alphahousecalgary.com
Social Media: www.facebook.com/AlphaHouseSociety;
twitter.com/alphahouseyyc

Note: Programs & services include: outreach; shelter; detox; & housing
Kathy Christiansen, Executive Director
kathy@alphahousecalgary.com

CALGARY: Aventa Addiction Treatment For Women
Affiliated with: Alberta Health Services
610 - 25 Ave. SW, Calgary, AB T2S 0L6

Tel: 403-245-9050 *Fax:* 403-245-9485
info@aventa.org
www.aventa.org
Social Media:
www.facebook.com/AventaAddictionTreatmentForWomen

Note: Provides addiction treatment services for women.
Kim Turgeon, Executive Director
kturgeon@aventa.org
Garth Boak, Financial Manager
gboak@aventa.org
Diane MacPherson, Communications Manager
dmacpherson@aventa.org

CALGARY: Calgary - 1177-11 Avenue SW
Affiliated with: Alberta Health Services
Stephenson Bldg., 1177 - 11th Ave. SW, Calgary, AB T2R 1K9

Tel: 403-297-3071 *Fax:* 403-297-3036
Toll-Free: 866-332-2322
www.albertahealthservices.ca

Note: Addiction prevention & adult counselling

CALGARY: Calgary Youth Addiction Services Centre
Affiliated with: Alberta Health Services
1005 - 17 St. NW, Calgary, AB T2N 2E5

Tel: 403-297-4664 *Fax:* 403-297-4668
Toll-Free: 866-332-2322
www.albertahealthservices.ca

CALGARY: Distress Centre Calgary (DCC)
Affiliated with: Alberta Health Services
#300, 1010 - 8th Ave. SW, Calgary, AB T2P 1J2

Tel: 403-266-1601
info@distresscentre.com
www.distresscentre.com
Info Line: 403-266-4357
Social Media: www.facebook.com/distresscentre;
twitter.com/Distress_Centre;
www.youtube.com/user/DistressCentreYYC

Note: Offers crisis support, professional counselling, & referrals to people in distress
Joan Roy, Executive Director
Bing Hu, Chief Financial Officer
Jerilyn Dressler, Director, Operations
Diane Jones Konihowski, Director, Fund Development & Communications

CALGARY: Fresh Start Recovery Centre
Affiliated with: Alberta Health Services
411 - 41 Ave. NE, Calgary, AB T2E 2N4

Tel: 403-387-6266 *Fax:* 403-235-1532
Toll-Free: 844-768-6266
info@freshstartrecovery.ca
www.freshstartrecovery.ca
Social Media: www.facebook.com/FreshStartRecovery;
twitter.com/FreshStartRC;
www.linkedin.com/company/fresh-start-recovery-centre
Year Founded: 1992
Number of Beds: 50 beds
Note: Residential alcohol & drug addiction treatment centre for men
Stacey Petersen, Executive Director
Bruce Holstead, Director, Operations
Pat Cole, Financial Administrator

CALGARY: Renfrew Recovery Detoxification Centre
Affiliated with: Alberta Health Services
1611 Remington Rd. NE, Calgary, AB T2E 5K6

Tel: 403-297-3337 *Fax:* 403-297-4592
Toll-Free: 866-332-2322
www.albertahealthservices.ca

CALGARY: Sunrise Native Addictions Services Society
Affiliated with: Alberta Health Services
Former Name: Native Addictions Services
Also Known As: SUNRISE
1231 - 34 Ave. NE, Calgary, AB T2E 6N4

Tel: 403-261-7921 *Fax:* 403-261-7945
nasgeneral@nass.ca
www.nass.ca

Year Founded: 1974
Number of Beds: 36
Area Served: Calgary & area
Number of Employees: 32
Note: Offers 12-step & Aboriginal-based addiction programming. Only treatment centre in Calgary that uses Aboriginal Spiritual Teachings as a core part of the program. Serves people 18 & over, of all nationalities.
Leslie Big Bull, Director, Operations
403-261-7921, lbigbull@nass.ca
Bryan Flack, Program Director
403-261-7921, bflack@nass.ca
Deborah Axworthy, Manager, Administration
403-261-7921, daxworthy@nass.ca

CANMORE: Canmore Boardwalk Building
Affiliated with: Alberta Health Services
743 Railway Ave., Canmore, AB T1W 1P2

Tel: 403-678-3133 *Fax:* 403-678-3138
Toll-Free: 866-332-2322
www.albertahealthservices.ca

Note: Addiction prevention & adult & youth counselling

CHESTERMERE: Chestermere Community Health Centre
Affiliated with: Alberta Health Services
288 Kinniburgh Blvd., Chestermere, AB T1X 0V8

Tel: 403-365-5400 *Toll-Free:* 877-652-4700
www.albertahealthservices.ca

Note: Provides mental health assessment & treatment as well as addiction prevention services

CLARESHOLM: Claresholm Centre for Mental Health & Addictions
Affiliated with: Alberta Health Services
PO Box 490, 139 - 43 Ave. West, Claresholm, AB T0L 0T0

Tel: 403-682-3563 *Fax:* 403-625-4318
claresholmcentre@albertahealthservices.ca
www.claresholmcentre.com

Year Founded: 1933
Number of Beds: 108 beds
Note: Programs & services include: active rehabilitation; concurrent disorders; extended treatment; & transitions

CLARESHOLM: Lander Treatment Centre
Affiliated with: Alberta Health Services
221 Fairway Dr., Claresholm, AB T0L 0T0

Tel: 403-625-1395 *Fax:* 403-625-1300
www.albertahealthservices.ca

Note: Adult residential addiction services

COLD LAKE: Cold Lake - 5013-51 Street
Affiliated with: Alberta Health Services
5013 - 51 St., Cold Lake, AB T9M 1P3

Tel: 780-594-7556 *Fax:* 780-594-2144
Toll-Free: 866-332-2322
www.albertahealthservices.ca

Note: Addiction prevention & adult & youth counselling

EDMONTON: Addiction Recovery Centre
Affiliated with: Alberta Health Services
10302 - 107 St. NW, Edmonton, AB T5J 1K2

Tel: 780-427-4291 *Fax:* 780-422-2881
www.albertahealthservices.ca

Note: Adult detoxification

EDMONTON: Addiction Services Edmonton
Affiliated with: Alberta Health Services
10010 - 102A Ave. NW, Edmonton, AB T5J 0G5
Tel: 780-427-2736 Fax: 780-427-4180
Toll-Free: 866-332-2322
www.albertahealthservices.ca

Note: Addiction prevention & mental health promotion

EDMONTON: Edmonton Addiction Youth Services
Affiliated with: Alberta Health Services
12325 - 140 St. NW, Edmonton, AB T5L 2C9
Tel: 780-422-7383
www.albertahealthservices.ca

EDMONTON: Forensic & Community Services
Affiliated with: Alberta Health Services
10225 - 106 St., Edmonton, AB T5J 1H5
Tel: 780-342-6400
www.albertahealthservices.ca

Note: Offers counselling as well as addiction &/or mental health treatment

EDMONTON: Henwood Treatment Centre
Affiliated with: Alberta Health Services
18750 - 18th St. NW, Edmonton, AB T5Y 6C1
Tel: 780-422-9069 Fax: 780-422-2223
www.albertahealthservices.ca

Note: Adult residential addiction services
Glenn Walmsley, Manager of Care

EDMONTON: Northeast Community Health Centre
Affiliated with: Alberta Health Services
14007 - 50 St., Edmonton, AB T5A 5E4
Tel: 780-342-4027
www.albertahealthservices.ca

Note: Addictions & mental health services

EDMONTON: Our House Addiction Recovery Centre
Affiliated with: Alberta Health Services
22210 Stony Plain Rd. NW, Edmonton, AB T5S 2C3
Tel: 780-474-8945 Fax: 780-479-2271
house@ourhouseedmonton.com
www.ourhouseedmonton.com
Social Media: www.facebook.com/107496326001549

Note: Offers a residential program for men over 18 years; addiction recovery programs for men & women; & education initiatives.
Patricia Bencz, Executive Director

EDMONTON: Poundmaker's Lodge Treatment Centres (PMLTC)
Affiliated with: Alberta Health Services
PO Box 34007 Stn. Kingsway Mall, Edmonton, AB T5G 3G4
Tel: 780-458-1884 Fax: 780-459-1876
Toll-Free: 866-458-1884
info@poundmaker.org
www.poundmakerslodge.ca
Social Media: www.facebook.com/poundmakers.lodge; twitter.com/pmltc14

Year Founded: 1973
Number of Beds: 64 beds
Number of Employees: 58
Specialties: Alcohol & drug treatment
Note: Aboriginal addiction treatment centre near Edmonton, Alberta. Provides holistic addiction treatment using concepts based in traditional First Nations, Metis, & Inuit beliefs as well as 12-step, abstinence based recovery. Serves adults aged 18 years & over from all walks of life.
Lacey Kaskamin, Coordinator, Community Engagement
780-458-1884, lacey-kaskamin@poundmaker.org
Linden Jessome, Executive Assistant
780-458-1884, linden-jessome@poundmaker.org
Darlene Marchuk, Clinical Manager
780-458-1884, darlene-marchuk@poundmaker.org

EDMONTON: Santa Rosa
Affiliated with: Alberta Health Services
6705 - 120 Ave., Edmonton, AB T5B 0C7
Tel: 780-644-3627
www.albertahealthservices.ca

Note: Youth detoxification & stabilization

FORT MCMURRAY: Fort McMurray Provincial Building
Affiliated with: Alberta Health Services
9915 Franklin Ave., Fort McMurray, AB T9H 2K4
Tel: 780-743-7187 Fax: 780-743-7112
Toll-Free: 866-332-2322
www.albertahealthservices.ca

Note: Addiction prevention, day treatment & adult & youth counselling

FORT SASKATCHEWAN: Fort Saskatchewan Community Hospital
Affiliated with: Alberta Health Services
Former Name: Fort Saskatchewan Health Centre
9401 - 86 Ave., Fort Saskatchewan, AB T8L 0C6
Tel: 780-342-2388 Fax: 780-342-3348
www.albertahealthservices.ca

Note: Provides addiction & mental health assessment & treatment services

GRANDE CACHE: Pine Plaza Building
Affiliated with: Alberta Health Services
PO Box 120, 702 Pine Plaza NW, Grande Cache, AB T0E 0Y0
Tel: 780-827-4998 Fax: 780-827-7207
www.albertahealthservices.ca
Info Line: 877-303-2642

Note: Addictions & mental health services

GRANDE PRAIRIE: Grande Prairie Aberdeen Centre
Affiliated with: Alberta Health Services
#300, 9728 Montrose Ave., Grande Prairie, AB T8V 5B6
Tel: 780-538-6330 Fax: 780-538-5256
Toll-Free: 866-332-2322
www.albertahealthservices.ca

GRANDE PRAIRIE: Northern Addictions Centre
Affiliated with: Alberta Health Services
11333 - 106 St., Grande Prairie, AB T8V 6T7
Tel: 780-538-5210 Fax: 780-538-6359
www.albertahealthservices.ca

Irene Gladue, Manager

HANNA: Hanna Provincial Building
Affiliated with: Alberta Health Services
401 Centre St., Hanna, AB T0J 1P0
Tel: 403-820-7863 Fax: 403-820-7865
Toll-Free: 866-332-2322
www.albertahealthservices.ca

Note: Addiction prevention & adult & youth counselling

HIGH LEVEL: Action North Recovery Centre
Affiliated with: Alberta Health Services
PO Box 872, 10502 103rd St., High Level, AB T0H 1Z0
Tel: 780-926-3113 Fax: 780-926-2060
www.actionnorth.org

Note: Residential addictions treatment facility

HINTON: Hinton Civic Centre Building
Affiliated with: Alberta Health Services
#102, 131 Civic Centre Rd., Hinton, AB T7V 2E8
Tel: 780-865-8263 Fax: 780-865-8314
Toll-Free: 866-332-2322
www.albertahealthservices.ca

Note: Addiction prevention & adult & youth counselling

JASPER: Jasper Provincial Building
Affiliated with: Alberta Health Services
631 Patricia St., Jasper, AB T0E 1E0
Tel: 780-852-3064 *Fax:* 780-865-8314
Toll-Free: 866-332-2322
www.albertahealthservices.ca

Note: Addiction prevention & adult & youth counselling

KILLAM: Flagstaff Family & Community Services
Affiliated with: Alberta Health Services
PO Box 450, 4809 - 49 Ave., Killam, AB T0B 2L0
Tel: 780-385-3976

Note: Adult & youth addiction counselling services
Lynne Jenkinson, Executive Director

LAKE LOUISE: Lake Louise - 200 Hector Street
Affiliated with: Alberta Health Services
200 Hector St., Lake Louise, AB T0L 1E0
Tel: 403-678-3133 *Fax:* 403-678-3138
www.albertahealthservices.ca

Note: Addiction prevention & adult & youth counselling; ambulatory community physiotherapy

LEDUC: Leduc Neighbourhood Centre
Affiliated with: Alberta Health Services
4901 - 50 Ave., Leduc, AB T9E 6W7
Tel: 780-980-7580 *Fax:* 780-980-7581
Toll-Free: 866-332-2322
www.albertahealthservices.ca

Note: Addiction & mental health services

LETHBRIDGE: Lethbridge Provincial Building
Affiliated with: Alberta Health Services
#103, 200 - 5th Ave. South, Lethbridge, AB T1J 4L1
Tel: 403-381-5260 *Fax:* 403-382-4518
www.albertahealthservices.ca

Note: Addictions & mental health services

LETHBRIDGE: Lethbridge Youth Treatment Centre
Affiliated with: Alberta Health Services
402 - 6th Ave. North, Lethbridge, AB T1H 6J9
Tel: 403-388-7600 *Fax:* 403-388-7619
www.albertahealthservices.ca

Note: Addictions counselling & treatment

MEDICINE HAT: Medicine Hat Recovery Centre
Affiliated with: Alberta Health Services
370 Kipling St. SE, Medicine Hat, AB T1A 1Y6
Tel: 403-529-9021 *Fax:* 403-529-9065
www.albertahealthservices.ca

Number of Beds: 18 beds
Note: Adult detoxification & addiction treatment

OKOTOKS: Okotoks Mental Health Centre
Affiliated with: Alberta Health Services
11 Cimarron Common, Okotoks, AB T1S 2E9
Tel: 403-995-2712 *Toll-Free:* 877-652-4700
www.albertahealthservices.ca

Note: Addiction prevention & mental health assessment & treatment services

OLDS: Olds Provincial Building
Affiliated with: Alberta Health Services
#212, 5025 - 50th St., Olds, AB T4H 1R9
Tel: 403-507-8174 *Fax:* 403-556-1584
www.albertahealthservices.ca

Note: Addictions & mental health services

OYEN: Oyen Community Health Services
Affiliated with: Alberta Health Services
315 - 3 Ave. East, Oyen, AB T0J 2J0
Tel: 403-529-3582 *Fax:* 403-529-3130
www.albertahealthservices.ca

Note: Addiction prevention & adult & youth counselling

PEACE RIVER: Peace River Provincial Building
Affiliated with: Alberta Health Services
Bag 900-1, 9621 - 96 Ave., Peace River, AB T8S 1T4
Tel: 780-624-6193 *Fax:* 780-624-6579
Toll-Free: 866-332-2322
www.albertahealthservices.ca

Note: Addictions prevention & adult & youth counselling

PONOKA: Ponoka Provincial Building
Affiliated with: Alberta Health Services
#223, 5110 - 49th Ave., Ponoka, AB T4J 1R6
Tel: 403-783-7903 *Fax:* 403-785-7926
www.albertahealthservices.ca

Note: Addictions & mental health services

RED DEER: Red Deer Provincial Building
Affiliated with: Alberta Health Services
4920 - 51 St., Red Deer, AB T4N 6K8
Tel: 403-340-5274 *Fax:* 403-340-4804
Toll-Free: 866-332-2322
www.albertahealthservices.ca

Note: Addictions prevention; adult & youth counselling & treatment

RED DEER: Safe Harbour Society for Health & Housing
Affiliated with: Alberta Health Services
5246 - 53 Ave., Red Deer, AB T4N 5K2
Tel: 403-347-0181 *Fax:* 403-347-7275
www.safeharboursociety.org

Year Founded: 2007
Number of Employees: 60
Note: Adult detox & shelter
Kath Hoffman, Executive Director
kath@safeharboursociety.org

SLAVE LAKE: Slave Lake - 101-3 Street SW
Affiliated with: Alberta Health Services
PO Box 1278, #104, 101 - 3rd St. SW, Slave Lake, AB T0G 2A4
Tel: 780-849-7127 *Fax:* 780-849-7394
www.albertahealthservices.ca

Note: Addiction prevention & adult & youth counselling

ST. PAUL: St. Paul Provincial Building
Affiliated with: Alberta Health Services
#116, 5025 - 49 Ave., St. Paul, AB T0A 3A4
Tel: 780-645-6346 *Fax:* 780-645-6249
Toll-Free: 866-332-2322
www.albertahealthservices.ca

Note: Addiction prevention & adult & youth counselling

STANDOFF: Kainai Wellness Centre
Blood Tribe Department of Health Inc.
PO Box 229, Standoff, AB T0L 1Y0
Tel: 403-737-3883 *Fax:* 403-737-2036
btdh.ca/staff/kainai-wellness-centre

Year Founded: 1985
Note: Provides programs & services for the Blood Tribe Community, including crisis intervention & prevention, mental health, alcohol & drug abuse programs, counselling, stress management, relaxation therapy, mental illness education, grief & loss recovery, & wellness.
Sandy Many Chief, Director
sandi.mc@btdh.ca

STETTLER: Stettler - 4837-50 Main Street
Affiliated with: Alberta Health Services
4837 - 50 Main St., Stettler, AB T0C 2L0
Tel: 403-742-7523 *Fax:* 403-742-7596
Toll-Free: 866-332-2322
www.albertahealthservices.ca

Note: Addiction prevention & adult & youth counselling

STONY PLAIN: WestView Health Centre
Affiliated with: Alberta Health Services
4405 South Park Dr., Stony Plain, AB T7Z 2M7
Tel: 780-963-6151 *Fax:* 780-963-7186
Toll-Free: 866-332-2322
www.albertahealthservices.ca

Note: Addiction prevention & mental health promotion services

STRATHMORE: Hilton Plaza
Affiliated with: Alberta Health Services
209 - 3 Ave., Strathmore, AB T1P 1K2
Tel: 403-361-7277 *Toll-Free:* 877-652-4700
www.albertahealthservices.ca

Note: Addiction prevention & adult & youth counselling

TABER: Taber Health Centre
Affiliated with: Alberta Health Services
4326 - 50 Ave., Taber, AB T1G 1N9
Tel: 403-223-7244 *Fax:* 403-223-7236
www.albertahealthservices.ca

Note: Offers assessment, treatment, counselling, & other addiction & mental health services.

THREE HILLS: Three Hills Provincial Building
Affiliated with: Alberta Health Services
Former Name: Three Hills Mental Health Centre
128 - 3 Ave. SE, Three Hills, AB T0M 2A0
Tel: 403-443-8532 *Fax:* 403-443-8541
www.albertahealthservices.ca

Note: Addictions (403-820-7863) & mental health services

VEGREVILLE: Vegreville Provincial Building
Affiliated with: Alberta Health Services
4809 - 50 St., Vegreville, AB T9C 1R1
Tel: 780-632-6617 *Fax:* 780-632-6618
vegaldrug@digitalweb.net
www.albertahealthservices.ca

Note: Addiction prevention & adult & youth counselling

WHITECOURT: Whitecourt Provincial Building
Affiliated with: Alberta Health Services
5020 - 52 Ave., Whitecourt, AB T7S 1N2
Tel: 780-778-7123 *Fax:* 780-778-7220
Toll-Free: 866-332-2322
www.albertahealthservices.ca

Note: Addiction prevention & adult & youth counselling

BRITISH COLUMBIA

BURNABY: The Burnaby Centre for Mental Health & Addiction (BCMHA)
Affiliated with: Interior Health Authority
3405 Willingdon Ave., Burnaby, BC V5G 3H4
Tel: 604-675-3950 *Fax:* 604-675-3955
burnabycentreinfo@interiorhealth.ca
www.interiorhealth.ca

Number of Beds: 100 beds
Note: Six to nine-month residential treatment program for BC residents with concurrent disorders

GRAND FORKS: Boundary Mental Health & Substance Use Services
Affiliated with: Interior Health Authority
7441 2nd St., Grand Forks, BC V0H 1H0
Tel: 250-442-0330
www.interiorhealth.ca

Note: Services include: adult community support; counselling; early psychosis intervention; eating disorders; intake, urgent response, & emergency; & seniors mental health.

HAZELTON: Hazelton Mental Health & Addictions
Affiliated with: Northern Health Authority
2506 Hwy. 62, Hazelton, BC V0J 1Y0
Tel: 250-842-5144 *Fax:* 250-842-2179
www.northernhealth.ca
Info Line: 888-562-1214

Note: Programs & services include: assessment & treatment; life skills training; recreational therapy; observation unit; perinatal depression; supportive recovery; & community response unit.

KAMLOOPS: Kamloops Mental Health & Substance Use
Affiliated with: Interior Health Authority
200 - 235 Lansdowne St., Kamloops, BC V2C 1X8
Tel: 250-377-6500
www.interiorhealth.ca

Note: Services include: adult community support; counselling; early psychosis intervention; eating disorders; intake, urgent response, & emergency; & seniors mental health.

KAMLOOPS: Phoenix Centre
922 - 3 Ave., Kamloops, BC V2C 6W5
Tel: 250-374-4634 *Fax:* 250-374-4621
Toll-Free: 877-318-1177
www.phoenixcentre.org

Number of Beds: 20 beds
Note: Detoxification centre
Sian Lewis, Executive Director
sian.lewis@phoenixcentre.org

KELOWNA: Kelowna Mental Health & Substance Use
Affiliated with: Interior Health Authority
505 Doyle Ave., Kelowna, BC V1Y 0C5
Tel: 250-469-7070
www.interiorhealth.ca

Note: Services include: adult community support; assessment; treatment; crisis intervention; counselling; & mental health support.

LILLOOET: Lillooet Mental Health
Affiliated with: Interior Health Authority
951 Murray St., Lillooet, BC V0K 1V0
Tel: 250-256-1343
www.interiorhealth.ca

Note: Services include: adult community support; counselling; early psychosis intervention; eating disorders; intake, urgent response, & emergency; & seniors mental health.

OLIVER: Desert Sun Counselling & Resource Centre
Affiliated with: Interior Health Authority
PO Box 1890, 762 Fairview Rd., Oliver, BC V0X 1C0
Tel: 250-498-2538 *Toll-Free:* 877-723-3911
www.desertsuncounselling.ca
Social Media: www.facebook.com/desertsuncounselling
Year Founded: 1998
Note: Services include: counselling; crisis help; parenting resources; seniors' resources; & community outreach.
Patricia Batchelor, Chair

PRINCE GEORGE: Legion Wing, Seniors Housing
Affiliated with: Northern Health Authority
2175 - 9th Ave., Prince George, BC V2M 5E3
Tel: 250-561-1499
www.northernhealth.ca

Note: Semi-independent housing for seniors experiencing dementia, or mental health/substance issues.

QUEEN CHARLOTTE: Queen Charlotte City Health Centre
Affiliated with: Northern Health Authority
302 - 2nd Ave., Queen Charlotte, BC V0T 1S0
Tel: 250-559-8765 *Fax:* 250-559-8765
www.northernhealth.ca

Note: Programs & services include: mental health & addictions; home care nursing; & home support.

QUESNEL: Quesnel Mental Health Team & QUESST Unit
Affiliated with: Northern Health Authority
543 Front St., Quesnel, BC V2J 2K7
Tel: 250-985-5608
www.northernhealth.ca

Number of Beds: 5 beds
Note: Short-term intensive services including assessment, stabilization, consultation, brief treatment, & discharge planning. QUESST stands for Quesnel Unit for Emergency Short Stay Treatment.

SALMON ARM: Mental Health/Addictions & Public Health
Affiliated with: Interior Health Authority
433 Hudson Rd., Salmon Arm, BC V1E 4S1
www.interiorhealth.ca

TUMBLER RIDGE: Tumbler Ridge Mental Health & Addictions
Affiliated with: Northern Health Authority
PO Box 1205, 220 Front St., Tumbler Ridge, BC V0C 2W0
Tel: 250-242-5505 *Fax:* 250-242-3595
www.northernhealth.ca

Note: Services include: case management; counselling; crisis response; education; intake; life skills support; medication management; & psychiatric consultation.

MANITOBA

ST NORBERT: The Behavioural Health Foundation, Inc. (BHF)
Affiliated with: Winnipeg Regional Health Authority
PO Box 250, 35, av de la Digue, St Norbert, MB R3V 1L6
info@bhf.ca
www.bhf.ca

Note: Long-term residential addictions treatment for men, women, teens & families
Jean Doucha, Executive Director
jeand@bhf.ca

WINNIPEG: Addictions Recovery Inc. (ARI)
Affiliated with: Winnipeg Regional Health Authority
93 Cathedral Ave., Winnipeg, MB R2W 0W7
Tel: 204-586-2550
info@addictionsrecovery.ca
www.addictionsrecovery.ca
Year Founded: 1979
Note: Provides an alcohol & drug addiction treatment program; runs two recovery homes in Winnipeg.

WINNIPEG: Esther House
Affiliated with: Winnipeg Regional Health Authority
PO Box 68022 Stn. Osborne Vill., Winnipeg, MB R3L 2V9
Tel: 204-582-4043
estherhs@mymts.net
www.estherhousewinnipeg.ca
Year Founded: 1997
Number of Beds: 6 beds
Note: Provides second-stage addiction recovery treatment for women. Works in cooperation with the Addictions Foundation of Manitoba.

WINNIPEG: The Laurel Centre
Affiliated with: Winnipeg Regional Health Authority
104 Roslyn Rd., Winnipeg, MB R3L 0G6
Tel: 204-783-5460 *Fax:* 204-774-2912
info@thelaurelcentre.com
thelaurelcentre.com

Note: Provides dual treatment for women with substance addictions & who are experiencing the traumatic effects of childhood/adolescent sexual abuse.
Suhad Bisharat, Executive Director

WINNIPEG: Main Street Project (MSP)
Affiliated with: Winnipeg Regional Health Authority
661 Main St., 2nd Fl., Winnipeg, MB R3B 1E3
Tel: 204-982-8245 *Fax:* 204-943-9474
admin@mainstreetproject.ca
www.mainstreetproject.ca
Social Media: www.facebook.com/mainstreetprojectinc; twitter.com/mainstreetwpg
Year Founded: 1972
Note: Programs & services include: emergency shelter & food; drug & alcohol detoxification unit; on-site counselling; transitional housing; & other critical services.
Rick Lees, Executive Director

WINNIPEG: Native Addictions Council of Manitoba (NACM)
Affiliated with: Winnipeg Regional Health Authority
160 Salter St., Winnipeg, MB R2W 4K1
Tel: 204-586-8395 *Fax:* 204-589-3921
www.nacm.ca
Year Founded: 1971
Note: Provides holistic treatment of addictions

WINNIPEG: Street Connections
Affiliated with: Winnipeg Regional Health Authority
496 Hargrave St., Winnipeg, MB R3A 0X7
Tel: 204-981-0742
outreach@wrha.mb.ca
www.streetconnections.ca

Note: Mobile harm reduction program specializing in harm reduction & free services to those in need. Programs & services include: general assistance (housing, addictions, food, legal, & more); counselling; nursing services; prenatal services; clean drug use supplies; needle exchange; & safe sex supplies.

WINNIPEG: Tamarack Recovery Centre Inc.
Affiliated with: Winnipeg Regional Health Authority
Former Name: Kia Zan Inc.
60 Balmoral St., Winnipeg, MB R3C 1X4
Tel: 204-775-3546 *Fax:* 204-772-9908
info@tamarackrecovery.org
www.tamarackrehab.org
Year Founded: 1974
Note: Provides abstinence-based addictions treatment & recovery services.
Lisa Cowan, Executive Director
204-772-9836

NEW BRUNSWICK

EDMUNDSTON: Services de toxicomanie
Affiliée à: Vitalité Health Network
345, boul Hébert, Edmundston, NB E3V 0E7
Tél: 506-735-2092
www.vitalitenb.ca

Nombre de lits: 10 lits
Note: Service de désintoxication interne
Johanne Lavoie, Directeur
johanne.lavoie@vitalitenb.ca

FREDERICTON: Fredericton Addiction Services
Affiliated with: Horizon Health Network
c/o Victoria Health Centre, 65 Brunswick St., Fredericton, NB E3B 1G5
Tel: 506-453-2132 *Fax:* 506-452-5533

MONCTON: Moncton Addiction Services
Affiliated with: Horizon Health Network
125 Mapleton Rd., Moncton, NB E1C 9G3
Tel: 506-856-2333 *Fax:* 506-856-2796
horizonnb.ca
Number of Beds: 20 beds
Note: Detoxification unit, methadone maintenance treatment program, addiction prevention & education, counselling, assessments

SAINT JOHN: Ridgewood Addiction Services
Affiliated with: Horizon Health Network
416 Bay St., Saint John, NB E2M 7L4
Tel: 506-674-4300 *Fax:* 506-674-4374
Number of Beds: 90 beds
Note: Comprehensive addiction treatment programs, detoxification, outpatient & short term residential services, addiction prevention & education, community reintegration.
Renee Fournier, Manager

NORTHWEST TERRITORIES

FORT LIARD: Fort Liard Mental Health & Addictions Program
Affiliated with: Northwest Territories Health & Social Services Authority
General Delivery, Fort Liard, NT X0G 0A0
Tel: 867-770-4770 *Fax:* 867-770-4813

FORT SIMPSON: Fort Simpson Mental Health & Addictions Program
Affiliated with: Northwest Territories Health & Social Services Authority
PO Box 246, Fort Simpson, NT X0E 0N0
Tel: 867-695-2293 *Fax:* 867-695-2920

NOVA SCOTIA

YARMOUTH: Addiction Services
Affiliated with: Nova Scotia Health Authority
Former Name: Western Drug Dependency Program
c/o Yarmouth Regional Hospital, 60 Vancouver St., Yarmouth, NS B5A 2P5
Tel: 902-742-2406 *Fax:* 902-742-0684

ONTARIO

BARRIE: Royal Victoria Hospital - Barrie Community Care Centre for Substance Abuse
70 Wellington St. West, Barrie, ON L4N 1K4
Tel: 705-728-9090 *Fax:* 705-728-7308
www.rvh.on.ca
Number of Beds: 41 beds
Note: Intoxification management, withdrawal management, assessments, family education, discharge planning
Angela McCuaig, Manager, Addictions Services

CORNWALL: Cornwall Withdrawal Management Services
Cornwall Community Hospital
840 McConnell Ave., Cornwall, ON K6H 5S5
Tel: 613-938-8506 *Fax:* 613-938-2867
www.cornwallhospital.ca/en/WithdrawalManagement

Note: Cornwall's Withdrawal Management Services hosts AA & NA meetings & group therapy for men & women sixteen years of age & over. Strategies & information are provided to prevent substance misuse. The organization is bilingual.

KINGSTON: Kingston Detoxification Centre
Hotel Dieu Hospital
240 Brock St., Kingston, ON K7L 5G2
Tel: 613-549-6461
www.hoteldieu.com

Note: The Detoxification Centre provides counselling, self-help groups, & referral to community services

KITCHENER: Waterloo Regional Withdrawal Management Centre
52 Glasgow St., Kitchener, ON N2G 1N6
Tel: 519-749-4318
www.grhosp.on.ca
Number of Beds: 28 beds
Note: Offers withdrawal management services.

SAULT STE MARIE: Sault Ste. Marie Withdrawal Management Services
Sault Area Hospital
911 Queen St. East, Sault Ste Marie, ON P6A 2B6
Tel: 705-942-1872 *Fax:* 705-759-6369
www.sah.on.ca
Number of Beds: 15 beds
Note: Detox centre
Jane Sippell, Director, Mental Health & Addictions
sippellj@sah.on.ca

ST CATHARINES: Niagara Regional Men's Withdrawal Management Service
Niagara Health System / Système de santé de Niagara
Affiliated with: Hamilton Niagara Haldimand Brant Local Health Integration Network
10 Adams St., St Catharines, ON L2R 2V8
Tel: 905-682-7211
Number of Beds: 18 beds
Note: The withdrawal management service offers crisis intervention, assessments, counselling, self-help groups, & treatment referrals for inpatients & outpatients.

ST CATHARINES: St Catharines Detoxification (Women's) Centre
6 Adams St., St Catharines, ON L2R 2V8
Tel: 905-687-9721 *Fax:* 905-687-9768
Number of Beds: 14 beds

SUDBURY: Withdrawal Management Services
Health Sciences North
336 Pine St., Sudbury, ON P3C 4E5
Tel: 705-671-7366

Note: Offers detox services & short-term crisis safe bed program

TORONTO: Centre for Addiction & Mental Health ARF Site
Former Name: Addiction Research Foundation
33 Russell St., Toronto, ON M5S 2S1
Tel: 416-595-6000 *Fax:* 416-595-9997
Toll-Free: 800-463-2338
info@camh.ca
www.camh.ca
Social Media: www.facebook.com/CentreforAddictionandMentalHealth; twitter.com/CAMHnews; www.youtube.com/camhtv; www.linkedin.com/company/camh

Note: Drug rehabilitation centre
David Cunic, Vice-President, Redevelopment & Support Services

TORONTO: Centre for Addiction & Mental Health (Corporate Office)
1001 Queen St. West, Toronto, ON M6J 1H4
Tel: 416-535-8501 *Toll-Free:* 800-463-2338
info@camh.ca
www.camh.ca
Social Media: www.facebook.com/CentreforAddictionandMentalHealth; twitter.com/CAMHnews; www.youtube.com/user/CAMHTV; www.linkedin.com/company/camh
Number of Beds: 530 inpatient beds
Note: Addiction treatment
Dr. Catherine Zahn, President & CEO

TORONTO: St. Michael's Hospital Withdrawal Management Services
135 Sherbourne St., Toronto, ON M5A 2R5
Fax: 416-864-5146
Toll-Free: 866-366-9513
www.stmichaelshospital.com

Number of Beds: 17 beds
Note: Detoxification centre
Tom Henderson, Manager

TORONTO: Toronto Western Hospital - Addiction Outpatient/Aftercare Clinic
University Health Network
Affiliated with: Toronto Central Local Health Integration Network
399 Bathurst St., Toronto, ON M5T 2S8
Tel: 416-603-5800 *Fax:* 416-603-5490
www.uhn.ca

Note: Assessment & referral, individual & group therapy, counseling, psychiatric consultation, education. Services in English, French, Portuguese, Polish

TORONTO: Withdrawal Management Centre
Michael Garron Hospital
985 Danforth Ave., Toronto, ON M4J 1M1
Tel: 416-461-2010 *Fax:* 416-461-1164
ptrep@tegh.on.ca (Patients); community@tegh.on.ca (Community)
www.tegh.on.ca
Number of Beds: 30 beds
Note: Specialties: Crisis intervention for adult males; Physical care for males in acute states of intoxication; Withdrawal from alcohol & other addictive substances; Addictions assessments; Counselling; Rehabilitation services; Education on substance abuse to family members

WINDSOR: Windsor Withdrawal Management Residential Service
Windsor Regional Hospital
1453 Prince Rd., Windsor, ON N9C 3Z4
Tel: 519-257-5225 *Fax:* 519-253-1752
www.wrh.on.ca
Number of Beds: 20 beds
Area Served: Counties of Essex, Kent, & Lambton, Ontario
Note: The agency assists men & women who are 16 years of age or older to access treatment for addiction. The service is funded by the Ministry of Health & Long-term Care.
Bill Marcotte, Service Director
bill_marcotte@wrh.on.ca

PRINCE EDWARD ISLAND

CHARLOTTETOWN: Provincial Addictions Treatment Facility
PO Box 2000, 2814 rte 215, Mt. Herbert, Charlottetown, PE C1A 7N8
Tel: 902-368-4120 *Fax:* 902-368-6229
Toll-Free: 888-299-8399
www.healthpei.ca
Number of Beds: 24 withdrawal management beds; 16 rehab beds
Specialties: Medically supervised detoxification

QUÉBEC

AMOS: Centre Normand
Affiliée à: CISSS de l'Abitibi-Témiscamingue
621, rue de l'Harricana, Amos, QC J9T 2P9
Tél: 819-732-8241 *Téléc:* 819-727-2210
www.cisss-at.gouv.qc.ca
Fondée en: 1981
Nombre de lits: 10 lits
Note: Offre des services de réadaptation aux personnes qui présentent une dépendance - à l'alcool, drogues illicites, médicaments, jeu; services de support psychosocial.

BEAUCEVILLE: Centre de réadaptation en alcoolisme et toxicomanie de Beauceville
Affiliée à: CISSS de Chaudière-Appalaches
Ancien nom: Centre de réadaptation en alcoolisme et toxicomanie de Chaudière-Appalaches
253, rte 108, Beauceville, QC G5X 2Z3
Tél: 418-774-3329 *Téléc:* 418-774-4423
Ligne sans frais: 888-774-3329
www.cisss-ca.gouv.qc.ca
Nombre de lits: 14 lits
Michel Laroche, Directeur, Programme santé mentale et dépendance

GATINEAU: Centre de réadaptation en dépendance de l'Outaouais
Ancien nom: Centre Jellinek; Pavillon Jelinek
25, rue Saint-François, Gatineau, QC J9A 1B1
Tél: 819-776-5584 *Téléc:* 819-776-0255
crdoutaouais@ssss.gouv.qc.ca
www.dependanceoutaouais.org
Nombre de lits: 33 places
Note: Centre de réadaptation des drogues, de l'alcool ou du jeu

MONTRÉAL: Centre de réadaptation en dépendance de Montréal - Institut universitaire
Ancien nom: Centre Dollard-Cormier
950, rue de Louvain est, Montréal, QC H2M 2E8
Tél: 514-385-1232
www.ciusss-centresudmtl.gouv.qc.ca
Nombre de lits: 55 lits
M. Jacques Couillard, Directeur général

ST-PHILIPPE: Foster Addiction Rehabilitation Centre
Affiliated with: CISSS de la Montérégie-Ouest
Former Name: Pavillon Foster
6 rue Foucreault, St-Philippe, QC J0L 2K0
Tel: 450-659-8911 *Fax:* 450-659-7173
www.crdfoster.org
Year Founded: 1964
Number of Beds: 20 lits
Note: Alcohol/drug rehabilitation
Pierre Guay, Directeur, Programmes santé mentale et dépendance

STE-ANNE-DES-MONTS: Centre de réadaptation en dépendance de la Haute-Gaspésie
Affiliée à: CISSS de la Gaspésie
Ancien nom: Centre de réadaptation L'Escale
52, rue du Belvédère, Ste-Anne-des-Monts, QC G4V 1X4
Tél: 418-763-5000 *Téléc:* 418-763-9024
www.cisss-gaspesie.gouv.qc.ca
Note: Pour personnes toxicomanes.

Sudden Infant Death Syndrome

Sudden Infant Death Syndrome (SIDS) is the sudden death of an infant or young child; the death is unexpected and shows no demonstrable cause. Almost all SIDS deaths occur when the infant is thought to be sleeping.

Cause
Despite extensive research, no cause for SIDS has been found, although evidence suggests that it may be related to the baby sleeping on his or her side or in a face-down position; a central nervous system abnormality; or a malfunction of the mechanisms that control body temperature, heart function or the breathing process. Possible risk factors include exposure to cigarette smoke, soft bedding, a cluttered sleeping area, an overheated environment, sharing a bed with a parent or sibling and being a sibling of a SIDS victim.

Symptoms
No symptoms have been identified that are specific to SIDS. If there is a pause in breathing that lasts for more than 10 seconds in a sleeping baby, an attempt should be made to waken the baby. A pause in breathing that lasts for more than 20 seconds is very dangerous.

Prevalence
In Canada, SIDS is the most common cause of death in healthy children under the age of one year. One of every 2,000 babies born in Canada dies of SIDS. Rare before one month of age and after one year of age, SIDS has a peak incidence between the second and fourth month of life.

Treatment Options

A pathologist examines the baby's body to determine if there were any abnormalities that could have caused the death. If no specific cause is identified, a diagnosis of SIDS is usually made.

Recent studies have indicated that having babies sleep on their backs reduces the risks of SIDS. The Canadian Paediatric Society, the Canadian Foundation for the Study of Infant Deaths, the Canadian Institute of Child Health and Health Canada all recommend that infants be placed on their backs for sleep. Other preventative measures include providing a smoke-free environment, breast-feeding, creating a safe sleep environment (free of clutter, toys and loose bedding) and placing the baby in a crib beside the parents' bed for the first six months of life. Between 1999 and 2004, the rate of SIDS dropped 50 percent in Canada. This decline is mostly attributed to recommendations that infants be placed to sleep on their backs.

Parents who lose a child to SIDS are grief-stricken and, because no definitive cause can be found for their seemingly healthy baby's death, usually have excessive feelings of guilt. Bereavement support is necessary not only during the days immediately following the infant's death, but also for at least several months.

National Associations

Baby's Breath
PO Box 21053, St Catharines ON L2M 7X2
Tel: 905-688-8884; *Fax:* 905-688-3300
Toll-Free: 800-363-7437
www.babysbreathcanada.ca
www.facebook.com/babysbreathca
twitter.com/babysbreathca
Previous Name: Canadian Foundation for the Study of Infant Deaths
Overview: A small national charitable organization founded in 1973
Mission: To support & represent families in Canada who are coping with the loss of an infant; To promote research on the health or medical conditions associated with infant deaths & stillbirths
Affliation(s): SIDS International
Chief Officer(s):
Wendy Potter, Chair
Publications:
• The Baby's Breath
Type: Newsletter; *ISSN:* 1192-9294
Profile: Foundation information & events, medical updates,
• Sam's Story [a publication of Baby's Breath]
Author: Fiona Chin-Yee
Profile: Resource for youngs SIDS siblings accompanied by a parents' guide

Infant & Toddler Safety Association (ITSA) / Association pour la sécurité des bébés et des tout petits
#154, 23 - 500 Fairway Rd. South, Kitchener ON N2C 1X3
Tel: 519-570-0181; *Fax:* 519-570-1078
Toll-Free: 888-570-0181
www.infantandtoddlersafety.ca
Overview: A small national charitable organization founded in 1980
Mission: To offer information & resources to promote & increase the safety of young children & prevent paediatric injury & death

Provincial Associations

QUÉBEC

Fondation des étoiles / Foundation of Stars
#205, 370, rue Guy, Montréal QC H3J 1S6
Tél: 514-595-5730; *Téléc:* 514-595-5745
Ligne sans frais: 800-665-2358
Courriel: info@fondationdesetoiles.ca
www.fondationdesetoiles.ca
www.linkedin.com/in/fondation-des-%C3%A9toiles-77a55063
www.facebook.com/FondationDesEtoiles
twitter.com/EnfantsEtoiles
instagram.com/fondation_des_etoiles

Aperçu: *Dimension:* moyenne; *Envergure:* provinciale; Organisme sans but lucratif; fondée en 1977
Mission: Amasser des fonds pour la recherche sur les maladies infantiles au Québec; ces fonds sont distribués aux quatre centres de recherche suivants: Centre de recherche de l'Hôpital Ste-Justine, Institut de recherche de l'Hôpital de Montréal pour enfants, Centre Hospitalier Universitaire de Québec et Centre Hospitalier Universitaire de Sherbrooke
Membre(s) du bureau directeur:
Josée Saint-Pierre, Présidente-directrice générale
   jsaint-pierre@fondationdesetoiles.ca
Étienne Lalonde, Directeur, Développement
   elalonde@fondationdesetoiles.ca

National Libraries

Baby's Breath
PO Box 21053, St Catharines, ON L2M 7X2
Tel: 905-688-8884; *Fax:* 905-688-3300
Toll-Free: 800-363-7437
www.babysbreathcanada.ca
Social Media: twitter.com/babysbreathca;
www.facebook.com/babysbreathca

Suicide

Suicide, which involves a complex interaction of psychological, neurological, medical, social and family factors, is a significant cause of early, preventable death in Canada.

Most professionals distinguish at least two suicide groups: those who actually kill themselves, or completed suicides; and those who attempt it, usually harming themselves, but survive. Those who succeed in killing themselves may suffer from one or more psychiatric disorders, most commonly depression, often along with alcohol or substance abuse. Some individuals plan suicide very carefully, taking steps to ensure that they will not be discovered and rescued, and they use lethal means, such as shooting themselves. Some act impulsively, reacting to a life disappointment by jumping off a nearby bridge. Those that survive often use means that make discovery and rescue probable, and are not likely to be lethal (for example, taking insufficient pills). Some people make repeated suicide attempts. For every completed suicide, there are an estimated 20 previous attempts. Each unsuccessful attempt increases the likelihood of a completed suicide in the future.

Cause

Nine out of 10 suicides are associated with some form of mental disorder, especially depression, schizophrenia, alcohol abuse, bipolar disorder and panic disorder. In addition, personality disorders have been diagnosed in one-third to one-half of people who kill themselves. These suicides often occur in younger people who live in an environment where drug and alcohol abuse, as well as violence, are common. The most common personality disorders associated with suicide are borderline personality disorder, antisocial personality disorder and narcissistic personality disorder. Among people with schizophrenia, especially those suffering from paranoid schizophrenia, suicide is the main reason for premature death; they have a lifetime risk of 10 percent.

A history of trauma or abuse is also a risk factor for suicide, as is a family history of suicide, loss of a job, loss of a loved one, lack of social support and barriers to accessible health care.

Some suicides result from insufficiently treated, severe, debilitating or terminal physical illness. The pain, restricted function and dread of dependence can all contribute to suicidal behaviour, especially in illnesses such as Huntington's disease, cancer, multiple sclerosis, spinal cord injuries and AIDS.

Some or many of the above risk factors are present in most completed suicides. But depression and suicide are not inevitable for people with severe general medical illnesses or disabilities. The recognition and treatment of depression, when it occurs, can prevent many suicides.

Symptoms

Most people who are contemplating suicide show warning signs before they attempt to kill themselves. Some of these signs may include substance abuse; dramatic mood changes; withdrawal; reckless behaviour; aggression; self-neglect; feelings of purposelessness, anxiety, hopelessness, helplessness and being trapped; loss of interest in activities that were previously enjoyed; and changes in sleeping or eating habits. People contemplating suicide may also make a will, give away cherished possessions, or directly or indirectly express sentiments such as, "I don't want to live anymore," or "Everyone will be better off without me."

In most cases, these signs do not, on their own, indicate that a person will commit suicide. However, the greater the number of signs presented, the higher the risk of suicide.

Prevalence

Suicide is the ninth leading cause of death in Canada and the second leading cause among 15- to 34-year-olds. About 246,596 Canadians died in 2012; 3,926 of these deaths were attributed to suicide. This may be far below the actual figure, however, since suicide is still stigmatized and often goes unreported.

Males are three times more likely than females to commit suicide. Females, however, are three to four times more likely than males to attempt suicide. They are less likely to die from suicide attempts because they usually use methods that are less fatal, such as poisoning. Men tend to use more lethal methods such as hanging and firearms. People who are married are the least likely to commit suicide; the rate of suicide for single people is 3.3 times higher. Among men, those who are single are much more likely to commit suicide, and among women, the rate is highest for widows. For both sexes, the highest rate of suicide occurs among those who are between the ages of 40 and 59. In 2012, 44 percent of all suicides in Canada were in this age group, 35 percent were in the 15 to 39 age group and 21 percent were among those over the age of 60. This is different from many other countries where elderly people are more likely than any other age group to commit suicide. The rate of suicide in First Nations youth is five to seven times higher that it is for non-Aboriginal youth.

In recent years, most deaths by suicide in Canada have been the result of hanging (including strangulation and suffocation). The next most common method of suicide has been poisoning, followed by firearm use. Those between the ages of 15 and 39 are most likely to die as a result of hanging. The use of this method of suicide decreases with age, while firearm use increases with age.

Treatment Options

Most suicides can be prevented if the warning signs are recognized and responded to in an appropriate manner. People who notice signs of suicidal thinking or behaviour in a family member or friend should encourage that individual to talk about how he or she is feeling, and urge the person to get the counselling or medical support they need as soon as possible.

To make a diagnosis, a professional must first make a careful assessment, taking all the risk factors into account, including the availability of weapons, pills and other lethal means, as well as suicidal thinking and whether or not the person has conveyed the intention to commit suicide. Someone who has no thought of death or has thoughts of death that are not connected with suicide is at a lower risk than someone who is thinking of suicide.

Among those who are thinking of it, those who have not worked out the means of committing suicide are at a lower risk than those who think of suicide and a specific method of carrying it out.

Treatment is partly based on the level of intervention that is believed to be required. If the person is seriously depressed, and is also anxious, tense, angry and in overwhelming psychological anguish, the risk is more acute. The first priority is to ensure the safety of the individual. Sometimes hospitalization is necessary.

After safety is assured, treatment is aimed at the underlying disorder. Professional treatment may include psychological support, medication and other therapies: group, art, dance/movement. Professional treatment should involve working with the family if possible and other medical staff. Regular reassessments should take place.

Early recognition of suicidal behaviour and thinking, prompt intervention, and appropriate and effective therapy could prevent many of the completed suicides which occur in Canada every year.

National Associations

Canadian Association for Suicide Prevention (CASP) / L'Association canadienne pour la prévention du suicide (ACPS)
285 Benjamin Rd., Waterloo ON N2J 3Z4
Tel: 519-884-1470
e-mail: casp@suicideprevention.ca
www.suicideprevention.ca
www.facebook.com/CanadianAssociationforSuicidePrevention
twitter.com/casp_ca
Overview: A small national charitable organization founded in 1985
Mission: To reduce the suicide rate; To minimize the harmful consequences of suicide
Chief Officer(s):
Karen Letofsky, President
Tana Nash, Executive Director

Your Life Counts (YLC)
Seaway Mall, #GG5B, 800 Niagara St. North, Welland ON L3C 5Z4
Tel: 289-820-5777
e-mail: info@yourlifecounts.org
www.yourlifecounts.org
www.facebook.com/YourLifeCounts
twitter.com/yourlifecounts
www.youtube.com/user/YOURLIFECOUNTSTV
Overview: A small national charitable organization founded in 2000
Mission: Works with youth, families, veterans and emergency services in the battle against trauma, addictions and overwhelming life situations that may lead to thoughts of suicide.
Chief Officer(s):
Kevin Bolibruck, Chair

Provincial Associations

ALBERTA

Centre for Suicide Prevention (CSP)
#320, 105 - 12 Ave. SE, Calgary AB T2G 1A1
Tel: 403-245-3900; *Fax:* 403-245-0299; *Crisis Hot-Line:* 403-266-4357
www.suicideinfo.ca
www.linkedin.com/company/centre-for-suicide-prevention
www.facebook.com/centreforsuicideprevention
twitter.com/cspyyc
suicideinfo.tumblr.com
Previous Name: Suicide Information & Education Centre
Overview: A medium-sized provincial charitable organization founded in 1982
Mission: To educate people about the risk of suicide & suicide prevention
Member of: Canadian Association for Suicide Prevention
Affiliation(s): Canadian Mental Health Association - Alberta Division

Chief Officer(s):
Mara Grunau, Executive Director
 mara@suicideinfo.ca
Hilary Sirman, Director, Impact & Engagement
 hilary@suicideinfo.ca
Crystal Walker, Coordinator, Communications
 crystal@suicideinfo.ca

QUÉBEC

Association québécoise de prévention du suicide (AQPS)
#230, 1135, Grande Allée iuest, Québec QC G1S 1E7
 Tel: 418-614-5909; *Fax:* 418-614-5906; *Crisis Hot-Line:* 866-277-3553
 e-mail: reception@aqps.info
 www.aqps.info
 www.facebook.com/preventiondusuicide
 twitter.com/AQPS_Quebec
 www.youtube.com/user/AQPSQuebec#p/a
Overview: A small provincial organization founded in 1986
Mission: L'Association québécoise de prévention du suicide réunit les organisations et les citoyens qui souhaitent voir diminuer significativement le nombre de décès par suicide au Québec.
Chief Officer(s):
Jérôme Gaudreault, Directeur général, 418-614-5909 Ext. 36
Catherine Rioux, Coordonnatrice des communications, 418-614-5909
 Ext. 33

Local Associations

ONTARIO

Community Torchlight Guelph/Wellington/Dufferin
PO Box 1027, Guelph ON N1H 6N1
 Tel: 519-821-3761; *Fax:* 519-821-8190; *Crisis Hot-Line:* 888-821-3760
 e-mail: info@communitytorchlight.com
 www.communitytorchlight.com
 www.linkedin.com/pub/community-torchlight/23/2a2/236
 twitter.com/CommunityTorch
Previous Name: Distress Centre Wellington/Dufferin; Guelph Distress Centre
Overview: A small local charitable organization founded in 1969 overseen by Distress Centres Ontario
Mission: To provide a free, 24-hour listening, referral & crisis assistance telephone service to Guelph & rural Wellington & Dufferin counties
Chief Officer(s):
Katherine Johnson, Manager, Services
 kjohnson@communitytorchlight.com
Judith Rosenberg, Coordinator, Community Development &
 Recruitment
 jrosenberg@communitytorchlight.com

Crisis Centre North Bay
PO Box 1407, North Bay ON P1B 8K6
 Tel: 705-472-6204; *Fax:* 705-472-6236
 e-mail: info@crisiscentre-nb.on.ca
 www.crisiscentre-nb.on.ca
Overview: A small local charitable organization founded in 1972 overseen by Distress Centres Ontario
Mission: To help people in crises by providing temporary room & board as well as rehabilitation services

Distress Centre Niagara Inc.
PO Box 25014, Stn. Pen Centre-Glendale Ave., St Catharines ON L2T 2C4
 Fax: 905-682-7959; *Crisis Hot-Line:* 905-688-3711
 e-mail: dcniagara@distresscentreniagara.com
 distresscentreniagara.com
Overview: A small local organization founded in 1970 overseen by Distress Centres Ontario
Mission: To provide a no-cost confidential telephone support service by trained volunteers to assist anyone in need in the Niagara area

Distress Centre North Halton
PO Box 85, Georgetown ON L7G 4T1
 Tel: 905-877-0655; *Fax:* 905-877-0655; *Crisis Hot-Line:* 905-877-1211
 e-mail: dcnhalton@bellnet.ca
 www.dchalton.ca

Overview: A small local organization founded in 1973 overseen by Distress Centres Ontario
Mission: To provide confidential listening, emotional support, referrals & information, & crisis intervention

Distress Centre of Durham Region (DCD)
306 Brock St. North, Whitby ON L1N 4H7
 Tel: 905-430-3511; *Crisis Hot-Line:* 800-452-0688
 e-mail: dcd@distresscentredurham.com
 www.distresscentredurham.com
 www.facebook.com/DurhamDistress
 twitter.com/DurhamDistress
Overview: A small local charitable organization founded in 1970
Mission: To help people in distress to cope, by providing emotional support, crisis/suicide management & community education
Member of: Distress Centres Ontario; Canadian Association of Suicide Prevention
Chief Officer(s):
Victoria Kehoe, Executive Director
 victoria@distresscentredurham.com

Distress Centre of Ottawa & Region (DCOR) / Centre de détresse d'Ottawa et la région
PO Box 3457, Stn. C, Ottawa ON K1Y 4J6
 Tel: 613-238-1089; *Fax:* 613-722-5217
 www.dcottawa.on.ca
 www.facebook.com/DistressCentreOR
 twitter.com/DistressCentreO
Also Known As: Distress Centre Ottawa
Previous Name: Distress Centre Ottawa/Carleton
Overview: A small local charitable organization founded in 1969 overseen by Distress Centres Ontario
Mission: The Distress Centre is a non-profit organization that provides 24/7 confidential telephone services for emotional support, suicide prevention/intervention, postvention, crisis intervention, information referral & education services. It is a registered charity, BN: 108079815RR0001
Affliation(s): American Association of Suicidology; Canadian Association for Suicide Prevention; International Association for Suicide Prevention

Distress Line Sarnia
Bldg. 1030, 1086 Modeland Rd., Sarnia ON N7S 6L2
 Tel: 519-336-0120; *Fax:* 519-336-8517
 Toll-Free: 800-831-3031; *Crisis Hot-Line:* 888-347-8737
 www.familycounsellingctr.com
Also Known As: Family Counselling Centre
Overview: A small local charitable organization founded in 1973 overseen by Distress Centres Ontario
Mission: To help strengthen people & their relationships with others
Member of: Distress Centres Ontario
Chief Officer(s):
Don Pitt, Executive Director
 don.pitt@familycounsellingctr.com

Oakville Distress Centre
PO Box 776, Oakville ON L6K 0A9
 Tel: 905-849-4559; *Crisis Hot-Line:* 905-849-4541
 e-mail: info@dchalton.ca
 www.dchalton.ca
 www.linkedin.com/company/distress-centre-oakville
 twitter.com/DCOakville
Overview: A small local charitable organization founded in 1974 overseen by Distress Centres Ontario
Mission: To provide telephone, crisis intervention, & support services for the community of Oakville, Milton, & surrounding areas; To develop & provide outreach & suicide prevention programs to meet the needs of the community

Tel-Aide Outaouais (TAO)
CP 7218, Succ. Vanier, Ottawa ON K1L 8E3
 Tél: 819-776-2649; *Téléc:* 888-765-7040
 Courriel: administration@telaideoutaouais.ca
 www.telaideoutaouais.ca
Aperçu: *Dimension:* petite; *Envergure:* locale; Organisme sans but lucratif; fondée en 1974

Mission: Offrir un service d'écoute téléphonique en français pour toute personne ayant besoin d'aide, de soutien et de référence; développer et offrir des services d'écoute en français pour la population de l'Outaouais et de l'Ontario; favoriser l'implication sociale de la communauté par le biais du bénévolat; sensibiliser et éduquer le public à la nécessité d'être à l'écoute des gens vivant dans la détresse; susciter et entretenir des partenariats avec des organismes du milieu de la santé et des services sociaux; promouvoir les services de Tel-Aide Outaouais auprès de la population
Membre de: Ontario Association of Distress Centres; Association québécois de suicidologie
Affiliation(s): Regroupement des organismes communautaires en santé mentale de l'Outaouais
Membre(s) du bureau directeur:
Jean-François Parent, Executive Director
  direction@telaideoutaouais.ca

Telephone Aid Line Kingston (TALK)
PO Box 1325, Kingston ON K7L 5C6
  Tel: 613-531-8529; *Fax:* 613-531-3312; *Crisis Hot-Line:* 613-544-1771
  e-mail: director@telephoneaidlinekingston.com
  www.telephoneaidlinekingston.com
  www.facebook.com/telephoneaidlinekingston
Overview: A small local organization founded in 1973 overseen by Distress Centres Ontario
Mission: To provide telephone & support services, as well as community outreach & education, to meet the needs of the community

QUÉBEC

Suicide Action Montréal (SAM)
2345, rue Bélanger, Montréal QC H2G 1C9
  Tel: 514-723-3594; *Fax:* 514-723-3605
  Toll-Free: 866-277-3553; *Crisis Hot-Line:* 514-723-4000
  e-mail: info@suicideactionmontreal.qc.ca
  www.suicideactionmontreal.org
Overview: A small local charitable organization founded in 1984
Affiliation(s): Canadian Association for Suicide Prevention
Chief Officer(s):
Suzanne Carrière, President

Provincial Libraries

Centre for Suicide Prevention
#320, 105 - 12 Ave. SE, Calgary, AB T2G 1A1
  Tel: 403-245-3900; *Fax:* 403-245-0299
  www.suicideinfo.ca/resources
  Social Media: twitter.com/cspyyc;
  www.facebook.com/centreforsuicideprevention;
  www.linkedin.com/company/centre-for-suicide-prevention
Collection: Video Collection (Circulation Alberta), Conference Proceedings
Mara Grunau, Executive Director
Robert Olson, Librarian

Tay-Sachs Disease

Cause
Tay-Sachs disease is a fatal genetic disorder that is caused by the absence of an enzyme (hexosaminidase A). Without this enzyme, fat (lipid) accumulates in the cerebral neurons (brain cells). This results in progressive destruction of the nervous system. Tay-Sachs disease is an autosomal recessive genetic disorder. This means that if two carriers have children, there is a one in four chance that the disease will be passed on.

Symptoms
The symptoms of Tay-Sachs usually present around six months of age. Early symptoms include mild muscle weakness, muscle spasms and feeding difficulties. As the disease progresses, the child may experience vision loss, seizures and loss of motor and mental function; the child will eventually become paralyzed and non-responsive. Death usually occurs by the age of five years. A rare form of the disease, late-onset Tay-Sachs, affects adolescents and adults. Symptoms may include weakness, clumsiness

and neurological and intellectual impairment. Unlike the childhood form of the disease, late-onset Tay-Sachs does not always shorten life expectancy.

Prevalence
Tay-Sachs disease is most prevalent in those of Eastern European (Ashkenazi) background or in French Canadians who live near the St. Lawrence River. In these individuals, the carrier rate is about 1 in 27 in comparison to the rate of 1 in 250 in the general population.

Treatment Options
Before birth, Tay-Sachs can be diagnosed through prenatal tests that detect the presence of the hexosaminidase A enzyme. In amniocentesis, a sample of the amniotic fluid is obtained for testing, and in chorionic villus sampling (CVS), the cells from a small sample of the placenta are tested. A blood test that measures the level of the hexosaminidase A enzyme can be used to diagnose Tay-Sachs in children and adults. A clinical sign of Tay-Sachs in babies is a cherry-red spot on the retina.

There is no cure for Tay-Sachs disease, so therapy is aimed at symptom management. Treatment for children with Tay-Sachs may include anti-seizure medication, chest physiotherapy, assistive feeding devices and physical therapy. Treatment for adults with the disorder may include speech therapy, assistive devices and mental health support.

Genetic and premarital counseling is important to those at high risk. Some carrier couples use assisted reproductive therapy to reduce the risk of giving birth to a child with Tay-Sachs. Researchers continue to investigate gene therapy, enzyme-replacement therapy and stem cell therapy in their search to find a cure for Tay-Sachs.

National Associations

Canadian Association of Genetic Counsellors (CAGC) / Association Canadienne des conseillers en génétique (ACCG)
PO Box 52083, Oakville ON L6J 7N5
  Tel: 905-847-1363; *Fax:* 905-847-3855
  Other Communication: president@cagc-accg.ca
  e-mail: CAGCOffice@cagc-accg.ca
  www.cagc-accg.ca
Overview: A small national organization
Mission: To promote high standards of practice; To encourage professional growth; To increase public awareness of the profession; To offer certification in genetic counselling

Canadian College of Medical Geneticists (CCMG) / Collège canadien de généticiens médicaux
#310, 4 Cataraqui St., Kingston ON K7K 1Z7
  Tel: 613-507-8345; *Fax:* 866-303-0626
  e-mail: info@ccmg-ccgm.org
  www.ccmg-ccgm.org
Overview: A small national licensing charitable organization founded in 1975
Mission: To establish & maintain professional & ethical standards for medical genetics services in Canada; To certify individuals who provide medical genetics services; to encourage research activities
Affiliation(s): Canadian Association of Genetic Counsellors (CAGC)
Chief Officer(s):
Gail Graham, President
Sean Young, Treasurer
Publications:
• CCMG [Canadian College of Medical Geneticists] Newsletter
Type: Newsletter
• CCMG [Canadian College of Medical Geneticists] Membership Directory
Type: Directory

International Associations

International Federation of Human Genetics Societies (IFHGS)
c/o Vienna Medical Academy, Alserstrasse 4, Vienna 1090 Austria
Tel: +43 1 405 13 83 22; *Fax:* +43 1 407 82 74
e-mail: ifhgs@medacad.org
www.ifhgs.org

Overview: A small international organization founded in 1996
Mission: To facilitate communication throughout the international community of human geneticists
Chief Officer(s):
Stephen Lam, President
ts_lam@dh.gov.hk

Thyroid Disease

Thyroid disease refers to a number of conditions that affect the thyroid, a small, butterfly-shaped gland located in the middle of the lower neck. Hormones T3 and T4, produced by the thyroid, deliver energy to cells of the body, thus controlling the body's metabolism. Conditions that result from an imbalance of these hormones include hypothyroidism, hyperthyroidism, thyroid nodules and thyroiditis. In Canada, one in ten people have a thyroid condition of some kind. Of this number, over 50 percent are undiagnosed. Thyroid disorders are four to seven times more common in women than in men.

Hypothyroidism

Hypothyroidism is a result of the thyroid gland producing insufficient amounts of the hormones T3 and T4. Consequently, the body uses energy more slowly than it should.

Causes
This condition can be caused by an inflammation of the thyroid gland (Hashimoto's thyroiditis); treatment of Graves' hyperthyroidism with radioactive iodine or by thyroid surgery; or surgical removal of the thyroid gland.

Symptoms
Symptoms of hypothyroidism may include constipation, fatigue, weakness, sensitivity to cold, memory and cognition problems, goitre (enlarged thyroid), poor appetite, dry skin and slow, weak heartbeat.

Prevalence
About 2 percent of Canadians are affected by hypothyroidism. Prevalence of the disorder increases with age.

Treatment Options
A diagnosis of hypothyroidism is confirmed if a blood test shows an elevated level of thyroid stimulating hormone (TSH) and high levels of thyroid antibodies. Newborns are tested for neonatal hypothyroidism by using a heelpad blood-spot test.

Hypothyroidism is treated with hormone replacement therapy. Patients take a form of thyroxine in pill form (Eltroxin, Synthroid or Euthyrox) for life. Ongoing monitoring of TSH levels is necessary since illness, pregnancy and major stress may affect the dosage of thyroxine needed.

Hyperthyroidism

Hyperthyroidism is a result of the thyroid gland producing excess amounts of the T3 and T4 hormones. Consequently, the body uses energy faster than it should.

Cause
The most common cause of this condition is Graves' disease, an autoimmune disease, in which antibodies speed up thyroid function.

Symptoms
Symptoms of hyperthyroidism may include heat intolerance, nervousness, irritability, muscle weakness, shakiness, hot, moist skin, goitre (enlarged thyroid), rapid heart rate, excessive sweating, diarrhea, tremor and bulging eyes.

Prevalence
Approximately 1 percent of Canadians are affected by Graves' disease. More women are affected than men.

Treatment Options
A physical examination of a patient with Graves' hyperthyroidism may reveal clinical signs that are characteristic of the disorder. Blood tests are usually ordered to measure the level of thyroid stimulating hormone (TSH) and thyroid antibodies. A radioactive iodine uptake test (a procedure where a patient swallows a dose of radioactive iodine and then the radioactivity over the thyroid gland is measured after 24 hours) and thyroid scan are also often used to confirm a diagnosis of hyperthyroidism.

Hyperthyroidism may be treated with antithyroid drugs (Propylthiouracil, Melthimazole), radioactive iodine to destroy the thyroid cells, or surgical removal of the thyroid gland (thyroidectomy).

Thyroid Nodules

Thyroid nodules are cysts, lumps, bumps and tumours that can be cancerous or benign. Nodules may be singular or multiple (multinodular goitre).

Symptoms
Thyroid nodules do not cause symptoms in most people. The nodules are usually painless. If they are over 2 cm, they can be felt through the skin.

Prevalence
Approximately 5 percent of the population has single thyroid nodules, however most people who are affected are not aware that they have this condition.

Treatment Options
An ultrasound of the thyroid is usually performed in order to identify the size, shape and consistency of the nodule. A biopsy of the thyroid nodule is also often performed to determine if the nodule is cancerous or benign.

Treatment depends on the nature of the nodule. If the nodule is benign, only surveillance is usually required. Sometimes thyroxine is prescribed in an effort to shrink the nodule. If the nodule is malignant, the thyroid gland is usually removed. Additional treatment may be required.

Hashimoto's Thyroiditis

Cause
Thyroiditis, or inflammation of the thyroid gland, is most commonly caused by Hashimoto's thyroiditis. This inflammatory disorder results in underactive thyroid function (hypothyroidism).

Symptoms
People with Hashimoto's thyroiditis often have no symptoms except for fatigue and, in the early stages of the disorder, an enlarged thyroid (goitre). About 10 percent of people also experience pain.

Prevalence
Hashimoto's thyroiditis most commonly affects women.

Treatment Options

Diagnosis of Hashimoto's thyroiditis is usually confirmed through a blood test that shows high levels of antibodies and high levels of thyroid stimulating hormone (TSH). Sometimes a thyroid biopsy is also performed.

Hypothyroidism is treated with hormone replacement therapy. Patients take a form of thyroxine in pill form (Eltroxin, Synthroid or Euthyrox). Ongoing monitoring of TSH levels is necessary to ensure that the thyroxine dosage remains adequate.

Although thyroid disease is a chronic condition, careful disease management allows affected individuals to live healthy, normal lives.

National Associations

Thyroid Foundation of Canada / La Fondation canadienne de la Thyroïde
PO Box 298, Bath ON K0H 1G0

Toll-Free: 800-267-8822
www.thyroid.ca

Overview: A medium-sized national charitable organization founded in 1980
Mission: To provide leadership to the fight against thyroid disease
Chief Officer(s):
Donna Miniely, President
Rinda Hartner, Treasurer

International Associations

American Thyroid Association (ATA)
#550, 6066 Leesburg Pike, Falls Church VA 22041 USA
Tel: 703-998-8890; *Fax:* 703-998-8893
Toll-Free: 800-849-7643
e-mail: thyroid@thyroid.org
www.thyroid.org
www.linkedin.com/company/american-thyroid-association
www.facebook.com/ThyroidAssociation
twitter.com/thyroidfriends
www.youtube.com/user/thyroidorg

Overview: A medium-sized international organization founded in 1923
Mission: To promote health & understanding of thyroid biology; To encourage innovation in research on physiology, diseases, & thyroid molecular & cell biology; To guide public policies on the causes, diagnosis, & management of thyroid diseases & related disorders; To advocate for thyroid specialists; To encourage interaction & collaboration among members; To work with other thyroid societies to address public health & scientific issues
Member of: International Thyroid Congress
Chief Officer(s):
John C. Morris, President
Victor J. Bernet, Chief Operating Officer & Secretary
Barbara (Bobbi) R. Smith, Executive Director
    thyroidexec@thyroid.org
Adonia C. Coates, Director, Meetings & Program Services
    acoates@thyroid.org
Publications:
• Clinical Thyroidology [a publication of the American Thyroid Association]
Type: Journal; *Frequency:* 3 pa; *Editor:* Jerome M. Hershman; *Price:* Free
Profile: A summary of & expert commentary on recently published clinical & preclinical thyroid literature from around the world
• Signal [a publication of the American Thyroid Association]
Type: Newsletter; *Frequency:* 3 pa; *Editor:* Barbara Smith
Profile: American Thyroid Association happenings, such as policies, leaders, & meetings, as well as thyroid-related issues
• Thyroid [a publication of the American Thyroid Association]
Type: Journal; *Frequency:* Monthly; *Editor:* Peter Kopp; *Price:* Free withmembership in the American thyroid association
Profile: A peer-reviewed journal, covering subjects such as the molecular biology of the thyroid gland & the clinical management of thyroid disorders

Tick-Borne Diseases

Ticks transmit disease to humans by being carriers for a variety of microorganisms. The most common tick-borne illness in Canada is Lyme disease. Cases of Rocky Mountain spotted fever have also been reported.

Lyme Disease

Cause

Lyme disease was first recognized and so named in 1975 because of a cluster of cases found in Lyme, Connecticut. It is caused by the bacterium Borrelia burgdorferi, and is spread by the bite of an infected blacklegged (deer) tick. In Canada, there are infected tick populations in the southern regions of Ontario, Manitoba and Quebec, in parts of New Brunswick and Nova Scotia, and in southern British Columbia.

Symptoms

The disease in its earliest stages causes an expanding red rash (erythema migrans) in at least 75 percent of patients. The rash usually begins three days to one week after a tick bite, and can last for up to eight weeks. Flu-like symptoms—headaches, fever, fatigue, swollen lymph nodes—are common. The rash may be followed by progressive joint pain and swelling. Dysfunction of the heart (8 percent) and nervous system (15 percent) develop weeks to months later. Further progression causes arthritis and more serious neurological problems. It is rare for people to die from Lyme disease.

Although only one third of patients remember a tick bite, more than 60 percent develop the tell-tale rash.

Treatment Options

Diagnosis of Lyme disease requires a blood test to confirm the physical symptoms.

Oral antibiotics may be sufficient for the disease caught in the early stages. A two to four week treatment of doxycycline, amoxicillin or ceftriaxone cures most cases of Lyme disease. Long-standing, disseminated disease responds best to intravenous antibiotics.

A vaccine may provide partial protection from Lyme disease for those regularly engaged in high-risk activities (such as property maintenance), although other conditions may complicate this treatment.

Rocky Mountain Spotted Fever

Cause

Rocky Mountain spotted fever, also known as tick fever, is caused by the Rickettsia bacteria. In Canada, the disease is transmitted by a bite from an infected Rocky Mountain wood tick.

Symptoms

Like Lyme disease, Rocky Mountain spotted fever begins with flu-like symptoms—chills, fever and loss of appetite. A rash of small, reddish bumps, which gives the disease its name, begins on the wrist and ankle and spreads to the rest of the body. In its early stages, Rocky Mountain spotted fever is sometimes confused with meningitis. Serious complications of the disease may include heart and kidney failure and neurological problems.

If left untreated, Rocky Mountain spotted fever commonly lasts for two to three weeks. It has a mortality rate of 20 to 30 percent in untreated patients, and 3 to 4 percent in treated patients.

Treatment Options

Rocky Mountain spotted fever is usually diagnosed through a blood test. Aggressive antibiotic treatment should begin as early as possible.

Prevention of tick-borne disease requires avoidance of tick bites, by using insect repellants and protective clothing, plus daily checks for ticks during periods of exposure. If an attached tick is found, it should be removed promptly.

National Associations

Canadian Lyme Disease Foundation / Fondation canadienne de la maladie de lyme
2495 Reece Rd., Westbank BC V4T 1N1
Tel: 250-768-0978; *Fax:* 250-768-0946
www.canlyme.org
www.facebook.com/143033619666
twitter.com/canlyme

Also Known As: CanLyme
Overview: A small national charitable organization
Mission: To advance research about Lyme Disease in Canada
Affliation(s): International Lyme & Associated Diseases Society (ILADS)
Chief Officer(s):
Jim Wilson, President & Founder
jimwilson@telus.net

Tourette Syndrome

Tourette syndrome (TS) is a neurological disorder characterized by tics—involuntary, rapid, sudden movements or vocalizations that occur repeatedly in the same way.

Cause

Although the cause of TS is unknown, researchers have identified factors which may be involved in producing the disease. Persons with TS may show subtle abnormalities in the structure of certain parts of the brain. The disease may reflect abnormal metabolism of a neurotransmitter (a chemical that brain cells use to signal one another) called dopamine. Relatives of affected persons have an increased risk of disease, suggesting a genetic component. Finally, in some cases, the brain's function may be affected by antibodies triggered by infection with a bacterium called Group A Strep.

Symptoms

The multiple motor and vocal tics that characterize Tourette syndrome can appear separately or simultaneously. Tics may occur many times daily, or intermittently, with periodic changes in their number, frequency, type and location. Sometimes they may disappear for weeks.

Most commonly, the initial symptom of Tourette syndrome is a facial tic such as mouth twitching or rapid eye blinking. Sometimes, the first sign of the disorder is throat clearing or sniffing. The vocalizations of Tourette syndrome can also consist of grunts, obscenities, or other words the individual otherwise would not make. They are disruptive and can be profoundly embarrassing. Between 10 percent and 40 percent of people with Tourette syndrome also have echolalia (automatically repeating words spoken by others) or echopraxia (imitating someone else's movements). Fewer than 10 percent have coprolalia (the involuntary utterance of obscenities). Stress generally leads to an increase in symptoms.

There seems to be a clear association between Tourette syndrome, and obsessive compulsive disorder (OCD). As many as 20 to 30 percent of people with OCD report having, or having had, tics, and between 5 and 7 percent of those with OCD also have Tourette syndrome. In studies of patients with Tourette syndrome, it was found that 36 to 52 percent also met the criteria for OCD. There is evidence that Tourette syndrome and OCD share a genetic basis, or some underlying physiological disturbance. The genetic evidence is further strengthened by the concordance rate in twins (the likelihood that if one member of the pair has the disorder, the other will also develop it): in identical twins, who have the same genes, the concordance is 53 percent, whereas in fraternal twins, who are no more closely related than other siblings, it is 8 percent.

Other conditions commonly associated with Tourette syndrome are hyperactivity, distractibility, impulsivity, difficulty in learning, emotional disturbances and social problems. The disorder may cause social uneasiness, shame, self-consciousness and depression. The person may be rejected by others and may develop anxiety about the tics, negatively affecting social, school and work functioning. In severe cases, the disorder may interfere with everyday activities like reading and writing.

The disorder usually lasts for the life of the person, but the severity, frequency and variability of the tics often diminish during adolescence and adulthood.

Prevalence

Tourette syndrome is about 10 times more prevalent in children and adolescents than in adults; the median age for the development of tics is seven years. Roughly one person in 2,000 will demonstrate this behaviour at some time in his or her life. Boys are three or four times as likely as girls to develop TS.

Treatment Options

Diagnosis of TS is usually based on symptoms described in a detailed medical history. There are no specific tests used to diagnose the disorder. Sometimes blood tests, a computerized tomography (CT) scan of the brain or electroencephalogram (EEG) (to check electrical activity in the brain) are used to rule out other conditions that could be causing the symptoms. For diagnosis to be confirmed, the following criteria must be met: multiple motor, as well as one or more vocal, tics have been present during the illness, not necessarily at the same time; the tics occur many times during a day (often in bouts) nearly every day or intermittently for more than one year, and during this period there was never a tic-free period of more three consecutive months; the disturbance causes clear distress or difficulties in social, work or other areas; the onset is before age 18; the involuntary movements or vocalizations are not due to the direct effects of a substance (such as stimulants) or a general medication condition.

Children who are not bothered by their tics should not be treated with drugs. Medications are reserved for those whose tics lead to symptoms which impair behavioural, physiologic or social function. Simple tics respond to benzodiazepines (tranquilizers). Selective serotonin reuptake inhibitors (SSRIs) have also been effective in some cases. For more severe cases, haloperidol, an antipsychotic, may be used. It acts directly on the brain source of the tic, counteracting the overactivity, and can have a calming effect, but should be started slowly. Unfortunately, it sometimes causes other movement disorders after prolonged use. Whether drug treatment is used or not, patients and their families may need counselling to deal with the disease's secondary effects, for example, bullying at school or conflict within the family. During periods of high stress, relaxation techniques and biofeedback may be useful. Other alternative therapies like acupuncture and yoga may also be of some benefit. In many cases, comprehensive behavioural intervention for tics (CBIT) is very effective. With this approach, people with Tourette syndrome are shown ways to prevent themselves from engaging in a tic so that over time, the tic is extinguished.

Fortunately, Tourette syndrome often becomes much less severe in adult life, without any treatment. In some cases, tics can disappear entirely. When they persist, even mild tics can be distressing, especially in social situations. However, most people with TS lead normal lives. Research is focused on locating the gene marker for TS, and developing improved medications to treat the disorder.

National Associations

Tourette Syndrome Foundation of Canada (TSFC) / La Fondation canadienne du syndrome de Tourette
#245, 5955 Airport Rd., Mississauga ON L4V 1R9
Tel: 905-673-2255; *Fax:* 905-673-2638
Toll-Free: 800-361-3120
www.tourette.ca
www.youtube.com/TSFCanada
Also Known As: Tourette Canada
Overview: A large national charitable organization founded in 1976
Mission: To educate & increase public awareness about Tourette Syndrome
Member of: Canadian Brain Tissue Bank; Canadian Centre for Philanthropy; Volunteers Canada; Canadian Coalition for Genetic Fairness
Affliation(s): Health Charities Council of Canada
Chief Officer(s):
Ramona Jennex, President
Publications:
• It's Your Move!
Type: Course
Profile: Personal development program aimed at helping youth with Tourette deal with their challenges
• Understanding Tourette Syndrome
Type: Handbook
Profile: Comprehensive information regarding Tourette Syndrome
• The Green Leaflet [a publication of the Tourette Syndrome Foundation of Canada]
Type: Newsletter; *Frequency:* 3 pa
• NewsFlash [a publication of the Tourette Syndrome Foundation of Canada]
Type: Newsletter
• Tourette Syndrome Foundation of Canada Annual Report
Type: Yearbook; *Frequency:* Annually
• Twitch Times [a publication of the Tourette Syndrome Foundation of Canada]
Type: Newsletter; *Frequency:* Monthly

Transplant-Related Conditions

In recent decades, transplantation of solid organs (heart, liver, lung, kidney), bone marrow and stem cells has become an established part of medical care for advanced diseases in many patients who otherwise face organ failure and poor prognosis. While on one hand, transplantation may serve to cure the underlying disease, it nonetheless often entails chronic medical therapy that will likely include the use of immunosuppressants to prevent rejection; chronic medications; frequent and long-term medical follow-up; and diagnostic testing which may be invasive.

Symptoms
Symptoms of ill health in post-transplantation patients are most commonly related to the long-term use of immunosuppressive medications, a compromised immune system and organ or tissue rejection. The side effects of specific immunosuppressants vary, but may include acne, anemia, anxiety, mood swings, insomnia, arthritis, headache, nausea, diarrhea, vomiting, high blood pressure, kidney damage, osteoporosis, weight gain and tremors. Since immunosuppressants slow down the immune system, they can also make post-transplantation patients more susceptible to

infections. In the first month after a transplant, patients are more likely to suffer from pneumonia, human herpes simplex virus, a urinary tract infection or infections at the site of the surgical wound or IV line. In the following six months, cytomegalovirus (CMV), Epstein-Barr virus, pneumonia or a central nervous system infection may develop. From six months to a year after transplantation, hepatitis B or C and other opportunistic infections may take hold. It is also common for a post-transplantation patient to have at least one episode of acute (short-term) organ rejection in the year following a transplant. Symptoms of organ rejection may include fever, flu-like symptoms, swelling, reduced urine output, pulse rate changes, weight gain and pain or tenderness at the transplant site. Chronic organ rejection is associated with gradual loss of organ function. In some cases, acute rejection can lead to chronic rejection.

Prevalence
In Canada, more than 4,500 people were on the transplant waiting list in 2014. Approximately 2,356 transplants were performed.

Treatment Options
A number of clinical management protocols are utilized in the care of post-transplantation patients, and these vary depending on the type of transplant undertaken, the extent of the tissue match between donor and recipient, and the experience of the given transplantation centre. In general, however, most patients who receive a transplanted organ or cells will require some chronic therapy (short- or long-term) with immunosuppressive medications. These can be several or many and are given in an effort to control the patient's own immunologic response to receiving an organ or cells from another person. The body's natural response after recognizing such an exposure is to "fight" these cells and tissues with its own defence cells, which are designed to attack and kill foreign material. The immunosuppressive medications help modulate this response so that the transplanted organ is not damaged, injured or "rejected" by the recipient who needs the organ or cells to function in a healthier manner. Post-transplant immunosuppressants may include azathioprine, basiliximab, daclizumab, prednisone, cyclosporine, tacrolimus, mycophenolate mofetil and rapamycin.

Immunosuppressive therapy and protection of the transplanted organ must be balanced against the adverse creation of an immunocompromised state in the patient, placing him at greater risk for contracting infections that can be serious and even life-threatening. Given these circumstances, transplant patients require close working relationships with their medical team along with a true commitment to be compliant with these potentially difficult and complicated medical regimens.

To detect early signs of rejection or infection, post-transplant tests are usually conducted on a regular basis. Blood pressure, pulse, temperature and weight are monitored for every patient. Other tests are organ-specific and may include blood tests, ultrasounds, X-rays, biopsies, pulmonary function tests (to check lung function) and electrocardiograms and echocardiograms (to monitor heart function).

In addition to the medical therapy for patients who have received transplants, one must also consider the significant psychological and social aspects of having undergone such procedures. Strong social support systems and close attention to a healthy emotional and psychological status are important for successful therapy. Many transplant centres have extensive support services available to patients from which they and their families can benefit.

Transplant survival rates continue to improve in Canada-the three-year survival rate for lung transplant survivors is 80 percent while the five-year survival rate for heart transplant survivors is 75 percent—and researchers are investigating ways improve survival rates of transplant patients even more.

National Associations

Canadian Association of Transplantation
114 Cheyenne Way, Ottawa ON K2J 0E9

Toll-Free: 877-968-9449
e-mail: admin@cst-transplant.ca
www.cst-transplant.ca

Overview: A medium-sized national organization
Mission: Health professionals committed to facilitating & enhancing the transplant process
Chief Officer(s):
Steven Paraskevas, President

Canadian Blood & Marrow Transplant Group (CBMTG) / Société Canadienne de greffe de cellules souches hematopoietiques
#400, 570 West 7th Ave., Vancouver BC V5Z 1B3

Tel: 604-874-4944; *Fax:* 604-874-4378
e-mail: cbmtg@malachite-mgmt.com
www.cbmtg.org

Overview: A small national organization
Mission: To provide leadership in the field of blood & marrow transplantation (BMT); to recognize & promote advances in clinical care; to promote basic, translational & clinical research & education; to represent BMT issues to government agencies, health care organizations & the public; to collaborate with fellow organizations
Chief Officer(s):
Ana Torres, Executive Director
 ana.torres@malachite-mgmt.com
Publications:
• CBMTG [Canadian Blood & Marrow Transplant Group] Newsletter
Type: Newsletter; *Frequency:* Quarterly; *Editor:* Nancy Henderson
Profile: Professional news; case studies; clinical papers; questions; letters to the editor; industry news

Canadian Society of Transplantation (CST) / Société canadienne de transplantation
114 Cheyenne Way, Ottawa ON K2J 0E9

Toll-Free: 877-968-9449
e-mail: admin@cst-transplant.ca
www.cst-transplant.ca

Previous Name: Canadian Transplantation Society
Overview: A small national charitable organization
Mission: To provide leadership for the advancement of educational, scientific, & clinical aspects of transplantation in Canada
Chief Officer(s):
Atul Humar, President
Kathryn Tinckam, Secretary
Michael Mengel, Treasurer
Publications:
• CST [Canadian Society of Transplantation] News
Type: Newsletter; *Frequency:* 3 pa
Profile: Feature articles, plus information about the Canadian Society of Transplantation sent to all members

Canadian Transplant Association (CTA) / Association canadienne des greffes
PO Box 74, Tavistock ON N0B 2R0

Toll-Free: 877-779-5991
e-mail: cta@txworks.ca
www.organ-donation-works.org
www.linkedin.com/company/5165307
www.facebook.com/CanadianTransplantAssociationandGames
twitter.com/CTACanada

Previous Name: Canadian Transplant Games Association
Overview: A medium-sized national charitable organization founded in 1989
Mission: To promote a healthy lifestyle for transplant recipients
Chief Officer(s):
Dave Smith, President
 davidsmith@txworks.ca

Jennifer Holman, Vice-President, West
 jenniferholman@txworks.ca
Bianca Segatto, Vice-President, East
 bsegatto@txworks.ca
Robert Sallows, Secretary
 rsallows@txworks.ca
Michael Sullivan, Treasurer
 msullivan@txworks.ca
Neil Folkins, Director, Membership Development
 neilfolkins@txworks.ca
Publications:
• The Living Proof [a publication of the Canadian Transplant Association]
Type: Newsletter; *Frequency:* Quarterly; *Editor:* Jennifer Holman;
Price: Free with membership in the CanadianTransplant Association
Profile: Canadian Transplant Association news, including event information, awards & inspiring stories

 Alberta Region
 AB

www.organ-donation-works.org

 British Columbia Region
 BC

www.organ-donation-works.org

 Chief Officer(s):
 Margaret Benson, Regional Director, British Columbia
 mmbenson@txworks.ca

 New Brunswick (Eastern Provinces) Region
 NB

www.organ-donation-works.org

 Chief Officer(s):
 Mark Black, Regional Director, Eastern Provinces
 markblack@txworks.ca

 Ontario Region
 ON

www.organ-donation-works.org

 Chief Officer(s):
 Sandra Holdsworth, Director, Ontario Region
 sandraholdsworth@txworks.ca

 Québec Region
 c/o Gaston Martin, 101, rue Lavigne, Repentigny QC J6A 6B6
Tel: 450-654-3786
www.organ-donation-works.org

 Chief Officer(s):
 Gaston Martin, Director, Québec Region
 gaston@txworks.ca

 Saskatchewan Region
 SK

www.organ-donation-works.org

 Chief Officer(s):
 Phil Gleim, Regional Director
 philgleim@txworks.ca

Fondation Diane Hébert Inc
132, rue Blainville Est, Sainte-Thérèse-de-Blainville QC J7E 1M2

Tél: 450-971-1112; *Téléc:* 450-971-1818
Ligne sans frais: 877-971-1110
Courriel: fdh@macten.net

Aperçu: *Dimension:* moyenne; *Envergure:* nationale; Organisme sans but lucratif; fondée en 1987
Mission: Services directs offerts aux patients en attente de greffes, aux greffés et à leur famille autant sur le plan moral, physique ou financier; prêt d'équipements médicaux tels que chaises roulantes électriques; la Fondation vise aussi à sensibiliser la population au don d'organes
Membre de: Info Don D'Organes; Québec Transplant; Canadian Transplant Association

Provincial Associations

BRITISH COLUMBIA

British Columbia Transplant Society (BCTS)
West Tower, #350, 555 West 12th Ave., Vancouver BC V5Z 3X7
Tel: 604-877-2240; *Fax:* 604-877-2111
Toll-Free: 800-663-6189
e-mail: info@bct.phsa.ca
www.transplant.bc.ca
www.facebook.com/BCTransplant
twitter.com/bc_transplant
Overview: A medium-sized provincial organization founded in 1986
Mission: To lead & coordinate all activities related to organ transplantation & donation, ensuring high standards of quality & efficient management
Affiliation(s): University of British Columbia
Chief Officer(s):
Ed Ferre, Director, Program Development & External Relations
Peggy John, Manager, Communications
Linda Irwin, Manager, Health Information

ONTARIO

Trillium Gift of Life Network
#900, 522 University Ave., Toronto ON M5G 1W7
Tel: 416-363-4001; *Fax:* 416-363-4002
Toll-Free: 800-263-2833
www.giftoflife.on.ca
www.linkedin.com/company/1426658
www.facebook.com/TrilliumGiftofLife
twitter.com/TrilliumGift
Previous Name: Multiple Organ Retrieval & Exchange Program of Ontario
Overview: A medium-sized provincial organization founded in 1988
Mission: To enable every Ontario resident to make an informed decision to donate organs & tissue; To support healthcare professionals in implementing their wishes; To maximize organ & tissue donation in Ontario in a respectful & equitable manner through education, research, services & support
Chief Officer(s):
Ronnie Gavsie, President & CEO

Local Associations

BRITISH COLUMBIA

David Foster Foundation
212 Henry St., Victoria BC V9A 3H9
Tel: 250-475-1223; *Fax:* 250-475-1193
Toll-Free: 877-777-7675
e-mail: info@davidfosterfoundation.com
www.davidfosterfoundation.com
www.linkedin.com/company/david-foster-foundation
www.facebook.com/DavidFosterFoundation
twitter.com/davidfosterfdn
Overview: A small local charitable organization founded in 1986
Mission: To provide financial assistance to families of children undergoing transplant surgery; To raise public awareness regarding organ donation
Chief Officer(s):
Michael Ravenhill, CEO
mravenhill@davidfosterfoundation.com

International Associations

The Transplantation Society (TTS)
International Headquarters, #1401, 505 boul René-Lévesque ouest, Montréal QC H2Z 1Y7
Tel: 514-874-1717; *Fax:* 514-874-1716
e-mail: info@tts.org
www.tts.org
Overview: A medium-sized international organization
Mission: To provide global leadership in transplantation; To develop the science & clinical practice
Chief Officer(s):
Nancy L. Ascher, President

Marcelo Cantarovich, Vice-President
Elmi Muller, Senior Treasurer
Jean-Pierre Mongeau, Executive Director
jp.mongeau@tts.org
Robert Colarusso, Director, Technologies
technologies@tts.org
Geneviève Leclerc, Director, Meetings
genevieve.leclerc@tts.org
Eugenia Siu, Coordinator, Registration & Administration
eugenia.siu@tts.org
Publications:
• Transplantation: The Official Journal of The Transplantation Society
Type: Journal; *Frequency:* Semimonthly
Profile: Advances in transplantation, in areas such as cell therapy & islet transplantation, clinical transplantation, experimental transplantation,immunobiology & genomics, & xenotransplantation
• Tribune [a publication of The Transplantation Society]
Type: Newsletter; *Frequency:* 3 pa; *Editor:* Nancy K. Man
Profile: Society news, meeting reviews, & feature articles

Local Hospitals & Health Centres

ONTARIO

TORONTO: Sunnybrook Health Sciences Centre - St. John's Rehab
Affiliated with: Toronto Central Local Health Integration Network
285 Cummer Ave., Toronto, ON M2M 2G1
Tel: 416-226-6780 *Fax:* 416-226-6265
www.sunnybrook.ca
Number of Beds: 160 beds
Note: Provides specialized rehabilitation services & care in burn injuries, organ transplant rehabilitation, cancer, cardiovascular surgery, strokes & other neurological conditions, traumatic injuries & complex medical conditions. Teaching site for the University of Toronto & a research facility. A multicultural & multifaith environment dedicated to the values of care of the Sisters of St. John the Divine.
Barry A. McLellan, President & CEO

Tuberculosis

Cause

Tuberculosis (TB) is an infectious disease caused by mycobacteria that normally affect the lungs (pulmonary tuberculosis). It is spread through the air in one of the following ways by people who have active TB: talking, singing, laughing, playing a wind instrument (such as a flute), sneezing or coughing. Pregnant women with TB can pass the disease on to their babies (congenital TB), but this is rare. Some people are at higher risk of catching TB, including the homeless; individuals with HIV or AIDS; people who live in correctional facilities, crowded housing or long-term care residences; those with a compromised immune system; those who have worked, lived or travelled in countries where TB is common; and those who have lived or worked with someone who has active TB.

Symptoms

TB can be active or inactive (latent). The usual symptoms of an active TB infection of the lungs include persistent cough, chest pain, fever and coughing up of blood. TB infection can cause weight loss, night sweats and fatigue. Left untreated, TB may spread to the spine, causing bone breakdown with deformity; to the lining of the brain, causing tuberculous meningitis; or, in fact, to any organ of the body (extrapulmonary TB). A person with active TB disease is contagious. It is estimated that a person with untreated active TB infects an average of 10 to 15 other people each year.

Many people who have been infected by TB keep it successfully contained by their own immune systems. They show no symptoms, and are not contagious. However, there is some risk of the contained germ, even years later, overcoming the body's resistance and causing active disease. If an inactive TB infection is left untreated, it becomes active TB disease in about 5 to 10 percent of cases.

Prevalence

In Canada, TB is not a very common disease. In 2014, there were approximately 1,568 cases of tuberculosis in Canada. TB is most prevalent in Aboriginal people, as well as immigrants and refugees who have come to Canada from a country where TB is more common. Most of the cases reported are in individuals between the ages of 24 and 44.

Treatment Options

The tuberculin skin test is used to determine if a person has been infected with TB. If the skin test is positive, more tests are often ordered to confirm active TB disease, including a chest X-ray and test of lung fluid.

People who have inactive TB can almost always be cured after six to twelve months of therapy with isoniazid.

Active TB is treated with at least two of these commonly used drugs: isoniazid, rifampin, pyrazinamide and ethambutol. The types of drugs prescribed and the length of treatment depends on age, overall health and where the infection is located. Persons infected with HIV, because of their lowered resistance to disease, have more trouble clearing their TB infection, even if they use effective drugs faithfully. [0][0]Therefore, they should be treated for one year. Regardless of length of treatment, the germ may become resistant to the drug being used. Incomplete or interrupted treatment often leads to drug resistance. Germs that are resistant to multiple drugs may be passed to others, and are now a serious public health menace. People with drug-resistant TB usually require stronger medication for a longer time than other TB patients. Some may need to be hospitalized in isolation for part of their treatment.

Although the risk of developing TB is low for most people in Canada, and the disease can usually be cured with antibiotics, it is still a health problem in other parts of the world. Consequently, TB prevention and surveillance programs have been developed to make sure that Canadians continue to be protected from tuberculosis.

Provincial Associations

BRITISH COLUMBIA

TB Vets
1410 Kootenay St., Vancouver BC V5K 4R1

Tel: 604-874-5626
Toll-Free: 888-874-5626
e-mail: information@tbvets.org
www.tbvets.org
www.facebook.com/tbvets
twitter.com/tbvets
plus.google.com/115497261163706842951
Overview: A medium-sized provincial charitable organization founded in 1945
Mission: Operates a key return service, with proceeds & donations going to respiratory disease research, treatments & education; annually sends out over 350,000 keytags to BC residents
Chief Officer(s):
Eric Beddis, Chair
Kanys Merola, Executive Director
Publications:
• TB Vets e-newsletter
Type: Newsletter; *Frequency:* Quarterly

International Associations

Heiser Program for Research in Leprosy & Tuberculosis
c/o The New York Community Trust, 909 - 3rd Ave., New York NY 10022 USA

Tel: 212-686-0010; *Fax:* 212-532-8528
Overview: A small international charitable organization
Mission: To award grants to fund research into leoprosy, tuberculosis & their bacterial agents to find measures for prevention & cure.
Chief Officer(s):
Gilla Kaplan, Chair, Scientific Advisory Committee
Len McNally, Director
  lm@nyct-cfi.org

Tuberous Sclerosis

Tuberous sclerosis is a genetic disorder that causes benign (non-cancerous) tumours to form in different locations—primarily in the brain, skin, kidneys, heart, lungs and even eyes.

Cause

Tuberous sclerosis is caused by a mutation either in the TSC1 gene on chromosome 9, or the TSC2 gene on chromosome 16. About one-third of the cases of tuberous sclerosis are due to an altered gene inherited from an affected parent. The other two-thirds of cases are the result of a spontaneous gene mutation. People with tuberous sclerosis have a 50 percent chance of passing the disease on to their children.

Symptoms

Disease severity is highly variable, even within the same family. In some cases, symptoms are so mild that they are not even noticed, while in others the health problems associated with the disorder are severe. The symptoms of tuberous sclerosis vary depending on where the tumours or lesions develop. For example, many people with tuberous sclerosis have skin abnormalities, such as an area of decreased skin pigmentation, called an ash-leaf spot because of its shape. Multiple ash-leaf spots may appear on the trunk and limbs during infancy. At age three or four, tiny red bumps, adenoma sebaceum, resembling acne may appear on the nose and cheeks. Finally, a roughened spot with the consistency of orange peel, shagren patch, may appear over the lower spine. There are also neurological symptoms, such as epilepsy; behavioural problems; and intellectual disabilities associated with the disorder. Up to 80 percent of people with tuberous sclerosis have seizures, and around two-thirds of those with a severe mental handicap demonstrate autistic behaviour. Aggression, hyperactivity, obsessive-compulsive behaviour and depression may also be exhibited by some people with tuberous sclerosis. Lesions in the heart may cause rhythm disturbances, while those in the kidney or lung may result in organ failure.

Prevalence

It is estimated that tuberous sclerosis affects one in every 6,000 to 10,000 people.

Treatment Options

Diagnosis of tuberous sclerosis often begins with a physical examination. Skin abnormalities characteristic of tuberous sclerosis may be identified in this manner. Eye tests to detect retinal lesions may also be conducted. Magnetic resonance imaging (MRI) and computerized tomography (CT) scans are often used to locate tumours that would be otherwise difficult to identify. An echocardiogram, which produces images of the heart, and an electrocardiogram (ECG), which measures the electrical activity of the heart, may also be used to identify heart tumours.

There is no cure for tuberous sclerosis so treatment is based on symptoms and can include anti-seizure medication, removal of skin lesions, treatment of high blood pressure caused by kidney problems, special education, psychological counselling and, in some instances, surgery to remove growing tumours. Certain types of brain growths can be treated with a drug called everolimus. Research into other tumour-suppressing drugs is currently underway.

With careful monitoring and appropriate medical support, many people with tuberous sclerosis can lead full, productive lives and have a normal life span.

National Associations

Tuberous Sclerosis Canada Sclérose Tubéreuse (TSCST)
PO Box 35057, Essa Rd., Barrie ON L4N 5Z2
e-mail: tscanadast@gmail.com
www.tscanada.ca
www.facebook.com/TSCanadaST
Overview: A small national charitable organization founded in 1990
Mission: To provide information & support to tuberous sclerosis patients & their families; To promote & improve professional & public awareness, education & research regarding this disease
Affliation(s): Tuberous Sclerosis Alliance (USA); Tuberous Sclerosis Association (GB); Tuberous Sclerosis International (The Netherlands)
Chief Officer(s):
Cathy Evanochko, Co-Chair
Karen Shulist, Co-Chair

Turner Syndrome

Cause
Turner syndrome is a genetic disorder that only affects females. Rather than having two complete female sex (X) chromosomes, women and girls with Turner syndrome are missing all or part of the second X chromosome.

Symptoms
In infants, symptoms of Turner syndrome may include swollen hands and feet, webbing at the back and side of the neck and heart abnormalities. Teen girls with Turner syndrome often have a small stature and absent or incomplete sexual development. In women, additional symptoms may include infertility, hearing problems, drooping eyelids, cataracts, high blood pressure and diabetes. Girls and women with Turner syndrome may also have developmental, social and learning problems.

Prevalence
Turner syndrome occurs in 1 of every 2,000 to 2,500 live female births. It is estimated that there are more than 6,000 women and girls with Turner syndrome in Canada.

Treatment Options
Turner syndrome can be diagnosed before birth through a prenatal test such as amniocentesis (a procedure where a sample of amniotic fluid is obtained for chromosome analysis). Due to increased awareness of Turner syndrome in the health care community, most girls with this condition are diagnosed at birth or as toddlers. A physical exam of an infant may show clinical signs of Turner's syndrome such as neck webbing and swollen hands and feet. Other tests including blood tests (to check for hormone levels) and karyotyping (to examine the chromosomes in a cell sample) may also be performed to confirm the diagnosis.

Turner syndrome cannot be cured, but hormonal treatment may give the person a more normal life. Growth hormone injections can help a girl reach a taller adult height, and estrogen replacement can encourage the development of breasts and other sex characteristics. A few girls will develop menstrual periods spontaneously, and a few women will become pregnant; most, however, are infertile. Some women with Turner syndrome who want to become pregnant use in-vitro fertilization.

Psychological support for women with this condition is important. With careful monitoring and appropriate therapy, women with Turner syndrome can lead normal, productive lives.

National Associations

Canadian Lymphedema Framework (CLF)
#204, 4800 Dundas St. West, Toronto ON M9A 1B1
Tel: 647-693-1083
e-mail: admin@canadalymph.ca
www.canadalymph.ca
Overview: A small national charitable organization founded in 2009
Mission: To advance the treatment of lymphedema & related disorders in Canada; To promote lymphedema research, practices, & clinical development
Affliation(s): International Lymphodema Framework
Chief Officer(s):
Anna Kennedy, Executive Director

Turner's Syndrome Society (TSS) / Société du syndrome de Turner
#9, 30 Clearly Ave., Ottawa ON K2A 4A1
Tel: 613-321-2267; *Fax:* 613-321-2268
Toll-Free: 800-465-6744
e-mail: info@turnersyndrome.ca
www.turnersyndrome.ca
www.facebook.com/TurnerSyndromeSocietyOfCanada
Overview: A small national charitable organization founded in 1981
Mission: To improve the quality of life for individuals & families affected by Turner's Syndrome; to strive to accomplish this through providing public & professional awareness about the needs & concerns of individuals with Turner's Syndrome & their families through the development of communication networks to provide mutual support
Chief Officer(s):
Krista Kamstra-Cooper, President

Provincial Associations

ONTARIO

Lymphovenous Association of Ontario (LAO)
#203, 4800 Dundas Street West, Toronto ON M9A 1B1
Tel: 416-410-2250; *Fax:* 416-546-8991
Toll-Free: 877-723-0033
e-mail: lymphontario@yahoo.com
www.lymphontario.org
Overview: A small provincial charitable organization founded in 1996
Mission: To educate the public; To promote improved treatments for lymphovenous disorders; To support research for a cure
Affliation(s): Canadian Disability Organization; Canadian Organization for Rare Disorders
Chief Officer(s):
Denise Lang, President
Anne Blair, Vice-Chair

QUÉBEC

Association du Syndrome de Turner du Québec
1484, Montée Gagnon, Val-David QC J0T 2N0
Tél: 819-320-0409
Courriel: turnerquebec@gmail.com
www.syndrometurnerquebec.com
Aperçu: *Dimension:* petite; *Envergure:* provinciale; Organisme sans but lucratif; fondée en 1984
Mission: Faire connaître les personnes atteintes du S.T.; faire circuler l'information médicale; créer des nouveaux contacts
Membre(s) du bureau directeur:
Marie-Claude Doire, Présidente
Jocelyne Jeanneau, Coordonnatrice

Ulcerative Colitis

Ulcerative colitis is an inflammatory condition of the large bowel, or colon. Inflammation of the wall of the bowel leads to ulcerations of its surface. Most often, the disease first affects the rectum, and then moves upward through the rest of the colon. Ulcerative colitis is a chronic condition, but there are periods when symptoms disappear (remissions), only to act up again later (flare-ups).

Cause

The cause of ulcerative colitis is unknown, but research suggests that an overactive immune system working to defend the body against a bacterial or viral substance could be involved. Environmental factors may also come into play. People who live in urban regions are more commonly affected by ulcerative colitis than those who live in rural areas. There is also a strong genetic association. First degree relatives have a 3 to 9 percent lifetime risk of the disease.

Symptoms

Symptoms of ulcerative colitis may include weight loss, fatigue, fever, abdominal pain false urges to have a bowel movement and diarrhea, which may be bloody. Ulcerative colitis in patients who have a specific antibody in their system (HLA-B27) has a strong association with an arthritis called ankylosing spondylitis. Several kinds of liver and biliary tract disease, inflammation of the eye and certain characteristic skin rashes may occur. Growth may be limited in children with the condition.

After many years of active ulcerative colitis there is an increased risk of colon cancer. It is usually preceded by warning signs visible in a colonoscopy, so physicians generally begin an aggressive surveillance program after 8 to 10 years of disease.

Prevalence

There are approximately 104,000 people in Canada with ulcerative colitis. Most often, the condition is diagnosed in people between the ages of 20 and 40.

Treatment Options

To diagnose ulcerative colitis, a physician usually takes a detailed medical history and performs a physical examination. Additional testing is often required. Blood tests may be ordered to check for an increased white blood cell count which could suggest an immune system disease like colitis. A stool sample may be taken to check for blood loss, or evidence of a bacterial infection that could be causing the symptoms. A colonoscopy is also often used to help diagnose ulcerative colitis. In this procedure, a flexible tube with a small camera at the end is inserted up the rectum and into the colon to check for inflammation. In some cases, a barium enema may also be required. In this procedure, barium is used to coat the bowel so that an X-ray can be taken.

Treatment depends on the severity of symptoms. Mild cases may respond to simple anti-diarrheal medicines and dietary modifications. More severe cases are treated with either rectal or oral forms of anti-inflammatory drugs such as 5-ASA. Corticosteroids are sometimes necessary. Disease confined to the rectum can generally be managed with steroid enemas. Extensive disease requires oral steroid medication. Immunosuppressive drugs like azathioprine and 6-mercaptopurine are sometimes given if the disease is resistant to steroids or if steroid side effects are unacceptable. Approximately 30 percent of patients will eventually have their entire colon removed.

Currently, the only cure for ulcerative colitis is removal of the colon, but appropriate drug therapy can greatly improve the quality of life for people with this condition.

National Associations

Crohn's & Colitis Canada / Crohn's et Colitis Canada
#600, 60 St. Clair Ave. East, Toronto ON M4T 1N5
Tel: 416-920-5035; *Fax:* 416-929-0364
Toll-Free: 800-387-1479
e-mail: support@crohnsandcolitis.ca
www.crohnsandcolitis.ca
www.linkedin.com/company/crohn's-and-colitis-foundation-of-canada
www.facebook.com/crohnsandcolitis.ca
twitter.com/getgutsyCanada
www.youtube.com/user/getgutsy
Previous Name: Crohn's & Colitis Foundation of Canada; Canadian Foundation for Ileitis & Colitis
Overview: A medium-sized national charitable organization founded in 1974
Mission: To find a cure for Crohn's disease & ulcerative colitis; To raise funds for medical research; To educate individuals with inflammatory bowel disease, their families, health professionals, & the public
Chief Officer(s):
Mina Mawani, President & CEO
Tim Berry, Vice-President, Finance
Angie Specic, Vice-President, Marketing & Communications

Alberta/NWT Region
#3100, 246 Stewart Green SW, Calgary AB T3H 3C8
Toll-Free: 888-884-2232
Chief Officer(s):
Patricia Glenn, Regional Director
pglenn@crohnsandcolitis.ca

Atlantic Canada Region
PO Box 173, Lower Sackville NS B4C 2S9
Tel: 902-297-1649; *Fax:* 902-422-6552
Toll-Free: 800-265-1101
Chief Officer(s):
Edna Mendelson, Regional Director
emendelson@crohnsandcolitis.ca

British Columbia/Yukon Region
PO Box 47147, Stn. City Square, Vancouver BC V5Z 4L6
Toll-Free: 800-513-8202
e-mail: britishcolumbia@crohnsandcolitis.ca
Chief Officer(s):
Colleen Hauck, Regional Director
chauck@crohnsandcolitis.ca

Bureau du Québec
#420, 1980, rue Sherbrooke Ouest, Montréal QC H3H 1E8
Tél: 514-342-0666; *Téléc:* 514-342-1011
Ligne sans frais: 800-461-4683
Chief Officer(s):
Edna Mendelson, Directrice régionale
emendelson@crohnsandcolitis.ca

Manitoba/Saskatchewan/Nunavut Region
PO Box 20009, 3310 Portage Ave., Winnipeg MB R3K 2E5
Tel: 204-231-2115; *Fax:* 204-237-8214
Toll-Free: 866-856-8551
e-mail: centralcanada@ccfc.ca
Chief Officer(s):
Shair Wolsey, Regional Director
swolsey@crohnsandcolitis.ca

Ontario Region
#600, 60 St. Clair Ave. East, Toronto ON M4T 1N5
Tel: 613-806-7956; *Fax:* 416-929-0364
Toll-Free: 800-387-1479
Chief Officer(s):
Jacqueline Alvarez, Regional Director
jalvarez@crohnsandcolitis.ca

Local Associations

MANITOBA

Winnipeg Ostomy Association (WOA)
#204, 825 Sherbrook St., Winnipeg MB R3A 1M5

Tel: 204-234-2022
e-mail: woainfo@mts.net
www.ostomy-winnipeg.ca

Overview: A small local charitable organization founded in 1972 overseen by Canadian Ostomy Society
Mission: To assist people with ostomy & related surgeries in Winnipeg and the surrounding area
Chief Officer(s):
Lorrie Pismenny, President
Publications:
• Inside Out
Type: Newsletter; *Frequency:* 6 pa

QUÉBEC

Ileostomy & Colostomy Association of Montréal (ICAM) / Association d'iléostomie et colostomie de Montréal (AICM)
5151, boul de l'Assomption, Montréal QC H1T 4A9

Tel: 514-255-3041; *Fax:* 514-645-5464
www.aicm-montreal.org

Overview: A small local charitable organization founded in 1958
Mission: To act for the welfare for ostomates & their families
Affiliation(s): United Ostomy Association of Canada Inc.
Chief Officer(s):
Jean-Pierre Lapointe, President & Treasurer, 514-645-4023
Huguette Fortier, Secretary, 514-355-1245

International Associations

American Society of Colon & Rectal Surgeons
#550, 85 West Algonquin Rd., Arlington Heights IL 60005 USA

Tel: 847-290-9184; *Fax:* 847-427-9656
e-mail: ascrs@fascrs.org
www.fascrs.org
www.linkedin.com/company/the-american-society-of-colon-and-rectal-surg
www.facebook.com/fascrs
twitter.com/fascrs_updates

Overview: A medium-sized international organization
Mission: To advance the science & practice of the treatment of patients with diseases & disorders that affect the colon, rectum, & anus
Chief Officer(s):
Patricia L. Roberts, MD, President
David A. Margolin, MD, Vice-President
Tracy L. Hull, MD, Secretary
Neil H. Hyman, MD, Treasurer
Publications:
• ASCRS [American Society of Colon & Rectal Surgeons] News
Type: Newsletter; *Frequency:* Semiannually
Profile: Information from the society of interest to its members

Visual Impairment

Visual impairment covers a continuum from decreased visual acuity correctible by refractive means (glasses and contact lenses) to legal blindness, indicating less than 20/200 vision in the better eye, or an extremely limited field of vision. Total blindness represents the complete loss of sight. Millions of Canadians are affected by some form of visual impairment. The risk of visual impairment increases with age; more than one in eleven Canadians over the age of 65 and more than one in eight over the age of 75 are living with severe vision loss.

A wide variety of disorders of the eye can cause visual impairment, including muscular imbalance, infections, congenital disorders and those associated with premature birth. Occasionally visual impairment reflects a disease behind the eye, involving some part of the brain that receives and processes images from the eyes. Many health problems and eye injuries also lead to visual impairment. Retinitis pigmentosa, a degeneration of the light-sensing tissue at the back of the eye, also causes vision (especially night vision) deterioration. The four main causes of visual impairment in Canada are age-related macular degeneration, diabetic retinopathy, glaucoma and cataracts.

Age-Related Macular Degeneration

Age-related macular degeneration (AMD) is characterized by deterioration of the macula (a spot near the centre of the retina) that causes blurriness in the centre of the field of vision.

Cause

AMD develops as the eye ages and is more common in Caucasians. Other risk factors for the condition may include a family history of AMD, severe obesity, smoking, cardiovascular disease and elevated cholesterol.

Symptoms

AMD usually develops gradually and may affect one or both eyes. Symptoms of the condition may include difficulty reading or seeing in low light, difficulty recognizing faces, haziness or a blind spot in the centre of the field of vision, crooked central vision and decreased colour intensity.

Prevalence

Approximately one million Canadians have early-stage age-related macular degeneration, and by 2031 the number of people who become blind as a result of AMD is expected to double.

Treatment Options

Age-related macular degeneration is usually diagnosed by means of a thorough eye exam. Commonly, the back of the eye is examined to identify drusen (yellow deposits that form under the retina in people with AMD), and the centre of vision is tested for defects. An angiogram of the eye (a procedure in which a camera takes pictures of the blood vessels in the eye after they have absorbed coloured dye) and an optical coherence tomography (OCT) (used to display detailed images of the retina) are often ordered, as well.

A high dose of antioxidant vitamins and zinc is sometimes prescribed to help slow the progression of AMD. In advanced cases of AMD in both eyes, a telescopic lens is sometimes implanted in one eye to help improve distance and close-up vision.

Diabetic Retinopathy

Cause

In some diabetics the blood vessels that nourish the retina are fragile, which makes them more apt to bleed. If this happens, it can cause vision loss. Anyone who has diabetes can develop diabetic retinopathy. However, the following factors may increase the risk: smoking, high blood pressure, high cholesterol, pregnancy and uncontrolled blood sugar levels. The longer a person has diabetes, the greater the risk of developing diabetic retinopathy.

Symptoms

In the early stages of diabetic retinopathy, there are often no symptoms. As the condition progresses, patients may experience difficulty perceiving colours, and may have blurred vision, floaters, dark areas in the field of vision and vision loss.

Prevalence

Close to 500,000 Canadians have some form of diabetic retinopathy.

Treatment Options

The most common method of diagnosing diabetic retinopathy is through a dilated eye exam. In this procedure, drops are put in the eye to enlarge the pupil so that it is easier to get a good view of the inside of the eye. Other diagnostic tests may include an angiogram of the eye and an OCT.

Severe diabetic retinopathy may be treated by focal laser therapy (to stop blood and liquid leakage in the eye), scatter laser therapy (to shrink abnormal blood vessels in the eye) or vitrectomy (a procedure in which a tiny incision is made in the eye to remove blood and scar tissue).

Glaucoma

Cause
Glaucoma is characterized by abnormal pressure in the eye that causes deterioration of the optic nerve. Vision loss may result. Risk factors for glaucoma may include family history of the condition, long-term corticosteroid use, severe eye injury, certain types of eye surgery, other eye conditions (such as retinal detachment), medical conditions (diabetes, high blood pressure) and aging.

Symptoms
The most common forms of glaucoma are primary open-angle glaucoma and angle-closure glaucoma. Symptoms of primary open-angle glaucoma may include loss of peripheral vision and tunnel vision. Symptoms of angle-closure glaucoma may include blurred vision, eye pain (accompanied by nausea and vomiting), reddening of the eye and visual disturbances that come on suddenly.

Prevalence
Glaucoma causes vision impairment in 250,000 Canadians.

Treatment Options
Several tests are usually used to diagnose glaucoma including tonometry (a procedure to measure internal eye pressure), optic nerve damage test, peripheral vision test, pachymetry (to measure the thickness of the cornea) and gonioscopy (a procedure in which a lens is placed on the eye to visualize the drainage angle and thus determine the form of glaucoma).

The goal of glaucoma therapy is to reduce internal eye pressure. Most commonly, eye drops are prescribed to treat glaucoma. If the eye pressure is still high, an oral medication (usually a carbonic anhydrase inhibitor) may be prescribed as well. Sometimes surgery is performed to treat glaucoma and may include laser surgery (to open drainage canals) and filtering surgery (where a small piece of tissue at the base of the cornea is removed to allow fluid drainage). In some cases, drainage implants are inserted in the eyes to drain fluid.

Cataracts

A cataract is a clouding of the lens of the eye. Vision loss occurs because light rays cannot get through the cloudy lens to the retina.

Cause
In most cases, cataracts are caused when the lens tissue is changed through aging, injury or an inherited genetic disorder. Risk factors for developing cataracts may include advanced age, family history of cataracts, diabetes, smoking, obesity, eye injury, eye surgery, extended use of corticosteroids and excessive exposure to sunlight.

Symptoms
The symptoms of cataracts may include cloudy, blurred vision, difficulty seeing at night, fading of colours, double vision, seeing halos around lights and increased sensitivity to light.

Prevalence
Cataracts affect more than 2.5 million Canadians, and it is estimated that the figure will double by 2031.

Treatment Options
Eye exams used to diagnose cataracts may include a visual acuity test (eye chart), a slit-lamp exam (a special microscope uses a line of light to examine the front of the eye) and a retinal examination (a procedure in which drops are put in the eyes to dilate the pupils, therefore making examination of the retina easier).

The only treatment for cataracts is cataract surgery (a procedure in which the cloudy lens is removed and replaced with a plastic lens implant).

Regular eye exams and early diagnosis of eye disorders could help minimize vision loss for many Canadians. It is estimated that 75 percent of vision loss can either be treated or prevented. Lifestyle changes such as wearing sunglasses, keeping diabetes under control, eating a healthy diet, exercising on a regular basis and refraining from smoking can also help prevent vision loss.

National Associations

Accessible Media Inc. (AMI)
#200, 1090 Don Mills Rd., Toronto ON M3C 3R6
Tel: 416-422-4222; *Fax:* 416-422-1633
Toll-Free: 800-567-6755
e-mail: info@ami.ca
www.ami.ca
www.linkedin.com/company/accessible-media-inc-
www.facebook.com/AccessibleMediaInc
twitter.com/AccessibleMedia
www.youtube.com/user/accessiblemedia
Overview: A medium-sized national charitable organization
Mission: To bring media in an alternate form to those not able to follow in traditional ways
Affiliation(s): Achilles Canada; Canadian Council of the Blind; CNIB; Courage Canada; Sight Night; Foundation Fighting Blindness
Chief Officer(s):
David Errington, President & CEO
John Melville, Vice-President, Programming & Production
Line Gendreau, Vice-President, Finance
Terry Reid, Vice-President, Human Resources
Peter Burke, Vice-President, Marketing & Communications
Darrel Sauerlender, Vice-President, Technology Services
Chris O'Brien, Accessibility Officer

Alliance for Equality of Blind Canadians / Alliance pour l'Égalite des Personnes Aveugles du Canada
PO Box 20262, Stn. RPO Town Centre, Kelowna BC V1Y 9H2
Toll-Free: 800-561-4774
www.blindcanadians.ca
twitter.com/blindcanadians
Previous Name: National Federation of the Blind: Advocates for Equality
Overview: A medium-sized national charitable organization
Mission: To promote the inclusion of blind, deaf-blind & partially-sighted Canadians in all aspects of social life, from employment to participation in elections
Chief Officer(s):
Dar Wournell, President

American Optometric Association (AOA)
243 North Lindbergh Blvd., 1st Fl., St. Louis MO 63141-7881 USA
Tel: 314-991-4100; *Fax:* 314-991-4101
Toll-Free: 800-365-2219
e-mail: aoa@aoa.org
www.aoa.org
www.linkedin.com/company/american-optometric-association
www.facebook.com/American.Optometric.Association
twitter.com/aoaconnect
www.youtube.com/user/aoaweb
Previous Name: American Association of Opticians
Overview: A large national organization founded in 1898
Mission: To advance the quality, availability & accessibility of eye, vision & related health care; To represent the profession of optometry; To enhance & promote the independent & ethical decision making of its members; To assist doctors of optometry in practicing successfully in

accordance with the highest standards of patient care
Member of: World Council of Optometry
Affliation(s): Canadian Association of Optometrists
Chief Officer(s):
David Cockrell, President
   DACockrell@aoa.org
Publications:
• Optometry
Type: Journal; *Frequency:* Monthly

Banque d'yeux nationale, inc.
2705, boul Laurier, Sainte-Foy QC G1V 2G2
Tél: 418-654-2702; *Téléc:* 418-654-2247
Aperçu: *Dimension:* petite; *Envergure:* nationale; fondée en 1970
Membre(s) du bureau directeur:
Céline Lemay, Coordonnatrice

Blind Sailing Association of Canada (BSAC)
17 Boustead Ave., Toronto ON M6R 1Y7
Tel: 416-489-2433
e-mail: info@blindsailing.ca
www.blindsailing.ca
www.facebook.com/385889524843037
twitter.com/blindcansail
Overview: A small national organization founded in 2002
Mission: To provide opportunities for the blind to learn to sail, thus boosting skills, confidence & self-esteem
Member of: Ontario Sailing Association; Sail Canada

Braille Literacy Canada (BLC)
c/o CNIB Library, 1929 Bayview Ave., Toronto ON M4G 3E8
Tel: 416-480-7522; *Fax:* 416-480-7700
e-mail: info@blc-lbc.ca
www.canadianbrailleauthority.ca
www.linkedin.com/company/3502741
www.facebook.com/brailleliteracycanada
twitter.com/@brllitcan
Previous Name: Canadian Braille Authority
Overview: A small national organization founded in 1990
Mission: To promote braille as a primary medium for persons who are blind; To enables all Canadians who require braille to access information to have braille literacy; To sets up systems that allow blind persons to access print information in braille
Chief Officer(s):
Jen Goulden, President

Canadian Association of Optometrists (CAO) / Association canadienne des optométristes (ACO)
234 Argyle Ave., Ottawa ON K2P 1B9
Tel: 613-235-7924; *Fax:* 613-235-2098
Toll-Free: 888-263-4676
e-mail: info@opto.ca
www.opto.ca
www.linkedin.com/company/canadian-association-of-optometrists
www.facebook.com/CanadianOpto
twitter.com/CanadianOpto
Overview: A large national organization founded in 1941
Mission: To represent & assist the profession of optometry in Canada; To improve the quality, availability, & accessibility of vision & eye care
Affliation(s): Eye Health Council of Canada
Chief Officer(s):
Laurie Clement, Executive Director
   lclement@opto.ca
Doug Dean, Director, 613-235-7924 Ext. 215
   ovp@opto.ca
Debra Yearwood, Director, Marketing & Communications
   dyearwood@opto.ca
Danielle Paquette, Manager, Canadian Certified Optometric Assistant (CCOA) Program, 613-235-7924 Ext. 211
   dpaquette@opto.ca
Publications:
• Canadian Journal of Optometry [a publication of the Canadian Association of Optometrists]
Type: Journal; *Frequency:* q.; *Editor:* Dr. B. Ralph Chou, OD, MSc;
ISSN: 0045-5075; *Price:* Free with CAO membership, $70 (Canada) or $80 (USA/overseas) without CAO membership

Profile: Features articles on clinical practice, research, case studies, & practicemanagement tips

Canadian Blind Sports Association Inc. (CBSA) / Association canadienne des sports pour aveugles inc.
#325, 5055 Joyce St., Vancouver BC V5R 6B2
Tel: 604-419-0480; *Fax:* 604-419-0481
Toll-Free: 866-604-0480
e-mail: info@canadianblindsports.ca
www.canadianblindsports.ca
www.facebook.com/canadianblindsports
Overview: A medium-sized national charitable organization founded in 1976
Mission: To facilitate opportunities for Canadians who are legally blind to participate in amateur sport at the national/international level, & to thereby enhance a healthy lifestyle & individual well-being.
Affliation(s): International Blind Sports Association; Canadian Paralympic Committee; Active Living Alliance
Chief Officer(s):
Jane D. Blaine, Chief Executive Officer
   jane@canadianblindsports.ca

The Canadian Council of the Blind (CCB) / Le Conseil canadien des aveugles
#100, 20 James St., Ottawa ON K2P 0T6
Tel: 613-567-0311; *Fax:* 613-567-2728
Toll-Free: 877-304-0968
www.ccbnational.net
www.facebook.com/ccbnational
twitter.com/ccbnational
Overview: A medium-sized national charitable organization founded in 1944
Mission: To promote the well-being of individuals who are blind or vision-impaired through higher education, profitable employment, & social association; To create a closer relationship between blind & sighted friends; To organize a nation-wide organization of people who are blind & vision-impaired & groups of blind persons throughout Canada; To promote measures for the conservation of sight & the prevention of blindness
Affliation(s): World Blind Union
Chief Officer(s):
Louise Gillis, National President
Lori Fry, First Vice-President
Jim Tokos, Second Vice-President
Publications:
• Canadian Council of the Blind / Le Conseil Canadien des Aveugles Newsletter
Type: Newsletter; *Frequency:* Monthly
Profile: Available electronically or in large print format, the newsletter features articles on issues affecting the blind & visually impaired,products for the blind, competition results, & CCB updates & events
• White Cane Week Magazine
Type: Magazine; *Frequency:* Annually; *Accepts Advertising*; *Editor:* Mike Potvin
Profile: CCB news & information, White Cane Week review & events, & a resource guide for the blind & vision impaired

Canadian Deafblind Association (National) (CDBA) / Association canadienne de la surdicécité (Bureau National)
PO Box 421, #14, 1860 Appleby Line, Burlington ON L7L 7H7
Fax: 905-319-2027
Toll-Free: 866-229-5832
e-mail: info@cdbanational.com
www.cdbanational.com
www.facebook.com/cdbanational
twitter.com/CDBANational
Overview: A medium-sized national charitable organization
Mission: To promote awareness, education & support for people who are deafblind, in order to enhance their well-being
Chief Officer(s):
Carolyn Monaco, President
   carolyn.monaco@sympatico.ca
Tom McFadden, National Executive Director

   Alberta Chapter

AB

Tel: 780-554-6083
www.deafblindalberta.ca

Chief Officer(s):
Nicole Sander, Vice-President
 nicsander@me.com

British Columbia Chapter
227 - 6th St., New Westminster BC V3L 3A5
Tel: 604-528-6170; Fax: 604-528-6174
www.cdbabc.ca

Chief Officer(s):
Theresa Tancock, Coordinator, Family Services
 theresa@cdbabc.ca

Canadian Deafblind Association - New Brunswick Inc.
#495 B Prospect St., #H, Fredericton NB E3B 9M4
Tel: 506-452-1544; Fax: 506-451-8309; TTY: 506-452-1544
www.cdba-nb.ca
www.facebook.com/CDBANB

Chief Officer(s):
Kevin Symes, Executive Director
 k.symes@cdba-nb.ca

Ontario Chapter
50 Main St., Paris ON N3L 2E2
Tel: 519-442-0463; Fax: 519-442-1871
Toll-Free: 877-760-7439; TTY: 519-442-6641
e-mail: info@cdbaontario.com
www.cdbaontario.com
www.facebook.com/cdbaontario
twitter.com/CDBAOntario

Chief Officer(s):
Cathy Proll, Executive Director

Saskatchewan Chapter
83 Tucker Cres., Saskatoon SK S7H 3H7
Tel: 306-374-0022; Fax: 306-374-0004
e-mail: cdba.sk@shaw.ca

Chief Officer(s):
Dana Heinrichs, Executive Director

Canadian Examiners in Optometry (CEO) / Examinateurs canadiens en optométrie (ECO)
#403, 37 Sandiford Dr., Stouffville ON L4A 7X5
Tel: 905-642-1373; Fax: 905-642-3786
e-mail: administration@ceo-eco.org
www.ceo-eco.org

Overview: A medium-sized national organization
Mission: To assess the competence of individual optometrists in the practice of optometry; To provide assessment results to the individuals & to relevant regulators; To provide mechanisms to evaluate the quality of practice of optometrists in Canada

Canadian Guide Dogs for the Blind (CGDB)
National Office & Training Centre, PO Box 280, 4120 Rideau Valley Dr. North, Manotick ON K4M 1A3
Tel: 613-692-7777; Fax: 613-692-0650
e-mail: info@guidedogs.ca
www.guidedogs.ca

Overview: A medium-sized national charitable organization founded in 1984
Mission: To assist visually-impaired Canadians with their mobility by providing & training them in the use of professionally trained guide dogs
Member of: International Guide Dog Federation; Assistance Dogs International, Inc.
Chief Officer(s):
Jane Thornton, Co-Founder & Chief Operating Officer
Publications:
• Side by Side [a publication of the Canadian Guide Dogs for the Blind]
Type: Newsletter; Frequency: s-a.

Canadian National Institute for the Blind (CNIB) / INCA (INCA)
1929 Bayview Ave., Toronto ON M4G 3E8
Toll-Free: 800-563-2642
e-mail: info@cnib.ca
www.cnib.ca
www.facebook.com/myCNIB
twitter.com/CNIB
www.youtube.com/cnibnatcomm

Also Known As: The Canadian National Institute for the Blind/Institut national canadien pour les aveugles
Overview: A large national charitable organization founded in 1918
Mission: To ameliorate the condition of persons with vision loss in Canada; To prevent blindness; To promote sight enhancement services; To direct services to more than 100,000 Canadians with vision loss, provided through a network of more than 57 service centres, within 13 provincial & territorial operating divisions; To provide library services, research, advocacy, public education, & accessible design consulting; To produce materials in alternative formats, including Braille & DAISY talking books; To supply assistive technologies for persons with vision loss
Affliation(s): World Blind Union; International Agency for the Prevention of Blindness
Chief Officer(s):
John M. Rafferty, President
Craig Lillico, CFO, Treasurer, & Vice-President
Margaret McGrory, Executive Director & Vice-President, CNIB Library
Tim Alcock, Vice-President, Marketing & Fund Development
Keith Gordon, Vice-President, Research
Publications:
• The Canadian National Institute for the Blind Annual Review
 Frequency: Annually
• CNIB [Canadian National Institute for the Blind] Vision
Type: Newsletter; Frequency: 3 pa
Profile: A nationally distributed newsletter presenting Canadian vision health issues, for consumers & professionals
• Insight [a publication of the Canadian National Institute for the Blind]
Type: Newsletter; Frequency: Monthly; Price: Free
Profile: Vision health information, consumer products & assistive technologies, & upcoming events

Alberta-Northwest Territories Division
12010 Jasper Ave., Edmonton AB T5K 0P3
Tel: 780-488-4871; Fax: 780-482-0017
Toll-Free: 800-563-2642; TTY: 780-482-4089
e-mail: alberta@cnib.ca

Chief Officer(s):
John Mulka, Regional Vice-President, Western Canada

British Columbia-Yukon Division
#200, 5055 Joyce St., Vancouver BC V5R 6B2
Tel: 604-431-2121; Fax: 604-431-2099
Toll-Free: 800-563-2642
e-mail: bcyukon@cnib.ca

Chief Officer(s):
John Mulka, Regional Vice-President, Western Canada

Division du Québec
3044, rue Delisle, Montréal QC H4C 1M9
Tél: 514-934-4622; Téléc: 514-934-2131
Ligne sans frais: 800-563-2642

Chief Officer(s):
Marie-Camille Blais, Directrice générale, Québec

E.A. Baker Foundation for the Prevention of Blindness
1929 Bayview Ave., Toronto ON M4G 3E8
Tel: 416-486-2500; Fax: 416-480-7700
www.cnib.ca

Manitoba Division
1080 Portage Ave., Winnipeg MB R3G 3M3
Tel: 204-774-5421; Fax: 204-775-5090
e-mail: manitoba@cnib.ca

Chief Officer(s):
Glenn Hildebrand, Chair

New Brunswick Division
22 Church St., #T120-22, Moncton NB E1C 0P7
Tel: 506-857-4240; Fax: 506-857-3019
Toll-Free: 800-536-2642

Chief Officer(s):
Pamela Gow-Boyd, Regional Vice-President, Atlantic Canada

Newfoundland & Labrador Division
70 The Boulevard, St. John's NL A1A 1K2
Tel: 709-754-1180; *Fax:* 709-754-2018
Toll-Free: 800-563-2642

Chief Officer(s):
Pamela Gow-Boyd, Regional Vice President, Atlantic Canada

Nova Scotia-PEI Division
6136 Almon St., Halifax NS B3K 1T8
Tel: 902-453-1480
Toll-Free: 800-563-2642

Chief Officer(s):
Pamela Gow-Boyd, Regional Vice-President, Atlantic Canada

Ontario Division
1929 Bayview Ave., Toronto ON M4G 3E8
Tel: 416-486-2500; *Fax:* 416-480-7700
Toll-Free: 800-563-2642; *TTY:* 416-480-8645

Chief Officer(s):
Len Baker, Regional Vice-President, Ontario & Quebec

Saskatchewan Division
2160 Broad St., Regina SK S4P 1Y5
Tel: 306-525-2571; *Fax:* 306-565-3300
Toll-Free: 800-563-2642

Chief Officer(s):
Christall Beaudry, Executive Director

Canadian Ophthalmological Society (COS) / Société canadienne d'opthalmologie (SCO)
#110, 2733 Lancaster Rd., Ottawa ON K1B 0A9
Tel: 613-729-6779; *Fax:* 613-729-7209
e-mail: cos@cos-sco.ca
www.cos-sco.ca

Overview: A medium-sized national organization founded in 1937
Mission: To assure the provision of optimal eye care to all Canadians by promoting excellence in ophthalmology & providing services to support its members in practice
Member of: Canadian Standards Association
Affiliation(s): Canadian Medical Association; Concilium Ophthalmological Universale
Chief Officer(s):
Jennifer Brunet-Colvey, Chief Executive Officer
Rosalind O'Connell, Manager, Communications & Public Affairs
communications@cos-sco.ca

Canadian Orthoptic Council / Conseil canadien d'orthoptique
CHUL, 2705, boul Laurier, Sainte-Foy QC G1V 4G2
Fax: 418-654-2188
e-mail: info@orthopticscanada.org
www.orthopticscanada.org

Overview: A medium-sized national organization
Mission: To establish standards in the training of orthoptic students; To establish standards for orthoptic training centres; To provide examinations of orthoptic students in order to determine their proficiency in orthopotics & to award a certificate of competency to qualified students who pass the examinations; To require evidence of continuing education of certified orthoptists; To establish standards for the professional ethical conduct of certified orthoptists
Affliation(s): Canadian Medical Association; Canadian Ophthalmological Society
Chief Officer(s):
Louis-Etienne Marcoux, Secretary-Treasurer
Ann Haver, Administrative Coordinator

Canadian Retina Society / Société canadienne de la rétine
c/o Canadian Ophthalmological Society, 110 - 2733 Lancaster Rd., Ottawa ON K1B 0A9
Toll-Free: 800-267-5763
www.cos-sco.ca/cpd/canadian-retina-society-meeting

Overview: A medium-sized national organization
Mission: To promote & support retina specialists in Canada
Chief Officer(s):
Amin Kherani, President

Canadian Society of Ophthalmic Registered Nurses (CSORN) / Société canadienne des infirmières et infirmiers en opthalmologie
c/o Donna Punch, Kensington Eye Institute, #600, 340 College St., Toronto ON M5T 3A9
www.csorn.ca

Overview: A small national organization
Mission: To promote high standards of practice in ophthalmic nursing; To encourage good ocular care
Chief Officer(s):
Donna Punch, President, 416-928-2132 Ext. 3104
president@csorn.ca
Catherine Callaghan, Vice-President
vicepresident@csorn.ca
Adonis Manglapus, Secretary
secretary@csorn.ca
Linda Wong, Treasurer
treasurer@csorn.ca
Publications:
• Canadian Society of Ophthalmic Registered Nurses Newsletter
Type: Newsletter
Profile: CSORN activities, including conference previews & reviews, executive news, updates from provincial representatives, & ophthalmology news

Dog Guides Canada
152 Wilson St., Oakville ON L6K 0G6
Tel: 905-842-2891; *Fax:* 905-842-3373
Toll-Free: 800-768-3030; *TTY:* 905-842-1585
e-mail: info@dogguides.com
www.dogguides.com
www.facebook.com/LFCDogGuides
twitter.com/LFCDogGuides

Also Known As: Lions Foundation of Canada Dog Guides and Sibtech Creations
Previous Name: Canine Vision Canada
Overview: A medium-sized national organization founded in 1985
Mission: To provide Dog Guides to Canadians through various programs, including Canine Vision Canada, Hearing Ear Dogs of Canada, & Service Dog Guides
Member of: Lions Foundation of Canada
Chief Officer(s):
Sandy Turney, Executive Director
sandyturney@dogguides.com
Julie Jelinek, Director, Development
jjelinek@dogguides.com
Alex Ivic, Director, Programs
aivic@dogguides.com
Sarah Miller, Manager, Communications
smiller@dogguides.com

The Foundation Fighting Blindness (FFB)
890 Yonge St., 12th Fl., Toronto ON M4W 3P4
Tel: 416-360-4200; *Fax:* 416-360-0060
Toll-Free: 800-461-3331
e-mail: info@ffb.ca
www.ffb.ca
www.facebook.com/187447074652378
twitter.com/FFBCanada
www.youtube.com/user/FFBCanada

Previous Name: RP Research Foundation - Fighting Blindness
Overview: A medium-sized national charitable organization founded in 1974
Mission: To support & promote research directed to finding the causes, treatments & ultimately the cures for retinitis pigmentosa, macular degeneration & related retinal diseases
Member of: International RP Association; Canadian Coalition for Genetic Fairness
Affiliation(s): US RP Foundation
Chief Officer(s):
Sharon M. Colle, President & CEO
scolle@ffb.ca
Rahn Dodick, Treasurer
Malcolm Hunter, Corporate Secretary

Glaucoma Research Society of Canada / Société canadienne de recherche sur le glaucome
#215E, 1929 Bayview Ave., Toronto ON M4G 3E8

Tel: 416-483-0200
Toll-Free: 877-483-0204
e-mail: info@glaucomaresearch.ca
www.glaucomaresearch.ca

Overview: A small national charitable organization founded in 1988
Mission: The Glaucoma Research Society of Canada is a national registered charity committed to funding research into the causes, diagnosis, prevention and treatment of glaucoma.
Chief Officer(s):
Martin Chasson, President

John Milton Society for the Blind in Canada
#202, 40 St. Clair Ave. East, Toronto ON M4T 1M9

Tel: 416-960-3953; Fax: 416-960-3570

Overview: A small national charitable organization
Mission: To provide Christian materials in alternative formats to blind, deafblind, & visually impaired Canadians
Chief Officer(s):
Barry Brown, Executive Director
bbrown@jmsblind.ca

Lions Foundation of Canada
152 Wilson St., Oakville ON L6J 5E8

Tel: 905-842-2891; Fax: 905-842-3373
Toll-Free: 800-768-3030; TTY: 905-842-1585
e-mail: info@dogguides.com
www.dogguides.com
www.facebook.com/LFCDogGuides
twitter.com/LFCDogGuides

Overview: A small national charitable organization founded in 1983
Mission: To provide service to physically challenged Canadians in the areas of mobility, safety & independence
Affiliation(s): Lions Clubs of Canada
Chief Officer(s):
Sandy Turney, Executive Director, 905-842-2891 Ext. 224
sandyturney@dogguides.com
Julie Jelinek, Director of Development, 905-842-2891 Ext. 223
jjelinek@dogguides.com

National Association of Canadian Optician Regulators (NACOR)
#2708, 83 Garry St., Winnipeg MB R3C 4J9

Tel: 204-949-1950; Fax: 204-949-9153
Toll-Free: 866-949-1950
e-mail: general@nacor.ca
www.nacor.ca

Overview: A medium-sized national organization
Mission: To offer a platform that enables Canadian optician regulators to network & exchange information; To establish opticianry accreditation standards & processes; To assess & examine opticianry issues
Affliation(s): College of Opticians of British Columbia; Alberta Opticians Association; Saskatchewan Ophthalmic Dispensers Association; The Opticians of Manitoba; The College of Opticians of Ontario; Ordre des Opticiens d'ordonnances du Qubec; Board of Dispensing Opticians of Newfoundland and Labrador; Opticians Association of New Brunswick; Nova Scotia Board of Dispensing Opticians; P.E.I. Board of Dispensing Opticians

Opticians Association of Canada (OAC)
#2706, 83 Garry St., Winnipeg MB R3C 4J9

Tel: 204-982-6060; Fax: 204-947-2519
Toll-Free: 800-842-3155
e-mail: canada@opticians.ca
www.opticians.ca
www.linkedin.com/company/opticians-association-of-canada
www.facebook.com/215512795151373
twitter.com/OACexecutiveDr
www.youtube.com/user/opticianstv

Overview: A medium-sized national organization
Chief Officer(s):
Robert Dalton, Executive Director
rdalton@opticians.ca

Vision Institute of Canada (VIC)
#205, 4025 Yonge St., Toronto ON M2P 2E3

Tel: 416-224-2273; Fax: 416-224-9234
www.visioninstitutecanada.com

Previous Name: Optometric Institute of Toronto
Overview: A medium-sized national charitable organization founded in 1981
Mission: To improve the quality of vision care in the community; To provide eye & vision care to persons with special needs
Chief Officer(s):
Paul Chris, Executive Director
Catherine Chiarelli, Director, Clinical Services

Provincial Associations

ALBERTA

Alberta Association of Optometrists (AAD)
#100, 8407 Argyll Rd., Edmonton AB T6C 4B2

Tel: 780-451-6824; Fax: 780-452-9918
Toll-Free: 800-272-8843
www.optometrists.ab.ca
www.facebook.com/AskaDoctorofOptometry
twitter.com/AAOOptometrists
www.youtube.com/DoctorsofOptometry

Overview: A medium-sized provincial organization overseen by Canadian Association of Optometrists
Mission: To promote excellence in the practice of Optometry, to enhance public recognition of Optometry as the primary vision care provider in Alberta, and to advance the interests of the profession.
Chief Officer(s):
Brian Wik, Executive Director

Alberta College of Optometrists (ACO)
#102, 8407 Argyll Rd. NW, Edmonton AB T6C 4B2

Tel: 780-466-5999; Fax: 780-466-5969
Toll-Free: 800-668-2694
e-mail: admin@collegeofoptometrists.ab.ca
www.collegeofoptometrists.ab.ca

Overview: A small provincial licensing organization founded in 1993
Mission: To act as the regulatory body for the profession of optometry in Alberta
Chief Officer(s):
Gordon Hensel, Registrar & CEO
registrar@collegeofoptometrists.ab.ca

Alberta Sports & Recreation Association for the Blind (ASRAB)
#007, 15 Colonel Baker Pl. NE, Calgary AB T2E 4Z3

Tel: 403-262-5332; Fax: 403-265-7221
Toll-Free: 888-882-7722
e-mail: info@asrab.ab.ca
www.asrab.ab.ca

Overview: A small provincial charitable organization founded in 1975 overseen by Canadian Blind Sports Association Inc.
Mission: To provide recreation & sports opportunities for Albertans who are blind & partially sighted
Member of: CBSA
Chief Officer(s):
Linda MacPhail, Executive Director
execdirector@asrab.ab.ca

College of Opticians of Alberta (COA)
#201, 2528 Ellwood Dr. SW, Edmonton AB T6X 0A9

Tel: 780-429-2694; Fax: 780-426-5576
Toll-Free: 800-263-6026
www.opticians.ab.ca
www.facebook.com/pages/Opticians-of-Alberta/301105265172
twitter.com/CO_alberta

Previous Name: Alberta Opticians Association; Alberta Guild of Opthalmic Dispensers
Overview: A medium-sized provincial organization founded in 1965
Mission: To promote the advancement of knowledge, skills & competence of members & encourage education & training programs while representing members on all issues affecting the profession; to act as a regulatory body; to provide opportunities for opticians to improve their skills while advancing competency through education & cooperation with other eye care professions

Member of: Opticians Association of Canada
Affliation(s): National Accreditation Committee of Opticians
Chief Officer(s):
Maureen Hussey, Executive Director & Registrar
  mhussey@opticians.ab.ca

BRITISH COLUMBIA

British Columbia Blind Sports & Recreation Association (BCBSRA)
#170, 5055 Joyce St., Vancouver BC V5R 6B2
Tel: 604-325-8638; *Fax:* 604-325-1638
Toll-Free: 877-604-8638
e-mail: info@bcblindsports.bc.ca
www.bcblindsports.bc.ca
www.facebook.com/BCBlindSports
twitter.com/bc_blind

Also Known As: BC Blind Sports
Overview: A medium-sized provincial charitable organization founded in 1975 overseen by Canadian Blind Sports Association Inc.
Mission: To provide sports, physical recreation & fitness activities & programs for persons of all ages who are blind/visually impaired; to alleviate isolating & inhibiting effects of blindness/visual impairment; to improve physical capabilities & self-image of blind/visually impaired individuals by providing opportunities for them to learn; to encourage, promote & maintain interest in & cooperation with all such amateur sports & recreation organizations.
Chief Officer(s):
Brian Cowie, President
Tami Grenon, Vice-President

British Columbia Doctors of Optometry (BCDO)
#610, 2525 Willow St., Vancouver BC V5Z 3N8
Tel: 604-737-9907; *Fax:* 604-737-9967
Toll-Free: 888-393-2226
e-mail: info@optometrists.bc.ca
bc.doctorsofoptometry.ca
www.facebook.com/AskaDoctorofOptometry
www.youtube.com/user/DoctorsofOptometry
Overview: A medium-sized provincial organization founded in 1921 overseen by Canadian Association of Optometrists
Mission: To maintain standards; To represent membership to government & other health care professions; To raise public levels of awareness about optometry, good vision & eye care
Chief Officer(s):
Cheryl Williams, Chief Executive Officer
Gurpreet Leekha, President

College of Opticians of British Columbia (COBC)
#403, 1505 West 2nd Ave., Vancouver BC V6H 3Y4
Tel: 604-278-7510; *Fax:* 604-278-7594
Toll-Free: 888-771-6755
e-mail: reception@cobc.ca
www.cobc.ca
www.facebook.com/CollegeofOpticiansBC
twitter.com/CO_BritishC
www.youtube.com/user/LicensedOptician
Overview: A small provincial licensing organization founded in 1994
Mission: To govern the practice of opticianry in BC.
Chief Officer(s):
Raheem Savja, Chair
Connie Chong, Registrar & Executive Director
  cchong@cobc.ca

College of Optometrists of BC
#906, 938 Howe St., Vancouver BC V6Z 1N9
Tel: 604-623-3464; *Fax:* 604-623-3465
Toll-Free: 866-910-3464
e-mail: college@optometrybc.ca
www.optometrybc.com
Previous Name: Board of Examiners in Optometry in B.C.
Overview: A medium-sized provincial organization
Mission: To serve & protect the public interest by guiding the profession of optometry in British Columbia
Chief Officer(s):
Dale Dergousoff, Chair
Robin Simpson, Registrar

Stanka Jovicevic, Chief Administrative Officer
Publications:
• College of Optometrists of BC Annual Report
Type: Yearbook; *Frequency:* Annually
Profile: A year end summary
• College of Optometrists of BC Registrant Directory
Type: Directory
Profile: Public information in the Register includes a registrant's name, class, registration number, business address, & business telephone number
• The Examiner: The Official Newsletter of The College of Optometrists of BC
Type: Newsletter
Profile: Messages from the Chair & the Registrar, plus information about fees, bylaws, & new registrants

Eye Bank of BC (EBBC)
Jim Pattison Pavilion North - B205, 855 West 12th Ave, Vancouver BC V5Z 1M9
Tel: 604-875-4567; *Fax:* 604-875-5316
Toll-Free: 800-667-2060
e-mail: eyebankofbc@vch.ca
www.eyebankofbc.ca
www.facebook.com/EyeBankBC
twitter.com/VCHEyeBankBC
Overview: A medium-sized provincial charitable organization founded in 1983
Mission: To acquire human donor eye tissue for the purposes of corneal transplant, scelra grafts & medical research
Member of: Eye Bank Association of America
Affliation(s): Canadian National Institute for the Blind; Eye Bank Association of America; Canadian Ophthalmological Society
Chief Officer(s):
Linda Wong, Manager
Sonia Yeung, Medical Director

MANITOBA

Lions Eye Bank of Manitoba & Northwest Ontario, Incorporated
320 Sherbrook St., Winnipeg MB R3B 2W6
Tel: 204-772-1899; *Fax:* 204-943-6823
Toll-Free: 800-552-6820
e-mail: lfmnoi@mts.net
www.eyebankmanitoba.com
Overview: A small provincial charitable organization founded in 1984
Mission: To maintain professional staff to procure, process, & distribute human donor eye tissue for surgical transplantation in recipients of Manitoba & Norhwest Ontario
Member of: Eye Bank Association of America
Affliation(s): Lions Eye Bank
Chief Officer(s):
Chris Barnard, Chair
  cbarnard@mts.net

Manitoba Association of Optometrists (MAO)
#217, 530 Century St., Winnipeg MB R3H OY4
Tel: 204-943-9811; *Fax:* 204-943-1208
e-mail: mao@optometrists.mb.ca
www.optometrists.mb.ca
Previous Name: Manitoba Optometric Society
Overview: A medium-sized provincial organization founded in 1909 overseen by Canadian Association of Optometrists
Mission: To regulate the practice of optometry in Manitoba, in accordance with The Optometry Act & Regulation; To represent optometrists in Manitoba; To protect & promote the vision care needs & eye health of Manitobans
Member of: Canadian Association of Optometrists (CAO)
Chief Officer(s):
Neil Campbell, President
Laureen Goodridge, Executive Director
Lorne Ryall, Registrar

Manitoba Blind Sports Association (MBSA)

145 Pacific Ave., Winnipeg MB R3B 2Z6

Tel: 204-925-5694; *Fax:* 204-925-5792

e-mail: blindsport@shawbiz.ca

www.blindsport.mb.ca

Previous Name: Manitoba Sport & Recreation Association for the Blind

Overview: A medium-sized provincial organization founded in 1976 overseen by Canadian Blind Sports Association Inc.

Mission: To provide blind & visually impaired Manitobans with the opportunity to participate in sport at all levels of skill & ability

Opticians of Manitoba (OOM)

#215, 1080 Portage Ave., Winnipeg MB R3G 3M3

Tel: 204-222-8404; *Fax:* 204-222-5296

Toll-Free: 855-346-3715

e-mail: oom@optm.ca

www.opticiansofmanitoba.ca

www.facebook.com/1396718373891003

Overview: A small provincial organization founded in 1953

Mission: To protect the public through the self-regulation of the practice of Opticianry; To set standards of practice for the profession; To ensure that opticians practice safely & competently; To investigate concerns raised about registrants' practice

Chief Officer(s):

Carol Ellerbeck, Registrar

cellerbeck@opticians.ca

Publications:

• Opticians of Manitoba Newsletter

Type: Newsletter

NEW BRUNSWICK

New Brunswick Association of Optometrists (NBAO) / Association des optométristes du Nouveau-Brunswick

#1, 490 Gibson St., Fredericton NB E3A 4E9

Tel: 506-458-8759; *Fax:* 506-450-1271

e-mail: nbao@nbnet.nb.ca

www.nbao.ca

Overview: A medium-sized provincial organization overseen by Canadian Association of Optometrists

Mission: To represent Doctors of Optometry in New Brunswick

Chief Officer(s):

Krista McDevitt, President

Opticians Association of New Brunswick / Association des otpiciens du Nouveau-Brunswick

PO Box 6743, Stn. Brunswick Square, Saint John NB E2L 4S2

Tel: 506-642-2878; *Fax:* 506-642-7984

e-mail: nbgdo@nbnet.nb.ca

www.opticiansnb.com

Previous Name: New Brunswick Guild of Dispensing Opticians

Overview: A small provincial licensing organization founded in 1976

Mission: To regulate the practice of opticianry in New Brunswick; To oversee education of candidates for licensing

NEWFOUNDLAND AND LABRADOR

Newfoundland & Labrador Association of Optometrists (NLAO)

PO Box 8042, St. John's NL A1B 3M7

Tel: 709-765-1096; *Fax:* 709-739-8378

e-mail: nlao@bellaliant.net

www.nlao.org

Previous Name: Newfoundland Association of Optometrists

Overview: A medium-sized provincial organization overseen by Canadian Association of Optometrists

Mission: To provide an online resource for Doctors of Optometry & other health care providers in Newfoundland & Labrador

Chief Officer(s):

Ed Breen, Executive Director

NOVA SCOTIA

Atlantic Provinces Special Education Authority / Commission d'enseignement spécial des provinces de l'Atlantique

5940 South St., Halifax NS B3H 1S6

Tel: 902-424-8500; *Fax:* 902-423-8700; *TTY:* 902-424-8500

e-mail: apsea@apsea.ca

www.apsea.ca

Overview: A small provincial organization founded in 1975

Mission: To provide educational services to children & youth who are visually impaired & hard of hearing

Chief Officer(s):

Bertram Tulk, Superintendent

tulkb@apsea.ca

Publications:

• Seen and Heard [a publication of the Atlantic Provinces Special Education Authority]

Type: Newsletter

Profile: News & updates for members

Blind Sports Nova Scotia

NS

e-mail: info@blindsportsnovascotia.ca

www.blindsportsnovascotia.ca

twitter.com/blindsportsns

Overview: A small provincial organization overseen by Canadian Blind Sports Association Inc.

Mission: Blind Sports Nova Scotia is an organization that presents sport & recreational activities for visually impaired athletes in Nova Scotia.

Member of: Canadian Blind Sport Association; Sport Nova Scotia

Chief Officer(s):

Peter Parsons, Chair

Charlie MacDonald, Secretary

Nova Scotia Association of Optometrists (NSAO)

PO Box 9410, Stn. A, #700, 6009 Quinpool Rd., Halifax NS B3K 5S3

Tel: 902-435-2845; *Fax:* 902-425-2441

e-mail: info@ns.doctorsofoptometry.ca

ns.doctorsofoptometry.ca

Previous Name: Nova Scotia Optometrical Society

Overview: A medium-sized provincial licensing organization founded in 1905 overseen by Canadian Association of Optometrists

Mission: To foster excellence in the delivery of vision & eye health services in Nova Scotia; To act as the voice of optometry in Nova Scotia

ONTARIO

College of Opticians of Ontario (COO)

#902, 85 Richmond St. West, Toronto ON M5H 2C9

Tel: 416-368-3616; *Fax:* 416-368-2713

Toll-Free: 800-990-9793

e-mail: mail@coptont.org

www.coptont.org

Overview: A medium-sized provincial organization

Mission: To regulate & improve the practice of opticians in Ontario

Affliation(s): Federation of Health Regulatory Colleges of Ontario

Chief Officer(s):

Fazal Khan, Registrar

fkhan@coptont.org

College of Optometrists of Ontario / Ordre des optométristes de l'Ontario

#900, 65 St. Clair Ave. East, Toronto ON M4T 2Y3

Tel: 416-962-4071; *Fax:* 416-962-4073

Toll-Free: 888-825-2554

e-mail: info@collegeoptom.on.ca

www.collegeoptom.on.ca

www.facebook.com/collegeoptom

twitter.com/collegeoptom

Overview: A medium-sized provincial licensing organization founded in 1919

Mission: To serve the public interest by guiding the optometry profession; To ensure that safe, ethical & quality eye care is delivered; To maintain high standards within the field

Chief Officer(s):

Thomas Noël, President

Paula Garshowitz, Registrar
Louise Kassabian, Manager, Membership & Office Administration
lkassabian@collegeoptom.on.ca

Eye Bank of Canada - Ontario Division
Dept. of Ophthalmology, University of Toronto, 1929 Bayview Ave.,
Toronto ON M4G 0A1

Tel: 416-978-7355; *Fax:* 416-978-1522
e-mail: eye.bank@utoronto.ca
www.eyebank.utoronto.ca

Also Known As: Ontario Eye Bank
Overview: A small provincial charitable organization founded in 1955
Mission: To provide donated eye tissue for surgical use in those
whose vision can be restored or improved through corneal
transplantation or other eye surgery
Affliation(s): Canadian National Institute for the Blind; University of
Toronto
Chief Officer(s):
Fides Coloma, Manager

Ontario Association of Optometrists (OAO)
PO Box 16, #801, 20 Adelaide St. East, Toronto ON M5C 2T6
Tel: 905-826-3522; *Fax:* 905-826-0625
Toll-Free: 800-540-3837
e-mail: info@optom.on.ca
www.optom.on.ca
www.facebook.com/pages/Ontario-Association-of-Optometrists/281663
12427
twitter.com/ONOptometrists
www.youtube.com/user/OntarioOptometrists

Overview: A medium-sized provincial organization founded in 1909
overseen by Canadian Association of Optometrists
Mission: To advance the profession of optometry at the government,
regulatory, & public levels
Chief Officer(s):
Beth Witney, Chief Executive Officer, 905-826-3522 Ext. 221
Bethany Carey, Director, Member Services, 905-826-3522 Ext. 227
Melissa Secord, Director, Professional Affairs, 905-826-3522 Ext. 243
Sandra Ng, Manager, Policy & Government Relations, 905-826-3522
Ext. 225

Ontario Blind Sports Association (OBSA)
#104, 3 Concorde Gate, Toronto ON M3C 3N6
Tel: 416-426-7191; *Fax:* 416-426-7361
blindsports.on.ca
www.facebook.com/OntarioBlindSports

Overview: A small provincial charitable organization founded in 1984
overseen by Canadian Blind Sports Association Inc.
Mission: To organize sporting events & activities for blind & visually
impaired athletes in Ontario
Chief Officer(s):
Kyle Pelly, Executive Director, 416-426-7244
Greg Theriault, Manager, Programs
greg@blindsports.on.ca
Publications:
• Ontario Blind Sports Association Newsletter
Type: Newsletter
Profile: News & updates for members

Ontario Foundation for Visually Impaired Children Inc. (OFVIC)
PO Box 1116, Stn. D, Toronto ON M6P 3K2
Tel: 416-767-5977; *Fax:* 416-767-5530
e-mail: ofvic@look.ca

Overview: A small provincial organization
Chief Officer(s):
April Cornell, Executive Director

Ontario Opticians Association (OOA)
PO Box 23518, Stn. Dexter, 5899 Leslie St., Toronto ON M2H 3R9
Tel: 905-709-4141; *Fax:* 416-226-6879
Toll-Free: 877-709-4141
e-mail: info@ontario-opticians.com
www.ontario-opticians.com
www.facebook.com/ontarioopticiansassociation

Overview: A small provincial organization founded in 1946
Mission: To advance & protect the profession of opticianry
Member of: Opticians Association of Canada (OAC)
Chief Officer(s):

Martin Lebeau, President
Publications:
• Focus [a publication of the Ontario Opticians Association]
Type: Newsletter; *Price:* Free with Ontario Opticians Association
membership
Profile: Local & national issues, business advice, member benefits, &
upcoming events

PRINCE EDWARD ISLAND

Prince Edward Island Association of Optometrists (PEIAO)
PO Box 1812, Charlottetown PE C1A 7N5
Tel: 902-566-4418; *Fax:* 902-566-4694
e-mail: peiregistrar@peisympatico.ca
www.peioptometrists.ca

Previous Name: Prince Edward Island Optometrical Association
Overview: A medium-sized provincial organization founded in 1922
overseen by Canadian Association of Optometrists
Mission: To promote the professional interests of optometrists in
Prince Edward Island Association; To improve optometrists' proficiency
Chief Officer(s):
Jayne Toombs, President
Susan Judson, Vice-President
Alanna Stetson, Secretary
Joe E. Hickey, Treasurer

QUÉBEC

Association des médecins ophtalmologistes du Québec (AMOQ)
CP 216, Succ. Desjardins, 2, Complexe Desjardins, Montréal QC H5B
1G8
Tél: 514-350-5124; *Téléc:* 514-350-5174
Courriel: amoq@fmsq.org
www.amoq.org

Aperçu: *Dimension:* petite; *Envergure:* provinciale; Organisme sans
but lucratif; fondée en 1955 surveillé par Fédération des médecins
spécialistes du Québec
Mission: Promouvoir les intérêts professionnels et économiques de
ses membres; se préoccuper du maintien de la compétence; susciter et
appuier des activités scientifiques susceptibles de favoriser
l'avancement de l'ophtalmologie; se préoccuper de l'accessibilité aux
soins ophtalmologiques
Membre(s) du bureau directeur:
Côme Fortin, Président
Sylvie Gariépy, Directrice, Administration

Association des optométristes du Québec (AOQ) / Québec Optometric Association
#217, 1255 boul Robert-Bourassa, Montréal QC H3B 3B2
Tél: 514-288-6272; *Téléc:* 514-288-7071
Courriel: aoq@aoqnet.qc.ca
www.aoqnet.qc.ca
www.linkedin.com/company/association-des-optom-tristes-du-qu-bec
www.facebook.com/109631962406806

Aperçu: *Dimension:* moyenne; *Envergure:* provinciale; fondée en 1973
surveillé par Canadian Association of Optometrists
Mission: De développer meilleures conditions de pratique
économiques et professionnelles pour les optométristes du Québec
Membre(s) du bureau directeur:
Steven Carrier, Président
Maryse Nolin, Directrice générale

Association québécoise des parents d'enfants handicapés visuels (AQPEHV) / Quebec Association for Parents of Visually Impaired Children (QAPVIC)
#203, 10, boul Churchill, Greenfield Park QC J4V 2L7
Tél: 450-465-7225; *Téléc:* 450-465-5129
Ligne sans frais: 888-849-8729
www.aqpehv.qc.ca

Aperçu: *Dimension:* petite; *Envergure:* provinciale; fondée en 2004
Membre(s) du bureau directeur:
Roland Savard, Directeur général
direction.generale@aqpehv.qc.ca

Fondation de la banque d'yeux du Québec inc. / Québec Eye Bank Foundation

5415, boul de l'Assomption, Montréal QC H1T 2M4

Tél: 514-252-3886; *Téléc:* 514-252-3821

Aperçu: *Dimension:* petite; *Envergure:* provinciale; Organisme sans but lucratif; fondée en 1976

Mission: Financement de la recherche sur les maladies de l'oeil et plus particulièment de la cornée (greffe)

Fondation des aveugles du Québec (FAQ)

5112, rue Bellechasse, Montréal QC H1T 2A4

Tél: 514-259-9470; *Téléc:* 514-254-5079

Ligne sans frais: 855-249-5112

www.aveugles.org

www.linkedin.com/company/2968845

www.facebook.com/aveugles

twitter.com/Aveugles_Qc

www.youtube.com/user/fondationaveuglesqc

Aperçu: *Dimension:* petite; *Envergure:* provinciale

Mission: Soutenir les personnes handicapées de la vue, les conseiller et les aider à mener la vie la plus autonome possible à la maison, au travail et dans les loisirs; informer le public sur l'importance de la prévention quotidienne afin de conserver une bonne vision

Membre(s) du bureau directeur:

Ronald Beauregard, Directeur général

Ordre des opticiens d'ordonnances du Québec (OOOQ)

#601, 630, rue Sherbrooke Ouest, Montréal QC H3A 1E4

Tél: 514-288-7542; *Téléc:* 514-288-5982

Ligne sans frais: 800-563-6345

Courriel: ordre@opticien.qc.ca

www.oodq.qc.ca

Aperçu: *Dimension:* moyenne; *Envergure:* provinciale; Organisme de réglementation; fondée en 1940 surveillé par Office des professions du Québec

Mission: Assurer la protection du public; contrôler l'exercice de la profession par ses membres

Membre de: National Accreditation Committee of Opticians

Affliation(s): Conseil interprofessionnel du Québec (CIQ)

Membre(s) du bureau directeur:

Linda Samson, Présidente et directrice générale

Québec Federation of the Blind Inc. (QFB) / Fédération des aveugles du Québec inc.

7010, rue Sherbrooke ouest, Montréal QC H4B 1R3

Tel: 514-484-9232

e-mail: qfb@ssss.gouv.qc.ca

qfb.ca

Overview: A small provincial charitable organization founded in 1970

SASKATCHEWAN

Saskatchewan Association of Optometrists (SAO)

#108, 2366 Ave. C North, Saskatoon SK S7L 5X5

Tel: 306-652-2069; *Fax:* 306-652-2642

Toll-Free: 877-660-3937

e-mail: admin@saosk.ca

optometrists.sk.ca

twitter.com/SaskEyecare

Previous Name: Saskatchewan Optometric Association

Overview: A medium-sized provincial licensing organization founded in 1909 overseen by Canadian Association of Optometrists

Mission: To license the delivery of optometric care in Saskatchewan; To regulate doctors of optometry throughout the province; To ensure excellence in the delivery of vision & eye health services across Saskatchewan; To enforce high standards of optometric eye care, in order to protect the public; To act as the voice of optometry in Saskatchewan

Chief Officer(s):

Sheila Spence, Executive Director

ed@saosk.ca

Publications:

• Eye on SAO

Type: Newsletter; *Frequency:* Monthly; *Price:* Free with membership in the Saskatchewan Association of Optometrists

Saskatchewan Blind Sports Association Inc. (SBSA)

510 Cynthia St., Saskatoon SK S7L 7K7

Tel: 306-975-0888

Toll-Free: 877-772-7798

e-mail: sbsa.sk@shaw.ca

www.saskblindsports.ca

Overview: A small provincial organization founded in 1978 overseen by Canadian Blind Sports Association Inc.

Mission: To assist persons who are blind or with visual impairment to achieve excellence in sport, satisfaction in recreation, independence, self-reliance & full community participation

Chief Officer(s):

Glenn Hunks, Executive Director

Saskatchewan College of Opticians

#13 - 350, 103 St. East, Saskatoon SK S7N 1Z1

Tel: 306-652-0769; *Fax:* 306-652-0784

e-mail: office@scoptic.ca

www.scoptic.ca

Overview: A small provincial organization

Mission: To ensure that Saskatchewan opticians adhere to high standards of care; To improve the vision of the people of Saskatchewan

Chief Officer(s):

Deanne Oleksyn, President

Saskatchewan Lions Eye Bank

Eye Dept., Saskatoon City Hospital, PO Box 447, Kipling SK S0G 2S0

www.eyebank.sklions.ca

Overview: A small provincial charitable organization founded in 1982

Mission: To promote corneal/eye donations after death to be used for transplantation to restore vision to people who have been rendered blind due to corneal injury, disease or degeneration

Member of: Eye Bank Association of America

Affliation(s): CNIB

Chief Officer(s):

Garnet Davis, President

Local Associations

ONTARIO

BALANCE for Blind Adults

#302, 4920 Dundas St. West, Toronto ON M9A 1B7

Tel: 416-236-1796; *Fax:* 416-236-4280

e-mail: info@balancefba.org

www.balancefba.org

www.facebook.com/balanceforblindadults

twitter.com/balancefba

Overview: A medium-sized local charitable organization founded in 1986

Mission: To provide instruction & support to individuals with visual impairment to enable them to live independently & confidently in their community; To promote independence, decision making, & self-fulfillment

Chief Officer(s):

Susan Archibald, Executive Director

QUÉBEC

Association des sports pour aveugles de Montréal (ASAM)

4545, av Pierre-de Coubertin, Montréal QC H1V 0B2

Tél: 514-252-3178

Courriel: infoasaq@sportsaveugles.qc.ca

www.sportsaveugles.qc.ca/asam

www.facebook.com/ASAMONTREAL

Aperçu: *Dimension:* petite; *Envergure:* locale; Organisme sans but lucratif; fondée en 1983

Mission: Promouvoir l'accessibilité et la pratique des sports et loisirs aux personnes handicapées visuelles; organiser et structurer les différentes activités sportives; recruter et former des bénévoles accompagnateurs

Affliation(s): Association sportive des aveugles du Québec

Membre(s) du bureau directeur:

Nathalie Chartrand, Directrice générale

nchartrand@sportsaveugles.qc.ca

Le Bon Pilote inc.

#511, 445, rue Jean-Talon ouest, Montréal QC H3N 1R1

Tél: 514-593-5454; *Téléc:* 514-419-6954
Courriel: lebonpilote@videotron.ca
www.lebonpilote.com
www.linkedin.com/company/2609230
twitter.com/lebonpilote

Aperçu: *Dimension:* petite; *Envergure:* locale
Mission: Pour aider les personnes ayant une déficience visuelle en leur fournissant des services et en développant de nouveaux services pour faire avancer leur cause
Affiliation(s): Institut Nazareth & Louis-Braille; MAB-Mackay; Agence de la santé et des services sociaux de Montréal; Agence de la santé et des services sociaux de la Montérégie; Les BusBoys.com, site pour les employés / retraités de la STM
Membre(s) du bureau directeur:
John D. Gill, Directeur général, 514-531-5330
  johngill@videotron.ca

Institut Nazareth et Louis-Braille (INLB)

1111, rue St-Charles ouest, Longueuil QC J4K 5G4

Tél: 450-463-1710; *Téléc:* 450-463-0243
Ligne sans frais: 800-361-7063
Courriel: info.inlb@ssss.gouv.qc.ca
www.inlb.qc.ca
www.facebook.com/InstitutNazarethEtLouisBraille

Aperçu: *Dimension:* petite; *Envergure:* locale; fondée en 1861
Mission: Pour trouver de nouvelles façons d'aider les personnes ayant une déficience visuelle deviennent autonomes
Membre(s) du bureau directeur:
Richard Deschamps, Président-directeur général

Montréal Association for the Blind (MAB) / Association montréalaise pour les aveugles

Head Office, 7000 Sherbrooke Rd. West, Montréal QC H4B 1R3

Tel: 514-488-5552; *Fax:* 514-489-3477
e-mail: info@mabmackay.ca
www.mabmackay.ca

Overview: A medium-sized local organization founded in 1908
Mission: To offer rehabilitation services (low vision, social work, occupational therapy, activites of daily living, orientation & mobility, computer adaptation, early intervention etc.) to blind & visually impaired persons; to offer residential services to blind & visually impaired seniors. The MAB-Mackay Rehabilitation Centre, located at 3500, boul Decarie in Montréal, provides family-centred adaptation, rehabilitation & social integration services to persons with a visual disability, and/or deaf or hard of hearing.

Regroupement des aveugles et amblyopes du Montréal métropolitain (RAAMM)

#101, 5225 rue Berri, Montréal QC H2J 2S4

Tél: 514-277-4401; *Téléc:* 514-277-8961
Courriel: info@raamm.org
www.raamm.org

Aperçu: *Dimension:* petite; *Envergure:* locale; fondée en 1975
Mission: Faire la défense des droits pour les gens avec une déficience visuelle et fournir le service d'aide bénévole
Membre(s) du bureau directeur:
Pascale Dussault, Directrice générale
  direction@raamm.org

International Associations

Christian Blind Mission International (CBMI)

PO Box 800, 3844 Stouffville Rd., Stouffville ON L4A 7Z9

Tel: 905-640-6464; *Fax:* 905-640-4332
Toll-Free: 800-567-2264
e-mail: cbm@cbmcanada.org
www.cbmcanada.org
www.facebook.com/101857609865125
twitter.com/cbmCanada
www.youtube.com/user/cbmcanada; pinterest.com/cbmcanada

Overview: A medium-sized international charitable organization founded in 1978
Mission: With core values based on Christian faith, CBMI serves the blind & disabled in the developing world, irrespective of nationality, race, sex, or religion; prevents & treats blindness & other disabilities through medical care, rehabilitation training & integration programs; helps people to help themselves.
Member of: Canadian Council of Christian Charities
Chief Officer(s):
Jonathan Liteplo, Chair
Ed Epp, Executive Director

International Council of Ophthalmology (ICO)

#445, 711 Van Ness Ave., San Francisco CA 94102 USA

Tel: 415-521-1651; *Fax:* 415-521-1649
e-mail: info@icoph.org
www.icoph.org
www.linkedin.com/company/713250
www.facebook.com/InternationalCouncilOphthalmology
twitter.com/intlcounciloph

Overview: A small international charitable organization founded in 1857
Mission: To advocate the prevention & treatment of preventable blindness in developing nations; To support the International Agency for the Prevention of Blindness & Vision 2020: Right to Sight with WHO; To support educational competency in ophthalmologic education worldwide; To evaluate & coordinate standardization in ophthalmology; To support ophthalmologic interchange through supranational organizations & international congresses
Member of: International Federation of Ophthalmological Societies
Affliation(s): Canadian Ophthalmological Society
Chief Officer(s):
Hugh Taylor, AC, MD, President
Kathleen Miller, Executive Director
  kmiller@icoph.org

International Orthoptic Association (IOA)

c/o RPG Crouch Chapman LLP, 62 Wilson St., London EC2A 2BU United Kingdom

e-mail: webmaster@internationalorthoptics.org
www.internationalorthoptics.org
twitter.com/followioa

Overview: A large international organization founded in 1967
Mission: To promote the science of orthoptics throughout the world; To maintain & improve standards of education, training, & orthoptic practice
Chief Officer(s):
Karen McMain, President
  president@internationalorthoptics.org
Jan Roelof Polling, Deputy President
  netherlands@internationalorthoptics.org
Katherine J. Fray, Secretary
  secretary@internationalorthoptics.org
Jane Tapley, Treasurer
  treasurer@internationalorthoptics.org

International Society for Eye Research

655 Beach St., San Francisco CA 94109 USA

Tel: 415-561-8569; *Fax:* 415-561-8531
e-mail: mail@iser.org
www.iser.org
www.facebook.com/ISERPage
twitter.com/iserworld

Overview: A medium-sized international organization founded in 1968
Mission: To support & sustain excellent eye & vision research around the globe
Chief Officer(s):
John S. Penn, President
Publications:
• Experimental Eye Research
Type: Journal
Profile: Original research papers in the following sections: Aqueous Humor & Blood Flow; Cornea & Ocular Surface; Lens & Retina; & Choroid

Operation Eyesight Universal

#200, 4 Parkdale Cres. NW, Calgary AB T2N 3T8

Tel: 403-283-6323; *Fax:* 403-270-1899
Toll-Free: 800-585-8265
e-mail: info@operationeyesight.ca
www.operationeyesight.ca
www.linkedin.com/company/operation-eyesight
www.facebook.com/OperationEyesightUniversal
twitter.com/OpEyesight
www.youtube.com/user/OpEyesightUniversal

Overview: A large international charitable organization founded in 1963
Mission: To eliminate avoidable blindness through the development & support of permanent, self-sustaining, quality blindness prevention & sight restoration programs for those people in greatest need
Member of: International Agency for the Prevention of Blindness
Affliation(s): International Agency for the Prevention of Blindness; L.V. Prasad Eye Institute; Vision 2020
Chief Officer(s):
Brian Foster, Executive Director
Publications:
• SightLines
Type: Newsletter

Vancouver Regional Office
#200, 4 Parkdale Crescent NW, Calgary AB T2N 3T8

Tel: 403-283-6323; *Fax:* 403-270-1899
Toll-Free: 800-585-8265
e-mail: vancouver@operationeyesight.ca
www.linkedin.com/company/operation-eyesight
www.facebook.com/OperationEyesightUniversal
twitter.com/OpEyesight
www.youtube.com/user/OpEyesightUniversal

Chief Officer(s):
Brian Foster, Executive Director
Rob Ohlson, Chair

Seva Canada Society

#100, 2000 West 12th Ave., Vancouver BC V6J 2G2

Tel: 604-713-6622; *Fax:* 604-733-4292
Toll-Free: 877-460-6622
www.seva.ca
www.facebook.com/sevacanada
twitter.com/sevacanada
www.instagram.com/sevacanada

Previous Name: Seva Service Society
Overview: A small international charitable organization founded in 1982
Mission: To prevent blindness in developing countries through the implementation of local eye care programs
Member of: British Columbia Council for International Cooperation
Chief Officer(s):
Penny Lyons, Executive Director
Ken Bassett, Director, Program
Deanne Berman, Director, Marketing & Communications
Christine Smith, Director, Development
Lisa Demers, Manager, Operations & Program

World Blind Union / Union mondiale des aveugles

1929 Bayview Ave., Toronto ON M4G 3E8

Tel: 416-486-9698; *Fax:* 416-486-8107
e-mail: info@wbu.ngo
www.worldblindunion.org
www.facebook.com/BlindUnion
twitter.com/BlindUnion

Overview: A medium-sized international organization founded in 1984
Mission: To speak on behalf of blind & partially sighted persons of the world, representing 285 million blind & visually impaired persons from 190 countries
Member of: Vision Alliance
Chief Officer(s):
Fredric Schroeder, President
  president@wbu.ngo
Penny Hartin, Chief Executive Officer
  penny.hartin@wbu.ngo
Ajai Kumar Mittal, Secretary General

National Publications

Canadian Journal of Ophthalmology (CJO)

c/o Canadian Ophthalmological Society, #110, 2733 Lancaster Rd., Ottawa, ON K1B 0A9

Tel: 613-729-6779; *Fax:* 613-729-7209

Frequency: Bi-Monthly
Phil Hooper, Editor-in-Chief MD, FRSCSC

Canadian Journal of Optometry

Canadian Association of Optometrists, 234 Argyle Ave., Ottawa, ON K2P 1B9

Tel: 613-235-7924 *Toll-Free:* 888-263-4676
cjo@opto.ca

Frequency: 6 times a year
Official publication of the Canadian Association of Optometrists.
Dr. Ralph Chou, Editor-in-Chief

Clinical & Refractive Optometry

Previous Name: Practical Optometry
Owned By: Mediconcept Inc.
#518, 3484 Sources Blvd., Dollard des Ormeaux, QC H9B 1Z9

info@crojournal.com

Circulation: 3,000 *Frequency:* 6 times a year
Lawrence Goldstein, Publisher, lgoldstein@mediconcept.ca
Mary Di Lemme, Managing Editor, mdilemme@mediconcept.ca

Optical Prism

Nusand Publishing Inc., #1113, 225 the East Mall, Toronto, ON M9B 0A9

Tel: 416-233-2487; *Fax:* 416-233-1746
info@opticalprism.ca
Social Media: pinterest.com/opticalprism
twitter.com/opticalprism
www.facebook.co m/OpticalPrismMagazine

Frequency: 8 times a year
Robert May, Publisher, rmay@opticalprism.ca
Sarah McGoldrick, Managing Editor, smcgoldrick@opticalprism.ca

Opti-Guide

Breton Communications Inc., #202, 495, boul St-Martin ouest, Laval, QC H7M 1Y9

Tel: 450-629-6005; *Fax:* 450-629-6044
Toll-Free: 888-462-2112
info@bretoncom.com

Circulation: 5,481 *Frequency:* Annually
Martine Breton, President/Publisher, martine@bretoncom.com

Provincial/Local Publications

EnVue

Breton Communications Inc., #202, 495, boul St-Martin ouest, Laval, QC H7M 1Y9

Tél: 450-629-6005; *Téléc:* 450-629-6044
Ligne sans frais: 888-462-2112

Tirage: 3,680 *Fréquence:* 6 fois par an
Martine Breton, President
Lorraine Boutin, Rédactrice en chef

L'Optométriste

Association des optométristes du Québec, #217, 1255, boul. Robert-Bourassa, Montréal, QC H3B 3B2

Tél: 514-288-6272; *Téléc:* 514-288-7071
aoq@aoqnet.qc.ca

Fréquence: 6 fois par an

Local Schools

NOVA SCOTIA

Halifax: Atlantic Provinces Special Education Authority (APSEA)

5940 South St., Halifax, NS B3H 1S6, Canada

Tel: 902-424-8500; *Fax:* 902-424-0543
apsea@apsea.ca
www.apsea.ca
TTY: 902-424-8500

Note: The Atlantic Provinces Special Education Authority (APSEA) is an interprovincial cooperative agency established in 1975 by joint agreement among the Ministers of Education of New Brunswick, Newfoundland, Nova Scotia, and Prince Edward Island.
Bertram R. Tulk, Supt.

ONTARIO

Brantford: The W. Ross Macdonald School for the Blind
350 Brant Ave., Brantford, ON N3T 3J9
Tel: 519-759-0730; Toll-Free: 866-618-9092
www.psbnet.ca/eng/schools/wross

Enrollment: 217
Donald Neale, Principal, Blind/Low Vision Program
Martha Martino, Principal, Deaf/Blind Program

Ottawa: Centre Jules-Léger
281, av Lanark, Ottawa, ON K1Z 6R8
Tél: 613-761-9300; *Téléc:* 613-761-9301
Other Information: ATS: 613-761-9302
Note: Services aux enfants (et leurs familles) en difficultés d'apprentissage, avec ou sans déficit d'attention/hyperactivité, qui sont sourds ou malentendant, qui sont aveugles ou en basse vision, ou qui sont sourds et aveugles.
Ginette Faubert, Surintendante

National Libraries

Canadian National Institute for the Blind/ Institut national canadien pour les aveugles
1929 Bayview Ave., Toronto, ON M4G 3E8
Tel: 800-563-2642; *Fax:* 416-480-7700
Toll-Free: 800-268-8818
library@cnib.ca
www.cnib.ca/library
Social Media: www.youtube.com/user/cnibnatcomm;
twitter.com/cniblibrary; www.facebook.com/myCNIB

Collection: Reference collection of print books on blindness; talking books; braille music
Margaret McGrory, Vice-President & Executive Director, Library

Provincial Libraries

A.E. MacDonald Ophthalmic Library & William Callahan Reading Room
Toronto Western Hospital, 399 Bathurst St., #MP6-319, Toronto, ON M5T 2S8
Tel: 416-978-4321

AERO: Alternative Education Resources for Ontario
350 Brant Ave., Brantford, ON N3T 3J9
Tel: 519-759-2522
aero@alternativeresources.ca
alternativeresources.ca
Profile: AERO is a web-based digital repository operated by the Ministry of Education in partnership with the Ministry of Training, Colleges and Universities with the mandate to provide alternate learning formats to students with perceptual disabilities who attend publicly funded educational institutions in Ontario. **Collection:** Braille, large print, e-text, or daisy digital audio

Canadian National Institute for the Blind/ Institut national canadien pour les aveugles
3044, rue Delisle, Montréal, QC H4C 1M9
Tel: 514-934-4622

Christian Record Services Inc.
1148 King St. East, Oshawa, ON L1H 1H8
Tel: 905-436-6938; *Fax:* 905-436-7102
Toll-Free: 888-899-0006
crs@adventist.ca
www.ncbservices.ca
Collection: Materails in braille, large print & audio cassette

National Hospitals

ONTARIO

TORONTO: Eye Bank of Canada
Ontario Division
c/o Dept. of Ophthalmology, University of Toronto, 340 College St., #B100, Toronto, ON M5T 3A9
Tel: 416-978-7355 *Fax:* 416-978-1522
eye.bank@utoronto.ca
www.eyebank.utoronto.ca

Year Founded: 1955
Dr. David Rootman, Medical Director
Dr. William Dixon, Medical Co-director
Fides Coloma, Manager

Local Hospitals & Health Centres

QUÉBEC

MONTRÉAL: Centre de réadaptation Mab-Mackay (CRMM)
7000, rue Sherbrooke Ouest, Montréal, QC H4B 1R3
Tél: 514-488-5552 *Téléc:* 514-489-3477
info@mabmackay.ca
www.mabmackay.ca

Fondée en: 2006
Note: Fournit des services de réadaptation pour les personnes ayant une déficience visuelle et déficience auditive afin qu'ils puissent vivre de façon autonome. Le centre de réadaptation a été formé à la suite d'une fusion entre l'Association montréalaise pour les aveugles et le Centre de réadaptation Mackay.
Sara Saber-Freedman, Présidente
Christine Boyle, Directrice générale

Wilson Disease

Wilson disease is a rare genetic disorder that results from an inability to adequately excrete copper. The resulting accumulation of copper in the body's tissues and organs leads to disease of the brain and liver, and to a lesser extent, the kidney and red blood cells.

Cause
The disease is an autosomal recessive hereditary disease. This means that if two carriers of the defective gene have children, there is a one in four chance of the child having the disease.

Symptoms
Some people with Wilson disease may be symptom-free for years. Eventually, build-up of copper in the liver causes a hepatitis-like illness with loss of appetite, low grade fever, abdominal discomfort and jaundice. If not detected and treated, this process can lead to cirrhosis and fatal liver failure. In 40 to 50 percent of people, the illness affects the brain and can cause symptoms including unsteadiness, tremors, slurred speech and psychiatric disorders such as mania, depression or suicidal behaviour. Copper rings (Kayser-Fleischer rings) may appear in the eye in up to 10 percent of patients. Although they do not cause any symptoms, their appearance may help establish the diagnosis.

Prevalence
In Canada, approximately one person in 30,000 has this condition.

Treatment Options
Various tests may be used to diagnose Wilson disease including blood tests (to measure levels of serum copper and ceruloplasmin, a blood protein that contains copper), urinalysis (to measure copper in the urine), liver biopsy and slit lamp examination of the eye (to determine the presence of Kayser-Fleischer rings). Genetic testing for Wilson disease is now available, and can be used to diagnose the condition in brothers and sisters of an affected person, even before they show symptoms.

The critical therapy for Wilson disease is administration of a drug that helps the body release its copper stores. Zinc therapy and decoppering agents such as penicillamine and trientine are the drugs most commonly used to treat Wilson disease. If a person has severe hepatitis or liver failure, liver transplantation may be required.

If untreated, Wilson disease is fatal, generally before the age of 30. Continual, lifelong treatment is mandatory for any patient with confirmed Wilson disease, whether symptomatic or not. With careful adherence to the appropriate drug regimen, most people with Wilson disease have a normal life expectancy.

National Associations

Canadian Association for the Study of the Liver (CASL) / Association canadienne pour l'étude du foie
c/o BUKSA Strategic Conference Services, #307, 10328 - 81st Ave., Edmonton AB T6C 3T5
Tel: 780-436-0983
e-mail: casl@hepatology.ca
www.hepatology.ca

Overview: A small national organization
Mission: To eliminate liver disease
Affliation(s): International Association for the Study of the Liver (IASL)
Chief Officer(s):
Rick Schreiber, President
Kelly Burak, Secretary-Treasurer
Marc Bilodeau, President-Elect
Publications:
• Canadian Journal of Gastroenterology & Hepatology [a publication of the Canadian Association for the Study of the Liver]
Type: Journal; *Price:* Free with membership in the Canadian Association for the Study of the Liver

Canadian Liver Foundation (CLF) / Fondation canadienne du foie (FCF)
#801, 3100 Steeles Ave. East, Toronto ON L3R 8T3
Tel: 416-491-3353; *Fax:* 905-752-1540
Toll-Free: 800-563-5483
e-mail: clf@liver.ca
www.liver.ca
www.facebook.com/6584473365
twitter.com/CdnLiverFdtn
www.youtube.com/user/clfwebmaster

Overview: A large national charitable organization founded in 1969
Mission: To reduce the incidence & impact of all liver disease by funding liver research & education; promote liver health through programs & publications
Chief Officer(s):
Morris Sherman, Chairman
Elliot M. Jacobson, Sec.-Treas.
Publications:
• Canadian Liver Foundation Annual Report
Type: Yearbook; *Frequency:* Annually

Atlantic Canada Regional Office/Halifax Chapter
#103-406, 287 Lacewood Dr., Halifax NS B3M 3Y7
Tel: 902-423-8538; *Fax:* 902-423-8811
Toll-Free: 866-423-8538
e-mail: atlantic@liver.ca
Chief Officer(s):
Shayla Steeves, Regional Director

British Columbia/Yukon Regional Office
#109, 828 West 8th Ave., Vancouver BC V5Z 1E2
Tel: 604-707-6430; *Fax:* 604-681-6067
Toll-Free: 800-856-7266
Chief Officer(s):

Mark Mansfield, Regional Manager
mmansfield@liver.ca

Chatham/Kent Chapter
PO Box 23, Chatham ON N7M 5K1
Tel: 519-682-9805; *Fax:* 519-682-2184
e-mail: clfchatham@liver.ca
Chief Officer(s):
Sheila Hughes, Development Manager

Eastern Ontario Regional Office
#641, 1500 Bank St., Ottawa ON K1H 1B8
Toll-Free: 844-316-6990
Chief Officer(s):
Gary O'Byrne, Regional Manager
GOByrne@liver.ca

London Chapter
Royal Bank Bldg., #1206, 383 Richmond St., London ON N6A 3C4
Fax: 905-752-1540
Toll-Free: 800-563-5483
e-mail: clf@liver.ca

Manitoba Chapter
#210, 375 York Ave., Winnipeg MB R3C 3J3
Tel: 204-831-6231
Chief Officer(s):
Bianca Pengelly, Reginal Coordinator
bpengelly@liver.ca

Moncton Chapter
#110, 1127B Main St., Moncton NB E1C 1H1
e-mail: atlantic@liver.ca
Chief Officer(s):
Shayla Steeves, Regional Director

Montréal Chapter
#1430, 1000, rue de la Gauchetière Ouest, Montréal QC H3B 4W5
Tél: 514-876-4170; *Téléc:* 514-876-4172
Courriel: montrealevents@liver.ca
Chief Officer(s):
Betty Esperanza, Regional Director
besperanza@liver.ca

Southern Alberta/Calgary Regional Office
#309, 1010 - 1st Ave. NE, Calgary AB T2E 7W7
Tel: 403-276-3390; *Fax:* 403-276-3423
Toll-Free: 888-557-5516
Debralee Fernets, Regional Manager
debralee@liver.ca

Toronto/GTA Chapter
#801, 3100 Steeles Ave. East, Markham ON L3R 8T3
Tel: 416-491-3353; *Fax:* 905-752-1540
Toll-Free: 800-563-5483
e-mail: clf@liver.ca
Chief Officer(s):
Steven Foster, Regional Manager
sfoster@liver.ca

National Publications

Canadian Journal of Gastroenterology & Hepatology (CJGH) / Journal Canadien de Gastroenterologie
Owned By: Hindawi Publishing Corp.
#3070, 315 Madison Ave., New York, NY
cjgh@hindawi.com

Frequency: Monthly
Official journal of the Canadian Association of Gastroenterology and the Canadian Association for the Study of the Liver.
John Marshall, Editor-in-chief
Eric Yoshida, Editor-in-chief

National Associations

Accreditation Canada / Agrément Canada
1150 Cyrville Rd., Ottawa ON K1J 7S9

Tel: 613-738-3800; *Fax:* 613-738-7755
Toll-Free: 800-814-7769
www.accreditation.ca
www.linkedin.com/company/accreditation-canada
twitter.com/AccredCanada

Previous Name: Canadian Council on Health Services Accreditation; Canadian Council on Health Facilities Accreditation
Overview: A large national licensing charitable organization founded in 1958
Mission: To improve quality in health services through accreditation; To provide health care organizations with a voluntary, external peer review to assess the quality of their services
Chief Officer(s):
George Weber, Chair
Leslee Thompson, President & CEO
Publications:
• Accreditation Canada Annual Report
Type: Yearbook; *Frequency:* Annually
• Accreditation Standard
Type: Newsletter; *Frequency:* Semiannually; *ISBN:* 978-1-55149-086-1
Profile: Updates & information about accreditation for Accreditation Canada's client organizations
• Canadian Health Accreditation Report
Frequency: Annually; *ISBN:* 978-1-55149-073-1
Profile: Findings from accreditation surveys, highlights of challenges & successes in health care, & leading practices by health organizations across Canada
• In Touch: A Newsletter for Surveyors
Type: Newsletter
Profile: Information for surveyors
• Leadership in the Journey to Quality Heath Care: The History of Accreditation
Type: Book
Profile: Evolution of Accreditation Canada over the past fifty years
• Leading Practices
Frequency: Annually
Profile: Companion report to the annual Canadian Health Accreditation Report which presents a compilation of practices identified by surveyors
• Qmentum Quarterly
Type: Journal; *Frequency:* Quarterly; *Accepts Advertising*
Profile: Educational information for health & social services organizations to improve quality & patient safety
• The Value & Impact of Accreditation in Health Care: A Review of the Literature
Author: Wendy Nicklin; Sarah Dickson
• Within Our Grasp: A Healthy Workplace Action Strategy for Success & Sustainability in Canada's Healthcare System

Association des établissements privés conventionnés - santé services sociaux (AEPC)
#200, 1076, rue de Bleury, Montréal QC H2Z 1N2

Tél: 514-499-3630; *Télec:* 514-873-7063
Courriel: info@aepc.qc.ca
www.aepc.qc.ca
www.facebook.com/416653585019212
twitter.com/AEPC_SSS

Nom précédent: Association des centres hospitaliers et centres d'accueil privés du Québec
Aperçu: *Dimension:* moyenne; *Envergure:* nationale; Organisme sans but lucratif; fondée en 1979
Mission: Promouvoir l'amélioration continue de la qualité des soins et des services donnés au sein des entreprises membres; protéger et promouvoir l'entreprise privée dans le domaine de la santé et du bien-être
Membre(s) du bureau directeur:
Danny Macdonald, Directeur général par intérim

Association for Vaccine Damaged Children
67 Shier Dr., Winnipeg MB R3R 2H2
Overview: A small national organization founded in 1986
Mission: To inform parents of the risks of immunization; To support parents in any challenging situation with public health authorities
Chief Officer(s):

Mary James, Co-Founder
tjames4@shaw.ca

Association of Faculties of Medicine of Canada (AFMC) / L'Association des facultés de médecine du Canada (AFMC)
#800, 265 Carling Ave., Ottawa ON K1S 2E1

Tel: 613-730-0687; *Fax:* 613-730-1196
e-mail: username@afmc.ca
www.afmc.ca
twitter.com/afmc_e

Previous Name: Association of Canadian Medical Colleges
Overview: A medium-sized national charitable organization founded in 1943
Mission: To represent the interests of members in medical research policy formulation; to promote & advance academic medicine through the review & development of standards for medical education, through the development of national policies appropriate to the aims & purposes of Canadian faculties of medicine, through the fostering of research, & through representation of Canadian faculties of medicine to professional associations & governments
Afiliation(s): Canadian Medical Association; Association of Universities & Colleges of Canada
Chief Officer(s):
Genevieve Moineau, President & CEO

Association of Medical Microbiology & Infectious Disease Canada (AMMI Canada) / Association pour la microbiologie médicale et l'infectiologie Canada
192 Bank St., Ottawa ON K2P 1W8

Tel: 613-260-3233; *Fax:* 613-260-3235
e-mail: communications@ammi.ca
www.ammi.ca

Previous Name: Canadian Infectious Disease Society
Overview: A small national charitable organization founded in 1978
Mission: To represent the broad interests of researchers & physicians who specialize in the fields of infectious diseases & medical microbiology in Canada; To contribute to the health of people at risk of, or affected by, infectious diseases; To promote & facilitate research; To develop policies for the prevention, diagnosis, & management of infectious diseases
Chief Officer(s):
Riccarda Galioto, Chief Operating Officer
manager@ammi.ca
Paul Glover, Coordinator, Meetings & Membership
info@ammi.ca
Tamara Nahal, Coordinator, Communications
communications@ammi.ca
Publications:
• Association of Medical Microbiology & Infectious Disease Canada Annual Report
Type: Yearbook; *Frequency:* Annually
• Association of Medical Microbiology & Infectious Disease Canada Membership Directory
Type: Directory
• Canadian Journal of Infectious Disease & Medical Microbiology
Type: Journal; *Editor:* Dr. John M. Conly; *Price:* Free with membership in the Association of Medical Microbiology & Infectious Disease
• Members Connect [a publication of the Association of Medical Microbiology & Infectious Disease Canada]
Type: Newsletter; *Price:* Free with membership in theAssociation of Medical Microbiology & Infectious Disease
Profile: The newsletter of the Association of Medical Microbiology & Infectious Disease Canada

Barth Syndrome Foundation of Canada
#115, 162 Guelph St., Georgetown ON L7G 5X7

Tel: 905-873-2391
Toll-Free: 888-732-9458
www.barthsyndrome.ca
www.facebook.com/barthsyndromecanada

Overview: A medium-sized national charitable organization
Mission: To find research grants into the cause, treatments & cure for Barth Syndrome; To assist Canadian families & physicians dealing with the disease
Afiliation(s): Barth Syndrome Foundation Inc.
Chief Officer(s):
Susan Hone, President

Biophysical Society of Canada (BSC) / La société de biophysique du Canada
c/o Department of Physics, Simon Fraser University, 8888 University Dr., Burnaby BC V5A 1S6
www.biophysicalsociety.ca
Overview: A medium-sized national organization founded in 1985 overseen by Canadian Federation of Biological Societies
Mission: To promote biophysical research & education; to encourage cross-feeding of ideas between the physical & biological sciences; to foster & support scientific meetings, workshops & discussions in biophysics; to represent Canadian biophysics & biophysicists
Chief Officer(s):
John E. Baenziger, President

BIOTECanada
#600, 1 Nicholas St., Ottawa ON K1N 7B7
Tel: 613-230-5585
e-mail: info@biotech.ca
www.biotech.ca
www.linkedin.com/company/biotecanada
twitter.com/biotecanada
Previous Name: Canadian Institute of Biotechnology; Industrial Biotechnology Association of Canada
Overview: A medium-sized national organization founded in 1987
Mission: To provide a unified voice fostering an environment that responds to the needs of the biotechnology industry & research community, both nationally & internationally
Affliation(s): AAFC Grains Innovation Roundtable Steering Committee; ACOA Atlantic Innovation Fund; Algonquin College Biotechnology Program Advisory Board; BIO Business Solutions Advisory Board; BIO International Convention Program Committee; BIO International Convention International Committee; Biorefinery Knowledge Network; Canadian Agri-Food Policy Institute Advisory Committee; DFAIT Life Sciences Advisory Board; DFAIT International Readiness Committee; EDC Stakeholder Roundtable; Environment Canada Scientific Expert Group for NSN(o); Health Canada Food Regulatory Advisory Committee
Chief Officer(s):
David Main, Chair
Andrew Casey, President & CEO
andrew.casey@biotech.ca

Canada Health Infoway / Inforoute Santé du Canada
#1200, 1000, rue Sherbrooke ouest, Montréal QC H3A 3G4
Tel: 514-868-0550; Fax: 514-868-1120
Toll-Free: 866-868-0550
www.infoway-inforoute.ca
www.linkedin.com/company/canada-health-infoway
www.facebook.com/CanadaHealthInfoway
twitter.com/infoway
www.youtube.com/user/InfowayInforoute
Overview: A medium-sized national organization founded in 2001
Mission: To accelerate the development of compatible electronic health information systems, which provide healthcare professionals with rapid access to complete & accurate patient information, enabling better decisions about diagnosis & treatment
Chief Officer(s):
Michael Green, President & CEO

Halifax
#125, 200 Waterfront Dr., Bedford NS B4A 4J4
Tel: 902-832-0876; Fax: 902-835-4719
Toll-Free: 877-832-0876
www.infoway-inforoute.ca
Chief Officer(s):
Michael Green, President & CEO

Toronto
#1300, 150 King St. West, Toronto ON M5H 1J9
Tel: 416-979-4606; Fax: 416-593-5911
Toll-Free: 888-733-6462
www.infoway-inforoute.ca
Chief Officer(s):
Michael Green, President & CEO

Vancouver

Commerce Place, #1120, 400 Burrard St., Vancouver BC V6C 3A6
Tel: 604-682-0420; Fax: 604-682-8034
Toll-Free: 877-682-0420
www.infoway-inforoute.ca
Chief Officer(s):
Michael Green, President & CEO

Canadian Academy of Facial Plastic & Reconstructive Surgery (CAFPRS)
c/o Dr. Andres Gantous, #230, 30 The Queensway, Toronto ON M6R 1B5
Tel: 905-569-6965
Toll-Free: 800-545-8864
www.cafprs.com
Overview: A small national organization
Mission: To represent cosmetic & plastic surgeons in Canada
Chief Officer(s):
Mark Taylor, President
Andres Gantous, Secretary-Treasurer

Canadian Alopecia Areata Foundation (CANAAF)
227 Burton Grove, King City ON L7B 1C7
e-mail: info@canaaf.org
canaaf.org
Overview: A medium-sized national charitable organization founded in 2009
Mission: To give support to people suffering from Alopecia Areata
Chief Officer(s):
Colleen Butler, President
colleen@canaaf.org

Canadian Anesthesiologists' Society (CAS) / Société canadienne des anesthésiologistes (SCA)
#208, 1 Eglinton Ave. East, Toronto ON M4P 3A1
Tel: 416-480-0320; Fax: 416-480-0602
e-mail: anesthesia@cas.ca
www.cas.ca
twitter.com/CASUpdate
Overview: A large national organization founded in 1943
Mission: To advance the medical practice of anesthesia throughout Canada
Affliation(s): Canadian Anesthesia Research Foundation (CARF); CAS International Education Foundation (CAS IEF)
Chief Officer(s):
Susan O'Leary, President
Douglas DuVal, Vice-President
Stanley Mandarich, Executive Director
director@cas.ca
Salvatore Spadafora, Secretary
François Gobeil, Treasurer
Publications:
• Anesthesia News
Type: Newsletter; Frequency: Quarterly; Editor: Dr. Patricia Houston
Profile: Society updates, including events, prizes, & research
• Canadian Anesthesiologists' Society Annual Report
Type: Yearbook; Frequency: Annually
• Canadian Journal of Anesthesia / Journal canadien d'anesthésie
Type: Journal; Frequency: Monthly; Editor: Donald R. Miller, MD, FRCPC; ISSN: 0832-610X
Profile: Peer-reviewed clinical research, basic research, & expert reviews & opinions to assist anesthesiologists
• Guidelines to the Practice of Anesthesia
Price: $25

Canadian Apheresis Group (CAG) / Groupe canadien d'aphérèse
#199, 435 St. Laurent Blvd., Ottawa ON K1K 2Z8
Tel: 613-748-9613; Fax: 613-748-6392
e-mail: cag@cagcanada.ca
www.cagcanada.ca
Overview: A small national organization founded in 1980
Mission: To provide a forum for information exchange among apheresis practioners in Canada; To promote clinical research in apheresis
Chief Officer(s):
Gail Rock, Chair

Canadian Art Therapy Association (CATA) / L'association canadienne d'art thérapie
PO Box 658, Stn. Main, Parksville BC V9P 2G7

cata15.wildapricot.org
www.linkedin.com/company/3574360
www.facebook.com/142451825860747

Overview: A small national organization founded in 1977
Mission: To promote the development & maintenance of professional standards of art therapy training, registration, research, & practice in Canada; To heighten awareness of art therapy as an important mental health discipline
Chief Officer(s):
Mehdi Naimi, President
 catapresident@gmail.com
Michelle Winkel, Vice-President
 catavicepresident@gmail.com
Kayla Cardinal, Treasurer
 catasecretary@gmail.com
Haley Toll, Director, Communications
 catacommunicationschair@gmail.com
Publications:
• Canadian Art Therapy Association Directory
Type: Directory
Profile: Listings of professional & registered art therapists, who are members of the Canadian Art Therapy Association & who chose to be listed in the directory
• Canadian Art Therapy Association Journal
Type: Journal; *Frequency:* Semiannually; *Editor:* Marilyn Magnuson; *ISSN:* 0832-2473; *Price:* Free with membership CATA; $30 non-members in Canada; $35 in the U.S.A.; $40 intl.
• Canadian Art Therapy Association Newsletter
Type: Newsletter; *Frequency:* 3 pa

Canadian Association for Clinical Microbiology & Infectious Diseases (CACMID) / Association canadienne de microbiologie clinique et des maladies contagieuses
c/o National Microbiology Laboratory, 1015 Arlington St., Winnipeg MB R3E 3R2

Fax: 204-789-2097
www.cacmid.ca
www.facebook.com/CACMID
twitter.com/cacmid

Overview: A small national charitable organization founded in 1932
Mission: To enhance the cooperation of professionals specializing in clinical microbiology & infectious disease; To act as the voice for clinical microbiology & infectious disease professionals; To develop standards in the field of clinical microbiology
Chief Officer(s):
Jeff Fuller, President
 jeff.fuller@albertahealthservices.ca
Matthew W. Gilmour, Secretary-Treasurer
 Matthew.Gilmour@cacmid.ca
Publications:
• CACMID [Canadian Association for Clinical Microbiology & Infectious Diseases] Membership Directory
Type: Directory

Canadian Association for Community Living (CACL) / Association canadienne pour l'intégration communautaire
20-850 King St. West, Oshawa ON L1J 8N5

Tel: 416-661-9611; *Fax:* 905-436-3587
Toll-Free: 855-661-9611
e-mail: inform@cacl.ca
www.cacl.ca
www.facebook.com/canadianacl
twitter.com/cacl_acic
www.youtube.com/canadianacl

Previous Name: Canadian Association for the Mentally Retarded
Overview: A large national charitable organization founded in 1958
Mission: To ensure the following for people with intellectual disabilities: the same rights, & access to choice, services, & supports as others; the same opportunities to live in freedom & dignity with the necessary supports to do so; & the ability to articulate & realize their rights & aspirations
Member of: Inclusion International
Affiliation(s): People First of Canada; Council of Canadians with Disabilities (CCD); National Alliance for Children & Youth; Active Living Alliance; Canadian Council on Social Development (CCSD); Canadian Coalition for the Rights of Children (CCRC); Canadian Institute of Child Health (CICH); Canadian Caregiver Coalition; Canadian Down Syndrome Society (CDSS); Family Service Canada; DisAbled Women's Network Canada (DAWN)
Chief Officer(s):
Joy Bacon, President
Michael Bach, Executive Vice-President
 mbach@cacl.ca
Sue Talmey, Director, Finance & Administration
 stalmey@cacl.ca
Tara Brinston Levandier, Director, Policy & Program Operations
 tbrinston@cacl.ca
Gordon Porter, Director, Inclusive Education Initiatives
 inclusiveeducation@cacl.ca
Agata Zieba, Senior Officer, Communications
 azieba@cacl.ca
Publications:
• Coming Together [a publication of the Canadian Association for Community Living]
Type: Newsletter
Profile: The Canadian Association for Community Living's family newsletter, featuring stories of families
• Education Watch [a publication of the Canadian Association for Community Living]
Type: Newsletter; *Frequency:* Quarterly
Profile: Inclusive education across Canada
• INFO@ [a publication of the Canadian Association for Community Living]
Type: Newsletter; *Frequency:* Bimonthly
Profile: Up-to-date topics & issues within the Canadian Association for Community Living & its members & affiliates
• Institution Watch [a publication of the Canadian Association for Community Living]
Type: Newsletter
Profile: Produced by the People First of Canada - CACL Joint Task Force on Deinstitutionalization
• Invisible No More [a publication of the Canadian Association for Community Living]
Type: Book; *Number of Pages:* 160; *Author:* Vincenzo Pietropaolo
Profile: A photography book chronicling the lives of individuals with intellectual disabilities
• National Report Card on Inclusion [a publication of the Canadian Association for Community Living]
Type: Report; *Frequency:* Annual
Profile: The purpose is to track the progress of inclusion in Canadian society
• Povery Watch [a publication of the Canadian Association for Community Living]
Type: Newsletter; *Frequency:* Quarterly
Profile: A publication from the Canadian Association for Community Living's National Action Committee on Disability Supports, Income, & Employment

Canadian Association for Health Services & Policy Research (CAHSPR) / Association canadienne pour la recherche sur les services et les politiques de la santé (ACRSPS)
292 Somerset St. West, Ottawa ON K2P 0J6

Tel: 613-288-9239; *Fax:* 613-599-7805
e-mail: info@cahspr.ca
www.cahspr.ca
www.facebook.com/CAHSPR
twitter.com/CAHSPR
www.youtube.com/CAHSPR

Previous Name: Canadian Health Economics Research Association
Overview: A small national organization founded in 1983
Mission: To provide a multidisciplinary association fostering and supporting linkages between researchers and decision makers; knowledge translation and exchange; education and training; and advocacy for research and its more effective use in planning, practice and policy-making.
Chief Officer(s):
Steve Morgan, President
Adalsteinn (Steini) Brown, President-Elect
Publications:
• CAHSPR [Canadian Association for Health Services & Policy Research] Newsletter
Type: Newsletter; *Frequency:* Weekly

Profile: CAHSPR activities & upcoming events, career opportunities, links to course materials for student members, research & policy items of interest to members
• Healthcare Policy
Type: Journal; *Frequency:* Quarterly

Canadian Association for Immunization Research & Evaluation
950 West 28th Ave., Vancouver BC V5Z 4H4

Tel: 604-875-2422; *Fax:* 604-875-2635
e-mail: caire@cfri.ca
www.caire.ca

Overview: A small national organization
Mission: To promote vaccinology research in Canada; To represent the interests of individuals in the vaccinology research field; To stimulate public interest in vaccine studies & vaccine-preventable diseases; To disseminate information from research studies to health professionals & the public
Chief Officer(s):
Brian Ward, Interim Chair

Canadian Association for Medical Education (CAME) / Association canadienne pour l'éducation médicale (ACÉM)
#100, 2733 Lancaster Rd., Ottawa ON K1B 0A9

Tel: 613-730-0687; *Fax:* 613-730-1196
e-mail: came@afmc.ca
www.came-acem.ca

Overview: A medium-sized national organization founded in 1987
Mission: To improve medical education in Canada; To promote excellence & scholarship in medical education; To support educational development; To encourage research in medical education
Chief Officer(s):
Allyn Walsh, President
Shelley Ross, Secretary
Anurag Saxena, Treasurer
Ming-Ka Chan, Coordinator, Membership
Susan Lieff, Liaison Officer
Publications:
• CAME [Canadian Association for Medical Education] Newsletter
Type: Newsletter
Profile: Articles & commentaries of interest to Canadian medical educators
• CAME [Canadian Association for Medical Education] E-Bulletin
Type: Newsletter; *Frequency:* Monthly
Profile: Current association information, such as announcements, upcoming meetings, grant opportunities, & career postings

Canadian Association for Music Therapy (CAMT) / Association de musicothérapie du Canada (AMC)
#5, 1124 Gainsborough Rd., London ON N6H 5N1

Fax: 519-641-0431
Toll-Free: 800-996-2268
e-mail: info@musictherapy.ca
www.musictherapy.ca

Overview: A medium-sized national licensing organization founded in 1974
Mission: To promote excellence in music therapy practice & education in Canadian clinical, educational, & community settings
Affiliation(s): World Federation of Music Therapy
Publications:
• CAMT [Canadian Association for Music Therapy] Newsletter
Type: Newsletter; *Frequency:* Quarterly
• Canadian Association for Music Therapy Conference Proceedings
Frequency: Annually
Profile: Proceedings from each CAMT national conference
• The Canadian Association for Music Therapy Member Sourcebook
Type: Directory
• The Canadian Journal of Music Therapy
Type: Journal; *Frequency:* Annually; *Accepts Advertising; Editor:* Kevin Kirkland
Profile: Peer-reviewed papers about music therapy knowledge & practice

Music Therapy Association of British Columbia

c/o Capilano College, 2055 Purcell Way, North Vancouver BC V7N 3H5

Tel: 604-924-0046; *Fax:* 604-983-7559
Toll-Free: 800-424-0556
e-mail: info@mtabc.com
www.mtabc.com
www.facebook.com/141974696573
twitter.com/musictherapybc
www.youtube.com/channel/UCiLiJ0Aj_3TLcmCatxASwBg
Chief Officer(s):
Gemma Isaac, President
president@mtabc.com

Canadian Association for Population Therapeutics (CAPT)
c/o Peggy Kee, Sunnybrook Health Sciences Centre, 2075 Bayview Ave., #E240, Toronto ON M4N 3M5

Tel: 416-480-6100; *Fax:* 416-480-6025
www.capt-actp.com

Overview: A small national organization founded in 1996
Mission: To advance the sound development of population-based studies of therapeutic interventions; To provide a forum for the reporting, scientific discussion & dissemination of the data derived from population-based therapeutic research, as an information resource for medical decision-making in the best interests of the individual patient & the public well-being
Chief Officer(s):
Peggy Kee, Administrative Officer
peggy.kee@sunnybrook.ca

Canadian Association for School Health (CASH)
16629 - 62A Ave., Surrey BC V3S 9L5

Tel: 604-575-3199
e-mail: info@cash-aces.ca
www.cash-aces.ca

Overview: A small national organization
Mission: Provincial/area coalitions who promote the health of youth through a school-related health program called Comprehensive School Health (CSH); to develop & implements projects, activities & services that follow the CSH approach. This approach helps community agencies, parents, educators, & health professionals work together.
Member of: International School Health Network

Canadian Association of Ambulatory Care (CAAC)
#200, 100 Consilium Pl., Toronto ON M1H 3E3

e-mail: canadianambulatorycare@gmail.com
www.canadianambulatorycare.com
twitter.com/ambulatorycare
www.youtube.com/channel/UCWGw_1LKg2L-DO1AqMuifGQ
Overview: A small national organization founded in 2012
Mission: To enhance the ambulatory care field in Canada
Chief Officer(s):
Denyse Henry, Chief Executive Officer
caacceo1@gmail.com
Jatinder Bains, President
caacpresident@gmail.com
Julia Young, Vice-President, Finance & Sponsorship
caactreasurer1@gmail.com
Edna Pasaoa, Vice-President, Membership & Promotions
caacmembership@gmail.com
Sherrol Palmer, Vice-President, Education
caaceducation@gmail.com
Adam Saporta, Vice-President, Special Projects
caacspecialprojects1@gmail.com
Vinder Nat, Vice-President, Communications & Stakeholders Relations
caaccommunications@gmail.com
Ellie Lee, Vice-President, Web Design & Publications
caacrelations@gmail.com
Jing Zhou, Secretary

Canadian Association of Apheresis Nurses (CAAN) / Association Canadienne des Infirmiers et Infirmieres d'Apheresis
Canadian Apheresis Group, #199, 435 St. Laurent Blvd., Ottawa ON K1K 2Z8

Tel: 613-748-9613; *Fax:* 613-748-6392
e-mail: apheresisnurses@live.ca
www.apheresisnurses.org

Overview: A small national organization founded in 1992
Mission: To establish apheresis standards; To promote & collect information on all apheresis procedures including plasma exchange,

cytapheresis, photopheresis & stem cell collection
Member of: World Apheresis Association
Affliation(s): Canadian Apheresis Group; Canadian Nurses Association
Publications:
• Canadian Association of Apheresis Nurses Newsletter
Type: Newsletter

Canadian Association of Bariatric Physicians & Surgeons (CABPS) / L'Association canadienne des medecins et chirurgiens bariatrique (ACMCB)
#210, 2800 - 14th Ave., Markham ON L3R 0E4
Tel: 416-491-2886; *Fax:* 416-491-1670
e-mail: cabps@associationconcepts.ca
cabps.ca
www.linkedin.com/company/cabps
www.facebook.com/pages/CABPS/215143185313177#
twitter.com/Cabps_Obesity
Overview: A small national organization
Mission: Represents Canadian specialists interested in the treatment of obesity and severe obesity for the purposes of professional development and coordination and promotion of common goals.
Affliation(s): International Federation for the Surgery of Obesity and Metabolic Disorders
Chief Officer(s):
Mehran Anvari, President, 905-522-2951
anvari@mcmaster.ca

Canadian Association of Blue Cross Plans (CABCP) / Association Canadienne des Croix Bleue (ACCB)
PO Box 2005, #610, 185 The West Mall, Toronto ON M9C 5P1
Toll-Free: 866-732-2583
www.bluecross.ca
Also Known As: Blue Cross Canada
Overview: A small national licensing organization founded in 1955
Mission: To maintain & monitor standards of performance by association members; to ensure members manage effectively supplementary health, dental, life insurance, & disability income products on an individual and group basis
Affliation(s): Blue Cross (USA); Blue Shield (USA); International Federation of Health Funds

Alberta Blue Cross
Blue Cross Place, 10009 - 108th St. NW, Edmonton AB T5J 3C5
Tel: 780-498-8100
Toll-Free: 800-661-6995
www.ab.bluecross.ca
www.linkedin.com/company/16959
www.facebook.com/AlbertaBlueCross
twitter.com/ABBluecross
vimeo.com/albertabluecross
Chief Officer(s):
Ray R. Pisani, President/CEO
• Alberta Blue Cross Annual Report
Type: Yearbook; *Frequency:* Annually

Manitoba Blue Cross
PO Box 1046, Stn. Main, Winnipeg MB R3C 2X7
Tel: 204-775-0151; *Fax:* 204-786-5965
Toll-Free: 800-873-2583
www.mb.bluecross.ca
Chief Officer(s):
Andrew Yorke, President & CEO

Medavie Blue Cross/Atlantic Blue Cross Care/Service Croix Bleue de l'Atlantique
PO Box 220, 644 Main St., Moncton NB E1C 8L3
Toll-Free: 800-667-4511
www.medavie.bluecross.ca
www.facebook.com/MedavieBlueCross
twitter.com/MedavieBC
www.youtube.com/MedavieBlueCross
Chief Officer(s):
Pierre-Yves Julien, CEO

Ontario Blue Cross

#610, 185 The West Mall, Toronto ON M9C 5P1
Tel: 416-646-2585; *Fax:* 800-893-0997
Toll-Free: 866-732-2583
e-mail: bco.indhealth@ont.bluecross.ca
www.useblue.com
• Ontario Blue Cross Annual Report
Type: Yearbook; *Frequency:* Annually

Pacific Blue Cross
c/o British Columbia Life & Casualty Company (BC Life), PO Box 7000, Vancouver BC V6B 4E1
Tel: 604-419-2000; *Fax:* 604-419-2990
Toll-Free: 888-275-4672
www.pac.bluecross.ca
www.linkedin.com/company/pacific-blue-cross
www.facebook.com/pacificbluecross
twitter.com/pacbluecross
Chief Officer(s):
Jan K. Grude, President/CEO
Gerry Smith, Chair
• Pacific Blue Cross Annual Report
Type: Yearboook; *Frequency:* Annually

Québec Blue Cross/Croix Bleue du Québec
#9B, 550, rue Sherbrooke Ouest, Montréal QC H3A 3S3
Tel: 514-286-7686; *Fax:* 866-286-8358
Toll-Free: 877-909-7686
e-mail: info@qc.croixbleue.ca
www.qc.croixbleue.ca
• Québec Blue Cross Annual Report
Type: Yearbook; *Frequency:* Annually

Saskatchewan Blue Cross
PO Box 4030, 516 - 2nd Ave. North, Saskatoon SK S7K 3T2
Tel: 306-244-1192; *Fax:* 306-652-5751
Toll-Free: 800-667-6853
www.sk.bluecross.ca
www.linkedin.com/company/saskatchewan-blue-cross
www.facebook.com/sk.push2play
twitter.com/SKBlueCross
Chief Officer(s):
G.N. (Arnie) Arnott, President/CEO

Canadian Association of Child Neurology (CACN) / L'Association canadienne de neurologie pédiatrique (ACNP)
#709, 7015 Macleod Trail SW, Calgary AB T2H 2K6
Tel: 403-229-9544; *Fax:* 403-229-1661
www.cnsfederation.org
Overview: A small national organization founded in 1991 overseen by Canadian Neurological Sciences Federation
Mission: To advance knowledge about the development of the nervous system from conception, as well as the diseases of the nervous system in children; To improve treatment of young people with neurological handicaps
Publications:
• Canadian Association of Child Neurology Membership Directory
Type: Directory

Canadian Association of Community Health Centres (CACHC) / Association canadienne des centres de santé communautiare
#500, 340 College St., Toronto ON M5T 3A9
Tel: 416-922-5694; *Fax:* 866-404-6040
www.cachc.ca
www.linkedin.com/groups/Canadian-Assoc-Community-Health-Centres-432281
www.facebook.com/CACHC.ACCSC
twitter.com/CACHC_ACCSC
www.youtube.com/user/CACHCandACCSC
Overview: A medium-sized national organization founded in 1995
Mission: To support provincially-based community health centre organizations in Canada; to represent community health centre organizations nationally; to improve health services in Canadian communities; to promote community health centre organizations for the delivery of primary health care
Chief Officer(s):
Scott Wolfe, Executive Director
swolfe@cachc.ca
Jane Moloney, Chair
Michelle Hurtubise, Treasurer

Canadian Association of General Surgeons (CAGS) / Association canadienne des chirurgiens généraux (ACCG)
PO Box 1428, Stn. B, Ottawa ON K1P 5R4

Tel: 613-882-6510
e-mail: cags@cags-accg.ca
www.cags-accg.ca
www.facebook.com/220880261312881
twitter.com/CAGS_ACCG

Overview: A medium-sized national charitable organization founded in 1977
Mission: To assist all general surgeons with continuing education; facilitate & promote surgical research; develop policies & new ideas in the areas of clinical care, education & research
Affliation(s): Canadian Medical Association; Royal College of Physicians & Surgeons of Canada
Chief Officer(s):
Debrah Wirtzfeld, President
Jasmin Lidington, Executive Director
  jlidington@cags-accg.ca
Publications:
• CAGS [Canadian Association of General Surgeons] Newsletter
Type: Newsletter
Profile: Association news, conference highlights, & research

Canadian Association of Medical Biochemists (CAMB) / Association des médecins biochimistes du Canada (AMBC)
2083 Black Friars Rd., Ottawa ON K2A 3K6

Tel: 613-680-8526; *Fax:* 613-249-3557
e-mail: camb.ambc@gmail.com
www.camb-ambc.ca

Overview: A small national organization founded in 1975
Chief Officer(s):
Andrew don Wauchope, President

Canadian Association of Medical Device Reprocessing (CAMDR)
147 Parkside Dr., Oak Bluff MB R4G 0A6

e-mail: info@camdr.ca
www.camdr.ca

Overview: A small national organization
Mission: CAMDR seeks to address numerous issues including patient safety, infection prevention & control, technology assessments, vendor relations, organizational management, and education.
Chief Officer(s):
Abdool Karim, President

Canadian Association of Medical Radiation Technologists (CAMRT) / Association canadienne des technologues en radiation médicale (ACTRM)
#1300, 180 Elgin St., Ottawa ON K2P 2K3

Tel: 613-234-0012; *Fax:* 613-234-1097
Toll-Free: 800-463-9729
e-mail: info@camrt.ca
www.camrt.ca
www.linkedin.com/company/1432897
www.facebook.com/CAMRTactrm
twitter.com/CAMRT_ACTRM

Overview: A medium-sized national licensing organization founded in 1942
Mission: To act as the certifying body for medical radiation technologists & therapists throughout Canada
Member of: International Society of Radiographers & Radiological Technologists
Chief Officer(s):
François Couillard, Chief Executive Officer
  fcouillard@camrt.ca
Michelle Charest, Director, Finance & Administration
  mcharest@camrt.ca
Elaine Dever, Director, Education
  edever@camrt.ca
Mark Given, Director, Professional Practice
  mgiven@camrt.ca
Christopher Topham, Director, Advocacy & Communications
  ctopham@camrt.ca
Karen Morrison, Director, Membership & Events
  kmorrison@camrt.ca
Publications:
• CAMRT [Canadian Association of Medical Radiation Technologists] Newsletter

Type: Newsletter; *Frequency:* Quarterly; *Accepts Advertising*
Profile: Canadian Association of Medical Radiation Technologists articles, education activities, & events
• Canadian Association of Medical Radiation Technologists Annual Report
Type: Yearbook; *Frequency:* Annually
• Journal of Medical Imaging & Radiation Sciences
Type: Journal; *Frequency:* Quarterly; *Accepts Advertising*; *Editor:* Lisa Di Prospero
Profile: A peer-reviewed journal of articles on recent research, professional practices, new technology, & book reviews

Canadian Association of Neuropathologists (CANP) / Association canadienne de neuropathologistes
c/o Service d'Anatomo-pathologie, CHA Hopital de l'Enfant-Jesus, #1401, 18ieme rue, Québec QC G1J 1Z4

Tel: 418-649-5725; *Fax:* 418-649-5856
www.canp.ca

Overview: A small national charitable organization founded in 1960
Mission: To promote the professional & educational objectives of neuropathologists; To ensure high standards in the neuropathology field
Affliation(s): International Society of Neuropathology
Chief Officer(s):
Marc Del Bigio, President
Peter Gould, Secretary-Treasurer
  peter.gould@fmed.ulaval.ca

Canadian Association of Nuclear Medicine (CANM) / Association canadienne de médecine nucléaire (ACMN)
PO Box 4383, Stn. E, Ottawa ON K1S 5B4

Tel: 613-882-5097
e-mail: canm@canm-acmn.ca
www.canm-acmn.ca

Overview: A small national organization founded in 1971
Mission: To strive for excellence in the practice of diagnostic & therapeutic nuclear medicine; to promote the continued professional competence of nuclear medicine specialists; to establish guidelines of clinical practice; to encourage biomedical research
Affliation(s): Canadian Medical Association; Society of Nuclear Medicine - USA; Canadian Association of Radiation Protection
Chief Officer(s):
Andrew Ross, President
Francois Lamoureux, Vice-President
Glenn Ollenberger, Secretary-Treasurer

Canadian Association of Occupational Therapists (CAOT) / Association canadienne des ergothérapeutes (ACE)
#100, 34 Colonnade Rd., Ottawa ON K2E 7J6

Tel: 613-523-2268; *Fax:* 613-523-2552
Toll-Free: 800-434-2268
e-mail: insurance@caot.ca
www.caot.ca
www.facebook.com/CAOT.ca
twitter.com/CAOT_ACE

Overview: A large national organization founded in 1926
Mission: To develop & promote the profession of occupational therapy in Canada & abroad; To assist occupational therapists achieve excellence in their professional practice by offering services, products, events, & networking opportunities
Affliation(s): World Federation of Occupational Therapists
Chief Officer(s):
Janet M. Craik, Executive Director, 613-523-2268 Ext. 244
  jcraik@caot.ca
Mike Brennan, Chief Operating Officer, 613-523-2268 Ext. 238
  mbrennan@caot.ca
Havelin Anand, Director, Government Affairs & Policy, 613-523-2268 Ext. 230
  hanand@caot.ca
Vicky Wang, Director, Finance, 613-523-2268 Ext. 227
  finance@caot.ca
Publications:
• Canadian Association of Occupational Therapists Annual Report
Type: Yearbook; *Frequency:* Annually
Profile: A review of association activities during the past year, plus financial information
• Canadian Journal of Occupational Therapy [a publication of the Canadian Association of Occupational Therapists]

Type: Journal; *Frequency:* 5 pa; *Accepts Advertising; Editor:* Helene Polatajko; *ISSN:* 0008-4174
Profile: Professional peer-reviewed scientific journal promotingadvancement in research & education
• Enabling Occupation II: Advancing an Occupational Therapy Vision for Health, Well-being & Justice through Occupation
Author: Elizabeth Townsend, Helen Polatajko; *ISBN:* 978-1-895437-76-8
Profile: A study & practice guide, focussing on occupation-basedenablement
• Occupational Therapy Now [a publication of the Canadian Association of Occupational Therapists]
Type: Magazine; *Frequency:* bi-m.; *Accepts Advertising; Editor:* Janna MacLachlan
Profile: Practice magazine, with clinical applications of recent research & theory, evidence-basedpractice, & product reviews

Canadian Association of Pathologists (CAP) / Association canadienne des pathologistes (ACP)
#310, 4 Cataraqui St., Kingston ON K7K 1Z7
Tel: 613-507-8528
Toll-Free: 866-531-0626
e-mail: info@cap-acp.org
cap-acp.org
www.linkedin.com/in/capacp
www.facebook.com/canadian.association.pathologists
twitter.com/CAPACP
Overview: A medium-sized national charitable organization founded in 1949
Mission: To maintain high standards for patient practices and care for pathologists and laboratory medicine.
Chief Officer(s):
Martin Trotter, President
Heather Dow, Manager
Publications:
• The CAP [Canadian Association of Pathologists] Newsletter
Type: Newsletter; *Frequency:* Quarterly; *Accepts Advertising*
Profile: Available to members only
• CAP [Canadian Association of Pathologists] Membership Directory
Type: Directory; *Frequency:* Annually

Canadian Association of Physical Medicine & Rehabilitation (CAPM&R) / Association canadienne de médecine physique et de réadaptation
#310, 4 Cataraqui St., Kingston ON K7K 1Z7
Tel: 613-507-0480; *Fax:* 866-531-0626
e-mail: info@capmr.ca
www.capmr.ca
www.facebook.com/capmr.ca
twitter.com/CAPM_R
Overview: A medium-sized national organization
Mission: The CAPM&R represents and promotes the interests of the speciality of physiatry in Canada by providing and maintaina a national forum and network. It advances and increases awareness of the specialty through strategic alliances and partnerships, public policy, and professional and practice development.
Chief Officer(s):
Rodney Li Pi Shan, President
Heather Dow, Executive Director

Canadian Association of Physician Assistants (CAPA)
#704, 265 Carling Ave., Ottawa ON K1S 2E1
Tel: 613-248-2272; *Fax:* 613-521-2226
Toll-Free: 877-744-2272
e-mail: admin@capa-acam.ca
capa-acam.ca
www.facebook.com/CAPA.ACAM
twitter.com/CAPAACAM
Overview: A small national organization
Mission: To develop Canadian health care; To advocate for members; To promote the delivery of patient-centered quality health care
Chief Officer(s):
Patrick Nelson, Executive Director

Canadian Association of Physicians of Indian Heritage (CAPIH)
115 Charingcross St., Brantford ON N3R 2H8
Tel: 519-304-1718; *Fax:* 519-304-4635
Toll-Free: 888-982-2744
e-mail: info@capih.ca
www.capih.ca
Overview: A medium-sized national organization founded in 2005
Mission: To arrange continuing medical educations meetings & seminars; to provide resources, services & expertise within Canada & in the Third World as needed
Affliation(s): American Association of Physicians of Indian Origin (AAPI)
Chief Officer(s):
Kempe S. Gowda, President
Joseph Kurian, CEO

Canadian Association of Physicians with Disabilities
70 Hillsdale Ave. West, Toronto ON M5P 1G1
Tel: 416-485-9461; *Fax:* 416-485-9461
e-mail: feedback@capd.ca
www.capd.ca
Overview: A small national organization
Mission: CAPD provides a national forum for physicians with disabilities, opening avenues for exchange of ideas & information, particularly as these apply to clinical practice. It aims to improve the quality of care & of life for people with disabilities by influencing clinical education & research in matters pertaining to both patients & physicians with disabilities. It also acts as a vehicle to inform & educate the public at large regarding the many facets of disabilities & to be proactive in influencing policies & laws.
Affliation(s): Canadian Medical Association
Chief Officer(s):
Ophelia Lynn MacDonald, Contact

Canadian Association of Professionals with Disabilities
714 Warder Place, Victoria BC V9A 7H6
Tel: 250-361-9697
e-mail: info@canadianprofessionals.org
www.canadianprofessionals.org
Overview: A medium-sized national organization founded in 2003
Mission: To address issues affecting professionals with disabilities

Canadian Association of Radiologists (CAR) / L'Association canadienne des radiologistes
#600, 294 Albert St., Ottawa ON K1P 6E6
Tel: 613-860-3111; *Fax:* 613-860-3112
e-mail: info@car.ca
www.car.ca
Overview: A medium-sized national organization founded in 1937
Mission: Voluntary organization representing the goals & the interests of imaging specialists; to promote the clinical, educational, research & political goals of Canadian radiology to members, organized radiology, medical associations, government & the public
Affliation(s): Canadian Medical Association
Chief Officer(s):
Adele Fifield, CEO, 613-860-3111 Ext. 200
afifield@car.ca
Publications:
• Canadian Association of Radiologists Journal / Journal de l'Association canadienne de radiologiste
Type: Journal; *Frequency:* 5 pa; *Accepts Advertising; Editor:* Craig Coblentz, MD, FRCPC; *ISSN:* 0846-5371
Profile: Scientific review of radiology in Canada

Canadian Association of Research Administrators (CARA) / Association canadienne des administratrices et des administrateurs de recherche (ACAAR)
#1710, 350 Albert St., Ottawa ON K1R 1B1
Tel: 289-244-3744
e-mail: webinars@cara-acaar.ca
cara-acaar.ca
www.linkedin.com/groups/4978586/profile
twitter.com/@cara_acaar
Previous Name: Canadian Association of University Research Administrators
Overview: A small national organization founded in 1971 overseen by Association of Universities & Colleges of Canada
Mission: To advance the research administrator profession; To improve the efficiency & effectiveness of research administration at

post-secondary institutions; To advocate for its membership through representation & unity; To foster & encourage collaboration with organizations in related disciplines
Member of: Association of Universities & Colleges of Canada; Canadian Consortium for Research
Affiliation(s): National Council of University Research Administrators; Society of Research Administrators; Association of University Technology Managers; Canadian Association of University Business Officers; Canadian Association of Research Ethics Boards; Research Administrators' Group Network
Chief Officer(s):
Sarah Lampson, Executive Director, 289-442-2992
  executive_director@cara-acaar.ca

Canadian Association of Specialized Kinesiology
PO Box 214, Tamworth ON K0K 3G0
  Toll-Free: 888-490-1340
  e-mail: office@canask.org
  www.canask.org
  www.facebook.com/219459068073143
  twitter.com/CanASK1
Also Known As: CanASK
Overview: A small national organization
Mission: To link association members to international affiliates; To promote & support the specialized kinesiology community of Canada
Affliation(s): International Kinesiology College; Touch for Health Kinesiology Association (USA); The Energy Kinesiology Association (USA)
Chief Officer(s):
Heather Phillips, President
Publications:
• Canadian Association of Specialized Kinesiology Membership Directory
Type: Directory; *Frequency:* Annually
Profile: Listing of instructors, practitioners, general members, & student members
• Reaching Out [a publication of the Canadian Association of Specialized Kinesiology]
Type: Newsletter; *Frequency:* Quarterly
Profile: News & information about kinesiology subjects, proposed bylaws, book reviews, reports from kinesiologists, & articles from NorthAmerican conferences

Canadian Blood Services (CBS) / Société canadienne du sang
1800 Alta Vista Dr., Ottawa ON K1G 4J5
  Tel: 613-739-2300; *Fax:* 613-731-1411
  Toll-Free: 888-236-6283
  e-mail: feedback@blood.ca
  www.blood.ca
  www.linkedin.com/company/canadian-blood-services
  www.facebook.com/itsinyoutogive
  twitter.com/itsinyoutogive
  www.youtube.com/18882DONATE
Previous Name: Canadian Red Cross - Blood Services
Overview: A medium-sized national organization founded in 1998
Mission: To manage the blood supply for Canadians; To ensure blood safety
Chief Officer(s):
Leah Hollins, Chair
Graham D. Sher, Chief Executive Officer
Publications:
• BloodNotes [a publication of Canadian Blood Services]
Type: Newsletter
Profile: Information & educational articles for hospital customers
• Canadian Blood Services Annual Report
Type: Yearbook; *Frequency:* Annually

Ancaster
35 Stone Church Rd., Ancaster ON L9K 1S5
  Toll-Free: 888-236-6283
Chief Officer(s):
Dunbar Russel, Regional Representative, Ontario

Barrie
#100, 231 Bayview Dr., Barrie ON L4N 4Y5
  Toll-Free: 888-823-6283

Brandon

c/o Westman Collection Site, Town Centre, 800 Rosser Ave., Brandon MB R7A 6N5
  Toll-Free: 888-236-6283

Burlington
1250 Brant St., Burlington ON L7P 1X8
  Toll-Free: 888-236-6283

Calgary
737 - 13th Ave., Calgary AB T2R 1J1
  Toll-Free: 888-236-6283
Chief Officer(s):
Mike Shaw, Regional Representative, Alberta, Saskatchewan, Manitoba, Northwest Territories, & Nunavut

Charlottetown
85 Fitzroy St., Charlottetown PE C1A 1R6
  Toll-Free: 888-236-6283
Chief Officer(s):
Jeff Scott, Regional Representative, Atlantic

Corner Brook
3 Herald Ave., Corner Brook NL A2H 4B8
  Toll-Free: 888-236-6283

Edmonton
8249 - 114th St., Edmonton AB T6G 2R8
  Toll-Free: 888-236-6283

Guelph
130 Silvercreek Pkwy. North, Guelph ON N1H 7Y5
  Toll-Free: 888-236-6283

Halifax
#252, 7071 Bayers Rd., Halifax NS B3L 2C2
  Toll-Free: 888-236-6283
Chief Officer(s):
Jeff Scott, Regional Representative, Atlantic

Kelowna
#103, 1865 Dilworth Dr., Kelowna BC V1Y 9T1
  Toll-Free: 888-236-6283

Kingston
850 Gardiners Rd., Kingston ON K7M 3X9
  Toll-Free: 888-236-6283

Kitchener-Waterloo
94 Bridgeport Rd. East, Waterloo ON N2J 2J9
  Toll-Free: 888-263-3283

Lethbridge
Lethbridge Centre Mall, #220, 200 - 4 Ave. South, Lethbridge AB T1J 4C9
  Toll-Free: 888-236-6283

London
820 Wharncliffe Rd. South, London ON N6J 2N4
  Toll-Free: 888-236-6283
Chief Officer(s):
Dunbar Russel, Regional Representative, Ontario

Mississauga
#15, 785 Britannia Rd. West, Mississauga ON L5V 2Y1
  Toll-Free: 888-236-6283

Moncton
500 Mapleton Rd., Moncton NB E1G 0N3
  Toll-Free: 888-236-6283

Oshawa
1300 Harmony Rd. North, Oshawa ON L1K 2B1
  Toll-Free: 888-236-6283

Ottawa
1575 Carling Ave., Ottawa ON K1Z 7M3
  Tel: 613-560-7440
  Toll-Free: 888-236-6283
Chief Officer(s):
Dunbar Russel, Regional Representative, Ontario

Ottawa - Alta Vista Dr. - National Fundraising Office
1800 Alta Vista Dr., Ottawa ON K1G 4J5
  Tel: 613-739-2300; *Fax:* 613-739-2141
  Toll-Free: 888-236-6283
  campaignforcanadians.ca

Chief Officer(s):
Penny Holmes-Tuor, Manager
  penny.holmes-tuor@blood.ca

Peterborough
55 George St. North, Peterborough ON K9J 3G2
Toll-Free: 888-236-6283

Prince George
2277 Westwood Dr., Prince George BC V2N 4V6
Toll-Free: 888-236-6283

Red Deer
#5, 5020 - 68th St., Red Deer AB T4N 7B4
Toll-Free: 888-236-6283

Regina
2571 Broad St., Regina SK S4P 4H6
Toll-Free: 888-236-6283
Chief Officer(s):
Mike Shaw, Regional Representative, Alberta, Saskatchewan,
  Manitoba, Northwest Territories, & Nunavut

Saint John
405 University Ave., Saint John NB E2L 4G7
Toll-Free: 888-236-6283
Chief Officer(s):
Jeff Scott, Regional Representative, Atlantic

St Catharines
#395, 397 Ontario St., St Catharines ON L2N 4M8
Toll-Free: 888-236-6283

St. John's
7 Wicklow St., St. John's NL A1B 3Z9
Toll-Free: 888-236-6283
Chief Officer(s):
Jeff Scott, Regional Representative, Atlantic

Sarnia
Bayside Mall, 150 Christina St. North, Sarnia ON N7T 7W5
Toll-Free: 888-236-6283

Saskatoon
325 - 20th St. East, Saskatoon SK S7K 0A9
Toll-Free: 888-236-6283
Chief Officer(s):
Mike Shaw, Regional Representative, Alberta, Saskatchewan,
  Manitoba, Northwest Territories, & Nunavut

Sudbury
235 Cedar St., Sudbury ON P3B 1M8
Tel: 705-674-4003
Toll-Free: 888-236-6283
Chief Officer(s):
Dunbar Russel, Regional Representative, Ontario

Sudbury - National Contact Centre
235 Cedar St., Sudbury ON P3B 1M8
Tel: 705-674-4003; Fax: 705-674-7165
Toll-Free: 888-236-6283

Surrey
15285 - 101 Ave., Surrey BC V3R 8X8
Toll-Free: 888-236-6283

Sydney
850 Grand Lake Rd., Sydney NS B1P 5T9
Toll-Free: 888-236-6283

Toronto - Bay & Bloor
Manulife Centre, 55 Bloor St. West, 2nd Fl., Toronto ON M4W 1A5
Toll-Free: 888-236-6283

Toronto - College St.
67 College St., Toronto ON M5G 2M1
Toll-Free: 888-236-6283
Chief Officer(s):
Dunbar Russel, Regional Representative, Ontario

Toronto - King Street
163 King St. West, Main Fl., Toronto ON M5H 4H2
Toll-Free: 888-236-6283

Vancouver - Oak Street

4750 Oak St., Vancouver BC V6H 2N9
Tel: 604-707-3400
Toll-Free: 888-236-6283

Vancouver - Standard Life
888 Dunsmur St., 2nd Fl., Vancouver BC V6C 3K4
Toll-Free: 888-236-6283

Victoria
3449 Saanich Rd., Victoria BC V8X 1W9
Toll-Free: 888-236-6283

Windsor
3909 Grand Marais Rd. East, Windsor ON N8W 1W9
Toll-Free: 888-236-6283

Winnipeg
777 William Ave., Winnipeg MB R3E 3R4
Toll-Free: 888-236-6283
Chief Officer(s):
Mike Shaw, Regional Representative, Alberta, Saskatchewan,
  Manitoba, Northwest Territories, & Nunavut

Canadian Burn Survivors Community (CBSC)
110 Bambrick Rd., Middle Sackville NS B4E 0J4
www.canadianburnsurvivors.ca
www.facebook.com/298455086834875
Overview: A small national organization founded in 2006
Mission: To provide support to burn survivors
Chief Officer(s):
Barbara Anne Hodge, Chair

Canadian Cancer Survivor Network (CCSN)
#210, 1750 Courtwood Cres., Ottawa ON K2C 2B5
Tel: 613-898-1871
e-mail: info@survivornet.ca
survivornet.ca
www.facebook.com/CanadianSurvivorNet
twitter.com/survivornetca
Overview: A large national organization
Mission: To help cancer patients & their families cope with their situation; To educate the public about the costs of cancer
Chief Officer(s):
Jackie Manthorne, President & CEO
  jmanthorne@survivornet.ca

Canadian Caregiver Coalition (CCC-CCAN) / Coalition canadienne des aidants et aidantes naturels
110 Argyle Ave., Ottawa ON K2P 1B4
Tel: 613-233-5694; Fax: 613-230-4376
Toll-Free: 888-866-2273
e-mail: info@ccc-ccan.ca
www.ccc-ccan.ca
Overview: A medium-sized national organization
Mission: To join with caregivers, service providers, policy makers & other stakeholders to identify & respond to the needs of caregivers in Canada

Canadian Centre for Wellbeing
PO Box 83030, Stn. Victoria Park, Toronto ON M4B 3N2
Tel: 647-560-4824
e-mail: info@ccfw.ca
www.ccfw.ca
Previous Name: Canadian Centre for Stress & Well-Being
Overview: A small national organization founded in 1982
Mission: To provide education about stress management; To increase health & wellness

Canadian Centre on Disability Studies (CCDS)
56 The Promenade, Winnipeg MB R3B 3H9
Tel: 204-287-8411; Fax: 204-284-5343; TTY: 204-475-6223
e-mail: ccds@disabilitystudies.ca
www.disabilitystudies.ca
Overview: A small national charitable organization founded in 1995
Mission: To research, educate, & disseminate information on disability issues
Chief Officer(s):
Susan Hardie, Executive Director, 204-287-8411 Ext. 25
  shardie@disabilitystudies.ca

Publications:
• CCDS [Canadian Centre on Disability Studies] Bulletin
Type: Newsletter; *Frequency:* Quarterly

Canadian College of Emergency Medical Services (CCEMS)
c/o Edmonton General Hospital, 4712 - 91 Ave., Edmonton AB T6B 2L1

Tel: 780-451-4437
Toll-Free: 800-797-4437
e-mail: info@ccofems.org
www.ccofems.org
twitter.com/ccofems

Overview: A medium-sized national organization founded in 1988
Mission: To provide training & education for emergency medical services professionals
Chief Officer(s):
Greg Clarkes, President
greg@ccofems.org

Canadian College of Health Leaders (CCHL) / Collège canadien des leaders en santé (CCLS)
292 Somerset St. West, Ottawa ON K2P 0J6

Tel: 613-235-7218; *Fax:* 613-235-5451
Toll-Free: 800-363-9056
Other Communication: communications@cchse.org
e-mail: info@cchl-ccls.ca
www.cchl-ccls.ca
www.linkedin.com/company/canadian-college-of-health-leaders
www.facebook.com/CCHL.National
twitter.com/CCHL_CCLS
www.youtube.com/HealthLeadersCanada

Previous Name: Canadian College of Service Executives
Overview: A large national organization founded in 1970
Mission: To advance excellence in health leadership; To act as a collective voice for the profession
Member of: Health Action Lobby; Coalition for Public Health in the 21st Century
Chief Officer(s):
Ray J. Racette, President & Chief Executive Office, 613-235-7218 Ext. 227
rracette@cchl-ccls.ca
Jaime Cleroux, Vice-President, Corporate Partnership Excellence, 613-235-7218 Ext. 235
jcleroux@cchl-ccls.ca
Sylvie M. Deliencourt, Director, Certification, Leadership Development & Chapter Support, 613-235-7218 Ext. 233
sdeliencourt@cchl-ccls.ca
Carolyn Farrington, Chief Financial Officer, 613-235-7218 Ext. 228
cfarrington@cchl-ccls.ca
Kathy Ivey, Manager, Marketing & Communications, 613-235-7218 Ext. 229
kivey@cchl-ccls.ca
Publications:
• Canadian College of Health Service Annual Report
Type: Report; *Frequency:* a.
• Code of Ethics for Members of the Canadian College of Health Service Executives
Price: Free
Profile: A guide for professional & personal behaviour
• Communiqué [a publication of the Canadian College of Health Leaders]
Type: Newsletter; *Frequency:* monthly; *Accepts Advertising; Price:* Free with membership
Profile: College & member news, initiatives in health care, & career opportunities for members
• Healthcare Management FORUM
Type: Journal; *Frequency:* q.; *Accepts Advertising; Editor:* Ron Lindstrom; *ISSN:* 0840-4704; *Price:* Free for active members of the College; $90 individuals in Canada; $212institutions
Profile: Peer-reviewed articles about Canadian health services management issues, theory, & practice

Assiniboia (Saskatchewan) Regional Chapter
SK

www.cchl-ccls.ca

Chief Officer(s):
John Knoch, Chair
john.knoch@schr.sk.ca

Bluenose (Nova Scotia & Prince Edward Island) Regional Chapter
NS

www.cchl-ccls.ca

Chief Officer(s):
Heather Wolfe, Chair
heather.wolfe@cehha.nshealth.ca
• Canadian College of Health Service Executives, Bluenose Chapter, News Update
Type: Newsletter; *Frequency:* Quarterly
Profile: Chapter activities & upcoming events for Bluenose members
• Canadian College of Health Service Executives, Bluenose Chapter, Annual Report
Frequency: Annually
Profile: Review of chapter programs & services

British Columbia Interior Regional Chapter
BC

www.cchl-ccls.ca

Chief Officer(s):
Paul Gallant, Chair
paul@gallanthealthworks.com

British Columbia Lower Mainland Regional Chapter
BC

www.cchl-ccls.ca

Chief Officer(s):
Paul Gallant, Chair
paul@gallanthealthworks.com
Moe Baloo, Vice-Chair
mbaloo@providencehealth.bc.ca
Zahida Esmail, Treasurer
zahidaesmail@gmail.com
David Thomopson, National Board Rep
dthompson@providencehealth.bc.ca
• Canadian College of Health Leaders British Columbia Lower Mainland Regional Chapter Executive Mentoring Program Handbook
Type: Handbook
Profile: Information for mentors & mentees

Eastern Ontario Regional Chapter
ON

www.cchl-ccls.ca

Chief Officer(s):
Jennifer Proulx, Chair
jen@proulx.info
Joanne Bezzubetz, Vice-Chair
jbezzubetz@gmail.com
Paul Caines, Secretary
• Canadian College of Health Service Executives Eastern Ontario Chapter Newsletter
Type: Newsletter
Profile: Chapter activities & upcoming professional development events

Greater Toronto Area Regional Chapter
Toronto ON

www.cchl-ccls.ca

Chief Officer(s):
Sean J. Molloy, Chair
seanmolloyis@gmail.com

Hamilton & Area Regional Chapter
ON

www.cchl-ccls.ca

Chief Officer(s):
Bryan Herechuk, Chair
bherechu@stjosham.on.ca
Ajay Bhardwaj, Vice-Chair
ajaybhardwaj@hotmail.com
Dilys Haughton, Treasurer
dilys.haughton@hnhb.ccac-ont.ca
• Canadian College of Health Leaders Hamilton & Area Regional Chapter News
Type: Newsletter
Profile: Chpater happenings & upcoming events

LEADS Collaborative

Toll-Free: 800-363-9056
e-mail: leads@cchl-ccls.ca
www.leadscollaborative.ca
www.linkedin.com/company/leads-collaborative
www.facebook.com/LEADSleaders
twitter.com/LEADSleaders

Chief Officer(s):
Brenda Lammi, Director
blammi@leadscanada.net
Lynne Marleau, Coordinator, Administrative & Communications
lmarleau@leadscanada.net
Anne Marie Lecompte, Program Leader
amlecompte@leadscanada.net

Manitoba Regional Chapter
c/o Donald Solar, Parkview Place Care Centre, 440 Edmonton
St., Winnipeg MB R3B 2M4

Tel: 204-942-5291
www.cchl-ccls.ca

Chief Officer(s):
Israel Mendez, Chair
imendez.mba2007@ivey.ca
Donald Solar, Treasurer
donald.solar@reveraliving.com
Randy Lock, Secretary
randy.lock@shaw.ca

Midnight Sun (Yukon, Northwest Territories, & Nunavut)
Regional Chapter
NT

www.cchl-ccls.ca

Chief Officer(s):
Wayne Overbo, Chair
wayne_overbo@gov.nt.ca
Donna L. Allen, Treasurer
donna_allen@gov.nt.ca

NEON Lights (Northeastern Ontario) Regional Chapter
c/o Patty MacDonald, Canadian Mental Health Association, #100,
111 Elm St., Sudbury ON P3C 1T3

Tel: 705-675-7252
www.cchl-ccls.ca

Chief Officer(s):
Patty MacDonald, Chair
pmacdonald@cmha-sm.on.ca
Cathy Bailey, Secretary-Treasurer
cathy.bailey@ne.ccac-ont.ca
• NEON Lights Regional Chapter Chair Update
Type: Newsletter; *Frequency:* Irregular
Profile: News from the national Canadian College of Health Leaders, as well as local activities & professional development events

New Brunswick Regional Chapter
NB

www.cchl-ccls.ca

Chief Officer(s):
Connor Atchison, Secretary
atchison.connorm@gmail.com
Thomas Maston, Treasurer
tom.maston@gnb.ca
Nancy Roberts, Chair
Nancy.Roberts@gnb.ca

Newfoundland & Labrador Regional Chapter
NL

www.cchl-ccls.ca

Chief Officer(s):
Cathy Hoyles, Chair
cathy.hoyles@easternhealth.ca
Mollie Butler, Vice-Chair
mollie.butler@easternhealth.ca
Sharon Paulette Lehr, Treasurer
sharon.lehr@easternhealth.ca

Northern & Central Saskatchewan Regional Chapter
Saskatoon SK

www.cchl-ccls.ca

Chief Officer(s):
Sandra Blevins, Chair
sandra.blevins@saskatoonhealthregion.ca

Northern Alberta Regional Chapter
AB

www.cchl-ccls.ca

Chief Officer(s):
Brenda Rebman, Chair
brebman@futuresrpi.com
Jewel Buksa, Secretary
jewel@buksa.com
Corinne B. Schalm, Treasurer
cbschalm@gmail.com
• Leader to Leader
Type: Newsletter
Profile: Chapter information, reports, membership information, & upcoming events

Northern British Columbia Regional Chapter
BC

e-mail: chapters@cchl-ccls.ca
www.cchl-ccls.ca

Northwestern Ontario Regional Chapter
ON

www.cchl-ccls.ca

Québec Regional Chapter
QC

www.cchl-ccls.ca

Chief Officer(s):
Martin Beaumont, President
martin.beaumont.csssnl@ssss.gouv.qc.ca
Diane Boivin, Vice-President
dianeboivin1@videotron.ca
Linda August, Secretary
linda.august@ssss.gouv.qc.ca
William-Jean Côté, Treasurer
willcote@bell.net

Southern Alberta Regional Chapter
c/o Patty Wickson, Alberta Health Services, 10030 - 107 St. NW,
Edmonton AB T5J 3E4

www.cchl-ccls.ca

Chief Officer(s):
Jennifer McCue, Chair
Brenda Rebman, Director
brebman@futuresrpi.com
Patty Wickson, Contact, Administration
patty.wickson@albertahealthservices.ca
Arlene Weidner, Contact, Professional Development
aweidner@shaw.ca

Southwestern Ontario Regional Chapter
c/o Paul Heinrich, North Bay Regional Health Centre, PO Box
2500, 50 College Dr., North Bay ON P1B 5A4

Tel: 705-474-8600
www.cchl-ccls.ca

Chief Officer(s):
Julie Campbell, Chair
juliemaycampbell@gmail.com
Paul Heinrich, Director
paul.heinrich@nbrhc.on.ca
• Canadian College of Health Service Executives, Southwestern Ontario Regional Chapter, Newsletter
Type: Newsletter
Profile: Chapter reports & upcoming events, plus news from the national Canadian College of Health Service Executives

Starlight (Canadian Forces Health Services Group) Regional
Chapter

www.cchl-ccls.ca

Chief Officer(s):
Stephan Plourde, Chair
Steve_plourde@hotmail.com
William-Jean Côté, Secretary
willcote@bell.net

Vancouver Island Regional Chapter
BC

www.cchl-ccls.ca

Chief Officer(s):

Tim Orr, Chair
timothy.orr@viha.ca
Bart Johnson, Treasurer
bart.johnson@viha.ca

Canadian College of Physicists in Medicine (CCPM) / Collège canadien des physiciens en médecine
PO Box 72124, RPO Kanata North, Kanata ON K2K 2P4
Tel: 613-599-3491; *Fax:* 613-435-7257
e-mail: admin@medphys.ca
www.ccpm.ca

Overview: A small national organization founded in 1979
Mission: To identify, through certification, individuals who have acquired & maintained a standard of knowledge & skill essential to the practice of medical physics, in order to serve the public
Affiliation(s): Canadian Organization of Medical Physicists (COMP)
Chief Officer(s):
Nancy Barrett, Executive Director
nancy@medphys.ca
Horacio Patrocinio, CCPM Registrar
registrar@ccpm.ca
Matthew G. Schmid, President
mschmid@bccancer.bc.ca
Publications:
• InterACTIONS!
Type: Newsletter; *Frequency:* Quarterly; *Accepts Advertising*; *Editor:* Dr. Parminder Basran
Profile: News from the Canadian Organization of Medical Physicists & the Canadian College of Physicists in Medicine for members

Canadian College of Professional Counsellors & Psychotherapists (CCPCP)
PO Box 23045, Vernon BC V1T 9L8
Tel: 250-558-7700
Toll-Free: 866-704-4828
e-mail: inquiry@ccpcp.ca
www.ccpcp.ca

Overview: A small national organization founded in 2006
Mission: To represent College members & persons who seek counselling & psychotherapy services; To establish & enforce standards of practice
Chief Officer(s):
Kristi Novakowski, Registrar

Canadian Council of University Physical Education & Kinesiology Administrators (CCUPEKA) / Conseil canadien des administrateurs universitaires en éducation physique et kinésiologie (CCAUEPK)
c/o Dr. J. Starkes, Department of Kinesiology, McMaster University, Hamilton ON L8S 4K1
www.ccupeka.ca

Overview: A small national organization founded in 1971 overseen by Association of Universities & Colleges of Canada
Mission: To serve as an accrediting body for physical education & kinesiology programs at universities in Canada; To offer a voice for academics, through lobbying initiatives
Chief Officer(s):
Angela Belcastro, President

Canadian Critical Care Society (CCCS) / Société canadienne de soins intensifs
#6, 20 Crown Steel Dr., Toronto ON L3R 9X9
Tel: 905-415-3917; *Fax:* 905-415-0071
Toll-Free: 855-415-3917
e-mail: cccs@secretariatcentral.com
www.canadiancriticalcare.org
www.facebook.com/269898849687697

Overview: A medium-sized national organization
Mission: To promote & develop critical care medicine in Canada
Affliation(s): Canadian Medical Association; World Federation of Societies of Intensive & Critical Care Medicine
Chief Officer(s):
Alison Fox-Robichaud, President

Canadian Dupuytren Society / Société canadienne de Dupuytren
107 av de Marlin Crescent, Pointe-Claire QC H9S 5B2
Overview: A small national charitable organization
Mission: To raise awareness of Dupuytren's contracture
Chief Officer(s):
Paule Gauthier

Canadian Federation of Medical Students (CFMS) / Fédération des étudiants en médecine du Canada (FEMC)
#401, 267 O'Connor St., Ottawa ON K2P 1V3
Tel: 613-565-7740; *Fax:* 613-565-7742
e-mail: office@cfms.org
www.cfms.org
www.linkedin.com/company/canadian-federation-of-medical-students-cfms-
www.facebook.com/CFMSFEMC
twitter.com/CFMSFEMC

Overview: A medium-sized national organization founded in 1979
Mission: To support medical students by representing their voices among the national organizations that direct or influence the policy environment or delivery of medical education in Canada; To provide services that support the needs of member medical students; To communicate national medical education issues of importance to individual medical students & to facilitate communication & interaction of medical students among member schools
Member of: International Federation of Medical Students' Associations
Chief Officer(s):
Franco Rizzuti, President
president@cfms.org
Emily Hodgson, Vice-President, Communications
vpcommunications@cfms.org
Tavis Apramian, Vice-President, Education
vpeducation@cfms.org
Daniel Peretz, Vice-President, Finance
vpfinance@cfms.org
Sarah Silverberg, Vice-President, Government Affairs
vpgovtaffairs@cfms.org
Han Yan, Vice-President, Student Affairs
vpstudentaffairs@cfms.org
Jessica Bryce, Vice-President, Global Health
vpglobalhealth@cfms.org

Canadian Federation of Orthotherapists (CFO) / Fédération Canadienne des Orthothérapeutes (FCO)
1090 boul St-Charles, Drummondville QC J2C 4Z2
Fax: 514-525-2167
Toll-Free: 888-330-6776
e-mail: info@fco-cfo.ca
fco-cfo.ca

Overview: A large national organization founded in 1998
Mission: To maintain the integrity of the orthotherapist profession

Canadian Fitness & Lifestyle Research Institute (CFLRI) / Institut canadien de la recherche sur la condition physique et le mode de vie
#201, 185 Somerset St. West, Ottawa ON K2P 0J2
Tel: 613-233-5528; *Fax:* 613-233-5536
www.cflri.ca

Previous Name: Canada Fitness Survey (1985)
Overview: A medium-sized national charitable organization founded in 1980
Mission: To conduct research, monitor trends, & make recommendations to increase physical activity & improve health in Canada
Chief Officer(s):
Nancy Dubois, Chair
Christine Cameron, President
Makda Araia, Research Analyst
Publications:
• Capacity Study [a publication of the Canadian Fitness & Lifestyle Research Institute]
Frequency: Annually
Profile: Information to increase physical activity in the Canadian workplace
• Kids CANPLAY [a publication of the Canadian Fitness & Lifestyle Research Institute]
Profile: Information to encourage children to be active at home, at school, & in the community
• The Lifestyle Tips [a publication of the Canadian Fitness & Lifestyle Research Institute]
Profile: Practical suggestions for integrating physical activity into daily life
• Physical Activity Monitor [a publication of the Canadian Fitness & Lifestyle Research Institute]
Frequency: Irregular; *ISBN:* 1-895724-49-X

Profile: Report presents trends in physical activity among Canadian workers
• The Research File [a publication of the Canadian Fitness & Lifestyle Research Institute]
ISSN: 1188-6641
Profile: Ongoing series of research summaries about physical activity, for professionals

Canadian Foundation for Dietetic Research (CFDR)
#604, 480 University Ave., Toronto ON M5G 1V2
Tel: 416-642-9309; *Fax:* 416-596-0603
e-mail: info@cfdr.ca
www.cfdr.ca

Overview: A medium-sized national charitable organization
Mission: To provide grants for research in dietetics & nutrition
Chief Officer(s):
Sarah Hewko, Chair

Canadian Harm Reduction Network
#1904, 666 Spadina Ave., Toronto ON M5S 2H8
Tel: 416-928-0279; *Fax:* 416-966-9512
Toll-Free: 800-728-1293
e-mail: noharm@canadianharmreduction.com
www.canadianharmreduction.com
www.facebook.com/noharmcanada
twitter.com/noharmcanada
youtube.com/noharmcanada

Overview: A small national organization
Mission: To reduce the social, health & economic harms associated with drugs & drug policies
Affliation(s): Drug Policy Alliance

Canadian Health Coalition (CHC) / Coalition canadienne de la santé
#212, 251 Bank St., Ottawa ON K2P 1X3
Tel: 613-688-4973
e-mail: contact@healthcoalition.ca
www.healthcoalition.ca
twitter.com/healthcoalition
www.youtube.com/user/HealthCoalition

Overview: A large national organization founded in 1979
Mission: To create good health; To preserve & strengthen the Canada Health Act, the foundation of Medicare; To make the health care system democratic, accountable & representative; To provide a continuum of care from large institutions to the home; To protect our investment in the skills & abilities of our health care workers; To ensure fair wages for all health care providers; To eliminate profit-making from illness; To reduce over-prescribing & make drugs affordable; to stop fee-for-service payments; To expand methods of health care & the role of non-physician health providers
Chief Officer(s):
Adrienne Silnicki, National Coordinator
asilnicki@healthcoalition.ca

Canadian Health Food Association (CHFA) / Association canadienne des aliments de santé
#302, 235 Yorkland Blvd., Toronto ON M2J 4Y8
Tel: 416-497-6939; *Fax:* 416-497-3214
Toll-Free: 800-661-4510
e-mail: info@chfa.ca
www.chfa.ca
www.facebook.com/CanadianHealthFoodAssociation
twitter.com/cdnhealthfood
instagram.com/canadianhealthfoodassociation
Previous Name: Health Food Dealers Association
Overview: A medium-sized national organization founded in 1964
Mission: To act as the voice of the natural products industry; To promote natural & organic products as an integral part of health & well-being; To ensure the growth of the natural & organic industry
Chief Officer(s):
Don Smith, Chair
Helen Long, President
Publications:
• Canadian Health Food Association Annual Report
Type: Yearbook; *Frequency:* Annually
Profile: Activities of the association during the past year
• Canadian Health Food Association Asssociate Member Directory
Type: Directory; *Frequency:* Monthly
Profile: A membership directory exclusively for members

• Canadian Health Food Association e-News
Type: Newsletter; *Frequency:* Weekly; *Price:* Free with membership in the Canadian Health Food Association
Profile: Latest developments in the natural health & organic products industry
• Canadian Health Food Association Member Bulletins
Type: Newsletter; *Frequency:* Irregular; *Price:* Free with membership in the Canadian Health Food Association
Profile: Recent news in the natural health & organic products industry
• Canadian Health Food Association Retail Member Directory
Type: Directory; *Frequency:* Monthly
Profile: A listing with contact information
• Canadian Health Food Association Supplier Member Directory
Type: Directory; *Frequency:* Monthly
Profile: A membership directory exclusively for members
• Membership that Matters! [a publication of the Canadian Health Food Association]
Type: Newsletter; *Price:* Free with membership in the Canadian Health Food Association
Profile: Information for members to help their businesses prosper
• NATURALeHealthy [a publication of the Canadian Health Food Association]
Type: Newsletter; *Frequency:* Monthly; *Price:* Free with membership in the Canadian Health Food Association
• Research & Your Health
Type: Newsletter; *Frequency:* Quarterly; *Number of Pages:* 8; *Price:* Free with membership in the Canadian Health Food Association
Profile: Abstracts about the value of natural health products

Canadian Health Information Management Association (CHIMA)
99 Enterprise Dr. South, London ON N6N 1B9
Tel: 519-438-6700; *Fax:* 519-438-7001
Toll-Free: 877-332-4462
www.echima.ca
www.linkedin.com/groups/4445368/profile
www.facebook.com/OfficialCHIMA
twitter.com/E_CHIMA
Previous Name: Canadian Health Record Association
Overview: A medium-sized national organization founded in 1942
Mission: To contribute to the promotion of wellness & the provision of quality healthcare through excellence in health information management; to assure competency of practice through credentialling, standards & continuing education; to promote value of health information management professionals
Affliation(s): International Federation of Health Information Management Associations; American Health Information Management Association
Chief Officer(s):
Gail Crook, CEO & Registrar, 519-438-6700 Ext. 227
gail.crook@echima.ca
Tasha Clipperton, Coordinator, Member Services
tasha.clipperton@echima.ca
Publications:
• An Essential Guide to Clinical Documentation Improvement [publication of Canadian Health Information Management Association]
Type: Report; *Author:* C. Grant & A. Jamal
Profile: White Paper discussing optical clinical documentation practices
• An Essential Guide to Clinical Documentation Improvement [publication of Canadian Health Information Management Association]
Type: Report
Profile: White Paper discussing optical clinical documentation practices
• CHIMA [Canadian Health Information Management Association] Connection
Type: Newsletter; *Frequency:* Bimonthly
Profile: Industry news & events
• Human Resources Outlook 2014-2019 [a publication of Canadian Health Information Management Association]
Type: Report
Profile: Discusses key industry changes & their impact on Health Informatics & Health Information Management professions

Manitoba Chapter
MB
e-mail: mbnuchapter@echima.ca
mbnu.echima.ca
Chief Officer(s):

Ric Van Amelsvoort-Barran, Chair
rvanamelsvoortbarran@manitoba-ehealth.ca
Chantal Plaetinck, Secretary-Treasurer

**New Brunswick Chapter
NB**

e-mail: nbchapter@echima.ca
nb.echima.ca

Chief Officer(s):
Jeannette Blanchard, Chair
jeannette.blanchard@horizonnb.ca
Susanne Surette, Secretary-Treasurer

**Newfoundland & Labrador Chapter
NL**

e-mail: nlchapter@echima.ca
nl.echima.ca

Chief Officer(s):
Jennifer Gushue, Chair
jennifer.gushue@easternhealth.ca
Jennifer Butler, Secretary-Treasurer

**Ontario Chapter
ON**

e-mail: onchapter@echima.ca
on.echima.ca

Chief Officer(s):
Stephanie Tambeau, Chair
stambeaudia@gmail.com

**Canadian Healthcare Engineering Society (CHES) / Société
canadienne d'ingénierie des services de santé (SCISS)**
#310, 4 Cataraqui St., Kingston ON K7K 1Z7
Tel: 613-531-2661; *Fax:* 613-531-0626
e-mail: ches@eventsmgt.com
www.ches.org
Previous Name: Canadian Hospital Engineering Society
Overview: A medium-sized national organization founded in 1980
Mission: To be a forum for exchange of information & ideas related to
excellence in communication & professional development in healthcare
facilities management
Chief Officer(s):
Mitch Weimer, President

**Canadian Home Care Association (CHCA) / Association
canadienne de soins et services à domicile**
#302, 2000 Argentia Rd., Mississauga ON L5N 1W1
Tel: 905-567-7373
e-mail: chca@cdnhomecare.ca
www.cdnhomecare.ca
twitter.com/CdnHomeCare
www.youtube.com/user/cdnhomecare
Overview: A medium-sized national organization founded in 1990
Mission: To promote the development, integration, delivery, public
awareness & evaluation of quality home care services in Canada; To
provide national leadership to strengthen & unify the home care sector;
To collect & disseminate information about home care; To encourage
or commission research; To influence policy & legislation; To establish
a code of ethics
Chief Officer(s):
Réal Cloutier, President
Nadine Henningsen, Executive Director
nhenningsen@cdnhomecare.ca

**Canadian Institute for Health Information (CIHI) / Institut canadien
d'information sur la santé (ICIS)**
#600, 495 Richmond Rd., Ottawa ON K2A 4H6
Tel: 613-241-7860; *Fax:* 613-241-8120
Other Communication: help@cihi.ca
e-mail: communications@cihi.ca
www.cihi.ca
www.facebook.com/141785889231388
twitter.com/CIHI_ICIS
www.youtube.com/user/CIHICanada
Overview: A small national organization founded in 1994
Mission: To collect, analyze, & provide information about the health
system in Canada & the health of Canadians; To support persons who
use data for health & health-services research
Chief Officer(s):

David O'Toole, President & Chief Executive Officer, 613-694-6500
dotoole@cihi.ca
Brent Diverty, Vice-President, Programs, 613-694-6501
BDiverty@cihi.ca
Anne McFarlane, Vice-President, Western Canada & Developmental
Initiatives, 250-220-2211
AMcFarlane@cihi.ca
Louise Ogilvie, Vice-President, Corporate Services, 613-694-6503
LOgilvie@cihi.caca
Jeremy Veillard, Vice-President, Research & Analysis, 416-549-5361
JVeillard@cihi.ca
Publications:
• Canadian Institute for Health Information Annual Report
Type: Yearbook; *Frequency:* Annually
• CIHI [Canadian Institute for Health Information] Directions ICIS
[Institut canadien d'information sur la santé]
Type: Newsletter; *ISSN:* 1201-0383

CIHI Montréal
#300, 1010 Sherbrooke St. West, Montréal QC H3A 2R7
Tel: 514-842-2226; *Fax:* 514-842-3996
Chief Officer(s):
Caroline Heick, Executive Director, Ontario and Quebec,
416-549-5517
CHeick@cihi.ca

CIHI St. John's
#701, 140 Water St., St. John's NL A1C 6H6
Tel: 709-576-7006; *Fax:* 709-576-0952
Chief Officer(s):
Stephen O'Reilly, Executive Director, Atlantic Canada, 709-733-7064
SOReilly@cihi.ca

CIHI Toronto
#300, 4110 Yonge St., Toronto ON M2P 2B7
Tel: 416-481-2002; *Fax:* 416-481-2950
Chief Officer(s):
Caroline Heick, Executive Director, Ontario and Quebec,
416-549-5517
CHeick@cihi.ca

CIHI Victoria
#600, 880 Douglas St., Victoria BC V8W 2B7
Tel: 250-220-4100; *Fax:* 250-220-7090

**Canadian Institute of Cultural Affairs / Institut canadien des
affaires culturelles**
#405, 401 Richmond St. West, Toronto ON M5V 3A8
Tel: 416-691-2316
e-mail: ica@icacan.org
www.icacan.org
www.facebook.com/ICAInternational
Also Known As: ICA Canada
Overview: A small national charitable organization founded in 1976
Mission: To empower people to develop leadership capacity; To
contribute to positive social change
Chief Officer(s):
Nan Hudson, Executive Director
Publications:
• L'art de la discussion structurée 100 applications concrèt [a
publication of the Canadian Institute of Cultural Affairs]
Author: R. Brian Stanfield; *Price:* $38.00
• The Art of Focused Conversation [a publication of the Canadian
Institute of Cultural Affairs]
Author: R. Brian Stanfield; *ISBN:* 0-86571-416-9; *Price:* $21.95
• The Art of Focused Conversation for Schools [a publication of the
Canadian Institute of Cultural Affairs]
Author: Jo Nelson; *ISBN:* 0-86571-435-5; *Price:* $21.95
• The Courage to Lead: Transform Self, Transform Society [a
publication of the Canadian Institute of Cultural Affairs]
Author: R. Brian Stanfield; *ISBN:* 1-4759-1001-0; *Price:* $29.95
• More Than 50 Ways to Build Team Consensus [a publication of the
Canadian Institute of Cultural Affairs]
Author: R. Bruce Williams; *ISBN:* 0-932935-48-6; *Price:* $38.95
• The Social Progress Triangles [a publication of the Canadian Institute
of Cultural Affairs]
Author: Jon C. Jenkins & Maureen R. Jenkins; *Price:* $31.95

• Transformational Strategy [a publication of the Canadian Institute of Cultural Affairs]
Author: Bill Staples; *ISBN:* 1-4759-6839-6; *Price:* $29.95
• The Workshop Book [a publication of the Canadian Institute of Cultural Affairs]
Author: R. Brian Stanfield; *ISBN:* 0-86571-470-3; *Price:* $22.95

Canadian Institute of Food Science & Technology (CIFST) / Institut canadien de science et technologie alimentaires (ICSTA)
#1311, 3-1750 The Queensway, Toronto ON M9C 5H5
Tel: 905-271-8338; *Fax:* 905-271-8344
e-mail: cifst@cifst.ca
www.cifst.ca
www.linkedin.com/groups/7472160
twitter.com/cifst_icsta
www.youtube.com/channel/UCdSu2hoVWg-sYc2v5YZ3kIA
Overview: A medium-sized national organization founded in 1951
Mission: To advance food science & technology; To act as a voice for scientific issues related to the Canadian food industry
Affiliation(s): British Columbia Food Technologists
Chief Officer(s):
Michael Nickerson, President
Carol Ann Burrell, Executive Director, 905-271-8338, Fax: 905-271-8344
caburrell@cifst.ca
Publications:
• Canadian Food Insights [a publication of the Canadian Institute of Food Science & Technology]
Type: Magazine

Canadian Institute of Public Health Inspectors (CIPHI) / Institut Canadien des inspecteurs en santé publique (ICISP)
#720, 999 West Broadway Ave., Vancouver BC V5Z 1K5
Tel: 604-739-8180; *Fax:* 604-738-4080
Toll-Free: 888-245-8180
Other Communication: office@ciphi.ca
e-mail: questions@ciphi.ca
www.ciphi.ca
www.facebook.com/CIPHI.ICISP
twitter.com/ciphi_national
Previous Name: Canadian Institute of Sanitary Inspectors
Overview: A medium-sized national licensing organization founded in 1934
Mission: To protect the health of all Canadians; To advance the environmental & health sciences; To enhance the field of public health inspection through certification, information, & advocacy
Affiliation(s): National Environmental Health Association (NEHA)
Chief Officer(s):
Ann Thomas, National President
president@ciphi.ca
Publications:
• Canadian Institute of Public Health Inspectors National Newsletter
Type: Newsletter
• Environmental Health Review [a publication of the Canadian Institute of Public Health Inspectors]
Type: Journal; *Frequency:* Quarterly; *Editor:* Andrew Papadopoulos; *Price:* Free for Canadian Institute of Public Health Inspectors members

The Canadian Laser and Aesthetic Specialists Society (CLASS)
2334 Heska Rd., Pickering ON L1V 2P9
Fax: 905-837-1125
Toll-Free: 877-578-0336
www.class.ca
Previous Name: Canadian Laser Aesthetic Surgery Society
Overview: A small national organization founded in 1997
Mission: To disseminate information & promote quality in all forms of aesthetic laser surgery; To promote communication between medical specialties to further awareness, education, & professional development
Chief Officer(s):
Karen Edstrom, President

Canadian Life & Health Insurance Association Inc. (CLHIA) / Association canadienne des compagnies d'assurances de personnes inc. (ACCAP)
#2300, 79 Wellingston St. West, Toronto ON M5K 1G8
Tel: 416-777-2221; *Fax:* 416-777-1895
Toll-Free: 888-295-8112
Other Communication: Ottawa: 613-230-0031; Montreal: 514-854-9004
e-mail: info@clhia.ca
www.clhia.ca
twitter.com/clhia
Previous Name: Canadian Life Insurance Association
Overview: A large national organization founded in 1894
Mission: To represent the interests of member life & health insurance companies
Chief Officer(s):
Dean Connor, Chair
Paul Mahon, President
Publications:
• Canadian Life & Health Insurance Facts
Type: Report; *Frequency:* a.
Profile: Statistics on life & health insurance ownership & purchases, life & health insurance companies' income & expenses, pension plan coverages, assets & obligations, & operations inCanada
• A Guide to Disability Insurance
Type: Booklet; *Number of Pages:* 20
Profile: A guide to understanding options for income replacement in the event of disability
• A Guide to Life Insurance
Type: Booklet; *Number of Pages:* 36
Profile: Consumer publication about types of policies, agent services, riders & dividends, & premiums
• A Guide to Long-Term Care Insurance
Type: Booklet; *Number of Pages:* 12
Profile: Resource to assist consumers
• A Guide to Supplementary Health Insurance
Type: Booklet; *Number of Pages:* 20
Profile: Resource to assist consumers
• A Guide to the Coordination of Benefits
Type: Booklet; *Number of Pages:* 12
Profile: Assistance in navigating the claims process
• A Guide to Travel Health Insurance
Type: Booklet; *Number of Pages:* 12
Profile: A review of the supplementary health insurance needed by Canadians when they travel ouside the province or country
• In The Loop
Type: Newsletter; *Frequency:* monthly; *Price:* Free with Claim Section Industry Associate status
Profile: Industry updates
• Key Facts About Segregated Fund Contracts
Type: Booklet; *Number of Pages:* 12
Profile: A guide for investors
• Provincial Facts & Figures
Type: Report; *Frequency:* a.

Canadian Medical Association (CMA) / Association médicale canadienne (AMC)
1209 Michael St., Ottawa ON K1J 7T2
Tel: 613-731-8610; *Fax:* 613-236-8864
Toll-Free: 888-855-2555
Other Communication: cmatechsupport@cma.ca (Technical Support)
e-mail: cmamsc@cma.ca
www.cma.ca
www.linkedin.com/company/canadian-medical-association
www.facebook.com/CanadianMedicalAssociation
twitter.com/CMA_Docs
www.youtube.com/user/CanadianMedicalAssoc
Overview: A large national organization founded in 1867
Mission: To act as the national voice of physicians in Canada; To serve the Canadian medical community; To promote the highest standards of health & health care
Member of: World Medical Association
Affiliation(s): Assn. of Cdn. Medical Colleges; Cdn. Anesthesiologists' Soc.; Cdn. Assn. of Medical Biochemists; Cdn. Assn. of Physicians with Disabilities; Cdn. Assn. of Physicians for the Environment; Cdn. Assn. of Radiation Oncologists; Cdn. Fedn. of Medical Students; Cdn. Infectious Disease Soc.; Cdn. Neurological/Neurosurgical/Clinical Neurophysiologists Societies; Cdn. Ophthalmological Soc.; Cdn.

Orthopaedic Assn.; Cdn. Paediatric Soc.; Cdn. Psychiatric Assn; Cdn. Rheumatology Assn.; Cdn. Soc. of Addiction Medicine; Cdn. Soc. of Internal Medicine; Cdn. Soc. of Nuclear Medicine; Cdn. Soc. of Otolaryngoly

Chief Officer(s):
Cindy Forbes, President
Brian Brodie, Chair
Granger Avery, President-Elect

Publications:
• Canadian Health Magazine
Type: Magazine; *Frequency:* Quarterly; *Accepts Advertising*; *Editor:* Diana Swift; *Price:* $12 / year
Profile: A health & wellness resource for patients in a physician's waiting room
• Canadian Journal of Surgery (CJS)
Type: Journal; *Frequency:* Bimonthly; *Accepts Advertising*; *Editor:* E.J. Harvey, MD; G.L. Warnock, MD; *ISSN:* 0008-428X; *Price:* $35 Canadian students & residents; $175 Canadian individuals; $270 institutions
Profile: Continuing medical education for Canadian surgical specialists
• Canadian Medical Association Complete Home Medical Guide
Type: Book; *ISSN:* 1-55363-054-8; *Price:* $51.95 members
Profile: An 1104 page authoritative & user-friendly resource for physicians to recommend to patients
• Canadian Medical Association Conference Updates
Profile: The latest news from major clinical meetings
• Canadian Medical Association Journal (CMAJ)
Type: Journal; *Frequency:* Semimonthly; *Accepts Advertising*; *Editor:* Paul C. Hébert; *ISSN:* 0820-3946; *Price:* $35 / issue Canadian; $40 / issue USA
Profile: Peer-reviewed original research, review articles, practice updates, drug alerts, health news, & commentaries for clinicians, available online& in print
• CMA [Canadian Medical Association] Bulletin
Type: Newsletter; *Frequency:* Semimonthly; *Editor:* Patrick Sullivan; Steve Wharry
Profile: A communication from the Canadian Medical Association, with news stories of interest to Canadian physicians, inserted in the Canadian MedicalAssociation Journal
• CMA [Canadian Medical Association] Driver's Guide: Determining Medical Fitness to Operate Motor Vehicles
Type: Guide; *Price:* Free for Canadian Medical Association members
Profile: Examples of sections include the following: Functional assessment - emerging emphasis; Reporting - when & why; Drivingcessation; Aging; Vision; Respiratory diseases; Psychiatric illness; Cardiovascular diseases; Seat belts & air bags; Motorcycles & off-road vehicles; Aviation; Railway; & Appendices
• CMA [Canadian Medical Association] Leadership Series: MD Pulse
Type: Magazine; *Price:* $8.95 / copy members; $14.95 nonmembers
Profile: Results of the National Physician Survey, prepared by the Canadian Medical Association in collaboration with the College of Family Physicians of Canada & theRoyal College of Physicians & Surgeons of Canada
• CMA [Canadian Medical Association] Leadership Series: Primary Care Reform
Type: Magazine; *Editor:* Dr. Albert Schumacher
Profile: An outline of primary care reform initiatives throughout Canada
• CMA [Canadian Medical Association] Leadership Series: Elder Care - Issues & Options
Type: Magazine; *Price:* $8.95 / copy members; $14.95 nonmemebers
Profile: An examination of the medical, social, & ethical dimensions of care for older patients
• CMA [Canadian Medical Association] Leadership Series: Women's Health - Research & Practice Issues for Canadian Physicians
Type: Magazine; *Price:* $8.95 / copy members; $14.95 nonmemebers
Profile: Published by the Canadian Medical Association in partnership with the Centre for Research inWomen's Health
• CMA [Canadian Medical Association] Complete Book of Mother & Baby Care
Type: Book; *Number of Pages:* 264; *Editor:* Anne Biringer MD, CCFP,FCFP; *ISBN:* 978-1-55363-154-5; *Price:* $24 members
Profile: Care for a mother & her baby, from conception to age three
• Future Practice
Type: Magazine; *Frequency:* Irregular; *Editor:* Pat Rich
Profile: Information for physicians about health information technology in Canada

• History of the Canadian Medical Association, 1954-94
Type: Book; *Number of Pages:* 388; *Author:* John Sutton Bennett, MD; *ISBN:* 0-920169-83-X; *Price:* $19.95 members
Profile: A comprehensive account of important events that continue to affect medicine in Canada
• Honour Due: the Story of Dr. Leonora Howard King
Type: Book; *Number of Pages:* 236; *Author:* Margaret I. Negodaeff-Tomsik; *ISBN:* 0-920169-33-3; *Price:* $19.95 members
Profile: The story of the first Canadian to work as a physician in China
• Lessons Learned: Reflections of Canadian Physician Leaders
Type: Book; *Number of Pages:* 123; *Editor:* Chris Carruthers, MD; *ISBN:* 978-1-897490-09-9; *Price:* $16.95 members
• MD Lounge
Type: Magazine; *Editor:* Dr. Francine Lemire et al.
Profile: Information & advice to strengthen relations between general practitioners, family physicians, & other specialists, published by the Canadian Medical Association in partnership withThe Royal College of Physicians & Surgeons of Canada & the College of Family Physicians of Canada
• PMI [Physician Management Institute] Newsletter: Leadership for Physicians
Type: Newsletter
Profile: Information about leadership theories & techniques

The Canadian Medical Protective Association / Association canadienne de protection médicale
PO Box 8225, Stn. T, Ottawa ON K1G 3H7
Tel: 613-725-2000; *Fax:* 613-725-1300
Toll-Free: 800-267-6522
e-mail: inquiries@cmpa.org
www.cmpa-acpm.ca
www.linkedin.com/company/canadian-medical-protective-association
twitter.com/CMPAmembers
www.youtube.com/user/cmpamembers

Overview: A large national organization founded in 1901
Mission: Founded by a group of Canadian doctors for their mutual protection against legal actions based on allegations of malpractice or negligence
Chief Officer(s):
Edward Crosby, Chair
Hartley Stern, Executive Director & CEO
Publications:
• CMPA [The Canadian Medical Protective Association] Perspective
Type: Magazine; *Frequency:* q.

Canadian MedTech Manufacturers' Alliance (CMMA)
#900, 405 The West Mall, Toronto ON M9C 5J1
Tel: 416-620-1915; *Fax:* 416-620-1595
Toll-Free: 866-586-3332
www.medec.org
twitter.com/medec_canada

Merged from: Trillium Medical Technology Association & MEDEC
Overview: A medium-sized national organization founded in 2011
Mission: To encourage the development of medical technology & to help this technology grow in international markets
Chief Officer(s):
Brian Lewis, President & CEO
ceo@medec.org
Iris Crawford, Vice-President, Finance & Operations
Gerry Frenette, Executive Director, Public & Member Relations
Debbie Gates, Manager, Events & Education
Natasha Alves, Coordinator, Administration
Christina D'Costa, Coordinator, Business Development

Canadian Network of Toxicology Centres (CNTC) / Réseau canadien des centres de toxicologie
University of Guelph, 50 Stone Rd E, Guelph ON N1G 2W1
Tel: 519-824-4120

Overview: A medium-sized national organization founded in 1983
Mission: To be recognized & respected for excellence in research, training, analysis & communication of information focused on critical toxicology issues for ecosystem & human health; to achieve this through innovative, multi-disciplinary teamwork & partnerships between the public & private sector
Affiliation(s): Metals in the Environment Research Network
Chief Officer(s):
Leonard Ritter, Executive Director
lritter@uoguelph.ca

Publications:
• CNTC [Canadian Network of Toxicology Centres] News
Type: Newsletter
Profile: Communication among CNTC member scientists & the public to increase education about toxicology
• CNTC [Canadian Network of Toxicology Centres] Science Briefs
Type: Newsletter
• CNTC [Canadian Network of Toxicology Centres] Annual Report
Type: Yearbook; *Frequency:* Annually
• CNTC [Canadian Network of Toxicology Centres] Annual Symposium Report
Type: Yearbook; *Frequency:* Annually

Canadian Nutrition Society (CNS) / Société canadienne de nutrition (SCN)
1867 La Chapelle St., Ottawa ON K1C 6A8

Toll-Free: 888-414-7188
e-mail: info@cns-scn.ca
www.cns-scn.ca
www.linkedin.com/groups?gid=4660487
www.facebook.com/canadiannutritionsociety
twitter.com/@CNS_SCN

Merged from: Canadian Society for Clinical Nutrition; Canadian Society for Nutritional Sciences
Overview: A medium-sized national organization founded in 2010
Mission: To promote nutrition science & education; To act as a voice for those engaged in furthering nutrition
Chief Officer(s):
Sarah Robbins, President
   president@cns-scn.ca
David Ma, Vice-President, Research
Valerie Marchand, Vice-President, Health Professionals
Alison Duncan, Treasurer
Andrea Grantham, Executive Director
   andrea@cns-scn.ca
Kathy Hare, Financial Administrator
   kathy@cns-scn.ca
Publications:
• CNS [Canadian Nutrition Society] Newsletter
Type: Newsletter

Canadian Organization for Rare Disorders (CORD)
#600, 151 Bloor St. West, Toronto ON M5S 1S4

Tel: 416-969-7464; *Fax:* 416-969-7420
Toll-Free: 877-302-7273
e-mail: info@raredisorders.ca
raredisorders.ca
www.facebook.com/RareDisorders
twitter.com/Durhane

Overview: A small national charitable organization founded in 1995
Mission: To advocate for health policy that works for people with rare disorders; to promote research & services for all rare disorders in Canada; To increase access to genetic screening & genetic counselling for rare disorders
Member of: Canadian Coalition for Genetic Fairness
Chief Officer(s):
Durhane Wong-Rieger, President & CEO
   durhane@sympatico.ca
John Adams, Chair
Publications:
• THE LINK Newsletter
Type: Newsletter; *Frequency:* Annually
Profile: Articles, conferences, & CORD activities

Canadian Organization of Medical Physicists (COMP) / L'Organisation canadienne des physiciens médicaux (OCPM)
#202, 300 March Rd., Kanata ON K2K 2E2

Tel: 613-599-3491; *Fax:* 613-595-1155
www.comp-ocpm.ca
www.facebook.com/CanadianMedphys
twitter.com/MedphysCA

Overview: A small national organization founded in 1989
Mission: To encourage the application of physics in medicine; To develop & protect professional standards; To encourage certification by the Canadian College of Physicists in Medicine
Member of: International Organization of Medical Physicists
Affliation(s): Canadian College of Physicists in Medicine; American

Association of Physicists in Medicine; Institute of Physics and Engineering in Medicine
Chief Officer(s):
Michelle Hilts, President
Nancy Barrett, Executive Director, 613-599-1948
   nancy.barrett@comp-ocpm.ca
Gisele Kite, Administrator
   gisele.kite@comp-ocpm.ca
Publications:
• InterACTIONS
Type: Newsletter; *Frequency:* Quarterly; *Accepts Advertising;* *Editor:* Dr. Christopher Thomas
Profile: Newsletter of the Canadian Organization of Medical Physicists (COMP) & the Canadian College of Physicists in Medicine (CCPM) for their members
• Medical Physics
Type: Journal; *Price:* Free with COMP membership
• Physics in Medicine & Biology
Type: Journal; *Price:* $385

Canadian Orthopractic Manual Therapy Association
#207, 1150 - 100 Ave., Edmonton AB T5K 0J7

Tel: 780-482-7428; *Fax:* 780-488-2463
e-mail: info@orthopractic.org
www.orthopractic.org

Overview: A medium-sized national organization
Mission: To provide the public, fellow healthcare professionals, government & funding agencies with guidelines on the provision of safe & effective manual therapy including mobilization & manipulation

Canadian Paediatric Society (CPS) / Société canadienne de pédiatrie
#100, 2305 St. Laurent Blvd., Ottawa ON K1G 4J8

Tel: 613-526-9397; *Fax:* 613-526-3332
www.cps.ca
www.linkedin.com/company/canadian-paediatric-society
www.facebook.com/CanadianPaediatricSociety
twitter.com/canpaedsociety
www.youtube.com/canpaedsociety

Overview: A medium-sized national organization founded in 1922
Mission: To advocate for the health needs of children & youth; To provide continuing education to paediatricians; To establish national guidelines for paediatric care & practice
Member of: International Paediatric Association
Chief Officer(s):
Jonathan Kronick, President
Marie Adèle Davis, Executive Director
   madavis@cps.ca
Elizabeth Moreau, Director, Communications & Knowledge Translation
   elizabethm@cps.ca
Publications:
• CPS [Canadian Paediatric Society] News
Type: Newsletter; *Frequency:* 5 pa; *Accepts Advertising;* *Price:* Free with CPS membership
Profile: Current society activities for CPS members
• Paediatrics & Child Health [a publication of the Canadian Paediatric Society]
Type: Journal; *Accepts Advertising;* *Price:* Free with CPS membership
Profile: Educational information & research reports for clinicians, parents, & caregivers

Canadian Patient Safety Institute (CPSI) / Institut canadien pour la sécurité des patients
#1414, 10235 - 101 St., Edmonton AB T5J 3G1

Tel: 780-409-8090; *Fax:* 780-409-8098
Toll-Free: 866-421-6933
e-mail: info@cpsi-icsp.ca
www.patientsafetyinstitute.ca
www.linkedin.com/companies/canadian-patient-safety-institute
www.facebook.com/PatientSafety
twitter.com/Patient_Safety
www.youtube.com/patientsafetycanada

Overview: A small national organization founded in 2003
Mission: To work with patients, healthcare providers, organizations, regulatory bodies, & governments to provide safer healthcare for Canadians; To promote leading practices for patient safety within Canada's health system
Chief Officer(s):

Doug Cochrane, Chair
Hugh MacLeod, CEO
  hmacleod@cpsi-icsp.ca
Cecilia Bloxom, Director, Communications
  cbloxom@cpsi-icsp.ca
Publications:
• Patient Safety Matters: The CPSI Newsletter
Type: Newsletter
Profile: Institute updates, courses, appointments, profiles, funding, & upcoming events

Canadian Physiological Society (CPS) / Société canadienne de physiologie
c/o Department of Physiology, University of Alberta, Edmonton AB T6G 2R3
                                          www.cpsscp.ca
Overview: A medium-sized national charitable organization founded in 1935 overseen by Canadian Federation of Biological Societies
Mission: To disseminate & discuss scientific information of interest to researchers in physiology & biological sciences
Chief Officer(s):
Catherine Chan, Vice-President & Acting Secretary
  cbchan@ualberta.ca

Canadian Physiotherapy Association (CPA) / L'Association canadienne de physiothérapie
#270, 955 Green Valley Cres., Ottawa ON K2C 3V4
                          Tel: 613-564-5454; *Fax:* 613-564-1577
                                  Toll-Free: 800-387-8679
                          e-mail: information@physiotherapy.ca
                                          www.physiotherapy.ca
        www.linkedin.com/company/canadian-physiotherapy-association
                          www.facebook.com/CPA.ACP
                                          twitter.com/physiocan
Overview: A large national organization founded in 1920
Mission: To provide leadership & direction to the profession; To foster excellence in practice, education & research; To promote high standards of health in Canada
Affiliation(s): World Confederation for Physical Therapy; Alliance of Physiotherapy Regulatory Boards of Canada; Canadian University Physiotherapy Academic Council; Health Action Lobby (HEAL); Physiotherapy Foundation of Canada; Accreditation Council for Canadian Physiotherapy Academic Programs
Chief Officer(s):
Linda Woodhouse, President
Publications:
• Canadian Physiotherapy Association Annual Report
Type: Yearbook; *Frequency:* Annually
• Physiotherapy Canada
Type: Journal; *Frequency:* Quarterly; *Accepts Advertising*; *Editor:* Dina Brooks, BSc(PT), MSc, PhD; *Price:* Free to CPA members
Profile: The Canadian Physiotherapy Association's official peer-reviewed scientific & clinical studies journal
• Physiotherapy Practice
Type: Magazine; *Frequency:* 5 pa; *Accepts Advertising*; *Price:* Free to CPA members
Profile: Information for physiotherapy clinicians, including an annual Buyers Guide

Canadian Podiatric Medical Association (CPMA) / Association médicale podiatrique canadienne
#2063, 61 Broadway Blvd., Sherwood Park AB T8H 2C1
                                  Toll-Free: 888-220-3338
                          e-mail: askus@podiatrycanada.org
                                          www.podiatrycanada.org
Overview: A small national organization founded in 1924
Mission: To effectively serve & provide guidance to its members & the podiatry profession in Canada; to serve the public; to provide the authoritative national voice for podiatrists in Canada; to recognize a particular responsibility to contribute to the development of national positions & standards related to the podiatric medical profession through education, research, materials & personnel
Member of: Federation of International Podiatrists
Affiliation(s): Canadian Podiatric Education Foundation (CPEF)
Chief Officer(s):
Jayne Jeneroux, Executive Director
Publications:
• CPMA [Canadian Podiatric Medical Association] Newsletter

Type: Newsletter; *Frequency:* Semiannually; *Price:* Free with CPMA membership

Canadian Post-MD Education Registry (CAPER) / Système informatisé sur les stagiaires post-MD en formation clinique
#800, 265 Carling Ave., Ottawa ON K1S 2E1
                          Tel: 613-730-1204; *Fax:* 613-730-1196
                                  e-mail: caper@afmc.ca
                                          www.caper.ca
                                  twitter.com/CAPERCanada
Overview: A medium-sized national charitable organization founded in 1986
Mission: To provide accurate & timely data pertaining to Post-MD training & physician resources in Canada to assist medical schools, governments & other work longitudinal research pertaining to physicians training & supply
Affiliation(s): Association of Faculties of Medicine of Canada
Chief Officer(s):
Lynda Buske, Interim Director
  lbuske@caper.ca
Publications:
• CAPER [Canadian Post-MD Education Registry] Annual Census
Type: Report; *Frequency:* Annually; *ISSN:* 1712-9184
Profile: Annual census of post-M.D. trainees
• CAPER [Canadian Post-MD Education Registry] Provincial Reports
Type: Report; *Frequency:* Annually

Canadian Professional Association for Transgender Health (CPATH)
#201, 1770 Fort St., Ottawa ON V8R 1J5
                          Tel: 250-592-6183; *Fax:* 250-592-6123
                                  e-mail: info@cpath.ca
                                          www.cpath.ca
Overview: A medium-sized national organization founded in 2008
Mission: CPATH is an interdisciplinary professional organization which works to support the health, wellbeing, and dignity of trans and gender diverse people.
Chief Officer(s):
Devon MacFarlane, President

Canadian Public Health Association (CPHA) / Association canadienne de santé publique (ACSP)
#404, 1525 Carling Ave., Ottawa ON K1Z 8R9
                          Tel: 613-725-3769; *Fax:* 613-725-9826
                                  e-mail: info@cpha.ca
                                          www.cpha.ca
        www.linkedin.com/company/113746?trk=prof-exp-company-name
                          www.facebook.com/cpha.acsp
                                          twitter.com/CPHA_ACSP
                www.youtube.com/channel/UC_SDgqaCLW1YKWKYqlO4evg
Overview: A large national charitable organization founded in 1910
Mission: To represent public health in Canada; To support universal & equitable access to the necessary conditions to achieve health for all Canadians; To provide links to the international public health community
Affiliation(s): World Health Organization; World Federation of Public Health Associations
Chief Officer(s):
Ardene Robinson Vollman, PhD, RN, CCHN(C, Chair
Susan Jackson, PhD, MSc, BSc, Chair-Elect
Annie Duchesne, MScPH, Director
Jacqueline Gahagan, PhD, Director
James Mintz, BA, Director
Manasi Parikh, Director
Publications:
• The Canadian Journal of Public Health
Type: Journal; *Frequency:* Bimonthly; *Accepts Advertising*; *Editor:* Debra Lynkowski; *Price:* Free with membership in the Canadian Public Health Association
Profile: Articles on public health, including epidemiology, nutrition, family health, environmental health, sexually transmitted diseases, gerontology, behavioural medicine,rural health, health promotion, & public health policy
• Canadian Public Health Association Annual Report
Type: Yearbook; *Frequency:* Annually
• CPHA [Canadian Public Health Association] Health Digest
Frequency: Quarterly; *Editor:* Debra Lynkowski; *ISBN:* 0703-5624; *Price:* Free with membership inthe Canadian Public Health Association

Profile: Incorporates the international newsletter, Partners Around the World, plus articles from across Canada & around the world

Canadian Radiation Protection Association (CRPA) / Association canadienne de radioprotection (ACRP)
PO Box 83, Carleton Place ON K7C 3P3

Tel: 613-253-3779; *Fax:* 888-551-0712
e-mail: secretariat@crpa-acrp.ca
www.crpa-acrp.ca
www.linkedin.com/groups?gid=4296889

Overview: A small national organization founded in 1979
Mission: To develop scientific knowledge for protection from the harmful effects of radiation; To encourage research; To assist in the development of professional standards in the discipline
Affiliation(s): International Radiation Protection Association (IRPA).
Chief Officer(s):
Jeff Dovyak, President
Ray Ilson, Treasurer
Publications:
• CRPA [Canadian Radiation Protection Association] Bulletin
Type: Newsletter; *Frequency:* Quarterly
Profile: For Canadian Radiation Protection Association members only

Canadian Register of Health Service Psychologists (CRHSP) / Répertoire canadien des psychologues offrant des services de santé (RCPOSS)
72 Saint-Raymond Blvd., Gatineau QC J8Y 1S2

Tel: 819-771-1441; *Fax:* 819-771-1444
e-mail: info@crhspp.ca
www.crhspp.ca

Overview: A small national organization founded in 1985
Mission: To promote & protect public access to qualified health service providers in psychology
Chief Officer(s):
John MacDonald, Executive Director
Publications:
• Directory of Canadian Health Service Psychologists [a publication of the Canadian Register of Health Service Psychologists]
Type: Directory; *Price:* $26.25/AB, MB, NT, NU, PE, QC, SK, YT; $28/BC; $28.25/NB, NL, ON; $28.75 NS

Canadian Society for Aesthetic Plastic Surgery (CSAPS) / Société canadienne de chirurgie plastique et esthétique
70 Carson Ave., Whitby ON L1M 1J5

Tel: 905-665-9889; *Fax:* 905-665-7319
e-mail: info@csaps.ca
www.csaps.ca
www.facebook.com/csaps

Previous Name: Canadian Society for Aesthetic (Cosmetic) Plastic Surgery
Overview: A small national organization founded in 1972
Mission: To improve cosmetic surgery outcomes; To maintain high surgical standards of clinical practice
Chief Officer(s):
Eric Bensimon, President
Tara Hewitt, Executive Administrator
csapsoffice@gmail.com

Canadian Society for Clinical Investigation (CSCI) / Société canadienne de recherches cliniques (SCRC)
114 Cheyenne Way, Ottawa ON K2J 0E9

Fax: 613-491-0073
Toll-Free: 877-968-9449
e-mail: info@csci-scrc.ca
www.csci-scrc.ca

Overview: A medium-sized national organization founded in 1951
Mission: To promote research in the field of human health throughout Canada; to lobby for research funding; to support Canadian researchers in their endeavours & at all stages of their careers by supporting knowledge translation & fostering communities of health science researchers
Chief Officer(s):
Norman Rosenblum, President
Publications:
• Clinical & Investigative Medicine (CIM)
Type: Journal; *Frequency:* Bimonthly; *Editor:* David R. Bevan
Profile: Original research, policy changes that affect biological & medical science research, issues related to medical research funding, information for clinician-scientisttrainees

Canadian Society for Epidemiology & Biostatistics (CESB) / Société canadienne d'épidémiologie et de biostatistique (SCEB)
c/o Pamela Wilson, The Willow Group, 1485 Laperriere Ave., Ottawa ON K1Z 7S8

Tel: 613-722-8796; *Fax:* 613-729-6206
e-mail: secretariat@cseb.ca
cseb.ca
www.facebook.com/109122749151677
twitter.com/csebsceb
www.youtube.com/user/CSEBSCEB

Overview: A small national organization founded in 1990
Mission: To foster epidemiology & biostatistics research in Canada; To improve training in the disciplines of epidemiology & biostatistics in Canada
Chief Officer(s):
Susan Jaglal, President
Paul Arora, Secretary
Publications:
• Canadian Society for Epidemiology & Biostatistics Newsletter
Type: Newsletter
Profile: Information of interest to members of the Society

Canadian Society for Exercise Physiology (CSEP) / Société canadienne de physiologie de l'exercice (SCPE)
#370, 18 Louisa St., Ottawa ON K1R 6Y6

Tel: 613-234-3755; *Fax:* 613-234-3565
Toll-Free: 877-651-3755
e-mail: info@csep.ca
www.csep.ca
www.linkedin.com/company/csep-scpe
www.facebook.com/520719817945510
twitter.com/CSEPdotCA

Previous Name: Canadian Association of Sport Sciences
Overview: A medium-sized national organization founded in 1967
Mission: To promote the generation, synthesis, transfer, & application of knowledge & research related to exercise physiology, encompassing physical activity, fitness, health, nutrition, epidemiology & human performance; To act as the voice for exercise physiology in Canada
Chief Officer(s):
Phil Chilibeck, President/Chair
Publications:
• Active Living During Pregnancy: Physical Activitiy Guidelines for Mother & Baby
Type: Manual; *Number of Pages:* 40; *ISBN:* 978-1-896900-06-3; *Price:* $11.95
Profile: A resource for pregnant women who want to maintain activity during pregnancy
• Applied Physiology, Nutrition & Metabolism (APNM)
Type: Journal; *Editor:* Terry Graham, PhD; *Price:* Free with membership in the Canadian Society for Exercise Physiology
Profile: Original research articles, reviews, & commentaries on the application of physiology, nutrition, & metabolism to the study of humanhealth, physical activity, & fitness
• Canada's Physical Activity Guide to Healthy Active Living (Adults 20-55): PA Guide Handbook
Type: Handbook; *Number of Pages:* 32
Profile: Detailed advice & case studies about becoming more active, produced by the Public Health Agency of Canada (PHAC) & theCanadian Society for Exercise Physiology (CSEP)
• The Canadian Physical Activity, Fitness & Lifestyle Approach (CPAFLA)
Type: Manual; *Number of Pages:* 300; *ISBN:* 978-1-896900-16-2; *Price:* $70
Profile: CSEP Health & Fitness Program's health-related appraisal & counselling strategy
• Communiqué [a publication of the Canadian Society for Exercise Physiology]
Type: Newsletter; *Frequency:* Monthly; *Accepts Advertising; Price:* Free withmembership in the Canadian Society for Exercise Physiology
Profile: A member newsletter of the Canadian Society for Exercise Physiology, with job postings & information about forthcoming conferences
• CSEP [Canadian Society for Exercise Physiology] Member Directory
Type: Directory
Profile: A listing of the more 4,500 members of the Canadian Society for Exercise Physiology, to help users locate CSEP Certified Personal Trainers or CSEPCertified Exercise Physiologists

• The CSEP [Canadian Society for Exercise Physiology] Certified Exercise Physiologist Certification Guide
Type: Guide; *Number of Pages:* 144; *ISBN:* 978-1-896900-26-1; *Price:* $39.95
Profile: For candidates preparing for the theory & practical examination process to be recognized as CSEPCertified Exercise Physiologist

• CSEP [Canadian Society for Exercise Physiology] Certified Personal Trainer Study Guide
Type: Guide; *Number of Pages:* 52; *ISBN:* 978-1-896900-28-5; *Price:* $29.95
Profile: For candidates preparing to obtain the professional personal training certificate in Canada

• Inclusive Fitness & Lifestyle Services for all (dis)Abilities
Type: Manual; *Number of Pages:* 300; *ISBN:* 978-1-896900-10-0; *Price:* $55
Profile: Resources to provide fitness assessment & active living counselling services

• Physical Activity Guide for Children (6-9 Years of Age): Family Guide to Physical Activity for Children
Type: Guide; *Number of Pages:* 12
Profile: Advice about how children can be active, produced by the Public Health Agency of Canada (PHAC) & the CanadianSociety for Exercise Physiology (CSEP)

• Physical Activity Guide for Children (6-9 Years of Age): Teacher's Guide to Physical Activity for Children
Type: Guide; *Number of Pages:* 8
Profile: Advice for teachers about how children can be active, produced by the Public Health Agency of Canada (PHAC) & theCanadian Society for Exercise Physiology (CSEP)

• Physical Activity Guide for Older Adults (Over 55): PA Guide Handbook for Older Adults
Type: Handbook; *Number of Pages:* 32
Profile: Detailed advice with tips on increasing physical activity, produced by the Public Health Agency of Canada (PHAC) & the CanadianSociety for Exercise Physiology (CSEP)

• Physical Activity Guide for Youth (10-14 Years of Age): Family Guide to Physical Activity for Youth
Type: Guide; *Number of Pages:* 12
Profile: A support resource for families, produced by the Public Health Agency of Canada (PHAC) & the Canadian Society forExercise Physiology (CSEP)

• Physical Activity Guide for Youth (10-14 Years of Age): Teacher's Guide to Physical Activity for Youth
Type: Guide; *Number of Pages:* 8
Profile: A support resource for teachers, produced by the Public Health Agency of Canada (PHAC) & the Canadian Society forExercise Physiology (CSEP)

• Professional Fitness & Lifestyle Consultant (PFLC) Resource Manual
Type: Manual; *Number of Pages:* 250; *ISBN:* 978-1-896900-04-9; *Price:* $55
Profile: The practical requirements for certification as a CSEP Certified Exercise Physiologist

Canadian Society for Immunology (CSI)
c/o Dept. of Veterinary Microbiology, Univ. of Saskatchewan, 52 Campus Dr., Saskatoon SK S7N 5B4
Tel: 306-966-7214; *Fax:* 306-966-7244
Other Communication: membership@csi-sci.ca
e-mail: info@csi-sci.ca
www.csi-sci.ca
Overview: A small national charitable organization founded in 1966
Mission: To foster & support immunology research & education across Canada
Member of: Research Canada
Chief Officer(s):
Hanne Ostergaard, President
  hanne.ostergaard@ualberta.ca
Lori Coulthurst, Society Administrator

Canadian Society for the History of Medicine (CSHM) / Société canadienne d'histoire de la médecine (SCHM)
c/o University of Ottawa, #14022, 120 University, Ottawa ON K1N 6N5
Tel: 613-562-5700
www.cshm-schm.ca
Overview: A small national organization founded in 1950

Mission: To promote the study & communication of the history of health & medicine
Chief Officer(s):
Sasha Mullally, President
Peter Twohig, Vice-President
Isabelle Perreault, Secretary-Treasurer & Coordinator, Membership
Publications:
• Canadian Bulletin of Medical History / Bulletin canadien d'histoire de la médecine
Type: Journal; *Frequency:* Semiannually; *Editor:* Cheryl Krasnick Warsh; *ISSN:* 0823-2105
Profile: Peer-reviewed original papers on all aspects of the history of medicine, health care, & related disciplines

Canadian Society for Transfusion Medicine (CSTM) / Société canadienne de médecine transfusionnelle
#6, 20 Crown Steel Dr., Markham ON L3R 9X9
Tel: 905-415-3917; *Fax:* 905-415-0071
Toll-Free: 855-415-3917
Other Communication: Toll-Free Fax: 866-882-7093
e-mail: office@transfusion.ca
www.transfusion.ca
www.facebook.com/290163767690083
twitter.com/CanSocTransMed
Previous Name: Canadian Association of Immunohematologists
Overview: A medium-sized national organization founded in 1989
Mission: To promulgate throughout Canada a high level of ethics & professional standards; To create national & regional opportunities for the presentation & discussion of research & developments in these & allied fields; To initiate & maintain a program of continuing education; To promote good laboratory & good manufacturing practices; To establish mutually beneficial working relationships with relevant national & international societies & organizations; To be the primary voice for transfusion medicine in Canada
Chief Officer(s):
Darlene Mueller, President
  president@transfusion.ca

Canadian Society for Vascular Surgery (CSVS) / Société canadienne de chirurgie vasculaire
PO Box 58062, Ottawa ON K1C 7H4
Tel: 613-286-7583
e-mail: info@canadianvascular.ca
canadianvascular.ca
twitter.com/canadianvascul1
Overview: A small national organization
Mission: To promote vascular health for Canadians
Chief Officer(s):
Greg Browne, President
  drgregbrown@gmail.com
Publications:
• Canadian Society for Vascular Surgery e-Newsletter
Type: Newsletter

Canadian Society of Clinical Chemists (CSCC) / Société canadienne des clinico-chimistes
PO Box 1570, #310, 4 Cataraqui St., Kingston ON K7K 1Z7
Tel: 613-531-8899; *Fax:* 866-303-0626
e-mail: office@cscc.ca
www.cscc.ca
Overview: A medium-sized national organization founded in 1965
Mission: To establish standards for diagnostic services in the practice of clinical biochemistry & clinical laboratory medicine
Chief Officer(s):
David Kinniburgh, President
Elizabeth Hooper, Executive Director
Ivan Blasutig, Treasurer
Publications:
• Canadian Society of Clinical Chemists Member Handbook
Type: Yearbook; *Frequency:* Annually
• Clinical Biochemistry
Type: Journal; *Editor:* Edgard E. Delvin; *ISSN:* 0009-9120
Profile: Analytical & clinical investigative articles related to molecular biology, chemistry, biochemistry, immunology, clinical investigation, diagnosis, therapy, & monitoring humandisease, for chemists, immunologists, biologists, & biochemists

• The CSCC [Canadian Society of Clinical Chemists] News
Type: Newsletter
Profile: Society activities & information for CSCC members

Canadian Society of Clinical Perfusion (CSCP) / Société Canadienne de Perfusion Clinique (SCPC)
914 Adirondack Rd., London ON N6K 4W7

Fax: 866-648-2763
Toll-Free: 888-496-2727
www.cscp.ca
www.facebook.com/CSCP-Online-1523661604524664
twitter.com/cscp_online
instagram.com/cscp_online

Overview: A medium-sized national organization
Mission: To encourage & foster the development of the profession of clinical perfusion, through education & certification
Chief Officer(s):
Roger Stanzel, President
Cyril Serrick, Vice-President
Naresh Tinani, Executive Secretary
Bill Gibb, Treasurer
Publications:
• The Perfusionist: The Official Publication of the Canadian Society of Clinical Perfusion
Type: Journal; *Frequency:* 3 pa; *Accepts Advertising*; *Editor:* Andrew Beney, MSc, CPC, CCP
Profile: Approximately 350 issues are distributed to Canadian certified perfusionists, subscribingstudents, American perfusionists, & corporate members

Canadian Society of Hand Therapists (CSHT) / Societe canadienne des therapeutes de la main (SCTM)
#101, 10277 154 St., Surrey BC V3R 4J7

e-mail: secretary@csht.org
www.csht.org
www.facebook.com/324550384259629
twitter.com/handtherapists

Overview: A medium-sized national organization
Mission: To provide education, information, & enhanced care for the improvement of upper extremity rehabilitation
Chief Officer(s):
Trevor Fraser, President
president@csht.org

Canadian Society of Internal Medicine (CSIM) / Société canadienne de médecine interne (SCMI)
#300, 421 Gilmour St., Ottawa ON K2P 0R5

Tel: 613-422-5977; *Fax:* 613-249-3326
Toll-Free: 855-893-2746
e-mail: info@csim.ca
csim.ca
www.facebook.com/canadiansocietyofinternalmedicine
twitter.com/CSIMSCMI

Overview: A medium-sized national organization founded in 1984
Mission: To promote healthy living among Canadians; to provide leadership for physicians; to conduct research & education.
Affliation(s): Canadian Medical Association
Chief Officer(s):
Benjamin Chen, President
Publications:
• CJGIM (Canadian Journal of General Internal Medicine)
Type: Journal; *Frequency:* Quarterly
Profile: CSIM news, book reviews, articles, case reviews, history of medicine, & medical education

Canadian Society of Medical Evaluators (CSME)
#301, 250 Consumers Rd., Toronto ON M2J 4V6

Tel: 416-487-4040; *Fax:* 416-495-8723
Toll-Free: 888-672-9999
e-mail: info@csme.org
www.csme.org
www.facebook.com/101574806684190

Overview: A small national organization
Mission: To serve Canadian physicians who perform medical & medicolegal evaluations for patients or as a professional service to the legal profession, employers, the workplace safety & insurance board & the insurance industry
Chief Officer(s):

Renee Levine, Executive Director
rlevine@csme.org

Canadian Society of Microbiologists (CSM) / Société canadienne des microbiologistes
CSM-SCM Secretariat, 17 Dossetter Way, Ottawa ON K1G 4S3

Tel: 613-421-7229; *Fax:* 613-421-9811
e-mail: info@csm-scm.org
www.csm-scm.org
twitter.com/CSM_SCM

Overview: A medium-sized national organization founded in 1958
Mission: To advance microbiology in all its aspects; to facilitate interchange of ideas between microbiologists
Affliation(s): Youth Science Foundation; International Union of Microbiological Societies
Chief Officer(s):
Charles Dozois, President
Mohan Babu, Secretary-Treasurer
Publications:
• Canadian Society of Microbiologists Call for Abstracts
Type: Booklet; *Frequency:* Annually
Profile: Published in advance of the Annual General Meeting in November / December
• Canadian Society of Microbiologists Programme & Abstracts
Frequency: Annually
Profile: Published for the Annual General Meeting each May
• Canadian Society of Microbiologists Graduate Studies & Membership Directory
Type: Directory; *Frequency:* Biennially
• CSM [Canadian Society of Microbiologists] Newsletter
Type: Newsletter; *Frequency:* 3 pa

Canadian Society of Nutrition Management / Société canadienne de gestion de la nutrition
#300, 1370 Don Mills Rd., Toronto ON M3B 3N7

Fax: 416-441-0591
Toll-Free: 866-355-2766
e-mail: csnm@csnm.ca
www.csnm.ca
ca.linkedin.com/in/thecsnm
twitter.com/TheCSNM

Previous Name: Canadian Food Service Supervisors Association
Overview: A medium-sized national organization
Mission: To foster an environment in which members can achieve success in their chosen field
Chief Officer(s):
Natasha Mooney, President
president@csnm.ca
Heather Shannon, Secretary-Treasurer
treasurer-secretary@csnm.ca

Canadian Society of Professionals in Disability Management (CSPDM)
c/o Pacific Coast University for Workplace Health Sciences, 4755 Cherry Creek Rd., Port Alberni BC V9Y 0A7

Tel: 778-421-0821; *Fax:* 778-421-0823
www.cspdm.ca

Overview: A small national organization founded in 2006
Mission: To minimize the socio-economic impact of disabling injuries & illnesses on employees & employers by establishing & supporting the practice of consensus based disability management through professional standards of quality innovation & leadership in the field
Member of: International Association of Professionals in Disability Management
Chief Officer(s):
Sheena Cook, Coordinator, Membership Services, 778-421-0821 Ext. 210
sheena@cspdm.ca
Publications:
• CSPDM [Canadian Society of Professionals in Disability Management] Connections
Type: Newsletter; *Frequency:* Quarterly
Profile: Information & resources relevant to disability management

Canadian Sport Massage Therapists Association (CSMTA) / Association canadienne des massothérapeutes du sport
#236, 229 St. Clair St., Chatham ON N7L 3J4

Tel: 519-800-7134
e-mail: natoffice@csmta.ca
www.csmta.ca

Overview: A medium-sized national licensing organization founded in 1987
Mission: To provide leadership in the field of sport massage therapy & education in Canada through the establishment of professional standards & qualifications of its members, as a certifying body
Affiliation(s): Canadian Olympic Committee; Expert Provider Group
Chief Officer(s):
Jessica Sears, President
Monty Churchman, Vice-President
Mike Grafstein, Secretary
Jeanette Dobmeier, Treasurer
Brenda Caley, National Office Coordinator

Canadians for Health Research (CHR) / Les Canadiens pour la recherche médicale
PO Box 126, Westmount QC H3Z 2T1

Tel: 514-398-7478; *Fax:* 514-398-8361
www.chrcrm.org
www.facebook.com/300688209959308
twitter.com/chr_news

Overview: A medium-sized national charitable organization founded in 1976
Mission: To further understanding & communication among the public, the scientific community & government; To promote stability & quality in Canadian health research; to meet goals through the direct provision of information on request, & development & circulation of literature & special programming; To sponsor periodic conferences, workshops, a journalism award, & a student essay competition
Chief Officer(s):
Tim Lougheed, Chair
Publications:
• 30 Years of Health Research [a publication of Canadians for Health Research]
Type: Report
Profile: Series of monographs that report on 30 years of progress in scientific research
• The Diary [a publication of Canadians for Health Research]
Type: Newsletter; *Frequency:* Quarterly; *Price:* $250
Profile: Monitors animal-related issues nationally and internationally
• Future Health [a publication of Canadians for Health Research]
Type: Magazine; *Frequency:* Quarterly; *Price:* $25; $15 for schools and libraries
Profile: Contains highlights of Canadian health research
• Road to Discovery [a publication of Canadians for Health Research]
Type: Report
Profile: Published in conjunction with the Medical Research Council of Canada to promote student awareness of research in healthcare
• Salute to Excellence [a publication of Canadians for Health Research]
Type: Report
Profile: An outline of achievements of Canadian medical research from the 20th century
• A True Story [a publication of Canadians for Health Research]
Type: Report
Profile: Illustrated monograph that provides information on animals and medical research

Catholic Health Alliance of Canada / Alliance catholique canadienne de la santé
Annex C, Saint-Vincent Hospital, 60 Cambridge St. North, Ottawa ON K1R 7A5

Tel: 613-562-6262; *Fax:* 613-782-2857
www.chac.ca

Previous Name: Catholic Health Association of Canada; Catholic Hospital Association of Canada
Overview: A large national charitable organization founded in 1939
Mission: To strengthen & support the ministry of Catholic health care organizations & providers, through advocacy & governance
Chief Officer(s):
Mike Shea, President & CEO, 780-781-4075
  shea.chac@gmail.com

James Roche, Senior Director, Mission & Ethics, 613-562-6262 Ext. 2164
  jroche@bruyere.org
Publications:
• Catholic Health Alliance of Canada Annual Report
Type: Yearbook; *Frequency:* Annually
Profile: Financial & executive reports
• Facing Death, Discovering Life
Number of Pages: 78; *Author:* James Roche; *ISBN:* 9780920705360; *Price:* $10.95
• Forming Health Care Leaders: A Guide
Number of Pages: 143; *ISBN:* 9780920705421; *Price:* $12.50
• Health Ethics Guide
Number of Pages: 122; *ISBN:* 9780920705018; *Price:* $12.50 members
• Lift Up Your Hearts to the Lord
Number of Pages: 104; *ISBN:* 9780920705056; *Price:* $4 members
• Living With Hope in Times of Illness
Number of Pages: 30; *Editor:* Barry McGrorry; Greg J. Humbert; *ISBN:* 9780920705407; *Price:* $2
• Spirituality & Health: What's Good for the Soul Can Be Good for the Body, Too
Number of Pages: 74; *Author:* James Roche; *ISBN:* 9780920705247; *Price:* $9.95

Child Development Institute (CDI)
197 Euclid Ave., Toronto ON M6J 2J8

Tel: 416-603-1827; *Fax:* 416-603-6655
e-mail: info@childdevelop.ca
www.childdevelop.ca
ca.linkedin.com/company/child-development-institute
www.facebook.com/childdevelop
twitter.com/officialcdi
www.youtube.com/user/CDICanada

Overview: A medium-sized international charitable organization
Mission: An accredited children's mental health agency that develops innovative programming for children ages 0-12 and youth ages 13-18 and their families in the areas of Early Intervention Services, Family Violence Services and Healthy Child Development.
Chief Officer(s):
Tony Diniz, Chief Executive Officer
  tdiniz@childdevelop.ca
Shauna Klein, Director, Fund Development, Marketing and Communications
  sklein@childdevelop.ca

Children and Youth in Challenging Contexts Network (CYCC)
PO Box 15000, 6420 Coburg Rd., Halifax ON B3H 4R2

Tel: 902-494-4087
cyccnetwork.org
www.facebook.com/CYCCNetwork
twitter.com/CYCCNetwork
www.youtube.com/user/cyccnetwork

Overview: A medium-sized national organization
Mission: The CYCC Network is a knowledge mobilization network that was created to improve mental health and well-being for vulnerable and at-risk children and youth in Canada.
Chief Officer(s):
Lisa Lachance, Executive Director
  lisa.lachance@dal.ca

COACH - Canada's Health Informatics Association (COACH)
#301, 250 Consumers Rd., Toronto ON M2J 4V6

Tel: 416-494-9324; *Fax:* 416-495-8723
Toll-Free: 888-253-8554
e-mail: info@coachorg.com
www.coachorg.com
www.linkedin.com/company/coach-canada's-health-informatics-association
www.facebook.com/COACHORG
twitter.com/COACH_HI
www.youtube.com/channel/UCiaVmX9quqgI14MTxJ3Wh6Q

Overview: A large national organization founded in 1975
Mission: To improve the health of Canadians & enhance the management of Canada's health system by advancing the practice of health information management & effective utilization of associated technologies
Member of: International Medical Informatics Association

Chief Officer(s):
Don Newsham, Chief Executive Officer
Shannon Bott, Executive Director, Operations
Linda Miller, Executive Director, CHIEF: Canada's Health Informatics
  Executive Forum
Mike Barron, President
Jim Mickelson, Sec.-Tres., 778-772-0954

College of Family Physicians of Canada (CFPC) / Collège des médecins de famille du Canada
2630 Skymark Ave., Mississauga ON L4W 5A4
Tel: 905-629-0900; *Fax:* 888-843-2372
Toll-Free: 800-387-6197
e-mail: info@cfpc.ca
www.cfpc.ca
twitter.com/FamPhysCan
www.youtube.com/user/CFPCMedia

Overview: A large national organization founded in 1954
Mission: To improve the health of Canadians by promoting high standards of medical education & care in family practice, by contributing to public understanding of healthful living, by supporting ready access to family physician services, & by encouraging research & disseminating knowledge about family medicine
Chief Officer(s):
David White, MD, CCFP, FCFP, President
Guillaume Charbonneau, MD, CCFP, President-Elect
Francine Lemire, MD CM, CCFP, FC, Executive Director & CEO
Publications:
• Canadian Family Physician [a publication of the College of Family Physicians of Canada]
Type: Journal
Profile: Current issues & developments in family medicine
• eNews [a publication of the College of Family Physicians of Canada]
Type: Newsletter; *Frequency:* Monthly
• Kaléidoscope [a publication of the College of Family Physicians of Canada]
Type: Newsletter
Profile: Developments in family medicine research
• Section of Residents Newsletter [a publication of the College of Family Physicians of Canada]
Type: Newsletter
Profile: Information for family medicine residents

Alberta College of Family Physicians
Centre 170, #370, 10403 - 172 St., Edmonton AB T5S 1K9
Tel: 780-488-2395; *Fax:* 780-488-2396
Toll-Free: 800-361-0607
e-mail: info@acfp.ca
www.acfp.ca
twitter.com/ABFamDocs
Chief Officer(s):
John Chmelicek, President
  acfppres@acfp.ca
Terri Potter, Executive Director
  terri.potter@acfp.ca

British Columbia College of Family Physicians
#330, 1665 West Broadway, Vancouver BC V6J 1X1
Tel: 604-736-1877; *Fax:* 604-736-4675
e-mail: office@bccfp.bc.ca
www.bccfp.bc.ca
Chief Officer(s):
Christie Newton, President
Toby Kirshin, Executive Director
Ian Tang, Project Manager

Collège québécois des médecins de famille
#202, 3210, av Jacques-Bureau, Laval QC H7P 0A9
Tél: 450-973-2228; *Téléc:* 450-973-4329
Ligne sans frais: 800-481-5962
Courriel: adjointe@cqmf.qc.ca
www.cqmf.qc.ca
Chief Officer(s):
Maxine Dumas Pilon, Présidente
Nicole Cloutier, Directrice générale

Manitoba College of Family Physicians

#240, 1695 Henderson Hwy., Winnipeg MB R2G 1P1
Tel: 204-668-3667; *Fax:* 204-668-3663
Toll-Free: 844-668-3667
www.mcfp.mb.ca
Chief Officer(s):
Deirdre O'Flaherty, President
Tamara Buchel, Executive Director
  tamarabuchel@mcfp.mb.ca
Amanda Woodard, Administrator & Office Manager
  amandaw@cfpc.ca

New Brunswick College of Family Physicians
950 Picot Ave., Bathurst NB E2A 4Z9
Tel: 506-548-4707; *Fax:* 506-548-4761
e-mail: nbcfp@cfpc.ca
www.nbcfp.ca
www.facebook.com/Nbcfp
twitter.com/nbcfp_cmfnb
Chief Officer(s):
Melissa McQuaid, President
Ghislain Lavoie, Secretary-Treasurer

Newfoundland & Labrador Chapter
#2713A, 300 Prince Philip Dr., St. John's NL A1B 3V6
Tel: 709-864-6566
nl.cfpc.ca
Chief Officer(s):
Dave Thomas, President
Debbie Rideout, Administrator
  debbierideout@cfpc.ca

Nova Scotia College of Family Physicians
Mill Cove Plaza, #207, 967 Bedford Hwy., Bedford NS B4A 1A9
Tel: 902-499-0303; *Fax:* 902-832-1193
e-mail: admin@nsfamdocs.com
www.nsfamdocs.com
Chief Officer(s):
Peter Brennan, President
Cathie W. Carroll, Executive Director

Ontario College of Family Physicians
#2100, 400 University Ave., Toronto ON M5G 1S5
Tel: 416-867-9646; *Fax:* 416-867-9990
Toll-Free: 800-670-6237
e-mail: ocfp@cfpc.ca
www.ocfp.on.ca
twitter.com/OntarioCollege
Chief Officer(s):
Jessica Hill, Chief Executive Officer
Glenn Brown, President

Prince Edward Island Chapter
253 King St., Charlottetown PE C1A 1C4
Tel: 902-894-2605; *Fax:* 902-894-3975
e-mail: pei.cfp@pei.aibn.com
pei.cfpc.ca
Chief Officer(s):
Shannon Curtis, President
Rosemary Burke-Perry, Administrator

Saskatchewan College of Family Physicians
105-2174 Airport Dr., Saskatoon SK S7L 6M6
Tel: 306-665-7714; *Fax:* 306-665-0047
e-mail: scfp@cfpc.ca
sk.cfpc.ca
twitter.com/SKChapterCFPC
Chief Officer(s):
Danielle Cutts, President
C. James Stewart, Executive Director
  jstewart@cfpc.ca

Consumer Health Organization of Canada (CHOC)
#1901, 355 St. Clair Ave. West, Toronto ON M5P 1N5
Tel: 416-924-9800; *Fax:* 416-924-6404
e-mail: info@consumerhealth.org
www.consumerhealth.org
Overview: A medium-sized national organization founded in 1973
Mission: To encourage the prevention of all kinds of illness through knowledge; To help the individual, the family & the community to enjoy the benefits of a more wholesome lifestyle; To promote harmony &

cooperation between like-minded groups
Affiliation(s): National Health Federation in US
Chief Officer(s):
Libby Gardon, President

The Council of Canadians (COC) / Le Conseil des Canadiens
#300, 251 Bank St., Ottawa ON K2P 1X3
Tel: 613-233-2773; *Fax:* 613-233-6776
Toll-Free: 800-387-7177
e-mail: inquiries@canadians.org
www.canadians.org
www.facebook.com/CouncilofCDNS?rf=105965852767091
twitter.com/councilofcdns
www.youtube.com/councilofcanadians
Overview: A medium-sized national organization founded in 1985
Mission: With chapters across the country, The Council of Canadians is Canada's largest citizens' organization, working to protect Canadian independence in areas such as energy & environment, health care & fair trade. The Council provides a critical voice on key national issues: safeguarding our social programs, promoting economic justice, renewing Canada's democracy, asserting Canadian sovereignty, promoting alternatives to corporate-style free trade & preserving the environment
Chief Officer(s):
Maude Barlow, National Chairperson

Council of Canadians with Disabilities (CCD) / Conseil des Canadiens avec déficiences
#909, 294 Portage Ave., Winnipeg MB R3C 0B9
Tel: 204-947-0303; *Fax:* 204-942-4625; *TTY:* 204-943-4757
e-mail: ccd@ccdonline.ca
www.ccdonline.ca
www.facebook.com/ccdonline
twitter.com/ccdonline
www.youtube.com/ccdonline
Overview: A medium-sized national organization founded in 1976
Mission: To improve the status of disabled citizens in Canadian society; To promote self-help for persons with disabilities; To provide a democratic structure for disabled citizens to voice concerns; To monitor federal legislation; To share information & cooperate with disabled persons' organizations in Canada & in other countries; To establish a positive image of disabled Canadians
Member of: Disabled Peoples International
Affiliation(s): Consumer Organization of Disabled People of Newfoundland & Labrador; PEI Council of the Disabled; Nova Scotia League for Equal Opportunities; PUSH-Ontario; Manitoba League of the Physically Handicapped; Saskatchewan Voice of the Handicapped; Alberta Committee of Disabled Citizens; British Columbia Coalition of the Disabled; Association canadienne des sourds; DAWN Canada; National Network on Mental Health; Thalidomide Victims of Canada; National Education Association of Disabled Students; People First of Canada
Chief Officer(s):
Jewelles Smith, Chair
Carmela Hutchison, Secretary
Kory Earle, Treasurer

Dietitians of Canada (DC) / Les diététistes du Canada
#604, 480 University Ave., Toronto ON M5G 1V2
Tel: 416-596-0857; *Fax:* 416-596-0603
e-mail: contactus@dietitians.ca
www.dietitians.ca
Previous Name: Canadian Dietetic Association
Overview: A medium-sized national organization founded in 1935
Mission: To advance health, through food & nutrition; To act as the voice of the dietitian profession in Canada
Chief Officer(s):
Marsha Sharp, Chief Executive Officer
Corinne Eisenbraun, Director, Professional Development & Support
Janice Macdonald, Director, Communications
Publications:
• Canadian Journal of Dietetic Research & Practice
Type: Journal; *Frequency:* Quarterly; *Editor:* Dawna Royall; *ISSN:* 1486-3847
Profile: A peer-reviewed publication, featuring manuscripts of original research, professional practice, & reviews
• Dietitians of Canada Annual Report
Type: Yearbook; *Frequency:* Annually

DisAbled Women's Network of Canada / Réseau d'Action des Femmes Handicapées du Canada
#505, 110, rue Ste. Thérèse, Montréal QC H2Y 1E6
Tel: 514-396-0009; *Fax:* 514-396-6585
Toll-Free: 866-396-0074
www.dawncanada.net
www.facebook.com/dawnrafhcanada
twitter.com/DAWNRAFHCanada
www.youtube.com/user/DAWNRAFHCanada
Also Known As: DAWN-RAFH Canada
Overview: A small national organization founded in 1985
Mission: To end the poverty, isolation, discrimination & violence experienced by women with disabilities; To ensure the accessibility of services to women with disabilities; To address key issues concerning women with disabilities
Member of: National Action Committee on the Status of Women
Affiliation(s): Council of Canadians with Disabilities
Chief Officer(s):
Bonnie Brayton, National Executive Director
Selma Kouidri, Coordinator, Inclusion
inclusion@dawncanada.net
Hanane Khales, Coordinator, Communications
communications@dawncanada.net

Doctors without Borders Canada (MSF) / Médecins sans frontières Canada (MSF-C)
#402, 720 Spadina Ave., Toronto ON M5S 2T9
Tel: 416-964-0619; *Fax:* 416-963-8707
Toll-Free: 800-982-7903
e-mail: msfcan@msf.ca
www.msf.ca
www.linkedin.com/company/6952
www.facebook.com/msf.english
twitter.com/MSF_Canada
www.youtube.com/user/MSFCanada
Also Known As: MSF Canada
Overview: A small national charitable organization founded in 1991
Mission: To offer assistance to populations in distress, to victims of natural or man-made disasters & to victims of armed conflict, without discrimination & irrespective of race, religion, creed or political affiliation
Chief Officer(s):
Heather Culbert, President
Stephen Cornish, Executive Director

Québec Office
#220, 1470, rue Peel, Montréal QC H3A 1T1
Tél: 514-845-5621; *Téléc:* 514-845-3707
Ligne sans frais: 866-878-5621
Courriel: msfqc@msf.ca

Evangelical Medical Aid Society Canada (EMAS)
1295 North Service Rd., Burlington ON L7R 4M2
Tel: 905-319-3415
Toll-Free: 866-648-0664
e-mail: info@emascanada.org
www.emascanada.org
www.facebook.com/EMASCANADA
twitter.com/emascanada
Overview: A medium-sized international charitable organization founded in 1948
Mission: To provide medical care for those in need in a Christlike manner
Chief Officer(s):
Peter Agwa, Executive Director
Ellen Watson, Director, Administration
ellen@emascanada.org
Publications:
• EMASsary [a publication of Evangelical Medical Aid Society Canada]
Type: Newsletter; *Editor:* Ellen Watson

Fédération de la santé et des services sociaux (FSSS)
1601, av de Lorimier, Montréal QC H2K 4M5
Tél: 514-598-2210; *Téléc:* 514-598-2223
www.fsss.qc.ca
www.facebook.com/FSSSCSN
twitter.com/FSSSCSN
www.youtube.com/user/f3scsn
Aperçu: *Dimension:* grande; *Envergure:* nationale

Mission: De promouvoir et sauvegarder la santé, la sécurité et les intérêts des personnes employées des établissements affiliés ou en voie d'affiliation; de représenter ses membres auprès de la Confédération des syndicats nationaux en lui soumettant toutes questions d'intérêt général; de représenter ses membres, de concert avec le CSN, partout où les intérêts généraux des travailleuses et travailleurs le justifient; d'aider à conclure, en faveur des syndicats affiliés, des conventions collectives de travail et en favoriser l'application; de collaborer à l'éducation des travailleuses et travailleurs et à la formation de responsables et militantes et militants syndicaux; d'assurer les services à ses syndicats affiliés; de favoriser et d'établir des liens inter-syndicaux avec les autres travailleuses et travailleurs dans le secteur public et para-public et dans le secteur privé du Québec et du Canada

Membre de: Confédération des syndicats nationaux

Membre(s) du bureau directeur:

Jeff Begley, Président
 jeff.begley@csn.qc.ca

Denyse Paradis, Secrétaire-trésorière
 denyse.paradis@csn.qc.ca

Federation of Medical Regulatory Authorities of Canada (FMRAC) / Fédération des ordres des médecins du Canada
#103, 2283 St. Laurent Blvd., Ottawa ON K1G 5A2

Tel: 613-738-0372; *Fax:* 613-738-9169
e-mail: info@fmrac.ca
www.fmrac.ca

Overview: A medium-sized national licensing organization founded in 1968

Mission: To provide a national structure for the provincial & territorial medical regulatory authorities; To present & pursue issues of common concern & interest; To share, consider, & develop positions on such matters

Chief Officer(s):

Fleur-Ange Lefebvre, Executive Director & CEO
 falefebvre@fmrac.ca

Federation of Medical Regulatory Authorities of Canada (FMRAC) / Fédération des ordres des médecins du Canada (FOMC)
1021 Thomas Spratt Pl., Ottawa ON K1G 5L5

Tel: 613-738-0372; *Fax:* 613-738-9169
e-mail: info@fmrac.ca
www.fmrac.ca
twitter.com/FMRAC_ca

Overview: A medium-sized national organization

Mission: To provide a national structure for the provincial & territorial medical regulatory authorities to present & pursue issues of common concerns & interest; To share, consider, & develop positions on such matters; To develop services & benefits for its members

Chief Officer(s):

Fleur-Ange Lefebvre, Executive Director & CEO
 falefebvre@fmrac.ca

Louise Auger, Director, Professional Affairs
 lauger@fmrac.ca

Kim MacDonald, Manager, Member Services
 kmacdonald@fmrac.ca

Federation of Medical Women of Canada (FMWC) / Fédération des femmes médecins du Canada
#170, 774 Prom. Echo Dr., Ottawa ON K1S 5N8

Tel: 613-569-5881; *Fax:* 613-249-3906
Toll-Free: 877-771-3777
e-mail: fmwcmain@fmwc.ca
www.fmwc.ca

Overview: A large national organization founded in 1924

Mission: Committed to the professional, social, & personal advancement of women physicians & to the promotion of the well-being of women in the medical profession & in society at large

Affiliation(s): Canadian Medical Association; Medical Women's International Association

Chief Officer(s):

Marnta Gautam, President

Health Action Network Society (HANS)
#214, 5589 Rumble Rd., Burnaby BC V5J 3J1

Tel: 604-435-0512; *Fax:* 604-435-1561
Toll-Free: 855-787-1891
e-mail: hans@hans.org
www.hans.org
www.facebook.com/HANSHealthAction
twitter.com/JoinHANS

Overview: A medium-sized national charitable organization founded in 1984

Mission: To support complementary & alternative health care; To provide resources about preventive medicine & natural therapeutics; To facilitate delivery of integrated health care; To act as a voice for natural health consumers in Canada

Chief Officer(s):

Lorna Hancock, Director

Health Care Public Relations Association (HCPRA) / Association des relations publiques des organismes de la santé (ARPOS)
PO Box 36029, 1106 Wellington St., Ottawa ON K1Y 4V3

Tel: 613-729-2102; *Fax:* 613-729-7708
e-mail: info@hcpra.org
www.hcpra.org
twitter.com/HCPRA

Overview: A medium-sized national organization founded in 1973

Mission: To address the concerns of the public relations professionals in Canadian health care settings

Affliation(s): Association for Healthcare Philanthropy

Chief Officer(s):

Jane Adams, National Coordinator

HealthCareCAN / SoinsSantéCAN
#100, 17 York St., Ottawa ON K1N 5S7

Tel: 613-241-8005; *Fax:* 613-241-5055
Toll-Free: 855-236-0213
e-mail: info@healthcarecan.ca
www.healthcarecan.ca
www.linkedin.com/company/1363724?trk=cws-btn-overview-0-0
www.facebook.com/healthcarecan.soinssantecan
twitter.com/healthcarecan

Merged from: Canadian Healthcare Association; Association of Canadian Academic Healthcare Organizations

Overview: A large national charitable organization

Mission: To improve the delivery of health services in Canada through policy development, advocacy & leadership

Affliation(s): American Hospital Association; Canadian Council on Health Services Accreditation

Chief Officer(s):

Bill Tholl, Presiden & Chief Executive Officer, 613-241-8005 Ext. 202
 btholl@healthcarecan.ca

Help Fill a Dream Foundation of Canada
4085 Quadra St., #D, Victoria BC V8X 1K5

Tel: 250-382-3135; *Fax:* 250-382-2711
Toll-Free: 866-382-2711
e-mail: contact@helpfilladream.com
helpfilladream.com
www.facebook.com/helpfilladream
twitter.com/helpfilladream

Overview: A small national charitable organization founded in 1986

Mission: To fill the dreams of children under 19 years of age who have life-threatening illness in BC

Chief Officer(s):

Craig Smith, Executive Director

Immunize Canada / Immunisation Canada
c/o Canadian Public Health Association, #404, 1525 Carling Ave., Ottawa ON K1Z 8R9

Tel: 613-725-3769; *Fax:* 613-725-9826
www.immunize.ca
www.facebook.com/ImmunizeCanada
twitter.com/immunizedotca
www.youtube.com/user/ImmunizeCanada

Previous Name: Canadian Coalition for Immunization Awareness & Promotion

Overview: A small national organization founded in 2004

Mission: To contribute to the control, elimination, & eradication of vaccine preventable diseases in Canada; To increase awareness of the benefits & risks of immunization for all ages

Chief Officer(s):
Shelly McNeil, Chair
Nicole Le Saux, Vice-Chair

Independent Living Canada (ILC) / Vie autonome Canada (VAC)
#1170, 343 Preston St., Ottawa ON K1S 1N4
Tel: 613-563-2581; *Fax:* 613-563-3861
e-mail: info@ilcanada.ca
www.ilcanada.ca
Previous Name: Canadian Association of Independent Living Centres
Overview: A medium-sized national charitable organization founded in 1986
Mission: To represent & coordinate the network of independent living centres; To guide & support independent living centres in the delivery of programs & services
Chief Officer(s):
Diane Kreuger, National Chair
Paula Sanders, Secretary
Publications:
• Independent Living Canada Annual Report
Type: Yearbook; *Frequency:* Annually
• The Perspective: The National Independent Living News Bulletin
Type: Newsletter
Profile: Organizational updates, current events, articles, social policy & research, & fundraising intiatives

Inner Peace Movement of Canada
PO Box 1138, Stn. B, Ottawa ON K1R 5R2
Tel: 613-238-7844
Toll-Free: 877-969-0095
www.innerpeacemovementptyltd.com
Overview: A small national organization founded in 1969
Mission: To promote self-help techniques by following 4 steps, each step providing tools to allow for a deeper self-awareness as a spiritual being

Institute for Optimizing Health Outcomes
#600, 151 Bloor St. West, Toronto ON M5S 1S4
Tel: 416-969-7431
www.optimizinghealth.org
Previous Name: Anemia Institute for Research & Education
Overview: A small national organization
Mission: Promotes patient-centred programs, education, research & advocacy to improve care & support for persons at risk for, or living with, health conditions (including, but not limited to, anemia)
Affliation(s): Ontario Patient Self-Management Network

Institute for Safe Medication Practices Canada (ISMP Canada)
#501, 4711 Yonge St., Toronto ON M2N 6K8
Tel: 416-733-3131; *Fax:* 416-733-1146
Toll-Free: 866-544-7672
e-mail: info@ismp-canada.org
www.ismp-canada.org
Overview: A medium-sized national organization
Mission: To promote medication safety in the healthcare industry; To analyze & provide information about safe medication practices; To conduct research on patient safety; To assess medication incidents for future prevention
Chief Officer(s):
Sylvia Hyland, Chief Operating Officer
Publications:
• ISMP Canada [Institute for Safe Medication Practices Canada] Safety Bulletin
Frequency: Monthly
Profile: Information on medication safety & medication incidents

KickStart Disability Arts & Culture
PO Box 2749, Stn. Terminal, Vancouver BC V6B 3X2
Tel: 604-559-6626
e-mail: info@kickstart-arts.ca
www.kickstart-arts.ca
www.facebook.com/318968627521
Previous Name: Society for Disability Arts & Culture
Overview: A small national organization founded in 1998
Mission: Kickstart's mission is to produce and present works by artists with disabilities and to promote artistic excellence among artists with disabilities working in a variety of disciplines.
Chief Officer(s):
Nisse Gustafson, Operations Director

Emma Kivisild, Artistic Director

McGill Centre for Medicine, Ethics & Law
McGill University, 3690, rue Peel, Montréal QC H3A 1W9
Tel: 514-398-7400; *Fax:* 514-398-4668
Overview: A small national organization founded in 1986
Mission: To undertake & promote research across the fields of health law & bioethics
Chief Officer(s):
Margaret Somerville, Founding Director
margaret.somerville@mcgill.ca

Médecins francophones du Canada
8355, boul Saint-Laurent, Montréal QC H2P 2Z6
Tél: 514-388-2228; *Téléc:* 514-388-5335
Ligne sans frais: 800-387-2228
www.medecinsfrancophones.ca
Nom précédent: Association des médecins de langue française du Canada
Aperçu: *Dimension:* moyenne; *Envergure:* nationale; fondée en 1902
Membre(s) du bureau directeur:
Marie-Françoise Mégie, Présidente
Céline Monette, Directrice générale

Medical Council of Canada (MCC) / Le Conseil médical du Canada (CMC)
#100, 2283 St. Laurent Blvd., Ottawa ON K1G 5A2
Tel: 613-521-6012; *Fax:* 613-521-9509
e-mail: service@mcc.ca
www.mcc.ca
www.linkedin.com/company/medical-council-of-canada
www.facebook.com/MedicalCouncilOfCanada
twitter.com/MedCouncilCan
www.youtube.com/user/medicalcouncilcanada
Overview: A large national licensing organization founded in 1912
Mission: To establish & promote a qualification in medicine, known as the Licentiate of the Medical Council of Canada, such that the holders thereof are acceptable to medical licensing authorities for the issuance of a licence to practise medicine
Chief Officer(s):
Ian Bowmer, Executive Director
Publications:
• The Echo
Type: Newsletter; *Frequency:* Bi-Annual

Medical Devices Canada
#900, 405 The West Mall, Toronto ON M9C 5J1
Tel: 416-620-1915
Toll-Free: 866-586-3332
www.medec.org
Also Known As: MEDEC
Previous Name: Canadian Association of Manufacturers of Medical Devices; Canada's Medical Device Technology Companies
Overview: A large national organization founded in 1973
Mission: To achieve a business & regulatory environment favourable to the growth of the industry & ensuring the availability of new cost-effective medical technologies that benefit Canadians
Chief Officer(s):
Paul Bradley, Chair
Brian Lewis, President & CEO
ceo@medec.org
Publications:
• Pulse
Type: Newsletter

Medical Group Management Association of Canada
102 Allen Cove, Hinton AB T7V 2A6
Tel: 780-865-7956
e-mail: info@mgmac.org
www.mgmac.org
Overview: A small national organization
Mission: To provide support for clinic managers across Canada
Chief Officer(s):
Tom Malone, President
Karen Chezick, Secretary

Meningitis Relief Canada
266 Thorndale Rd., Brampton ON L6P 3H2
Tel: 647-702-7447; *Fax:* 905-915-7434
e-mail: info@meningitisrelief.com
www.meningitisrelief.com
www.facebook.com/MeningitisReliefCanada
Overview: A small national charitable organization
Mission: To raise awareness of meningitis in Canada; To prevent deaths caused by meningitis; To provide support & services for individuals & families affected by meningitis
Chief Officer(s):
Furakh Mir, President

The Michener Institute for Applied Health Sciences
222 St. Patrick St., Toronto ON M5T 1V4
Tel: 416-596-3101
Toll-Free: 800-387-9066
e-mail: info@michener.ca
www.michener.ca
www.facebook.com/TheMichenerInstitute
twitter.com/michenerinst
www.youtube.com/user/TheMichenerInstitute
Previous Name: Toronto Institute of Medical Technology
Overview: A medium-sized national organization founded in 1967
Mission: To design, develop & deliver the best educational programs, products & services in applied health sciences
Affiliation(s): 170 hospitals, labs, & clinics across Canada
Chief Officer(s):
Cliff Nordal, Chair
President Adamson, President & CEO

National Association of Physical Activity & Health (NAPAH)
e-mail: info@napah.ca
www.napah.ca
Overview: A medium-sized national organization
Mission: Committed to empowering Canadians in acheiving optimum wellness through physical activity & healthy lifestyles; To networking & affiliating with a diversity of groups, organizations & volunteers who are strong advocates for public policies that support long-term physical activity programs as prevention to combat increasing rates of obesity, cancer, diabetes & cardiovascular disease

National Educational Association of Disabled Students (NEADS) / Association nationale des étudiant(e)s handicapé(e)s au niveau postsecondaire
Carleton University, Unicentre, #514, 1125 Colonel By Dr., Ottawa ON K1S 5B6
Tel: 613-380-8065; *Fax:* 613-369-4391
Toll-Free: 877-670-1256
e-mail: info@neads.ca
www.neads.ca
www.facebook.com/myNEADS
Overview: A small national organization founded in 1986
Mission: To encourage the self-empowerment of post-secondary students with disabilities; To advocate for increased accessibility at all levels so that disabled students may gain equal access to a college or university education; To provide an information resource base on services for disabled students nationwide according to a file of material from post-secondary institutions
Affiliation(s): Association québécoise des étudiant(e)s handicapé(e)s au post-secondaire; Council of Canadians with Disabilites
Chief Officer(s):
Frank Smith, National Coordinator, 613-380-8065 Ext. 201
frank.smith@neads.ca

National Health Union (NHU) / Syndicat national de la santé (SNS)
#1202, 233 Gilmour St., Ottawa ON K2P 0P2
Tel: 613-237-2732; *Fax:* 613-237-6954
Toll-Free: 888-545-6305
www.nhu-sns.ca
Overview: A medium-sized national organization overseen by Public Service Alliance of Canada (CLC)
Mission: To protect members by ensuring safe working conditions & fair wage rights & benefits
Chief Officer(s):
Tony Tilley, President

Occupational & Environmental Medical Association of Canada (OEMAC) / Association canadienne de la médecine du travail et de l'environnement (ACMTE)
#503, 386 Broadway, Winnipeg MB R3C 3R6
Toll-Free: 888-223-3808
e-mail: info@oemac.org
oemac.org
Overview: A medium-sized national organization founded in 1983
Mission: To act as the voice of the Canadian occupational & environmental medicine sector
Affiliation(s): Canadian Medical Association; Canadian Board of Occupational Medicine; Royal College of Physicians & Surgeons of Canada
Chief Officer(s):
Daniel Gouws, President
president@oemac.org
Jonathan Strauss, Executive Director
Melanie Tsouras, Coordinator, Programs & Services
mtsouras@oemac.org
Chantal Champagne, Event Manager
cchampagne@oemac.org
Publications:
• Liaison [a publication of the Occupational & Environmental Medical Association of Canada]
Type: Newsletter; *Frequency:* Quarterly

Orthotics Prosthetics Canada (OPC)
National Office, #202, 300 March Rd., Ottawa ON K2K 2E2
Tel: 613-595-1919; *Fax:* 613-595-1155
e-mail: info@opcanada.ca
www.opcanada.ca
Previous Name: Canadian Association of Prosthetists & Orthotists
Merged from: Can. Ass'n for Prosthetics & Orthotics; Can. Board for Certification of Prosthetists & Orthotists
Overview: A medium-sized national organization founded in 1955
Mission: To promote high standards of patient care & professionalism in the prosthetic & orthotic profession throughout Canada; To represent members with government, related organizations, & the general public
Chief Officer(s):
Dan Mead, President
Dana Cooper, Executive Director
dana@opcanada.ca

Paramedic Association of Canada
#201, 4 Florence St, Ottawa ON K2P 0W7
Tel: 613-836-6581; *Fax:* 613-836-6581
Toll-Free: 844-836-6581
e-mail: info@paramedic.ca
www.paramedic.ca
www.linkedin.com/company/3173844
www.facebook.com/PACParamedic
twitter.com/PAC_Paramedic
plus.google.com/b/114891282468589944660
Overview: A medium-sized national organization founded in 1988
Mission: To represent the public & practitioner nationally on health related paramedic issues; To lobby government & to speak to the media; To establish national communications network for all practitioners
Affliation(s): Ambulance Paramedics of British Columbia; Alberta College of Paramedics; Saskatchewan College of Paramedics; Paramedic Association of Manitoba; Ontario Paramedic Association; Association Professionnelle des Paramédics du Québec; Paramedic Association of New Brunswick; Paramedic Association of Newfoundland & Labrador
Chief Officer(s):
Chris Hood, President
Dwayne Forsman, Sec.-Treas.
Pierre Poirier, Executive Director

Patients Canada
PO Box 68, #2010, 65 Queen St. West, Toronto ON M5H 2M5
Tel: 416-900-2975
e-mail: communications@patientscanada.ca
www.patientscanada.ca
www.facebook.com/patientscanada
Previous Name: Patients' Association of Canada
Overview: A medium-sized national charitable organization

SECTION II:
General Resources

Mission: To bring changes & improvements to health care policy & delivery in Canada; To represent patients in health care decision-making
Chief Officer(s):
Michael Decter, Chair

People First of Canada (PFC) / Personnes d'abord du Canada
#5, 120 Maryland St., Winnipeg MB R3G 1L1
Tel: 204-784-7362; *Fax:* 204-784-7364
e-mail: info@peoplefirstofcanada.ca
www.peoplefirstofcanada.ca
www.facebook.com/PeopleFirstofCanada
twitter.com/PeopleFirstCA
www.youtube.com/user/PeopleFirstofCanada
Previous Name: National People First
Overview: A medium-sized national charitable organization founded in 1981
Mission: To educate the public on issues faced by persons with intellectual disabilities; To promote equality; To work toward the deinstitutionalization of persons with intellectual disabilities
Chief Officer(s):
Shelley Fletcher, Executive Director
  sfletcher@peoplefirstofcanada.ca

Physical & Health Education Canada / Éducation physique et santé Canada
#301, 2197 Riverside Dr., Ottawa ON K1H 7X3
Tel: 613-523-1348; *Fax:* 613-523-1206
Toll-Free: 800-663-8708
e-mail: info@phecanada.ca
www.phecanada.ca
www.facebook.com/PHECanada
twitter.com/PHECanada
Also Known As: PHE Canada
Previous Name: Canadian Physical Education Association; Canadian Association for Health, Physical Education, Recreation, & Dance
Overview: A large national charitable organization founded in 1933
Mission: To promote quality school health programs & the healthy development of Canadian children & youth
Chief Officer(s):
Fran Harris, President
Chris Jones, Executive Director & CEO, 613-523-1348 Ext. 224
  Chris@phecanada.ca
Jodie Lyn-Harrison, Chief Administrative Officer, 613-523-1348 Ext. 223
  Jodie@phecanada.ca
Stephanie Talsma, Program Manager, 613-523-1348 Ext. 236
  Stephanie@phecanada.ca
Publications:
• In Touch Newsletter [a publication of the Physical & Health Education Canada]
Type: Newsletter
• phénEPS-PHEnex Journal [a publication of the Physical & Health Education Canada]
Type: Journal
Profile: Research, position papers, reviews & critical essays
• Physical & Health Education Journal
Type: Journal; *Frequency:* Quarterly
Profile: School physical education programs, quality school health programs, ready-to-use activities, resource reviews, & teaching strategies

---

Quintiles IMS Canada
16720 Route Transcanadienne, Kirkland QC H9H 5M3
Tel: 514-428-6000; *Fax:* 514-428-6086
www.quintileims.com
Previous Name: IMS Health Canada
Overview: A small national organization founded in 1960
Mission: To provide business intelligence & strategic consulting services for the pharmaceutical & health care industries
Chief Officer(s):
Murray Aitken, Executive Director

Radiation Safety Institute of Canada / Institut de radioprotection du Canada
Head Office & National Education Centre, #300, 165 Avenue Rd., Toronto ON M5R 3S4
Tel: 416-650-9090; *Fax:* 416-650-9920
Toll-Free: 800-263-5803
e-mail: info@radiationsafety.ca
www.radiationsafety.ca
www.linkedin.com/company/radiation-safety-institute-of-canada
www.facebook.com/143472245714096
twitter.com/RSICanada
Previous Name: Canadian Institute for Radiation Safety
Overview: A medium-sized national charitable organization founded in 1981
Mission: To be an independent source for knowledge about radiation safety in the environment, the community, & the workplace
Chief Officer(s):
Steve Horvath, President & Chief Executive Officer
Laura Boksman, Chief Scientist
Bruce Sylvester, Chief Financial Officer
Natalia Mozayani, Executive Director
Tara Hargreaves, Scientist & Coordinator, Training
Maria Costa, Administrative Assistant, Communications

  National Laboratories
  #102, 110 Research Dr., Saskatoon SK S7N 3R3
  Tel: 306-975-0566; *Fax:* 306-975-0494
  www.radiationsafety.ca

Resident Doctors of Canada (RDoC)
#412, 151 Slater St., Ottawa ON K1P 5H3
Tel: 613-234-6448; *Fax:* 613-234-5292
e-mail: communications@residentdoctors.ca
www.residentdoctors.ca
www.facebook.com/ResidentDoctorsCAN
twitter.com/residentdoctors
Previous Name: Canadian Association of Internes & Residents
Overview: A medium-sized national organization founded in 1973
Mission: To improve the quality of medical education & professionalism for resident physicians in Canada
Affliation(s): Royal College of Physicians & Surgeons of Canada; College of Family Physicians of Canada; Canadian Medical Association; Federation of Medical Licensing Authorities of Canada
Chief Officer(s):
Kimberly Williams, President
Irving Gold, Executive Director
  irving@residentdoctors.ca
Todd Coopee, Manager, Communications
  tcoopee@residentdoctors.ca
Maryan McCarrey, Manager, Policy & Research
  mmccarrey@residentdoctors.ca
Publications:
• Resident Doctors of Canada Annual Report
Type: Report; *Frequency:* Annually

The Royal College of Physicians & Surgeons of Canada (RCPSC) / Le Collège royal des médecins et chirurgiens du Canada (CRMCC)
774 Echo Dr., Ottawa ON K1S 5N8
Tel: 613-730-8177; *Fax:* 613-730-8830
Toll-Free: 800-668-3740
e-mail: feedback@royalcollege.ca
www.royalcollege.ca
www.facebook.com/TheRoyalCollege
twitter.com/Royal_College
Overview: A large national charitable organization founded in 1929
Mission: To oversee the medical education of specialists in Canada; To set the highest standards in postgraduate medical education, through national certification examinations & lifelong learning programs; To promote sound health policy
Affliation(s): Canadian Medical Association; College of Family Physicians of Canada; Association of Canadian Medical Colleges; National Specialty Societies; Federation of Medical Licensing Authorities of Canada
Chief Officer(s):
Andrew Padmos, CEO

SIGMA Canadian Menopause Society
#103, 1089 West Broadway, Vancouver BC V6H 1E5
Tel: 604-736-7267
e-mail: info@sigmamenopause.com
www.sigmamenopause.com
twitter.com/sigmamenopause
Overview: A medium-sized national organization founded in 2008
Mission: To act as a group of family physicians, specialists &
healthcare professionals interested in menopausal & postmenopausal
health; To provide educational initiatives & information services to
women going through menopause, in order to advance women's health
Chief Officer(s):
Elaine Jolly, OC, MD, FRCSC, President
Christine Derzko, MD, FRCS(C), Vice-President
Nesé Yuksel, B.Sc.Pharm, Pha, Secretary
Michael Fortier, MD, FRCS(C), Treasurer
Chui Kin Yuen, MD, FRCS(C), FA, Executive Director

Société Santé en français (SSF)
#223, rue Main, #L396, Ottawa ON K1S 1C4
Tél: 613-244-1889; *Téléc:* 613-244-0283
Courriel: info@santefrancais.ca
www.santefrancais.ca
www.linkedin.com/company/soci-t-sant-en-fran-ais
www.facebook.com/santefrancais
twitter.com/santefrancais
Aperçu: *Dimension:* moyenne; *Envergure:* nationale; fondée en 2002
surveillé par Fédération des communautés francophones et acadienne
du Canada
Mission: Pour améliorer l'accès et la qualité des services de soins de
santé en français au Canada
Affiliation(s): Réseau de santé en français de
Terre-Neuve-et-Labrador; Réseau Santé en français I.-P.-É; Réseau
Santé - Nouvelle-Écosse; Réseau-action Communautaire;
Réseau-action Formation et recherche; Réseau-action Organisation
des services; Société Santé et Mieux-être en français du
Nouveau-Brunswick; Réseau francophone de santé du Nord de
l'Ontario; Réseau santé en français du Moyen-Nord de l'Ontario;
Réseau franco-santé du Sud de l'Ontario; Réseau des services de
santé en français de l'Est de l'Ontario; Conseil communauté en santé
du Manitoba; Réseau Santé en français de la Saskatchewan
Membre(s) du bureau directeur:
Aurel Schofield, Président
Michel Tremblay, Directeur général, 613-244-1889 Ext. 230
m.tremblay@santefrancais.ca

Society of Obstetricians & Gynaecologists of Canada (SOGC) /
Société des obstétriciens et gynécologues du Canada
780 Echo Dr., Ottawa ON K1S 5R7
Tel: 613-730-4192; *Fax:* 613-730-4314
Toll-Free: 800-561-2416
e-mail: info@sogc.org
www.sogc.org
www.facebook.com/sogc.org
twitter.com/SOGCorg
Overview: A medium-sized national organization founded in 1944
Mission: To promote excellence in the practice of obstetrics &
gynaecology; To produce national clinical guidelines for medical
education on women's health issues; To promote optimal,
comprehensive women's health care
Chief Officer(s):
George Carson, President
Jennifer Blake, Chief Executive Officer
Publications:
• Health News [a publication of the Society of Obstetricians &
Gynaecologists of Canada]
Type: Newsletter
Profile: SOGC media reports & health news
• Healthy Beginnings [a publication of the Society of Obstetricians &
Gynaecologists of Canada]
Profile: A guide to pregnancy & childbirth
• Journal of Obstetrics & Gynaecology Canada (JOGC)
Type: Journal; *Frequency:* Monthly; *Price:* Free with membership in the
Society ofObstetricians & Gynaecologists of Canada
Profile: A peer-reviewed journal of obstetrics, gynaecology, & women's
health, featuring original research articles,case reports, & reviews

• Sex Sense [a publication of the Society of Obstetricians &
Gynaecologists of Canada]
Profile: A guide to contraception
• SOGC [Society of Obstetricians & Gynaecologists of Canada] News
Type: Newsletter; *Frequency:* 10 pa
Profile: Society work & events, plus information about recent legislation
& developments in women's health care
• What You Should Know About The Society of Obstetricians &
Gynaecologists of Canada

Society of Rural Physicians of Canada (SRPC) / Société de la
médecine rurale du Canada
PO Box 893, 269 Main St., Shawville QC J0X 2Y0
Fax: 819-647-2485
Toll-Free: 877-276-1949
e-mail: info@srpc.ca
www.srpc.ca
Overview: A small national organization founded in 1993
Mission: To provide equitable medical care for rural communities; to
provide sustainable working conditions for rural physicians
Affiliation(s): Canadian Medical Association; World Organization of
Rural Doctors
Chief Officer(s):
John Soles, President
Lee Teperman, Administrative Officer

Society of Toxicology of Canada (STC) / Société de toxicologie du
Canada
PO Box 55094, Montréal QC H3G 2W5
e-mail: stcsecretariat@mcgill.ca
www.stcweb.ca
www.facebook.com/societyoftoxicologyofcanada
Overview: A medium-sized national organization founded in 1964
Mission: To promote acquisition, facilitate dissemination & encourage
utilization of knowledge in the science of toxicology
Affliation(s): Canadian Federation of Biological Societies; International
Union of Toxicology
Chief Officer(s):
Mike Wade, President
Veronica Atehortua, Information Executive Secretary

Sport Physiotherapy Canada (SPC)
#75, 2192 Queen St. East, Toronto ON M4E 1E6
Tel: 647-722-3461
e-mail: info@sportphysio.ca
www.sportphysio.ca
www.facebook.com/sportphysiocanada
twitter.com/sportphysiocan
www.youtube.com/user/physiotherapycan
Previous Name: Sport Physiotherapy Division of the Canadian
Physiotherapy Association
Overview: A small national organization founded in 1972
Mission: To promote professional development of members; To
ensure high-quality health care for Canada's athletes
Member of: Canadian Physiotherapy Association; Sport Medicine
Council of Canada
Chief Officer(s):
Ashley Lewis, Executive Director
alewis@sportphysio.ca
Ereka Roach, Coordinator, Member Services
program@sportphysio.ca

Tetra Society of North America
#318, 425 Carrall St., Vancouver BC V6B 6E3
Tel: 604-688-6464; *Fax:* 604-688-6463
Toll-Free: 877-688-8762
www.tetrasociety.org
Overview: A small national charitable organization founded in 1992
Mission: To link volunteer engineers & technicians with persons with
disabilities to create custom assistive devices to help them achieve
greater independence
Member of: Sam Sullivan Disability Foundation, Volunteer Vancouver
Chief Officer(s):
Pat Tweedie, National Coordinator, Program
ptweedie@tetrasociety.org
Eric Molendyk, Coordinator, BC Chapter
eric@tetrasociety.org
Matthew Wild, Coordinator, Communications
matthew@disabilityfoundation.org

Thalidomide Victims Association of Canada (TVAC) / Association canadienne des victimes de la thalidomide (ACVT)
#102, 7744 Sherbrooke St. East, Montréal QC H1L 1A1
Tel: 514-355-0811; *Fax:* 514-355-0860
Toll-Free: 877-355-0811
e-mail: tvac.acvt@sympatico.ca
www.thalidomide.ca
Overview: A medium-sized national charitable organization founded in 1988
Mission: To monitor the drug thalidomide & to meet the needs of thalidomide survivors; To empower & enhance the quality of life of Canadians living with the effects of thalidomide
Affiliation(s): Council of Canadians with Disabilities; Canadian Centre for Philanthropy
Chief Officer(s):
Mercedes Benegbi, Executive Director

Vaccination Risk Awareness Network Inc. (VRAN)
PO Box 169, Winlaw BC V0G 2J0
e-mail: info@vaccinechoicecanada.com
www.vran.org
www.facebook.com/330700720307290
twitter.com/vran_canada
Overview: A small national organization
Mission: To provide information about the potential risks & side-effects of vaccines; To foster a multi-disciplinary approach to child & family health; To uphold the right of persons to exercise informed consent
Publications:
• Vaccination Risk Awareness Network Newsletter
Type: Newsletter; *Frequency:* 3 pa; *Price:* Free with membership in the Vaccination Risk Awareness Network
Profile: Information about the educational & outreach work of the organization

Vecova Centre for Disability Services & Research
3304 - 33 St. NW, Calgary AB T2L 2A6
Tel: 403-284-1121; *Fax:* 403-284-1146
e-mail: info@vecova.ca
www.vecova.ca
www.linkedin.com/company/vecova
www.facebook.com/Vecova
twitter.com/Vecova
www.youtube.com/user/Vecovadisability
Previous Name: Vocational & Rehabilitation Research Institute
Overview: A large national charitable organization founded in 1966
Mission: To be leaders in innovative services & research that support persons with disabilities to live as contributing & valued members of the community
Member of: Alberta Association of Rehabilitation Centres
Affiliation(s): University of Calgary
Chief Officer(s):
John Lee, CEO
Neil MacKenzie, Chair

Welcome Friend Association (WFA)
PO Box 242, 76 Dawson St., Thessalon ON P0R 1L0
Fax: 705-998-2612
Toll-Free: 888-909-2234
Other Communication: rainbowcamp.ca
e-mail: info@welcomefriend.ca
www.welcomefriend.ca
www.facebook.com/welcomefriendassociation
twitter.com/WelcomeFriend
Overview: A medium-sized national organization founded in 2009
Mission: To educate & promote awareness in society regarding gender, sexual identities, & expressions; To support individuals facing gender & sexual issues; To increase understanding of the queer community; To work towards a society that includes & respects all persons regardless of gender or sexual orientation
Chief Officer(s):
Harry Stewart, Chair
hstewart@welcomefriend.ca

YWCA Canada / Association des jeunes femmes chrétiennes du Canada
104 Edward St., 1st Fl., Toronto ON M5G 0A7
Tel: 416-962-8881; *Fax:* 416-962-8084
e-mail: national@ywcacanada.ca
www.ywcacanada.ca
www.facebook.com/ywcacanada
twitter.com/YWCA_Canada
www.instagram.com/ywcacanada
Also Known As: Young Women's Christian Association of Canada
Overview: A large national charitable organization founded in 1893
Mission: To coordinate the YWCA movement in Canada, & advocate for the equity & equality rights of women; To raise awareness on the prevention of violence against women, and the need for universal, accessible and quality child care
Affiliation(s): Selective: Canadian Policy Research Network; National Council of Women; National Youth Serving Organizations; Women's Future Fund; Canadian Centre for Philanthropy; National Action Committee on the Status of Women
Chief Officer(s):
Paulette Senior, Chief Executive Officer
Ann Decter, Director, Advocacy & Public Policy
adecter@ywcacanada.ca
Raine Liliefeldt, Director, Membership Services & Development
rliliefeldt@ywcacanada.ca

Community YWCA of Muskoka
440 Ecclestone Dr., Bracebridge ON P1L 1Z6
Tel: 705-645-9827; *Fax:* 705-645-4804
www.ywcamuskoka.com
www.facebook.com/muskoka.yw
twitter.com/YWCAMuskoka
Chief Officer(s):
Hannah Lin, Executive Director

YWCA Niagara Region
183 King St., St Catharines ON L2R 3J5
Tel: 905-988-3528; *Fax:* 905-988-3739
e-mail: info@ywcaniagararegion.ca
www.ywcaniagararegion.ca
www.facebook.com/YWCANiagaraRegion
twitter.com/YWCA_Niagara
Chief Officer(s):
Elisabeth Zimmermann, Executive Director
ezimmermann@ywcaniagararegion.ca

YWCA Northeast Avalon
PO Box 21291, St. John's NL A1A 5G6
Tel: 709-726-9622; *Fax:* 709-576-0410
www.ynortheastavalon.com
www.linkedin.com/groups?about=&gid=1903327
www.facebook.com/pages/YMCA-of-Northeast-Avalon/348363604436
twitter.com/YMCAofNEA
Chief Officer(s):
Jason Brown, CEO/President
jbrown@ynortheastavalon.com

YWCA of Banff
PO Box 520, 102 Spray Ave., Banff AB T1L 1A6
Tel: 403-762-3560; *Fax:* 403-762-3204
e-mail: info@ywcabanff.ca
www.ywcabanff.ab.ca
www.facebook.com/YWCABanff
twitter.com/ywcabanff
Chief Officer(s):
Connie MacDonald, Executive Director

YWCA of Brandon
148 - 11th St., Brandon MB R7A 4J4
Tel: 204-571-3680; *Fax:* 204-571-3687
e-mail: ywca2@wcgwave.ca
www.ywcabrandon.com
www.facebook.com/YWCABrandon
twitter.com/YWCABrandon
Chief Officer(s):
Karen Peto, Executive Director
kpeto@wcgwave.ca

YWCA of Calgary

320 - 5th Ave. SE, Calgary AB T2G 0E5
Tel: 403-263-1550; *Fax:* 403-263-4681; *Crisis Hot-Line:* 403-266-0707
e-mail: communications@ywcaofcalgary.com
www.ywcaofcalgary.com
www.facebook.com/pages/YWCA-of-Calgary/10150115104400262
twitter.com/ywcaofcalgary
www.youtube.com/ywcaofcalgary

Chief Officer(s):
Sue Tomney, Chief Executive Officer

YWCA of Durham
33 McGrigor St., Oshawa ON L1H 1X8
Tel: 905-576-6356; *Fax:* 905-576-0816
www.ywcadurham.org

Chief Officer(s):
Kim Beatty, President

YWCA of Edmonton
Empire Building, #400, 10080 Jasper Ave., Edmonton AB T5J 1V9
Tel: 780-423-9922; *Fax:* 780-488-6077
e-mail: information@ywcaofedmonton.org
www.ywcaofedmonton.org
www.facebook.com/pages/YWCA-Edmonton/109755395744949
twitter.com/ywcaedmonton
www.flickr.com/photos/ywcaedmonton

Chief Officer(s):
Hilary Anaka, President

YWCA of Guelph
130 Woodland Glen Dr., Guelph ON N1G 4M3
Tel: 519-824-5150; *Fax:* 519-824-4729
e-mail: contact@guelphy.org
www.guelphy.org
www.facebook.com/pages/YMCA-YWCA-of-Guelph/306629139364333
twitter.com/YGuelph

Chief Officer(s):
Jim Bonk, CEO
jim_bonk@ymca.ca

YWCA of Halifax
1239 Barrington St., Halifax NS B3J 1Y2
Tel: 902-423-6162; *Fax:* 902-444-3568
www.ywcahalifax.com
www.facebook.com/ywcahalifax
twitter.com/YWCAHalifax
www.youtube.com/user/YWCAHalifax

Chief Officer(s):
Miia Suokonautio, Executive Director
m.suokonautio@ywcahalifax.com

YWCA of Hamilton
75 MacNab St. South, Hamilton ON L8P 3C1
Tel: 905-522-9922
www.ywcahamilton.org
www.facebook.com/YWCAHamilton

Chief Officer(s):
Denise Christopherson, Chief Executive Officer
dchristopherson@ywcahamilton.org

YWCA of Kitchener-Waterloo
153 Frederick St., Kitchener ON N2H 2M2
Tel: 519-576-8856; *Fax:* 519-576-0129
e-mail: general@ywcakw.on.ca
www.ywcakw.on.ca
www.facebook.com/ywcakw
twitter.com/YWCA_KW

Chief Officer(s):
Tracy Van Kalsbeek, President

YWCA of Lethbridge & District
604 - 8th St. South, Lethbridge AB T1J 2K1
Tel: 403-329-0088; *Fax:* 403-327-9112; *Crisis Hot-Line:* 403-320-1881
e-mail: inquiries@ywcalethbridge.org
www.ywcalethbridge.org
www.facebook.com/pages/YWCA-of-Lethbridge-and-District/21516367559

Chief Officer(s):
Kristine Cassie, CEO

YWCA of Moncton

#T310, 22 Church St., Moncton NB E1C 0P7
Tel: 506-855-4349; *Fax:* 506-855-3320
e-mail: info@ywcamoncton.com
www.ywcamoncton.com
www.facebook.com/ywcamoncton
twitter.com/ywcamoncton
www.ywcamoncton.tumblr.com

Chief Officer(s):
Jewell Mitchell, Executive Director
jmitchell@ywcamoncton.com

YWCA of Montréal
1355, boul René-Lévesque Ouest, Montréal QC H3G 1T3
Tel: 514-866-9941; *Fax:* 514-866-4866
e-mail: info@ydesfemmesmtl.org
www.ydesfemmesmtl.org
www.linkedin.com/company/fondation-y-des-femmes-de-montr-al
www.facebook.com/pages/Le-Y-des-femmes-de-Montreal/122110488922
twitter.com/YWCA_mtl
www.youtube.com/user/YWCAMTL

Chief Officer(s):
Hélène Lépine, Présidente-directrice générale

YWCA of Peterborough, Victoria & Haliburton
216 Simcoe St., Peterborough ON K9H 2H7
Tel: 705-743-3526; *Fax:* 705-745-4654; *TTY:* 705-743-4015; *Crisis Hot-Line:* 800-461-7656
e-mail: info@ywcapeterborough.org
www.ywcapeterborough.org
www.facebook.com/ywcapeterborough
twitter.com/YWCAPtbo

Chief Officer(s):
Lynn Zimmer, Executive Director
lzimmer@ywcapeterborough.org

YWCA of Pictou County
2756 Westville Rd., RR#3, New Glasgow NS B2H 5C6
Tel: 902-752-0202; *Fax:* 902-755-3446
e-mail: frontdesk@pcymca.ca
www.pcymca.ca
www.facebook.com/YMCAPictouCounty

Chief Officer(s):
Dave MacIntyre, Chief Executive Officer

YWCA of Prince Albert
1895 Central Ave., Prince Albert SK S6V 4W8
Tel: 306-763-8571; *Fax:* 306-763-8165
ywcaprincealbert.ca

Chief Officer(s):
Donna Brooks, Chief Executive Officer
donnabrooks.ywca@sasktel.net

YWCA of Regina
1940 McIntyre St., Regina SK S4P 2R3
Tel: 306-525-2141; *Fax:* 306-525-2171
e-mail: ywcaregina@ywcaregina.com
www.ywcaregina.com

Chief Officer(s):
Deanna Elias-Henry, Executive Director
deanna@ywcaregina.com

YWCA of Saint John
130 Broadview Ave., Saint John NB E2L 5C5
Tel: 506-693-9622; *Fax:* 506-634-4180
www.saintjohny.com
www.facebook.com/SaintJohnY
twitter.com/Y_SaintJohn

Chief Officer(s):
Shilo Boucher, CEO/President

YWCA of St. Thomas Elgin
16 Mary St. West, St Thomas ON N5P 2S3
Tel: 519-631-9800; *Fax:* 519-631-6411
Toll-Free: 800-461-0954
e-mail: ywcastthomaselgin@bellnet.ca
www.ywcastthomaselgin.org
www.facebook.com/pages/YWCA-St-Thomas-Elgin/174545902575534
twitter.com/YWCAStThomas

Chief Officer(s):

Marla Champion, Executive Director

YWCA of Saskatoon
510 - 25th St. East, Saskatoon SK S7K 4A7
Tel: 306-244-0944; *Fax:* 306-653-2468
e-mail: info@ywcasaskatoon.com
www.ywcasaskatoon.com
www.facebook.com/ywcasaskatoon
twitter.com/YWCASaskatoon

Chief Officer(s):
Deb Parker-Loewen, President

YWCA of Sudbury
370 St. Raphael St., Sudbury ON P3B 4K7
Tel: 705-673-4754; *Fax:* 705-688-1727
ywcasudbury.ca

Chief Officer(s):
Marlene Gorman, Executive Director
m.gorman@ywcasudbury.ca

YWCA of Thompson
39 Nickel Rd., Thompson MB R8N 0Y5
Tel: 204-778-6341; *Fax:* 204-778-5308
www.ywcathompson.ca
www.facebook.com/pages/YWCA-Thompson/282578048442942

Chief Officer(s):
Elaine McGregor, Executive Director
ywcaexdir@mymts.net

YWCA of Vancouver
535 Hornby St., Vancouver BC V6C 2E8
Tel: 250-895-5800
e-mail: enquire@ywcavan.org
www.ywcavan.org
www.linkedin.com/company/ywca-metro-vancouver
www.facebook.com/pages/YWCA-Vancouver/268163004562
twitter.com/YWCAVAN
www.youtube.com/user/YWCAVancouver

Chief Officer(s):
Janet Austin, CEO

YWCA of Western Ontario
382 Waterloo St., London ON N6B 2N8
Tel: 519-667-3306; *Fax:* 519-433-8527
www.ymcawo.ca
www.facebook.com/CentreBranchYMCALondon
twitter.com/yourYMCAWO
www.youtube.com/mylondony

Chief Officer(s):
Shaun Elliott, CEO

YWCA of Winnipeg
3550 Portage Ave., Winnipeg MB R3K 0Z8
Tel: 204-947-3044
www.ywinnipeg.ca
www.facebook.com/ywinnipeg
twitter.com/YWinnipeg
www.youtube.com/user/YWinnipeg

Chief Officer(s):
Kent Paterson, President & CEO

YWCA of Yellowknife
PO Box 1679, Yellowknife NT X1A 2P3
Tel: 867-920-2777; *Fax:* 867-873-9406
e-mail: info@ywcanwt.ca
www.ywcanwt.ca
www.facebook.com/122130201165447
twitter.com/YWCAYK

Chief Officer(s):
Lyda Fuller, Executive Director

YWCA Québec
855, av Holland, Québec QC G1S 3S5
Tél: 418-683-2155; *Téléc:* 418-683-5526
Courriel: info@ywcaquebec.qc.ca
www.ywcaquebec.qc.ca
www.facebook.com/ywcaquebec
twitter.com/ywcaqc

Chief Officer(s):
Katia de Pokomandy-Morin, Directrice générale
directiongenerale@ywcaquebec.qc.ca

YWCA Toronto
87 Elm St., Toronto ON M5G OA8
Tel: 416-961-8100; *Fax:* 416-961-7739
Toll-Free: 888-843-9922
e-mail: info@ywcatoronto.org
www.ywcatoronto.org
www.facebook.com/pages/YWCA-Toronto/29472659546
twitter.com/YWCAToronto

Chief Officer(s):
Heather McGregor, CEO

YWCAs of Cambridge & Kitchener-Waterloo
#203, 460 Frederick St., Kitchener ON N2H 2P5
Tel: 519-584-7479; *Fax:* 519-576-6223
e-mail: info@ckwymca.ca
www.ymcacambridgekw.ca
www.linkedin.com/company/ymcas-of-cambridge-&-kitchener-waterloo
www.facebook.com/YMCAsofCandKW
twitter.com/ymcasofcandkw
www.youtube.com/YMCAsofCandKW

Chief Officer(s):
John Haddock, Chief Executive Officer

Provincial Associations

ALBERTA

Alberta Association of Rehabilitation Centres (AARC)
#19, 3220 - 5 Ave. NE, Calgary AB T2A 5N1
Tel: 403-250-9495; *Fax:* 403-291-9864
e-mail: acds@acds.ca
www.acds.ca

Overview: A medium-sized provincial organization founded in 1972
Mission: To support organizations that provide services & supports to people with disabilities; To act as a voice for the field of community rehabilitation to the political & administrative arms of government; To focus on human resource initiatives for the services sector; To provide in-service training opportunities for people employed in the field; To accredit & certify service in Alberta
Chief Officer(s):
Ann Nicol, CEO, 403-250-9495 Ext. 238
Helen Ficocelli, President
Bob Diewold, Vice-President

Alberta College of Medical Diagnostic & Therapeutic Technologists
#800, 4445 Calgary Trail NW, Edmonton AB T6H 5R7
Tel: 780-487-6130; *Fax:* 780-432-9106
Toll-Free: 800-282-2165
e-mail: info@acmdtt.com
acmdtt.com
twitter.com/acmdtt

Also Known As: ACMDTT
Previous Name: Alberta Association of Medical Radiation Technologists
Overview: A medium-sized provincial organization founded in 2004 overseen by Canadian Association of Medical Radiation Technologists
Mission: To act in accordance with the Province of Alberta Health Professions Act, Medical Diagnostic & Therapeutic Technologists Profession Regulation, & by the ACMDTT Bylaws; To abide by & promote ethical practice as described in the ACMDTT Code of Ethics for diagnostic & therapeutic professionals; To promote standards of practice within the discipline; To advance the profession in Alberta; To ensure that the public receives safe & ethical diagnostic & therapeutic care
Member of: Alliance of Medical Radiation Technologists Regulators of Canada; Alberta Federation of Regulated Health Professions; Canadian National Network of the Profession of Medical Radiological Technology; Canadian Association of Medical Radiation Technologists
Chief Officer(s):
Karen Stone, Chief Executive Officer & Registrar
kstone@acmdtt.com
Pree Tyagi, Deputy Registrar
ptyagi@acmdtt.com
Publications:
• Alberta College of Medical Diagnostic & Therapeutic Technologists Annual Report
Type: Yearbook; *Frequency:* Annually

Profile: A yearly report on the activities of the College, including complaints, hearings, & appeals, & audited financial information
• Alberta College of Medical Diagnostic & Therapeutic Technologists Member Directory
Type: Directory
• Internal Matters [a publication of the Alberta College of Medical Diagnostic & Therapeutic Technologists]
Type: Newsletter; *Frequency:* Quarterly
Profile: Updates from the College, including branch, education, & awards information

Alberta College of Paramedics (ACP)
#220, 2755 Broadmoor Blvd., Sherwood Park AB T8H 2W7
Tel: 780-449-3114; *Fax:* 780-417-6911
Toll-Free: 877-351-2267
e-mail: acp@collegeofparamedics.org
www.collegeofparamedics.org
Overview: A small provincial licensing organization
Mission: To carry out operations in accordance with the Health Disciplines Act; to govern & regulate the practice of paramedicine in Alberta; to maintain & enforce the Code of Ethics, to ensure safe & ethical care for Alberta's citizens; to establish & enforce standards of practice for the profession, to ensure competent care for the protection of the public interest
Chief Officer(s):
Sheldon Thunstrom, President
Tim Essington, Registrar/Executive Director
tim.essington@collegeofparamedics.org
Becky Donelon, Deputy Registrar
becky.donelon@collegeofparamedics.org
Carl Damour, Manager, Education & Equivalency
carl.damour@collegeofparamedics.org
Becky Donelon, Manager, Continuing Education & Standards
becky.donelon@collegeofparamedics.org
Heather Verbaas, Manager, Communications
heather.verbaas@collegeofparamedics.org
Bill Carstairs, Manager, Finance, 780-410-4138
bill.carstairs@collegeofparamedics.org
Publications:
• Alberta College of Paramedics Annual Report
Type: Yearbook; *Frequency:* Annually
• Alberta College of Paramedics Continuing Competency Program Handbook
Type: Handbook
• Emergency Medical Dialogue (EMD)
Frequency: 3 pa
Profile: Alberta College of Paramedics updates from the pre-hospital field, for practitioners
• The Pulse: News from the Alberta College of Paramedics
Type: Newsletter; *Frequency:* Monthly
Profile: Updates & announcements for the Emergency Medical Services profession

Alberta Committee of Citizens with Disabilities (ACCD)
#106, 10423 - 178 St. NW, Edmonton AB T5S 1R5
Tel: 780-488-9088; *Fax:* 780-488-3757
Toll-Free: 800-387-2514
e-mail: accd@accd.net
www.accd.net
www.facebook.com/accdisabilities
twitter.com/accdisabilities
Overview: A medium-sized provincial charitable organization founded in 1973
Mission: To promote full participation in society for Albertans with disabilities
Member of: Alberta Disability Forum
Affliation(s): Council of Canadians with Disabilities
Chief Officer(s):
Beverley D. Matthiessen, Executive Director

Alberta Medical Association (AMA)
12230 - 106 Ave. NW, Edmonton AB T5N 3Z1
Tel: 780-482-2626; *Fax:* 780-482-5445
Toll-Free: 800-272-9680
e-mail: amamail@albertadoctors.org
www.albertadoctors.org
www.linkedin.com/company/alberta-medical-association
www.facebook.com/AlbertaMedicalAssociation
twitter.com/Albertadoctors
www.youtube.com/user/ABMedAssoc
Overview: A medium-sized provincial organization founded in 1905 overseen by Canadian Medical Association
Mission: To advocate on behalf of its physician members; to provide leadership & support for their role in the provision of quality health care
Chief Officer(s):
Richard Johnston, President
Michael A. Gormley, Executive Director
mike.gormley@albertadoctors.org
Cameron N. Plitt, Chief Financial Officer
cameron.plitt@albertadoctors.org

Alberta Public Health Association (APHA)
c/o Injury Prevention Centre, University of Alberta, #4075 RTF, 8308 - 114 St., Edmonton AB T6G 2E1
e-mail: apha.comm@gmail.com
www.apha.ab.ca
Overview: A medium-sized provincial charitable organization founded in 1943 overseen by Canadian Public Health Association
Mission: To protect public health through advocacy, partnerships, & education
Chief Officer(s):
Lindsay McLaren, President

Alberta Society of Radiologists (ASR)
#220, 10339 - 124th St., Edmonton AB T5N 3W1
Tel: 780-443-2615
www.radiologists.ab.ca
Overview: A small provincial organization founded in 1957
Mission: To represent radiologists & radiology residents in Alberta
Chief Officer(s):
Chris Hayduk, Executive Director
execdir@radiologists.ab.ca

Christian Health Association of Alberta (CHAA)
PO Box 4173, 132 Warwick Rd., Edmonton AB T6E 4P8
Tel: 780-488-8074; *Fax:* 780-475-7968
e-mail: chaaa@compusmart.ab.ca
www.chaaa.ab.ca
Also Known As: Catholic Health Association of Alberta & Affiliates
Previous Name: Catholic Health Care Conference of Alberta
Overview: A medium-sized provincial charitable organization founded in 1943 overseen by Catholic Health Association of Canada
Mission: Represents the shared vision & values of those seeking to make visible Jesus the Healer; provides support & leadership to members & the community through education, advocacy & collaboration
Member of: Catholic Health Association of Canada
Chief Officer(s):
Glyn J. Smith, Administrator

College of Physicians & Surgeons of Alberta (CPSA)
#2700, 10020 - 100 St. NW, Edmonton AB T5J 0N3
Tel: 780-423-4764; *Fax:* 780-420-0651
Toll-Free: 800-561-3899
e-mail: publicinquiries@cpsa.ab.ca
www.cpsa.ca
Overview: A medium-sized provincial licensing organization founded in 1905 overseen by Federation of Regulatory Authorities of Canada
Mission: To serve the public & guide the medical profession; To identify factors affecting competent medical practice; To promote quality improvement in medical practice; To ensure practitioners meet our registration standards; To resolve complaints involving practitioners fairly & effectively
Chief Officer(s):
James Stone, President

SECTION II: General Resources

College of Podiatric Physicians of Alberta (CPPA)
#2020, 61 Broadway Blvd., Sherwood Park AB T8H 2C1
Tel: 780-922-7609
www.albertapodiatry.com
Overview: A small provincial organization founded in 1932
Mission: To act in accordance with the Podiatry Act, under the Statutes of Alberta; To advance the profession of podiatry in Alberta
Member of: American Podiatric Medical Association, Inc., Region 7
Chief Officer(s):
Jayne Jeneroux, Executive Director
Bradley Sonnema, President
president@albertapodiatry.com

Covenant Health (Alberta) (ACHC)
3033 66 St. NW, Edmonton AB T6K 4B2
Tel: 780-735-9000
www.covenanthealth.ca
Previous Name: Catholic Health of Alberta
Overview: A small provincial organization
Chief Officer(s):
Patrick Dumelie, CEO

EmployAbilities
10909 Jasper Ave., 4th Fl., Edmonton AB T5J 3L9
Tel: 780-423-4106
e-mail: employ@employabilities.ab.ca
www.employabilities.ab.ca
www.facebook.com/EmployAbilities
twitter.com/employabilities
Overview: A medium-sized provincial charitable organization
Mission: To promote & enhance employment & learning opportunities for persons with disabilities
Chief Officer(s):
Ollie Triska, President

Health Sciences Association of Alberta (HSAA) / Association des sciences de la santé de l'Alberta (ind.)
10212 - 112 St., Edmonton AB T5K 1M4
Tel: 780-488-0168; *Fax:* 780-488-0534
Toll-Free: 800-252-7904
www.hsaa.ca
www.facebook.com/349561555109272
twitter.com/HSAAlberta
Overview: A medium-sized provincial organization founded in 1971
Mission: To conduct activities as a labour union to enhance the quality of life for HSAA members & society
Member of: National Union of Public and General Employees
Chief Officer(s):
Elisabeth Ballermann, President
elisabethb@hsaa.ca
Lynette McAvoy, Executive Director
lynettem@hsaa.ca
Publications:
• Challenger [a publication of the Health Sciences Association of Alberta]
Type: Magazine; *Frequency:* Quarterly; *Accepts Advertising*
Profile: Feature articles, labour relations updates, HSAA activities, affiliate & member news, forthcoming workshops & events

Poison & Drug Information Service
Foothills Medical Centre, 1403 - 29th St. NW, Calgary AB T2N 2T9
Tel: 403-944-6900
Toll-Free: 800-332-1414
www.albertahealthservices.ca/5423.asp
Also Known As: PADIS
Previous Name: Alberta Poison Centre
Overview: A small provincial organization
Mission: To provide information & advice on poisons, medications, & chemicals
Member of: Canadian Association of Poison Control Centres
Chief Officer(s):
Ryan Chuang, Associate Medical Director

Professional Association of Residents of Alberta (PARA) / Association professionnelle des résidents de l'Alberta
Garneau Professional Center, #340, 11044 - 82 Ave., Edmonton AB T6G 0T2
Tel: 780-432-1749; *Fax:* 780-432-1778
Toll-Free: 877-375-7272
e-mail: para@para-ab.ca
www.para-ab.ca
www.facebook.com/ProfessionalAssociationofResidentPhysiciansofAB
twitter.com/para_ab
Overview: A medium-sized provincial organization founded in 1975 overseen by Resident Doctors of Canada
Mission: To represent physicians completing further training in residency programs; To promote excellence in education & patient care; To advocate for health care issues & for improvement in working conditions, salary, & benefits for resident physicians of Alberta
Affliation(s): Canadian Association of Internes & Residents
Chief Officer(s):
Catherine Cheng, President
Rob Key, Chief Executive Officer
rob.key@para-ab.ca
Kiersten Doblanko, Specialist, Communications
kiersten.doblanko@para-ab.ca

Réseau santé albertain
#304A, 8627, rue Marie-Anne-Gaboury, Edmonton AB T6C 3N1
Tél: 780-466-9816
Courriel: info@reseausantealbertain.ca
www.reseausantealbertain.ca
www.facebook.com/162905357095396
twitter.com/inforsab
www.youtube.com/user/reseausantealbertain
Aperçu: Dimension: petite; *Envergure:* provinciale surveillé par Société santé en français
Membre(s) du bureau directeur:
Pauline Légaré, Directrice générale par intérim
pauline.legare@reseausantealbertain.ca

BRITISH COLUMBIA

Ambulance Paramedics of British Columbia
#105, 21900 Westminster Hwy., Richmond BC V6V 0A8
Tel: 604-273-5722; *Fax:* 604-273-5762
Toll-Free: 866-273-5766
e-mail: info@apbc.ca
www.paramedicsofbc.com
www.facebook.com/APBC873
twitter.com/apbc873
www.youtube.com/user/APBCCUPE873
Overview: A small provincial organization
Mission: To provide emergency medical care to the sick & injured in British Columbia
Member of: Paramedic Association of Canada

BC Association for Individualized Technology and Supports (BCITS)
#103, 366 East Kent Ave. South, Vancouver BC V5X 4N6
Tel: 604-326-0175; *Fax:* 604-326-0176
Toll-Free: 866-326-1245
e-mail: info@bcits.org
www.bcits.org
Overview: A medium-sized provincial charitable organization
Mission: To help meet the needs of people with severe disabilities who require assistive technologies & supports
Chief Officer(s):
Christine Gordon, Chair
Ruth Marzetti, Executive Director
Richard Bing, Office Administrator

British Columbia Association of Healthcare Auxiliaries
#200, 1333 West Broadway, Vancouver BC V6H 4C6
Tel: 236-999-4752
e-mail: info@bchealthcareaux.org
www.bchealthcareaux.org
Overview: A medium-sized provincial organization founded in 1945
Mission: To promote education & high standards of performance in order to ensure success for member auxiliaries
Chief Officer(s):
Judith McBride, Executive Director

British Columbia Association of Kinesiologists (BCAK)
#102, 211 Columbia St., Vancouver BC V6A 2R5
Tel: 604-601-5100; *Fax:* 604-681-4545
e-mail: office@bcak.bc.ca
www.bcak.bc.ca
www.linkedin.com/groups/BCAK-British-Columbia-Association-Kinesiol
ogis
www.facebook.com/BC.Association.of.Kinesiologists
twitter.com/BCKinesiology
Overview: A small provincial organization founded in 1991
Mission: To uphold the standards of the profession of kinesiology; to promote the applications of kinesiology to other professionals & to the community; to assist in professional development; to encourage the exchange of ideas
Chief Officer(s):
Bassam Khaleel, President
Happy Jhaj, Vice-President
Craig Aspinall, Treasurer
Edwards Reynolds, Executive Director

British Columbia Association of Medical Radiation Technologists (BCAMRT)
Central Office, #102, 211 Columbia St., Vancouver BC V6A 2R5
Tel: 604-682-8171; *Fax:* 604-681-4545
Toll-Free: 800-990-7090
e-mail: office@bcamrt.bc.ca
www.bcamrt.bc.ca
Overview: A medium-sized provincial organization founded in 1951 overseen by Canadian Association of Medical Radiation Technologists
Mission: To manage the professional affairs of medical radiation technologists in British Columbia; To advocate for the profession of medical radiation technology across the province
Chief Officer(s):
Louise Rimanic, President

British Columbia Association of Professionals with Disabilities
714 Warder Place, Victoria BC V9A 7H6
Tel: 250-361-9697
e-mail: info@bcprofessionals.org
www.bcprofessionals.org
Overview: A small provincial organization founded in 2003
Mission: Provincially incorporated non-profit association dedicated to maximizing the inclusion, job retention, and advancement of current and future professionals with disabilities
Affliation(s): Canadian Association of Professionals with Disabilities

British Columbia Association of School Psychologists (BCASP)
c/o Barbara Nichols, 7715 Loedel Cres., Prince George BC V2N 0A5
e-mail: executives@bcasp.ca
www.bcasp.ca
Overview: A small provincial organization
Mission: To represent the interests of school psychologists and to further the standards of school psychology practice in order to promote effective service to all students and their families.
Chief Officer(s):
Douglas Agar, President
president@bcasp.ca

British Columbia Centre for Ability
2805 Kingsway, Vancouver BC V5R 5H9
Tel: 604-451-5511; *Fax:* 604-451-5651
e-mail: info@bc-cfa.org
www.bc-cfa.org
www.linkedin.com/company/bc-centre-for-ability
twitter.com/bccfa
Previous Name: Neurolodical Centre & Children's Centre for Ability; Vancouver Neurological Association
Overview: A small provincial charitable organization founded in 1969
Mission: To enhance the quality of life for children, youth & adults with disabilities & their families in ways that build on their potential & promotes inclusion in all aspects of social life
Member of: United Way
Chief Officer(s):
Angela Kwok, Executive Director

British Columbia Centre for Ability Association (BCCFA)
2805 Kingsway, Vancouver BC V5R 5H9
Tel: 604-451-5511; *Fax:* 604-451-5651
www.bc-cfa.org
www.linkedin.com/company/bc-centre-for-ability
twitter.com/bccfa
www.youtube.com/channel/UCIjOVwg7zWgpD5WLT6RNzzA
Previous Name: Children's Rehabilitation & Cerebral Palsy Association; Children's Centre for Ability
Overview: A medium-sized provincial charitable organization founded in 1970
Mission: To provide community-based services that promote inclusion & improve the quality of life for children, youth & adults with disabilities & their families
Member of: United Way
Chief Officer(s):
Jennifer Baumbusch, President

British Columbia Centre of Excellence for Women's Health (BCCEWH)
c/o British Columbia Women's Hospital & Health Centre, PO Box 48, 4500 Oak St., #E209, Vancouver BC V6H 3N1
Tel: 604-875-2633; *Fax:* 604-875-3716
www.bccewh.bc.ca
Overview: A small provincial charitable organization founded in 1995
Mission: To ensure that women's health & wellness are considered by clinicians & policy makers
Chief Officer(s):
Nancy Poole, Director
Leanna Rose, Director, Finance & Operations
Publications:
• British Columbia Centre of Excellence for Women's Health Research Bulletin
Profile: Research findings produced by the four Centres of Excellence for Women's Health
• Women-Health eNews
Type: Newsletter
Profile: Information for researchers, policy makers, & activists

British Columbia Drug & Poison Information Centre (DPIC)
BC Centre for Disease Control, #0063, 655 West 12th Ave., Vancouver BC V5Z 4R4
Tel: 604-707-2789; *Fax:* 604-707-2807; *Crisis Hot-Line:* 800-567-8911
e-mail: info@dpic.ca
www.dpic.org
www.facebook.com/231889396821389
twitter.com/BCDPIC
Overview: A small provincial organization founded in 1975
Mission: To support healthcare providers in British Columbia, by providing a consultative service
Publications:
• Drug Information Perspectives
Type: Newsletter; *Editor:* Barbara Cadario
Profile: Issues on topics such as Dementia Therapy, Rivastigmine, Rasagiline, & Varenicline
• Drug Information Reference
Price: $65
Profile: Basic clinical facts. evaluations of commonly used drugs, investigational uses, nursing instructions, & clinical trial summaries

British Columbia Podiatric Medical Association (BCPMA)
#220, 445 Mountain Hwy., North Vancouver BC V7J 2L1
Tel: 604-985-3338; *Fax:* 604-682-2766
e-mail: info@bcpodiatrists.ca
www.bcpodiatrists.ca
Overview: A small provincial organization
Chief Officer(s):
Howard Green, President

British Columbia Surgical Society (BCSS)
#115, 1665 West Broadway, Vancouver BC V6J 5A4
Tel: 604-638-2843; *Fax:* 604-638-2938
www.bcss.ca
Overview: A small provincial organization founded in 1947
Mission: To further the teaching, practice, & science of the branches of surgery; to advance patient care
Chief Officer(s):
Nam Nguyen, President

British Columbia Ultrasonographers' Society (BCUS)
127 - 62nd Ave. East, Vancouver BC V5X 2E7

www.bcus.org

Overview: A small provincial organization founded in 1981
Mission: To promote & encourage the science & art of diagnostic medical sonography; provide a forum to promote the discussion of matters affecting the field; provide a place for professional growth
Chief Officer(s):
Vickie Lessoway, Executive Director

Catholic Health Association of British Columbia (CHABC)
9387 Holmes St., Burnaby BC V3N 4C3

Tel: 604-524-3427; *Fax:* 604-524-3428
e-mail: smhouse@shawlink.ca
chabc.bc.ca

Overview: A medium-sized provincial organization founded in 1940 overseen by Catholic Health Association of Canada
Mission: To witness to the healing ministry and abiding presence of Jesus. Inspired by the Gospel, this Association strives to have a universal concern for health as a condition for full human development.
Member of: Catholic Health Alliance of Canada; Health Employers Association of British Columbia
Affliation(s): Euthanasia Prevention Coalition; Canadian Association of Parish Nurse Ministries
Chief Officer(s):
Dianne Doyle, President

College of Occupational Therapists of British Columbia (COTBC)
#402, 3795 Carey Rd., Victoria BC V8Z 6T8

Tel: 250-386-6822; *Fax:* 250-386-6824
Toll-Free: 866-386-6822
e-mail: info@cotbc.org
www.cotbc.org
www.linkedin.com/company/college-of-occupational-therapists-of-britis
h
www.facebook.com/OTCollegeBC
twitter.com/OTCollegeBC

Overview: A small provincial licensing organization
Mission: To establish standards of practice & conduct; To enhance quality assurance; To monitor quality of practice & continuing competence; To improve competence of occupational therapists; To investigate complaints; To enforce standards
Chief Officer(s):
Kathy Corbett, Registrar
kcorbett@cotbc.org
Cindy McLean, Deputy Registrar
cmclean@cotbc.org
Mary Clark, Director, Quality Assurance Program & Communications
mclark@cotbc.org

College of Physicians & Surgeons of British Columbia (CPSBC)
#300, 699 Howe St., Vancouver BC V6C 0B4

Tel: 604-733-7758; *Fax:* 604-733-3503
Toll-Free: 800-461-3008
www.cpsbc.ca
www.linkedin.com/company/2905395
twitter.com/cpsbc_ca

Overview: A medium-sized provincial licensing organization founded in 1886 overseen by Federation of Regulatory Authorities of Canada
Chief Officer(s):
L.C. Jewett, President
Heidi Oetter, Registrar

Disability Alliance British Columbia
#204, 456 West Broadway, Vancouver BC V5Y 1R3

Tel: 604-875-0188; *Fax:* 604-875-9227
Toll-Free: 800-663-1278; *TTY:* 604-875-8835
e-mail: feedback@disabilityalliancebc.org
www.disabilityalliancebc.org
www.facebook.com/DisabilityAllianceBC
twitter.com/DisabAllianceBC
www.youtube.com/user/TheBCCPD

Previous Name: British Columbia Coalition of People with Disabilities
Overview: A medium-sized provincial organization founded in 1977
Mission: To raise public & political awareness of issues concerning people with disabilities; To facilitate full participation of disabled people in society by promoting independence & the self-help model; To lobby government on policies & attitudes which affect people with disabilities
Affliation(s): Council of Canadians with Disabilities
Chief Officer(s):
Pat Danforth, President
Sheryl Burns, Secretary

Doctors of BC
#115, 1665 West Broadway, Vancouver BC V6J 5A4

Tel: 604-736-5551; *Fax:* 604-638-2917
Toll-Free: 800-665-2262
e-mail: communications@doctorsofbc.ca
www.doctorsofbc.ca
ca.linkedin.com/company/1154933
www.facebook.com/bcsdoctors
twitter.com/doctorsofbc

Previous Name: British Columbia Medical Association
Overview: A medium-sized provincial organization founded in 1900 overseen by Canadian Medical Association
Mission: To promote a social, economic, & political climate in which members can provide the citizens of British Columbia with the highest standard of health care while achieving maximum professional satisfaction & fair economic reward
Chief Officer(s):
Allan Seckel, Chief Executive Officer
Alan Ruddiman, President
president@doctorsofbc.ca
Publications:
• BC Medical Journal
Type: Journal; *Editor:* D.R. Richardson, MD

Environmental Health Association of British Columbia (EHABC)
PO Box 30033, RPO Reyolds, Victoria BC V8X 5E1

Tel: 250-658-2027
Other Communication: ehabc.wordpress.com
e-mail: info@ehabc.org
www.ehabc.org
www.facebook.com/353025931439290

Overview: A medium-sized provincial charitable organization founded in 1993
Mission: To raise awareness within the medical community, educational institutions, & the general public to prevent further cases of environmental sensitivity from occurring
Affliation(s): EHA Nova Scotia; EHA Québec; EHA Ontario; EHA Alberta

Family Caregivers of British Columbia
#6, 3318 Oak St., Victoria BC V8X 1R1

Tel: 250-384-0408; *Fax:* 250-361-2660
Toll-Free: 877-520-3267
www.familycaregiversbc.ca
www.facebook.com/FamilyCaregiversBC
twitter.com/caringbc

Previous Name: Family Caregivers' Network Society
Overview: A small provincial charitable organization founded in 1989
Mission: To provide support, education, & information for family caregivers in British Columbia
Chief Officer(s):
Barb MacLean, Executive Director
Alyshia Vogt, President
Publications:
• Caregiver Connection [a publication of the Family Caregivers of British Columbia]
Type: Newsletter; *Frequency:* Quarterly
Profile: Articles about family caregiving issues
• Facilitator's Manual: Educational Activities to Support Family Caregivers
Price: $75
Profile: Featuring facilitation techniques, outlines for workshops, & learning activities for healthcare provider training programs
• Medical Information Package
Price: Free with membership in theFamily Caregivers of British Columbia; $3 non-members
Profile: Including a medical information record, information about incapacity planning, plus information from the British Columbia Transplant Society & the Heart & Stroke Foundation
• Network News [a publication of the Family Caregivers of British Columbia]
Type: Newsletter; *Frequency:* Bimonthly; *Price:* Free with membership

in the Family Caregivers of British Columbia
Profile: Informative articles about caregiving issues & notices of upcoming events
• Resource Guide for Family Caregivers
Type: Handbook; *Number of Pages:* 160; *Price:* $15 members; $20 non-members
Profile: Practical information to help caregivers make decisions

Health Employers Association of British Columbia (HEABC)
#200, 1333 West Broadway, Vancouver BC V6H 4C6
Tel: 604-736-5909; *Fax:* 604-736-2715
e-mail: contact@heabc.bc.ca
www.heabc.bc.ca
www.linkedin.com/company/heabc
twitter.com/heabcnews
www.youtube.com/user/BCHealthCareAwards
Overview: A medium-sized provincial organization founded in 1993 overseen by Canadian Healthcare Association
Mission: To serve a diverse group of over 250 publicly funded healthcare employers; To deliver high quality labour relations services; To advance the efficiency & productivity of human resources system-wide
Chief Officer(s):
David Logan, President & CEO
Lyn Kocher, Executive Director

Health Record Association of British Columbia (HRABC)
c/o Faye Jones, 397 Rindle Ct., Kelowna BC V1W 5G5
www.hrabc.net
Overview: A small provincial organization founded in 1949
Mission: To contribute to the promotion of wellness & the provision of quality healthcare through excellence in information management
Member of: National Health Information Management Alliance
Affliation(s): Canadian Health Information Management Association
Chief Officer(s):
Dawn Lawrie, President
Faye Jones, Treasurer

Health Sciences Association of British Columbia (HSABC)
180 East Columbia St., New Westminster BC V3L 0G7
Tel: 604-517-0994; *Fax:* 604-515-8889
Toll-Free: 800-663-2017
www.hsabc.org
www.facebook.com/HSABC
twitter.com/hsabc
www.youtube.com/channel/UCzmTkWmoWZR-yE8MTb0lJ2A
Overview: A large provincial organization founded in 1971
Mission: To negotiate collective agreements for members; To preserve & promote public health care in Canada
Member of: National Union of Public and General Employees
Chief Officer(s):
Val Avery, President
webpres@hsabc.org
Janice Morrison, Vice-President
Marg Beddis, Secretary-Treasurer

Hospital Employees' Union (HEU) / Syndicat des employés d'hôpitaux
5000 North Fraser Way, Burnaby BC V5J 5M3
Tel: 604-438-5000; *Fax:* 604-739-1510
Toll-Free: 800-663-5813
e-mail: info@heu.org
www.heu.org
twitter.com/HospEmpUnion
Overview: A large provincial organization founded in 1944
Mission: To unite & associate together all employees employed in hospital, medical or related work for the purpose of securing concerted action in whatever may be regarded as conducive to their best interests; to embrace the concept of equality of treatment for all in hospital, medical or related employment, with respect to wages & job opportunities, recognizing their obligation to provide high-quality care; to defend & preserve the right of all persons to high standards of medical & hospital treatment
Member of: CUPE; Canadian & BC Health Coalitions; BC Federation of Labour
Affliation(s): Labour Councils
Chief Officer(s):
Victor Elkins, President
Bonnie Pearson, Secretary & Business Manager

Publications:
• The Guardian
Type: Magazine; *Frequency:* 3-4 pa

Meningitis BC
20 Hallman St., Kitimat BC V8C 2R1
Tel: 250-632-5946
www.meningitisbc.org
www.facebook.com/meningitisbc.org
Overview: A small provincial organization
Mission: To educate the public about meningitis & prevention by vaccination; To promote meningitis awareness initiatives; To advocate for the use of MCV4 & 4CMenB vaccines in the public immunization program

Occupational First Aid Attendants Association of British Columbia (OFAAA)
#108, 2323 Boundary Rd., Vancouver BC V5M 4V8
Tel: 604-294-0244; *Fax:* 604-294-0289
Toll-Free: 800-667-4566
e-mail: ofaaa@ofaaa.bc.ca
www.ofaaa.bc.ca
www.facebook.com/119440864766772
twitter.com/OFAAABC
Previous Name: Industrial First Aid Attendants Association of British Columbia
Overview: A small provincial charitable organization founded in 1935
Mission: To enhance the professional status of first aid attendants & to promote accessibility to high standards of first aid for the workers of the province of British Columbia
Chief Officer(s):
Allan Zdunic, President
azdunich@ofaaa.bc.ca

Prosthetics & Orthotics Association of British Columbia (POABC)
PO Box 30594, Stn. Brentwood Mall, #47A, 4567 Lougheed Hwy., Burnaby BC V5C 2A0
e-mail: info@poabc.ca
www.poabc.ca
www.facebook.com/poabc.ca
Overview: A small provincial organization founded in 1974 overseen by Orthotics Prosthetics Canada
Mission: To promote quality patient care & professionalism in the field of prosthetics & orthotics in British Columbia
Chief Officer(s):
Scott Hedlund, President
Randy Kramer, Vice-President
Gord Dillon, Secretary
Travis Finlayson, Treasurer

Public Health Association of British Columbia (PHABC)
#210, 1027 Pandora Ave., Victoria BC V8V 3P6
Tel: 250-595-8422; *Fax:* 250-595-8622
e-mail: staff@phabc.org
www.phabc.org
Overview: A medium-sized provincial organization founded in 1953 overseen by Canadian Public Health Association
Mission: To constitute a special resource in BC for the betterment & maintenance of the population's health at the community & personal level

Resident Doctors of British Columbia
#2399, 650 West Georgia St., Vancouver BC V6B 4N7
Tel: 604-876-7636
Toll-Free: 888-877-2722
e-mail: info@residentdoctorsbc.ca
www.residentdoctorsbc.ca
www.facebook.com/ResidentDoctorsBC
twitter.com/ResidentDocsBC
Overview: A medium-sized provincial organization overseen by Resident Doctors of Canada
Mission: To bargain collectively on behalf of residents in British Columbia; To foster the personal well-being of members
Affliation(s): Canadian Association of Internes & Residents
Chief Officer(s):
David Kim, President
Gagandeep Dhaliwal, Vice-President
Boluwaji Ogunyemi, Director, Communications
Clark Funnell, Director, Finance

Pria Sandhu, Executive Director
Brandi MacLean, Office Administrator

Réso Santé Colombie Britannique (RSCB)
#201, 2929, rue Commercial, Vancouver BC V5N 4C8
Tél: 604-629-1000
Courriel: info@resosante.ca
www.resosante.ca
www.linkedin.com/company/résosanté-colombie-britannique
www.facebook.com/resosante
twitter.com/resosante
Aperçu: *Dimension:* petite; *Envergure:* provinciale; fondée en 2003
surveillé par Société santé en français
Mission: Promouvoir des services de la santé et du bien-être en
français en Colombie-Britannique
Membre(s) du bureau directeur:
Benjamin Stoll, Directeur général
bstoll@resosante.ca

MANITOBA

Catholic Health Association of Manitoba (CHAM) / Association catholique manitobaine de la santé (ACMS)
SBGH Education Bldg., 409 Taché Ave., #N5067, Winnipeg MB R2H 2A6
Tel: 204-235-3136; *Fax:* 204-235-3811
www.cham.mb.ca
Overview: A medium-sized provincial charitable organization founded
in 1943 overseen by Catholic Health Alliance of Canada
Mission: To carry out the healing ministry of the Catholic Church in the
delivery of both health & social services in Manitoba; To treat the
people of Manitoba with compassion & respect for all; To recognize the
spiritual dimension integral to health & healing
Member of: Catholic Health Alliance of Canada
Affiliation(s): Bishops of Manitoba; Diocese of Churchill-Hudson Bay,
Northwest Territories
Chief Officer(s):
Wilmar Chopyk, Executive Director
wchopyk@cham.mb.ca
Publications:
• CHAM [Catholic Health Association of Manitoba] Newsletter
Type: Newsletter
Profile: Educational information for members & CHAM activities

College of Physicians & Surgeons of Manitoba (CPSM)
#1000, 1661 Portage Ave., Winnipeg MB R3J 3T7
Tel: 204-774-4344; *Fax:* 204-774-0750
Toll-Free: 877-774-4344
e-mail: cpsm@cpsm.mb.ca
cpsm.mb.ca
Also Known As: CPS Manitoba
Overview: A medium-sized provincial licensing organization founded in
1871 overseen by Federation of Regulatory Authorities of Canada
Chief Officer(s):
Brent Kvern, President
Anna Ziomek, Registrar
theregistrar@cpsm.mb.ca

College of Podiatrists of Manitoba (COPOM)
#512, 428 Portage Ave., Winnipeg MB R3C 0E2
Tel: 204-942-3256
www.copom.org
Overview: A small provincial licensing organization
Mission: The College is a provincial regulatory body that protects the
public by ensuring podiatrists in Mantioba follow the standards of
practice defined in The Podiatry Act, 2001.
Chief Officer(s):
Iain Palmer, Chair
Martin Colledge, Registrar
Registrar@copom.org

Conseil communauté en santé du Manitoba (CCS)
#400, 400, av Taché, Saint-Boniface MB R2H 3C3
Tél: 204-235-3293; *Téléc:* 204-237-0984
Courriel: santeenfrancais@santeenfrancais.com
www.santeenfrancais.com
Aperçu: *Dimension:* petite; *Envergure:* provinciale; fondée en 2004
surveillé par Société santé en français
Mission: Promouvoir l'accès à des services de qualité en français

Membre(s) du bureau directeur:
Annie Bédard, Directrice générale
abedard2@santeenfrancais.com

Doctors Manitoba
20 Desjardins Dr., Winnipeg MB R3X 0E8
Tel: 204-985-5888; *Fax:* 204-985-5844
Toll-Free: 888-322-4242
e-mail: general@docsmb.org
www.docsmb.org
Previous Name: Manitoba Medical Association
Overview: A medium-sized provincial organization founded in 1908
overseen by Canadian Medical Association
Mission: To unite & advocate for Manitoba physicians; To encourage
the highest standards of health care for the people of Manitoba
Chief Officer(s):
Robert Cram, Chief Executive Officer, 204-985-5843
rcram@docsmb.org
Rick Sawyer, Chief Administrative Officer, 204-985-5842
rsawyer@docsmb.org
Publications:
• Rounds [a publication of Doctors Manitoba]
Type: Magazine; *Frequency:* 4 pa.; *Accepts Advertising*
Profile: Features member profiles & industry news

Injured Workers Association of Manitoba Inc. (IWAM)
Injured & Disabled Centre, 734 Polson Ave., Winnipeg MB R2X 1M2
Tel: 204-586-8183
Overview: A small provincial charitable organization founded in 1971
Mission: To reduce the resulting psychological impact of workplace
injuries on workers & families by assisting them to understand the
policies & procedures of the Workers Compensation Board or other
disability related insurance policies; free services include consultations,
information & referrals to appropriate resources
Member of: Canadian Injured Workers Alliance

International Mennonite Health Association Inc. (IMHA)
15 Coleridge Park Dr., Winnipeg MB R3K 0B2
Tel: 204-831-1699; *Fax:* 204-985-3226
e-mail: info@africancanadianhealth.ca
www.intermenno.net
Overview: A small international charitable organization
Mission: Providing resources and services to Mennonite and Brethren
in Christ health programs in developing countries.
Chief Officer(s):
Murray Nickel, President
nickel.murray@gmail.com

Manitoba Association of Health Care Professionals (MAHCP) / Association des professionnels de la santé du Manitoba
#101, 1500 Notre Dame Ave., Winnipeg MB R3E 0P9
Tel: 204-772-0425; *Fax:* 204-775-6829
Toll-Free: 800-315-3331
e-mail: info@mahcp.ca
mahcp.com
www.facebook.com/manitobaahcp
twitter.com/MAHCP_MB
Overview: A medium-sized provincial organization
Mission: To protect, advocate for & advance the rights of its members
through labour relations activities
Chief Officer(s):
Bob Moroz, President
bobm@mahcp.ca
Lee Manning, Executive Director
lee@mahcp.ca

Manitoba Association of Medical Radiation Technologists (MAMRT)
#202, 819 Sargent Ave., Winnipeg MB R3E 0B9
Tel: 204-774-5346; *Fax:* 204-774-5346
e-mail: admin@mamrt.ca
www.mamrt.ca
Overview: A small provincial organization founded in 1929 overseen
by Canadian Association of Medical Radiation Technologists
Mission: To support medical radiation technologists & therapists
throughout Manitoba
Chief Officer(s):
Jenna Bruderer, President
Salin Guttormsson, Executive Director

Jordan Veale, Director, Communications
Jason Lewis, Director, Finance & Administration
Corey Baschuk, Office Administrator
Publications:
• MAMRT News: A Newsletter of the Manitoba Association of Medical Radiation Technologists
Type: Newsletter; *Frequency:* 3 pa; *Accepts Advertising*
Profile: Information from the association for members

Manitoba Association of School Psychologists Inc.
#562, 162 - 2025 Corydon Ave., Winnipeg MB R3P 0N5
www.masp.mb.ca
Overview: A small provincial organization founded in 1981
Mission: To promote & support school psychology in Manitoba; to develop a network of communication among practitioners of school psychology in Manitoba; to encourage & provide information to educators & the public regarding the practice of school psycholology & other related educational issues
Chief Officer(s):
Barry Mallin, President

Manitoba Medical Students' Association (MMSA)
c/o Faculty of Medicine, University of Manitoba, #260, 727 McDermot Ave., Winnipeg MB R3E 3P5
Tel: 204-789-3424; *Fax:* 204-789-3929
mmsa.online
twitter.com/UofMMSA
Overview: A small provincial organization
Mission: To represent & promote the interests of students at the Max Rady College of Medicine at the University of Manitoba
Chief Officer(s):
Matthew Kochan, Contact, Communications
kochanm3@myumanitoba.ca

Manitoba Poison Control Centre
Children's Hospital Health Sciences Centre, 840 Sherbrook St., Winnipeg MB R3A 1S1
Tel: 204-787-2444; *Crisis Hot-Line:* 204-787-2591
Overview: A small provincial organization
Mission: To provide poison information, by physicians, for the public & health care advisers
Member of: Canadian Association of Poison Control Centres

Manitoba Public Health Association (MPHA)
c/o Klinic Community Health Centre, 870 Portage Ave., Winnipeg MB R3G 0P1
e-mail: manitobapha@mts.net
www.manitobapha.ca
Overview: A small provincial organization founded in 1940 overseen by Canadian Public Health Association
Mission: To influence health, social, environmental, & economic policy decisions, in order to improve the well-being of people in Manitoba; To ensure that health promotion, health protection, & disease protection are part of services
Member of: Canadian Public Health Association (CPHA)
Chief Officer(s):
Barb Wasilewski, President

MBTelehealth Network
John Buhler Research Centre, #772, 715 McDermot Ave., Winnipeg MB R3E 3P4
Tel: 204-272-3063; *Fax:* 204-975-7787
Toll-Free: 866-667-9891
www.mbtelehealth.ca
Overview: A small provincial organization
Mission: To promote the use of information technology to link people to health care expertise at a distance
Chief Officer(s):
Liz Loewen, Director, Coordination of Care

Paramedic Association of Manitoba (PAM)
#230, 530 Century St., Winnipeg MB R3H 0Y4
Fax: 866-222-6471
Toll-Free: 866-726-1210
e-mail: info@paramedicsofmanitoba.ca
www.paramedicsofmanitoba.ca
www.facebook.com/262118083807029
twitter.com/PAM_manitoba
Overview: A small provincial organization founded in 2001

Mission: To promote excellence in pre-hospital emergency health care & excellence in the profession of paramedicine
Member of: Paramedic Association of Canada
Chief Officer(s):
Jodi Possia, Chair
chairman@paramedicsofmanitoba.ca
Christy Beazley, Director, Public Relations
cbeazley@paramedicsofmanitoba.ca

Professional Association of Residents & Interns of Manitoba (PARIM) / Association professionnelle des résidents et internes du Manitoba
Health Sciences Centre, 820 Sherbrook St., #GF132, Winnipeg MB R3A 1R9
Tel: 204-787-3673; *Fax:* 204-787-2692
e-mail: parim.office@gmail.com
www.parim.org
Also Known As: PARI Manitoba
Overview: A small provincial organization founded in 1975 overseen by Resident Doctors of Canada
Mission: To represent the concerns of all residents & interns in Manitoba; To advocate for the well-being of residents & interns; To promote quality medical education & excellent patient care
Affiliation(s): Canadian Association of Internes & Residents
Chief Officer(s):
Leslie Anderson, Co-President
Maha Haddad, Co-President
Jessica Burleson, Executive Director
jburleson@hsc.mb.ca

The Regional Health Authorities of Manitoba (RHAM)
#2, 203 Duffield St., Winnipeg MB R3J 0H6
Tel: 204-833-1720; *Fax:* 204-940-2042
www.rham.mb.ca
Previous Name: Manitoba Health Organizations
Overview: A medium-sized provincial organization founded in 1998 overseen by Canadian Healthcare Association
Mission: To establish programs that help to improve Manitoba health authorities
Chief Officer(s):
Gayle Hryshko, Interim Executive Director
ghryshko@wrha.mb.ca
Debbie St. Amant, Coordinator, Finance & Administration
dstamant@rham.mb.ca

Society for Manitobans with Disabilities Inc. (SMD)
825 Sherbrook St., Winnipeg MB R3A 1M5
Tel: 204-975-3010; *Fax:* 204-975-3073
Toll-Free: 866-282-8041; *TTY:* 204-784-3012
e-mail: info@smd.mb.ca
smd.mb.ca
Overview: A large provincial charitable organization founded in 1946 overseen by Easter Seals Canada
Mission: To promote the full participation & equality of people with disabilities: To provide a full range of rehabilitation services; To facilitate the development of a receptive & supportive environment
Affiliation(s): Autism Society Manitoba

Central Regional Office
#100, 30 Stephen St., Morden MB R6M 2G5
Tel: 204-822-7412; *Fax:* 204-822-7413
Toll-Free: 800-269-5451; *TTY:* 204-822-7412
smd.mb.ca

Eastman Regional Office
#5, 227 Main St., Steinbach MB R5G 1Y7
Tel: 204-326-5336; *Fax:* 204-326-9762
Toll-Free: 800-497-8196; *TTY:* 204-346-3998
smd.mb.ca

Interlake Regional Office
382 Main St., Selkirk MB R1A 1T8
Tel: 204-785-9338; *Fax:* 204-785-9340
Toll-Free: 888-831-4213; *TTY:* 204-482-5638
smd.mb.ca

Northern Regional Office

#303, 83 Churchill Dr., Thompson MB R8N 0L6
Tel: 204-778-4277; *Fax:* 204-778-4461
Toll-Free: 888-367-0268; *TTY:* 204-778-4277
smd.mb.ca

Parkland Regional Office
#411, 27 - 2 Ave. SW, Dauphin MB R7N 3E5
Tel: 204-622-2293; *Fax:* 204-622-2260
Toll-Free: 800-844-2307; *TTY:* 204-622-2293
smd.mb.ca

SMD Self-Help Clearinghouse
825 Sherbrook St., Winnipeg MB R3A 1M5
Tel: 204-975-3010; *Fax:* 204-975-3073
Toll-Free: 866-282-8041; *TTY:* 204-975-3012
smd.mb.ca

Westman Regional Office
#140, 340 - 9th St., Brandon MB R7A 6C2
Tel: 204-726-6157; *Fax:* 204-726-6499
Toll-Free: 800-813-3325; *TTY:* 204-726-6157
smd.mb.ca

Wheelchair Services
1857 Notre Dame Ave., Winnipeg MB R3E 3E7
Tel: 204-975-3250; *Fax:* 204-975-3240
Toll-Free: 800-836-5551; *TTY:* 800-856-7934
e-mail: wreception@smd.mb.ca
smd.mb.ca

NEW BRUNSWICK

Canadian Public Health Association - NB/PEI Branch
NB
e-mail: nbpei.pha@gmail.com
Overview: A small provincial organization founded in 1952 overseen by Canadian Public Health Association
Mission: To maintain & improve the level of personal & community health
Chief Officer(s):
Tracey Rickards, President
Anne Lebans, Secretary-Treasurer

Catholic Health Association of New Brunswick (CHANB) / L'Association catholique de la santé du Nouveau-Brunswick
1773 Water St., Miramichi NB E1N 1B2
Tel: 506-778-5302; *Fax:* 506-778-5303
e-mail: nbcha@nb.aibn.com
www.chanb.com
Overview: A small provincial organization founded in 1986 overseen by Catholic Health Association of Canada
Mission: The Catholic Health Association of New Brunswick is a provincial Christian organization promoting health care in the tradition of the Catholic Church. The Association fosters healing in all its aspects: Physical, psychological, social and spiritual
Member of: Catholic Health Alliance of Canada
Chief Officer(s):
Robert Stewart, Executive Director
rstewart@health.nb.ca

College of Physicians & Surgeons of New Brunswick / Collège des médecins et chirurgiens du Nouveau-Brunswick
#300, 1 Hampton Rd., Rothesay NB E2E 5K8
Tel: 506-849-5050; *Fax:* 506-849-5069
Toll-Free: 800-667-4641
e-mail: info@cpsnb.org
www.cpsnb.org
Overview: A medium-sized provincial licensing organization founded in 1981 overseen by Federation of Regulatory Authorities of Canada
Chief Officer(s):
Lisa Jean Sutherland, President

New Brunswick Association of Medical Radiation Technologists (NBAMRT)
Memramcook Institute, #129, 488, rue Centrale, Memramcook NB E4K 3S6
Tel: 506-758-9673
www.nbamrt.ca
Previous Name: New Brunswick Association of Radiation Technologists; Canadian Association of Medical Radiation Technologists - New Brunswick

Overview: A small provincial organization founded in 1957 overseen by Canadian Association of Medical Radiation Technologists
Mission: To register medical radiation techologists in New Brunswick
Chief Officer(s):
Melanie Roybedy, Registrar

New Brunswick Medical Society (NBMS) / Société médicale du Nouveau-Brunswick
21 Alison Blvd., Fredericton NB E3C 2N5
Tel: 506-458-8860; *Fax:* 506-458-9853
e-mail: nbms@nb.aibn.com
www.nbms.nb.ca
www.facebook.com/CareFirstLasanteenpremier
twitter.com/nb_docs
Overview: A medium-sized provincial organization founded in 1867 overseen by Canadian Medical Association
Mission: To advance medical science in all its branches; to promote improvement of medical services; to prevent disease in cooperation with health officers & all others engaged in such work; to maintain high scientific & professional status for its members; to promote medical science & related arts & sciences
Chief Officer(s):
Camille Haddad, President

Paramedic Association of New Brunswick (PANB) / L'Association des paramédics du Nouveau-Brunswick
298 Main St., Fredericton NB E3A 1C9
Tel: 506-459-2638; *Fax:* 506-459-6728
Toll-Free: 888-887-7262
e-mail: info@panb.ca
www.panb.ca
twitter.com/PANB_Paramedic
Overview: A small provincial organization
Mission: To develop & promote the highest ethical, educational, & clinical standards for all levels of Prehospital Care Professionals in New Brunswick
Member of: Paramedic Association of Canada
Chief Officer(s):
Chris Hood, Executive Director/Registrar
chris.hood@panb.ca
Chantale Hayes, Assistant Registrar/Office Manager
chantale.hayes@panb.ca

Société Santé et Mieux-être en français du Nouveau-Brunswick (SSMEFFNB)
CP 1764, Moncton NB E1C 9X6
Tél: 506-389-3351; *Téléc:* 506-389-3366
Courriel: ssmefnb@nb.aibn.com
www.ssmefnb.ca
www.facebook.com/SSMEFNB
twitter.com/SSMEFNB
Aperçu: *Dimension:* petite; *Envergure:* provinciale surveillé par Société santé en français
Membre(s) du bureau directeur:
Gilles Vienneau, Directeur général

NEWFOUNDLAND AND LABRADOR

Association of Allied Health Professionals: Newfoundland & Labrador (Ind.) (AAHP) / Association des professionnels unis de la santé: Terre-Neuve et Labrador (ind.)
6 Mount Carson Ave., Mount Pearl NL A1N 3K4
Tel: 709-722-3353; *Fax:* 709-722-0987
Toll-Free: 800-728-2247
e-mail: info@aahp.nf.ca
www.aahp.nf.ca
Overview: A small provincial organization founded in 1975

College of Physicians & Surgeons of Newfoundland & Labrador
#W100, 120 Torbay Rd., St. John's NL A1A 2G8
Tel: 709-726-8546; *Fax:* 709-726-4725
e-mail: cpsnl@cpsnl.ca
www.cpsnl.ca
Previous Name: Newfoundland Medical Board
Overview: A medium-sized provincial licensing organization founded in 1893 overseen by Federation of Regulatory Authorities of Canada
Mission: To protect the public; to regulate the practice of medicine & medical practitioners
Chief Officer(s):
Linda Inkpen, Registrar

Arthur Rideout, Chair
Publications:
• College of Physicians & Surgeons of Newfoundland & Labrador
Annual Report
Type: Yearbook; *Frequency:* Annually
• Practice Dialogue [a publication of the College of Physicians &
Surgeons of Newfoundland & Labrador]
Type: Newsletter
Profile: Published under authority of the Registrar

**Newfoundland & Labrador Association of Medical Radiation
Technologists (NLAMRT)**
PO Box 29141, Stn. Torbay Rd. Post Office, St. John's NL A1A 5B5
Tel: 709-777-6036
www.nlamrt.ca

Overview: A small provincial organization founded in 1951 overseen
by Canadian Association of Medical Radiation Technologists
Mission: To represent all working medical radiation technologists in
Newfoundland & Labrador
Chief Officer(s):
Nicole Jenkins, President
njenkins668@hotmail.com

Newfoundland & Labrador Medical Association (NLMA)
164 MacDonald Dr., St. John's NL A1A 4B3
Tel: 709-726-7424; *Fax:* 709-726-7525
Toll-Free: 800-563-2003
e-mail: nlma@nlma.nl.ca
www.nlma.nl.ca
www.facebook.com/nlma.nl.ca
twitter.com/_nlma
www.youtube.com/user/nlmavideo

Overview: A medium-sized provincial organization founded in 1924
overseen by Canadian Medical Association
Mission: To represent & support physicians in Newfoundland &
Labrador; provide leadership in the promotion of good health & the
provision of quality health care to the people of the province
Chief Officer(s):
Wendy Graham, President
president@nlma.nl.ca
Robert Thompson, Executive Director, 709-726-7424 Ext. 302
rthompson@nlma.nl.ca

Newfoundland & Labrador Public Health Association (NLPHA)
PO Box 8172, St. John's NL A1B 3M9
Tel: 709-364-1589
e-mail: info@nlpha.ca
www.nlpha.ca

Overview: A small provincial organization founded in 1978 overseen
by Canadian Public Health Association
Mission: To advocate for the physical, emotional, social, &
environmental well-being of Newfoundland & Labrador's people &
communities
Member of: Canadian Public Health Association (CPHA)
Chief Officer(s):
Lynn Vivian-Book, President
Elizabeth Wright, Secretary
Pat Murray, Treasurer
Publications:
• Newfoundland & Labrador Public Health Association Newsletter
Type: Newsletter; *Editor:* Douglas Howse

Paramedic Association of Newfoundland & Labrador (PANL)
PO Box 8086, St. John's NL A1B 3M9
Toll-Free: 855-561-3698
e-mail: contact_us@panl.ca
www.panl.ca

Overview: A small provincial organization founded in 2005
Mission: To improve prehospital patient care in Newfoundland &
Labrador
Member of: Paramedic Association of Canada

**Professional Association of Internes & Residents of
Newfoundland (PAIRN) / Association professionnelle des internes
et résidents de Terre-Neuve**
**c/o Student Affairs, Health Sciences Complex, Memorial
University, #2713, 300 Prince Philip Dr., St. John's NL A1B 3V6**
Tel: 709-777-7118; *Fax:* 709-777-6968
e-mail: pairn@mun.ca
www.pairn.ca

Overview: A small provincial organization overseen by Resident
Doctors of Canada
Mission: To collaborate with local & national health care organizations
to advocate on behalf of internes, resident physicians, & fellows of
Newfoundland & Labrador; To advocate for the acknowledgement of
the resident's role in medical education
Affiliation(s): Canadian Association of Internes & Residents;
Newfoundland & Labrador Medical Association; Canadian Medical
Association
Chief Officer(s):
Sarah Kean, President
Robert Mercer, Vice-President
Heather O'Reilly, Secretary
Erika Hansford, Treasurer

Réseau santé en français Terre-Neuve-et-Labrador
**Centre scolaire et communautaire des Grads-Vants, #233, 65 ch
Ridge, St. John's NL A1B 4P5**
Tél: 709-575-2862; *Téléc:* 709-722-9904
Courriel: reseausante@fftnl.ca
www.francotnl.ca

Aperçu: *Dimension:* petite; *Envergure:* provinciale surveillé par Société
santé en français
Mission: Améliorer l'offre de services de santé en français
Membre(s) du bureau directeur:
Roxanne Leduc, Contact

NORTHWEST TERRITORIES

Association of Psychologists of the Northwest Territories
PO Box 1320, Yellowknife NT X1A 2L9
Tel: 867-920-8058
e-mail: psych@theedge.ca

Overview: A small provincial organization
Affiliation(s): Canadian Provincial Association of Psychologists (CPAP)
Chief Officer(s):
Robert O'Rourke, President

**Canadian Public Health Association - NWT/Nunavut Branch
(NTNUPHA)**
PO Box 1709, Yellowknife NT X1A 2P3
Overview: A small provincial organization overseen by Canadian
Public Health Association
Mission: To represent public health professionals
Chief Officer(s):
Cheryl Case, President

Northwest Territories Medical Association (NWTMA)
PO Box 1732, Yellowknife NT X1A 2P3
Tel: 867-920-4575; *Fax:* 867-920-4575
e-mail: nwtmedassoc@ssimicro.com
www.nwtma.ca

Overview: A medium-sized provincial organization overseen by
Canadian Medical Association
Mission: To advocate on behalf of its members & citizens for access to
quality health care; To provide leadership & guidance to its members
Member of: Canadian Medical Association
Chief Officer(s):
Steve Kraus, President

NWT Disabilities Council (NWTCPD)
#116, 5102 50th Ave., Yellowknife NT X1A 3S8
Tel: 867-873-8230; *Fax:* 867-873-4124
Toll-Free: 800-491-8885
e-mail: admin@nwtdc.net
www.nwtdc.net
www.facebook.com/436138019806132
Previous Name: Northwest Territories Council for the Disabled; NWT
Council for Disabled Persons
Overview: A medium-sized provincial charitable organization founded
in 1978

Mission: To encourage & support the self-determination of people with disabilities
Affiliation(s): Council of Canadians with Disabilities
Chief Officer(s):
Denise McKee, Executive Director
ed@nwtdc.net
Jennifer Winsor, Office Manager
finance@nwtdc.net

Réseau TNO Santé en français
CP 1325, 5016, 48 rue, Yellowknife NT X1A 2N9
Tél: 867-920-2919; *Téléc:* 867-873-2158
Courriel: santetno@franco-nord.com
www.reseautnosante.ca
twitter.com/SanteTno
Aperçu: *Dimension:* petite; *Envergure:* provinciale surveillé par Société santé en français
Mission: Contribuer à l'amélioration de l'accès à des services de santé de qualité en français
Membre(s) du bureau directeur:
Audrey Fournier, Coordonnatrice

NOVA SCOTIA

College of Physicians & Surgeons of Nova Scotia (CPSNS)
#5005, 7071 Bayers Rd., Halifax NS B3L 2C2
Tel: 902-422-5823; *Fax:* 902-422-7476
Toll-Free: 877-282-7767
e-mail: info@cpsns.ns.ca
www.cpsns.ns.ca
www.linkedin.com/company/2497006
www.facebook.com/291670920671
Previous Name: Provincial Medical Board of Nova Scotia
Overview: A medium-sized provincial licensing organization founded in 1872 overseen by Federation of Regulatory Authorities of Canada
Mission: To govern the practice of medicine in the public interest
Chief Officer(s):
James MacLachlan, President

Doctors Nova Scotia
25 Spectacle Lake Dr., Dartmouth NS B3B 1X7
Tel: 902-468-1866; *Fax:* 902-468-6578
Toll-Free: 800-563-3427
e-mail: info@doctorsns.com
www.doctorsns.com
twitter.com/Doctors_NS
Previous Name: Medical Society of Nova Scotia
Overview: A medium-sized provincial organization founded in 1861 overseen by Canadian Medical Association
Mission: To maintain the integrity of the medical profession; To represent members; To promote high quality health care & disease prevention in Nova Scotia
Member of: Canadian Medical Association
Chief Officer(s):
Nancy MacCready-Williams, CEO
John Sullivan, President

Entrepreneurs with Disabilities Network (EDN)
PO Box 44, #504, 5475 Spring Garden Rd., Halifax NS B3J 3T2
ednns.ca
www.facebook.com/EntrepreneurswithDisabilitiesNetwork
twitter.com/EDNns
Overview: A small provincial organization founded in 2004
Mission: To encourage entrepreneurship to people with disabilities; to understand the needs of entrepreneurs with disabilities & to represent them; to work on behalf of entrepreneurs with disabilities to advise government, business service providers & others on how best to serve them
Affiliation(s): Centre for Entrepreneurship Education & Development Inc.
Chief Officer(s):
Brian Aird, Executive Director
Publications:
• EDN [Entrepreneurs with Disabilities Network] Newsletter
Type: Newsletter; *Frequency:* q.

Environmental Health Association of Nova Scotia (EHANS)
PO Box 31323, Halifax NS B3K 5Y5
Toll-Free: 800-449-1995
e-mail: ehans@environmentalhealth.ca
www.environmentalhealth.ca
www.facebook.com/165405756830794
Previous Name: Nova Scotia Allergy & Environmental Health Association
Overview: A small provincial organization founded in 1985
Mission: To offer assistance to individuals affected by environmental health issues; To prevent illness caused by environmental factors through the promotion of health policies & practices
Chief Officer(s):
Eric Slone, President

Health Association Nova Scotia
2 Dartmouth Rd., Halifax NS B4A 2K7
Tel: 902-832-8500; *Fax:* 902-832-8505
www.healthassociation.ns.ca
twitter.com/HealthAssnNS
Previous Name: Nova Scotia Association of Health Organizations
Overview: A medium-sized provincial organization founded in 1960 overseen by Canadian Healthcare Association
Mission: To promote an effective, efficient & integrated quality health system for all Nova Scotians through leadership in influencing the development of public policy, representing & advocating members' interests & providing services to assist its members meet the health care needs of their communities
Member of: Canadian Alliance for Long Term Care
Chief Officer(s):
Gerald Pottier, Chair
Mary Lee, President/CEO, 902-832-8500 Ext. 236
Alex Cross, Communications Assistant, 902-832-8500 Ext. 295
alex.cross@healthassociation.ns.ca

Bedford Office
Clinical Engineering, 2 Dartmouth Rd., Bedford NS B4A 2K7
Tel: 902-832-8500; *Fax:* 902-832-8507
e-mail: contactus@healthassociation.ns.ca
Chief Officer(s):
Steve Smith, Director, Clinical Engineering
steve.smith@healthassociation.ns.ca

Central Region Office
Clinical Engineering, 150 Exhibition St., Kentville NS B4N 5E3
Tel: 902-678-7090; *Fax:* 902-578-0565
Chief Officer(s):
Ed Ezekiel, Coordinator, Central Region
edward.ezekiel@healthassociation.ns.ca

Northern Region Office
Clinical Engineering, 835 East River Rd., New Glasgow NS B2H 3S6
Tel: 902-752-5487; *Fax:* 902-755-6297
Chief Officer(s):
John Inch, CET, CBET, Coordinator, Northern Region
john.inch@healthassociation.ns.ca

Southern Region Office
Clinical Engineering, 90 Glenn Allen Dr., Bridgewater NS B4V 3S6
Tel: 902-527-5234; *Fax:* 902-543-1662
Chief Officer(s):
Philip Bradfield, CET, CBET, Technical Support & Development Officer
phil.bradfield@healthassociation.ns.ca

Health Association of African Canadians (HAAC)
c/o Black Cultural Centre for Nova Scotia, 10 Cherry Brook Rd., Cherry Brook NS B2Z 1A8
Tel: 902-405-4222
e-mail: info@haac.ca
www.haac.ca
Overview: A medium-sized provincial organization founded in 2000
Mission: To promote & improve the health of African Canadians in Nova Scotia through community engagement, education, policy recommendations, partnerships, & research participation
Chief Officer(s):
Donna Smith-Darrell, Co-Chair
Sharon Davis-Murdoch, Co-Chair

Nova Scotia Association of Medical Radiation Technologists (NSAMRT)
Park Lane Terraces, PO Box 142, #502, 5657 Spring Garden Rd., Halifax NS B3J 3R4

Tel: 902-434-6525; *Fax:* 902-832-8676
Toll-Free: 866-788-6525
e-mail: info@nsamrt.ca
www.nsamrt.ca

Overview: A small provincial organization overseen by Canadian Association of Medical Radiation Technologists
Mission: To uphold standards of practice in the field of medical radiation technology in Nova Scotia, in order to ensure the public is given optimal care
Chief Officer(s):
Julie Avery, Executive Director
julieavery@nsamrt.ca

Public Health Association of Nova Scotia (PHANS)
PO Box 33074, Halifax NS B3L 4T6
www.phans.ca

Overview: A small provincial charitable organization overseen by Canadian Public Health Association
Mission: To build public health capacity & to make progress on the determinants of health in Nova Scotia
Affliation(s): Canadian Public Health Association

Réseau Santé - Nouvelle-Écosse
#222, 2 rue Bluewater, Bedford NS B4B 1G7

Tél: 902-222-5871
Courriel: reseau@reseausantene.ca
www.reseausantene.ca
www.facebook.com/reseausantenouvelleecosse
twitter.com/ReseauSanteNE

Aperçu: *Dimension:* petite; *Envergure:* provinciale surveillé par Société santé en français
Mission: Promouvoir et d'améliorer l'accessibilité en français aux services de santé et de mieux-être de qualité
Membre(s) du bureau directeur:
Jeanne-Françoise Caillaud, Directrice générale

NUNAVUT

Réseau de Santé en Français au Nunavut (SAFRAN)
CP 1516, Iqaluit NU X0A 0H0

Tél: 867-222-2107
Courriel: resefan.nu@gmail.com
www.resefan.ca

Aperçu: *Dimension:* petite; *Envergure:* provinciale; fondée en 2004 surveillé par Société santé en français
Mission: Contribuer à l'amélioration de la santé des francophones du Nunavut
Membre(s) du bureau directeur:
Carine Chalut, Directrice générale

ONTARIO

Alberta Association of Prosthetists & Orthotists
c/o Orthotics Prosthetics Canada, #202, 300 March Rd., Ottawa ON K2K 2E2

e-mail: secretary@albertaoandp.com
www.albertaoandp.com

Overview: A small provincial organization overseen by Orthotics Prosthetics Canada
Mission: To represent members in Alberta's prosthetic & orthotic field; To promote high standards of patient care & professionalism
Chief Officer(s):
Jon Allen, President
Nolan Hayday, Vice-President
Ryan Cochrane, Secretary

ARCH Disability Law Centre
#110, 425 Bloor St. East, Toronto ON M4W 3R5

Tel: 416-482-8255; *Fax:* 416-482-2981
Toll-Free: 866-482-2724; *TTY:* 416-482-1254
e-mail: archlib@lao.on.ca
www.archdisabilitylaw.ca
www.facebook.com/ARCHDisabilityLawCentre
twitter.com/ARCHDisability
www.youtube.com/channel/UCZI_6YpK8XB7LJ_dQxdonIg

Previous Name: A Legal Resource Centre for Persons with Disabilities
Overview: A medium-sized provincial charitable organization founded in 1980
Mission: To defend & advance the equality rights of persons with disabilities; assisting individuals with disabilities to understand their rights & how to enforce them; working with groups representing people with disabilities throughout Ontario; representing in precedent setting cases where client cannot be represented appropriately by other legal services; summary advice & referral - lawyers who specialize in areas of law as they relate to disability provide free, confidential, basic legal advice & referral to other sources of assistance
Chief Officer(s):
Ivana Petricone, Executive Director

Armenian Canadian Medical Association of Ontario (ACMAO)
2030 Victoria Park Ave., Toronto ON M1R 1V2

Tel: 416-443-9971; *Fax:* 416-443-8865
e-mail: acmaoexecutive@gmail.com
www.acmao.ca

Overview: A small provincial charitable organization founded in 1988
Mission: The Armenian Canadian Medical Association of Ontario (ACMAO) is a multidisciplinary organization of health care professionals in Ontario,
Chief Officer(s):
Avedis Bogosyan, President

Association of Family Health Teams of Ontario (AFHTO)
#800, 60 St. Clair Ave. East, Toronto ON M4T 1N5

Tel: 647-234-8605
e-mail: info@afhto.ca
www.afhto.ca
www.facebook.com/afhto
twitter.com/afhto

Overview: A medium-sized provincial organization
Mission: To promote the expansion of high-quality, comprehensive, well-integrated interprofessional primary care for the benefit of all Ontarians
Chief Officer(s):
Kavita Mehta, Chief Executive Officer
kavita.mehta@afhto.ca
Sombo Saviye, Office Manager
sombo.saviye@afhto.ca
Paula Myers, Coordinator, Membership, Communications & Conference
paula.myers@afhto.ca

Association of International Physicians & Surgeons of Ontario (AIPSO)
#850, 36 Toronto St., Toronto ON M5C 2C5

e-mail: imdontario@yahoo.ca
aipso.webs.com

Overview: A small provincial organization founded in 1998
Mission: To assist internationally trained physicians & surgeons by facilitating access to the licensing process in Canada; To ensure the integration of internationally-trained physicians & surgeons into the Canadian health care system
Chief Officer(s):
Amin Lakhani, President
aylakhani@hotmail.com
Publications:
• Association of International Physicians & Surgeons of Ontario Members Directory
Type: Directory

Association of Local Public Health Agencies (ALPHA)
#1306, 2 Carlton St., Toronto ON M5B 1J3

Tel: 416-595-0006; *Fax:* 416-595-0030
e-mail: info@alphaweb.org
www.alphaweb.org

Previous Name: Association of Local Official Health Agencies (ALOHA)
Overview: A medium-sized provincial organization founded in 1986
Mission: To provide leadership in public health management to health units in Ontario; To assist local public health units in the provision of efficient & effective services
Affliation(s): ANDSOOHA - Public Health Nursing Management; Association of Ontario Public Health Business Administrators; Association of Public Health Epidemiologists in Ontario; Association of Supervisors of Public Health Inspectors of Ontario; Health Promotion

Ontario; Ontario Association of Public Health Dentistry; Ontario Society of Nutrition Professionals in Public Health
Chief Officer(s):
Linda Stewart, Executive Director
  linda@alphaweb.org
Gordon Fleming, Manager, Public Health Issues
  gordon@alphaweb.org
Susan Lee, Manager, Administrative & Association Services
  susan@alphaweb.org
Publications:
• Public Health Pulse
Type: Newsletter; *Frequency:* Quarterly
Profile: Association activities, affiliate information, conference highlights, & upcoming events

Association of Ontario Health Centres (AOHC) / Association des centres de santé de l'Ontario (ACSO)
#500, 970 Lawrence Ave. West, Toronto ON M6A 3B6
Tel: 416-236-2539; *Fax:* 416-236-0431
e-mail: mail@aohc.org
www.aohc.org
www.facebook.com/AOHC.ACSO
twitter.com/aohc_acso
Overview: A medium-sized provincial charitable organization founded in 1982
Mission: To promote community based primary care, health promotion, & illness prevention services, focusing on the broader determinants of health such as education, employment, poverty, isolation, & housing
Member of: Canadian Alliance of Community Health Centre Associations; Ontario Health Providers Alliance; Ontario Public Health Association
Affiliation(s): Healthy Communities; Ontario Rural Council; Health Determinants Partnership; Canadian Health Network
Chief Officer(s):
Adrianna Tetley, Chief Executive Officer, 416-236-2539 Ext. 222
  adrianna@aohc.org
Leah Stephenson, Director, Special Projects, 416-236-2539 Ext. 244
  leah.stephenson@aohc.org
Sandra Wong, Manager, Corporate Services, 416-236-2539 Ext. 241
  sandra@aohc.org
Publications:
• Bridging the Gap [a publication of the Association of Ontario Health Centres]
Type: Report
Profile: 2014 report released in conjunction with the Coalition of Community Health & Resource Centres of Ottawa (CHRC) to evaluate the wellbeing ofOttawa using the Canadian Index of Wellbeing framework
• Leading Transformative Change: [a publication of the Association of Ontario Health Centres]
Type: Report
Profile: A report on the 2012-2015 AOHC strategic plan
• Measuring What Matters [a publication of the Association of Ontario Health Centres]
Type: Report
Profile: A report on how the Canadian Index of Wellbeing can improve the quality of life in Ontario

Atlantic Association of Prosthetists & Orthotists
c/o Orthotics Prosthetics Canada, #202, 300 March Rd., Ottawa ON K2K 2E2
Overview: A small provincial organization overseen by Orthotics Prosthetics Canada
Mission: To promote quality patient care & a high standard of professionalism in the prosthetic & orthotic profession in the Atlantic region
Chief Officer(s):
Elizabeth Harris, President

Canadian Association of Occupational Therapists - British Columbia (CAOT-BC)
c/o National Office, #100, 34 Colonnade Rd., Ottawa ON K2E 7J6
Tel: 613-523-2268; *Fax:* 613-523-2552
Toll-Free: 800-434-2268
www.caot.ca/default.asp?pageid=4125
twitter.com/Caot_bc
Overview: A medium-sized provincial organization

Mission: To promote the profession of occupational therapy throughout the province & represent its members to regional health boards & government, health professional groups & the public; to foster the growth & development of the profession in BC; to provide a variety of services to its members including continuing education, reentry & participation in professional issues
Member of: Canadian Association of Occupational Therapists
Chief Officer(s):
Giovanna Boniface, Managing Director
  gboniface@caot.ca

Catholic Health Sponsors of Ontario
#1801, 1 Yonge St., Toronto ON M5E 1W7
Tel: 416-740-0444
e-mail: chco@chco.ca
www.chco.ca
Overview: A medium-sized provincial organization overseen by Catholic Health Association of Canada
Mission: To sponsor member institutions & strengthen Catholic health care in Ontario
Chief Officer(s):
John P. Ruetz, President & CEO
  john.ruetz@chco.ca
Sarah Quackenbush, Consultant, Mission Education
  squackenbush@csjssm.ca

College of Chiropodists of Ontario (COCOO)
#2102, 180 Dundas St. West, Toronto ON M5G 1Z8
Tel: 416-542-1333; *Fax:* 416-542-1666
Toll-Free: 877-232-7653
www.cocoo.on.ca
Overview: A small provincial licensing organization
Mission: To protect public interest by ensuring competent care is given by chiropodists & podiatrists in Ontario
Chief Officer(s):
Sohail Mall, President

College of Medical Radiation Technologists of Ontario / Ordre des technologues en radiation médicale de l'Ontario
#300, 375 University Ave., Toronto ON M5G 2J5
Tel: 416-975-4353; *Fax:* 416-975-4355
Toll-Free: 800-563-5847
e-mail: info@cmrto.org
www.cmrto.org
www.linkedin.com/company/college-of-medical-radiation-technologists-of
www.facebook.com/pages/CMRTO/897367403625523
Overview: A medium-sized provincial organization
Mission: To serve & protect the people of Ontario through self-regulation of the profession
Chief Officer(s):
Linda Gough, Registrar & CEO
  lgough@cmrto.org

College of Optometrists of Ontario / Ordre des optométristes de l'Ontario
#900, 65 St. Clair Ave. East, Toronto ON M4T 2Y3
Tel: 416-962-4071; *Fax:* 416-962-4073
Toll-Free: 888-825-2554
e-mail: info@collegeoptom.on.ca
www.collegeoptom.on.ca
www.facebook.com/collegeoptom
twitter.com/collegeoptom
Overview: A medium-sized provincial licensing organization founded in 1919
Mission: To serve the public interest by guiding the optometry profession; To ensure that safe, ethical & quality eye care is delivered; To maintain high standards within the field
Chief Officer(s):
Thomas Noël, President
Paula Garshowitz, Registrar
Louise Kassabian, Manager, Membership & Office Administration
  lkassabian@collegeoptom.on.ca

College of Physicians & Surgeons of Ontario (CPSO)
80 College St., Toronto ON M5G 2E2
Tel: 416-967-2603; *Fax:* 416-961-3330
Toll-Free: 800-268-7096
e-mail: feedback@cpso.on.ca
www.cpso.on.ca
www.linkedin.com/groups/College-Physicians-Surgeons-Ontario-4760466
www.facebook.com/144601285573797
twitter.com/cpso_ca
www.youtube.com/user/theCpso
Overview: A large provincial licensing organization founded in 1866 overseen by Federation of Regulatory Authorities of Canada
Mission: To ensure the best quality care for the people of Ontario by the doctors of Ontario
Chief Officer(s):
Carol Leet, President
Rocco Gerace, Registrar
Publications:
• Dialogue
Type: Magazine
• Methadone News: Patient Forum
Type: Newsletter

College of Registered Psychotherapists of Ontario (CRPO)
163 Queen St. East, 4th Fl., Toronto ON M5A 1S21
Tel: 416-862-4801; *Fax:* 416-974-4079
Toll-Free: 888-661-4801
e-mail: info@crpo.ca
www.crpo.ca
Overview: A small provincial licensing organization
Mission: To regulate the profession of psychotherapy & to maintain professional, ethical standards.
Chief Officer(s):
Joyce Rowlands, Registrar

Family Service Ontario / Services à la famille - Ontario
#630, 190 Attwell Dr., Toronto ON M9W 6H8
Tel: 416-231-6003; *Fax:* 416-231-2405
www.familyserviceontario.org
www.facebook.com/pages/Family-Service-Ontario/328478643913963
twitter.com/FamServOntario
Overview: A medium-sized provincial charitable organization founded in 1974
Mission: To support & assist member family service agencies
Affilation(s): Ontario Association of Credit Counselling Services; Family Services Canada; Catholic Charities; United Way; Canadian Council of Social Development
Chief Officer(s):
John Ellis, Executive Director

Federation of Health Regulatory Colleges of Ontario (FHRCO) / Ordres de réglementation des professionnels de la santé de l'Ontario (ORPSO)
PO Box 244, #301, 396 Osborne St., Beaverton ON L0K 1A0
Tel: 416-493-4076; *Fax:* 866-814-6456
e-mail: info@regulatedhealthprofessions.on.ca
www.regulatedhealthprofessions.on.ca
Overview: A medium-sized provincial organization
Mission: To regulate health professionals in Ontario; To protect the public's right to safe, effective, & ethical health care
Chief Officer(s):
Shenda Tanchak, President
Beth Ann Kenny, Executive Coordinator

Hospital Auxiliaries Association of Ontario (HAAO)
#2800, 200 Front St. West, Toronto ON M5V 3L1
Tel: 416-205-1407; *Fax:* 416-205-1596
www.haao.com
www.facebook.com/193203857388754
Overview: A medium-sized provincial charitable organization founded in 1910
Mission: To advocate for community partnerships to support health care in Ontario; To promote volunteer services

Manitoba Association of Prosthetists & Orthotists
c/o Orthotics Prosthetics Canada, #202, 300 March Rd., Ottawa ON K2K 2E2
Overview: A small provincial organization overseen by Orthotics Prosthetics Canada
Mission: To promote quality care for prosthetic & orthotic patients in Manitoba; To encourage professionalism in Manitoba's prosthetic & orthotic field
Chief Officer(s):
Daniel Mazur, Contact

Medical Device Reprocessing Association of Ontario (MDRAO)
PO Box 225, Timmins ON P4N 7C9
Tel: 705-268-4763; *Fax:* 705-268-4421
e-mail: mdrao@ntl.sympatico.ca
www.mdrao.ca
www.linkedin.com/groups/5036123
www.facebook.com/CSAO-237386583016742
twitter.com/CSAOCanada
Previous Name: Central Service Association of Ontario
Overview: A medium-sized provincial organization founded in 1963
Mission: To promote standards of practice & education in the medical device reprocessing industry; To provide opportunities for all members
Chief Officer(s):
Louis Konstant, President
Rohan Jagasar, Vice-President
Stephenie Naugler, Director, Communications

Ontario Agencies Supporting Individuals with Special Needs (OASIS)
c/o Community Living South Muskoka, 15 Depot Dr., Bracebridge ON P1L 0A1
Tel: 705-645-5494
e-mail: administrativesupport@oasisonline.ca
www.oasisonline.ca
www.facebook.com/oasis.ontario
twitter.com/oasisontario
Overview: A medium-sized provincial organization
Mission: To facilitate the sharing of ideas, resources, systems & information; to liaise with government on behalf of member organizations with the goal of improving the development of cost effective quality supports for individuals with developmental disabilities
Chief Officer(s):
David Barber, President
Amanda Brown, Administrative Contact

Ontario Art Therapy Association (OATA)
#103, 611 Wonderland Rd. N, London ON N6H 5N7
e-mail: president@oata.ca
www.oata.ca
Overview: A small provincial licensing organization founded in 1978
Mission: To provide for the development, the promotion & the maintenance of the field of art therapy in Ontario; to grant registration to its professional members upon successful completion of a rigorous process & documentation of training & experience
Chief Officer(s):
Susan Richardson, President
  president@oata.ca

Ontario Association of Medical Radiation Sciences (OAMRS)
#415A, 175 Longwood Rd. South, Hamilton ON L8P 0A1
Tel: 289-674-0034; *Fax:* 289-674-0037
Toll-Free: 800-387-4674
www.oamrs.org
www.linkedin.com/company/oamrs—ontario-association-of-medical-radiati
www.facebook.com/OAMRS1
twitter.com/OAMRS1
Merged from: Ont. Assn. of Medical Radiation Technologists; Ont. Society of Diagnostic Medical Sonographers
Overview: A medium-sized provincial organization founded in 2012 overseen by Canadian Association of Medical Radiation Technologists
Mission: To advocate on behalf of the profession of medical radiation science practitioners to government bodies
Chief Officer(s):
Greg Toffner, President & CEO
  toffnerg@oamrs.org
Publications:
• Filter: The Journal of The Ontario Association of Medical Radiation

Sciences
Type: E-Newsletter; *Frequency:* Bimonthly; *Accepts Advertising*
Profile: Information for technologists who specialize in radiography, C.T., P.E.T., M.R.I, radiation therapy, ultrasound, & nuclear medicine

Ontario Association of Pathologists (OAP)
#310, 4 Cataraqui St., Kingston ON K7K 1Z7
Tel: 613-507-7663
e-mail: oap@eventsmgt.com
www.ontariopathologists.org
www.linkedin.com/company/ontario-association-of-pathologists
www.facebook.com/OntarioPathologists
Overview: A small provincial organization founded in 1937
Mission: To advance pathology & its allied sciences; To maintain a high standard of proficiency & ethics among its members; To promote research in pathology; To promote the interests of members
Chief Officer(s):
Russell Price, President
Satish Chawla, Secretary-Treasurer

Ontario Association of Prosthetists & Orthotists (OAPO)
15 Britannia Ave., Toronto ON M6N 3T6
Other Communication: E-mails: mediarelations@oapo.org; committee@oapo.org
e-mail: info@oapo.org
oapo.org
Overview: A small provincial organization overseen by Orthotics Prosthetics Canada
Mission: To promote professionalism & high standards of care in the prosthetic & orthotic field in Ontario
Chief Officer(s):
Eric Bapty, Director

Ontario Association of Radiology Managers (OARM)
26 Gateway Crt., Whitby ON L1R 3M9
Tel: 905-655-5645
e-mail: headoffice@oarm.org
www.oarm.org
Overview: A medium-sized provincial organization founded in 1983
Mission: To serve as an education & communication platform for radiology managers in Ontario
Chief Officer(s):
Mike Mukesh Sharma, President

Ontario Healthcare Housekeepers' Association Inc. (OHHA)
2053 County Road 22, Bath ON K0H 1G0
Tel: 613-352-5696; *Fax:* 613-352-5840
www.ohha.org
www.facebook.com/ontariohealthcarehousekeepersassociationinc
twitter.com/healthcarehskpr
Previous Name: Ontario Health Care Housekeepers Association Inc.
Overview: A small provincial organization founded in 1957
Affiliation(s): Ontario Hospital Association, CSSA, OLTCA, ISSA
Chief Officer(s):
Wendy Boone-Watt, Executive Director
executivedirector@ohha.org

Ontario Healthy Communities Coalition (OHCC) / Coalition des communautés en santé de l'Ontario
#1810, 2 Carlton St., Toronto ON M5B 1J3
Tel: 416-408-4841; *Fax:* 416-408-4843
Toll-Free: 800-766-3418
www.ohcc-ccso.ca
www.facebook.com/OntarioHealthyCommunitiesCoalition
twitter.com/OntarioHCC
www.youtube.com/user/ohccccso
Overview: A medium-sized provincial charitable organization founded in 1992
Mission: To achieve social, environmental, economic & physical well-being for individuals, communities & local governments throughout Ontario
Chief Officer(s):
Lorna McCue, Executive Director

Ontario Hospital Association (OHA)
#2800, 200 Front St. West, Toronto ON M5V 3L1
Tel: 416-205-1300; *Fax:* 416-205-1301
Toll-Free: 800-598-8002
e-mail: info@oha.com
www.oha.com
www.linkedin.com/company/ontario-hospital-association
www.facebook.com/onthospitalassn
twitter.com/OntHospitalAssn
www.youtube.com/onthospitalassn
Overview: A medium-sized provincial organization founded in 1924 overseen by Canadian Healthcare Association
Mission: To build a strong, innovative, & sustainable health care system that meets patient care needs throughout Ontario; To promote an efficent & effective health care system
Chief Officer(s):
Jamie McCracken, Chair
Anthony Dale, President & CEO
Warren DiClemente, Chief Operating Officer & VP, Educational Services
Elizabeth Carlton, Vice-President, Policy & Public Affairs
Hazim Hassan, Vice-President, Business Planning & Strategy
Publications:
• Healthcare Governance Update
Type: Newsletter
Profile: Information from the Governance Centre of Excellence to maintain & increase trustees' knowledge of health care governance issues
• Healthscape [a publication of Ontario Hospital Association]
Type: Newsletter
• Hospital Perspectives
Type: Newsletter; *ISSN:* 1198-0192
Profile: Articles about innovations in health care
• Labour Relations Bulletin [a publication of Ontario Hospital Association]
Type: Newsletter
• OHA [Ontario Hospital Association] Executive Report
Type: Newsletter; *Frequency:* Weekly; *Price:* Free with membership in the Ontario Hospital Association
Profile: Current health care news
• Ontario Hospital Association Annual Report
Type: Yearbook; *Frequency:* Annually

Ontario Kinesiology Association (OKA)
#100, 6700 Century Ave., Mississauga ON L5N 6A4
Tel: 905-567-7194; *Fax:* 905-567-7191
e-mail: info@oka.on.ca
www.oka.on.ca
www.linkedin.com/groups?home=&gid=1264707
www.facebook.com/ontariokinesiologyassociation
twitter.com/ONKinesiology
Overview: A medium-sized provincial organization founded in 1982
Mission: To promote the application of the science of human movement to other professionals & to the community; to uphold the standards of the profession of kinesiology; to assist kinesiologists in the performance of their duties & responsibilities
Member of: Canadian Kinesiology Alliance
Chief Officer(s):
Jennifer Chapman, President

Ontario Medical Association (OMA)
#900, 150 Bloor St. West, Toronto ON M5S 3C1
Tel: 416-599-2580; *Fax:* 416-340-2944
Toll-Free: 800-268-7215
Other Communication: membership@oma.org
e-mail: info@oma.org
www.oma.org
www.linkedin.com/company/ontario-medical-association
www.facebook.com/Ontariosdoctors
twitter.com/OntariosDoctors
www.youtube.com/user/OntMedAssociation
Overview: A large provincial organization founded in 1880 overseen by Canadian Medical Association
Mission: To represent the clinical, political, & economic interests of Ontario physicians; To promote an accessible, quality health-care system
Chief Officer(s):

Tom Magyarody, Chief Executive Officer
Danielle Milley, Senior Advisor, Media Relations, 416-599-2580
  danielle.milley@oma.org
Publications:
• Ontario Medical Review [a publication of the Ontario Medical
Association]
Type: Journal; *Editor:* Kim Secord
• Scrub-In [a publication of the Ontario Medical Association]
Type: Magazine; *Frequency:* 3 pa.; *ISSN:* 1923-953X
Profile: Contains medical student-generated content written for a
student audience

Ontario Medical Students Association (OMSA)
**c/o Ontario Medical Association, #900, 150 Bloor St. West, Toronto
ON M5S 3C1**

Tel: 416-599-2580
Toll-Free: 800-268-7215
www.omsa.ca
www.facebook.com/OntarioMedicalStudents
twitter.com/OMSAofficial
www.instagram.com/OMSAofficial

Overview: A medium-sized provincial organization founded in 1974
overseen by Ontario Medical Association
Mission: To represent the concerns & views of medical students in
Ontario
Member of: Ontario Medical Association
Affiliation(s): Canadian Medical Association
Chief Officer(s):
Ali Damji, Co-Chair
  chair@omsa.ca
Justin Cottrell, Co-Chair
  co-chair@omsa.ca

Ontario Paramedic Association (OPA)
PO Box 1628, Blind River ON P0R 1B0

Toll-Free: 888-672-5463
e-mail: info@ontarioparamedic.ca
www.ontarioparamedic.ca
www.facebook.com/sendaparamedic
twitter.com/OntParamedic
vimeo.com/ontarioparamedic

Overview: A small provincial organization founded in 1996
Mission: To act as a voice for both professional & patient care issues;
To advocate for improvements in patient care
Member of: Paramedic Association of Canada (PAC)
Chief Officer(s):
Geoff MacBride, President
Publications:
• OPA [Ontario Paramedic Association] News
Type: Newsletter; *Accepts Advertising; Editor:* Elizabeth Anderson;
Price: Free with Ontario Paramedic Association membership
Profile: Association newsletter contained in Canadian Emergency News

Ontario Personal Support Worker Association (OPSWA)
Cambridge ON

Tel: 519-654-9878
e-mail: admin@opswa.com
www.opswa.com
www.facebook.com/pages/Ontario-PSW-Association/14136082755692
05
twitter.com/OntarioPSWAssoc
instagram.com/OPSWA

Overview: A small provincial organization
Mission: To continuously strive to improve the professional status of
the Personal Support Workers of Ontario through advocacy for
excellence & consistency in training, services, working conditions &
value to those they serve.
Chief Officer(s):
Miranda Ferrier, President

Ontario Podiatric Medical Association (OPMA)
#900, 45 Sheppard Ave. East, Toronto ON M2N 5W9

Tel: 416-927-9111; *Fax:* 416-927-9111
Toll-Free: 866-424-6762
e-mail: contact@opma.ca
www.opma.ca
www.facebook.com/756620137694740

Overview: A small provincial organization

Mission: To act as the voice of podiatry & podiatrists in Ontario; To
advance the profession of podiatry in Ontario; To ensure timely access
to high quality foot care services in Ontario in order to serve & protect
the public
Member of: American Podiatric Medical Association, Inc., Region 5
Chief Officer(s):
Bruce Ramsden, President
Sheldon Freelan, Vice-President
Martin Brain, Secretary
Peter Higenell, Treasurer

Ontario Public Health Association (OPHA) / Association pour la santé publique de l'Ontario
#502, 44 Victoria St., Toronto ON M5C 1Y2

Tel: 416-367-3313; *Fax:* 416-367-2844
e-mail: admin@opha.on.ca
www.opha.on.ca
www.linkedin.com/company/ontario-public-health-association
www.facebook.com/opha1949
twitter.com/OPHA_Ontario
twitter.com/nutritionrc

Overview: A medium-sized provincial charitable organization founded
in 1949 overseen by Canadian Public Health Association
Mission: To provide leadership on issues affecting public health in
Ontario, such as preserving the environment, promoting disease
prevention, narrowing health disparities & reducing poverty; To
strengthen the influence of persons involved in public & community
health across Ontario
Chief Officer(s):
Ellen Wodchis, President
Pegeen Walsh, Executive Director
Barb Prud'homme, Coordinator
  barbp@opha.on.ca
Publications:
• Ontario Public Health Association E-Bulletin
Type: Newsletter; *Frequency:* Monthly
Profile: Current topics in public health & information about the
association's workgroups & partnerships
• Public Health Today
Type: Magazine; *Price:* Free with membership in the Ontario Public
Health Association

Ontario Public Service Employees Union (OPSEU) / Syndicat des employées et employés de la fonction publique de l'Ontario
100 Lesmill Rd., Toronto ON M3B 3P8

Tel: 416-443-8888; *Fax:* 416-443-9670
Toll-Free: 800-268-7376
e-mail: opseu@opseu.org
www.opseu.org
www.facebook.com/OPSEU?v=app_4949752878
twitter.com/OPSEU
www.youtube.com/user/OPSEUSEFPO

Previous Name: Civil Service Association of Ontario
Overview: A large provincial organization founded in 1911
Mission: To negotiate collective agreements; to conduct membership
education; to lobby governments to maintain & improve public services;
to defend the principle of social unionism by speaking out on public
policy issues such as taxes, free trade, privatization, health care, social
services, occupational health & safety, & employment equity.
Member of: National Union of Public and General Employees
Affliation(s): Canadian Labour Council; Ontario Federation of Labour
Chief Officer(s):
Warren (Smokey) Thomas, President
Publications:
• Autumn View
Type: Newsletter; *Frequency:* Quarterly
• In Solidarity
Type: Newsletter; *Frequency:* Quarterly

Ontario Regional Poison Information Centre (ORPIC)
**The Hospital for Sick Children, 555 University Ave., Toronto ON
M5G 1X8**

Tel: 416-813-5900
Toll-Free: 800-268-9017; *TTY:* 416-597-0215
www.ontariopoisoncentre.com

Overview: A small provincial organization founded in 1978
Mission: To provide telephone information & advice about exposures
to poisonous substances; operates 24 hour, 7 day a week through local

SECTION II:
General Resources

& toll free numbers
Member of: Canadian Association of Poison Control Centres
Chief Officer(s):
Lutfi Haj-Assaad, Director, Child Health Services

Ontario Society of Chiropodists (OSC)
#100, 6700 Century Ave., Mississauga ON L5N 6A4

Tel: 905-567-3094; *Fax:* 905-567-7191
Toll-Free: 877-823-1508
e-mail: info@ontariochiropodist.com
www.ontariochiropodist.com

Overview: A small provincial organization founded in 1985
Mission: To provide extensive & regular postgraduate education
programs to ensure that the chiropodist remains a first rate foot care
specialist
Chief Officer(s):
Sarah Robinson, President

Ontario Society of Medical Technologists (OSMT)
#402, 234 Eglinton Ave. East, Toronto ON M4P 1K5

Tel: 416-485-6768; *Fax:* 416-485-7660
Toll-Free: 800-461-6768
e-mail: osmt@osmt.org
www.osmt.org
www.linkedin.com/company/ontario-society-of-medical-technologists
www.facebook.com/217098608317170
twitter.com/osmt2011

Overview: A medium-sized provincial organization founded in 1963
overseen by Canadian Society For Medical Laboratory Science
Mission: To represent the professional interests of medical
technologists & medical laboratory assistants/technicians in relations
with government & the public; to provide continuing education &
technical consulting services
Member of: Canadian Society for Medical Laboratory Science
Chief Officer(s):
Blanca McArthur, Executive Director, 416-485-6768 Ext. 25
bmcarthur@osmt.org
Publications:
•
• Advocate
Type: Magazine; *Frequency:* q.; *Accepts Advertising; Editor:* Blanca
McArthur
Profile: The magazine features articles that pertain to medical
technologists, including case studies & educational reports

Ontario Society of Occupational Therapists (OSOT)
#210, 55 Eglinton Ave. East, Toronto ON M4P 1G8

Tel: 416-322-3011; *Fax:* 416-322-6705
Toll-Free: 877-676-6768
e-mail: osot@osot.on.ca
www.osot.on.ca
www.linkedin.com/company/ontario-society-of-occupational-therapists
www.facebook.com/161471573904550
twitter.com/osotvoice

Overview: A medium-sized provincial organization founded in 1920
Mission: To promote & represent the profession of occupational
therapy in the areas of government affairs, education, professional
issues & public relations in Ontario
Affliation(s): Canadian Association of Occupational Therapists
Chief Officer(s):
Christie Benchley, Executive Director, 416-322-3011 Ext. 224
cbrenchley@osot.on.ca
Rob Linkiewicz, Manager, Operations, 416-322-3011 Ext. 231
rlinkiewicz@osot.on.ca
Seema Sindwani, Manager, Professional Development & Practice
Support, 416-322-3011 Ext. 238
ssindwani@osot.on.ca

Ontario Society of Periodontists (OSP)
#300, 1370 Don Mills Rd., Toronto ON M3B 3N7

Tel: 416-424-6632; *Fax:* 416-441-0591
Toll-Free: 855-336-8556
e-mail: info@osp.on.ca
www.osp.on.ca

Overview: A medium-sized provincial organization
Mission: To be the official voice of Ontario periodontists; to serve the
providers and recipients of periodontal care
Member of: Ontario Dental Association

Chief Officer(s):
Shari Bricks, Managing Director
shari@osp.on.ca
Stephen Gangbar, President
president@osp.on.ca

Ontario Society of Psychotherapists (OSP)
#1, 189 Queen St. East, Toronto ON M5A 1S2

Tel: 416-923-4050; *Fax:* 416-968-6818
e-mail: mail@psychotherapyontario.org
psychotherapyontario.com
twitter.com/psychotherapyon

Overview: A small provincial organization
Mission: The Ontario Society of Psychotherapists is committed to the
continuing development of ethically responsible and self-reflective
psychotherapists
Chief Officer(s):
Christina Becker, President

Professional Association of Residents of Ontario (PARO)
#1901, 400 University Ave., Toronto ON M5G 1S5

Tel: 416-979-1182; *Fax:* 416-595-9778
Toll-Free: 877-979-1183
e-mail: paro@paroteam.ca
www.myparo.ca

Overview: A small provincial organization overseen by Resident
Doctors of Canada
Mission: To improve the quality of life for young doctors training in
Ontario; To advocate for acknowledgment of the resident's role in
medical education; To ensure that patients receive excellent care
Member of: Resident Doctors of Canada
Chief Officer(s):
Robert Conn, CEO
Stephanie Kenny, President

Réseau du mieux-être francophone du Nord de l'Ontario
CP 270, 469, rue Bouchard, Sudbury ON P3E 2K8

Tél: 705-674-9381
Ligne sans frais: 866-489-7484
www.reseaudumieuxetre.ca
www.facebook.com/rmefno
twitter.com/rmefno

Aperçu: *Dimension:* petite; *Envergure:* provinciale surveillé par Société
santé en français
Mission: Favorisant l'offre de services de santé en français
Membre(s) du bureau directeur:
Diane Quintas, Directrice générale
dquintas@rmefno.ca

Réseau franco-santé du Sud de l'Ontario (RFSSO)
CP 90057, 1000, rue Golf Links, Ancaster ON L9K 0B4

Tél: 416-413-1717
Ligne sans frais: 888-549-5775
www.francosantesud.ca
www.facebook.com/RFSSO
twitter.com/RFSSO

Aperçu: *Dimension:* petite; *Envergure:* provinciale; fondée en 2004
surveillé par Société santé en français
Mission: Contribue au développement des services de santé en
français
Membre(s) du bureau directeur:
Julie Lantaigne, Directrice générale
jlantaigne@francosantesud.ca

Saskatchewan Association of Prosthetists & Orthotists (SAPO)
**c/o Orthotics Prosthetics Canada, #202, 300 March Rd., Ottawa ON
K2K 2E2**
Overview: A small provincial organization founded in 1999 overseen
by Orthotics Prosthetics Canada
Mission: To represent the prosthetic & orthotic field in Saskatchewan

The Therapeutic Touch Network of Ontario (TTNO)
#4, 290 The West Mall, 2nd Fl., Toronto ON M9C 1C6

Tel: 416-231-6824
e-mail: ttno.membership@bellnet.ca
www.therapeutictouchontario.org
twitter.com/TTNOntario

Previous Name: The Therapeutic Touch Network (Ontario)
Overview: A small provincial licensing organization founded in 1994

Mission: To promote the practice & acceptance of Therapeutic Touch as developed by Dolores Krieger & Dora Kunz
Chief Officer(s):
Sharron Parrott, Chair
Publications:
• In Touch
Type: Newsletter

PRINCE EDWARD ISLAND

College of Physicians & Surgeons of Prince Edward Island
14 Paramount Dr., Charlottetown PE C1E 0C7
Tel: 902-566-3861; *Fax:* 902-566-3986
cpspei.ca
Previous Name: Medical Council of Prince Edward Island
Overview: A small provincial licensing organization founded in 1988 overseen by Federation of Regulatory Authorities of Canada
Mission: To act as the regulatory body for physicians in the province, responsible for licensing all medical doctors, maintaining medical standards, handling complaints from the public, & delivering disciplinary action
Chief Officer(s):
Cyril Moyse, Registrar
cmoyse@cpspei.ca
Melissa MacDonald, Office Manager
mmacdonald@cpspei.ca

Health Association of PEI (HAPEI)
10 Pownal St., Charlottetown PE C1A 3V6
Tel: 902-368-3901
Previous Name: Hospital Association of PEI
Overview: A small provincial organization founded in 1961 overseen by Canadian Healthcare Association
Mission: To influence the change & development of the health delivery system; to provide services which assist members in managing their human, financial & physical resources.

Medical Society of Prince Edward Island (MSPEI)
2 Myrtle St., Stratford PE C1B 2W2
Tel: 902-368-7303; *Fax:* 902-566-3934
www.mspei.org
twitter.com/MSPEI_Docs
Overview: A medium-sized provincial organization founded in 1855 overseen by Canadian Medical Association
Mission: To promote health & improvement of medical services; To prevent disease; To represent members at national bodies & government; To consider all matters concerning the professional welfare of members
Chief Officer(s):
Lea Bryden, Chief Executive Officer
lea@mspei.org
Erica Jenkins, Office Coordinator
erica@mspei.org

Prince Edward Island Association of Medical Radiation Technologists (PEIAMRT)
60 Riverside Dr., Charlottetown PE C1A 8T5
e-mail: peiamrt@gmail.com
www.peiamrt.com
Overview: A small provincial organization founded in 1982 overseen by Canadian Association of Medical Radiation Technologists
Mission: To act in accordance with the Public Health Act, "Radiation Safety Regulations"; To promote excellence in health care
Chief Officer(s):
Tyler Ferrish, President
tjferrish@ihis.org
Susan Colwill, Registrar

Prince Edward Island Society for Medical Laboratory Science (PEIMLS)
PO Box 20061, Stn. Sherwood, 161 St. Peters Rd., Charlottetown PE C1A 9E3
peismls.com
www.facebook.com/320495861437823
twitter.com/peismls
Overview: A medium-sized provincial organization founded in 1953 overseen by Canadian Society for Medical Laboratory Science
Mission: To promote, maintain & protect professional identity & interests of medical laboratory technologist & of the profession; to promote development of continuing education; to provide information on current developments in medical laboratory technology
Chief Officer(s):
Carolyn McCarville, President
Andrea Dowling, Vice-President
Gerard Fernando, Treasurer

Réseau Santé en français I.-P.-É
CP 58, 48, ch Mill, Wellington PE C0B 2E0
Tél: 902-854-7444; *Téléc:* 902-854-7255
Courriel: info@santeipe.ca
www.santeipe.ca
www.facebook.com/RSFIPE
Aperçu: *Dimension:* petite; *Envergure:* provinciale surveillé par Société santé en français
Mission: Améliorer l'accès à des programmes et services de santé de qualité en français
Membre(s) du bureau directeur:
Élise Arsenault, Directrice
elisearsenault@gov.pe.ca

United Way of Prince Edward Island / Centraide PEI
PO Box 247, 180 Kent St., 2nd Fl., Charlottetown PE C1A 7K4
Tel: 902-894-8202; *Fax:* 902-894-9643
Toll-Free: 877-902-4438
www.peiunitedway.com
www.facebook.com/peiunitedway
twitter.com/uwpei
www.youtube.com/channel/UCQAZJYD21v35hI9ggOoAJ9w
Overview: A small provincial charitable organization founded in 1962 overseen by United Way of Canada - Centraide Canada
Mission: To provide funds needed to meet community needs & build stronger communities
Chief Officer(s):
Carol O'Hanley, President
Andrea MacDonald, CEO
amacdonald@peiunitedway.com

QUÉBEC

Alliance des communautés culturelles pour l'égalité dans la santé et les services sociaux (ACCÉSSS)
#408, 7000, av Du Parc, Montréal QC H3N 1X1
Tél: 514-287-1106; *Téléc:* 514-287-7443
Ligne sans frais: 866-744-1106
Courriel: accesss@accesss.net
accesss.net
www.facebook.com/pages/ACCÉSSS/273142908412
Aperçu: *Dimension:* petite; *Envergure:* provinciale; fondée en 1984
Mission: Offre des services facilitant l'intégration et l'adaptation des services sociaux et de santé aux personnes issues de communautés ethnoculturelles; représente les intérêts des communautés ethnoculturelles auprès des instances décisionnelles en matières de santé et services sociaux; mène des recherches sur les besoins d'adaptation et d'adéquation des services sociaux et de santé en vue de leur pleine utilisation par les personnes issues des communautés ethnoculturelles
Membre(s) du bureau directeur:
Carmen Gonzalez, Présidente
Jérôme Di Giovanni, Directeur général
jerome.digiovanni@accesss.net

Alliance du personnel professionnel et technique de la santé et des services sociaux (APTS)
#1050, 1111 rue Saint-Charles Ouest, Longueuil QC J4K 5G4
Tél: 450-670-2411; *Téléc:* 450-679-0107
Ligne sans frais: 866-521-2411
Courriel: info@aptsq.com
www.aptsq.com
www.facebook.com/SyndicatAPTS
twitter.com/APTSQ
www.youtube.com/channel/UC1srtPhluOjUv_ohjlMhM0g
Nom précédent: Centrale des professionnelles et professionnels de la santé
Aperçu: *Dimension:* grande; *Envergure:* provinciale; Organisme sans but lucratif; fondée en 2004
Mission: Regrouper les organisations syndicales représentant toutes les catégories des personnes salariées professionnelles ou

paramédicales travaillant dans le domaine de la santé; défendre, promouvoir et sauvegarder les intérêts collectifs des membres
Membre(s) du bureau directeur:
Carolle Dubé, Présidente
Dominique Aubertin, Directrice générale

Association d'oto-rhino-laryngologie et de chirurgie cervico-faciale du Québec
CP 216, #3000, 2, Complexe Desjardins, Montréal QC H5B 1G8
Tél: 514-350-5125; *Téléc:* 514-350-5165
Courriel: assorl@fmsq.org
www.orlquebec.org
Aperçu: *Dimension:* petite; *Envergure:* provinciale; Organisme sans but lucratif; fondée en 1959 surveillé par Fédération des médecins spécialistes du Québec
Mission: Valoriser le statut professionnel de ses membres, promouvoir leurs intérêts scientifiques, économiques et professionnels, et contribuer au développement de l'oto-rhino-laryngologie
Membre(s) du bureau directeur:
Janik Sarrazin, Président
Jocelyne Fortin, Directrice, Administration

Association des arts thérapeutes du Québec (AATQ)
#307B, 911, rue Jean-Talon Est, Montréal QC H2R 1V5
Tél: 514-990-5415
Courriel: info@aatq.org
aatq.org
Aperçu: *Dimension:* petite; *Envergure:* provinciale; fondée en 1981
Membre(s) du bureau directeur:
Sylvie Goyette, Président

Association des cadres supérieurs de la santé et des services sociaux du Québec (ACSSSS)
#1494, rue Victoria, Greenfield Park QC J4V 1M2
Tél: 450-465-0360; *Téléc:* 450-465-0444
Courriel: cadres.superieurs@acssss.qc.ca
www.acssss.qc.ca
www.linkedin.com/company/association-des-cadres-supérieurs-de-la-santé
www.facebook.com/1438926259719098
www.youtube.com/user/ACSSSSQC
Aperçu: *Dimension:* petite; *Envergure:* provinciale; fondée en 1959
Affiliation(s): La Coalition de l'encadrement en matière de retraite d'assurance; Commission administrative des régimes de retraite et d'assurances; Commission administrative des régimes de retraite et d'assurances Québec
Membre(s) du bureau directeur:
Carole Trempe, Directrice générale
carole.trempe.acssss@ssss.gouv.qc.ca

Association des conseils des médecins, dentistes et pharmaciens du Québec (ACMDP) / Association of Councils of Physicians, Dentists & Pharmacists of Québec
#212, 560, boul Henri-Bourassa ouest, Montréal QC H3L 1P4
Tél: 514-858-5885; *Téléc:* 514-858-6767
Courriel: acmdp@acmdp.qc.ca
www.acmdp.qc.ca
Aperçu: *Dimension:* moyenne; *Envergure:* provinciale; Organisme sans but lucratif; fondée en 1946
Mission: Offrir l'information, la motivation, et la formation médico-administrative nécessaire aux Conseils des médecins, dentistes, et pharmaciens membres afin qu'ils accomplissent adéquatement leurs tâches
Membre(s) du bureau directeur:
Martin Arata, Président-Directeur général
Publications:
• Conseiller express [publication de l'Association des conseils des médecins, dentistes et pharmaciens du Québec]
Type: Infolettre
• Guides de formation [publication de l'Association des conseils des médecins, dentistes et pharmaciens du Québec]
• Mémoire [publication de l'Association des conseils des médecins, dentistes et pharmaciens du Québec]

Association des directeurs généraux des services de santé et des services sociaux du Québec (ADGSSSQ) / Association of Executive Directors of Québec Health & Social Services
#B-10, 425, boul de Maisonneuve Ouest, Montréal QC H3A 3G5
Tél: 514-281-1896; *Téléc:* 514-281-5054
www.adgsssq.qc.ca

Aperçu: *Dimension:* moyenne; *Envergure:* provinciale; Organisme de réglementation; fondée en 1973
Mission: L'Association des directeurs généraux des services de santé et des services sociaux du Québec est une société dont l'objet premier est r l'étude, la défense et le développement des intérêts économiques, sociaux et moraux de ses membres _
Membre(s) du bureau directeur:
André Côté, Président-directeur général
Michel Lapointe, Président

Association des fondations d'établissements de santé du Québec (AFÉSAQ)
#A301, 455, boul Base-de-Roc, Joliette QC J6E 5P3
Tél: 450-760-2325; *Téléc:* 450-760-2326
Ligne sans frais: 888-760-2325
www.afesaq.qc.ca
Aperçu: *Dimension:* petite; *Envergure:* provinciale
Mission: Pour représenter les intérêts des associations de soins de santé et les associations de services sociaux
Membre(s) du bureau directeur:
Roland Granger, Président-directeur général
rgranger@afesaq.qc.ca

Association des Gestionnaires de l'information de la santé du Québec (AGISQ)
#104, 5104, boul Bourque, Sherbrooke QC J1N 2K7
Tél: 819-823-6670; *Téléc:* 819-823-0799
Courriel: info@agisq.ca
www.agisq.ca
www.facebook.com/pages/Agisq/392680864114521
Nom précédent: Association québécoise des archivistes médicales; Association des archivistes médicales de la province de Québec
Aperçu: *Dimension:* moyenne; *Envergure:* provinciale; Organisme sans but lucratif; fondée en 1960
Mission: Promouvoir les connaissances scientifiques, techniques, professionnelles, morales, sociales et légales se rattachant directement ou indirectement à la profession d'archiviste médicale; promouvoir la formation et le perfectionnement des membres; promouvoir la profession dans les différents établissements de santé, organismes gouvernementaux, paragouvernementaux et privés; favoriser les échanges et les communications entre les membres; offrir des services-conseils; accomplir toute activité qui peut être nécessaire à l'atteinte des objectifs fixés
Membre(s) du bureau directeur:
Lise Chagnon, Directrice générale
Alexandre Allard, Président
Monica Ouellet, Vice-Président
Marie-Eve Sirois, Trésorière

Association des gestionnaires des établissements de santé et des services sociaux (AGESSS) / Association for Manager of Health Facilities & Social Services
#101, 601, rue Adoncour, Longueuil QC J4G 2M6
Tél: 450-651-6000; *Téléc:* 450-651-9750
Ligne sans frais: 800-361-6526
Courriel: reception@agesss.qc.ca
www.agesss.qc.ca
Aperçu: *Dimension:* moyenne; *Envergure:* provinciale; fondée en 1969
Mission: Représenter ses membres; promouvoir et défendre l'intérêt de ses membres; tenir ses membres informés; gérer ses biens pour assurer sa survie et l'efficacité de son action
Affliation(s): Desjardins Sécurité financière; laPersonelle; RACAR; La Capitale; Le Point
Membre(s) du bureau directeur:
Yves Bolduc, Président-directeur général
Chantal Marchand, Vice-Président
Johanne Simard, Trésorière

Association des intervenantes et des intervenants en soins spirituels du Québec (AIISSQ)
6910, rue St-Denis, Montréal QC H2S 2S0
Tél: 514-259-9229; *Téléc:* 514-259-3741
Courriel: secretariat@aiissq.org
www.aiissq.org
Nom précédent: Association québécoise de la pastorale de la santé
Aperçu: *Dimension:* petite; *Envergure:* provinciale; Organisme sans but lucratif; fondée en 2005
Mission: Formation professionnelle des membres et promotion de leurs intérêts spirituels et professionnels; représentation des membres

auprès d'instances civiles et religieuses reconnues
Membre de: Association canadienne des périodiques catholiques
Affliation(s): Association canadienne pour la pratique et l'éducation pastorale; Association catholique canadienne de la santé; Carrefour Humanisation - Santé
Membre(s) du bureau directeur:
Lorraine Rooke, Présidente
   presidence@aiissq.org
Fernand Patry, Vice-président
   vice-presidence@aiissq.org

Association des intervenants en toxicomanie du Québec inc. (AITQ)
505, rue Ste-Hélène, 2e étage, Longueuil QC J4K 3R5

Tél: 450-646-3271; *Téléc:* 450-646-3275
Courriel: info@aitq.com
www.aitq.com
www.facebook.com/480553332024591
Aperçu: *Dimension:* moyenne; *Envergure:* provinciale; Organisme sans but lucratif; fondée en 1977
Mission: Regrouper les intervenants professionnels et bénévoles oeuvrant dans le domaine de la toxicomanie et du jeu excessif
Membre(s) du bureau directeur:
Carmen Trottier, Directrice générale
   ctrottier@aitq.com

Association des médecins biochimistes du Québec (AMBQ)
CP 216, Succ. Desjardins, #3000, 2, Complexe Desjardins, Montréal QC H5B 1G8

Tél: 514-350-5105
Courriel: ambq@fmsq.org
www.ambq.med.usherbrooke.ca
Aperçu: *Dimension:* petite; *Envergure:* provinciale surveillé par Fédération des médecins spécialistes du Québec
Mission: Promouvoir l'utilisation optimale des tests de laboratoire au Québec en offrant, au professionnel de la santé et au patient, les meilleurs services de diagnostic et de dépistage de maladies grâce à des techniques biochimiques et immunologiques
Membre(s) du bureau directeur:
Jean Dubé, Président

Association des médecins généticiens du Québec
#3000, 2, Complexe Desjardins, Montréal QC H5B 1G8
Tél: 514-350-5141; *Téléc:* 514-350-5116
www.medecingeneticien.ca
Aperçu: *Dimension:* petite; *Envergure:* provinciale surveillé par Fédération des médecins spécialistes du Québec
Membre(s) du bureau directeur:
Bruno Maranda, M.D., Président
Sandrine Guillot, Directrice
   sguillot@fmsq.org

Association des médecins spécialistes en médecine nucléaire du Québec (AMSMNQ)
CP 216, Succ. Desjardins, #3000, 2, Complexe Desjardins, Montréal QC H5B 1G8

Tél: 514-350-5133; *Téléc:* 514-350-5151
Ligne sans frais: 800-561-0703
Courriel: amsmnq@fmsq.org
www.medecinenucleaire.com
Aperçu: *Dimension:* petite; *Envergure:* provinciale surveillé par Fédération des médecins spécialistes du Québec
Mission: Pour former ses membres et maintenir un haut niveau de professionnalisme
Membre(s) du bureau directeur:
François Lamoureux, Président
Jean Guimond, Vice-président
Michelle Laviolette, Directrice administrative

Association des médecins spécialistes en santé communautaire du Québec (AMSSCQ)
CP 216, #3000, 2, Complexe Desjardins, Montréal QC H5B 1G8
Tél: 514-350-5138; *Téléc:* 514-350-5151
Courriel: asmpq@fmsq.org
www.amscq.org
Aperçu: *Dimension:* petite; *Envergure:* provinciale; fondée en 1982 surveillé par Fédération des médecins spécialistes du Québec
Mission: De promouvoir les intérêts professionnels et économiques de ses membres

Membre(s) du bureau directeur:
Isabelle Samson, Présidente
Valery Gasse, Coordonnatrice

Association des orthésistes et prothésistes du Québec (AOPQ)
715-A, ch des Pères, Magog QC J1X 5R9
Tél: 514-396-9303; *Téléc:* 514-396-9304
Ligne sans frais: 888-323-8834
Courriel: info@aopq.ca
www.aopq.ca
Nom précédent: Association nationale des orthésistes du pied
Aperçu: *Dimension:* petite; *Envergure:* provinciale
Mission: Protéger et à développer des intérêts professionnels, moraux, sociaux et économiques des membres

Association des pathologistes du Québec (APQ)
CP 216, Succ. Desjardins, #3000, 2, Complexe Desjardins, Montréal QC H5B 1G8

Tél: 514-350-5102; *Téléc:* 514-350-5152
Ligne sans frais: 800-561-0703
Courriel: patho@fmsq.org
www.apq.qc.ca
Aperçu: *Dimension:* petite; *Envergure:* provinciale surveillé par Fédération des médecins spécialistes du Québec
Mission: Promouvoir les intérêts professionnels et économiques de ses membres
Membre de: Fédération des médecins spécialistes du Québec
Membre(s) du bureau directeur:
Christian Lussier, Président
Danielle Joncas, Directrice, Administration

Association des pédiatres du Québec
CP 216, Succ. Desjardins, #3000, 2, Complexe Desjardins, Montréal QC H5B 1G8

Tél: 514-350-5127; *Téléc:* 514-350-5177
Courriel: pediatrie@fmsq.org
www.pediatres.ca
Aperçu: *Dimension:* moyenne; *Envergure:* provinciale surveillé par Fédération des médecins spécialistes du Québec
Membre de: Fédération des Médcins Spécialistes du Québec (FMSQ)
Affliation(s): Association des allergologues et immunologues du Québec; Association des anesthésiologistes du Québec; Association des médecins biochimistes du Québec; Association des cardiologues du Québec; Association des chirurgiens cardio-vasculaires et thoraciques du Québec; Association québécoise de chirurgie; Association des chirurgiens vasculaires du Québec; Association des spécialistes en chirurgie plastique et esthétique du Québec; Association des dermatologistes du Québec; Association des médecins endocrinologues du Québec; Association des gastro-entérologues du Québec
Membre(s) du bureau directeur:
May Dagher, Directrice, Administration

Association des Perfusionnistes du Québec Inc. (APQI)
CP 32172, Succ. Saint-André, Montréal QC H2L 4Y5
www.apqi.com
Aperçu: *Dimension:* petite; *Envergure:* provinciale
Membre(s) du bureau directeur:
Alina Parapuf, Présidente, 514-415-7622
Audrey Chapman, Vice-Présidente, 514-406-2186
Catherine André-Guimont, Trésorière
Thierry Lamarre-Renaud, Secrétaire, 514-406-4676

Association des physiatres du Québec (APQ)
CP 216, Succ. Desjardins, #3000, 2, Complexe Desjardins, Montréal QC H5B 1G8

Tél: 514-350-5119; *Téléc:* 514-350-5147
Courriel: apq@fmsq.org
www.fmsq.org
Aperçu: *Dimension:* petite; *Envergure:* provinciale surveillé par Fédération des médecins spécialistes du Québec
Mission: Pour ouvrer à la prévention, au diagnostic et au traitement médical des douleurs et des troubles de l'appareil locomoteur (la colonne vertébrale, les os, les muscles, les tendons, les articulations, les vaisseaux et le cerveau)
Membre de: Fédération des Médecins Spécialistes du Québec (FMSQ)
Membre(s) du bureau directeur:
Marc Filiatrault, Président

Elsa Fournier, Directrice, Administration

Association des professionnels en santé du travail (APST)
1370, rue Notre-Dame Ouest, Montréal QC H3C 1K8
Tél: 514-282-4231; *Téléc:* 514-282-4292
Courriel: admin@santedutravail.ca
www.santedutravail.ca
Nom précédent: Association des infirmières et infirmiers en santé du travail du Québec
Aperçu: *Dimension:* moyenne; *Envergure:* provinciale; Organisme sans but lucratif; fondée en 1978
Mission: Assurer la protection du statut; consolider l'autonomie professionnelle et définir les besoins de ses membres; promouvoir et maintenir la qualité des services professionnels dispensés; favoriser l'actualisation des connaissances dans un contexte de constante évolution; intensifier le lien entre ses membres et la santé et sécurité au travail
Membre de: Association canadienne des infirmiers et infirmières en santé du travail
Membre(s) du bureau directeur:
Carl Brouillette, Président
Bruno-Gil Breton, Vice-président
Benoît Blossier, Administrateur

Association des radiologistes du Québec
CP 216, Succ. Desjardins, #3000, 2, Complexe Desjardins, Montréal QC H5B 1G8
Tél: 514-350-5129; *Téléc:* 514-350-5179
Courriel: bureau@arq.qc.ca
www.arq.qc.ca
twitter.com/SCFRQuebec
Aperçu: *Dimension:* petite; *Envergure:* provinciale surveillé par Fédération des médecins spécialistes du Québec
Mission: Regrouper les médecins spécialisés en radiologie; défendre leurs intérêts et promouvoir leur spécialité
Membre(s) du bureau directeur:
Vincent Oliva, Président
Lisette Pipon, Directrice, Administration

Association des radio-oncologues du Québec (AROQ)
CP 216, Succ. Desjardins, #3000, 2, Complexe Desjardins, Montréal QC H5B 1G8
Tél: 514-350-5130; *Téléc:* 514-350-5126
Courriel: aroq@fmsq.org
www.aroq.ca
Aperçu: *Dimension:* petite; *Envergure:* provinciale surveillé par Fédération des médecins spécialistes du Québec
Mission: De fournir un forum où ses membres peuvent échanger des idées afin d'aider à améliorer leurs méthodes de traitement
Membre(s) du bureau directeur:
Khalil Sultanem, Président

Association des spécialistes en chirurgie plastique et esthétique du Québec (ASCPEQ)
CP 216, Succ. Desjardins, 2, Complexe Desjardins, Montréal QC H5B 1G8
Tél: 514-350-5109; *Téléc:* 514-350-5246
Courriel: ascpeq@fmsq.org
www.ascpeq.org
Aperçu: *Dimension:* petite; *Envergure:* provinciale surveillé par Fédération des médecins spécialistes du Québec
Mission: L'Association entend se consacrer essentiellement au développement continu de l'art et de la science de la chirurgie plastique et esthétique, entre autres par la diffusion de renseignements pertinents auprès du public, par la promotion d'une relation médecin-patient fondée sur la communication, la compréhension et le respect mutuel, ainsi que par une contribution active aux programmes d'éducation et de formation continue et par une participation critique aux débats relatifs au rôle et à la place des professionnels de la santé au sein de la société québécoise
Affiliation(s): La Société canadienne des chirurgiens plasticiens, The Toronto Aesthetic Meeting, The Toronto Breast Symposium, La Société canadienne de chirurgie plastique esthétique, The Canadian Association for Accreditation of Ambulatory Surgical Facilities
Membre(s) du bureau directeur:
Éric Bensimon, Président

Association des spécialistes en médecine d'urgence du Québec
Tour de l'Est, #3000, 2, Complexe Desjardins, Montréal QC H5B 1G8
Tél: 514-350-5115; *Téléc:* 514-350-5116
www.asmuq.org
Aperçu: *Dimension:* moyenne; *Envergure:* provinciale surveillé par Fédération des médecins spécialistes du Québec
Membre(s) du bureau directeur:
François Dufresne, Président

Association des spécialistes en médecine interne du Québec
Tour Est, 2, Complexe Desjardins, 30e étage, Montréal QC H5B 1G8
Tél: 514-350-5118; *Téléc:* 514-350-5168
asmiq.org
Aperçu: *Dimension:* moyenne; *Envergure:* provinciale; Organisme sans but lucratif
Membre de: Fédération des médecins spécialistes du Québec
Membre(s) du bureau directeur:
Mario Dallaire, Président

Association médicale du Québec (AMQ) / Québec Medical Association (QMA)
#3200, 380, rue Saint-Antoine Ouest, Montréal QC H2Y 3X7
Tél: 514-866-0660; *Téléc:* 514-866-0670
Ligne sans frais: 800-363-3932
Courriel: admin@amq.ca
www.amq.ca
www.facebook.com/Association.medicale.du.Quebec
twitter.com/amquebec
Aperçu: *Dimension:* moyenne; *Envergure:* provinciale; Organisme sans but lucratif; fondée en 1922 surveillé par Canadian Medical Association
Mission: Rassembler et soutenir les médecins du Québec afin de garantir à la population québécoise des conditions et des soins de santé de qualité
Membre(s) du bureau directeur:
Normand Laberge, Directeur général
  normand.laberge@amq.ca

Association pour la santé publique du Québec (ASPQ) / Québec Public Health Association
#102, 4529, rue Clark, Montréal QC H2T 2T3
Tél: 514-528-5811; *Téléc:* 514-528-5590
Courriel: info@aspq.org
www.aspq.org
fr-ca.facebook.com/AssociationPourLaSantePubliqueDuQuebecaspq
twitter.com/ASPQuebec
Aperçu: *Dimension:* moyenne; *Envergure:* provinciale; Organisme sans but lucratif; fondée en 1943 surveillé par Canadian Public Health Association
Mission: Favoriser un regard critique sur les enjeux de santé publique au Québec en constituant un regroupement volontaire, autonome, multidisciplinaire et multisectoriel de personnes et d'organisations provenant des milieux tant institutionnels et professionnels que communautaires; offre un espace à ses membres pour développer des prises de position communes ou concertées, appuyer des politiques favorables à la santé et au bien-être et développer des coalitions et des projets en collaboration avec d'autres partenaires de santé publique ou du milieu
Membre(s) du bureau directeur:
Lilianne Bertrand, Présidente
Lucie Granger, Directrice générale, 514-528-5811 Ext. 225
  lgranger@aspq.org

Association Québécoise de chirurgie
CP 216, Succ. Desjardins, #3000, 2, Complexe Desjardins, Montréal QC H5B 1G8
Tél: 514-350-5107; *Téléc:* 514-350-5157
Courriel: info@chirurgiequebec.ca
www.chirurgiequebec.ca
www.facebook.com/DPCAQC
twitter.com/AQCChirurgieQub
Nom précédent: Association des chirurgiens généraux du Québec
Aperçu: *Dimension:* moyenne; *Envergure:* provinciale surveillé par Fédération des médecins spécialistes du Québec
Mission: Objectifs sont la protection et défense des intérêts professionnels collectifs des chirurgiens et l'enseignement chirurgical continu

Membre(s) du bureau directeur:
Mario Viens, Président
Chantale Jubinville, Directrice

Association québécoise pour le loisir des personnes handicapées (AQLPH)
858, rue Laviolette, Trois-Rivières QC G9A 5J1
Tél: 819-693-3339
Courriel: info@aqlph.qc.ca
www.aqlph.qc.ca
Aperçu: Dimension: moyenne; Envergure: provinciale; fondée en 1978
Mission: Promouvoir le droit à un loisir de qualité (éducatif, sécuritaire, valorisant et de détente); promouvoir la participation et la libre expression de la personne face à son loisir; promouvoir l'accès à tous les champs d'application du loisir (tourisme, plein air, sport et activité physique, loisir scientifique, socio-éducatif et socioculturel) pour toutes les personnes handicapées du Québec sans restriction d'âge, de sexe, ni de type d'handicap
Membre de: Alliance de vie active pour les canadiens; Canadiennes ayant un handicap
Membre(s) du bureau directeur:
Marc St-Onge, Directeur

AlterGo
#340, 525, rue Dominion, Montréal QC H3J 2B4
Tél: 514-933-2739; Téléc: 514-933-9384
Courriel: info@altergo.ca
www.altergo.ca
Membre(s) du bureau directeur:
Élise Blais, Présidente

ARLPH Abitibi-Témiscamingue
330, rue Perreault est, Rouyn-Noranda QC J9X 3C6
Tél: 819-762-8121
www.ulsat.qc.ca/arlphat/
Membre(s) du bureau directeur:
Laurent Juteau, Coordonateur Programme
ljuteau@ulsat.qc.ca

ARLPH Centre du Québec
La Place Rita St-Pierre, #236, 59, rue Monfette, Victoriaville QC G6P 1J8
Tél: 819-758-5464; Téléc: 819-758-4375
Courriel: arlphcq@cdcbf.qc.ca
www.arlphcq.com
Membre(s) du bureau directeur:

ARLPH Chaudière-Appalaches
5501, rue St-Georges, Lévis QC G6V 4M7
Tél: 418-833-4495; Téléc: 418-833-7214
Courriel: arlphca@videotron.ca
www.arlphca.com
Membre(s) du bureau directeur:
Amélie Richard, Directrice régionale

ARLPH Côte-Nord
#218, 859, rue Bossé, Baie-Comeau QC G5C 3P8
Tél: 418-589-5774; Téléc: 418-589-4612
Ligne sans frais: 888-330-8757
Courriel: info@urlscn.qc.ca
www.urlscn.qc.ca
Membre(s) du bureau directeur:
Pierre LeBreux, Directeur général
lebreux.pierre@urlscn.qc.ca

ARLPH de la Capitale-Nationale
CP 1000, Succ. M, 4545, av Pierre-De Coubertin, Montréal QC H1V 3R2
Tél: 514-252-3144
Courriel: info@aqlph.qc.ca
www.aqlph.qc.ca
Membre(s) du bureau directeur:
Guylaine Laforest, Directrice

ARLPH Estrie
5182, boul Bourque, Sherbrooke QC J1N 1H4
Tél: 819-864-0864; Téléc: 819-864-1864
Courriel: csle@abacom.com
www.csle.qc.ca/fr/arlpphe
Membre(s) du bureau directeur:
Claire Gaudreault, Directrice régionale

ARLPH Lanaudière
200, rue de Salaberry, Joliette QC J6E 4G1
Tél: 450-752-2586; Téléc: 450-759-8749
Ligne sans frais: 800-752-2586
Courriel: arlphl@cepap.ca
Membre(s) du bureau directeur:
Paulette Goulet, Présidente

ARLPH Laurentides
#100, 300, rue Longpré, Saint-Jérôme QC J7Y 3B9
Tél: 450-431-3388; Téléc: 450-436-2277
Courriel: arlphl@videotron.ca
www.arlphl.org
Membre(s) du bureau directeur:
Kevin Hoskins, Président
Bernard Oligny, Directeur général

ARLPH Laval
#215A, 387, boul. des Prairies, Laval QC H7N 2W4
Tél: 450-668-2354; Téléc: 450-668-2226
Courriel: info@arlphl.qc.ca
www.arlphl.qc.ca
Membre(s) du bureau directeur:
Rachid Ababou, Président
Louise Langevin, Directrice régionale

URLS Bas St-Laurent
#304, 38, rue St-Germain est, Rimouski QC G5L 1A2
Tél: 418-723-5036; Téléc: 418-722-8906
Courriel: info@urls-bsl.qc.ca
www.urls-bsl.qc.ca
www.facebook.com/urlsbsl
twitter.com/urlsbsl
Membre(s) du bureau directeur:
Lucille Porlier, Directrice générale
lucilleporlier@urls-bsl.qc.ca

URLS Gaspésie/Iles de la Madeleine
CP 99, 8, boul. Perron Est, Caplan QC G0C 1H0
Tél: 418-388-2121; Téléc: 418-388-2133
Courriel: informations@urlsgim.com
www.urlsgim.com
www.facebook.com/urlsgim
Membre(s) du bureau directeur:
Nicolas Méthot, Directeur général
nicolas.methot@urlsgim.com

URLS Mauricie
260, rue Dessureault, Trois-Rivières QC G8T 9T9
Tél: 819-691-3075; Téléc: 819-373-6046
Courriel: urls@urlsmauricie.com
www.urlsmauricie.com
Membre(s) du bureau directeur:
Jean-Marc Gauthier, Directeur général

URLS Outaouais
#209, 390 av de Buckingham, Gatineau QC J8L 2G7
Tél: 819-663-2575; Téléc: 819-281-6369
Courriel: info@loisirsportoutaouais.com
www.urlso.qc.ca
Membre(s) du bureau directeur:
Frédérique Delisle, Directrice générale
direction@loisirsportoutaouais.com

Zone loisir Montérégie
3800, boul Casavant ouest, Saint-Hyacinthe QC J2S 8E3
Tél: 450-771-0707
Courriel: infozlm@zlm.qc.ca
www.zlm.qc.ca
Membre(s) du bureau directeur:
Jean Lemonde, Directeur général
jlemonde@zlm.qc.ca

Centraide Abitibi Témiscamingue et Nord-du-Québec
1009, 6e rue, Val-d'Or QC J9P 3W4
Tél: 819-825-7139; Téléc: 819-825-7155
Courriel: courrier@centraide-atnq.qc.ca
www.centraide-atnq.qc.ca
www.facebook.com/Centraide.ATNQ

Aperçu: *Dimension:* moyenne; *Envergure:* provinciale; Organisme sans but lucratif; fondée en 1983 surveillé par United Way of Canada - Centraide Canada
Affiliation(s): Chambre de Commerce; Comité prévention des crimes
Membre(s) du bureau directeur:
Huguette Boucher, Directrice générale

Centre Anti-Poison du Québec
1270, ch Sainte-Foy, 4e étage, Québec QC G1S 2M4
Tél: 418-654-2731; *Téléc:* 418-654-2747
Ligne sans frais: 800-463-5060
Aperçu: *Dimension:* petite; *Envergure:* provinciale
Membre de: Canadian Association of Poison Control Centres
Membre(s) du bureau directeur:
Hélène Levasseur, Chef de service

Collège des médecins du Québec (CMQ)
2170, boul René-Lévesque Ouest, Montréal QC H3H 2T8
Tél: 514-933-4441; *Téléc:* 514-933-3112
Ligne sans frais: 888-633-3246
Courriel: info@cmq.org
www.cmq.org
www.facebook.com/257741694238490
twitter.com/CMQ_org
Aperçu: *Dimension:* moyenne; *Envergure:* provinciale; Organisme sans but lucratif; fondée en 1847
Mission: Promouvoir une médecine de qualité pour protéger le public et contribuer à l'amélioration de la santé des Québécois
Membre de: Conseil interprofessionnel du Québec
Affiliation(s): Federation of Medical Licensing Authorities of Canada
Membre(s) du bureau directeur:
Charles Bernard, Président-directeur général
Yves Robert, Secrétaire

Confédération des Organismes de Personnes Handicapées du Québec (COPHAN)
#300, 2030, boul Pie-IX, Montréal QC H1V 2C8
Tél: 514-284-0155; *Téléc:* 514-284-0775
Courriel: info@cophan.org
www.cophan.org
Nom précédent: Confédération des organismes provinciaux de personnes handicapées du Québec
Aperçu: *Dimension:* moyenne; *Envergure:* provinciale; Organisme sans but lucratif; fondée en 1985
Mission: Milite pour la défense des droits et la promotion des intérêts des personnes ayant des limitations fonctionnelles, de tous âges
Membre de: Conseil de canadiens avec déficiences
Membre(s) du bureau directeur:
Richard Lavigne, Directeur général
direction@cophan.org
Véronique Vézina, Présidente

Corporation des services d'ambulance du Québec
#205, 455, rue Marais, Québec QC G1M 3A2
Tél: 418-681-4448; *Téléc:* 418-681-4667
Ligne sans frais: 800-463-6773
www.csaq.org
Aperçu: *Dimension:* petite; *Envergure:* provinciale; fondée en 1972
Mission: Pour offrir une gamme de services et d'avantages à ses membres et à défendre les intérêts de ces derniers auprès des différentes instances gouvernementales, auprès de ses membres au Québec.
Affiliation(s): Association des hôpitaux du Québec
Membre(s) du bureau directeur:
Denis Perrault, Directeur général
denis.perrault@csaq.org

Fédération des médecins omnipraticiens du Québec (FMOQ) / Québec Federation of General Practitioners
2, Place Alexis Nihon, 3500, boul. de Maisonneuve ouest, 20e étage, Westmount QC H3Z 3C1
Tél: 514-878-1911
Ligne sans frais: 800-361-8499
Courriel: info@fmoq.org
www.fmoq.org
twitter.com/FMOQ
Aperçu: *Dimension:* moyenne; *Envergure:* provinciale; fondée en 1963
Mission: Étude et défense des intérêts économiques, sociaux, moraux et scientifiques des associations et de leurs membres; promouvoir et développer le rôle de l'omnipraticien dans les sphères de la vie économique, sociale, scientifique et culturelle en définissant d'une façon objective le statut propre à l'omnipraticien
Membre de: World Organization of National Colleges; Academies & Academic Associations of General Practitioners/Family Physicians
Membre(s) du bureau directeur:
Louis Godin, Président-directeur général
lgodin@fmoq.org

Fédération des médecins résidents du Québec inc. (ind.) (FMRQ) / Québec Federation of Residents (Ind.)
#510, 630, rue Sherbrooke ouest, Montréal QC H3A 1E4
Tél: 514-282-0256; *Téléc:* 514-282-0471
Ligne sans frais: 800-465-0215
Courriel: fmrq@fmrq.qc.ca
www.fmrq.qc.ca
www.facebook.com/fmrqc
twitter.com/fmrq
Aperçu: *Dimension:* moyenne; *Envergure:* provinciale; fondée en 1966
Mission: D'étudier, de défendre et de développer des intérêts économiques, sociaux, moraux et scientifiques des syndicats et des leurs membres
Membre(s) du bureau directeur:
Patrice Savignac Dufour, Executive Director
psavignacdufour@fmrq.qc.ca
Patrick Labelle, Director, Administrative Services
plabelle@fmrq.qc.ca

Fédération des médecins spécialistes du Québec (FMSQ)
CP 216, Succ. Desjardins, #3000, 2, Complexe Desjardins, Montréal QC H5B 1G8
Tél: 514-350-5000; *Téléc:* 514-350-5100
Ligne sans frais: 800-561-0703
www.fmsq.org
www.facebook.com/laFMSQ
twitter.com/FMSQ
Aperçu: *Dimension:* moyenne; *Envergure:* provinciale; fondée en 1965
Mission: Défendre et promouvoir les intérêts économiques, professionnels et scientifiques des médecins spécialistes
Membre(s) du bureau directeur:
Diane Francoeur, Présidente

Fédération des professionnèles (FPCSN) / Quebec Federation of Managers & Professional Salaried Workers (CNTU)
#150, 1601, av de Lorimier, Montréal QC H2K 4M5
Tél: 514-598-2143; *Téléc:* 514-598-2491
Ligne sans frais: 888-633-2143
www.fpcsn.qc.ca
Nom précédent: Fédération des professionnelles et professionnels salarié(e)s et des cadres du Québec
Aperçu: *Dimension:* moyenne; *Envergure:* provinciale; Organisme sans but lucratif; fondée en 1964
Mission: Regroupe plus de 7000 professionnèles oeuvrant dans différents secteurs d'activités: santé et services sociaux, organismes gouvernementaux, éducation, secteur municipal, médecines alternatives, secteur juridique, intégration à l'emploi, professionnèles autonomes, organismes communautaires
Membre de: Confédération des syndicats nationaux
Membre(s) du bureau directeur:
Ginette Langlois, Présidente
ginette.langlois@csn.qc.ca
Lucie Dufour, Secrétaire générale
lucie.dufour@csn.qc.ca

Fédération des syndicats de la santé et des services sociaux (F4S-CSQ)
9405, rue Sherbrooke est, Montréal QC H1L 6P3
Tél: 514-356-8888; *Téléc:* 514-356-2845
Courriel: info@f4s.gs
www.f4s.gs
Aperçu: *Dimension:* petite; *Envergure:* provinciale
Mission: S'assurer que ses membres travaillent dans des conditions de sécurité; de représenter les intérêts de ses membres au cours des conventions collectives
Membre(s) du bureau directeur:
Claude Demontigny, Président
demontigny.claude@csq.qc.net

Fondation pour l'aide aux travailleuses et travailleurs accidentés (FATA)
6839-A, rue Drolet, Montréal QC H2S 2T1
Tél: 514-271-0901; Téléc: 514-271-6078
Courriel: fata@fata.qc.ca
www.fata.qc.ca
Aperçu: Dimension: petite; Envergure: provinciale
Mission: Promouvoir des intérêts de travailleuses et de travailleurs affectés par des accidents ou des maladies du travail

Kéroul, Tourisme pour personnes à capacité physique restreinte / Keroul, Tourism & culture for people with restricted physical ability
4545, av Pierre-de Coubertin, Montréal QC H1V 0B2
Tél: 514-252-3104; Téléc: 514-254-0766
Courriel: infos@keroul.qc.ca
www.keroul.qc.ca
www.facebook.com/keroul1979
Aperçu: Dimension: moyenne; Envergure: provinciale; fondée en 1979
Mission: Rendre le tourisme et la culture accessibles aux personnes à capacité physique restreinte
Affliation(s): Regroupement loisir Québec
Membre(s) du bureau directeur:
André Leclerc, Président-directeur général et fondateur
  aleclerc@keroul.qc.ca
Lyne Ménard, Directrice adjointe
  lmenard@keroul.qc.ca

Ordre des chiropraticiens du Québec
7950, boul Métropolitain est, Montréal QC H1K 1A1
Tél: 514-355-8540; Téléc: 514-355-2290
Ligne sans frais: 888-655-8540
Courriel: info@ordredeschiropraticiens.qc.ca
www.ordredeschiropraticiens.qc.ca
www.youtube.com/user/Ordrechirosqc
Aperçu: Dimension: petite; Envergure: provinciale; Organisme sans but lucratif; fondée en 1973
Mission: Organisme paragouvernemental qui assure la protection du public & octroie les permis de pratique; fondation de recherche chiropratique
Membre(s) du bureau directeur:
Pierre Paquin, Coordonnateur

Ordre des Podiatres du Québec
#1000, 7151, rue Jean-Talon Est, Anjou QC H1M 3N8
Tél: 514-288-0019; Téléc: 514-288-5463
Ligne sans frais: 888-514-7433
Courriel: podiatres@ordredespodiatres.qc.ca
www.ordredespodiatres.qc.ca
Aperçu: Dimension: petite; Envergure: provinciale
Membre(s) du bureau directeur:
Charles Faucher, Président
Martine Gosselin, Directrice générale

Ordre des techniciens et techniciennes dentaires du Québec (OTTDQ)
#900, 500, rue Sherbrooke Ouest, Montréal QC H3A 3C6
Tél: 514-282-3837; Téléc: 514-844-7556
www.ottdq.com
www.facebook.com/OTTDQ
Aperçu: Dimension: petite; Envergure: provinciale; Organisme de réglementation
Mission: De réglementer la profession des techniciens dentaires afin de protéger le public et d'assurer la meilleure qualité de service possible est fournie
Membre(s) du bureau directeur:
Linda Carbone, Secrétaire

Ordre des technologues en imagerie médicale, en radio-oncologie et en élétrophysiologie médicale du Québec
#401, 6455, rue Jean-Talon, Saint-Léonard QC H1S 3E8
Tél: 514-351-0052
Ligne sans frais: 800-361-8759
www.otimroepmq.ca
Nom précédent: Ordre des technologues en radiologie du Québec
Aperçu: Dimension: moyenne; Envergure: provinciale; Organisme de réglementation; fondée en 1941
Mission: De surveiller l'exercice de la profession par ses membres, contribuer à leur développement professionnel & assurer au public des services de qualité en matière d'imagerie médicale & de radio-oncologies
Membre de: Canadian Association of Medical Radiation Technologists
Membre(s) du bureau directeur:
Danielle Boué, Présidente

Ordre professionnel des technologistes médicaux du Québec (OPTMQ)
281, av Laurier est, Montréal QC H2T 1G2
Tél: 514-527-9811; Téléc: 514-527-7314
Ligne sans frais: 800-567-7763
Courriel: info@optmq.org
www.optmq.org
Nom précédent: Corporation professionnelle des technologistes médicaux du Québec
Aperçu: Dimension: moyenne; Envergure: provinciale; Organisme de réglementation; fondée en 1973 surveillé par Canadian Society for Medical Laboratory Science
Mission: Protection du public en vérifiant la pratique des membres, en effectuant un contrôle lors de l'émission du permis, par la discipline et l'inspection professionnelle
Membre de: Conseil Interprofessionnel du Québec
Membre(s) du bureau directeur:
Doris Levasseur Bourbeau, Présidente
Alain Collette, Avocat, secrétaire et directeur général
  acollette@optmq.org

Québec Black Medical Association
#180, 2021 av Atwater, Montréal QC H3H 2P2
Tel: 514-937-8822
www.qbma.ca
Overview: A medium-sized provincial organization
Mission: The Québec Black Medical Association aims to enable young people from the Black community to pursue careers as health professionals and to advance medical practice and research in Quebec.
Chief Officer(s):
Edouard Tucker, President

Syndicat des professionnels et des techniciens de la santé du Québec (SPTSQ) / Québec Union of Health Professionals & Technicians
7595, boul St-Michel, Montréal QC H2A 3A4
Tél: 514-723-0422; Téléc: 514-723-5248
Ligne sans frais: 800-567-2022
Courriel: secretariat@stepsq.org
stepsq.org
www.facebook.com/STEPSQ
twitter.com/STEPSQ
Aperçu: Dimension: moyenne; Envergure: provinciale; fondée en 1963
Mission: Défense des intérêts socio-économiques de ses membres
Affliation(s): Centrale des professionnelles et professionnels de la santé
Membre(s) du bureau directeur:
Nancy Corriveau, Présidente
  nancy.corriveau@stepsq.org

Syndicat professionnel des médecins du gouvernement du Québec (ind.) (SPMGQ) / Professional Union of Government of Québec Physicians (Ind.)
1390, rue du Père-Jamet, Sainte-Foy QC G1W 3G5
Tél: 418-266-4670
Aperçu: Dimension: petite; Envergure: provinciale; Organisme sans but lucratif; Organisme de réglementation; fondée en 1966
Mission: Représenter les médecins à l'emploi du gouvernement du Québec
Membre(s) du bureau directeur:
Christine Gagné, Présidente

SASKATCHEWAN

Catholic Health Association of Saskatchewan (CHAS)
1702 - 20 St. West, Saskatoon SK S7M 0Z9
Tel: 306-655-5330; Fax: 306-655-5333
e-mail: cath.health@chassk.ca
www.chassk.ca
Overview: A medium-sized provincial charitable organization founded in 1943 overseen by Catholic Health Association of Canada
Mission: To provide leadership in mission, ethics, spiritual care, & social justice in Saskatchewan; To promote the sanctity of life & the

dignity of all
Member of: Catholic Health Alliance of Canada
Chief Officer(s):
Chris Donald, President
Sandra Kary, Executive Director
    sandra@chassk.ca
Terrie Michaud, Vice-President
Anne Reddekopp, Secretary-Treasurer
Sandy Normand, Coordinator, Mission Education
    snormand@chassk.ca

College of Physicians & Surgeons of Saskatchewan (CPSS)
#101, 2174 Airport Dr., Saskatoon SK S7L 6M6
                    Tel: 306-244-7355; *Fax:* 306-244-0090
                                Toll-Free: 800-667-1668
                        e-mail: cpssinfo@cps.sk.ca
                                    www.cps.sk.ca
Overview: A medium-sized provincial organization founded in 1905
overseen by Federation of Regulatory Authorities of Canada
Mission: To be responsible for licensing properly qualified medical
practitioners, developing & ensuring the standards of practice in all
fields of medicine, investigating & disciplining of all doctors whose
standards of medical care, ethical or professional conduct are
questioned
Chief Officer(s):
Karen Shaw, Registar & Chief Executive Officer
    karen.shaw@cps.sk.ca
Micheal Howard-Tripp, Deputy Registrar & Medical Manager
    micheal.howard-tripp@cps.sk.ca
Barb Porter, Director, Physician Registration
    cpssreg@cps.sk.ca

Health Sciences Association of Saskatchewan (HSAS) / Association des sciences de la santé de la Saskatchewan (ind.)
#42, 1736 Quebec Ave., Saskatoon SK S7K 1V9
                    Tel: 306-955-3399; *Fax:* 306-955-3396
                                Toll-Free: 888-565-3399
                        e-mail: hsasstoon@hsas.ca
                                    www.hsas.ca
                www.facebook.com/124779960928913
                www.youtube.com/user/HealthScienceSask
Overview: A medium-sized provincial organization founded in 1972
Mission: To conduct activities as an independent union representing
its members who are health sciences professionals in Saskatchewan
Chief Officer(s):
Karen Wasylenko, President
    president@hsa-sk.com
Bill Feldbruegge, Vice-President
    mt@hsas.ca
Maureen Kraemer, Secretary
    sw1@hsas.ca

Réseau Santé en français de la Saskatchewan (RSFS)
#220, 308 4e av Nord, Saskatoon SK S7K 2L7
                    Tél: 306-653-7445; *Téléc:* 306-664-6447
                                    www.rsfs.ca
                www.facebook.com/rsfsaskatchewan
Aperçu: *Dimension:* petite; *Envergure:* provinciale; fondée en 2003
surveillé par Société santé en français
Mission: D'assurer un meilleur accès à des programmes et services
sociaux et de santé en français
Membre(s) du bureau directeur:
Roger Gauthier, Directeur
    rsfs@shaw.ca

Saskatchewan Association of Chiropodists (SAC)
100 - 2nd Ave. NE, Moose Jaw SK S6H 1B8
                    Tel: 306-691-6405; *Fax:* 306-691-3608
                        e-mail: asta@fhhr.ca
Also Known As: Podiatry Association of Saskatchewan
Overview: A small provincial organization founded in 1943
Mission: To participate in the improvement of podiatry; To increase the
scope & availability of practitioners in Saskatchewan; To encourage
continuing post-graduate education in order to keep up with current
trends

Saskatchewan Association of Health Organizations (SAHO)
#500, 2002 Victoria Ave., Regina SK S4P 0R7
                    Tel: 306-347-1740; *Fax:* 306-347-1043
                                    www.saho.ca
Overview: A small provincial charitable organization founded in 1993
overseen by Canadian Healthcare Association
Mission: To serve members through services, support, & programs
Publications:
• Health Matters
Type: Magazine; *Frequency:* Quarterly
Profile: Issues in the health care system

Saskatchewan Association of Medical Radiation Technologists (SAMRT)
#218, 408 Broad St., Regina SK S4R 1X3
                    Tel: 306-525-9678; *Fax:* 306-525-9680
                        e-mail: info@samrt.org
                                    samrt.org
Previous Name: Saskatchewan Society of X-Ray Technicians
Overview: A small provincial organization founded in 1940 overseen
by Canadian Association of Medical Radiation Technologists
Mission: To serve & protect the public by regulating the practice of the
profession of medical radiation technology
Chief Officer(s):
Peter Derrick, President
Bashir Jalloh, Vice-President
Chelsea Wilker, Executive Director
    chelseawilker@samrt.org
Publications:
• SAMRT Newsletter
Type: Newsletter; *Frequency:* Quarterly
Profile: Reports from the Saskatchewan Association of Medical
Radiation Technologists, upcoming seminars, plus updates on
legislation & bylaws, health & safety, & professional practice

Saskatchewan Association of Rehabilitation Centres (SARC)
111 Cardinal Cres., Saskatoon SK S7L 6H5
                    Tel: 306-933-0616; *Fax:* 306-653-3932
                        e-mail: contact@sarcan.sk.ca
                                    www.sarcsarcan.ca
                www.facebook.com/487285284623365
                                    twitter.com/sarc_sk
Overview: A medium-sized provincial charitable organization founded
in 1968
Mission: To provide vision, leadership & support to agencies through
advocacy, education, provision & development of employment
opportunities
Member of: Saskatchewan Association of Rehabilitation Centres

Saskatchewan College of Paramedics (SCoP)
#202, 1900 Albert St., Regina SK S4P 4K8
                    Tel: 306-585-0145; *Fax:* 306-543-6161
                                Toll-Free: 877-725-4202
                        e-mail: office@collegeofparamedics.sk.ca
                                www.collegeofparamedics.sk.ca
Overview: A small provincial organization
Member of: Paramedic Association of Canada
Chief Officer(s):
Jacquie Messer-Lepage, Executive Director & Registrar
    jmesserlepage@collegeofparamedics.sk.ca
Daniel Lewis, President
Jason Trask, Vice-President

Saskatchewan College of Physical Therapists (SCPT)
#102, 320 - 21st St. West, Saskatoon SK S7M 4E6
                    Tel: 306-931-6661; *Fax:* 306-931-7333
                                Toll-Free: 877-967-7278
                                    www.scpt.org
Previous Name: Saskatchewan College of Physical Therapy
Overview: A small provincial licensing organization overseen by
Canadian Alliance of Physiotherapy Regulators
Member of: Canadian Alliance of Physiotherapy Regulators
Chief Officer(s):
Lynn Kuffner, Acting Executive Director & Registrar
    ed@scpt.org

Saskatchewan College of Podiatrists (SCOP)
2105 Retallack St., Regina SK S4T 2K5
Tel: 306-352-9091; *Fax:* 306-352-9124
e-mail: registrar@scop.ca
www.scop.ca
Overview: A small provincial licensing organization founded in 2003
Mission: To regulate the practice of podiatry; Establish standards of practice; Establish educational requirements; Establish continuing education; Educate the public on the practice of podiatry
Chief Officer(s):
Ata Stationwala, President
Axel Rohrmann, Registrar

Saskatchewan Emergency Medical Services Association (SEMSA)
#105, 111 Research Dr., Saskatoon SK S7N 3R2
Tel: 306-382-2147; *Fax:* 306-955-5353
e-mail: semsa@semsa.org
www.semsa.org
Overview: A medium-sized provincial organization founded in 1959
Mission: To strengthen & advance EMS in Saskatchewan by ensuring high-quality, accountable patient care
Chief Officer(s):
Larise Skoretz, Administrator
Gerry Schriemer, President

Saskatchewan Medical Association (SMA)
#201, 2174 Airport Dr., Saskatoon SK S7L 6M6
Tel: 306-244-2196; *Fax:* 306-653-1631
Toll-Free: 800-667-3781
e-mail: sma@sma.sk.ca
www.sma.sk.ca
www.facebook.com/SMAdocs
twitter.com/SMA_docs
Overview: A medium-sized provincial organization founded in 1906 overseen by Canadian Medical Association
Mission: To represent physicians in Saskatchewan; To advance the professional, educational, & economic welfare of physicians in the province
Chief Officer(s):
Intheran Pillay, President
Bonnie Brossart, Chief Executive Officer
Joanne Sivertson, Vice-President
Siva Karunakaran, Honourary Treasurer
Publications:
• SMA [Saskatchewan Medical Association] News
Type: Newsletter
Profile: Association issues & events

Saskatchewan Prevention Institute (SPI)
1319 Colony St., Saskatoon SK S7N 2Z1
Tel: 306-651-4300; *Fax:* 306-651-4301
e-mail: info@skprevention.ca
www.skprevention.ca
www.facebook.com/SaskatchewanPreventionInstitute
www.youtube.com/user/PreventionInstitute1
Previous Name: Saskatchewan Institute on Prevention of Handicaps
Overview: A small provincial charitable organization founded in 1980
Mission: To reduce the occurrence of disabling conditions in children
Member of: Saskatchewan Health Care Association; Canadian College of Health Service Executives
Chief Officer(s):
Noreen Agrey, Executive Director, 306-651-4302
nagrey@skprevention.ca

Saskatchewan Public Health Association Inc.
PO Box 845, Regina SK S4P 3B1
e-mail: saskpha@gmail.com
Overview: A small provincial organization overseen by Canadian Public Health Association
Mission: To constitute a resource in Saskatchewan for the improvement & maintenance of health
Chief Officer(s):
Greg Riehl, President

Saskatchewan Voice of People with Disabilities, Inc. (SVOPD)
#201, 2206 Dewdney Ave., Regina SK S4R 1H3
Tel: 306-569-3111; *Fax:* 306-569-1889
Toll-Free: 877-569-3111; *TTY:* 306-569-3111
e-mail: voice@saskvoice.com
www.saskvoice.com
www.facebook.com/SaskVoice
Also Known As: Sask Voice
Previous Name: Saskatchewan Voice of the Handicapped
Overview: A medium-sized provincial charitable organization founded in 1973
Mission: To act as a voice for people with disabilities throughout Saskatchewan; To participate in the life of society without discrimination; To increase employment opportunities, accessible housing & tranportation, & family support services
Member of: Council of Canadians with Disabilities

YUKON TERRITORY

Partenariat communauté en santé (PCS)
#328, 302, rue Strickland, Whitehorse YT Y1A 2K1
Tél: 867-668-2663; *Téléc:* 867-668-3511
Courriel: pcsyukon@francosante.ca
www.francosante.org
Aperçu: *Dimension:* petite; *Envergure:* provinciale; fondée en 2003 surveillé par Société santé en français
Mission: Favorise l'offre de services de santé en français
Membre(s) du bureau directeur:
Sandra St-Laurent, Directrice

Yukon Medical Association
5 Hospital Rd., Whitehorse YT Y1A 3H7
Tel: 867-393-8749
e-mail: office@yukondoctors.ca
www.yukondoctors.ca
Overview: A medium-sized provincial organization overseen by Canadian Medical Association
Mission: A voluntary association of Yukon doctors; advocates on behalf of members; promotes professionalism in medical practice & accessibility to quality health care for Yukoners
Affiliation(s): British Columbia Medical Association
Chief Officer(s):
Ken Quong, President
yma@yukondoctors.ca

Local Associations

ALBERTA

Accessible Housing Society
Deerfoot Junction III, #215, 1212 - 31st Ave. NE, Calgary AB T2E 7S8
Tel: 403-282-1872; *Fax:* 403-284-0304
e-mail: info@accessiblehousing.ca
www.accessiblehousing.ca
www.facebook.com/AccessibleHousing
twitter.com/AccessibleYYC
Overview: A small local charitable organization founded in 1974
Mission: To create opportunities for safe, affordable, barrier-free housing for people experiencing mobility problems
Chief Officer(s):
Jeff Dyer, Executive Director
jeff@accessiblehousing.ca
Publications:
• Accessible Housing Society Newsletter
Type: Newsletter

Calgary & Area Medical Staff Society (CAPA)
c/o Alberta Medical Association, 350, 708 - 11 Ave. SW, Calgary AB T2R 0E4
Tel: 403-205-2093
e-mail: audrey.harlow@albertadoctors.org
www.camss.ca
Previous Name: Calgary & Area Physician's Association
Overview: A small local organization
Mission: Represents physicians working in the Calgary Health Region in hospitals or in the community
Chief Officer(s):

Dave Lowery, Communications Director
Steve Patterson, President
  steve.patterson@albertahealthservices.ca
Publications:
• Vital Signs
Type: Magazine; *Frequency:* Monthly; *Editor:* Dave Lowery

Calgary Firefighters Burn Treatment Society (CFFBTS)
2234 - 30 Ave. NE, Calgary AB T2E 7K9
Tel: 403-701-2876; *Fax:* 403-271-0744
e-mail: info@cfbts.org
cfbts.org
www.facebook.com/hotstuffcalgary
twitter.com/hotstuffcalgary
Overview: A medium-sized local charitable organization founded in 1978
Mission: To raise funds for burn victims in burn units throughout Calgary & Southern Alberta
Chief Officer(s):
Jim Fisher, President
  president@cfbts.org
Publications:
• Calgary Firefighters Burn Treatment Society Newsletter
Type: Newsletter

Developmental Disabilities Resource Centre of Calgary (DDRC)
4631 Richardson Way SW, Calgary AB T3E 7B7
Tel: 403-240-3111; *Fax:* 403-240-3230
e-mail: info@ddrc.com
www.ddrc.ca
www.linkedin.com/company/ddrc_2
www.facebook.com/DDRCCalgary
twitter.com/DDRC_Calgary
instagram.com/ddrc_calgary
Overview: A medium-sized local charitable organization founded in 1952
Mission: To facilitate personal choice & build the community's capacity to include person's with developmental disabilities
Member of: Alberta Association for Community Living
Chief Officer(s):
Helen Cowie, Chief Executive Officer
Publications:
• Connection [a publication of the Developmental Disabilities Resource Centre of Calgary]
Type: Newsletter; *Frequency:* Biannually
• Developmental Disabilities Resource Centre of Calgary Annual Report
Type: Report; *Frequency:* Annually

Edmonton Zone Medical Staff Association (EZMSA)
Edmonton AB
Tel: 780-735-2924; *Fax:* 780-735-9091
Overview: A small local organization
Mission: Represents physicians working in the Capital Region of Alberta (Edmonton) in a number of forums including the Regional Medical Advisory Committee, Physician's Liason Committee & the Minister of Health for Alberta
Chief Officer(s):
Robert Broad, President, 780-735-2924
Laurie Wear, Administrator
  laurie.wear@covenanthealth.ca

Falher Friendship Corner Association (FFCA)
PO Box 453, Falher AB T0H 1M0
Tel: 780-837-2153; *Fax:* 780-837-2254
Overview: A small local organization
Mission: To promote the welfare of people with handicaps & their families
Member of: Alberta Association for Community Living

Grande Prairie & Region United Way
#213, 11330 - 106 St., Grande Prairie AB T8V 7X9
Tel: 780-532-1105; *Fax:* 780-532-3532
e-mail: info@unitedwayabnw.org
www.gpunitedway.org
www.facebook.com/UnitedWayABNW
twitter.com/UnitedWayABNW
www.youtube.com/user/GrowUnitedBreakfast

Overview: A small local organization overseen by United Way of Canada - Centraide Canada
Mission: To bring people together to strengthen the community; To strengthen the capacity of community & other local agencies to bring about positive change
Chief Officer(s):
Brenda Yamkowy, Executive Director
  brenda@gpunitedwayabnw.org

Lakeland United Way
Marina Mall, PO Box 8125, #3, 901 - 10 St., Cold Lake AB T9M 1N1
Tel: 780-826-0045; *Fax:* 780-639-2699
www.lakelandunitedway.com
Overview: A small local charitable organization founded in 1987 overseen by United Way of Canada - Centraide Canada
Chief Officer(s):
Ajaz Quraishi, President
  president@lakelandunitedway.com

Lloydminster & District United Way
4419 - 52nd Ave., Lloydminster AB T9V 0Y8
Tel: 780-875-3743; *Fax:* 780-875-3793
Other Communication: office@lloydminster.unitedway.ca
e-mail: luw@telusplanet.net
www.lloydminster.unitedway.ca
Overview: A small local organization overseen by United Way of Canada - Centraide Canada
Mission: To strengthen the community by supporting local agencies

Red Deer Action Group
#202, 4805 - 48 St., Red Deer AB T4N 1S6
Tel: 403-343-1198; *Fax:* 403-343-8945
e-mail: rdag@telus.net
www.rdactiongroup.ca
Previous Name: Red Deer Action Group for the Physically Disabled
Overview: A small local charitable organization founded in 1976
Mission: To work toward providing a better quality of life for people with disabilities
Affliation(s): Alberta Committee for Citizens with Disabilities
Chief Officer(s):
Jean Stinson, President

Rehabilitation Society of Southwestern Alberta
Ability Resource Centre, 1610 - 29th St. North, Lethbridge AB T1H 5L3
Tel: 403-329-3911; *Fax:* 403-329-3581
e-mail: staff@rehab.ab.ca
www.abilityresource.ca
Overview: A small local charitable organization
Mission: To support adults living with disabilities & provide them with a means of accessing opportunities; to facilitate personal growth; to promote inclusion
Chief Officer(s):
Guy McNab, President
Paige McCann Sauter, Executive Director
  paige@rehab.ab.ca

JobLinks Employment Centre
416 - 8th St. South, Lethbridge AB T1J 2J7
Tel: 403-317-4550; *Fax:* 403-317-4552
e-mail: joblinks@rehab.ab.ca
www.job-links.ca

United Way Alberta Northwest
#213, 11330 106 St., Grande Prairie AB T8V 7X9
Tel: 780-532-1105
e-mail: info@unitedwayabnw.org
www.unitedwayabnw.org
www.facebook.com/UnitedWayABNW
twitter.com/UnitedWayABNW
www.youtube.com/user/GrowUnitedBreakfast
Overview: A small local organization overseen by United Way of Canada - Centraide Canada
Mission: To change community conditions & improve the lives of people in need
Chief Officer(s):
Sheldon Rowe, Chair
Brenda Yamkowy, Executive Director
  brenda@unitedwayabnw.org

Jodie Johnson, Director, Resource Development
  resource@unitedwayabnw.org
Marnie Young, Director, Resource Development
  resource@unitedwayabnw.org
Joanne Cousins, Administrator

United Way of Calgary & Area
#600, 105 - 12 Ave SE, Calgary AB T2G 1A1
Tel: 403-231-6265; *Fax:* 403-355-3135
e-mail: uway@calgaryunitedway.org
www.calgaryunitedway.org
www.linkedin.com/companies/united-way-of-calgary-and-area
www.facebook.com/calgaryunitedway
twitter.com/UnitedWayCgy
www.instagram.com/unitedwaycgy
Overview: A small local organization overseen by United Way of
Canada - Centraide Canada
Mission: To invest in 250 programs offered by 130 agencies in
Calgary, Airdrie, Cochrane, High River, Okotoks & Strathmore
Chief Officer(s):
Lucy Miller, President

United Way of Central Alberta
4811 - 48th St., Red Deer AB T4N 1S6
Tel: 403-343-3900; *Fax:* 403-309-3820
e-mail: info@caunitedway.ca
www.caunitedway.ca
Overview: A small local charitable organization founded in 1965
overseen by United Way of Canada - Centraide Canada
Mission: To improve lives & build community by engaging individuals
& mobilizing collective action
Chief Officer(s):
Robert J. Mitchell, Chief Executive Officer

United Way of Fort McMurray
The Redpoll Centre, #200, 10010 Franklin Ave., Fort McMurray AB
T9H 2K6

Tel: 780-791-0077
e-mail: info@fmunitedway.com
fmunitedway.com
www.facebook.com/142299649181047
twitter.com/FMUnitedWay
www.youtube.com/user/fmunitedwaycampaign
Overview: A small local charitable organization founded in 1978
overseen by United Way of Canada - Centraide Canada
Mission: To provide effective support for social health & welfare
services in the community of Fort McMurray
Chief Officer(s):
Ben Dutton, President
Diane Shannon, Executive Director
  dshannon@fmunitedway.com
Russell Thomas, Director, Communications & Community Impact
  communications@fmunitedway.com

United Way of Lethbridge & South Western Alberta
1277 - 3 Ave. South, Lethbridge AB T1J 0K3
Tel: 403-327-1700; *Fax:* 403-317-7940
e-mail: together@lethbridgeunitedway.ca
www.lethbridgeunitedway.ca
www.facebook.com/unitedwaylethy
twitter.com/unitedwaylethy
Overview: A small local charitable organization overseen by United
Way of Canada - Centraide Canada
Mission: To build a better community by organizing the capacity of
people to care for one another
Chief Officer(s):
Jeff McLarty, Executive Director
  jmclarty@lethbridgeunitedway.ca

United Way of South Eastern Alberta
928 Allowance Ave., Medicine Hat AB T1A 7G7
Tel: 403-526-5544; *Fax:* 403-526-5244
www.utdway.ca
www.facebook.com/UnitedWaySEAB
twitter.com/UnitedWaySEAB
Previous Name: United Way of Medicine Hat, Redcliff & District
Overview: A small local organization overseen by United Way of
Canada - Centraide Canada
Chief Officer(s):

Melissa Fandrick, Coordinator, Community Investment
  communityinvestment@utdway.ca

United Way of the Alberta Capital Region
15132 Stony Plain Rd., Edmonton AB T5P 3Y3
Tel: 780-990-1000; *Fax:* 780-990-0203
e-mail: united@myunitedway.ca
myunitedway.ca
www.facebook.com/myUnitedWay
twitter.com/myunitedway
www.youtube.com/uwacr
Overview: A large local charitable organization founded in 1941
overseen by United Way of Canada - Centraide Canada
Mission: To bring people & resources together to build caring, vibrant
communities
Chief Officer(s):
Mona Hale, Chair
Anne Smith, Secretary/Treasurer
Publications:
• WE Magazine
Type: Magazine

Variety Club of Southern Alberta
Calgary AB
Tel: 403-228-6168
e-mail: info@varietyalberta.ca
www.varietyalberta.ca
www.facebook.com/VarietyAlberta
Overview: A small local charitable organization founded in 1982
Mission: To provide disabled & disadvantaged children with the means
to enjoy quality life experiences; to support research for below the knee
amputee children; to provide assistance & bursaries to children in
special situations
Affiliation(s): Variety Children's Lifeline

YWCA of Banff Programs & Services
PO Box 520, 102 Spray Ave., Banff AB T1L 1A6
Tel: 403-762-3560; *Fax:* 403-760-3202
e-mail: info@ywcabanff.ca
www.ywcabanff.ca
www.facebook.com/YWCABanff
twitter.com/YWCABanff
Previous Name: Planned Parenthood Banff; Banff YWCA Community
Resource Centre
Overview: A small local charitable organization founded in 1987
Mission: To provide safe, affordable housing & prevent family violence
through education, programming, events, resource management &
crisis intervention
Affiliation(s): Society Against Family Violence
Chief Officer(s):
Wendy Kuiper, President
Connie MacDonald, Chief Executive Director

BRITISH COLUMBIA

Campbell River & District United Way
PO Box 135, Campbell River BC V9W 5A7
Tel: 250-702-2911
e-mail: bvbayly@uwcnvi.ca
Overview: A small local organization overseen by United Way of
Canada - Centraide Canada
Mission: To raise & distribute funds to member agencies that are
providing support and services to residents in the Campbell River area
Member of: United Way of Canada

Care Institute of Safety & Health Inc.
1770 East 18th Ave., Vancouver BC V5N 5P6
Tel: 604-873-6018; *Fax:* 604-873-4443
Toll-Free: 800-923-4566
www.care-institute.com
Overview: A small local organization
Mission: To provide safety training for individuals & organizations
Chief Officer(s):
Elaine Shigetomi, President & CEO

Carefree Society
2832 Queensway St., Prince George BC V2L 4M5
Tel: 250-562-1394; *Fax:* 250-562-1393
e-mail: carefree_society@telus.net
www.carefreesociety.org

Also Known As: handyDART
Overview: A small local charitable organization founded in 1971
Mission: To provide transportation services for the disabled
Affliation(s): BC Transit

Children's Health Foundation of Vancouver Island
2390 Arbutus Rd., Victoria BC V8N 1V7
Tel: 250-519-6977; *Fax:* 250-519-6715
childrenshealthvi.org
www.linkedin.com/company/2291213
twitter.com/childrensvi
www.youtube.com/user/QAFoundation
Overview: A small local charitable organization founded in 1922
Mission: To support children in need by raising funds towards improving their health and well being
Chief Officer(s):
Veronica Carroll, Chief Executive Officer
veronica.carroll@viha.ca
Frances Melville, Director, Operations
frances.melville@viha.ca

Comox Valley United Way
PO Box 3097, Stn. Main, Courtenay BC V9N 5N3
Tel: 250-338-1151
www.uwcnvi.ca
Overview: A small local organization overseen by United Way of Canada - Centraide Canada

Cowichan United Way
1 Kenneth Place, Duncan BC V9L 5G3
Tel: 250-748-1312; *Fax:* 250-748-7652
Toll-Free: 877-748-1312
e-mail: office@cowichan.unitedway.ca
www.cowichan.unitedway.ca
www.facebook.com/UnitedWayCowichan
twitter.com/uwcowichan
Overview: A small local charitable organization founded in 1976 overseen by United Way of Canada - Centraide Canada
Mission: To fundraise for charities; To provide guidance & counsel to charitable organization; To take leadership role in raising awareness of community needs
Chief Officer(s):
Mike Murphy, President
Heather Gardiner, Interim Advisor
hgardiner@cowichan.unitedway.ca

McCreary Centre Society (MCS)
3552 Hastings St. East, Vancouver BC V5K 2A7
Tel: 604-291-1996; *Fax:* 604-291-7308
e-mail: mccreary@mcs.bc.ca
www.mcs.bc.ca
Previous Name: Friends of the McCreary Centre Society
Overview: A small local charitable organization founded in 1977
Mission: To raise awareness & understanding of youth health & related issues; To address the health needs of young people through the development of projects & initiatives
Member of: Canadian Health Network
Chief Officer(s):
Annie Smith, Executive Director

North Shore Disability Resource Centre Association (NSDRC)
3158 Mountain Hwy., North Vancouver BC V7K 2H5
Tel: 604-985-5371; *Fax:* 604-985-7594; *TTY:* 604-985-5371
e-mail: nsdrc@nsdrc.org
www.nsdrc.org
www.facebook.com/227106267339398
twitter.com/NSDRCcbsProg
Previous Name: North Shore Association for the Physically Handicapped
Overview: A medium-sized local charitable organization founded in 1976
Mission: To provide programs & services based on the belief that all people are important to their community; To work to ensure that people with disabilities can participate actively as members of the community; To work toward a community which is free from physical, financial, & attitudinal barriers
Member of: BC Association for Community Living; United Way of the Lower Mainland

Affliation(s): BC Federation of Private Child Care Agencies; United Way of the Lower Mainland; BC Coalition of People with Disabilities
Chief Officer(s):
Liz Barnett, Executive Director
lizb@nsdrc.org

Planned Lifetime Advocacy Network (PLAN)
#260, 3665 Kingsway, Vancouver BC V5R 5W2
Tel: 604-439-9566; *Fax:* 604-439-7001
www.plan.ca
www.facebook.com/JoinPLAN
twitter.com/plannedlifetime
www.youtube.com/user/PLANvids
Overview: A small local organization
Mission: To help families with disabled relatives plan for their future
Affliation(s): PLAN Toronto; Thunderbay Family Network; PLAN Edmonton; Lethbridge Association for Community Living; PLAN Calgary; Lifetime Networks Ottawa; Planned Lifetime Networks; LifeSPAN; PLAN Okanagan; Regina RDACL PLAN; Family Link; PLAN of Arizona
Chief Officer(s):
Tim Ames, Executive Director
tames@plan.ca
Adam Trombley, Manager, Communications & Member Engagement

Powell River & District United Way
PO Box 370, #205, 4750 Joyce Ave., Powell River BC V8A 5C2
Tel: 604-485-2791
e-mail: admin@unitedwayofpowellriver.ca
www.unitedwayofpowellriver.ca
www.facebook.com/322827261966
twitter.com/PRUnitedway
Overview: A small local charitable organization founded in 1976 overseen by United Way of Canada - Centraide Canada
Chief Officer(s):
Ashley Hull, President
hullashley@gmail.com

Prince George United Way
1600 - 3rd Ave., Prince George BC V2L 3G6
Tel: 250-561-1040; *Fax:* 250-562-8102
e-mail: info@unitedwaynbc.ca
www.pguw.bc.ca
www.facebook.com/unitedwaynorthernbc
Overview: A small local charitable organization founded in 1969 overseen by United Way of Canada - Centraide Canada
Mission: To promote the organized capacity of persons to care for one another through voluntarism, leadership & education; To ensure the effective raising & allocation of charitable funds for community-based social services; To foster the effective provision of services that are in the best interest of the community
Chief Officer(s):
Trevor Williams, Executive Director
trevorw@unitedwaynbc.ca
Rob Jarvis, Chair

Richmond Caring Place Society (RCPS)
#140, 7000 Minoru Blvd., Richmond BC V6Y 3Z5
Tel: 604-279-7000; *Fax:* 604-279-7008
e-mail: admin.caringplace@shaw.ca
www.richmondcaringplace.ca
Overview: A small local organization founded in 1994
Mission: RCPS operates Richmond Caring Place, a facility that serves as one convenient location housing several, non-profit, community service agencies. The agencies have common access to meeting rooms & can collaborate on programs with ease due to proximity. Agencies include: Alzheimer Society of BC; Canadian Cancer Society; Canadian Hemochromatosis Society; BC Centre for Ability; Richmond Hospice Association; & more. RCPS is a registered charity, BN: 130560139RR0001.
Chief Officer(s):
Gary M. Hagel, Chair

Social Planning Council for the North Okanagan (SPCNO)
c/o Community Futures North Okanagan, 3105 - 33rd St., Vernon BC V1T 9P7
Tel: 250-540-8572
e-mail: info@socialplanning.ca
www.socialplanning.ca

Previous Name: North Okanagan Social Planning Council
Overview: A small local charitable organization founded in 1969
Mission: To facilitate & coordinate community planning & development by encouraging communication & cooperation amongst social, educational & health services in the North Okanagan
Chief Officer(s):
Annette Sharkey, Executive Director

South Peace Community Resources Society (SPCRS)
PO Box 713, 10110 - 13th St., Dawson Creek BC V1G 4H7
Tel: 250-782-9174; *Fax:* 250-782-4167
Toll-Free: 866-712-9174
e-mail: reception@spcrs.ca
www.spcrs.ca
www.facebook.com/spcrs.dawsoncreek
twitter.com/SPCRS
Overview: A small local charitable organization founded in 1974
Mission: To meet the social, educational & personal needs of the community by providing services that develop skills for living; To provide community & residential services; to meet the needs of children, youth & families, women who have experienced violence, victims of crime, adults with mental handicaps, children with special needs, couples & individuals experiencing trauma or difficulties in their life
Member of: British Columbia Association for Community Living; Federation of Child & Family Services; BC/Yukon Society of Transition Houses; BC Association for Specialized Victims Assistance Programs & Counselling
Chief Officer(s):
Stefan Pavlis, Executive Director

Theatre Terrific Society
#430, 111 West Hastings St., Vancouver BC V6B 1H4
Tel: 604-222-4020; *Fax:* 604-669-2662
e-mail: info@theatreterrific.ca
www.theatreterrific.ca
twitter.com/TheatreTerrific
www.youtube.com/user/theatreterrific
Overview: A small local charitable organization founded in 1985
Mission: To provide theatrical opportunities to people with disabilities
Member of: Alliance for Arts & Culture
Affliation(s): Volunteer Vancouver; Greater Vancouver Professional Theatre Association
Chief Officer(s):
Susanna Uchatius, Artistic Director

Thompson, Nicola, Cariboo United Way
177 Victoria St., Kamloops BC V2C 1Z4
Tel: 250-372-9933; *Fax:* 250-372-5926
Toll-Free: 855-372-9933
e-mail: office@unitedwaytnc.ca
www.unitedwaytnc.ca
www.linkedin.com/company/thompson-nicola-cariboo-united-way
www.facebook.com/unitedwaytnc
twitter.com/unitedwaytnc
www.youtube.com/unitedwaytnc
Previous Name: United Way of Kamloops & Region
Overview: A small local organization founded in 1960 overseen by United Way of Canada - Centraide Canada
Mission: To enable all citizens to join in a community wide effort to fund & provide in consort with others, effective delivery of health & social services & programs in response to the needs of the community
Member of: United Way of Canada - Centraide Canada
Chief Officer(s):
Danalee Baker, Executive Director
danalee@unitedwaytnc.ca

United Way Central & Northern Vancouver Island
#9, 327 Prideaux St., Nanaimo BC V9R 2N4
Tel: 250-591-8731; *Fax:* 250-591-7340
e-mail: info@uwcnvi.ca
www.uwcnvi.ca
www.linkedin.com/company/united-way-central-&-northern-vancouver-islan
www.facebook.com/UWCNVI
twitter.com/UWCNVI
www.youtube.com/user/UnitedWayCNVI
Previous Name: United Way of Nanaimo & District

Overview: A small local charitable organization founded in 1958 overseen by United Way of Canada - Centraide Canada
Mission: To improve lives by engaging individuals & mobilizing collective action
Member of: Nanaimo & Ladysmith Chambers of Commerce
Chief Officer(s):
Signy Madden, Executive Director
signy@uwcnvi.ca
Publications:
• Younited [a publication of the United Way Central & Northern Vancouver Island]
Type: Newsletter; *Frequency:* irregular
Profile: An information resource for United Way donors, volunteers, & supporters

United Way of East Kootenay
PO Box 657, 930 Baker St., Cranbrook BC V1C 4J2
Tel: 250-426-8833; *Fax:* 250-426-5455
e-mail: office@cranbrook.unitedway.ca
www.cranbrook.unitedway.ca
www.facebook.com/ourunitedway
Overview: A small local charitable organization founded in 1969 overseen by United Way of Canada - Centraide Canada
Mission: To ensure the effective raising & allocation of charitable funds for community based social services that are in the best interest of the community
Chief Officer(s):
Donna Brady Fields, Executive Director

United Way of North Okanagan Columbia Shuswap
3304 - 30th Ave., Vernon BC V1T 2C8
Tel: 250-549-1346; *Fax:* 250-549-1357
Toll-Free: 866-448-3489
e-mail: unitedwaynocs@shaw.ca
www.unitedwaynocs.com
www.facebook.com/226411234037024
twitter.com/unitedwaynocs
Previous Name: North Okanagan United Way
Overview: A small local charitable organization founded in 1961 overseen by United Way of Canada - Centraide Canada
Mission: To promote a healthy, caring inclusive community; To strenghten our community's capacity to address social issues
Member of: Vernon Chamber of Commerce
Chief Officer(s):
Linda Yule, Executive Director

United Way of the Central Okanagan & South Okanagan/Similkameen
#202, 1456 St. Paul St., Kelowna BC V1Y 2E6
Tel: 250-860-2356; *Fax:* 250-868-3206
e-mail: info@unitedwaycso.com
unitedwaycso.com
www.facebook.com/unitedwaycso
twitter.com/UnitedWayCSO
www.youtube.com/user/UnitedWayCSO
Overview: A medium-sized local charitable organization founded in 1950 overseen by United Way of Canada - Centraide Canada
Mission: To increase the organized capacity of people in our community to care for one another
Chief Officer(s):
Shelley Gilmore, Executive Director

United Way of the Fraser Valley (UWFV)
Sweeney Neighbourhood Centre, #208, 33355 Bevan Ave., Abbotsford BC V2S 0E7
Tel: 604-852-1234; *Fax:* 604-852-2316
Toll-Free: 888-251-7777
e-mail: info@uwfv.bc.ca
www.facebook.com/unitedwayfraservalley
twitter.com/unitedwayfv
Overview: A small local charitable organization founded in 1985 overseen by United Way of Canada - Centraide Canada
Mission: To promote the organized capacity of people to care for one another
Member of: United Way of Canada; Abbotsford Chamber of Commerce; Chilliwack Chamber of Commerce
Chief Officer(s):
Wayne Green, Executive Director
wayne@uwfv.bc.ca

United Way of the Lower Mainland
4543 Canada Way, Burnaby BC V5G 4T4
Tel: 604-294-8929; *Fax:* 604-293-0220
www.uwlm.ca
www.linkedin.com/groups?about=&gid=4196396
www.facebook.com/UnitedWayoftheLowerMainland
twitter.com/uwlm
www.youtube.com/user/UnitedWayVancouver
Overview: A small local organization overseen by United Way of Canada - Centraide Canada
Chief Officer(s):
Michael McKnight, President & CEO
michaelm@uwlm.ca

United Way of Trail & District
803B Victoria St., Trail BC V1R 3T3
Tel: 250-364-0999; *Fax:* 250-364-1564
www.traildistrictunitedway.com
Overview: A small local charitable organization founded in 1928 overseen by United Way of Canada - Centraide Canada
Mission: To raise funds which are allocated to 26 affiliated non-profit organizations
Chief Officer(s):
Jodi LeSergent, President

The Vancouver Art Therapy Institute
1575 Johnston St., Vancouver BC V6H 3R9
Tel: 604-681-8284; *Fax:* 604-331-8262
e-mail: info@vati.bc.ca
www.vati.bc.ca
Overview: A small local charitable organization founded in 1982
Mission: To train art therapists at the graduate level; To provide art therapy as a service; To educate the public about the effciency of art therapy
Member of: Canadian Art Therapy Association; BC Art Therapy Association
Chief Officer(s):
Tatjana Jansen, Executive Director

Vancouver Island Society for Disabled Artists
#304, 1550 Church Ave., Victoria BC V8P 2H1
Tel: 250-472-2917
Overview: A small local organization founded in 1995
Mission: To support artists with disabilities by creating an art gallery in Victoria British Columbia so artists can showcase their art work
Chief Officer(s):
Garry Curry, President
Alistair Green

Victoria Medical Society (VMS)
Eric Martin Pavillion, #190, 2334 Trent St., Victoria BC V8R 4Z3
Tel: 250-598-6021; *Fax:* 250-370-8274
e-mail: administrator@victoriamedicalsociety.org
www.victoriamedicalsociety.org
Overview: A small local organization founded in 1895
Mission: To promote good health & act as an advocate on health issues; to promote good & appropriate medical practice in accord with the Code of Ethics; to promote the good name of medicine; to promote medical education; to promote fellowship & good relations within the profession & with the public; to help, as much as possible, any member in distress from any cause; to advocate for any doctor or group of doctors subjected to injustice; to mediate, when requested, in disputes & differences between local medical groups or individuals (mediation & advocacy does not apply to cases under the jurisdiction of the College of Physicians & Surgeons of BC); to cooperate with the BCMA, CMA & College of Physicians & Surgeons of BC
Affliation(s): BC College of Physicians & Surgeons; BC Medical Association
Chief Officer(s):
C. Peter Innes, President
vicmedso@telus.net

Victoria Youth Empowerment Society
533 Yates St., Victoria BC V8W 1K7
Tel: 250-383-3514; *Fax:* 250-383-3812
e-mail: office_manager@vyes.ca
www.vyes.ca
Merged from: Alliance Club; Association for Street Kids
Overview: A small local charitable organization founded in 1992

Mission: To assist youth to remove themselves from the high risk environment of the street & make the transition to healthier & more constructive life situations; To help youth make positive choices which will prevent involvement in at risk behaviour or connection with the street scene
Member of: Federation of Child & Family Services of BC; United Way

MANITOBA

Child & Family Services of Western Manitoba (C&FS Western)
800 McTavish Ave., Brandon MB R7A 7L4
Tel: 204-726-6030; *Fax:* 204-726-6775
Toll-Free: 800-483-8980
e-mail: info@cfswestern.mb.ca
www.cfswestern.mb.ca
Previous Name: Children's Aid Society of Western Manitoba
Overview: A medium-sized local charitable organization founded in 1899
Mission: To ensure children are safe in strong loving families within caring communities
Member of: Child Welfare League of Canada
Chief Officer(s):
Phil Shaman, President
Candace Kowalchuk, Specialist, Human Resources
hr@cfswestern.mb.ca
Susan Cable, Coordinator, Community Education
commed@cfswestern.mb.ca

Neepawa & District United Way
PO Box 1545, Neepawa MB R0J 1H0
Tel: 204-476-3410
e-mail: unitedwayneepawa@mymts.net
www.neepawaunitedway.org
Overview: A small local organization overseen by United Way of Canada - Centraide Canada
Mission: Local United Way Chapter raising funds to help community organization.

Portage Plains United Way
PO Box 953, 20 Saskatchewan Ave. East, Portage la Prairie MB R1N 3C4
Tel: 204-857-4440; *Fax:* 204-239-1740
e-mail: info@portageplainsuw.ca
www.portageplainsuw.ca
www.facebook.com/353759031400503
twitter.com/PortagePlainsUW
Overview: A small local charitable organization founded in 1968 overseen by United Way of Canada - Centraide Canada
Mission: To unite the community & enhance the quality of life for those in need
Chief Officer(s):
Mandy Dubois, Executive Director
Jennifer Sneesby, Office Manager

Rainbow Resource Centre
170 Scott St., Winnipeg MB R3L 0L3
Tel: 204-474-0212; *Fax:* 204-478-1160
Toll-Free: 855-437-8523
www.rainbowresourcecentre.org
www.facebook.com/RainbowResourceCentre
twitter.com/RainbowResCtr
www.instagram.com/rainbowresourcecentre
Also Known As: Gays for Equality
Previous Name: Campus Gay Club (University of Manitoba)
Overview: A small local charitable organization founded in 1972
Mission: To work toward an equal & diverse society, free of homophobia & discrimination, by encouraging visibility & fostering health & self-acceptance through education, support, resources & outreach
Chief Officer(s):
Mike Tutthill, Executive Director

Samaritan House Ministries Inc.
820 Pacific Ave., Brandon MB R7A 0J1
Tel: 204-726-0758
e-mail: info@samaritanhouse.net
samaritanhouse.net
www.facebook.com/210774752373958
twitter.com/SHM_Brandon

Overview: A small local charitable organization founded in 1987
Mission: To provide support & services to at-risk populations - the homeless, those living in poverty, people with literacy challenges or persons leaving abusive relationships
Chief Officer(s):
Thea Dennis, Executive Director

United Way of Brandon & District Inc.
Scotia Towers, 201 - 1011 Rosser Ave., Brandon MB R7A 0L5
Tel: 204-571-8929; *Fax:* 204-727-8939
e-mail: office@brandonuw.ca
www.brandonuw.ca
www.facebook.com/UnitedWayBrandon
Also Known As: Brandon & District United Way
Overview: A small local organization founded in 1966 overseen by United Way of Canada - Centraide Canada
Chief Officer(s):
Cynamon Mychasiw, CEO

United Way of Morden & District Inc.
PO Box 758, 379 Stephen St., Morden MB R6M 1A7
Tel: 204-822-6992
e-mail: mordendistrictuw@gmail.com
www.unitedwaymorden.com
Overview: A small local organization overseen by United Way of Canada - Centraide Canada
Mission: To partner with charitable agencies & organizations to improve the lives of residents in Morden & the surrounding area
Chief Officer(s):
Lisa Gander, President

United Way of Winnipeg / Winnipeg Centraide
580 Main St., Winnipeg MB R3B 1C7
Tel: 204-477-5360; *Fax:* 204-453-6198
e-mail: info@unitedwaywinnipeg.mb.ca
www.unitedwaywinnipeg.ca
www.facebook.com/unitedwaywinnipeg
twitter.com/unitedwaywpg
www.youtube.com/user/uwaywinnipeg
Overview: A small local organization founded in 1965 overseen by United Way of Canada - Centraide Canada
Mission: To support & strengthen the organized capacity of people to care for one another
Chief Officer(s):
Marilyn McLaren, Chair

Winkler & District United Way
PO Box 1528, Winkler MB R6W 4B4
Tel: 204-325-6321
e-mail: unitedwaywinkler@gmail.com
www.unitedwaywinkler.com
www.facebook.com/609225769188170
Overview: A small local organization overseen by United Way of Canada - Centraide Canada
Mission: To serve & improve the community
Chief Officer(s):
Lori Penner, President

Winnipeg Association of Public Service Officers (WAPSO) / Association des agents de services au public de Winnipeg
#2705, 83 Garry St., Winnipeg MB R3C 4J9
Tel: 204-925-4120; *Fax:* 201-925-4128
www.wapso.ca
www.facebook.com/WinnipegAssociationofPublicServiceOfficers
www.flickr.com/photos/112212984@N04
Overview: A medium-sized local organization founded in 1969
Mission: To represent the interests of its workers during collective bargaining; to ensure its members a high standard quality of work life.
Chief Officer(s):
Robert Young, Executive Director
Andrew Weremy, President
Alex Regiec, 1st Vice-President
Michael Robinson, 2nd Vice-President

NEW BRUNSWICK

United Way of Greater Moncton & Southeastern New Brunswick (UWGMSENB) / Centraide de la région du Grand Moncton et du Sud-Est du NB Inc. (CGMSENB)
22 Church St., #T210, Moncton NB E1C 0P7
Tel: 506-858-8600; *Fax:* 506-858-0584
e-mail: office@moncton.unitedway.ca
www.gmsenbunitedway.ca
www.facebook.com/UnitedWayGMSENBCentraideGMSENB
twitter.com/unitedwaygmsenb
www.flickr.com/photos/unitedwaygmsenb
Previous Name: United Way/Centraide of the Moncton Region
Overview: A small local charitable organization founded in 1953 overseen by United Way of Canada - Centraide Canada
Mission: To strengthen Southeastern New Brunswick's communities
Chief Officer(s):
Debbie McInnis, Executive Director
dmcinnis@moncton.unitedway.ca

United Way of Greater Saint John Inc.
#301, 28 Richmond St., Saint John NB E2L 3B2
Tel: 506-658-1212; *Fax:* 506-633-7724
e-mail: contactus@unitedwaysaintjohn.com
www.unitedwaysaintjohn.com
www.facebook.com/21724743048
twitter.com/SJUnitedWay
www.youtube.com/UnitedWaySJ
Overview: A small local charitable organization founded in 1958 overseen by United Way of Canada - Centraide Canada
Chief Officer(s):
Wendy MacDermott, Executive Director
wendy@unitedwaysaintjohn.com

United Way/Centraide (Central NB) Inc.
#1A, 385 Wilsey Rd., Fredericton NB E3B 5N6
Tel: 506-459-7773; *Fax:* 506-451-1104
e-mail: office@unitedwaycentral.com
www.unitedwaycentral.com
www.facebook.com/148382218531358
twitter.com/JessieUnitedWay
Previous Name: United Way/Centraide Fredericton Inc.
Overview: A small local charitable organization founded in 1960 overseen by United Way of Canada - Centraide Canada
Mission: To be a leader in helping to create & sustain a caring & healthy community
Chief Officer(s):
Blair McLaughlin, President
Jeff Richardson, Executive Director
jeff@unitedwaycentral.com

NEWFOUNDLAND AND LABRADOR

Libra House Inc.
PO Box 449, Stn. B, Happy Valley-Goose Bay NL A0P 1E0
Tel: 709-896-8022; *Fax:* 709-896-8223
Toll-Free: 877-896-3014; *Crisis Hot-Line:* 709-896-3014
e-mail: librahouse@nf.aibn.com
www.librahouse.ca
Overview: A small local organization founded in 1983
Mission: To provide crisis shelter services for abused women & their children; To offer support & education to women
Member of: Provincial Association Against Family Violence
Chief Officer(s):
Janet O'Donnell, Executive Director

NOVA SCOTIA

Adsum for Women & Children
2421 Brunswick St., Halifax NS B3K 2Z4
Tel: 902-423-5049; *Fax:* 902-423-9336; *Crisis Hot-Line:* 902-423-4443
e-mail: adsum@adsumforwomen.org
www.adsumforwomen.org
www.facebook.com/pages/Adsum-for-Women-Children/111571128907431
twitter.com/AdsumForWomen
www.youtube.com/user/adsumforwomen
Previous Name: Association for Women's Residential Facilities
Overview: A medium-sized local charitable organization founded in 1983

Mission: To administer Adsum House; To provide emergency shelter for homeless women & children
Chief Officer(s):
Sheri Lecker, Executive Director
sheri.lecker@adsumforwomen.org

Community Involvement of the Disabled (CID)
#5, 28 Hillview Ave., Sydney NS B1P 2H4
Tel: 902-564-9817; *Fax:* 902-564-5758
Overview: A small local charitable organization founded in 1977
Mission: Advocacy for persons with disabilities
Member of: Nova Scotia League for Equal Opportunities

Cumberland Equal Rights for the Disabled (CERD)
PO Box 75, Maccan NS B0L 1B0
Tel: 902-545-2065
Overview: A small local organization
Affiliation(s): Nova Scotia League for Equal Opportunities; Disabled Individuals Alliance
Chief Officer(s):
Linda Styles, Contact

Disabled Individuals Alliance (DIAL)
Bethune Bldg., #262, 1278 Tower Rd., Halifax NS B3H 2Y9
Tel: 902-422-6888; *Fax:* 902-425-0766
e-mail: MAJ@ns.sympatico.ca
www.nsnet.org/dial
Overview: A small local organization founded in 1978
Mission: DIAL (Disabled Individuals Alliance) is a cross-disability consumer group formed to bring together persons with varying disabilities and interested non-disabled individuals, enabling the disabled as a whole to speak out with a unified voice as to their common needs and goals.
Member of: Nova Scotia League for Equal Opportunities

Handicapped Organization Promoting Equality
PO Box 562, 84 Main St., Yarmouth NS B5A 4B4
Tel: 902-742-6579; *Fax:* 902-742-1281
e-mail: hopecentre@ns.sympatico.ca
www.facebook.com/HOPECentreanddialaride
Also Known As: HOPE
Overview: A small local charitable organization founded in 1981
Mission: To provide life skill courses for adults & programs for children with special needs
Affiliation(s): Nova Scotia League for Equal Opportunities

New Leaf Enterprises
3670 Kempt Rd., Halifax NS B3K 4X8
Tel: 902-453-6000
www.easterseals.ns.ca
Overview: A small local organization founded in 1960 overseen by Easter Seals Nova Scotia
Mission: To create a collaborative social setting in order to help adults with physical disabilities develop job skills
Member of: Easter Seals Nova Scotia; DIRECTIONS Council for Vocational Services Society
Chief Officer(s):
Veronica Dale, Executive Director
v.dale@easterseals.ns.ca

Richmond County Disabled Association (RCD)
PO Box 379, Petit de Grat NS B0E 2L0
Tel: 902-226-1353
Overview: A small local organization
Affiliation(s): Nova Scotia League For Equal Opportunities
Chief Officer(s):
Kenneth L. David, Contact

Shelburne Association Supporting Inclusion (SASI)
PO Box 59, 151 Water St., Shelburne NS B0T 1W0
Tel: 902-875-1083; *Fax:* 902-875-1056
e-mail: sasi@eastlink.ca
www.supportinginclusion.ca
Overview: A small local charitable organization founded in 1985
Mission: To improve the quality of life for individuals with disabilities & mental health difficulties through person-centred programs
Member of: DIRECTIONS Council for Vocational Services Society
Chief Officer(s):
Martha Holmes, Chair

Publications:
• Shelburne Association Supporting Inclusion Newsletter
Type: Newsletter

United Way of Cape Breton
245 Charlotte St., Sydney NS B1P 6W4
Tel: 902-562-5226; *Fax:* 902-562-5721
www.unitedwaycapebreton.com
www.facebook.com/UnitedWayOfCapeBreton
Overview: A small local organization overseen by United Way of Canada - Centraide Canada
Mission: To improve the quality of life of Cape Breton's residents
Chief Officer(s):
Lynne McCarron, Executive Director

United Way of Cumberland County
PO Box 535, #206, 16 Church St., Amherst NS B4H 4A1
Tel: 902-667-2203; *Fax:* 902-667-3819
www.amherst.unitedway.ca
Previous Name: United Way of Amherst
Overview: A small local organization overseen by United Way of Canada - Centraide Canada
Chief Officer(s):
Curt Gunn, President

United Way of Halifax Region
Royal Bank Bldg., 46 Portland St., 7th Fl., Dartmouth NS B2Y 1H4
Tel: 902-422-1501; *Fax:* 902-423-6837
www.unitedwayhalifax.ca
www.linkedin.com/company/united-way-of-halifax-region
www.facebook.com/UnitedWayHalifaxRegion
twitter.com/UWHalifax
Previous Name: Metro United Way (Halifax-Dartmouth)
Overview: A medium-sized local charitable organization founded in 1924 overseen by United Way of Canada - Centraide Canada
Mission: To strengthen neighbourhoods & communities by providing programs & services that link people & resources, encourage participation & increase giving
Chief Officer(s):
Sara Napier, President & CEO
snapier@unitedwayhalifax.ca

United Way of Pictou County
PO Box 75, 342 Stewart St., New Glasgow NS B2H 5E1
Tel: 902-755-1754; *Fax:* 902-755-0853
e-mail: info@pictoucountyunitedway.ca
www.pictoucountyunitedway.ca
www.facebook.com/UWPictouCounty
twitter.com/UWPictouCo
Overview: A small local charitable organization founded in 1960 overseen by United Way of Canada - Centraide Canada
Mission: To strengthen communities by facilitating programs & services that link people & resources; encourage participation; increase giving
Chief Officer(s):
Jessica Smith, Executive Director
jessica@pictoucountyunitedway.ca

ONTARIO

Access Counselling & Family Services
#200, 460 Brant St., Burlington ON L7R 4B6
Tel: 905-637-5256; *Fax:* 905-637-8221
Toll-Free: 866-457-0234
e-mail: info@accesscounselling.ca
www.accesscounselling.ca
Overview: A small local charitable organization founded in 1968 overseen by Family Service Ontario
Mission: To serve members of the community in times of crisis, assisting people to cope with conflict, grief, loss, violence, abuse.
Member of: United Way Burlington
Chief Officer(s):
Susan Jewett, Executive Director

African Community Health Services
#207, 110 Spadina Ave., Toronto ON M5V 2K4
Tel: 416-591-7600
Overview: A small local organization
Mission: To offer health & social support services to African immigrants & African Canadians

Agincourt Community Services Association (ACSA)
#100, 4155 Sheppard Ave. East, Toronto ON M1S 1T4
Tel: 416-321-6912; *Fax:* 416-321-6922
e-mail: info@agincourtcommunityservices.com
www.agincourtcommunityservices.com
www.linkedin.com/company/agincourt-community-services-association
www.facebook.com/AgincourtCommunityServices
twitter.com/AginComServices
Previous Name: Information Agincourt; Information Scarborough
Overview: A small local charitable organization founded in 1970 overseen by InformOntario
Mission: A charitable, multi-service neighbourhood agency that exists to identify & provide services, information & programs in response to the diverse needs & interest of the multicultural community; strives to improve the quality of life for individuals & families by mobilizing volunteers, providing links & partnerships between those who wish to help & those who need services
Chief Officer(s):
Vinitha Gengatharan, Chairperson

Amherstburg Community Services
179 Victoria St., Amherstburg ON N9V 3N5
Tel: 519-736-5471; *Fax:* 519-736-1391
e-mail: staffacs@bellnet.ca
www.amherstburg-cs.com
Overview: A small local organization founded in 1973 overseen by InforOntario
Mission: To study the social, health, educational, recreational and other human needs of the Amherstburg area, and services available to satisfy those needs; To promote the orderly development of well-balanced community services.
Chief Officer(s):
Kathy DiBartolomeo, Executive Director
edacs@bellnet.ca

Amputee Society of Ottawa & District
#1404, 505 Smyth Rd., Ottawa ON K1H 8M2
Tel: 613-737-7350; *Fax:* 613-737-7056
Overview: A small local organization
Mission: Provides support to new amputees from trained amputee visitors, information on community services available to amputees and ongoing contact with amputees via a visitor program
Chief Officer(s):
Betty Lanigan, President
bblanigan@hotmail.com

Ancaster Community Services (ACS)
300 Wilson St. East, Ancaster ON L9G 2B9
Tel: 905-648-6675
www.ancastercommunityservices.ca
www.facebook.com/AncasterCommunityServices.ca
Previous Name: Ancaster Information Centre & Community Services Inc.
Overview: A small local charitable organization founded in 1969 overseen by InformOntario
Chief Officer(s):
Melanie Barlow, Interim Executive Director

ASK! Community Information Centre (LAMP)
185 - 5th St., Toronto ON M8V 2Z5
Tel: 416-252-6471; *Fax:* 416-252-4474
www.lampchc.org
www.facebook.com/LAMPCHEALTHC
Previous Name: YMCA ASK! & YMCA ASCC
Overview: A small local organization founded in 1969 overseen by InformOntario
Mission: To offer a range of programs & services to support residents & workers of southern Etobicoke (South/West Toronto); To offer community information, referral, legal advice, immigrant program, & refugee support
Member of: Federation of Community Information Centres of Toronto; Lakeshore Area Multi-Servcies Program
Chief Officer(s):
Russ Ford, Executive Director

Assisted Living Southwestern Ontario (ALSO)
3141 Sandwich St., Windsor ON N9C 1A7
Tel: 519-969-8188; *Fax:* 519-969-0390
e-mail: info@alsogroup.org
www.appdgroup.org
Previous Name: Association for Persons with Physical Disabilities of Windsor & Essex County
Overview: A small local organization founded in 1985
Mission: Provides personal care, homemaking services and assistance with tasks of daily living to adults with permanent physical disabilities.
Chief Officer(s):
Lyn Calder, Executive Director

Association of Jewish Chaplains of Ontario
c/o Beth Emeth Bais Yehuda Synagogue, 100 Elder St., Toronto ON M3H 5G7
Tel: 416-633-3838; *Fax:* 416-633-3153
e-mail: info@beby.org
www.beby.org
www.facebook.com/BEBY.Toronto
twitter.com/BethEmeth
Overview: A small local organization
Mission: To draw together those who are active in pastoral care of Jewish people & their families, for fellowship, mutual support & education; to facilitate the understanding of the role & function that a professional performs in the pastoral care of Jewish people in hospitals, seniors' homes, correctional institutions, synagogues & schools; to develop & define standards for Jewish pastoral care providers; to develop & provide training & ensure the availability of competent pastor care where needed
Affliation(s): Toronto Board of Rabbis
Chief Officer(s):
Bernard Schwartz, President
Pearl Grundland, Executive Director

Brant United Way (BUW)
125 Morrell St., Brantford ON N3T 4J9
Tel: 519-752-7848; *Fax:* 519-752-7913
e-mail: info@brantunitedway.org
www.brantunitedway.org
www.facebook.com/pages/Brant-United-Way/33874902961
twitter.com/brantunitedway
Overview: A small local charitable organization founded in 1953 overseen by United Way of Canada - Centraide Canada
Mission: To help people in their time of need
Chief Officer(s):
Sherry Haines, Executive Director

Burn Survivors Association
c/o Camp BUCKO, #15549, 265 Port Union Rd., Toronto ON M1C 4Z7
Tel: 647-343-2267
Toll-Free: 877-272-8256
www.campbucko.ca
twitter.com/camp_bucko
Also Known As: Camp BUCKO
Overview: A small local charitable organization founded in 1979
Mission: To provide support & information for burn survivors & their families; To offer a safe & caring camp program for children, from ages 7 to 17, with burn injuries
Publications:
• Survivor [a publication of the Burn Survivors Association]
Type: Newsletter
Profile: Information & reviews of Camp BUCKO experiences

Caledon Community Services (CCS)
Royal Cortyards, Upper Level, 18 King St. East, Bolton ON L7E 1E8
Tel: 905-584-2300; *Fax:* 905-951-2303
e-mail: info@ccs4u.org
www.ccs4u.org
www.facebook.com/pages/Caledon-Community-Services/17402156736
0
twitter.com/CaledonCS
www.youtube.com/user/CaledonCServices
Overview: A small local charitable organization founded in 1971 overseen by InformOntario

Mission: CCS is a health & social service organization with volunteer-delivered programs to provide the Caledon community with support in times of difficulty & change.
Member of: Ontario Community Support Association; Association of Community Information Centres in Ontario
Affiliation(s): Social Planning Council of Peel; Volunteer Centre of Peel
Chief Officer(s):
Monty Laskin, Chief Executive Officer

Carizon Family & Community Services
400 Queen St. South, Kitchener ON N2G 1W7
Tel: 519-743-6333; *Fax:* 519-743-3496
e-mail: info@carizon.ca
www.carizon.ca
www.linkedin.com/company/carizon-family-and-community-services
www.facebook.com/carizonupdates
twitter.com/@carizon
Previous Name: kidsLINK; Mosaic Counselling & Family Services; Catholic Family Counselling Centre; Catholic Social Services; Catholic Welfare Bureau
Overview: A small local charitable organization founded in 1952 overseen by Ontario Association of Credit Counselling Services
Mission: To provide full-service professional counselling services in Kitchener & the surrounding region
Member of: Canadian Association of Credit Counselling Services; Ontario Association of Credit Counselling Services; United Way of Kitchener-Waterloo & Area; Family Service Ontario
Chief Officer(s):
Stephen Swatridge, CEO
Lesley Barraball, Director, Children's Mental Health Services
Jennifer Berry, Director, Communications
Ted Conlin, Director, Business
Jean Davies, Director, Pathways to Education
Debbie Engel, Director, Community Services
Dale Gellatly, Director, Community Engagement

St. Agatha Office
PO Box 190, 1855 Notre Dame Dr., St Agatha ON N0B 2L0
Tel: 519-746-5437

Catholic Family Service of Ottawa (CFS Ottawa) / Service familial catholique d'Ottawa (SFC Ottawa)
310 Olmstead St., Ottawa ON K1L 7K3
Tel: 613-233-8478; *Fax:* 613-233-9881
e-mail: info@cfsottawa.ca
www.cfsottawa.ca
Previous Name: Catholic Family Service of Ottawa-Carleton
Overview: A small local charitable organization founded in 1940 overseen by Family Service Ontario
Mission: CFS Ottawa offers a range of social services in English & French to all residents of the Ottawa-Carleton area. Services include counselling, support to the victims or witnesses of family violence or sexual abuse, advocacy, community development. It is a registered charity, BN: 118841105RR0001.
Member of: Family Service Canada
Chief Officer(s):
Isabelle Massip, President
Franca DiDiomete, Executive Director

Catholic Family Services of Hamilton (CFS)
#201, 447 Main St. East, Hamilton ON L8N 1K1
Tel: 905-527-3823; *Fax:* 905-546-5779
Toll-Free: 877-527-3823
e-mail: intake@cfshw.com
www.cfshw.com
www.linkedin.com/company/catholic-family-services-of-hamilton
www.facebook.com/Catholic.Family.Services.Hamilton
twitter.com/CFSHW
www.youtube.com/channel/UCeLsGYd3vHt5PGRkS8JJFjA
Previous Name: Catholic Family Services of Hamilton-Wentworth
Overview: A small local organization founded in 1944 overseen by Ontario Association of Credit Counselling Services
Mission: To provide individual, marriage, family, & credit counselling services in the Hamilton & Burlington communities
Member of: Ontario Association of Credit Counselling Service
Affliation(s): Ontario Community Support Association; ONTCHILD; Family Services Ontario; Canadian Association for Community Care; Continuing Gerontological Education Cooperative; Older Persons' Mental Health & Addictions Network; Ontario Association on

Developmental Disabilities; Ontario Case Managers Association; Ontario Gerontology Association; Ontario Partnership on Aging Development Disabilities
Chief Officer(s):
Linda Dayler, Executive Director & Secretary
Paula Forbes, Associate Director

Catholic Family Services of Peel Dufferin (CFSPD)
Emerald Centre, #400, 10 Kingsbridge Garden Circle, Mississauga ON L5R 3K6
Tel: 905-450-1608; *Fax:* 905-897-2467
Other Communication: Services en Français 905-450-1608 ext 169
e-mail: info@cfspd.com
www.cfspd.com
www.facebook.com/208938825992
Previous Name: Peel Dufferin Catholic Services
Overview: A small local charitable organization founded in 1981 overseen by Family Service Ontario
Mission: CFSPD is a multi-service counselling agency that supports families coping with difficulties, notably violence, trauma & abuse. Services are available in many languages to help people deal with such problems as depression, anxiety, grief, marital difficulties, parent-child conflict, developmental transitions & cutural adjustments. Offices in Mississauga & Brampton have walk-in clinics. The Society is a registered charity, BN: 119087823RR0001.
Member of: Catholic Charities; Archdiocese of Toronto; United Way of Peel Region
Chief Officer(s):
Ana Hill, Manager, Operations, 905-450-1608 Ext. 404
anahill@cfspd.com

Brampton Branch
#201, 60 West Dr., Brampton ON L6T 3T6
Tel: 905-450-1608; *Fax:* 905-450-8902

Caledon Branch
#D8, 18 King St. East, Bolton ON L7E 1E8
Tel: 905-450-1608; *Fax:* 905-450-8902

Orangeville Branch
Dufferin Child & Family Services, 655 Riddell Rd., Orangeville ON L9W 4Z5
Toll-Free: 888-940-0584

Catholic Family Services of Simcoe County (CFSSC)
20 Anne St. S, Barrie ON L4N 2C6
Tel: 705-726-2503; *Fax:* 705-726-2570
e-mail: info@cfssc.ca
www.cfssc.ca
www.facebook.com/CFSSC
twitter.com/CounselorSimcoe
Previous Name: Catholic Family Life Centre-Simcoe South; North Simcoe Catholic Family Life Centre
Overview: A small local charitable organization founded in 1979 overseen by Family Service Ontario
Mission: To offer professional social services to all residents of Simcoe South; services will be directed to the treatment of troubled families & individuals, as well as to strengthening & enriching family life & individual functioning in all their dimensions & contexts
Chief Officer(s):
Michelle Bergin, Executive Director
mbergin@cfssc.ca

Catholic Family Services of Toronto (CFS Toronto) / Services familiaux catholiques de Toronto
Catholic Pastoral Centre, #200, 1155 Yonge St., Toronto ON M4T 1W2
Tel: 416-921-1163; *Fax:* 416-921-1579
e-mail: info@cfstoronto.com
www.cfstoronto.com
Previous Name: Catholic Welfare Bureau
Overview: A medium-sized local charitable organization founded in 1922
Mission: To help individuals & families develop their potential by providing wellness programs & treatment services
Member of: Catholic Charities of the Archdiocese of Toronto
Affliation(s): Family Service Canada; Family Service Ontario
Chief Officer(s):
Ivana Zanardo, President
Denis Costello, Executive Director & Secretary

North Toronto Office
#300, 5799 Yonge St., Toronto ON M2M 3V3
Tel: 416-222-0048; *Fax:* 416-222-3321

Centre for Independent Living in Toronto (CILT)
#902, 365 Bloor St. East, Toronto ON M4W 3L4
Tel: 416-599-2458; *Fax:* 416-599-3555; *TTY:* 416-599-5077
e-mail: cilt@cilt.ca
www.cilt.ca

Overview: A small local charitable organization
Mission: To help people with disabilities learn independent living skills & integrate into the community
Member of: Canadian Association of Independent Living Centers (CAILC); United Way of Greater Toronto
Chief Officer(s):
Meenu Sikand, President

Centre francophone de Toronto (CFT)
#303, 555, rue Richmond ouest, Toronto ON M5V 3B1
Tél: 416-922-2672; *Téléc:* 416-203-1165
Courriel: infos@centrefranco.org
www.centrefranco.org
www.facebook.com/Centre.francophone.de.Toronto
twitter.com/CentrefrancoT
www.youtube.com/channel/UCK-ySdR14i29fBcm-xBVFYw

Nom précédent: Conseil des organismes francophones du Toronto Métropolitain; Centre francophones du Toronto Métropolitain
Aperçu: *Dimension:* moyenne; *Envergure:* locale; Organisme sans but lucratif; fondée en 1977
Mission: Permettre à la population francophone du grand Toronto d'avoir accès à des services d'information, d'orientation et d'encadrement susceptibles de promouvoir la dimension humaine, culturelle et communautaire des multiples visages de la francophonie
Affiliation(s): Assemblée des centres culturels de l'Ontario; Centraide
Membre(s) du bureau directeur:
Lise Marie Baudry, Directrice générale

The Change Foundation
PO Box 42, #2501, 200 Front St. West, Toronto ON M5V 3M1
Tel: 416-205-1353; *Fax:* 416-205-1440
e-mail: asunnak@changefoundation.com
www.changefoundation.ca
www.linkedin.com/company/the-change-foundation
twitter.com/TheChangeFdn
www.youtube.com/user/thechangefoundation

Overview: A large local organization founded in 1996
Mission: To promote, support & improve health & health care delivery through four activity areas: applied research, grants for Change Initiatives, & knowledge transfer through development & education programs
Chief Officer(s):
Cathy Fooks, President & CEO
cfooks@changefoundation.com
Christa Haanstra, Executive Lead, Strategic Communications

Chinese Family Services of Ontario
#229, 3330 Midland Ave., Toronto ON M1V 5E7
Tel: 416-979-8299; *Fax:* 416-979-2743
Toll-Free: 866-979-8298; *TTY:* 416-979-5898
e-mail: info@chinesefamilyso.com
www.chinesefamilyso.com

Previous Name: Chinese Family Life Services Project
Overview: A small local charitable organization founded in 1988 overseen by Ontario Council of Agencies Serving Immigrants
Mission: To offer service that help Chinese immigrants settle in Canada
Chief Officer(s):
Patrick Au, Executive Director

Community Action Resource Centre (CARC)
1652 Keele St., Toronto ON M6M 3W3
Tel: 416-652-2273; *Fax:* 416-652-8992
www.communityarc.ca
www.facebook.com/CommunityActionResourceCentre
twitter.com/communityarc

Merged from: Community Information Centre for the City of York & Connect Information Post
Overview: A small local charitable organization founded in 2004 overseen by InformOntario

Mission: Mobilizing resources and providing supportive social services for the empowerment of individuals and groups.

Community Connection (CDIC)
PO Box 683, 275 - 1st St., Collingwood ON L9Y 4E8
Tel: 705-444-0040; *Fax:* 705-445-1516
e-mail: info@communityconnection.ca
www.communityconnection.ca

Also Known As: Collingwood & District Information Centre
Overview: A medium-sized local charitable organization founded in 1969 overseen by InformOntario
Mission: To offer free & confidential information & referral services to anyone needing help
Member of: InformCanada; Alliance of Information & Referral Systems; Volunteer Canada; InformOntario; Community Information Online Consortium; Child Youth and Family Services Coalition of Simcoe County
Affliation(s): United Way

Community Information Fairview (CIF)
PO Box 210, 1800 Sheppard Ave. East, Toronto ON M2J 5A7
Tel: 416-493-0752; *Fax:* 416-493-0823
e-mail: communityinfofairview@rogers.com

Overview: A small local organization founded in 1971
Mission: To provide accessible space within Fairview Mall to better serve the community; To assure equality of access to CIF services to the best of our abilities; To provide full access to people with physical & mental impairments; to improve & build partnerships with other community organizations & the private sector; To assist community development activities; To assist other community organizations to attain their goals; To promote the development of a Community Resource Centre
Member of: Federation of Community Information Centres of Toronto; Inform Canada

Community Living Elgin (CLE)
400 Talbot St., St Thomas ON N5P 1B8
Tel: 519-631-9222; *Fax:* 519-633-4392
e-mail: info@communitylivingelgin.com
www.communitylivingelgin.com

Previous Name: Elgin Association for Community Living
Overview: A small local charitable organization founded in 1958
Mission: To provide support & services, primarily to people with developmental disabilities & their families to enable them to participate at full potential within the community
Member of: Community Living Ontario
Chief Officer(s):
Bob Ashcroft, President
Michelle Palmer, Interim Executive Director
m.palmer@communitylivingelgin.com

Community Resource Centre (Killaloe) Inc. (CRC)
PO Box 59, Killaloe ON K0J 2A0
Tel: 613-757-3108; *Fax:* 613-757-0208
Toll-Free: 888-757-3108
e-mail: director@crc-renfrewcounty.com
www.crc-renfrewcounty.com

Also Known As: The Resource Centre
Overview: A small local charitable organization founded in 1987 overseen by InformOntario
Mission: To improve the quality of life in the community by supporting and encouraging improved family life, cooperation, right livelihood and social development.
Member of: Ontario Association of Family Resource Programs; FRP Canada
Affliation(s): Ontario Community Action Program for Children; Canada Prenatal Nutrition Coation

Counselling & Support Services of S.D. & G. / Centre de counselling familial de Cornwall et Comtés unis
26 Montreal Rd., Cornwall ON K6H 1B1
Tel: 613-932-4610; *Fax:* 613-932-5765
e-mail: admin@css-sdg.ca
www.css-sdg.ca

Previous Name: Family Counselling Centre of Cornwall & United Counties
Overview: A small local organization founded in 1938 overseen by Ontario Association of Credit Counselling Services

Mission: To offer professional credit & family counselling as well as support services to persons in Cornwall & the United Counties; To support adults with a developmental disability to live within the community & to achieve their potential
Member of: United Way; Family Service Ontario
Chief Officer(s):
Raymond Houde, Executive Director

Counselling Services of Belleville & District (CSBD)
12 Moira St. East, Belleville ON K8P 2R9
                                   Tel: 613-966-7413; *Fax:* 613-966-2357
                                   e-mail: csbd@csbd.on.ca
                                   www.csbd.on.ca
Overview: A small local charitable organization founded in 1978 overseen by Family Service Ontario
Mission: To offer behavioural assessment & counselling, advocacy & support to families & individuals.
Affiliation(s): YMCA, for summer camps

Covenant House Toronto
20 Gerrard St. East, Toronto ON M5B 2P3
                                   Tel: 416-598-4898; *Fax:* 416-204-7030
                                   Toll-Free: 800-435-7308
                                   www.covenanthouse.on.ca
                                   www.linkedin.com/company/covenant-house-toronto
                                   www.facebook.com/covenanthousetoronto
                                   twitter.com/covenanthouseto
                                   www.youtube.com/user/covenanthousetoronto
Overview: A large local charitable organization founded in 1982
Mission: To provide a crisis shelter for homeless & runaway youth, who are 16 to 21 years of age; to offer assessment, counselling, & referral services
Affiliation(s): Covenant House International
Chief Officer(s):
Duncan Hannay, Chair
Bruce Rivers, Executive Director
Rose Cino, Contact, Communications
  cino@covenanthouse.on.ca
Publications:
• Good Samaritan News [a publication of Covenant House Toronto]
Type: Newsletter

Disability Awareness Consultants (DAC)
146 Haslam St., Toronto ON M1N 3N7
                                   Tel: 416-267-5939
                                   disabilityawarenessconsultants.com
Previous Name: Handidactis
Overview: A small local organization founded in 2006
Mission: To offer training & awareness programs to company employees so they can work comfortably with clients & coworkers who have disabilities; To help companies comply with the Accessibility for Ontarians with Disabilities Act; To conduct site audits in order to build barrier-free environments
Chief Officer(s):
Lauri Sue Robertson, President & Owner
  laurisue@bell.net
William F. Robertson, Vice-President, Operations

Distress Centres of Toronto
PO Box 243, Stn. Adelaide, Toronto ON M5C 2J4
  Tel: 416-598-0166; *TTY:* 416-408-0007; *Crisis Hot-Line:* 416-408-4357
                                   e-mail: info@torontodistresscentre.com
                                   www.torontodistresscentre.com
                                   www.facebook.com/1536691786591642
                                   twitter.com/DC_TO
Overview: A small local organization founded in 1967
Mission: To assist emotionally distressed individuals deal with those issues they are currently unable to manage
Affiliation(s): Ontario Association of Distress Centres
Chief Officer(s):
Karen Letofsky, Executive Director, 416-598-0168
  karen@torontodistresscentre.com

East Wellington Community Services (EWCS)
PO Box 786, 45 Main St., Erin ON N0B 1T0
                                   Tel: 519-833-9696; *Fax:* 519-833-7563
                                   www.eastwellingtoncommunityservices.com
                                   www.facebook.com/east.wellington
Previous Name: East Wellington Advisory Group for Family Services

Overview: A small local charitable organization founded in 1984
Mission: To provide essential services to the community in order to support families, individuals, children, & seniors
Member of: Inform Ontario; Community Support Association
Chief Officer(s):
Rebeca Greco, President
Kari Simpson, Chief Executive Officer
  kari.s@ew-cs.com

Eli Bay Relaxation Response Institute
226 Wychwood Ave., Toronto ON M6C 2T3
                                   Tel: 416-932-2784
                Other Communication: Presentation & Workshop e-mail:
                                   info@kmprod.com
                                   www.elibay.com
Also Known As: The Relaxation Response Ltd.
Overview: A small local organization founded in 1978
Mission: To empower individuals & organizations with mind-body skills proven to effectively release stress anywhere & anytime
Chief Officer(s):
Eli Bay, Founder

Employees' Union of St. Mary's of the Lake Hospital - CNFIU Local 3001 / Association des employés, l'Hôpital Saint Mary's of the Lake (FCNSI)
340 Union St., Kingston ON K7L 5A2
                                   Tel: 613-544-5220; *Fax:* 613-544-8527
Overview: A small local organization

Essex Community Services (ECS)
#7, 35 Victoria Ave., Essex ON N8M 1M4
                                   Tel: 519-776-4231; *Fax:* 519-776-4966
                                   e-mail: ecs@essexcs.on.ca
                                   www.essexcs.on.ca
Previous Name: Community Information - Essex
Overview: A small local charitable organization founded in 1975 overseen by InformOntario
Mission: The organization provides a number of services to members of the community, including door-to-door transporation assistance for seniors, coat collection for children, income tax clinic, job bank, community resource library.
Affiliation(s): Inform Canada
Chief Officer(s):
Kelly Stack, Executive Director
  director@essexcs.on.ca

Family & Children's Services of Lanark, Leeds & Grenville
438 Laurier Blvd., Brockville ON K6V 6C5
                                   Tel: 613-498-2100; *Fax:* 613-498-2108
                                   Toll-Free: 800-481-7834
                                   www.casbrock.com
Merged from: Children's Aid Society of Lanark & Smiths Falls; Family & Children's Services of Leeds & Grenville
Overview: A small local organization overseen by Family Service Ontario
Mission: To protect children & ensure the safety of those in need; to provide care for those children under concern, as well as guidance & counselling to families to prevent circumstances requiring the protection of children.

  Gananoque Office
  #300, 375 William St., Gananoque ON K7G 1T2
                                   Tel: 613-382-8220; *Fax:* 613-382-3579

  Kemptville Office
  PO Box 1299, 5 Clothier St. East, Kemptville ON K0G 1J0
                                   Tel: 613-258-1460; *Fax:* 613-258-4459

Family Counselling & Support Services for Guelph-Wellington (FCSS)
109 Surrey St. East, Guelph ON N1H 3P7
                                   Tel: 519-824-2431
                                   Toll-Free: 800-307-7078
                                   e-mail: info@familyserviceguelph.on.ca
                                   www.familyserviceguelph.on.ca
Previous Name: Guelph-Wellington Counselling Centre
Overview: A small local charitable organization founded in 1987 overseen by Ontario Association of Credit Counselling Services
Mission: To provide professional counselling, support, educational, & advocacy services for the citizens of the Guelph-Wellington region

Member of: Credit Counselling Canada; Ontario Association of Credit Counselling Services
Affiliation(s): Family Service Ontario; Family Service Canada
Publications:
• Family Counselling & Support Services for Guelph-Wellington Annual Report
Type: Yearbook; *Frequency:* Annually

Family Day Care Services (Toronto)
#400, 155 Gordon Baker Rd., Toronto ON M2H 3N5
Tel: 416-922-9556; *Fax:* 416-922-5335
www.familydaycare.com
twitter.com/familydaygta
Previous Name: Protestant Children's Home
Overview: A large local charitable organization founded in 1851 overseen by Family Service Ontario
Mission: To meet the needs of children & families; To aid in optimum development of the child, be it physical care, social, emotional or cognitive development; To assist & support the family unit to function more effectively economically, socially & emotionally
Member of: Home Child Care Association of Ontario
Chief Officer(s):
S. Gopikrishna, President
Joan Arruda, CEO

Family Service Centre of Ottawa-Carleton / Centre de service familial d'Ottawa-Carleton
312 Parkdale Ave., Ottawa ON K1Y 4X5
Tel: 613-725-3601; *Fax:* 613-725-5651; *TTY:* 613-725-6175
e-mail: fsfo@familyservicesottawa.org
www.familyservicesottawa.org
www.facebook.com/familyservicesottawa
Overview: A medium-sized local organization founded in 1914 overseen by Family Service Ontario
Mission: To strengthen all aspects of family & community living through the provision of family focused, professional social services in the areas of counselling, family life education, social planning & advocacy
Affiliation(s): Family Service Canada
Chief Officer(s):
Kathryn Ann Hill, Executive Director

Family Service Thames Valley (FSTV)
125 Woodward Ave., London ON N6J 2H1
Tel: 519-433-0159
e-mail: fstv@familyservicethamesvalley.com
www.familyservicethamesvalley.com
Previous Name: Credit Counselling Thames Valley; Family Service London
Overview: A small local organization founded in 1967 overseen by Ontario Association of Credit Counselling Services
Mission: To provide counselling & support services for individuals, families, & organizations in London & its surrounding communities; To promote wise money management by consumers
Chief Officer(s):
Louise Pitre, Executive Director

Family Service Toronto (FST)
#202, 128A Sterling Rd., Toronto ON M6R 2B7
Tel: 416-595-9618
www.familyservicetoronto.org
www.linkedin.com/company/family-service-toronto
www.facebook.com/FamilyServiceToronto
twitter.com/FamilyServiceTO
www.youtube.com/user/FamilyServiceToronto
Previous Name: Family Service Association of Toronto
Overview: A small local charitable organization founded in 1914
Mission: To help individuals & families affected by socio-economic circumstances or mental health issues
Member of: Family Service Ontario; United Way
Affiliation(s): Family Service Canada
Chief Officer(s):
Ted Betts, President
Margaret Hancock, Executive Director

Family Services Windsor-Essex Counselling & Advocacy Centre
1770 Langlois Ave., Windsor ON N8X 4M5
Tel: 519-966-5010; *Fax:* 519-256-5258
Toll-Free: 888-933-1831
e-mail: info@fswe.ca
www.familyserviceswe.ca
Previous Name: Windsor Catholic Family Service Bureau
Overview: A small local charitable organization
Mission: To strengthen the ability of individuals, families & communities to reach their potential

Family Services York Region (Georgina)
PO Box 8, 25202 Warden Ave., Sutton West ON L0E 1R0
Tel: 905-476-3611; *Fax:* 905-476-6601
Previous Name: Georgina Family Life Centre
Overview: A small local charitable organization founded in 1972 overseen by Family Service Ontario
Mission: To counsel families & individuals through times of stress; to enrich the quality of life in individuals, marriage & family relationships; to help family members develop life skills which will enable them to live fuller & happier lives; to provide grief counselling
Member of: United Way

Findhelp Information Services
PO Box 203, #125, 543 Richmond St. West, Toronto ON M5V 1Y6
Tel: 416-392-4605; *Fax:* 416-392-4404
Toll-Free: 800-836-3238; *TTY:* 888-340-1001
e-mail: info@findhelp.ca
www.211toronto.ca
www.facebook.com/pages/211-Central/137803876305769
twitter.com/211Central
Also Known As: 211 Toronto
Overview: A small local charitable organization founded in 1952 overseen by InformOntario
Mission: To provide comprehensive information & referral services in English, French & other languages; resources for information & referral professionals; call centre; newcomer services; Possibilities online employment resource centre; training & outreach
Member of: Alliance of Information & Referral Systems
Affiliation(s): United Way of Greater Toronto

Flamborough Information & Community Services (FICS)
857 Millgrove Side Rd., Waterdown ON L0R 2H0
Tel: 905-689-7880
e-mail: fics@infoflam.on.ca
www.infoflam.on.ca
www.facebook.com/FlamboroughInformationAndCommunityServices
Overview: A small local charitable organization founded in 1977 overseen by InformOntario
Mission: To empower residents through information & referral services; to enhance quality of life by identifying unmet needs, liaising with the community & facilitating social services
Member of: Inform Hamilton
Chief Officer(s):
Shelley Scott, Executive Director

Foodshare Toronto
90 Croatia St., Toronto ON M6H 1K9
Tel: 416-363-6441; *Fax:* 416-363-0474
e-mail: info@foodshare.net
www.foodshare.net
www.facebook.com/FoodShareTO
twitter.com/FoodShareTO
www.youtube.com/user/FoodShareTO
Previous Name: Foodshare (Metro) Toronto
Overview: A medium-sized local charitable organization founded in 1985
Mission: Working with communities to improve access to affordable & healthy food, from field to table
Chief Officer(s):
Debbie Field, Executive Director
debbie@foodshare.net

Guelph-Wellington Women in Crisis
PO Box 1451, Guelph ON N1H 6N9
Tel: 519-836-1110; *Fax:* 519-836-1979; *Crisis Hot-Line:* 519-836-5710
e-mail: feedback@gwwomenincrisis.org
www.gwwomenincrisis.org
www.facebook.com/pages/Guelph-Wellington-Women-in-Crisis/476967
22728
twitter.com/gwwic
www.youtube.com/user/gwwic
Previous Name: Sexual Assault Centre of Guelph
Overview: A small local organization founded in 1979
Mission: To end violence against women & children in all its forms
Member of: Ontario Association of Interval & Transition Houses;
Ontario Coalition of Rape Crisis Center

Haldimand-Norfolk Information Centre (HNIC)
643 Park Rd. North, Brantford ON N3T 5L8
Tel: 519-758-8228
haldimand.cioc.ca
Overview: A small local charitable organization founded in 1974
overseen by InformOntario
Mission: To provide human service information to community
Member of: On-Line Ontario

Halton Family Services (HFS)
235 Lakeshore Rd. East, Oakville ON L6J 7R4
Tel: 905-845-3811; *Fax:* 905-845-3537
e-mail: info@haltonfamilyservices.org
www.haltonfamilyservices.org
Overview: A small local charitable organization founded in 1954
overseen by Ontario Association of Credit Counselling Services
Mission: To assist individuals, couples, & families in Oakville & the
Halton region cope with challenges, by providing a professional
counselling service; To operate the Halton-Peel Consumer Credit
Counselling Service, to help persons find solutions to their financial
problems
Member of: Ontario Association of Credit Counselling Services
Publications:
• Halton Family Services Annual Report
Type: Yearbook; *Frequency:* Annually

Hamilton Niagara Haldimand Brant Community Care Access Centre (HNHB CCAC)
#4, 195 Henry St., Bldg. 4, Brantford ON N3S 5C9
Tel: 519-759-7752
Toll-Free: 800-810-0000
healthcareathome.ca
Overview: A small local organization
Mission: To provide access to community health care services
Chief Officer(s):
Melody Miles, CEO

Hatzoloh Toronto
#219, 534 Lawrence Ave. West, Toronto ON M6A 1A2
Tel: 416-398-2300
e-mail: office@hatzolohtoronto.org
www.hatzolohtoronto.ca
Overview: A small local organization
Mission: To offer emergency medical services to Toronto's Jewish
community
Chief Officer(s):
Yisroel Dovid Goldstein, Executive Director

Hospice Niagara
#2, 403 Ontario St., St Catharines ON L2N 1L5
Tel: 905-984-8766; *Fax:* 905-984-8242
e-mail: info@hospiceniagara.ca
www.hospiceniagara.ca
www.facebook.com/pages/Hospice-Niagara/157424072710
twitter.com/HospiceNiagara
Overview: A small local charitable organization founded in 1993
Mission: To improve the quality of life for individuals with a life-limiting,
progressive illness
Member of: Hospice Palliative Care Ontario
Chief Officer(s):
Carol Nagy, Executive Director, 905-984-8766 Ext. 225
cnagy@hospiceniagara.ca

Info Northumberland
#700, 600 William St., Cobourg ON K9A 5J4
Tel: 905-372-8913; *Fax:* 905-372-4417
Toll-Free: 800-396-6626
e-mail: Northumberland@fourinfo.com
www.fourinfo.com
twitter.com/fourinfo2
Also Known As: SHARE INFO Community Information Centre Inc.
Previous Name: Cobourg Community Information Centre Inc.
Overview: A small local charitable organization founded in 1979
overseen by InformOntario
Mission: To aid all citizens of Northumberland County giving them,
upon request, information &/or referring them to the proper organization
or service; To assess trends which meet needs of the community by
careful evaluation of demands made by citizens
Member of: Community Information Online Consortium

Information Barrie
Barrie Public Library, 60 Worsley St., Barrie ON L4M 1L6
Tel: 705-728-1010; *Fax:* 705-728-4322
e-mail: infobarrie@barrie.ca
library.barrie.ca/about/information-barrie
Overview: A small local organization founded in 1977 overseen by
InformOntario
Mission: To provide community information & referral; To work with
other community agencies
Member of: Inform Canada; InformOntario
Affiliation(s): Information Providers Coalition (Simcoe County); 211
Simcoe County; Community Connection (Collingwood & Dist.);
Information Orillia; Contact (Alliston)
Chief Officer(s):
Cathy Bodle, Coordinator

Information Brock
PO Box 131, 30 Allan St., Cannington ON L0E 1E0
Tel: 705-432-2636
Previous Name: Brock Information Centre
Overview: A small local organization founded in 1963 overseen by
InformOntario
Mission: Free & confidential information & referral service; on-site thrift
shop
Member of: InformOntario

Information Burlington
c/o Burlington Public Library, 2331 New St., 2nd Floor, Burlington ON L7R 1J4
Tel: 905-639-3611; *Fax:* 905-681-7277
e-mail: infoburlington@bpl.on.ca
www.bpl.on.ca/resources/community-info
Overview: A small local organization founded in 1971 overseen by
InformOntario
Mission: To offer a free, confidential information service to the citizens
of Burlington; To connect people with the community & government
services they need; To ensure that the public is aware of the
programmes & services offered in the community
Member of: InformOntario
Affiliation(s): Halton Information Providers
Chief Officer(s):
Glynis Maxwell, Coordinator

Information by Markham
101 Town Centre Blvd., Markham ON L3R 9W3
Tel: 905-415-7500
e-mail: imarkham@markham.ca
www.informationmarkham.ca
www.facebook.com/InformationMarkham
Overview: A small local organization founded in 1972 overseen by
InformOntario
Mission: To deliver quality information services to our clients; To
enhance community life & promote Markham & York Region
Affiliation(s): Community Information & Volunteer Centre - York Region
Chief Officer(s):
Dianne Murray, Executive Director

Information Niagara
#10, 235 Martindale Rd., St Catharines ON L2W 1A5
Tel: 905-682-6611; *Fax:* 905-682-4314
Toll-Free: 800-263-3695
e-mail: info@incommunities.ca
www.informationniagara.com
www.facebook.com/InformationNiagara
twitter.com/211CentralSouth

Also Known As: 211 Central South
Overview: A small local charitable organization founded in 1974 overseen by InformOntario
Mission: The organization offers community information & referral services, including an online searchable information database & another database of volunteers. It also maintains an interpretation service for a wide range of languages.
Member of: United Way
Chief Officer(s):
Terri Bruce, Information Services Manager, 905-682-1900 Ext. 221
terri@informationniagara.com

Information Orillia
c/o Orillia Public Library, 33 Mississauga St. West, Orillia ON L3V 3A6
Tel: 705-326-7743
e-mail: info@informationorillia.org
www.informationorillia.org
www.facebook.com/Info.Orillia
twitter.com/InfoOrillia

Overview: A small local organization founded in 1969 overseen by InformOntario
Mission: To bring people & services together in Orillia & surrounding townships by information & referral
Member of: InformCanada; InformOntario
Afliation(s): Coalition of Information Providers of Simcoe County
Chief Officer(s):
Shannon O'Donnell, Executive Director

Information Sarnia Lambton (ISL)
PO Box 354, Sarnia ON N7T 7J2
Tel: 519-542-1949
www.informationsarnialambton.org
www.facebook.com/pages/Information-Sarnia-Lambton/167455956644103

Overview: A small local organization founded in 1960 overseen by InformOntario
Mission: To maintain a database of social & human service organizations in Lambton County

Information Tilbury & Help Centre
PO Box 309, 20 Queen St. North, Tilbury ON N0P 2L0
Tel: 519-682-2268; *Fax:* 519-682-3771
Overview: A small local charitable organization founded in 1982 overseen by InformOntario
Mission: To act as a "middle person" connecting people with services or volunteers who can help & to become involved with the community when & where needed; to provide the community with mediation information & referrals to community services by accessing individual & community needs by formulating programs services & resources in cooperation with existing organizations
Chief Officer(s):
Karen Kirkwood-Whyte, Executive Director
karen@uwock.ca

Lakehead Social Planning Council (LSPC)
Victoria Mall, #28, 125 Syndicate Ave. South, Thunder Bay ON P7E 6H8
Tel: 807-624-1720; *Fax:* 807-625-9427
Toll-Free: 866-624-1729; *TTY:* 888-622-4651
e-mail: info@lspc.ca
lspc-circ.on.ca
Overview: A small local charitable organization founded in 1963
Mission: To strengthen Thunder Bay by providing collaborative community responses to social issues, research & access to human service information; to bring people together, promote social & economic justice, develop programs & services, link people to services; to research social, economic, environmental & health issues
Member of: Inform Ontario; Ontario Social Development Council; Canadian Council on Social Development

Chief Officer(s):
Marie Klassen, Director, Services

Lakeshore Community Services (LCS)
PO Box 885, 499 Notre Dame St., Belle River ON N0R 1A0
Tel: 519-728-1435; *Fax:* 519-728-4713
Toll-Free: 855-728-1433
www.lakeshorecommunity.net
www.facebook.com/542559895805728
twitter.com/CscEssexCounty
Previous Name: Community Information Centre Belle River
Overview: A small local organization overseen by InformOntario
Mission: The Mission of LCS is to service the Community of Lakeshore responsibly by providing information about and access to health, government, and community and support services and through this research social needs.
Chief Officer(s):
Tracey Bailey, Executive Director

LAMP Community Health Centre
185 - 5th St., Toronto ON M8V 2Z5
Tel: 416-252-6471; *Fax:* 416-252-4474
e-mail: volunteering@lampchc.org
www.lampchc.org
www.facebook.com/pages/LAMP-Community-Health-Centre/273206986162658
twitter.com/LAMPCHC_info
www.pinterest.com/lampchc
Also Known As: Lakeshore Area Multi-Services Project Inc.
Overview: A large local charitable organization founded in 1976
Mission: To meet the community's health needs through integrated programs & services
Chief Officer(s):
Barbara Pidcock, Chair
Russ Ford, Executive Director
Publications:
• LAMP Community Health Centre Newsletter
Type: Newsletter

Neighbourhood Centre
c/o Secord Community Centre, 91 Barrington Ave., Toronto ON M4C 4Y9
Tel: 416-698-1626
e-mail: info@neighbourhoodcentre.org
neighbourhoodcentre.org
Overview: A small local organization overseen by InformOntario
Mission: The Neighbourhood Centre is a community place for inquiry and dialogue as well as the Taylor-Massey's community information and referral centre.
Chief Officer(s):
Claire Barcik, Executive Director
ed@neighbourhoodcentre.org

Nellie's Shelter
PO Box 98118, 970 Queen St. East, Toronto ON M4M 1J8
Tel: 416-461-8903; *Fax:* 416-461-0970; *Crisis Hot-Line:* 416-461-1084
e-mail: community@nellies.org
www.nellies.org
www.facebook.com/nelliesshelter
twitter.com/nelliesshelter
www.youtube.com/nelliesshelter
Overview: A small local charitable organization founded in 1974
Mission: To advocate for social justice for all women & children
Chief Officer(s):
Margarita Mendez, Executive Director, 416-461-9849, Fax: 416-461-0970

North Renfrew Family Services Inc. (NRFS)
PO Box 1334, 109 Banting Dr., Deep River ON K0J 1P0
Tel: 613-584-3358; *Fax:* 613-584-5520
e-mail: nrfs@drdh.org
bright-ideas-software.com/NRFS
Overview: A small local charitable organization founded in 1968 overseen by Family Service Ontario
Mission: To provide referral & counselling services for individuals & families in North Renfrew
Member of: Renfrew County United Way
Afliation(s): Family Service Ontario
Chief Officer(s):

Kelly Hawley, Executive Director

Northumberland United Way
#700, 600 William St., Cobourg ON K9A 3A5

Tel: 905-372-6955; *Fax:* 905-372-4417
Toll-Free: 800-833-0002
e-mail: office@nuw.unitedway.ca
www.mynuw.org
www.facebook.com/northumberlandunitedway
twitter.com/nlanduw
www.youtube.com/user/NlandUnitedWay

Overview: A small local organization founded in 1969 overseen by United Way of Canada - Centraide Canada
Mission: To raise & allocate funds in an efficient manner & to promote the effective delivery of services in response to current & emerging social needs in Northumberland County
Chief Officer(s):
Lynda Kay, CEO
lkay@nuw.unitedway.ca

Northwood Neighbourhood Services
#400, 1860 Wilson Ave., Toronto ON M9M 3A7

Tel: 416-748-0788; *Fax:* 416-748-0525
e-mail: info@northw.ca
www.northw.ca

Overview: A small local charitable organization founded in 1982 overseen by Ontario Council of Agencies Serving Immigrants
Mission: To provide programs & services within the community that will empower individuals, families & groups to achieve, maintain & enhance a state of physical, mental & social well being
Chief Officer(s):
François Yabit, Executive Director
fyabit@northw.ca
Azaria Wolday, Manager, Settlement & Sponsorship
awolday@northw.ca

The Olde Forge Community Resource Centre (OFCRC) / Centre de ressources communautaires Olde Forge
2730 Carling Ave., Ottawa ON K2B 7J1

Tel: 613-829-9777
oldeforge.ca

Overview: A small local charitable organization founded in 1970
Mission: To provide an information & referral service; To operate a support service to enable senior citizens to remain in their own homes as long as possible
Member of: Ontario Community Support Association
Chief Officer(s):
Anita Bloom, Executive Director, 613-829-9777 Ext. 224

Ottawa Safety Council (OSC) / Conseil de sécurité d'Ottawa
#105, 2068 Robertson Rd., Nepean ON K2H 5Y8

Tel: 613-238-1513; *Fax:* 613-238-8744
e-mail: info@ottawasafetycouncil.ca
www.ottawasafetycouncil.ca
www.facebook.com/OttawaSafetyCouncil
twitter.com/SafetyOttawa

Previous Name: Ottawa-Carleton Safety Council
Overview: A small local charitable organization founded in 1957
Mission: To assist the citizens of Ottawa to protect themselves & others from injury, property destruction due to accidents, & accidental death
Chief Officer(s):
Julie Vogt, Interim Executive Director, 613-238-1513 Ext. 223
julie.vogt@ottawasafetycouncil.ca
Publications:
• Ottawa Safety Council Newsletter
Type: Newsletter
Profile: Council reports & program updates

Peel Family Services
#501, 151 City Centre Dr., Mississauga ON L5B 1M7

Tel: 905-270-2250; *Fax:* 905-270-2869; *TTY:* 905-270-7357
e-mail: fsp@fspeel.org
www.fspeel.org
www.facebook.com/pages/Family-Services-of-Peel/163434633676036
twitter.com/fspeelca

Also Known As: Family Services of Peel
Overview: A medium-sized local charitable organization founded in 1971 overseen by Family Service Ontario

Mission: To provide support & community services to families in the Peel region.
Member of: Family Service Canada; Ontario Association of Credit CounsellingServices
Chief Officer(s):
Chuck MacLean, Executive Director

Peterborough Social Planning Council (PSPC)
Peterborough Square, 360 George St. North, Lower Level, Peterborough ON K9H 7E7

Tel: 705-743-5915
www.pspc.on.ca

Overview: A small local organization founded in 1977
Mission: To facilitate citizen participation in forming strong, healthy, & just communities in the City & County of Peterborough, Ontario; To act as a catalyst for positive social change; To promote social justice
Chief Officer(s):
Brenda Dales, Executive Director
Dawm Berry Merriam, Research & Policy Analyst

Reach Canada
400 Coventry Rd., 3rd Fl, Ottawa ON K1K 2C7

Tel: 613-236-6636; *Fax:* 613-236-6605
Toll-Free: 800-465-8898; *TTY:* 613-236-9478
e-mail: reach@reach.ca
www.reach.ca
www.facebook.com/ReachCanada
twitter.com/reachcanada1

Previous Name: Reach Equality & Justice for People with Disabilities; Resource, Education & Advocacy Centre for the Handicapped
Overview: A small local organization founded in 1981
Mission: To provide legal referral services & educational programs for people with disabilities
Chief Officer(s):
Renette Sasouni, President

Reena
927 Clark Ave. West, Thornhill ON L4J 8G6

Tel: 905-889-6484; *Fax:* 905-889-3827
e-mail: info@reena.org
www.reena.org
www.facebook.com/ReenaFoundation
twitter.com/ReenaFoundation

Previous Name: Reena Foundation
Overview: A medium-sized local charitable organization founded in 1975
Mission: To integrate developmentally disabled people towards independent living within community, with emphasis on Judaic programming
Affiliation(s): Jewish Federation of Greater Toronto
Chief Officer(s):
Lorne Sossin, Chair
Bryan Keshen, President & CEO
bkeshen@reena.org

Renfrew County United Way
224 Pembroke St. West, Pembroke ON K8A 5N2

Tel: 613-735-0436; *Fax:* 613-735-2663
Toll-Free: 888-592-2213
e-mail: info@renfrewcountyunitedway.ca
www.renfrewcountyunitedway.ca
www.facebook.com/182315931870874

Merged from: United Way/Centraide of the Upper Ottawa Valley Inc. and The Deep River District United Way
Overview: A small local charitable organization founded in 1971 overseen by United Way of Canada - Centraide Canada
Mission: To identify & address the needs of our community by organizing the resources of community members to care for one another
Affiliation(s): Arnprior Community Council; Upper Ottawa Valley Chamber of Commerce; Pembroke Downtown Development Commission
Chief Officer(s):
Shelley Rolland-Porucks, Chair
Gail Logan, Executive Director

Réseau des services de santé en français de l'Est de l'Ontario
#300, 1173, ch Cyrville, Ottawa ON K1J 7S6

Tél: 613-747-7431; *Téléc:* 613-747-2907
Ligne sans frais: 877-528-7565
Courriel: reseau@rssfe.on.ca
www.rssfe.on.ca

Aperçu: Dimension: petite; *Envergure:* locale; fondée en 1998 surveillé par Société santé en français
Mission: Améliorer l'offre active et l'accès à un continuum de services de santé de qualité en français
Membre(s) du bureau directeur:
Jacinthe Desaulniers, Directrice générale
jdesaulniers@rssfe.on.ca

Scarborough Centre for Healthy Communities (SCHC)
#2, 629 Markham Rd., Toronto ON M1H 2A4

Tel: 416-642-9445
www.schcontario.ca
ca.linkedin.com/company/scarborough-centre-for-healthy-communities
www.facebook.com/ScarboroughCentreforHealthyCommunities
twitter.com/schcont
www.youtube.com/schcont

Overview: A medium-sized local charitable organization
Mission: To offer home support, transportation, medical, & family support programs for individuals & families
Chief Officer(s):
Janice Dusek, Chair & President

Service familial de Sudbury (SFS) / Sudbury Family Service
c/o Sudbury Counselling Centre, 260, rue Cedar, Sudbury ON P3B 1M7

Tél: 705-524-9629; *Téléc:* 705-524-1530; *Crisis Hot-Line:* 705-675-4760
Courriel: info@counsellingccs.com
www.counsellingccs.com

Aperçu: Dimension: petite; *Envergure:* locale; Organisme sans but lucratif; fondée en 1971 surveillé par Family Service Ontario
Mission: Amélioration de la qualité de vie et la résolution des problèmes psychosociaux des individus, des familles, des groupes & de la communauté
Affliation(s): Conseil de Développement social
Membre(s) du bureau directeur:
Lynne Lamontagne, Directrice générale
llamontagne@counsellingccs.com

South Etobicoke Community Legal Services (SECLS)
#210, 5353 Dundas St. West, Toronto ON M9B 6H8

Tel: 416-252-7218; *Fax:* 416-252-1474
e-mail: secls@southetobicokelegal.ca
www.southetobicokelegal.ca

Overview: A small local charitable organization founded in 1982
Mission: To protect & promote the legal welfare of community members by offering services, unique to the community, through a network of volunteers & staff members, where language, financial hardship or disability will not act as barriers
Member of: Association of Community Legal Clinics of Ontario
Affliation(s): Toronto Refugees Affairs Council; Federation of Metro Tenants Ontario Council of Agencies Serving Immigrants

South Simcoe Community Information Centre
Town Square, PO Box 932, 39 Victoria St. East, Alliston ON L9R 1W1

Tel: 705-435-4900; *Fax:* 705-435-1106
e-mail: contact@contactsouthsimcoe.ca
www.contactsouthsimcoe.ca
www.facebook.com/CONTACTCommunityServices

Overview: A small local organization founded in 1977 overseen by InformOntario
Mission: To work to create a community that is informed of available resources through the provision of information & referral, access to information technologies & partnership with others
Chief Officer(s):
Liz Beattie, Co-Executive Director
Sandra Mawby, Co-Executive Director

South-East Grey Support Services (SEGSS)
PO Box 12, 24 Toronto St., Flesherton ON N0C 1E0

Tel: 519-924-3339; *Fax:* 519-924-3575
www.southeastgreysupportservices.com
www.facebook.com/329076267124425

Overview: A small local organization founded in 1961
Mission: Provides and advocates for a full range of community-based services for individuals with intellectual disabilities including accommodation, employment, day program, planning and family supports.
Member of: Community Living Ontario
Publications:
• Grey Bruce Facilitation Network Newsletter [a publication of South-East Grey Support Services]
Type: Newsletter

Spectra Helpline
#402, 7700 Hurontario St., Brampton ON L6Y 4M3

Tel: 289-569-1200; *Fax:* 888-658-8577; *Crisis Hot-Line:* 905-459-7777
e-mail: info@spectrahelpline.org
www.spectrahelpline.org
www.linkedin.com/company/spectra-community-support-services
www.facebook.com/SpectraHelpline
twitter.com/spectrasupport

Previous Name: Telecare Distress Centre Brampton
Overview: A small local charitable organization founded in 1973 overseen by Distress Centres Ontario
Mission: To provide a 24-hour-a-day telephone service to people in need; To aim to be a listening ministry, not a problem-solving, advice-giving institution
Affiliation(s): Telecare Teleministries of Canada Inc.; Life Line International
Chief Officer(s):
Alison Caird, Executive Director

Sudbury Community Service Centre Inc. / Centre de services communautaires de Sudbury
1166 Roy Ave., Sudbury ON P3A 3M6

Tel: 705-560-0430; *Fax:* 705-560-0440
Toll-Free: 800-685-1521
e-mail: scsc@vianet.ca
www.sudburycommunityservicecentre.ca
www.youtube.com/channel/UCfXnydiEvAc1pf8QzXFbc1A

Overview: A small local charitable organization founded in 1972 overseen by Ontario Association of Credit Counselling Service
Mission: To provide support services to individuals with developmental disabilities & their families; To assist persons who are experiencing financial difficulties in the Greater Sudbury Area, as well as the Espanola & Parry Sound areas, through Credit Counselling Sudbury
Member of: Ontario Association of Credit Counselling Services

Temporomandibular Joint Society of Canada (TMJSC)
#7, 119 Henderson Ave., Thornhill ON L3T 2L3

Tel: 416-414-2445
e-mail: tmjscanada@gmail.com

Overview: A small local organization founded in 2015
Mission: TJSC (Temporomandibular Joint Society of Canada) is devoted to furthering TMJ disease/disfunction /disorders support, education, and awareness in Canada for both those afflicted and those who provide professional care for them.
Chief Officer(s):
Anita Frank, Executive Director, 416-414-2445
tmjscanada@gmail.com

Tikinagan Child & Family Services
PO Box 627, 65 King St., Sioux Lookout ON P8T 1B1

Tel: 807-737-3466; *Fax:* 807-737-3543
Toll-Free: 800-465-3624
www.tikinagan.org

Previous Name: Tikinagan North Child & Family Services
Overview: A small local organization founded in 1984
Mission: To provide child protection services to First Nations communities
Member of: Association of Native Child & Family Services Agencies of Ontario
Chief Officer(s):
Thelma Morris, Executive Director

SECTION II:
General Resources

Timmins Family Counselling Centre, Inc. / Centre de Counselling Familial de Timmins inc.
#310, 60 Wilson Ave., Timmins ON P4N 2S7
Tel: 705-267-7333; Fax: 705-268-6850
www.timminsfamilycounselling.com
Overview: A small local charitable organization founded in 1979
Mission: To provide high quality therapeutic services in regards to maintaining & improving the functioning of families, couples & the individual; aims to promote education & development in the community & intercedes for the client's rights with a goal of impro0ing the quality of life in Timmins & its surrounding areas
Chief Officer(s):
Nathalie Parnell, Executive Director

Toronto Community Care Access Centre
#305, 250 Dundas St. West, Toronto ON M5T 2Z5
Tel: 416-506-9888; Fax: 416-506-0374
Toll-Free: 866-243-0061
e-mail: feedback@toronto.ccac-ont.ca
healthcareathome.ca/torontocentral
ca.linkedin.com/company/toronto-central-community-care-access-centre
twitter.com/tcccac
www.youtube.com/torontoccac
Previous Name: Home Care Program for Metropolitan Toronto
Overview: A medium-sized local organization founded in 1964
Mission: To coordinate & deliver health & social care to all people in Metro Toronto who are sick or disabled; to enhance the quality of their lives & enable them to remain at home; to provide & coordinate an appropriate range of services to meet the diverse needs (health & social) of individuals & families
Member of: Canadian Home Care Association; Ontario Home Care Programs Association
Chief Officer(s):
Stacey Daub, CEO
William Yetman, Chair

Toronto Paramedic Association
c/o Toronto Emergency Medical Services, 4330 Dufferin St., Toronto ON M3H 5R9
Tel: 416-410-9453
torontoparamedic.com
www.facebook.com/pages/Toronto-Paramedic-Association/155191410832
twitter.com/tpanews
Overview: A small local organization founded in 1992
Mission: To support the paramedic community and focus on paramedic advancements in patient care.
Member of: Ontario Paramedic Association

Travellers' Aid Society of Toronto (TAS)
13 Mountalan Ave., Toronto ON M4J 1H3
Tel: 416-366-7788; Fax: 416-466-6552
e-mail: TAID668@gmail.com
www.travellersaid.ca
Also Known As: Travellers'Aid
Overview: A small local charitable organization founded in 1903
Mission: To provide a base of needed information for travellers as well as shelter & other help in crisis situations
Member of: Tourism Toronto; Volunteer Centre of Toronto/Etobicoke; Green Tourism; Travellers Assistance Services of Toronto
Affliation(s): Travellers Aid International

211 Ontario North
Victoria Mall, #38, 125 Syndicate Ave., Thunder Bay ON P7E 6H8
Tel: 807-624-1729
Toll-Free: 866-586-5638; TTY: 888-622-4651
e-mail: info@lspc.ca
www.211OntarioNorth.ca
Overview: A small local organization founded in 2008 overseen by InformOntario
Mission: To provide accurate, up-to-date information on community services, organizations, clubs, events & activities; To assist organizations & the general public in accessing information & the resources they require & identify gaps in services; To work with individuals & groups to meet their needs & improve community well-being
Affliation(s): A program of the Lakehead Social Planning Council
Chief Officer(s):

Kristen Tomcko, Supervisor

United Way Elgin-St. Thomas
#103, 10 Mondamin St., St Thomas ON N5P 2V1
Tel: 519-631-3171; Fax: 519-631-9253
www.stthomasunitedway.ca
www.facebook.com/UnitedWayElginStThomas
Previous Name: Elgin-St.Thomas United Way Services
Overview: A small local charitable organization founded in 1957 overseen by United Way of Canada - Centraide Canada
Mission: To be a leader in improving the quality of life for all people in Elgin County.
Member of: St. Thomas & District Chamber of Commerce; Canadian Association of Gift Planners
Chief Officer(s):
James Todd, President
Melissa Schneider, Campaign/Communications Coordinator

United Way for the City of Kawartha Lakes (UWVC)
50 Mary St. West, Lindsay ON K9V 2N6
Tel: 705-878-5081; Fax: 705-878-0475
e-mail: office@ckl.unitedway.ca
www.ckl-unitedway.ca
www.facebook.com/UWCKL
twitter.com/unitedwayckl
Previous Name: United Way of Victoria County (UWVC)
Overview: A medium-sized local charitable organization founded in 1983 overseen by United Way of Canada - Centraide Canada
Mission: To promote the organized capacity of people & groups in the City of Kawartha Lakes to care for each other
Chief Officer(s):
Penny Barton Dyke, Executive Director
pbartondyke@ckl.unitedway.ca

United Way of Burlington & Greater Hamilton
177 Rebecca St., Hamilton ON L8R 1B9
Tel: 905-527-4543; Fax: 905-527-5152
e-mail: uway@uwaybh.ca
www.uwaybh.ca
www.facebook.com/unitedwaybh
twitter.com/UnitedWayBH
www.youtube.com/user/UnitedWayBH
Previous Name: United Way of Burlington, Hamilton-Wentworth
Overview: A small local charitable organization overseen by United Way of Canada - Centraide Canada
Mission: To empower a diverse community to achieve positive social development
Chief Officer(s):
Jeff Vallentin, CEO

Burlington Office
#107, 3425 Harvester Rd., Burlington ON L7N 3N1
Tel: 905-635-3138; Fax: 905-632-1918
e-mail: uway@uwaybh.ca
Chief Officer(s):
Jeff Vallentin, CEO

United Way of Cambridge & North Dumfries
#2, 135 Thompson Dr., Cambridge ON N1T 2E4
Tel: 519-621-1030; Fax: 519-621-6220
www.uwcambridge.on.ca
www.facebook.com/UWCND
twitter.com/uwcambridge
www.youtube.com/user/UWcambridge
Overview: A small local charitable organization founded in 1940 overseen by United Way of Canada - Centraide Canada
Mission: To enhance the quality of life in Cambridge & North Dumfries by caring for & contributing to community needs
Chief Officer(s):
Ron Dowhaniuk, CEO
ron@uwcambridge.on.ca

United Way of Chatham-Kent County
PO Box 606, 425 McNaughton Ave. West, Chatham ON N7M 5K8
Tel: 519-354-0430; *Fax:* 519-354-9511
e-mail: info@uwock.ca
uwock.ca
www.facebook.com/UnitedWayofChathamKent
twitter.com/UnitedWayCK
www.youtube.com/user/UnitedWayChathamKent
Previous Name: United Way of Kent County
Overview: A small local charitable organization founded in 1948 overseen by United Way of Canada - Centraide Canada
Mission: To build the organized capacity of people to care for one another
Chief Officer(s):
Alison Patrick, President
Karen Kirkwood-Whyte, CEO

United Way of Cochrane-Timiskaming
PO Box 984, Timmins ON P4N 7H6
Tel: 705-268-9696
www.facebook.com/85026973282
Overview: A small local charitable organization founded in 1967 overseen by United Way of Canada - Centraide Canada
Mission: To promote the organized capacity of people to care for one another
Chief Officer(s):
Jennifer Gorman, Coordinator, Resource Development

United Way of Durham Region
345 Simcoe St. South, Oshawa ON L1H 4J2
Tel: 905-436-7377
Toll-Free: 866-463-6910
www.unitedwaydr.com
Overview: A small local organization founded in 1940 overseen by United Way of Canada - Centraide Canada
Mission: To strengthen the Durham region communities & improve the quality of life of its residents
Chief Officer(s):
Cindy Murray, Chief Executive Officer
Robert Howard, Director, Campaign & Communications
Karie Stephenson, Manager, Finance & Office
Michele Watson, Manager, Information Services Program
Jessica Hanson, Manager, Communications & Data
Barb Fannin, Coordinator, Community Investment

  Ajax Office
  Ajax ON
Tel: 905-686-0606

United Way of Greater Simcoe County
1110 Hwy. 26, Midhurst ON L9X 1N6
Tel: 705-726-2301; *Fax:* 705-726-4897
e-mail: info@uwsimcoemuskoka.ca
www.unitedwaygsc.ca
www.facebook.com/UWSimcoeMuskoka
twitter.com/UWSimcoeMuskoka
www.youtube.com/user/UnitedWaySimcoeCty
Previous Name: United Way of Barrie/South Simcoe
Overview: A small local charitable organization founded in 1960 overseen by United Way of Canada - Centraide Canada
Mission: To improve quality of life & build community by helping those most in need
Member of: Barrie Chamber of Commerce
Chief Officer(s):
Dale Biddell, CEO, 705-726-2301 Ext. 2033
dbiddell@uwsimcoemuskoka.ca

United Way of Guelph, Wellington & Dufferin
85 Westmount Rd., Guelph ON N1H 5J2
Tel: 519-821-0571; *Fax:* 519-821-7847
www.unitedwayguelph.com
www.linkedin.com/company/united-way-of-guelph-&-wellington
www.facebook.com/unitedwayguelph
twitter.com/uwguelph
Previous Name: Guelph & Wellington United Way Social Planning Council
Overview: A small local charitable organization founded in 1945 overseen by United Way of Canada - Centraide Canada
Mission: To meet the needs of the community & improve lives

Chief Officer(s):
Ken Dardano, Executive Director
ken@unitedwayguelph.com

United Way of Haldimand-Norfolk
PO Box 472, 45 Kent St. North, Simcoe ON N3Y 4L5
Tel: 519-426-5660; *Fax:* 519-426-0017
e-mail: reception@unitedwayhn.on.ca
www.unitedwayhn.on.ca
www.facebook.com/UnitedwayofHn
twitter.com/UnitedWayofHN
Previous Name: Norfolk Community Chest
Overview: A small local charitable organization founded in 1946 overseen by United Way of Canada - Centraide Canada
Mission: To improve people's lives & to strengthen the community
Chief Officer(s):
Brittany Burley, Executive Director
brittany.burley@unitedwayhn.on.ca

United Way of Halton Hills
PO Box 286, Georgetown ON L7G 4Y5
Tel: 905-877-3066; *Fax:* 905-877-3067
e-mail: office@unitedwayofhaltonhills.ca
www.unitedwayofhaltonhills.ca
Overview: A small local charitable organization founded in 1986 overseen by United Way of Canada - Centraide Canada
Mission: To provide leadership in the raising & allocation of funds to meet human needs & to improve social conditions in the community
Chief Officer(s):
Janet Foster, Executive Director

United Way of Kingston, Frontenac, Lennox & Addington
417 Bagot St., Kingston ON K7K 3C1
Tel: 613-542-2674; *Fax:* 613-542-1379
e-mail: uway@unitedwaykfla.ca
www.unitedwaykfla.ca
www.facebook.com/unitedwaykfla
twitter.com/unitedwaykfla
www.youtube.com/unitedwaykfla
Overview: A small local charitable organization overseen by United Way of Canada - Centraide Canada
Mission: To strengthen the community by supporting social service & health agencies
Chief Officer(s):
Bhavana Varma, President & CEO
bvarma@unitedwaykfla.ca

United Way of Kitchener-Waterloo & Area
Marsland Centre, #801, 20 Erb St. West, Waterloo ON N2L 1T2
Tel: 519-888-6100
e-mail: info@uwaykw.org
www.uwaykw.org
www.facebook.com/uwaykw
twitter.com/UnitedWayKW
www.youtube.com/user/UwayKW
Overview: A small local charitable organization founded in 1941 overseen by United Way of Canada - Centraide Canada
Mission: To improve quality of life in the community
Member of: Kitchener-Waterloo Chamber of Commerce
Chief Officer(s):
Ingrid Pregel, President
Jan Varner, CEO
jvarner@uwaykw.org

United Way of Lanark County
15 Bates Dr., Carleton Place ON K7C 4J8
Tel: 613-253-9074; *Fax:* 888-249-9075
www.lanarkunitedway.com
www.linkedin.com/company/united-way-of-lanark-county
www.facebook.com/UnitedWayLanarkCounty
twitter.com/UWLanarkCounty
Overview: A small local organization overseen by United Way of Canada - Centraide Canada
Mission: To mobilize people to strengthen the community & enact social change
Chief Officer(s):
Fraser Scantlebury, Executive Director
fscantlebury@lanarkunitedway.com

United Way of Leeds & Grenville
PO Box 576, 42 George St., Brockville ON K6V 5V7
Tel: 613-342-8889; *Fax:* 613-342-8850
e-mail: info@uwlg.org
www.uwlg.org
www.facebook.com/UnitedWayLG
www.youtube.com/user/UnitedWayLeedsGrenv
Overview: A small local licensing charitable organization founded in 1957 overseen by United Way of Canada - Centraide Canada
Mission: To unite people to improve quality of life & build healthy communities
Chief Officer(s):
Melissa Hillier, Executive Director

United Way of London & Middlesex
409 King St., London ON N6B 1S5
Tel: 519-438-1721; *Fax:* 519-438-9938
www.unitedwaylm.ca
www.linkedin.com/company/unitedwaylm
www.facebook.com/unitedwaylm
twitter.com/unitedwaylm
Overview: A small local charitable organization founded in 1965 overseen by United Way of Canada - Centraide Canada
Mission: To exercise leadership in coordinating people & organizations to assist those in need in our community
Chief Officer(s):
Kelly Ziegner, Chief Executive Officer
kziegner@unitedwaylm.ca
Suzanne Bembridge, Director, Finance & Operations
sbembridge@unitedwaylm.ca

United Way of Milton
PO Box 212, 1 Chris Hadfield Way, Milton ON L9T 4N9
Tel: 905-875-2550; *Fax:* 905-875-2402
e-mail: campaign@miltonunitedway.ca
www.miltonunitedway.ca
www.linkedin.com/groups?gid=2558626
www.facebook.com/UnitedWayMilton
twitter.com/unitedwaymilton
www.youtube.com/unitedwaymilton
Overview: A small local charitable organization founded in 1982 overseen by United Way of Canada - Centraide Canada
Mission: To serve the people of the Milton area by working with recognized charitable agencies to ensure human services that enhance the quality of life in the community
Chief Officer(s):
Kate Holmes, CEO

United Way of Niagara Falls & Greater Fort Erie
7150 Montrose Rd., Niagara Falls ON L2H 3N3
Tel: 905-735-0490
www.unitedwayniagara.org
www.facebook.com/UnitedWayNiagara
twitter.com/UWNiagara
Overview: A small local organization founded in 1942 overseen by United Way of Canada - Centraide Canada
Mission: To support the people in Fort Erie, Niagara Falls, Pelham, Port Colborne, Wainfleet, & Welland; To bring about positive change to the community
Chief Officer(s):
Tamara Coleman-Lawrie, Executive Director
tamara.coleman-lawrie@unitedwayniagara.org

United Way of Oakville (UWO)
#200, 466 Speers Rd., Oakville ON L6K 3W9
Tel: 905-845-5571; *Fax:* 905-845-0166
e-mail: info@uwoakville.org
www.uwoakville.org
www.linkedin.com/company/united-way-oakville
www.facebook.com/UnitedWayOakville
twitter.com/uwoakville
www.youtube.com/user/UnitedWayofOakville
Overview: A medium-sized local charitable organization founded in 1955 overseen by United Way of Canada - Centraide Canada
Mission: To bring people & resources together to strengthen the Oakville community
Chief Officer(s):
John Armstrong, Chair

Brad Park, Chief Executive Officer
brad@uwoakville.org
Tara Neal, Office Administrator
tara@uwoakville.org

United Way of Oxford
#447 Hunter St., Woodstock ON N4S 4G7
Tel: 519-539-3851
e-mail: info@unitedwayoxford.ca
www.unitedwayoxford.ca
www.facebook.com/UnitedWayOxford
twitter.com/UnitedWayOxford
www.youtube.com/channel/UCup-8AJZ2pJFCCeZbJ4t87w
Overview: A small local organization overseen by United Way of Canada - Centraide Canada
Mission: To build strong communities & help improve the lives of residents, especially those affected by poverty, mental health issues, or other social challenges
Member of: United Way of Ontario
Chief Officer(s):
Kelly Gilson, Executive Director
kelly@unitedwayoxford.ca
Anne Wismer, Manager, Operations
anne@unitedwayoxford.ca

United Way of Peel Region
PO Box 58, #408, 90 Burnhamthorpe Rd. West, Mississauga ON L5B 3C3
Tel: 905-602-3650; *Fax:* 905-602-3651; *TTY:* 905-602-3653
www.unitedwaypeel.org
www.linkedin.com/company/657177
www.facebook.com/unitedwaypeel
twitter.com/Unitedwaypeel
www.youtube.com/user/unitedwaypeel
Overview: A large local charitable organization founded in 1967 overseen by United Way of Canada - Centraide Canada
Mission: United Way of Peel Region was established in 1967 and serves the communities of Mississauga, Brampton and Caledon, improving social conditions so that everyone can thrive. United Way provides a strong voice for social change that strengthens communities and improves lives.
Chief Officer(s):
Shelley White, President/ CEO
swhite@unitedwaypeel.org
Shirley Crocker, Vice President, Finance & Administration
scrocker@unitedwaypeel.org
Carol Kotacka, Interim Vice President, Communications & Marketing
ckotacka@unitedwaypeel.org
Anita Stellinga, Vice President, Community Investment
astellinga@unitedwaypeel.org

United Way of Perth-Huron
32 Erie St., Stratford ON N5A 2M4
Tel: 519-271-7730; *Fax:* 519-273-9350
Toll-Free: 877-818-8867
e-mail: info@perthhuron.unitedway.ca
www.perthhuron.unitedway.ca
www.linkedin.com/groups?gid=3966504
www.facebook.com/UWPH1
twitter.com/UnitedWayPH
www.youtube.com/user/UnitedWPH
Previous Name: United Way of Stratford-Perth
Overview: A small local charitable organization founded in 1967 overseen by United Way of Canada - Centraide Canada
Mission: To improve people's lives & meet the needs of the community by mobilizing agencies, individuals, & resources
Affiliation(s): Perth County Community Development Council; Local Voices
Chief Officer(s):
Ryan Erb, Executive Director
rerb@perthhuron.unitedway.ca
Carolynne Champagne, Vice-President, Resource Development & Communications
cchampagne@perthhuron.unitedway.ca
Jeanine Clarke, Director, Finance & Property
jclarke@perthhuron.unitedway.ca
Susan Faber, Director, Communications & Community Information
sfaber@perthhuron.unitedway.ca

United Way of Peterborough & District
277 Stewart St., Peterborough ON K9J 3M8
Tel: 705-742-8839; *Fax:* 705-742-9186
e-mail: office@uwpeterborough.ca
www.uwpeterborough.ca
www.facebook.com/15103169591
twitter.com/UnitedWayPtbo
Overview: A medium-sized local charitable organization founded in 1941 overseen by United Way of Canada - Centraide Canada
Mission: To improve lives & build community by engaging individuals & mobilizing collective action; to provide resources, services & programs for community leadership
Chief Officer(s):
Jim Russell, CEO
jrussell@uwpeterborough.ca

United Way of Quinte
PO Box 815, Belleville ON K8N 5B5
Tel: 613-962-9531; *Fax:* 613-962-4165
www.unitedwayofquinte.ca
www.facebook.com/UnitedWayofQuinte
twitter.com/unitedwayquinte
Previous Name: United Way of Belleville & District
Overview: A small local charitable organization founded in 1959 overseen by United Way of Canada - Centraide Canada
Mission: To provide leadership in a collaborative endeavor with our member agencies & others to increase the capacity of our community to respond to human service needs
Member of: United Way Ontario
Chief Officer(s):
Danny Nickle, Chair
Judi Gilbert, Executive Director
jgilbert@unitedwayofquinte.ca
Tambra Patrick-MacDonald, Director, Finance & Administration
tmacdonald@unitedwayofquinte.ca

United Way of St Catharines & District
63 Church St., #LC1, St Catharines ON L2R 3C4
Tel: 905-688-5050; *Fax:* 905-688-2997
e-mail: office@stcatharines.unitedway.ca
www.unitedwaysc.ca
www.facebook.com/148938585140989
twitter.com/uwaysc
Overview: A small local charitable organization founded in 1953 overseen by United Way of Canada - Centraide Canada
Mission: To increase the organized capacity of people to care for one another
Chief Officer(s):
Frances Hallworth, Executive Director
fhallworth@stcatharines.unitedway.ca

United Way of Sarnia-Lambton
PO Box 548, 420 East St. North, Sarnia ON N7T 6Y5
Tel: 519-336-5452; *Fax:* 519-383-6032
e-mail: info@theunitedway.on.ca
www.theunitedway.on.ca
Overview: A small local charitable organization founded in 1959 overseen by United Way of Canada - Centraide Canada
Mission: To generate resources enabling the community to respond to human care priorities in Sarnia-Lambton
Chief Officer(s):
Dave Brown, Executive Director
dave@theunitedway.on.ca

United Way of Sault Ste Marie & District
7A Oxford St., Sault Ste Marie ON P6B 1R7
Tel: 705-256-7476; *Fax:* 705-759-5899
e-mail: uwssm@ssmunitedway.ca
www.ssmunitedway.ca
www.facebook.com/unitedwaysault
Overview: A small local organization founded in 1957 overseen by United Way of Canada - Centraide Canada
Mission: To improve the health, well-being, & quality of life of individuals & families in the community; To fight against poverty & address community issues
Member of: Chamber of Commerce of Sault Ste Marie
Affliation(s): United Way of Ontario; Regional Professional Advisory Council

Chief Officer(s):
Gary Vipond, CEO

United Way of Stormont, Dundas & Glengarry / Centraide de Stormont, Dundas & Glengarry
PO Box 441, Stn. Case Postale, Cornwall ON K6H 5T2
Tel: 613-932-2051; *Fax:* 613-932-7534
e-mail: info@unitedwaysdg.com
www.unitedwaysdg.com
www.facebook.com/209841445745076
twitter.com/unitedwaysdg
Previous Name: United Way of Cornwall & District
Overview: A small local charitable organization founded in 1944 overseen by United Way of Canada - Centraide Canada
Mission: To improve lives & build community by supporting agencies, programs & services in the area
Chief Officer(s):
Nolan Quinn, President
Lori Greer, Executive Director
lori@unitedwaysdg.com
Stephanie Lalonde, Coordinator, Campaign & Communication
stephanie@unitedwaysdg.com

United Way of Windsor-Essex County
300 Giles Blvd. East, #A1, Windsor ON N9A 4C4
Tel: 519-258-0000; *Fax:* 519-258-2346
e-mail: info@weareunited.com
www.weareunited.com
www.facebook.com/unitedway.windsoressex
twitter.com/UnitedWayWE
Overview: A small local charitable organization overseen by United Way of Canada - Centraide Canada
Mission: To bring people & resources together to improve the community
Chief Officer(s):
Lorraine Goddard, CEO
lgoddard@weareunited.com

United Way South Niagara (UWSN) / Centraide de Niagara Sud
Seaway Mall, 800 Niagara St., 2nd Fl, Welland ON L3C 5Z4
Tel: 905-735-0490; *Fax:* 905-735-5432
e-mail: office@southniagara.unitedway.ca
www.unitedwaysouthniagara.ca
www.facebook.com/pages/United-Way-of-South-Niagara/22780191029
2
twitter.com/UnitedWaySN
www.youtube.com/UWSouthNiagara
Overview: A medium-sized local charitable organization founded in 1964 overseen by United Way of Canada - Centraide Canada
Chief Officer(s):
Tamara Coleman-Lawrie, Executive Director

United Way Toronto & York Region
26 Wellington St. East, 12th Fl., Toronto ON M5E 1S2
Tel: 416-777-2001; *Fax:* 416-777-0962; *TTY:* 866-620-2993
www.unitedwaytyr.com
www.linkedin.com/company/unitedwaytyr
www.facebook.com/unitedwaytyr
twitter.com/unitedwaytyr
instagram.com/unitedwaytyr
Previous Name: United Way Toronto; Red Feather United Appeal; United Way of Greater Toronto
Overview: A medium-sized local organization founded in 1956 overseen by United Way of Canada - Centraide Canada
Mission: To meet urgent human needs & improve social conditions by mobilizing the community's volunteer & financial resources in a common cause of caring
Chief Officer(s):
Vince Timpano, Chair
Daniele Zanotti, President & CEO

United Way/Centraide Ottawa (UW/CO)
363 Coventry Rd., Ottawa ON K1K 2C5
Tel: 613-228-6700; *Fax:* 613-228-6730
e-mail: info@unitedwayottawa.ca
www.unitedwayottawa.ca
www.linkedin.com/company/united-way-centraide-ottawa
www.facebook.com/unitedwayottawa
twitter.com/UnitedWayOttawa
www.youtube.com/user/unitedwayottawa
Previous Name: United Appeal of Ottawa-Carleton
Overview: A small local organization founded in 1933
overseen by United Way of Canada - Centraide Canada
Mission: To bring people & resources together to build a strong,
healthy, safe community for all; to build & support a network of high
priority, results-oriented community services; to offer leadership in
bringing the community together; to excel in fundraising; to invest
resources & charitable funds in partnership with the community; to
inform & engage community stakeholders
Chief Officer(s):
Michael Allen, President/CEO

United Way/Centraide Sudbury & District
#E6, 105 Elm St., Sudbury ON P3C 1T3
Tel: 705-560-3330
www.unitedwaysudbury.com
www.facebook.com/UWSudNip
twitter.com/UWSudNip
Overview: A small local charitable organization founded in 1982
overseen by United Way of Canada - Centraide Canada
Mission: To increase the organized capacity of people to care for one
another through effective fundraising & allocation of these funds
Chief Officer(s):
Michael Cullen, Executive Director
edirector@unitedwaysudbury.com

VHA Home HealthCare
#600, 30 Soudan Ave., Toronto ON M4S 1V6
Tel: 416-489-2500; *Fax:* 416-482-8773
Toll-Free: 888-314-6622
www.vha.ca
www.facebook.com/VHAHomeHealthCare
twitter.com/VHACaregiving
www.youtube.com/user/VHAHomeHealthCare
Also Known As: Visiting Homemakers Association
Overview: A large local charitable organization founded in 1925
Mission: To be a leading not-for-profit provider of community-based,
client-centred health & support services in the Greater Toronto Area
Member of: United Way
Chief Officer(s):
Adwoa K. Buahene, Chair
Carol Annett, President/CEO

Volunteer Centre of Guelph/Wellington
#1, 46 Cork St. East, Guelph ON N1H 2W8
Tel: 519-822-0912; *Fax:* 519-822-1389
Toll-Free: 866-693-3318
e-mail: info@volunteerguelphwellington.on.ca
www.volunteerguelphwellington.on.ca
www.linkedin.com/company/volunteer-centre-of-guelph-wellington
www.facebook.com/VolunteerGW
twitter.com/volunteergw
Previous Name: Guelph Information
Overview: A small local charitable organization founded in 2001
overseen by InformOntario
Mission: The Centre strives to build a vibrant, volunteer-based
community. It offers programs to assist non-profit organizations find &
maintain a force of capable volunteer workers.
Chief Officer(s):
Christine Oldfield, Executive Director, 519-822-0912 Ext. 222
coldfield@volunteerguelphwellington.on.ca

The Women's Centre
#229, 1515 Rebecca St., Oakville ON L6G 5G8
Tel: 905-847-5520; *Fax:* 905-847-7413
e-mail: admin@haltonwomenscentre.org
www.haltonwomenscentre.org
www.facebook.com/pages/The-Halton-Womens-Centre/191885775004
twitter.com/HalWomensCentre
www.flickr.com/photos/haltonwomenscentre
Also Known As: Halton Women's Centre
Overview: A small local organization founded in 1991
Mission: To make a positive difference in the lives of women in
transition, crisis or distress

Woolwich Community Services (WCS)
5 Memorial Ave., Elmira ON N3B 2P8
Tel: 519-669-5139; *Fax:* 519-669-4210
e-mail: wcs@execulink.com
www.woolwichcommunityservices.com
Overview: A small local organization founded in 1974 overseen by
InformOntario
Mission: To help people find solutions to social, legal, health,
government & environmental problems; To define unmet needs in the
community & communicate with appropriate agencies or organizations
about such needs; To initiate action toward solutions when appropriate
agencies do not exist in the community, including direct assistance,
organizing & coordinating

York Region Family Services (Markham)
#203, 4261 Hwy. 7, Unionville ON L3R 1L5
Tel: 905-415-9719; *Fax:* 905-415-9706
Toll-Free: 888-820-9986
www.fsyr.ca
Also Known As: FSYR Markham
Overview: A medium-sized local organization founded in 1968
overseen by Family Service Ontario
Mission: To assist people experiencing emotional, behavioural,
relational &/or financial challenges through counselling, educational &
assessment programs & services designed to improve functioning &
coping skills in daily life
Member of: Ontario Psychological Association; Ontario Association of
Credit Counselling Services
Affiliation(s): Canadian Register of Health Service Providers in
Psychology; United Way of York Region
Chief Officer(s):
Elisha Laker, Executive Director
elaker@fsyr.ca

QUÉBEC

**Association de balle des jeunes handicapés de
Laval-Laurentides-Lanaudière (ABJHLLL)**
2020, av Laplante, Laval QC H7S 1E7
Tél: 450-689-4668
Également appelé: Association de balle des jeunes handicapés de
Laval/ABJHL
Aperçu: *Dimension:* petite; *Envergure:* locale; Organisme sans but
lucratif; fondée en 1995
Mission: Etablir et opérer des équipes de balle pour la détente de
l'esprit et du corps de jeunes handicapés physiques et/ou intellectuels,
garçons et filles, principalement des régions de Laval, Laurentides et
Lanaudière. Organiser et maintenir toute autre activités social, sportive
et culturelle connexe pour promouvoir les buts de la corporations
Membre de: La petite ligue de baseball du Québec (Division
Challenger)
Membre(s) du bureau directeur:
Tony Condello, Responsable
tcondello@videotron.ca

**Association de loisirs pour personnes handicapées psychiques de
Laval (ALPHPL)**
6600, av 29e, Laval QC H7R 3M3
Tél: 450-627-4525; *Téléc:* 450-627-4370
Courriel: alphpl@videotron.ca
www.alphpl.org
Aperçu: *Dimension:* petite; *Envergure:* locale; Organisme sans but
lucratif; fondée en 1983
Mission: Promouvoir l'évolution sociale des personnes handicapées
psychiques en stimulant leurs intérêts pour des activités physiques,
socio-culturelles et des loisirs; les soutenir dans leur apprentissage,

l'entraînement et l'utilisation des ressources et équipements socio-communautaires; créer un sentiment d'appartenance du participant dans son milieu
Membre de: Association régionale pour personnes handicapées des Laurentides; Association québécoise pour la réadaptation psychosociale; Regroupement des ressources alternatives en santé mentale du Québec; l'Association canadienne pour la santé mentale
Membre(s) du bureau directeur:
François Bullock, Directeur général

Association des goélands de Longueuil
#203, 425 Leblanc ouest, Longueuil QC J4J 1L2
Tél: 450-674-3490
Aperçu: *Dimension:* petite; *Envergure:* locale
Mission: Pour réunir les personnes ayant des handicaps physiques et de leur fournir des services de loisirs et de l'information

Association des handicapés adultes de la Côte-Nord / Association of Disabled Adults on the North Shore (AHACNI)
#103, 859, rue Bossé, Baie-Comeau QC G5C 3P8
Tél: 418-589-2393; *Téléc:* 418-589-2953
www.ahacn.org
Aperçu: *Dimension:* petite; *Envergure:* locale; fondée en 1978
Mission: Pour répondre aux besoins des personnes handicapées et une lésion cérébrale traumatique, et leurs familles, sur la Rive-Nord de Québec
Membre de: Regroupement des associations de personnes traumatisées craniocérébrales du Québec / Coalition of Associations of Craniocerebral Trauma in Quebec
Membre(s) du bureau directeur:
Stéphanie Jourdain, Directrice générale

Association des handicapés adultes de la Mauricie (AHAM)
1322, rue Ste-Julie, Trois-Rivières QC G9A 1Y6
Tél: 819-374-9566; *Téléc:* 819-374-2230
Courriel: aham1322@yahoo.com
www.ahamauricie.org
Aperçu: *Dimension:* petite; *Envergure:* locale; fondée en 1951
Mission: Promouvoir et sauvegarder les droits et privilèges des personnes handicapées; offrir également des services de prêt de fauteuils roulants, de béquilles, et de marchettes
Membre(s) du bureau directeur:
Francois Dubois, Président
Stephane Drolet, Vice-Président

Association des médecins cliniciens enseignants de Laval (AMCEL)
c/o Hôpital Laval, 2360, ch Ste-Foy, Québec QC G1V 4H2
Tél: 418-656-4810; *Téléc:* 418-656-4825
Courriel: amcel@criucpq.ulaval.ca
Aperçu: *Dimension:* petite; *Envergure:* locale; fondée en 1975
Mission: Défense des intérêts de ses membres (médécins-professeurs à l'Université Laval)

Association des médecins cliniciens enseignants de Montréal (AMCEM)
a/s Dr. Jean-Luc Senécal, 1255, boul du Mont-Royal, Montréal QC H2V 2H7
Aperçu: *Dimension:* petite; *Envergure:* locale; fondée en 1969
Membre(s) du bureau directeur:
Jean-Luc Senécal, Président

Association des médecins omnipraticiens de Montréal (AMOM)
2 Place Alexis Nihon, #2000, 3550 boul. De Maisonneuve Ouest, Westmount QC H3Z 3C1
Tél: 514-878-1911; *Téléc:* 514-878-2608
Autres numéros: 514-878-9219
Courriel: contact@amom.net
www.amom.net
www.facebook.com/1592356060980998
twitter.com/AMOMTL
www.youtube.com/channel/UCeavcJVodU-j6Cdq7eRuAWA
Aperçu: *Dimension:* petite; *Envergure:* locale; fondée en 1961
Mission: L'AMOM représente plus de 1900 médecins généralistes oeuvrant dans les différentes sphères de l'omnipratique, de l'urgentologie à la gériatrie en passant par la médecine familiale
Affiliation(s): Fédération des médecins omnipraticiens du Québec
Membre(s) du bureau directeur:
Michel Vachon, Président, 514-376-7702, Fax: 514-376-2639
mvachon@amom.net

Association des parents d'enfants handicapés du Témiscamingue inc.
#1, 3, rue Industrielle, Ville-Marie QC JV9 1S3
Tél: 819-622-1126; *Téléc:* 819-622-0021
Courriel: apeht@cablevision.qc.ca
Aperçu: *Dimension:* petite; *Envergure:* locale
Mission: Offrir des services d'aide aux personnes vivant avec un handicap physique et intellectuel ainsi qu'à leurs familles.
Affiliation(s): Association du Québec pour l'intégration sociale

Association des personnes handicapées de Charlevoix inc. (APHC)
#428, 367, rue St-Étienne, La Malbaie QC G5A 1M3
Tél: 418-665-0015; *Téléc:* 418-665-6787
www.aphcharlevoix.com
www.facebook.com/aphcharlevoix
Nom précédent: Association des handicapées de Charlevoix
Aperçu: *Dimension:* petite; *Envergure:* locale; fondée en 1978
Mission: Regrouper régionalement les personnes handicapées du Comté de Charlevoix afin de permettre leur intégration pleine et entière à la collectivité dans toutes les sphères d'activités du milieu, et à tous les niveaux
Membre(s) du bureau directeur:
Yves Lavoie, Président
Sylvie Breton, Coordonnatrice

Association des personnes handicapées de la Rive-Sud Ouest (APHRSO)
100, rue Ste-Marie, La Prairie QC J5R 1E8
Tél: 450-659-6519; *Téléc:* 450-659-6510
Courriel: info@aphrso.org
www.aphrso.org
www.facebook.com/aphrso
Aperçu: *Dimension:* petite; *Envergure:* locale; Organisme sans but lucratif; fondée en 1980
Mission: Promotion, intégration et défense des droits des personnes handicapées
Affiliation(s): Groupement des Associations personnes handicapées Rive-Sud Montréal
Membre(s) du bureau directeur:
Priscille Arel, Présidente
Nancy Côté, Directrice

Association des personnes handicapées de la Vallée du Richelieu (APHVR)
308, rue Montsabré, #D209, Beloeil QC J3G 2H5
Tél: 450-464-7445; *Téléc:* 450-464-6049
Courriel: informations@aphvr.org
www.aphvr.org
Aperçu: *Dimension:* petite; *Envergure:* locale; fondée en 1981
Mission: Aider ses membres à accroître leur qualité de vie et informer le public sur les problèmes rencontrés par les personnes handicapées
Membre(s) du bureau directeur:
Louis McDuff, Président

Association des personnes handicapés visuels de l'Estrie, inc (AHVEI)
838, rue St-Charles, Sherbrooke QC J1H 4Z2
Tél: 819-566-4848; *Téléc:* 819-566-5913
Courriel: aphve@cooptel.qc.ca
www.aphve.com
Aperçu: *Dimension:* petite; *Envergure:* locale; Organisme sans but lucratif; fondée en 1991
Mission: Favoriser l'intégration sociale des personnes handicapées visuelles; promouvoir les droits et intérêts des personnes handicapées visuelles; sensibiliser la population à la problématique du handicap visuel
Affiliation(s): Regroupement des aveugles et amblyopes du Québec
Membre(s) du bureau directeur:
Denis Barrette, Président
Publications:
• Journal Nouveau Regard
Type: Newsletter; *Frequency:* Quarterly; *Editor:* Marie Claude Guay, Hélène Dubois

Association pour la promotion des droits des personnes handicapées
CP 814, 2435, rue Saint-Jean-Bâptiste, Jonquière QC G7X 7W6
Tél: 418-548-5832; *Téléc:* 418-548-5291
Courriel: apdph@videotron.ca

Aperçu: *Dimension:* petite; *Envergure:* locale; Organisme sans but lucratif; fondée en 1972

Mission: Trouver des solutions et des moyens aux problèmes rencontrés relatifs à la santé, à l'éducation, aux loisirs et à l'intégration sociale des personnes handicapées; sensibiliser la population; informer et assister les parents et les personnes handicapées et offrir des activités de loisirs adaptés aux besoins des personnes handicapées

Affiliation(s): Association du Québec pour l'intégration sociale

Membre(s) du bureau directeur:
Geneviève Siméon, Directrice générale

Association pour la santé environnementale du Québec (ASEQ) / Environmental Health Association of Québec (EHA Québec)
CP 364, Saint-Sauveur QC J0R 1R0

Tél: 450-240-5700; *Téléc:* 450-227-9648
Courriel: office@aseq-ehaq.ca
www.aeha-quebec.ca
www.facebook.com/184591904921401
twitter.com/aseq_ehaq

Aperçu: *Dimension:* petite; *Envergure:* locale

Mission: La mission de l'ASEQ est la protection de l'environnement et la santé humaine au plan individuel et collectif en sensibilisant, soutenant et éduquant la population en regard les produits toxiques et les pesticides. Numéro d'enregistrement d'organisme de bienfaisance: BN 810116624RR0001.

Affiliation(s): EHA Nova Scotia; EHA Ontario; EHA Alberta; EHA BC

Membre(s) du bureau directeur:
Rohini Peris, Président

Association pour le développement de la personne handicapée intellectuelle du Saguenay (ADHIS)
766, rue du Cénacle, Chicoutimi QC G7H 2J2

Tél: 418-543-0093; *Téléc:* 866-896-0820
Courriel: adhis@bellnet.ca
www.adhis.ca

Aperçu: *Dimension:* petite; *Envergure:* locale; fondée en 1976

Mission: Travailler à la défense des droits des personnes vivant avec une déficience intellectuelle, apporter du support aux parents et voir à l'amélioration de la qualité de vie des personnes

Affiliation(s): Association du Québec pour l'intégration sociale

Membre(s) du bureau directeur:
Sylvie Jean, Directrice générale

Auxiliaires bénévoles de l'Hôpital de Chibougamau
51, 3e Rue, Chibougamau QC G8P 1N1

Tél: 418-748-2676

Aperçu: *Dimension:* petite; *Envergure:* locale

Membre(s) du bureau directeur:
Priscilla Ratthé, Présidente, 418-748-6453

Batshaw Youth & Family Centres
5 Weredale Pk., Westmount QC H3Z 1Y5

Tel: 514-989-1885
www.batshaw.ca

Overview: A small local organization founded in 1992

Mission: To intervene with children and families in situations of abuse, neglect, abandonment & when youth have serious behaviour problems, providing psychosocial, rehabilitation & social integration services.

Chief Officer(s):
Judy Martin, President
Lesley Hill, Executive Director

Bouffe pour tous/Moisson Longueuil
911, boul Roalnd-Therrien, Longueuil QC J4J 4L3

Tél: 450-670-5449

Aperçu: *Dimension:* petite; *Envergure:* locale

Mission: Faciliter l'approvisionnement en d'enrées alimentaires aux familles démunies et personnes seules depuis plus de 12 ans; familles monoparentales, gens sans emploi, gens aux prises avec des problèmes de drogues ou de violence

---

Centraide Bas St-Laurent
#303, 1555, boul. Jacques Cartier, Mont-Joli QC G5H 2W1

Tél: 418-775-5555; *Téléc:* 418-775-5525
www.centraidebsl.org
www.facebook.com/Centraidebsl

Aperçu: *Dimension:* petite; *Envergure:* locale; Organisme sans but lucratif; fondée en 1982 surveillé par United Way of Canada - Centraide Canada

---

Mission: Organisme sans but lucratif de lutte à la pauvreté et de soutien aux personnes démunies

Membre(s) du bureau directeur:
Eve Lavoie, Directrice générale

Centraide Centre du Québec
154, rue Dunkin, Drummondville QC J2B 5V1

Tél: 819-477-0505; *Téléc:* 819-477-6719
Ligne sans frais: 888-477-0505
Courriel: bureau@centraide-cdq.ca
www.centraide-cdq.ca
www.facebook.com/pages/Centraide_cdq/152071968150658
twitter.com/centraide_cdq

Nom précédent: Centraide Coeur du Québec

Aperçu: *Dimension:* petite; *Envergure:* locale; Organisme sans but lucratif; fondée en 1979 surveillé par United Way of Canada - Centraide Canada

Mission: Rassembler les personnes et les ressources du Centre-du-Québec afin de contribuer au développement social de la communauté et d'améliorer la qualité de vie de ses membres les plus vulnérables et ce, en lien avec les organismes communautaires.

Membre(s) du bureau directeur:
Isabelle Dionne, Directrice générale
idionne@centraide-cdq.ca

Centraide du Grand Montréal / Centraide of Greater Montréal
493, rue Sherbrooke Ouest, Montréal QC H3A 1B6

Tél: 514-288-1261; *Téléc:* 514-350-7282
Courriel: info@centraide-mtl.org
centraide-mtl.org
www.facebook.com/centraide.du.grand.montreal
twitter.com/centraidemtl
www.youtube.com/user/CentraideMtl

Aperçu: *Dimension:* grande; *Envergure:* locale; fondée en 1975 surveillé par United Way of Canada - Centraide Canada

Mission: To maximize financial & volunteer resources in order to promote mutual aid, social commitment, & self-reliance as effective means of improving the quality of life of the community, & especially of its neediest members

Membre(s) du bureau directeur:
Lili-Anna Peresa, Présidente et Directrice générale

Centraide Duplessis
#101, 185, rue Napoléon, Sept-Iles QC G4R 4R7

Tél: 418-962-2011
Courriel: administration@centraideduplessis.org
www.centraideduplessis.org
www.facebook.com/centraide.duplessis

Aperçu: *Dimension:* petite; *Envergure:* locale surveillé par United Way of Canada - Centraide Canada

Membre(s) du bureau directeur:
Denis Miousse, Directeur général
direction@centraideduplessis.org

Centraide Estrie
1150, rue Belvédère sud, Sherbrooke QC J1H 4C7

Tél: 819-569-9281; *Téléc:* 819-569-5195
Courriel: reception.centraide@qc.aibn.com
www.centraideestrie.com
www.facebook.com/Centraide-Estrie-177152949010458
www.youtube.com/channel/UCM2Tm-5MS5gAIJ4UWEfg5jA

Aperçu: *Dimension:* petite; *Envergure:* locale; Organisme sans but lucratif; fondée en 1975 surveillé par United Way of Canada - Centraide Canada

Mission: Vise à soutenir les organismes bénévoles et communautaires engagés directement auprès des clientèles les plus démunies et vulnérables

Membre(s) du bureau directeur:
Claude Forgues, Directeur général
centraide_estrie@qc.aibn.com

Centraide Gaspésie Iles-de-la-Madeleine
#216, 230, rte du Parc, Sainte-Anne-des-Monts QC G4V 2C4

Tél: 418-763-2171
Courriel: mejcentraide@globetrotter.net
www.centraidegim.ca
www.facebook.com/centraide.gaspesie

Aperçu: *Dimension:* petite; *Envergure:* locale; fondée en 1988 surveillé par United Way of Canada - Centraide Canada

Mission: Soulager la misère et la souffrance humaine
Membre(s) du bureau directeur:
Stéphan Boucher, Directeur général

Centraide Gatineau-Labelle-Hautes-Laurentides
CP 154, 343, rue de la Madone, Mont-Laurier QC J9L 3G9
Tél: 819-623-4090; *Téléc:* 819-623-7646
Courriel: bureau@centraideglhl.ca
www.maregioncentraide.com
www.facebook.com/Centraide.Gatineau.Labelle.Hautes.Laurentides
Aperçu: Dimension: moyenne; *Envergure:* locale; fondée en 1985
surveillé par United Way of Canada - Centraide Canada
Membre(s) du bureau directeur:
Laure Voilquin, Directrice générale

Centraide Haute-Côte-Nord/Manicouagan
#301, 858, rue de Puyjalon, Baie-Comeau QC G5C 1N1
Tél: 418-589-5567; *Téléc:* 418-295-2567
www.centraidehcnmanicouagan.ca
Nom précédent: Centraide Côte-Nord/Secteur ouest
Aperçu: Dimension: moyenne; *Envergure:* locale; Organisme sans but
lucratif surveillé par United Way of Canada - Centraide Canada
Membre(s) du bureau directeur:
Carole Lemieux, Directrice générale

Centraide KRTB-Côte-du-Sud
100, 4e av, La Pocatière QC G0R 1Z0
Tél: 418-856-5105; *Téléc:* 418-856-4385
Courriel: centraideportage@bellnet.ca
www.facebook.com/CentraideKrtbCoteDuSud
Nom précédent: Centraide Portage-Taché
Aperçu: Dimension: petite; *Envergure:* locale surveillé par United Way
of Canada - Centraide Canada
Mission: D'aider les gens, d'affecter les ressources en fonction des
besoins, d'améliorer la qualité de vie de chacun et de renforcer le
soutien communautaire
Membre(s) du bureau directeur:
Sylvain Roy, Directeur général

Centraide Lanaudière
674, rue St-Louis, Joliette QC J6E 2Z6
Tél: 450-752-1999
www.centraide-lanaudiere.com
www.facebook.com/275362692481275
Aperçu: Dimension: moyenne; *Envergure:* locale; Organisme sans but
lucratif; fondée en 1977 surveillé par United Way of Canada - Centraide
Canada
Mission: Promouvoir l'entraide, le partage et l'engagement bénévole et
communautaire
Membre de: Centraide Canada
Membre(s) du bureau directeur:
Nicole Campeau, Directrice générale

Centraide Laurentides
#107, 880, Michèle-Bohec, Blainville QC J7C 5E2
Tél: 450-436-1584; *Téléc:* 450-951-2772
www.centraidelaurentides.org
www.facebook.com/CentraideLaurentides
twitter.com/CentraideLauren
www.youtube.com/user/centraidelaurentides
Aperçu: Dimension: petite; *Envergure:* locale; Organisme sans but
lucratif; fondée en 1962 surveillé par United Way of Canada - Centraide
Canada
Mission: Contribuer, par la promotion du partage et de l'engagement
bénévole et communautaire, à la construction d'une société d'entraide
vouée à l'amélioration de la qualité de vie des personnes en difficulté
Membre(s) du bureau directeur:
Suzanne M. Piché, Directrice générale, 450-436-1584 Ext. 225
spiche@centraidelaurentides.org

Centraide Mauricie
90, Des Casernes, Trois-Rivières QC G9A 1X2
Tél: 819-374-6207; *Téléc:* 819-374-6857
Courriel: centraide.mauricie@centraidemauricie.ca
www.centraidemauricie.ca
www.linkedin.com/company/centraide-mauricie
www.facebook.com/centraide.mauricie
twitter.com/centraidem

Aperçu: Dimension: petite; *Envergure:* locale; Organisme sans but
lucratif; fondée en 1956 surveillé par United Way of Canada - Centraide
Canada
Mission: Travailler à un changement social pour une société plus
juste, plus humaine et plus démocratique à travers la promotion de
l'entraide, la solidarité et l'engagement bénévole afin de répondre aux
besoins socio-économiques de notre communauté.
Membre de: Assemblée des Centraide du Québec
Membre(s) du bureau directeur:
Julie Colbert, Directrice générale, 819-374-6207 Ext. 227
julie.colbert@centraidemauricie.ca

Centraide Outaouais
74, boul. Montclair, Gatineau QC J8Y 2E7
Tél: 819-771-7751; *Téléc:* 819-771-0301
Ligne sans frais: 800-325-7751
Courriel: information@centraideoutaouais.com
www.centraideoutaouais.com
www.facebook.com/CentraideOutaouais
twitter.com/CentraidOuais
www.youtube.com/user/centraideoutaouais
Nom précédent: Centraide de l'ouest québécois
Aperçu: Dimension: moyenne; *Envergure:* locale; Organisme sans but
lucratif; fondée en 1944 surveillé par United Way of Canada -
Centraide Canada
Mission: Mobiliser le gens et rassembler les ressources pour
améliorer la qualité de vie de personnes plus vulnérables et contribuer
au développement de collectivités solidaires
Membre(s) du bureau directeur:
Nathalie Lepage, Directrice générale
lepagen@centraideoutaouais.com

Centraide Québec
#101, 3100, av du Bourg-Royal, Québec QC G1C 5S7
Tél: 418-660-2100; *Téléc:* 418-660-2111
Courriel: centraide@centraide-quebec.com
www.centraide-quebec.com
www.linkedin.com/company/centraide-qu-bec-et-chaudi-re-appalaches
www.facebook.com/centraidequebec
twitter.com/CentraideQc
www.youtube.com/user/CentraideQuebec
Aperçu: Dimension: moyenne; *Envergure:* locale; Organisme sans but
lucratif; fondée en 1945 surveillé par United Way of Canada - Centraide
Canada
Mission: Levées de fonds et attribution de subventions à 166
organismes communautaires pour aider les personnes les plus
démunies
Membre(s) du bureau directeur:
Bruno Marchand, Président/Directeur général

Centraide Richelieu-Yamaska
320, av de la Concorde nord, Saint-Hyacinthe QC J2S 4N7
Tél: 450-773-6679; *Téléc:* 450-773-4734
Ligne sans frais: 844-773-6679
Courriel: bureau@centraidery.org
www.centraidery.org
www.facebook.com/Centraiderichelieuyamaska
twitter.com/centraidery
Aperçu: Dimension: petite; *Envergure:* locale surveillé par United Way
of Canada - Centraide Canada
Mission: D'améliorer les conditions de vie des plus démuni(e)s de son
territoire
Membre(s) du bureau directeur:
Daniel Laplante, Directeur général
dan.laplante@centraidery.org

Centraide Saguenay-Lac St-Jean
#107, 475, boul. Talbot, Chicoutimi QC G7H 4A3
Tél: 418-543-3131; *Téléc:* 418-543-0665
Courriel: info@centraideslsj.ca
www.centraidesaglac.ca
Aperçu: Dimension: moyenne; *Envergure:* locale; Organisme sans but
lucratif; fondée en 1978 surveillé par United Way of Canada - Centraide
Canada
Mission: Rassembler et développer des ressources financières et
bénévoles afin d'aider les diverses communautés du
Saguenay-Lac-St-Jean à organiser et à promouvoir l'entreaide,
l'engagement social et la prise en charge afin d'améliorer la qualité de

vie de sa collectivité et de ses membres les plus démunis et les plus vulnérables

Membre(s) du bureau directeur:
Martin St-Pierre, Directeur général
   martin.stpierre@centraideslsj.ca
Johanne Bouchard, Secrétaire

Centraide sud-ouest du Québec
#161, 11 rue de l'Église, Salaberry-de-Valleyfield QC J6T 1J5
Tél: 450-371-2061; *Téléc:* 450-377-2309
Courriel: centraide@oricom.ca
www.centraidesudouest.org
www.facebook.com/195796617125646

Aperçu: *Dimension:* moyenne; *Envergure:* locale; Organisme sans but lucratif; fondée en 1982 surveillé par United Way of Canada - Centraide Canada
Mission: Grâce à votre don, il y a du changement possible. En effet, la misère qu'elle soit physique, morale, psychologique ou matérielle peut toucher tout le monde, peu importe la classe sociale. Donner à Centraide Sud-Ouest, c'est susciter un changement positif dans notre communauté
Membre(s) du bureau directeur:
Steve Hickey, Directeur général

Centre de réadaptation Constance-Lethbridge (CRCL) / Constance Lethbridge Rehabilitation Centre
7005, boul de Maisonneuve Ouest, Montréal QC H4B 1T3
Tél: 514-487-1770
Ligne sans frais: 866-487-1891
www.constance-lethbridge.qc.ca
www.linkedin.com/company/centre-de-readaptation-constance-lethbridge-r
www.facebook.com/ConstanceLethbridge

Aperçu: *Dimension:* moyenne; *Envergure:* locale; fondée en 1945 surveillé par Easter Seals Canada
Mission: Offrir des services spécialisés et ultraspécialisés à des adultes ayant une déficience motrice, en externe ou à domicile, de réadaptation, d'adaptation, de préparation et de support à l'intégration sociale ou professionnelle aux clientèles ayant des problèmes orthopédiques, neurologiques et rhumatologiques; offrir aussi une expertise d'évaluation de la conduite automobile, d'évaluation et d'orientation des capacités de travail de la personne handicapée
Affiliation(s): Confédération québécoise des centres d'hébergement et de réadaptation
Publications:
• Centre de réadaptation Constance-Lethbridge rapport annuel
Type: Rapport; *Frequency:* Annuel

Centre Montérégien de réadaptation (CMR)
5300, ch. de Chambly, Saint-Hubert QC J3Y 3N7
Tél: 450-676-7447; *Téléc:* 450-676-0047
Ligne sans frais: 800-667-4369; *TTY:* 450-676-9841
Autres numéros: ATME sans frais: 1-866-676-1411
Courriel: 16cmr@ssss.gouv.qc.ca
www.cmrmonteregie.ca

Aperçu: *Dimension:* petite; *Envergure:* locale; fondée en 1991
Mission: Pour aider à la réhabilitation des personnes handicapées physiques et les troubles du langage
Membre(s) du bureau directeur:
Eve Morrisette, Présidente
Hélène Duval, Directrice générale, 450-676-7447 Ext. 2400

La coopérative de Solidarité de Répit et d'Etraide (COOP SORE)
170, rue des Épinettes, Morin-Heights QC J0R 1H0
Tél: 450-226-2466; *Téléc:* 450-226-2211
Courriel: sore@cgocable.ca
coopsore.org

Aperçu: *Dimension:* petite; *Envergure:* locale; Organisme sans but lucratif
Mission: De créer une communauté de soignants où les idées et les informations sont fournies afin d'apporter de nouveaux éléments à leur emploi en aidant les personnes âgées
Membre(s) du bureau directeur:
Nicole Poirier, Présidente
Claire Lefebvre, Coordonnatrice

Head & Hands / A deux mains
5833, rue Sherbrooke ouest, Montréal QC H4A 1X4
Tel: 514-481-0277; *Fax:* 514-481-2336
e-mail: info@headandhands.ca
www.headandhands.ca
www.facebook.com/headandhands
twitter.com/headandhands
www.youtube.com/user/HeadandHands

Overview: A small local charitable organization founded in 1970
Mission: Medical, social, and legal services with an approach that is harm-reductive, holistic, and non-judgmental.
Chief Officer(s):
Jon McPhedran Waitzer, Director
   admin@headandhands.ca
Juniper Belshaw, Contact, Fundraising and Development
   membres@headandhands.ca

Mouvement contre le viol et l'inceste (MCVI)
CP 50009, Succ. Jarry, Montréal QC H2P 0A1
Tél: 514-278-9383; *Téléc:* 514-278-9385
Courriel: mcvi@contreleviol.org
www.mcvicontreleviol.org
www.facebook.com/mcvicontreleviol

Aperçu: *Dimension:* petite; *Envergure:* locale; Organisme sans but lucratif; fondée en 1976
Mission: Contrer la violence sexuelle dont sont victimes les femmes et les enfants
Affiliation(s): Regroupement québécois des Centre d'aide et de lutte contre les agressions à caractère sexuel

Viol-secours inc.
3293 - 1e av, Québec QC G1L 3R2
Tél: 418-522-2120; *Téléc:* 418-522-2130
Courriel: info@violsecours.qc.ca
www.violsecours.qc.ca

Aperçu: *Dimension:* petite; *Envergure:* locale; Organisme sans but lucratif; fondée en 1976
Mission: Venir en aide à toute femme, adolescente ou enfant ayant subi une situation d'agression à caractère sexuel en offrant divers services: intervention téléphonique, accompagnement médico-légal et juridique, suivi individuel et de groupe
Affiliation(s): Regroupement québécois des CALACS

SASKATCHEWAN

Battlefords United Way Inc.
#203, 891 - 99th St., North Battleford SK S9A 0N8
Tel: 306-445-1717
e-mail: buw@sasktel.net
www.battlefordsunitedway.ca

Overview: A small local charitable organization founded in 1967 overseen by United Way of Canada - Centraide Canada
Mission: To improve lives & build community by engaging individuals & mobilizing collective action
Chief Officer(s):
Brendon Boothman, Chair
Jana Blais, Treasurer

Swift Current United Way
Swift Current Business Centre, 145 1st Ave. NE, Swift Current SK S9H 2B1
Tel: 306-773-4828
e-mail: unitedway@sasktel.net
www.swiftcurrentunitedway.ca
www.facebook.com/swiftunitedway
twitter.com/swiftunitedway
www.instagram.com/swiftunitedway

Overview: A small local organization overseen by United Way of Canada - Centraide Canada
Mission: To strengthen the social & economic conditions of the community; To improve the lives of all residents of Swift Current & Southern Saskatchewan
Chief Officer(s):
Stacey Schwartz, Executive Director

United Way of Estevan
PO Box 611, Estevan SK S4A 2A5

Tel: 306-634-7375
e-mail: admin@unitedwayestevan.com
www.unitedwayofestevan.com
www.facebook.com/unitedwayestevan
twitter.com/uwestevan

Overview: A small local organization founded in 1967 overseen by United Way of Canada - Centraide Canada
Mission: To strengthen the community
Chief Officer(s):
Christa Morhart, President

United Way of Regina
1440 Scarth St., Regina SK S4R 2E9

Tel: 306-757-5671; *Fax:* 306-522-7199
www.unitedwayregina.ca
www.facebook.com/UnitedWayRegina
twitter.com/unitedwayregina
www.instagram.com/unitedwayregina

Overview: A small local charitable organization founded in 1935 overseen by United Way of Canada - Centraide Canada
Mission: To mobilize individuals, agencies & resources to improve lives & strengthen the community
Chief Officer(s):
Robyn Edwards-Bentz, CEO
    redwardsbentz@unitedwayregina.ca
Tanya Murray, Director, Operations
    tmurray@unitedwayregina.ca

United Way of Saskatoon & Area
#100, 506 - 25 St. East, Saskatoon SK S7K 4A7

Tel: 306-975-7700
e-mail: office@unitedwaysaskatoon.ca
www.unitedwaysaskatoon.ca
www.facebook.com/UnitedWaySaskatoonAndArea
twitter.com/UnitedWayStoon

Overview: A small local organization overseen by United Way of Canada - Centraide Canada
Mission: To improve social conditions & build a strong community
Chief Officer(s):
Jocelyn Zurakowski, Interim CEO

Weyburn & District United Way
PO Box 608, Weyburn SK S4H 2K7

www.weyburnunitedway.com
Overview: A small local charitable organization overseen by United Way of Canada - Centraide Canada
Mission: To improve lives & strengthen the community
Chief Officer(s):
Sandra Alexander, Executive Director

Yorkton & District United Way Inc.
180 Broadway St. West, #A, Yorkton SK S3N 0M6
Overview: A small local charitable organization founded in 1982 overseen by United Way of Canada - Centraide Canada
Mission: To unite & facilitate community fundraising; To strengthen the community

International Associations

Africa Inland Mission International (Canada) (AIM) / Mission à l'intérieur de l'Afrique (Canada)
1641 Victoria Park Ave., Toronto ON M1R 1P8

Tel: 416-751-6077; *Fax:* 416-751-3467
Toll-Free: 877-407-6077
ca.aimint.org
www.facebook.com/aimcanada
twitter.com/aimcan

Also Known As: AIM Canada
Overview: A medium-sized international charitable organization founded in 1895
Mission: To evangelize within Eastern & Central Africa & Islands around India Ocean; To establish churches; To provide training leadership for those churches; To provide medical, educational, & agricultural services
Member of: Africa Inland Mission International, Bristol, England; Interdenominational Foreign Mission Association

American Academy of Neurology (AAN)
201 Chicago Ave., Minneapolis MN 55415 USA

Tel: 612-928-6000; *Fax:* 612-454-2746
Toll-Free: 800-879-1960
e-mail: memberservices@aan.com
www.aan.com
www.linkedin.com/groups/2386034
www.facebook.com/AmericanAcademyofNeurology
twitter.com/AANMember
www.youtube.com/AANChannel

Overview: A large international organization
Mission: To advance the art & science of neurology; To promote the best possible care for patients with neurological disorders
Chief Officer(s):
Catherine M. Rydell, Executive Director & CEO
    crydell@aan.com
Jason Kopinski, Deputy Executive Director
    jkopinski@aan.com
Timothy Engel, Chief Financial Officer
    tengel@aan.com
Angela Babb, Chief Communications Officer
    ababb@aan.com
Chris Becker, Chief Business Development Officer
    cbecker@aan.com
Lynee Koester, Project Manager, Health Policy
    lkoester@aan.com
Publications:
• AANnews [a publication of the American Academy of Neurology]
Type: Newsletter; *Frequency:* Monthly; *Price:* Free with American Academy of Neurology membership
Profile: American Academy of Neurology & practice information
• American Academy of Neurology Patient Education Series
Type: Books
Profile: Information & treatment options for patients & caregivers
• Continuum: Lifelong Learning in Neurology
 Frequency: Bimonthly; *Editor:* Steven L. Lewis, MD
Profile: A self-study continuing medical education publication
• Neurology
Type: Journal; *Editor:* Robert A. Gross, MD, PhD, FAAN
Profile: The official scientific journal of the American Academy of Neurology, directed to physicians concerned with diseases & conditions of the nervous system
• Neurology Now
Type: Magazine; *Frequency:* Bimonthly
Profile: Updated & important information for neurology patients, families, & caregivers
• Neurology Today
Type: Newspaper; *Frequency:* Biweekly
Profile: Clinical, policy, research, & practice news, for neurologists

American Industrial Hygiene Association (AIHA)
#777, 3141 Fairview Park Dr., Falls Church VA 22042 USA

Tel: 703-849-8888; *Fax:* 703-207-3561
www.aiha.org
www.linkedin.com/company/aiha
www.facebook.com/aihaglobal
twitter.com/AIHA
www.youtube.com/user/IHValue

Overview: A medium-sized international organization founded in 1939
Mission: To serve the needs of occupational & environmental health professionals; To achieve high professional standards; To promote certification of industrial hygienists
Chief Officer(s):
Lawrence Sloan, Chief Executive Officer
Publications:
• American Industrial Hygiene Association Member Directory
Type: Directory
• Journal of Occupational & Environmental Hygiene
Type: Journal; *Accepts Advertising*; *Editor:* Mark Nicas
Profile: A peer-reviewed publication to enhance the knowledge & practice of occupational & environmental hygiene & safety
• The Synergist
Type: Magazine; *Frequency:* Monthly; *Accepts Advertising*; *Editor:* Ed Rutkowski
Profile: Information about the occupational & environmental health & safety fields & the industrial hygiene profession, including industry trends, government activities, technical information, &association news

American Medical Association
330 North Wabash Ave., Chicago IL 60610-5885 USA
Tel: 312-464-4430
Toll-Free: 800-621-8335
www.ama-assn.org
www.linkedin.com/groups?home=&gid=76194
www.facebook.com/AmericanMedicalAssociation
twitter.com/AmerMedicalAssn
plus.google.com/107410187242660838577
Overview: A large international organization founded in 1847
Chief Officer(s):
James L. Madara, Exec. Vice President & CEO
Publications:
• JAMA [The Journal of the American Medical Association]
Type: Journal

American Society for Parenteral & Enteral Nutrition (ASPEN)
#412, 8630 Fenton St., Silver Spring MD 20910 USA
Tel: 301-587-6315; *Fax:* 301-587-2365
e-mail: aspen@nutritioncare.org
www.nutritioncare.org
www.linkedin.com/company/american-society-for-parenteral-&-enteral-nut
www.facebook.com/nutritioncare.org
twitter.com/aspenweb
Overview: A medium-sized international organization founded in 1976
Mission: To advance the science & practice of nutrition support therapy; To improve patient care
Chief Officer(s):
Debra BenAvram, Chief Executive Officer
debrab@nutritioncare.org
Colleen Harper, Chief Operating Officer
colleenh@nutritioncare.org
Fatema Gharzai, Director, Membership & Marketing
fatemag@nutritioncare.org
Publications:
• Journal of Parenteral & Enteral Nutrition
Type: Journal; *Frequency:* Bimonthly; *Accepts Advertising*; *Price:* Free with membership in the American Society for Parenteral & EnteralNutrition
Profile: Original peer-reviewed studies about basic & clinical research in the field of nutrition & metabolic support
• Nutrition in Clinical Practice
Type: Journal; *Frequency:* Bimonthly; *Accepts Advertising*; *Price:* Free with membership in the American Society for Parenteral & Enteral Nutrition
Profile: Multidisciplinary peer-reviewed articles for the clinical practice professional

American Society of Neuroradiology (ASNR)
#205, 800 Enterprise Dr., Oak Brook IL 60523 USA
Tel: 630-574-0220; *Fax:* 630-574-0661
www.asnr.org
www.facebook.com/TheASNR
twitter.com/TheASNR
Overview: A medium-sized international organization
Mission: To develop standards for the training & practice of neuroradiologists; To promote understanding of neuroradiology among patients & other professionals & public agencies
Chief Officer(s):
Mary Beth Hepp, Executive Director & CEO
Angelo Artemakis, Director, Communications
aartemakis@asnr.org
Ken Cammarata, Director, Specialty Societies & Member Services
kcammarata@asnr.org
Tina Cheng, Director, Finance & Information Systems
Publications:
• American Journal of Neuroradiology
Type: Journal; *Frequency:* 10 pa; *Number of Pages:* 200
Profile: Peer-reviewed original research papers, review articles, & technical notes

American Society of Plastic Surgeons (ASPS)
444 East Algonquin Rd., Arlington Heights IL 60005 USA
Tel: 847-228-9900
e-mail: media@plasticsurgery.org
www.plasticsurgery.org
www.facebook.com/PlasticSurgeryASPS
twitter.com/ASPS_News
Overview: A medium-sized international organization founded in 1931
Mission: To advance quality care to plastic surgery patients; To promote high standards of training, professionalism, ethics, physician practice, & research
Affiliation(s): Plastic Surgery Educational Foundation (PSEF)
Chief Officer(s):
Debra Johnson, President
Michael D. Costelloe, Executive Vice-President
Heather Gates, Director, Communications
Publications:
• Plastic & Reconstructive Surgery: Journal of the American Society of Plastic Surgeons
Type: Journal; *Frequency:* Monthly; *Editor:* Rod J. Rohrich, M.D.; *ISSN:* 0032-1052

American Society of Regional Anesthesia & Pain Medicine (ASRA)
#401, 4 Penn Center West, Pittsburgh PA 15276 USA
Tel: 412-471-2718
Toll-Free: 855-795-2772
e-mail: asraassistant@asra.com
www.asra.com
www.linkedin.com/groups?gid=4797719
www.facebook.com/228281927234196
twitter.com/asra_society
Overview: A medium-sized international organization founded in 1923
Mission: To assure excellence in patient care utilizing regional anesthesia & pain medicine; To investigate the scientific basis of the specialty
Chief Officer(s):
Oscar De Leon-Casasola, President
Angie Stengel, Executive Director
astengel@asra.com
Publications:
• ASRA [American Society of Regional Anesthesia & Pain Medicine] News
Type: Newsletter; *Frequency:* Quarterly; *Editor:* Colin McCartney, M.B., F.R.C.A.
Profile: Society news, articles, & meeting reviews
• ASRA [American Society of Regional Anesthesia & Pain Medicine] E-News
Type: Newsletter
Profile: Society announcements, including information about meetings, workshops, awards
• Regional Anesthesia & Pain Medicine
Type: Journal; *Frequency:* Bimonthly; *Editor:* Joseph M. Neal, M.D.
Profile: Peer-reviewed scientific & clinical studies

Association of Telehealth Service Providers (ATSP)
#400, 4702 SW Scholls Ferry Rd., Portland OR 97225-2008 USA
Tel: 503-922-0988; *Fax:* 315-222-2402
www.atsp.org
Overview: A small international organization founded in 1996
Mission: To improve health care through growth of the telehealth industry
Chief Officer(s):
William Engle, Executive Director

Canadian Physicians for Aid & Relief (CPAR)
1425 Bloor St. West, Toronto ON M6P 3L6
Tel: 416-369-0865; *Fax:* 416-369-0294
Toll-Free: 800-263-2727
e-mail: info@cpar.ca
www.cpar.ca
www.linkedin.com/company/canadian-physicians-for-aid-and-relief
www.facebook.com/cparcan
twitter.com/cpar
www.youtube.com/channel/UC_7_sOan_HyDiTpvn07BH3A
Overview: A large international charitable organization founded in 1984
Mission: To help impoverished communities in developing nations become prosperous, while maintaining harmony with the environment;

To tackle all aspects of poverty; To emphasize healthy community empowerment & integrated community based development; To achieve a world in which the basic needs of all individuals & communities are met

Member of: Ontario Council for International Cooperation
Chief Officer(s):
Dusanka Pavlica, Executive Director
Aruna Aysola, Director, Development & Communications
Kathy Johnston, Manager, Human Resources
   kjohnston@cpar.ca

Canadian Red Cross (CRC) / La Société la Croix-Rouge canadienne
170 Metcalfe St., Ottawa ON K2P 2P2
Tel: 613-740-1900; *Fax:* 613-740-1911
Toll-Free: 800-418-1111
e-mail: WeCare@redcross.ca
www.redcross.ca
www.facebook.com/canadianredcross
twitter.com/redcrossCanada
www.youtube.com/user/canadianredcross

Overview: A large international charitable organization founded in 1896
Mission: To help people deal with situations that threaten: their survival & safety, their security & well-being, their human dignity, in Canada & around the world; To improve the lives of vulnerable people by mobilizing the power of humanity
Member of: International Red Cross & Red Crescent Societies
Affliation(s): International Committee of the Red Cross; International Federation of Red Cross & Red Crescent Societies (Geneva)
Chief Officer(s):
Conrad Sauvé, Secretary General & Chief Executive Officer
Jimmy Mui, Chief Financial Officer
Samuel Schwisberg, General Counsel & Corporate Secretary
Publications:
• Be Ready, Be Safe
Type: Booklet; *Number of Pages:* 60; *ISBN:* 978-1-55104-506-1
Profile: An activity booklet for 12 & 13 year old children
• Bug Out Activity Booklet: Get the Facts on Germs
Type: Booklet
Profile: Booklets for ages 6 to 8, 9 to 11, & 12 to 13, plus a family guide for ages 4 to 13
• Bug Out Facilitator Guide: Get the Facts on Germs
Type: Guide
Profile: Booklets for educators & caregivers of children from ages 6 to 8, 9 to 11, & 12 to 13
• Canadian Red Cross Society Annual Report
Type: Yearbook; *Frequency:* Annually
Profile: A review of Canadian & international disaster management, health & homecare services, humanitarian issues, donations, & financial information
• Canadian Red Cross Society: Working to Serve Humanity 2010-2015
Type: Report; *Number of Pages:* 20
Profile: A strategic plan for the future
• Drowning Research: Water Safety Poll
Type: Survey; *ISBN:* 0
Profile: Canadian parents concerned about safety in backyard pools
• Expect the Unexpected Facilitator's Guide
Type: Guide
Profile: Guides for educators using the Emergency Preparedness Program with students aged 7 to 8, 9 to 11, & 12 to 13
• Facing Fear: Helping Young People Deal with Terrorism & Tragic Events
Type: Guide; *ISBN:* 1-55104-277-0
Profile: Booklets with activities & lesson plans for students aged 5 to 7, 8 to 10, 11 to 13, & 14 to 16
• Facing the Unexpected, Be Prepared
Type: Booklet; *Number of Pages:* 44; *ISBN:* 978-1-55104-504-7
Profile: An activity booklet for children ages 10 & 11
• Integrating Emergency Management & High-Risk Populations: Survey Report & Action Recommendations
Type: Report; *Number of Pages:* 58
Profile: Prepared for Public Safety Canada by Canadian Red Cross
• It Can Happen, Be Ready
Type: Booklet; *Number of Pages:* 36; *ISBN:* 978-1-55104-502-3
Profile: An activity booklet for 7 & 8 year old children

• Let's Plan for The Unexpected
Type: Booklet; *Number of Pages:* 52; *ISBN:* 978-1-55104-508-5
Profile: An activity booklet for families
• Social Media During Emergencies
Type: Survey
Profile: Exploring how to use social media during an emergency
• Survive the Peace: Landmine Education & Community Involvement Guide
Type: Guide; *Number of Pages:* 54
Profile: Background information about the landmine crisis, learning activities, & ways to take action
• Your Emergency Preparedness Guide
Type: Guide; *Number of Pages:* 36
Profile: A publication from Public Safety Canada, in collaboration with the Canadian Red Cross, the Canadian Association of Chiefs of Police, the Canadian Association of Fire Chiefs, St. JohnAmbulance, & The Salvation Army, available in print, audio, Braille, large print, diskette, & CD

Atlantic Zone Office
Burnside Industrial Park, 133 Troop Ave., Dartmouth NS B3B 2A7
Tel: 902-423-3680; *Fax:* 902-422-6247

Division du Québec
6, place du Commerce, Verdun QC H3E 1P4
Tél: 514-362-2930; *Téléc:* 514-362-9991
Chief Officer(s):
Michel Léveillé, Directeur

Ontario Zone Office
5700 Cancross Ct., Mississauga ON L5R 3E9
Tel: 905-890-1000
Toll-Free: 877-356-3226

Western Zone Office
#100, 1305 - 11 Ave. SW, Calgary AB T3C 3P6
Tel: 403-541-6100; *Fax:* 403-541-6129

Canadian Society for International Health (CSIH) / Société canadienne de la santé internationale
#726, 1 Nicholas St., Ottawa ON K1N 7B7
Tel: 613-241-5785
e-mail: csih@csih.org
www.csih.org
www.linkedin.com/groups/CSIH-Global-Health-Forum-3671985
www.facebook.com/CSIH.org
twitter.com/globalsante

Previous Name: Canadian Society for Tropical Medicine & International Health
Overview: A medium-sized international charitable organization founded in 1977
Mission: To promote international health & development through mobilization of Canadian resources; To advocate & facilitate research, education, & service activities in international health; To further Canadian strengths of progressive health policy & programming in all fields where global & domestic health concerns meet; To contribute to the evolving global understanding of health & development
Member of: Canadian Coalition for Global Health Research
Chief Officer(s):
Kate Dickson, Co-Chair
L. Duncan Saunders, Co-Chair
Eva Slawecki, Acting Director, 613-241-5785 Ext. 325
Publications:
• Synergy Online
Type: Newsletter; *Frequency:* Monthly
Profile: International health & development information, news bulletins, awards, conference information, & job listings

Collaboration Santé Internationale (CSI)
1001, ch de la Canardière, Québec QC G1J 5G5
Tél: 418-522-6065; *Téléc:* 418-522-5530
Courriel: csi@csiquebec.org
www.csiquebec.org
www.facebook.com/csiquebec

Aperçu: *Dimension:* grande; *Envergure:* internationale; Organisme sans but lucratif; fondée en 1968
Mission: Soutenir nos Canadiens impliqués dans les dispensaires et les hôpitaux des pays en voie de développement en leur fournissant le matériel de travail; recueillir, sélectionner, et expédier dans les pays du

tiers-monde, par l'intermédiaire de Canadiens qui oeuvrent dans le domaine de la santé, des médicaments et de l'équipement médical et hospitalier; parrainer des projets de construction et d'aménagement de dispensaires et d'hôpitaux et soutenir des équipes de médecins et de techniciens spécialisés dans le domaine de la santé publique
Membre de: Association Québecoise des Organismes de Coopération Internationale; Conseil Canadien pour la Coopération Internationale; Canadian International Development Agency
Membre(s) du bureau directeur:
Stéphane Galibois, Président
Publications:
• Bulletin de Collaboration Santé Internationale
Type: Bulletin; *Frequency:* semi-annuel; *Price:* Free

Confederation of Meningitis Organizations
Newminster House, Baldwin St., Bristol BS1 1LT UK
Tel: 44-333-405-6264
e-mail: info@comomeningitis.org
www.comomeningitis.org
www.facebook.com/ConfederationOfMeningitisOrganisations
twitter.com/COMOmeningitis
www.youtube.com/user/COMOmeningitis
Overview: A small international organization
Mission: To prevent meningitis & to lessen the impact of the disease worldwide through education & advocacy
Chief Officer(s):
Chris Head, President

Disabled Peoples' International (DPI) / Organisation mondiale des personnes handicapées
PO Box 70073, Stn. Place Bell, 160 Elgin St., Ottawa ON K2P 2M3
www.dpi.org
Overview: A small international charitable organization founded in 1981
Mission: To promote the human rights of disabled people through full participation, equalization of opportunity & development
Affliation(s): United Nations; International Labour Organization
Chief Officer(s):
Rachel Kachaje, Chair
rachel.kachaje@dpi.org

Healthcare Information & Management Systems Society (HIMSS)
#1700, 33 West Monroe St., Chicago IL 60603-5616 USA
Tel: 312-664-4467; Fax: 312-664-6143
www.himss.org
www.linkedin.com/company/himss
www.facebook.com/HIMSSpage
twitter.com/himss
www.youtube.com/himss
Overview: A large international organization
Mission: To provide worldwide leadership in the optimal use of healthcare information technology & management systems in order to improve healthcare
Chief Officer(s):
Sebastian Krolop, Chair
H. Stephen Lieber, President & Chief Executive Officer
slieber@himss.org
Blain Newton, Executive Vice-President
blain.newton@himssanalytics.org
Carla Smith, Executive Vice-President
csmith@himss.org
John Whelan, Executive Vice-President, Media
john.whelan@himssmedia.com
Publications:
• The Digital Office
Type: Newsletter; *Frequency:* Monthly; *Price:* Free with HIMSS membership
Profile: Information about health information technology & electronic medical records
• Financial Edge
Type: Newsletter; *Frequency:* Monthly; *Price:* Free with HIMSS membership
Profile: HIMSS' financial systems e-newsletter, with current issues & trends related to financial systems & other technologies in healthcare
• Healthcare IT News
Type: Newspaper; *Frequency:* Monthly; *Price:* Free with HIMSS membership

Profile: Features the HIMSS Insider newsletter, plus information about advocacy, education, & HIMSS happenings
• HIMSS [Healthcare Information & Management Systems Society] Weekly Insider
Type: Newsletter; *Frequency:* Weekly; *Price:* Free with HIMSS membership
Profile: Current news from HIMSS, member profiles, & interviews
• HIMSS [Healthcare Information & Management Systems Society] Conference Proceedings
Frequency: Annually
Profile: Proceedings from the annual HIMSS conference & exhibition
• HIMSS [Healthcare Information & Management Systems Society] Clinical Informatics Insights
Type: Newsletter; *Frequency:* Monthly; *Price:* Free with HIMSS membership
Profile: Comprehensive articles about informatics across the continuum of care
• HIMSS [Healthcare Information & Management Systems Society] Pulse on Public Policy
Type: Newsletter; *Frequency:* Monthly; *Price:* Free with HIMSS membership
Profile: Information for HIMSS members, policymakers, regulators, & interested stakeholders
• HIMSS [Healthcare Information & Management Systems Society] HIELights
Type: Newsletter; *Frequency:* Monthly; *Price:* Free with HIMSS membership
Profile: Issues pertaining to health information exchange & regional health information organizations
• Journal of Healthcare Information Management
Type: Journal; *Frequency:* Quarterly; *Accepts Advertising*; *Price:* Free with HIMSS membership
Profile: Peer-reviewed journal for healthcare information & management systems professionals

Human Anatomy & Physiology Society (HAPS)
PO Box 2945, 251 S.L. White Blvd., LaGrange GA 30241-2945 USA
Tel: 800-448-4277; Fax: 706-883-8215
e-mail: info@hapsconnect.org
www.hapsweb.org
www.linkedin.com/groups/972787
twitter.com/humanaandpsoc
Overview: A medium-sized international organization
Mission: To promote excellence in the teaching of human anatomy & physiology
Chief Officer(s):
Terry Thompson, President
tthompson@hapsconnect.org
Peter English, Executive Director
peter@hapsconnect.org
Brittney Roberts, Coordinator, Membership
Publications:
• HAPS [Human Anatomy & Physiology Society] EDucator
Frequency: Quarterly
Profile: Teaching tips for anatomy & physiology instructors

Infectious Diseases Society of America (IDSA)
#300, 1300 Wilson Blvd., Arlington VA 22209 USA
Tel: 703-299-0200; Fax: 703-299-0204
e-mail: membership@idsociety.org
www.idsociety.org
www.linkedin.com/company/357844
www.facebook.com/IDSociety
twitter.com/idsinfo
www.flickr.com/photos/idsociety
Overview: A large international organization
Mission: To improve the health of individuals, communities, & society; To promote excellence in education, research, public health, prevention, & patient care
Chief Officer(s):
William G. Powderly, MD, FIDSA, President
Cynthia L. Sears, MD, FIDSA, Vice-President
Larry K. Pickering, MD, FIDSA, Secretary
Helen W. Boucher, MD, FIDSA, Treasurer
Publications:
• Clinical Infectious Diseases
Type: Journal

Profile: State-of-the-art clinical articles, medical & legal issues, review articles, & studies in infectious disease research

• IDSA [Infectious Diseases Society of America] News
Type: Newsletter
Profile: Society activities, education, research, & prevention & treatment advances

• Journal of Infectious Diseases
Type: Journal
Profile: Original research about the pathogenesis, diagnosis, & treatment of infectious diseases

International Association for Medical Assistance to Travellers (IAMAT)
#036, 67 Mowat Ave., Toronto ON M6K 3E3

Tel: 416-652-0137; *Fax:* 416-652-1983
www.iamat.org
www.facebook.com/IAMATHealth
twitter.com/IAMAT_Travel
www.flickr.com/photos/iamat_photo_contest/

Overview: A medium-sized international charitable organization founded in 1960
Mission: To make competent care available to the traveller around the world; to make direct grants to medical institutions
Member of: Foundation for the Support of International Medical Training (Canada)
Chief Officer(s):
Assunta Uffer-Marcolongo, President
Tullia Marcolongo, Director, Programs & Development
Nadia Sallete, Director, Membership Services

Guelph Office
2162 Gordon St., Guelph ON N1L 1G6

International Commission on Radiological Protection (ICRP)
280 Slater St., Ottawa ON K1P 5S9

Tel: 613-947-9750; *Fax:* 613-944-1920
e-mail: admin@icrp.org
www.icrp.org
www.facebook.com/ICRP1
twitter.com/ICRP

Overview: A small international charitable organization founded in 1928
Mission: To advance for the public benefit the science of radiological protection, in particular by providing recommendations & guidance on all aspects of protection against ionisary radiation
Chief Officer(s):
Christopher Clement, Scientific Secretary
sci.sec@icrp.org

International Confederation for Plastic Reconstructive & Aesthetic Surgery (IPRAS)
Zita Congress SA, PO Box 155, 1st km Peanias Markopoulou Ave, Peania Attica 190 02 Greece

Tel: (30) 211 100 1777; *Fax:* (30) 210 664 2216
e-mail: ipras@iprasmanagement.com
www.ipras.org
www.facebook.com/ipras.org

Overview: A large international organization founded in 1955
Mission: To promote plastic surgery both scientifically & clinically; To further education
Chief Officer(s):
Marita Eisenmann-Klein, President
Publications:
• Globalplast
Type: Newsletter; *Frequency:* Annually
• IPRAS [International Confederation for Plastic, Reconstructive & Aesthetic Surgery] Journal
Type: Journal

International Federation for Cell Biology (IFCB)

www.ifcbiol.org
Overview: A medium-sized international organization founded in 1972
Mission: To promote cooperation & to contribute to the advancement of cell biology in all its branches
Affliation(s): International Union of Biological Sciences; International Cell Research Organization
Chief Officer(s):
Nobutaka Hirokawa, President, Japan
hirokawa@m.u-tokyo.ac.jp

Hernandez F. Carvalho, Secretary General, Brazil
hern@unicamp.br

International Federation of Health Information Management Associations (IFHIMA)
c/o University of Erlangen-Nuremberg, DRG Controlling, Quality Mngmnt, Schwabachanlage 6, Erlangen D 91054 Germany

www.ifhima.org
Previous Name: International Federation of Health Records Organizations
Overview: A medium-sized international organization
Mission: To improve health/medical record practices in member countries; to be a forum for the exchange of information relating to health records & information technology
Member of: World Health Organization
Affliation(s): Canadian Health Record Association
Chief Officer(s):
Angelika Haendel, President
angelika.haendel@uk-erlangen.de

International Federation of Red Cross & Red Crescent Societies / Fédération Internationale des Sociétés de la Croix-Rouge & du Croissant-Rouge
PO Box 303, Geneva CH-1211 19 Switzerland

Tel: 41-22-730-42-22; *Fax:* 41-730-4200
www.ifrc.org
www.facebook.com/IFRC
twitter.com/Federation
www.youtube.com/user/ifrc

Overview: A small international organization founded in 1919
Mission: To provide assistance & relief operations without discrimination
Affliation(s): Canadian Red Cross Society
Chief Officer(s):
Tadateru Konoé, President
Elhadj As Sy, Secretary General

International Hospital Federation (IHF) / Fédération internationale des hôpitaux
P.A. Hôpital de Loëx, Route de Loëx 151, Bernex 1233 Switzerland

Tel: 41-22-850-94-20; *Fax:* 41-22-757-10-16
e-mail: info@ihf-fih.org
www.ihf-fih.org

Overview: A medium-sized international charitable organization founded in 1947
Mission: To provide the opportunity for exchange of information, education, experience relevant to the provision of high-quality health services in member countries; to promote modern management techniques to improve efficiency; to participate in & encourage research & experimentation in hospital & health service planning & management; to collect & disseminate international health service data; to serve as advocate for hospital & related health service organizations in world health affairs
Affliation(s): World Health Organization
Chief Officer(s):
Eric de Roodenbeke, CEO

International Institute of Concern for Public Health (IICPH)
PO Box 40017, 292 Dupont St., Toronto ON M5R 0A2

Tel: 905-906-6128
e-mail: info@concernforhealth.org
concernforhealth.org

Overview: A medium-sized international charitable organization founded in 1984
Mission: To engage in advocacy on health issues; to assist in promoting & protecting people in their work & living environment in Ontario; to provide expertise on health, scientific & environmental issues
Member of: Ontario Environment Network; Earth Appeal; Nuclear Waste Watch

International Medical Informatics Association (IMIA)
c/o Health On the Net, Chemin du Petit-Bel-Air 2, Chêne-Bourg, Geneva CH-1225 Switzerland

Tel: 41-22-3727249
e-mail: imia@imia-services.org
www.imia-medinfo.org
www.facebook.com/pages/IMIA/191053744240749
Overview: A small international organization founded in 1989

Mission: To promote informatics in health care & biomedical research; To advance international cooperation; To stimulate research, development & education; To disseminate & exchange information

Chief Officer(s):

Elaine Huesing, Chief Executive Officer
  elaine.huesing@shaw.ca

International Occupational Safety & Health Information Network / Centre international d'informations de sécurité et de santé au travail

International Labour Office/CIS, 4 route des Morillons, Geneva CH-1211 Switzerland

Tel: 41-22-799-61-11; *Fax:* 41-22-798-86-85
www.ilo.org/cis/

Also Known As: Centro Internacional de Informacion sobre Seguridad y Salud en el Trabajo

Overview: A small international organization founded in 1959

Mission: To collect & disseminate world information that can contribute to the prevention of occupational accidents & diseases

Affiliation(s): Canadian Centre for Occupational Health & Safety; Canada Safety Council; Institut de recherche en santé et en sécurité de travail - Québec

International Society for Environmental Epidemiology (ISEE)

c/o ISEE Secretariat, JSI Research & Training Institute, 44 Farnsworth St., Boston MA 2210 USA

Tel: 617-482-9485; *Fax:* 617-482-0617
www.iseepi.org

Overview: A small international organization founded in 1989

Mission: To provide a forum for the discussion of problems unique to the study of health & the environment, such as environmental exposures, health effects, methodology, environment-gene interactions, & ethics & law

Member of: International Society of Exposure Analysis

Chief Officer(s):

Verónica Vieira, Secretary-Treasurer
  vvieira@uci.edu
Francine Laden, President
  francine.laden@channing.harvard.edu
Francine Laden, Sec.-Treas.
  francine.laden@channing.harvard.edu

Publications:

• Epidemiology

Type: Journal; *Frequency:* Bimonthly; *Editor:* Allen J. Wilcox; *ISSN:* 1044-3983

Profile: A peer-reviewed scientific journal featuring original research on the full spectrum of epidemiologic topics

• International Society for Environmental Epidemiology Directory of Members

Type: Directory

Profile: Includes all ISEE members

International Society for Magnetic Resonance in Medicine (ISMRM)

#620, 2300 Clayton Rd., Concord CA 94520 USA

Tel: 510-841-1899; *Fax:* 510-841-2340
e-mail: info@ismrm.org
www.ismrm.org
www.linkedin.com/company/ismrm
www.facebook.com/ISMRM
twitter.com/ismrm

Previous Name: Society of Magnetic Resonance

Merged from: Society of Magnetic Resonance in Medicine; Society of Magnetic Resonance Imaging

Overview: A medium-sized international organization founded in 1994

Mission: To further the development & application of magnetic resonance techniques in medicine & biology; To promote research, development, & applications in the field

Chief Officer(s):

Roberta A. Kravitz, Executive Director
  roberta@ismrm.org
Kerry Crockett, Associate Executive Director
  kerry@ismrm.org
Candace Spradley, Director, Education
  candace@ismrm.org
Stephanie M. Haaf, Director, Membership & Study Groups
  stephanie@ismrm.org
Mariam Barzin, Director, Finance
  mariam@ismrm.org

Mary Keydash, Director, Marketing
  mary@ismrm.org
Anne-Marie Kahrovic, Director, Meetings
  anne-marie@ismrm.org
Kristina King, Registrar & Coordinator, Accounting
  kristina@ismrm.org

Publications:

• Journal of Magnetic Resonance Imaging

Type: Journal; *Editor:* Mark E. Schweitzer, MD

Profile: Basic & clinical research, plus educational & review articles related to the diagnostic applications of magnetic resonance

• Magnetic Resonance in Medicine

Type: Journal; *Editor:* Matt A. Bernstein

Profile: Original investigations concerned with the development & use of nuclear magnetic resonance & electron paramagnetic resonance techniques for medical applications

• MR Pulse

Type: Newsletter

Profile: Society updates & announcements

International Society for Telemedicine & eHealth

c/o AMTS Luzern, Luzerner Kantonsspital, Luzern 16 CH - 6000 Switzerland

e-mail: telemedicine@skynet.be
www.isft.net

Overview: A small international organization

Mission: To facilitate the international dissemination of knowledge & experience in telemedicine & e-health & to provide access to recognized experts in the field worldwide

Chief Officer(s):

Andy Fischer, President
  president@isfteh.org

International Society for the History of Medicine - Canadian Section (ISHM) / Société internationale d'histoire de la médecine (SIHM)

c/o Isabelle Perreault, Université d'Ottawa, Pavillon FSS, #14022, 120 Université, Ottawa ON K1N 6N5

Tel: 613-562-5700
e-mail: iperreault@uottawa.ca

Overview: A small international charitable organization founded in 1921

Mission: To hold biennial conferences; to publish proceedings, abstracts & periodical

Chief Officer(s):

Isabelle Perreault, PhD, Secretary-Treasurer, Canada

Publications:

• Canadian Bulletin of Medical History

Type: Journal; *Frequency:* Semiannually; *Editor:* Kristin Burnett, Jayne Elliott; *Price:* Free to members

International Society of Physical & Rehabilitation Medicine (ISPRM)

7, rue François-Versonnex, Geneva 1207 Switzerland

Tel: 41-22-908-04-83; *Fax:* 41-22-732-26-07
www.isprm.org
twitter.com/ISPRM

Previous Name: International Federation of Physical Medicine & Rehabilitation

Overview: A medium-sized international organization founded in 1999

Mission: To work with practitioners to improve the quality of life of people with impairments & disabilities

Member of: World Health Organization

Chief Officer(s):

Lorraine de Montmollin, Executive Director
  isprmoffice@kenes.com
Jianan Li, President
  presidentjiananli@isprm.org
Francesca Gimigliano, Secretary
  secretary@isprm.org
John Olver, Treasurer
  treasurer@isprm.org

Publications:

• International Society of Physical & Rehabilitation Medicine Congress Abstracts

• The Journal of Rehabilitation Medicine

Type: Journal; *Frequency:* 8 pa; *Editor:* Professor Gunnar Grimby

Profile: International peer-review scientific journal of original articles,

reviews, case reports, brief communications, special reports, letters to the editor, &editorials
• News & Views [a publication of the International Society of Physical & Rehabilitation Medicine]
Type: Newsletter; *Frequency:* Monthly; *Editor:* Nicholas Christodoulou

International Society of Radiographers & Radiological Technologists (ISRRT)
143 Bryn Pinwydden, Cardiff CF23 7DG Wales
Tel: 44-(0)-29-20735038; *Fax:* 44-(0)-29-540551
www.isrrt.org
Overview: A large international charitable organization founded in 1959
Mission: To advance radiation medicine technology through international communication & sponsorship of professional activities
Affiliation(s): World Health Organization; United Nations

International Society of Surgery (ISS) / La Société internationale de Chirurgie (SIC)
c/o Allveco AG, Seltisbergerstrasse 16, Lupsingen CH-4419 Switzerland
Tel: 41-61-815-9666; *Fax:* 41-61-811-4775
e-mail: surgery@iss-sic.ch
www.iss-sic.com
www.facebook.com/iss.sic
Overview: A medium-sized international organization founded in 1902
Mission: To contribute to the advancement of the science & art of surgery by researching & discussing surgical problems, through congresses, courses, & publications
Chief Officer(s):
Jean-Claude Givel, Secretary General
givel@cabchirvisc.ch
Victor Bertschi, Administrative Director
victor.bertschi@iss-sic.ch
Publications:
• International Society of Surgery Newsletter
Type: Newsletter; *Frequency:* Semiannually
• World Journal of Surgery: The Official Journal of the International Society of Surgery/Société Internationale de Chirurgie
Type: Journal; *Editor:* John G. Hunter, M.D.; *ISSN:* 0364-2313
Profile: Authoritative scientific reports in the fields of clinical &experimental surgery, surgical education, & socioeconomic aspects of surgical care

International Union of Societies for Biomaterials Science & Engineering (IUSBSE)
c/o Prof. Nicholas A. Peppas, The University of Texas at Austin, 1 University Station, #C-0400, Austin TX 78712-0231 USA
Tel: 512-471-6644; *Fax:* 512-471-8227
www.worldbiomaterials.org
Overview: A medium-sized international organization
Mission: To advance biomaterials, surgical implants, prosthetics, artificial organs, tissue engineering, & regenerative medicine
Chief Officer(s):
Nicholas A. Peppas, President
peppas@che.utexas.edu

Israel Medical Association-Canadian Chapter (IMA)
#309, 788 Marlee Ave., Toronto ON M6B 3K1
Tel: 416-781-9562; *Fax:* 416-781-3166
Overview: A small international charitable organization founded in 1958
Mission: Devoted to promotion of professional & cultural ties between physicians in Israel & their colleagues abroad
Affiliation(s): Israel Medical Association World Fellowship
Chief Officer(s):
Rose Geist, President
rgeist@thc.on.ca

Medical Women's International Association (MWIA)
7555 Morley Dr., Burnaby BC V5E 3Y2
Tel: 604-522-1960; *Fax:* 604-522-1960
www.mwia.net
twitter.com/MedWIA
Overview: A small international organization founded in 1919
Mission: To offer medical women the opportunity to meet so as to confer upon questions concerning the health & well-being of humanity; to overcome gender-related differences in health & healthcare between women & men, girls & boys throughout the world; to overcome

gender-related inequalities in the medical profession; to promote health for all throughout the world with particular interest in women, health & development
Affiliation(s): Federation of Medical Women of Canada
Chief Officer(s):
Shelley Ross, Secretary General

Missionary Sisters of The Precious Blood of North America
St Bernard's Convent, 685 Finch Ave. West, Toronto ON M2R 1P2
Tel: 416-630-3298; *Fax:* 416-630-9114
www.preciousbloodsisters.com
www.facebook.com/156106151112902
Overview: A small international organization founded in 1885
Mission: Involved in early childhood education & teaching in the elementary, secondary, & college levels. Also work in health care services as nurses, doctors, administrators, physical & occupational therapists, hospital chaplains, caregivers for the elderly, with AIDs patients & in nutrition education. Serves in social work, parish ministry, domestic work, gardening, religious education, work with the mentally & physically handicapped, retreat work, art, & in ministry to the Hispanic & First Nations people.

National Alopecia Areata Foundation (NAAF)
#200B, 65 Mitchel Blvd., San Rafael CA 94903 USA
Tel: 415-472-3780; *Fax:* 415-480-1800
e-mail: info@naaf.org
www.naaf.org
www.facebook.com/NAAFUSA
twitter.com/NAAF_Org
www.youtube.com/user/naaforg
Overview: A medium-sized international charitable organization founded in 1981
Mission: To support research to find a cure or acceptable treatment for aropecia areata; to support those with the disease & educate the public about aropecia areata
Member of: National Health Council; National Organization of Rare Disorders; BBB Wise Giving Alliance Accredited Charities; Dermatology Nurses' Association; Coalition of Skin Diseases; Research America
Affiliation(s): Society for Investigative Dermatology; American Academy of Dermatology; National Institute for Arthritis & Musculoskeletal & Skin Diseases
Chief Officer(s):
Dory Kranz, President/CEO

National Organization for Rare Disorders, Inc. (NORD)
55 Kenosia Ave., Danbury CT 06810 USA
Tel: 203-744-0100; *Fax:* 203-798-2291
www.rarediseases.org
twitter.com/rarediseases
www.youtube.com/raredisorders
Overview: A large international organization founded in 1983
Mission: To identify, treat & cure rare diseases through programs of education, services & research
Affiliation(s): 127 national voluntary agencies for rare disorders
Chief Officer(s):
Sheldon M. Schuster, Chair
Peter L. Saltonstall, President & CEO

Parents Without Partners Inc. (PWP)
1100-H Brandywine Blvd., Zanesville OH 43701-7303 USA
Toll-Free: 800-637-7974
www.parentswithoutpartners.org
www.facebook.com/parentswithoutpartnersinternational
Overview: A large international organization founded in 1957
Mission: To provide single parents & their children with an opportunity for enhancing personal growth, self-confidence & sensitivity towards others by offering an environment for support, friendship & the exchange of parenting techniques
Chief Officer(s):
Janet Gallinati, President
Intl.pres@parentswithoutpartners.org

Physicians for Global Survival (Canada) (PGS) / Médecins pour la survie mondiale (Canada)
30 Cleary Ave., Ottawa ON K2A 4A1

Tel: 613-233-1982
e-mail: pgsadmin@web.ca
www.pgs.ca
www.facebook.com/pages/Physicians-For-Global-Survival/1340224545
68
www.youtube.com/user/pgsottawa

Previous Name: Canadian Physicians for the Prevention of Nuclear War
Overview: A small international charitable organization founded in 1980
Mission: Committed to the abolition of nuclear weapons, the prevention of war, the promotion of non-violent means of conflict resolution & social justice in a sustainable world
Affiliation(s): International Physicians for the Prevention of Nuclear War (IPPNW)
Chief Officer(s):
Juan Carolos Chirgwin, President

Rotary International
One Rotary Center, 1560 Sherman Ave., Evanston IL 60201-3698 USA

Toll-Free: 866-976-8279
www.rotary.org
www.linkedin.com/groups?gid=858557
www.facebook.com/pages/Rotary-International/7268844551
twitter.com/rotary
www.youtube.com/user/RotaryInternational

Overview: A large international organization
Mission: To support its member clubs in fulfilling the Object of Rotary by fostering unity among member clubs, strengthening & expanding rotary around the world, communicating worldwide the work of Rotary & providing a system of international administration
Chief Officer(s):
Gary C.K. Huang, President

St. John Ambulance / Ambulance Saint-Jean
#400, 1900 City Park Dr., Ottawa ON K1J 1A3

Tel: 613-236-7461
Toll-Free: 888-840-5646
www.sja.ca
www.facebook.com/St.John.Ambulance.TO
twitter.com/sja_canada
www.youtube.com/channel/UCKqDpzz1BjDqUgImjquTC7w

Also Known As: The Priory of Canada of the Most Venerable Order of the Hospital of St. John of Jerusalem
Overview: A medium-sized international charitable organization founded in 1883
Mission: To enable Canadians to improve their health, safety & quality of life by providing training & community service. Courses in CPR, emergency first aid, & safety training are offered, as well as community service programs (medical first response, therapy dog services, emergency preparedness, youth programs), & first aid kits
Chief Officer(s):
Robert White, Chancellor
Jerry Rankin, Interim Chief Operating Officer

Alberta Council
12304 - 118 Ave., Edmonton AB T5L 5G8

Tel: 780-452-6565
Toll-Free: 800-665-7114
ab.sjatraining.ca

Chief Officer(s):
Maureen Gray, Contact
maureen.gray@stjohn.ab.ca

British Columbia & Yukon Council
6111 Cambie St., 2nd Fl., Vancouver BC V5Z 3B2

Tel: 604-321-7242
Toll-Free: 866-321-2651
bc.sjatraining.ca

Chief Officer(s):
Sandy Gerber, Director, Marketing
sandy.gerber@bc.sja.ca

Federal District Council (Ottawa Area)

#101, 1050 Morrison Dr., Ottawa ON K2H 8K7

Tel: 613-722-2002; Fax: 613-722-7024
e-mail: registrations@fd.sja.ca

Chief Officer(s):
Steven Gaetz, CEO

Manitoba Council
1 St John Ambulance Way, Winnipeg MB R3G 3H5

Tel: 204-784-7000; Fax: 204-786-2295
Toll-Free: 800-471-7771
e-mail: info@mb.sja.ca
mb.sjatraining.ca

Chief Officer(s):
Richard Fetherston, Coordinator, Sales & Marketing
richard.fetherston@mb.sja.ca

New Brunswick Council
PO Box 3599, Stn. B, 200 Miles St., Fredericton NB E3A 5J8

Fax: 506-452-8699
Toll-Free: 800-563-9998
nb.sjatraining.ca

Chief Officer(s):
Lisa Murphy, Director, Operations
lisa.murphy@nb.sja.ca

Newfoundland Council
8 Thomas Byrne Dr., Mount Pearl NL A1N 0E1

Tel: 709-726-4200; Fax: 709-726-4117
Toll-Free: 800-801-0181
nl.sjatraining.ca

Chief Officer(s):
Glenda Janes, CEO, 709-757-3374
glenda.janes@nl.sja.ca

Nova Scotia/PEI Council
72 Highfield Park Dr., Dartmouth NS B3A 4X2

Tel: 902-463-5646; Fax: 902-469-9609
Toll-Free: 800-565-5056
ns.sjatraining.ca

Chief Officer(s):
Steven Gaetz, CEO

NWT & Nunavut Council
5023 - 51st St., Yellowknife NT X1A 1S5

Tel: 867-873-5658
e-mail: info@mb.sja.ca
ntnu.sjatraining.ca

Chief Officer(s):
Richard Fetherston, Coordinator, Sales & Marketing
richard.fetherston@mb.sja.ca

Ontario Council
#800, 15 Toronto St., Toronto ON M5C 2E3

Tel: 416-923-8411; Fax: 416-923-4856
Toll-Free: 800-268-7581
ont.sjatraining.ca

Chief Officer(s):
Brian Cole, CEO
bcole@on.sja.ca

Québec Council
#10, 110, boul Crémazie ouest, Montréal QC H2P 1B9

Téléc: 514-842-4807
Ligne sans frais: 877-272-7607
Courriel: medias@qc.sja.ca

Chief Officer(s):
Karoline Bergeron, Conseillère principale, Services à la collectivité

Saskatchewan Council
2625 - 3rd Ave., Regina SK S4T 0C8

Tel: 306-522-7226; Fax: 306-525-4177
Toll-Free: 888-273-0003
sk.sjatraining.ca

Chief Officer(s):
Michael Brenholen, Director, Operations
michael.brenholen@sk.sja.ca

Yukon Branch
128 Copper Rd., #C, Whitehorse YT Y1A 2Z6

Tel: 867-668-5001; Fax: 867-667-5050
e-mail: yukon@yt.sja.ca

Les Soeurs de Sainte-Anne
1950, rue Provost, Lachine QC H8S 1P7
Tél: 514-637-3783; *Téléc:* 514-637-5400
Courriel: accueil@ssacong.org
www.ssacong.org

Aperçu: *Dimension:* petite; *Envergure:* internationale; Organisme sans but lucratif; fondée en 1850
Mission: Impliquée dans l'éducation, les soins de santé, l'animation pastorale et sociale en divers milieux
Membre(s) du bureau directeur:
Marie Ellen King, Supérieure générale
Madeleine Lanoue, Secrétaire générale

United Way of America
701 North Fairfax St., Alexandria VA 22314 USA
Tel: 703-836-7112
www.liveunited.org
www.facebook.com/UnitedWay
twitter.com/live_united
www.youtube.com/user/UnitedWayPSAs

Overview: A large international organization
Mission: United Way of America is the national organization dedicated to leading the United Way movement
Chief Officer(s):
Brian A. Gallagher, President & CEO

World Confederation for Physical Therapy (WCPT)
Victoria Charity Centre, 11 Belgrave Rd., London SW1V 1RB United Kingdom
Tel: 44-20-7931-6465; *Fax:* 44-20-7931-6494
e-mail: info@wcpt.org
www.wcpt.org
www.linkedin.com/company/world-confederation-for-physical-therapy-w cpt
www.facebook.com/116826698351147
twitter.com/WCPT1951
www.youtube.com/user/theWCPT

Overview: A small international charitable organization founded in 1951
Mission: To better global health by encouraging high standards of physical therapy research, education & practice, by supporting communication & by collaborating with national & international organizations
Affliation(s): Canadian Physiotherapy Association
Chief Officer(s):
Jonathon Kruger, Chief Executive Officer
Tracy Bury, Director, Professional Policy
Mia Lockner, Manager, Communications & Office
Publications:
• WCPT [World Confederation for Physical Therapy] News
Type: Newsletter; *Frequency:* Quarterly
Profile: News from member organizations, regions & subgroups, reports on WCPT initiatives, executive committee & general meeting decisions, & opinion articles on internationalissues relevant to the profession

World Health Organization (WHO) / Organisation mondiale de la santé (OMS)
20 Appia Ave., Geneva 1211 Switzerland
Tel: 41-22-791-21-11; *Fax:* 41-22-791-31-11
www.who.int
www.linkedin.com/company/world-health-organization
www.facebook.com/WorldHealthOrganization
twitter.com/WHONEWS
www.youtube.com/who

Overview: A large international organization founded in 1948
Mission: To attain for all peoples the highest possible level of health
Chief Officer(s):
Mohamed Shareef, Chairman, Executive Board
Margaret Chan, Director General
Publications:
• International Classification of Diseases [a publication of the World Health Organization]
Profile: A diagnostic tool for epidemiology, health management & clinical purposes
• International Health Regulations [a publication of the World Health Organization]

Profile: Rules to enhance national, regional & global public health security
• The International Pharmacopoeia [a publication of the World Health Organization]
Profile: To harmonize global quality specifications for selected pharmaceutical products, excipients & dosage forms
• International Travel & Health [a publication of the World Health Organization]
Type: Report
Profile: Information on health risks for travellers
• The World Health Report [a publication of the World Health Organization]
Type: Report
Profile: An expert assessment of global health
• World Health Statistics [a publication of the World Health Organization]
Type: Report
Profile: Recent health statistics for member states

World Health Organization Partnership for Health in the Criminal Justice Sytem
c/o WHO Regional Office for Europe, Marmorvej 51, Copenhagen DK-2100 Denmark
Tel: 45-45-33-70-00; *Fax:* 45-45-33-70-01
e-mail: hpp@euro.who.int
www.euro.who.int

Previous Name: World Health Organization Health in Prisons Programme; International Council of Prison Medical Services
Overview: A small international organization founded in 1995
Chief Officer(s):
Lars Moller, Programme Manager, Alcohol & Illicit Drugs
lmo@euro.who.int

World Safety Organization (WSO)
WSO World Management Centre, PO Box 518, Warrensburg MO 64093 USA
Tel: 660-747-3132; *Fax:* 660-747-2647
e-mail: info@worldsafety.org
www.worldsafety.org
www.facebook.com/WorldSafetyOrganization
twitter.com/WorldSafetyOrg

Overview: A medium-sized international organization founded in 1875
Mission: To protect people, property, resources & the environment; To internationalize occupational & environmental safety through exchange of knowledge, programs, etc.
Member of: Consultative Status Category II (non-governmental) with Economic & Social Council of the United Nations
Chief Officer(s):
Vlado Senkovich, President & Director General
Edward E. Hogue, Vice-President & Deputy Director General
Lon S. McDaniel, Chief Executive Officer
Charles H. Baker, Chief Operations Officer

National Publications

Alive
Owned By: Alive Publishing Group
#100, 12751 Vulcan Way, Richmond, BC V6V 3C8
Fax: 800-663-6597
Toll-Free: 800-663-6580
Social Media: plus.google.com/+aliveHealthMag
twitter.com/alivehealth
www.faceboo k.com/alive.health.wellness

Circulation: 200,000 *Frequency:* Monthly
Topics include health, wellness, natural health.
Ryan Benn, Publisher

Best Health
Owned By: Reader's Digest Magazines (Canada) Ltd.
PO Box 974 Main, Markham, ON L3P 0K6
Toll-Free: 866-659-2887
Social Media: pinterest.com/besthealthmag/
twitter.com/besthealthmag
www.facebook .com/besthealth

Circulation: 100,000 *Frequency:* 7 times a year
Beth Thompson, Editor-in-Chief

Canadian Family Physician
College of Family Physicians of Canada, 2630 Skymark Ave.,
Mississauga, ON L4W 5A4

Tel: 905-629-0900; Fax: 905-629-0893
Toll-Free: 800-387-6197
CFPmedia@cfpc.ca
Social Media: twitter.com/CanFamPhysician

Frequency: Monthly
Kathryn Taylor, Managing Editor

Canadian Healthcare Technology
#207, 1118 Centre St., Thornhill, ON L4J 7R9

Tel: 905-709-2330; Fax: 905-709-2258
info2@canhealth.com

Circulation: 8,400 Frequency: 8 times a year
Jerry Zeidenberg, Publisher/Editor

Canadian Journal of Anesthesia / Journal Canadien d'Anesthésie
c/o Canadian Anesthesiologists' Society, #208, 1 Eglinton Ave.
East, Toronto, ON M4P 3A1

Tel: 416-480-0602; Fax: 416-480-0320
anesthesia@cas.ca
Social Media: twitter.com/CASUpdate

Frequency: Monthly
Hilary Grocott, Editor-in-chief
Gregory Bryson, Deputy Editor-in-chief

The Canadian Journal of Continuing Medical Education
Owned By: STA Communications Inc.
#310, 6500 Trans-Canada Hwy., Pointe-Claire, QC H9R 0A5

Tel: 514-695-7623; Fax: 514-695-8554
Circulation: 38,399 Frequency: 10 times a year
Paul Brand, Editor

The Canadian Journal of Diagnosis
Owned By: STA Communications Inc.
#310, 6500 Trans-Canada Hwy., Pointe-Claire, QC H9R 0A5

Tel: 514-695-7623; Fax: 514-695-8554
Circulation: 38,399 Frequency: Monthly
Robert Passaretti, Publisher

**Canadian Journal of Emergency Medicine (CJEM/JCMU) / Journal
canadien de la médecine d'urgence**
Owned By: Cambridge University Press
University Printing House, Shaftesbury Rd., Cambridge, UK CB2
8BS

cjem@rogers.com
Circulation: 4,000 Frequency: 6 times a year
Dr. James Ducharme, Editor-in-Chief

**Canadian Journal of Infectious Diseases & Medical Microbiology
(CJIDMM)**
Owned By: Hindawi Publishing Corp.
#3070, 315 Madison Ave., New York, NY, USA 10017

cjidmm@hindawi.com
Frequency: Quarterly
Official journal of Medical Microbiology and Infectious Disease Canada
(AMMI Canada).

Canadian Journal of Medical Laboratory Science (CJMLS)
Cdn. Society for Medical Laboratory Science, 33 Wellington St.
North, Hamilton, ON L8R 1M7

Tel: 905-528-8642; Fax: 905-528-4968
Toll-Free: 800-263-8277
info@csmls.org
Frequency: Quarterly
Journal available only to members

**The Canadian Journal of Occupational Therapy (CJOT) / Revue
canadienne d'ergothérapie**
Canadian Association of Occupational Therapists, #100, 34
Colonnade Rd., Ottawa, ON K2E 7J6

Tel: 613-523-2268; Fax: 613-523-2552
Toll-Free: 800-434-2268
publications@caot.ca
Social Media: twitter.com/CAOT_ACE
www.facebook.com/CAOT.ca

Circulation: 7,000 Frequency: 5 times a year

Jane Davis, Executive Editor
Helene Polatajko, Scientific Editor

**Canadian Journal of Public Health (CJPH) / Revue canadienne de
santé publique**
Canadian Public Health Association, #404, 1525 Carling Ave.,
Ottawa, ON K1Z 8R9

Tel: 613-725-3769; Fax: 613-725-9826
Frequency: Bi-Monthly
Dr. Louise Potvin, Editor-in-Chief

**Canadian Journal of Rural Medicine (CJRM) / Journal canadien de
la médecine rurale**
Owned By: Society of Rural Physicians of Canada
PO Box 22015, 45 Overlea Blvd., Toronto, ON M4H 1N9

Tel: 416-961-7775; Fax: 416-961-8271
Toll-Free: 877-276-1949
Circulation: 7,000 Frequency: 4 times a year
The official publication of the Society of Rural Physicians of Canada.
Suzanne Kingsmill, Managing Editor, manedcjrm@gmail.com

**Canadian Journal of Surgery (CJS/JCC) / Journal canadien de
chirurgie**
Owned By: Canadian Medical Association
1867 Alta Vista Dr., Ottawa, ON K1G 5W8

Toll-Free: 888-855-2555
Frequency: 6 times a year
A peer reviewed journal meeting the medical education needs of
Canada's surgical specialists.
Wendy Carroll, Managing Editor, wendy.carroll@cma.ca

Canadian Paramedicine
Previous Name: Canadian Emergency News
PO Box 579, Drumheller, AB T0J 0Y0

Fax: 888-264-2854
Toll-Free: 800-567-0911
cp@emsnews.com
Social Media: twitter.com/CdnParamedicine
www.facebook.com/CanadianParamedicine

Frequency: 6 times a year
Lyle Blumhagen, Publisher/Editor

**Clinical & Investigative Medicine (CIM) / Médecine clinique et
expérimentale**
Owned By: Canadian Society for Clinical Investigation
CSCI Head Office, 114 Cheyenne Way, Ottawa, ON K2J 0E9

Circulation: 1,000 Frequency: 6 times a year
Dr. Bob Bortolussi, Editor, robert.bortolussi@dal.ca

Doctor's Review
Owned By: Parkhurst Publishing
400 McGill St., 4th Fl., Montréal, QC H2Y 2G1

Tel: 514-397-8833; Fax: 514-397-0228
Toll-Free: 800-663-7403
Social Media: twitter.com/doctorsreview
www.facebook.com/doctorsreview

Circulation: 43,000 Frequency: 10 times a year
Monthly travel & lifestyle journal.
David Elkins, Publisher

FMWC Newsletter
Federation of Medical Women of Canada, 1021 Thomas Spratt Pl.,
Ottawa, ON K1G 5L5

Tel: 613-569-5881; Fax: 613-249-3906
Toll-Free: 877-771-3777
fmwcmain@fmwc.ca
Circulation: 1,000 Frequency: 3 times a year
Dr. Anne Niec, President

Future Health
c/o Canadians for Health Research, PO Box 126, Westmount, QC
H3Z 2T1

Tel: 514-398-7478; Fax: 514-398-8361
Circulation: 2,000 Frequency: Quarterly
Tim Lougheed, Chair, Canadians for Health Research

Guide to Canadian Healthcare Facilities
Previous Name: Canadian Hospital Association Buyer's Guide
c/o HealthCareCAN, #100, 17 York St., Ottawa, ON K1N 5S7
Tel: 613-241-8005; *Fax:* 613-241-5055
Toll-Free: 855-236-0213
guide@healthcarecan.ca
Social Media: twitter.com/healthcarecan
www.facebook.com/healthcarecan.soinssantecan
Circulation: 1,300 *Frequency:* Annually
Claire Samuelson, Editor

HEALTHbeat
Owned By: McCrone Publications
#319, 9768 - 170 St., Edmonton, AB T5T 5L4
Toll-Free: 800-727-0782
Circulation: 40,000 *Frequency:* 12 times a year
Jan Henry, Publisher, jan@mccronehealthbeat.com

Healthcare Information Management & Communications Canada
Owned By: Healthcare Computing & Communications Canada, Inc.
12 - 9196 Tronson Rd., Vernon, BC V1H 1E8
Tel: 780-489-4521; *Fax:* 780-489-3290
healthcare@shaw.ca
Circulation: 6,000 *Frequency:* 3 times a year
Dave Wattling, Associate Editor

Healthcare Management FORUM / Forum gestion des soins de santé
Canadian College of Health Leaders, 292 Somerset St. West, Ottawa, ON K2P 0J6
Tel: 613-235-7218; *Fax:* 613-235-5451
Toll-Free: 800-363-9056
Frequency: Quarterly
Ron Lindstrom, Editor-in-Chief

Hospital News, Canada
#401, 610 Applewood Cres., Vaughan, ON L4K 0E3
Tel: 905-532-2600
info@hospitalnews.com
Social Media: www.facebook.com/HospitalNews
Frequency: Monthly
Stefan Dreesen, Publisher, stefan@hospitalnews.com
Kristie Jones, Editor, editor@hospitalnews.com

The Journal of Current Clinical Care
71 Dewlane Dr., Toronto, ON M2R 2P9
contactus@healthplexus.net
Social Media: www.facebook.com/172966859396867
Frequency: 6 times a year
Mark Varnovitski, Publisher
D'Arcy Little, Medical Director

Journal of Medical Imaging & Radiation Sciences / Le Journal Canadien des Techniques en Radiation Médicale
Canadian Assn. of Medical Radiation Technologists, #1300, 180 rue Elgin St., Ottawa, ON K2P 2K3
Tel: 613-234-0012; *Fax:* 613-234-1097
Toll-Free: 800-463-9729
editor@camrt.ca
Frequency: 4 times a year
CAMRT Journal available only to members.
Lisa Di Prospero, Editor in Chief

Médecine/sciences
109, av Aristide Briand, Montrouge Cedex, France 92541
Tirage: 2 007 *Fréquence:* 10 fois par an
Hervé Chneiweiss, Rédacteur en chef

The Medical Post
Owned By: EnsembleIQ
#1510, 2300 Yonge St., Toronto, ON M4P 1E4
Tel: 416-256-9908
Social Media: twitter.com/MedicalPost
Circulation: 47,000 *Frequency:* 14 times a year
Colin Leslie, Editor

Occupational Therapy Now / Actualités ergothérapiques
Canadian Association of Occupational Therapists, #100, 34 Colonnade Rd., Ottawa, ON K2E 7J6
Tel: 613-523-2268; *Fax:* 613-523-2552
Toll-Free: 800-434-2268
otnow@caot.ca
Social Media: twitter.com/CAOT_ACE
www.facebook.com/CAOT.ca
Circulation: 6,500 *Frequency:* 6 times a year
Flora To-Miles, Managing Editor

Parkhurst Exchange
Owned By: Parkhurst Publishing
400, rue McGill, 4e étage, Montréal, QC H2Y 2G1
Tel: 514-397-8833; *Fax:* 514-397-0228
Toll-Free: 800-663-7403
Circulation: 39,453 *Frequency:* 12 times a year
Monthly GP/FP journal.
Dr. Steven Blitzer, Medical Editor-in-Chief

Physiotherapy Canada
Owned By: University of Toronto Press
5201 Dufferin St., Toronto, ON M3H 5T8
Tel: 416-667-7810; *Fax:* 416-667-7881
editor@physiotherapy.ca
Frequency: 4 times a year
Dina Brooks, Scientific Editor PhD, dina.brooks@utoronto.ca

The Plastic Surgery / Chirurgie plastique
Previous Name: Canadian Journal of Plastic Surgery
Owned By: Pulsus Group Inc.
2902 South Sheridan Way, Oakville, ON L6J 7L6
Tel: 905-829-4770; *Fax:* 905-829-4799
pulsus@pulsus.com
Frequency: 4 times a year
Official journal of the Canadian Society of Plastic Surgeons, the Canadian Society for Aesthetic (Cosmetic) Plastic Surgery, Groupe pour l'Avancement de la Microchirurgie Canada, and the Canadian Society for Surgery of the Hand (Manus Canada).
Edward Buchel, Editor

Rehab & Community Care Medicine
Previous Name: Rehab & Community Care Management
Owned By: BCS Communications
#803, 255 Duncan Mill Rd., Toronto, ON M3B 3H9
Tel: 416-421-7944; *Fax:* 416-421-8418
Toll-Free: 800-798-6282
Social Media: www.facebook.com/RehabMagazine
Frequency: Quarterly
Caroline Tapp-McDougall, Publisher & Editor-in-Chief, caroline@bcsgroup.com
Helmut Dostal, Managing Editor, dostal@bcsgroup.com

Vitality Magazine
356 Dupont St., Toronto, ON M5R 1V9
Tel: 416-964-0528
editorial@vitalitymagazine.com
vitalitymagazine.com
Social Media: www.facebook.com/VitalityMagazine;
twitter.com/vitalityonline
Circulation: 60,000 *Frequency:* 10 times a year
Julia Woodford, Editor

Provincial/Local Publications

L'Actualité Médicale
Détenteur: EnsembleIQ
#800, 1200, av McGill College, Montréal, QC H3B 4G7
Ligne sans frais: 844-246-3190
Fréquence: 23 fois par an
Caroline Bélisle, Directrice de marque, 514-843-2569, cbelisle@ensembleiq.com

The Alberta Doctors' Digest
Alberta Medical Association, 12230 - 106 Ave. NW, Edmonton, AB T5N 3Z1

Tel: 780-482-2626; *Fax:* 780-482-5445
Toll-Free: 800-272-9680
amamail@albertadoctors.org
Social Media: twitter.com/Albertadoctors

Frequency: Bi-Monthly
Dr. Dennis W. Jirsch, Editor

British Columbia Medical Journal
#115, 1665 West Broadway, Vancouver, BC V6J 5A4

Tel: 604-638-2815; *Fax:* 604-638-2917
journal@doctorsofbc.ca
Social Media: twitter.com/BCMedicalJrnl
www.facebook.com/BCMedicalJournal

Circulation: 10,500 *Frequency:* 10 times a year
Provides clinical & review articles written by physicians who debate medicine & medical politics in letters as well as long essays
Jay Draper, Editor, jdraper@doctorsofbc.ca

doctorNS
Previous Name: Medical Society of Nova Scotia DoctorsNS
Doctors Nova Scotia, 25 Spectacle Lake Dr., Dartmouth, NS B3B 1X7

Tel: 902-468-1866; *Fax:* 902-468-6578
Toll-Free: 800-563-3427
info@doctorsns.com
Social Media: twitter.com/Doctors_NS

Circulation: 3,300 *Frequency:* 10 times a year
Melissa Murray, Production Manager, 902-481-4923,
melissa.murray@doctorsns.com

Family Health
10006 - 101 St., Edmonton, AB T5J 0S1

Circulation: 95,000 *Frequency:* 4 times a year
Robert Clarke, Publisher

Fédération des Médecins Omnipraticien du Québec (FMOQ)
2, Place Alexis Nihon, #2000, 3500 boul de Maisonneuve ouest, 20e étage, Westmount, QC H3Z 3C1

Tél: 514-878-1911; *Téléc:* 514-878-4455
Ligne sans frais: 800-361-8499
mpsaintgelais@fmoq.org
Médias sociaux: www.youtube.com/lafmoq
twitter.com/OMNIPRATICIENS
www.facebook.com/ lafmoq

Tirage: 14,000 *Fréquence:* Mensuel
Louise Roy, Rédacteur M.D.

Health, Wellness & Safety Magazine (HWS)
Owned By: Business Link Media Group
#200, 36 Hiscott St., St Catharines, ON L2R 1C8

Tel: 905-646-9366; *Fax:* 905-646-5486
info@hwsmag.com
Social Media: twitter.com/HWSmag
www.facebook.com/HWSmag

Frequency: Bi-monthly
Distributed to health, wellness & safety professionals in the Niagara, Hamilton, Burlington & Oakville regions.
Adam Shields, Co-Publisher, adam@businesslinkmedia.com
Jim Shields, Co-Publisher, jim@businesslinkmedia.com

Impact Magazine
2007 - 2nd St. SW, Calgary, AB T2S 1S4

Tel: 403-228-0605
info@impactmagazine.ca

Circulation: 90,000 *Frequency:* Bi-monthly
Elaine Kupser, Publisher, elaine@impactmagazine.ca
Chris Welner, Editor, editor@impactmagazine.ca

Nutrition - Science en Evolution
Anciennement: Diététique en Action
Ordre professionnel des diététistes du Québec, #1855, 550, rue Sherbrooke ouest, Montréal, QC H3A 1B9

Tél: 514-393-3733; *Téléc:* 514-393-3582
Ligne sans frais: 888-393-8528
opdq@opdq.org

Fréquence: 3 fois par ans

Paule Bernier, Présidente

Ontario Medical Review (OMR)
Ontario Medical Assn., #900, 150 Bloor St. West, Toronto, ON M5S 3C1

Tel: 416-599-2580; *Fax:* 416-340-2944
Toll-Free: 800-268-7215
Social Media: twitter.com/OntariosDoctors
www.facebook.com/Ontariosdoctors

Circulation: 33,000 *Frequency:* 11 times a year
Jeff Henry, Editor, jeff.henry@oma.org
Elizabeth Petruccelli, Managing Editor, elizabeth.petruccelli@oma.org
Kim Secord, Circulation Manager, kim.secord@oma.org

Vitalité Québec Mag
#200, 3210 Jacques-Bureau, Laval, QC H7P 0A9

Tél: 450-973-4863; *Téléc:* 450-973-7856
vitalitemag@qc.aira.com
Médias sociaux:
www.facebook.com/vitalite.quebec

Tirage: 40 000 *Fréquence:* 10 fois par an
Pierre Martineau, Président, pm@videotron.ca
Dino Halikas, Rédacteur en chef, dino@nobilis.ca

National Libraries

Canadian Association of Medical Radiation Technologists
#1300, 180 rue Elgin St., Ottawa, ON K2P 2K3

Tel: 613-234-0012; *Fax:* 613-234-1097
Toll-Free: 800-463-9729
info@camrt.ca
www.camrt.ca
Social Media: twitter.com/camrt_actrm;
www.facebook.com/CAMRTactrm;
www.linkedin.com/company/1432897

Collection: Archives Medical radiation technology, X-ray/radiation therapy; Nuclear medicine; Magnetic resonance
François Couillard, Chief Executive Officer
fcouillard@camrt.ca

Canadian Forces Health Services Group Headquarters/ Quartier général du Groupe des Services de Santé des Forces canadiennes
1745 Alta Vista Dr., Ottawa, ON K1A 0K6

Fax: 613-945-6938
librarycfhs-bibliothequessfc@forces.gc.ca

Canadian Foundation for Healthcare Improvement
#700, 1565 Carling Ave., Ottawa, ON K1Z 8R1

Tel: 613-728-2238; *Fax:* 613-728-3527
info@cfhi-fcass.ca
www.cfhi-fcass.ca
Social Media: www.youtube.com/user/cfhifcass;
twitter.com/CFHI_FCASS;
www.facebook.com/CanFoundationforHealthImprovement

Canadian Medical Association (CMA)/ Association médicale canadienne
1867 Alta Vista Dr., Ottawa, ON K1G 5W8

Tel: 613-731-9331; *Fax:* 613-731-2076
cmalibrary@cma.ca
www.cma.ca

Collection: Gordon Fahrni Archives, History of CMA activities 1867 to present

Canadian Memorial Chiropractic College
6100 Leslie St., Toronto, ON M2H 3J1

Tel: 416-482-2340; *Fax:* 416-482-4816
www.cmcc.ca/Page.aspx?pid=377

Collection: Chiropractic History
Margaret Butkovic, Library Director
416-482-2340 ext. 159
Kent Murnaghan, Reference Librarian
416-482-2340 ext. 205
Steve Zoltai, Collection Development Librarian
Todd Vasey, Library Technician (Cataloguing)
Deanne Collier, Library Technician
Shabana Siddiqui, Library Technician (Serials)

Canadian Science Centre for Human & Animal Health (CSCHAH)
1015 Arlington St., Winnipeg, MB R3E 3P6

www.phac-aspc.gc.ca

Canadian Society for International Health/ Société canadienne de la santé internationale
#726, 1 Nicholas St., Ottawa, ON K1N 7B7

Tel: 613-241-5785
info@csih.org
www.csih.org

Social Media: twitter.com/globalsante; www.facebook.com/CSIH.org
Collection: Print & electronic media related to international health & development
Eva Slawecki, Executive Director
eslawecki@csih.org
613-241-5785 ext. 325

Canadian Society for Medical Laboratory Science
33 Wellington St. North, Hamilton, ON L8R 1M7

Tel: 905-528-8642; *Fax:* 905-528-4968
Toll-Free: 800-263-8277
info@csmls.org
www.csmls.org

Social Media: twitter.com/csmls
Collection: Self-study educational materials for professional development in the areas of medical laboratory science, management & life skills; audio-visual materials; laboratory standards
Michele Perry, Manager, Learning Services
Lucy Agro, Administrator, Learning Services

Canadian Women's Health Network/ Le Réseau canadien pour la santé des femmes
#203, 419 Graham Ave., Winnipeg, MB R3C 0M3

cwhn@cwhn.ca
www.cwhn.ca
Social Media: twitter.com/CdnWomensHealth;
www.facebook.com/CWHN.RCSF
Collection: Women's health publications from Canada & around the world

College of Family Physicians of Canada
Taylor Library, University of Western Ontario, #106K, London, ON N6A 5B7

Tel: 519-661-3170; *Fax:* 519-661-3880
clfm@uwo.ca
www.cfpc.ca/LibraryServices

Health Canada/ Santé Canada
70 Colombine Driveway, Ottawa, ON K1A 0K9

Tel: 613-957-2991; *Fax:* 613-941-5366
Toll-Free: 866-225-0709
info@hc-sc.gc.ca
www.hc-sc.gc.ca

Profile: The library serves the information needs of employees at Health Canada & the Public Health Agency of Canada. The print collection is located in closed stacks at the National Research Council's facility in Ottawa, & access is administered by Infotrieve Canada Inc. **Collection:** Print materials; extensive electronic collections of ejournals, ebooks, & databases (available by intranet only)
Lynda Gamble, Portfolio Manager
Kathryn Jackson, Portfolio Manager

Integrated Orthomolecular Network

www.ionhealth.ca

The Royal College of Physicians & Surgeons of Canada
774 Echo Dr., Ottawa, ON K1S 5N8

Tel: 613-730-8177; *Fax:* 613-730-8830
Toll-Free: 800-668-3740
www.royalcollege.ca

Collection: Corporate Archives History of Canadian Medicine; Book and monographs by Fellows, Osler Collection, Antiquarian Collection, John M. Last Collection

Provincial Libraries

Aberdeen Hospital
c/o Pictou County Health Authority, 835 East River Rd., New Glasgow, NS B2H 3S6

Tel: 902-752-7600; *Fax:* 902-752-2507
arh.library@pcha.nshealth.ca
www.pcha.nshealth.ca/aberdeen

A.E. MacDonald Ophthalmic Library & William Callahan Reading Room
Toronto Western Hospital, 399 Bathurst St., #MP6-319, Toronto, ON M5T 2S8

Tel: 416-978-4321

Alberta Health Services
North Tower, Seventh St. Plaza, 10030 - 107 St. NW, 14th Fl., Edmonton, AB T5J 3E4

Tel: 780-342-2000; *Fax:* 780-342-2060
Toll-Free: 888-342-2471
www.albertahealthservices.ca

Collection: Online articles & resources on the following subjects: cancer; new patients; tobacco reduction

Alexandra Marine & General Hospital
120 Napier St., Goderich, ON N7A 1W5

Tel: 519-524-8689; *Fax:* 519-524-5579
www.amgh.ca

Profile: The Health Records Department maintains the hospital library & handles hospital health records.
Sulav Pant, Director, Finance & Health Records
sulav.pant@amgh.ca

Allyn & Betty Taylor Library
Natural Sciences Centre, University of Western Ontario, #1, 1151 Richmond St., London, ON N6A 3K7

Tel: 519-661-3168
taylib@uwo.ca
www.lib.uwo.ca/taylor/
Social Media: twitter.com/westernulibsTAY; www.facebook.com/taylib
Kim Cornell, Assistant University Librarian, Allyn & Betty Taylor Library
kcornel@uwo.ca
519-679-2111 ext. 86362
Deborah Meert-Williston, Head, Research & Instructional Services
dmeertwi@uwo.ca
519-661-2111 ext. 86383
Lauren Munn, Manager, Resource Support Services
lmunn@uwo.ca
519-661-2111 ext. 86360

ARCH Disability Law Centre
55 University Ave., 15th Fl., Toronto, ON M5J 2H7

Tel: 416-482-8255; *Fax:* 416-482-2981
Toll-Free: 866-482-2724
TTY: 416-482-125
archlib@lao.on.ca
www.archdisabilitylaw.ca

Roberto Lattanzio, Executive Director
Doreen Way, Office Manager

Archives des Augustines du Monastère de l'Hôpital Général de Québec
260, boul Langelier, Québec, QC G1K 5N1

Tél: 418-529-0931
www.augustines.ca

Collection: Anciennes éditions à partir du XVII siècle
Juliette Cloutier, Archiviste
418-529-0931 ext. 217

Atlantic Health Knowledge Partnership (AHKP)
c/o Patrick Ellis, Librarian, W.K. Kellogg Health Sciences Library, Dalhousie University, 5850 College St., Halifax, NS B3H 1X5

Tel: 902-494-2458; *Fax:* 902-494-3750
kellogg.library@dal.ca

Profile: Members of the Atlantic Health Knowledge Partnership consortium are institutions based in Nova Scotia & Newfoundland & Labrador. To improve the effective use of resources, electronic products are reviewed & purchased by the member institutions.
Ann Barrett, Interim Head, Health Sciences Library
ann.barrett@dal.ca

Banff Mineral Springs Hospital
305 Lynx St., Banff, AB T1L 1H7
Tel: 403-760-2222; *Fax:* 403-762-4193

Battlefords Union Hospital
1092 - 107th St., North Battleford, SK S9A 1Z1
Tel: 306-446-6600; *Fax:* 306-445-6561
buhlibrary@bathd.sk.ca

Bibliothèque des sciences de la santé
#L-623, Pavillon Roger-Gaudry, 2900, boul, Édouard-Montpetit,
Montréal, QC H3T 1J4
Tél: 514-343-7664; *Téléc:* 514-343-6457
prsant@bib.umontreal.ca
bib.umontreal.ca/SA

Monique St-Jean, Directrice des bibliothèques des sciences de la santé
monique.st-jean@umontreal.ca
514-343-7810
Sylvie Desbiens, Chef de service
s.desbiens@umontreal.ca
514-343-6111 ext. 3583
Natalie Clairoux, Bibliothécaire
natalie.clairoux@umontreal.ca
514-343-6111 ext. 3585
Monique Clar, Bibliothécaire
monique.clar@umontreal.ca
514-343-6111 ext. 0866
Patrice Dupont, Bibliothécaire
patrice.dupont@umontreal.ca
514-343-6111 ext. 0865
Sarah-Julie Richard, Technicienne en documentation
sarah-julie.richard@umontreal.ca
514-343-6111 ext. 3580

Bibliothèque des sciences de la santé
Pavillons X1 et X2, 3001, 12e av Nord, Sherbrooke, QC J1H 5N4
Tél: 819-564-5296; *Téléc:* 819-820-6817
Ligne sans frais: 866-325-2433
bibliotheque.sante@usherbrooke.ca
www.usherbrooke.ca/biblio

Kathy Rose, Bibliothécaire
kathy.rose@usherbrooke.ca
819-821-8000 ext. 75852
Josée Toulouse, Bibliothécaire
josee.toulouse@usherbrooke.ca
819-821-8000 ext. 63575

Biomedical Branch Library
Gordon & Leslie Diamond Health Centre, 2775 Laurel St., 2nd Fl.,
Vancouver, BC V5Z 1M9
Tel: 604-875-4505; *Fax:* 604-875-4689
bmb.library@ubc.ca
www.library.ubc.ca/bmb

Dean Giustini, Reference Librarian
dean.giustini@ubc.ca
604-875-4111 ext. 62392

Bluewater Health
89 Norman St., Sarnia, ON N7T 6S3
Tel: 519-464-4400; *Fax:* 519-464-4407
www.bluewaterhealth.ca

Jill Campbell, Manager, Learning Services
jcampbell@bluewaterhealth.ca

Bracken Health Sciences Library
Botterell Hall, Queen's University, 18 Stuart St., Kingston, ON K7L
3N6
Tel: 613-533-3176; *Fax:* 613-533-6892
Toll-Free: 877-209-5641
Reference: bracken.library@queensu.ca
library.queensu.ca/health

Paola Durando, Acting Head
paola.durando@queensu.ca
613-533-6000 ext. 74733
Anne Smithers, Head, Collection Development & Assessment
smithers@queensu.ca
613-533-6000 ext. 74530

Sandra Halliday, Acting co-head, Health Sciences Librarian
halliday@queensu.ca
613-533-6000 ext. 77568
Amanada Ross-White, Librarian, Clinical Outreach Services
amanda.ross-white@queensu.ca
613-533-6000 ext. 78136
Elizabeth MacDonald-Pratt, Senior Information Services Technician
pratte@queensu.ca
Jane Reeves, Reference Assistant, Information Services
reevesj@queensu.ca
Hilda Thompson, Information Services Technician
thompsnh@queensu.ca
613-533-6000 ext. 32510
Sandra McKeown, Health Sciences Librarian
sandra.mckeown@queensu.ca
613-533-6000 ext. 75284
Sarah Wickett, Health Informatics Librarian
wicketts@queensu.ca
613-533-6000 ext. 77078

Bridgepoint Health
14 St. Matthews Rd., Toronto, ON M4M 2B5
Tel: 416-461-8252
Collection: Vertical File, Audio-Visual Cassettes, Internet Bookmarks
Patricia Petruga, Clinical Librarian

British Columbia Health & Human Services
1515 Blanshard St., 1st Fl., Victoria, BC V8W 3C8
Tel: 250-952-2196; *Fax:* 250-952-2180
hlth.library@gov.bc.ca
www2.gov.bc.ca/gov/content/health

Burnaby Hospital
3935 Kincaid St., Burnaby, BC V5G 2X6
Tel: 604-412-6255; *Fax:* 604-412-6177

Julie Mason, Librarian
julie.mason@fraserhealth.ca

Cambridge Memorial Hospital
700 Coronation Blvd., Cambridge, ON N1R 3G2
Tel: 519-621-2330; *Fax:* 519-740-4938
TTY: 519-621-918
libraryservices@cmh.org
www.cmh.org

Carbonear General Hospital
86 Highland Rd. South, Carbonear, NL A1Y 1A4
Tel: 709-945-5111; *Fax:* 709-945-5158
www.easternhealth.ca

Catholic Health Association of Saskatchewan
1702 - 20th St. West, Saskatoon, SK S7M 0Z9
Tel: 306-655-5330; *Fax:* 306-655-5333
cath.health@chassk.ca
www.chassk.ca

Sandra Kary, Executive Director
sandra@chassk.ca
306-655-5332
Sandy Normand, Mission Education Coordinator
snormand@chassk.ca
306-655-5331

Central Newfoundland Regional Health Centre
50 Union St., Grand Falls-Windsor, NL A2A 2E1
Tel: 709-292-2500
www.centralhealth.nl.ca

Kelly Adams, Chief Operating Officer
kelly.adams@centralhealth.nl.ca

Centre de documentation du Centre hospitalier de l'Université de Montréal
1560, rue Sherbrooke est, Montréal, QC H2L 4M1
Tél: 514-890-8000; *Téléc:* 514-412-7569
biblio.chum@ssss.gouv.qc.ca
www.bibliothequeduchum.ca
Mèdia social: www.youtube.com/user/bibliothequeduchum/videos;
twitter.com/cdchum

Centre de documentation du Centre hospitalier de l'Université de Montréal
1058, rue St-Denis, Montréal, QC H2X 3J4

Tel: 514-890-8000
biblio.chum@ssss.gouv.qc.ca

Collection: Hépatologie, médecine interne

Centre de documentation du Centre hospitalier de l'Université de Montréal
Pavillon Olier, #2-428, 3840, rue St-Urbain, 4e étage, Montréal, QC H2W 1T8

Tél: 514-890-8000
biblio.chum@ssss.gouv.qc.ca
bibliothequeduchum.ca

Centre de recherche du CHUL-CHUQ/ CHUQ-CHUL Research Centre
CHUQ Research Centre, Université Laval, 2705 boul Laurier, #TR-72, Québec, QC G1V 4G2

Tél: 418-654-2296; *Téléc:* 418-654-2298
sec.drs@crchuq.ulaval.ca
www.crchudequebec.ulaval.ca

Centre de santé et de services sociaux de Gatineau, Hôpital de Hull
116, boul Lionel-Emond, Gatineau, QC J8Y 1W7

Tél: 819-595-6050; *Téléc:* 819-595-6098
www.csssgatineau.qc.ca

Dianne Couture, Services de bibliothèque
dianne_couture@ssss.gouv.qc.ca

Centre de santé et de services sociaux de Sept-Iles
45, rue Père Divet, Sept-Iles, QC G4R 3N7

Tél: 418-962-9761; *Téléc:* 418-961-2768

Centre de santé et des services sociaux du Nord de Lanaudière
1000, boul Ste-Anne, #RC-C-01, Saint-Charles-Borromée, QC J6E 6J2

Tél: 450-759-8222; *Téléc:* 450-759-7343
csssnl.bibliotheque@ssss.gouv.qc.ca
www.csssnl.qc.ca/Bibliotheque

Nancy Gadoury, Bibliothécaire
nancy.gadoury@ssss.gouv.qc.ca

Centre hospitalier de Charlevoix
74, rue Ambroise-Fafard, Baie-Saint-Paul, QC G3Z 2J6

Tél: 418-435-5150; *Téléc:* 418-435-0212

Centre Hospitalier de Lamèque
29, rue de l'Hôpital, Lamèque, NB E8T 1C5

Tél: 506-344-2261; *Téléc:* 506-344-3403

Centre hospitalier Pierre-Janet
20, rue Pharand, Gatineau, QC J9A 1K7

Tél: 819-771-7761; *Téléc:* 819-771-2908

Centre hospitalier Pierre-Le Gardeur
911, montée des Pionniers, Lachenaie, QC J6V 2H2

Tél: 450-654-7525; *Téléc:* 450-585-9724
Ligne sans frais: 888-654-7525
documentation@cssssl.ca

Centre hospitalier régional de Trois-Rivières
1991, boul du Carmel, Trois-Rivières, QC G8Z 3R9

Tél: 819-697-3333; *Téléc:* 819-379-9850
www.cssstr.qc.ca

Centre hospitalier régional du Grand-Portage
75, rue St-Henri, Rivière-du-Loup, QC G5R 2A4

Tél: 418-868-1000; *Téléc:* 418-868-1032
www.csssrivieredeloup.qc.ca

Centre hospitalier universitaire de Sherbrooke Hôtel-Dieu
#1110, 580, rue Bowen sud, Sherbrooke, QC J1G 2E8

Tél: 819-346-1110; *Téléc:* 819-822-6745
usherbrooke.ca/biblio/sans-gabarit/pole/chus

Gilberte Poirier, Responsable
gilbertepoirier.chus@ssss.gouv.qc.ca
819-346-1110 ext. 21126

Centre hospitalier Vallée-de-l'Or et de soins psychiatriques régionaux
725, 6e rue, Val-d'Or, QC J9P 3Y1

Tél: 819-825-5858; *Téléc:* 819-825-5950

Centre intégré de santé et de services sociaux de l'Outaouais
116, boul Lionel-Émond, Gatineau, QC J8Y 1W7

Tél: 819-966-6050; *Téléc:* 819-966-6098
santeoutaouais.qc.ca

Dianne Couture, Technicienne en documentation
dianne_couture@ssss.gouv.qc.ca
819-966-6050

Le Centre intégré de santé et de services sociaux de la Montérégie-Est
2750, boul Laframboise, Saint-Hyacinthe, QC J2S 4Y8

Tél: 450-771-3333; *Téléc:* 450-771-3304
peb.csssry@rrsss16.gouv.qc.ca
santeme.quebec

Centre intégré de santé et de services sociaux de Laval
1755, boul René-Laënnec, Laval, QC H7M 3L9

Tél: 450-975-5493; *Téléc:* 450-975-5572
biblio.csssl@ssss.gouv.qc.ca
catalogue.cssslaval.qc.ca
Mèdia social: twitter.com/bibliocsssl

Josée Noël, Technicienne en documentation et webmestre
450-975-5493 ext. 55493

Centre intégré de santé et de services sociaux des Laurentides
#252, 500, boul des Laurentides, Saint-Jérome, QC J7Z 4M2

Tél: 450-569-2974; *Téléc:* 450-569-2961
www.santelaurentides.gouv.qc.ca

Centre intégré universitaire de santé et de services sociaux de la Capitale-Nationale
2400, av D'Estimauville, Québec, QC G1E 7G9

Tél: 418-666-7000; *Téléc:* 418-666-2776
www.ciusss-capitalenationale.gouv.qc.ca

Sylvie Bélanger, Technicienne de la documentation
sylvie.belanger.ciussscn@ssss.gouv.qc.ca

Centre intégré universitaire de santé et de services sociaux du Saguenay-Lac-Saint-Jean
305, rue St-Vallier, Chicoutimi, QC G7H 5H6

Tél: 418-541-1234; *Téléc:* 418-541-1145
www.santesaglac.com

Charles S. Curtis Memorial Hospital
#178, 200 West St., St Anthony, NL A0K 4S0

Tel: 709-454-3333
www.lghealth.ca/index.php?pageid=38

Chatham-Kent Health Alliance
80 Grand Ave. West, Chatham, ON N7L 1B7

Tel: 519-352-6400
www.ckha.on.ca

CHU Sainte-Justine
3175, ch de la Côte Ste-Catherine, Montréal, QC H3T 1C5

Tél: 514-345-4931
www.chusj.org

Mélanie Durocher, Technicienne en documentation

CHUQ-CHUL
2705, boul Laurier, #RC-315, Québec, QC G1V 4G2

Tél: 418-525-4444; *Téléc:* 418-654-2143
www.chudequebec.ca

CHUQ-Hôpital Saint-François d'Assise
10, rue de l'Espinay, Québec, QC G1L 3L5

Tél: 418-525-4408; *Téléc:* 418-525-4483
biblio.sfa@ens.chuq.qc.ca
www.chudequebec.ca

Collection: Médecine

CHUQ-L'Hôtel-Dieu du Québec
11, côte du Palais, Québec, QC G1R 2J6

Tél: 418-525-4444; *Téléc:* 418-691-5468
biblio.hdq@ens.chuq.qc.ca

CHUS Hôtel-Dieu
#1110, 580, rue Bowen sud, Sherbrooke, QC J1G 2E8
Tél: 819-346-1110; *Téléc:* 819-822-6745
bibliotheque.chus@ssss.gouv.qc.ca
www.chus.qc.ca

CIUSSS de la Mauricie-et-du-Centre-du Québec (Hôpital Sainte-Croix)
570, rue Hériot, Drummondville, QC J2B 1C1
Tél: 819-478-6464; *Téléc:* 819-478-6440
biblio_hsc@ssss.gouv.qc.ca
www.ciusssmcq.ca

CIUSSS de la Mauricie-et-du-Centre-du-Québec, Hôtel-Dieu d'Arthabaska
5, rue des Hospitalières, Victoriaville, QC G6P 6N2
Tél: 819-357-2030; *Téléc:* 819-357-4314

Clinton Public Hospital
98 Shipley St., Clinton, ON N0M 1L0
Tel: 519-482-3440
www.hpha.ca
Profile: The Clinton Public Hospital Site is a member of the Huron Perth Healthcare Alliance.
Jane Crawford, Contact, Huron Perth Healthcare Alliance Library Services
jane.crawford@hpha.ca
519-272-8210 ext. 2250

Collège des médecins du Québec
#3500, 1250, boul René-Lévesque ouest, Montréal, QC H3B 0G2
Tél: 514-933-4441; *Téléc:* 514-933-3112
info@cmq.org
www.cmq.org
Marie-Eve Barsalou, Archiviste
514-933-4441 ext. 5308

College of Physicians & Surgeons of BC
#300, 669 Howe St., Vancouver, BC V6C 0B4
Tel: 604-733-6671; *Fax:* 604-737-8582
Toll-Free: 800-461-3008
medlib@cpsbc.ca
www.cpsbc.ca/library
J. Galt Wilson, Senior Deputy Registrar

College of Physicians & Surgeons of Ontario
80 College St., Toronto, ON M5G 2E2
Tel: 416-967-2600; *Fax:* 416-961-3330
Toll-Free: 800-268-7096
www.cpso.on.ca
Collection: Committee meeting minutes; Memorabilia of the College from 1866 to the present; Physicians' registration; Policy; Regulations; Discipline
Ellen Tulchinsky, Librarian
etulchinsky@cpso.on.ca

Commission des norms, de l'équité, de la santé et de la sécurité du travail
1199, rue de Bleury, 4e étage, Montréal, QC H3B 3J1
Ligne sans frais: 844-838-0808
documentation@cnesst.gouv.qc.ca
www.centredoc.cnesst.gouv.qc.ca
Collection: Cis/Bit Sur CD-ROM, Rapports d'enquête d'accident accessibles en ligne

Concordia Hospital
1095 Concordia Ave., Winnipeg, MB R2K 3S8
Tel: 204-661-7163; *Fax:* 204-661-7282
chlibrary@umanitoba.ca
libguides.lib.umanitoba.ca/concordia
Melissa Raynard, Hospital Librarian
204-661-7440
Thomas Quinlan, Library Assistant
204-661-7163

Consortium of Ontario Academic Health Libraries (COAHL)
c/o Kim Cornell, Librarian, A. & B. Taylor Library, Natural Sciences Centre, The University of Western Ontario, London, ON N6A 5B7
www.coahl.weebly.com

Patty Fink, Chair
pattyfink@nosm.ca
Kim Cornell, Secretary
kcornel@uwo.ca

Constance-Lethbridge Rehabilitation Centre/ Centre de Réadaptation Constance-Lethbridge Bibliothèque
7005, boul de Maisonneuve ouest, Montréal, QC H4B 1T3
Tél: 514-487-1770; *Toll-Free:* 866-487-1891
www.constance-lethbridge.qc.ca
Collection: Over 5,000 books & journals; Material to support CLRC programs

Covenant Health
#0634, 1100 Youville Dr. West, Edmonton, AB T6L 5X8
Tel: 780-735-7300; *Fax:* 780-735-7202
covenantlibrary@covenanthealth.ca
www.covenanthealth.ca
Sharna Polard, Manager, Library Services
sharna.polard@covenanthealth.ca
780-735-7251
Roger Salus, Medical Library Technician
roger.salus@covenanthealth.ca
780-735-7301
Paulette Pelland, Library Technician
paulette.pelland@covenanthealth.ca
780-735-7313
Lyndsey Lisitza, Program Assistant
lyndsey.lisitza@covenanthealth.ca
780-735-7300

Credit Valley Hospital
2200 Eglinton Ave. West, Mississauga, ON L5M 2N1
Tel: 905-813-2411; *Fax:* 905-813-3969
Collection: Consumer health collection
Penka Stoyanova, Senior Librarian
penka.stoyanova@trilliumhealthpartners.ca
905-813-1100 ext. 6479

CSSS de la Haute-Yamaska
205, boul Leclerc, Granby, QC J2G 1T7
Tél: 450-375-8000

CSSS de St-Jérôme
290, rue Montigny, Saint-Jérome, QC J7Z 5T3
Tél: 450-432-2777; *Ligne sans frais:* 866-963-2777

CSSS Hôpital Le Royer
635, boul Joliet, Baie-Comeau, QC G5C 1P1
Tél: 418-589-3701; *Téléc:* 418-587-9654

CSSS Pierre-Boucher Hopital Pierre-Boucher
1333, boul Jacques-Cartier Est, Longueuil, QC J4M 2A5
Tél: 450-468-8111

Dalhousie University Libraries
6225 University Ave., Halifax, NS B3H 4H8
Tel: 902-494-3617; *Fax:* 902-494-2062
Other Numbers: Reference: 902-494-3611
libraries.dal.ca
Social Media: www.youtube.com/user/DalhousieLibraries;
twitter.com/DalLibraries; www.facebook.com/36011919042
Collection: Kipling Collection, Morse Collection, J.J. Stewart Collection, Canadian Small Press Collection, Bacon Collection, Cockerell Collection, Canadiana
Sarah Stevenson, Interim Head
sarah.stevenson@dal.ca
Michael Moosberger, Archivist

Dartmouth General Hospital Site
#2205, 325 Pleasant St., Dartmouth, NS B2Y 4G8
Tel: 902-465-8519; *Fax:* 902-465-8494
www.cdha.nshealth.ca

Dickson Building Site
#5106, 1276 South Park St., Halifax, NS B3H 2Y9
Tel: 902-473-8497; *Fax:* 902-473-7456
www.cdha.nshealth.ca
Katie McLean, Site Supervisor
katie.mclean@nshealth.ca
902-473-3118

Direction de santé publique - CIUSSS du Centre-Sud-de-l'île-de-Montréal
1301, rue Sherbrooke Est, Montréal, QC H2L 1M3

Tél: 514-528-2400
www.dsp.santemontreal.qc.ca

Doctors of BC
#115 - 1665 West Broadway, Vancouver, BC V6J 5A4

museum@doctorsofbc.ca
www.bcmamedicalmuseum.org

Profile: The collection currently holds 2600 items, some having been acquired from the Vancouver Medical Association. The artifacts show the medical history of British Columbia from the past 150 years.
Collection: Anaesthesiology, Anatomy & Pathology, Audio-Visual, Dentistry, Diagnostic (Clinical/Laboratory), Gynaecology/Obsterics/Contraception, Materia Medica & Pharmacology, Military, Nursing & Physician Furnishings/Sundries, Nutrition/Diet, Ophthamology, Oriental Medicine, Orthopaedics, Otalaryngology, Pharmacy-ware, Proctology, Public Health & Hygene, Radiomedicine, Surgery, Therapeutics, Urology

Douglas Memorial Hospital Site
230 Bertie St., Fort Erie, ON L2A 1Z2

Tel: 905-378-4647
Other Numbers: Health Records Fax: 905-871-9078

Dr. Everett Chalmers Regional Hospital
700 Priestman St., Fredericton, NB E3B 5N5

Tel: 506-452-5432; *Fax:* 506-452-5585
library.fredricton@horizonnb.ca
en.horizonnb.ca/facilities-and-services/facilities

Collection: Classics of Medicine Series

Édifice Hôtel-Dieu de Roberval
450, rue Brassard, Roberval, QC G8H 1B9

Tél: 418-275-0110; *Téléc:* 418-275-6202
www.csssdomaineduroy.com

Electronic Health Library of BC (e-HLbc)
e-HLbc Administrative Centre, W.A.C. Bennett Library, Simon Fraser Univ., #7600, 8888 University Dr., Burnaby, BC V5A 1S6

Tel: 778-782-5440; *Fax:* 778-782-3023
info@ehlbc.ca
www.ehlbc.ca

Leigh Anne Palmer, Coordinator
leighannep@ehlbc.ca
778-782-6297
Jennifer Bancroft, Librarian
jenniferb@ehlbc.ca
778-782-7002

Etobicoke General Hospital
101 Humber College Blvd., Toronto, ON M9V 1R8

Tel: 416-747-3400; *Fax:* 416-747-3484

Family & Community Medicine Library
500 University Ave., 5th Fl., Toronto, ON M5G 1V7

Tel: 416-978-5606
dfcm.library@utoronto.ca
www.dfcm.utoronto.ca/landing-page/library

Collection: 800 volumes; 40 periodical titles; 700 manuscripts; resources in Family Medicine education & research
Robyn Butcher, Librarian
416-978-5606

Fédération des médecins omnipraticiens du Québec
3500, boul de Maisonneuve Ouest, Montréal, QC H3Z 3C1

Tél: 514-878-1911; *Ligne sans frais:* 800-361-8499
info@fmoq.org
www.fmoq.org

Ghislain Germain, Directeur et archiviste

Fédération des médecins spécialistes du Québec
Tour Est, 2, Complexe Desjardins, porte 3000, Montréal, QC H5B 1G8

Tél: 514-350-5000; *Téléc:* 514-350-5100
Ligne sans frais: 800-561-0703
www.fmsq.org

Julie Voiselle, Directrice, Services administratifs et ressources humaines

Five Hills Health Region
455 Fairford St. East, Moose Jaw, SK S6H 1H3

Tel: 306-694-0374; *Fax:* 306-694-0270
inquiries@fhhr.ca
www.fhhr.ca

Gerstein Science Information Centre
Sigmund Samuel Library Bldg., 9 King's College Circle, Toronto, ON M5S 1A5

Tel: 416-978-2280
ask.gerstein@utoronto.ca
gerstein.library.utoronto.ca

Collection: Technical reports, Microfiche, Landmarks of Science
Bonnie Horne, Science Librarian
b.horne@utoronto.ca
416-978-5329

Grace Hospital
300 Booth Dr., Winnipeg, MB R3J 3M7

Tel: 204-837-0127; *Fax:* 204-897-9486
Other Numbers: 204-837-0518
gghlibrary@umanitoba.ca
libguides.lib.umanitoba.ca/grace
Social Media: twitter.com/healthlibrary

Lori Giles-Smith, Hospital Librarian
204-837-0127

Grand River Hospital Health Sciences Library
835 King St. West, Kitchener, ON N2G 1G3

Tel: 519-749-4300; *Fax:* 519-749-4208
info@grhosp.on.ca
www.grhosp.on.ca

Profile: Library services helps staff, affiliated students, and volunteers find and use information. Helps with research and improving search skills.

Greater Niagara General Hospital Site
5546 Portage Rd., Niagara Falls, ON L2E 6X2

Tel: 905-378-4647
Other Numbers: Health Records Fax: 905-358-0829

Grey-Bruce Health Services
1800 - 8th St. East, Owen Sound, ON N4K 6M9

Tel: 519-376-2121
library@gbhs.on.ca
www.gbhs.on.ca

Christine Fenton-Stone, Library Technician
519-376-2121 ext. 2043

Guelph General Hospital
115 Delhi St., Guelph, ON N1E 4J4

Tel: 519-837-6440; *Fax:* 519-837-6467
TTY: 519-837-643
info@gghorg.ca
www.gghorg.ca

Collection: Health records

Halton Healthcare Services Corporation
3001 Hospital Gate, Oakville, ON L6M 0L8

Tel: 905-845-2571; *Fax:* 905-338-4454
www.haltonhealthcare.on.ca

Jeanna Hough, Manager
jhough@haltonhealthcare.on.ca

Hamilton Health Sciences
#125, 293 Wellington St. North, Hamilton, ON L8L 8E7

Tel: 905-527-4322
libraryg@hhsc.ca
www.hhsc.ca

Hamiota District Health Centre
177 Birch Ave. East, Hamiota, MB R0M 0T0

Tel: 204-764-2412; *Fax:* 204-764-2049
www.hamiota.com/health_centre.html

Health Knowledge Network (HKN)
University of Calgary, Health Sciences Bldg., #1492, 3330 Hospital Dr. NW, Calgary, AB T2N 4N1

hkn@ucalgary.ca
www.hkn.ca

Vivian Stieda, HKN General Manager
vstieda@ucalgary.ca

Health Quality Council (HQC)
Atrium Bldg., Innovation Pl., #241, 111 Research Dr., Saskatoon, SK S7N 3R2

Tel: 306-668-8810; *Fax:* 306-668-8820
info@hqc.sk.ca
www.hqc.sk.ca
Social Media: www.youtube.com/user/SaskHQC; twitter.com/hqcsask; www.facebook.com/healthqualitycouncil
Greg Basky, Director, Communications
gbasky@hqc.sk.ca

Health Quality Council of Alberta
#210, 811 - 14 St. NW, Calgary, AB T2N 2A4

Tel: 403-297-8162; *Fax:* 403-297-8258
info@hqca.ca
www.hqca.ca
Social Media: www.youtube.com/user/HealthQltyCouncilAB; twitter.com/HQCA
Charlene McBrien-Morrison, Executive Director

Health Science Information Consortium of Toronto
c/o Lori Anne Oja, Gerstein Science Information Centre, University of Toronto, 9 King's College Circle, Toronto, ON M5S 1A5

Tel: 416-978-5217; *Fax:* 416-971-2637
hsict.library.utoronto.ca
Lori Anne Oja, Executive Director
Neil Romanosky, Chair

Health Sciences Library/ Bibliothèque des sciences de la santé
Roger-Guindon Hall, #1020, 451 Smyth Rd., Ottawa, ON K1H 8M5

Tel: 613-562-5407
bibliorgnlibrary@uottawa.ca
biblio.uottawa.ca/health-sciences-library
Jessica McEwan, Acting Library Director
613-562-5418

Health Sciences Library
1280 Main St. West, Hamilton, ON L8S 4K1

Tel: 905-525-9140; *Fax:* 905-528-3733
hslib@mcmaster.ca
hsl.mcmaster.ca
Social Media: www.youtube.com/user/machealthscilibrary; twitter.com/machealthscilib; www.facebook.com/machealthscilibrary
Collection: History of Medicine (Canadian, World Wars), Archives
Jennifer McKinnell, Director
mckinn@mcmaster.ca
905-525-9140 ext. 24381
Neera Bhatnagar, Head, Public Services
bhatnag@mcmaster.ca
Andrea McLellan, Head, Collections & Technical Services
mclell@mcmaster.ca

Health Sciences Library
Health Sciences Centre, #1450, 3330 Hospital Dr. NW, Calgary, AB T2N 4N1

Tel: 403-220-6855; *Fax:* 403-282-7992
hslibr@ucalgary.ca
library.ucalgary.ca/hsl
Collection: Family Medicine, History of Medicine
Heather Ganshorn, Interim Head
heather.ganshorn@ucalgary.ca
403-220-6858

Health Sciences Library
#E1400 Academic Health Sciences Bldg., 104 Clinic Pl., Saskatoon, SK S7N 2Z4

Tel: 306-966-5991; *Fax:* 306-966-5918
ill.ssum@usask.ca
library.usask.ca/hsl
Collection: Baltzan Medical Canadiana, Brodie History of Medicine
Gwen Chan, Supervisor
gwen.chan@usask.ca
306-966-6025
Debbie Chomyshen, Interlibrary Loan
debbie.chomyshen@usask.ca
306-966-5995

Health Sciences Library
Memorial University of Newfoundland, 300 Prince Philip Dr., St. John's, NL A1B 3V6

Tel: 709-864-4904; *Fax:* 709-864-4968
www.library.mun.ca/hsl
Social Media: twitter.com/MUNHSL; www.facebook.com/munhsl
Collection: History of Medicine Collection
Janet Bangma, Associate University Librarian, Health Sciences
janet.bangma@mun.ca
709-864-6027
Lindsey Alcock, Head of Public Services
lalcock@mun.ca
709-864-6072

Health Sciences North/ Horizon Santé-Nord
North Tower, Ramsey Lake Health Centre, 41 Ramsey Lake Rd., 1st Fl., Sudbury, ON P3E 5J1

Tel: 705-523-7100; *Fax:* 705-523-7317
Other Numbers: Patient Library, Ext. 2351
library@hsnsudbury.ca
www.hsnsudbury.ca/portalen/library
Irma Sauvola, Librarian Supervisor
isauvola@hsnsudbury.ca
705-523-7100 ext. 1098

Hôpital Anna-Laberge
200, boul Brisebois, Châteauguay, QC J6K 4W8

Tél: 450-699-2425; *Téléc:* 450-699-2510
documentation.csssjr16@ssss.gouv.qc.ca

Hôpital de Gatineau
909, boul de la Verendrye, Gatineau, QC J8P 7H2

Tél: 819-966-6100

Hôpital de Verdun
4000, boul Lasalle, Montréal, QC H4G 2A3

Tél: 514-362-1000

Hôpital du Centre-de-la-Mauricie
50, 119e rue, Shawinigan, QC G9P 5K1

Tél: 819-536-7500
www.etrehumain.ca

Hôpital du Haut-Richelieu
920, boul du Séminaire Nord, Saint-Jean-sur-Richelieu, QC J3A 1B7

Tél: 450-359-5000; *Téléc:* 450-359-5363
Ligne sans frais: 866-967-4825
biblio.cssshrr16@ssss.gouv.qc.ca
Carole Hébert, Responsable
450-359-5000 ext. 5055

Hôpital du Sacré-Coeur de Montréal
Pavillon principal, G-3000, 5400, boul Gouin Ouest, Montréal, QC H4J 1C5

Tél: 514-338-2222; *Téléc:* 514-338-3154
www.hscm.ca
Profile: Le mandat de la bibliothèque Norman-Bethune est de fournir à tout le personnel les ressources et les services documentaires permettant de répondre aux besoins d'information professionnelle pour soutenir la démarche clinique, l'enseignement, la recherche et la formation professionnelle continue. **Collection:** Collection d'imprimés, de photographies et d'objets sur Norman Bethune

Hôpital du St-Sacrement
1050, ch Ste-Foy, Québec, QC G1S 4L8

Tél: 418-682-7511
www.chudequebec.ca
Sylvie Marcoux, Technicienne en documentation
sylvie.marcoux.cha@ssss.gouv.qc.ca

Hôpital Jean-Talon
1385, rue Jean-Talon est, Montréal, QC H2E 1S6

Tél: 514-495-6767; *Téléc:* 514-495-6738
Collection: La Collection d'illustrations medicaux CIBA

Hôpital Montfort/ Montfort Hospital
#2D113, 713, ch Montréal, Ottawa, ON K1K 0T2

Tél: 613-746-4621
www.hopitalmontfort.com

Hôpital Notre-Dame-du-Lac
58, rue de l'Église, Témiscouata-sur-le-Lac, QC G0L 1X0
Tél: 418-899-6751; *Téléc:* 418-899-2809

Hôpital Sainte-Anne
305, boul des Anciens-Combattants, Sainte-Anne-de-Bellevue, QC H9X 1Y9
Tél: 514-457-3440; *Téléc:* 514-457-8450
Ligne sans frais: 800-361-9287
informations.comtl@ssss.gouv.qc.ca
www.ciusss-ouestmtl.gouv.qc.ca

Hôpital Santa Cabrini
5655, rue St Zotique est, Montréal, QC H1T 1P7
Tél: 514-252-4897; *Téléc:* 514-252-6432
centrededoc.santc@ssss.gouv.qc.ca
www.santacabrini.qc.ca
Josée Berthelette, Technicienne en documentation

Horizon Health Network
135 MacBeath Ave., Moncton, NB E1C 6Z8
Tel: 506-857-5447; *Fax:* 506-857-5785
www.horizonnb.ca

Hornepayne Community Hospital
278 Front St., Hornepayne, ON P0M 1Z0
Tel: 807-868-2442; *Fax:* 807-868-2697
www.hornepaynecommunityhospital.ca
Heather Jaremy-Berube, Chief Executive Officer

Hôtel-Dieu de Sorel
400, av Hôtel-Dieu, Sorel-Tracy, QC J3P 1N5
Tél: 450-746-6000; *Téléc:* 450-746-6082
Renée Fontaine, Bibliothécaire
renee.fontaine@rrsss16.gouv.qc.ca

Hôtel-Dieu Shaver Health & Rehabilitation Centre
541 Glenridge Ave., St Catharines, ON L2T 4C2
Tel: 905-685-1381; *Fax:* 905-687-4871
www.hoteldieushaver.org
Jane Rufrano, Chief Executive Officer

Humber River Regional Hospital
1235 Wilson Ave., Toronto, ON M3M 0B2
Tel: 416-242-1000; *Fax:* 416-242-1047
pfrc@hrh.ca
www.hrh.ca/patientandfamilyresourcecentre
Collection: Health resources

Infrastructure Health & Safety Association
#400, 5110 Creekbank Rd., Mississauga, ON L4W 0A1
Tel: 905-625-0100; *Fax:* 905-652-8998
Toll-Free: 800-263-5024
info@ihsa.ca
www.ihsa.ca
Collection: Print & Audio-Visual materials

Institut de réadaptation Gingras-Lindsay de Montréal/ Montreal Gingras-Lindsay Rehabilitation Institute
Pavillon Lindsay, 6363 ch Hudson, Montréal, QC H3S 1M9
Tél: 514-340-2085; *Téléc:* 514-340-2716
biblio.irglm@ssss.gouv.qc.ca
www.irglm.qc.ca
Profile: Centre de documentation spécialisé dans le domaine de réadaptation **Collection:** 4 000 monographies; 50 titres de journaux; 6 bases de données
Lucie Pelletier, Bibliotechnicienne

Institut de recherches cliniques de Montréal/ Clinical Research Institute of Montreal
110, av des Pins ouest, Montréal, QC H2W 1R7
Tél: 514-987-5500
info@ircm.qc.ca
www.ircm.qc.ca

Institut national de santé publique du Québec
945, rue Wolfe, #A4-44, Québec, QC G1V 5B3
Tél: 418-650-5115; *Téléc:* 418-654-2148
catalogue.santecom.qc.ca
Média social: twitter.com/INSPQ; www.facebook.com/inspq;
Magali Leverd, Technicienne en documentation

Institut Nazareth et Louis-Braille
1111, rue St-Charles ouest, Longueuil, QC J4K 5G4
Tél: 450-463-1710; *Téléc:* 450-463-0243
www.inlb.qc.ca
Collection: Ouvrages de référence; Monographies; Rapports; Périodiques spécialisés; bases de données; Portails; Livres en Braille; Ludothèque: jouets, jeux adaptés
Francine Baril, Responsable
450-463-1710 ext. 242

Interior Health Authority
Royal Inland Hospital, 311 Columbia St., Kamloops, BC V2C 2T1
Tel: 250-314-2234; *Fax:* 250-314-2189
www.interiorhealth.ca

Jewish Rehabilitation Hospital/ Hôpital juif de réadaptation
3205, Place Alton Goldbloom, Laval, QC H7V 1R2
Tel: 450-688-9550; *Fax:* 450-488-3673
www.hjr-jrh.qc.ca
Collection: Journals about rehabilitation specialties
Loredana Caputo, Librarian
450-688-9550 ext. 226

John W. Scott Health Sciences Library
#2K3.28 Walter C. Mackenzie Health Sciences Centre, University of Alberta, Edmonton, AB T6G 2R7
Tel: 780-492-7947
jwsinfo@ualberta.ca
www.library.ualberta.ca/aboutus/health
Social Media: twitter.com/jwslibrary; www.facebook.com/jwslibrary
Marlene Dorgan, Head, Health Sciences Library
780-492-7945

Joseph Brant Memorial Hospital
1230 North Shore Blvd., Burlington, ON L7S 1W7
Tel: 905-632-3737
www.josephbranthospital.ca

Juravinski Hospital Library
699 Concession St., Hamilton, ON L8V 1C3
Tel: 905-527-4322
libraryh@hhsc.ca

Kaye Edmonton Clinic
11402 University Ave., Edmonton, AB T6G 1Z1
Tel: 780-407-5136; *Fax:* 780-407-5652

Kingston Frontenac Lennox & Addington Public Health Library
221 Portsmouth Ave., Kingston, ON K7M 1V5
Tel: 613-549-1232; *Fax:* 613-549-7896
Toll-Free: 800-267-7875
www.kflaph.ca
Social Media: twitter.com/kflaph; www.facebook.com/kflapublichealth

Knowledge Resource Service
#1450, 3330 Hospital Dr. NW, Calgary, AB T2N 4N1
Tel: 403-220-6855
hslibr@ucalgary.ca
library.ucalgary.ca/hsl

Labrador-Grenfell Health - Labrador Health Centre
227 Hamilton River Rd., Happy Valley-Goose Bay, NL A0P 1C0
Fax: 709-896-4032
Toll-Free: 855-897-2267
www.lghealth.ca

Lakehead University
955 Oliver Rd., Thunder Bay, ON P7B 5E1
Tel: 807-343-8205; *Fax:* 807-343-8007
circdesk@lakeheadu.ca
library.lakeheadu.ca
Social Media: twitter.com/LakeheadLibTBay;
www.facebook.com/LakeheadLibTBay
Karen Keiller, University Librarian
kkeiller@lakeheadu.ca
807-343-8205
Louise Wuorinen, Librarian, Collections Development
louise.wuorinen@lakeheadu.ca
807-343-8856

Valerie Gibbons, Librarian, Services & Assessment
valerie.gibbons@lakeheadu.ca
807-343-8165
Moira Davidson, Librarian, Scholarly Communications
moira.davidson@lakeheadu.ca
807-343-8315
Gisella Scalese, Librarian, Instructional Technology
gisella.scalese@lakeheadu.ca
807-343-8719
Trudy Russo, Librarian, Special Collections
trusso@lakeheadu.ca
807-343-8728
Jason Zou, Librarian, Digital Initiatives
qzou@lakeheadu.ca
807-343-8251
Janice Mutz, Librarian, User Experience
jmutz@lakeheadu.ca
807-343-8147
Sara Janes, University Archivist
sjanes1@lakeheadu.ca
807-343-8272

Lakeridge Health - Oshawa
1 Hospital Ct., Oshawa, ON L1G 2B9
Tel: 905-576-8711
www.lakeridgehealth.on.ca
Profile: Library services supports clinical decision-making, research & education for medical & hospital colleagues, including medical students & students from many health disciplines. **Collection:** Printed & virtual resources, including point-of-care tools, such as UpToDate, LexiComp, E-CPS
Debbie Arsenault, Coordinator
darsenault@lakeridgehealth.on.ca
905-576-8711 ext. 3754

Leamington District Memorial Hospital
194 Talbot St. West, Leamington, ON N8H 1N9
Tel: 519-326-2373
www.leamingtonhospital.com
Barbara Colaizzi, Manager, Health Information Management

Listowel Memorial Hospital
255 Elizabeth St. East, Listowel, ON N4W 2P5
Tel: 519-291-3120; *Fax:* 519-291-5440
www.lwha.ca

London Health Sciences Centre
800 Commissioners Rd. East, London, ON N6A 5W9
Tel: 519-685-8500
www.lhsc.on.ca
Darren Hamilton, Manager

Mackenzie Richmond Hill Hospital
10 Trench St., Richmond Hill, ON L4C 4Z3
Tel: 905-883-1212
www.mackenziehealth.ca
Kimberley Aslett, Librarian

Magrath Community Health Centre
37E - 2nd Ave. North, Magrath, AB T0K 1J0
Tel: 403-758-4422; *Fax:* 403-758-3332
www.albertahealthservices.ca
Collection: Safety & injury prevention information

Markham Stouffville Hospital
381 Church St., Markham, ON L3P 7P3
Tel: 905-472-7061
TTY: 905-472-758
www.msh.on.ca
Juliana Muema, Librarian
jmuema@msh.on.ca

McGill University
McLennan Library Bldg., 3459, rue McTavish, Montréal, QC H3A 0C9
Tel: 514-398-4677; *Fax:* 514-398-7356
doadmin.library@mcgill.ca
www.mcgill.ca/library
Social Media: twitter.com/mcgilllib; www.facebook.com/mcgill.library

Collection: e-Journals; e-Books; CDs & audiocassettes; DVDs & videocasettes; Microforms
C. Colleen Cook, PhD, Trenholme Dean of Libraries
Bruna Ceccolini, Assistant to the Trenholme Dean of Libraries

McGill University Health Centre
Rm B.RC.0078, 1001, boul Decarie, Montréal, QC H4A 3J1
Tel: 514-934-1934; *Fax:* 514-843-1483
library.glen@muhc.mcgill.ca
muhclibraries.ca/libraries/glen
Bénédicte Nauche, Librarian, Coordinator MUHC Medical Libraries
benedicte.nauche@muhc.mcgill.ca
514-934-1934 ext. 35292
Elena Guadagno, Librarian
elena.guadagno@muhc.mcgill.ca
514-934-1934 ext. 22554
Vincent Caetano, Documentation Technician
vincent.caetano@muhc.mcgill.ca
514-934-1934 ext. 22374
Myra Davies, Documentation Technician
myra.davies@muhc.mcgill.ca
514-934-1934 ext. 22374

McMaster University
1280 Main St. West, Hamilton, ON L8S 4L8
Tel: 905-525-9140
library@mcmaster.ca
library.mcmaster.ca
Social Media: www.youtube.com/maclibraries; twitter.com/maclibraries; www.facebook.com/maclibraries
Collection: Bertrand Russell Archives, Eighteenth Century British & European Imprints, Canadian Archives (Social History, Labour Studies), Pacifism, Maps
Vivian Lewis, University Librarian
lewisvm@mcmaster.ca
905-525-9140 ext. 23883
Anne Pottier, Associate University Librarian, Library Services
pottier@mcmaster.ca
905-525-9140 ext. 22410
Dale Askey, Associate University Librarian, Library & Learning Technologies
askeyd@mcmaster.ca
905-525-9140 ext. 21880
Marlene Mastragostino, Administrator
mastrag@mcmaster.ca
905-525-9140 ext. 24355

Medical Society of Prince Edward Island
2 Myrtle St., Stratford, PE C1B 2W2
Tel: 902-368-7303; *Fax:* 902-566-3934
Toll-Free: 888-368-7303
mspei.org
Lea Bryden, Chief Executive Officer
lea@mspei.org

Medicine Hat Regional Hospital
666 - 5th St. SW, Medicine Hat, AB T1A 4H6
Tel: 403-529-8000

Memorial University of Newfoundland
234 Elizabeth Ave., St. John's, NL A1B 3Y1
Tel: 709-864-7423; *Fax:* 709-864-2153
qe2ill@mun.ca
www.library.mun.ca/qeii
Social Media: twitter.com/MUNQEII; facebook.com/QEIILibrary
Collection: Centre for Newfoundland Studies
Susan Cleyle, University Librarian
scleyle@mun.ca
Louise White, Associate University Librarian
louisew@mun.ca

Michael Garron Hospital - Toronto East Health Network
825 Coxwell Ave., Toronto, ON M4C 3E7
Tel: 416-461-8272; *Fax:* 416-469-6106
library@tegh.on.ca
www.tegh.on.ca

The Michener Institute for Applied Health Sciences
222 St Patrick St., 2nd Fl., Toronto, ON M5T 1V4
Tel: 416-596-3123; *Toll-Free:* 800-387-9066
lrc@michener.ca
www.michener.ca/lrc
Social Media: twitter.com/michenerlrc

Juanita Richardson, Librarian
JRichardson@michener.ca
416-596-3101 ext. 3454

Misericordia Community Hospital
#1NW-32, 16940 - 87th Ave. NW, Edmonton, AB T5R 4H5
Tel: 780-735-2708; *Fax:* 780-735-2509
mislibrary@covenanthealth.ca

Tara Sommerfeld, Library Technician
tara.sommerfeld@covenanthealth.ca

Misericordia Health Centre
691 Wolseley Ave., 1st Fl., Winnipeg, MB R3G 1C3
Tel: 204-788-8109; *Fax:* 204-889-4174
Toll-Free: 888-315-9257
mhclibrary@umanitoba.ca
libguides.lib.umanitoba.ca/misericordia
Social Media: twitter.com/healthlibrary/;
www.facebook.com/98627719719
Profile: The Sister St. Odilon Library is a branch of the Neil John
Maclean Health Sciences Library. It is a resource to the health care
providers of the Misericordia Health Care facility.
Angela Osterreicher, Acting Hospital Librarian
204-788-8108

Miss Margaret Robins Archives
76 Grenville St., Toronto, ON M5S 1B2
Tel: 416-323-6400; *Fax:* 416-323-6122
wch.archives@wchospital.ca
Collection: Photographs; historical records; Academic papers

Mohawk-McMaster Institute for Applied Health Sciences
#104, 1400 Main St. West, Hamilton, ON L8S 1C7
Tel: 905-540-4247; *Fax:* 905-528-5307
Collection: Nursing, Radiography, Ultrasound, Occupational Therapy,
Physical Therapy, Pharmacy, Medical Laboratory Technology
Fiona Inglis, Outreach & Instruction Librarian
905-540-4247 ext. 6720
Amy Morgan, Library Services Technician
905-540-4247 ext. 6719
Nancy Whetstone, Technician, Information Services
905-540-4247 ext. 6716
Arlene Smith, Technician, Information Services
905-540-4247 ext. 6718

Montréal General Hospital/ L'Hôpital général de Montréal
1650, av Cedar, #E6-157, Montréal, QC H3G 1A4
Tel: 514-934-1934; *Fax:* 514-934-8250
library.mgh@muhc.mcgill.ca
www.muhclibraries.ca/libraries/mgh
Bénédicte Nauche, Librarian & Coordinator
benedicte.nauche@muhc.mcgill.ca
514-934-1934 ext. 35292
Tara Landry, Librarian
tara.landry@muhc.mcgill.ca
514-934-1934 ext. 43057
Taline Ekmekjian, Librarian
taline.ekmekjian@muhc.mcgill.ca
514-934-1934 ext. 43056
Daniel Lavigne, Documentation Technician
daniel.lavigne@muhc.mcgill.ca
514-934-1934 ext. 43058

Mount Sinai Hospital
#18-234, 600 University Ave., Toronto, ON M5G 1X5
Tel: 416-586-4800
library.msh@sinaihealthsystem.ca
www.mountsinai.on.ca/education/library
Sandra Kendall, Director, Library Services

Neil John Maclean Health Sciences Library
Brodie Centre, 727 McDermot Ave., Winnipeg, MB R3E 3P5
Tel: 204-789-3342; *Fax:* 204-789-3922
healthlibrary@umanitoba.ca
libguides.lib.umanitoba.ca/njmhsl
Collection: History of Medicine, Aboriginal Health, Archives of the
Faculty of Medicine
Ada Ducas, Medical Librarian
204-789-3821

**Newfoundland & Labrador Department of Health & Community
Services**
125 Trans Canada Hwy., Gander, NL A1V 1P7
www.health.gov.nl.ca/health/index.html

The Niagara Health System
1200 - 4th Ave., St Catharines, ON L2S 0A9
Tel: 905-378-4647; *Fax:* 905-323-3800
www.niagarahealth.on.ca
Collection: Hospital Archives
Janice Russell, Library Technician

Norfolk General Hospital
365 West St., Simcoe, ON N3Y 1T7
www.ngh.on.ca
Social Media: twitter.com/NorfolkGeneralH;
www.facebook.com/NGHSimcoe/NGHSimcoe

North York General Hospital - General Site
4001 Leslie St., 1st Fl., Toronto, ON M2K 1E1
Tel: 416-756-6142; *Fax:* 416-756-6605
library@nygh.on.ca
www.nygh.on.ca/Default.aspx?cid=1261&lang=1
Profile: Library Services provides clinical, research, & education
information for North York General Hospital's staff, residents, &
students.

Northern Health Library
**University Hospital of Northern BC, 1475 Edmonton St., Prince
George, BC V2M 1S2**
Tel: 250-565-2219
Other Numbers: 250-565-2152
library@northernhealth.ca
library.northernhealth.ca
Collection: Canadian Health Research Collection, ACP Journal Club
Anne Allgaier, Librarian
Danell Clay, Library Technician

Northern Ontario School of Medicine
**Medical School Bldg., Lakehead University, #2007, 955 Oliver Rd.,
Thunder Bay, ON P7B 5E1**
Tel: 807-766-7375; *Fax:* 807-766-7361
askthelibrary@nosm.ca
www.nosm.ca/about_us/library
Social Media: www.youtube.com/user/NOSMtv;
twitter.com/NOSMLibrary; www.facebook.com/NOSMLibrary
Jennifer Dumond, Education Services Librarian
jennifer.dumond@nosm.ca
Sophie Regalado, Research Support Librarian
sophie.regalado@nosm.ca
Donna Brown, Library Technician
donna.brown@nosm.ca
Marian Diamond, Library Coordinator
marian.diamond@nosm.ca

Northern Ontario School of Medicine
**Laurentian University, #MS120, 935 Ramsey Lake Rd., Sudbury, ON
P3E 2C6**
Tel: 705-662-7282; *Fax:* 705-662-7269
askthelibrary@nosm.ca
www.nosm.ca/library
Social Media: twitter.com/NOSMLibrary;
www.facebook.com/NOSMLibrary
Patty Fink, Director, Library Services
patty.fink@nosm.ca
Alanna Campbell, Public Services Librarian
alanna.campbell@nosm.ca

Kaitlin Haley, Health Sciences Librarian
  kaitlin.haley@nosm.ca
Michael McArthur, Access Services Librarian
  michael.mcarthur@nosm.ca
Carol Delorme, Library Technician
  carol.delorme@nosm.ca

Notre Dame Bay Memorial Health Centre
Twillingate, NL A0G 4M0
                              Tel: 709-884-2131; *Fax:* 709-884-2586

Nova Scotia Health Authority
#2201, 1796 Summer St., Halifax, NS B3H 3A7
                              Tel: 902-473-4296; *Fax:* 902-473-7168
                  www.cdha.nshealth.ca/health-sciences-library
Joanne Hodder, Manager, Library Services
  joanner.hodder@nshealth.ca
  902-473-4383

Nova Scotia Hospital Site
Hugh Bell Bldg., #200, 300 Pleasant St., Dartmouth, NS B2Y 3Z9
                              Tel: 902-464-3254; *Fax:* 902-464-4804
                                        www.cdha.nshealth.ca
Lara Killian, Site Supervisor
  lara.killian@nshealth.ca

Ontario Medical Association
#900, 150 Bloor St. West, Toronto, ON M5S 3C1
                              Tel: 416-599-2580; *Fax:* 416-340-2944
                                        Toll-Free: 800-268-7215
                                                      info@oma.org
                                                      www.oma.org

Ontario Ministry of Health & Long-Term Care
1075 Bay St., Toronto, ON M5S 2B1
                              Tel: 416-212-0820; *Fax:* 416-212-5232
                                                    TTY: 800-387-555
                                                www.health.gov.on.ca
Social Media: twitter.com/ONThealth; www.facebook.com/ONThealth

Ordre des infirmières et infirmiers du Québec
4200, rue Molson, Montréal, QC H1Y 4V4
                    Tél: 514-935-2501; *Ligne sans frais:* 800-363-6048
                                                      svrd@oiiq.org
                                                      www.oiiq.org
Véronic Fortin, Chef de service, Veille et ressources documentaires

Orillia Soldiers' Memorial Hospital
170 Colborne St. West, Orillia, ON L3V 2Z3
                                              Tel: 705-325-2201
                                              library@osmh.on.ca
                                              www.osmh.on.ca

Osler Library of the History of Medicine
McIntyre Medical Bldg., 3655, Promenade Sir William Osler, 3rd Fl.,
Montréal, QC H3G 1Y6
                              Tel: 514-398-4475; *Fax:* 514-398-5747
                                        osler.library@mcgill.ca
                                  www.mcgill.ca/library/branches/osler
Social Media: twitter.com/OslerLibrary; www.facebook.com/osler.library
Collection: Original collection of Sir William Osler, Archives,
Nineteenth Century French Medical Theses
Christopher Lyons, Head Librarian
  christopher.lyons@mcgill.ca
  514-398-4475 ext. 09847

Ottawa Hospital/ Hôpital d'Ottawa
501 Smyth Rd., #M1404, Ottawa, ON K1H 8L6
                              Tel: 613-737-8899; *Fax:* 613-737-8521
                                        learningservices@toh.ca
                                        www.ottawahospital.on.ca
     Social Media: www.youtube.com/user/TheOttawaHospital;
          twitter.com/OttawaHospital; www.facebook.com/OttawaHospital
Collection: Sexual abuse; Special cancer collection

Ottawa Public Health Library
100 Constellation Cres., Nepean, ON K2G 6J8
                              Tel: 613-580-6744; *Fax:* 613-580-9639
                                                    Toll-Free: 866-426-8885
                                                      healthsante@ottawa.ca
                  ottawa.ca/en/residents/public-health/ottawa-public-health
                              Social Media: twitter.com/ottawahealth

Peel Public Health
7120 Hurontario St., Mississauga, ON L5M 2C2
                              Tel: 905-791-7800; *Fax:* 905-564-2683
                                        peelhealthlibrary@peelregion.ca
                                        www.peelregion.ca/health/library
                              Social Media: twitter.com/PeelHealthLib
Rebecca Strange, Librarian Specialist

Peter Lougheed Knowledge Centre
#0634, 3500 - 26 Ave. NE, Calgary, AB T1Y 6J4
                              Tel: 403-943-4737; *Fax:* 403-219-3559
                                        krs@albertahealthservices.ca
                                        krs.albertahealthservices.ca

Peterborough Regional Health Centre
1 Hospital Dr., Peterborough, ON K9J 7C6
                                              Tel: 705-743-2121
                                              www.prhc.on.ca
Peter McLaughlin, President & CEO

Port Colborne General Hospital Site
260 Sugarloaf St., Port Colborne, ON L3K 2N7
                                              Tel: 905-378-4647
                  Other Numbers: Health Records Fax: 905-834-0016

Prairie Mountain Health
150 McTavish Ave. East, Brandon, MB R7A 2B3
                              Tel: 204-578-4080; *Fax:* 204-578-4984
                                              library@pmh-mb.ca
                  prairiemountainhealth.ca/index.php/health-resource-centre
Wendy Wareham, Supervisor, Health Resource Centre

Premiers' Council on the Status of Disabled Persons/ Conseil du
premier ministre sur la condition des personnes handicapées
#140, 250 King St., Fredericton, NB E3B 9M9
                              Tel: 506-444-3000; *Fax:* 506-444-3001
                                                    Toll-Free: 800-442-4412
                                                      pcsdp@gnb.ca
                                                      www.gnb.ca/council
                              Social Media: twitter.com/nbPCSDP
Brian Saunders, Executive Director

Providence Care - St. Mary's of the Lake
340 Union St., Kingston, ON K7L 5A2
                                              Tel: 613-584-7222
                                              www.providencecare.ca
Collection: The Kingston Task Force on Elder Abuse Collection,
Spirituality & Aging Collection, Archives
Karen Gagnon, Director, Library Services
  gagnonk@providencecare.ca

Providence Healthcare
3276 St. Clair Ave. East, Toronto, ON M1L 1W1
                                              Tel: 416-285-3666
                                              info@providence.on.ca
                                              www.providence.on.ca

Public Health Ontario
#300, 480 University Ave., Toronto, ON M5G 1V2
                                              Tel: 647-260-7100
                                              library@oahpp.ca
                                              www.publichealthontario.ca
Beata Pach, Manager, Library Services
  beata.pach@oahpp.ca

Québec Ministère de la santé et des services sociaux
1075, ch Sainte-Foy, Québec, QC G1S 2M1
                              Tél: 418-266-7171; *Téléc:* 418-266-7197
                                              www.msss.gouv.qc.ca

Queen Elizabeth Hospital
60 Riverside Dr., 3rd Fl., Charlottetown, PE C1A 8T5
Tel: 902-894-2371; *Fax:* 902-894-2424
QEHLibrary@ihis.org
www.qehlibrarypei.ca
Collection: Journals; e-books; Health databases; Clinical practice guidelines
Julie Cole, Library Manager
jacole@ihis.org
Melissa Stanley, Library Clerk
mmstanley@ihis.org

Queen Elizabeth II Hospital
10409 - 98th St., Grande Prairie, AB T8V 2E8
Tel: 780-538-7100

Queensway-Carleton Hospital
3045 Baseline Rd., Nepean, ON K2H 8P4
Tel: 613-721-2000; *Toll-Free:* 888-824-9111
www.qch.on.ca

Quinte Health Care - Belleville General
265 Dundas St. East, Belleville, ON K8N 5A9
Tel: 613-969-7400; *Fax:* 613-968-8234
Toll-Free: 800-483-2811
info@qhc.on.ca
www.qhc.on.ca
Social Media: www.facebook.com/Quinte-Health-Care-173689537296
Collection: Health Sciences

Red Deer Regional Hospital Centre
South Complex, 3942 - 50A Ave., Lower Level, Red Deer, AB T4N 4E7
Tel: 403-343-4557; *Fax:* 403-343-4910
krs@albertahealthservices.ca

Regina Qu'Appelle Health Region
Regina General Hospital, 1440 - 14th Ave., Regina, SK S4P 0W5
Tel: 306-766-4142; *Fax:* 306-766-3839
library@rqhealth.ca
rqhealth.ca/knowledge-and-technology/health-sciences-library-1
Collection: Texts; Journals; Electronic resources; Audiovisual materials
Fay Hutchinson, Archivist
fay.hutchinson@rqhealth.ca
306-766-4148

Regina Qu'Appelle Health Region - Wascana Rehabilitation Centre
2180 - 23 Ave., Regina, SK S4S 0A5
Tel: 306-766-5441; *Fax:* 306-766-5460
library@rqhealth.ca
www.rqhealth.ca/inside/hlthy_live_learn/library_page.shtml
Profile: Provides reference & research services, and extends borrowing privileges to RQHR staff & physicians, and students of medicine. Public may use the library during specified hours

Regina Qu'Appelle Health Region Library Services - Regina General Hospital
#0B, 1440 - 14th Ave., Regina, SK S4P 0W5
Tel: 306-766-4142; *Fax:* 306-766-3839
library@rqhealth.ca
www.rqhealth.ca
Profile: Provides reference & research services, and extends borrowing privileges to RQHR staff & physicians, and students of medicine. Public may use the library during specified hours **Collection:** RQHR Archives houses student records from Regina General Hospital School of Nursing
Susan Baer, Director
susan.baer@rqhealth.ca

Réseau de santé Vitalité - Beauséjour Zone
330, av Université, Moncton, NB E1C 2Z3
Tél: 506-862-4247; *Téléc:* 506-862-4246
info@vitalitenb.ca
www.vitalitenb.ca
Collection: Oncologie

Rockyview General Hospital Knowledge Centre
7007 - 14 St. SW, 4th Fl., Calgary, AB T2V 1P9
Tel: 403-943-3373; *Fax:* 403-943-3486
krs@albertahealthservices.ca
krs.albertahealthservices.ca

Rouge Valley Health System
2867 Ellesmere Rd., Toronto, ON M1E 4B9
Tel: 416-281-7101; *Fax:* 416-281-7360
library@rougevalley.ca
www.rougevalley.ca
Natalia Tukhareli, Librarian
ntukhareli@rougevalley.ca

Royal Alexandra Hospital
Active Treatment Centre, #1418, 10240 Kingsway Ave. NW, Edmonton, AB T5H 3V9
Tel: 780-735-5832; *Fax:* 780-735-4136
rahlibrary@albertahealthservices.ca
Morgan Truax, Team Lead
morgan.truax@albertahealthservices.ca
Fazia Baksh, Library Technician
fazia.baksh@albertahealthservices.ca
Sophie Bradley, Library Technician
sophie.bradley@albertahealthservices.ca

Royal Columbian Hospital
330 Columbia St. East, New Westminster, BC V3L 3W7
Tel: 604-520-4281; *Fax:* 604-520-4755
feedback@fraserhealth.ca
www.fraserhealth.ca
Brooke Ballantyne Scott, Librarian
brooke.scott@fraserhealth.ca
604-520-4755
Allison Lambert, Library Technician
allison.lambert@fraserhealth.ca
604-520-4281

Royal Victoria Regional Health Centre (Barrie)
201 Georgian Dr., Barrie, ON L4M 6M2
Tel: 705-728-9802; *Fax:* 705-739-5693
healthlibrary@rvh.on.ca
www.rvh.on.ca
Collection: Professional & consumer health resources
Barb Strudwick, Coordinator
strudwickb@rvh.on.ca

St. Boniface General Hospital
351 Taché Ave., Winnipeg, MB R2H 2A6
Tel: 204-237-2807; *Fax:* 204-235-3339
sbghlib@umanitoba.ca
libguides.lib.umanitoba.ca/sbh
Ada Ducas, Head
204-237-2808
Andrea Szwajcer, Clinical Librarian
204-247-2991

St Catharines General Hospital Site
1200 - 4th Ave., St Catharines, ON L2S 0A9
Tel: 905-378-4647
Other Numbers: Health Records Fax: 905-684-1136

St Clare's Mercy Hospital
154 LeMarchant Rd., St. John's, NL A1C 5B8
Tel: 709-777-5000

St John's Rehabilitation Hospital
285 Cummer Ave., #S325, Toronto, ON M2M 2G1
Tel: 416-480-4562; *Fax:* 416-226-6265
www.sunnybrook.ca/content/?page=st-johns-rehab
Farid Miah, Manager, Library Services

St Joseph's Health Care, London
268 Grosvenor St., London, ON N6A 4V2
Tel: 519-646-6000; *Fax:* 519-646-6228
stjoseph_library@sjhc.london.on.ca
www.sjhc.london.on.ca
Brad Dishan, Medical Librarian
brad.dishan@sjhc.london.on.ca
519-646-6100 ext. 65727

St Joseph's Health Centre (Toronto)
30 The Queensway, Toronto, ON M6R 1B5
Tel: 416-530-6726
www.stjoestoronto.ca
Collection: Hospital Administration; Pastoral Care
Ana Jeremic, Manager, Library Services

St Joseph's Hospital (Hamilton)
Juravinski Innovation Tower, 50 Charlton Ave. East, #T2305,
Hamilton, ON L8N 4A6
Tel: 905-522-1155; Fax: 905-540-6504
library@stjoes.ca
www.stjoes.ca
Social Media: www.youtube.com/stjoesfoundation;
twitter.com/stjoeshamilton
Jean Maragno, Director, Library Services
jmaragno@stjoes.ca
905-522-1155 ext. 33410
Lois Cottrell, Library Technician
905-522-1155 ext. 33440

St Joseph's Hospital (Hamilton)
West 5th Campus, 100 West 5th St., Level 2 Atrium, Hamilton, ON
L9C 0E3
Tel: 905-522-1155; Fax: 905-575-6035
cmhslib@stjoes.ca
www.stjoes.ca
Profile: The Library Resource Centre is a member of the Hamilton &
District Health Library Network. Resource sharing occurs among
McMaster University libraries & teaching & community hospitals in the
Hamilton area. **Collection:** Books, medical journals, & audiovisual
materials on the subject of mental health, including research, patient
care, & education.

St Joseph's Hospital (Saint John)
130 Bayard Dr., Saint John, NB E2L 3L6
Tel: 506-632-5555; Fax: 506-632-5551
www.horizonnb.ca

St Martha's Regional Hospital
25 Bay St., Antigonish, NS B2G 2G5
Tel: 902-863-2830; Fax: 902-867-1059
www.gasha.nshealth.ca/facilities/hospitals/stmarthas

St. Mary's General Hospital
911 Queen's Blvd., 10th Fl., Kitchener, ON N2M 1B2
Tel: 519-749-6549; Fax: 519-749-6426
www.smgh.ca
Profile: The library is available to staff & volunteers all day, every day.
The librarian is available by appointment. **Collection:** Health related
journals & databases; Fiction collection for patients & visitors
Laura Paprocki, Medical Librarian
lpaprock@smgh.ca

St. Mary's Hospital Centre/ Centre Hospitalier de St. Mary
3830, av Lacombe, Montréal, QC H3T 1M5
Tel: 514-345-3511
www.smhc.qc.ca
Collection: References books & materials on research

St Marys Memorial Hospital
267 Queen St. West, St Marys, ON N4X 1B6
Tel: 519-284-1332
www.hpha.ca
Profile: St Marys Memorial Hospital Site is a member of the Huron
Perth Healthcare Alliance.
Jane Crawford, Contact, Library Services, Huron Perth Healthcare
Alliance
jane.crawford@hpha.ca

St Michael's Hospital
East Bldg., Li Ka Shing International Healthcare Education Centre,
209 Victoria St., 3rd Fl., Toronto, ON M5B 1T8
Tel: 416-864-5059
hslibrary@smh.ca
www.stmichaelshospital.com/education/library.php

St Paul's Health Sciences Library
Providence Bldg., #1555, 1081 Burrard St., Vancouver, BC V6Z 1Y6
Tel: 604-822-4440
woodward.library.ubc.ca/services-at-hospitals/st-pauls-hospital

St. Paul's Hospital
#B0.2.07, 1702 - 20th St. West, Saskatoon, SK S7M 0Z9
Tel: 306-655-5224; Fax: 306-655-5209
library@saskatoonhealthregion.ca
libguides.saskatoonhealthregion.ca/medlib
Suzanne Shepaard, Director

Saint-Thomas Community Health Centre/ Centre de santé
communautaire Saint-Thomas
9040 - 84 St., Edmonton, AB T6C 1E4
Tel: 780-434-2778; Fax: 780-466-8702
www.cscst.ca
Francesca Sebastian, Office Manager

Saskatchewan Health Information Resources Program (SHIRP)
Leslie & Irene Dube Health Sciences Library, Academic Health
Sciences Bldg., #E1400, 104 Clinic Pl., Saskatoon, SK S7N 2Z4
Tel: 306-966-1291; Fax: 306-966-5918
info@shirp.ca
www.shirp.ca
Susan Murphy, Administrative Head
Susan.Murphy@usask.ca
306-966-6022
Valerie Moore, SHIRP Librarian
valerie.moore@usask.ca
306-966-8739

Saskatchewan Hospital Branch Library
PO Box 39, 1 Jersey St., North Battleford, SK S9A 2X8
Tel: 306-446-6863; Fax: 306-446-6810
saskhospital.lib@lakeland.lib.sk.ca
www.lakelandlibrary.ca

Saskatoon City Hospital
Saskatoon City Hospital, #1923, 701 Queen St., Saskatoon, SK S7K
0M7
Tel: 306-655-7677; Fax: 306-655-8727
library@saskatoonhealthregion.ca
www.saskatoonhealthregion.ca
Lauren Seal, Librarian
306-655-7899

Sault Area Hospital
750 Great Northern Rd., Sault Ste Marie, ON P6B 0A8
Tel: 705-759-3434
library@sah.on.ca
www.sah.on.ca
Ron Gagnon, President & CEO

The Scarborough Hospital - General Campus
3050 Lawrence Ave. East, Toronto, ON M1P 2V5
Tel: 416-431-8200; Fax: 416-431-8232
library@tsh.to
tsh.to
Judy Ng, Library Technician
jung@tsh.to

Schulich Library of Physical Sciences, Life Sciences, &
Engineering
Macdonald-Stewart Library Bldg., 809 Sherbrooke St. West,
Montréal, QC H3A 0C1
Tel: 514-398-4769; Fax: 514-398-3903
schulich.library@mcgill.ca
www.mcgill.ca/library/branches/schulich
Social Media: blogs.library.mcgill.ca/schulich/
Collection: Books & journals in the physical sciences & engineering
subject areas; e-Journals; Databases
Natalie Waters, Acting Head Librarian
natalie.waters@mcgill.ca
Giovanna Badia, Liaison Librarian, Chemical Engineering & Earth &
Planetary Sciences
giovanna.badia@mcgill.ca
April Colosimo, Liaison Librarian, Chemistry, Mathematices, Statistics,
& Physics
april.colosimo@mcgill.ca
Tara Mawhinney, Liaison Librarian, Atmospheric & Oceanic Science,
Civil Engineering
tara.mawhinney@mcgill.ca

Jennifer Zhao, Liaison Librarian, Electrical & Computer Engineering & Geography
jennifer.zhao@mcgill.ca
Jill Boruff, Liaison Librarian, Consumer Health, Physical Therapy & Psychiatry
jill.boruff@mcgill.ca
Francesca Frati, Liaison Librarian, Nursing
francesca.frati@mcgill.ca
Genevieve Gore, Liaison Librarian, Epidemiology, Family Medicine & Pediatrics
genevieve.gore@mcgill.ca
Andrea Miller-Nesbitt, Liaison Librarian, Anatomy, Biochemistry, Pharmacology & Physiology
andrea.miller-nesbitt@mcgill.ca
Martin Morris, Liaison Librarian, Dentistry, Diagnostic Radiology & Pathology
martin.morris@mcgill.ca
Nazi Torabi, Liaison Librarian, Internal Medicine, Medical Education & Surgery
nazi.torabi@mcgill.ca

Seaforth Community Hospital
24 Centennial Dr., Seaforth, ON N0K 1W0
Tel: 519-527-1650
www.hpha.ca
Profile: Seaforth Community Hospital Site is a member of the Huron Perth Healthcare Alliance.
Jane Crawford, Contact, Huron Perth Healthcare Alliance Library Services
jane.crawford@hpha.ca
519-272-8210 ext. 2250

Secrétariat Permanent: Bibliothèque de la santé, Université de Montréal
Pavillon Roger-Gaudry, 2900, boul Édouard-Montpetit, 6e étage, #L-623, Montréal, QC H3T 1J4
Tél: 514-343-6826; *Téléc:* 514-343-6457
www.bib.umontreal.ca/nous-joindre/SA.htm
Monique St-Jean, Directrice des bibliothèques des sciences de la santé
514-343-7810

Seven Oaks General Hospital
#2LB01, 2300 McPhillips St., Winnipeg, MB R2V 3M3
Tel: 204-632-3124; *Fax:* 204-694-8240
soghlibrary@umanitoba.ca
sogh.ca/hospital-services/library
Social Media: twitter.com/healthlibrary;
Nicole Askin, Hospital Librarian
Nicole.Askin@umanitoba.ca
Stefania Zimarino, Library Assistant
204-632-3124

Le siège social du CSSS de Rimouski-Neigette, Hôpital régional - Rimouski
150, av Rouleau, Rimouski, QC G5L 5T1
Tél: 418-724-3000; *Téléc:* 418-724-8139
www.chrr.qc.ca
Mèdia social: twitter.com/CSSS_Rimouski_N;
www.facebook.com/pages/CSSS-de-Rimouski-Neigette/185128391529883

Simcoe Muskoka District Health Unit
15 Sperling Dr., Barrie, ON L4M 6K9
Tel: 705-721-7520; *Toll-Free:* 877-721-7520
www.simcoemuskokahealth.org/HealthUnit/Library.aspx

Sioux Lookout Meno-Ya-Win Health Centre
1 Meno Ya Win Way, Sioux Lookout, ON P8T 1B4
Tel: 807-737-3030
www.slmhc.on.ca

Sir Mortimer B. Davis Jewish General Hospital/ Hôpital général juif
3755, côte Ste-Catherine, #A-200, Montréal, QC H3T 1E2
Tel: 514-340-8222; *Fax:* 514-340-7552
www.jgh.ca/hsl
Collection: General medical; Judaica & Medical Ethics
Sabrina Page, Library Technician
sabrina.page.ccomtl@ssss.gouv.qc.ca
514-340-8222 ext. 25931

Society for Manitobans with Disabilities
825 Sherbrook St., Winnipeg, MB R3A 1M5
Tel: 204-975-3010; *Fax:* 204-975-3073
Toll-Free: 866-282-8041
TTY: 204-975-308
www.smd.mb.ca
Collection: Online resources

South Health Campus Knowledge Centre
Wellness Centre, 1st Fl., 4448 Front St., Calgary, AB T3M 1M4
Tel: 403-956-3930

South West Health
60 Vancouver St., Yarmouth, NS B5A 2P5
Tel: 902-742-3541; *Fax:* 902-742-0369
www.swndha.nshealth.ca

Southlake Regional Health Centre
596 Davis Dr., Newmarket, ON L3Y 2P9
Tel: 905-895-4521
www.southlakeregional.org
Patrick Clifford, Director, Research/Innovation
pclifford@southlakeregional.org
905-895-4521 ext. 2387

Sport Information Resource Centre (SIRC)
#100, 85 Plymouth St., Ottawa, ON K1S 3E2
Tel: 613-231-7472; *Fax:* 613-231-3739
Toll-Free: 800-665-6413
info@sirc.ca
www.sirc.ca
Social Media: twitter.com/SIRCtweets;
www.facebook.com/sirc.sportresearch;
www.linkedin.com/company/sirc_2
Debra Gassewitz, President & CEO
debrag@sirc.ca

Stratford General Hospital
46 General Hospital Dr., Stratford, ON N5A 2Y6
Tel: 519-272-8210
Profile: Stratford General Hospital is a member of the Huron Perth Healthcare Alliance.
Jane Crawford, Contact, Library Services, Huron Perth Healthcare Alliance
jane.crawford@hpha.ca

Student Health & Development Resource Library
Student Services Bldg., Wilfrid Laurier University, 75 University Ave. West, 1st Fl., Waterloo, ON N2L 3C5
Tel: 519-884-0710
waterloo.mylaurier.ca/development/info/services/library.htm
Collection: Health related materials.

Sun Country Health Region
PO Box 2003, Weyburn, SK S4H 2Z9
Tel: 306-842-8665
info@schr.sk.ca
www.suncountry.sk.ca
Collection: Relaxation tapes; videos

Sunnybrook Health Sciences Centre
Bayview Campus, 2075 Bayview Ave., #EG29, Toronto, ON M4N 3M5
Tel: 416-480-4562
sunnybrook.ca/content/?page=Care_Serv_Lib

Sunrise Health Region Library Services
270 Bradbrooke Dr., Yorkton, SK S3N 2K6
Tel: 306-782-2401
www.sunrisehealthregion.sk.ca
Collection: Palliative Care, Breastfeeding
Lorelei Stusek, Vice-President, Corporate Services

Surrey Memorial Hospital
13750 - 96th Ave., Surrey, BC V3V 1Z2
Tel: 604-585-5666
library@fraserhealth.ca
www.fraserhealth.ca
Michelle Purdon, Manager, Library Services
michelle.purdon@fraserhealth.ca
604-851-4700 ext. 64683

Surrey Place Centre
2 Surrey Pl., Toronto, ON M5S 2C2
Tel: 416-925-5141; *Fax:* 416-923-8476
www.surreyplace.on.ca
Katinka English, Manager
katinka.english@surreyplace.on.ca

Thunder Bay District Health Unit
999 Balmoral St., Thunder Bay, ON P7B 6E7
Tel: 807-625-5901; *Fax:* 807-623-2369
Toll-Free: 888-294-6630
www.tbdhu.com
Collection: Books, reports, brochures, teacher kits & audio-visual
materials related to public health
Tracy Zurich, Librarian

Thunder Bay Regional Health Sciences Centre
980 Oliver Rd., Thunder Bay, ON P7B 6V4
Tel: 807-684-6230; *Fax:* 807-684-5830
library@tbh.net
www.tbrhsc.net
Rita Marchesin, Chief Librarian
marchesr@tbh.net
807-684-6230

Timmins & District Hospital
700 Ross Ave. East, Timmins, ON P4N 8P2
Tel: 705-267-2131
www.tadh.com
Blaise MacNeil, President & CEO

Toronto General Hospital
Eaton North Wing, #1-418, 200 Elizabeth St., Toronto, ON M5G 2C4
Tel: 416-340-3429; *Fax:* 416-340-4384

Toronto Public Health
277 Victoria St., 6th Fl., Toronto, ON M5B 1W2
Tel: 416-338-7865; *Fax:* 416-338-0049
hlibrary@toronto.ca
www.toronto.ca/health
Bruce Gardham, Senior Librarian
bgardha@toronto.ca
416-338-8284

Toronto Rehabilitation Institute
#2-055, 550 University Ave., Toronto, ON M5G 2A2
Tel: 416-597-3422
uhnlibraries@uhn.ca
www.uhn.ca/TorontoRehab

Toronto Western Hospital
Fraser Fell Pavilion, #5-505, 399 Bathurst St., Toronto, ON M5T 2S8
Tel: 416-603-5750; *Fax:* 416-603-5326

Toward Optimized Practice (TOP)
#200, 12315 Stony Plain Rd., Edmonton, AB T5N 3Y8
Tel: 780-482-0319; *Fax:* 866-895-5661
Toll-Free: 866-505-3302
top@topalbertadoctors.org
www.topalbertadoctors.org
Social Media: www.youtube.com/user/TOPABDoctors;
twitter.com/TOP_AB

Trillium Health Centre - Mississauga Site
100 Queensway West, Mississauga, ON L5B 1B8
Tel: 905-848-7100
www.trilliumhealthpartners.ca
Penka Stoyanova, Senior Librarian
penka.stoyanova@trilliumhealthpartners.ca
905-813-1100 ext. 6479

Université de Sherbrooke
Pavillon Georges-Cabana, Université de Sherbrooke, 2500, boul de l'Université, Sherbrooke, QC J1K 2R1
Tél: 819-821-7550; *Téléc:* 819-821-7096
Ligne sans frais: 866-506-2433
www.usherbrooke.ca/biblio
Mèdia social: www.youtube.com/bibliosusherbrooke;
www.facebook.com/BibliothequesUdeS

Sylvie Fournier, Directrice générale
sylvie.fournier2@usherbrooke.ca
819-821-8000 ext. 63556
France Paul, Directrice, Documents administratifs et archives
france.paul@usherbrooke.ca
819-821-8000 ext. 63340

University Archives & Special Collections
c/o Killam Memorial Library, 6225 University Ave., 5th Fl., Halifax, NS B3H 4H8
Tel: 902-494-3615; *Fax:* 902-494-2062
archives@dal.ca
libraries.dal.ca/collection/archives.html
Social Media: www.facebook.com/dalhousiearchives
Collection: Material relating to the University; private manuscripts &
records representing Business, Theatre, Labour, Archives of the
Neptune Theatre, Medicine, Oceans, NS Literature, Rare Books, Small
Canadian Literary Press, University Thesis, Special Collections of
Rudyard Kipling & Francis Bacon, Music Collection
Michael Moosberger, University Archivist & Associate University
Librarian
michael.moosberger@dal.ca
902-494-5176
Creighton Barrett, Digital Archivist
creighton.barrett@Dal.ca
902-494-6490
Kelly Casey, Archives Assistant
Kelly.Stevens@Dal.Ca
902-494-6612
Dianne Landry, Archives Assistant
dianne.landry@dal.ca
902-494-6794

University Health Network
610 University Ave., 5th Fl., Toronto, ON M5G 2M9
Tel: 416-946-4482; *Fax:* 416-946-2084
uhnlibraries@uhn.ca
www.uhn.ca
Bogusia Trojan, Director, Library & Information Services
Ani Orchanian-Cheff, Archivist

University of Alberta
Cameron Library, University of Alberta, Edmonton, AB T6G 2J8
Tel: 780-492-8440; *Fax:* 780-492-2721
sciref@ualberta.ca
www.library.ualberta.ca
Social Media: twitter.com/Cameron_Library
Gerald Beasley, Vice-Provost & Chief Librarian
gbeasley@ualberta.ca
780-492-5170
Margaret Law, Director, External Relations
Kathleen De Long, Senior Human Resources Officer

University of British Columbia
1961 East Mall, Vancouver, BC V6T 1Z1
Tel: 604-822-6375; *Fax:* 604-822-3893
www.library.ubc.ca
Social Media: www.flickr.com/photos/ubclibrary; twitter.com/ubclibrary;
www.facebook.com/UBCLibrary
Collection: Pacific Northwest History, Canadiana, English 19th
Century Literature (Colbeck), History of Cartography, Cartographic
Archives, Early Japanese Maps (Bean), English & American Children's
Literature from 18th Century to 1930's, University Archives, UBC
Theses, History of Medicine & Science, Oriental Collection including
The P'u-pan Collection, Harry Hawthorne Angling Collection, Literature
(Colbeck), Canadiana Maps (Rogers-Tucker), The Chung Collection,
The H.C.S. Stravinsky Collection
Melody Burton, Interim University Librarian
university.librarian@ubc.ca
604-822-4903
Allan Bell, Associate University Librarian, Digital Programs & Services
allan.bell@ubc.ca
604-827-4830
Sheldon Armstrong, Associate University Librarian, Collection
Development
sheldon.armstrong@ubc.ca
604-822-5300

Lea Starr, Associate University Librarian, Research Services
lea.starr@ubc.ca
604-822-2826

University of Calgary
410 University Ct. NW, Calgary, AB T2N 1N4
Tel: 403-220-8895; *Fax:* 403-282-6024
libinfo@ucalgary.ca
library.ucalgary.ca
Social Media: twitter.com/UCalgaryLibrary;
www.facebook.com/UCalgaryLibraries
Thomas Hickerson, Vice-Provost (Libraries)
tom.hickerson@ucalgary.ca
403-220-3765
Barb Murray, Manager, Office of Vice-Provost (Libraries & Cultural
Resources)
bmurray@ucalgary.ca
403-220-3765
Mary McConnell, Associate University Librarian, Content Development
mmcconne@ucalgary.ca
403-220-3725

University of Manitoba Libraries
Elizabeth Dafoe Library, University of Manitoba, 25 Chancellors
Circle, Winnipeg, MB R3T 2N2
Tel: 204-474-9881; *Fax:* 204-474-7583
libwww@umanitoba.ca
www.umanitoba.ca/libraries/

Mary-Jo Romaniuk, University Librarian
mary-jo.romaniuk@umanitoba.ca
204-474-8749
Donna Breyfogle, Associate University Librarian, Collections
donna_breyfogle@umanitoba.ca
Vera Keown, Associate University Librarian, Academic Engagement
Services
vera_keown@umanitoba.ca
204-474-7842
Krys Rowinski, Manager, Administrative Services
krys_rowinski@umanitoba.ca

University of Ottawa/ Université d'Ottawa
Morisset Hall, 65 University Private, Ottawa, ON K1N 6N5
Tel: 613-562-5213
Other Numbers: Circulation: 613-562-5212
referenc@uottawa.ca
www.biblio.uottawa.ca
Collection: e-Books; eJournals; Government publications; Databases
Leslie Weir, University Librarian
lweir@uottawa.ca

University of Toronto Libraries
130 St George St., Toronto, ON M5S 1A5
Tel: 416-978-8450
library.info@utoronto.ca
www.library.utoronto.ca
Social Media: twitter.com/uoftlibraries
Larry Alford, Chief Librarian
larry.alford@utoronto.ca
416-978-2292
Alastair Boyd, Head, Cataloguing
416-978-8934
Caitlin Tillman, Associate Chief Librarian, Collections & Materials
Management
416-946-3856
Sian Meikle, Director, Information Technology Services
416-978-7649

University of Victoria School of Health Information Science
Health Information Science, U. of Victoria, #A202, 3800 Finnerty
Rd., Victoria, BC V8P 5C2
Tel: 250-721-8575; *Fax:* 250-472-4751
his@uvic.ca
www.uvic.ca/hsd/hinf
Collection: Colloquium recordings, archived seminars,& CIHR
workshops available online
Andre Kishniruk, Director
andrek@uvic.ca
250-472-5132

Vancouver Coastal Health Authority
520 West 6th Ave., Vancouver, BC V5Z 1A1
Tel: 604-730-7656
vchlibraryservices@vch.ca
www.vch.ca/your-health/library-services/library-services

Vancouver Island Health Authority
1952 Bay St., Victoria, BC V8R 1J8
Tel: 250-370-8699; *Fax:* 250-370-8274
Toll-Free: 877-370-8699
info@viha.ca
www.viha.ca/library
Cliff Cornish, Manager, Library Services
Joyce Constantine, Librarian

Vancouver Island Health Authority
c/o Nanaimo Regional General Hospital, 1200 Dufferin Cres.,
#G250, Nanaimo, BC V9S 2B7
Tel: 250-755-7691; *Fax:* 250-755-7662
librarianci@viha.ca
Teresa Prior, Librarian

Victoria General Hospital (Winnipeg)
2340 Pembina Hwy., Winnipeg, MB R3T 2E8
Tel: 204-477-3307; *Fax:* 204-269-7936
www.vgh.mb.ca
Social Media: twitter.com/VGHLibrary
Melissa Raynard, Acting Hospital Librarian
204-477-3284

Vitalité Health Network/ Réseau de sante vitalité
#600, 275 Main St., Bathurst, NB E2A 1A9
Tel: 506-544-2133; *Fax:* 506-544-2145
Toll-Free: 888-472-2220
www.santevitalitehealth.ca

West Park Healthcare Centre
82 Buttonwood Dr., Toronto, ON M6M 2J5
Tel: 416-243-3600; *Fax:* 416-243-8947
www.westpark.org
Collection: 3000 monographs; 50 journals
John Tagg, Librarian
john.tagg@westpark.org

Western Health Care Corporation
PO Box 2005, Corner Brook, NL A2H 6J7
Tel: 709-637-5000; *Fax:* 709-637-5268
library@westernhealth.nl.ca
westernhealth.nl.ca/index.php/learning/library-services
Kimberly Hancock, Team Leader
kimhancock@westernhealth.nl.ca
709-637-5000 ext. 5218
Barbara Gallant, Librarian
lbgallant@grenfell.mun.ca
709-637-5000 ext. 5395
Lisa Miller, Clerical Support
lisamiller@westernhealth.nl.ca
709-637-5000 ext. 5395

Western Ontario Health Knowledge Network
c/o Kim Cornell, Allyn & Betty Taylor Library, Western University
Libraries, Natural Science Centre, Western University, London, ON
N6A 5B7
www.wohkn.ca

William Osler Health Centre
Brampton Memorial Hospital Campus, 2100 Bovaird Dr. East,
Brampton, ON L6R 3J7
Tel: 905-494-2120; *Fax:* 905-494-6641
www.williamoslerhs.ca
Janice Thompson, Library Technician
janice.thompson@williamoslerhs.ca

Windsor Essex County Health Unit
1005 Ouellette Ave., Windsor, ON N9A 4J8
Tel: 519-258-2146; *Fax:* 519-258-6003
Toll-Free: 800-265-5822
www.wechu.org
Collection: Booklets; brochures; manuals; reports; fact sheets;
pamphlets & handouts; news letters; posters & flyers

Lorie Gregg, Director, Corporate Services
519-258-2146 ext. 1392

Windsor Regional Hospital - Metropolitan Campus
1995 Lens Ave., Windsor, ON N8W 1L9
Tel: 519-254-5577; Fax: 519-985-2640
www.wrh.on.ca
Toni Janik, Coordinator, Library Services
toni.janik@wrh.on.ca

Windsor Regional Hospital - Ouellette Campus
1030 Ouellette Ave., Windsor, ON N9A 1E1
Tel: 519-973-4411; Fax: 519-973-0642
www.wrh.on.ca
Collection: Books; journals; eJournals; eBooks; online databases & products

Wingham & District Hospital
270 Carling Terrace, Wingham, ON N0G 2W0
Tel: 519-357-3210; Fax: 519-357-3522
www.lwha.ca

W.K. Kellogg Health Sciences Library
Sir Charles Tupper Bldg., Dalhousie University, 5850 College St., Halifax, NS B3H 1X5
Tel: 902-494-2458; Fax: 902-494-3798
Other Numbers: Reference: 902-494-2482; Circulation: 902-494-2479
Social Media: www.facebook.com/kellogghealthscienceslibrary
Collection: Dr Charles Cogswell's Medical Library, 1864
Ann Barrett, Interim Head
902-494-1669
Penelope David, Technical Services Contact
902-494-3740
Nadine Day-Boutilier, Access Services/Document Delivery/Reference Librarian
902-494-2479

Women's College Hospital
#2410, 76 Grenville St., Toronto, ON M5S 1B2
Tel: 416-323-6036; Fax: 416-323-6122
www.womenscollegehospital.ca
Collection: Hospital Archives
Mary Anne Howse, Manager, Library Services
maryanne.howse@wchospital.ca

Women's Health Knowledge Centre
North Tower, Foothills Medical Centre, 1441 - 29th St. NW, Calgary, AB T2N 4J8
Tel: 403-944-2267; Fax: 403-944-4772

Woodstock General Hospital
310 Juliana Dr., Woodstock, ON N4V 0A4
Tel: 519-421-4233; Fax: 519-421-4236
info@wgh.on.ca
www.wgh.on.ca
Linda Wilcox, Librarian

Woodward Library
2198 Health Sciences Mall, Vancouver, BC V6T 1Z3
Tel: 604-822-4440; Fax: 604-822-5596
wd.ref@ubc.ca
woodward.library.ubc.ca
Collection: History of Life Sciences collection; Various records relating to Canadian, British & European scientists

York Region Public Health Services
17250 Yonge St., Newmarket, ON L3Y 6Z1
Tel: 905-895-4511; Fax: 905-895-3166
www.york.ca
Maria Aulicino, Librarian & Resource Coordinator
Maria.Aulicino@york.ca

Yukon Department of Health & Social Services
PO Box 2703, Whitehorse, YT Y1A 2C6
Tel: 867-667-5919; Fax: 867-393-6457
Toll-Free: 800-661-0408
www.hss.gov.yk.ca
Social Media: www.youtube.com/user/hssyukongovernment; twitter.com/HSSYukon; www.facebook.com/yukonhss
Collection: Acts & regulations; forms & applications; guidelines; permits; reports

National Government

Canadian Centre for Occupational Health & Safety (CCOHS) / Centre canadien d'hygiène et de sécurité au travail (CCHST)
135 Hunter St. East, Hamilton, ON L8N 1M5
Tel: 905-572-2981
Fax: 905-572-4500
Toll-Free: 800-668-4284
www.ccohs.ca
twitter.com/ccohs
www.facebook.com/CCOHS
www.youtube.com/ccohs

Provides occupational health & safety & environmental information in the form of publications, responses to inquiries & a computerized information service available in various formats. Topics include: environmental acts & regulations; occupational & environmental health data; toxic effects of chemical substances; transport of dangerous goods; chemical evaluation; hazardous substances; & domestic substances listed under the Canadian Environmental Protection Act; biological hazards; ergonomics

Chair, Council of Governors, Gary Robertson

Acting President & CEO; Vice-President, Operations, Gareth Jones
Tel: 905-572-2981 ext: 4537

Chief Financial Officer; Vice-President, Finance, Frank Leduc
Tel: 905-572-2981 ext: 4401

Director, Marketing Communications, Lynda Brown
Tel: 905-572-2981 ext: 4472

Manager, Inquiries & Client Services, Renzo Bertolini
Tel: 905-572-2981 ext: 4477

Manager, General Health & Safety, Gerry Culina
Tel: 905-572-2981 ext: 4527

Manager, Chemical Services, Lorraine Davison
Tel: 905-572-2981 ext: 4466

Manager, Training & Education Services, Christopher Moore
Tel: 905-572-2981 ext: 4462

Canadian Institutes of Health Research (CIHR) / Instituts de recherche en santé du Canada (IRSC)
160 Elgin St., 9th Fl., Ottawa, ON K1A 0W9
Tel: 613-954-1968
Fax: 613-954-1800
Toll-Free: 888-603-4178
support@cihr-irsc.gc.ca
www.cihr-irsc.gc.ca
Other Communication: Reception: 613-941-2672
twitter.com/cihr_irsc
www.facebook.com/HealthResearchInCanada
linkedin.com/company/canadian-institutes-of-health-research
www.youtube.com/user/HealthResearchCanada

Promotes health research excellence in Canada through training & funding programs in basic, clinical, health systems & services, & population health research. Research is carried out in universities, in the health sciences faculties, affiliated hospitals & institutions & other faculties where research projects are highly relevant to human health. University-Industry programs create the opportunity for collaboration between Canadian companies & researchers conducting research in Canadian universities or affiliated institutions. Also manages the health-related Networks of Centres of Excellence & operates 13 "virtual" institutes, which link & support researchers pursuing common goals in specific areas of focus.

President, Alain Beaudet
Tel: 613-954-1808

Chief Scientific Officer & Vice-President, Research, Knowledge Translation & Ethics, Dr. Jane E. Aubin
Tel: 613-954-1805
VPResearch@cihr-irsc.gc.ca

Chief Financial Officer & Vice-President, Resource Planning & Management, Thérèse Roy, CPA, CA
Tel: 613-954-1946
therese.roy@cihr-irsc.gc.ca

Vice-President, External Affairs and Business Development, Michel Perron
Tel: 613-957-6134
michel.perron@cihr-irsc.gc.ca

Associate Vice-President, Program Operations, Jeff Latimer
Tel: 613-960-6218
jeff.latimer@cihr-irsc.gc.ca

Director General, Program Design & Delivery, Peggy Borbey
Tel: 613-954-0582

Director General, Communications & Public Outreach, Christina Cefaloni
Tel: 613-954-1812

Director General, College of Reviewers, Sarah Connor Gorber
Tel: 613-954-0616

Acting Director General, Science, Knowledge Translation & Ethics, Dr. Michelle Peel
Tel: 613-954-6242

Executive Director, Secretariat on Responsible Conduct of Research, Susan Zimmerman
Tel: 613-947-7148

Institute of Aboriginal Peoples' Health (IAPH) / Institut de la santé des Autochtones (ISA)
Health Sciences North Research Institute, 41 Ramsay Lake Rd., Sudbury, ON P3E 5J1
Toll-Free: 888-603-4178
iaph.isa@cihr-irsc.gc.ca
www.cihr-irsc.gc.ca/e/8668.html
The purpose of IAPH is to improve & promote the health of First Nations, Inuit & Métis peoples in Canada.
Scientific Director, Dr. Carrie Bourassa
Tel: 705-523-7300 ext: 2118
Fax: 705-523-7326
Carrie.Bourassa@cihr-irsc.gc.ca

Institute of Aging (IA) / Institut du vieillissement (IV)
Centre de recherche, CRIUGM, 4545, ch Queen-Mary, Montréal, QC H3W 1W5
Fax: 514-360-2439
Toll-Free: 888-603-4178
www.cihr-irsc.gc.ca/e/8671.html
IA looks at the effects of aging, & the effects of different diseases & conditions on aging, rather than focusing on particular diseases.
Scientific Director, Yves Joanette, PhD, FCAHS
Tel: 514-360-2431
yves.joanette@umontreal.ca

Institute of Cancer Research (ICR) / Institut du cancer (IC)
Heritage Medical Research Bldg., University of Calgary, #372, 3330 Hospital Dr. NW, Calgary, AB T2N 4N1
Toll-Free: 888-603-4178
cihr.icr@ucalgary.ca
www.cihr-irsc.gc.ca/e/12506.html
ICR funds cancer research in Canada.
Scientific Director, Stephen M. Robbins, PhD
Tel: 403-220-7091
Fax: 403-210-9641
srobbins@ucalgary.ca

Institute of Circulatory & Respiratory Health (ICRH) / Institut de la santé circulatoire et respiratoire (ISCR)
University of Alberta, Office of the VP (Research), 602 College Plaza, 8215 112 St. NW, Edmonton, AB T6G 2C8
Tel: 780-492-0272
Fax: 780-248-1317
Toll-Free: 888-603-4178
icrh-iscr@cihr-irsc.gc.ca
www.cihr-irsc.gc.ca/e/8663.html
ICRH supports research into the heart, lung, brain, blood, blood vessels, critical care & sleep. Areas of focus include causes, mechanisms, prevention, screening, diagnosis, treatment, support systems & palliation for a range of conditions.
Scientific Director, Dr. Brian Rowe
Tel: 780-407-6707
Fax: 613-954-1800

Institute of Gender & Health (IGH) / Institut de la santé des femmes et des hommes (ISFH)
Centre de Recherche, CRIUGM, 4565 Chemin Queen-Mary, Montréal, QC H3W 1W5
Fax: 514-312-9005
Toll-Free: 888-603-4178
www.cihr-irsc.gc.ca/e/8673.html
IGH researches the influence of gender & sex on the health of women & men in order to identify & address important health issues.
Scientific Director, Dr. Cara Tannenbaum
Tel: 514-312-9036
cara.tannenbaum@umontreal.ca

Institute of Genetics (IG) / Institut de génétique (IG)
McGill University, #279, 3649, promenade Sir William Osler, Montréal, QC H3G 0B1
Fax: 514-398-1684
Toll-Free: 888-603-4178
cihr-ig.biology@mcgill.ca
www.cihr-irsc.gc.ca/e/13147.html
IG supports research into all aspects of genetics, especially basic biochemistry & cell biology related to health & disease.
Scientific Director, Paul Lasko, PhD
Tel: 514-398-3416
paul.lasko@mcgill.ca

Institute of Health Services & Policy Research (IHSPR) / Institut des services et des politiques de la santé (ISPS)
3666, rue McTavish, Montréal, QC H3A 1Y2
Toll-Free: 888-603-4178
info.ihspr@mcgill.ca
www.cihr-irsc.gc.ca/e/13733.html
IHSPR is mandated to improve the way health care services are organized, regulated, managed, financed, paid for, used & delivered.
Scientific Director, Dr. Robyn Tamblyn
rtamblyn.ihspr@mcgill.ca

Institute of Human Development, Child & Youth Health (IHDCYH) / Institut du développement et de la santé des enfants et des adolescents (IDSEA)
Mount Sinai Hospital, #19-231D, 600 University Ave., Toronto, ON M5G 1X5
Toll-Free: 888-603-4178
ihdcyh-idsea@cihr-irsc.gc.ca
www.cihr-irsc.gc.ca/e/8688.html
Secondary Address: #8-500, 700 University Ave.
Toronto Location, Ontario Power Generation Bldg.
Toronto, ON M5G 1X6
IHDCYH focuses on reproduction, early development, childhood & adolescence.
Scientific Director, Dr. Shoo K. Lee
Tel: 416-586-4800 ext: 6370
Shoo.Lee@sinaihealthsystem.ca

Institute of Infection & Immunity (III) / Institut des maladies infectieuses et immunitaires (IMII)
Centre de recherche du CHU de Québec, 2705, boul Laurier, #TR-62, Québec, QC G1V 4G2

Tel: 418-577-4688
Fax: 418-577-4689
Toll-Free: 888-603-4178
HIVAIDS-VIHSIDA@cihr-irsc.gc.ca
www.cihr-irsc.gc.ca/e/13533.html

III supports research into infectious diseases & the body's immune system.
Scientific Director, Marc Ouellette
  Tel: 418-525-4444 ext: 48016
  Fax: 418-577-4689
  marc.ouellette@crchul.ulaval.ca

Institute of Musculoskeletal Health & Arthritis (IMHA) / Institut de l'appareil locomoteur et de l'arthrite (IALA)
Brodie Centre, University of Manitoba, #290, 727 McDermot Ave., Winnipeg, MB R3E 3P5

Fax: 204-789-3943
Toll-Free: 888-603-4178
imha@cihr-irsc.gc.ca
www.cihr-irsc.gc.ca/e/13217.html

IMHA focuses on conditions related to bones, joints, muscles, connective tissue, skin & teeth.
Scientific Director, Dr. Hani El-Gabalawy
  Tel: 204-318-3552
  Fax: 204-789-3943
  Hani.Elgabalawy@umanitoba.ca

Institute of Neurosciences, Mental Health & Addiction (INMHA) / Institut des neurosciences, de la santé mentale et des toxicomanies (INSMT)
Djavad Mowafaghian Centre for Brain Health, UBC, #3402, 2215 Wesbrook Mall, Vancouver, BC V6T 1Z3

Fax: 604-822-0361
Toll-Free: 888-603-4178
INMHA-INSMT@cihr-irsc.gc.ca
www.cihr-irsc.gc.ca/e/8602.html

INMHA supports research into mental health, neurological health, vision, hearing & cognitive functioning.
Scientific Director, Dr. Anthony G. Phillips
  Tel: 604-822-4624
  Fax: 604-822-7756
  aphillips@psych.ubc.ca

Institute of Nutrition, Metabolism & Diabetes (INMD) / Institut de la nutrition, du métabolisme et du diabète (INMD)
Banting Bldg., Hospital for Sick Children, #311, 100 College St., Toronto, ON M5G 1L5

Fax: 416-978-1334
Toll-Free: 888-603-4178
inmd.comms@sickkids.ca
www.cihr-irsc.gc.ca/e/13521.html

INMD focuses on research related to diet, digestion, excretion & metabolism, & conditions associated with hormone, digestive system, kidney & liver function.
Scientific Director, Dr. Philip Sherman
  Tel: 416-978-1315
  sd.inmd@sickkids.ca

Institute of Population & Public Health (IPPH) / Institut de la santé publique et des populations (ISPP)
57 Louis Pasteur, Ottawa, ON K1N 6N5

Fax: 613-562-5713
Toll-Free: 888-603-4178
ipph-ispp@globalstrategylab.org
www.cihr-irsc.gc.ca/e/13777.html

IPPH focuses on the interactions (biological, social, cultural, environmental) that determine the health of individuals, communities & global populations. Research includes environment & health issues, such as radiation, contaminants, ecosystems & air quality.
Scientific Director, Steven J. Hoffman
  Tel: 613-562-5800 ext: 3256
  steven.hoffman@globalstrategylab.org

Correctional Service Canada (CSC) / Service correctionnel Canada
340 Laurier Ave. West, Ottawa, ON K1A 0P9

Tel: 613-992-5891
Fax: 613-943-1630
www.csc-scc.gc.ca
twitter.com/csc_scc_en
www.youtube.com/user/CSCsccEN

An agency within Public Safety & Emergency Preparedness Canada responsible for the administration of sentences with respect to convicted offenders sentenced to two or more years as decided by the federal courts, & certain provincial inmates who have been transferred to a federal institution. CSC is also responsible for the supervision of inmates who have been granted conditional release by the authority of the National Parole Board.

Minister, Public Safety & Emergency Preparedness, Hon. Ralph Goodale, P.C., B.A., LL.B.
Tel: 613-947-1153
Fax: 613-996-9790
ralph.goodale@parl.gc.ca

Commissioner, Don Head
Tel: 613-995-5781
Fax: 613-943-1630

Senior Deputy Commissioner, Transformation, Anne Kelly
Tel: 613-947-0643
Fax: 613-943-1630

Associate Assistant Commissioner, Public Affairs Directorate, Amy Jarrette
Tel: 613-996-5476
Fax: 613-947-1184

Director General, Aboriginal Initiatives Directorate, Lisa Allgaier
Tel: 613-995-5465
Fax: 613-943-0493

Health Services / Services de santé
Assistant Commissioner, Jenifer Wheatley
  Tel: 613-995-8023
  Fax: 613-992-9995
Director General, Clinical Services, Henry de Souza
  Tel: 613-947-1013
  Fax: 613-995-6277
National Coordinator, Institutional Mental Health Initiatives, Natalie Gabora-Roth
  Tel: 613-316-7285
  Fax: 613-995-6277
Manager, Quality Improvement & Strategic Priorities, Audrey Castonguay
  Tel: 613-947-9541
  Fax: 613-992-9995
Manager, Institutional & Community Mental Health Services, Ginette Clarke
  Tel: 613-992-5866
  Fax: 613-992-9995
Manager, Infectious Diseases Program, Sylvie-Ann Lavigne
  Tel: 613-943-5333
  Fax: 613-992-9995
Manager, Epidemiology Services, Jonathan Smith
  Tel: 613-947-9541
  Fax: 613-992-9995
Senior Nursing Advisor, Clinical Services, Lucie Poliquin
  Tel: 613-943-2784
  Fax: 613-992-9995

Health Canada / Santé Canada
Tunney's Pasture, Ottawa, ON K1A 0K9

Tel: 613-957-2991
Fax: 613-941-5366
Toll-Free: 866-225-0709
TTY: 800-465-7735
info@hc-sc.gc.ca
www.hc-sc.gc.ca
Other Communication: Information on Medical Marijuana:
1-866-337-7705; omc-bcm@hc-sc.gc.ca
twitter.com/healthcanada
www.facebook.com/HealthyCdns
www.youtube.com/user/healthcanada

In partnership with provincial & territorial governments, Health Canada (HC) develops health policy, enforces health regulations, promotes disease prevention, & enhances healthy living for all Canadians. HC ensures that health services are available & accessible to First Nations & Inuit communities. It works closely with other federal departments, agencies & health stakeholders to reduce health & safety risks to Canadians. Through its Health Intelligence Network, HC works with other levels of government & the health care system in the surveillance, prevention, control & research of disease outbreaks across Canada & around the world. It also monitors health & safety risks related to the sale & use of drugs, food, chemicals, pesticides, medical devices & certain consumer products. HC negotiates agreements regarding hazardous materials in the workplace, performs medical assessments for pilots & air traffic controllers, & conducts environmental health assessments. As of April 1, 2013, Health Canada assumed the responsibilities & functions under the Hazardous Materials Information Review Act, formerly carried out by the Hazardous Materials Information Review Commission.

Minister, Health, Hon. Jane Philpott, P.C.
Tel: 613-992-3640
Fax: 613-992-3642
Jane.Philpott@parl.gc.ca

Deputy Minister, Simon Kennedy
Tel: 613-957-0212

Director, Parliamentary Affairs, Peter Cleary
Tel: 613-957-0200

Director, Communications, David Clements
Tel: 613-957-0200

Director, Policy, Caroline Pitfield
Tel: 613-957-0200

Press Secretary, Andrew MacKendrick
Tel: 613-957-0200

Departmental Liaison (PHAC & CIHR), Marianne DeVito
Tel: 613-957-0200

Health Canada Regulations Section / Section de la réglementation
General Counsel & Director, Claude Lesage
Tel: 613-952-9645

Legal Services / Services juridiques
www.hc-sc.gc.ca/ahc-asc/branch-dirgen/ls-sj/index-eng.php
Executive Director & Senior General Counsel, Shalene Curtis-Micallef
Tel: 613-957-3766
Manager & Senior Administrative Officer, Ginette Morin
Tel: 613-941-5343

Communications & Public Affairs Branch / Direction générale des affaires publiques et des communications
The Communications & Public Affairs Branch integrates national & regional perspectives into all of its policies & strategies, communications & consultation functions. The Branch plays a key role in delivering Health Canada's commitment to transparency. Through the branch, Health Canada aims to continue improving communications & the flow of information to & from stakeholders, clients, partners, media & the Canadian public.
Acting Assistant Deputy Minister, Jennifer Hollington
Tel: 613-960-2176

Director General, Public Affairs Directorate, Renee Couturier
Tel: 613-957-0215
Director General, Ministerial Services & Integrated Communications Directorate, Marian Hubley
Tel: 613-960-6040
Acting Director General, Public Health Strategic Communications Directorate, Sara MacKenzie
Tel: 613-952-8155
Executive Director, Health, Regulatory Strategic Commuications Division, Ken Polk
Tel: 613-948-8916
Director, The Blueprint Group, Carol Della Penta
Tel: 613-941-2683
Director, Strategic Advice & Planning, Darrin Denne
Tel: 613-948-7624
Director, Regional Communications & Executive Correspondence Division, Franca Gatto
Tel: 613-948-6420
Director, Media Relations & Ministerial Services, Louise Payette
Tel: 613-957-2987
Director, Public Engagement, Research & Analysis, Yanik Perigny
Tel: 613-957-1556
Director, Shared Services Integration, John Pierlot
Tel: 613-952-1009
Director, Food & Drugs Act Liaison Office, Serena Siqueira
Tel: 613-948-3238
Director, Marketing, Partnerships, & Creative Services Division, Sheri Todd
Tel: 613-948-8444
Senior Communications Advisor, Blossom Leung
Tel: 613-957-6219

Corporate Services Branch (CSB) / Direction générale aux services de gestion
The CSB provides corporate support & services across the Department in the following areas: human resources management; official languages; real property & facilities management; occupational health, safety emergency & security management; information technology & information management; executive correspondence; & access to information & privacy requests/issues.
Assistant Deputy Minister, Debbie Beresford-Green
Tel: 613-946-3200
Chief Information Officer, Information Management, Kirk Shaw
Tel: 613-595-1307
Director General, Human Resources, Robert Ianiro
Tel: 613-957-3236
Director General, Planning, Integration & Management Services Directorate, Jean-Francois Luc
Tel: 613-946-8132
Director General, Business Renewal & Enterprise Architecture Directorate, Scott McKenna
Tel: 902-426-4600
Director General, Specialized Health Services Directorate, Nancy Porteous
Tel: 613-957-7669
Director General, Real Property & Security Directorate, Martin Tomkin
Tel: 613-952-6190
Executive Director, National Real Property Management Division, Paul Bortolotti
Tel: 613-952-0936
Executive Director, Service Management Division, Karl Ghiara
Tel: 613-595-1287
Executive Director, Executive Group Services Division, Peter Hooey
Tel: 613-668-7893
Executive Director, Workplace Wellbeing & Workforce Development, Delroy Lawrence
Tel: 613-954-2248
Executive Director, Corporate Policies & Programs, Regional Operations Division, Caroline Legare
Tel: 613-941-4214
Executive Director, Solutions Centre, Tracey Sampson
Tel: 613-595-1371

Deputy Minister's Office / Bureau de la Sous-Ministre
Deputy Minister, Simon Kennedy
Tel: 613-957-0212

Associate Deputy Minister, Christine Donoghue
Tel: 613-954-5904

Ombudsman & Executive Director, Organizational Ombudsman, Luc Begin
Tel: 613-948-8259

Director, Values & Ethics, Organizational Ombudsman, Sylvie Houde, PhD
Tel: 613-941-7313

First Nations & Inuit Health Branch (FNIHB) / Direction générale de la santé des Premières nations et des Inuits (DGSPNI)

Assists First Nations & Inuit communities & people to address health inequalities & diseases threats through health surveillance & population health interventions. Ensures the availability of, or access to, health services for First Nations & Inuit people. Devolves control & management of community-based health services to First Nations & Inuit communities & organizations. The Environmental Health Division addresses conditions in the environment that could affect the health of community members, such as drinking water quality, mould, food safety, facilities inspections, transportation of dangerous goods. The Environmental Research Division conducts, coordinates & funds contaminants-related research, coordinates the replacement or upgrading of diesel-fuel tanks & remediation of fuel oil-contaminated sites, lab services for testing of PCBs & mercury, drinking water-related research & testing.

Senior Assistant Deputy Minister, Sony Perron
Tel: 613-957-7701

Assistant Deputy Minister, Regional Operations, Valerie Gideon
Tel: 613-946-1722

Chief Medical Officer of Health & Executive Director, Population & Public Health, Tom Wong
Tel: 613-952-9616

Director General, Non-Insured Health Benefits Directorate, Scott Doidge
Tel: 613-954-8825

Director General, Strategic Policy, Planning & Information, Mary-Luisa Kapelus
Tel: 613-954-2445

Director General, Delivery, Active Response & Coordination, Aruna Sadana
Tel: 613-954-0765

Director General, Branch, Anthony Sangster
Tel: 613-818-1243

Executive Director, Primary Health Care, Robin Buckland
Tel: 613-957-6359

Executive Director, Operational Services & Systems Division, Jean Pruneau
Tel: 613-960-3656

Executive Director, Internal Client Services Directorate, Susan Russell
Tel: 613-952-3151

Acting Executive Director, Policy & Partnerships, Tasha Stefanis
Tel: 613-941-1606

Director, Environmental Public Health Division, Ivy Chan
Tel: 613-948-7773

Director, Primary Health Care Systems, Leila Gillis
Tel: 613-952-7492

Director, Communicable Disease Control, Erin E. Henry
Tel: 613-957-1151

Director, Home, Community & Preventative Care Division, Jacques Néron
Tel: 613-948-5445

Health Products & Food Branch (HPFB) / Direction générale des produits de santé et des aliments (DGPSA)

HPFB's mandate is to take an integrated apporach to the management of risks & benefits related to health products & food by minimizing health factors to Canadians while maximizing the safety provided by the regulatory system for health products & food; & to promote conditions that enable Canadians to make healthy choices & provide information so that they can make informed decisions about their health. The Environmental Impact Initiative develops strategy & policy in response to the Canadian Environmental Protection Act requirement that all new substances for use in Canada must be assessed for direct & indirect impact on human health & the environment.

Assistant Deputy Minister, Pierre Sabourin
Tel: 613-957-1804

Senior Medical Officer, Centre for Evaluation of Radiopharmaceuticals & Biotherapeutics, Jerieta Waltin-James
Tel: 613-790-4541

Director General, Natural & Non-Prescription Health Products Directorate, Manon Bombardier
Tel: 613-952-2558

Director General, Veterinary Drugs Directorate, Daniel Chaput
Tel: 613-954-1873

Director General, HPFB Inspectorate - Ottawa, Robin Chiponski
Tel: 613-957-6836

Director General, Office of Nutrition Policy & Promotion, Dr. Hasan Hutchinson
Tel: 613-957-8330

Director General, Veterinary Drugs Directorate, Mary-Jane Ireland
Tel: 613-941-8718

Director General, Therapeutic Products Directorate, Marion Law
Tel: 613-957-6466

Director General, Food Directorate, Karen McIntyre
Tel: 613-957-1820

Director General, Policy, Planning & International Affairs Directorate, Ed Morgan
Tel: 613-952-8149

Director General, Biologics & Genetic Therapies Directorate, Cathy Parker
Tel: 613-946-0099

Interim Director General, Marketed Health Products Directorate, Dr. John Patrick Stewart
Tel: 613-941-8889

Director General, Resource Management & Operations Directorate, Deryck Trehearne
Tel: 613-957-6690

Senior Executive Director, Therapeutic Products Directorate, Kimby Barton
Tel: 613-952-4619

Executive Director, Business Transformation, Umang Bali
Tel: 613-954-6741

Acting Director, Bureau of Strategic Planning & Business Services, Dina Aly
Tel: 613-946-9280

Director, Bureau of Policy, Science & International Programs, Marilena Bassi
Tel: 613-957-6451

Director, Marketed Pharmaceuticals & Medical Devices Bureau, Dr. Marc Berthiaume
Tel: 613-952-6239

Director, Marketed Biologicals, Biotechnology & Natural Health Products Bureau, Dr. Megan Bettle
Tel: 613-954-0731

Director, Bureau of Cardiology, Allergy & Neurological Sciences, Dr. Leo Bouthillier
Tel: 613-954-6498

Director, Office of Submissions & Intellectual Property, Therapeutic Products, Anne Bowes
Tel: 613-941-0842
Fax: 613-946-5610

Director, Bureau of Food Surveillance & Science Integration, Dr. Danielle Bruie
Tel: 613-957-1923

Director, Operational Management & Scientific Learning Division, Meggan Davis
Tel: 613-960-2491

Director, International Affairs, Louise Dery
Tel: 613-948-7787

Director, Centre for Biologics Evaluation, Dr. Lindsay Elmgren
Tel: 613-957-1061

Director, Bureau of Microbial Hazards, Dr. Jeff Farber, PhD
Tel: 613-957-0880

Acting Director, Resource & Facilities Management Division, Carolle Gagne
Tel: 613-960-8032

Acting Director, Policy & International Collaboration, Liz Anne Gillham-Eisen
Tel: 613-960-5315

Director, Bureau of Policy, Intergovernmental & International Affairs, Mae Johnson
Tel: 613-957-8417

Director, Centre for Evaluation of Radiopharmaceuticals &
Biotherapeutics, Agnes V. Klein
Tel: 613-954-5706

Director, Planning & Evaluation, Kim LaForce
Tel: 613-948-6319

Director, Therapeutic Effectiveness & Policy Bureau, Lisa Lange
Tel: 613-946-6509

Director, Bureau of Chemical Safety, Barbara Lee
Tel: 613-957-0973
Fax: 613-952-7756

Director, Office of Clinical Trials, Dr. Carole Legare
Tel: 613-954-6494

Director, Bureau of Gastroenterolgy, Infection & Viral Diseases, Ceila
Lourenco, PhD
Tel: 613-941-2588

Acting Director, Bureau of Microbial Hazards, Denise MacGillivray
Tel: 613-957-0881

Acting Director, Office of Legislative & Regulatory Modernization, Lynn
Mainland
Tel: 613-946-6586

Director, Human Safety Division, Manisha Mehrotra, PhD
Tel: 613-946-6586

Director, Consumer Health Product Modernisation, Amanda Moir
Tel: 613-355-2413

Director, Bureau of Program Policy, Risk Management & Stakeholder
Engagement, Amanda Moir, PhD
Tel: 613-948-3515

Director, Bureau of Strategic Issues & Planning, Hamida Rahim
Tel: 613-941-3447

Director, Bureau of Pharmaceutical Sciences, Bruce Randall
Tel: 613-948-1782

Director, Bureau of Licensing Services & Systems, Stephanie Reid
Tel: 613-948-6279

Acting Director, Centre for Evaluation of Radiopharmaceuticals &
Biotherapeutics, Dr. Anthony Ridgway
Tel: 613-790-8171

Director, Bureau of Metabolism, Oncology & Reproductive Sciences,
Kelly Robinson
Tel: 613-941-1154

Director, Office of Legislation & Regulatory Modernization, Bruno
Rodrigue
Tel: 613-946-6586

Director, Office of Regulatory Affairs, Georgette Roy
Tel: 613-957-1488
Fax: 613-952-7756

Director, Marketed Health Products Safety & Effectiveness Information
Bureau, Sophie Sommerer
Tel: 613-946-1138

Director, Environmental Impact Initiative, Gordon Stringer
Tel: 613-960-3747

Director, Business Integration & Risk Management, Marianne Tang
Tel: 613-957-6468

Director, Bureau of Nutritional Sciences, William Yan, PhD
Tel: 613-948-8478

Healthy Environments & Consumer Safety (HECSB) / Direction générale, santé environnementale et sécurité des consommateurs (DGSESC)

The HECSB mission is to help Canadians to maintain & improve their health by promoting healthy & safe living, working & recreational environments & by reducing the harm caused by tobacco, alcohol, controlled substances, environmental contaminants, & unsafe consumer & industrial products.

Assistant Deputy Minister, Hilary Geller
Tel: 613-946-6701

Director General, Tobacco Control Directorate, Beth Pieterson
Tel: 613-946-9009

Director General, Controlled Substances Directorate, Ana Renart
Tel: 613-960-2496

Director General, Environmental & Radiation Health Sciences, Tim
Singer
Tel: 613-954-3859

Director General, Consumer Product Safety Directorate, James Van
Loon
Tel: 613-957-1422

Director, Radiation Protection Bureau, Brian Ahier
Tel: 613-954-6647

Director, New Substances Assessment & Control Bureau, Maya Berci
Tel: 613-946-1843

Director, Office of Science Policy, Liaison and Coordination, Tara
Bower
Tel: 613-957-6371

Director, Tobacco Products Regulatory Office, Denis Choiniere
Tel: 613-941-1560

Director, Consumer Product Safety Directorate, Katie Greenwood
Tel: 613-960-8029

Director, Tobacco Office of Research & Surveillance, Sonia Johnson,
PhD
Tel: 613-946-4223

Acting Director, Office of Workforce Initiatives, Elpiniki Karalis
Tel: 613-957-3132

Acting Director, Consumer & Clinical Radiation Protection Bureau,
Narine Martel
Tel: 613-954-9584

Director, Controlled Substances Directorate, Dr. Kirsten Mattison
Tel: 613-954-8451

Director, Office of Sustainable Development, Amber McCool
Tel: 613-946-8107

Acting Director, Environmental Health Science & Research Bureau,
Michele Regimbald-Krnel
Tel: 613-941-6681

Acting Director, Program Development Bureau, Heather A. Watson
Tel: 613-957-4469

Safe Environments Programme (SEP) / Programme de la sécurité des milieux (PSM)

Other Communication: URL:
www.hc-sc.gc.ca/ahc-asc/branch-dirgen/hecs-dgsesc/sep-psm/index-eng.php

Investigates, monitors & assesses health risks in the work, home & natural environments. Areas investigated & regulated include: medical devices, chemicals & biotechnology products in the environment, drinking water, air quality, tobacco, hazardous products & toxic waste, as well as anything that emits radiation from natural & human sources. Aims to protect Canadians from health hazards associated with natural & man-made environments through assessment & investigation of the health effects of environmental pollutants & health hazards associated with radiation sources & hazardous products.

Director General, Safe Environments Directorate, David Morin
Tel: 613-954-0291

Director, Risk Management Bureau, Andrew Beck
Tel: 613-948-2585

Director, New Substances Assessment & Control Bureau, Maya Berci
Tel: 613-946-1843

Director, Water & Air Quality Bureau, John Cooper
Tel: 613-948-2568

Director, Chemicals & Environmental Health Management Bureau,
Suzanne Leppinen
Tel: 613-941-8071

Director, Existing Substances Risk Assessment Bureau, Christine
Norman
Tel: 613-948-7451

Director, Governance & Integrated Planning, Anastasia Poulin
Tel: 613-957-1609

Director, Climate Change & Innovation Bureau, Carolyn Tateishi
Tel: 613-952-8773

Workplace Hazardous Materials System (WHIMS) / Système d'information sur les matières dangereuses utilisées au travail (SIMDUT)

Fax: 613-952-1994
www.hc-sc.gc.ca/ewh-semt/occup-travail/whmis-simdut/index_e.php

A nationwide hazard communication system providing information on hazardous materials used in the workplace. Key elements of the system are cautionary labelling on containers of hazardous materials, material safety data sheets (MSDSs) that contain more detailed information, & worker training. Suppliers must ensure that products are appropriately labelled & that MSDSs are provided to purchasers. Employers are required to make MSDSs available to their employees & provide workers with training on WHMIS & the safe use of hazardous materials. WHMIS supports the workers' right to know the hazards of the materials they use. WHMIS requirements are administered through federal & provincial coordinators. WHMIS was updated in 2015 to incorporate the Globally Harmonized System of Classification and

Labelling for chemicals (GHS), bringing it in line with systems used in the United States & other Canadian partners.

Director, Rosslynn Miller-Lee
 Tel: 613-941-3583

Acting Manager, Assessment, Compliance & Enforcement Division, Julie Calendino
 Tel: 613-952-5208

Pest Management Regulatory Agency (PMRA) / Agence de réglementation de la lutte antiparasitaire (ARLA)
2720 Riverside Dr., Ottawa, ON K1A 0K9

Tel: 613-736-3799
Fax: 613-736-3798
Toll-Free: 800-267-6315
TTY: 800-465-7735
pmra.infoserv@hc-sc.gc.ca
www.hc-sc.gc.ca/cps-spc/pest/index-eng.php
Other Communication: Agency URL:
www.hc-sc.gc.ca/ahc-asc/branch-dirgen/pmra-arla/index-eng.php

Created in 1995, The PMRA determines if proposed pesticides can be used safely when label directions are followed & will be effective for their intended use. If there is reasonable certainty from scientific evaluation that no harm to human health, future generations or the environment will result from exposure to or use of a pesticide, its registration for use in Canada will be approved. Once the pesticides are on the market, the PMRA monitors their use through a series of education, compliance & enforcement programs. Pesticides are also reviewed every fifteen years or sooner as new information is discovered & as science evolves. Companies are also required to report any incident they receive about their products, just as the public is encouraged to report any incidents to these companies or through the Incident Reporting Program. The PMRA administers the Pest Control Products Act on behalf of the Minister of Health.

Executive Director, Richard Aucoin
 Tel: 613-736-3701

Chief Registrar & Director General, Registration Directorate, Peter Brander
 Tel: 613-736-3704

Director General, Health Evaluation Directorate, Peter Chan, PhD
 Tel: 613-736-3510

Director General, Value Assessment & Re-evaluation Management Directorate, Margherita Conti
 Tel: 613-736-3485

Director General, Compliance, Lab Services & Regional Operations Directorate, Diana Dowthwaite
 Tel: 613-736-3484

Director, Policy, Communications & Regulatory Affairs, Jason Flint
 Tel: 613-736-3660

Acting Director General, Environmental Assessment Directorate, Scott Kirby
 Tel: 613-736-3715

Acting Director, Re-evaluation Program, Dr. Bio Aikawa
 Tel: 613-736-3780

Director, Health Effects Division 1 - Antimicrobial, Insecticide, Microbial & Biochemical, Yavinder Bhuller
 Tel: 613-736-3390

Director, Strategic Planning, Financial & Business Operations, Anne Lapierre
 Tel: 613-736-3411

Director, Health Effects Division II - Fungicides & Herbicides, Connie Moase, PhD
 Tel: 613-736-3517

Director, Submission & Information Management Division, Joanna O'Reilly
 Tel: 613-736-3570

Director, Review & Science Integration Division, Neilda Sterkenburg
 Tel: 613-736-3851
 Fax: 613-736-3666

Regulatory Operations & Regions Branch / Direction générale des opérations réglementaires et des régions
Assistant Deputy Minister, Anne Lamar
 Tel: 613-954-0690

Director General, Laboratories, Guy Aucoin
 Tel: 450-928-4100

Director General, Medical Devices & Clinical Compliance, Todd Cain
 Tel: 613-941-3344

Director General, Controlled Substances & Environmental Health, Ward Chickoski
 Tel: 780-495-3857

Director General, Planning & Operations Directorate, Debbie Holbrook
 Tel: 613-957-3152

Director General, Consumer Product Safety Tobacco Pesticides, Krista Locke
 Tel: 902-407-7810
 Other Communications: Secure Phone: 902-426-8248

Director General, Policy & Regulatory Strategies, Greg Loyst
 Tel: 613-948-4274

Director General, Health Product Compliance, Steven Schwendt
 Tel: 613-957-6836

Director, Drug Analysis Service Laboratories, Benoit Archambault
 Tel: 450-928-4037

Acting Director, Border Centres & Cell-Based Therapeutics, Alex Basiji
 Tel: 416-973-1452

Director, Community of Federal Regulators & Departmental Regulatory Affairs, Brenda Czich
 Tel: 613-948-8431

Director, Health Products & Food Laboratories, Jim Daskalopoulos
 Tel: 416-954-2209

Director, Centre for Regulatory & Compliance Strategies, Kim Dayman-Rutkus
 Tel: 613-954-6785

Director, Consumer Product Safety, Peggy Farnsworth
 Tel: 514-496-6923

Director, Environmental Health Programs & Internationally Protected Persons, Teressa Laforest
 Tel: 902-426-8457

Acting Director, Controlled Substances, Gladis Lemus
 Tel: 604-250-2887

Director, Health Product Compliance & Risk Management, Ken Moore
 Tel: 416-954-3592

Director, Office of Regulatory Initiatives, Nathalie Nye
 Tel: 613-960-5614

Director, Health Product Inspection & Licencing, Etienne Ouimette
 Tel: 613-954-2996

Director, Tobacco & Pesticides, Mary Frances Wright
 Tel: 780-495-2625

Strategic Policy Branch (SPB) / Direction générale de la politique stratégique (DGPS)
The SPB plays a lead role in health policy, communications & consultations. The SPB's objective is to promote national coordination & development of a strong, shared knowledge base to address health & health care priorities for all Canadians. They also aim to facilitate successful health system adaptation to changes in technology, society, industry & the environment, such that Canadians will continue to be protected from health risks, have access to quality health care, & gain positive health benefits from information & innovation.

Assistant Deputy Minister, Abby Hoffman
 Tel: 613-946-1791

Director General, Policy Coordination & Planning Directorate, Cheryl Grant
 Tel: 613-957-1940

Director General, Health Care Programs & Policy Directorate, Helen McElroy
 Tel: 613-954-0834

Director General, Strategic Pharmaceutical Initiatives, Kendal Weber
 Tel: 613-960-9712

Acting Executive Director, Office of Pharmaceuticals Management Strategies, Frances Hall
 Tel: 613-952-6451

Executive Director, Health Programs & Strategic Initiatives, Cindy Moriarty
 Tel: 613-946-9375

Executive Director, Office of Pharmaceuticals Management Strategies, Karen Reynolds
 Tel: 613-957-1692

Executive Director, Science Policy, Laird Roe
 Tel: 613-941-3003

Executive Director, Health Accord Secretariat, Jocelyne Voisin
 Tel: 613-957-9945

Director, Health Care System Division, Gavin Brown
 Tel: 613-957-8994

Director, Federal-Provincial-Territorial Relations Division, Luke Carter
Tel: 613-946-0345

Director, Canada Health Act Division, Gigi Mandy
Tel: 613-954-8685

Director, Drugs Program, Joanne McCabe
Tel: 613-957-8337

Director, Cabinet & Parliamentary Affairs Division, Reesha Namasivayam
Tel: 613-952-0563

National Research Council Canada (NRC) / Conseil national de recherches Canada (CNRC)
Building M-58, 1200 Montreal Rd., Ottawa, ON K1A 0R6

Tel: 613-993-9101
Fax: 613-952-9907
Toll-Free: 877-672-2672
TTY: 613-949-3042
info@nrc-cnrc.ca
www.nrc-cnrc.gc.ca
Other Communication: Media Relations, Toll-free Phone: 1-855-282-1637; E-mail: media@nrc-cnrc.gc.ca
twitter.com/nrc_cnrc
www.linkedin.com/company/8417
www.youtube.com/researchcouncilcan

The National Research Council is the Government of Canada's agency for research & development. Reporting to Parliament is through the Minister of Industry. The Council works with partners & clients to meet industrial & societal needs, in accordance with the *National Research Council Act*.

Technical & advisory services are available to assist enterprises solve technical problems. The following are some examples of the specialized services available: analytical chemistry services, calibration services, cold regions techologies & services, molecular biology services, environmental hydraulics services, marine performance & evaluation services, flight test & evaluation services, surface transportation services, medical diagnostics, nuclear magnetic resonance services, & protein purification services.

The National Research Council encourages & engages in research & business partnerships. Licensing opportunities are available for research & development solutions.

President, Iain Stewart

Vice-President, Business & Professional Services, Maria Aubrey

Vice-President, Emerging Technologies - Platforms, François Cordeau

Vice-President, Industrial Research Assistance Program (IRAP), David Lisk

Vice-President, Human Resources, Isabelle Gingras

Vice-President, Corporate Services & Chief Financial Officer, Dale MacMillan

Vice-President, Engineering, Ian Potter

Vice-President, Life Sciences, Roman Szumski

Vice-President, Policy, Roger Scott-Douglas

Secretary General, Dick Bourgeois-Doyle

National Research Council Canada - National Science Library / Bibliothèque scientifique nationale
Bldg. M-55, 1200 Montreal Rd., Ottawa, ON K1A 0R6

Tel: 613-998-8544
Toll-Free: 800-668-1222
science-libraries.canada.ca/eng/national-science-library
www.facebook.com/cisti.icist

Formerly known as the Canada Institute for Scientific & Technical Information (l'Institut canadien de l'information scientifique et technique), the National Science Library was founded in 1924. Under the *National Research Council Act* the NRC is mandated to operate & maintain a national library. The Library supports Canada's research, innovation, & health communities by supplying resources & services to

aid in discoveries & commercialization.

The main library, located in Ottawa, is open to the public (all branch libraries across Canada were closed by the end of 2012). Library users have online access to the NRC-CISTI Public Catalogue in order to search for & order print & electronic holdings in the areas of science, technology, engineering, & medicine. Interlibrary Loan services are handled by Infotrieve. The Library features the following online services: DataCite Canada; DOCLINE in Canada; PubMed Central Canada; & the NRC Archives. The Archives service offers information about the development of scientific research at the Council & the history of science in Canada.

The National Science Library is governed by a Director General & an Advisory Board that comprises national & international stakeholders from the library, publishing, academic, & business sectors. Board members are appointed by the Council of the National Research Council Canada.

In 2017, the National Science Library joined the Federal Science Library online portal.

Director General, Knowledge Management, Kathleen M. O'Connell
Tel: 613-993-2341
kathleen.oconnell@canada.ca

Director, Information & Analysis Services, Jean Archambault
Tel: 450-306-1094
Fax: 450-306-1094
jean.archambeault@canada.ca

Director, Information Management Services Directorate, Alexandra Freeland
alexandra.freeland2@canada.ca

Natural Sciences & Engineering Research Council of Canada (NSERC) / Conseil des recherches en sciences naturelles et en génie du Canada (CRSNG)
350 Albert St., 16th Fl., Ottawa, ON K1A 1H5

Tel: 613-995-4273
Fax: 613-992-5337
Toll-Free: 855-275-2861
www.nserc-crsng.gc.ca
twitter.com/nserc_crsng
www.facebook.com/nserccanada
www.linkedin.com/company-beta/357122
www.youtube.com/user/NSERCTube

Science & Engineering Research Canada (NSERC) is a federal agency whose role is to make investments in people, discovery & innovation for the benefit of all Canadians. With an annual budget of more than $860 million, it supports more than 20,000 university students & postdoctoral fellows in their advanced studies. NSERC promotes discovery by funding more than 10,000 university professors every year & helps make innovation happen by encouraging more than 500 Canadian companies to participate & invest in university research projects.

President, Mario Pinto
Tel: 613-995-5840
pres@nserc-crsng.gc.ca

Vice-President & Chair, Daniel F. Muzyka

Chief Financial Officer & Vice-President, Common Administrative Services, Patricia Sauvé-McCuan
Tel: 613-995-3914
Fax: 613-944-1760
Patricia.Sauve-McCuan@nserc-crsng.gc.ca

Vice-President, Research Grants & Scholarships, Pierre Charest
Tel: 613-995-5833
Pierre.Charest@nserc-crsng.gc.ca

Vice-President, Communications, Corporate & International Affairs Directorate, Alfred LeBlanc
Tel: 613-943-5317
Alfred.Leblanc@nserc-crsng.gc.ca

Vice-President, Research Partnerships, Bettina Hamelin
Tel: 613-992-1585
Bettina.Hamelin@nserc-crsng.gc.ca

Acting Associate Vice-President, Networks of Centres of Excellence, Jean Saint-Vil

Tel: 613-995-6010
Jean.Saint-Vil@nserc-crsng.gc.ca

Director General, Human Resources, Jennifer Gualtieri
Tel: 613-944-9264
Jennifer.Gualtieri@nserc-crsng.gc.ca

Director General & Chief Information Officer, Information & Innovation Solutions, Philippe Johnston
Tel: 613-996-8820
Philippe.Johnston@nserc-crsng.gc.ca

Director General & Deputy Chief Financial Officer, Finance & Awards Administration Division, Nathalie Manseau
Tel: 613-996-8269
Nathalie.Manseau@nserc-crsng.gc.ca

Director, Mathematical, Environmental & Physical Sciences, Elizabeth Boston
Tel: 613-943-0310
Elizabeth.Boston@nserc-crsng.gc.ca

Director, Innovative Collaborations, Science Promotion & Program Ops, Norman Marcotte
Tel: 613-996-2832
norman.marcotte@nserc-crsng.gc.ca

Director, Communications, Christian Riel
Tel: 613-995-5993
Christian.Riel@nserc-crsng.gc.ca

Director, Scholarships & Fellowships, Serge Villemure
Tel: 613-996-2832
serge.villemure@nserc-crsng.gc.ca

Networks of Centres of Excellence of Canada (NCE) / Réseaux de centres d'excellence (RCE)
350 Albert Street, 16th Fl., Ottawa, ON K1A 1H5

Tel: 613-995-6010
Fax: 613-992-7356
info@nce-rce.gc.ca
www.nce-rce.gc.ca
twitter.com/nce_rce
www.facebook.com/networksofcentresofexcellence
www.linkedin.com/company/networks-of-centres-of-excellence

The Networks of Centres of Excellence (NCE) is mandated to persue discoveries in the fields of natural sciences, engineering, social sciences & health sciences, in order to transform them into products, services & processes that improve the lives of Canadians. In partnership with Innovation, Science & Economic Development & Health Canada, NCE is jointly administered by The Canadian Institutes of Health Research (CIHR), the Natural Sciences & Engineering Research Council (NSERC) & the Social Sciences & Humanities Research Council (SSHRC).

Chair, Management Committee, Bettina Hamelin

Acting Associate Vice-President, NCE Secretariat, Jean Saint-Vil
Tel: 613-992-5512
Jean.Saint-Vil@nce-rce.gc.ca

Deputy Director, Networks of Centres of Excellence (NCE) Program, Carmen Gervais
Tel: 613-996-9403
Carmen.Gervais@nce-rce.gc.ca

Deputy Director, Centres of Excellence for Commercialization & Research (CECR) & Business-Led Networks of Centres of Excellence (BL-NCE), Denis Godin
Tel: 613-947-8894
Denis.Godin@nce-rce.gc.ca

Acting Manager, Communications, Hans Posthuma
Tel: 613-943-8752
Hans.Posthuma@nce-rce.gc.ca

Patented Medicine Prices Review Board / Conseil d'examen du prix des médicaments brevetés
Standard Life Centre, #1400, 333 Laurier Ave. West, PO Box L40 Ottawa, ON K1P 1C1

Tel: 613-954-8299
Fax: 613-952-7626
Toll-Free: 877-861-2350
TTY: 613-957-4373
PMPRB.Information-Renseignements.CEPMB@pmprb-cepmb.gc.ca
www.pmprb-cepmb.gc.ca
twitter.com/PMPRB_CEPMB

The Patented Medicine Prices Review Board (PMPRB) is an independent quasi-judicial body established by Parliament in 1987 under the Patent Act (Act). The PMPRB is responsible for regulating the prices that patentees charge, the "factory-gate" price, for prescription & non-prescription patented drugs sold in Canada, to wholesalers, hospitals or pharmacies, for human and veterinary use to ensure that they are not excessive. The PMPRB regulates the price of each patented drug product, including each strength of each dosage form of each patented medicine sold in Canada.

Chair, Vacant

Vice-Chair, Mitchell Levine

Executive Director, Douglas Clark
Tel: 613-957-3656
Fax: 613-952-7626

Director, Board Secretariat & Communications, Guillaume Couillard
Tel: 613-954-8299
Fax: 613-952-7626

Director, Corporate Services, Devon Menard
Tel: 613-952-3304
Fax: 613-952-7626

Director, Policy & Economic Analysis Branch, Tanya Potashnik
Tel: 613-952-9406
Fax: 613-952-7626

Director, Regulatory Affairs & Outreach, Ginette Tognet
Tel: 613-954-8297
Fax: 613-952-7626

Statistics Canada / Statistique Canada
150 Tunney's Pasture Driveway, Ottawa, ON K1A 0T6

Tel: 514-283-8300
Fax: 514-283-9350
Toll-Free: 800-263-1136
TTY: 800-363-7629
STATCAN.infostats-infostats.STATCAN@canada.ca
www.statcan.ca
twitter.com/statcan_eng
www.facebook.com/statisticscanada
www.youtube.com/statisticscanada

Agency of the federal government, headed by the Chief Statistician of Canada which reports to Parliament through the Minister of Industry. As Canada's central statistical agency, it has a mandate to collect, compile, analyse, abstract & publish statistical information relating to the commercial, industrial, financial, social, economic & general activities & condition of the people of Canada; coordinates activities with its federal & provincial partners in the national statistical system to avoid duplication of effort & to ensure the consistency & usefulness of statistics. The agency profiles & measures both social & economic changes in Canada. It presents a comprehensive picture of the national economy through statistics on manufacturing, agriculture, retail sales, services, prices, productivity changes, trade, transportation, employment & unemployment, & aggregate measures such as gross domestic product. It also presents a comprehensive picture of social conditions through statistics on demography, health, areas. In Nov. 2015, Prime Minister Trudeau reintroduced the long-form census, which had been replaced by the Conservatives in 2010 with the National Household Survey.

Chief Statistician of Canada, Anil Arora

Tel: 613-951-9757
Anil.Arora@canada.ca

Director General, Karen Mihorean
Tel: 613-951-9869
Fax: 613-951-4842
karen.mihorean@canada.ca

Census, Operations & Communications
Assistant Chief Statistician, Connie Graziadei
Tel: 613-951-7081
Fax: 613-951-1394
connie.graziadei@canada.ca
Other Communications: Alternate Phone: 613-290-0794
Director General, Communications & Dissemination Branch, Gabrielle Beaudoin
Tel: 613-951-2808
Fax: 613-951-2827
gabrielle.beaudoin@canada.ca
Other Communications: Alternate Phone: 613-218-0854

Social, Health & Labour Statistics
Director General, Health, Justice & Special Surveys, Lynn Barr-Telford
Tel: 613-951-1518
Fax: 613-951-7333
lynn.barr-telford@canada.ca

Provincial Government

Alberta Advanced Education
Legislature Bldg., #403, 10800 - 97 Ave., Edmonton, AB T5K 2B6
Tel: 780-422-5400
Toll-Free: -310-0000
www.iae.alberta.ca

On Oct. 22, 2015, Premier Notley created Alberta Economic Development & Trade, drawing from parts of Innovation & Advanced Education, and leaving Advanced Education as its own portfolio. The key responsibilities of Advanced Education include post-secondary matters, apprenticeship & industry training & adult learning.
The following are some specific activities: funding public post-secondary institutions in Alberta; developing program standards with industry; counselling apprentices & employers; certifying apprentices & occupational trainees; providing student financial assistance; funding education providers; & funding apprentices.

Minister, Advanced Education, Hon. Marlin Schmidt
Tel: 780-427-5777
Fax: 780-422-8733
ae.minister@gov.ab.ca

Deputy Minister, Rod Skura
Tel: 780-415-4744
rod.skura@gov.ab.ca

Executive Director, Human Resources, Gerry Jacubo
Tel: 780-422-5324
Fax: 780-427-3316
gerry.jacubo@gov.ab.ca

Director, Communications, John Muir
Tel: 780-422-1562
Fax: 780-427-0821
john.muir@gov.ab.ca

Apprenticeship & Student Aid Division
Commerce Place, 10155 - 102 St., 6th Fl., Edmonton, AB T5J 4L5
Assistant Deputy Minister, Andy Weiler
Tel: 780-644-7732
andy.weiler@gov.ab.ca
Executive Director, Student Aid, Maggie DesLauriers
Tel: 780-422-4498
Fax: 780-422-4517
maggie.deslauriers@gov.ab.ca
Acting Executive Director, Operations & Client Connections, John St. Arnaud
Tel: 780-427-5770
Fax: 780-422-7376
john.starnaud@gov.ab.ca

Acting Director, Assessment, Certification & Examination Services, Irene Darius
Tel: 780-427-8376
Fax: 780-422-7376
irene.darius@gov.ab.ca

Alberta Economic Development & Trade
Commerce Place, 10155 - 102 St., 12th Fl., Edmonton, AB T5J 4G8
economic.alberta.ca
Created in 2015, Economic Development & Trade focuses on the following priorities: Economic Development & Small & Medium-Sized Enterprises; Science & Innovation (including the Alberta Innovated programs); & Trade & Investment Attraction (including Alberta's international offices).
The following international offices work to promote trade & to attract investment & other interests such as culture & education: Alberta Beijing Office; Alberta Hong Kong Office; Alberta New Delhi Office; Alberta Japan Office; Alberta South Korea Office; Alberta Guangzhou Office; Alberta Mexico Office; Alberta Shanghai Office; Alberta Singapore Office; Alberta Taiwan Office; Alberta United Kingdom Office; & Alberta Washington, D.C. Office.

Minister, Economic Development & Trade, Hon. Deron Bilous
Tel: 780-644-8554
Fax: 780-644-8572
edt.ministeroffice@gov.ab.ca

Deputy Minister, Jason Krips
Tel: 780-415-0900
Fax: 780-415-6114
jason.krips@gov.ab.ca

Executive Director, Office of the Deputy Minister, Alisa Neuman
Tel: 780-643-2968
alisa.neuman@gov.ab.ca

Director, Communications, Gregory Jack
Tel: 780-422-2524
Fax: 780-422-2635
gregory.jack@gov.ab.ca

Science & Innovation Division
Phipps-McKinnon Bldg., 10020 - 101A Ave., 5th Fl., Edmonton, AB T5J 3G2
Assistant Deputy Minister, John Brown
Tel: 780-638-3725
john.brown@gov.ab.ca
Executive Director, Innovation System Engagement Branch, Lisa Bowes
Tel: 780-422-3117
lisa.bowes@gov.ab.ca
Executive Director, Science & Research - Special Initiatives, Daphne Cheel
Tel: 780-422-0054
daphne.cheel@gov.ab.ca
Executive Director, Science & Innovation Policy & Strategy, Lee Kruszewski
Tel: 780-638-3795
lee.kruszewski@gov.ab.ca
Executive Director, Technology Partnerships & Investments Branch, Brent Lakeman
Tel: 780-643-6511
brent.lakeman@gov.ab.ca
Senior Director, Emerging Technologies & Industries Unit, Mathew Anil
Tel: 780-415-8751
mathew.anil@gov.ab.ca
Senior Director, Governance & Accountability, Frances Arnieri Ballas
Tel: 780-422-1853
frances.arnieriballas@gov.ab.ca
Senior Director, Life Sciences Industries Unit, Hubert Eng
Tel: 780-427-0649
hubert.eng@gov.ab.ca
Senior Director, Research Capacity Planning, Kate Murie
Tel: 780-422-0158
kate.murie@gov.ab.ca

Senior Director, ICT Industries Unit, Tim Olsen
 Tel: 780-644-4970
 tim.olsen@gov.ab.ca
Senior Director, Emerging Science & Technology Initiatives, Lori Querengesser
 Tel: 780-427-6616
 lori.querengesser@gov.ab.ca
Senior Director, Science Policy & Evaluation, David Schwarz
 Tel: 780-641-9418
 david.schwarz@gov.ab.ca
Senior Director, Innovation Policy & Strategy, Alex Umnikov
 Tel: 780-427-6620
 alex.umnikov@gov.ab.ca
Senior Director, Integrated Science & Research Initiatives, Chris Van Tighem
 Tel: 780-427-5229
 chris.vantighem@gov.ab.ca

Alberta Health
PO Box 1360 Stn. Main, Edmonton, AB T5J 2N3
 Tel: 780-427-7164
 Toll-Free: -310-0000
 TTY: 800-232-7215
 www.health.alberta.ca
 twitter.com/goahealth
 www.flickr.com/photos/albertahealth

Formerly Alberta Health & Wellness, Alberta Health is involved in the following activities: establishing legislation, policy, & standards; supporting the health system; allocating resources; & administering provincial programs.
In 2012, Alberta Health absorbed elements of the former Alberta Seniors. In 2014, Premier Jim Prentice made Seniors a separate department again.

Minister, Health, Hon. Sarah Hoffman
 Tel: 780-427-3665
 Fax: 780-415-0961
 health.minister@gov.ab.ca

Associate Minister, Health, Hon. Brandy Payne
 Tel: 780-427-3665
 Fax: 780-415-0961

Deputy Minister, Carl Amrhein
 Tel: 780-422-0747
 Fax: 780-427-1016
 carl.amrhein@gov.ab.ca

Associate Deputy Minister, Andre Tremblay
 andre.tremblay@gov.ab.ca

Assistant Deputy Minister, External & Stakeholder Relations Division, Justin Riemer
 Tel: 780-427-6302
 justin.riemer@gov.ab.ca

Director, Communications, Cameron Traynor
 Tel: 780-427-5344
 Fax: 780-427-1171
 cameron.traynor@gov.ab.ca

Senior Nursing Advisor, Vacant
 Tel: 780-427-5488
 Fax: 780-638-3811

Office of the Chief Medical Officer of Health (OCMOH)
ATB Place, 10025 Jasper Ave., 24th Fl., Edmonton, AB T5J 1S6
 Tel: 780-427-5263
 Fax: 780-427-7683
 www.health.alberta.ca/about/chief-medical-officer.html

The Office of the Chief Medical Officer of Health offers guidelines to Alberta Health Services about public health policy. The Office also provides information to the public about communicable diseases & public health programs.
The Chief Medical Officer of Health works under the authority of the Public Health Act to promote & protect the health of the people of Alberta.

Chief Medical Officer of Health, Dr. Karen Grimsrud
 Tel: 780-415-2809
 karen.grimsrud@gov.ab.ca
Deputy Chief Medical Officer of Health, Dr. Martin Lavoie
 Tel: 780-644-7557
 martin.lavoie@gov.ab.ca
Deputy Medical Officer of Health, Dr. Kristin Klein
 Tel: 780-641-8636
 kristin.klein@gov.ab.ca
Senior Public Health Advisor, Dean Blue
 Tel: 780-415-2816
 dean.blue@gov.ab.ca
FPT Epidemiologist, Sabrina Plitt
 Tel: 780-644-7658
 sabrina.plitt@gov.ab.ca

Health Information Systems Division
ATB Place, 10025 Jasper Ave., 21st Fl., Edmonton, AB T5J 1S6
Assistant Deputy Minister, Kim Wieringa
 Tel: 780-415-2492
 Fax: 780-422-5176
 kim.wieringa@gov.ab.ca
Executive Director, Information Management Branch, Quinn Mah
 Tel: 780-422-1251
 quinn.mah@gov.ab.ca
Executive Director, Information Technology & Operations, Blaine Steward
 Tel: 780-415-1562
 Fax: 780-644-3091
 blaine.steward@gov.ab.ca
Executive Director, Strategic IMT Services Branch, Martin Tailleur
 Tel: 780-415-1427
 martin.tailleur@gov.ab.ca
Director, Provincial Registries & Systems, Glenn Burton
 Tel: 780-415-1479
 glenn.burton@gov.ab.ca
Acting Director, eHealth Information Governance, Robert Silversides
 Tel: 780-638-4017
 bob.silversides@gov.ab.ca

Health Workforce Planning & Accountability Division
ATB Place, 10025 Jasper Ave., 10th Fl., Edmonton, AB T5J 1S6
Assistant Deputy Minister, Miin Alikhan
 Tel: 780-427-1572
 Fax: 780-415-8455
 miin.alikhan@gov.ab.ca
Acting Executive Director, Provider Compensation & Strategic Partnerships Branch, Michael Ducie
 Tel: 780-638-3193
 michael.ducie@gov.ab.ca
Executive Director, Health Human Resources Planning & Strategy Branch, Shawn Knight
 Tel: 780-422-0981
 shawn.knight@gov.ab.ca
Executive Director, Health Insurance Programs Branch, Donna Manuel
 Tel: 780-644-3149
 donna.manuel@gov.ab.ca
Acting Director, Alternative Compensation Design Unit, Jeremy Anthony
 Tel: 780-643-6980
 jeremy.anthony@gov.ab.ca
Director, Health Professions, Policy & Partnerships, Andrew Douglas
 Tel: 780-422-8860
 andrew.douglas@gov.ab.ca
Director, Registration Business Services, Joanne Gallacher
 Tel: 780-415-1563
 joanne.gallacher@gov.ab.ca
Director, Insured Services & Compensation Design, Fedja Lazarevic
 Tel: 780-415-2459
 fedja.lazarevic@gov.ab.ca
Director, Claims Management & Special Programs Deptartment, Carol Taylor
 Tel: 780-427-0362
 carol.taylor@gov.ab.ca
Director, Policy, Special Projects & Communications, Dalton Wenstob
 Tel: 780-415-0211
 dalton.wenstob@gov.ab.ca

Health Service Delivery Division
ATB Place, 10025 Jasper Ave., 18th Fl., Edmonton, AB T5J 1S6
Assistant Deputy Minister, Kathy Ness
Tel: 780-644-7666
Fax: 780-422-0134
kathy.ness@gov.ab.ca
Provincial MES Medical Director, Hal Canham
Tel: 780-422-2061
hal.canham@gov.ab.ca
Executive Director, Primary Health Care Branch, Shannon Berg
Tel: 780-641-9067
Fax: 780-427-8055
shannon.berg@gov.ab.ca
Executive Director, Addiction & Mental Health Branch, Michelle Craig
Tel: 780-641-8644
michelle.craig@gov.ab.ca
Executive Director, Continuing Care Branch, Corinne Schalm
Tel: 780-644-3621
Fax: 780-422-1515
corinne.schalm@gov.ab.ca
Director, Addiction Unit, Everington Coreen
Tel: 780-643-9353
coreen.everington@gov.ab.ca
Director, Innovation Unit, Darren Joslin
Tel: 780-427-3538
darren.joslin@gov.ab.ca
Director, Disaster Recovery Unit, Diane McNeil
Tel: 780-415-2754
diane.mcneil@gov.ab.ca
Director, Funding & Information Planning Unit, Dennis H. Schrieber
Tel: 780-644-3291
dennis.h.schrieber@gov.ab.ca
Director, Mental Health Unit, Sharlene Stayberg
Tel: 780-415-2609
sharlene.stayberg@gov.ab.ca

Health Standards, Quality & Performance
ATB Place, North Tower, 10025 Jasper Ave., 22nd Fl., Edmonton, AB T5J 1S6
Acting Assistant Deputy Minister, Dr. Alan Casson
Tel: 780-644-1450
Fax: 780-638-3811
alan.casson@gov.ab.ca
Executive Director & Provincial Health Analytics Officer, Analytics & Performance Reporting Branch, Larry Svenson
Tel: 780-422-4767
larry.svenson@gov.ab.ca
Director, Health Systems Planning Unit, Sherri Kashuba
Tel: 780-422-6489
sherri.kashuba@gov.ab.ca
Director, Methods & Analysis Unit, Katherine Lyman
Tel: 780-415-1521
katherine.lyman@gov.ab.ca
Director, Epidemiology & Surveillance Unit, Shaun Malo
Tel: 780-422-4771
shaun.malo@gov.ab.ca
Director, Data Services Unit, Peter C. Marshall
Tel: 780-422-0889
peter.c.marshall@gov.ab.ca
Director, Customer Relationship Management (CRM) & Data Access Unit, David Onyschuk
Tel: 780-415-0218
david.onyschuk@gov.ab.ca
Director, Data Management Unit, Sonya Stasiuk
Tel: 780-644-1102
sonya.stasiuk@gov.ab.ca

Ministry Operations & Financial & Corporate Services Division
ATB Place, 10025 Jasper Ave., 16th Fl., Edmonton, AB T5J 1S6
Assistant Deputy Minister, Vacant
Tel: 780-422-1045
Fax: 780-422-3672
Senior Executive Director, Financial Planning Branch, Charlene Wong
Tel: 780-427-7100
charlene.wong@gov.ab.ca

Executive Director, Corporate Services, Stephen Arthur
Tel: 780-415-0201
stephen.arthur@gov.ab.ca
Executive Director, Health Facilities Planning, Wayne Campbell
Tel: 780-638-3546
Fax: 780-422-3672
wayne.campbell@gov.ab.ca
Executive Director, Human Resources, Marina Christopherson
Tel: 780-641-9521
Fax: 780-422-1700
marina.christopherson@gov.ab.ca
Executive Director, Health Economics & Funding Branch, Dee-Jay King
Tel: 780-427-8596
Fax: 780-427-1577
dee-jay.king@gov.ab.ca
Executive Director & Senior Financial Officer, Financial Reporting Branch, Scott McIntyre
Tel: 780-427-6011
scott.mcintyre@gov.ab.ca
Director, Procurement & Contracting Services, Julie Lundgren
Tel: 780-643-0922
julie.lundgren@gov.ab.ca
Director, Organizational Effectiveness, Torri Parkin
Tel: 780-415-0488
torri.parkin@gov.ab.ca
Director, Continuing Care Capital Programs, Trish Spurr
Tel: 780-427-8381
trish.spurr@gov.ab.ca

Pharmaceuticals & Supplementary Health Benefits Division
ATB Place, 10025 Jasper Ave., 11th Fl., Edmonton, AB T5J 1S6
Assistant Deputy Minister, Michele Evans
Tel: 780-427-8019
Fax: 780-422-3646
michele.evans@gov.ab.ca
Executive Director, Health Insurance Programs, Donna Manuel
Tel: 780-644-3149
Fax: 780-644-1445
donna.manuel@gov.ab.ca
Acting Executive Director, Chad Mitchell
Tel: 780-422-9632
chad.mitchell@gov.ab.ca
Director, Supplementary Health Benefits Unit, Mark Harasymuk
Tel: 780-422-6985
mark.harasymuk@gov.ab.ca
Director, Provincial Services, Glenna Laing
Tel: 780-644-3034
glenna.laing@gov.ab.ca
Director, Professional & Industry Relations Unit, Andrea Nagle
Tel: 780-427-0866
andrea.nagle@gov.ab.ca
Director, Policy & Advisory Unit, Bob Sprague
Tel: 780-422-4415
bob.sprague@gov.ab.ca

Alberta Aids to Daily Living (AADL)
Milner Building, 10040 - 104 St., 10th Fl., Edmonton, AB T5J 0Z2
Tel: 780-427-0731
Fax: 780-422-0968
Toll-Free: -310-0000
www.health.alberta.ca/services/aids-to-daily-living.html
AADL provides financial assistance to Albertans with long-term disabilities, chronic or terminal illnesses, who live at home, in lodges, or in group homes.

Strategic Planning & Policy Development Division
ATB Place, North Tower, 10025 Jasper Ave., 19th Fl., Edmonton, AB T5J 1S6
Acting Executive Director, Health System Monitoring Branch, Alex Boudreau
Tel: 780-638-4304
alex.boudreau@gov.ab.ca
Executive Director, Executive Operations, Robyn Cochrane
Tel: 780-415-1541
robyn.cochrane@gov.ab.ca
Executive Director, Intergovernmental Relations Branch, Scott F. Harris
Tel: 780-638-4315
scott.f.harris@gov.ab.ca

Executive Director, Research & Innovation Branch, Bart Johnson
Tel: 780-427-8102
bart.johnson@gov.ab.ca
Executive Director, Strategic Policy, Lara McClelland
Tel: 780-638-4389
lara.mcclelland@gov.ab.ca
Director, Centre of Organizational Learning (COOL), George Flynn
Tel: 780-415-9852
george.flynn@gov.ab.ca
Director, Health Research Policy & Partnerships Unit, Christie Lutsiak
Tel: 780-422-9358
christie.lutsiak@gov.ab.ca
Director, Health Technologies & Services Policy Unit, Ruth Mitchell
Tel: 780-427-4260
ruth.mitchell@gov.ab.ca
Director, Research & Planning Unit, Anita Paras
Tel: 780-415-2784
anita.paras@gov.ab.ca
Director, Clinical Innovation & Policy Unit, Kimberley Simmonds
Tel: 780-422-1940
kimberley.simmonds@gov.ab.ca

Alberta Office of the Public Interest Commissioner (PIC)
#700, 9925 - 109 St., Edmonton, AB T5K 2J8

Tel: 780-641-8659
Toll-Free: 855-641-8659
info@pic.alberta.ca
yourvoiceprotected.ca
Secondary Address: #2560, 801 - 6th Ave. West
Calgary, AB T2P 3W2
The Office of the Public Interest Commissioner investigates disclosures of wrongdoing & complaints of reprisals for employees of government ministries, agencies, boards & commissions, & other public entities.

Public Interest Commissioner & Alberta Ombudsman, Peter Hourihan
Tel: 780-641-8659
peter.hourihan@ombudsman.ab.ca
Note: Alberta Ombudsman Peter Hourihan was appointed as the province's first Public Interest Commissioner in April 2013.

Director, Ted Miles
Tel: 780-641-8659
ted.miles@pic.alberta.ca

British Columbia Centre for Disease Control (BCCDC)
655 West 12th Ave., Vancouver, BC V5Z 4R4

Tel: 604-707-2400
Fax: 604-707-2401
admininfo@bccdc.ca
www.bccdc.ca
Other Communication: Media/Communications, Phone: 604-707-2412
twitter.com/cdcofbc
The BCCDC is both a provincial & national leader in public health as it detects, treats, & prevents diseases in its patients. Not only does it offer direct services for people with diseases & health concerns, but it also provides analytical & policy support to health authorities at all levels of government.

Executive Medical Director, Dr. Mark Tyndall

Interm Medical Director, Communicable Disease Prevention & Control Service, Dr. Eleni Galanis

Medical Director, Environmental Health Services, Dr. Tom Kosatsky

Medical Director, Immunization Programs & Vaccine Preventable Diseases, Dr. Monika Naus

British Columbia Ministry of Children & Family Development (MCFD)
Customer Service Centre, PO Box 9770 Stn. Prov Govt, Victoria, BC V8W 9S5

Tel: 250-387-7027
Fax: 250-356-5720
Toll-Free: 877-387-7027
TTY: 800-667-4770
MCF.CorrespondenceManagement@gov.bc.ca
www.gov.bc.ca/mcf
Other Communication: Helpline for Children: 310-1234; Emergencies outside office hours: 1-800-663-9122
The Ministry of Children & Family Development works to support healthy child development, to maximize the potential of children & youth, & to achieve meaningful outcomes for children, youth, & families. A client-centered approach is used to deliver services. The following services are available to families throughout British Columbia: adoption services; early childhood development & child care services; child safety, family support, & children in care services; services for children & youth with special needs; mental health services for children & youth; & youth justice services.

Minister, Children & Family Development, Hon. Stephanie Cadieux
Tel: 250-387-9699
Fax: 250-387-9722
MCF.Minister@gov.bc.ca
PO Box 9057 Prov Govt Sta.
Victoria, BC V8W 9E2

Deputy Minister, Lori Wanamaker
Tel: 250-387-1541
Fax: 250-356-2920
mcf.deputyminister@gov.bc.ca
PO Box 9721 Prov Govt Sta.
Victoria, BC V8W 9S2

Aboriginal Services
PO Box 9777 Stn. Prov Govt, Victoria, BC V8W 9S5
Tel: 250-356-9791
Fax: 250-387-1732
Executive Director, Divisional Operations, Shane DeMeyer
Tel: 250-387-7081
Director, Practice, Cindy Ghostkeeper
Tel: 250-565-6645

Provincial Services
PO Box 9717 Stn. Prov Govt, Victoria, BC V8W 9S1
Tel: 250-387-0978
Fax: 250-356-2079
Executive Director, Youth Custody Services, Lenora Angel
Tel: 604-356-1970
Fax: 604-356-2079
PO Box 9719 Prov Govt Sta.
Victoria, BC V8W 9S5
Provincial Director, Youth Forensic Psychiatric Services, Andre Picard
Tel: 778-452-2202
Fax: 778-452-2201
Provincial Clinical Director, Youth Forensic Psychiatric Services, Dr. Kulwant Riar
Tel: 778-452-2205
Fax: 778-452-2201
Office Manager, Provincial Services for Deaf & Hard of Hearing, Elaine Bains
Tel: 604-660-1800
Fax: 604-660-1859
psdhh@gov.bc.ca
Other Communications: TTY: 604-660-1807
TTY: 800-667-4770

Policy & Provincial Services
PO Box 9738 Stn. Prov Govt, Victoria, BC V8W 9S2
Tel: 250-387-5954
Fax: 250-387-2481
Assistant Deputy Minister, Christine Massey
Tel: 250-387-7090
Fax: 250-387-2481

Executive Director, Child Care Programs & Services Branch, Jonathan Barry
Tel: 250-387-7762
Toll-free: 888-338-6622
Fax: 250-387-2997
Executive Director, CW, Permanency, QA & Aboriginal Policy, Cheryl May
Tel: 250-356-5581
Executive Director, Children & Youth with Special Needs Policy, Aleksandra Stevanovic
Tel: 250-387-1828
Aleksandra.Stevanovic@gov.bc.ca
Executive Director, Child & Youth Mental Health Policy, Sandy Wiens
Tel: 250-216-3657
Fax: 250-356-0580
MCF.ChildYouthMentalHealth@gov.bc.ca
Director, Child & Youth Mental Health Policy, Robert Lampard
Tel: 250-356-5201
Director, Aboriginal Policy, Lise LeLievre
Tel: 250-356-2777
Director, Vancouver After Hours, Lesley Renshaw
Tel: 604-660-4927
Toll-free: 800-663-9122
Director, Child Welfare Policy, James Wale
Tel: 250-387-7075
James.Wale@gov.bc.ca
Director, Policy Initiatives & Coordination, Sonja Yli-Kahila
Tel: 250-953-4360
Sonja.YliKahila@gov.bc.ca

Provincial Office for the Early Years
PO Box 9721 Stn. Prov Govt, Victoria, BC V8W 9S2
Tel: 250-387-5942
Fax: 250-356-0311

Acting Executive Director, Emily Horton
Tel: 250-413-7608
Director, Danielle Smith
Tel: 250-387-9714
Director, Stakeholder Engagement & Coordination, Jan White
Tel: 778-679-9646

Provincial Office of Domestic Violence & Strategic Priorities
PO Box 9768 Stn. Prov Govt, Victoria, BC V8W 9S5
Tel: 250-356-9808
Fax: 250-387-8000

Acting Assistant Deputy Minister, Tami Currie
Tel: 250-356-5332
Executive Director, Strategic Priorities Branch, Linda Bradford
Tel: 250-387-7423
Executive Director, Provincial Office of Domestic Violence, Catherine Talbott
Tel: 250-387-7044
Director, System & Service Coordination, Provincial Office of Domestic Violence, Clark Russell
Tel: 250-952-0893

Office of the Provincial Director of Child Welfare
PO Box 9721 Stn. Prov Govt, Victoria, BC V8W 9S2
Tel: 250-356-9791
Fax: 250-356-6534

Assistant Deputy Minister & Provincial Director, Child Welfare, Cory Heavener
Tel: 250-356-9791
Deputy Director, Child Welfare, Alex Scheiber
Tel: 250-387-7418
Executive Director, Guardianship, Adoption & Permanency Planning, Anne Clayton
Tel: 250-387-2281
MCF.AdoptionsBranch@gov.bc.ca
Director, Adoption Services, Renaa Bacy
Tel: 250-387-7069
MCF.AdoptionsBranch@gov.bc.ca

British Columbia Ministry of Health
PO Box 9639 Stn. Prov Govt, Victoria, BC V8W 9P1
Toll-Free: 800-663-7867
hlth.health@gov.bc.ca
www.gov.bc.ca/health
Other Communication: Media Inquiries, Phone: 250-952-1887, Fax: 250-952-1883

The Ministry of Health is responsible for ensuring quality, timely, & cost effective health services for all citizens of British Columbia. To guide & enhance British Columbia's health services, the ministry works with health authorities, agencies, care providers, & other groups.

Minister, Health, Hon. Terry Lake
Tel: 250-953-3547
Fax: 250-356-9587
hlth.minister@gov.bc.ca

Deputy Minister, Health, Stephen Brown
Tel: 250-952-1590
Fax: 250-952-1909
hlth.dmoffice@gov.bc.ca

Parliamentary Secretary to the Minister of Health for Seniors, Darryl Plecas
Tel: 250-952-7275
Fax: 250-387-9100
darryl.plecas.mla@leg.bc.ca

Director, Executive Operations, Jordan Will
Tel: 250-952-1908

Manager, Correspondence & Documents Management Unit, Jo Tyson
Tel: 250-952-1912

Corporate Services
Fax: 250-952-1909

Associate Deputy Minister, Sabine Feulgen
Tel: 250-952-1764
Assistant Deputy Minister, Health Sector Information, Analysis & Reporting, Teri Collins
Tel: 250-952-2569
Assistant Deputy Minister, Finance & Corporate Services, Manjit Sidhu
Tel: 250-952-2066
Assistant Deputy Minister, Health Sector IM/IT, Deborah Shera
Tel: 250-952-6202
Assistant Deputy Minister, Medical Beneficiary & Pharmaceutical Services, Barbara Walman
Tel: 250-952-1464
Executive Lead, Strategic Management & Organizational Development, Debbie Godfrey
Tel: 250-952-1026
Director, Health & Corporate Services, Jennifer Michell
Tel: 250-952-1685

Health Services
Tel: 250-952-2402
Fax: 250-952-1390

Associate Deputy Minister, Lynn Stevenson
Tel: 250-952-2402
Assistant Deputy Minister, Partnerships & Innovation Division, Heather Davidson
Tel: 250-952-2159
Assistant Deputy Minister, Primary & Community Care Division, Doug Hughes
Tel: 250-952-1049
Assistant Deputy Minister, Population & Public Health, Arlene Paton
Tel: 250-952-1731
Assistant Deputy Minister, Health Sector Workforce Division, Ted Patterson
Tel: 250-952-3166
Ted.Patterson@gov.bc.ca
Assistant Deputy Minister, Hospital, Diagnostic & Clinical Services Division, Ian Rongve
Tel: 250-953-4504
Executive Director, Wendy Trotter
Tel: 250-952-2378

Chief Nursing Advisor, David Byres
Tel: 250-952-2464
David.Byres@gov.bc.ca
Director, Program Integration, Anne Stearn
Tel: 250-952-3572

HealthLink BC
PO Box 9600 Stn. Prov Govt, Victoria, BC V8W 9P1

Fax: 250-952-6509
healthlinkbc@gov.bc.ca
www.HealthLinkBC.ca

Other Communication: HealthLink BC hotline: 8-1-1; TTY: 7-1-1
HealthLink BC allows residents of British Columbia to access health care information by phone or online, and incorporates the following previously existing services: BC HealthGuide, BC HealthFiles, BC NurseLine & Pharmacist service, & Dial-a-Dietitian.
Executive Director, Marie Root
Tel: 604-215-5118
Fax: 250-952-6509
Director, Navigation Services, Pooyan Khorsandi
Tel: 604-215-5156
Director, Dietitian Services, Barbara Leslie
Tel: 604-215-5138
Director, Nursing Services, Leanne Thain
Tel: 604-215-8100

Office of the Provincial Health Officer
PO Box 9648 Stn. Prov Govt, Victoria, BC V8W 9P4

Tel: 250-952-1330
Fax: 250-952-1570

Provincial Health Officer, Dr. Perry Kendall
Perry.Kendall@gov.bc.ca
Deputy Provincial Health Officer, Dr. Bonnie Henry
Provincial Drinking Water Officer, Joanne Edwards
Tel: 250-952-1572
Director, Epidemiology, Xibiao Ye
Tel: 250-952-1457
Aboriginal Health Physician Advisor, Dr. Shannon Waters
Tel: 250-952-2406

Office of the Seniors Advocate
PO Box 9651 Stn. Prov Govt, Victoria, BC V8W 9P4

Tel: 250-952-3034
Toll-Free: 877-952-3181
info@seniorsadvocatebc.ca
www.seniorsadvocatebc.ca

Seniors Advocate, Isobel Mackenzie
Tel: 250-952-2503
Deputy Seniors Advocate, Nancy Gault
Tel: 250-952-2999
Executive Director, Bruce Ronayne
Tel: 250-952-2998
Director, Communications, Sara Darling
Tel: 250-952-3035
Director, Systemic Review Monitoring, Anita Nadziejko
Tel: 250-952-1177

British Columbia Ministry of Social Development & Social Innovation
PO Box 9058 Stn. Prov Govt, Victoria, BC V8W 9E1

Toll-Free: 800-663-7867
TTY: 800-661-8773
EnquiryBC@gov.bc.ca
www.gov.bc.ca/sdsi

The main responsibilities of the Ministry of Social Development & Social Innovation include supporting community living services that assist persons with developmental disabilities; providing employment programs & services to unemployed & underemploye persons; & delivering income assistance to persons in need.

Minister, Social Development & Social Innovation, Hon. Michelle Stilwell
Tel: 250-356-7750
Fax: 250-356-7292
SDSI.minister@gov.bc.ca

Deputy Minister, Sheila Taylor
Tel: 250-387-3471

Fax: 250-387-5775
PO Box 9934 Prov Govt Sta.
Victoria, BC V8W 9R2

Advocate for Service Quality, Leanne Dospital

Executive Director, Corporate Planning & Strategic Initiatives, Mark S. Medgyesi
Tel: 250-387-2001

Manager, Executive Operations, Karen MacMillan
Tel: 250-387-2807
Fax: 250-387-5775

Acting Manager, Executive Correspondence Services, Adriana Di Castri
Tel: 250-387-7660
Fax: 250-387-5775

Employment & Labour Market Services Division
PO Box 9762 Stn. Prov Govt, Victoria, BC V8W 1A4

Tel: 250-953-3921
Fax: 250-953-3928

Assistant Deputy Minister, Nichola Manning
Tel: 250-953-3921
Fax: 250-953-3928

Services to Adults with Developmental Disabilities
PO Box 9875 Stn. Prov Govt, Victoria, BC V8W 9R1

Toll-Free: 855-356-5609

Acting Executive Director, Paula Grant
Tel: 250-953-4538
Director, Integrated Services & Supports - Prince George/Kamloops, Rob Rail
Tel: 250-645-4011
Rob.Rail@gov.bc.ca
Director, Corporate/Vancouver Island, Lynn Forbes
Tel: 250-387-2098
Lynn.Forbes@gov.bc.ca
Director, Fraser Region/Provincial Practice Lead, Sonia Hall
Tel: 604-575-7586
Sonia.Hall@gov.bc.ca
Manager, Program Development & Performance, Lauren Nackman
Senior Policy Project Manager, Integrated Services Support Team (ISST), Allan Hyggen
Tel: 250-356-1635
Fax: 250-217-9888
ISST@gov.bc.ca

Research, Innovation & Policy Division
PO Box 9936 Stn. Prov Govt, Victoria, BC V8W 9R2

Tel: 250-356-5065
Fax: 250-387-5775

Assistant Deputy Minister, Molly Harrington
Tel: 250-356-5065
Fax: 250-387-2418
Executive Director, Research Branch, Robert Bruce
Tel: 250-356-6787
Fax: 250-387-8164
Robert.Bruce@gov.bc.ca
Executive Director, Strategic Policy, Ian Ross
Tel: 250-953-3923
Fax: 250-387-8164
Ian.Ross@gov.bc.ca
Executive Director, Social Innovation, Robin McLay
Tel: 250-356-1074
Fax: 250-387-5775
Executive Director, Accessibility Secretariat, Susan Mader
Tel: 250-356-0923
Susan.Mader@gov.bc.ca
Acting Director, Reconsideration & Appeals Section, Melissa Bauer
Tel: 250-387-1164
RB@gov.bc.ca
Executive Director, Accessibility Secretariat, Susan Mader
Tel: 250-356-0923
Fax: 250-387-8164
Susan.Mader@gov.bc.ca

Director, Policy, Shannon Pendergast
Tel: 250-356-5002
Fax: 250-387-8164

British Columbia Vital Statistics Agency
PO Box 9657 Stn. Prov Govt, Victoria, BC V8W 9P3
Tel: 250-952-2681
Fax: 250-952-9097
VSOFFCEO@gov.bc.ca
www2.gov.bc.ca/gov/content/life-events

The Vital Statistics Agency operates under the Ministry of Health, & offers the following services: Birth registration; marriage certificates; death certificates; wills; name changes; & geneaology.

Registrar General, Jack Shewchuk
Tel: 250-952-9039
Fax: 250-952-9097
Jack.Shewchuk@gov.bc.ca

Director, Information Technology Services, Suzanne Jennings
Tel: 250-952-9084
Suzanne.Jennings@gov.bc.ca

Team Lead, Confidential Services, Renae Kinnee
Tel: 250-952-9057
Fax: 250-952-9044
Renae.Kinnee@gov.bc.ca
Other Communications: Alt. E-mail: VSCS@gov.bc.ca

Office Manager, Melanie Arscott
Tel: 250-952-9075
Fax: 250-952-9097
Melanie.Arscott@gov.bc.ca

Manitoba Education & Training
#168, Legislative Bldg., 450 Broadway, Winnipeg, MB R3C 0V8
Tel: 204-945-3720
Fax: 204-945-1291
minedu@leg.gov.mb.ca
www.edu.gov.mb.ca

Manitoba Education & Advanced Learning was renamed Education & Training after the 2016 general election.

Minister, Education & Training, Hon. Ian Wishart
Tel: 204-945-3720
Fax: 204-945-1291
minedu@leg.gov.mb.ca

Deputy Minister, Bramwell (Bram) Strain
Tel: 204-945-1648

Manitoba Healthy Child Office
332 Bannatyne Ave., 3rd Fl., Winnipeg, MB R3A 0E2
Tel: 204-945-2266
Toll-Free: 888-848-0140
healthychild@gov.mb.ca
www.gov.mb.ca/healthychild

Office provides leadership & encourages actions that address health concerns & reduces the need for medical care for children. Following the 2016 general election, the Manitoba Healthy Child Office became part of Manitoba Education & Training.

Assistant Deputy Minister; Associate Secretary to Healthy Child Committee of Cabinet, Rob Santos
Tel: 204-945-8670
Executive Director, Programs & Administration, Susan Tessler
Tel: 204-945-1275
Director, Policy Development, Research & Evaluation, Leanne Boyd
Tel: 204-945-5447
Director, Parenting Initiatives, Steven Feldgaier
Tel: 204-945-3084
Manager, FASD Initiatives, Holly Gammon
Tel: 204-945-2215

Manitoba Families
Legislative Building, #357, 450 Broadway, Winnipeg, MB R3C 0V8
Tel: 204-945-3744
Toll-Free: 866-626-4862
TTY: 204-945-4796
www.gov.mb.ca/fs

Manitoba Family Services was renamed to Manitoba Families following the 2016 general election. The department supports citizens in need to achieve fuller participation in society & greater self-suffiency & independence. Helps keep children, families & communities safe & secure & promotes healthy citizen development & well-being. Mission is accomplished through: provision of financial support; provision of supports & services for adults & children with disabilities; provision of child protection & related services; assistance to people facing family violence or family disruption; provision of services & supports to promote the healthy development & well-being of children & families; assistance to Manitobans to access safe, appropriate & affordable housing; fostering community capacity & engaging the broader community to participate in & contribute to decision-making; & respectful & appropriate delivery of programs & services.

Minister, Families, Hon. Scott Fielding
Tel: 204-945-4337
Fax: 204-945-5149
minfs@leg.gov.mb.ca

Deputy Minister, Vacant

Administration & Finance
777 Portage Ave., 3rd Fl., Winnipeg, MB R3G 0N3
Tel: 204-945-3242
fadmin@gov.mb.ca

Acting Assistant Deputy Minister, Brian Brown
Tel: 204-945-5943
Executive Director, Project Management & Information & Technology, Sherry Zajac
Tel: 204-945-0032
Director, Financial & Administrative Services, Wayne Pestun
Tel: 204-945-4005
Project Manager, Agency Accountability & Support Unit, Rick Dykes
Tel: 204-945-1109
Non-Profit Organization Manager, Agency Accountability & Support Unit, Dennis Ceicko
Tel: 204-945-4869

Child & Family Services
777 Portage Ave., Winnipeg, MB R3G 0N3
Tel: 204-945-6964
cfsd@gov.mb.ca
www.gov.mb.ca/fs/childfam/index.html

Assistant Deputy Minister, Diane Kelly
Tel: 204-945-4575
Chief Executive Officer, General Child & Family Services Authority, Debbie Besant
Director, Bringing Families Together Project, Christy Holnbeck
Tel: 204-801-0964
Manager, Operations, Char Davian
Tel: 204-945-8813
Operations Manager, All Nations Coordinated Response Network (ANCR), Terry Driedger
Tel: 204-944-4200
Acting Manager of Administration, Child Protection, Sharon Field
Tel: 204-945-0840
Acting Manager, Quality Assurance & Evaluation, Chris Nash
Tel: 204-945-1413
Specialist, Community Development, Sharon Krysko
Tel: 204-945-2152
Provincial Adoption Clerk, Stephanie Turmaine
Tel: 204-945-6958

Community Engagement & Corporate Services
cfsd@gov.mb.ca

Assistant Deputy Minister, Jennifer Rattray
Tel: 204-945-6374
Acting Executive Director, Children's disABILITY Services, Tracy Moore
Tel: 204-945-3255

Acting Executive Director, Corporate Services & Administration, Michelle Stephen-Wiens
Tel: 204-945-5810
Director, Early Learning & Child Care Program, Margaret Ferniuk
Tel: 204-945-2668
Vulnerable Persons' Commissioner, JoAnne Reinsch
Tel: 204-945-0564

Community Service Delivery
#119, 114 Garry St., Winnipeg, MB R3C 4V4

Tel: 204-945-1634
csd@gov.mb.ca

Assistant Deputy Minister, Michelle Dubik
Tel: 204-945-2204
Acting Executive Director, Rural & Northern Services, Dan Knight
Tel: 204-945-4998
Acting Director, Strategic Planning & Program Support, Cees deVries
Tel: 204-945-0454
Acting Director, Provincial Services, Esther Kiernan
Tel: 204-945-6854
Acting Assistant Director, Adult Disability Programs, Andrea Thibault-McNeill
Tel: 204-945-6131
Program Specialist, Community Living disABILITY Services, Craig Wynands
Tel: 204-945-5599

Manitoba Developmental Centre
840 - 3rd St. NE, Portage la Prairie, MB R1N 3C6

Tel: 204-856-4200
csd@gov.mb.ca
www.gov.mb.ca/fs/pwd/mdc

Chief Executive Officer, Tom Sidebottom
Tel: 204-856-4237
Director, Habilitation/Specialty Program, Melanie Ferg
Tel: 204-856-4223
Director, Operations, Michele Roteliuk
Tel: 204-856-4219
Acting Manager, Environmental Services, Shelly Strong
Tel: 204-856-4333

Manitoba Health, Seniors & Active Living
#100, 300 Carlton St., Winnipeg, MB R3B 3M9

Tel: 204-945-3744
Toll-Free: 866-626-4862
mgi@gov.mb.ca
www.gov.mb.ca/health/index.html

Renamed Health, Seniors & Active Living after the 2016 general election, the department is responsible for the overall quality of the health system in the province, for maintaining the health system, & for ensuring that the health needs of Manitobans are met. Services are provided through regional delivery systems, hospitals & other health care facilities. The Department also makes insured benefits claims payments for residents of Manitoba related to the cost of medical, hospital, personal care, pharmacare & other health services. To lead the way to quality health care, built with creativity, compassion, confidence, trust & respect; empower Manitobans through knowledge, choices & access to the best possible health resources; & build partnerships & alliances for healthy & supportive communities. To foster innovation in the health care system. This is accomplished through: developing mechanisms to assess & monitor quality of care, utilization & cost effectiveness; fostering behaviours & environments which promote health; & promoting responsiveness & flexibility of delivery systems, & alternative & less expensive services.

Minister, Health, Seniors & Active Living, Hon. Kelvin Goertzen
Tel: 204-945-3731
Fax: 204-945-0441
minhsal@leg.gov.mb.ca

Deputy Minister, Karen Herd
Tel: 204-945-3771
Fax: 204-945-4564
dmhlt@leg.gov.mb.ca

Acting Chief Provincial Public Health Officer, Dr. Elise Weiss, M.D., C.C.F.P., F.C.F.P., M.Sc.
Tel: 204-788-6636

Administration & Finance
Assistant Deputy Minister & Chief Financial Officer, Dan Skwarchuk
Tel: 204-788-2525
Comptroller, Tony Messner
Tel: 204-786-7135
Executive Director, Finance, Rhonda Hogg
Tel: 204-788-7138
Executive Director, Health Information Management, Deborah Malazdrewicz
Tel: 204-786-7149
Executive Director, Management Services, Scott Murray
Tel: 204-786-7230
Acting Director, Regional Finance, Charlyene Cosens
Tel: 204-786-7260

Health Workforce Secretariat
Assistant Deputy Minister, Beth Beaupre
Tel: 204-786-6674
Executive Director, Contracts & Negotiations, Pearl Reimer
Tel: 204-788-6374
Director, Health Human Resource Planning, Sean Brygidyr
Tel: 204-788-6767
Director, Fee for Service/Insured Benefits, Gayle Martens
Tel: 204-788-6623
Medical Consultant, Medical Consulting Group, T. Ali Khan
Tel: 204-786-7198
Audit & Investigations Officer, Roch St-Vincent
Tel: 204-786-7343

Provincial Policy & Programs
Assistant Deputy Minister, Bernadette Preun
Tel: 204-788-6439
Executive Director, Capital Planning, Norman Blackie
Tel: 204-788-6691
Executive Director, Provincial Drug Programs, Patricia Caetano
Tel: 204-786-7333
Executive Director, Information Systems, Bryan Payne
Tel: 204-786-7232
Director, Corporate Services, Jeff Gunter
Tel: 204-788-6749
Acting Director, Drug Management Policy, Jeff Onyskiw
Tel: 204-788-6436
Manager, Protection for Persons in Care, Chris Campbell
Tel: 204-786-7264
Acting Manager, Pharmacare, Lisa Leong
Tel: 204-788-2561
Coordinator, French Language Services, Richard Loiselle
Tel: 204-788-6698
Fax: 204-772-2943

Public Health & Primary Health Care
300 Carlton St., 4th Floor, Winnipeg, MB R3B 3M9

Tel: 204-788-6666
www.gov.mb.ca/health/publichealth
Other Communication: Primary Care, Phone: 204-788-6732; Fax: 204-943-5305; E-mail: phc@gov.mb.ca; URL: www.gov.mb.ca/health/primarycare
Mission is to encourage the prevention of illness & injury, coordinate access to health care, & strengthen existing primary health care services with new initiatives
Assistant Deputy Minister, Avis Gray
Tel: 204-788-6656
Acting Executive Director, Public Health Branch; Program Manager, Population Health & Health Equity, Claire Betker
Tel: 204-788-7246
Executive Director, Primary Health Care Branch, Barbara Wasilewski
Tel: 204-788-7176
Director, Communicable Disease Control, Richard Baydack
Tel: 204-788-6715
Director, Northern Nursing Stations, Kim Hutcheson
Tel: 204-788-6642
Lead Epidemiologist & Director, Epidemiology & Surveillance, Carla Loeppky
Tel: 204-788-7392
Director, Environment Health & Emergency Preparedness, Peter Parys
Tel: 204-788-6745
Manager, Health Protection Unit, Mike LeBlanc
Tel: 204-788-6726

Regional Policy & Programs

Assistant Deputy Minister, Jean Cox
  Tel: 204-786-7301
Acting Chief Provincial Psychiatrist, Hugh Andrew
  Tel: 204-788-6677
Chief Provincial Psychiatrist, Richard Zloty
  Tel: 204-788-6677
Executive Director, Continuing Care, Lorraine Dacombe Dewar
  Tel: 204-788-6649
Executive Director, Acute, Tertiary & Specialty Care, Brie DeMone
  Tel: 204-788-6331
Executive Director, Health Emergency Management, Teresa Mrozek
  Tel: 204-945-6382
Executive Director, Provincial Cancer & Diagnostic Services Branch, Robert Shaffer
  Tel: 204-788-6670
Executive Director, Urban Regional Support Services, Vacant
Provincial Medical Director, Emergency Medical Services, Anthony Herd
  Tel: 204-945-6501
Director, Medical Transportation Coordination Centre, John Jones
  Tel: 204-571-8863
Director, Diagnostic Services, Provincial Cancer & Diagnostic Services Branch, Michele Mathae-Hunter
  Tel: 204-788-6628
Director, Office of Provincial Transplant & Transfusion Services, Wendy Peppel
  Tel: 204-786-7374
Disaster Management Specialist, Office of Disaster Management, Jennifer Chiarotto
  Tel: 204-945-7434

Manitoba Liquor & Lotteries (MBLL)
830 Empress St., Winnipeg, MB R3G 3H3

Tel: 204-957-2500
Fax: 204-284-3500
Toll-Free: 800-265-3912
www.mbll.ca
twitter.com/ImpactTeamMB
www.linkedin.com/company/manitoba-lotteries
www.youtube.com/liquormarts

The Crown Corporation was formed with the merger of the Manitoba Liquor Control Commission & Manitoba Lotteries Corporation in 2014. This coincided with the creation of the Liquor & Gaming Authority of Manitoba.
Manitoba Liquor & Lotteries operates the following: Liquor Marts & Liquor Mart Express stores; Club Regent Casino; McPhillips Station Casino; Video Lotto & PlayNow.com; & distributes & sells Western Canada Lottery products through a network of lottery ticket retailers.

Vice-President, Corporate Governance & Business Transformation, Brent Hlady

Vice-President, Liquor Operations, Robert Holmberg

Vice-President, Gaming Operations, Dan Sanscartier

Senior Executive Director, Strategic Gaming & Liquor Development, Secretary to the Council, Kerry Wolfe

Premier's Council on the Status of Disabled Persons / Conseil du Premier ministre sur la condition des personnes handicapées
Place 2000, Room 140, PO Box 6000 Fredericton, NB E3B 5H1

Tel: 506-444-3000
Fax: 506-444-3001
Toll-Free: 800-442-4412
pcsdp@gnb.ca
www.gnb.ca/council
twitter.com/nbPCSDP
www.facebook.com/PCSDP

The role of the Premier's Council on the Status of Disabled Persons is to provide advice to the provincial government of New Brunswick & the public about issues of interest & concern that affect the status of persons with disabilities.

Premier, Hon. Brian Gallant

Tel: 506-453-2144
Brian.Gallant@gnb.ca

Chair, Jeff Sparks

Executive Director, Brian Saunders

Office Manager, Kristin Colwell
kristin.colwell@gnb.ca

New Brunswick Department of Health / Santé
HSBC Place, PO Box 5100 Fredericton, NB E3B 5G8

Tel: 506-457-4800
Fax: 506-453-5243
Health.Sante@gnb.ca
www.gnb.ca/health
twitter.com/NBHealth

The mission of New Brunswick's Department of Health is to work with New Brunswickers in achieving well-being, by promoting self-sufficiency & personal responsibility, & providing approved services as required.
The development & delivery of health programs & services to New Brunswick residents is supported by a range of internal department functions, such as administration, planning & evaluation, & program support. The department provides services to prevent illness & disability. Education & awareness-raising initiatives promote the health & well-being of New Brunswickers of all ages, so that they can achieve their best potential, while enjoying an independent & healthy lifestyle for as long as possible.
Public Health services are delivered through the province's seven health regions, under the management of Regional Directors. A Chief Medical Officer of Health & a Deputy Chief Medical Officer of Health oversee the development of policy & regulations, & provide medical operational support to the regional Medical Officers of Health. Public Health Services support healthy growth & development, foster healthy lifestyles, control communicable diseases, & protect the public from adverse health consequences of exposure to chemical, physical & biological agents.

Minister, Health, Hon. Victor Éric Boudreau
  Tel: 506-457-4800
  Fax: 506-453-5442
  victor.boudreau@gnb.ca

Deputy Minister, Tom Maston
  Tel: 506-453-2542
  Tom.Maston@gnb.ca

Director, Communications, Véronique Taylor
  Tel: 506-444-4583
  Veronique.Taylor@gnb.ca

Office of the Chief Medical Officer of Health Division / Bureau du médecin-hygiéniste en chef

Tel: 506-444-2112
Fax: 506-453-5243

Acting Chief Medical Officer & Deputy Chief Medical Officer of Health, Jennifer Russell
  Tel: 506-453-2280
  jennifer.russell@gnb.ca
Executive Director, Planning & Operations, Janique Robichaud-Savoie
  Tel: 506-453-6962
  Janique.Robichaud-savoie@gnb.ca
Director, Public Health Practice & Population Health, Kimberly Blinco
  Tel: 506-453-6874
  kimberley.blinco@gnb.ca
Director, Communicable Disease & Control, Shelley Landsburg
  Tel: 506-444-3044
  Shelley.Landsburg@gnb.ca
Director, Healthy Environments, Karen White Masry
  Tel: 506-453-2427
  karen.white-masry@gnb.ca

Corporate Services Division / Services ministériels

Tel: 506-453-2745
Fax: 506-444-4698

Assistant Deputy Minister, Renée Laforest
 Tel: 506-453-2745
 dh-ms@gnb.ca
Executive Director, Financial Services, Patsy Mackinnon
 Tel: 506-453-2117
 Patsy.MacKinnon@gnb.ca
Director, Health Analytics, James Ayles
 Tel: 506-453-2793
 james.ayles@gnb.ca
Director, Health Facility Planning, Charles Chouinard
 Tel: 506-453-2117
 Charles.Chouinard2@gnb.ca
Director, Emergency Preparedness & Response, Cathy Goodfellow
 Tel: 506-444-4788
 cathy.goodfellow@gnb.ca
Director, Health Information Management, Debbie Peters
 Tel: 506-453-4079
 debbie.peters@gnb.ca

Health Services & Francophone Affairs / Services de santé et Affaires francophones

Associate Deputy Minister, Claude Allard
 Tel: 506-453-2582
 Claude.Allard2@gnb.ca
Executive Director, Primary Health Care, Nancy Roberts
 Tel: 506-453-6349
 Nancy.Roberts@gnb.ca
Director, Home Care, John Bustard
 Tel: 506-444-5360
 jean.bustard@gnb.ca
Director, Emergency Health Services, John Estey
 Tel: 506-453-6349
 john.estey@gnb.ca

Policy, Planning, Medicare & Pharmaceutical Services / Politiques, Planification, Assurance-maladie et Services pharmaceutiques

Tel: 506-453-2582
Fax: 506-453-5523

Assistant Deputy Minister, Mark Wies
 Tel: 506-453-2582
 Mark.Wies@gnb.ca
Executive Director, Program Alignment & Performance, René Boudreau
 Tel: 506-457-4800
 rene.boudreau@gnb.ca
Executive Director, Pharmaceutical Services, Leanne Jardine
 Tel: 506-453-3884
 leanne.jardine@gnb.ca
Chief Privacy Officer, Corporate Privacy, Sara Miller
 Tel: 506-453-8663
 Sara.Miller@gnb.ca
Director, Federal/Provincial/Territorial Relations & Atlantic Collaboration, Dale Dell
 Tel: 506-457-4800
 dave.dell@gnb.ca
Director, Formulary Management, Pharmaceutical Services, Tina Leclerc
 Tel: 506-457-3564
 Tina.LeClerc@gnb.ca
Director, Medicare & Physician Services, Michel Léger
 Tel: 506-453-2793
 Michel.Leger@gnb.ca
Director, Health Workforce Planning, Eric Levesque
 Tel: 506-453-2793
 Eric.Levesque2@gnb.ca
Director, Drug Utilization, Pharmaceutical Services, Heidi Liston
 Tel: 506-444-3326
 heidi.liston@gnb.ca
Director, Business Management, Pharmaceutical Services, Kevin Pothier
 Tel: 506-444-5961
 Kevin.Pothier@gnb.ca

Service New Brunswick / Service Nouveau Brunswick
Westmorland Pl., PO Box 1998 Fredericton, NB E3B 5G4

Tel: 506-457-3581
Fax: 506-444-2850
snb@snb.ca
www.snb.ca

Other Communication: SNB TeleServices Within NB: 1-888-762-8600; Outside NB: 506-684-7901

Service New Brunswick provides the following services to the public: Service New Brunswick TeleServices (Call Centre); delivery of federal, provincial & municipal government services; Land Registry; Personal Property Registry; Corporate Registry; Property Assessment & Taxation System; & maintaining land information infrastructure.
On Oct. 1, 2015, the new Service New Brunswick was launched, bringing together the former Service New Brunswick, Department of Government Services, FacilicorpNB & New Brunswick Internal Services Agency under one organization.

Minister Responsible, Hon. Ed Doherty
 Tel: 506-453-6100
 ed.doherty@snb.ca

Chair, Elizabeth Webster

Chief Executive Officer, Roy Alan
 Tel: 506-444-2897
 alan.roy@snb.ca

Chief Operating Officer, Technology & Health Services, Derrick Jardine
 Tel: 506-663-2510
 derrick.jardine@snb.ca

Health Services / Services de santé

Tel: 506-457-3581
Fax: 506-444-2850

Vice-President, David Dumont
 Tel: 506-663-2510
 david.dumont@snb.ca
Executive Director, Clinical Engineering, Charles Beaulieu
 Tel: 506-737-5781
 Charles.Beaulieu@snb.ca
Executive Director, Strategic Procurement (Health), Ann Dolan
 Tel: 506-663-2538
 ann.dolan@snb.ca
Executive Director, Supply Chain, Michel Levesque
 Tel: 506-869-6140
 Michel.Levesque@snb.ca
Executive Director, Laundry & Linen Services, Terry Watters
 Tel: 506-674-0058
 Terry.Watters@snb.ca
Director, Maintenance - Linen Services, James Belliveau
 Tel: 506-457-3581
 James.Belliveau@snb.ca
Director, Sourcing Renewal, Nancy Butler-Rioux
 Tel: 506-544-2505
 Nancy.Butlerrioux@snb.ca
Director, Logistics, Greg Demerchant
 Tel: 506-452-5623
 greg.demerchant@snb.ca
Director, Procurement (Vitalité), Annick Godin-Bourque
 Tel: 506-869-2720
 Annick.GodinBourque@snb.ca
Director, Procurement (Horizon), Jana Kirkpatrick
 Tel: 506-649-2661
 Jana.Kirkpatrick@snb.ca

Technology Services / Services technologiques
435 Brookside Dr., Fredericton, NB E3A 8V4

Tel: 506-444-4600
Fax: 506-444-3784
Toll-Free: 888-487-5050
NBISA-ASINB@gnb.ca

Vice-President, Pam Gagnon
 Tel: 506-457-3582
 Pam.Gagnon@snb.ca

Executive Director, Health Application Services, Tania Davies
  Tania.Davies@snb.ca
Director, Horizon Health Network Application Services, Sharon Jamer
  Tel: 506-375-2743
  Sharon.Jamer@snb.ca
Director, Provincial Health Services, Dawn O'Donnell
  Tel: 506-457-4800
  dawn.o'donnell@snb.ca
Director, Vitalité Health Network Application Services, Ghislain Roy
  Tel: 506-789-5901
  Ghislain.Roy@snb.ca

New Brunswick Department of Social Development / Développement social
Sartain MacDonald Bldg., 551 King St., PO Box 6000 Fredericton, NB E3B 5H1

  Tel: 506-453-2001
  Fax: 506-453-2164
  sd-ds@gnb.ca
  www.gnb.ca/socialdevelopment
  twitter.com/WellnessNB
  www.facebook.com/WellnessNBMieuxEtreNB

The Department of Social Development oversees services to the following citizens of New Brunswick: seniors & persons with disabilities who need long-term care & nursing home services; children who require assistance to prepare for school; abused & neglected children & adults; families in need of affordable day care; & persons in need of affordable housing & social assistance. As of June 6, 2016 the department will be managed by both the minister of families & children as well as the minister of seniors & long term care.

Minister, Families & Children, Hon. Stephen Horsman
Stephen.Horsman@gnb.ca

Minister, Seniors & Long-Term Care, Hon. Lisa Harris
lisa.harris@gnb.ca

Deputy Minister, Craig Dalton
Tel: 506-453-2590
craig.dalton@gnb.ca

Director, Corporate Communications, Dave Maclean
Tel: 506-444-2501
Dave.Maclean@gnb.ca

Families & Children / Familles et des enfants
  Tel: 506-453-2181
  Fax: 506-453-2164
Assistant Deputy Minister, Lisa Doucette
  Tel: 506-453-2181
  Lisa.Doucette@gnb.ca
Director, Community & Individual Development, Amélie Deschênes
  Tel: 506-444-4213
  Amélie.Deschenes@gnb.ca
Director, Child & Youth Services, William Innes
  Tel: 506-453-3622
  bill.innes@gnb.ca
Director, Wellness, Marlien McKay
  Tel: 506-444-4633
  marlien.mckay@gnb.ca

Program Delivery / Prestation des programmes
  Tel: 506-453-2379
  Fax: 506-453-2164
Assistant Deputy Minister, Jean Rioux
  Tel: 506-453-2379
  jean.rioux@gnb.ca
Director, Provincial Program Delivery, Marc Gagnon
  Tel: 506-856-3364
  Marc.Gagnon@gnb.ca

Seniors & Long Term Care / Aînés et Soins de longue durée
  Tel: 506-453-2940
  Fax: 506-453-2164
  seniors@gnb.ca
  www.gnb.ca/seniors

Assistant Deputy Minister, Steven Hart
  Tel: 506-453-2181
  Steven.Hart@gnb.ca
Director, Long Term Care & Disability Support Services, Joan McGowan
  Tel: 506-457-6811
  joan.McGowan@gnb.ca
Director, Nursing Homes Services, Janet Thomas
  Tel: 506-453-3821
  janet.thomas@gnb.ca

WorkSafeNB (WHSCC) / Travail sécuritaire NB
1 Portland St., PO Box 160 Saint John, NB E2L 3X9
  Tel: 506-632-2200
  Toll-Free: 877-647-0777
  communications@ws-ts.nb.ca
  www.worksafenb.ca
  Other Communication: Toll-Free Fax: 888-629-4722
  twitter.com/WorkSafeNB
  www.linkedin.com/company/worksafenb
  www.youtube.com/user/WorksafeNB

WorkSafeNB is a crown corporation, responsible for the application of the New Brunswick Occupational Health & Safety Act, the Workers' Compensation Act of New Brunswick, & the Workplace Health, Safety & Compensation Commission Act of New Brunswick on behalf of the workers & employers of this province. WorkSafeNB provides insurance for the workers it represents.

Chair, Dorine Pirie

Acting President & CEO, Tim Petersen

Vice-President, WorkSafe Services, Shelly Dauphinee

Acting Vice-President, Corporate Services, Carolyn MacDonald

Corporate Secretary & General Counsel, Michael McGovern

Director, Communications, Manon Arsenault

Newfoundland & Labrador Department of Health & Community Services (HCS)
West Block, Confederation Bldg., PO Box 8700 St. John's, NL A1B 4J6

  Tel: 709-729-4984
  healthinfo@gov.nl.ca
  www.health.gov.nl.ca
  Other Communication: Immunization Records, Phone: 709-729-0724

Provides a leadership role in health & community service programs & policy development for the Province. This involves working in partnership with a number of key stakeholders including regional boards, community organizations, professional associations, post-secondary educational institutions, unions, consumer & other government departments.

Minister, Hon. Dr. John Haggie
Tel: 709-729-3124
Fax: 709-729-0121
johnhaggie@gov.nl.ca

Deputy Minister, Health, Beverley Clarke
Tel: 709-729-3125
johnabbott@gov.nl.ca

Parliamentary Assistant, Bernard Davis
Tel: 709-729-3335
Fax: 709-729-0121
bernarddavis@gov.nl.ca

Assistant Deputy Minister, Michelle Jewer
Tel: 709-729-0620
Fax: 709-729-0640
michellejewer@gov.nl.ca

Assistant Deputy Minister, Denise Tubrett
Tel: 709-729-0580

Fax: 709-729-0640
dtubrett@gov.nl.ca

Director, Communications, Tina Williams
Tel: 709-729-1377
Fax: 709-728-2837
tinawilliams@gov.nl.ca

Corporate Services Branch

Regional Director, Audit & Claims Integrity, Glenn Budgell
Tel: 709-292-4009
Fax: 709-292-4052
gbudgell@gov.nl.ca
Director, Information Management, Michael Bannister
Tel: 709-729-3421
michaelbannister@gov.nl.ca
Budgeting Manager, Financial Services, Chad Antle
Tel: 709-729-2113
ChadAntle@gov.nl.ca
Budgeting Manager, Financial Services, Linda Boland
Tel: 709-729-7956
Fax: 709-729-3151
lindaboland@gov.nl.ca
Manager, Financial Operations, Tony Martin
Tel: 709-729-2304
TonyMartin@gov.nl.ca
Manager, e-Health Transformation, Kevin Durdle
Tel: 709-729-1596
KevinDurdle@gov.nl.ca

Policy & Planning Branch

Assistant Deputy Minister, Michael Harvey
Tel: 709-729-3103
michaelharvey@gov.nl.ca
Director, Planning, Performance Monitoring & Evaluation, Andrea
Kearley
Tel: 709-729-6866
andreakearley@gov.nl.ca

Population Health Branch

Assistant Deputy Minister, Karen Stone
Tel: 709-729-3103
karens@gov.nl.ca
Chief Medical Officer of Health, Dr. David Allison
Tel: 709-729-3433
davidallison@gov.nl.ca
Director, Environmental Public Health, Darryl Johnson
Tel: 709-729-3422
Fax: 709-729-0730
djohnson@gov.nl.ca
Director, Disease Control, Cathy O'Keefe
Tel: 709-729-5019
Fax: 709-729-5824
cokeefe@gov.nl.ca

Professional Services

Assistant Deputy Minister, Heather Hanrahan
Tel: 709-729-1716
heatherhanrahan@gov.nl.ca
Provincial Director, Physician Services, Angela Batstone
Tel: 709-729-7686
angelabatstone@gov.nl.ca
Director, Pharmaceutical Services Division, Keith Sheppard
Tel: 709-758-7977
keithsheppard@gov.nl.ca
Acting Director, Health Workforce Planning, Andrew Wells
Tel: 709-729-2501
andrewwells@gov.nl.ca
Director, Dental Services, Dr. Ed Williams
Tel: 709-758-1503
edwilliams@gov.nl.ca

Regional Services Branch

Acting Director, Long-Term Care & Community Support Services,
Annette Bridgeman
Tel: 709-729-7628
annettebridgeman@gov.nl.ca
Director, Acute Health Services, Emergency Management & Nursing
Policy, Beverly Griffiths

Tel: 709-729-0717
bgriffiths@gov.nl.ca

Newfoundland & Labrador Workplace Health, Safety & Compensation Commission (WorkplaceNL)
146 - 148 Forest Rd., PO Box 9000 St. John's, NL A1A 3B8
Tel: 709-778-1000
Fax: 709-738-1714
Toll-Free: 800-563-9000
general.inquiries@whscc.nl.ca
www.whscc.nf.ca
Other Communication: Grand Falls toll-free: 800-563-3448; Corner
Brook toll-free: 800-563-2772
www.facebook.com/127058107367289
www.youtube.com/user/safeworknl
Utilizing skilled, professional employees, in partnership with workplace
parties, the commission facilitates safe & healthy workplaces by
assisting employers & workers to prevent accidents, & manage
workplace injuries/illnesses & return-to-work processes. Operating as
the administrator of the workers' compensation insurance program, the
commission provides a reasonable level of benefits to injured workers
& their dependents based on reasonable assessment rates for
employers, while maintaining or exceeding service level performance
when compared to other jurisdictions in Canada.

Minister Responsible, WorkplaceNL, Hon. Eddie Joyce
Tel: 709-729-3048
Fax: 709-729-0943
ejoyce@gov.nl.ca

Interim Chair, Elizabeth Forward

Chief Executive Officer, Dennis Hogan

Chief Financial & Information Officer, Paul Kavanagh

General Counsel & Corporate Secretary, Ann Martin

Executive Director, Employer Services, Brian Delaney

Executive Director, Workers Services, Tom Mahoney

Director, Human Resources, Glenda Peet

Director, Communications, Carla Riggs

Northwest Territories Department of Health & Social Services (HSS)
5015 - 49th St., PO Box 1320 Yellowknife, NT X1A 2L9
www.hss.gov.nt.ca
Other Communication: Media Relations, Phone: 867-920-8927; Health
Care Coverage/Vital Statistics: 1-800-661-0830
www.youtube.com/user/HSSCommunications
The Department of Health & Social Services is mandated to provide a
broad range of health & social programs & services to the residents of
the NWT. Seven regional Health & Social Services Authorities plan,
manage & deliver a full spectrum of community & facility-based
services for health care & social services. Community health programs
include daily sick clinics, public health clinics, home care, school health
programs & educational programs. Visiting physicians & specialists
routinely visit the communities.

**Minister, Health & Social Services; Minister Responsible,
Seniors & Persons with Disabilities,** Hon. Glen Abernethy
Tel: 867-767-9141 ext: 11135
glen_abernethy@gov.nt.ca

Deputy Minister, Debbie DeLancey
Tel: 867-767-9060 ext: 49005
debbie_delancey@gov.nt.ca

Assistant Deputy Minister, Corporate Services, Derek Elkin
Tel: 867-767-9050 ext: 49001

Assistant Deputy Minister, Health Programs, Kim Riles
Tel: 867-767-9050 ext: 49002

Chief Public Health Officer, Dr. André Corriveau
Tel: 867-767-9063 ext: 49215

Deputy Chief Public Health Officer, Dr. Kami Kandola
Tel: 867-767-9063 ext: 49216

Director, Corporate Planning, Reporting & Evaluation, Lisa Cardinal
Tel: 867-767-9053 ext: 49050
Fax: 867-873-0484

Director, Strategic Human Resource Planning Division, Beth Collinson
Tel: 867-767-9059 ext: 49150

Director, Infrastructure Planning, Perry Heath
Tel: 867-767-9057 ext: 49125

Director, Innovation & Project Management, Dave Nightingale
Tel: 867-767-9058 ext: 49139

Communications Officer, Dorothy Westerman
Tel: 867-767-9052 ext: 49035
Fax: 867-873-0204

Aboriginal Health & Community Wellness
Fax: 867-873-3585
Director, Aboriginal Health & Community Wellness, Sabrina Broadhead
Tel: 867-876-0640
Territorial Nutritionist, Vacant
Tel: 867-767-9064 ext: 49231
Manager, Health & Wellness Promotion, Ethel Blake
Tel: 867-767-9064 ext: 49230
Manager, Community Wellness Initiatives, Guy Erasmus
Tel: 867-767-9064 ext: 49247
Manager, Cancer Initiatives, Crystal Milligan
Tel: 867-767-9064 ext: 49238
Senior Advisor, Aboriginal Health, Karen Blondin Hall
Tel: 867-767-9064 ext: 49224
Senior Advisor, Anti-Poverty, Kyla Kakfwi-Scott
Tel: 867-767-9064 ext: 49248
Senior Advisor, Early Childhood Development, Nina Larsson
Tel: 867-767-9064 ext: 49228

Finance
Director, Finance, Jeannie Mathison
Tel: 867-767-9056 ext: 49100
Assistant Director, Financial Planning & Analysis, Elizabeth Johnson
Tel: 867-767-9056 ext: 49110
Manager, Control & Procurement Services, Joe Tkachuk
Tel: 867-767-9056 ext: 49105

Information Services
Fax: 867-873-0484
Chief Information Officer, Michele Herriot
Tel: 867-767-9054 ext: 49065
Registrar General, Jenetta Day
Tel: 867-777-7422
Director, Health Services Administration, Nick Saturnino
Tel: 867-777-7400
Manager, Project Management Services, Kitty Dang
Tel: 867-767-9054 ext: 49089
Manager, Informatics Strategy, Derek Sing
Tel: 867-767-9054 ext: 49067
Manager, Information Systems, Roger Soulodre
Tel: 867-767-9054 ext: 49071
Manager, Health Care Eligibility & Insurance Programs, Roslyn Watters
Tel: 867-777-7404

Northwest Territories Health & Social Services Authority (NTHSSA)
PO Box 1320 Yellowknife, NT X1A 2L9

Tel: 867-767-9090
hss_transformation@gov.nt.ca
www.nthssa.ca

The NTHSSA was formed in Aug. 2016 as a result of the amalgamation of six regional health authorities: Beaufort-Delta Health & Social Services Authority, Dehcho Health & Social Services Authority, Fort Smith Health & Social Services Authority, Sahtu Health & Social Services Authority, Stanton Territorial Health Authority, & Yellowknife Health & Social Services Authority. The authority maintains regional operations in those areas.
Chief Executive Officer, Sue Cullen
Tel: 867-767-9090 ext: 40000
Territorial Medical Director, Dr. Sarah Cook
Tel: 867-767-9090 ext: 40000
Chief Medical Information Officer, Dr. Ewan Affleck
Tel: 867-873-7609
Executive Director, Stanton Renewal, Gloria Badari
Tel: 867-767-9127 ext: 35002
Executive Director, Clinical Integration, Les Harrison
Tel: 867-767-9106 ext: 40000
Executive Director, Corporate & Support Services, Kevin Taylor
Tel: 867-767-9107 ext: 40000
Director, Quality, Safety & Client Experience, Natalie Campbell
Tel: 867-872-6256
Director, Health Services, Joanne Engram
Tel: 867-767-9090 ext: 40027
Director, Information & Health Technology, Marta Moir
Tel: 867-767-9107 ext: 40170
Director, Child, Family & Community Wellness, Nathalie Nadeau
Tel: 867-767-9106 ext: 40050
Manager, Communications, David Maguire
Tel: 867-767-9107 ext: 40150

Policy, Legislation & Communications
Fax: 867-873-0204
Director, Policy, Legislation & Communications, Denise Canuel
Tel: 867-767-9052 ext: 49018
Chief Health Privacy Officer, Natasha Brotherston
Tel: 867-767-9052 ext: 49040
Manager, Communications, Damien Healy
Tel: 867-767-9052 ext: 49034
Manager, Policy & Legislation, Colette Perry
Tel: 867-767-9052 ext: 49020
Manager, Official Languages, Sean Whitcomb
Tel: 867-767-9052 ext: 49045

Population Health
Fax: 867-873-0442
Director, Population Health, Laura Seddon
Tel: 867-767-9066 ext: 49253
Chief Environmental Health Officer, Peter Workman
Tel: 867-767-9066 ext: 49260
Territorial Epidemiologist, Epidemiology & Disease Registries, Heather Hannah
Tel: 867-767-9066 ext: 49285
Manager, Public Health Registries Unit, Marc Arseneau
Tel: 867-767-9066 ext: 49286
Manager, Communicable Disease Control, Colin Eddie
Tel: 867-767-9066 ext: 49275

Seniors & Continuing Care Services
Fax: 867-920-3088
Director, Victorine Lafferty
Tel: 867-767-9030 ext: 49205
Acting Manager, Continuing Care & Health Systems Planning Unit, Sandra Mann
Tel: 867-767-9030 ext: 49208
Manager, Strategic Initiatives Unit, Stacy Ridgely
Tel: 867-767-9030 ext: 49900

Territorial Health Services
Fax: 867-873-0196
Director, Territorial Health Services, Jo-Anne Hubert
Tel: 867-767-9062 ext: 49190
Manager, Primary Community & Acute Care Services, Kate Thompson
Tel: 867-767-9062 ext: 49195
Health Planner, Health Emergency Management, Stephen Moss
Tel: 867-767-9062 ext: 49196

Territorial Social Programs
Assistant Deputy Minister, Families & Communities, Patricia Kyle
Tel: 867-767-9061 ext: 49009
Public Guardian, Office of the Public Guardian, Beatrice Raddi
Tel: 867-767-9155 ext: 49460

Manager, Mental Health & Addictions, Sara Chorostowski
Tel: 867-767-9061 ext: 49178
Manager, Out of Territory Placements, Brian Kolback
Tel: 867-767-9061 ext: 49163
Fax: 867-920-6159
Manager, Child & Family Services, Bethan Williams-Simpson
Tel: 867-767-9061 ext: 49165

Nova Scotia Department of Community Services
Nelson Place, 5675 Spring Garden Rd., 8th Fl., PO Box 696 Halifax, NS B3J 2T7

Toll-Free: 877-424-1177
www.novascotia.ca/coms
twitter.com/NS_DCS

The Department of Community Services is committed to a sustainable social service system that promotes the independence, self-reliance & security of the people it serves.

Minister; Minister, Voluntary Sector, Hon. Joanne Bernard
Fax: 902-424-3287
dcsmin@gov.ns.ca

Deputy Minister, Lynn Carey Hartwell
Tel: 902-424-3224

Associate Deputy Minister, Nancy MacLellan
Tel: 902-424-5181

Director, Prevention & Early Intervention, Natalie Downey
Tel: 902-424-0780

Director, Programs & Stakeholder Relations, Patricia Gorham
Tel: 902-424-3306

Director, Placement Services, Janet Nearing
Tel: 902-424-5367

Project Director, Community Services, Katherine Isnor
Tel: 902-424-4260

Children, Youth & Families
www.novascotia.ca/coms/families
Executive Director, Children & Family Services, Leonard Doiron
Tel: 902-424-3867
Director, Child Protection Services, Wendy Marie Leiper
Tel: 902-424-7433

Disability Support Program (DSP)
www.novascotia.ca/coms/disabilities
The DSP serves children, youth & adults with intellectual disabilities, long-term mental illness, & physical disabilities in a range of community-based, residential & vocational/day programs.
Director, Disability Support System Planning, Judith Ann LaPierre
Tel: 902-424-6296

Nova Scotia Department of Health & Wellness
Barrington Tower., 1894 Barrington St., PO Box 488 Halifax, NS B3J 2R8

Tel: 902-424-5818
Toll-Free: 800-387-6665
TTY: 800-670-8888
novascotia.ca/dhw

Other Communication: TeleHealth Network: 1-800-889-5949
Mission: Working together to empower individuals, families, partners, & communities to promote, improve, & maintain the health of Nova Scotians through a proactive & sustainable health care system.

Minister, Hon. Leo Glavine
Tel: 902-424-3377
Fax: 902-424-0559
Health.Minister@novascotia.ca

Deputy Minister, Denise Perret

Associate Deputy Minister, Tracey Barbrick
Tel: 902-424-7337

Senior Executive Director, Corporate Services, David Bartol
Tel: 902-424-4991

Senior Executive Director, System Strategy, Ruby Knowles
Tel: 902-424-3221

Executive Director, EHS & Primary Health Care, Ian Bower
Tel: 902-464-6098

Director, Acute Care, Lewis Bedford
Tel: 902-424-4878

Director, Health Intergovernmental Affairs, Vijay Bhashyakarla
Tel: 902-424-2842

Director, Formulary & Clinical Practice, Kathleen Coleman
Tel: 902-424-4837

Director, Health Workforce Policies, Cynthia Cruickshank
Tel: 902-424-8838

Director, Accountability & Performance Management, Barbara Harvie
Tel: 902-424-0059

Director, Legislative Policy, Dean Hirtle
Tel: 902-424-1797

Director, Health Economics, Michael Joyce
Tel: 902-427-6879

Director, Insured Services, Harold McCarthy
Tel: 902-424-7538

Director, Master Agreement Fee for Service, Angela Purcell

Director, Emergency Managment Centre, Russell Stuart
Tel: 902-424-0000

Health Services

IWK Health Centre
#5850/5980 University Ave., PO Box 9700 Halifax, NS B3K 6R8

Tel: 902-470-8888
Toll-Free: 888-470-5888
feedback@iwk.nshealth.ca
www.iwk.nshealth.ca
twitter.com/IWKHealthCentre
www.facebook.com/iwkhealthcentre
www.youtube.com/iwkhealthcentre

Chair, Bob Hanf
President & CEO, Tracy Kitch
Chief Financial Officer, Stephen D'Arcy
Vice-President, People & Organization Development, Steve Ashton
Vice-President, Strategy & Organizational Performance, Mary-Ann Hiltz
Vice-President, Medicine & Academic Affairs, Dr. Krista Jangaard
Chief Nure Executive & Vice-President, Patient Care, Jocelyn Vine

Nova Scotia Health Authority
#201, 90 Lovett Lake Ct., Halifax, NS B3S 0H6

Toll-Free: 844-491-5890
wearelistening@nshealth.ca
www.nshealth.ca

Other Communication: Mental Health Crisis Line: 1-888-429-8167
twitter.com/healthns
www.facebook.com/NovaScotiaHealthAuthority
All former Nova Scotia health districts merged in 2015, forming the Nova Scotia Health Authority. The organization oversees 8 regional hospitals & 1 specialty hospital, 135 community health centres, 33 auxiliaries & 37 community health boards.
Chair, Steven Parker
President & CEO, Janet Knox

Infection Prevention & Control Nova Scotia (IPCNS)
1894 Barrington St., 5th Fl., PO Box 488 Halifax, NS B3J 2R8

Tel: 902-424-5818
Toll-Free: 800-387-6665
TTY: 800-670-8888
ipc.gov.ns.ca

Established in 2009, IPCNS provides educational resources, monitors provincial data, supports other departments that provide health-related services, and develops documents that direct health care workers in infection prevention and control issues.

Office of the Chief Public Health Officer
PO Box 488 Halifax, NS B3J 2R8

Tel: 902-424-2358
Fax: 902-424-4716
novascotia.ca/dhw/publichealth/cpho.asp

The Office of the Chief Public Health Officer is responsible for the Department of Health's legislated responsibility to protect & promote the public's health in the following areas: communicable disease control, environmental health, emergency preparedness & response. In addition, staff in the Office of the Chief Public Health Officer, in collaboration with academic expertise at Dalhousie University, function as an expert resource in community health science & an epidemiological resource for the department, the health districts, & other relevant government & community groups.

Chief Public Health Officer/Chief Medical Officer of Health, Dr. Robert Strang
Tel: 902-424-2358
Fax: 902-424-0550

Acting Deputy Chief Medical Officer of Health, Dr. Gaynor Watson-Creed
Tel: 902-424-2358
Fax: 902-424-0550

Nunavut Territory Department of Health
PO Box 1000 Stn. 1000, Iqaluit, NU X0A 0H0

Tel: 867-975-5700
Fax: 867-975-5705
Toll-Free: 800-661-0833
www.gov.nu.ca/health

The Environmental Health Specialist provides recommendations & direction, consultation, development of standards, monitoring, maintenance & evaluation of all environmental health programs within Nunavut. Reviews the Public Health Act & Regulations & environmental health standards & policies & makes recommendations for revisions. Guides the regional environmental health officers in development & implementation of programs & policies in prevention of diseases caused by environmental factors, including food, water, waste disposal, housing & the sanitation of public places, including schools, day cares & other institutional facilities. Guides the Regional Environmental Health Officers in water & food-borne related illness investigations & food recalls. Guides the regions in the monitoring of drinking water supplies. Assists with development of health education & promotional materials & activities related to environmental health.

Minister; Minister Responsible, Suicide Prevention, Hon. George Hickes
Tel: 867-975-5074
Fax: 867-975-2034
ghickes@gov.nu.ca

Deputy Minister, Colleen Stockley
Tel: 867-975-5702
cstockley@gov.nu.ca

Assistant Deputy Minister, Rosemary Keenainak
Tel: 867-975-5798
rkeenainak@gov.nu.ca

Assistant Deputy Minister, Operations, Jacquie Pepper-Journal
Tel: 867-975-5956
JPepper-Journal@gov.nu.ca

Assistant Deputy Minister, Operations, Kathy Perrin
Tel: 867-975-5708
kperrin@gov.nu.ca

Chief Medical Officer of Health, Dr. Kim Barker
Tel: 867-975-5769
kbarker@gov.nu.ca

Deputy Chief Medical Officer of Health, Dr. Barry Pakes
Tel: 867-975-5743
BPakes@gov.nu.ca

Territorial Director, Medical Affairs, Kevin Compton
Tel: 867-975-7146
kcompton@gov.nu.ca

Territorial Director, Pharmacy, Donna Mulvey
Tel: 867-975-8600 ext: 6302
DMulvey@gov.nu.ca

Executive Director, Corporate Services, Greg Babstock
Tel: 867-975-5736
GBabstock@gov.nu.ca

Executive Director, Population Health, Gogi Greeley
Tel: 867-975-5002
GGreeley@gov.nu.ca

Executive Director, Health Operations, Nancy Laframboise
Tel: 867-975-5724
NLaframboise@gov.nu.ca

Executive Director, Lynn Ryan MacKenzie
Tel: 867-975-5992
lmackenzie1@gov.nu.ca

Director, Support Services, Katrina Burt
Tel: 867-975-8600 ext: 2309
kburt@gov.nu.ca

Physician & Director, Medical Education, Dr. Madeleine Cole
Tel: 867-979-7300
mcole@gov.nu.ca

Director, Professional Practice, Barbara Harvey
Tel: 867-982-7655
BHarvey@gov.nu.ca

Acting Director, Policy & Planning, Linnea Ingebrigston
Tel: 867-975-5717
LIngebrigtson@gov.nu.ca

Director, Mental Health, Victoria Madsen
Tel: 867-975-5290
vmadsen@gov.nu.ca

Director, Medical Affairs & Telehealth, Dr. William MacDonald
Tel: 867-975-8600 ext: 5009
wmacdonald2@gov.nu.ca

Director, Clinical Services, Darlene McPherson
Tel: 867-975-8600 ext: 5008
DMcPherson@gov.nu.ca

Acting Director, Population Health, Gary Nelson
Tel: 867-645-8071
GNelson@gov.nu.ca

Director, Operations OHSNI, Judy Plourde

Director, Human Resources, Lisa Richter
Tel: 867-975-5738
lrichter@gov.nu.ca

Acting Director, Health IT, Jessica Rideout
Tel: 867-975-5934
JRideout@gov.nu.ca

Acting Director, Health Programs, Monique Skinner

Tel: 867-983-4070
mskinner@gov.nu.ca

Environmental Health Consultant, Wanda Joy
Tel: 867-975-5782
wjoy@gov.nu.ca

Ontario Ministry of Health & Long-Term Care
Hepburn Block, 80 Grosvenor St., 10th Fl, Toronto, ON M7A 2C4
Tel: 416-327-4327
Toll-Free: 800-268-1153
TTY: 800-387-5559
www.health.gov.on.ca
twitter.com/ONThealth
www.facebook.com/217753654940869
www.youtube.com/user/ontariomohltc

The Ministry is responsible for administering the health care system & providing services to the Ontario public through such programs as health insurance, drug benefits, assistive devices, care for the mentally ill, long-term care, home care, community & public health, & health promotion & disease prevention. It also regulates hospitals & nursing homes, operates psychiatric hospitals & medical laboratories, & co-ordinates emergency health services.

Minister, Hon. Dr. Eric Hoskins
Tel: 416-327-4300
Fax: 416-326-1571
ehoskins.mpp@liberal.ola.org

Deputy Minister, Dr. Bob Bell
Tel: 416-327-4496
Fax: 416-326-1570
Robert.Bell@ontario.ca

Parliamentary Assistant, John Fraser
Tel: 416-327-0205
Fax: 416-325-3862
jfraser.mpp.co@liberal.ola.org

Chief of Staff to the Minister, Derrick Araneda
Tel: 416-212-3763
Derrick.Araneda@ontario.ca

Associate Deputy Minister, Delivery & Implementation, Nancy Naylor
Tel: 416-326-0232
Fax: 416-327-5186
nancy.naylor@ontario.ca

Associate Deputy Minister, Policy & Transformation, Sharon Lee Smith
Tel: 416-212-4030
sharonlee.smith@ontario.ca

Assistant Deputy Minister, Communications & Marketing, Jean-Claude Camus
Tel: 416-327-4352
jean-claude.camus@ontario.ca

Chief Health Innovation Strategist, William Charnetski
Tel: 416-325-3718
William.Charnetski@ontario.ca

Director, Communications, Minister's Office, Maria Babbage
Tel: 416-327-9728
maria.babbage@ontario.ca

Director, Legal Services Branch, Janice B. Crawford
Tel: 416-327-8565
Fax: 416-327-8605
janice.crawford@ontario.ca

Director, Policy & Delivery, Deputy Minister's Office, Wiesia Kubicka
Tel: 416-325-7999
Fax: 416-326-1570
wiesia.kubicka@ontario.ca

Director, Operations & Stakeholder Relations, Dara McLeod
Tel: 416-326-3985
Dara.McLeod@ontario.ca

Director, Policy, Minister's Office, Alyson Rowe
Tel: 416-326-3982
Alyson.Rowe@ontario.ca

Chief Medical Officer of Health (CMOH)
393 University Ave., 21st Fl., Toronto, ON M5G 2M2
Tel: 416-212-3831
Fax: 416-325-8412
health.gov.on.ca/en/common/ministry/cmoh.aspx

Chief Medical Officer of Health & Associate Chief Medical Officer of Health, Infrastructure and System (Transition), Dr. David Williams, BSc., MD, MHSc, FRCPS
dr.david.williams@ontario.ca
Associate Chief Medical Officer of Health, Environmental Health, Vacant
Associate Chief Medical Officer of Health, Health Promotion, Chronic Diseases & Injury Prevention, Vacant
Associate Chief Medical Officer of Health, Communicable & Infectious Disease, Vacant
Manager, Gillian MacDonald
Tel: 416-327-2738
gillian.macdonald2@ontario.ca
Senior Communications Consultant, Catherine Fraser
Tel: 416-326-0033
Catherine.Fraser@ontario.ca
Senior Policy & Strategic Advisor, Mikayla Wicks
Tel: 416-325-3911
Mikayla.Wicks@ontario.ca

Corporate Services Division
Hepburn Block, 80 Grosvenor St., 11th Fl., Toronto, ON M7A 1R3
Tel: 416-327-4266
Fax: 416-314-5915

Assistant Deputy Minister & Chief Administrative Officer, Justine Jackson
Tel: 416-327-4387
Justine.Jackson@ontario.ca
Director, Supply Chain & Facilities Branch, Shelley Gibson
Tel: 416-327-0782
Fax: 416-327-7312
shelley.gibson@ontario.ca
Director, HR Strategic Business Unit, Rhonda Lindo
Tel: 416-327-8747
Fax: 416-327-7580
rhonda.lindo@ontario.ca
Director, Business Innovation Office, Simon Trevarthen
Tel: 416-327-2299
simon.trevarthen@ontario.ca
Other Communications: Alt. E-mail: bio.mohltc@ontario.ca

Direct Services Division
56 Wellesley St. West, 2nd Fl., Toronto, ON M5S 2S3
Fax: 416-212-9710

Assistant Deputy Minister, Patricia Li
Tel: 416-327-4845
patricia.li@ontario.ca
Director, Psychiatric Patient Advocate Office & Acting Director, Assistive Devices Program, Nancy Dickson
Tel: 613-545-4366
Fax: 416-327-7008
nancy.dickson@ontario.ca
www.ppao.gov.on.ca
Other Communications: Alt. E-mail: ppao.moh@ontario.ca
Director, Claims Services, Josephine Fuller
Tel: 613-548-6333
Toll-free: 800-268-1154
Fax: 416-548-6320
josephine.fuller@ontario.ca
Acting Director, Emergency Health Services (Land & Air), Donna Piasentini
Tel: 416-327-7909
Toll-free: 800-461-6431
Fax: 416-327-7879

donna.piasentini@ontario.ca
www.health.gov.on.ca/english/public/program/ehs/ehs_mn.html
Acting Senior Manager, Enhancing Emergency Services in Ontario 2.0
Office, Steven Haddad
Tel: 416-212-2178
steven.haddad@ontario.ca

Health Capital Division
#601, 1075 Bay St., 6th Fl., Toronto, ON M5S 2B1
Tel: 416-326-2943

Assistant Deputy Minister, Peter Kaftarian
Tel: 416-314-0402
peter.kaftarian@ontario.ca
Director, Long-Term Care Home Renewal Branch, Brenda Blackstock
Tel: 416-212-1374
brenda.blackstock@ontario.ca
Director, Health Capital Investment Branch, James Stewart
Tel: 416-326-1088
james.stewart@ontario.ca
Manager, Capital Project Management Office, Gary Freedman
Tel: 416-327-7069
gary.freedman@ontario.ca
Manager, Capital Programs & Standards, Ezra Isaacson
Tel: 416-326-0743
ezra.isaacson@ontario.ca
Manager, Capital Financial Services, Fareen Madhani
Tel: 416-326-0742
fareen.madhani@ontario.ca

Health Services Information & Information Technology Cluster
56 Wellesley St. West, 10th Fl., Toronto, ON M5S 2S3
Tel: 416-314-0234
Fax: 416-314-4182

Associate Deputy Minister & Chief Information Officer, Lorelle Taylor
Tel: 416-314-1279
Fax: 416-314-0234
lorelle.taylor@ontario.ca
Acting Director, Digital Health Solutions & Innovation Branch, Chris
Pentleton
Tel: 416-212-1815
chris.pentleton@ontario.ca
Executive Lead, Health Services Cluster, Karen McKibbin
Tel: 416-326-7169
karen.mckibbin@ontario.ca
Acting Head, Business Consulting Branch, Louise Doyon
Tel: 416-314-2946
Fax: 416-315-4182
louise.doyon@ontario.ca
Acting Manager, Planning, Architecture & Financial Management
Branch, Swetlana Signarowski
Tel: 416-212-6409
Fax: 416-315-4182
Swetlana.Signarowski@ontario.ca

Health System Accountability & Performance Division
Hepburn Block, 80 Grosvenor St., 5th Fl., Toronto, ON M7A 1R3
Fax: 416-212-1859

Assistant Deputy Minister, Tim G. Hadwen
Tel: 416-212-1134
tim.hadwen@ontario.ca
Acting Director, LHIN Renewal Branch, Alison Blair
Tel: 416-212-4433
alison.blair@ontario.ca
Director, Primary Health Care Branch, Phil Graham
Tel: 416-212-0832
Phil.Graham@ontario.ca
Director, Home & Community Care, Amy Olmstead
Tel: 416-327-7056
amy.olmstead@ontario.ca
Director, LHIN Liaison, Jane Sager
Tel: 416-314-1864
Fax: 416-326-9734
jane.sager@ontario.ca

Health System Information Management
1075 Bay St., 13th Fl., Toronto, ON M5S 2B1
Tel: 416-212-1852
Fax: 416-327-8835
hsim@ontario.ca

Associate Deputy Minister & Chief Information Officer, Lorelle Taylor
Tel: 416-314-1279
lorelle.taylor@ontario.ca
Executive Director, Information Management, Data & Analytics Office,
Michael Hillmer
Tel: 416-327-8854
michael.hillmer@ontario.ca
Director, Health Data, Aileen Chan
Tel: 416-325-2311
Fax: 416-327-8951
aileen.chan@ontario.ca
Director, Health Analytics Branch, Ashif Damji
Tel: 416-327-6483
Fax: 416-326-6560
ashif.damji@ontario.ca
Director, eHealth Strategy & Investment Branch, Greg Hein
Tel: 416-325-9075
Fax: 416-326-9967
greg.hein@ontario.ca
Director, Special Projects, Vacant
Tel: 416-212-2301
Fax: 416-212-3542

Health System Quality & Funding Division
Hepburn Block, 80 Grosvenor St., 5th Fl., Toronto, ON M7A 1R3
Assistant Deputy Minister, Melissa Farrell
Tel: 416-327-8533
Melissa.Farrell@ontario.ca
Director, Health Sector Models Branch, Sherif Kaldas
Tel: 416-327-2396
sherif.kaldas@ontario.ca
Director, Hospitals Branch, Melanie Kohn
Tel: 416-326-6026
Melanie.Kohn@ontario.ca
Director, Policy & Innovation Branch, Jillian Paul
Tel: 416-325-5600
jillian.paul@ontario.ca
Director, HQO Liaison & Program Development Branch, Fredrika
Scarth
Tel: 416-327-3932
fredrika.scarth@ontario.ca
Acting Manager, Divisional Business Integration Services Unit, Cathy
Cheng
Tel: 416-212-4595
cathy.cheng@ontario.ca

Health Workforce Planning & Regulatory Affairs Division
56 Wellesley St. West, 12th Fl., Toronto, ON M5S 2S3
Tel: 416-212-6115
Fax: 416-327-1878

Assistant Deputy Minister, Denise Cole
Tel: 416-212-7688
denise.cole@ontario.ca
Director, Health System Labour Relations & Regulatory Policy, Allison
Henry
Tel: 416-327-8543
Fax: 416-325-8897
allison.henry@ontario.ca
Director, Health Workforce Policy, David Lamb
Tel: 416-212-2089
Fax: 416-327-0167
david.lamb@ontario.ca
Acting Director, Nursing Policy & Innovation Branch, Marsha Pinto
Tel: 416-212-4835
Fax: 416-327-1878
marsha.pinto@ontario.ca

Long-Term Care Homes Division
1075 Bay St., 11th Fl., Toronto, ON M5S 2B1
Tel: 416-327-7461
Fax: 416-327-7603

Acting Assistant Deputy Minister, Brian Pollard
Tel: 416-212-9069
brian.pollard@ontario.ca

Acting Director, Licensing & Policy Branch & Acting Manager, Aging & Long-Term Care, Michelle-Ann Hylton
Tel: 416-212-8996
Michelle-Ann.Hylton@ontario.ca

Director, Long-Term Care Inspections Branch, Karen Simpson
Tel: 613-364-2250
karen.simpson@ontario.ca

Manager, Licensing & Long-Term Care Programs, Margaret Allore
Tel: 416-325-8881
margaret.allore@ontario.ca

Manager, Licensing & X-ray Inspection, Leo Tse
Tel: 416-327-8277
leo.tse@ontario.ca

Negotiations & Accountability Management Division
Hepburn Block, 80 Grosvenor St., 5th Fl., Toronto, ON M7A 1R3
Tel: 416-212-7012

Assistant Deputy Minister, Lynn Guerriero
Tel: 416-212-7012
Lynn.Guerriero@ontario.ca

Senior Medical Advisor, Medical Advisory Unit, Dr. Garry Salisbury
Tel: 613-536-3078
garry.salisbury@ontario.ca

Director, Negotiations, David W. Clarke
Tel: 613-212-4904
Fax: 416-327-7519
david.w.clarke@ontario.ca

Director, Laboratories & Genetics Branch, Bonnie Reib
Tel: 416-212-1777
Fax: 416-327-7519
Bonnie.Reib@ontario.ca

Director, Health Services, Pauline Ryan
Tel: 613-536-3015
Toll-free: 866-684-8620
Fax: 613-536-3188
pauline.ryan@ontario.ca

Acting Director, Provincial Programs, Neeta Sarta
Tel: 416-326-3834
Neeta.Sarta@ontario.ca

Manager, Health Facilities & Provider Accountability, Kathryn Boone
Tel: 613-536-3157
kathryn.boone@ontario.ca

Manager, AIDS & Hepatitis C Programs, Susan Furino
Tel: 416-327-7431
susan.furino@ontario.ca

Manager, Provincial Agencies Trillium Gift of Life Network (TGLN) / Blood & Specialized Programs, Dai Kim
Tel: 416-326-6471
dai.kim@ontario.ca

Manager, OHIP Eligibility & OOC/OOP Prior Approvals, Brad Murphy
Tel: 613-536-3044
brad.murphy@ontario.ca

Manager, Provincial Agencies Cancer Care Ontario (CCO) / Related Programs, Vena Persaud
Tel: 416-212-0778
vena.persaud@ontario.ca

Manager, Specialist Physician Contracts Unit, Fawne Stratford-Devai
Tel: 416-327-7262
fawne.stratford-devai@ontario.ca

Manager, Priority & Acute Programs, Kristin Taylor
Tel: 416-212-6801
kristin.taylor@ontario.ca

Ontario Public Drug Programs Division
Hepburn Block, 80 Grosvenor St., 9th Fl., Toronto, ON M7A 1R3
Tel: 416-212-4724
Fax: 416-325-6647
www.health.gov.on.ca/en/public/programs/drugs

Assistant Deputy Minister & Executive Officer, Suzanne McGurn
Tel: 416-327-0902
suzanne.mcgurn@ontario.ca

Acting Director, Exceptional Access Program Branch / Drug Programs Delivery Branch, David Schachow
Tel: 416-327-8118

Fax: 416-327-8912
david.schachow@ontario.ca

Director, Drug Programs Policy & Strategy Branch, Angie Wong
Tel: 416-327-8315
angie.wong@ontario.ca

Manager, Drug Benefits Management Unit, Karina Lee
Tel: 416-327-8124
karina.lee@ontario.ca

Manager, Exceptional Access Program, David Pao
Tel: 416-326-1624
david.pao@ontario.ca

Population & Public Health Division
College Park, #1903, 777 Bay St., 19th Fl., Toronto, M7A 1S5
Fax: 416-212-2200

Assistant Deputy Minister, Roselle Martino
Tel: 416-327-9555
roselle.martino@ontario.ca

Acting Director, Healthy Living Policy & Programs Branch, Dianne Alexander
Tel: 416-212-7637
dianne.alexander@ontario.ca

Director, Disease Prevention Policy & Programs Branch, Nina Arron
Tel: 416-212-4873
nina.arron@ontario.ca

Director, Health Protection Policy & Programs Branch, Laura Pisko
Tel: 416-327-7445
laura.pisko@ontario.ca

Director, Emergency Management Branch, Clint Shingler
Tel: 416-327-8865
clint.shingler@ontario.ca

Director, Accountability & Liaison Branch, Elizabeth Walker
Tel: 416-212-6359
elizabeth.walker@ontario.ca

Director, Planning & Performance Branch, Jackie Wood
Tel: 416-212-7785
jackie.wood@ontario.ca

Manager, Environmental Health Policy & Programs Unit, Tony Amalfa
Tel: 416-327-7624
tony.amalfa@ontario.ca

Manager, Immunization Policy & Programs Unit, Michael Di Tomasso
Tel: 416-314-6955
michael.ditomasso@ontario.ca

Manager, Indigenous & Intergovernmental Unit, Susy Faria
Tel: 416-325-4657
susy.faria@ontario.ca

Manager, Funding & Oversight Unit, Brent Feeney
Tel: 416-212-6397
brent.feeney@ontario.ca

Manager, Addiction & Substances Policy & Programs Unit, Chris Harold
Tel: 416-326-5253
Chris.Harold@ontario.ca

Manager, Infectious Diseases Policy & Programs Unit, Melissa Helferty
Tel: 416-326-3107
melissa.helferty@ontario.ca

Strategic Policy & Planning Division
Hepburn Block, 80 Grosvenor St., Toronto, M7A 1R3
Tel: 416-327-8295

Assistant Deputy Minister, Patrick Dicerni
Tel: 416-327-7261
patrick.dicerni@ontario.ca

Director, Mental Health & Addictions Branch, Marg Connor
Tel: 416-327-8996
marg.connor@ontario.ca

Director, Strategic Policy Branch, Sean Court
Tel: 416-327-7531
Sean.Court@ontario.ca

Director, Policy Coordination & Intergovernmental Relations Branch, Louis Dimitracopoulos
Tel: 416-327-3314
anne.hayes@ontario.ca

Acting Director, Research, Analysis & Evaluation Branch, Anne Hayes
Tel: 416-327-3314
anne.hayes@ontario.ca

Director, Health Equity Branch, Joanne Plaxton
Tel: 416-212-5218
joanne.plaxton@ontario.ca
Director, Capacity Planning & Priorities Branch, Michael Robertson
Tel: 416-327-7615
michael.robertson@ontario.ca
Acting Manager, Mental Health & Addictions Policy Unit, Nina Acco Weston
Tel: 416-327-8319
Nina.AccoWeston@ontario.ca
Manager, Indigenous Health Policy, Lisa Alphonse
Tel: 416-327-0951
lisa.alphonse@ontario.ca
Manager, Housing, Forensic Mental Health & Community Services Unit, Miriam Johnston
Tel: 416-314-1189
miriam.johnston@ontario.ca
Manager, Health Equity Policy Unit, Joanne Thanos
Tel: 416-326-2420
joanne.thanos@ontario.ca

Workplace Safety & Insurance Board (WSIB)
200 Front St. West, Ground Fl., Toronto, ON M5V 3J1
Tel: 416-344-1000
Fax: 416-344-4684
Toll-Free: 800-387-0750
TTY: 800-387-0050
www.wsib.on.ca

Other Communication: Toll-Free Fax: 1-888-313-7373; eServices Inquiries, Phone: 1-888-243-1569; Collections, Phone: 1-800-268-0929
twitter.com/wsib
www.linkedin.com/company/wsib
www.youtube.com/ontariowsib

The Workplace Safety & Insurance Board is involved in Ontario's occupational health & safety system. The Board's responsibilities are as follows: administering no-fault workplace insurance in Ontario for employers & workers; providing disability benefits; monitoring the quality of healthcare; & assisting workers who have been injured on the job or persons who have contracted an occupational disease in an early & safe return to work.

Chair, Elizabeth Witmer
Tel: 416-344-3775

President & CEO, Thomas Teahen
Thomas_Teahen@wsib.on.ca

Prince Edward Island Department of Health & Wellness
Shaw Bldg., 105 Rochford St. North, 4th Fl., Charlottetown, PE C1A 7N8
Tel: 902-368-6414
Fax: 902-368-4121
healthweb@gov.pe.ca
www.gov.pe.ca/health

The Department of Health & Wellness carries out the following responsibilities: ensuring quality health care to the citizens of Prince Edward Island; providing leadership in policy, programs, & operations; maintaining & improving the health of citizens; playing a leadership role in innovation; coordinating the implementation of the Healthy Living Strategy; providing regulatory services to the health system; acting as a central contact for Aboriginal organizations; & promoting cooperation on governmental matters related to Aboriginal affairs.

Minister, Hon. Robert L. Henderson
Tel: 902-368-6414
Fax: 902-368-4121
rlhenderson@gov.pe.ca

Deputy Minister, Dr. Kim Critchley
Tel: 902-368-5290
kacritchley@gov.pe.ca

Senior Communications Officer, Autumn Tremere
Tel: 902-368-5610
agtremere@gov.pe.ca

Chief Public Health Office
Sullivan Bldg., 16 Fitzroy St., Charlottetown, PE C1A 7N8
Tel: 902-368-4996
The Chief Health Office administers & enforces the Public Health Act. The office also delivers services in the following areas: environmental health, epidemiology, reproductive care, & vital statistics.
Chief Public Health Officer, Dr. Heather G. Morrison
Tel: 902-368-4996
Fax: 902-620-3354
hgmorrison@gov.pe.ca
Deputy Chief Public Health Officer, Dr. David S. Sabapathy
Tel: 902-368-4996
Fax: 902-620-3354
dsabapathy@gov.pe.ca
Provincial Epidemiologist, Dr. Carolyn J. Sanford
Tel: 902-368-4964
Fax: 902-620-3354
cjsanford@gov.pe.ca
Senior Environmental Health Officer, Kelly D. Hughes
Tel: 902-368-4795
kdhughes@ihis.org
Manager, Health Promotion, Laura Lee Noonan
Tel: 902-620-3517
lanoonan@gov.pe.ca
Coordinator, Communicable Disease Program, Stacey L. Burns
Tel: 902-368-4934
Fax: 902-620-3354
slburns@ihis.org
Coordinator, Immunization & Vaccine Preventable Disease Program, Christine Drummond
Tel: 902-368-4934
cmdrummond@ihis.org

Health Policy & Programs
The Health Policy & Programs Division supports the Department of Health & Wellness. It includes the Health Recruitment & Retention section.
Acting Director, Kevin Barnes
Tel: 902-368-4865
Fax: 902-368-4224
kcbarnes@gov.pe.ca
Consultant, Pharmacy, Roy Cairns
Tel: 902-368-4907
Fax: 902-368-4905
brcairns@gov.pe.ca
Consultant, Dietetic Services, Diane M. Clow
Tel: 902-368-6262
Fax: 902-569-7656
mdclow@ihis.org
Legislative Specialist, Nichola M. Hewitt
Tel: 902-368-6681
Fax: 902-368-4224
nmhewitt@gov.pe.ca
Inspector, Cindy Carragher
Tel: 902-894-2202
cjcarragher@ihis.org

Sport, Recreation & Physical Activity
Tel: 902-368-4789
Fax: 902-368-4224
www.teampei.ca
twitter.com/Team_PEI
www.facebook.com/Team-PEI-Canada-Games-176351129056630
The main role of this division is to encourage citizens of Prince Edward Island to be active. Sport, recreation, & other physical activities are promoted.
Consultation services & grants are available for community, regional, & provincial groups.
Director, John Morrison
Tel: 902-894-0283
Fax: 902-368-4224
jwmorris@gov.pe.ca
Officer, Special Projects, Terry Bernard
Tel: 902-368-4549
Fax: 902-368-4548
thbernard@gov.pe.ca

Health PEI
16 Garfield St., PO Box 2000 Charlottetown, PE C1A 7N8
Tel: 902-368-6130
Fax: 902-368-6136
healthinput@gov.pe.ca
www.healthpei.ca
twitter.com/Health_PEI

When the Health Services Act was proclaimed in 2010, Health PEI took on responsibility for the operation & delivery of health services in the province.

The main goals of Health PEI are to improve access to quality health care across Prince Edward Island & to develop more consistent standards & practices for health services

Chair, Phyllis Horne, M.Ed.
Tel: 902-368-4637
Fax: 902-368-4974
phorne@gov.pe.ca

Chief Executive Officer, Dr. Michael Mayne
Tel: 902-368-4935
Fax: 902-368-4974
mbmayne@gov.pe.ca

Chief, Nursing, Allied Health & Patient Experience, Marion H. Dowling
Tel: 902-894-2356
Fax: 902-894-2416
mhdowling@gov.pe.ca

Executive Director, Quality & Safety, Rick Adams
Tel: 902-368-5804
Fax: 902-368-6136
radams@gov.pe.ca

Executive Director, Human Resources, Tanya Tynski
Tel: 902-368-6257
Fax: 902-368-4969
tmtynski@gov.pe.ca

Senior Communications Officer, Amanda J. Hamel
Tel: 902-368-6135
Fax: 902-368-4969
ajhamel@gov.pe.ca

Corporate Services & Pharmacare
Sullivan Bldg., 16 Fitzroy St., Charlottetown, PE C1A 7N8
Tel: 902-368-4947
Toll-Free: 877-577-3737
www.healthpei.ca/pharmacare

Chief Operating Officer, Denise M. Lewis Fleming
Tel: 902-368-6125
Fax: 902-368-6136
dmlewis@gov.pe.ca
Chief Information Officer & Director, Health Information & Performance, Mark Spidel
Tel: 902-620-3165
Fax: 902-368-6136
maspidel@gov.pe.ca
Senior Director, QEH Operations, Norman MacDonald
Tel: 902-894-2375
Fax: 902-894-2279
ncmacdonald@gov.pe.ca
Director, Materials Management, Todd G. Gillis
Tel: 902-894-2097
Fax: 902-894-2384
gtgillis@ihis.org
Director, Planning, Evaluation & Audit, Kellie C. Hawes
Tel: 902-569-0506
Fax: 902-368-6136
kchawes@ihis.org
Director, eHealth Clinical Operations, Robin Laird
Tel: 902-620-3869
Fax: 902-620-3388
rlaird@ihis.org
Administrative Officer, Pharmacare Program, Amanda D. Clair
Tel: 902-620-3288

Fax: 902-368-6443
adclair@ihis.org

Emergency Health Services, Long-Term Care & Hospital Services East
www.healthpei.ca/hospitals

Chief Administrative Officer, Jamie MacDonald
Tel: 902-894-2350
Fax: 902-894-2416
jamiemacdonald@gov.pe.ca
Director, Facilities Management, Kevin Barry
Tel: 902-894-2032
Fax: 902-894-2386
kpbarry@gov.pe.ca
Medical Director, Emergency Services, Dr. Scott Cameron
slcameron@ihis.org
Director, Support Services, Terry Campbell
Tel: 902-894-2353
Fax: 902-894-2416
tscampbell@gov.pe.ca
Medical Director, Program, Dr. George Carruthers
drgeorgecarruthers@gmail.com
Medical Director, Diagnostic Imaging, Dr. Siddharth Chhibber
schhibber@ihis.org
Director, Medical Affairs & Legal Services, Dr. Lori L. Ellis
Tel: 902-620-3692
Fax: 902-620-3072
llellis@gov.pe.ca
Medical Director, CPOE & Clinical Informatics, Dr. Tim Fitzpatrick
tjfitzpatrick@ihis.org
Director, Environmental Services, Ken Hughes
kjhughes@gov.pe.ca
Director, Long-Term Care, Andrew MacDougall
asmacdougall@gov.pe.ca
Director, Nursing, Queen Elizabeth Hospital & Community Hospitals East, Sandra MacKay
sgmackay@ihis.org
Acting Director, Provincial Diagnostic Imaging Services, Gailyne MacPherson
Tel: 902-894-2979
Fax: 902-894-2276
tgmacpherson@gov.pe.ca
Medical Director, Provincial Laboratory Services, Dr. Kristen Mead
Tel: 902-894-2316
Fax: 902-894-2385
kamead@ihis.org
Director, Support Services, Marsha Pyke
Tel: 902-438-4530
Fax: 902-438-4381
mlpyke@gov.pe.ca
Director, Hospital Services, Kelley Rayner
Tel: 902-894-2364
Fax: 902-894-2416
kjrayner@gov.pe.ca
Director, Pharmacy Services, Iain D. Smith
Tel: 902-894-0292
Fax: 902-894-2911
idsmith@gov.pe.ca
Director, Emergency Health & Planning Services, James Sullivan
Tel: 902-368-6719
Fax: 902-620-3072
jasullivan@gov.pe.ca
Provincial Technical Director, Laboratory Services, Brian Timmons
Tel: 902-569-7647
Fax: 902-894-2385
bdtimmons@ihis.org
Administrator, Community Hospitals East, Edna Miller
Tel: 902-687-7150
Fax: 902-687-7175
emiller@ihis.org

Family & Community Medicine & Hospital Services West
www.healthpei.ca/hospitals

Chief Administrative Officer, Arlene Gallant-Bernard
Tel: 902-438-4514
Fax: 902-438-4381
algallant-bernard@gov.pe.ca

Director, Hospital Services & Provincial Renal Program, Cheryl Banks
Tel: 902-438-4519
cabanks@gov.pe.ca
Director, Primary Care & Chronic Disease, Marilyn A. Barrett
Tel: 902-569-7640
Fax: 902-569-0579
mabarrett@gov.pe.ca
Director, Nursing, Lisa Campbell
Tel: 902-859-3910
lhcampbell@ihis.org
Director, Public Health & Children's Developmental Services, Kathy Jones
Tel: 902-894-0247
Fax: 902-569-0579
kljones@gov.pe.ca
Director, Prince County Hospital Foundation, Heather Matheson
Tel: 902-432-2834
Fax: 902-432-2551
hematheson@ihis.org
Director, Home Care, Palliative & Geriatric Care, Mary Sullivan
Tel: 902-569-7646
Fax: 902-368-6136
mksullivan@gov.pe.ca
Acting Director, Nursing, Kelley Wright
Tel: 902-438-4516
Fax: 902-438-4381
kmwright@gov.pe.ca
Manager, Environmental Services, Tyler Ellis
Tel: 902-438-4265
Fax: 902-438-4381
tdellis@ihis.org
Provincial Coordinator, Geriatrics Services, Elaine Campbell
Tel: 902-432-2861
Fax: 902-432-2859
eecampbell@ihis.org
Provincial Coordinator, Cancer, Marla Delaney
Tel: 902-368-6714
Fax: 902-569-0579
mdelaney@ihis.org
Provincial Coordinator, Dialysis, Lanea Harris
Tel: 902-368-6738
Fax: 902-368-6136
lcharris@ihis.org
Coordinator, Physician Services, Kelly Waite
Tel: 902-438-4518
Fax: 902-438-4381
kdwaite@ihis.org
Administrator, Community Hospitals West, Paul Young
Tel: 902-853-8663
Fax: 902-853-8658
psyoung@ihis.org

Mental Health & Addictions Services
www.healthpei.ca/mentalhealth
Other Communication: Island Helpline: 1-800-218-2885
Chief Administrative Officer, Verna Ryan
Tel: 902-368-6197
Fax: 902-569-0579
vryan@gov.pe.ca
Director, Nursing & Manager, Clinical Services, Kathy Anderson
Tel: 902-368-5413
Fax: 902-368-4195
klanderson@gov.pe.ca
Manager, Administration & Finance, David Berrigan
Tel: 902-368-5405
Fax: 902-368-5467
daberrigan@ihis.org
Manager, Community Mental Health & Addictions West, Shirley Cole
Tel: 902-432-2592
Fax: 902-432-2585
sjcole@gov.pe.ca
Manager, Lacey House - Central, Joyce Gallant
Tel: 902-368-4083
Fax: 902-368-6229
jlgallant@ihis.org
Program Manager, Child & Youth Mental Health & Addictions, Sean Morrison

Tel: 902-620-3745
msmorrison@gov.pe.ca
Manager, Addictions Programming, Shauna Reddin
Tel: 902-620-3550
Fax: 902-368-4969
smreddin@gov.pe.ca
Manager, Addictions East, Leslie Warren
Tel: 902-368-6129
Fax: 902-368-6229
lawarren@gov.pe.ca

Ministère de la Santé et des Services sociaux / Health & Social Services
Direction des communications, 1075, ch Sainte-Foy, 15e étage, Québec, QC G1S 2M1

Tél: 418-644-4545
Ligne sans frais: 877-644-4545
TTY: 800-361-9596
www.msss.gouv.qc.ca
Autres nombres: Montréal: 514-644-4545

Ministre, L'hon. Gaétan Barrette
Tél: 418-266-7171
Téléc: 418-266-7197
ministre@msss.gouv.qc.ca

Ministre déléguée, Réadaptation, à la Protection de la jeunesse, à la Santé publique et aux Saines habitudes de vie, L'hon. Lucie Charlebois
Tél: 418-266-7181
Téléc: 418-266-7199
ministre.deleguee@msss.gouv.qc.ca

Directeur, Cabinet du ministre, Daniel Desharnais
Tél: 418-266-7171

Directrice, Cabinet du ministre délégué, Natacha Joncas-Boudreau
Tél: 418-266-7181

Cabinet du Sous-ministre / Office of the Deputy Minister
Sous-ministre, Michel Fontaine
Tél: 418-266-8989
Directeur général, Cancérologie, Jean Latreille
Tél: 418-266-6940
Directrice, Bureau du sous-ministre, Domonique Breton
Tél: 418-266-8989
Directeur, Secrétariat général, André Giguère
Tél: 418-266-8989
Directeur, Communications, Marie-Claude Gagnon
Tél: 418-266-8905
Directrice, Affaires juridiques, Patricia Lavoie
Tél: 418-266-8950
Directrice, Audit interne, Isabelle Savard
Tél: 418-266-8989

Coordination réseau et ministérielle / Network & Departmental Coordination
Sous-ministre adjoint, Pierre Lafleur
Tel: 418-266-8850
Directeur général adjoint, Coordination et à la sécurité civile, Martin Simard
Tél: 418-266-6822
Directeur, Inspection et des enquêtes, Jean-François Therrien
Tel: 418-527-5211
Directeur, Gestion intégrée de l'information et de la performance, Sylvie Vézina
Tel: 418-266-8399
Directeur, Ententes de gestion et d'imputabilité et des relations institutionnelles, Yves Villeneuve
Tél: 418-266-2362

Finances, infrastructures et budget / Finance, Infrastructure & Budget
Sous-ministre adjoint, François Dion
Tél: 418-266-5965
Directeur général adjointe, Infrastructures, Luc Desbiens
Tél: 418-266-5830

Directrice générale adjointe, Gestion financière et des politiques de financement, Guylaine Lajoie
Tél: 418-266-5920

Directrice, Expertise et de la normalisation, Céline Drolet
Tél: 418-266-7108

Directeur, Équipement, de la logistique et de la conservation des infrastructures, Jacques Gagné
Tél: 418-266-5835

Directrice, Investissements et du financement, Caroline Imbeau
Tél: 418-266-5850

Directeur, Politiques de financement et de l'allocation des ressources, Normand Latagne
Tél: 418-266-7111

Directeur, Gestion financière - réseau, Pierre Martin
Tél: 418-266-5940

Directrice, Services administratifs - informatique; Directrice (par intérim), Gestion budgétaire et comptable ministérielle, Anne Martineau
Tél: 418-529-4898

Planification, évaluation et qualité / Planning, Evaluation and Quality

Sous-ministre adjoint, Luc Castonguay
Tél: 418-266-5990

Directeur général adjointe, Évaluation et de la qualité; Directeur (par intérim), Éthique et de la qualité, Éric Fournier
Tél: 418-266-7025

Directeur (par intérim), Affaires pharmaceutiques et du médicament, Dominic Bélanger
Tél: 418-266-8815

Directeur, Évaluation, Harold Côté
Tél: 418-266-8782

Directrice, Planification et orientations stratégiques, Lynda Fortin
Tél: 418-266-7088

Directeur, Affaires autochtones, Martin Rhéaume
Tél: 418-266-6811

Directrice, Recherche, innovation et transfert des connaissances, Manon St-Pierre
Tél: 418-266-7056

Directrice (par intérim), Affaires intergouvernementales et de la coopération internationale, Sara Veilleux
Tél: 418-266-8740

Personnel réseau et ministériel / Personal & Corporate Network

Sous-ministre adjoint, Marco Thibault
Tél: 418-266-8400

Directeur général adjointe, Ressources humaines et ressources matérielles ministérielles, Daniel Charbonneau
Tél: 418-266-8717

Directrice générale adjointe, Relations de travail et professionnelles; Directrice, Personnel syndiqué, Josée Doyon
Tél: 418-266-8408

Directrice, Ressources matérielles ministérielles, Marie-Claude Beauchamp
Tél: 418-266-8760

Directrice, Planification de la main-d'oeuvre salariée et médicale et du soutien au changement, Martyne Charland
Tél: 418-266-8835

Directrice (par intérim), Personnel hors établissement et de la classification réseau, Kim Lacerte
Tél: 418-266-8410

Directeur, Professionels de la santé et personnel d'encadrement, Yves Lapointe
Tél: 418-266-8420

Directeur, Relations professionnelles avec les Fédérations médicales, Manon Paquin
Tél: 418-266-8430

Directeur, Analyse et du soutien informationnel, Philippe St-Hilaire
Tél: 418-266-8450

Santé publique / Public Health

Sous-ministre adjoint; Directeur général adjoint (par intérim), Santé publique; Directeur (par intérim), Protection de la santé publlique, Horacio Arruda
Tél: 418-266-6700

Directeur, Prévention et de la promotion de la santé, André Dontigny
Tél: 418-266-6714

Services de santé et médecine universitaire / Health Services & Academic Medicine

Sous-ministre associé; Directeur, Affaires universitaires, Michel A. Bureau
Tél: 418-266-6930

Directrice nationale, Soins et services infirmiers, Sylvie Dubois
Tél: 418-266-8485

Directrice, Soutien à l'organisation clinique; Directrice (par intérim), Gestion des effectifs medicaux, Lise Caron
Tél: 418-266-6946

Directeur, Santé mentale, André Delorme
Tél: 418-266-6835

Directeur, Organisation des services de première ligne intégrés, Antoine Groulx
Tél: 418-266-6969

Directeur, Biovigilance et de la biologie médicales, Denis Ouellet
Tél: 418-266-6710

Directeur, Soins spécialisés, Daniel Riverin
Tél: 418-266-5827

Services sociaux / Social Services

Sous-ministre adjointe; Directrice (par intérim), Projet pour la mise en oeuvre de la Loi sur la représentation des RI-RTF, Lyne Jobin
Tél: 418-266-6800

Directrice générale adjointe, Services aux aînés, Natalie Rosebush
Tél: 418-266-6855

Directrice, Orientations des services aux aînés, Danielle Benoit
Tél: 418-266-6860

Directrice, Qualité des milieux de vie, Sylvie Cayer
Tél: 418-266-8775

Directrice, Dépendances et de l'itinérance, Lynne Duguay
Tél: 418-266-6830

Directeur, Services sociaux généraux et des activités communautaires, Mario Fréchette
Tél: 418-266-6936

Directeur, Organisation des services en déficience et en réadaptation physique, Daniel Garneau
Tél: 418-266-6874

Directrice, Secrétariat à l'adoption internationale, Josée-Anne Goupil
Tél: 514-873-4747

Directeur, Jeunes et des familles, Pascale Lemay
Tél: 418-226-6840

Directeur, Soutien à domicile, Élise Paquette
Tél: 418-266-6893

Technologies de l'information / Information Technology

Sous-ministre associé, Richard Audet
Tél: 418-529-4898

Directeur général adjoint, Planification et de la coordination, Alain Chouinard
Tél: 418-529-4898

Directeur général adjoint, Licences et des actifs informationnels, Denis Deslauriers
Tél: 514-597-2066

Directeur général adjoint, Orientations et architecture, Renald Lemieux
Tél: 514-597-2066

Directrice générale adjointe, Projets d'unification et des systèmes ministériels, Nathalie Surprenant
Tél: 418-529-4898

Directrice générale adjointe, Opérations technologiques, Agathe Tremblay
Tél: 418-527-5211

Directeur, Gestion des licenses et de l'assurance qualité, Stéphane Brossard
Tél: 514-597-2066

Directrice, Pilotage, France Émond
Tél: 418-529-4898

Directeur, Architecture, Boris Gueissaz-Teufel
Tél: 418-529-4898

Directrice, Soutien à la gouvernance, Danielle Lavoie
Tél: 418-529-4898

Directrice, Infrastructures technologiques et sécurité operationnelle, Caroline Lemelin
Tél: 418-527-5211

Directrice, Centre de services, Caroline Martin
Tél: 418-527-5211

Directeur, Systèmes aux services de santé et administratifs, Alexandre Poirier
Tél: 418-529-4898
Directeur, Coordination, des investissements majeurs et de la sécurité de l'information, Dave Roussy
Tél: 418-527-5211

Commission de la santé et de la sécurité du travail du Québec (CSST) / Québec Occupational Health & Safety Commission
524, rue Bourdages, CP 1200 Succ Terminus, Québec, QC G1K 7E2

Téléc: 418-266-4015
Ligne sans frais: 844-838-0808
www.csst.qc.ca
Autres nombres:
www.linkedin.com/company/commission-de-la-sant-et-s-curit-du-travail-csst-
twitter.com/laCSST
www.facebook.com/laCSST
www.youtube.com/user/LaCSST

A pour mission de soutenir aux travailleurs & aux employeurs dans leurs démarches pour éliminer les dangers présents dans leur milieu de travail, inspecter des lieux de travail, & promouvoir la santé & sécurité du travail

Présidente & Chef de la direction, Manuelle Oudar

Vice-président, Normes du travail, Michel Beaudoin

Vice-présidente, Opérations, Josée Dupont

Vice-président, Finances et administration, Carl Gauthier

Vice-président, Ressources informationnelles, matérielles et immobilières, Christian Goulet

Vice-présidente, Partenariat et l'expertise-conseil, Claude Sicard

Directrice générale, Ressources humaines, Anouk Gagné

Directeur général (par intérim), Prévention-inspection, Louis Genest

Directrice générale, Opérations centralisées, Louise Handfield

Directeur général, Solutions en ressources informationnelles, Bertrand Lauzon

Directeur général, Affaires juridiques, Jean-François Paquet

Directeur, Gestion immobilière, Marcel Renaud

Saskatchewan Health (HE)
T.C. Douglas Bldg., 3475 Albert St., Regina, SK S4S 6X6
Tel: 306-787-0146
Toll-Free: 800-667-7766
info@health.gov.sk.ca
www.health.gov.sk.ca
Other Communication: Family Health Benefits: 1-800-266-0695; HealthLine: 1-877-800-0002; Health Registration / Health Card: 1-800-667-7551; Prescription Drug Plan: 1-800-667-7581
Saskatchewan Health offers the following programs & services: continuing care to help people live independently; e-health & information systems for access to medical information; emergency services; health benefits; recruitment & retention of healthcare providers; promotion of mental health & treatment for mental illness & addictions; personal health services; prescription drug coverage; public health programs; privacy of health information; services for people with long term disabilities or illnesses; surgery & diagnostics initiatives; & vital statistics.

Minister, Health, Hon. Jim Reiter
Tel: 306-787-7345
Fax: 306-787-0237
he.minister@gov.sk.ca
Office of the Minister of Health, Legislative Building

#204, 2405 Legislative Dr.
Regina, SK S4S 0B3

Minister Responsible, Rural & Remote Health, Hon. Greg Ottenbreit
Tel: 306-798-9014
Fax: 306-798-9013
minister.rrhe@gov.sk.ca
Office of the Minister Responsible for Rural & Remote Health, Legislative Building
#208, 2405 Legislative Dr.
Regina, SK S4S 0B3

Deputy Minister, Max Hendricks
Tel: 306-787-3041
Fax: 306-787-4533
max.hendricks@health.gov.sk.ca

Chief of Staff, Morgan Bradshaw
Tel: 306-787-9091
Fax: 306-787-0237
morgan.bradshaw@gov.sk.ca

Assistant Deputy Minister, Kimberly Kratzig
Tel: 306-787-0513
Fax: 306-787-4533
kimberly.kratzig@health.gov.sk.ca

Assistant Deputy Minister, Karen Lautsch
Tel: 306-787-3186
Fax: 306-787-4533
karen.lautsch@health.gov.sk.ca

Assistant Deputy Minister, Tracey Smith
Tel: 306-787-3147
Fax: 306-787-4533
tracey.smith@health.gov.sk.ca

Assistant Deputy Minister, Mark Wyatt
Tel: 306-787-4695
Fax: 306-787-4533
mark.wyatt@health.gov.sk.ca

Director, Patient Safety Unit, Valerie Phillips
Tel: 306-787-3542
vphillips@health.gov.sk.ca

Acute & Emergency Services
Tel: 306-787-3204
Fax: 306-787-6113

Executive Director, Deborah Jordan
Tel: 306-787-7854
Fax: 306-787-6113
djordan@health.gov.sk.ca
Director, Quality & Continuous Improvement, Terry Blackmore
Tel: 306-787-3219
Fax: 306-787-6113
terry.blackmore@health.gov.sk.ca
Director, Hospitals & Specialized Services, Luke Jackiw
Tel: 306-787-3656
ljackiw@health.gov.sk.ca
Director, Cancer Services & EMS, Evan Ulmer
Tel: 306-787-1101
Fax: 306-787-6113
evan.ulmer@health.gov.sk.ca

Communications Branch
Tel: 306-787-3696
Fax: 306-787-8310
Toll-Free: 800-667-7766

Executive Director, Joan Petrie
Tel: 306-787-8433
Fax: 306-787-8310
joan.petrie@gov.sk.ca
Director, Program Services, Carolyn Hamilton
Tel: 306-787-2743

Fax: 306-787-8310
carolyn.hamilton@gov.sk.ca
Director, Internal Communications, Karen Prokopetz
Tel: 306-787-2036
Fax: 306-787-8310
karen.prokopetz@gov.sk.ca
Director, Regional Services, Julianne Jack
Tel: 306-787-7296
Fax: 306-787-8310
julianne.jack@gov.sk.ca

Community Care Branch

Tel: 306-787-7239
Fax: 306-787-7095

Executive Director, Janice Colquhoun
Tel: 306-787-6092
Fax: 306-787-7095
janice.colquhoun@health.gov.sk.ca
Director, Research, Evaluation & Central Support, Heather Murray
Tel: 306-787-3236
Fax: 306-787-7095
hmurray@health.gov.sk.ca
Director, Continuing Care & Rehabilitation, Linda Restau
Tel: 306-787-7901
Fax: 306-787-7095
lrestau@health.gov.sk.ca
Director, Licensing, Dawn Skalicky-Souliere
Tel: 306-787-1718
Fax: 306-787-7095
Director, Mental Health & Addictions, Kathy Willerth
Tel: 306-787-5020
Fax: 306-787-7095
kwillerth@health.gov.sk.ca

Drug Plan & Extended Benefits Branch

Tel: 306-787-3317
Fax: 306-787-8679
dp.sys.support@health.gov.sk.ca

Executive Director, Kevin Wilson
Tel: 306-787-3301
Fax: 306-787-8679
kwilson@health.gov.sk.ca
Director, Professional Practice, Perry Behl
Tel: 306-787-6970
Fax: 306-787-8679
perry.behl@health.gov.sk.ca
Director, Pharmaceutical Policy & Appropriateness, Nick Doulias
Tel: 306-787-3110
Fax: 306-787-8679
nick.doulias@health.gov.sk.ca
Director, Client Services, Extended Benefits & Policy, Dave Morhart
Tel: 306-787-1129
Fax: 306-787-8679
dave.morhart@health.gov.sk.ca
Director, Financial & Information Services, Jill Raddysh
Tel: 306-787-3031
Fax: 306-787-8679
jill.raddysh@health.gov.sk.ca

Financial Services Branch

Tel: 306-787-4923
Fax: 306-787-0218

Executive Director, Billie-Jo Morrissette
Tel: 306-787-5025
Fax: 306-787-0218
billie-jo.morrissette@health.gov.sk.ca
Director, Operations & Internal Audit, Cindy Fedak
Tel: 306-787-7738
Fax: 306-787-0218
cindy.fedak@health.gov.sk.ca
Director, Corporate & Regional Financial Planning, Jill Kaczmar
Tel: 306-787-2392
Fax: 306-787-0218
jill.kaczmar@health.gov.sk.ca
Manager, Regional Financial Services Unit, Heather Darrah
Tel: 306-787-0110
Fax: 306-787-0218
heather.darrah@health.gov.sk.ca

Medical Services Branch

Tel: 306-787-3475
Fax: 306-787-3761
Toll-Free: 800-667-7523

Acting Executive Director, Gord Tweed
Tel: 306-787-3423
Fax: 306-787-3761
gord.tweed@health.gov.sk.ca
Acting Director, Fee For Service and Statistics, Policy, Research & Negotiations, Ingrid Kirby
Tel: 306-787-3761
Fax: 306-787-8851
ingrid.kirby@health.gov.sk.ca
Director, Insured Services, Jennifer Lindenbach
Tel: 306-787-3425
Fax: 306-787-3761
jennifer.lindenbach@health.gov.sk.ca
Acting Director, Non-Fee For Service, Policy, Research & Negotiations, Kim Statler
Tel: 306-787-8938
Fax: 306-787-3761
kim.statler@health.gov.sk.ca
Director, Strategic Financial Planning & Support, Joy Vanstone
Tel: 306-787-2982
Fax: 306-787-3761
jvanstone@health.gov.sk.ca

Partnerships & Workforce Planning

Tel: 306-787-3143
Fax: 306-787-4534

Executive Director, Duane Mombourquette
Tel: 306-787-2869
Fax: 306-787-4534
duane.mombourquette@health.gov.sk.ca
Chief Nursing Officer, Mary Martin-Smith
Tel: 306-787-7195
Fax: 306-787-4534
mary.martin-smith@health.gov.sk.ca
Director, Labour Relations, Valerie Bayer
Tel: 306-787-8309
Fax: 306-787-4534
valerie.bayer@health.gov.sk.ca
Director, Workforce Policy & Planning, Andy Churko
Tel: 306-787-3072
Fax: 306-798-0023
andy.churko@health.gov.sk.ca
Director, Health Information & Privacy, Lisa Dietrich
Tel: 306-787-3565
Fax: 306-787-2974
lisa.dietrich@health.gov.sk.ca
Acting Director, Intergovernmental, First Nations & Métis Relations & Regional Planning and Support, Mark Goossens
Tel: 306-787-3145
mark.goossens@health.gov.sk.ca

Population Health Branch

Tel: 306-787-8847
Fax: 306-787-3237

Chief Medical Health Officer, Dr. Saqib Shahab
Tel: 306-787-4722
Fax: 306-787-3237
Chief Population Health Epidemiologist, Dr. Valerie Mann
Tel: 306-787-4086
Fax: 306-787-3823
vmann@health.gov.sk.ca
Executive Director, Donna Magnusson
Tel: 306-787-8847
Fax: 306-787-3237
donna.magnusson@health.gov.sk.ca
Director, Surveillance & Central Support, Patty Beck
Tel: 306-787-3237
Fax: 306-787-1405
patty.beck@health.gov.sk.ca
Director, Disease Prevention, Suzanne Fedorowich
Tel: 306-787-1580
Fax: 306-787-3823
suzanne.fedorowich@health.gov.sk.ca

Director, Tobacco Litigation, Angela Fornelli
Tel: 306-787-3973
Fax: 306-787-3237
angela.fornelli@health.gov.sk.ca
Director, Environmental Health, Tim Macaulay
Tel: 306-787-7128
Fax: 306-787-3237
tim.macaulay@health.gov.sk.ca

Primary Health Services Branch

Tel: 306-787-0889
Fax: 306-787-0890

Executive Director, Margaret Baker
Tel: 306-798-0670
Fax: 306-787-8679
margaret.baker@health.gov.sk.ca
Director, Primary Health Services, Jason Liggett
Tel: 306-787-1001
Fax: 306-787-0890
jason.liggett@health.gov.sk.ca
Director, Health Promotion, Tanya Schilling
Tel: 306-798-7491
Fax: 306-787-0890
tanya.schilling@health.gov.sk.ca

Saskatchewan Disease Control Laboratory
5 Research Dr., Regina, SK S4S 0A4

Tel: 306-787-3131
Fax: 306-787-1525

Executive Director, Patrick O'Byrne
Tel: 306-787-3129
Fax: 306-787-1525
patrick.obyrne@health.gov.sk.ca
Medical Director, Dr. Greg Horsman
Tel: 306-787-8316
Fax: 306-787-1525
ghorsman@health.gov.sk.ca
Clinical Director, Dr. Paul Levett
Tel: 306-787-3135
Fax: 306-787-1525
paul.levett@health.gov.sk.ca
Director, Provincial Molecular Diagnostics, Dr. Nick Antonishyn
Tel: 306-787-7744
Fax: 306-798-3137
nick.antonishyn@health.gov.sk.ca
Director, Environmental Services, Dr. Phillip Bailey
Tel: 306-787-3140
Fax: 306-787-1525
pbailey@health.gov.sk.ca
Director, Bacteriology & Assistant Clinical Director, Dr. David Farrell
Tel: 306-798-4154
Fax: 306-787-1525
david.farrell@health.gov.sk.ca
Director, Virology, Dr. Amanda Lang
Tel: 306-798-4153
Fax: 306-787-1525
amanda.lang@health.gov.sk.ca

Strategy & Innovation Branch

Tel: 306-787-7291
Fax: 306-787-2974

Executive Director, Pauline M. Rousseau
Tel: 306-787-3951
Fax: 306-787-2974
paulinem.rousseau@health.gov.sk.ca
Director, Continuous Improvement Office, Claudia Burke
Tel: 306-787-7507
Fax: 306-787-2974
claudia.burke@health.gov.sk.ca
Director, Health System Planning, Lori Evert
Tel: 306-787-3163
Fax: 306-787-2974
lori.evert@health.gov.sk.ca
Director, Health System Policy & Innovation, Michelle Schmalenberg
Tel: 306-787-5744
Fax: 306-787-2974
michelle.schmalenberg@health.gov.sk.ca

Director, Executive Management Information & Analytics, Doug Scott
Tel: 306-787-0626
Fax: 306-787-2974
doug.scott@health.gov.sk.ca
Director, Capital Asset Planning, Brad Williams
Tel: 306-787-3232
Fax: 306-787-2974
brad.williams@health.gov.sk.ca

Physician Recruitment Agency of Saskatchewan (SaskDocs)
#100, 311 Wellman Lane, Saskatoon, SK S7T 0J1

Tel: 306-933-5000
Fax: 306-933-5115
Toll-Free: 888-415-3627
info@saskdocs.ca
www.saskdocs.ca
twitter.com/saskdocs
www.facebook.com/saskdocs
linkedin.com/company/physician-recruitment-agency-of-saskatchewan
The Physician Recruitment Agency of Saskatchewan is a Crown corporation established in 2009. Its mandate is to provide resources for physicians & their families wanting to live & work in Saskatchewan. It partners with students, medical trainees, physicians, international medical graduates, communities, health facilities & others, & aims to match communities with the right physicians.

Chair; Assistant Deputy Minister, Health, Karen Lautsch
Tel: 306-787-3186
Fax: 306-787-4533
karen.lautsch@health.gov.sk.ca

Acting Chief Executive Officer/Director, Erin Brady
Tel: 306-933-5074
Fax: 306-933-5115
erin.brady@saskdocs.ca

Director, Corporate Operations, Erin Brady
Tel: 306-933-5074
erin.brady@saskdocs.ca

Manager, Communications, James Winkel
Tel: 306-933-5094
james.winkel@saskdocs.ca

Coordinator, Recruitment (HCIS), Leah Graver
Tel: 306-933-7744
leah.graver@saskdocs.ca

Recruitment Consultant, Rhoda Yakubowski
Tel: 306-933-5108
rhoda.yakubowski@saskdocs.ca

Yukon Health & Social Services
PO Box 2703 Whitehorse, YT Y1A 2C6

Tel: 867-667-3673
Fax: 867-667-3096
Toll-Free: 800-661-0408
hss@gov.yk.ca
www.hss.gov.yk.ca
twitter.com/HSSYukon
www.facebook.com/yukonhss
www.youtube.com/user/hssyukongovernment
Committed to quality health & social services for Yukoners by helping individuals acquire the skills to live responsible, healthy & independent lives; & providing a range of accessible, affordable services that assist individuals, families & communities to reach their full potential.

Minister, Hon. Pauline Frost
pauline.frost@gov.yk.ca

Deputy Minister, Bruce McLennan
Tel: 867-667-5770
Bruce.McLennan@gov.yk.ca

Chief Medical Officer of Health, Brendan Hanley
Tel: 867-456-6136
brendan.hanley@gov.yk.ca

Director, Communications & Social Marketing, Patricia Living
Tel: 867-667-3673
patricia.living@gov.yk.ca

Director, Human Resources, Cheryl Van Blaricom
Tel: 867-667-3031
cheryl.vanblaricom@gov.yk.ca

Continuing Care
#201, 1 Hospital Rd., Whitehorse, YT Y1A 3H7

Tel: 867-667-5945
Fax: 867-456-6545
www.hss.gov.yk.ca/continuing.php

Other Communication: Toll-Free Phone: 800-661-0408, ext. 5945
Provides residential, home care & regional therapy services for the citizens of the Yukon Territory.
Assistant Deputy Minister, Cathy Morton-Bielz
Tel: 867-667-8922
Fax: 867-456-6545
cathy.morton-bielz@gov.yk.ca
Director, Clinical Psychology, Reagan Gale
Tel: 867-667-5968
Director, Safety & Clinical Excellence, Adeline Griffin
Tel: 867-667-8750
adeline.griffin@gov.yk.ca
Director, Care & Community, Liris Smith
Tel: 867-456-6839
liris.smith@gov.yk.ca
Director, Extended Care Services, Sharon Specht
Tel: 867-393-7574
sharon.specht@gov.yk.ca
Manager, Intermediate & Complex Extended Care, Katharina McArthur
Tel: 867-393-8642
katharina.mcarthur@gov.yk.ca
Manager, Community Care, Cathy McNeil
Tel: 867-667-3607
cathy.mcneil@gov.yk.ca

Corporate Services

Fax: 867-393-6457
www.hss.gov.yk.ca/corporate.php

Plays a key role in ensuring that Yukon residents have accurate, up-to-date information about the territory's health & social programs, services & systems.
Assistant Deputy Minister, Birgitte Hunter
Tel: 867-667-8309
birgitte.hunter@gov.yk.ca
Director, Corporate Planning & Risk Management, Kathy Frederickson
Tel: 867-667-5943
kathy.fredrickson@gov.yk.ca
Director, Policy & Program Development, Brian Kitchen
Tel: 867-667-5688
Fax: 867-667-3096
brian.kitchen@gov.yk.ca
Manager, Emergency Services, Chris Balzer
Tel: 867-667-5887
chris.balzer@gov.yk.ca

Health Services
#201, 1 Hospital Rd., Whitehorse, YT Y1A 3H7

Fax: 867-667-3096
www.hss.gov.yk.ca/healthservices.php

Responsible for a variety of health care, disease prevention & treatment services which assist eligible Yukon residents in attaining maximum individual independence within their community.
Assistant Deputy Minister, Health Services, Sherri Wright
Tel: 867-667-5689
Fax: 867-667-3096
sherri.wright@gov.yk.ca
Deputy Registrar, Vital Statistics, Karen Carriere
Tel: 867-667-5207
karen.carriere@gov.yk.ca
Director, Community Health Programs, Cathy Stannard
Tel: 867-667-8340
Fax: 867-456-6502
cathy.stannard@gov.yk.ca

Director, Community Nursing, Sheila Thompson
Tel: 867-667-8325
sheila.thompson@gov.yk.ca
Manager, Health Promotion Unit, Ian Parker
Tel: 867-456-6576
ian.parker@gov.yk.ca
Manager, Insured Health & Hearing Services, Dorothea Talsma
Tel: 867-667-5628
dorothea.talsma@gov.yk.ca
Manager, Chronic Conditions Support Program, Emily Wale
Tel: 867-393-7487
emily.wale@gov.yk.ca
Manager/Clinician, Hearing Services, Leah Wittrock
Tel: 867-667-5913
Fax: 867-667-5922
leah.wittrock@gov.yk.ca

Social Services

www.hss.gov.yk.ca/socialservices.php

Consists of Adult Community Services, Alcohol & Drug Services, Family & Children's Services, Regional Services, Senior Services, Seniors & Elder Abuse, Services for People With Disabilities, & Social Assistance.
Assistant Deputy Minister, BrendaLee Doyle
Tel: 867-667-3702
brendalee.doyle@gov.yk.ca
Director, Family & Children's Services Branch, Elaine Schroeder
Tel: 867-667-3471
Fax: 867-393-6239
elaine.schroeder@gov.yk.ca
Manager, Community & Program Support, Kelly Cooper
Tel: 867-456-3948
Fax: 867-393-6926
kelly.cooper@gov.yk.ca
Manager, Services to Persons with Disabilities, Jean Kellogg
Tel: 867-393-7169
jean.kellogg@gov.yk.ca

Yukon Workers' Compensation Health & Safety Board (YWCHSB)
401 Strickland St., Whitehorse, YT Y1A 5N8

Tel: 867-667-5645
Fax: 867-393-6279
Toll-Free: 800-661-0443
worksafe@gov.yk.ca
wcb.yk.ca

Other Communication: 24-Hour Emergency Line: 867-667-5450
The Yukon Workers' Compensation Health & Safety Board (YWCHSB) administers workers' compensation & occupational health & safety in the Yukon.

Minister responsible, Hon. Jeanie Dendys
jeanie.dendys@gov.yk.ca

President & Chief Executive Officer, Kurt Dieckmann
Tel: 867-667-5975
Fax: 867-393-6419
kurt.dieckmann@gov.yk.ca

Vice-President & Chief Financial Officer, Jim Stephens
Tel: 867-689-0970
Fax: 867-393-6279
jim.stephens@gov.yk.ca

Chief Mine Safety Officer, Michael Henney
Tel: 867-667-8739
michael.henney@gov.yk.ca

Director, Claimant Services, Karen Branigan
Tel: 867-667-8186
karen.branigan@gov.yk.ca

Acting Director, Occupational Health & Safety, Bruce Milligan
Tel: 867-667-3726
bruce.milligan@gov.yk.ca

Director, Human Resources, Karen Pearson

Tel: 867-667-8190
karen.pearson@gov.yk.ca

Director, Corporate Services, Clarence Timmons
Tel: 867-667-8695
clarence.timmons@gov.yk.ca

Local Schools

ALBERTA

Athabasca: Athabasca University (AU)
1 University Dr., Athabasca, AB T9S 3A3
Tel: 780-675-6100; Fax: 780-675-6437
Toll-Free: 800-788-9041
www.athabascau.ca
www.facebook.com/AthabascaU
twitter.com/Athabascau
www.linkedin.com/company/19365
www.youtube.com/user/AthabascaUniversity
Full Time Equivalency: 30660 Note: An open university offering any student access to university-level study.
Mark Fabbro, Registrar, 780-675-6165
 markf@athabascau.ca
Dr. Neil Fassina, President
Dr. Cindy Ives, Interim Vice-President, Academic
 cindyi@athabascau.ca
Estelle Lo, Vice-President, Finance & Administration
Pamela Walsh, Vice-President, Advancement
Mike Battistel, Chief Information Officer
Elaine Fabbro, Director, Library & Scholarly Resources

Faculty of Health Disciplines
1 University Dr., Athabasca, AB T9S 3A3
Toll-Free: 800-788-9041
fhdcontact@athabascau.ca
fhd.athabascau.ca/index.php
Margaret Edwards, Dean

Calgary: University of Calgary
2500 University Dr. NW, Calgary, AB T2N 1N4, Canada
Tel: 403-220-5110
www.ucalgary.ca
www.facebook.com/97582259854
twitter.com/UCalgary
www.linkedin.com/company/university-of-calgary
Full Time Equivalency: 31495
Number of Employees: 1800 faculty; 3000 staff
Elizabeth Cannon, B.Sc., M.Sc., Ph.D., President & Vice-Chancellor
Susan Belcher, Secretary
Nuvyn L. Peters, Vice-President, Development
Linda Dalgetty, Vice-President, Finance & Services
Bart Becker, Vice-President, Facilities
Karen Jackson, General Counsel
Diane Kenyon, Vice-President, University Relations
Dru Marshall, Vice-President Academic & Provost
Ed McCauley, Vice-President, Research

Medicine
Foothills Campus
3330 Hospital Dr. NW, Calgary, AB T2N 4N1
Tel: 403-220-6842
medicine.ucalgary.ca
www.facebook.com/ucalgarymedicine
twitter.com/UofCMedicine
www.youtube.com/UCalgaryMedicine
Dr. Jon Meddings, Dean
 meddings@ucalgary.ca

Nursing
Tel: 403-220-6262
nursing.ucalgary.ca
twitter.com/ucalgarynursing
www.youtube.com/ucalgarynursing
Dianne Tapp, M.N., Ph.D., Dean

Kinesiology
Tel: 403-220-3407
www.ucalgary.ca/knes
www.facebook.com/UofCKinesiology
twitter.com/uofcknes
Penny Werthner, Dean

Edmonton: Grant MacEwan University
Also known as: MacEwan University
P.O. Box 1796
Edmonton, AB T5J 2P2, Canada
Toll-Free: 888-497-4622
info@macewan.ca
www.macewan.ca
www.facebook.com/MacEwanUniversity
twitter.com/macewanu
www.linkedin.com/edu/school?id=21055
www.youtube.com/macewanchannel
Deborah Saucier, President

Edmonton: University of Alberta
116 St. & 85 Ave., Edmonton, AB T6G 2R3
Tel: 780-492-3111
chat@ualberta.ca
www.ualberta.ca
www.facebook.com/ualberta
twitter.com/ualberta
www.youtube.com/user/UniversityofAlberta
Full Time Equivalency: 37830
Ralph Young, Chancellor
David H. Turpin, CM, PhD, LLD, FRSC, President, 780-492-3212
Dew Steve, PhD, Provost & Vice-President, Academic
 provost@ualberta.ca
Phyllis Clark, Vice-President, Finance & Administration, 780-492-2657
Don Hickey, PEng, Vice-President, Facilities
Lorne Babiuk, Vice-President, Research, 780-492-5353
 lorne.babiuk@ualberta.ca
Debra Pozega Osburn, PhD, Vice-President, University Relations, 780-492-1583
 debra.osburn@ualberta.ca
Heather McCaw, Vice-President, Advancement Services, 780-492-7400
 giving@ualberta.ca

Faculty of Medicine & Dentistry
Walter C. Mackenzie Health Sciences Centre
8440 - 112 St. NW, Edmonton, AB T6G 2R7
Tel: 780-492-6621; Fax: 780-492-7303
meddent@ualberta.ca
www.ualberta.ca/medicine
www.facebook.com/UofAMedicineDentistry
twitter.com/UAlberta_FoMD
www.linkedin.com/school/15095830
www.youtube.com/user/FoMDcommsteam
Richard N. Fedorak, Dean

Faculty of Nursing
Level 3, Edmonton Clinic Health Academy
11405 - 87 Ave., Edmonton, AB T6G 1C9
Fax: 780-492-2551
Toll-Free: 888-492-8089
www.ualberta.ca/nursing
www.facebook.com/UofANursing
Dr. Anita Molzahn, Ph.D., Dean

Faculty of Pharmacy & Pharmaceutical Sciences
2-35 Medical Sciences
8613 - 114 St., Edmonton, AB T6G 2H7
Tel: 780-492-3362
www.ualberta.ca/pharmacy
Neal Davies, Dean
 ndavies@ualberta.ca

Faculty of Rehabilitation Medicine
3-48 Corbett Hall
8205 - 114 St., Edmonton, AB T6G 2G4
Tel: 780-492-2903; *Fax:* 780-492-1626
info@rehabmed.ualberta.ca
www.ualberta.ca/rehabilitation
www.facebook.com/UofARehabMedicine
twitter.com/UofARehabMed
www.youtube.com/user/RehabMedicineUofA
Bob Haennel, Ph.D., Dean

<u>Schools</u>
School of Public Health
3-300 Edmonton Clinic Health Academy
11405 - 87 Ave., Edmonton, AB T6G 1C9
Tel: 780-492-9954; *Fax:* 780-492-0364
school.publichealth@ualberta.ca
www.ualberta.ca/public-health
twitter.com/UofAPublicHlth
www.youtube.com/user/SPHUofA
Kue Young, Dean
kue.young@ualberta.ca

Alberta Institute for Human Nutrition (AIHN)
4-002 Li Ka Shing Centre
Edmonton, AB T6G 2E1
Tel: 780-492-6668

Lethbridge: **University of Lethbridge**
4401 University Dr., Lethbridge, AB T1K 3M4, Canada
Tel: 403-329-2111
www.uleth.ca
www.facebook.com/ulethbridge.ca
twitter.com/ulethbridge
www.linkedin.com/company/university-of-lethbridge
www.youtube.com/user/ulethbridge
Full Time Equivalency: 8212
Number of Employees: 1157
Mike Mahon, Ph.D., President & Vice-Chancellor
president@uleth.ca
Lesley Brown, Vice-President, Research
l.brown@uleth.ca
Andrew Hakin, Vice-President, Academic & Provost
hakin@uleth.ca
Nancy Walker, Vice-President, Finance & Administration
nancy.walker@uleth.ca

Faculty of Health Sciences
Tel: 403-329-2699
health.sciences@uleth.ca
www.uleth.ca/healthsciences
Christopher Hosgood, Dean

BRITISH COLUMBIA

Abbotsford: **University of the Fraser Valley**
33844 King Rd., Abbotsford, BC V2S 7M8
Tel: 604-504-7441; *Fax:* 604-855-7614
Toll-Free: 888-504-7441
info@ufv.ca
www.ufv.ca
www.facebook.com/goUFV
www.twitter.com/goUFV
www.linkedin.com/company/university-of-the-fraser-valley_2
www.youtube.com/user/goUFV
Full Time Equivalency: 15446
Dr. Gwen Point, Chancellor
Dr. Mark Evered, President & Vice-Chancellor, 604-864-4608
Dr. Eric Davis, Provost & Vice-President, Academic, 604-864-4630
eric.davis@ufv.ca
Jackie Hogan, Vice-President, Administration
Al Wiseman, University Secretary
al.wiseman@ufv.ca
Dr. Lucy Lee, Dean, Faculty of Science, 604-851-6346
lucy.lee@ufv.ca

Faculty of Health Sciences
45190 Caen Ave., Chilliwack, BC V2R 0N3
www.ufv.ca/health

Joanne MacLean, Dean, 604-795-2816
joanne.maclean@ufv.ca

Burnaby: **CDI College of Business, Technology, & Health Care (CDI)**
Collège CDI de la Technologie et de la Santé
Headquarters
#500, 5021 Kingsway, Burnaby, BC V5H 4A5
Toll-Free: 1-800-675-4392
www.cdicollege.com
www.facebook.com/CDICollege
twitter.com/CDICollege
www.youtube.com/CDICareerCollege
Note: Graduates of the college are trained to work in the business, technology, & healthcare sectors.
Bohdan J. Bilan, Vice-President, Academics

Burnaby: **Simon Fraser University**
8888 University Dr., Burnaby, BC V5A 1S6, Canada
Tel: 604-291-3111
www.sfu.ca
Other Information: Student Services: 778-782-6930
www.facebook.com/simonfraseruniversity
twitter.com/sfu
www.linkedin.com/company/simon-fraser-university
www.youtube.com/user/SFUNews
Full Time Equivalency: 35398
Anne E. Giardini, Chancellor
Andrew Petter, President & Vice-Chancellor
Dr. Jon Driver, Vice-President, Academic
Philip Steenkamp, Vice-President, External Relations
Pat Hibbitts, Vice-President, Finance & Administration
Judith Osborne, Vice-President, Legal Affairs & University Secretary
Mark Walker, Registrar
Gwen Bird, University Librarian & Dean
Joy Johnson, Vice-President, Research
Cathy Daminato, Vice-President, Advancement & Alumni Engagement

Health Sciences
Tel: 778-782-4821; *Fax:* 778-782-5927
fhs@sfu.ca
www.sfu.ca/fhs.html
John O'Neil, Dean

Castlegar: **Selkirk College**
Castlegar Campus
301 Frank Beinder Way, Castlegar, BC V1N 4L3
Tel: 250-365-7292; *Fax:* 250-365-6568
Toll-Free: 888-953-1133
www.selkirk.ca
www.facebook.com/SelkirkCollege
twitter.com/selkirkcollege
www.youtube.com/selkirkcollege
Note: The regional community college consists of the following schools: Kootenay School of the Arts; School of Adult Basic Education & Transitional Training; School of Business & Aviation; School of Digital Media & Music; School of Environment & Geomatics; School of Health & Human Services; School of Hospitality & Tourism; School of Industry & Trades Training; School of Renewable Resources; School of University Arts & Sciences & Selkirk International.
Allison Alder, Chair
Angus Graeme, President & Chief Executive Officer

Kamloops: **Thompson Rivers University**
P.O. Box 3010
900 McGill Rd., Kamloops, BC V2C 0C8
Tel: 250-828-5000; *Fax:* 250-828-5086
admissions@tru.ca
www.tru.ca
www.facebook.com/thompsonriversu
www.twitter.com/thompsonriversu
www.youtube.com/user/truwebbies
Full Time Equivalency: 13443
Number of Employees: 1,543 staff; 415 faculty *Note:* With distance-learning, enrolment figures swell to over 25,000 students.
Wally Oppal, Chancellor
Dr. Alan Shaver, President & Vice-Chancellor, 250-828-5001
president@tru.ca
Dr. Christine Bovis-Cnossen, Provost & Vice-President, Academic

Matt Milovick, Vice-President, Administration & Finance, 250-377-6123
Christopher Seguin, Vice-President, Advancement, 250-574-0474
  cseguin@tru.ca
Dr. Irwin DeVries, Interim Associate Vice-President, Open Learning
Paul Michel, Executive Director, Aboriginal Education

School of Nursing
Ken Lepin Bldg.
900 McGill Rd., #S204, Kamloops, BC V2C 0C8

Tel: 250-828-5401; *Fax:* 250-371-5909
www.tru.ca/nursing

Donna Murnaghan, Dean
  dmurnaghan@tru.ca

Kelowna: Okanagan College
1000 KLO Rd., Kelowna, BC V1Y 4X2

Tel: 250-862-5480; *Fax:* 250-862-5434
Toll-Free: 866-638-0058
cscentral@okanagan.bc.ca
www.okanagan.bc.ca
www.facebook.com/okanagancollege.ca
twitter.com/OkanaganCollege
www.linkedin.com/company/okanagan-college
www.youtube.com/user/OkanaganCollege

Enrollment: 5000
Jim Hamilton, President
  jhamilton@okanagan.bc.ca
Roy Daykin, Vice-President, Employee & Corporate Services
  rdaykin@okanagan.bc.ca
Andrew Hay, Vice-President, Education
  ahay@okanagan.bc.ca
Charlotte Kushner, Vice-President, Students
  ckushner@okanagan.bc.ca

Langley: Trinity Western University
7600 Glover Rd., Langley, BC V2Y 1Y1

Tel: 604-888-7511; *Fax:* 604-513-2061
Toll-Free: 888-468-6898
admissions@twu.ca
www.twu.ca
www.facebook.com/trinitywestern
twitter.com/TrinityWestern
instagram.com/trinitywestern

Full Time Equivalency: 4000
Bob Kuhn, President
  president@twu.ca
W. Robert Wood, Provost
Scott Fehrenbacher, Senior Vice-President, External Relations
Bob Nice, Senior Vice-President, Business Affairs
Jim Poulsen, Vice-President, Finance
  poulsen@twu.ca
Janis Ryder, Executive Director, Human Resources
  janis.ryder@twu.ca
Grant McMillan, Registrar, 604-513-2070
  registrar@twu.ca

School of Human Kinetics, Sport & Leisure Management

Tel: 604-513-2114
www.twu.ca/academics/school-human-kinetics
www.facebook.com/trinity.hkin

Blair Whitmarsh, Dean
  blair.whitmarsh@twu.ca

School of Nursing

Tel: 604-513-2050; *Fax:* 604-513-2012
www.twu.ca/academics/school-nursing
Dr. Sonya Grypma, Dean, 604-513-2121
  dean.nursing@twu.ca

Nanaimo: Vancouver Island University (VIU)
Nanaimo Campus
900 - 5th St., Nanaimo, BC V9R 5S5

Tel: 250-753-3245; *Toll-Free:* 888-920-2221
info@viu.ca
www.viu.ca
twitter.com/VIUniversity
www.linkedin.com/school/287349
www.youtube.com/user/viuchannel

Full Time Equivalency: 16000

Dr. Ralph Nilson, President & Vice-Chancellor
Dr. David Witty, Provost & Vice-President, Academic
Shelley Legin, Chief Financial Officer & Vice-President, Administration
William Litchfield, Interim Executive Director, University Relations
Marie Armstrong, University Secretary

North Vancouver: Capilano University
North Vancouver Campus
2055 Purcell Way, North Vancouver, BC V7J 3H5

Tel: 604-986-1911; *Fax:* 604-984-4985
www.capilanou.ca
TTY: 604-990-7848
www.facebook.com/capilanou
www.twitter.com/capilanou
www.youtube.com/user/CapilanoUniversity

Full Time Equivalency: 7000
David T. Fung, Chancellor
Paul Dangerfield, President & Vice-Chancellor, 604-984-4933
  president@capilanou.ca
Richard Gale, Vice-President, Academic & Provost, 604-984-1740
  richardgale@capilanou.ca
Jacqui Stewart, Acting Vice-President, Finance & Administration, 604-984-4937
  jacquistewart@capilanou.ca
Mike Knudson, Associate Vice-President, Human Resources
  mikeknudson@capilanou.ca
Irene Chanin, Executive Director, Advancement
  irenechanin@capilanou.ca
Mark Clifford, Director, Contract Services & Purchasing
  mcliffor@capilanou.ca
Mike Proud, Director, Finance
  mproud@capilanou.ca
Karen McCredie, Registrar, 604-984-4900
  kmccredi@capilanou.ca

Faculty of Education, Health & Human Development

www.capilanou.ca/education-health-development
Brad Martin, Dean
  bradmartin@capilanou.ca

Prince George: University of Northern British Columbia (UNBC)
3333 University Way, Prince George, BC V2N 4Z9

Tel: 250-960-5555; *Fax:* 250-960-5794
www.unbc.ca
www.facebook.com/UNBC
twitter.com/UNBC
www.youtube.com/UNBCnews

Full Time Equivalency: 4020
Number of Employees: 190 Full-time faculty; 176 Part-time faculty; 394 Non-academic staff
The Hon. James Moore, Chancellor
Daniel J. Weeks, President & Vice-Chancellor
Robert Knight, Vice-President, Finance & Business Operations
Geoffrey Payne, Interim Vice-President, Research
Dan Ryan, Interim Vice-President, Academic & Provost
Tim Tribe, Vice-President, Advancement
Colleen Smith, Associate Vice-President, Financial Services, 250-960-5519
  colleen.smith@unbc.ca
Greg Condon, Chief Information Officer, 250-960-5289
  greg.condon@unbc.ca
Shelley Rennick, Director, Facilities Management, 250-960-6413

Faculties
Arts, Social & Health Sciences
Dr. John Young, Acting Dean

Surrey: Kwantlen Polytechnic University
12666 - 72nd Ave., Surrey, BC V3W 2M8

Tel: 604-599-2000; *Fax:* 604-599-2068
studentinfo@kpu.ca
www.kpu.ca
www.facebook.com/kwantlenu
twitter.com/kwantlenu
instagram.com/kwantlenu

Full Time Equivalency: 19000
Number of Employees: 1400
George Melville, Chancellor

Alan R. Davis, President & Vice-Chancellor, 604-599-2078
Salvador Ferreras, Provost & Vice-President, Academic
  salvador.ferreras@kpu.ca
Jane Fee, Vice-Provost, Students
  jane.fee@kpu.ca
Zena Mitchell, Registrar, 604-599-2463
  zena.mitchell@kpu.ca
Keri van Gerven, University Secretary, 604-599-2078
  keri.vangerven@kpu.ca
Scott Gowen, Director, Supply & Business Services, 604-599-2134
  supply@kwantlen.ca

Faculty of Health
South Bldg.
#2810, 20901 Langley Bypass, Langley, BC V3A 4H9
                              Tel: 604-599-2263
                              www.kpu.ca/health

Dr. David Florkowski, Dean
  david.florkowski@kpu.ca

Surrey: West Coast College of Health Care
#204, 9648 - 128 St., Surrey, BC V3T 2X9
            Tel: 604-951-6644; *Toll-Free:* 1-800-807-8558
                      admin@westcoastcollege.com
                      www.westcoastcollege.com
    www.facebook.com/pages/West-Coast-College/173782172655449
Note: West Coast College of Health Care provides health & human
services training. Programs include instruction to become a medical
laboratory assistant, a pharmacy technician, & a veterinary assistant.
The college is accredited by the Private Career Training Institutions
Agency of British Columbia.
Jill Arnold, Director

Vancouver: University of British Columbia (UBC)
2329 West Mall, Vancouver, BC V6T 1Z4, Canada
                              Tel: 604-822-2211
                              www.ubc.ca
                Other Information: Telex: 04-51233
                www.facebook.com/universityofbc?fref=ts
                      twitter.com/ubcaplaceofmind
        www.linkedin.com/company/4373?trk=NUS_CMPY_TWIT
                      www.youtube.com/user/ubc
Full Time Equivalency: 58284
Number of Employees: 15,171 faculty and staff
Stuart Belkin, Chair
Lindsay Gordon, Chancellor
Santa J. Ono, President, 604-822-8300
  presidents.office@ubc.ca
A. Simpson, Vice-President Finance, 604-822-2823
  kirin.jeffrey@ubc.ca
Barbara Miles, Vice-President, Development & Alumni Engagement,
  604-822-1585
  barbara.miles@ubc.ca
Philip Steenkamp, Vice-President, External, Legal & Community
  Relations, 604-822-5017
Professor Helen M. Burt, Interim Vice-President, Research &
  International, 604-822-1467
  helen.burt@ubc.ca
Louise Cowin, Vice President, Students
  vpstudents@exchange.ubc.ca
Kate Ross, Associate Vice-President, Enrolment Services & Registrar,
  604-822-2951
  kate.ross@ubc.ca

Faculty of Dentistry
#350, 2194 Health Sciences Mall, Vancouver, BC V6T 1Z3
            Tel: 604-822-5773; *Fax:* 604-822-4532
                      www.dentistry.ubc.ca

Dr. Charles Shuler, Dean
  cshuler@dentistry.ubc.ca

Faculty of Medicine
#317, 2194 Health Sciences Mall, Vancouver, BC V6T 1Z3
            Tel: 604-822-2421; *Fax:* 604-822-6061
                      fomdo.reception@ubc.ca
                      www.med.ubc.ca
                www.facebook.com/UBCmed
                      twitter.com/UBCMedicine
            www.youtube.com/user/UBCmedicine

Dermot Kelleher, Dean

Faculty of Pharmaceutical Sciences
2405 Wesbrook Mall, Vancouver, BC V6T 1Z3

                              pharmsci.ubc.ca
                www.facebook.com/ubcpharmacy
                      twitter.com/ubcpharmacy
  www.linkedin.com/company/ubc-faculty-of-pharmaceutical-sciences
Michael Coughtrie, Dean

School of Audiology & Speech Sciences
2177 Wesbrook Mall, Vancouver, BC V6T 1Z3
            Tel: 604-822-5591; *Fax:* 604-822-6569
                  inquiry@audiospeech.ubc.ca
                      www.audiospeech.ubc.ca
                www.facebook.com/ubc.sass
                      twitter.com/UBC_Sass

Valter Ciocca, Director
  director@audiospeech.ubc.ca

School of Kinesiology
210-6081 University Blvd., Vancouver, BC V6T 1Z1
            Tel: 604-822-9192; *Fax:* 604-822-6842
                      ubc.kin@ubc.ca
                      kin.educ.ubc.ca
                www.facebook.com/ubckin
                      twitter.com/ubckin
            www.youtube.com/user/UBCKinesiology

Robert Boushel, Director
  robert.boushel@ubc.ca

School of Nursing
2211 Wesbrook Mall, #T201, Vancouver, BC V6T 2B5
            Tel: 604-822-7417; *Fax:* 604-822-7466
                      www.nursing.ubc.ca
                www.facebook.com/ubcnursing
                      twitter.com/ubcnursing
        www.linkedin.com/company/ubc-school-of-nursing
Suzanne Campbell, Director
  suzanne.campbell@ubc.ca

School of Population & Public Health
2206 East Mall, Vancouver, BC V6T 1Z3
            Tel: 604-822-2772; *Fax:* 604-822-4994
                      info@spph.ubc.ca
                      www.spph.ubc.ca
                www.facebook.com/ubc.spph
                      twitter.com/ubcspph
                www.youtube.com/ubcspph1

Carolyn Gotay, Co-Director
  carolyn.gotay@ubc.ca
Chris Lovato, Co-Director
  chris.lovato@ubc.ca

College of Health Disciplines
            Tel: 604-822-5571; *Fax:* 604-822-2495

Louise Nasmith, Principal
  louise.nasmith@ubc.ca

Victoria: Royal Roads University
2005 Sooke Rd., Victoria, BC V9B 5Y2, Canada
            Tel: 250-391-2511; *Fax:* 250-391-2500
                Toll-Free: 1-800-788-8028
                      www.royalroads.ca
                www.facebook.com/royalroadsu
                      twitter.com/royalroads
            www.linkedin.com/company/19123
            www.youtube.com/user/RoyalRoadsUni
Full Time Equivalency: 4640 *Note:* Royal Roads University offers:
Doctoral degrees in Social Sciences; Masters degrees in Arts,
Business Admin., Science; Bachelor degrees in Arts, Commerce,
Science; Graduate Certificates; Graduate Diplomas.
Wayne Standlund, Chair & Chancellor
Dr Allan Cahoon, President & Vice-Chancellor
Dr. Stephen Grundy, Vice-President, Academic & Provost,
  250-391-2545

Victoria: **University of Victoria**
3800 Finnerty Rd., Victoria, BC V8P 5C2, Canada

Tel: 250-721-7211; *Fax:* 250-721-7212
Toll-Free: 888-721-8620
www.uvic.ca
Other Information: 250-721-7599
www.facebook.com/universityofvictoria
twitter.com/uvic
www.linkedin.com/company/university-of-victoria
www.youtube.com/UVic

Full Time Equivalency: 20330
Shelagh Rogers, Chancellor
Jamie Cassels, Q.C., President
  pres@uvic.ca
David Castle, PhD, Vice-President, Research
  vpr@uvic.ca
Carmen Charette, Vice-President, External Relations
  ncernoia@uvic.ca
Gayle Gorrill, B.B.A., C.A., C.B.V., Vice-President, Finance &
  Operations
  vpfo@uvic.ca
Valerie Kuehne, B.Sc.N., M.Ed., M.A., Ph., Vice-President, Academic &
  Provost (Acting)
  provost@uvic.ca
Julia Eastman, B.A., M.A., Ph.D., University Secretary
  usec@uvic.ca

Centres/Institutes
Centre for Addictions Research BC (CARBC)
P.O. Box 1700 CSC
Victoria, BC V8W 2Y2

Tel: 250-472-5445; *Fax:* 250-472-5321
carbc@uvic.ca
www.uvic.ca/research/centres/carbc
www.facebook.com/CARBC.UVic
twitter.com/CARBC_Uvic
www.youtube.com/user/CARBCUVic

Tim Stockwell, Director
  timstock@uvic.ca

Centre for Biomedical Research
P.O. Box 1700 CSC
Victoria, BC V8W 2Y2

Tel: 250-472-4067; *Fax:* 250-472-4075
cfbr@uvic.ca
cbr.uvic.ca
twitter.com/UVicCBR

Dr. E. Paul Zehr, Director

Centre for Indigenous Research & Community-Led Engagement
(CIRCLE)
P.O. Box 1700 CSC
Victoria, BC V8W 2Y2

Tel: 250-472-5456; *Fax:* 250-472-5450
circle@uvic.ca
www.uvic.ca/research/centres/circle
www.facebook.com/CIRCLE.UVic
twitter.com/CIRCLE_UVic
www.youtube.com/UVic

Charlotte Loppie, Director

MANITOBA

Brandon: **Brandon University**
270 - 18th St., Brandon, MB R7A 6A9, Canada

Tel: 204-728-9520; *Fax:* 204-726-4573
www.brandonu.ca
www.facebook.com/brandonu.ca
twitter.com/brandonunews
www.linkedin.com/company/51014?trk=tyah

Full Time Equivalency: 2940
Dr. Gervan Fearon, President & Vice-Chancellor
  president@brandonu.ca
Scott J.B. Lamont, Vice-President, Administration & Finance
  lamont@brandonu.ca
Dr. Heather Duncan, Acting Vice-President, Academic & Provost
  duncanh@brandonu.ca

Schools
Faculty of Health Studies

Tel: 204-727-7409; *Fax:* 204-571-8568
healthstudies@brandonu.ca
www.brandonu.ca/health-studies

W. Dean Care, Dean

Portage la Prairie: **Gladys Cook Educational Centre**
P.O. Box 1342
2 River Rd., Portage la Prairie, MB R1N 3A9

Tel: 204-239-3029; *Fax:* 204-239-3025

Grades: 1-12

Winnipeg: **University of Manitoba**
66 Chancellors Circle, Winnipeg, MB R3T 2N2

Tel: 204-474-8880; *Toll-Free:* 800-432-1960
www.umanitoba.ca
www.facebook.com/umanitoba
twitter.com/umanitoba
www.linkedin.com/company/university-of-manitoba
www.youtube.com/user/YouManitoba

Full Time Equivalency: 29987
Harvey Secter, Chancellor
Dr. David T. Barnard, B.Sc., M.Sc., Ph.D., Dip., President &
  Vice-Chancellor
John Kearsey, Vice-President, External
Digvir Jayas, Ph.D., Vice-President, Research & International
Dr. Janice Ristock, Vice-President, Academic & Provost
Dr. Joanne C. Keselman, Interim Vice-President, Administration
David Collins, Vice-Provost, Integrated Planning & Academic Programs
  david.collins@umanitoba.ca
Susan Gottheil, Vice-Provost, Students
  susan.gottheil@umanitoba.ca
Dr. Todd Mondor, Vice-Provost, Graduate Education
  todd.mondor@umanitoba.ca
Jeff Leclerc, B.Ed., University Secretary
  jeff.leclerc@umanitoba.ca

Faculty of Dentistry
780 Bannatyne Ave., #D113, Winnipeg, MB R3T 2N2

Tel: 204-789-3631; *Fax:* 204-789-3912
info_dent@umanitoba.ca
umanitoba.ca/healthsciences/dentistry

Dr. Anthony Iacopino, Dean

Faculty of Medicine
260 Brodie Centre
727 McDermot Ave., Winnipeg, MB R3E 3P5

Tel: 204-789-3557; *Fax:* 204-789-3928
med.communications@umanitoba.ca
umanitoba.ca/faculties/health_sciences/medicine
www.facebook.com/RadyFaculty
twitter.com/UM_RadyFHS

Brian Postl, Dean

Faculty of Nursing
Helen Glass Centre for Nursing
89 Curry Pl., Winnipeg, MB R3T 2N2

Tel: 204-474-7452; *Fax:* 204-474-7682
Toll-Free: 800-432-1960
nursing@umanitoba.ca
umanitoba.ca/nursing
www.facebook.com/NursingatUofM

Beverly O'Connell, Dean
  beverly.oconnell@umanitoba.ca

Faculty of Pharmacy
Apotex Centre
750 McDermot Ave., Winnipeg, MB R3E 0T5

Tel: 204-474-9306; *Fax:* 204-789-3744
pharmacy@umanitoba.ca
umanitoba.ca/faculties/health_sciences/pharmacy
Xiaochen Gu, Acting Dean

Students Association for Health, Physical Education & Recreation Studies
194 Extended Education Complex
Winnipeg, MB R3T 2N2

Tel: 204-474-8892
sahpercouncil@gmail.com
umanitoba.ca/faculties/kinrec/undergrad/sahper
www.facebook.com/sahper.council
twitter.com/sahpercouncil

Crystal Teichrieb, President

Winnipeg: **University of Winnipeg**
515 Portage Ave., Winnipeg, MB R3B 2E9, Canada

Tel: 204-786-7811; *Fax:* 204-783-4996
www.uwinnipeg.ca
www.facebook.com/uwinnipeg
twitter.com/UWinnipeg
www.linkedin.com/edu/school?id=10811
www.youtube.com/user/uwinnipeg

Full Time Equivalency: 10106
Robert Silver, Chancellor
Annette Trimbee, President & Vice-Chancellor, 204-786-9214
president@uwinnipeg.ca
Neil Besner, Vice-Pres., Academic & Provost, 204-988-7104
n.besner@uwinnipeg.ca
Bill Balan, Vice-Pres., Finance & Administration, 204-786-9229
b.balan@uwinnipeg.ca
Laurel Repski, Vice-Pres., Human Resources, 204-789-1451
l.repski@uwinnipeg.ca
Sherman Kreiner, Vice-Pres., Student Life, 204-988-7116
s.kreiner@uwinnipeg.ca

Gupta Faculty of Kinesiology & Applied Health

Fax: 204-783-7866
kinesiology@uwinnipeg.ca
uwinnipeg.ca/kinesiology

David Fitzpatrick, Dean of Kinesiology, 204-786-9943
d.fitzpatrick@uwinnipeg.ca

NEW BRUNSWICK

Fredericton: **University of New Brunswick**
P.O. Box 4400
Fredericton, NB E3B 5A3

Tel: 506-453-4666
www.unb.ca
www.facebook.com/uofnb
twitter.com/unb
www.youtube.com/unbtube

Full Time Equivalency: 11000
Dr. H.E.A. (Eddy) Campbell, President & Vice-Chancellor
George MacLean, Vice-President, Academic
Bob Skillen, Vice-President, Advancement
Dr. David Burns, Vice-President, Research
Karen Cunningham, Vice-President, Administration & Finance
Sarah DeVarenne, University Secretary
sjd@unb.ca

Faculty of Kinesiology
P.O. Box 4400
Fredericton, NB E3B 5A3

Tel: 506-453-4666
kin@unb.ca
www.unb.ca/fredericton/kinesiology

Wayne Albert, Dean

Faculty of Nursing
P.O. Box 4400
Fredericton, NB E3B 5A3

Tel: 506-458-7670; *Fax:* 506-453-3512
registrar@unb.ca
www.unb.ca/fredericton/nursing

Pat Seaman, Acting Dean

NEWFOUNDLAND & LABRADOR

St. John's: **Memorial University of Newfoundland (MUN)**
P.O. Box 4200
St. John's, NL A1C 5S7

Tel: 709-737-8000; *Fax:* 709-864-3514
www.mun.ca
www.facebook.com/MemorialUniversity
twitter.com/MemorialU
www.linkedin.com/company/memorial-university-of-newfoundland
www.youtube.com/user/MemorialUVideos

Full Time Equivalency: 18470
Susan Knight, Chancellor
smknight@mun.ca@mun.ca
Dr. Gary Kachanoski, President & Vice-Chancellor
Dr. Noreen Golfman, Provost & Vice-President, Academic
Kent Decker, Vice-President, Administration & Finance
Dr. Ray Gosine, Vice-President, Research
Sheila Singleton, Registrar
ssinglet@mun.ca

Faculty of Medicine

Tel: 709-864-6358; *Fax:* 709-864-6294
www.med.mun.ca
www.facebook.com/MUNMedicine
twitter.com/MUNMed
www.youtube.com/user/MUNmedicine

Dr. James Rourke, Dean

School of Human Kinetics & Recreation

Tel: 709-864-8130; *Fax:* 709-864-3979
www.mun.ca/hkr
www.facebook.com/SchoolofHumanKineticsandRecreation

Dr. Heather Carnahan, Dean

School of Nursing
300 Prince Phillip Dr., St. John's, NL A1B 3V6

Tel: 709-777-2165
www.nurs.mun.ca
www.facebook.com/196576727034976
twitter.com/MUN_Nursing

Dr. Alice Gaudine, Dean

School of Pharmacy

Tel: 709-777-8300; *Fax:* 709-777-7044
pharminfo@mun.ca
www.mun.ca/pharmacy
www.facebook.com/schoolofpharmacy
twitter.com/SchoolofPharm

Dr. Carlo Marra, Dean

Stephenville: **College of the North Atlantic (CNA)**
P.O. Box 5400
Stephenville, NL A2N 2Z6, Canada

Toll-Free: 888-982-2268
info@cna.nl.ca
www.cna.nl.ca
www.facebook.com/CNANewfoundlandLabrador
twitter.com/cna_news
www.youtube.com/user/CNamarketing

Full Time Equivalency: 25000
Bob Gardiner, Interim President & CEO
William Radford, Chief Learning Officer & Senior Vice-President,
Academic, 709-643-7732
Elizabeth Kidd, COO & Vice-President, Corporate Services,
709-643-7704
Robin Walters, Vice-President, Industry & Community Engagement,
709-643-3012

School of Health Sciences
Jane Gamberg, Dean, 709-758-7624
jane.gamberg@cna.nl.ca
Irene O'Brien, Dean, Qatar
irene.obrien@cna-qatar.edu.qa

NOVA SCOTIA

Halifax: Dalhousie University
P.O. Box 15000
Halifax, NS B3H 4R2

Tel: 902-494-2211; *Fax:* 902-494-1630
communications.marketing@dal.ca
www.dal.ca
www.facebook.com/DalhousieUniversity
twitter.com/Dalnews
www.youtube.com/user/DalhousieU

Full Time Equivalency: 18500 *Note:* Dalhousie University is a comprehensive teaching & research university located in Atlantic Canada. Dalhousie places special emphasis on Ocean Studies & Health Studies & has a growing involvement in Advanced Technical Studies.
A. Anne McLellan, Chancellor
Richard Florizone, President & Vice-Chancellor, 902-494-2511
  richard.florizone@dal.ca
Dr. Martha Crago, Vice-President, Research, 902-494-6513
  martha.crago@dal.ca
Peter Fardy, Vice-President, Advancement
Ian Nason, Vice-President, Finance & Administration, 902-494-3862
  ian.nason@dal.ca
Dr. Carolyn Watters, Vice-President, Academic & Provost,
  902-494-2586
  carolyn.watters@dal.ca
Dr. Arig al Shaibah, Vice-Provost, Student Affairs, 902-494-8021
  arig.alshaibah@dal.ca

Faculty of Dentistry
P.O. Box 15000
5981 University Ave., Halifax, NS B3H 4R2

Tel: 902-494-2824; *Fax:* 902-494-2527
admissions.dentistry@dal.ca
www.facebook.com/daldentistry

Dr. Thomas Boran, Dean, 902-494-2274
  thomas.boran@dal.ca

Faculty of Health Professions
P.O. Box 15000
#316, 5968 College St.

Tel: 902-494-3327; *Fax:* 902-494-1966
www.dal.ca/faculty/healthprofessions.html

Alice Aiken, Dean, 902-494-3856
  alice.aiken@dal.ca

Faculty of Medicine
1459 Oxford St., Halifax, NS B3H 4R2

Tel: 902-494-6592; *Fax:* 902-494-7119
medicine.dal.ca

Dr. David Anderson, Dean
  dean.medicine@dal.ca

College of Pharmacy
5968 College St., Halifax, NS B3H 4R2

Tel: 902-494-2378; *Fax:* 902-494-1396
pharmacy@dal.ca

Susan Mansour, Director, 902-494-3504
  susan.mansour@dal.ca

School of Health & Human Performance
P.O. Box 15000
Halifax, NS B3H 4R2

Tel: 902-494-2152; *Fax:* 902-494-5120
Toll-Free: 866-325-4247
hahp@dal.ca

Dr. Jacqueline Gahagan, Interim Director

School of Health Administration
P.O. Box 15000
5850 College St., Halifax, NS B3H 4R2

Tel: 902-494-7097; *Fax:* 902-494-6849
healthadmin@dal.ca

Dr. Joseph M. Byrne, Director
  byrne@dal.ca

School of Human Communication Disorders
P.O. Box 15000
5850 College St., #2C01, Halifax, NS B3H 4R2

Tel: 902-494-7052; *Fax:* 902-494-5151
hucd@dal.ca

Joy Armson, Director, 902-494-5154
  j.armson@dal.ca

School of Nursing
P.O. Box 15000
5869 University Ave., Halifax, NS B3H 4R2

Tel: 902-494-2535; *Fax:* 902-494-3487

Kathleen MacMillan, Director

School of Occupational Therapy
Forrest Bldg.
#215, 5869 University Ave., Halifax, NS B3H 4R2

Tel: 902-494-8804; *Fax:* 902-494-1229
occupational.therapy@dal.ca
www.facebook.com/dalsot

Lynn Shaw, Director

School of Physiotherapy
Forrest Bldg.
5869 University Ave., 4th Fl., Halifax, NS B3H 4R2

Tel: 902-494-2524; *Fax:* 902-494-1941
physiotherapy@dal.ca

Anne Fenety, Director

Healthy Populations Institute (HPI)
P.O. Box 15000
1318 Robie St., Halifax, NS B3H 3E2

Tel: 902-494-2240; *Fax:* 902-494-3594
hpi@dal.ca
www.dal.ca/dept/hpi.html

Maureen Summers, Managing Director

Neuroscience Institute

Tel: 902-494-2051; *Fax:* 902-494-1212
neuroscience.institute@dal.ca
neuroscience.dal.ca

Dr. Victor Rafuse, Director
  vrafuse@dal.ca

ONTARIO

Guelph: University of Guelph
50 Stone Rd. East, Guelph, ON N1G 2W1

Tel: 519-824-4120; *Fax:* 519-767-1693
www.uoguelph.ca
www.facebook.com/uofguelph
twitter.com/uofg
www.linkedin.com/company/university-of-guelph
www.youtube.com/uofguelph

Full Time Equivalency: 27890
David Mirvish, Chancellor
Franco Vaccarino, President & Vice-Chancellor
  president@uoguelph.ca
Charlotte Yates, Provost & Vice-President (Academic)
Daniel Atlin, Vice-President (External)
Malcolm Campbell, Vice-President (Research)
Don O'Leary, Vice-President (Finance, Administration & Risk)
Rebecca Graham, Chief Information Officer & Chief Librarian
Deanna McQuarrie, Interim Registrar

College of Social & Applied Human Sciences (CSAHS)

Tel: 519-824-4120; *Fax:* 519-766-4797
csahs@uoguelph.ca
www.uoguelph.ca/csahs
www.facebook.com/195767463900558
twitter.com/CSAHS_UoG
www.youtube.com/user/CSAHSUofG

John Smithers, Interim Dean
  csahsdean@uoguelph.ca

Hamilton: Grand Health Academy
760 King St. East, Hamilton, ON L8M 1A6

Tel: 905-577-7707; *Fax:* 905-577-7738
www.grandhealthacademy.com
www.facebook.com/grandhealthacademy
twitter.com/GHA_school

Note: Established in 1992, Grand Health Academy offers programs that prepare students to become personal support workers, food service workers, pharmacy assistants, & rehabilitation assistants.

Hamilton: McMaster University
1280 Main St. West, Hamilton, ON L8S 4L8, Canada

Tel: 905-525-9140
www.mcmaster.ca
www.facebook.com/mcmasteruniversity
twitter.com/mcmasteru
www.linkedin.com/company/mcmaster-university
www.youtube.com/mcmasterutv

Full Time Equivalency: 29411
Suzanne Labarge, Chancellor, 905-525-9140, ext. 24340
Patrick Deane, President & Vice-Chancellor, 905-525-9140, ext. 24340

CanChild Centre for Childhood Disability Research
Institute for Applied Health Sciences
#408, 1400 Main St. West, Hamilton, ON L8S 1C7

Tel: 905-525-9140; *Fax:* 905-529-7687
canchild@mcmaster.ca
www.canchild.ca
www.facebook.com/canchild.ca
twitter.com/canchild_ca
vimeo.com/canchild

Dr. Jan Willem Gorter, Director

Centre for Evaluation of Medicines (CEM)
Centre for Evaluation of Medicines
#2000, 25 Main St. West, Hamilton, ON L8P 1H1

Tel: 905-523-7284; *Fax:* 905-523-9222
www.research.mcmaster.ca/research-chairs-and-institutes/cfeom
Mitchell Levine, Director
levinem@mcmaster.ca

Centre for Health Economics & Policy Analysis (CHEPA)
CRL Bldg.
#282, 1280 Main St. West, Hamilton, ON L8S 4K1

Tel: 905-525-9140; *Fax:* 905-546-5211
chepa@mcmaster.ca
www.chepa.org

Michel Grignon, Director
grignon@mcmaster.ca

Centre for Microbial Chemical Biology (CMCB)
1200 Main St. West, #MDCL-2330, Hamilton, ON L8S 4K1

Tel: 905-525-9140; *Fax:* 905-528-5330
www.cmcbmcmaster.ca

Tracey Campbell, Research Manager
campbtl@mcmaster.ca

Centre for Minimal Access Surgery (CMAS)
50 Charlton Ave. East, #T2141, Hamilton, ON L8N 4A6

Tel: 905-522-1155; *Fax:* 905-521-6194
info@cmas.ca
www.cmas.ca
www.facebook.com/CMASHamilton
twitter.com/cmashamilton

Marie Fairgrieve, Manager

Centre for Surgical Invention & Innovation (CSII)
39 Charlton Ave. East, Hamilton, ON L8N 1Y3

Tel: 905-522-1155
www.csii.ca
www.facebook.com/174502995911995
twitter.com/CSiiCECR

Debra Vivian, Director, Communications
dvivian@stjosham.on.ca

Farncombe Family Digestive Health Research Institute
Heath Sciences Centre
1280 Main St. West, #3N4, Hamilton, ON L8S 4K1

Tel: 905-525-9140
farncombe.mcmaster.ca

Dr. Stephen Collins, Director
scollins@mcmaster.ca

Firestone Institute for Respiratory Health
St. Joseph's Healthcare
50 Charlton Ave. East, Hamilton, ON L8N 4A6

Tel: 905-522-1155
www.firh.ca

Marnie Buchanan, Clinical Manager
mbuchana@stjosham.on.ca

Gilbrea Centre for Studies in Aging
L.R. Wilson Hall
#2025-2028, 1280 Main St. West, Hamilton, ON L8S 4K1

Tel: 905-525-9140; *Fax:* 905-525-4198
gilbrea@mcmaster.ca
www.aging.mcmaster.ca
www.facebook.com/TheGilbreaCentre
twitter.com/GilbreaCentre
www.linkedin.com/in/gilbreacentre
www.youtube.com/user/TheGilbreaCentre

Amanda Grenier, Director
grenier@mcmaster.ca

McMaster Immunology Research Centre
MDCL
#4010, 1280 Main St. West, Hamilton, ON L8S 4K1

Tel: 905-525-9140; *Fax:* 905-522-6750
mirc.mcmaster.ca
www.facebook.com/169351976425223
twitter.com/MacImmunology
www.youtube.com/user/immunologyresearch

Dr. Carl Richards, Director
richards@mcmaster.ca

McMaster Institute of Applied Radiation Sciences (McIARS)
1280 Main St. West, Hamilton, ON L8S 4L8

Tel: 905-525-9140
www.research.mcmaster.ca/research-chairs-and-institutes/mciars
David Novog, Director
novog@mcmaster.ca

McMaster Institute for Healthier Environments (MIHE)
1280 Main St. West, Hamilton, ON L8S 4L8

Tel: 905-525-9140
www.mcmaster.ca/mihe

Jim Dunn, Director

McMaster Institute for Molecular Biology & Medicine (MOBIX)
Health Sciences Centre
1200 Main St. West, #3N4F, Hamilton, ON L8N 3Z5

Tel: 905-525-9140
mobixlab@mcmaster.ca
www.science.mcmaster.ca/mobixlab

Galina Kataeva, Manager

Stem Cell & Cancer Research Institute (SCC-RI)
Michael DeGroote Centre for Learning & Discovery
1280 Main St. West, Hamilton, ON L8S 4K1

Tel: 905-525-9140
sccri@mcmaster.ca
sccri.mcmaster.ca
twitter.com/McMasterSCCRI

Mick Bhatia, Director

Medical Imaging Informatics Research Centre at McMaster (MIIRC@M)
1280 Main St. West, Hamilton, ON L8S 4L8

Tel: 905-521-2100
www.miircam.ca

David A. Koff, Director
david.koff@miircam.ca

Michael G. DeGroote Institute for Infectious Disease Research
MDCL
#2301, 1280 Main St. West, Hamilton, ON L8S 4K1

Tel: 905-525-9140; *Fax:* 905-528-5330
www.mcmasteriidr.ca
www.facebook.com/McMasterIIDR
twitter.com/McMasterIIDR
www.youtube.com/user/McMasterIIDR

Dr. Gerry Wright, Director
wrightge@mcmaster.ca

Michael G. DeGroote Institute for Pain Research & Care
MDCL
#2101, 1280 Main St. West, Hamilton, ON L8S 4K1
Tel: 905-525-9140; *Fax:* 905-523-1224
npc@mcmaster.ca
fhs.mcmaster.ca/paininstitute

Dr. Norm Buckley, Scientific Director
buckleyn@mcmaster.ca

Population Health Research Institute (PHRI)
237 Barton St. East, Hamilton, ON L8L 2X2
Tel: 905-521-2100
information@phri.ca
www.phri.ca

Dr. Salim Yusuf, Executive Director
yusufs@mcmaster.ca

Surgical Outcomes Research Centre (SOURCE)
#202, 39 Charlton Ave. East, Hamilton, ON L8N 1Y3
Tel: 905-523-0019; *Fax:* 905-523-0229
www.fhs.mcmaster.ca/source

Dr. Achilleas Thoma, Director
athoma@mcmaster.ca

Thrombosis & Atherosclerosis Research Institute (TaARI)
David Braley Research Institute
237 Bartin St. East, #C5-121, Hamilton, ON L8L 2X2
Tel: 905-521-2100; *Fax:* 905-575-2646
info@taari.ca
www.taari.ca

Annette Rosati, Administrator
annette.rosati@taari.ca

Kingston: Queen's University
99 University Ave., Kingston, ON K7L 3N6, Canada
Tel: 613-533-2000
admission@queensu.ca
www.queensu.ca
www.facebook.com/queensuniversity
twitter.com/queensu
www.linkedin.com/company/queen's-university
www.youtube.com/QueensUCanada

Full Time Equivalency: 24582
Jim Leech, Chancellor
Dr. Daniel Woolf, Principal & Vice-Chancellor
Mike Young, Rector
Alan Harrison, Vice-Principal Academic & Provost
Thomas Harris, Vice-Principal Advancement
John Metcalfe, University Registrar
Lon Knox, Secretary of the Senate, University & Board
Caroline Davis, Vice-Principal Finance & Administration
Dr. Steven Liss, Vice-Principal, Research
Michael Fraser, Vice-Principal University Relations

Faculty of Health Sciences
Decanal Office
18 Barrie St., Kingston, ON K7L 3N6
Tel: 613-533-2544
healthsci.queensu.ca

Dr. Richard Reznick, Dean
deanfhs@queensu.ca

School of Nursing (SON)
Cataraqui Bldg.
92 Barrie St., Kingston, ON K7L 3N6
Tel: 613-533-2668; *Fax:* 613-533-6770
nursing@queensu.ca
nursing@queensu.ca
www.facebook.com/Queensu.SON
twitter.com/QueensuSON
www.linkedin.com/groups/Queens-University-School-Nursing-8189529
instagram.com/queensnursing

Jennifer Medves, Director

School of Kinesiology & Health Sciences (SKHS)
SKHS Bldg.
28 Division St., Kingston, ON K7L 3N6
Tel: 613-533-2666; *Fax:* 613-533-2009
www.queensu.ca/skhs
www.facebook.com/SchoolOfKinesiologyAndHealthStudies

Jean Côté, Director

School of Rehabilitation Therapy
Louise D. Action Bldg.
31 George St., Kingston, ON K7L 3N6
Tel: 613-533-6103; *Fax:* 613-533-6776
rehab@queensu.ca
www.rehab.queensu.ca
www.facebook.com/QueensSRT
twitter.com/QueensSRT

Richard Reznick, Director

Canadian Institute for Military & Veteran Health Research
301 Kingston Hall
103 Stuart St., Kingston, ON K7L 3N6
Tel: 613-533-3329; *Fax:* 613-533-3405
www.cimvhr.ca
www.facebook.com/CIMVHR
twitter.com/CIMVHR_ICRSMV

Stéphanie Bélanger, Co-Scientific Director
Heidi Cramm, Co-Scientific Director

Queen's Cancer Research Institute (QCRI)
#302, 10 Stuart St., Kingston, ON K7L 3N6
Tel: 613-533-6507
qcri.queensu.ca

David M. Berman, Director
bermand@queensu.ca

Centre for Health Services & Policy Research
Abramsky Hall
21 Arch St., 3rd Fl., Kingston, ON K7L 3N6
Tel: 613-533-6387; *Fax:* 613-533-6353
chspr@queensu.ca
healthsci.queensu.ca/research/chspr

Michael Green, Director
michael.green@dfm.queensu.ca

Centre for Neuroscience Studies (CNS)
Botterell Hall
18 Stuart St., Kingston, ON K7L 3N6
Tel: 613-533-6360; *Fax:* 613-533-6840
neuroscience.queensu.ca

Doug Munoz, Director
doug.munoz@queensu.ca

Centre for Studies in Primary Care (CSPC)
P.O. Box 8888
220 Bagot St., Kingston, ON K7L 5E9
Tel: 613-533-9300; *Fax:* 613-533-9302
Toll-Free: 866-599-8090
www.queensu.ca/cspc
twitter.com/CSPC_QueensU

Richard Birtwhistle, Director
richard.birtwhistle@dfm.queensu.ca

Centre for Innovation in Healthcare Policy
Robert Sutherland Hall
138 Union St., Kingston, ON K7L 3N6
Tel: 613-533-3020
www.queensu.ca/sps/cihp
www.youtube.com/moniesonhealth

A. Scott Carson, Executive Director

Human Mobility Research Centre (HMRC)
Kingston General Hospital
76 Stuart St., Kingston, ON K7L 2V7
Tel: 613-548-2430; *Fax:* 613-549-2529
hmrc@queensu.ca
www.queensu.ca/hmrc

Brian Amsden, Co-Director, Regenerative Medicine
Ryan Bicknell, Co-Director, Clinical Studies
Tim Bryant, Co-Director, Biomechanical Design & Rehabilitation
James Stewart, Co-Director, Computer Assisted Therapies

London: Western University
Also known as: University of Western Ontario
1151 Richmond St., London, ON N6A 3K7, Canada

Tel: 519-661-2111
media@uwo.ca
www.uwo.ca
www.facebook.com/WesternUniversity
twitter.com/westernu
www.linkedin.com/company/westernuniversity
www.youtube.com/user/WesternUniversity

Full Time Equivalency: 28386
Number of Employees: 3,868
Dr. Amit Chakma, President & Vice-Chancellor, 519-661-3106
  achakma@uwo.ca
Janice Deakin, Provost & Vice-President, 519-661-3110
  provostvpa@uwo.ca
Gitta Kulczycki, Vice-President, Resources & Operations,
  519-661-3114
  gitta@uwo.ca
John Capone, Vice-President, Research, 519-661-3812
  vpr@uwo.ca
Kelly Cole, Vice-President, External, 519-661-4120
  kelly.cole@uwo.ca
Jennifer Meister, Ombudsperson, 519-661-3573, ext. 82602
  jmeiste@uwo.ca
Irene Birrell, Secretary, 519-661-2056
  ibirrell@uwo.ca
Lynn Logan, Associate Vice-President, Financial Services,
  519-661-2111, ext. 85416
  llogan2@uwo.ca
Elizabeth Krische, Director of Purchasing, 519-661-2038, ext. 84576
  ekrische@uwo.ca
Debbie Jones, Director, Information Technology Services,
  519-850-2470, ext. 82470
  debbie@uwo.ca
Helen Connell, Associate Vice-President, Communications & Public
  Affairs, 519-850-2446, ext. 85469
  hconnell@uwo.ca
Susan Grindrod, Associate Vice-President, Housing & Ancillary
  Services, 519-661-3549
  grindrod@housing.uwo.ca

Faculty of Health Sciences
200 Arthur and Sonia Labatt Health Sciences Bldg.
London, ON N6A 5B9

Tel: 519-661-2111
www.uwo.ca/fhs
www.facebook.com/fhswestern
twitter.com/westernuFHS
instagram.com/westernufhs
Jim Weese, Dean, Faculty of Health Sciences, 519-661-2111, ext.
  84239
  jweese1@uwo.ca

Schulich School of Medicine & Dentistry
Clinical Skills Building
London, ON N6A 5C1

Tel: 519-661-3459
www.schulich.uwo.ca
www.facebook.com/SchulichMedicineAndDentistry
twitter.com/SchulichMedDent
Dr. Michael J. Strong, Dean, Schulich School of Medicine & Dentistry

Affiliations
Brescia University College
1285 Western Rd., London, ON N6G 1H2

Tel: 519-432-8353; *Fax:* 519-858-5137
brescia@uwo.ca
www.brescia.uwo.ca
www.facebook.com/BresciaUniversityCollege
twitter.com/bresciauc
www.linkedin.com/company/brescia-university-college
www.youtube.com/bresciauc
Dr. Susan Mumm, Principal, 519-432-8353, ext. 28263
  bucprincipal@uwo.ca
Donna M. Rogers, Vice-Principal & Academic Dean, 519-432-8353,
  ext. 28263
  donna.rogers@uwo.ca

Canadian Centre for Activity & Aging
CCAA
1490 Richmond St., London, ON N6G 2M3

Tel: 519-661-1603; *Fax:* 519-661-1612
Toll-Free: 866-661-1603
ccaa@uwo.ca
www.uwo.ca/actage
www.facebook.com/actage
www.youtube.com/user/CCAAUWO
Clara Fitzgerald, Program Director

Centre for Population, Aging & Health
#5230 Social Science Centre
London, ON N6A 5C2

Fax: 519-661-3220
cpah@uwo.ca
sociology.uwo.ca/cpah
David Shoesmith, Director

Mississauga: Good Samaritan School for Exceptional Learners
Also known as: Good Samaritan Private School
6341 Mississauga Rd., Mississauga, ON L5N 1A7

Tel: 905-219-9969
Grades: JK-12; Adult Ed.

North Bay: Nipissing University
P.O. Box 5002
100 College Dr., North Bay, ON P1B 8L7

Tel: 705-474-3450; *Fax:* 705-474-1947
nuinfo@nipissingu.ca
www.nipissingu.ca
TTY: 877-688-5507
www.facebook.com/NipissingU
twitter.com/NipissingU
www.youtube.com/user/nipissinguniversity

Full Time Equivalency: 5200
Paul Cook, Chancellor
Mike DeGagné, President & Vice-Chancellor
Dr. Harley d'Entremont, Provost & Vice-President, Academic &
  Research
Cheryl Sutton, Vice-President, Finance & Administration
  cheryls@nipissingu.ca
Jamie Graham, Registrar & Assistant Vice-President, Institutional
  Planning
Tanya Lukin-Linklater, Director, Aboriginal Initiatives
Karen Charles, Manager, Accounting & Purchasing Services, ext. 4435
  karench@nipissingu.ca

Oshawa: University of Ontario Institute of Technology (UOIT)
2000 Simcoe St. North, Oshawa, ON L1H 7K4, Canada

Tel: 905-721-8668; *Fax:* 905-721-3178
admissions@uoit.ca
www.uoit.ca
facebook.com/myuoit
twitter.com/uoit
www.linkedin.com/company/uoit
www.youtube.com/uoit

Full Time Equivalency: 9990
Hon. Perrin Beatty, B.A., Chancellor
Tim McTiernan, President & Vice-Chancellor
Deborah Saucier, Provost & Vice-President, Academic
  provost@uoit.ca
Susan McGovern, Vice-President, External Relations, 905-721-8668,
  ext. 3135
  susan.mcgovern@uoit.ca
Murray Lapp, Vice-President, Human Resources & Services,
  905-721-8668, ext. 5666
  murray.lapp@uoit.ca
Michael Owen, Vice-President, Research, Innovation & International,
  905-721-8668, ext. 5661
  michael.owen@uoit.ca
Pamela Drayson, B.A., M.A., Ph.D., Chief Librarian, 905-721-8668, ext.
  2348
  pamela.drayson@uoit.ca
Brad MacIsaac, Registrar, 905-721-8668, ext. 5688
  brad.macisaac@uoit.ca

Health Sciences

Tel: 905-721-3166; *Fax:* 905-721-3179
healthsciences@uoit.ca
www.healthsciences.uoit.ca
Ellen Vogel, R.D., F.D.C., Ph.D., Dean, 905-721-8668, ext. 2518
ellen.vogel@uoit.ca

Ottawa: **Algonquin College of Applied Arts & Technology**
1385 Woodroffe Ave., Ottawa, ON K2G 1V8, Canada

Tel: 613-727-4723
www.algonquincollege.com
www.facebook.com/algonquincolleg
twitter.com/AlgonquinColleg
www.linkedin.com/company/14808
www.youtube.com/user/algonquinvideos
Full Time Equivalency: 19000
Cheryl Jensen, President

School of Health & Community Studies

Tel: 613-727-4723
www3.algonquincollege.com/healthandcommunity
twitter.com/AChealthstudies
Barbara Foulds, Dean

Ottawa: **Carleton University**
1125 Colonel By Dr., Ottawa, ON K1S 5B6

Tel: 613-520-7400; *Fax:* 613-520-7858
www.carleton.ca
www.facebook.com/carletonuniversity
twitter.com/Carleton_U
www.youtube.com/user/carletonuvideos
Full Time Equivalency: 28845
Number of Employees: 865 academic staff; 1059 management & support staff; 777 contract instructors; 1739 TAs
Charles Chi, Chancellor
Peter Ricketts, Provost & Vice-President, 613-520-2600, ext. 3806
provost@carleton.ca
Michel Piché, Vice-President, Finance & Administration, 613-520-2600, ext. 3804
michel.piche@carleton.ca
Rafik Goubran, Acting Vice-President, Research & International

Institute of Cognitive Science
#2202A, Dunton Tower, Carleton University
1125 Colonel By Dr., Ottawa, ON K1S 5B6

Tel: 613-520-2600; *Fax:* 613-520-3985
www.carleton.ca/ics
twitter.com/CogSciCU
Dr. Jo-Anne LeFevre, Director, 613-520-2600, ext. 2693
jo-anne.lefevre@carleton.ca

Ottawa Medical Physics Institute (OMPI)

ompi_aao@physics.carleton.ca
www.physics.carleton.ca/ompi
Dr. Malcolm McEwen, Director
malcolm.mcewen@nrc-cnrc.gc.ca

Centre for Research on Health: Science, Technology & Policy
Tel: 613-520-2600

Center for Applied Cognitive Research (CACR)
Loeb Bldg.
1125 Colonel By Dr., #B550, Ottawa, ON K1S 5B6

Tel: 613-520-2600; *Fax:* 613-520-3515
www.carleton.ca/cacr
Jo-Anne LeFevre, Director
jlefevre@connect.carleton.ca

Ottawa: **Ican College of Computers and Healthcare**
1825 Woodward Dr., Ottawa, ON K2C 0P9, Canada

Tel: 613-519-0703
www.icancollegeottawa.ca

Ottawa: **Saint Paul University**
Université Saint-Paul
223 Main St., Ottawa, ON K1S 1C4, Canada

Tel: 613-236-1393; *Fax:* 613-782-3005
Toll-Free: 1-800-637-6859
www.ustpaul.ca
www.facebook.com/143697609023948
twitter.com/ustpaul_ca
www.linkedin.com/company/saint-paul-university
www.youtube.com/user/uspottawa
Full Time Equivalency: 820
Chantal Beauvais, Rector
rectrice-rector@ustpaul.ca
Jean-Marc Barrette, Vice-Rector, Academic & Research
Normand Beaulieu, Vice-Rector, Administration

Faculty of Human Sciences

Tel: 613-236-1393; *Toll-Free:* 800-637-6859
humansciences@ustpaul.ca
Manal Guirguis-Younger, Dean

Ottawa: **University of Ottawa**
Université d'Ottawa
Also known as: uOttawa
75 Laurier Ave. East, Ottawa, ON K1N 6N5, Canada

Tel: 613-562-5700; *Fax:* 613-562-5103
Toll-Free: 1-877-868-8292
www.uottawa.ca
www.facebook.com/uottawa
twitter.com/uottawa
www.linkedin.com/edu/school?id=10858
www.youtube.com/uOttawa
Full Time Equivalency: 42700
Number of Employees: 5,000
Calin Rovinescu, Chancellor
Jacques Frémont, President & Vice-Chancellor
Michel Laurier, Vice-President, Academic & Provost, 613-562-5737
vpacademic@uOttawa.ca
Mona Nemer, Vice-President, Research
Louis de Melo, Vice-President, External Relations
Marc Joyal, Vice-President, Resources
Diane Davidson, Vice-President, Governance

Health Sciences
Hélène Perrault, Dean

Medicine
Jacques Bradwejn, Dean

Peterborough: **Trent University**
1600 West Bank Dr., Peterborough, ON K9J 7B8, Canada

Tel: 705-748-1011; *Toll-Free:* 1-855-698-7368
communications@trentu.ca
www.trentu.ca
www.facebook.com/trentuniversity
twitter.com/TrentUniversity
www.linkedin.com/company/trent-university
www.youtube.com/user/trentUniversity
Full Time Equivalency: 8006
Bryan P. Davies, Chair
Don Tapscott, Chancellor
Leo Groarke, President
Gary Boire, Vice-President Academic & Provost
Steven Pillar, Vice-President Administration
Tracy Al-Idrissi, Registrar
Deb deBruijn, University Secretary

St Catharines: **Brock University**
1812 Sir Isaac Brock Way, St Catharines, ON L2S 3A1

Tel: 905-688-5550; *Fax:* 905-688-2789
www.brocku.ca
www.facebook.com/brockuniversity
twitter.com/brockuniversity
www.linkedin.com/school/14912
www.youtube.com/brockuvideo
Full Time Equivalency: 18000
Number of Employees: 594 faculty
Shirley Cheechoo, Chancellor
Tom Traves, Interim President & Vice-Chancellor

Thomas Dunk, Interim Provost & Vice-President, Academic
  tdunk@brocku.ca
Brian Hutchings, Vice-President, Administration
Joffre Mercier, Vice-President, Research
Geraldine Jones, Registrar
Chuck MacLean, Director, Procurement Services, ext. 3746
  cmaclean@brocku.ca

Faculty of Applied Health Sciences

facebook.com/brockfahs
twitter.com/brockfahs
www.youtube.com/user/brockappliedhealthsc
Peter Tiidus, Dean, 905-688-5550, ext. 3385
  peter.tiidus@brocku.ca

Sudbury: Huntington University
935 Ramsey Lake Rd., Sudbury, ON P3E 2C6, Canada
Tel: 705-673-4126; *Fax:* 705-673-6917
Toll-Free: 800-461-6366
info@huntingtonuniversity.com
huntingtonu.ca
www.facebook.com/pages/Huntington-University/162876393781377
twitter.com/HuntingtonUni
instagram.com/huntingtonuniversity
Note: Liberal Arts University specializing in Communication Studies, Ethics, Gerontology, Religious studies and Theology.

Centres/Institutes
Centre for Holistic Health
935 Ramsey Lake Rd., Sudbury, ON P3E 2C6

Canadian Institute for Studies in Aging (CISA)
935 Ramsey Lake Rd., Sudbury, ON P3E 2C6
Lorraine Mercer, Director
  lmercer@huntingtonu.ca

Sudbury: Laurentian University (Sudbury) (LU)
Université Laurentienne (Sudbury)
935 Ramsey Lake Rd., Sudbury, ON P3E 2C6, Canada
Tel: 705-675-1151; *Toll-Free:* 800-461-4030
explore@laurentian.ca
www.laurentian.ca
www.facebook.com/laurentian
twitter.com/laurentianu
www.linkedin.com/company/laurentian-university
www.youtube.com/laurentianuniversity
Full Time Equivalency: 9515 *Note:* Teaching is in French & English. Certain faculties offer parallel programs in both languages.
Dominic Giroux, MBA, President
Robert Kerr, Vice-President & Provost
Carol McAulay, Vice-President
Rui Wang, Vice-President
Terez Klotz, Execurive Director, Human Resources & Org Dev
Serge Demers, Registrar
Chris Mercer, Executive Director, Student Life
Sara Kunto, University Secretary & General Counsel

Human Kinetics
Céline Boudreau-Larivière, Director

Nursing
nursing@laurentian.ca
Sylvie Laroque, Director

Centre for Rural & Northern Health Research
935 Ramsey Lake Rd., Sudbury, ON P3E 2C6
laurentian.ca/centre-rural-and-northern-health-research

Evaluating Children's Health Outcomes Research Centre
935 Ramsey Lake Rd., Sudbury, ON P3E 2C6
laurentian.ca/node/378
Nancy Young, Director

International Centre for Interdisciplinary Research in the Human Sciences
935 Ramsey Lake Rd., Sudbury, ON P3E 2C6
laurentian.ca/ICIRHS

David Robinson, Director

Thunder Bay: Lakehead University
955 Oliver Rd., Thunder Bay, ON P7B 5E1, Canada
Tel: 807-343-8110; *Fax:* 807-343-8023
www.lakeheadu.ca
www.facebook.com/lakeheaduniversity
twitter.com/mylakehead
www.linkedin.com/company/lakehead-university
www.youtube.com/lakeheaduniversity
Full Time Equivalency: 7848
Number of Employees: 2567
Derek Burney, Chancellor
Brian Stevenson, President & Vice-Chancellor
Andrea Tarsitano, Registrar
Anne Deighton, University Librarian
Rita Blais, Associate Vice-President, Financial Services
Kathy Pozihun, Vice-President, Administration & Finance
Moira McPherson, Provost & Vice-President, Academic
Andrew Dean, Vice-President, Research, Economic Development & Innovation
Kerrie-Lee Clarke, Vice-Provost
Deb Comuzzi, Vice-President, External Relations

Northern Ontario School of Medicine
www.nosm.ca
Roger Strasser, Dean

Schools
Kinesiology
Joey Farrell, Director

Nursing
Karen Poole, Director

Centre for Education and Research on Aging & Health
955 Oliver Rd., Thunder Bay, ON P7B 5E1
Tel: 807-766-7271; *Fax:* 807-766-7222
cerah@lakeheadu.ca
cerah.lakeheadu.ca
Ian Newhouse, Director
  ian.newhouse@lakeheadu.ca

Thunder Bay: Northern Ontario School of Medicine (NOSM)
West Campus, Lakehead University
955 Oliver Rd., Thunder Bay, ON P7B 5E1, Canada
Tel: 807-766-7300; *Fax:* 807-766-7370
Toll-Free: 1-800-461-8777
communications@nosm.ca
www.nosm.ca
www.facebook.com/thenosm
twitter.com/nosmtweets
www.youtube.com/user/NOSMtv
Note: 4-year MD program
Moira McPherson, Chair
Roger Strasser, Dean & CEO

Toronto: CJ Health Care College - Scarborough Campus
#401, 1371 Neilson Rd., Toronto, ON M1B 4Z8, Canada
Tel: 416-283-8252; *Fax:* 416-283-3796
admin.scar@cjcollege.com
www.cjcollege.com
Note: Health care related program.
Altheia Jordan, Manager

Toronto: Finding The Way Learning Centre & Bright Start Academy (FTW)
#318, 4630 Dufferin St., Toronto, ON M3H 5S4
Tel: 416-514-1415; *Fax:* 416-514-1410
registration@brightstartacademy.info
www.brightstartacademy.info
www.facebook.com/BSAandFTW
twitter.com/ftwlcautism
Grades: Pre.-9 *Note:* The Academy offers a behaviour & education program for children with autism & learning difficulties.
Allie Offman, Executive Director & Principal

Toronto: Kohai Educational Centre
41 Roehampton Ave., Toronto, ON M4P 1P9
Tel: 416-489-3636; *Fax:* 416-489-3662
kohai@bellnet.ca
www.kohai.ca
www.facebook.com/Kohai.Educational.Centre
www.twitter.com/Kohai41
Grades: Pre.-12 *Note:* Programs & education for students with genetic disorders, behaviour problems, & language disorders.
Barbara Brown, Principal

Toronto: New Skills College of Health, Business, & Technology
1500 Birchmount Rd., Toronto, ON M1P 2G5
Tel: 416-269-8878; *Fax:* 416-266-3898
www.newskillscollege.ca
Note: The New Skills College is a member of the Ontario Association of Career Colleges. The college provides training for health care personnel. Examples of programs include training for food handlers, personal attendants, & medical office assistants.
Julia Li, President, 416-266-8878
Paul Preikschas, Program Manager, 416-269-2666, ext. 221

Toronto: University of Toronto
Also known as: U of T
Old Name: King's College
563 Spadina Cres., Toronto, ON M5S 2J7
Tel: 416-978-2011
www.utoronto.ca
Other Information: 416-978-7669
www.facebook.com/universitytoronto
twitter.com/uoft
www.linkedin.com/company/university-of-toronto
www.youtube.com/user/universitytoronto
Full Time Equivalency: 83012 *Note:* Founded in 1827, the University of Toronto has over 700 undergraduate programs across three campuses in the Greater Toronto Area, & offers the most courses of any University in Canada. The University contributes to the country's research landscape in both the scientific & medical fields. The library network is the largest collection in the country. U of T is home to more students & faculty than any other in Canada.
The Hon. Michael Wilson, Chancellor
Meric S. Gertler, President
Cheryl Regehr, Vice-President & Provost
Sioban Nelson, Vice-Provost, Academic Programs
Jill Matus, Vice-Provost, Students & First-Entry Divisions
Locke Rowe, Vice-Provost, Graduate Research & Education
Catharine Whiteside, Vice-Provost, Relations with Health Care Institutions
Scott Mabury, Vice-President, University Operations
Lucy Fromowitz, Assistant Vice-President, Student Life
Sally Garner, Executive Director, Planning & Budget
Joan E. Foley, University Ombudsperson
Bryn MacPherson, Assistant Vice-President
Shirley Hoy, Chair of the Governing Council
Sheila Brown, CFO
Judith Wolfson, Vice-President, University Relations

Faculty of Dentistry
124 Edward St., Toronto, ON M5G 1G6
Tel: 416-979-4900; *Fax:* 416-979-4936
www.dentistry.utoronto.ca
www.facebook.com/UofTDentistry
twitter.com/UofTDentistry
Daniel Haas, Dean

Faculty of Medicine
Medical Sciences Bldg.
#2109, 1 King's College Circle, Toronto, ON M5S 1A8
Tel: 416-978-6585
discovery.commons@utoronto.ca
medicine.utoronto.ca
www.facebook.com/UofTMedicine
twitter.com/uoftmedicine
instagram.com/uoftmedicine
www.youtube.com/user/UofTMed
Trevor Young, MD, PhD, FRCPC, FCAHS, Dean

Lawrence S. Bloomberg Faculty of Nursing
#130, 155 College St., Toronto, ON M5T 1P8
Tel: 416-978-2392
communications.nursing@utoronto.ca
bloomberg.nursing.utoronto.ca
www.facebook.com/UofTNursing
twitter.com/UofTNursing
www.youtube.com/user/uoftnursing
Linda Johnston, Dean
dean.nursing@utoronto.ca

Leslie Dan Faculty of Pharmacy
144 College St., Toronto, ON M5S 3M2
Tel: 416-978-2889; *Fax:* 416-978-8511
adm.phm@utoronto.ca
www.pharmacy.utoronto.ca
twitter.com/UofTPharmacy
Heather Boon, Dean

Faculty of Kinesiology & Physical Education
#2080, 55 Harbord St., Toronto, ON M5S 2W6
Tel: 416-978-5909
www.kpe.utoronto.ca
twitter.com/UofTKPE
Ira Jacobs, Dean
dean.kpe@utoronto.ca

Centre for the Study of Pain
#300, 155 College St., Toronto, ON M5T 1P8
Tel: 416-946-8270
sites.utoronto.ca/pain
twitter.com/UofT_Pain
Nancy Mitchell, Contact
nancy.mitchell@utoronto.ca

Institute for Life Course & Aging
#328, 263 McCaul St., Toronto, ON M5T 1W7
Tel: 416-978-0377
aging@utoronto.ca
www.aging.utoronto.ca
www.facebook.com/agingutoronto.ca
twitter.com/lifecourseUofT
Esme Fuller-Thomson, Director

Institute of Medical Science (IMS)
Medical Sciences Bldg.
#2374, 1 King's College Circle, Toronto, ON M5S 1A8
Tel: 416-946-8286; *Fax:* 416-971-2253
dir.medscience@utoronto.ca
www.ims.utoronto.ca
www.facebook.com/uoftims
twitter.com/UofTIMS
Mingyao Liu, Director

Dental Research Institute
124 Edward St., Toronto, ON M5G 1G6
Tel: 416-979-4900
www.dentistry.utoronto.ca/dental-research-institute
Bernhard Ganss, Associate Dean, Research
b.ganss@utoronto.ca
Farah Thong, Manager, Research & Business Development
farah.thong@dentistry.utoronto.ca

Centre for Forensic Science & Medicine
Medical Science Bldg.
#6231, 1 King's College Circle, Toronto, ON M5S 1A8
Tel: 416-946-0136
www.forensics.utoronto.ca
Michael Pollanen, Director
michael.pollanen@ontario.ca

Institute of Health Policy, Management & Evaluation
#425, 155 College St., Toronto, ON M5T 3M6
Tel: 416-978-4326; *Fax:* 416-978-7350
ihpme@utoronto.ca
ihpme.utoronto.ca
twitter.com/IHPMEGSU
Adalsteinn Brown, Director
adalsteinn.brown@utoronto.ca

McLaughlin Centre
Peter Gilgan Centre for Research & Learning
686 Bay St., 13th Fl., Toronto, ON M5G 0A4

Tel: 416-813-7654
www.mclaughlin.utoronto.ca

Stephen Scherer, Director
stephen.scherer@sickkids.ca

Institute for Optical Sciences (IOS)
#331, 60 St. George St., Toronto, ON M5S 1A7

Tel: 416-978-1457; Fax: 416-978-3936
www.optics.utoronto.ca

Cynthia Goh, Director
cgoh@optics.utoronto.ca

Tanz Centre for Research in Neurodegenerative Diseases
Krembil Discovery Tower
60 Leonard Ave., #4KD481, Toronto, ON M5T 2S8

Tel: 416-507-6838; Fax: 416-603-6435
crnd.admin@utoronto.ca
tanz.med.utoronto.ca

Peter St. George-Hyslop, Director

Toronto: York University
4700 Keele St., Toronto, ON M3J 1P3, Canada

Tel: 416-736-2100
www.yorku.ca
www.facebook.com/yorkuniversityhome
twitter.com/YorkUnews
www.linkedin.com/company/york-university
www.youtube.com/user/YorkUniversity

Full Time Equivalency: 55000
Number of Employees: 7000 administrative staff
Rick E. Waugh, Chair of the Board
Gregory Sorbara, Chancellor
Mahmoud Shoukri, B.Sc., M.Eng., Ph.D., President & Vice-Chancellor
Rhonda Lenton, Vice-President & Academic Provost
Jeff O'Hagan, Vice-President Advancement
Gary Brewer, Vice-President Finance & Administration
Robert Haché, Vice-President Research & Innovation
Maureen Armstron, University Secretary & General Counsel
Janet Morrison, Vice-Provost, Students
Trudy Pound-Curtis, BCom., FCA, CFO & Assistant Vice-President Finance
Bob Gagne, Chief Information Officer, 416-736-5818
bgagne@yorku.ca
Carol Altilia, Registrar, 416-736-2100, ext. 55262
roinfo@yorku.ca

Faculty of Health

Tel: 416-736-5124; Fax: 416-736-5760
healthdn@yorku.ca
health.info.yorku.ca
www.facebook.com/yorkuniversityfacultyofhealth
twitter.com/YorkUHealth
www.youtube.com/user/FacultyofHealth
Harvey Skinner, Dean

The Centre for Vision Research (CVR)

Tel: 416-736-5659; Fax: 416-736-5857
manini@cvr.yorku.ca
www.cvr.yorku.ca

Laurence Harris, Director & Professor

York Institute for Health Research

Tel: 416-736-5941; Fax: 416-736-5986
yihr@yorku.ca
www.yorku.ca/yihr
www.facebook.com/102017273196330
twitter.com/York_YIHR
Jianhong Wu, Director

Toronto: Zareinu Educational Centre of Metropolitan Toronto
Administration Office
#301, 4630 Dufferin St., Toronto, ON M3H 5S4

Tel: 416-661-1800; Fax: 416-661-1801
info@zareinu.org
zareinu.org
www.facebook.com/ZareinuEducationalCentre

Grades: Pre.-12 Note: Zareinu Educational Centre is a treatment centre & Jewish day school for children with physical & developmental disabilities.
Dr. Mitchell Parker, Principal & Clinical Director
Phyllis Resnick, Contact, School Administration
Sarah Weitz, Contact, School Administration

Waterloo: University of Waterloo
200 University Ave. West, Waterloo, ON N2L 3G1, Canada

Tel: 519-888-4567
www.uwaterloo.ca
Other Information: 519-888-4911
www.facebook.com/university.waterloo
twitter.com/uWaterloo
www.linkedin.com/company/university-of-waterloo
www.youtube.com/uwaterloo

Full Time Equivalency: 31362
V. Prem Watsa, Chancellor
Kevin Lynch, Chair
Feridun Hamdullahpur, C.C., A.B., L.L.B., President & Vice-Chancellor
Ian Orchard, Vice-President Academic & Provost
George Dixon, Vice-President University Research
Chris Read, Associate Provost, Students
Kenneth McGillivray, Vice-President Advancement
Jim Frank, Interim Associate Provost, Graduate Studies
Logan Atkinson, University Secretary & General Counsel
Nello Angerilli, Associate Vice-President, International
Ray Darling, Registrar

Faculties
Faculty of Applied Health Sciences

Tel: 519-888-4567; Fax: 519-746-6776
ahsrecep@uwaterloo.ca
uwaterloo.ca/applied-health-sciences
www.facebook.com/waterloo.appliedhealthsciences
twitter.com/ahswaterloo
instagram.com/uwaterlooahs
James Rush, Interim Dean
jwerush@uwaterloo.ca

St. Jerome's University
290 Westmount Rd. North, Waterloo, ON N2L 3G3

Tel: 519-884-8111; Fax: 519-884-5759
www.sju.ca
www.facebook.com/stjeromesuniversity
twitter.com/StJeromesUni
www.linkedin.com/groups/2548753
instagram.com/stjeromesuni

Note: Federated with the University of Waterloo, St. Jerome's University is a public Catholic university. Education in the Arts & Mathematics is provided.
James Beingessner, Chancellor
Dr. Katherine Bergman, President & Vice-Chancellor
Dr. Scott Kline, Dean & Vice-President, Academic
Darren D. Becks, Vice-President, Administration
Rod Barr, Chair
Graham Brown, Principal
ggbrown@uwaterloo.ca
Peter Frick, Academic Dean
pfrick@uwaterloo.ca
Cathy Newell Kelly, Director
cnkelly@uwaterloo.ca
Donna Ellis, Director
Jo-Anne Absolon, Coordinator
abserv@uwaterloo.ca

Waterloo: Wilfrid Laurier University
75 University Ave. West, Waterloo, ON N2L 3C5, Canada

Tel: 519-884-0710
chooselaurier@wlu.ca
www.wlu.ca
www.facebook.com/LaurierNow
twitter.com/LaurierNews
www.linkedin.com/company/wilfrid-laurier-university
www.youtube.com/lauriervideo

Full Time Equivalency: 18541
Dr. Max Blouw, President & Vice-Chancellor
Dr. Deborah MacLatchy, Vice-President Academic & Provost

Jim Butler, Vice-President Finance & Administration
Ruth MacNeil, Acting Registrar
Robert Donelson, Vice-President Development & Alumni Relations
David McMurray, Vice-President Student Affairs

Windsor: St. Clair College
South Campus
2000 Talbot Rd. West, Windsor, ON N9A 6S4
Tel: 519-966-1656; *Fax:* 519-972-3811
Toll-Free: 1-800-387-0524
info@stclaircollege.ca
www.stclaircollege.ca
www.facebook.com/StClairCollege
www.twitter.com/stclaircollege
www.youtube.com/stclairmarketing

Full Time Equivalency: 8300 *Note:* The College consists of the following schools of specialization: School of Liberal Arts & Sciences; School of Business & Information Technology; School of Academic Studies; School of Community Studies; School of Media, Art & Design; School of Engineering Technologies; School of Health Sciences; & School of Skilled Trades.
Dan Wilson, Chair
Patricia France, President, 519-972-2701
pfrance@stclaircollege.ca
Michael Silvaggi, Registrar, 519-972-2727, ext. 4260
msilvaggi@stclaircollege.ca

Centres/Institutes
Centre For Applied Health Sciences
2000 Talbot Rd. West, Windsor, ON N9A 6S4
www.stclaircollege.ca/healthsciences
Dr. Ken Blanchette, Chair, School of Health Sciences
kblanchette@stclaircollege.ca

Windsor: University of Windsor
401 Sunset Ave., Windsor, ON N9B 3P4, Canada
Tel: 519-253-3000; *Fax:* 519-973-7050
www.uwindsor.ca
www.facebook.com/uwindsor
www.twitter.com/uwindsor
www.linkedin.com/groups?gid=38761
www.youtube.com/uwindsor

Full Time Equivalency: 16500
Dr. Alan Wildeman, President & Vice-Chancellor
Edward Lumley, Chancellor

Faculty of Human Kinetics
www1.uwindsor.ca/hk
Dr. Michael A. Khan, Dean

Faculty of Nursing
Toldo Health Education Centre
#336, 401 Sunset Ave., Windsor, ON N9B 3P4
Tel: 519-253-3000; *Fax:* 519-973-7084
nurse@uwindsor.ca
www1.uwindsor.ca/nursing
twitter.com/UWinNursing
Dr. Linda Patrick, RN, BScN, MA, MSc, PhD, Dean

PRINCE EDWARD ISLAND

Charlottetown: University of Prince Edward Island
550 University Ave., Charlottetown, PE C1A 4P3, Canada
Tel: 902-566-0439; *Fax:* 902-566-0420
home.upei.ca
www.facebook.com/UniversityofPEI
twitter.com/upei
www.youtube.com/UofPEI

Full Time Equivalency: 3500
Tom Cullen, Chair of the Board
Don McDougall, Chancellor
Alaa Abd-El-Aziz, President & Vice-Chancellor
presidentea@upei.ca
Robert Gilmour, Vice-President, Research & Graduate Studies
research@upei.ca
Christian Lacroix, Vice-President, Academic
ecardy@upei.ca

Jackie Podger, Vice-President, Administration & Finance
kharrison@upei.ca
Dana Sanderson, Chief Information Officer
dsanderson@upei.ca
Kathleen Kielly, Registrar & Director, Enrolment Services
kkielly@upei.ca
Mark Leggott, University Librarian
mleggott@upei.ca
Roger Cook, Procurement Services Manager
rcook@upei.ca

School of Nursing
Tel: 902-566-0733
nursing@upei.ca
nursing.upei.ca
Dr. Rosemary Herbert, Dean

QUÉBEC

Montréal: McGill University
845 Sherbrooke St. West, Montréal, QC H3A 0G4
Tel: 514-398-4455
info.publicaffairs@mcgill.ca
www.mcgill.ca
www.facebook.com/McGillUniversity
twitter.com/mcgillu
www.linkedin.com/company/mcgill-university
plus.google.com/+mcgilluniversity/posts

Full Time Equivalency: 40493
Michael Meighen, Chancellor
Stuart Cobbett, Chair of Board
Suzanne Fortier, Principal & Vice-Chancellor
Christopher Manfredi, Provost & Vice-Principal, Academic
Louis Arseneault, Vice-Principal, Communications & External Relations
Yves Beauchamp, Vice-Principal, Administration & Finance
Rosie Goldstein, Vice-Principal, Research & Innovation
Marc Weinstein, Vice-Principal, University Advancement
Angelique Mannella, Associate Vice-Principal, Innovation & Partnerships
Edyta Rogowska, Secretary-General

Faculty of Dentistry
#500, 2001 McGill College Ave., Montréal, QC H3A 1G1
Tel: 514-398-7203; *Fax:* 514-398-8900
undergrad.dentistry@mcgill.ca
www.mcgill.ca/dentistry
Paul Allison, Dean

Faculty of Medicine
McIntyre Medical Bldg.
3655 Promenade Sir William Osler, Montréal, QC H3G 1Y6
Tel: 514-398-1768; *Fax:* 514-398-3595
recep.med@mcgill.ca
www.mcgill.ca/medicine
David Eidelman, Dean

Communication Sciences & Disorders
2001 McGill College Ave., 8th Fl., Montréal, QC H3A 1G1
Tel: 514-398-4137; *Fax:* 514-398-8123
scsd@mcgill.ca
www.mcgill.ca/scsd
www.facebook.com/50YearsSchoolOfCommunicationSciencesAndDisorders
Dr. Marc D. Pell, Associate Dean & Director
director.scsd@mcgill.ca

School of Dietetics & Human Nutrition
Macdonald-Stewart Bldg.
21111 Lakeshore Rd., Ste-Anne-de-Bellevue, QC H9X 3V9
Tel: 514-398-7773; *Fax:* 514-398-7739
nutrition.dietetics@mcgill.ca
www.mcgill.ca/nutrition
Linda Wykes, Director
linda.wykes@mcgill.ca

School of Physical & Occupational Therapy (SPOT)
3654 Promenade Sir William Osler, Montreal, QC H3G 1Y5
Tel: 514-398-4500; *Fax:* 514-398-6360
www.mcgill.ca/spot
www.facebook.com/McgillSchoolofPhysicalandOccupationalTherapy
instagram.com/mcgill_spot
Dr. Annette Majnemer, Director

McGill Centre for the Convergence of Health & Economics (MCCHE)
3430 McTavish St., Montréal, QC H3A 1X9
Tel: 514-398-3299; *Fax:* 514-398-3876
www.mcgill.ca/desautels/mcche
twitter.com/Desautels_MCCHE
Dora Koop, Managing Director

Research Institute of the McGill University Health Centre
Also known as: Research Institute of the MUHC
#500, 2155 Guy St., Montréal, QC H3H 2R9
Tel: 514-934-1934
ri.it@muhc.mcgill.ca
www.rimuhc.ca/web/research-institute-muhc
Bruce Mazer, Executive Director

Québec: Université Laval
2325, rue de l'Université, Québec, QC G1V 0A6, Canada
Tél: 418-656-2131; *Ligne sans frais:* 1-877-785-2825
renseignements@ulaval.ca
www.ulaval.ca
www.facebook.com/ulaval.ca
twitter.com/universitelaval
www.linkedin.com/company/universite-laval
www.youtube.com/ulavaltv
Full Time Equivalency: 45400 *Note:* Première université francophone d'Amerique, ouverte sur le monde et animée d'une culture de l'exigence, l'Université Laval contribue au développement de la société par laformation de personnes compétentes, responsables et promotrice de changement, par l'avancement et le partage des connaissances, dans un environnement dynamique de recherche et de création
Denis Brière, Recteur
Richard Fournier, Directeur

Centres/Institutes
Centre de recherche de l'Institut universitaire en santé mentale de Québec
2601, ch de la Canardière, Québec, QC G1J 2G3
Tél: 418-663-5971; *Téléc:* 418-663-9540
info@crulrg.ulaval.ca
www.crulrg.ulaval.ca
Réjean Cantin, Président

Centre de recherche sur le cancer (CRC)
9, rue McMahon, Québec, QC G1R 3S3
Tél: 418-525-4444; *Téléc:* 418-691-5439
secretaire@crc.ulaval.ca
www.crc.ulaval.ca
Luc Beaulieu, Directeur

Centre de recherche du CHU de Québec
2705, boul Laurier, Québec, QC G1V 4G2
Tél: 418-654-2296; *Téléc:* 418-654-2298
sec.drs@crchuq.ulaval.ca
www.crchudequebec.ulaval.ca
Serge Rivest, Directeur

Sherbrooke: Bishop's University
2600 College St., Sherbrooke, QC J1M 1Z7
Tel: 819-822-9600; *Fax:* 819-822-9661
www.ubishops.ca
www.facebook.com/ubishops
twitter.com/ubishops
www.linkedin.com/school/34318
www.youtube.com/user/bishopsuniversity
Full Time Equivalency: 2371
Michael Goldbloom, Principal & Vice-Chancellor
principal@ubishops.ca
Victoria Meikle, Secretary General & Vice-Principal, Government & Planning

SASKATCHEWAN

Regina: University of Regina
3737 Wascana Pkwy., Regina, SK S4S 0A2
Tel: 306-585-4111; *Fax:* 306-585-5203
registrar@uregina.ca
www.uregina.ca
www.facebook.com/UniversityofRegina
twitter.com/UofRegina
www.linkedin.com/company/university-of-regina
Full Time Equivalency: 14360
Number of Employees: 2800
Dr. Jim Tomkins, Chancellor
Dr. Vianne Timmins, B.A., B.Ed., M.Ed., Ph.D., President & Vice-Chancellor
Dr. Thomas Chase, Provost & Vice-President, Academic
Dave Button, M.Sc., P.Eng., PMP, Vice-President, Administration
David Malloy, Vice-President, Research
Kelly Kummerfield, B.Admin., Associate Vice-President, Human Resources
Dr. Dena McMartin, Associate Vice-President, Academic & Research
Dale Schoffer, Associate Vice-President, Finance
John D. Smith, Associate Vice-President, Student Affairs
Nelson Wagner, Associate Vice-President, Facilities Management
Glenys Sylvestre, University Secretary
glenys.sylvestre@uregina.ca
James D'Arcy, Registrar
the.registrar@uregina.ca

Faculty of Kinesiology & Health Studies
3737 Wascana Pkwy., Regina, SK S4S 0A2
Tel: 306-585-4360; *Fax:* 306-585-4854
kinesiology@uregina.ca
www.uregina.ca/kinesiology
Dr. Harold Riemer, Dean
khs.dean@uregina.ca

Centres/Institutes
Centre on Aging & Health
Regina, SK S4S 0A2
Tel: 306-337-8477; *Fax:* 306-337-3204
cah@uregina.ca
www2.uregina.ca/cah
twitter.com/UofRAgingCentre
Scott Wilson, Administrator
scott.j.wilson@uregina.ca

Indigenous Peoples' Health Research Centre (IPHRC)
237 2 Research Dr., Regina, SK S4S 7H1
Tel: 306-337-2461; *Fax:* 306-585-5694
www.iphrc.ca
www.facebook.com/IPHRC
twitter.com/iphrcsask
Kathy McNutt, Acting Director
kathy.mcnutt@uregina.ca

Saskatoon: University of Saskatchewan
Administration Bldg.
105 Administration Pl., Saskatoon, SK S7N 5A2
Tel: 306-966-4343
www.usask.ca
www.facebook.com/usask
twitter.com/usask
www.linkedin.com/company/university-of-saskatchewan
instagram.com/usask
Full Time Equivalency: 20080
Blaine C. Favel, Chancellor
Peter Stoicheff, President & Vice-Chancellor
Ernie Barber, Interim Provost & Vice-President
Greg Fowler, Vice-President, Finance & Resources
Elizabeth Williamson, University Secretary
Russell Isinger, Registrar
Jim Basinger, Assoc. Vice-President, Research
jim.basinger@usask.ca
Karen Chad, Ph.D., Vice-President, Research
Jeff Dumba, Assoc. Vice-President, Financial Services & Controller
Ivan Muzychka, Assoc. Vice-President, Communications
Patti McDougall, Vice-Provost, Teaching & Learning

Mark Roman, Assoc. Vice-President, Information & Communications Tech

College of Dentistry

Toll-Free: 877-363-7275
dentistry@usask.ca
www.usask.ca/dentistry

Gerry Uswak, Dean, 306-966-5122
gerry.uswak@usask.ca

College of Kinesiology
87 Campus Dr., Saskatoon, SK S7N 5B2

Tel: 306-966-1060; *Fax:* 306-966-6464
kinesiology.usask.ca

Chad London, Dean
chad.london@usask.ca

College of Medicine
Health Sciences Bldg.
107 Wiggins Rd., #5D40, Saskatoon, SK S7N 5E5

Tel: 306-966-2673
medicine.reception@usask.ca
www.medicine.usask.ca

Dr. Preston Smith, M.D., Ph.D., FRCPC, Dean

College of Nursing
104 Clinic Pl., Saskatoon, SK S7N 2Z4

Tel: 306-966-6221; *Fax:* 306-966-6621
Toll-Free: 844-966-6269
www.usask.ca/nursing
www.facebook.com/usaskNursing
twitter.com/uofsnursing
www.youtube.com/user/usasknursing

Beth Horsburgh, Interim Dean
beth.horsburgh@usask.ca

College of Pharmacy & Nutrition
Thorvaldson Bldg.
#116, 110 Science Pl., Saskatoon, SK S7N 5C9

Tel: 306-966-6327; *Fax:* 306-966-6377
pharmacy-nutrition.usask.ca
www.facebook.com/usaskPharmNut

Kishor Wasan, Dean

School of Physical Therapy
#3400, 104 Clinic Pl., Saskatoon, SK S7N 2Z4

Tel: 306-966-6579; *Fax:* 306-966-6575
pt.generaloffice@usask.ca
www.medicine.usask.ca/pt

Elizabeth Harrison, Associate Dean

Centre for Integrative Medicine
HSC E-Wing, College of Medicine
107 Wiggins Rd., Saskatoon, SK S7N 5E5

Tel: 306-966-7935
integrative.medicine@usask.ca
twitter.com/usask

Michael Epstein, Managing Director

Local Hospitals & Health Centres

ALBERTA

AIRDRIE: Airdrie Regional Health Centre
Affiliated with: Alberta Health Services
604 Main St. South, Airdrie, AB T4B 3K7

Tel: 403-912-8400 *Fax:* 403-912-8410
www.albertahealthservices.ca

ANZAC: Anzac Community Health Services
Affiliated with: Alberta Health Services
240 Christina Dr., Anzac, AB T0P 1J0

Tel: 780-334-2023 *Fax:* 780-791-6288
www.albertahealthservices.ca

Note: Services: immunization; public health nursing

ATHABASCA: Athabasca Community Health Services
Affiliated with: Alberta Health Services
3401 - 48 Ave., Athabasca, AB T9S 1M7

Tel: 780-675-2231 *Fax:* 780-675-3111
www.albertahealthservices.ca

ATHABASCA: Athabasca Healthcare Centre
Affiliated with: Alberta Health Services
3100 - 48 Ave., Athabasca, AB T9S 1M9

Tel: 780-675-6000 *Fax:* 780-675-7050
www.albertahealthservices.ca
Social Media: www.facebook.com/179579998746821;
twitter.com/AHS_media; www.youtube.com/ahschannel
Number of Beds: 26 acute care beds; 1 palliative care bed; 23 continuing care beds
Note: Programs & services include: emergency services; diagnostic imaging; laboratory services; acute care; obstetrics; pediatrics; continuing care; rehabilitation; recreation services; palliative care; & x-ray.
Mary Proskie, Site Manager

BANFF: Banff - Mineral Springs Hospital
Covenant Health
Affiliated with: Alberta Health Services
PO Box 1050, 305 Lynx St., Banff, AB T1L 1H7

Tel: 403-762-2222 *Fax:* 403-762-4193
www.covenanthealth.ca
Social Media: www.facebook.com/Banff.MSH
Year Founded: 1930
Note: Programs & services include: emergency services; surgery; acute care; maternal & child care; physiotherapy; occupational therapy; recreation therapy; music therapy; mental health services; continuing care; outpatient clinics; & palliative care.
Shelley Buchan, Site Administrator

BANFF: Banff Community Health Centre
Affiliated with: Alberta Health Services
Former Name: Banff National Park Health Unit Office
303 Lynx St., Banff, AB T1L 1B3

Tel: 403-762-2990 *Fax:* 403-762-5570
www.albertahealthservices.ca

BARRHEAD: Barrhead Community Health Services
Affiliated with: Alberta Health Services
6203 - 49 St., Barrhead, AB T7N 1A1

Tel: 780-674-3408 *Fax:* 780-674-3941
www.albertahealthservices.ca

BARRHEAD: Barrhead Healthcare Centre
Affiliated with: Alberta Health Services
4815 - 51 Ave., Barrhead, AB T7N 1M1

Tel: 780-674-2221 *Fax:* 780-674-3541
www.albertahealthservices.ca
Social Media: www.facebook.com/179579998746821;
twitter.com/AHS_media; www.youtube.com/ahschannel
Number of Beds: 34 beds
Note: Programs & services include: emergency services; diagnostic imaging; laboratory services; obstetrics; community cancer centre; rehabilitation services; social work; diet counselling; education programs; outpatient clinics; & palliative care.

BASHAW: Bashaw Community Health Centre
Affiliated with: Alberta Health Services
5308 - 53 St., Bashaw, AB T0B 0H0

Tel: 780-372-3731 *Fax:* 780-372-4050
www.albertahealthservices.ca

Note: Programs & services include: diagnostic imaging; laboratory; occupational therapy; physical therapy; dietitian; & respiratory services
Lora Miller, Site Manager

BASSANO: Bassano Health Centre
Affiliated with: Alberta Health Services
608 - 5 Ave., Bassano, AB T0J 0B0

Tel: 403-641-6100 *Fax:* 403-641-2157
www.albertahealthservices.ca
Social Media: www.facebook.com/179579998746821;
twitter.com/AHS_media; www.youtube.com/ahschannel
Year Founded: 1914
Number of Beds: 4 acute care beds; 8 continuing care beds; 1 palliative

care bed; 1 respite care bed
Note: Programs & services include: emergency services; diagnostic imaging; acute care; physiotherapy; occupational therapy; physiotherapy; mental health services; nutrition services; social work; continuing care; respite care; & palliative care.

BEAUMONT: Beaumont Public Health Centre
Affiliated with: Alberta Health Services
4918 - 50 Ave., Beaumont, AB T4X 1J9
Tel: 780-929-4822
www.albertahealthservices.ca

Note: Services include: addiction & mental health; immunization; public health; & tuberculosis testing.

BEAVERLODGE: Beaverlodge Community Health Services
Affiliated with: Alberta Health Services
Former Name: Beaverlodge Public Health Centre
412 - 10A St., Beaverlodge, AB T0H 0C0
Tel: 780-354-2647 *Fax:* 780-354-8410
www.albertahealthservices.ca

BEAVERLODGE: Beaverlodge Municipal Hospital
Affiliated with: Alberta Health Services
PO Box 480, 422 - 10A St., Beaverlodge, AB T0H 0C0
Tel: 780-354-2136 *Fax:* 780-354-8355
www.albertahealthservices.ca
Social Media: www.facebook.com/179579998746821;
twitter.com/AHS_media; www.youtube.com/ahschannel
Number of Beds: 18 acute care beds
Note: Programs & services include: emergency services; general radiography; medical laboratory; acute care; obstetrics; physiotherapy; occupational therapy; & palliative care.
Janet Wallace, Site Manager

BENTLEY: Bentley Care Centre
Affiliated with: Alberta Health Services
4834 - 52 Ave., Bentley, AB T0C 0J0
Tel: 403-748-4115 *Fax:* 403-748-2727
www.albertahealthservices.ca

Note: Programs & services include: continuing care services; physiotherapy; occupational therapy; recreational therapy; & palliative care.

BLACK DIAMOND: Black Diamond Public Health Unit at Oilfields General Hospital
Affiliated with: Alberta Health Services
717 Government Rd., Black Diamond, AB T0L 0H0
Tel: 403-933-6505 *Fax:* 403-933-2031
www.albertahealthservices.ca

Note: Community health services

BLACK DIAMOND: Oilfields General Hospital
Affiliated with: Alberta Health Services
717 Government Rd., Black Diamond, AB T0L 0H0
Tel: 403-933-2222 *Fax:* 403-933-2031
www.albertahealthservices.ca
Social Media: www.facebook.com/179579998746821;
twitter.com/AHS_media; www.youtube.com/ahschannel

Note: Programs & services include: addiction services; adult day support program; diagnostic imaging; laboratory services; occupational therapy; physical therapy; & speech language pathology.
Carla Ralph, Site Manager

BLAIRMORE: Crowsnest Pass Health Centre
Affiliated with: Alberta Health Services
2001 - 107 St., Blairmore, AB T0K 0E0
Tel: 403-562-5011 *Fax:* 403-562-8992
www.albertahealthservices.ca
Social Media: www.facebook.com/179579998746821;
twitter.com/AHS_media; www.youtube.com/AHSChannel

Note: Programs & services include: emergency; diagnostic imaging services; laboratory; surgery; neonatal intensive care nursery; pediatrics; critical care services; acute care; rehabilitation services, including occupational therapy & therapeutic recreation; Southern Alberta Renal Program; continuing care; & palliative care.

Diane Nummi, Manager, Continuing Care

BLAIRMORE: Crowsnest Pass Provincial Building
Affiliated with: Alberta Health Services
12501 - 20 Ave., Blairmore, AB T0K 0E0
Tel: 403-562-5030 *Fax:* 403-562-7379
www.albertahealthservices.ca

Note: Environmental public health

BONNYVILLE: Bonnyville Community Health Services
Affiliated with: Alberta Health Services
4904 - 50 Ave., Bonnyville, AB T9N 2G4
Tel: 780-826-3381 *Fax:* 780-826-6470
www.albertahealthservices.ca

BONNYVILLE: Bonnyville Healthcare Centre
Covenant Health
Affiliated with: Alberta Health Services
5001 Lakeshore Dr., Bonnyville, AB T9N 2J7
Tel: 780-826-3311 *Fax:* 780-826-6527
www.covenanthealth.ca/hospitals-care-centres/bonnyville-health-centre
Social Media: www.facebook.com/179579998746821;
twitter.com/AHS_media; www.youtube.com/ahschannel
Year Founded: 1986
Number of Beds: 63 beds
Number of Employees: 317
Note: Programs & services include: emergency services; regional laboratory services; diagnostic imaging; pathology; surgery; acute care; community cancer centre; cardiac stress testing; obstetrics; rehabilitation; medical accupunture; occupational therapy; respiratory therapy; continuing care; & palliative care.
Alex Smyl, Administrator

BOW ISLAND: Bow Island Health Centre
Affiliated with: Alberta Health Services
938 Centre St., Bow Island, AB T0K 0G0
Tel: 403-545-3200 *Fax:* 403-545-2281
www.albertahealthservices.ca
Social Media: www.facebook.com/179579998746821;
twitter.com/AHS_media; www.youtube.com/ahschannel
Number of Beds: 10 acute care beds; 20 continuing care beds
Note: Programs & services include: emergency services; diagnostic imaging & laboratory services; acute care; physiotherapy; occupational therapy; continuing care; & respite services.

BOW ISLAND: Bow Island Provincial Building
Affiliated with: Alberta Health Services
Former Name: Bow Island Public Health/Home Care
802 - 6 St. East, Bow Island, AB T0K 0G0
Tel: 403-545-2296 *Fax:* 403-529-3562
www.albertahealthservices.ca

BOYLE: Boyle Healthcare Centre
Affiliated with: Alberta Health Services
5004 Lakeview Rd., Boyle, AB T0A 0M0
Tel: 780-689-3731 *Fax:* 780-689-3951
www.albertahealthservices.ca
Social Media: www.facebook.com/179579998746821;
twitter.com/AHS_media; www.youtube.com/ahschannel
Year Founded: 1966
Number of Beds: 19 acute care beds; 1 palliative care bed
Note: Programs & services include: emergency services; diagnostic imaging; laboratory services; acute care services; nutrition services; community health; social work; & palliative care.
Mary Proskie, Site Manager

BOYLE: Boyle Healthcare Centre
Affiliated with: Alberta Health Services
5004 Lakeview Rd., Boyle, AB T0A 0M0
Tel: 780-689-2677 *Fax:* 780-689-2835
www.albertahealthservices.ca

Note: Home care office
Mary Proskie, Site Manager

BRETON: Breton Health Centre
Affiliated with: Alberta Health Services
4919 - 49th Ave., Breton, AB T0C 0P0
Tel: 780-696-4713 *Fax:* 780-696-4747
www.albertahealthservices.ca

Year Founded: 1994
Number of Beds: 23 long-term care beds
Note: Programs & services include: laboratory services; occupational therapy; physical therapy; speech language pathology; nutrition; continuing care; & palliative care.

BROOKS: Brooks Community Health Care
Affiliated with: Alberta Health Services
440 - 3rd St. East, Brooks, AB T1R 1B3
Tel: 403-501-3232
www.albertahealthservices.ca

BROOKS: Brooks Health Centre
Affiliated with: Alberta Health Services
440 - 3rd St. East, Brooks, AB T1R 0G5
Tel: 403-501-3232 *Fax:* 403-362-6039
www.albertahealthservices.ca
Social Media: www.facebook.com/179579998746821;
twitter.com/AHS_media; www.youtube.com/ahschannel
Number of Beds: 40 acute care beds; 75 long term care beds
Note: Programs & services include: emergency services; ambulatory care; acute care; obstetrics; pediatrics; physiotherapy; occupational therapy; recreational therapy; Healthy Living Program / cardiac rehabilitation; diabetes education; community health; continuing care; & palliative care.

BROOKS: Brooks Home Care
Affiliated with: Alberta Health Services
311 - 9 St. SE, Brooks, AB T1R 1B7
Tel: 403-362-7766 *Fax:* 403-362-7778
www.albertahealthservices.ca

BUFFALO LAKE SETTLEMENT: Buffalo Lake Settlement Community Health Services
Affiliated with: Alberta Health Services
Buffalo Lake Dr., Buffalo Lake Settlement, AB T0A 0R0
Tel: 780-689-4771
www.albertahealthservices.ca

CADOTTE LAKE: Woodland Cree Health Centre
Affiliated with: Alberta Health Services
General Delivery, Cadotte Lake, AB T0H 0N0
Tel: 780-629-8963
www.albertahealthservices.ca

Note: Services: immunization; public health nursing

CALGARY: Acadia Community Health Centre
Affiliated with: Alberta Health Services
151 - 86 Ave. SE, Calgary, AB T2H 3A5
Tel: 403-944-7200 *Fax:* 403-253-5129
www.albertahealthservices.ca

CALGARY: Calgary Women's Health Centre
Affiliated with: Alberta Health Services
1441 29 St. NW, Calgary, AB T2N 4J8
Tel: 403-944-2270 *Fax:* 403-944-2271
www.albertahealthservices.ca

Note: Provides breast health & nutrition counselling services.

CALGARY: East Calgary Health Centre
Affiliated with: Alberta Health Services
4715 - 8 Ave. SE, Calgary, AB T2A 3N4
Tel: 403-955-1250 *Fax:* 403-955-1299
www.albertahealthservices.ca

Sue Ramsden, Site Manager

CALGARY: Foothills Medical Centre
Affiliated with: Alberta Health Services
1403 - 29 St. NW, Calgary, AB T2N 2T9
Tel: 403-944-1110
www.albertahealthservices.ca
Social Media: www.facebook.com/179579998746821;
twitter.com/AHS_media; www.youtube.com/ahschannel
Year Founded: 1966
Note: Programs & services include: emergency services; trauma services; diagnostic imaging; acute care; gynecology; newborn care; cardiology; gastrointestinal services; hematology; adult neuropsychology service; neurology; psychiatry; renal services;

Movement Disorders Program; respiratory services; social work; & addiction services.

CALGARY: North Hill Community Health Centre
Affiliated with: Alberta Health Services
1527 - 19 St. NW, Calgary, AB T2N 2K2
Tel: 403-944-7400 *Fax:* 403-944-7447
www.albertahealthservices.ca

CALGARY: Peter Lougheed Centre
Affiliated with: Alberta Health Services
3500 - 26 Ave. NE, Calgary, AB T1Y 6J4
Tel: 403-943-4555
www.albertahealthservices.ca
Social Media: www.facebook.com/179579998746821;
twitter.com/AHS_media; www.youtube.com/AHSChannel
Year Founded: 1988
Number of Beds: 600 beds
Note: Programs & services include: Aboriginal services; abortion; angiography; anticoagulation management; bronchoscopy; cardiology; clinics; CT imaging; mental health services; surgery; diabetes, hypertension & cholesterol; diagnostic imaging; electroencephalography; emergency; enterostomal therapy; fluoroscopy; gastrointestinal; general medicine; general radiography; hematology; hemodialysis; intensive care; laboratory; magnetic resonance imaging; neurology; nuclear medicine; nutrition; occupational therapy; oncology; palliative care; pharmacy; psychiatry; speech language pathology; social work; & ultrasound.

CALGARY: Ranchlands Village Mall
Affiliated with: Alberta Health Services
Former Name: High Level General Hospital; Northwest Health Centre
Northwest Community Health Centre, #109, 1829 Ranchlands Blvd. NW, Calgary, AB T3G 2A7
Tel: 403-943-9700 *Fax:* 403-943-9735
www.albertahealthservices.ca

Note: Programs & services include: cardiology; immunization; laboratory; & nutrition counselling.

CALGARY: Rockyview General Hospital
Affiliated with: Alberta Health Services
7007 - 14 St. SW, Calgary, AB T2V 1P9
Tel: 403-943-3000
www.albertahealthservices.ca
Social Media: www.facebook.com/179579998746821;
twitter.com/AHS_media; www.youtube.com/AHSChannel
Number of Beds: 650 beds
Note: Programs & services include: emergency; acute care; CT imaging; cardiac intensive care/coronary care units; colorectal surgery; cystoscopy; diagnostic imaging; electroencephalography; endoscopy; geriatric assessment & rehabilitation; & obstetrics/gynecology outpatient.
Nancy Guebert, Vice-President

CALGARY: Shaganappi Complex
Affiliated with: Alberta Health Services
3415 - 8th Ave. SW, Calgary, AB T3C 0E8
Tel: 403-944-7373 *Fax:* 403-246-0326
www.albertahealthservices.ca

Note: Programs & services include: immunization; school health program; & Well Child services

CALGARY: Sheldon M. Chumir Health Centre
Affiliated with: Alberta Health Services
1213 - 4 St. SW, Calgary, AB T2R 0X7
Tel: 403-955-6200
www.albertahealthservices.ca

Note: Programs & services include: addiction & mental health; Community Accessible Rehabilitation; computed tomography; diagnostic imaging; general radiography; hemodialysis; laboratory; public health; sexual & reproductive health; speech language pathology; travel health; tuberculosis testing; & urgent care.
Sherry Heather, Site Manager

CALGARY: South Calgary Health Centre
Affiliated with: Alberta Health Services
31 Sunpark Plaza SE, Calgary, AB T2X 3W5
Tel: 403-943-9300
www.albertahealthservices.ca

Note: Open 365 days a year
Sue Ramsden, Site Manager

CALGARY: South Health Campus (SHC)
Affiliated with: Alberta Health Services
4448 Front St. SE, Calgary, AB T3M 1M4
Tel: 403-956-1111
www.albertahealthservices.ca/facilities/shc
Social Media: www.facebook.com/179579998746821;
twitter.com/ahs_media; www.youtube.com/user/AHSChannel
Year Founded: 2012
Note: Programs & services include: clinics; angiography;
bronchoscopy; cardiology; child & adolescent addiction & mental
health; CT services; surgery; diabetes; diagnostic imaging;
electroencephalography; electromyography; emergency; endocrinology;
gastrointestinal; general medicine; radiography; hematology; infectious
diseases; intensive care; magnetic resonance; neurology; nuclear
medicine; nutrition; obstetrics; orthopedics; pediatric; pharmacy;
psychiatric; respiratory/pulmonary; rheumatology; speech language
pathology; & ultrasound.

CALGARY: Thornhill Library / Community Health Centre
Affiliated with: Alberta Health Services
Former Name: Thornhill District Office
6617 Centre St. North, Calgary, AB T2K 4Y5
Tel: 403-944-7500 *Fax:* 403-275-9064
www.albertahealthservices.ca

Note: Programs & services include: fluoride protection; immunization;
school health & oral health; & tuberculosis testing

CALGARY: Village Square Community Health Centre
Affiliated with: Alberta Health Services
2623 - 56 St. NE, Calgary, AB T1Y 6E7
Tel: 403-944-7000 *Fax:* 403-285-6304
www.albertahealthservices.ca

Note: Programs & services include: prenatal program; postpartum
services; school health; & Well Child services

CALLING LAKE: Calling Lake Community Health Services
Affiliated with: Alberta Health Services
General Delivery, Calling Lake, AB T0G 0K0
Tel: 780-331-3760 *Fax:* 780-331-2200
www.albertahealthservices.ca

CAMROSE: Camrose Public Health / Rehab
Affiliated with: Alberta Health Services
5510 - 46 Ave., Camrose, AB T4V 4P8
Tel: 780-679-2980 *Fax:* 780-679-2999
www.albertahealthservices.ca

CAMROSE: St. Mary's Hospital
Covenant Health
Affiliated with: Alberta Health Services
4607 - 53 St., Camrose, AB T4V 1Y5
Tel: 780-679-6100 *Fax:* 780-679-6196
www.covenanthealth.ca/hospitals-care-centres/st-marys-hospital
Social Media: www.facebook.com/179579998746821;
twitter.com/AHS_media; www.youtube.com/ahschannel
Year Founded: 1924
Number of Beds: 76 beds
Population Served: 15000
Number of Employees: 389
Note: Programs & services include: emergency; cardiology; diabetic
education; diagnostic imaging (CT scans, fluoroscopy, radiology,
mammography, ultrasound); community cancer clinic; women's health;
pediatrics; palliative care; respiratory therapy; occupational therapy;
mental health; & urology.
Cherylyn Antymniuk, Site Administrator

CANMORE: Canmore General Hospital
Affiliated with: Alberta Health Services
1100 Hospital Pl., Canmore, AB T1W 1N2
Tel: 403-678-5536 *Fax:* 403-678-9874
www.albertahealthservices.ca
Social Media: www.facebook.com/179579998746821;
twitter.com/AHS_media; www.youtube.com/ahschannel
Year Founded: 1984
Number of Employees: 350
Note: Programs & services include: emergency services; diagnostic
imaging; laboratory services; surgical services; obstetrics; newborn
care; acute care; cardiology; audiology; chemotherapy treatments;
wound centre; occupational therapy; physical therapy; recreation
therapy; speech language pathology; mental health; Indigenous Liaison
Hospital services; diabetes prevention; adult day support program;
respite care; long term care; & palliative care.
Kim Chalcroft, Manager, Long-Term Care

CANMORE: Canmore Provincial Building
Affiliated with: Alberta Health Services
Former Name: Canmore Public Health Office
800 Railway Ave., Canmore, AB T1W 1P1
Tel: 403-678-5656 *Fax:* 403-678-5068
www.albertahealthservices.ca

Note: Public health programs

CARDSTON: Cardston Health Centre
Affiliated with: Alberta Health Services
PO Box 1440, 144 - 2nd St. West, Cardston, AB T0K 0K0
Tel: 403-653-5234 *Fax:* 403-653-4399
www.albertahealthservices.ca
Social Media: www.facebook.com/179579998746821;
twitter.com/AHS_media; www.youtube.com/AHSChannel

Note: Programs & services include: continuing care; diagnostic
imaging; emergency; general radiography; laboratory; occupational
therapy; physical therapy; & speech language pathology.

CARDSTON: Cardston Health Unit
Affiliated with: Alberta Health Services
Former Name: Cardston Community Health Centre
576 Main St., Cardston, AB T0K 0K0
Tel: 403-653-5230 *Fax:* 403-653-2926
www.albertahealthservices.ca

Note: Services include: Children's Allied Health Services; prenatal
education; public health nursing; & oral health.

CASTOR: Castor Community Health Centre
Affiliated with: Alberta Health Services
4909 - 50 Ave., Castor, AB T0C 0X0
Tel: 403-882-3404 *Fax:* 403-882-2387
www.albertahealthservices.ca

CASTOR: Our Lady of the Rosary Hospital
Covenant Health
Affiliated with: Alberta Health Services
5402 - 47 St., Castor, AB T0C 0X0
Tel: 403-882-3434 *Fax:* 403-882-2751
www.covenanthealth.ca/hospitals-care-centres/our-lady-of-the-rosary-h
ospital
Social Media: www.facebook.com/179579998746821;
twitter.com/AHS_media; www.youtube.com/ahschannel
Number of Beds: 26 beds
Number of Employees: 85
Note: One of the provincial heritage sites in Castor. Programs &
services include: addiction services; emergency; occupational therapy
(acute & continuing care); speech language pathology; diagnostic
imaging; laboratory; long-term care; palliative care; & pharmacy.
Brenda Brigley, Clinical Manager

CLARESHOLM: Claresholm Community Health Centre
Affiliated with: Alberta Health Services
5221 - 2nd St. West, Claresholm, AB T0L 0T0
Tel: 403-625-4061 *Fax:* 403-625-4062
www.albertahealthservices.ca

CLARESHOLM: Claresholm General Hospital
Affiliated with: Alberta Health Services
221 - 43 Ave. West, Claresholm, AB T0L 0T0
Tel: 403-682-3700 Fax: 403-682-3789
www.albertahealthservices.ca
Social Media: www.facebook.com/179579998746821;
twitter.com/AHS_media; www.youtube.com/AHSChannel
Year Founded: 1972
Number of Beds: 16 beds
Note: Programs & services include: emergency services; diagnostic imaging; cardiology electrocardiogram services; Holter monitoring; acute care; physiotherapy; respite care; & palliative care.

CLARESHOLM: Willow Creek Continuing Care Centre
Affiliated with: Alberta Health Services
4221 - 8 St. West, Claresholm, AB T0L 0T0
Tel: 403-625-3361 Fax: 403-625-3822
www.albertahealthservices.ca
Number of Beds: 100 beds
Note: Continuing care facility

COALDALE: Coaldale Health Centre
Affiliated with: Alberta Health Services
Former Name: Coaldale Community Health
2100 - 11 St., Coaldale, AB T1M 1L2
Tel: 403-345-3075 Fax: 403-345-2681
www.albertahealthservices.ca
Social Media: www.facebook.com/179579998746821;
twitter.com/AHS_media; www.youtube.com/ahschannel

Note: Programs & services include: continuing care; diagnostic imaging; general radiography; laboratory; occupational & physical therapy; primary care; speech language pathology; & therapeutic recreation.

COCHRANE: Cochrane Community Health Centre
Affiliated with: Alberta Health Services
60 Grande Blvd., Cochrane, AB T4C 0S4
Tel: 403-851-6000
www.albertahealthservices.ca

COLD LAKE: Cold Lake Community Health Services
Affiliated with: Alberta Health Services
4720 - 55 St., Cold Lake, AB T9M 1V8
Tel: 780-594-4404 Fax: 780-594-2404
www.albertahealthservices.ca

COLD LAKE: Cold Lake Healthcare Centre
Affiliated with: Alberta Health Services
314 - 25 St., Cold Lake, AB T9M 1G6
Tel: 780-639-3322 Fax: 780-639-2255
www.albertahealthservices.ca
Social Media: www.facebook.com/179579998746821;
twitter.com/AHS_media; www.youtube.com/ahschannel
Number of Beds: 30 continuing care beds; 24 acute care beds
Note: Programs & services include: emergency services; diagnostic imaging services; laboratory services; surgical services; acute care; ambulatory care; obstetrics; pediatrics; eating disorder services; rehabilitation services, including physiotherapy, occupational therapy, recreation therapy, & respiratory therapy; continuing care; dementia care; respite services; & palliative care.
Catherine Garon, Site Manager

CONSORT: Consort Community Health Centre
Affiliated with: Alberta Health Services
5410 - 52 Ave., Consort, AB T0C 1B0
Tel: 403-577-3770 Fax: 403-577-2235
www.albertahealthservices.ca

CONSORT: Consort Hospital & Care Centre
Affiliated with: Alberta Health Services
5402 - 52 Ave., Consort, AB T0C 1B0
Tel: 403-577-3555 Fax: 403-577-3950
www.albertahealthservices.ca
Social Media: www.facebook.com/179579998746821;
twitter.com/AHS_media; www.youtube.com/ahschannel

Note: Programs & services include: emergency services; diagnostic imaging; laboratory services; acute care; occupational therapy; physiotherapy; continuing care; & palliative care.

CORONATION: Coronation Community Health Centre
Affiliated with: Alberta Health Services
4909 Royal St., Coronation, AB T0C 1C0
Tel: 403-578-3200 Fax: 403-578-2702
www.albertahealthservices.ca

CORONATION: Coronation Hospital & Care Centre
Affiliated with: Alberta Health Services
Also Known As: Coronation Hospital
5000 Municipal Rd., Coronation, AB T0C 1C0
Tel: 403-578-3803 Fax: 403-578-3474
www.albertahealthservices.ca
Social Media: www.facebook.com/179579998746821;
twitter.com/AHS_media; www.youtube.com/ahschannel
Number of Beds: 10 acute beds; 19 assisted living beds
Note: Programs & services include: emergency services; diagnostic imaging; laboratory services; acute care; occupational therapy; physical therapy; speech language pathology; continuing care; supportive living; Seniors Mental Health Program; & palliative care.

DAYSLAND: Daysland Health Centre
Affiliated with: Alberta Health Services
5920 - 51st Ave., Daysland, AB T0B 1A0
Tel: 780-374-3746 Fax: 780-374-2111
www.albertahealthservices.ca
Social Media: www.facebook.com/179579998746821;
twitter.com/AHS_media; www.youtube.com/ahschannel
Number of Beds: 16 acute care beds; 10 rehabilitation beds
Note: Programs & services include: emergency services; laboratory services; surgery; acute care; obstetrics; rehabilitation services, including occupational therapy, physiotherapy, & respiratory therapy; pediatric speech language services; respite care; & palliative care.
Paul Vieira, Site Manager

DEVON: Devon General Hospital
Affiliated with: Alberta Health Services
101 Erie St. South, Devon, AB T9G 1A6
Tel: 780-987-8200
www.albertahealthservices.ca
Social Media: www.facebook.com/179579998746821;
twitter.com/AHS_media; www.youtube.com/ahschannel
Number of Beds: 9 acute care beds; 10 continuing care beds; 2 respite beds
Note: Programs & services include: emergency services; laboratory services; radiology services; acute care; rehabilitation services; mental health therapy; public health; tuberculosis testing & immunization; diabetes education; nutrition information; social work; adult day program; home care; & continuing care.
Tod Pharis, Site Manager

DIDSBURY: Didsbury District Health Services
Affiliated with: Alberta Health Services
1210 - 20 Ave., Didsbury, AB T0M 0W0
Tel: 403-335-9393
www.albertahealthservices.ca
Social Media: www.facebook.com/179579998746821;
twitter.com/AHS_media; www.youtube.com/ahschannel

Note: Programs & services include: emergency services; laboratory services; diagnostic imaging; acute care; rehabilitation, including occupational therapy & physiotherapy; speech language pathology; clinical nutrition services; public health services; respite care; long term care; & palliative care.

DRAYTON VALLEY: Drayton Valley Community Health Centre
Affiliated with: Alberta Health Services
4110 - 50 Ave., Drayton Valley, AB T7A 0B3
Tel: 780-542-4415 Fax: 780-621-4998
www.albertahealthservices.ca

DRAYTON VALLEY: Drayton Valley Hospital & Care Centre
Affiliated with: Alberta Health Services
4550 Madsen Ave., Drayton Valley, AB T7A 1N8
Tel: 780-542-5321 Fax: 780-621-4966
www.albertahealthservices.ca
Social Media: www.facebook.com/179579998746821;
twitter.com/AHS_media; www.youtube.com/ahschannel
Number of Beds: 34 acute care beds; 50 long term care beds
Population Served: 23000
Note: Programs & services include: emergency services; diagnostic

imaging; laboratory services; acute care; obstetrics; Northern Alberta Renal Program; occupational therapy, physiotherapy, & recreation therapy; diabetes education; nutrition services; long-term care; & palliative care.
Valerie Larsen, Manager, Acute Care

DRUMHELLER: Drumheller Health Centre
Affiliated with: Alberta Health Services
351 - 9 St. NW, Drumheller, AB T0J 0Y1
Tel: 403-823-6500 *Fax:* 403-823-5076
www.albertahealthservices.ca
Social Media: www.facebook.com/179579998746821;
twitter.com/AHS_media; www.youtube.com/ahschannel

Note: Programs & services include: emergency services; diagnostic imaging; acute care; obstetrics; cardiac rehabilitation program; occupational therapy, physical therapy, & recreation therapy; mental health services; nutrition services; public health; asthma education; continuing care; respite care; home care; & palliative care.
Nancy Guntrip, Site Director

DRUMHELLER: Drumheller Health Centre
Affiliated with: Alberta Health Services
351 - 9 St. NW, Drumheller, AB T0J 0Y1
Tel: 403-820-6004
www.albertahealthservices.ca

EAST PRAIRIE METIS SETTLEMENT: East Prairie Metis Settlement
Affiliated with: Alberta Health Services
East Prairie Metis Settle, AB T0G 1E0
Tel: 780-523-2594
www.albertahealthservices.ca

Note: Services: immunization; oral health

ECKVILLE: Eckville Community Health Centre
Affiliated with: Alberta Health Services
PO Box 150, 5120 - 51 Ave., Eckville, AB T0M 0X0
Tel: 403-746-2201 *Fax:* 403-746-2185
www.albertahealthservices.ca

Note: Programs & services include: continuing care counselling; diagnostic imaging; general radiography; home care; immunization; laboratory; occupational therapy; oral health; palliative care; physical therapy; prenatal education; public health; speech language pathology; & tuberculosis testing.

EDMONTON: Alberta Health Services (AHS)
Seventh Street Plaza, North Tower, 14th Fl., 10030 - 107 St. NW, Edmonton, AB T5J 3E4
Tel: 780-342-2000 *Fax:* 780-342-2060
Toll-Free: 888-342-2471
ahsinfo@albertahealthservices.ca
www.albertahealthservices.ca
Info Line: 811
Social Media: www.facebook.com/179579998746821;
twitter.com/AHS_media; www.youtube.com/ahschannel
Year Founded: 2009
Number of Beds: 23,742 continuing care beds; 8,471 acute care beds; 208 palliative & hospice beds; 2,439 mental health beds
Population Served: 4000000
Note: Provincial governance board, overseeing hospitals, other health facilities, & ground ambulance service in Alberta. The agency employs over 108,000 employees.
Verna Yiu, President & CEO
Dr. David Mador, Vice-President & Medical Director, Northern Alberta
Deb Gordon, Vice-President & Chief Health Operations Officer, Northern Alberta
Brenda Huband, Vice-President & Chief Health Operations Officer, Central & Southern Alberta

EDMONTON: Belvedere Medical Clinic
12720 - 66 St., Edmonton, AB T5C 0A3
Tel: 780-761-8529
www.mddoctors.ca

EDMONTON: Bonnie Doon Public Health Centre
Affiliated with: Alberta Health Services
8314 - 88 Ave. NW, Edmonton, AB T6C 1L1
Tel: 780-342-1520
www.albertahealthservices.ca
Lisa Sereda, Operations Manager

EDMONTON: Boyle McCauley Health Centre
Affiliated with: Alberta Health Services
10628 - 96 St., Edmonton, AB T5H 2J2
Tel: 780-422-7333 *Fax:* 780-422-7343
www.bmhc.net
Social Media: www.facebook.com/BoyleMcCauleyHealthCentre.BMHC;
twitter.com/BMHC_HealthCare

Note: Programs & services include: acupuncture; chiropractic clinic; dental; foot care; medical; mental health; optometry; & women's health clinic
Cecilia Blasetti, Executive Director
cecilia.blasetti@albertahealthservic
Karin Frederiksen, Clinic Coordinator
kfrederiksen@bmhc.net

EDMONTON: Capilano Medical Centre
Medigroup Inc.
Affiliated with: Alberta Health Services
5818 Terrace Rd., Edmonton, AB T6A 3Y8
Tel: 780-761-3330
medigroup.ca

EDMONTON: East Edmonton Health Centre
Affiliated with: Alberta Health Services
7910 - 112 Ave. NW, Edmonton, AB T5B 0C2
Tel: 780-342-4799
www.albertahealthservices.ca

Note: Programs & services include: addiction & mental health; community prenatal program; diagnostic imaging; family care clinic; general radiography; immunization; laboratory; public health; school dental, health, & oral health services; tuberculosis testing; & urgent care
Karen DeViller, Site Director
karen.deviller@albertahealthservices

EDMONTON: Eastwood Medical Clinic
Affiliated with: Alberta Health Services
7919 - 118 Ave., Edmonton, AB T5B 0R5
Tel: 780-756-3666

EDMONTON: Glenrose Rehabilitation Hospital
Affiliated with: Alberta Health Services
10230 - 111 Ave. NW, Edmonton, AB T5G 0B7
Tel: 780-735-7999
www.ahs.ca/grh
Social Media: www.facebook.com/179579998746821;
twitter.com/AHS_media; www.youtube.com/AHSChannel
Year Founded: 1964
Number of Beds: 244 beds
Note: Rehabilitation centre for both adults & children; research & training centre for rehabilitation fields.
Lisa Froese, Site Director
Isabel Henderson, Senior Operating Officer
Dr. Gary Faulkner, Director, Rehabilitation Research & Technology Development

EDMONTON: Grey Nuns Community Hospital
Covenant Health
Affiliated with: Alberta Health Services
Former Name: Grey Nuns Community Hospital & Health Centre
1100 Youville Dr. West, Edmonton, AB T6L 5X8
Tel: 780-735-7000
www.covenanthealth.ca/hospitals-care-centres/grey-nuns-community-hospital
Social Media: www.facebook.com/179579998746821;
twitter.com/AHS_media; www.youtube.com/ahschannel
Number of Beds: 351 beds
Note: Programs & services include: emergency; general & vascular surgery; intensive & cardiac care; children's health; women's health; diagnostics; & mental health.

EDMONTON: Kensington Medical Clinic
Medigroup Inc.
Affiliated with: Alberta Health Services
12620A - 132 Ave., Edmonton, AB T5L 3P9

Tel: 780-990-1820
medigroup.ca

EDMONTON: Lois Hole Hospital for Women
Royal Alexandra Hospital
Affiliated with: Alberta Health Services
10240 Kingsway Ave., Edmonton, AB T5H 3V9

Tel: 780-735-4111
www.albertahealthservices.ca
Social Media: www.facebook.com/LoisHoleHospitalForWomen

Note: Programs & services include: clinical care (high-risk obstetrics, gynecological services & surgery); & innovation, research, education & prevention in women's health issues. Located within the Royal Alexandra Hospital.
Janie Tyrrell, Executive Director, Women's Health

EDMONTON: Millwoods Public Health Centre
Affiliated with: Alberta Health Services
7525 - 38 Ave. NW, Edmonton, AB T6K 3X9

Tel: 780-342-1660
www.albertahealthservices.ca

EDMONTON: Misericordia Community Hospital
Covanent Health
Affiliated with: Alberta Health Services
Former Name: Misericordia Community Hospital & Health Centre
16940 - 87 Ave., Edmonton, AB T5R 4H5

Tel: 780-735-2000
www.albertahealthservices.ca
Social Media: www.facebook.com/179579998746821;
twitter.com/AHS_media; www.youtube.com/ahschannel
Number of Beds: 259 beds
Note: Programs & services include: emergency care; surgery; orthopedics; urology; plastic surgery; intensive & coronary care; pediatrics; geriatrics; mental health; women's health; diagnostics; & ambulatory care. The hospital is also home to the Institute for Reconstructive Sciences in Medicine (iRSM) & the Mother Rosalie Health Services Centre.

EDMONTON: Mother Rosalie Health Services Centre
Misericordia Community Hospital
Affiliated with: Alberta Health Services
16930 - 87 Ave., Edmonton, AB T5R 4H5

Tel: 780-735-2413 *Fax:* 780-735-2414
www.albertahealthservices.ca

Note: Programs & services include: diabetes education; urodynamics; child health; outpatient psychiatry; & physiotherapy.

EDMONTON: Northeast Community Health Centre
Affiliated with: Alberta Health Services
14007 - 50 St., Edmonton, AB T5A 5E4

Tel: 780-342-4000
www.albertahealthservices.ca

EDMONTON: Northgate Centre
Affiliated with: Alberta Health Services
9499 - 137 Ave., Edmonton, AB T5E 5R8

Tel: 780-342-2800 *Fax:* 780-457-5638
www.albertahealthservices.ca

Note: Programs & services include: immunization; health education; assessments & screenings; referral; & community resources

EDMONTON: Royal Alexandra Hospital
Affiliated with: Alberta Health Services
10240 Kingsway Ave., Edmonton, AB T5H 3V9

Tel: 780-735-4111
www.albertahealthservices.ca
Social Media: www.facebook.com/179579998746821;
twitter.com/AHS_media; www.youtube.com/ahschannel
Number of Beds: 678 beds
Note: Programs & services include: emergency; acute care of the elderly; clinics; otolaryngology; angiography; child & adolescent psychiatry; colonoscopy; diagnostic imaging; electroencephalography;

gastroscopy; radiology; intensive care; mental health; nutrition counselling; ophthalmology; plastics surgery; rehabilitation services; sexual assault response team; ultrasound; & urology. Located in this hospital is the Lois Hole Hospital for Women.

EDMONTON: Rutherford Health Centre
Affiliated with: Alberta Health Services
11153 Ellerslie Rd. SW, Edmonton, AB T6W 0E9

Tel: 780-342-6800
www.albertahealthservices.ca

Note: Programs & services include: addiction & mental health; immunization; public health; school health & oral health services; & tuberculosis testing

EDMONTON: St. Joseph's Auxiliary Hospital
Covenant Health
Affiliated with: Alberta Health Services
10707 - 29 Ave. NW, Edmonton, AB T6J 6W1

Tel: 780-430-9110 *Fax:* 780-430-9777
www.covenanthealth.ca
Year Founded: 1927
Number of Beds: 202 beds
Note: Continuing care hospital
Sandi Clarke, Program Manager, Care & Nursing

EDMONTON: Seventh Street Plaza
Affiliated with: Alberta Health Services
10030 - 107 St., Edmonton, AB T5J 3E4

Tel: 780-735-0010
www.albertahealthservices.ca

Note: Programs & services include: birth control centre; immunization; & travel health

EDMONTON: Stollery Children's Hospital
University of Alberta Hospital
Affiliated with: Alberta Health Services
8440 - 112 St., Edmonton, AB T6G 2B7

Tel: 780-407-8822
www.albertahealthservices.ca
Area Served: Northern & Central Alberta; parts of Manitoba
Specialties: Organ transplantation
Note: Western Canada's referral centre for pediatric cardiac surgery. Programs & services include: clinics; audiology; Child & Adolescent Protection Centre; chronic pain service; Diabetes Education Centre; diagnostic imaging; endocrinology; gastroenterology & nutrition; hematology; home nutrition support/dietician; infectious diseases; medicine; Neonatal Intensive Care Unit; Northern Alberta Children's Cancer Program; Northern Alberta Pediatric Sleep Program; occupational & physical therapy; otolaryngology; palliative care; Pediatric Comprehensive Epilepsy Program; feeding & swallowing service; hemophilia; intensive care; Medicine/Surgical Ambulatory Unit; neurology; social work; speech language pathology; & surgery.

EDMONTON: Tipaskan Medical Clinic
#3236, 3206 - 82 St., Edmonton, AB T6K 3Y3

Tel: 780-761-3335
www.mddoctors.ca

EDMONTON: Twin Brooks Public Health Centre
Affiliated with: Alberta Health Services
1110 - 113 St. NW, Edmonton, AB T6J 7J4

Tel: 780-342-1560
www.albertahealthservices.ca

Note: Programs & services include: immunization; health education; assessments & screenings; referral; & community resources

EDMONTON: West Jasper Place Public Health Centre
Affiliated with: Alberta Health Services
9720 - 182 St., Edmonton, AB T5T 3T9

Tel: 780-342-1234 *Fax:* 780-484-9516
www.albertahealthservices.ca

Note: Programs & services include: fluoride protection; immunization; public health; school dental, nursing, & health services; & tuberculosis testing

EDMONTON: Westmount Medical Clinic
Medigroup Inc.
Affiliated with: Alberta Health Services
11035 Groat Rd., Edmonton, AB T5M 3J9
Tel: 780-705-4090
medigroup.ca

EDMONTON: Woodcroft Public Health Centre
Affiliated with: Alberta Health Services
Westmount Shopping Centre, 111 Ave. & Groat Rd., Edmonton, AB T5M 4B7
Tel: 780-342-1600 *Fax:* 780-451-5886
www.albertahealthservices.ca

EDSON: Edson Community Health Services
Affiliated with: Alberta Health Services
5028 - 3 Ave., Edson, AB T7E 1X4
Tel: 780-723-4421 *Fax:* 780-723-6299
www.albertahealthservices.ca

EDSON: Edson Healthcare Centre
Affiliated with: Alberta Health Services
3837 - 6 Ave., Edson, AB T7E 0C5
Tel: 780-723-3331 *Fax:* 780-723-7787
www.albertahealthservices.ca
Social Media: www.facebook.com/179579998746821;
twitter.com/AHS_media; www.youtube.com/AHSChannel

Note: Programs & services include: emergency; diagnostic imaging; laboratory services; surgical services & recovery; acute care; ambulatory care; obstetrics; pediatrics; rehabilitation services; social work; respite care; community health; pharmacy; & palliative care.

EDSON: Edson Healthcare Centre
Affiliated with: Alberta Health Services
4716 - 5 Ave., Edson, AB T7E 1S8
Tel: 780-723-2229 *Fax:* 780-723-2135
Toll-Free: 855-371-4122
www.albertahealthservices.ca

ELIZABETH METIS SETTLEMENT: Elizabeth Settlement Community Health Services
Affiliated with: Alberta Health Services
Elizabeth Metis Settlement, AB T9M 1V8
Tel: 780-594-3383 *Fax:* 780-594-3384
www.albertahealthservices.ca

Note: Programs & services include: home care; immunization; Indigenous Health Program; oral health; postpartum support; sexual health; & tuberculosis testing

ELK POINT: Elk Point Community Health Services
Affiliated with: Alberta Health Services
5310 - 50th Ave., Elk Point, AB T0A 1A0
Tel: 780-724-3532 *Fax:* 780-724-2867
www.albertahealthservices.ca

ELK POINT: Elk Point Healthcare Centre
Affiliated with: Alberta Health Services
5310 - 50th Ave., Elk Point, AB T0A 1A0
Tel: 780-724-3847 *Fax:* 780-724-3085
www.albertahealthservices.ca
Social Media: www.facebook.com/179579998746821;
twitter.com/AHS_media; www.youtube.com/ahschannel
Number of Beds: 12 beds
Note: Programs & services include: pharmacy; recreation therapy; rehabilitation services; & x-ray.
Kristen Peleshok, Site Manager

ELNORA: Elnora Community Health Centre
Affiliated with: Alberta Health Services
PO Box 659, 425 - 8 Ave., Elnora, AB T0M 0Y0
Tel: 403-773-3636 *Fax:* 403-773-3949
www.albertahealthservices.ca

FAIRVIEW: Fairview Health Complex
Affiliated with: Alberta Health Services
10628 - 110 St., Fairview, AB T0H 1L0
Tel: 780-835-6100 *Fax:* 780-835-5789
www.albertahealthservices.ca
Social Media: www.facebook.com/179579998746821;
twitter.com/AHS_media; www.youtube.com/ahschannel
Number of Beds: 22 beds
Note: Programs & services include: Early Intervention Program; emergency services; intensive care unit; acute care; obstetrics; pediatrics; rehabilitation services, including occupational therapy, physiotherapy, & therapeutic recreation; mental health services; prenatal education & counselling; Environmental Public Health Program; Newborn Hearing Screening Program; Respiratory Health Program; social work; nutrition services; continuing care; & palliative care.
Jamie Halliday, Site Administrator

FISHING LAKE METIS SETTLEMENT: Fishing Lake Metis Settlement Community Health Services
Affiliated with: Alberta Health Services
Fishing Lake Metis Settlement, AB T0A 1A0
Tel: 780-943-3058 *Fax:* 780-943-2213
www.albertahealthservices.ca

Note: Programs & services include: home care; immunization; Indigenous Health Program; oral health; postpartum support; sexual health; & tuberculosis testing

FORT MACLEOD: Fort Macleod Community Health
Affiliated with: Alberta Health Services
744 - 26 St. South, Fort MacLeod, AB T0L 0Z0
Tel: 403-553-5351 *Fax:* 403-553-4567
www.albertahealthservices.ca

Note: Programs & services include: environmental public health; prenatal education; & public health nursing.

FORT MACLEOD: Fort Macleod Health Centre
Affiliated with: Alberta Health Services
744 - 26 St. South, Fort MacLeod, AB T0L 0Z0
Tel: 403-553-5311 *Fax:* 403-553-4567
www.albertahealthservices.ca

Angela McLeod, Site Manager

FORT MCMURRAY: Fort McMurray Community Health Services
Affiliated with: Alberta Health Services
113 Thickwood Blvd., Fort McMurray, AB T9H 5E5
Tel: 780-791-6247 *Fax:* 780-791-6282
www.albertahealthservices.ca

Note: Services: immunization; public health nursing

FORT MCMURRAY: Northern Lights Regional Health Centre
Affiliated with: Alberta Health Services
7 Hospital St., Fort McMurray, AB T9H 1P2
Tel: 780-791-6161 *Fax:* 780-791-6167
www.albertahealthservices.ca
Social Media: www.facebook.com/179579998746821;
twitter.com/AHS_media; www.youtube.com/ahschannel

Note: Programs & services include: emergency; laboratory; x-ray; mental health; general surgery; ambulatory care; rehabilitation; home care; speech language; & community health.
David Matear, Senior Operating Director

FORT SASKATCHEWAN: Fort Saskatchewan Community Hospital
Affiliated with: Alberta Health Services
Former Name: Fort Saskatchewan Health Centre
9401 - 86 Ave., Fort Saskatchewan, AB T8L 0C6
Tel: 780-998-2256
www.albertahealthservices.ca
Social Media: www.facebook.com/179579998746821;
twitter.com/AHS_media; www.youtube.com/ahschannel
Number of Beds: 32 beds
Note: Programs & services include: emergency; surgery; public health; home care addiction & mental health; audiology; respiratory therapy; occupational therapy; & nutritional counselling.
Heather Ward, Director

FORT SASKATCHEWAN: Sherrit Health Centre
Affiliated with: Alberta Health Services
Former Name: Fort Saskatchewan Health
9401 - 86 Ave., Fort Saskatchewan, AB T8L 0C6
Tel: 780-342-2366 *Fax:* 780-342-3342
www.albertahealthservices.ca

FORT VERMILION: Fort Vermilion Community Health Centre
Affiliated with: Alberta Health Services
4804 - 50 St., Fort Vermilion, AB T0H 1N0
Tel: 780-927-3391
www.albertahealthservices.ca

Note: Programs & services include: mental health; home care; STI program; speech & language; travel health; & tuberculosis testing

FORT VERMILION: St. Theresa General Hospital
Affiliated with: Alberta Health Services
4506 - 46 Ave., Fort Vermilion, AB T0H 1N0
Tel: 780-927-3761 *Fax:* 780-927-6207
www.albertahealthservices.ca
Social Media: www.facebook.com/179579998746821;
twitter.com/AHS_media; www.youtube.com/ahschannel
Number of Beds: 36 acute care beds; 10 long-term care beds
Note: Programs & services include: emergency; clinical nutrition; continuing care; diagnostic imaging; interpretive services; laboratory; maternity; mental health; occupational therapy; palliative care; pediatrics; physical therapy; & spiritual care.

FOX CREEK: Fox Creek Healthcare Centre
Affiliated with: Alberta Health Services
600 - 3rd St., Fox Creek, AB T0H 1P0
Tel: 780-622-3545 *Fax:* 780-622-3474
www.albertahealthservices.ca
Social Media: www.facebook.com/179579998746821;
twitter.com/AHS_media; www.youtube.com/ahschannel
Number of Beds: 4 acute care beds
Note: Programs & services include: clinics; community health; diagnostic imaging; emergency services; environmental services; general radiography; laboratory services; acute care; pediatrics; diabetes education; mental health; nutrition; oral health; home care; palliative care; Parenting Preschoolers; pharmacy; speech language pathology; travel health services; & tuberculosis testing.

FOX CREEK: Fox Creek Healthcare Centre
Affiliated with: Alberta Health Services
Former Name: Aspen Health Services
600 - 3rd St., Fox Creek, AB T0H 1P0
Tel: 780-622-3730 *Fax:* 780-622-3474
www.albertahealthservices.ca

GIBBONS: Gibbons Health Unit
Affiliated with: Alberta Health Services
4720 - 50 Ave., Gibbons, AB T0A 1N0
Tel: 780-342-2660
www.albertahealthservices.ca

GIFT LAKE: Gift Lake Community Health Services
Affiliated with: Alberta Health Services
Main St., Gift Lake, AB T0G 1B0
Tel: 780-767-2101 *Fax:* 780-767-2490
www.albertahealthservices.ca

GLENDON: Glendon Community Health Services
Affiliated with: Alberta Health Services
Former Name: Glendon Community Health Clinic
2 St. Railway Ave., Glendon, AB T0A 1P0
Tel: 780-635-3861 *Fax:* 780-635-4213
www.albertahealthservices.ca

Note: Programs & services include: general medicine; immunization; laboratory; social work; & tuberculosis testing.

GRANDE CACHE: Grande Cache Community Health Complex
Affiliated with: Alberta Health Services
10200 Shand Ave., Grande Cache, AB T0E 0Y0
Tel: 780-827-3701 *Fax:* 780-827-2859
www.albertahealthservices.ca
Social Media: www.facebook.com/179579998746821;
twitter.com/AHS_media; www.youtube.com/ahschannel

Number of Beds: 10 acute care beds; 4 continuing care beds
Note: Programs & services include: cardiology; continuing care; diagnostic imaging; emergency; environmental; general radiography; laboratory services; nutrition; occupational & physical therapy; palliative care; pediatrics; & respiratory health.

GRANDE CACHE: Grande Cache Provincial Building
Affiliated with: Alberta Health Services
Public Health Centre, 10001 Hoppe Ave., Grande Cache, AB T0E 0Y0
Tel: 780-827-3504 *Fax:* 780-827-2728
www.albertahealthservices.ca

GRANDE PRAIRIE: Community Village
Affiliated with: Alberta Health Services
10116 - 102 Ave., Grande Prairie, AB T8V 1A1
Tel: 780-532-4494
admin@thecommunityvillage.ca
www.thecommunityvillage.ca

Note: Offers immunization clinics, wellness clinics, nurse practitioner, & other services
Bev Moylan, Program Manager
bev.moylan@albertahealthservices.ca

GRANDE PRAIRIE: Grande Prairie College & Community Health Centre
Affiliated with: Alberta Health Services
10620 - 104 Ave., Grande Prairie, AB T8V 8J8
Tel: 780-814-5800 *Fax:* 780-538-4400
www.albertahealthservices.ca

Note: Programs & services include: physician; nurse practitioner; dietitian; nutrition; mental health; diagnostic imaging; immunization; laboratory; & sexual health

GRANDE PRAIRIE: Grande Prairie Provincial Building
Affiliated with: Alberta Health Services
Former Name: Public Health Centre
10320 - 99 St., Grande Prairie, AB T8V 6J4
Tel: 780-513-7500
www.albertahealthservices.ca

GRANDE PRAIRIE: Grande Prairie Virene Building (Home Care)
Affiliated with: Alberta Health Services
10121 - 97 Ave., Grande Prairie, AB T8V 0N5
Tel: 780-532-4447 *Fax:* 780-532-2477
Toll-Free: 855-371-4122
www.albertahealthservices.ca

GRANDE PRAIRIE: Queen Elizabeth II Hospital
Affiliated with: Alberta Health Services
10409 - 98 St., Grande Prairie, AB T8V 2E8
Tel: 780-538-7100
www.albertahealthservices.ca
Social Media: www.facebook.com/179579998746821;
twitter.com/AHS_media; www.youtube.com/ahschannel
Year Founded: 1978
Number of Beds: 167 beds
Population Served: 250000
Note: Programs & services include: Indigenous health; acute care; hip & knee clinics; angiography; cardiology; computed tomography; continuing care; day surgery; diagnostic imaging; EEG; echocardiography; emergency; fluoroscopy; general radiography; hemodialysis; intensive care; laboratory; obstetrics; magnetic resonance imaging; mammography; medicine; nuclear medicine; occupational therapy; orthopedics; pediatrics; pharmacy; respiratory; social work; ultrasound; & urology.

GRIMSHAW: Grimshaw/Berwyn & District Community Health Centre
Affiliated with: Alberta Health Services
5621 Wilcox Rd., Grimshaw, AB T0H 1W0
Tel: 780-332-6500 *Fax:* 780-332-1177
www.albertahealthservices.ca
Social Media: www.facebook.com/179579998746821;
twitter.com/AHS_media; www.youtube.com/AHSChannel

Note: Programs & services include: clinics; community health; continuing care; diagnostic imaging; emergency; environmental;

general radiography; home care; laboratory; palliative care; physical therapy; social work; travel health services; & tuberculosis testing.

HANNA: Hanna Health Centre
Affiliated with: Alberta Health Services
904 Centre St. North, Hanna, AB T0J 1P0
Tel: 403-854-3331 Fax: 403-854-3253
www.albertahealthservices.ca
Social Media: www.facebook.com/179579998746821;
twitter.com/AHS_media; www.youtube.com/ahschannel
Number of Beds: 18 acute care beds; 49 continuing care beds
Note: Programs & services include: acute care; continuing care; emergency; minor surgery; obstetrics; mental health; & palliative care.
Sandra Rubbelke, Site Manager

HANNA: Hanna Health Centre
Affiliated with: Alberta Health Services
Former Name: Hanna Health Unit
PO Box 730, 904 Centre St. North, Hanna, AB T0J 1P0
Tel: 403-854-5236 Fax: 403-854-3253
www.albertahealthservices.ca

HARDISTY: Hardisty Health Centre
Affiliated with: Alberta Health Services
PO Box 269, 4531 - 47 Ave., Hardisty, AB T0B 1V0
Tel: 780-888-3742 Fax: 780-888-2427
www.albertahealthservices.ca
Social Media: www.facebook.com/179579998746821;
twitter.com/AHS_media; www.youtube.com/ahschannel
Number of Beds: 5 acute care beds; 14 long-term care beds; 1 respite bed
Note: Programs & services include: acute care; clinics; child & adolescent services; diagnostic imaging; emergency; general radiography; laboratory services; long-term care; mental health; nutrition; occupational & physical therapy; palliative care; pulmonary/respiratory; respite care; speech language services; & Vital Heart Response/STEMI Program.

HIGH LEVEL: Northwest Health Centre
Affiliated with: Alberta Health Services
11202 - 100 Ave., High Level, AB T0H 1Z0
Tel: 780-841-3200 Fax: 780-926-7378
www.albertahealthservices.ca
Social Media: www.facebook.com/179579998746821;
twitter.com/AHS_media; www.youtube.com/ahschannel

Note: Programs & services include: acute care; community health; community nutrition; continuing care; emergency; mental health; laboratory; public health; palliative care; & x-ray.

HIGH PRAIRIE: High Prairie Health Complex
Affiliated with: Alberta Health Services
4620 - 53 Ave., High Prairie, AB T0G 1E0
Tel: 780-523-6440 Fax: 780-523-6642
www.albertahealthservices.ca
Social Media: www.facebook.com/179579998746821;
twitter.com/AHS_media; www.youtube.com/ahschannel
Number of Beds: 30 acute care beds; 67 continuing care beds
Note: Programs & services include: acute care; continuing care; emergency; rehabilitation; palliative care; pediatrics; radiology; recreational therapy; & speech-language pathology.
Roxanne Stuckless, Director, Clinical Operations

HIGH PRAIRIE: High Prairie Public Health Centre
Affiliated with: Alberta Health Services
4620 - 53 Ave., High Prairie, AB T0G 1E0
Tel: 780-523-6450 Fax: 780-523-6458
www.albertahealthservices.ca

Note: Services: immunization & public health nursing

HIGH RIVER: High River General Hospital
Affiliated with: Alberta Health Services
560 - 9 Ave. SW, High River, AB T1V 1B3
Tel: 403-652-2200 Fax: 403-652-0199
www.albertahealthservices.ca
Social Media: www.facebook.com/179579998746821;
twitter.com/AHS_media; www.youtube.com/ahschannel
Year Founded: 1982
Number of Beds: 32 active treatment beds; 75 long-term care beds

Note: Programs & services include: cancer treatment & care; cardiology; CT imaging; continuing care; diagnostic imaging; emergency services; gynecological surgery; holter monitoring; laboratory; nutrition; & physical therapy.

HIGH RIVER: High River Public Health Centre
Affiliated with: Alberta Health Services
310 Macleod Trail SW, High River, AB T1V 1M7
Tel: 403-652-5450 Fax: 403-652-5455
www.albertahealthservices.ca

HINTON: Hinton Healthcare Centre
Affiliated with: Alberta Health Services
1280 Switzer Dr., Hinton, AB T7V 1V2
Tel: 780-865-3333 Fax: 780-865-1099
www.albertahealthservices.ca
Social Media: www.facebook.com/179579998746821;
twitter.com/AHS_media; www.youtube.com/ahschannel
Number of Beds: 23 beds; 1 palliative bed
Note: Programs & services include: acute care; community cancer centre; diabetic nephropathy; pharmacy; rehabilitation; ultrasound; x-ray, CT scan; & MRI.
Fiona Murray-Galbraith, Site Manager

INNISFAIL: Innisfail Health Centre
Affiliated with: Alberta Health Services
5023 - 42 St., Innisfail, AB T4G 1A9
Tel: 403-227-7800 Fax: 403-227-8781
www.albertahealthservices.ca
Social Media: www.facebook.com/179579998746821;
twitter.com/AHS_media; www.youtube.com/ahschannel

Note: Programs & services include: addiction & mental health services; child & adolescent services; community health; continuing care; diagnostic imaging; emergency; general radiography; laboratory services; long-term care; nutrition; occupational & physical therapy; oral health program; palliative care; pharmacy; public health; pulmonary function testing; rehabilitation; respite care; speech language pathology; spiritual care; & tuberculosis testing.

JASPER: Seton - Jasper Healthcare Centre
Affiliated with: Alberta Health Services
PO Box 310, 518 Robson St., Jasper, AB T0E 1E0
Tel: 780-852-3344 Fax: 780-852-3413
www.albertahealthservices.ca
Social Media: www.facebook.com/179579998746821;
twitter.com/AHS_media; www.youtube.com/ahschannel
Number of Beds: 12 active treatment beds; 16 long-term care beds
Note: Programs & services include: emergency; acute care services; diagnostic imaging; eating disorder services; mental health services; occupational therapy; palliative care; physiotherapy; & social work.
Lorna Chisholm, Site Manager

JASPER: Seton - Jasper Healthcare Centre
Affiliated with: Alberta Health Services
Former Name: Jasper Community Health Services
Public Health Centre, PO Box 310, 518 Robson St., Jasper, AB T0E 1E0
Tel: 780-852-4759
www.albertahealthservices.ca

KIKINO: Kikino Metis Settlement Community Health Services
Affiliated with: Alberta Health Services
Kikino, AB T0A 2B0
Tel: 780-623-7797 Fax: 780-623-4212
www.albertahealthservices.ca

KILLAM: Killam Health Care Centre
Covenant Health
Affiliated with: Alberta Health Services
5203 - 49 Ave., Killam, AB T0B 2L0
Tel: 780-385-3741 Fax: 780-385-3904
www.covenanthealth.ca/hospitals-care-centres/killam-health-centre
Social Media: www.facebook.com/179579998746821;
twitter.com/AHS_media; www.youtube.com/AHSChannel
Year Founded: 1930
Number of Beds: 50 beds
Number of Employees: 103
Note: Programs & services include: adult day support; Asthma Education Program; continuing care; diagnostic imaging; emergency;

general radiography; laboratory; long-term care; palliative care; respiratory/pulmonary; respite care; & Vital Heart Response/STEMI Program.
Geri Clark, Chief Executive Officer

KINUSO: Kinuso Community Health Services
Affiliated with: Alberta Health Services
230 Centre St., Kinuso, AB T0G 1K0
Tel: 780-775-3501 *Fax:* 780-775-3944
www.albertahealthservices.ca

KITSCOTY: Kitscoty Community Health Centre
Affiliated with: Alberta Health Services
4922 - 49 Ave., Kitscoty, AB T0B 2P0
Tel: 780-846-2824 *Fax:* 780-846-2731
www.albertahealthservices.ca

LA CRETE: La Crete Continuing Care Centre
Affiliated with: Alberta Health Services
Former Name: La Crete Health Centre
10601 - 100 Ave., La Crete, AB T0H 2H0
Tel: 780-928-3242 *Fax:* 780-928-4237
www.albertahealthservices.ca

Note: Offers community health services as well as continuing care.

LAC LA BICHE: Lac La Biche Provincial Building
Affiliated with: Alberta Health Services
Former Name: Lac La Biche Community Health Services
PO Box 297, 9503 Beaverhill Rd., Lac La Biche, AB T0A 2C0
Tel: 780-623-4471
www.albertahealthservices.ca

LAC LA BICHE: William J. Cadzow - Lac La Biche Healthcare Centre
Affiliated with: Alberta Health Services
9110 - 93 St., Lac La Biche, AB T0A 2C0
Tel: 780-623-4404 *Fax:* 780-623-5904
www.albertahealthservices.ca
Social Media: www.facebook.com/179579998746821; twitter.com/AHS_media; www.youtube.com/ahschannel
Number of Beds: 23 acute care beds; 42 long-term care beds; 1 palliative bed; 1 respite bed
Note: Programs & services include: ambulatory services; clinics; continuing care; day surgery; diagnostic imaging; emergency; environmental; general medicine; general radiography; hemodialysis; laboratory; nutrition; obstetrics; occupational & physical therapy; palliative care; pastoral care; pediatrics; pharmacy; respiratory; respite care; social work; special care unit; stress testing; & therapeutic recreation.

LACOMBE: Lacombe Community Health Centre
Affiliated with: Alberta Health Services
5010 - 51 St., Lacombe, AB T4L 1W2
Tel: 403-782-3218 *Fax:* 403-782-2866
www.albertahealthservices.ca

Note: Programs & services include: community health; continuing care; home care; clinics; oral health; prenatal education; public health; rehabilitation; travel health; & tuberculosis testing.

LACOMBE: Lacombe Hospital & Care Centre
Affiliated with: Alberta Health Services
5430 - 47 Ave., Lacombe, AB T4L 1G8
Tel: 403-782-3336 *Fax:* 403-782-2818
www.albertahealthservices.ca
Social Media: www.facebook.com/179579998746821; twitter.com/AHS_media; www.youtube.com/ahschannel
Number of Beds: 24 beds; 75 long-term care beds; 2 palliative care suites; 5 transition beds
Note: Programs & services include: acute care; continuing care; crisis response team (rural); diagnostic imaging; emergency; general radiography; laboratory; long-term care; nutrition; obstetrics; occupational & physical therapy; palliative care; pharmacy; pulmonary; speech language pathology; spiritual care; surgery; & ultrasound.

LAMONT: Lamont Health Care Centre
Affiliated with: Alberta Health Services
PO Box 479, 5216 - 53 St., Lamont, AB T0B 2R0
Tel: 780-895-2211 *Fax:* 780-895-7305
www.lamonthealthcarecentre.com

Year Founded: 1912
Number of Beds: 14 acute beds; 101 continuing care beds; 2 palliative care beds; 2 respite beds; 6 day surgery beds; 2 surgical suites
Population Served: 10000
Note: Programs & services include: acute & continuing care; emergency; general radiography; occupational therapy; mental health services; rehabilitation; & palliative care. Affiliated with the United Church of Canada.
Harold James, CEO

LAMONT: Lamont Health Care Centre
Affiliated with: Alberta Health Services
PO Box 479, 5216 - 53 St., Lamont, AB T0B 2R0
Tel: 780-895-2211 *Fax:* 780-895-7305
www.lamonthealthcarecentre.com

Note: Affiliated with the United Church of Canada.
Harold James, Executive Director

LEDUC: Leduc Community Hospital
Affiliated with: Alberta Health Services
Former Name: Leduc Community Hospital & Health Centre
4210 - 48 St., Leduc, AB T9E 5Z3
Tel: 780-986-7711
www.albertahealthservices.ca
Social Media: www.facebook.com/179579998746821; twitter.com/AHS_media; www.youtube.com/ahschannel
Number of Beds: 34 acute beds; 22 subacute beds; 14 transition beds
Note: Programs & services include: inpatient medical & surgical care; general & specialized day surgery; rehabilitation programs; laboratory services; diagnostic imaging; outpatient clinics; emergency; audiology; echocardiography; endoscopy; fluoroscopy; radiography; infectious diseases; nutrition; pediatrics; Pulmonary Rehabilitation Program; Sexual Assault Response Team; social work; & ultrasound.
Dr. Bob Simard, Medical Director

LEDUC: Leduc Public Health Centre
Affiliated with: Alberta Health Services
4219 - 50 St., Leduc, AB T9E 8C9
Tel: 780-980-4644 *Fax:* 780-980-4666
www.albertahealthservices.ca

Note: Programs & services include: immunization; health education; assessments & screenings; & referral

LETHBRIDGE: Chinook Regional Hospital
Affiliated with: Alberta Health Services
Former Name: Lethbridge Regional Hospital
960 - 19 St. South, Lethbridge, AB T1J 1W5
Tel: 403-388-6111 *Fax:* 403-388-6011
www.albertahealthservices.ca
Social Media: www.facebook.com/179579998746821; twitter.com/AHS_media; www.youtube.com/AHSChannel
Year Founded: 1988
Number of Beds: 270 beds
Population Served: 150000
Note: Programs & services include: acute geriatrics; angiography; breast health program; cardiology; CT imaging; surgery; diagnostic imaging; echocardiography; emergency; fluoroscopy; clinics; general radiography; hemodialysis; laboratory; children & adolescent mental health program; labour delivery & maternal child services; magnetic resonance imaging; occupational therapy; palliative care; post partum & gynecology; pediatrics; social work; speech language pathology; therapeutic recreation; & ultrasound.
Diane Shanks, Director, Critical Care & Emergency

LETHBRIDGE: Lethbridge Community Health Centre
Affiliated with: Alberta Health Services
801 - 1 Ave. South, Lethbridge, AB T1J 4L5
Tel: 403-388-6666 *Fax:* 403-328-5934
www.albertahealthservices.ca

Note: Includes prenatal education

LETHBRIDGE: St. Michael's Health Centre
Covenant Health
Affiliated with: Alberta Health Services
1400 - 9 Ave. South, Lethbridge, AB T1J 4V5
Tel: 403-382-6400 *Fax:* 403-382-6413
www.covenanthealth.ca

Year Founded: 1929
Number of Beds: 210 beds
Note: A long-term care (continuing care) facility focusing on assisted living, palliative care, & post-acute rehabilitative program; offers the Bridges program (care for the elderly in their own home).

MAGRATH: Magrath Community Health Centre
Affiliated with: Alberta Health Services
Former Name: Magrath Hospital
PO Box 550, 37E - 2 Ave. North, Magrath, AB T0K 1J0
Tel: 403-758-4422 *Fax:* 403-758-3332
www.albertahealthservices.ca

Note: Programs & services include: diagnostic imaging; general radiography; laboratory; occupational therapy; physical therapy; public health nursing; respiratory therapy; & speech language pathology.

MANNING: Manning Community Health Centre
Affiliated with: Alberta Health Services
600 - 2 St. NE, Manning, AB T0H 2M0
Tel: 780-836-3391 *Fax:* 780-836-7352
www.albertahealthservices.ca
Social Media: www.facebook.com/179579998746821; twitter.com/AHS_media; www.youtube.com/ahschannel
Number of Beds: 10 acute care beds; 16 long-term care beds
Note: Programs & services include: acute care; clinics; cardiology; community health services; continuing care; diabetes prevention & wellness program; diagnostic imaging; early childhood development; eating disorder services; emergency; environmental; general radiography; home care; laboratory; mental health; newborn hearing screening program; nutrition; occupational & physical therapy; oral health; palliative care; pediatrics; pharmacy; prenatal education; P.A.R.T.Y. (Prevent Alcohol & Risk Related Trauma in Youth); respiratory; social work; therapeutic recreation; travel health; tuberculosis testing; & ultrasound.
Jo Kelemen, Site Manager

MANNING: Manning Community Health Centre
Affiliated with: Alberta Health Services
Former Name: Peace Country Health Unit
PO Box 1260, 600 - 2 St. NE, Manning, AB T0H 2M0
Tel: 780-836-7361
www.albertahealthservices.ca
Jo Kelemen, Site Manager

MANNVILLE: Mannville Care Centre
Affiliated with: Alberta Health Services
5007 - 46 St., Mannville, AB T0B 2W0
Tel: 780-763-3621 *Fax:* 780-763-3678
Toll-Free: 855-371-4122
www.albertahealthservices.ca
Number of Beds: 23 beds
Note: Services include: continuing care; early intervention program; home care; laboratory; palliative care; & respite care.

MASKWACIS: Maskwacis Health Services
PO Box 100, Maskwacis, AB T0C 1N0
Tel: 780-585-3830 *Fax:* 780-585-2203
www.maskwacishealth.ca
Social Media: twitter.com/Maskwacishealth

Note: Programs & services include: community health; environmental health; HIV/AIDS education; medical clinic; optical; dental; pharmacy; home care; diabetes; counselling & support services; National Native Alcohol & Drug Awareness Program; & Indian Residential School Support Program.

MAYERTHORPE: Mayerthorpe Healthcare Centre
Affiliated with: Alberta Health Services
4417 - 45 St., Mayerthorpe, AB T0E 1N0
Tel: 780-786-2261 *Fax:* 780-786-2023
www.albertahealthservices.ca
Social Media: www.facebook.com/179579998746821; twitter.com/AHS_media; www.youtube.com/ahschannel
Number of Beds: 25 active beds; 30 auxiliary beds
Note: Programs & services include: acute care; continuing care; community health; emergency; pharmacy; rehabilitation; x-ray; & laboratory.

MAYERTHORPE: Mayerthorpe Healthcare Centre
Affiliated with: Alberta Health Services
4417 - 45 St., Mayerthorpe, AB T0E 1N0
Tel: 780-786-2488 *Fax:* 780-786-2023
www.albertahealthservices.ca

MCLENNAN: Public Health Centre
Affiliated with: Alberta Health Services
Former Name: Peace Country Health Unit - McLennan
c/o Sacred Heart Community Health Centre, 350 - 3 Ave. NW, McLennan, AB T0H 2L0
Tel: 780-324-3750
www.albertahealthservices.ca

MCLENNAN: Sacred Heart Community Health Centre
Affiliated with: Alberta Health Services
Former Name: McLennan Sacred Heart Community Health Centre
350 - 3 Ave. NW, McLennan, AB T0H 2L0
Tel: 780-324-3730 *Fax:* 780-324-4206
www.albertahealthservices.ca
Social Media: www.facebook.com/179579998746821; twitter.com/AHS_media; www.youtube.com/ahschannel
Number of Beds: 120 beds
Note: Programs & services include: acute care; emergency; Indigenous Health Program; intensive care; laboratory; rehabilitation; palliative care; & pediatrics.
Barbara Mader, Site Manager

MEDICINE HAT: Medicine Hat Community Health Services
Affiliated with: Alberta Health Services
2948 Dunmore Rd. SE, Medicine Hat, AB T1A 8E3
Tel: 403-502-8200 *Fax:* 403-528-2250
www.albertahealthservices.ca

MEDICINE HAT: Medicine Hat Regional Hospital
Affiliated with: Alberta Health Services
666 - 5 St. SW, Medicine Hat, AB T1A 4H6
Tel: 403-529-8000 *Fax:* 403-529-8950
www.albertahealthservices.ca
Social Media: www.facebook.com/179579998746821; twitter.com/AHS_media; www.youtube.com/ahschannel
Number of Beds: 190 acute care beds; 135 long-term care beds
Note: Programs & services include: acute care; supportive rehab; laboratory; surgery; mental health; critical care; pediatrics; emergency; ambulatory care; obstetrics; neonatal intensive care; geriatric services; community health; home care; & x-ray.
Linda Iwasiw, Senior Operating Officer

MILK RIVER: Milk River Health Centre
Affiliated with: Alberta Health Services
Former Name: Milk River Hospital
PO Box 90, 517 Centre Ave. East, Milk River, AB T0K 1M0
Tel: 403-647-3500 *Fax:* 403-647-2337
www.albertahealthservices.ca

Note: Programs & services include: diagnostic imaging; emergency; general radiography; laboratory; nutrition counselling; occupational therapy; physical therapy; prenatal education; public health nursing; respiratory therapy; & speech language pathology.

MORINVILLE: Morinville Provincial Building
Affiliated with: Alberta Health Services
Former Name: Morinville Public Health Centre; Morinville Health Services
10008 - 107 St., Morinville, AB T8R 1L3
Tel: 780-342-2600 *Fax:* 780-939-7126
www.albertahealthservices.ca

Note: Public health services

MUNDARE: Mary Immaculate Hospital
Covenant Health
Affiliated with: Alberta Health Services
PO Box 349, Mundare, AB T0B 3H0
Tel: 780-764-3730 *Fax:* 780-764-2112
www.covenanthealth.ca/hospitals-care-centres/mary-immaculate-hospital
Social Media: www.facebook.com/179579998746821; twitter.com/AHS_media; www.youtube.com/ahschannel

Year Founded: 1929
Number of Beds: 30 continuing care beds
Number of Employees: 70
Note: Programs & services include: ambulatory care; continuing care; occupational therapy; palliative care; & spiritual care.
Anthony Brannen, Site Administrator

NANTON: Nanton Community Health Centre
Affiliated with: Alberta Health Services
2214 - 20th St., Nanton, AB T0L 1R0
Tel: 403-646-2218 *Fax:* 403-646-3046
www.albertahealthservices.ca

Note: Programs & services include: adult day support program; electrocardiogram; immunization; laboratory; mental health; occupational therapy; physiotherapy; & tuberculosis testing

OKOTOKS: Okotoks Health & Wellness Centre
Affiliated with: Alberta Health Services
11 Cimarron Common, Okotoks, AB T1S 2E9
Tel: 403-995-2600 *Fax:* 403-995-2663
www.albertahealthservices.ca

OLDS: Olds Campus Community Health Centre
Affiliated with: Alberta Health Services
Ralph Klein Bldg., #2029, 4500 - 50th St., Olds, AB T4H 1R6
Tel: 403-559-2150 *Fax:* 403-559-2151
www.albertahealthservices.ca

Note: Programs & services include: early intervention program; environmental; immunization; oral health; prenatal education; public health; travel health; & tuberculosis testing

OLDS: Olds Hospital & Care Centre
Affiliated with: Alberta Health Services
3901 - 57 Ave., Olds, AB T4H 1T4
Tel: 403-556-3381 *Fax:* 403-556-2199
www.albertahealthservices.ca
Social Media: www.facebook.com/179579998746821; twitter.com/AHS_media; www.youtube.com/ahschannel
Number of Beds: 30 acute care beds; 3 palliative care beds; 50 LTC beds; 4 surgical beds; 2 coronary care beds; 2 labour & delivery beds; 4 day surgery beds
Note: Programs & services include: clinics; continuing care; crisis response team (rural); diagnostic imaging; emergency; general radiography; hemodialysis; laboratory services; long-term care; nutrition; obstetrics; occupational & physical therapy; palliative care; pharmacy; pulmonary/respiratory; seniors mental health program; speech language pathology; spiritual care; surgical; & Vital Heart Response/STEMI Program.
Wayne Krejci, Site Manager

OLDS: Olds Provincial Building
Affiliated with: Alberta Health Services
Former Name: Olds Community Health Centre
5025 - 50th St., Olds, AB T4H 1R9
Tel: 403-556-8441 *Fax:* 403-556-6842
www.albertahealthservices.ca

Note: Public health programs

ONOWAY: Onoway Community Health Services
Affiliated with: Alberta Health Services
4919 Lac St. Anne Trail, Onoway, AB T0E 1V0
Tel: 780-967-6200 *Fax:* 780-967-4433
www.albertahealthservices.ca

OYEN: Big Country Hospital
Affiliated with: Alberta Health Services
312 - 3 Ave. East, Oyen, AB T0J 2J0
Tel: 403-664-4300
www.albertahealthservices.ca
Social Media: www.facebook.com/179579998746821; twitter.com/AHS_media; www.youtube.com/ahschannel
Number of Beds: 10 acute care beds; 30 continuing care beds; 1 palliative care suite
Note: Programs & services include: acute care; continuing care; diagnostic imaging; emergency; general radiography; laboratory; labour delivery & maternal child services; occupational & physical therapy; respiratory services; respite services; & therapeutic recreation.

OYEN: Oyen Community Health Services
Affiliated with: Alberta Health Services
PO Box 296, 315 - 3 Ave. East, Oyen, AB T0J 2J0
Tel: 403-664-3651 *Fax:* 403-664-2934
www.albertahealthservices.ca

Note: Programs & services include: addiction; early hearing detection & intervention; home care; physical therapy; public health nursing; & travel health

PADDLE PRAIRIE: Paddle Prairie Health Centre
Affiliated with: Alberta Health Services
PO Box 46, Paddle Prairie, AB T0H 2W0
Tel: 780-841-3342 *Fax:* 780-926-7394
Toll-Free: 855-371-4122
www.albertahealthservices.ca

PEACE RIVER: Peace River Community Health Centre
Affiliated with: Alberta Health Services
10101 - 68 St., Peace River, AB T8S 1T6
Tel: 780-624-7500 *Fax:* 780-618-3472
www.albertahealthservices.ca
Social Media: www.facebook.com/179579998746821; twitter.com/AHS_media; www.youtube.com/AHSChannel
Number of Beds: 30 acute care beds; 40 long-term care beds
Note: Programs & services include: acute care; CT; continuing care; diagnostic imaging; early childhood intervention; emergency; environmental public health; fluoroscopy; general radiography; home care; Indigenous health program; laboratory; mammography; nutrition; occupational therapy; oral health; palliative care; pharmacy; physical therapy; respiratory therapy; sexual health; social work; speech language pathology; therapeutic recreation; tuberculosis testing; & ultrasound.
Robert Kielly, Site Manager

PEERLESS LAKE: Trout/Peerless Lake Community Health Services
Affiliated with: Alberta Health Services
PO Box 90, Peerless Lake, AB T0G 2W0
Tel: 780-869-2362 *Fax:* 780-869-2053
www.albertahealthservices.ca

PICTURE BUTTE: Piyami Health Centre
Affiliated with: Alberta Health Services
Former Name: Picture Butte Hospital
300-A Rogers Ave., Picture Butte, AB T0K 1V0
Tel: 403-388-6751
www.albertahealthservices.ca

Note: Programs & services include: ambulatory care; diagnostic imaging; general radiography; laboratory; occupational therapy; physical therapy; public health nursing; respiratory therapy; & speech language pathology.

PINCHER CREEK: Pincher Creek Community Health Centre
Affiliated with: Alberta Health Services
1222 Bev McLachlin Dr., Pincher Creek, AB T0K 1W0
Tel: 403-627-1234 *Fax:* 403-627-2771
www.albertahealthservices.ca

PINCHER CREEK: Pincher Creek Health Centre
Affiliated with: Alberta Health Services
Former Name: Pincher Creek Hospital
1222 Bev McLachlin Dr., Pincher Creek, AB T0K 1W0
Tel: 403-627-1234 *Fax:* 403-627-5275
www.albertahealthservices.ca
Social Media: www.facebook.com/179579998746821; twitter.com/AHS_media; www.youtube.com/ahschannel
Number of Beds: 16 acute care beds; 3 long-term beds
Note: Programs & services include: audiology; diagnostic imaging; emergency; general radiography; laboratory; nutrition; & pediatrics.
Jordan Koch, Site Manager

PONOKA: Ponoka Community Health Centre
Affiliated with: Alberta Health Services
5900 Hwy. 2A, Ponoka, AB T4J 1P5
Tel: 403-783-4491 *Fax:* 403-783-3825
www.albertahealthservices.ca

PONOKA: Ponoka Hospital & Healthcare Centre
Affiliated with: Alberta Health Services
5800 - 57 Ave., Ponoka, AB T4J 1P1
Tel: 403-783-3341 *Fax:* 403-783-6907
www.albertahealthservices.ca
Social Media: www.facebook.com/179579998746821;
twitter.com/AHS_media; www.youtube.com/ahschannel
Number of Beds: 75 beds (34 acute care beds)
Note: Programs & services include: acute care; continuing care;
emergency; general medicine; laboratory; obstetrics; surgery;
pediatrics; & radiology.

PROVOST: Provost Health Centre
Affiliated with: Alberta Health Services
5002 - 54 Ave., Provost, AB T0B 3S0
Tel: 780-753-2291 *Fax:* 780-753-6132
www.albertahealthservices.ca
Social Media: www.facebook.com/179579998746821;
twitter.com/AHS_media; www.youtube.com/ahschannel
Number of Beds: 15 acute care; 36 continuing care beds; 15 surgical
beds; 4 day surgery beds; 2 labour & delivery beds; 1 coronary care
beds
Note: Programs & services include: acute care; continuing care; day
support; emergency; respite & palliative care; surgery; obstetrics; &
x-ray.
Lana Clark, Manager

PROVOST: Provost Provincial Building
Affiliated with: Alberta Health Services
Former Name: Hughenden Public Health: Home Care
5419 - 44 St., Provost, AB T0B 3S0
Tel: 780-753-6180 *Fax:* 780-753-2064
www.albertahealthservices.ca

RAINBOW LAKE: Rainbow Lake Community Health Services
Affiliated with: Alberta Health Services
Former Name: Rainbow Lake Health Centre
PO Box 177, 6A Commercial Rd., Rainbow Lake, AB T0H 2Y0
Tel: 780-956-3646
www.albertahealthservices.ca
Note: Programs & services include: addiction & mental health;
environmental; nutrition counselling; & tuberculosis testing.

RAYMOND: Raymond Health Centre
Affiliated with: Alberta Health Services
Former Name: Raymond Hospital
150 North 4th St. East, Raymond, AB T0K 2S0
Tel: 403-752-4561 *Fax:* 403-752-3554
www.albertahealthservices.ca
Social Media: www.facebook.com/179579998746821;
twitter.com/AHS_media; www.youtube.com/ahschannel

Note: Programs & services include: continuing care; diagnostic
imaging; emergency; general radiography; laboratory; nutrition;
occupational & physical therapy; & therapeutic recreation.

RED DEER: Red Deer - 49th Street Community Health Centre
Affiliated with: Alberta Health Services
4755 - 49th St., Red Deer, AB T4N 1T6
Tel: 403-314-5225 *Fax:* 403-314-5230
www.albertahealthservices.ca

RED DEER: Red Deer - Bremner Ave. Community Health Centre
Affiliated with: Alberta Health Services
2845 Bremner Ave., Red Deer, AB T4R 1S2
Tel: 403-341-2100 *Fax:* 403-346-2610
www.albertahealthservices.ca

Note: Programs & services include: asthma education program;
continuing care counselling; enterostomal therapy; home care; mobility
clinic; nutrition counselling; & rehabilitation

RED DEER: Red Deer - Johnstone Crossing Community Health Centre
Affiliated with: Alberta Health Services
300 Jordan Pkwy., Red Deer, AB T4P 0G8
Tel: 403-356-6300 *Fax:* 403-356-6440
www.albertahealthservices.ca

Note: Programs & services include: early intervention program;
environmental; immunization; oral health; prenatal education; dietitian
counselling; public health; respiratory therapy; travel health; &
tuberculosis testing

RED DEER: Red Deer Regional Hospital Centre
Affiliated with: Alberta Health Services
3942 - 50A Ave., Red Deer, AB T4N 4E7
Tel: 403-343-4422
www.albertahealthservices.ca
Social Media: www.facebook.com/179579998746821;
twitter.com/AHS_media; www.youtube.com/ahschannel
Number of Beds: 390 acute care beds; 40 mental health beds
Note: Programs & services include: Indigenous health; mental health
(adult & child); angiography; laboratory; bronchoscopy; cardiology;
clinics; CT scan; crisis response team; diagnostic imaging;
echocardiography; electroencephalography; electromyography;
emergency; Fibromyalgia group; fluoroscopy; general radiography;
hemodialysis; MRI; neonatal intensive care; nuclear medicine; nuclear
stress testing; nutrition; obstetrics; palliative care; pediatrics; perinatal
bereavement program; pharmacy; physical therapy;
pulmonary/respiratory; rehabilitation; specialized geriatric services;
speech language pathology; spiritual care; stress echocardiography;
surgery; & ultrasound.
Dr. Evan Lundall, Medical Director

RED EARTH CREEK: Red Earth Creek Community Health Services
Affiliated with: Alberta Health Services
Red Earth Creek, AB T0G 1X0
Tel: 780-649-2242 *Fax:* 780-649-2029
www.albertahealthservices.ca

REDWATER: Redwater Health Centre
Affiliated with: Alberta Health Services
4812 - 58 St., Redwater, AB T0A 2W0
Tel: 780-942-3932 *Fax:* 780-942-2373
www.albertahealthservices.ca
Number of Beds: 14 acute care beds; 7 continuing care beds

REDWATER: Redwater Health Centre
Affiliated with: Alberta Health Services
4812 - 58 St., Redwater, AB T0A 2W0
Tel: 780-942-3932 *Fax:* 780-942-2373
www.albertahealthservices.ca
Social Media: www.facebook.com/179579998746821;
twitter.com/AHS_media; www.youtube.com/AHSChannel
Year Founded: 1973
Number of Beds: 14 acute care beds; 7 long-term care beds; 1
palliative care bed
Note: Programs & services include: addiction & mental health;
continuing care; diagnostic imaging; emergency; environmental;
general radiography; laboratory; nutrition; social work; & spiritual care.

RIMBEY: Rimbey Community Health Centre
Affiliated with: Alberta Health Services
4709 - 51 Ave., Rimbey, AB T0C 2J0
Tel: 403-843-2288 *Fax:* 403-843-3050
www.albertahealthservices.ca

RIMBEY: Rimbey Hospital & Care Centre
Affiliated with: Alberta Health Services
PO Box 440, 5228 - 50 St., Rimbey, AB T0C 2J0
Tel: 403-843-2271
www.albertahealthservices.ca
Social Media: www.facebook.com/179579998746821;
twitter.com/AHS_media; www.youtube.com/AHSChannel

Note: Programs & services include: addiction & mental health; child &
adolescent services; continuing care counselling; crisis response team
(rural); diagnostic imaging; emergency; general radiography;
laboratory; long-term care; nutrition; obstetrics; occupational & physical
therapy; palliative care; pharmacy; respite care; speech language
pathology; & spiritual care.

ROCKY MOUNTAIN HOUSE: Rocky Mountain House Health Centre
Affiliated with: Alberta Health Services
5016 - 52 Ave., Rocky Mountain House, AB T4T 1T2
Tel: 403-845-3347 *Fax:* 403-845-7030
www.albertahealthservices.ca
Social Media: www.facebook.com/179579998746821;
twitter.com/AHS_media; www.youtube.com/ahschannel
Number of Beds: 30 continuing care beds
Note: Programs & services include: Indigenous health; addiction &
mental health; child & adolescent services; community health centres;
continuing care counselling; crisis response team (rural); diagnostic
imaging; emergency; environmental public health; general radiography;
hemodialysis; home care; laboratory; long-term care; nutrition;
obstetrics; occupational & physical therapy; oral health; palliative care;
pharmacy; prenatal education; public health; respiratory; speech
language pathology; surgery; tuberculosis testing; ultrasound; & Vital
Heart Response/STEMI Program.
Shirley Hope, Site Manager

ROCKY MOUNTAIN HOUSE: Rocky Mountain House Health Centre
Affiliated with: Alberta Health Services
5016 - 52 Ave., Rocky Mountain House, AB T4T 1T2
Tel: 403-845-3030 *Fax:* 403-845-4975
www.albertahealthservices.ca

SEDGEWICK: Sedgewick Home Care / Public Health / Rehab
Affiliated with: Alberta Health Services
4822 - 50 St., Sedgewick, AB T0B 4C0
Tel: 780-384-3652 *Fax:* 780-384-3699
www.albertahealthservices.ca

SHERWOOD PARK: Strathcona Community Hospital
Affiliated with: Alberta Health Services
Former Name: Health First Strathcona
9000 Emerald Dr., Sherwood Park, AB T8H 0J3
Tel: 780-449-5380
www.albertahealthservices.ca
Social Media: www.facebook.com/179579998746821;
twitter.com/AHS_media; www.youtube.com/ahschannel
Year Founded: 2014
Note: Programs & services include: addiction & mental health; CT
scans; diabetes program; diagnostic imaging; emergency; laboratory;
rehabilitation; radiography; & ultrasound.

SHERWOOD PARK: Strathcona County Health Centre
Affiliated with: Alberta Health Services
2 Brower Dr., Sherwood Park, AB T8H 1V4
Tel: 780-342-4600 *Fax:* 780-449-1338
www.albertahealthservices.ca

SLAVE LAKE: Slave Lake Healthcare Centre
Affiliated with: Alberta Health Services
309 - 6 St. NE, Slave Lake, AB T0G 2A2
Tel: 780-805-3500 *Fax:* 780-805-3577
www.albertahealthservices.ca
Social Media: www.facebook.com/179579998746821;
twitter.com/AHS_media; www.youtube.com/ahschannel
Number of Beds: 24 inpatient beds; 20 long-term care beds; 9
emergency beds; 2 special care beds; 1 palliative care bed
Note: Programs & services include: emergency; acute care; continuing
care; mental health; pharmacy; renal dialysis; rehabilitation; obstetrics;
occupational therapy; pediatrics; respiratory therapy; social work;
ultrasound; & x-ray.

SLAVE LAKE: Slave Lake Healthcare Centre
Affiliated with: Alberta Health Services
Public Health Centre, 309 - 6 St. NE, Slave Lake, AB T0G 2A2
Tel: 780-849-3947 *Fax:* 780-805-3550
www.albertahealthservices.ca

SMOKY LAKE: George McDougall - Smoky Lake Healthcare Centre
Affiliated with: Alberta Health Services
PO Box 340, 4212 - 55 Ave., Smoky Lake, AB T0A 3C0
Tel: 780-656-3034 *Fax:* 780-656-5010
www.albertahealthservices.ca
Social Media: www.facebook.com/179579998746821;
twitter.com/AHS_media; www.youtube.com/ahschannel
Number of Beds: 12 active beds; 23 auxiliary beds
Note: Programs & services include: emergency services; diagnostic
imaging; laboratory services; ambulatory services; acute care;

rehabilitation; occupational therapy; physical therapy services;
therapeutic recreation; community health services; nutrition services;
social work; continuing care; & palliative care.

SMOKY LAKE: George McDougall - Smoky Lake Healthcare Centre
Affiliated with: Alberta Health Services
4212 - 55 Ave., Smoky Lake, AB T0A 3C0
Tel: 780-656-3595 *Fax:* 780-656-2242
www.albertahealthservices.ca

SPIRIT RIVER: Central Peace Health Complex
Affiliated with: Alberta Health Services
5010 - 45th Ave., Spirit River, AB T0H 3G0
Tel: 780-864-3993 *Fax:* 780-864-3495
www.albertahealthservices.ca
Social Media: www.facebook.com/179579998746821;
twitter.com/AHS_media; www.youtube.com/ahschannel
Year Founded: 1972
Number of Beds: 10 acute care beds; 16 continuing care beds
Note: Programs & services include: emergency care; laboratory
services; acute care; newborn hearing screening program; pediatrics;
rehabilitation; physical therapy; nutrition counselling; continuing care;
& palliative care.

SPIRIT RIVER: Spirit River Community Health Services
Affiliated with: Alberta Health Services
Former Name: Mistahia Health Unit - Spirit River
5003 - 45 Ave., Spirit River, AB T0H 3G0
Tel: 780-864-3063 *Fax:* 780-864-4187
www.albertahealthservices.ca

SPRUCE GROVE: Spruce Grove Health Unit
Affiliated with: Alberta Health Services
505 Queen St., Spruce Grove, AB T7X 2V2
Tel: 780-342-1301 *Fax:* 780-342-1328
www.albertahealthservices.ca

Note: Programs & services include: early intervention program;
laboratory; public health; & school dental & health services

SPRUCE GROVE: Stan Woloshyn Building
Affiliated with: Alberta Health Services
205 Diamond Ave., Spruce Grove, AB T7X 3A8
Tel: 780-342-1380 *Fax:* 780-960-0369
www.albertahealthservices.ca

Note: Primarily provides environmental health services

ST ALBERT: St. Albert Public Health Centre
Affiliated with: Alberta Health Services
23 Sir Winston Churchill Ave., St. Albert, AB T8N 2S7
Tel: 780-459-6671 *Fax:* 780-460-7062
www.albertahealthservices.ca

Note: Programs & services include: environmental public health;
immunization; school dental, nursing, & health services; & travel health

ST ALBERT: Sturgeon Community Hospital
Affiliated with: Alberta Health Services
Former Name: Sturgeon Community Hospital & Health Centre
201 Boudreau Rd., St Albert, AB T8N 6C4
Tel: 780-418-8200
www.albertahealthservices.ca
Social Media: www.facebook.com/179579998746821;
twitter.com/AHS_media; www.youtube.com/ahschannel
Year Founded: 1992
Number of Beds: 167 beds
Note: Programs & services include: emergency; cardiac rehabilitation;
diagnostic imaging (CT scans, radiology, fluoroscopy); intensive care
unit; nutrition counselling; obstetrics; physical therapy/occupational
therapy; prenatal program; sexual assault response team; spiritual
care; & surgery.
Wendy Tanaka-Collins, Site Director

ST PAUL: St. Paul Community Health Services
Affiliated with: Alberta Health Services
5610 - 50 Ave., St Paul, AB T0A 3A1
Tel: 780-645-3396 *Fax:* 780-645-6609
www.albertahealthservices.ca

ST PAUL: St. Therese - St. Paul Healthcare Centre
Affiliated with: Alberta Health Services
4713 - 48 Ave., St. Paul, AB T0A 3A3
Tel: 780-645-3331 *Fax:* 780-645-1702
www.albertahealthservices.ca
Social Media: www.facebook.com/179579998746821;
twitter.com/AHS_media; www.youtube.com/ahschannel

Note: Programs & services include: emergency; diagnostic imaging
(ultrasound, x-ray); eating disorder services; obstetrics; pharmacy;
rehabilitation; renal dialysis; & laboratory.
Michelle Blanchette, Site Manager

STETTLER: Stettler Community Health Centre
Affiliated with: Alberta Health Services
5911 - 50 Ave., Stettler, AB T0C 2L0
Tel: 403-742-3326 *Fax:* 403-742-1353
www.albertahealthservices.ca

STETTLER: Stettler Hospital & Care Centre
Affiliated with: Alberta Health Services
5912 - 47 Ave., Stettler, AB T0C 2L0
Tel: 403-742-7400 *Fax:* 403-742-1244
www.albertahealthservices.ca
Social Media: www.facebook.com/179579998746821;
twitter.com/AHS_media; www.youtube.com/ahschannel

Note: Programs & services include: continuing care; diagnostic
imaging; mental health; obstetrics; occupational therapy (for acute &
continuing care); palliative care; pharmacy; physical therapy; renal
dialysis; respiratory therapy; sleep program; & speech language
pathology.

STONY PLAIN: WestView Health Centre
Affiliated with: Alberta Health Services
4405 South Park Dr., Stony Plain, AB T7Z 2M7
Tel: 780-968-3600
www.albertahealthservices.ca
Social Media: www.facebook.com/179579998746821;
twitter.com/AHS_media; www.youtube.com/AHSChannel
Number of Beds: 16 inpatient beds; 50 continuing care beds
Note: Programs & services include: acute care; continuing care;
emergency; diagnostic imaging; laboratory; day surgery; obstetrics;
public health; environmental; community care; rehabilitation;
dental; & mental health.
Ellen Billay, Site Director

STRATHMORE: Strathmore District Health Services
Affiliated with: Alberta Health Services
200 Brent Blvd., Strathmore, AB T1P 1J9
Tel: 403-361-7000 *Fax:* 403-361-7048
www.albertahealthservices.ca
Social Media: www.facebook.com/179579998746821;
twitter.com/AHS_media; www.youtube.com/ahschannel
Number of Beds: 25 acute care beds
Note: Programs & services include: Adult Day Support Program;
diagnostic imaging; cardiology; laboratory; occupational therapy;
palliative care; pharmacy; physical therapy; respiratory services; respite
care; & speech language pathology.

STRATHMORE: Strathmore Public Health Office
Affiliated with: Alberta Health Services
650 Westchester Rd., Strathmore, AB T1P 1H8
Tel: 403-361-7200 *Fax:* 403-361-7244
www.albertahealthservices.ca

SUNDRE: Sundre Community Health Centre
Affiliated with: Alberta Health Services
212 - 6 Ave. NE, Sundre, AB T0M 1X0
Tel: 403-638-4063 *Fax:* 403-638-4460
www.albertahealthservices.ca

SUNDRE: Sundre Hospital & Care Centre
Affiliated with: Alberta Health Services
709 - 1 St. NE, Sundre, AB T0M 1X0
Tel: 403-638-3033 *Fax:* 403-636-6284
www.albertahealthservices.ca
Social Media: www.facebook.com/179579998746821;
twitter.com/AHS_media; www.youtube.com/ahschannel

Number of Beds: 14 acute care beds
Note: Programs & services include: emergency; nutrition; continuing
care counseling; diagnostic imaging; laboratory; obstetrics;
occupational therapy; palliative care; pharmacy; physical therapy; &
speech language pathology.
Larry Gratton, Site Manager

SWAN HILLS: Swan Hills Healthcare Centre
Affiliated with: Alberta Health Services
PO Box 261, 29 Freeman Dr., Swan Hills, AB T0G 2C0
Tel: 780-333-7000 *Fax:* 780-333-7009
www.albertahealthservices.ca
Social Media: www.facebook.com/179579998746821;
twitter.com/AHS_media; www.youtube.com/AHSChannel
Year Founded: 1985
Number of Beds: 24 hospital beds
Note: Programs & services include: ambulatory services; clinics;
community health; diagnostic imaging; early childhood development;
eating disorder services; emergency; environmental; general medicine;
general radiography; home care; laboratory; mental health; nutrition;
oral health; palliative care; pharmacy; P.A.R.T.Y. (Prevent Alcohol &
Risk Related Trauma in Youth); sexual health; & social work.

SWAN HILLS: Swan Hills Healthcare Centre
Affiliated with: Alberta Health Services
**Public Health Centre, PO Box 261, 29 Freeman Dr., Swan Hills, AB
T0G 2C0**
Tel: 780-333-7077 *Fax:* 780-333-7009
www.albertahealthservices.ca

SYLVAN LAKE: Sylvan Lake Community Health Centre
Affiliated with: Alberta Health Services
4602 - 49 Ave., Sylvan Lake, AB T4S 1M7
Tel: 403-887-2241 *Fax:* 403-887-2610
www.albertahealthservices.ca

TABER: Taber Community Health
Affiliated with: Alberta Health Services
4326 - 50th Ave., Taber, AB T1G 1N9
Tel: 403-223-7230
www.albertahealthservices.ca

TABER: Taber Health Centre
Affiliated with: Alberta Health Services
Former Name: Taber Hospital
4326 - 50 Ave., Taber, AB T1G 1N9
Tel: 403-223-7211 *Fax:* 403-223-1703
www.albertahealthservices.ca
Social Media: www.facebook.com/179579998746821;
twitter.com/AHS_media; www.youtube.com/AHSChannel

Note: Programs & services include: addiction services; continuing care;
emergency; diagnostic imaging; environmental; laboratory; mental
health services; nutrition; occupational therapy; pediatrics; radiography;
speech language pathology; & therapeutic recreation.

THORHILD: Thorhild Community Health Services
Affiliated with: Alberta Health Services
302 - 2 Ave., Thorhild, AB T0A 3J0
Tel: 780-398-3879 *Fax:* 780-398-2671
www.albertahealthservices.ca

Note: Programs & services include: early childhood intervention
program; fluoride protection; home care; laboratory; oral health;
postpartum support; sexual health; social work; & tuberculosis testing

THORSBY: Thorsby Public Health Centre
Affiliated with: Alberta Health Services
4825 Hankin St., Thorsby, AB T0C 2P0
Tel: 780-789-4800 *Fax:* 780-789-4811
www.albertahealthservices.ca

THREE HILLS: Three Hills Health Centre
Affiliated with: Alberta Health Services
1504 - 2nd St. North, Three Hills, AB T0M 2A0
Tel: 403-443-2444 *Fax:* 403-443-5565
www.albertahealthservices.ca
Social Media: www.facebook.com/179579998746821;
twitter.com/AHS_media; www.youtube.com/ahschannel

Note: Programs & services include: community health; continuing care;

diagnostic imaging; early intervention program; emergency; fluoride protection for toddlers; general radiography; home care & Alberta Aids to Daily Living; laboratory; long-term care; nutrition; obstetrics; occupational & physical therapy; oral health; palliative care; pharmacy; prenatal education; public health; pulmonary; rehabilitation; respite care; speech language pathology; surgery; travel health services; tuberculosis testing; & ultrasound.
Ruth Wold, Site Manager

TOFIELD: Tofield Health Centre
Affiliated with: Alberta Health Services
5543 - 44 St., Tofield, AB T0B 4J0
Tel: 780-662-3263 *Fax:* 780-662-3835
www.albertahealthservices.ca
Social Media: www.facebook.com/179579998746821;
twitter.com/AHS_media; www.youtube.com/AHSChannel
Number of Beds: 50 beds
Note: Programs & services include: emergency; acute care; asthma education program; continuing care; home care; laboratory; occupational therapy; palliative care; physiotherapy; postnatal services; radiography; respiratory therapy; respite care; speech language services; & surgery.

TROCHU: St. Mary's Health Care Centre
Covenant Health
Affiliated with: Alberta Health Services
451 de Chauney Ave., Trochu, AB T0M 2C0
Tel: 403-442-3955
www.covenanthealth.ca
Number of Beds: 56 beds
Number of Employees: 72
Note: Programs & services include: continuing care counselling; diagnostic imaging; general radiography; interpretive services; laboratory; long-term care; occupational therapy; & palliative care.

TWO HILLS: Two Hills Health Centre
Affiliated with: Alberta Health Services
4401 - 53 Ave., Two Hills, AB T0B 4K0
Tel: 780-657-3344 *Fax:* 780-657-2508
www.albertahealthservices.ca
Social Media: www.facebook.com/179579998746821;
twitter.com/AHS_media; www.youtube.com/AHSChannel
Year Founded: 1986
Number of Beds: 15 acute care beds; 56 long term care beds; 6 emergency beds; 12 SaGE beds
Note: Programs & services include: emergency; acute care; community health; nutrition; continuing care; home care; general radiography; laboratory; occupational therapy; oral health; palliative care; pharmacy; prenatal education; respiratory therapy; respite care; & stroke & geriatric empowerment unit.

TWO HILLS: Two Hills Health Centre
Affiliated with: Alberta Health Services
4401 - 53 Ave., Two Hills, AB T0B 4K0
Tel: 780-657-3361 *Fax:* 780-657-2508
www.albertahealthservices.ca

VALLEYVIEW: Valleyview Community Health Services
Affiliated with: Alberta Health Services
Former Name: Mistahia Health Unit, Valleyview; Valleyview District Home Care Office
5112 - 50 Ave., Valleyview, AB T0H 3N0
Tel: 780-524-3338
www.albertahealthservices.ca

VALLEYVIEW: Valleyview Health Centre
Affiliated with: Alberta Health Services
Former Name: Valleyview Health Complex
4802 Highway St., Valleyview, AB T0H 3N0
Tel: 780-524-3356 *Fax:* 780-524-2107
www.albertahealthservices.ca
Social Media: www.facebook.com/179579998746821;
twitter.com/AHS_media; www.youtube.com/AHSChannel
Number of Beds: 35 acute care beds; 25 extended care beds; 20 continuing care beds
Note: Programs & services include: Indigenous health; cardiology; continuing care; diagnostic imaging; early intervention; emergency; environmental; general radiography; laboratory; newborn hearing screening program; nutrition; occupational & physical therapy; palliative

care; pediatrics; pharmacy; respiratory; social work; therapeutic recreation; & tuberculosis testing.
Tracy Brown, Site Manager

VAUXHALL: Vauxhall Community Health
Affiliated with: Alberta Health Services
406 - 1 Ave. North, Vauxhall, AB T0K 2K0
Tel: 403-223-7229 *Fax:* 403-654-2134
www.albertahealthservices.ca

VEGREVILLE: St. Joseph's General Hospital
Covenant Health
Affiliated with: Alberta Health Services
5241 - 43 St., Vegreville, AB T9C 1R5
Tel: 780-632-2811 *Fax:* 780-603-4401
www.covenanthealth.ca/hospitals-care-centres/st-josephs-general-hospital
Social Media: www.facebook.com/179579998746821;
twitter.com/AHS_media; www.youtube.com/AHSChannel
Year Founded: 1910
Number of Beds: 25 beds
Number of Employees: 169
Note: Programs & services include: emergency; medicine; laboratory; diagnostic imaging (x-ray, ultrasound); dialysis; diabetic education; occupational & physical therapy; respiratory therapy; palliative care; & day support.
Anthony Brannen, Site Administrator

VEGREVILLE: Vegreville Community Health Centre
Affiliated with: Alberta Health Services
5318 - 50 St., Vegreville, AB T9C 1R1
Tel: 780-632-3331 *Fax:* 780-632-4334
www.albertahealthservices.ca

VERMILION: Vermilion Health Centre
Affiliated with: Alberta Health Services
5720 - 50 Ave., Vermilion, AB T9X 1K7
Tel: 780-853-5305 *Fax:* 780-853-4786
www.albertahealthservices.ca
Social Media: www.facebook.com/179579998746821;
twitter.com/AHS_media; www.youtube.com/AHSChannel
Number of Beds: 25 acute care beds; 48 continuing care beds; 4 day surgery beds
Note: Programs & services include: acute care; clinics; diagnostic imaging; emergency; general radiography; laboratory; long-term care; nutrition; occupational & physical therapy; palliative care; pharmacy; pulmonary/respiratory; surgery; ultrasound; & Vital Heart Response/STEMI Program.
Debora Okrainetz, Area Director

VERMILION: Vermilion Provincial Building
Affiliated with: Alberta Health Services
Former Name: Vermilion Public Health, Home Care, Rehab
4701 - 52 St., Vermilion, AB T9X 1J9
Tel: 780-853-5270 *Fax:* 780-853-7362
www.albertahealthservices.ca

VIKING: Viking Community Health Centre
Affiliated with: Alberta Health Services
Former Name: Viking Health Centre
5224 - 50 St., Viking, AB T0B 4N0
Tel: 780-336-4782
www.albertahealthservices.ca

VIKING: Viking Health Centre
Affiliated with: Alberta Health Services
PO Box 60, 5110 - 57 Ave., Viking, AB T0B 4N0
Tel: 780-336-4786 *Fax:* 780-336-4983
www.albertahealthservices.ca
Social Media: www.facebook.com/179579998746821;
twitter.com/AHS_media; www.youtube.com/AHSChannel
Number of Beds: 16 acute care beds
Note: Programs & services include: emergency; acute care; continuing care; palliative care; surgery; mental health services; nutrition; obstetrics; rehabilitation; respiratory therapy; & x-ray.
Sharon Burden, Site Manager

VILNA: Vilna Community Health Services
Affiliated with: Alberta Health Services
Former Name: Our Lady's Health Centre
5103 - 48 St., Vilna, AB T0A 3L0
Tel: 780-636-3533 *Fax:* 780-656-2242
www.albertahealthservices.ca

Note: Programs & services include: early childhood intervention program; environmental; laboratory; social work; & tuberculosis testing.

VULCAN: Vulcan Community Health Centre
Affiliated with: Alberta Health Services
610 Elizabeth St. South, Vulcan, AB T0L 2B0
Tel: 403-485-3333 *Fax:* 403-485-2336
www.albertahealthservices.ca
Social Media: www.facebook.com/179579998746821;
twitter.com/AHS_media; www.youtube.com/AHSChannel
Number of Beds: 8 acute care beds; 15 long-term care beds
Note: Programs & services include: adult day program; continuing care; diabetes education; diagnostic imaging; emergency; general medicine; general radiography; surgery; Healthy Moms, Healthy Babies Program; Home Parenteral Therapy Program; laboratory; mental health; nutrition; pharmacy; & respiratory therapy.

VULCAN: Vulcan Health Unit
Affiliated with: Alberta Health Services
Vulcan Community Health Centre, 610 Elizabeth St., Vulcan, AB
T0L 2B0
Tel: 403-485-2285 *Fax:* 403-485-2639
www.albertahealthservices.ca

WABASCA: Wabasca/Desmarais Community Health Services
Affiliated with: Alberta Health Services
867 Stoney Point Rd., Wabasca, AB T0G 2K0
Tel: 780-891-3931 *Fax:* 780-891-3011
www.albertahealthservices.ca

WABASCA: Wabasca/Desmarais Healthcare Centre
Affiliated with: Alberta Health Services
Former Name: Wabasca/Desmarais General Hospital
881 Mistassiniy Rd., Wabasca, AB T0G 2K0
Tel: 780-891-3007 *Fax:* 780-891-3784
www.albertahealthservices.ca
Social Media: www.facebook.com/179579998746821;
twitter.com/AHS_media; www.youtube.com/ahschannel
Number of Beds: 10 beds
Note: Serves the Wabasca, Desmarais, Sandy Lake, Chipewyan Lake & Bigstone Cree Nation area. Programs & services: emergency; laboratory; rehabilitation; & x-ray.

WAINWRIGHT: Wainwright Health Centre
Affiliated with: Alberta Health Services
530 - 6 Ave., Wainwright, AB T9W 1R6
Tel: 780-842-3324 *Fax:* 780-842-4290
www.albertahealthservices.ca
Social Media: www.facebook.com/179579998746821;
twitter.com/AHS_media; www.youtube.com/AHSChannel
Number of Beds: 22 inpatient beds; 60 long-term care beds; 2 intensive care beds; 3 labour & delivery beds; 6 day surgery beds
Note: Programs & services include: acute care; asthma education program; emergency; continuing care; palliative care; surgery; obstetrics; cardiac education; speech language services; respiratory therapy; physical therapy; ultrasound; & x-ray.
Cheryl Huxley, Site Manager

WAINWRIGHT: Wainwright Provincial Building
Affiliated with: Alberta Health Services
810 - 14 Ave., Wainwright, AB T9W 1R2
Tel: 780-842-4077 *Fax:* 780-842-3151
www.albertahealthservices.ca

WESTLOCK: Westlock Community Health Services
Affiliated with: Alberta Health Services
10024 - 107 Ave., Westlock, AB T7P 2E3
Tel: 780-349-3316 *Fax:* 780-349-5725
www.albertahealthservices.ca

WESTLOCK: Westlock Healthcare Centre
Affiliated with: Alberta Health Services
10220 - 93 St., Westlock, AB T7P 2G4
Tel: 780-349-3301 *Fax:* 780-349-6973
www.albertahealthservices.ca
Social Media: www.facebook.com/179579998746821;
twitter.com/AHS_media; www.youtube.com/AHSChannel
Number of Beds: 62 beds
Note: Programs & services include: ambulatory services; day surgery; diagnostic imaging; emergency; environmental; fluoroscopy; general medicine; general radiography; laboratory; MRI; obstetrics; occupational therapy; orthopedic; palliative care; pastoral care; pediatrics; respiratory; special care; & ultrasound.
Sherry Gough, Manager

WETASKIWIN: Wetaskiwin Community Health Centre
Affiliated with: Alberta Health Services
5610 - 40 Ave., Wetaskiwin, AB T9A 3E4
Tel: 780-361-4333 *Fax:* 780-361-4335
www.albertahealthservices.ca

WETASKIWIN: Wetaskiwin Hospital & Care Centre
Affiliated with: Alberta Health Services
Former Name: Crossroads Hospital & Health Centre - Wetaskiwin
6910 - 47 St., Wetaskiwin, AB T9A 3N3
Tel: 780-361-7100 *Fax:* 780-361-4107
Toll-Free: 866-361-7101
www.albertahealthservices.ca
Social Media: www.facebook.com/179579998746821;
twitter.com/AHS_media; www.youtube.com/AHSChannel
Number of Beds: 83 acute care beds; 105 long-term care beds
Note: Programs & services include: Indigenous Health Program; bronchoscopy; cardiology; CT imaging; continuing care; Northern Alberta Renal Program; diagnostic imaging; emergency; fluoroscopy; general radiography; hemodialysis; laboratory; nutrition; obstetrics; occupational therapy; physical therapy; palliative care; pharmacy; respiratory/pulmonary; respite care; sleep program; speech language pathology; surgery; & ultrasound.
Brenda Zilkie, Area Manager

WHITECOURT: Whitecourt Community Health Services
Affiliated with: Alberta Health Services
4707 - 50 Ave., Whitecourt, AB T7S 1P1
Tel: 780-706-3173 *Fax:* 780-706-7154
www.albertahealthservices.ca

WHITECOURT: Whitecourt Healthcare Centre
Affiliated with: Alberta Health Services
20 Sunset Blvd., Whitecourt, AB T7S 1M8
Tel: 780-778-2285 *Fax:* 780-778-5161
www.albertahealthservices.ca
Social Media: www.facebook.com/179579998746821;
twitter.com/AHS_media; www.youtube.com/AHSChannel
Number of Beds: 24 beds; 2 special care beds; 1 palliative care bed
Note: Programs & services include: acute care; special care; palliative care; emergency; pharmacy; rehabilitation; ultrasound; x-ray; ambulatory; audiology; clinics; community health services; day surgery; diagnostic imaging; early childhood development; Early Intervention Program; eating disorder services; environmental services; general medicine; general radiography; home care; laboratory; nutrition; obstetrics; occupational therapy; physical therapy; pastoral care; pediatrics; prenatal education; P.A.R.T.Y. (Prevent Alcohol & Risk Related Trauma in Youth); respiratory; sexual health; social work; stress testing; travel health; tuberculosis testing; & ultrasound.
Allan Shemanko, Site Manager

WINFIELD: Winfield Community Health Centre
Affiliated with: Alberta Health Services
Former Name: Crossroads Health Unit - Winfield
PO Box 114, 10 - 2 Ave. West, Winfield, AB T0C 2X0
Tel: 780-682-4755 *Fax:* 780-682-4750
www.albertahealthservices.ca

WORSLEY: Worsley Community Health Services
Affiliated with: Alberta Health Services
General Delivery, Worsley, AB T0H 3W0
Tel: 780-685-3752
www.albertahealthservices.ca

ZAMA CITY: Zama City Community Health Services
Affiliated with: Alberta Health Services
General Delivery, Zama City, AB T0H 4E0
Tel: 780-683-2220
www.albertahealthservices.ca

Note: Services: immunization; public health nursing

BRITISH COLUMBIA

100 MILE HOUSE: 100 Mile District General Hospital
Affiliated with: Interior Health Authority
South Cariboo Health Centre, 555 Cedar Ave. South, 100 Mile House, BC V0K 2E0
Tel: 250-395-7600 *Fax:* 250-395-7578
www.interiorhealth.ca
Social Media: www.facebook.com/InteriorHealth;
twitter.com/Interior_Health; www.youtube.com/InteriorHealthAuth;
www.linkedin.com/company/interior-health-authority

Note: Programs & services include: antepartum care; BC Early Hearing program; Breathe Well program; chemotherapy; dental surgery; diabetes education; electrocardiogram; emergency; endoscopy; gastroenterology; general medicine, rehabilitation, & surgery; hematology; HIV testing; Holter monitor; hospice; intrapartum care; laboratory; maternity; nutrition; oncology; palliative care; physiotherapy; postpartum care; psychiatry; pulmonary rehabilitation; radiology; spiritual care; surgical daycare; swallowing intervention; Telehealth; transfusion; & vasectomy.
Tracy Haddow, Program Director, Hospice
tracy.hospice@shaw.ca

100 MILE HOUSE: South Cariboo Health Centre
Affiliated with: Interior Health Authority
555 Cedar Ave. South, 100 Mile House, BC V0K 2E0
Tel: 250-395-7676
www.interiorhealth.ca

Note: Programs & services include: acquired brain injury services; adult day services; BC Early Hearing Program; caregiver support; case management; community care clinic; community nursing; community nutrition; diabetes education; hearing; home support; immunization; postpartum care; prenatal services; rehabilitation; social work; speech-language pathology; & Tuberculin Skin Testing

ABBOTSFORD: Abbotsford Health Protection Office
Affiliated with: Fraser Health Authority
2776 Bourquin Cres. West, Abbotsford, BC V2S 6A4
Tel: 604-870-7900 *Fax:* 604-870-7901

ABBOTSFORD: Abbotsford Home Health Office
Affiliated with: Fraser Health Authority
34194 Marshall Rd., Abbotsford, BC V2S 5E4
Tel: 604-556-5000 *Fax:* 604-556-5010

ABBOTSFORD: Abbotsford Public Health Unit
Affiliated with: Fraser Health Authority
34194 Marshall Rd., Abbotsford, BC V2S 5E4
Tel: 604-864-3400 *Fax:* 604-864-3410

ABBOTSFORD: Abbotsford Regional Hospital & Cancer Centre
Affiliated with: Fraser Health Authority
32900 Marshall Rd., Abbotsford, BC V2S 0C2
Tel: 604-851-4700
feedback@fraserhealth.ca
www.fraserhealth.ca
Social Media: www.facebook.com/FraserHealthAuthority;
twitter.com/Fraserhealth; www.youtube.com/user/fraserhealth;
www.linkedin.com/company/fraser-health-authority
Number of Beds: 300 beds
Note: Programs & services include: acute care; ambulatory care; angiography; antepartum care; audiology; bone densitometry; cardiac; clinics; CT scans; echocardiography; emergency; enterostomal therapy; fluoroscopy; forensic nursing; general medicine, radiography & surgery; geriatric; hemodialysis; inpatient psychiatric unit; intensive care; interventional radiography; MRI; mammography; maternity; medical oncology; nuclear medicine; outpatient services; pediatrics; pharmacy; postpartum; pulmonary function lab; sleep lab; spiritual care; & ultrasound.
Valerie Spurrell, Executive Director

ABBOTSFORD: Menno Hospital
Affiliated with: Fraser Health Authority
32945 Marshall Rd., Abbotsford, BC V2S 1K1
Tel: 604-859-7631 *Fax:* 604-859-6931
www.mennoplace.ca
Number of Beds: 150 beds
Note: Residential care facility offering 24 hour nursing care, physician, dietitian, occupational therapy, physiotherapy, pharmacy, & recreation services.
Karen Baillie, CEO
Kathrin McMath, Executive Director, Finance & Operations
Hilde Wiebe, Executive Director, Care Services
Jeanette Lee, Director, Human Resources
Sharon Simpson, Director, Communications & Stakeholder
Engagement

AGASSIZ: Agassiz Health Protection Office
Affiliated with: Fraser Health Authority
7243 Pioneer Ave., Agassiz, BC V0M 1A0
Tel: 604-793-7160

AGASSIZ: Agassiz Home Health Office
Affiliated with: Fraser Health Authority
7243 Pioneer Ave., Agassiz, BC V0M 1A0
Tel: 604-793-7160 *Fax:* 604-796-8587

AGASSIZ: Agassiz Mental Health Office
Affiliated with: Fraser Health Authority
7243 Pioneer Ave., Agassiz, BC V0M 1A0
Tel: 604-793-7160 *Fax:* 604-796-8587

AGASSIZ: Agassiz Public Health Unit
Affiliated with: Fraser Health Authority
7243 Pioneer Ave., Agassiz, BC V0M 1A0
Tel: 604-793-7160 *Fax:* 604-796-8587

ALERT BAY: Cormorant Island Health Centre
Affiliated with: Vancouver Island Health Authority
49 School Rd., Alert Bay, BC V0N 1A0
Tel: 250-974-5585
info@viha.ca
www.viha.ca
Social Media: www.facebook.com/VanIslandHealth;
twitter.com/vanislandhealth

Note: Programs & services include: emergency; acute care; residential care; ambulatory outpatient services; laboratory; medical imaging; palliative care; emergency obstetrics; visiting specialists; & medical detox.
Sarah Kowalenko, Communications & Public Relations Assistant, VIHA
250-740-6951, sarah.kowalenko@viha.ca

ALEXIS CREEK: Alexis Creek Health Centre
Affiliated with: Interior Health Authority
2592 Morton Rd., Alexis Creek, BC V0L 1A0
Tel: 250-394-4313
www.interiorhealth.ca

Note: Services include: adult day services; caregiver support; case management; community care clinic; nursing; nutrition; home support; laboratory; rehabilitation; social work; & Telehealth

ARMSTRONG: Armstrong Community Services
Affiliated with: Interior Health Authority
3800 Patten Dr., Armstrong, BC V0E 1B2
Tel: 250-546-4752
www.interiorhealth.ca

ARMSTRONG: Pleasant Valley Health Centre
Affiliated with: Interior Health Authority
3800 Patten Dr., Armstrong, BC V0E 1B2
Tel: 250-546-4700
www.interiorhealth.ca

Note: Programs & services include: acquired brain injury services; adult community support services; adult day services; caregiver support; case management; child & youth immunization program; community care clinic; community nursing; counselling; diabetes education; early psychosis intervention; eating disorders; electrocardiogram; general medicine; home support; immunization; laboratory; nutrition; oncology; ophthalmology; palliative care; physiotherapy; postpartum care;

prenatal; Publicly Funded Tuberculin Skin Testing; radiology; rehabilitation; social work; surgical daycare; & wound care.

ASHCROFT: Ashcroft Hospital & Community Health Care Centre
Affiliated with: Interior Health Authority
700 Ash-Cache Creek Hwy., Ashcroft, BC V0K 1A0
Tel: 250-453-2211 *Fax:* 250-453-9685
Toll-Free: 877-499-6599
www.interiorhealth.ca
Social Media: www.facebook.com/InteriorHealth;
twitter.com/Interior_Health;
www.linkedin.com/company/interior-health-authority
Year Founded: 1970
Number of Beds: 24 extended care beds; 4 emergency beds; 1 respite bed
Note: Programs & services include: diabetes education program; laboratory & radiology; urgent care; ambulatory care; community services; long-term residential care; & on-site doctors' offices.

ATLIN: Atlin Health Centre
Affiliated with: Northern Health Authority
Former Name: Red Cross Outpost Hospital
PO Box 330, 164 3rd St., Atlin, BC V0W 1A0
Tel: 250-651-7677 *Fax:* 250-651-7687
www.northernhealth.ca

Note: Non-emergency services on a walk-in basis; two nurses

BAMFIELD: Bamfield Health Centre
Affiliated with: Vancouver Island Health Authority
PO Box 40, 353 Bamfield Rd., Bamfield, BC V0R 1B0
Tel: 250-728-3312

Kathryn Kilpatrick, Manager
Kathryn.Kilpatrick@viha.ca

BARRIERE: Barriere Health Centre
Affiliated with: Interior Health Authority
4537 Barriere Town Rd., Barriere, BC V0E 1E0
Tel: 250-672-9731
www.interiorhealth.ca

BLUE RIVER: Blue River Health Centre
Affiliated with: Interior Health Authority
Former Name: Red Cross Outpost Hospital
858 Main St., Blue River, BC V0E 1J0
Tel: 250-673-8311
www.interiorhealth.ca

Note: Services include: adult day services; case management; Choice in Support for Independent Living; community care clinic; nursing; nutrition; home support; laboratory; Publicly Funded Tuberculin Skin Testing; rehabilitation; social work; Telehealth

BURNABY: Burnaby Health Protection Office
Affiliated with: Fraser Health Authority
#300, 4946 Canada Way, Burnaby, BC V5G 4H7
Tel: 604-918-7683 *Fax:* 604-918-7520

BURNABY: Burnaby Home Health Office
Affiliated with: Fraser Health Authority
4946 Canada Way, Burnaby, BC V5G 4H7
Tel: 604-918-7447 *Fax:* 604-918-7631

BURNABY: Burnaby Hospital
Affiliated with: Fraser Health Authority
3935 Kincaid St., Burnaby, BC V5G 2X6
Tel: 604-434-4211 *Fax:* 604-412-6190
feedback@fraserhealth.ca
www.fraserhealth.ca
Social Media: www.facebook.com/FraserHealthAuthority;
twitter.com/Fraserhealth;
www.linkedin.com/company/fraser-health-authority
Number of Beds: 295 beds
Note: Programs & services include: acute care; ambulatory care; antepartum care; cardiac; CT scan; concurrent disorders; echocardiography; emergency; fluoroscopy; general medicine; radiography & surgery; geriatric; inpatient psychiatry unit; intensive care; interventional radiography; MRI; mammography; maternity; medical oncology; neonatal intensive care; nuclear medicine; ophthalmology services; orthopaedic surgery; outpatient services; pharmacy; postpartum care; pulmonary function lab; & ultrasound.

Sheila Finamore, Executive Director

BURNABY: Burnaby Public Health Unit
Affiliated with: Fraser Health Authority
4946 Canada Way, Burnaby, BC V5G 4H7
Tel: 604-918-7605 *Fax:* 604-918-7630

BURNABY: Willingdon Care Centre
Affiliated with: Fraser Health Authority
Former Name: Willingdon Private Hospital
4435 Grange St., Burnaby, BC V5H 1P4
Tel: 604-433-2455 *Fax:* 604-433-5804
Number of Beds: 95 beds

BURNS LAKE: Lakes District Hospital & Health Centre
Affiliated with: Northern Health Authority
PO Box 7500, 741 Centre St., Burns Lake, BC V0J 1E0
Tel: 250-692-2400 *Fax:* 250-692-2403
www.northernhealth.ca
Number of Beds: 16 beds
Note: Programs & services include: acute care; emergency; diagnostic imaging; laboratory; public health; mental health & addictions; home & community care; pharmacy; & rehabilitation.

CAMPBELL RIVER: Campbell River & District Regional Hospital
Affiliated with: Vancouver Island Health Authority
Also Known As: Campbell River Hospital
375 - 2nd Ave., Campbell River, BC V9W 3V1
Tel: 250-850-2141
info@viha.ca
www.viha.ca
Social Media: www.facebook.com/VanIslandHealth;
twitter.com/vanislandhealth

Note: Programs & services include: Aboriginal health nurse; diabetes education; heart function clinic; heart health services; laboratory; medical imaging; nutrition; pacemaker clinic; rehabilitation; & surgery.
Christina Rozema, Site Director

CASTLEGAR: Castlegar & District Community Health Centre
Castlegar & District Hospital Foundation
Affiliated with: Interior Health Authority
709 - 10th St., Castlegar, BC V1N 2H7
Tel: 250-365-7711
www.interiorhealth.ca

Note: Programs & services include: acquired brain injury services; addictions treatment programs; adult day services; BC Early Hearing Program; caregiver support; case management; community care clinic; community nursing; community nutrition; community respiratory therapy; diabetes education; electrocardiogram; emergency; harm reduction services; HIV testing; Holter monitor; home support; immunization; postpartum care; prenatal services; Publicly Funded Tuberculin Skin Testing; pulmonary diagnostics; radiology; rehabilitation; social work; Telehealth; & ultrasound.

CELISTA: Scotch Creek Medical Clinic
Affiliated with: Interior Health Authority
#2, 3874 Squilax-Anglemont Rd., Celista, BC V2C 2T1
Tel: 250-955-0660
www.interiorhealth.ca

Note: Programs & services include: acquired brain injury services; adult day services; caregiver support; case management; community care clinic; community nursing; community nutrition; home support; rehabilitation; & social work

CHASE: Chase Health Centre
Affiliated with: Interior Health Authority
825 Thompson Ave., Chase, BC V0E 1M0
Tel: 250-679-3312 *Fax:* 250-679-5329
www.interiorhealth.ca

CHASE: Chase Primary Health Care Clinic
Affiliated with: Interior Health Authority
826 Thompson Ave., Chase, BC V0E 1M0
Tel: 250-679-1400
www.interiorhealth.ca

Note: Programs & services include: acquired brain injury services; adult day services; caregiver support; community care clinic; community nursing; community nutrition; emergency health services; home support; primary health care; pulmonary rehabilitation; rehabilitation; & social work

CHEMAINUS: Chemainus Health Care Centre
Affiliated with: Vancouver Island Health Authority
9909 Esplanade St., Chemainus, BC V0R 1K1
Tel: 250-737-2040 *Fax:* 250-246-3844
Number of Beds: 75 beds
Note: Diagnostic & treatment centre, multilevel care facility
Sue Kurucz, Manager, Residential Care

CHETWYND: Chetwynd Health Unit
Affiliated with: Northern Health Authority
PO Box 507, 5500 Hospital Rd., Chetwynd, BC V0C 1J0
Tel: 250-788-7200 *Fax:* 250-788-7247
www.northernhealth.ca

CHETWYND: Chetwynd Hospital & Health Centre
Affiliated with: Northern Health Authority
PO Box 507, 5500 Hospital Rd., Chetwynd, BC V0C 1J0
Tel: 250-788-2236 *Fax:* 250-788-7247
www.northernhealth.ca
Social Media: www.facebook.com/NorthernHealth;
twitter.com/northern_health; www.youtube.com/northernhealthbc;
www.linkedin.com/company/northern-health-authority
Number of Beds: 7 long-term care beds; 5 acute care beds
Note: Programs & services include: Aboriginal liaison; emergency; medical inpatient; palliative; public health nursing; home & community nursing; home support; & respiratory therapy.

CHILLIWACK: Chilliwack General Hospital
Affiliated with: Fraser Health Authority
45600 Menholm Rd., Chilliwack, BC V2P 1P7
Tel: 604-795-4141 *Fax:* 604-795-4110
feedback@fraserhealth.ca
www.fraserhealth.ca
Social Media: www.facebook.com/FraserHealthAuthority;
twitter.com/Fraserhealth; www.youtube.com/user/fraserhealth;
www.linkedin.com/company/fraser-health-authority
Number of Beds: 135 beds
Note: Programs & services include: acute care; ambulatory care; angiography; antepartum care; cardiac; CT scan; emergency; enterostomal therapy; fluoroscopy; general medicine, radiography & surgery; geriatric; home detox; inpatient psychiatry unit; intensive care; interventional radiography; mammography; maternity; medical oncology; ophthalmology; orthopaedic surgery; outpatient services; pantomography; pharmacy; postpartum; pulmonary function lab; spiritual care; substance use; & ultrasound.
Tracy Irwin, Executive Director
Carol Peters, Aboriginal Health Liaison
carol.peters@fraserhealth.ca

CHILLIWACK: Chilliwack Health Protection Office
Affiliated with: Fraser Health Authority
45470 Menholm Rd., Chilliwack, BC V2P 1M2
Tel: 604-702-4950

CHILLIWACK: Chilliwack Home Health Office
Affiliated with: Fraser Health Authority
45470 Menholm Rd., Chilliwack, BC V2P 1M2
Tel: 604-702-4800 *Fax:* 604-702-4801

CHILLIWACK: Chilliwack Mental Health Office
Affiliated with: Fraser Health Authority
45470 Menholm Rd., Chilliwack, BC V2P 1M2
Tel: 604-702-4860 *Fax:* 604-702-4861

CHILLIWACK: Chilliwack Public Health Unit
Affiliated with: Fraser Health Authority
45470 Menholm Rd., Chilliwack, BC V2P 1M2
Tel: 604-702-4900 *Fax:* 604-702-4901

CLEARWATER: Clearwater Community Health
Affiliated with: Interior Health Authority
640 Park Dr., Clearwater, BC V0E 1N0
Tel: 250-674-3141
www.interiorhealth.ca

Note: Programs & services include: acquired brain injury services; adult day services; caregiver support; community care clinic; community

nursing; community nutrition; home support; immunization; postpartum care; prenatal services; rehabilitation; & social work

CLEARWATER: Dr. Helmcken Memorial Hospital (DHM)
Affiliated with: Interior Health Authority
640 Park Dr., RR#1, Clearwater, BC V0E 1N0
Tel: 250-674-2244 *Fax:* 250-674-2477
www.interiorhealth.ca
Social Media: www.facebook.com/InteriorHealth;
twitter.com/Interior_Health; www.youtube.com/InteriorHealthAuth;
www.linkedin.com/company/interior-health-authority
Number of Beds: 6 beds
Note: Programs & services include: community care; emergency; end of life/palliative care; extended care; general medicine; general rehabilitation; geriatric medicine; hematology; hospice; laboratory; nutrition; orthotics; physiotherapy; radiology; telehealth; & wound care.

CLINTON: Clinton Health & Wellness Centre
Affiliated with: Interior Health Authority
1510 Cariboo Hwy., Clinton, BC V0K 1K0
Tel: 250-459-2080 *Toll-Free:* 855-459-2080
www.interiorhealth.ca

COMOX: St. Joseph's General Hospital
Affiliated with: Vancouver Island Health Authority
2137 Comox Ave., Comox, BC V9M 1P2
Tel: 250-339-2242 *Fax:* 250-339-1432
administration@sjghcomox.ca
www.sjghcomox.ca
Year Founded: 1913
Number of Beds: 241 beds
Note: Programs & services include: colposcopy; daycare; diabetes; diagnostic imaging (mammography, radiology, ultrasound); emergency; extended care; intensive care; laboratory; maternity; nursing; nutritional; oncology; paediatrics; physical medicine; psychiatry; social work; & surgery.
Jane Murphy, President & CEO
Paul Herselman, Medical Director
Cathie Sturam, Site Director, Acute Care

COQUITLAM: Lakeshore Care Centre
The Care Group
Affiliated with: Fraser Health Authority
657 Gatensbury St., Coquitlam, BC V3J 5G9
Tel: 604-939-9277 *Fax:* 604-939-6518
tcgcare.com
Number of Beds: 56 beds
Barb Mendt, Office Manager
lakecare@telus.net
Dana Botelho, Care Coordinator
lakeshoredoc@tcgcare.com

CRANBROOK: Associates Medical Clinic
Affiliated with: Interior Health Authority
123 - 10th Ave. South, Cranbrook, BC V1C 2N1
Tel: 250-426-4231
www.interiorhealth.ca

Note: Services include: pregnancy options & sexual health counselling; immunizations; & referrals

CRANBROOK: Cranbrook Health Centre
Affiliated with: Interior Health Authority
20 - 23rd Ave. South, Cranbrook, BC V1C 5V1
Tel: 250-420-2200
www.interiorhealth.ca

Note: Programs & services include: acquired brain injury services; adult day services; asthma education; caregiver support; case management; community care clinic; community nursing; dietitian/nutrition; dental; diabetes education; environmental; harm reduction supplies & services; hearing services; home oxygen program; home support; immunization; postpartum care; prenatal services; Publicly Funded Tuberculin Skin Testing; rehabilitation; respiratory therapy; social work; & speech-language pathology

SECTION II:
General Resources

CRANBROOK: Cranbrook Wellness Centre
Affiliated with: Interior Health Authority
20 - 23rd Ave. South, Cranbrook, BC V1C 5V1
Tel: 250-489-6414
www.interiorhealth.ca

Note: Programs & services include: Breathe Well Program; Healthy Heart Program; Heart Function Clinic; pulmonary rehabilitation; & TIA Rapid Access Clinic

CRANBROOK: East Kootenay Regional Hospital (EKRH)
Affiliated with: Interior Health Authority
13 - 24th Ave. North, Cranbrook, BC V1C 3H9
Tel: 250-426-5281 *Fax:* 250-426-5285
Toll-Free: 866-288-8082
www.interiorhealth.ca
Social Media: www.facebook.com/InteriorHealth;
twitter.com/Interior_Health; www.youtube.com/InteriorHealthAuth;
www.linkedin.com/company/interior-health-authority

Note: Programs & services include: antepartum care; bone density; cardioversion; chemotherapy; chronic obstructive pulmonary disease services; community care; convalescent care; CT scan; dental surgery; diagnostic bronchoscopy; diagnostic cardiology; ear, nose & throat; echocardiogram, ECG/EKG; emergency; end of life/palliative care; endoscopy; enterostomal therapy; fluoroscopy; general medicine; general rehabilitation; general surgery; hematology; holter monitor; intensive care; intrapartum care; laboratory; mammography; maternity; microbiology; MRI; nuclear medicine; nutrition; oncology; ophthalmology; orthotics; pediatrics; pharmacy; physiotherapy; postpartum care; pulmonary diagnostics; radiology; respiratory therapy; speech-language pathology; spiritual care; telehealth; transfusion; ultrasound; urology; vasectomy; & wound care. Also hosts the Mary Pack Arthritis Program, a service of Vancouver Coastal Health.
Erica Phillips, Administrator, Acute Health Service

CRAWFORD BAY: East Shore Community Health Centre
Affiliated with: Interior Health Authority
15985 Hwy. 3A, Crawford Bay, BC V0B 1E0
Tel: 250-227-9006
www.interiorhealth.ca

CRESTON: Creston Health Unit
Affiliated with: Interior Health Authority
312 - 15th Ave. North, Creston, BC V0B 1G0
Tel: 250-428-3873
www.interiorhealth.ca

Note: Programs & services include: acquired brain injury services; adult day services; caregiver support; case management; community care clinic; community nursing; community nutrition; dental; environmental; home support; immunization; postpartum care; prenatal services; rehabilitation; social work; & Tuberculin Skin Testing

CRESTON: Creston Valley Hospital & Health Care (CVH)
Affiliated with: Interior Health Authority
312 - 15th Ave. North, Creston, BC V0B 1G0
Tel: 250-428-2286 *Fax:* 250-428-4860
www.interiorhealth.ca
Social Media: www.facebook.com/InteriorHealth;
twitter.com/Interior_Health; www.youtube.com/InteriorHealthAuth;
www.linkedin.com/company/interior-health-authority
Number of Beds: 16 beds
Note: Programs & services include: adult day services; antepartum care; community care; community nursing; community nutrition; community respiratory therapy; convalescent care; diabetes education program; dental surgery; ear, nose & throat; ECG/EKG; emergency; end of life/palliative care; endoscopy; enterostomal therapy; general medicine; general rehabilitation; general surgery; hematology; holter monitor; home support; hospice; intrapartum care; laboratory; maternity; pharmacy; physiotherapy; postpartum care; psychiatry; radiology; social work; telehealth; transfusion; ultrasound; vasectomy; vision; & wound care.
Carolyn Hawton, Site Manager

CUMBERLAND: Cumberland Health Care Centre
Affiliated with: Vancouver Island Health Authority
PO Box 400, 2696 Windermere Ave., Cumberland, BC V0R 1S0
Tel: 250-331-8505 *Fax:* 250-336-2100

Number of Beds: 75 beds

DAWSON CREEK: Dawson Creek & District Hospital
Affiliated with: Northern Health Authority
11100 - 13th St., Dawson Creek, BC V1G 3W8
Tel: 250-782-8501 *Fax:* 250-783-7301
www.northernhealth.ca
Social Media: www.facebook.com/NorthernHealth;
twitter.com/northern_health; www.youtube.com/northernhealthbc;
www.linkedin.com/company/northern-health-authority
Number of Beds: 31 acute care beds; 15 adult psychiatric beds
Note: Programs & services include: emergency; ICU; medical & surgical inpatient care; day surgery; maternity; respiratory therapy; rehab therapy; diabetic education; primary care; general surgery; diagnostics (laboratory & medical imaging); cancer care; & visiting specialists in urology, dermatology, & pediatrics.

DAWSON CREEK: Dawson Creek Health Unit
Affiliated with: Northern Health Authority
1001 - 110th Ave., Dawson Creek, BC V1G 4X3
Tel: 250-719-6500 *Fax:* 250-719-6513
www.northernhealth.ca

DEASE LAKE: Stikine Health Centre
Affiliated with: Northern Health Authority
PO Box 386, 7171 Hwy. 37, Dease Lake, BC V0C 1L0
Tel: 250-771-4444 *Fax:* 250-771-3911
www.northernhealth.ca

DELTA: Delta Health Protection Office
Affiliated with: Fraser Health Authority
11245 - 84 Ave., Delta, BC V4C 2L9
Tel: 604-507-5478 *Fax:* 604-507-5492

DELTA: Delta Hospital
Affiliated with: Fraser Health Authority
5800 Mountain View Blvd., Delta, BC V4K 3V6
Tel: 604-946-1121
feedback@fraserhealth.ca
www.fraserhealth.ca
Social Media: www.facebook.com/FraserHealthAuthority;
twitter.com/Fraserhealth; www.youtube.com/user/fraserhealth;
www.linkedin.com/company/fraser-health-authority
Number of Beds: 58 acute care beds
Note: Programs & services include: acute care; cardiac; CT scan; emergency; electrocardiogram; general medicine, radiography & surgery; mammography; outpatient services; pharmacy; pulmonary function testing; palliative care; respiratory therapy; & ultrasound.
Rhonda Veldhoen, Executive Director

DELTA: Delta-South Home Health Office
Affiliated with: Fraser Health Authority
4470 Clarence Taylor Cres., Delta, BC V4K 3W3
Tel: 604-952-3552 *Fax:* 604-946-6953

DUNCAN: Cowichan District Hospital (CDH)
Affiliated with: Vancouver Island Health Authority
3045 Gibbins Rd., Duncan, BC V9L 1E5
Tel: 250-737-2030
info@viha.ca
www.viha.ca
Social Media: www.facebook.com/VanIslandHealth;
twitter.com/vanisalandhealth
Number of Beds: 95 beds
Note: Programs & services include: Aboriginal health nurse; acute inpatient psychiatric services; diabetes education; eye health; heart health; laboratory; medical imaging; mental health; nutrition; rehabilitation; spiritual care; & surgery.
Sarah Kowalenko, Communications & Public Relations Assistant, VIHA
    250-740-6951, sarah.kowalenko@viha.ca
Helen Dunlop, Aboriginal Liaison Nurse, Cowichan & Duncan
    250-746-6184, helen.dunlop@cowichantribes.com

EDGEWOOD: Edgewood Health Centre
Affiliated with: Interior Health Authority
Former Name: Red Cross Outpost Nursing Station
322 Monashee Ave., Edgewood, BC V0G 1J0
Tel: 250-269-7313 *Fax:* 250-269-7520
www.interiorhealth.ca

ELKFORD: Elkford Health Centre
Affiliated with: Interior Health Authority
212 Alpine Way, Elkford, BC V0B 1H0

Tel: 250-865-2247
www.interiorhealth.ca

ENDERBY: Enderby Community Health Centre
Affiliated with: Interior Health Authority
707 - 3rd Ave., Enderby, BC V0E 1V0

Tel: 250-838-2450
www.interiorhealth.ca

Note: Primary health care centre

FERNIE: Elk Valley Hospital
Affiliated with: Interior Health Authority
1501 - 5th Ave., Fernie, BC V0B 1M0

Tel: 250-423-4453 *Fax:* 250-423-3732
www.interiorhealth.ca
Social Media: www.facebook.com/InteriorHealth;
twitter.com/Interior_Health; www.youtube.com/InteriorHealthAuth;
www.linkedin.com/company/interior-health-authority
Number of Beds: 20 beds
Note: Programs & services include: antepartum care; community care;
convalescent care; dental surgery; ear, nose & throat; ECG/EKG;
emergency; end of life/palliative care; endoscopy; enterostomal
therapy; gastroenterology; general medicine; general rehabilitation;
general surgery; hematology; holter monitor; hospice; intrapartum care;
laboratory; maternity; mental health & substance abuse; nutrition;
pharmacy; physiotherapy; postpartum care; radiology; telehealth;
transfusion; urology; vasectomy; & wound care.

FERNIE: Fernie Health Centre
Affiliated with: Interior Health Authority
1501 - 5th Ave., Fernie, BC V0B 1M0

Tel: 250-423-8288
www.interiorhealth.ca

Note: Programs & services include: acquired brain injury services; adult
day services; caregiver support; case management; community care
clinic; community nursing; community nutrition; diabetes education;
home support; immunization; postpartum care; prenatal services;
Publicly Funded Tuberculin Skin Testing; rehabilitation; & social work

FORT LANGLEY: Simpson Manor
Affiliated with: Fraser Health Authority
PO Box 40, Fort Langley, BC V1M 2R4

Tel: 604-888-0711 *Fax:* 604-888-1218
inquiries@simpsonManor.ca
www.simpsonmanor.ca

Note: intermediate & extended care

FORT NELSON: Fort Nelson Health Unit
Affiliated with: Northern Health Authority
Bag 1000, 5217 Airport Dr., Fort Nelson, BC V0C 1R0

Tel: 250-774-7092 *Fax:* 250-774-7096
www.northernhealth.ca

FORT NELSON: Fort Nelson Hospital
Affiliated with: Northern Health Authority
PO Box 1000, 5315 Liard Street, Fort Nelson, BC V0C 1R0

Tel: 250-774-8100 *Fax:* 250-774-8110
www.northernhealth.ca
Social Media: www.facebook.com/NorthernHealth;
twitter.com/northern_health; www.youtube.com/northernhealthbc;
www.linkedin.com/company/northern-health-authority
Number of Beds: 25 acute care beds; 8 long-term care beds
Note: Programs & services include: acute care; child & youth programs;
counselling services; dental clinic; drug & alcohol programs; health unit;
laboratory & x-ray; obstetrics; surgeries; specialists (pediatricians &
OB-GYN); & complementary massage therapy, acupuncture &
physiotherapy.

FORT ST JAMES: Fort St. James Health Unit
Affiliated with: Northern Health Authority
#121, 250 Stuart Dr. NE, Fort St James, BC V0J 1P0

Tel: 250-996-7178 *Fax:* 250-996-2216
www.northernhealth.ca

FORT ST JAMES: Stuart Lake Hospital
Affiliated with: Northern Health Authority
PO Box 1060, 600 Stuart Dr. East, Fort St James, BC V0J 1P0

Tel: 250-996-8201 *Fax:* 250-996-8777
www.northernhealth.ca
Social Media: www.facebook.com/NorthernHealth;
twitter.com/northern_health; www.youtube.com/northernhealthbc;
www.linkedin.com/company/northern-health-authority
Number of Beds: 12 beds
Note: Programs & services include: acute care; emergency; medicine;
mental health & addictions counselling; laboratory; & x-ray.
Amanda Edge, Head Nurse

FORT ST JOHN: Fort St. John Health Unit
Affiliated with: Northern Health Authority
10115 - 110 Ave., Fort St John, BC V1J 6M9

Tel: 250-263-6000 *Fax:* 250-263-6086
www.northernhealth.ca

FORT ST JOHN: Fort St. John Hospital & Peace Villa
Affiliated with: Northern Health Authority
Former Name: Fort St. John Hospital & Health Centre
8407 - 112 Ave., Fort St John, BC V1J 0J5

Tel: 250-262-5200 *Fax:* 250-261-7650
www.northernhealth.ca
Social Media: www.facebook.com/NorthernHealth;
twitter.com/northern_health; www.youtube.com/northernhealthbc;
www.linkedin.com/company/northern-health-authority
Number of Beds: 55 acute care beds; 124 residential care beds
Population Served: 21000
Note: Programs & services include: Aboriginal liaison; acute care;
diagnostics; surgery; medicine; ICU; maternity; mental health &
addictions; palliative care; community cancer centre; community
hemodialysis; social work; & visiting specialists. Also connected to the
Fort St. John Health Unit, North Peace Villa & Heritage Manor II.

FORT ST JOHN: Fort St. John Unattached Patient Clinic
Affiliated with: Northern Health Authority
10011 - 96th St., Fort St John, BC V1J 3P3

Tel: 250-262-5210
www.northernhealth.ca

FRASER LAKE: Fraser Lake Community Health Centre
Affiliated with: Northern Health Authority
PO Box 1000, 130 Chowsunket St., Fraser Lake, BC V0J 1S0

Tel: 250-699-6225 *Fax:* 250-699-6987
www.northernhealth.ca

GOLD RIVER: Gold River Health Centre
Affiliated with: Vancouver Island Health Authority
601 Trumpeter Dr., Gold River, BC V0P 1G0

Tel: 250-283-2626 *Fax:* 250-283-7436

Note: Urgent care centre; laboratory; addiction services; child health
care.

GOLDEN: Golden & District General Hospital
Affiliated with: Interior Health Authority
835 - 9th Ave. South, Golden, BC V0A 1H0

Tel: 250-344-5271 *Fax:* 250-344-2511
www.interiorhealth.ca
Social Media: www.facebook.com/InteriorHealth;
twitter.com/Interior_Health; www.youtube.com/InteriorHealthAuth;
www.linkedin.com/company/interior-health-authority
Number of Beds: 8 beds
Note: Programs & services include: antepartum care; community care;
community respiratory therapy; convalescent care; diabetes education
program; ear, nose & throat; ECG/EKG; emergency; end of
life/palliative care; endoscopy; general medicine; general rehabilitation;
general surgery; hematology; holter monitor; hospice; intrapartum care;
laboratory; maternity; nutrition; orthopedics; postpartum care;
psychiatry; pulmonary diagnostics; radiology; telehealth; transfusion;
ultrasound; vasectomy; & wound care.

GOLDEN: Golden Health Centre
Affiliated with: Interior Health Authority
835 - 9th Ave. South, Golden, BC V0A 1H0

Tel: 250-344-3001
www.interiorhealth.ca

Note: Programs & services include: adult day services; caregiver support; case management; community care clinic; community nursing; community nutrition; home support; immunization; postpartum care; prenatal services; rehabilitation; social work; speech-language pathology; & Tuberculin Skin Testing

GRAND FORKS: Boundary Community Health Centre
Affiliated with: Interior Health Authority
7441 - 2nd St., Grand Forks, BC V0H 1H0

Tel: 250-443-3150
www.interiorhealth.ca

GRAND FORKS: Boundary Hospital
Affiliated with: Interior Health Authority
7649 - 22nd St., Grand Forks, BC V0H 1H2

Tel: 250-443-2100 *Fax:* 250-442-8331
www.interiorhealth.ca
Social Media: www.facebook.com/InteriorHealth;
twitter.com/Interior_Health; www.youtube.com/InteriorHealthAuth;
www.linkedin.com/company/interior-health-authority
Number of Beds: 12 acute care beds
Note: Programs & services include: chemotherapy; community care; community respiratory therapy; diabetes education program; ECG/EKG; emergency; end of life/palliative; extended care; general medicine; holter monitor; hospice; laboratory; mental health & substance abuse; nutrition; oncology; physiotherapy; pulmonary diagnostics; radiology; telehealth; transfusion; ultrasound; & wound care.

GRAND FORKS: Grand Forks Public Health
Affiliated with: Interior Health Authority
7441 2nd St., Grand Forks, BC V0H 1H0

Tel: 250-443-3150
www.interiorhealth.ca

Note: Programs & services include: dental; environmental; food safety; immunization; postpartum care; & prenatal services

GRANISLE: Granisle Community Health Centre
Affiliated with: Northern Health Authority
PO Box 219, 1 Hagen St., Granisle, BC V0J 1W0

Tel: 250-697-2251 *Fax:* 250-697-6221
www.northernhealth.ca

HAZELTON: Hazelton Community Health
Affiliated with: Northern Health Authority
Bag 999, 2510 Hwy. 62, Hazelton, BC V0J 1Y0

Tel: 250-842-4640 *Fax:* 250-842-4642
www.northernhealth.ca

HAZELTON: Wrinch Memorial Hospital
Affiliated with: Northern Health Authority
PO Box 999, 2510 Hwy. 62, Hazelton, BC V0J 1Y0

Tel: 250-842-5211 *Fax:* 250-842-5865
www.northernhealth.ca
Number of Beds: 10 acute care beds; 9 complex care beds; 1 respite bed; 1 psychiatric observation room
Population Served: 7000
Number of Employees: 70
Note: Programs & services include: acute care; complex care; diabetes education; doctors clinic; emergency room; home & community care; laboratory (ultrasound & x-ray); pharmacy; physiotherapy & occupational therapy; & visiting specialists.

HOPE: Fraser Canyon Hospital
Affiliated with: Fraser Health Authority
1275 - 7th Ave., Hope, BC V0X 1L4

Tel: 604-869-5656 *Fax:* 604-860-7732
feedback@fraserhealth.ca
www.fraserhealth.ca
Social Media: www.facebook.com/FraserHealthAuthority;
twitter.com/Fraserhealth; www.youtube.com/user/fraserhealth;
www.linkedin.com/company/fraser-health-authority
Number of Beds: 10 beds
Note: Programs & services include: acute care; ambulatory care; emergency; general medicine & radiography; hospice residence; outpatient services; & spiritual care.
Petra Pardy, Executive Director

HOPE: Fraser Hope Lodge
Affiliated with: Fraser Health Authority
1275 - 7th Ave., Hope, BC V0X 1L4

Tel: 604-860-7706 *Fax:* 604-860-7708
Number of Beds: 50 beds

HOUSTON: Houston Health Centre
Affiliated with: Northern Health Authority
PO Box 538, 3202 - 14 St., Houston, BC V0J 1Z0

Tel: 250-845-2294 *Fax:* 250-845-7884
www.northernhealth.ca

HUDSON'S HOPE: Hudson's Hope Health Centre
Affiliated with: Northern Health Authority
Former Name: Hudson's Hope Gething Diagnostic & Treatment Centre
PO Box 599, 10309 Kyllo St., Hudson's Hope, BC V0C 1V0

Tel: 250-783-9991 *Fax:* 250-783-9125
www.northernhealth.ca
Number of Beds: 2 emergency beds
Population Served: 1000

INVERMERE: Invermere & District Hospital
Affiliated with: Interior Health Authority
850 - 10th Ave., Invermere, BC V0A 1K0

Tel: 250-342-9201
www.interiorhealth.ca
Social Media: www.facebook.com/InteriorHealth;
twitter.com/Interior_Health; www.youtube.com/InteriorHealthAuth;
www.linkedin.com/company/interior-health-authority
Number of Beds: 8 acute care beds; 30 residential beds
Note: Programs & services include: antepartum care; community care; community respiratory therapy; convalescent care; diabetes education program; ear, nose & throat; ECG/EKG; end of life/palliative care; general medicine; general rehabilitation; hematology; holter monitor; hospice; intrapartum care; laboratory; maternity; nutrition; postpartum care; psychiatry; pulmonary diagnostics; radiology; transfusion; & wound care.

INVERMERE: Invermere Health Centre
Affiliated with: Interior Health Authority
PO Box 2069, 850 - 10th Ave., Invermere, BC V0A 1K0

Tel: 250-342-2360
www.interiorhealth.ca

Note: Programs & services include: adult day services; caregiver support; case management; community care clinic; community nursing; community nutrition; emergency; environmental health; home support; immunization; postpartum care; prenatal services; rehabilitation; social work; speech language pathology; & Tuberculin Skin Testing

KAMLOOPS: Kamloops Primary Care Clinic
Affiliated with: Interior Health Authority
#36, 450 Lansdowne St., Kamloops, BC V2C 1Y3

Tel: 250-851-7954
www.interiorhealth.ca

Note: Programs & services include: Breathe Well program; primary health care; & pulmonary rehabilitation

KAMLOOPS: Kamloops Public Health Unit
Affiliated with: Interior Health Authority
519 Columbia St., Kamloops, BC V2C 2T8

Tel: 250-851-7300 *Toll-Free:* 866-847-4372
www.interiorhealth.ca

Note: Programs & services include: adult day services; caregiver support; case management; community care clinic; community nursing; community nutrition; dental; environmental; hearing; home support; immunization; nutrition; postpartum care; prenatal services; Publicly Funded Tuberculin Skin Testing; recreational water safety; rehabilitation; social work; & speech-language pathology

KAMLOOPS: North Shore X-Ray Clinic
Affiliated with: Interior Health Authority
789 Fortune Dr., #B3, Kamloops, BC V2B 2L3

Tel: 250-314-2420
www.interiorhealth.ca

Note: Services include bone density & radiology

KAMLOOPS: Royal Inland Hospital
Affiliated with: Interior Health Authority
311 Columbia St., Kamloops, BC V2C 2T1
Tel: 250-374-5111 *Fax:* 250-314-2333
Toll-Free: 877-288-5688
www.interiorhealth.ca
Social Media: www.facebook.com/InteriorHealth;
twitter.com/Interior_Health; www.youtube.com/InteriorHealthAuth;
www.linkedin.com/company/interior-health-authority
Number of Beds: 224 beds
Note: Programs & services include: acute neurology; antepartum care; cardioversion; chemotherapy; chronic obstructive pulmonary disease services; community care; community respiratory therapy; convalescent care; CT scan; dental surgery; diabetes education program; diagnostic bronchoscopy; ear, nose & throat; echocardiogram; ECG/EKG; emergency; end of life/palliative; endoscopy; enterostomal therapy; fluoroscopy; gastroenterology; general medicine, rehabilitation & surgery; geriatric medicine; hematology; holter monitor; hospice; intensive care; intrapartum care; laboratory; mammography; maternity; mental health & substance abuse; microbiology; MRI; neonatal intensive care; nutrition; oncology; ophthalmology; orthotics; otolaryngology surgery; pediatrics; pharmacy; physiotherapy; plastic surgery; postpartum care; pulmonary diagnostics; radiology; respiratory therapy; sleep disorders; speech-language pathology; spiritual care; telehealth; transfusion; ultrasound; urology; vascular & thoracic; vasectomy; & wound care.
Deb Donald, Aboriginal Patient Liaison

KASLO: Kaslo Physiotherapy
Affiliated with: Interior Health Authority
673A Ave., Kaslo, BC V0G 1M0
Tel: 250-353-2742
www.interiorhealth.ca

KASLO: Kaslo Primary Health Centre
Affiliated with: Interior Health Authority
673A Ave., Lower Level, Kaslo, BC V0G 1M0
Tel: 250-353-2291
www.interiorhealth.ca

Note: Programs & services include: adult day services; caregiver support; case management; community care clinic; community nursing; community nutrition; home support; immunization; postpartum care; prenatal services; primary health care; rehabilitation; social work; & Tuberculin Skin Testing

KASLO: Victorian Community Health Centre of Kaslo
Affiliated with: Interior Health Authority
Former Name: Victoria Hospital of Kaslo
673 A Ave., Kaslo, BC V0G 1M0
Tel: 250-353-2211 *Fax:* 250-353-2738
www.interiorhealth.ca

Note: Programs & services include: acquired brain injury services; addictions day treatment program; adult day services; caregiver support; case management; community care clinic; community nursing; community nutrition; emergency health; home support; radiology; rehabilitation; social work; & Telehealth.
Aimee Watson, Regional Director

KELOWNA: Capri Community Health Centre
Affiliated with: Interior Health Authority
Capri Centre Mall, #118, 1835 Gordon Dr., Kelowna, BC V1Y 3H4
Tel: 250-980-1400
www.interiorhealth.ca

KELOWNA: Interior Health Authority
505 Doyle Ave., Kelowna, BC V1Y 0C5
Tel: 250-469-7070 *Fax:* 250-469-7068
www.interiorhealth.ca
Info Line: 811
Social Media: www.facebook.com/InteriorHealth;
twitter.com/Interior_Health; www.youtube.com/user/InteriorHealthAuth;
www.linkedin.com/company/interior-health-authority
Year Founded: 2001
Number of Beds: 6,584 residential care & assisted living beds; 1,391 hospital beds
Area Served: 215,000 sq km
Population Served: 740000

Number of Employees: 19000
Note: Serves cities such as Kelowna, Kamloops, Cranbrook, Trail, Penticton & Vernon, as well as rural & remote communities. Services include: Acute care, health promotion & prevention, community care, residential care, mental health & substance use, & public health.
John O'Fee, Board Chair
Chris Mazurkewich, President & CEO
Dr. Trevor Corneil, Chief Medical Health Officer & Vice-President, Population Health
Donna Lommer, Chief Financial Officer & Vice-President, Support Services
Susan Brown, COO & Vice-President, Hospitals & Communities
Dr. Alan Stewart, Vice-President, Medicine & Quality
Mal Griffin, Vice-President, Human Resources
Jamie Braman, Vice-President, Communications & Public Engagement
Norma Malanowich, Chief Information Officer & Vice-President, Clinical Support Services

KELOWNA: Kelowna General Hospital
Affiliated with: Interior Health Authority
2268 Pandosy St., Kelowna, BC V1Y 1T2
Tel: 250-862-4000 *Fax:* 250-862-4020
Toll-Free: 888-877-4442
www.interiorhealth.ca
Social Media: www.facebook.com/InteriorHealth;
twitter.com/Interior_Health; www.youtube.com/InteriorHealthAuth;
www.linkedin.com/company/interior-health-authority
Number of Beds: 341 acute care beds
Note: Programs & services include: acute neurology; acute psychiatry; angioplasty; antepartum care; arthritis rehabilitation; cardiac angiogram; cardioversion; chemotherapy; chronic obstructive pulmonary disease services; community care; community respiratory therapy; convalescent care; CT scan; dental surgery; diabetes education program; diagnostic bronchoscopy; diagnostic cardiology; ear, nose & throat; echocardiogram; ECG/EKG; emergency; end of life/palliative; endocrinology; endoscopy; enterostomal therapy; fluoroscopy; gastroenterology; general medicine, rehabilitation & surgery; geriatric medicine; hematology; holter monitor; hospice; intensive care; intrapartum care; laboratory; mammography; maternity; mental health & substance abuse; microbiology; MRI; nuclear medicine; nutrition; oncology; ophthalmology; orthotics; otolaryngology surgery; pediatrics; pharmacy; physiotherapy; plastic surgery; postpartum care; psoriasis & phototherapy; radiology; respiratory therapy; sleep disorders; speech-language pathology; spiritual care; telehealth; transfusion; ultrasound; urology; vascular & thoracic surgery; vasectomy; vision; & wound care.
John Cabral, Director, Health Services

KELOWNA: Kelowna Research Centre
Affiliated with: Interior Health Authority
2309 Abbott St., Kelowna, BC V1Y 1T2
Tel: 250-862-9777
www.interiorhealth.ca

Note: Services include: assessment & case management; nursing; rehabilitation; home support; & palliative care

KELOWNA: Kelowna Transplant Clinic
Affiliated with: Interior Health Authority
2268 Pandosy St., Kelowna, BC V1Y 1T2
Tel: 250-862-4156
www.interiorhealth.ca

Note: Follow-up care for organ transplant recipients, primarily renal transplant.

KELOWNA: May Bennett Wellness Centre
Affiliated with: Interior Health Authority
Former Name: May Bennett Home
135 Davie Rd., Kelowna, BC V1X 1Y8
Tel: 250-980-1400
www.interiorhealth.ca

Note: Services include: adult day services; caregiver support; case management; Choice in Support for Independent Living; community care clinic; nursing; nutrition; diabetes education; home support; rehabilitation; & social work

KELOWNA: Outreach Urban Health Centre
Affiliated with: Interior Health Authority
455 Leon Ave., Kelowna, BC V1V 6J3
Tel: 250-868-2230
www.interiorhealth.ca

Note: Primary health centre

KELOWNA: Rutland Aurora Health Centre
Affiliated with: Interior Health Authority
#102, 285 Aurora Cres., Kelowna, BC V1X 7N6
Tel: 250-491-1100
www.interiorhealth.ca

KELOWNA: Rutland Health Centre
Affiliated with: Interior Health Authority
155 Gray Rd., Kelowna, BC V1X 1W6
Tel: 250-980-4825
www.interiorhealth.ca

Note: Programs & services include: immunization; postpartum care; & prenatal services

KELOWNA: Surgical Optimization Clinic (Hip & Knee)
Affiliated with: Interior Health Authority
#118, 1835 Gordon Dr., Kelowna, BC V1Y 3H5
Tel: 250-980-1515
www.interiorhealth.ca

KEREMEOS: South Similkameen Health Centre
Affiliated with: Interior Health Authority
700 - 3rd St., Keremeos, BC V0X 1N3
Tel: 250-499-3000
www.interiorhealth.ca

Note: Community services (250-499-3029). Programs & services include: acquired brain injury services; adult day services; caregiver support; case management; community care clinic; community nursing; community nutrition; diabetes education; electrocardiogram; emergency; Holter monitor; home support; immunization; postpartum care; prenatal services; Publicly Funded Tuberculin Skin Testing; radiology; rehabilitation; social work; & Telehealth

KIMBERLEY: Kimberley Health Centre & Home Support
Affiliated with: Interior Health Authority
260 - 4th Ave., Kimberley, BC V1A 2R6
Tel: 250-427-2215
www.interiorhealth.ca

Note: A primary health care centre also providing home-based services, such as assessment & case management, nursing, rehabilitation, home support, & palliative care.

KINCOLITH: Kincolith Nursing Station
1303 Fireman St., Kincolith, BC V0V 1B0
Tel: 250-326-4242

KITIMAT: Kitimat General Hospital & Health Centre
Affiliated with: Northern Health Authority
920 Lahakas Blvd. South, Kitimat, BC V8C 2S3
Tel: 250-632-2121 *Fax:* 250-632-8726
www.northernhealth.ca
Social Media: www.facebook.com/NorthernHealth;
twitter.com/northern_health; www.youtube.com/northernhealthbc;
www.linkedin.com/company/northern-health-authority
Number of Beds: 22 acute care beds; 36 multi-level care beds
Note: Programs & services include: acute care; medicine; pediatrics; surgery; obstetrics; emergency; physiotherapy; radiology; laboratory; home support/home nursing; long-term care case management; orthopedics; & visiting specialists in urology, ENT surgery, dermatology, neurology, ophthalmology, & radiology.
Jonathan Cooper, Administrator, Health Services

LADYSMITH: Ladysmith Community Health Centre
Affiliated with: Vancouver Island Health Authority
Former Name: Ladysmith & District General Hospital
PO Box 10, 1111 - 4 Ave., Ladysmith, BC V9G 1A1
Tel: 250-739-5777 *Fax:* 250-740-2689
info@viha.ca
www.viha.ca
Social Media: www.facebook.com/135150073228437;
twitter.com/vanislandhealth

Heather Dunne, Site Manager
Heather.Dunne@viha.ca

LAKE COUNTRY: Public Health Satellite Office
Affiliated with: Interior Health Authority
10080 Main St., Lake Country, BC V4V 1T8
www.interiorhealth.ca

LANGLEY: Langley Memorial Hospital
Affiliated with: Fraser Health Authority
Former Name: Langley Health Services
22051 Fraser Hwy., Langley, BC V3A 4H4
Tel: 604-514-6000 *Fax:* 604-534-8283
feedback@fraserhealth.ca
www.fraserhealth.ca
Social Media: www.facebook.com/FraserHealthAuthority;
twitter.com/Fraserhealth; www.youtube.com/user/fraserhealth;
www.linkedin.com/company/fraser-health-authority
Number of Beds: 166 acute care beds; 224 extended care beds
Note: Programs & services include: acute care; ambulatory care; antepartum care; CT scan; echocardiography; emergency; fluoroscopy; general medicine, radiography & surgery; hospice residence; inpatient psychiatry unit; intensive care; interventional radiography; maternity; outpatient services; pediatrics; pharmacy; postpartum care; spiritual care; & ultrasound.
Jason Cook, Executive Director

LILLOOET: Lillooet Home & Community Centre
Affiliated with: Interior Health Authority
951 Murray St., Lillooet, BC V0K 1V0
Tel: 250-256-4233
www.interiorhealth.ca

LILLOOET: Lillooet Hospital & Health Centre
Affiliated with: Interior Health Authority
Former Name: Lillooet District Hospital & Community Health Programs
951 Murray St., Lillooet, BC V0K 1V0
Tel: 250-256-4233 *Fax:* 250-256-1336
Toll-Free: 855-656-4233
www.interiorhealth.ca
Social Media: www.facebook.com/InteriorHealth;
twitter.com/Interior_Health; www.youtube.com/InteriorHealthAuth;
www.linkedin.com/company/interior-health-authority
Number of Beds: 6 acute care beds
Note: Programs & services include: antepartum care; community care; dental surgery; diabetes education program; ECG/EKG; emergency; end of life/palliative care; endoscopy; general medicine; general surgery; holter monitor; home support; hospice; intrapartum care; laboratory; maternity; mental health & substance issues; nutrition; physiotherapy; postpartum care; prenatal; radiology; rehabilitation; social work; telehealth; vasectomy; & wound care.

LOGAN LAKE: Logan Lake Primary Health Care
Affiliated with: Interior Health Authority
Former Name: Logan Lake Health Centre
5 Beryl Dr., Logan Lake, BC V0K 1W0
Tel: 250-523-9414
www.interiorhealth.ca

LUMBY: Lumby Health Unit
Affiliated with: Interior Health Authority
2135 Norris Ave., Lumby, BC V0E 2G0
Tel: 250-547-9741
www.interiorhealth.ca

Note: Programs & services include: acquired brain injury services; adult day services; caregiver support; case management; community care clinic; community nursing; community nutrition; home support;

immunization; postpartum care; prenatal services; Publicly Funded Tuberculin Skin Testing; rehabilitation; & social work

LUMBY: Whitevalley Community Resource Centre
Affiliated with: Interior Health Authority
2114 Shuswap Ave., Lumby, BC V0E 2G0

Tel: 250-547-8866

LYTTON: St. Bartholomew's Health Centre
Affiliated with: Interior Health Authority
575A Main St., Lytton, BC V0K 1Z0

Tel: 250-455-2221 *Fax:* 250-455-6621
Toll-Free: 855-955-2221
www.interiorhealth.ca

Note: Programs & services include: acquired brain injury services; adult day services; caregiver support; case management; community care clinic; community nursing; community nutrition; electrocardiogram; emergency; home support; Publicly Funded Tuberculin Skin Testing; radiology; rehabilitation; social work; & Telehealth.

MACKENZIE: MacKenzie & District Hospital & Health Centre
Affiliated with: Northern Health Authority
Former Name: Mackenzie & District Hospital
PO Box 249, 45 Centennial Dr., MacKenzie, BC V0J 2C0

Tel: 250-997-3263 *Fax:* 250-997-3940
www.northernhealth.ca
Social Media: www.facebook.com/NorthernHealth;
twitter.com/northern_health; www.youtube.com/northernhealthbc;
www.linkedin.com/company/northern-health-authority
Number of Beds: 5 beds
Population Served: 4539
Note: Programs & services include: emergency; medicine; medical imaging; laboratory; home care nursing; public health; & mental health & addictions.
Barb Crook, Administrator

MAPLE RIDGE: Holyrood Manor
Revera Inc.
Affiliated with: Fraser Health Authority
22710 Holyrood Ave., Maple Ridge, BC V2X 3E6

Tel: 604-467-8831 *Fax:* 604-467-8262
holyrood@reveraliving.com
www.reveraliving.com
Social Media: www.facebook.com/400950748267;
twitter.com/Revera_Inc; www.youtube.com/user/ReveraInc;
www.linkedin.com/company/revera-inc
Number of Beds: 125 beds
Thomas G. Wellner, President & CEO, Revera Living

MAPLE RIDGE: Ridge Meadows Hospital
Affiliated with: Fraser Health Authority
Former Name: Ridge Meadows Hospice Society
PO Box 5000, 11666 Laity St., Maple Ridge, BC V2X 7G5

Tel: 604-463-4111 *Fax:* 604-463-1888
feedback@fraserhealth.ca
www.fraserhealth.ca
Social Media: www.facebook.com/FraserHealthAuthority;
twitter.com/Fraserhealth;
www.linkedin.com/company/fraser-health-authority
Number of Beds: 125 acute care beds; 148 residential care beds; 20 psychiatric beds; 10 convalescent beds; 10 hospice beds
Note: Programs & services include: acute care; ambulatory care; antepartum care; cardiac; CT scan; emergency; fluoroscopy; general medicine, radiography, rehabilitation & surgery; inpatient psychiatry; intensive care; interventional radiography; mammography; maternity; medical daycare; medical oncology; outpatient services; pediatrics; pharmacy; postpartum; pulmonary; spiritual care; & ultrasound.
Kathy Doull, Executive Director

MASSET: Masset Community Health
Affiliated with: Northern Health Authority
PO Box 215, 2520 Harrison Ave., Masset, BC V0T 1M0

Tel: 250-626-4727 *Fax:* 250-626-5279
www.northernhealth.ca

MASSET: Northern Haida Gwaii Hospital & Health Centre
Affiliated with: Northern Health Authority
PO Box 319, 2520 Harrison Ave., Masset, BC V0T 1M0

Tel: 250-626-4700 *Fax:* 250-626-4709
www.northernhealth.ca
Number of Beds: 4 acute care beds; 4 long-term care beds
Note: Programs & services include: acute care; emergency; general medicine; surgery; community health; public health; & mental health.

MCBRIDE: McBride & District Hospital
Affiliated with: Northern Health Authority
1136 - 5th Ave., McBride, BC V0J 2E0

Tel: 250-569-2251 *Fax:* 250-569-2232
www.northernhealth.ca
Social Media: www.facebook.com/NorthernHealth;
twitter.com/northern_health; www.youtube.com/northernhealthbc;
www.linkedin.com/company/northern-health-authority
Number of Beds: 3 acute care beds; 8 long-term care beds
Note: Programs & services include: acute care; diagnostic imaging; emergency; laboratory; long-term care; mental health & addictions counselling; physiotherapy; & public health.

MCBRIDE: McBride Health Unit
Affiliated with: Northern Health Authority
1126 - 5th Ave., McBride, BC V0J 2E0

Tel: 250-569-2251 *Fax:* 250-569-2232
www.northernhealth.ca
Info Line: 888-562-1214

MERRITT: Merritt Public Health
Affiliated with: Interior Health Authority
3451 Voght St., Merritt, BC V1K 1C6

Tel: 250-378-3400
www.interiorhealth.ca

Note: Programs & services include: immunization; postpartum care; prenatal services; & Tuberculin Skin Testing

MERRITT: Nicola Valley Hospital & Health Centre
Affiliated with: Interior Health Authority
Former Name: Nicola Valley General Hospital
3451 Voght St., Merritt, BC V1K 1C6

Tel: 250-378-2242 *Fax:* 250-378-3287
www.interiorhealth.ca
Social Media: www.facebook.com/InteriorHealth;
twitter.com/interior_health; www.youtube.com/InteriorHealthAuth;
www.linkedin.com/company/interior-health-authority
Number of Beds: 8 beds
Note: Programs & services include: diabetes education program; emergency; rehabilitation & physiotherapy; public health; mental health; home & community care nursing; home support; laboratory; & x-ray.

MIDWAY: Midway Health Unit
Affiliated with: Interior Health Authority
540 - 7th Ave., Midway, BC V0H 1M0

Tel: 250-449-2887
www.interiorhealth.ca

Note: Programs & services include: acquired brain injury services; adult day services; caregiver support; case management; community care clinic; community nursing; community nutrition; home support; immunization; postpartum care; prenatal services; rehabilitation; social work; & Tuberculin Skin Testing

MISSION: Mission Memorial Hospital
Affiliated with: Fraser Health Authority
7324 Hurd St., Mission, BC V2V 3H5

Tel: 604-826-6261 *Fax:* 604-826-9513
feedback@fraserhealth.ca
www.fraserhealth.ca
Social Media: www.facebook.com/FraserHealthAuthority;
twitter.com/Fraserhealth; www.youtube.com/user/fraserhealth;
www.linkedin.com/company/fraser-health-authority
Number of Beds: 20 beds; 2 palliative care beds
Note: Programs & services include: acute care; ambulatory care; emergency; general medicine & radiography; hospice residence; orthopaedic surgery; outpatient laboratory; residential care; spiritual care; & ultrasound.
Valerie Spurrell, Executive Director

SECTION II:
General Resources

NAKUSP: Arrow & Slocan Lakes Community Services
Affiliated with: Interior Health Authority
205 - 6th Ave., Nakusp, BC V0G 1R0

Tel: 250-265-3674
www.interiorhealth.ca

Note: Services: addictions treatment
Tim Payne, Executive Director

NAKUSP: Arrow Lakes Hospital
Affiliated with: Interior Health Authority
97 - 1st Ave. NE, Nakusp, BC V0G 1R0

Tel: 250-265-3622 Fax: 250-265-4435
www.interiorhealth.ca
Social Media: www.facebook.com/InteriorHealth;
twitter.com/Interior_Health; www.youtube.com/InteriorHealthAuth;
www.linkedin.com/company/interior-health-authority
Number of Beds: 14 beds
Note: Programs & services include: community care; community respiratory therapy; diabetes education program; emergency; end of life/palliative care; extended care; general medicine; hospice; laboratory; mental health & substance abuse; nutrition/dietitian; physiotherapy; pulmonary diagnostics; radiology; telehealth; transfusion; & wound care.

NAKUSP: Nakusp Health Unit
Affiliated with: Interior Health Authority
97 - 1st Ave. NE, Nakusp, BC V0G 1R0

Tel: 250-265-3608
www.interiorhealth.ca

Note: Programs & services include: acquired brain injury services; adult day services; caregiver support; case management; community care clinic; community nursing; community nutrition; home support; immunization; postpartum clinic; prenatal services; rehabilitation; social work; & Tuberculin Skin Testing

NANAIMO: Columbian Centre Society
2356 Rosstown Rd., Nanaimo, BC V9T 3R7

Tel: 250-758-8711 Fax: 250-751-1128
info@columbiancentre.org
www.columbiancentre.org

Number of Beds: 10 beds
Tom Grauman, Administrator

NANAIMO: Nanaimo Regional General Hospital
Affiliated with: Vancouver Island Health Authority
1200 Dufferin Cres., Nanaimo, BC V9S 2B7

Tel: 250-755-7691 Toll-Free: 250-947-8214
www.viha.ca
Social Media: www.facebook.com/VanIslandHealth;
twitter.com/vanislandhealth

Number of Beds: 220+ beds
Note: Programs & services include: Aboriginal health nurse; acute inpatient psychiatric services; cardiac risk reduction; diabetes education; eye health; heart function; heart health; laboratory; medical imaging; neurophysiology; nutrition; pacemaker; pain program; rehabilitation; spiritual care; & surgery.
Carol Nelson, Aboriginal Liaison Nurse
  carol.nelson@viha.ca

NELSON: Kootenay Lake Hospital
Affiliated with: Interior Health Authority
3 View St., Nelson, BC V1L 2V1

Tel: 250-352-3111 Fax: 250-354-2320
Toll-Free: 866-352-3111
www.interiorhealth.ca
Social Media: www.facebook.com/InteriorHealth;
twitter.com/Interior_Health; www.youtube.com/InteriorHealthAuth;
www.linkedin.com/company/interior-health-authority
Number of Beds: 30 beds
Note: Services offered include: antepartum care; chemotherapy; chronic obstructive pulmonary disease services; community care; community respiratory therapy; convalescent care; CT scan; dental surgery; diabetes education program; echocardiogram; ECG/EKG; emergency; end of life/palliative care; endoscopy; general medicine & rehabilitation; geriatric medicine; hematology; holter monitor; hospice; intrapartum care; laboratory; mammography; maternity; microbiology; nutrition; oncology; ophthalmology; pediatrics; pharmacy;

physiotherapy; postpartum care; pulmonary diagnostics & rehabilitation; radiology; telehealth; transfusion; & ultrasound.

NELSON: Nelson Health Centre
Affiliated with: Interior Health Authority
333 Victoria St., Nelson, BC V1L 4K3

Tel: 250-505-7200
www.interiorhealth.ca

Note: Programs & services include: acquired brain injury services; addictions treatment programs; caregiver support; case management; community care clinic; community nursing; community nutrition; dental; environmental; home support; immunization; nutrition; postpartum care; prenatal services; Publicly Funded Tuberculin Skin Testing; rehabilitation; social work; & speech-language pathology

NEW DENVER: Slocan Community Health Centre
Affiliated with: Interior Health Authority
401 Galena Ave., New Denver, BC V0G 1S0

Tel: 250-358-7911 Fax: 250-358-7117
www.interiorhealth.ca

Number of Beds: 30 beds
Note: Primary health care centre. Services include: caregiver support; community care clinic; electrocardiogram; emergency; home support; radiology; rehabilitation; social work; & therapy.

NEW WESTMINSTER: Honour House
Honour House Society
Former Name: Blue Spruce Cottage
509 St. George St., New Westminster, BC V3L 1L1

Tel: 778-397-4399 Fax: 778-397-4396
admin@honourhouse.ca
www.honourhouse.ca

Year Founded: 2010
Number of Beds: 11 beds
Number of Employees: 2
Note: Honour House provides a free of charge, temporary home for Canadian Armed Forces, Veterans, Emergency Services Personnel & their families while they travel to receive medical care & treatment in the Metro Vancouver Area.
Craig Longstaff, General Manager
  craig@honourhouse.ca

NEW WESTMINSTER: Royal Columbian Hospital
Affiliated with: Fraser Health Authority
330 East Columbia St., New Westminster, BC V3L 3W7

Tel: 604-520-4253
feedback@fraserhealth.ca
www.fraserhealth.ca
Social Media: www.facebook.com/FraserHealthAuthority;
twitter.com/Fraserhealth

Year Founded: 1862
Number of Beds: 402 acute care beds
Note: Programs & services include: emergency; acute care; care for the elderly; angiography; antepartum care; bone densitometry; cardiac; bronchoscopy services; ultrasound; fluoroscopy; radiography; surgery unit; hemodialysis; psychiatry; intensive care unit; MRI; mammography; oncology; neonatal intensive care; neurological services; orthopaedic surgery; paediatrics; pantomography; physiotherapy; plastic surgery; & vascular & thoracic surgery.
Darlene MacKinnon, Executive Director

OLIVER: Oliver Health Centre
Affiliated with: Interior Health Authority
930 Spillway Rd., Oliver, BC V0H 1T0

Tel: 250-498-5080
www.interiorhealth.ca

Note: Programs & services include: acquired brain injury services; adult day services; caregiver support; case management; community care clinic; community nursing; community nutrition; home support; immunization; postpartum care; prenatal services; Publicly Funded Tuberculin Skin Testing; rehabilitation; social work; & speech-language pathology

OLIVER: South Okanagan General Hospital
Affiliated with: Interior Health Authority
911 McKinney Rd., Oliver, BC V0H 1T0
Tel: 250-498-5000 *Fax:* 250-498-5004
www.interiorhealth.ca
Social Media: www.facebook.com/InteriorHealth;
twitter.com/Interior_Health; www.youtube.com/InteriorHealthAuth;
www.linkedin.com/company/interior-health-authority
Number of Beds: 18 beds
Note: Programs & services include: chronic obstructive pulmonary
disease services; community care; diabetes education program;
ECG/EKG; emergency; end of life/palliative care; extended care;
fluoroscopy; general medicine; hematology; holter monitor; hospice;
laboratory; nutrition; pharmacy; physiotherapy; radiology; telehealth; &
wound care.
Lori Motluk, Administrator, Acute Care
Sara Evans, Manager, Acute Care

OSOYOOS: Osoyoos Health Centre
Affiliated with: Interior Health Authority
4816 - 89 St., Osoyoos, BC V0H 1V1
Tel: 250-495-6433
www.interiorhealth.ca

PARKSVILLE: Oceanside Health Centre
Affiliated with: Vancouver Island Health Authority
489 Alberni Hwy., Parksville, BC V9P 1J9
Tel: 250-951-9550
www.viha.ca/locations/oceanside

Note: Services include: urgent care; primary care; medical imaging;
laboratory; Telehealth; environmental health; & medical day care
Nancy Kroes, Coordinator, Integrated Services

PENTICTON: Penticton Health Centre
Affiliated with: Interior Health Authority
740 Carmi Ave., Penticton, BC V2A 8P9
Tel: 250-770-3434
www.interiorhealth.ca

Note: Programs & services include: acquired brain injury services; adult
day services; BC Early Hearing Program; caregiver support; case
management; community care clinic; community nursing; community
nutrition; dental; diabetes education; harm reduction services; home
support; immunization; nutrition; postpartum care; prenatal services;
Publicly Funded Tuberculin Skin Testing; pulmonary rehabilitation;
rehabilitation; social work; & speech-language pathology

PENTICTON: Penticton Regional Hospital (PRH)
Affiliated with: Interior Health Authority
550 Carmi Ave., Penticton, BC V2A 3G6
Tel: 250-492-4000 *Fax:* 250-492-9068
www.interiorhealth.ca
Social Media: www.facebook.com/InteriorHealth;
twitter.com/Interior_Health; www.youtube.com/InteriorHealthAuth;
www.linkedin.com/company/interior-health-authority
Number of Beds: 137 beds
Note: Programs & services include: acute neurology & psychiatric
services; antepartum care; cardioversion; chemotherapy; chronic
obstructive pulmonary disease services; community care; community
respiratory therapy; CT scan; diabetes education program; diagnostic
bronchoscopy; diagnostic cardiology; ear, nose & throat;
echocardiogram; ECG/EKG; emergency; endoscopy; enterostomal
therapy; extended care; fluoroscopy; gastroenterology; general
medicine, rehabilitation & surgery; hematology; holter monitor; hospice;
intensive care; intrapartum care; laboratory; mammography; maternity;
mental health & substance abuse; microbiology; MRI; nutrition;
oncology; ophthalmology; orthotics; otolaryngology surgery; pediatrics;
pharmacy; physiotherapy; postpartum care; pulmonary diagnostics;
radiology; respiratory therapy; speech-language pathology; spiritual
care; telehealth; transesophageal echocardiogram (TEE); transfusion;
ultrasound; urology; vasectomy; & wound care. Also offers the Mary
Pack Arthritis Program, a service of Vancouver Coastal Health.

PORT ALBERNI: West Coast General Hospital
Affiliated with: Vancouver Island Health Authority
3949 Port Alberni Hwy., Port Alberni, BC V9Y 4S1
Tel: 250-731-1370
info@viha.ca
www.viha.ca
Social Media: www.facebook.com/VanIslandHealth;
twitter.com/vanislandhealth
Number of Beds: 52 acute care beds; 32 extended care beds
Note: Programs & services include: Aboriginal health; diabetes
education; laboratory; nutrition; rehabilitation; & surgery.
Sarah Kowalenko, Communications & Public Relations Assistant, VIHA
250-740-6951, sarah.kowalenko@viha.ca
Vanessa Gallic, Aboriginal Liaison Nurse
vanessa.gallic@viha.ca

PORT ALICE: Port Alice Health Centre
Affiliated with: Vancouver Island Health Authority
Former Name: Port Alice Hospital
1090 Marine Dr., Port Alice, BC V0N 2N0
Tel: 250-284-3555
info@viha.ca
www.viha.ca

PORT COQUITLAM: Community Integration Services Society
2175 Mary Hill Rd., Port Coquitlam, BC V3C 3A2
Tel: 604-461-2131 *Fax:* 778-285-5520
oadmin@gociss.org
www.gociss.org
Year Founded: 1990
Note: Helps adults with disabilities gain skills to become more active
members of society.
Shari Mahar, Executive Director
604-568-4753, smahar@gociss.org

PORT HARDY: Port Hardy Hospital
Affiliated with: Vancouver Island Health Authority
9120 Granville St., Port Hardy, BC V0N 2P0
Tel: 250-902-6011
info@viha.ca
www.viha.ca
Social Media: www.facebook.com/VanIslandHealth;
twitter.com/vanislandhealth
Number of Beds: 17 beds
Note: Programs & services include: Aboriginal health; acute care;
emergency; residential care; ambulatory outpatient services; laboratory;
medical detox; palliative care; emergency obstetrics; visiting
specialists; & x-ray.
Sarah Kowalenko, Communications & Public Relations Assistant, VIHA
sarah.kowalenko@viha.ca

PORT MCNEILL: Port McNeill & District Hospital
Affiliated with: Vancouver Island Health Authority
Also Known As: Port McNeill Hospital
2750 Kingcome Pl., Port McNeill, BC V0N 2R0
Tel: 250-956-4461
info@viha.ca
www.viha.ca
Social Media: www.facebook.com/VanIslandHealth;
twitter.com/vanislandhealth
Number of Beds: 11 acute care beds
Note: Services include: acute care; ambulatory outpatient services;
diabetes education; emergency; laboratory; medical detox; medical
imaging; nutrition; palliative care; regional obstetrics; & visiting
specialists.
Sarah Kowalenko, Communications & Public Relations Assistant, VIHA
250-740-6951, sarah.kowalenko@viha.ca

PORT MOODY: Eagle Ridge Hospital (ERH)
Affiliated with: Fraser Health Authority
475 Guildford Way, Port Moody, BC V3H 3W9
Tel: 604-461-2022 *Fax:* 604-461-9972
feedback@fraserhealth.ca
www.fraserhealth.ca
Social Media: www.facebook.com/FraserHealthAuthority;
twitter.com/Fraserhealth; www.youtube.com/user/fraserhealth;
www.linkedin.com/company/fraser-health-authority
Year Founded: 1984
Number of Beds: 175 beds

Note: Programs & services include: acute care; ambulatory care; cardiac; CT scan; emergency; fluoroscopy; general medicine, radiography & surgery; high intensity rehabilitation unit; outpatient services; pharmacy; spiritual care; & ultrasound.
Heather Findlay, Executive Director

PRINCE GEORGE: Centre for Healthy Living
Affiliated with: Northern Health Authority
1788 Diefenbaker Dr., Prince George, BC V2N 4V7
Tel: 250-649-7011
www.northernhealth.ca

PRINCE GEORGE: Highland Community Centre
Affiliated with: Northern Health Authority
#101, 155 McDermid Dr., Prince George, BC V2M 4T8
Tel: 250-565-7317 *Fax:* 250-565-7410
www.northernhealth.ca

PRINCE GEORGE: Northern Health Authority
Former Name: Northern Interior Health Board
Corporate Office, #600, 299 Victoria St., Prince George, BC V2L 5B8
Tel: 250-565-2649 *Fax:* 250-565-2640
hello@northernhealth.ca
www.northernhealth.ca
Info Line: 811
Social Media: www.facebook.com/NorthernHealth;
twitter.com/northern_health; www.youtube.com/northernhealthbc;
www.linkedin.com/company/northern-health-authority
Number of Beds: 1,106 HCC residential care beds; 599 hospital beds
Area Served: 600,000 sq km in northern British Columbia
Population Served: 300000
Number of Employees: 7000
Note: Services administered through 3 service delivery areas:
Northwest, Northeast, Northern Interior.
Charles Jago, Board Chair
Cathy Ulrich, President & CEO
Penny Anguish, Chief Operating Officer, Northern Interior
Chris Simms, Interim Chief Operating Officer, Northwest
Angela De Smit, Chief Operating Officer, Northeast

PRINCE GEORGE: Northern Interior Health Unit - Prince George
Affiliated with: Northern Health Authority
1444 Edmonton St., Prince George, BC V2M 6W5
Tel: 250-565-7311 *Fax:* 250-565-5702
www.northernhealth.ca

Note: Programs & services: mental health; public health

PRINCE GEORGE: Prince George Family Resource Centre
Affiliated with: Northern Health Authority
1200 Lasalle Ave., Prince George, BC V2L 4J8
Tel: 250-614-9449 *Fax:* 250-614-9448
www.northernhealth.ca

PRINCE GEORGE: University Hospital of Northern British Columbia (UHNBC)
Affiliated with: Northern Health Authority
Former Name: Prince George Regional Hospital
1475 Edmonton St., Prince George, BC V2M 1S2
Tel: 250-565-2000 *Fax:* 250-565-2343
www.northernhealth.ca
Social Media: www.facebook.com/NorthernHealth;
twitter.com/Northern_Health;
www.linkedin.com/company/northern-health-authority
Number of Beds: 219 beds
Note: Hospital & clinical academic campus run by the University of British Columbia & University of Northern British Columbia.

PRINCE RUPERT: Prince Rupert Community Health
Affiliated with: Northern Health Authority
300 - 3rd Ave. West, Prince Rupert, BC V8J 1L4
Tel: 250-622-6380 *Fax:* 250-622-6391
www.northernhealth.ca

Michael Melia, Administrator, Health Services

PRINCE RUPERT: Prince Rupert Regional Hospital
Affiliated with: Northern Health Authority
1305 Summit Ave., Prince Rupert, BC V8J 2A6
Tel: 250-624-2171 *Fax:* 250-624-2195
www.northernhealth.ca
Social Media: www.facebook.com/NorthernHealth;
twitter.com/northern_health; www.youtube.com/northernhealthBC;
www.linkedin.com/company/northern-health-authority
Number of Beds: 25 beds
Note: Programs & services include: acute care; diagnostics; ultrasound; CAT scan; surgery; emergency; day care; extended care; diabetes education; rehabilitation; & specialists in pediatrics, radiology, obstetrics, gynecology, surgery, internal medicine, podiatry & orthopedics.

PRINCETON: Princeton General Hospital
Affiliated with: Interior Health Authority
98 Ridgewood Dr., Princeton, BC V0X 1W0
Tel: 250-295-3233
www.interiorhealth.ca
Social Media: www.facebook.com/InteriorHealth;
twitter.com/Interior_Health; www.youtube.com/InteriorHealthAuth;
www.linkedin.com/company/interior-health-authority
Number of Beds: 6 acute care beds
Note: Programs & services include: community care; convalescent care; diabetes education program; drug & alcohol resources; ECG/EKG; emergency; end of life/palliative care; general medicine; holter monitor; hospice; laboratory; psychiatry; radiology; telehealth; transfusion; & wound care.
Cherie Whittaker, Manager

PRINCETON: Princeton Health Centre
Affiliated with: Interior Health Authority
98 Ridgewood Dr., Princeton, BC V0X 1W0
Tel: 250-295-4442
www.interiorhealth.ca

Note: Programs & services include: acquired brain injury services; adult day services; caregiver support; case management; community care clinic; community nursing; community nutrition; diabetes education; home support; immunization; postpartum care; prenatal services; rehabilitation; social work; & Tuberculin Skin Testing

QUEEN CHARLOTTE: Haida Gwaii Hospital & Health Centre
Affiliated with: Northern Health Authority
Former Name: Queen Charlotte Islands General Hospital
PO Box 9, 3209 Oceanview Dr., Queen Charlotte, BC V0T 1S0
Tel: 250-559-4900 *Fax:* 250-559-4312
www.northernhealth.ca
Social Media: www.facebook.com/NorthernHealth;
twitter.com/northern_health; www.youtube.com/northernhealthBC;
www.linkedin.com/company/northern-health-authority
Number of Beds: 8 acute care beds
Population Served: 4500
Note: Programs & services include: community care; diagnostic imaging; home care; laboratory; mental health & addictions; pharmacy; & public health.

QUEEN CHARLOTTE: Queen Charlotte Islands Community Health
Affiliated with: Northern Health Authority
3211 - 3rd Ave., Queen Charlotte, BC V0T 1S0
Tel: 250-559-2350
www.northernhealth.ca

QUESNEL: GR Baker Memorial Hospital
Affiliated with: Northern Health Authority
543 Front St., Quesnel, BC V2J 2K7
Tel: 250-985-5600 *Fax:* 250-992-5652
www.northernhealth.ca
Social Media: www.facebook.com/NorthernHealth;
twitter.com/northern_health; www.youtube.com/northernhealthBC;
www.linkedin.com/company/northern-health-authority
Year Founded: 1955
Number of Beds: 38 acute care beds; 40 extended care beds; 5 crisis stabilization beds; 4 ICU beds
Note: Programs & services include: cardiology; urology; & surgery (ENT & general). Facilities include the Dunrovin Park Lodge Care Facility & Maple House.
Kim McIvor, Manager, Support Services

QUESNEL: Quesnel Health Unit - Nursing
Affiliated with: Northern Health Authority
511 Reid St., Quesnel, BC V2J 2M8
Tel: 250-991-7571 Fax: 250-991-7577
www.northernhealth.ca
Debbie Strang, Administrator, Health Services

QUESNEL: Quesnel Health Unit - Preventative
Affiliated with: Northern Health Authority
523 Front St., Quesnel, BC V2J 2K7
Tel: 250-983-6810 Fax: 250-992-1031
www.northernhealth.ca
Debbie Strang, Administrator, Health Services

REVELSTOKE: Queen Victoria Health Centre
Affiliated with: Interior Health Authority
1200 Newlands Rd., Revelstoke, BC V0E 2S0
Tel: 250-837-2131
www.interiorhealth.ca

Note: Programs & services include: acquired brain injury services; adult day services; caregiver support; case management; community care clinic; community nursing; community nutrition; home support; Publicly Funded Tuberculin Skin Testing; rehabilitation; & social work

REVELSTOKE: Queen Victoria Hospital & Health Centre
Affiliated with: Interior Health Authority
1200 Newlands Rd., Revelstoke, BC V0E 2S0
Tel: 250-837-2131 Fax: 250-837-4788
www.interiorhealth.ca
Social Media: www.facebook.com/InteriorHealth;
twitter.com/Interior_Health; www.youtube.com/InteriorHealthAuth;
www.linkedin.com/company/interior-health-authority
Number of Beds: 48 residential beds; 10 acute beds
Note: Programs & services include: antepartum care; chemotherapy; dental surgery; diabetes education program; ECG/EKG; emergency; end of life/palliative care; endoscopy; fluoroscopy; general medicine, rehabilitation & surgery; hematology; holter monitor; hospice; intrapartum care; laboratory; maternity; mental health & substance abuse; nutrition; physiotherapy; postpartum care; radiology; spiritual care; telehealth; transfusion; & ultrasound.
Julie Lowes, Site Manager

REVELSTOKE: Revelstoke Public Health
Affiliated with: Interior Health Authority
1200 Newlands Rd., Revelstoke, BC V0E 2S0
Tel: 250-814-2244
www.interiorhealth.ca

Note: Programs & services include: acquired brain injury services; adult day services; BC Early Hearing Program; caregiver support; case management; community care clinic; community nursing; community nutrition; home support; immunization; postpartum care; prenatal services; rehabilitation; social work; & Tuberculin Skin Testing

REVELSTOKE: Revelstoke Speech & Language Clinic
Affiliated with: Interior Health Authority
1001 Mackenzie Ave., Revelstoke, BC V0E 2S0
Tel: 250-837-4285
www.interiorhealth.ca

Note: Offers speech-language pathology services

ROCK CREEK: Rock Creek Health Centre
Affiliated with: Interior Health Authority
100 Rock Creek Cutoff Rd., Rock Creek, BC V0H 1Y0
Tel: 250-446-2272
www.interiorhealth.ca

Note: Programs & services include: acquired brain injury services; adult day services; caregiver support; case management; community care clinic; community nursing; community nutrition; home support; Publicly Funded Tuberculin Skin Testing; rehabilitation; & social work

SAANICHTON: Saanich Peninsula Hospital
Affiliated with: Vancouver Island Health Authority
2166 Mount Newton Cross Rd., Saanichton, BC V8M 2B2
Tel: 250-544-7676 Toll-Free: 877-370-8699
www.viha.ca
Social Media: www.facebook.com/VanIslandHealth;
twitter.com/vanislandhealth
Number of Beds: 48 acute care beds; 144 extended care beds
Note: Programs & services include: eye health; heart health; laboratory; medical imaging; nutrition; rehabilitation; residential; spiritual care; & surgery.
Sarah Kowalenko, Communications & Public Relations Assistant, VIHA
250-740-6951, sarah.kowalenko@viha.ca

SALMO: Salmo Health & Wellness Centre
Affiliated with: Interior Health Authority
413 Baker Ave., Salmo, BC V0G 1Z0
Tel: 250-357-0104
www.interiorhealth.ca

Note: Programs & services include: acquired brain injury services; adult day services; caregiver support; case management; community care clinic; community nursing; community nutrition; home support; immunization; postpartum care; prenatal services; Publicly Funded Tuberculin Skin Testing; rehabilitation; & social work

SALMON ARM: Salmon Arm Health Centre
Affiliated with: Interior Health Authority
851 - 16th St. NE, Salmon Arm, BC V1E 4N7
Tel: 250-833-4100
www.interiorhealth.ca

Note: Programs & services include: acquired brain injury services; adult day services; BC Early Hearing Program; caregiver support; case management; community care clinic; community nursing; community nutrition; environmental health; harm reduction services; home support; immunization; postpartum care; prenatal services; Publicly Funded Tuberculin Skin Testing; rehabilitation; social work; & speech-language pathology

SALMON ARM: Salmon Arm Physiotherapy
Affiliated with: Interior Health Authority
#1, 2770 - 10th Ave., Salmon Arm, BC V1E 2E8
www.interiorhealth.ca

SALMON ARM: Shuswap Home & Community Care
Affiliated with: Interior Health Authority
2770 - 10th Ave. NE, #B, Salmon Arm, BC V1E 4N6
Tel: 250-832-6643
www.interiorhealth.ca

SALMON ARM: Shuswap Lake General Hospital
Affiliated with: Interior Health Authority
PO Box 520, 601 - 10th St. NE, Salmon Arm, BC V1E 4N6
Tel: 250-833-3600 Fax: 250-833-3611
www.interiorhealth.ca
Social Media: www.facebook.com/InteriorHealth;
twitter.com/Interior_Health; www.youtube.com/InteriorHealthAuth;
www.linkedin.com/company/interior-health-authority
Number of Beds: 40 beds
Note: Programs & services include: antepartum care; cardioversion; chemotherapy; CT scan; dental surgery; diabetes education program; echocardiogram; ECG/EKG; emergency; end of life/palliative; endoscopy; gastroenterology; general medicine, rehabilitation & surgery; hematology; holter monitor; hospice; intensive care; intrapartum care; laboratory; maternity; nutrition; oncology; pharmacy; physiotherapy; postpartum care; pulmonary diagnostics & rehabilitation; radiology; speech-language pathology; spiritual care; telehealth; transfusion; ultrasound; urology; vascular & thoracic; & vasectomy.
Mark Pugh, Manager

SALT SPRING ISLAND: The Lady Minto Gulf Islands Hospital
Affiliated with: Vancouver Island Health Authority
Former Name: Lady Minto Hospital
135 Crofton Rd., Salt Spring Island, BC V8K 1T1
Tel: 250-538-4800 *Fax:* 250-538-4870
info@viha.ca
www.viha.ca
Social Media: www.facebook.com/VanIslandHealth;
twitter.com/vanislandhealth
Number of Beds: 19 acute care beds; 31 extended care beds
Note: Programs & services include: emergency; acute care; heart
health; residential care; obstetrics; psychiatry; laboratory; medical
imaging; spiritual care; endoscopy; pharmacy; physiotherapy; & internal
medicine.
Bill Relph, Manager, Rural Services

SICAMOUS: Sicamous Health Centre
Affiliated with: Interior Health Authority
1133 Hwy. 97A, Sicamous, BC V0E 2V0
Tel: 250-836-4835
www.interiorhealth.ca

Note: Programs & services include: acquired brain injury services; adult
day services; caregiver support; case management; community care
clinic; community nursing; community nutrition; home support;
immunization; Publicly Funded Tuberculin Skin Testing; rehabilitation;
& social work

SMITHERS: Bulkley Valley District Hospital
Affiliated with: Northern Health Authority
PO Box 370, 3950 - 8th Ave., Smithers, BC V0J 2N0
Tel: 250-847-2611 *Fax:* 250-847-2446
www.northernhealth.ca
Social Media: www.facebook.com/NorthernHealth;
twitter.com/northern_health; www.youtube.com/northernhealthBC;
www.linkedin.com/company/northern-health-authority
Number of Beds: 25 beds
Area Served: Communities from Houston in the east to Hazelton in the
west
Note: Programs & services include: acute care; emergency; medical;
surgical; maternity; & palliative care.

SMITHERS: Smithers Community Health
Affiliated with: Northern Health Authority
Bag 5000, 3793 Alfred Ave., Smithers, BC V0J 2N0
Tel: 250-847-6400 *Fax:* 250-847-5908
www.northernhealth.ca

SMITHERS: Smithers Home & Community Care
Affiliated with: Northern Health Authority
PO Box 370, 3950 - 8th Ave., Smithers, BC V0J 2N0
Tel: 250-847-6234 *Fax:* 250-847-6239
www.northernhealth.ca
Cormac Hikisch, Administrator, Health Services

SORRENTO: Sorrento & Area Community Health Centre
Affiliated with: Interior Health Authority
1250 TransCanada Hwy., Sorrento, BC V0E 2W0
Tel: 250-803-5251
www.interiorhealth.ca

Note: Offers primary health care services
Marilyn Clark, Chair

SPARWOOD: Sparwood Mental Health
Affiliated with: Interior Health Authority
570 Pine Ave., Sparwood, BC V0B 2G0
Tel: 250-425-2064
www.interiorhealth.ca

Note: Programs & services include: adult community support;
counselling; Early Psychosis Intervention; eating disorders; & seniors
mental health

SPARWOOD: Sparwood Primary Health Care
Affiliated with: Interior Health Authority
570 Pine Ave., Sparwood, BC V0B 2G0
Tel: 250-425-6212 *Fax:* 250-425-2313
www.interiorhealth.ca

Note: Programs & services include: acquired brain injury services; adult
day services; BC Early Hearing program; caregiver support; case
management; child & youth immunization program; community care
clinic; community nursing; community nutrition; diabetes education;
electrocardiogram; emergency health; home support; immunization;
postpartum care; prenatal; primary health care; pulmonary diagnostics;
radiology; rehabilitation; social work; Telehealth; & Tuberculin Skin
Testing.

STEWART: Stewart Health Centre
Affiliated with: Northern Health Authority
PO Box 8, 904 Brightwell St., Stewart, BC V0T 1W0
Tel: 250-636-2221 *Fax:* 250-636-2715
www.northernhealth.ca

Note: Programs & services include: public health; infant & child care;
walk-in emergency; & doctor's clinic.

SUMMERLAND: Summerland Health Centre
Affiliated with: Interior Health Authority
12815 Atkinson Rd., Summerland, BC V0H 1Z0
Tel: 250-404-8000
www.interiorhealth.ca

Note: Programs & services include: acquired brain injury services; adult
day services; caregiver support; case management; community care
clinic; community nursing; community nutrition; dental; diabetes
education; ear, nose, & throat services; electrocardiogram; extended
care unit; general medicine; home support; immunization; laboratory
outpatient services; ophthalmology; otolaryngology surgery;
post-anaesthetic care; postpartum care; prenatal services; Publicly
Funded Tuberculin Skin Testing; radiology; rehabilitation; social work;
speech-language pathology; & surgical daycare

SURREY: Fraser Health Authority
Central City Tower, #400, 13450 - 102nd Ave., Surrey, BC V3T 0H1
Tel: 604-587-4600 *Fax:* 604-587-4666
Toll-Free: 877-935-5669
feedback@fraserhealth.ca
www.fraserhealth.ca
Info Line: 811
Social Media: www.facebook.com/FraserHealthAuthority;
twitter.com/Fraserhealth;
www.linkedin.com/company/fraser-health-authority
Number of Beds: 7,760 residential care beds
Area Served: Burnaby to Hope to Boston Bar in British Columbia
Population Served: 1800000
Number of Employees: 25000
Note: Communities served include around 38,100 First Nations people,
associated with 32 bands; provides mental health care, public health,
home, & community care services.
Karen Matty, Board Chair
Michael Marchbank, President & CEO
Dr. Victoria Lee, Chief Medical Health Officer & Vice-President,
Population Health
Brenda Liggett, Chief Financial Officer
Philip Barker, Vice-President, Planning, Informatics & Analytics
Linda Dempster, Vice-President, Patient Experience
Vivian Giglio, Vice-President, Regional Hospitals & Communities
Naseem Nuraney, Vice-President, Communications & Public Affairs
Cameron Brine, Vice-President, People & Organization Development
Dr. Roy Morton, Vice-President, Medicine

SURREY: Guildford Public Health Unit
Affiliated with: Fraser Health Authority
10233 - 153 St., Surrey, BC V3R 0Z7
Tel: 604-587-4750 *Fax:* 604-587-4777

SURREY: Surrey Memorial Hospital
Affiliated with: Fraser Health Authority
13750 - 96 Ave., Surrey, BC V3V 1Z2
Tel: 604-581-2211 *Fax:* 604-588-3320
feedback@fraserhealth.ca
www.fraserhealth.ca
Social Media: www.facebook.com/FraserHealthAuthority;
twitter.com/Fraserhealth;
www.linkedin.com/company/fraser-health-authority

Number of Beds: 499 beds
Note: Programs & services include: emergency; adolescent psychiatry; angiography; antepartum care; diagnostic imaging (CT scans, bone densitometry, fluoroscopy, mammography, MRI, radiology, ultrasound); cardiology; outpatient services; dental surgery; acute tertiary palliative care; intensive care; neonatal intensive care; ophthalmology; otolaryngology; paediatrics; pharmacy; plastic surgery; postpartum care; psychiatry; sleep lab; speech language pathology; spiritual care; urological surgery; & vascular & thoracic surgery.
Cathie Heritage, Executive Director
Dr. Urbain Ip, Medical Director

TAHSIS: Tahsis Health Centre
Affiliated with: Vancouver Island Health Authority
1085 Maquinna Dr., Tahsis, BC V0P 1X0
Tel: 250-934-6322 *Fax:* 250-934-6404
www.viha.ca

Note: Services include: child health clinic; communicable disease control program; family practice medical care; home care nursing; home support; laboratory; & urgent care.
Enid O'Hara, Manager, Rural Services
250-283-2626, Fax: 250-283-7561, enid.ohara@viha.ca

TATLA LAKE: West Chilcotin Health Centre
Affiliated with: Interior Health Authority
16452 Hwy. 20, Tatla Lake, BC V0L 1V0
Tel: 250-476-1114 *Fax:* 250-476-1266
www.interiorhealth.ca

TERRACE: Mills Memorial Hospital
Affiliated with: Northern Health Authority
4720 Haugland Ave., Terrace, BC V8G 2W7
Tel: 250-635-2211 *Fax:* 250-638-4017
www.northernhealth.ca
Social Media: www.facebook.com/northernhealth; twitter.com/northern_health; www.youtube.com/northernhealthBC; www.linkedin.com/company/northern-health-authority
Number of Beds: 39 acute care beds
Note: Programs & services include: acute care; community based programs; CT & nuclear medicine; obstetrics/gynecology; psychiatry; surgery; urology; ophthalmology; otolaryngology; anaesthetics; radiology; nuclear medicine; pathology; ENT; podiatrists; pediatrics; & internal medicine.

TERRACE: Terrace Health Unit
Affiliated with: Northern Health Authority
3412 Kalum St., Terrace, BC V8G 4T2
Tel: 250-631-4200 *Fax:* 250-638-2264
www.northernhealth.ca

TOFINO: Tofino General Hospital
Affiliated with: Vancouver Island Health Authority
PO Box 190, 261 Neill St., Tofino, BC V0R 2Z0
Tel: 250-725-4010
info@viha.ca
www.viha.ca
Social Media: www.facebook.com/VanIslandHealth; twitter.com/vanislandhealth
Year Founded: 1954
Number of Beds: 10 acute care beds
Note: Programs & services include: acute care; emergency; emergency obstetrics; outpatient ambulatory care; Telehealth; medical imaging; laboratory services; outpatient blood collection; & rehabilitation.
Kathryn Kilpatrick, Manager
250-725-4005, kathryn.kilpatrick@viha.ca

TRAIL: Kiro Wellness Centre
Affiliated with: Interior Health Authority
1500 Columbia Ave., Trail, BC V1R 1J9
Tel: 250-364-6219
www.interiorhealth.ca

Note: Programs & services include: acquired brain injury services; addictions treatment programs; adult day services; caregiver support; case management; community care clinic; community nursing; community nutrition; dental; environmental; home support; immunization; postpartum care; prenatal services; Publicly Funded

Tuberculin Skin Testing; pulmonary rehabilitation; rehabilitation; social work; & speech-language pathology

TRAIL: Kootenay Boundary Regional Hospital
Affiliated with: Interior Health Authority
Former Name: Trail Regional Hospital
1200 Hospital Bench, Trail, BC V1R 4M1
Tel: 250-368-3311 *Fax:* 250-364-3422
Toll-Free: 866-368-3314
info@kbrh.ca
www.kbrh.ca
Number of Beds: 75 beds
Note: Programs & services include: antepartum care; arthritis rehabilitation; cardioversion; chemotherapy; chronic obstructive pulmonary disease services; community care; convalescent care; CT scan; dental surgery; diabetes education program; ear, nose & throat; echocardiogram; ECG/EKG; emergency; end of life/palliative care; endoscopy; enterostomal therapy; extended care; fluoroscopy; general medicine, rehabilitation & surgery; geriatric medicine; hematology; holter monitor; hospice; intensive care; intrapartum care; laboratory; mammography; maternity; mental health & substance abuse; microbiology; MRI; nuclear medicine; nutrition; oncology; ophthalmology; orthotics; otolaryngology surgery; pediatrics; physiotherapy; plastic surgery; postpartum care; psoriasis & phototherapy; psychiatry; pulmonary diagnostics; radiology; respiratory therapy; speech-language pathology; spiritual care; telehealth; transfusion; ultrasound; urology; vasectomy; & wound care.
Jane Cusden, Interim Administrator, Health Services

TRAIL: Kootenay Boundary Transplant Clinic
Affiliated with: Interior Health Authority
1200 Hospital Bench, Trail, BC V1R 4M1
Tel: 250-364-3494
www.interiorhealth.ca

Note: Follow-up care for organ transplant recipients, primarily renal transplant.

TUMBLER RIDGE: Tumbler Ridge Community Health Unit
Affiliated with: Northern Health Authority
PO Box 1090, 220 Front St., Tumbler Ridge, BC V0C 2W0
Tel: 250-242-4262 *Fax:* 250-242-4009
www.northernhealth.ca

TUMBLER RIDGE: Tumbler Ridge Health Care Centre
Affiliated with: Northern Health Authority
PO Box 80, 220 Front St., Tumbler Ridge, BC V0C 2W0
Tel: 250-242-5271 *Fax:* 250-242-3889
www.northernhealth.ca
Gail Neumann, Site Manager
gail.neumann@northernhealth.ca

VALEMOUNT: Valemount Community Health Centre
Affiliated with: Northern Health Authority
PO Box 697, 1445 - 5 Ave., Valemount, BC V0E 2Z0
Tel: 250-566-9138 *Fax:* 250-566-4319
www.northernhealth.ca

VANCOUVER: BC Women's Hospital & Health Centre
Affiliated with: Provincial Health Services Authority
4500 Oak St., Vancouver, BC V6H 3N1
Tel: 604-875-2424 *Toll-Free:* 888-300-3088
comm@cw.bc.ca
www.bcwomens.ca
Info Line: 604-875-2929
Social Media: twitter.com/BCWomensHosp

Note: Hospital Specialties: Health care for women, newborn, & families; Gynecological & reproductive health services; Sexual assault service; HIV care of women & children; Birth control & abortion support & counselling; Substance dependency; Psychology; Social work; Aboriginal Health Program; Osteoporosis
Dr. Jan Christilaw, Site Executive

VANCOUVER: Provincial Health Services Authority (PHSA)
#700, 1380 Burrard St., Vancouver, BC V6Z 2H3

Tel: 604-675-7400 Fax: 604-708-2700
phsacomm@phsa.ca
www.phsa.ca
Info Line: 811
Social Media: twitter.com/PHSAofBC;
www.youtube.com/ProvHealthServAuth;
www.linkedin.com/company/provincial-health-services-authority

Note: PHSA operates provincial agencies including BC Children's Hospital, BC Transplant, & BC Cancer Agency. It is also responsible for specialized provincial health services like chest surgery & trauma services.
Tim Manning, Board Chair
Carl Roy, President & CEO
Arden Krystal, Executive Vice-President, Patient & Employee Experience
Thomas Chan, Chief Financial Officer
Nick Foster, Vice-President, Consolidated Services & Special Projects
Dave Cunningham, Chief Communications Officer
Sandra MacKay, Chief Freedom of Information & Privacy Officer, & General Counsel
Linda Lupini, Executive Vice-President, PHSA & BCEHS
Carla Gregor, Vice-President, Acute Specialty Services
Oliver Grüter-Andrew, Chief Information Officer
Colleen Hart, Vice-President, Provincial Population Health, Chronic Conditions & Specialized Populations

VANCOUVER: Vancouver Coastal Health (VCH)
Corporate Office, 601 West Broadway, 11th Fl., Vancouver, BC V5Z 4C2

Tel: 604-736-2033 Toll-Free: 866-884-0888
www.vch.ca
Info Line: 811
Social Media: www.facebook.com/VCHhealthcare;
twitter.com/vchhealthcare; www.youtube.com/user/VCHhealthcare

Population Served: 1000000
Note: Vancouver Coastal Health provides health care services through a network of hospitals, primary care clinics, community health centres & residential care homes. Search VCH health care services in Vancouver, Richmond, North & West Vancouver & along the Sea-to-Sky Highway, Sunshine Coast & BC's Central Coast: www.vch.ca/locations-services.

VANDERHOOF: St. John Hospital
Affiliated with: Northern Health Authority
3255 Hospital Rd., Vanderhoof, BC V0J 3A0

Tel: 250-567-2211 Fax: 250-567-9713
www.northernhealth.ca
Social Media: www.facebook.com/NorthernHealth;
twitter.com/Northern_Health; www.youtube.com/northernhealthBC;
www.linkedin.com/company/northern-health-authority
Year Founded: 1941
Number of Beds: 24 acute care; 8 bassinets
Population Served: 5000
Number of Employees: 180
Note: Programs & services include: emergency; labour & delivery; diagnostic imaging (x-ray, ultrasound); orthopedic surgery; general surgeries; physiotherapy; & visiting specialists.

VANDERHOOF: Vanderhoof Health Unit
Affiliated with: Northern Health Authority
3299 Hospital Rd., Vanderhoof, BC V0J 3A2

Tel: 250-567-6900 Fax: 250-567-6170
www.northernhealth.ca

VERNON: Vernon - Ortho Clinic
Affiliated with: Interior Health Authority
3210 - 25th Ave., Vernon, BC V1T 2T1

www.interiorhealth.ca

VERNON: Vernon Community Care Health Services
Affiliated with: Interior Health Authority
4505 - 25th St., Vernon, BC V1T 4S8

Tel: 250-541-2200
www.interiorhealth.ca

Note: Programs & services include: acquired brain injury services; adult day services; caregiver support; case management; community care clinic; community nursing; community nutrition; home support; rehabilitation; respiratory therapy; & social work

VERNON: Vernon Downtown Primary Care Centre
Affiliated with: Interior Health Authority
3306A - 32nd Ave., Vernon, BC V1T 2M6

Tel: 250-541-1097
www.interiorhealth.ca

Note: Programs & services include: case management; health outreach; needle distribution; primary care mental health; & primary health care

VERNON: Vernon Health Unit
Affiliated with: Interior Health Authority
1440 - 14th Ave., Vernon, BC V1B 2T1

Tel: 250-549-5700
www.interiorhealth.ca

VERNON: Vernon Jubilee Hospital (VJH)
Affiliated with: Interior Health Authority
2101 - 32 St., Vernon, BC V1T 5L2

Tel: 250-545-2211
www.interiorhealth.ca
Social Media: www.facebook.com/InteriorHealth;
twitter.com/Interior_Health; www.youtube.com/InteriorHealthAuth;
www.linkedin.com/company/interior-health-authority
Number of Beds: 148 beds
Note: Programs & services include: acute neurology; antepartum care; arthritis rehabilitation; cardioversion; chemotherapy; chronic obstructive pulmonary disease services; community care; CT scan; dental surgery; diabetes education program; ear, nose & throat; echocardiogram; ECG/EKG; emergency; end of life/palliative care; endoscopy; enterostomal therapy; extended care; fluoroscopy; general medicine, rehabilitation & surgery; hematology; holter monitor; intensive care; intrapartum care; laboratory; mammography; maternity; mental health & substance abuse; microbiology; nuclear medicine; nutrition; oncology; ophthalmology; orthopaedic surgery; otolaryngology surgery; pediatrics; pharmacy; physiotherapy; postpartum care; pulmonary diagnostics & rehabilitation; radiology; respiratory therapy; social work; speech-language pathology; spiritual care; telehealth; transesophageal echocardiogram (TEE); transfusion; ultrasound; urology; vasectomy; & wound care.
Richard Harding, Administrator, Health Services

VICTORIA: Aberdeen Hospital
Affiliated with: Vancouver Island Health Authority
1450 Hillside Ave., Victoria, BC V8T 2B7

Tel: 250-370-5626 Toll-Free: 866-995-3299
info@viha.ca
www.viha.ca/hcc/residential/locations/aberdeen.htm

Note: Extended care hospital
Sarah Kowalenko, Communications & Public Relations Assistant, VIHA
250-740-6951, sarah.kowalenko@viha.ca

VICTORIA: Glengarry Hospital
Affiliated with: Vancouver Island Health Authority
Former Name: Glengarry Extended Care Hospital
1780 Fairfield Rd., Victoria, BC V8S 1G7

Tel: 250-370-5626 Toll-Free: 866-995-3299
info@viha.ca
www.viha.ca/hcc/residential/locations/glengarry.htm
Year Founded: 1963
Number of Beds: 165 units
Note: Extended care hospital

VICTORIA: Mount Tolmie Extended Care Hospital
Affiliated with: Vancouver Island Health Authority
3690 Richmond Rd., Victoria, BC V8P 4R6

Tel: 250-370-5757 Toll-Free: 866-995-3299
info@viha.ca
www.viha.ca/hcc/residential/locations/mount_tolmie.htm
Number of Beds: 72 units
Note: Extended care hospital

VICTORIA: Priory Hospital
Affiliated with: Vancouver Island Health Authority
567 Goldstream Ave., Victoria, BC V9B 2W4
Tel: 250-370-5626 Toll-Free: 866-995-3299
info@viha.ca
www.viha.ca/hcc/residential/locations/priory_hiscock_heritage_woods.htm
Social Media: www.facebook.com/VanIslandHealth;
twitter.com/vanislandhealth

Number of Beds: 140 units
Note: Extended care hospital

VICTORIA: Royal Jubilee Hospital
Affiliated with: Vancouver Island Health Authority
1952 Bay St., Victoria, BC V8R 1J8
Tel: 250-370-8000 Toll-Free: 877-370-8699
info@viha.ca
www.viha.ca
Social Media: www.facebook.com/135150073228437;
twitter.com/vanislandhealth

Note: Acute care, cystic fibrosis clinic, rehabilitation services, breast physiotherapy, breast surgical oncology. Located in Memorial Pavilion.
Dr. Brendan Carr, President & CEO, VIHA

VICTORIA: Vancouver Island Health Authority
Former Name: Capital Health Region
Also Known As: Island Health
1952 Bay St., Victoria, BC V8R 1J8
Tel: 250-370-8699 Toll-Free: 877-370-8699
info@viha.ca
www.viha.ca
Info Line: 811
Social Media: www.facebook.com/VanIslandHealth;
twitter.com/vanislandhealth

Area Served: Vancouver Island & the islands of the George Strait
Population Served: 765000
Number of Employees: 18000
Don Hubbard, Board Chair
Dr. Brendan Carr, President & CEO
Dr. Richard Stanwick, Chief Medical Health Officer
Jeremy Etherington, Chief Medical Officer & Executive Vice-President
Catherine Mackay, Chief Operating Officer & Executive Vice-President
Kim Kerrone, Chief Financial Officer & Vice-President, Corporate Services
Dawn Nedzelski, Chief Nursing Officer & Chief, Professional Practice
Catherine Claiter-Larsen, Chief Information Officer & Vice-President
Kathy MacNeil, Executive Vice-President, Quality, Safety & Experience
Toni O'Keeffe, Vice-President & Chief, Communications & Public Relations

VICTORIA: Victoria General Hospital
Affiliated with: Vancouver Island Health Authority
1 Hospital Way, Victoria, BC V8Z 6R5
Tel: 250-727-4212 Toll-Free: 877-370-8699
www.viha.ca
Social Media: www.facebook.com/135150073228437;
twitter.com/vanislandhealth

Note: Programs & services include: Aboriginal health nurses; breast health; diabetes education; eye health; heart health; Jeneece Place; laboratory; medical imaging; neurosciences; nutrition; rehabilitation; spiritual care; stroke rapid assessment; & surgery.
Dr. Brendan Carr, President & CEO, VIHA

VICTORIA: Wayside House
550 Foul Bay Rd., Victoria, BC V8S 4H1
Tel: 250-598-4521 Fax: 250-598-4547
inquiries@waysidehousevictoria.org
www.waysidehousevictoria.org

Number of Beds: 9 beds
Barb Colwill, Office Manager
holm.c@hotmail.com

WEST KELOWNA: West Kelowna Health Centre
Affiliated with: Interior Health Authority
#106, 2300 Carrington Rd., West Kelowna, BC V4T 2N6
Tel: 250-980-5150
www.interiorhealth.ca

Note: Programs & services include: acquired brain injury services; adult day services; caregiver support; case management; community care clinic; community nursing; community nutrition; dental; diabetes education; home support; immunization; postpartum care; prenatal services; Publicly Funded Tuberculin Skin Testing; rehabilitation; & social work

WEST VANCOUVER: First Nations Health Authority (FNHA)
#501, 100 Park Royal South, West Vancouver, BC V7T 1A2
Tel: 604-693-6500 Fax: 604-913-2081
Toll-Free: 866-913-0033
info@fnha.ca
www.fnha.ca
Info Line: 855-550-5454
Social Media: www.facebook.com/firstnationshealthauthority;
twitter.com/FNHA; www.youtube.com/user/fnhealthcouncil;
www.linkedin.com/company/first-nations-health-authority
Year Founded: 2013
Area Served: 5 regions; 955,186 sq km
Note: Assumed the following responsibilities, formerly handled by Health Canada's First Nations Inuit Health Branch - Pacific Region: to plan, design, manage, & fund the delivery of First Nations health programs & services in BC. Health services include: primary care services; children, youth & maternal health; mental health & addictions programming; health & wellness planning; health infrastructure & human resources; environmental health & research; First Nations health benefits; & eHealth technology.
Areas served include the following regions: Fraser Salish; Interior; North; Vancouver Coastal; & Vancouver Island.
Lydia Hwitsum, Board Chair
Joe Gallagher, Chief Executive Officer
Joseph Mendez, Chief Information Officer & Vice-President, Innovation & Information Management Services
Dr. Evan Adams, Chief Medical Officer
Richard Jock, Chief Operating Officer
John Mah, Vice-President, First Nations Health Benefits
Greg Shea, Executive Director

WHITE ROCK: Peace Arch Hospital
Affiliated with: Fraser Health Authority
15521 Russell Ave., White Rock, BC V4B 2R4
Tel: 604-531-5512
feedback@fraserhealth.ca
www.fraserhealth.ca
Social Media: www.facebook.com/FraserHealthAuthority;
twitter.com/Fraserhealth; www.youtube.com/user/fraserhealth;
www.linkedin.com/company/fraser-health-authority
Number of Beds: 146 beds
Note: Programs & services include: acute care; adult community support; ambulatory care; angiography; antepartum care; cardiac; CT scan; diagnostic bronchoscopy; echocardiography; emergency; fluoroscopy; general medicine, radiography, rehabilitation & surgery; geriatrics; hospice residence; inpatient psychiatry unit; intensive care; MRI; mammography; maternity; nuclear medicine; outpatient services; pharmacy; postpartum care; pulmonary function lab; spiritual care; & ultrasound.
Rhonda Veldhoen, Executive Director

WILLIAMS LAKE: Cariboo Memorial Health Centre
Affiliated with: Interior Health Authority
517 North 6th Ave., Williams Lake, BC V2G 2G8
Tel: 250-392-4411
www.interiorhealth.ca

Note: Programs & services include: adult day services; nursing; nutrition; home support; rehabilitation; & social work

WILLIAMS LAKE: Cariboo Memorial Hospital
Affiliated with: Interior Health Authority
517 North 6th Ave., Williams Lake, BC V2G 2G8
Tel: 250-392-4411 Fax: 250-392-2157
www.interiorhealth.ca
Social Media: www.facebook.com/InteriorHealth;
twitter.com/Interior_Health; www.youtube.com/InteriorHealthAuth;
www.linkedin.com/company/interior-health-authority
Number of Beds: 31 beds
Note: Programs & services include: antepartum care; chemotherapy;

community care; community respiratory therapy; CT scan; dental surgery; diabetes education program; diagnostic bronchoscopy; echocardiogram; ECG/EKG; emergency; end of life/palliative care; endoscopy; general medicine; general rehabilitation; general surgery; hematology; holter monitor; intensive care; intrapartum care; laboratory; mammography; maternity services; mental health & substance abuse; nutrition; oncology; pediatrics; physiotherapy; postpartum care; pulmonary diagnostics/rehabilitation; radiology; spiritual care; telehealth; transfusion; ultrasound; & vasectomy.
Barbara Mack, Aboriginal Patient Liaison
 250-302-3266, barbara.mack@interiorhealth.ca

MANITOBA

ALONSA: Alonsa Community Health
Affiliated with: Prairie Mountain Health
General Delivery, 27 Railway Ave. South, Alonsa, MB R0H 0A0
Tel: 204-767-3000 *Fax:* 204-767-3001
www.prairiemountainhealth.ca

Note: Services include: home care; mental health; primary health care; & public health

ARBORG: Arborg & District Health Centre
Affiliated with: Interlake-Eastern Regional Health Authority
234 Gislason Dr., Arborg, MB R0C 0A0
Tel: 204-376-2781

ARBORG: Arborg & District Hospital
Affiliated with: Interlake-Eastern Regional Health Authority
Former Name: Arborg & District Health Centre
PO Box 10, 234 Gislason Dr., Arborg, MB R0C 0A0
Tel: 204-376-5247 *Fax:* 204-376-5669
www.ierha.ca

Number of Beds: 13 acute care beds
Note: Services offered include: acute care; diagnostic imaging; emergency; laboratory; occupational therapy; palliative care; physiotherapy; rehabilitation; medical clinic; spiritual care.

ASHERN: Lakeshore General Hospital
Affiliated with: Interlake-Eastern Regional Health Authority
PO Box 110, 1 Steenson Dr., Ashern, MB R0C 0E0
Tel: 204-768-2461 *Fax:* 204-768-2337
www.ierha.ca

Number of Beds: 16 acute care beds
Note: Programs & services include: acute care; dental clinic; diagnostic imaging; laboratory; hemodialysis; emergency/out patient; EMS/ambulance; palliative care; rehabilitation; spiritual care; dietitian; First Nations liaison worker

BALDUR: Baldur Health Centre
Affiliated with: Prairie Mountain Health
PO Box 128, 531 Elizabeth St., Baldur, MB R0K 0B0
Tel: 204-535-2373 *Fax:* 204-535-2116
www.prairiemountainhealth.ca

Number of Beds: 20 long-term care beds
Note: Programs & services include: transitional care; laboratory; public health; mental health; home care; physicians clinic; adult day program; palliative care; occupational & physiotherapy; dietitian; & Meals on Wheels.

BEAUSEJOUR: Beausejour HEW Primary Health Care Centre
Affiliated with: Interlake-Eastern Regional Health Authority
31 - 1st St., Beausejour, MB R0E 0C0
Tel: 204-268-2288

BEAUSEJOUR: Beausejour Hospital in Beausejour Health Centre
Affiliated with: Interlake-Eastern Regional Health Authority
PO Box 1178, 151 First St. South, Beausejour, MB R0E 0C0
Tel: 204-268-1076 *Fax:* 204-268-1207
www.ierha.ca

Number of Beds: 30 acute care beds
Note: Programs & services include: acute care; diagnostic imaging; laboratory; emergency/out patient; occupational therapy; physiotherapy; palliative care; regional staff educator; regional staff pharmacist; rehabilitation; & spiritual care.

BEAUSEJOUR: Beausejour Primary Health Care Centre
Affiliated with: Interlake-Eastern Regional Health Authority
151 - 1st St. South, Beausejour, MB R0E 0C0
Tel: 204-268-4966

BENITO: Benito Health Centre
Affiliated with: Prairie Mountain Health
PO Box 490, 200 - 1st St. SE, Benito, MB R0L 0C0
Tel: 204-539-2815
www.pmh-mb.ca

Note: Includes home care services (204-539-2075)

BIRTLE: Birtle Health Centre
Affiliated with: Prairie Mountain Health
PO Box 2000, 843 Gertrude St., Birtle, MB R0M 0C0
Tel: 204-842-3317 *Fax:* 204-842-3375
www.prairiemountainhealth.ca

Number of Beds: 20 personal care beds
Note: Programs & services include: transitional care; diagnostic; EMS/ambulance; public health; mental health; home care; physicians clinic; palliative care; occupational & physiotherapy; dietitian; elderly persons housing unit (30 suites); & congregate meal program.

BOISSEVAIN: Boissevain Health Centre
Affiliated with: Prairie Mountain Health
PO Box 889, 305 Mill Rd., Boissevain, MB R0K 0E0
Tel: 204-534-2451 *Fax:* 204-534-6487
www.prairiemountainhealth.ca

Number of Beds: 11 acute care beds
Note: Programs & services include: acute care; diagnostic; emergency; public health; mental health; home care; physicians clinic; palliative care; occupational & physiotherapy; dietitian; & respite care.
Donalu Graham, Manager, Care Team

BRANDON: 7th Street Health Access Centre
Affiliated with: Prairie Mountain Health
Also Known As: ACCESS Brandon
20 - 7th St., Brandon, MB R7A 6M8
Tel: 204-578-4800 *Fax:* 204-578-4950
www.pmh-mb.ca

Note: ACCESS Centres offer health & social services. Programs & services at this location include: nurse practitioner; community health nurse; adult community mental health worker; community social worker; addictions services; housing resource worker; cultural facilitators; consumer peer support educator; & Community Volunteer Income Tax Program.
Vicky Legassie, Manager, Primary Health Care

BRANDON: Brandon Regional Health Centre
Affiliated with: Prairie Mountain Health
Former Name: Brandon General Hospital
150 McTavish Ave. East, Brandon, MB R7A 2B3
Tel: 204-578-4000
www.prairiemountainhealth.ca

Number of Beds: 300+ beds
Note: Services include: inpatient & outpatient care; rehabilitation; diagnostics; & clinics.
Penny Gilson, CEO, Prairie Mountain Health
Dr. Shaun Gauthier, Vice-President, Medical & Diagnostic Services

CAMPERVILLE: Camperville Health Centre
Affiliated with: Prairie Mountain Health
PO Box 177, Camperville, MB R0L 0J0
Tel: 204-524-2169
www.prairiemountainhealth.ca

Note: Services include: home care; mental health; primary health care; & public health

CARBERRY: Carberry Plains Health Centre
Affiliated with: Prairie Mountain Health
PO Box 2000, 340 Toronto St., Carberry, MB R0K 0H0
Tel: 204-834-2144 *Fax:* 204-834-3333
www.prairiemountainhealth.ca

Note: Programs & service include: acute care; diagnostic; emergency; EMS/ambulance; public health; mental health; home care; physicians clinic; primary care nurse; dietitian; Meals on Wheels; palliative care; & occupational & physiotherapy. Also has a Personal Care Home on site.

CARTWRIGHT: Davidson Memorial Health Centre
Affiliated with: Prairie Mountain Health
Former Name: Cartwright & District Hospital
PO Box 118, 345 Davidson St., Cartwright, MB R0K 0L0
Tel: 204-529-2483 Fax: 204-529-2562
www.prairiemountainhealth.ca

Note: Programs & services include: transitional care; home care; mental health; public health; & Meals on Wheels.

CHURCHILL: Churchill Health Centre
Affiliated with: Winnipeg Regional Health Authority
162 Laverandrye Ave., Churchill, MB R0B 0E0
Tel: 204-675-8881 Fax: 204-675-2243
www.churchillhealthcentre.com
Social Media: www.facebook.com/ChurchillHealthCentre
Area Served: Churchill; Kivalliq Region of Nunavut
Note: Health & social services include: acute care; primary care clinic; diagnostic; dental clinic/oral surgery; clinical & retail pharmacy; optometry; physiotherapy; chiropractic; massage therapy; mental health; public health; probation; addictions; children & family; child & youth receiving home; home care; Children's Centre; & Telehealth. Services provided through the J.A. Hildes Northern Medical Unit, Department of Community Medicine, University of Manitoba, include: anaesthesia; orthopedics; surgery; geriatrics; internal medicine; gynaecology; ophthalmology; otolaryngology; paediatrics; colposcopy; psychiatry; pediatric dental surgery; & urology.
Laura Wessman, Chief Operating Officer
  lwessman@wrha-ch.ca
Charlene Cornwallis-Bate, Director, Integrated Health & Integrated Services
  ccharlene@wrha-ch.ca
Bobbi Sigurdson, Director, Corporate Services
  bsigurdson2@wrha-ch.ca

CORMORANT: Cormorant Health Care Centre
Affiliated with: Northern Regional Health Authority
PO Box 42, Cormorant, MB R0B 0G0
Tel: 204-357-2161 Fax: 204-357-2259
www.northernhealthregion.ca

CRANBERRY PORTAGE: Cranberry Portage Wellness Centre
Affiliated with: Northern Regional Health Authority
PO Box 186, Cranberry Portage, MB R0B 0H0
Tel: 204-472-3338 Fax: 204-472-3389
www.northernhealthregion.ca

CRANE RIVER: Crane River Health Services
Affiliated with: Prairie Mountain Health
PO Box 156, Crane River, MB R0L 0M0
Tel: 204-732-2286
www.prairiemountainhealth.ca

Note: Programs & services include: home care; mental health; primary health care; public health; & diabetes/heart/chronic disease program

DAUPHIN: Dauphin Community Health Services
Affiliated with: Prairie Mountain Health
625 - 3rd St. SW, Dauphin, MB R7N 1R7
Tel: 204-638-2118 Fax: 204-629-3418
www.pmh-mb.ca

Note: Includes home care services (204-638-2105). Other services include: mental health; child health; immunization; infection prevention & control; prenatal; sexual health; & school health programs

DAUPHIN: Dauphin Regional Health Centre (DRHC)
Affiliated with: Prairie Mountain Health
625 - 3rd St. SW, Dauphin, MB R7N 1R7
Tel: 204-638-3010 Fax: 204-629-3418
www.pmh-mb.ca
Number of Beds: 90 beds
Note: Programs & services include: cancer care; dialysis; emergency; inpatient rehab; maternity; outpatient therapy; palliative care; surgery.

DELORAINE: Deloraine Health Centre
Affiliated with: Prairie Mountain Health
PO Box 447, 109 Kellett St. South, Deloraine, MB R0M 0M0
Tel: 204-747-2745
www.prairiemountainhealth.ca

Number of Beds: 16 personal care beds (Delwynda Court PCH); 30 personal care beds (Bren-del-Win Lodge)
Note: Programs & services include: acute care; diagnostic; emergency; public health; mental health; home care; Manitoba Telehealth; community bath program; adult day program; Meals on Wheels; physicians clinic; palliative care; occupational & physiotherapy; dietitian; & community cancer program.

DUCK BAY: Duck Bay Community Health
Affiliated with: Prairie Mountain Health
PO Box 133, Duck Bay, MB R0L 0N0
Tel: 204-524-2176
www.prairiemountainhealth.ca

Note: Programs & services include: diabetes/heart/chronic disease program; home care; mental health; primary health care; & public health

EBB & FLOW: Bacon Ridge Community Health
Affiliated with: Prairie Mountain Health
General Delivery, Post Office Bldg., Ebb & Flow, MB R0L 0R0
Tel: 204-448-2229
www.prairiemountainhealth.ca

Note: Services include: home care; mental health; primary health care; & public health

ERICKSON: Erickson Health Centre
Affiliated with: Prairie Mountain Health
PO Box 25, 60 Queen Elizabeth Rd., Erickson, MB R0J 0P0
Tel: 204-636-7777 Fax: 204-636-2471
www.prairiemountainhealth.ca
Number of Beds: 9 transitional care beds
Note: Programs & services include: transitional care; diagnostic; EMS/ambulance; public health; mental health; home care; physicians; primary care nurse; Meals on Wheels; & community bath program.

ERIKSDALE: Eriksdale - E.M. Crowe Memorial Hospital
Affiliated with: Interlake-Eastern Regional Health Authority
PO Box 130, 40 Railway Ave., Eriksdale, MB R0C 0W0
Tel: 204-739-2611 Fax: 204-739-2065
www.ierha.ca
Number of Beds: 13 acute care beds
Note: Programs & services include: acute care; diagnostic imaging; laboratory; emergency/out patient; palliative care; physiotherapy; rehabilitation; & spiritual care.

ETHELBERT: Ethelbert Health Centre
Affiliated with: Prairie Mountain Health
PO Box 156, 31 Railway Ave., Ethelbert, MB R0L 0T0
Tel: 204-742-4400
www.pmh-mb.ca

Note: Services include: diabetes/heart/chronic disease program; family physician; home care; mental health; primary health care; & public health

FLIN FLON: Flin Flon General Hospital Inc.
Affiliated with: Northern Regional Health Authority
Third Ave. & Church St., Flin Flon, MB R8A 1N2
Tel: 204-687-7591 Fax: 204-687-8494
www.northernhealthregion.ca
Number of Beds: 42 acute care beds
Note: Hospital Specialty: Acute care

FLIN FLON: Northern Regional Health Authority
Also Known As: Northern Health Region
84 Church St., Flin Flon, MB R8A 1L8
Tel: 204-687-1300 Fax: 204-687-6405
Toll-Free: 888-340-6742
www.northernhealthregion.ca
Year Founded: 2012
Area Served: 396,000 sq km
Population Served: 74983
Note: Northern Regional Health Authority is an amalgamation of NOR-MAN Regional Health Authority & Burntwood Regional Health Authority.
Cal Huntley, Board Chair
Helga Bryant, Chief Executive Officer & Chief Nursing Officer

Dr. Deborah Mabin, Chief Medical Officer & Vice-President, Medical Services

Shawn Hnidy, Chief Financial Officer & Vice-President, Corporate Services

Rusty Beardy, Vice-President, Indigenous Health Services & Relations

Wanda Reader, Chief Human Resources Officer & Vice-President, Human Resources

Joy Tetlock, Vice-President, Planning & Innovation

GILBERT PLAINS: Gilbert Plains Health Centre
Affiliated with: Prairie Mountain Health
PO Box 368, 100 Cutforth St. North, Gilbert Plains, MB R0L 0X0
Tel: 204-548-2161
www.prairiemountainhealth.ca

Note: Physician clinic attached to Gilbert Plains Personal Care Home. Services include: emergency/ambulance; home care; mental health; primary health care; & public health.

GILLAM: Gillam Hospital Inc.
Affiliated with: Northern Regional Health Authority
PO Box 2000, 115 Gillam Dr., Gillam, MB R0B 0L0
Tel: 204-652-2600 Fax: 204-652-2536
www.northernhealthregion.ca

Number of Beds: 7 acute care beds
Note: Programs & services include: emergency services; laboratory services; acute care; public health; long term care; x-ray; medical clinic; visiting specialists (optometry, chiropractic & pediatrics); full-time Public Health Nurse; Mental Health Worker; Probation Officer; Employment & Income Assistance Counsellor; & Addictions Foundation Rehabilitation Counsellor.

GIMLI: Gimli Community Health Centre (GCHC)
Affiliated with: Interlake-Eastern Regional Health Authority
PO Box 250, 120 - 6th Ave., Gimli, MB R0C 1B0
Tel: 204-642-5116 Fax: 204-642-5860
www.ierha.ca

Year Founded: 2004
Number of Beds: 26 acute care beds
Note: The centre contains the following: Johnson Memorial Hospital; Community Health Office; & Gimli Clinic.
Programs & services include: acute care; adult day program; chemotherapy; community cancer program; diagnostic imaging; laboratory; emergency/out patient; EMS/ambulance; hemodialysis; occupational therapy; palliative care; physiotherapy; medical clinic; & spiritual care.

GLENBORO: Glenboro Health Centre
Affiliated with: Prairie Mountain Health
Former Name: Glenboro Health District Hospital
PO Box 310, 219 Murray Ave., Glenboro, MB R0K 0X0
Tel: 204-827-2438 Fax: 204-827-2199
www.prairiemountainhealth.ca

Number of Beds: 20 personal care beds
Note: Programs & services include: acute care; diagnostic; EMS/ambulance; public health; mental health; home care; physicians clinic; palliative care; occupational & physiotherapy; dietitian; & Meals on Wheels. Also includes a Personal Care Home on site.

GRANDVIEW: Grandview Community Health
Affiliated with: Prairie Mountain Health
PO Box 339, 644 Mill St., Grandview, MB R0L 0Y0
Tel: 204-546-5150
www.prairiemountainhealth.ca

GRANDVIEW: Grandview District Hospital
Affiliated with: Prairie Mountain Health
PO Box 339, 644 Mill St., Grandview, MB R0L 0Y0
Tel: 204-546-2425
www.pmh-mb.ca

Number of Beds: 18 beds
Note: Programs & services include: acute medicine; EKG; laboratory testing; outpatient services; palliative care; telehealth; x-ray; & 24-hour emergency services.

HAMIOTA: Hamiota Health Centre
Affiliated with: Prairie Mountain Health
177 Birch Ave., Hamiota, MB R0M 0T0
Tel: 204-764-2412 Fax: 204-764-2049
www.prairiemountainhealth.ca

Number of Beds: 30 personal care home beds
Note: Programs & services include: acute care; community cancer program; diagnostic; EMS/ambulance; public health; mental health; home care; Manitoba Telehealth; physicians clinic; primary care nurse; palliative care; occupational & physiotherapy; dietitian; Meals on Wheels; Lilac Elderly Person Housing (30 units); & congregate meal program.

HARTNEY: Hartney Health Centre
Affiliated with: Prairie Mountain Health
Former Name: Hartney Medical Nursing Unit
PO Box 280, 617 River Ave., Hartney, MB R0M 0X0
Tel: 204-858-2054 Fax: 204-858-2303
www.prairiemountainhealth.ca

Number of Beds: 20 personal care beds
Note: Programs & services include: rehabilitation; long-term care; public health; mental health; & home care. Also includes a Personal Care Home on site.

HODGSON: Percy E. Moore Hospital
Affiliated with: Interlake-Eastern Regional Health Authority
PO Box 190, Hodgson, MB R0C 1N0
Tel: 204-372-8444 Fax: 204-372-6991
www.ierha.ca

Year Founded: 1973
Number of Beds: 16 beds
Area Served: RM of Fisher, Peguis, Fisher River, & Kinonjeoshtegon
Population Served: 10000
Note: The hospital is operated by First Nations & Inuit Health of Health Canada.

ILFORD: Ilford Community Health Centre
Affiliated with: Northern Regional Health Authority
53 First St., Ilford, MB R0B 0S0
Tel: 204-288-4348 Fax: 204-288-4248
www.northernhealthregion.ca

KILLARNEY: Tri-Lake Health Centre
Affiliated with: Prairie Mountain Health
PO Box 5000, 86 Ellis Dr., Killarney, MB R0K 1G0
Tel: 204-523-4661 Fax: 204-523-8948
www.prairiemountainhealth.ca

Number of Beds: 60 personal care beds
Note: Programs & services include: acute care; diagnostic; EMS/ambulance; public health; mental health; home care; Manitoba Telehealth; physicians clinic; palliative care; occupational & physiotherapy; dietitian; & Meals on Wheels.

LA BROQUERIE: Southern Health-Santé Sud
La Broquerie Regional Office, PO Box 470, 94 Principale St., La Broquerie, MB R0A 0W0
www.southernhealth.ca

Area Served: 27,025 sq km
Note: Regional offices are located in La Broquerie, Morden, Notre Dame de Lourdes & Southport. For a complete list of health sites overseen by Southern Health-Santé Sud, please see the following URL: www.southernhealth.ca/healthsites.php.

LAC DU BONNET: Lac du Bonnet District Health Centre
Affiliated with: Interlake-Eastern Regional Health Authority
89 McIntosh St., Lac du Bonnet, MB R0E 1A0
Tel: 204-345-8647

Note: Diagnostics; physiotherapy; counselling; clinic.
Lorri Beer, Regional Manager, Physician Services

LEAF RAPIDS: Leaf Rapids Health Centre
Affiliated with: Northern Regional Health Authority
PO Box 370, Leaf Rapids, MB R0B 1W0
Tel: 204-473-2441 Fax: 204-473-8273
www.northernhealthregion.ca

Year Founded: 1973

LUNDAR: Lundar Health Centre
Affiliated with: Interlake-Eastern Regional Health Authority
97 - 1st St. South, Lundar, MB R0C 1Y0
Tel: 204-762-6076

Note: Nurse Practitioner Clinic (one day a week)

LUNDAR: Lundar Medical Clinic
38 Main St., Lundar, MB R0C 1Y0
Tel: 204-762-5609

Note: Private clinic

LYNN LAKE: Lynn Lake District Hospital
Affiliated with: Northern Regional Health Authority
PO Box 2030, 2040 Camp St., Lynn Lake, MB R0B 0W0
Tel: 204-356-2474 *Fax:* 204-356-8023
www.northernhealthregion.ca
Number of Beds: 11 acute care beds
Marianne Jantz, Manager

MCCREARY: McCreary Community Health
Affiliated with: Prairie Mountain Health
PO Box 208, McCreary, MB R0J 1B0
Tel: 204-835-5010 *Fax:* 204-835-5011
www.pmh-mb.ca

Note: Offers public health services

MCCREARY: McCreary/Alonsa Health Centre
Affiliated with: Prairie Mountain Health
PO Box 250, 613 Provincial Trunk Hwy. 50, McCreary, MB R0J 1B0
Tel: 204-853-2482 *Fax:* 204-853-2713
www.pmh-mb.ca
Number of Beds: 12 transitional care beds
Note: Programs & services include: diagnostic; home care; outpatient; palliative care; & clinics.

MELITA: Melita Health Centre
Affiliated with: Prairie Mountain Health
PO Box 459, 147 Summit Ave., Melita, MB R0M 1L0
Tel: 204-522-3403
www.prairiemountainhealth.ca
Number of Beds: 20 long-term care beds
Note: Programs & services include: acute care; EMS/ambulance; diagnostic; emergency; public health; mental health; home care; physicians clinic; palliative care; occupational & physiotherapy; dietitian; & Meals on Wheels.

MINNEDOSA: Minnedosa Health Centre
Affiliated with: Prairie Mountain Health
PO Box 960, 334 1st St. SW, Minnedosa, MB R0J 1E0
Tel: 204-867-2701 *Fax:* 204-867-2239
www.prairiemountainhealth.ca
Number of Beds: 27 acute care beds
Note: Programs & services include: acute care; general surgery; diagnostic; EMS/ambulance; public health; mental health; home care; physicians clinic; occupational & physiotherapy; dietitian; & Meals on Wheels.

NEEPAWA: Neepawa Health Centre
Affiliated with: Prairie Mountain Health
Former Name: Neepawa District Memorial Hospital
PO Box 1240, 500 Hospital St., Neepawa, MB R0J 1H0
Tel: 204-476-2394 *Fax:* 204-476-5007
www.prairiemountainhealth.ca
Number of Beds: 38 beds
Note: Programs & services include: acute care; general surgery; obstetrics; diagnostic; ultrasound; EMS/ambulance; home care; palliative care; occupational & physiotherapy; dietitian; & Meals on Wheels.

NORWAY HOUSE: Norway House Health Services Inc. (NHHS)
PO Box 250, Norway House, MB R0B 1B0
Tel: 204-359-6704 *Fax:* 204-359-6161
www.nhcn.ca/health_division
Year Founded: 2003
Area Served: 19,435 acre reserve
Note: Provides health services to the community of the Norway House Cree Nation. Oversees Pinaow Wachi Personal Care Home, Kinosao Sipi Dental Centre, Norway House Community Clinic & Norway House Hospital/Norway House Nursing Station (with Northern Regional Health Authority).

NORWAY HOUSE: Norway House Nursing Station
Norway House Health Services Inc.
Affiliated with: Northern Regional Health Authority
Also Known As: Norway House Hospital
PO Box 730, Norway House, MB R0B 1B0
Tel: 204-359-8230 *Fax:* 204-359-6599
www.northernhealthregion.ca

Number of Employees: 20
Note: Programs & services include: dialysis; laboratory; x-ray; & dietary.

OPASKWAYAK: Beatrice Wilson Health Centre
Affiliated with: Northern Regional Health Authority
245 Waller Rd., Opaskwayak, MB R0B 2J0
Tel: 204-627-7410 *Fax:* 204-623-1491
www.northernhealthregion.ca

PELICAN RAPIDS: Pelican Rapids Community Health
Affiliated with: Prairie Mountain Health
General Delivery, Council Office, Pelican Rapids, MB R0L 1L0
Tel: 204-587-2058 *Fax:* 204-587-2036
www.pmh-mb.ca

PIKWITONEI: Pikwitonei Health Centre
Affiliated with: Northern Regional Health Authority
General Delivery, Pikwitonei, MB R0B 1E0
Tel: 204-458-2402 *Fax:* 204-458-2468
www.northernhealthregion.ca

PINAWA: Pinawa Hospital
Affiliated with: Interlake-Eastern Regional Health Authority
PO Box 220, 30 Vanier Dr., Pinawa, MB R0E 1L0
Tel: 204-753-2334 *Fax:* 204-753-2219
www.ierha.ca
Year Founded: 1964
Number of Beds: 17 acute care beds
Note: Programs & services include: acute care; community cancer care; dietitians; diagnostics; EMS/ambulance; medical clinic; occupational therapy; physiotherapy; palliative care; rehabilitation; & spiritual care.

PINAWA: Pinawa Primary Health Care Centre
Affiliated with: Interlake-Eastern Regional Health Authority
30 Vanier Dr., Pinawa, MB R0E 1L0
Tel: 204-753-2351

PINE FALLS: Pine Falls Hospital in Pine Falls Health Complex
Affiliated with: Interlake-Eastern Regional Health Authority
PO Box 2000, 37 Maple St., Pine Falls, MB R0E 1M0
Tel: 204-367-4441 *Fax:* 204-367-8981
www.ierha.ca
Number of Beds: 23 acute care beds
Note: Programs & services include: dietitians; diagnostic imaging; laboratory; hemodialysis; occupational therapy; palliative care; physiotherapy; rehabilitation; & spiritual care.

PINE FALLS: Pine Falls Primary Health Care Centre
Affiliated with: Interlake-Eastern Regional Health Authority
37 Maple St., Pine Falls, MB R0E 1M0
Tel: 204-367-2278

RESTON: Reston Health Centre
Affiliated with: Prairie Mountain Health
PO Box 250, 523 1st St. North, Reston, MB R0M 1X0
Tel: 204-877-3925 *Fax:* 204-877-3998
www.prairiemountainhealth.ca
Number of Beds: 20 personal care beds
Note: Programs & services include: transitional care; public health; mental health; home care; long-term care; occupational & physiotherapy; primary health care; & Meals on Wheels.

RIVERS: Riverdale Health Centre
Affiliated with: Prairie Mountain Health
PO Box 428, 512 Quebec St., Rivers, MB R0K 1X0
Tel: 204-328-5321 *Fax:* 204-328-7130
www.prairiemountainhealth.ca
Number of Beds: 20 personal care beds
Note: Programs & services include: rehabilitation unit; diagnostic; public health; mental health; home care; physicians clinics; palliative

care; occupational & physiotherapy; dietitian; Meals on Wheels & elderly persons housing (12 units).
Greg Paddock, Area Manager

RIVERTON: Riverton Clinic
Affiliated with: Interlake-Eastern Regional Health Authority
Riverton, MB R0C 2R0

Tel: 204-378-2460

ROBLIN: Roblin Community Health Service
Affiliated with: Prairie Mountain Health
PO Box 940, 15 Hospital St., Roblin, MB R0L 1P0

Tel: 204-937-2151 *Fax:* 204-937-5992
www.pmh-mb.ca

Note: Includes home care (204-937-6271), community rehabilitation, & mental health services

ROBLIN: Roblin Health Centre
Affiliated with: Prairie Mountain Health
PO Box 940, 15 Hospital St., Roblin, MB R0L 1P0

Tel: 204-937-2142 *Fax:* 204-937-8892
www.prairiemountainhealth.ca

Number of Beds: 25 beds
Note: Programs & services include: acute care; diagnostic; EKG; emergency; laboratory; outpatient services; palliative care; Manitoba Telehealth; & x-ray.

ROSSBURN: Rossburn District Health Centre
Affiliated with: Prairie Mountain Health
PO Box 40, 166 Parkview Dr., Rossburn, MB R0J 1V0

Tel: 204-859-2413 *Fax:* 204-859-2526
www.prairiemountainhealth.ca

Number of Beds: 20 personal care beds
Note: Programs & services include: transitional care; diagnostic; public health; mental health; home care; physician clinic; primary care nurse; palliative care; occupational & physiotherapy; & dietitian.

RUSSELL: Russell Health Centre
Affiliated with: Prairie Mountain Health
426 Alexandria Ave., Russell, MB R0J 1W0

Tel: 204-773-2125 *Fax:* 204-773-2142
www.prairiemountainhealth.ca

Note: Programs & services include: acute care; community cancer program; diagnostic; EMS/ambulance; public health; mental health; home care; Manitoba Telehealth; physicians clinic; palliative care; occupational & physiotherapy; dietitian; Meals on Wheels; & pharmacy.

SELKIRK: Clandeboye Medical Clinic & Interlake Surgical Associates
210 Clandeboye Ave., Selkirk, MB R1A 0X1

Tel: 204-785-2555 *Fax:* 204-482-4525
www.clandeboyeclinic.ca

Note: Interlake Surgical Associates Phone: 204-785-5507. Clandeboye Medical Clinic specializes in general & family practice. Interlake Surgical Associates specializes in general, endoscopic, & laparoscopic surgery.

SELKIRK: Eveline Street Clinic
Affiliated with: Interlake-Eastern Regional Health Authority
66 Eveline St., Selkirk, MB R1A 1K6

Tel: 204-785-5550

Note: Alternate phone: 204-785-5552

SELKIRK: Interlake-Eastern Regional Health Authority
Former Name: Interlake Regional Health Authority, North Eastman Regional Health Authority
Corporate Office, 233A Main St., Selkirk, MB R1A 1S1

Tel: 204-785-4700 *Fax:* 204-482-4300
Toll-Free: 855-347-8500
info@ierha.ca
www.ierha.ca
Social Media: twitter.com/IERHA_MB

Area Served: 61,000 sq km
Population Served: 124000
Number of Employees: 3100
Note: Interlake-Eastern RHA is an amalgamation of Interlake Regional Health Authority & North Eastman Regional Health Authority.

Ed Bergen, Board Chair
Ron Van Denakker, Chief Executive Officer
Dr. Tim Hilderman, Medical Officer of Health
Dr. Karen Robinson, Medical Officer of Health
Dr. Myron Thiessen, Chief Medical Officer & Vice-President, Primary Health Care
Cynthia Ostapyk, Vice-President, Finance
Karen Stevens-Chambers, Chief Allied Health Officer & Vice-President, Community Services
Marion Ellis, Chief Nursing Officer & Vice-President, Acute Care

SELKIRK: Red River Walk-In Clinic
Affiliated with: Interlake-Eastern Regional Health Authority
367 Eveline St., Selkirk, MB R1A 1N2

Tel: 204-482-8953

SELKIRK: Selkirk & District General Hospital
Affiliated with: Interlake-Eastern Regional Health Authority
PO Box 5000, 100 Easton Dr., Selkirk, MB R1A 2M2

Tel: 204-482-5800 *Fax:* 204-785-9113
www.ierha.ca

Year Founded: 1907
Number of Beds: 51 beds
Note: Programs & services include: acute care; chemotherapy; community cancer care; diagnostic imaging & ultrasound; dialysis; emergency/out patient; EMS/ambulance; obstetrical program; occupational therapy; palliative care; physiotherapy; regional surgical services; & spiritual care.

SELKIRK: Selkirk Medical Centre
Affiliated with: Interlake-Eastern Regional Health Authority
353 Eveline St., Selkirk, MB R1A 1N1

Note: Physicians at this location should be contacted directly

SELKIRK: Selkirk QuickCare Clinic
Affiliated with: Interlake-Eastern Regional Health Authority
#3, 1020 Manitoba Ave., Selkirk, MB R1A 4M2

Tel: 204-482-4399

Note: Part of Manitoba's QuickCare Clinic initiative; for diagnosing & treating minor health issues

SELKIRK: Selkirk Travel Health Clinic
Affiliated with: Interlake-Eastern Regional Health Authority
#202, 237 Manitoba Ave., Selkirk, MB R1A 0Y4

Tel: 204-785-4891

Note: Appointments available only on Wednesdays

SHERRIDON: Sherridon Health Centre
Affiliated with: Northern Regional Health Authority
General Delivery, Sherridon, MB R0B 1L0

Tel: 204-468-2012 *Fax:* 204-468-2167
www.northernhealthregion.ca

SHOAL LAKE: Shoal Lake/Strathclair Health Centre
Affiliated with: Prairie Mountain Health
PO Box 490, 526 Mary St., Shoal Lake, MB R0J 1Z0

Tel: 204-759-2336 *Fax:* 204-759-2230
www.prairiemountainhealth.ca

Number of Beds: 40 personal care beds
Note: Programs & services include: acute care; diagnostic; EMS/ambulance; public health; mental health; home care; physicians clinic; palliative care; occupational & physiotherapy; dietitian; Meals on Wheels; & Elderly Persons Housing.

SNOW LAKE: Snow Lake Health Centre
Affiliated with: Northern Regional Health Authority
100 Lakeshore Dr., Snow Lake, MB R0B 1M0

Tel: 204-358-2300 *Fax:* 204-358-7310
www.northernhealthregion.ca

Kelly Wiwcharuk, Nurse Manager

SOURIS: Prairie Mountain Health
PO Box 579, 192 - 1st Ave. West, Souris, MB R0K 2C0
Tel: 204-483-5000 *Fax:* 204-483-5005
Toll-Free: 888-682-2253
www.prairiemountainhealth.ca
Social Media: www.facebook.com/prairiemountainhealth;
twitter.com/prairiemthealth

Year Founded: 2012
Number of Beds: 2,003 long term care beds; 795 acute care beds; 91 transitional care beds
Population Served: 168477
Number of Employees: 8700
Note: Prairie Mountain Health is an amalgamation of Brandon Regional Health Authority, Assiniboine Regional Health Authority & Parkland Regional Health Authority. Services include: public health, home care, long term care, mental health services, comprehensive health services (cancer care, cardiac, birthing & neonatal, rehabilitation, & surgery).
Catheryn Pederson, Board Chair
Penny Gilson, Chief Executive Officer

SOURIS: Souris Health Centre
Affiliated with: Prairie Mountain Health
PO Box 10, 155 Brindle Ave., Souris, MB R0K 2C0
Tel: 204-483-2121 *Fax:* 204-483-2310
www.prairiemountainhealth.ca
Number of Beds: 25 acute care beds; 42 long-term care beds; 1 respite bed
Note: Programs & services include: acute care; EMS; general surgery; diagnostic; public health; mental health; home care; physicians clinic; palliative care; occupational & physiotherapy; dietitian; & Meals on Wheels.

ST. LAURENT: St. Laurent Health Centre
Affiliated with: Interlake-Eastern Regional Health Authority
1 Parish Lane, St. Laurent, MB R0C 0E7
Tel: 204-646-2504

Note: Nurse Practitioner Clinic (one day a week)

STE ROSE: Ste Rose Community Health Services
Affiliated with: Prairie Mountain Health
PO Box 149, 603 - 1st Ave. East, Ste Rose, MB R0L 1S0
Tel: 204-447-4080
www.prairiemountainhealth.ca

Note: Services include: home care; mental health; & public health

STE ROSE DU LAC: Ste Rose General Hospital
Affiliated with: Prairie Mountain Health
Also Known As: Ste Rose Health Centre
PO Box 149, 480 - 3rd Ave. SE, Ste Rose du Lac, MB R0L 1S0
Tel: 204-447-2131 *Fax:* 204-447-2250
www.prairiemountainhealth.ca
Number of Beds: 25 beds
Note: Programs & services include: acute care; EKG; emergency; laboratory; outpatient services; palliative care; x-ray; rehabilitation; & public health.
Michelle Quennelle, Executive Director

STONEWALL: Hope Medical Clinic
Affiliated with: Interlake-Eastern Regional Health Authority
#4B, 408 Main St., Stonewall, MB R0C 2Z0
Tel: 204-467-7595

STONEWALL: Interlake Medical Clinic
Affiliated with: Interlake-Eastern Regional Health Authority
#2, 330 - 3rd Ave. South, Stonewall, MB R0C 2Z0
Tel: 204-467-5717

STONEWALL: Rockwood Medical Clinic
Affiliated with: Interlake-Eastern Regional Health Authority
#5, 405 - 3rd Ave. South, Stonewall, MB R0C 2Z0
Tel: 204-467-9707

STONEWALL: Stonewall & District Health Centre
Affiliated with: Interlake-Eastern Regional Health Authority
589 - 3rd Ave., Stonewall, MB R0C 2Z0
Tel: 204-467-5514 *Fax:* 204-467-4431
www.ierha.ca
Number of Beds: 14 acute care beds; 1 palliative care bed; 3 observation beds

Note: Centre contains: hospital; community health office; & clinic. Programs & services include: diagnostic imaging; laboratory; emergency/out patient; EMS/ambulance; occupational therapy; palliative care; physiotherapy; rehabilitation; & spiritual care.

SWAN RIVER: Swan River Community Health Services
Affiliated with: Prairie Mountain Health
PO Box 1028, 1013 Main St., Swan River, MB R0L 1Z0
Tel: 204-734-6660
www.prairiemountainhealth.ca

Note: Services include: acute care; outpatient; diagnostic; emergency/ambulance; rehabilitation; home care; mental health; long-term care; primary health care; public health; & Manitoba Telehealth

SWAN RIVER: Swan Valley Health Centre
Affiliated with: Prairie Mountain Health
PO Box 1450, 1011 Main St., Swan River, MB R0L 1Z0
Tel: 204-734-3441
www.prairiemountainhealth.ca
Year Founded: 2005
Number of Beds: 52 acute care beds
Note: Programs & services include: public health; home care; diagnostics; dialysis; physiotherapy; speech therapy; surgery; mental health; emergency; chemotherapy; Manitoba Telehealth; occupational therapy; respiratory therapy; rehabilitation; long term care; & Meals on Wheels.

TEULON: Teulon - Hunter Memorial Hospital
Affiliated with: Interlake-Eastern Regional Health Authority
PO Box 89, 162 - 3rd Ave. SE, Teulon, MB R0C 3B0
Tel: 204-886-2433 *Fax:* 204-886-2653
www.ierha.ca
Number of Beds: 20 acute care beds
Note: Programs & services include: acute care; diagnostic imaging; laboratory; emergency/out patient; EMS/ambulance; physiotherapy/occupational therapy; dietary; palliative care; & rehabilitation.

TEULON: Teulon - Private Clinic
34 Main St., Teulon, MB R0C 3B0
Tel: 204-886-3039

THE PAS: St. Anthony's General Hospital
Affiliated with: Northern Regional Health Authority
Also Known As: The Pas Health Complex
PO Box 240, 67 - 1 St. West, The Pas, MB R9A 1K4
Tel: 204-623-6431 *Fax:* 204-623-9263
www.northernhealthregion.ca
Year Founded: 1969
Number of Beds: 40 acute care beds; 8 in-patient acute care adult psychiatric beds

THICKET PORTAGE: Thicket Portage Community Health Centre
Affiliated with: Northern Regional Health Authority
398 Evens Ave., Thicket Portage, MB R0B 1R0
Tel: 204-286-3254 *Fax:* 204-286-3216
www.northernhealthregion.ca

THOMPSON: Burntwood Community Health Resource Centre
Affiliated with: Northern Regional Health Authority
50 Selkirk Ave., Thompson, MB R8N 0M7
Tel: 204-677-1777 *Fax:* 204-677-1755

Note: Family doctor.

THOMPSON: Thompson General Hospital
Affiliated with: Northern Regional Health Authority
871 Thompson Dr. South, Thompson, MB R8N 0C8
Tel: 204-677-2381 *Fax:* 204-778-1413
www.northernhealthregion.ca
Number of Beds: 79 acute care beds; 10 in-patient acute care adult psychiatric beds
Note: Programs & services include: emergency; community mental health; cancer services/chemotherapy; consultation clinic; diagnostic (lab & radiology); general medicine; Northern Patient Transportation Program (NPTP); nutritional services; obstetrics; pediatrics; physiotherapy; surgery & telehealth.

TREHERNE: Tiger Hills Health Centre
Affiliated with: Prairie Mountain Health
PO Box 130, 64 Clark St., Treherne, MB R0G 2V0
Tel: 204-723-2133 *Fax:* 204-723-2869
www.prairiemountainhealth.ca
Number of Beds: 22 personal care beds; 13 acute care beds
Note: Programs & services include: acute care; diagnostic; emergency; public health; mental health; home care; physician clinic; palliative care; occupation & physiotherapy; dietitian; Meals on Wheels; & Elderly Persons Housing (21 units).

VIRDEN: Virden Health Centre
Affiliated with: Prairie Mountain Health
PO Box 400, 480 King St., Virden, MB R0M 2C0
Tel: 204-748-1230 *Fax:* 204-748-2053
www.prairiemountainhealth.ca
Number of Beds: 25 acute care beds
Note: Programs & services include: acute care; diagnostic; EMS/ambulance; laboratory; Manitoba Telehealth; physician clinic; palliative care; occupational & physiotherapy; & dietitian.

WABOWDEN: Wabowden Community Health Centre
Affiliated with: Northern Regional Health Authority
88 Lakeside Dr., Wabowden, MB R0B 1S0
Tel: 204-689-2600 *Fax:* 204-689-2180
www.northernhealthregion.ca

WATERHEN: Waterhen Health Centre
Affiliated with: Prairie Mountain Health
PO Box 10, 104 North Mallard Rd., Waterhen, MB R0L 2C0
Tel: 204-628-3329
www.prairiemountainhealth.ca
Note: Services include: emergency/ambulance; home care; mental health; primary health care; & public health

WAWANESA: Wawanesa Health Centre
Affiliated with: Prairie Mountain Health
Former Name: Wawanesa & District Memorial Health Centre
PO Box 309, 506 George St., Wawanesa, MB R0K 2G0
Tel: 204-824-2335 *Fax:* 204-824-2148
www.prairiemountainhealth.ca
Number of Beds: 20 personal care beds
Note: Programs & services include: transitional care; diagnostic; public health; mental health; home care; physician clinic; primary care nurse; occupational & physiotherapy; dietitian; & Meals on Wheels.

WHITEMOUTH: Whitemouth Primary Health Care Centre
Affiliated with: Interlake-Eastern Regional Health Authority
75 Hospital St., Whitemouth, MB R0E 2G0
Tel: 204-348-2291

WINNIPEG: ACCESS Downtown
Affiliated with: Winnipeg Regional Health Authority
640 Main St., Winnipeg, MB R3B 0L8
Tel: 204-940-3638
www.wrha.mb.ca
Note: ACCESS Centres offer health & social services; programs & services vary by community

WINNIPEG: ACCESS NorWest
Affiliated with: Winnipeg Regional Health Authority
785 Keewatin St., Winnipeg, MB R2X 3B9
Tel: 204-938-5900
www.wrha.mb.ca
Note: ACCESS Centres offer health & social services; programs & services vary by community. This branch is in the same location as NorWest Co-op Community Health.

WINNIPEG: ACCESS River East
Affiliated with: Winnipeg Regional Health Authority
975 Henderson Hwy., Winnipeg, MB R2K 4L7
Tel: 204-938-5000
www.wrha.mb.ca
Note: ACCESS Centres offer health & social services; programs & services vary by community

WINNIPEG: ACCESS Transcona
Affiliated with: Winnipeg Regional Health Authority
845 Regent Ave. West, Winnipeg, MB R2C 3A9
Tel: 204-938-5555
www.wrha.mb.ca
Note: ACCESS Centres offer health & social services; programs & services vary by community

WINNIPEG: ACCESS Winnipeg West
Affiliated with: Winnipeg Regional Health Authority
280 Booth Dr., Winnipeg, MB R3J 3R5
Tel: 204-940-2040
www.wrha.mb.ca
Note: ACCESS Centres offer health & social services; programs & services vary by community. St. James clients (204-940-2397); Assiniboine South clients (204-940-2453).

WINNIPEG: Centre de santé Saint-Boniface
Affiliated with: Winnipeg Regional Health Authority
170 Goulet St., Winnipeg, MB R2H 0R7
Tel: 204-940-1155 *Fax:* 204-237-9057
access@centredesante.mb.ca
www.centredesante.mb.ca
Note: Bilingual primary health centre. Programs & services include: medical; nutrition; mental health; community support; & Health Links - Info Santé.
Monique Constant, Executive Director

WINNIPEG: Concordia Hospital
Affiliated with: Winnipeg Regional Health Authority
1095 Concordia Ave., Winnipeg, MB R2K 3S8
Tel: 204-667-1560 *Fax:* 204-667-1049
www.concordiahospital.mb.ca
Year Founded: 1928
Number of Beds: Includes the 140-bed Concordia Place Personal Care Home
Number of Employees: 1100
Specialties: Orthopaedics - lower & upper joint replacement
Note: Programs & services include: diagnostic imaging; laboratory services (204-661-7174); surgery (a major centre for hip & knee replacements); intensive care; A.M.I. (Acute Myocardial Infarcation) Program; occupational therapy (204-661-7216); physiotherapy (204-661-7354); respiratory therapy (204-661-7346); oncology haematology service; social work (204-661-7185); cardiac teaching program (nurse home visit); & lifeline personal response & support services.
Valerie Wiebe, President & COO

WINNIPEG: Downtown East Community Office
Affiliated with: Winnipeg Regional Health Authority
#2, 640 Main St., Winnipeg, MB R3B 0L8
Tel: 204-940-8441
www.wrha.mb.ca
Note: Provides services related to: healthy parenting & early childhood development; healthy children & youth; nutrition promotion; communicable disease prevention & management; immunization; & more. This office is in the same location as ACCESS Downtown.

WINNIPEG: Downtown West Community Office
Affiliated with: Winnipeg Regional Health Authority
755 Portage Ave., Winnipeg, MB R3G 0N2
Tel: 204-940-6669
www.wrha.mb.ca

WINNIPEG: Fort Garry Community Office
Affiliated with: Winnipeg Regional Health Authority
2735 Pembina Hwy., Winnipeg, MB R3T 2H5
Tel: 204-940-2015
www.wrha.mb.ca
Note: Provides services related to: healthy parenting & early childhood development; healthy children & youth; nutrition promotion; communicable disease prevention & management; immunization; & more.

WINNIPEG: Grace Hospital
Affiliated with: Winnipeg Regional Health Authority
Former Name: The Salvation Army Grace General Hospital
300 Booth Dr., Winnipeg, MB R3J 3M7

Tel: 204-837-0111
pr@ggh.mb.ca
www.gracehospital.ca

Year Founded: 1904
Number of Beds: 251 beds
Note: Programs & services include: emergency & critical care; surgery; mental health; Aboriginal health services; & hospice care.

WINNIPEG: Health Action Centre
Affiliated with: Winnipeg Regional Health Authority
640 Main St., Winnipeg, MB R3B 0L8

Tel: 204-940-1626 *Fax:* 204-942-7828
www.wrha.mb.ca

WINNIPEG: Health Sciences Centre (HSC)
Affiliated with: Winnipeg Regional Health Authority
820 Sherbrook St., Winnipeg, MB R3A 1R9

Tel: 204-787-3661 *Fax:* 204-787-1233
Toll-Free: 877-499-8774
info@hsc.mb.ca
www.hsc.mb.ca
Social Media: www.facebook.com/184583582309;
www.twitter.com/hsc_winnipeg

Year Founded: 1973
Area Served: Manitoba, northwestern Ontario & Nunavut
Number of Employees: 8000
Specialties: Transplants, burns, neurosciences & pediatric care
Note: A teaching hospital & the designated Trauma Centre for Manitoba. Programs & services include: Aboriginal health services; adult mental health; anesthesia; child & adolescent mental health; child health; clinical health psychology; critical care; diagnostic imaging; dialysis; emergency; medicine; oncology; rehab; geriatrics; surgery; & women's health.
Kathy Doerksen, Chief Nursing Officer
Dr. Perry Gray, Vice-President & Chief Medical Officer

WINNIPEG: Hope Centre Health Care Inc.
Affiliated with: Winnipeg Regional Health Authority
240 Powers St., Winnipeg, MB R2W 5L1

Tel: 204-589-8354 *Fax:* 204-586-4260
www.wrha.mb.ca
Year Founded: 1982

WINNIPEG: Hôpital St-Boniface Hospital
Affiliated with: Winnipeg Regional Health Authority
Former Name: St. Boniface General Hospital
409 Taché Ave., Winnipeg, MB R2H 2A6

Tel: 204-233-8563
sbghweb@sbgh.mb.ca
www.sbgh.mb.ca
Social Media: twitter.com/sbh_winnipeg;
www.youtube.com/stbonifacehosp

Year Founded: 1871
Number of Employees: 4000
Note: Catholic tertiary care facility & teaching hospital affiliated with the University of Manitoba & dedicated to the values of care of the Sisters of Charity of Montreal (Grey Nuns). Programs & services include: Aboriginal health services; emergency services; family medicine; mental health; geriatrics & rehabilitation; surgery; women's health; & paediatrics.
Dr. Bruce Roe, Chief Medical Officer & Executive Director, Clinical Programs
204-237-2317

WINNIPEG: Klinic Community Health Centre
Affiliated with: Winnipeg Regional Health Authority
870 Portage Ave., Winnipeg, MB R3G 0P1

Tel: 204-784-4090 *Fax:* 204-772-7998
www.klinic.mb.ca

Nicole Chammartin, Executive Director
nchammartin@klinic.mb.ca

WINNIPEG: MFL Occupational Health Centre, Inc.
Affiliated with: Winnipeg Regional Health Authority
#102, 275 Broadway, Winnipeg, MB R3C 4M6

Tel: 204-949-0811 *Fax:* 204-956-0848
Toll-Free: 888-843-1229
mflohc@mflohc.mb.ca
www.mflohc.mb.ca
Social Media: www.facebook.com/OccupationalHealthCentre;
www.linkedin.com/company/mfl-occupational-health-centre

Year Founded: 1983
Note: Specializes in occupational health (health issues related to work experiences), improvement of workplace health & safety conditions, & elimination of hazards.
Mike Kelly, Executive Director
204-926-7900, mkelly@mflohc.mb.ca

WINNIPEG: Misericordia Health Centre (MHC)
Affiliated with: Winnipeg Regional Health Authority
99 Cornish Ave., Winnipeg, MB R3C 1A2

Tel: 204-774-6581 *Fax:* 204-783-6052
info@misericordia.mb.ca
www.misericordia.mb.ca
Social Media: www.facebook.com/MisericordiaMB;
twitter.com/MisericordiaMB; instagram.com/misericordiamb

Year Founded: 1898
Number of Beds: 250 beds; 100 personal care home beds
Note: Research & teaching health centre, with programs & services including: ambulatory care; Buhler Eye Care Centre; Community IV Program; diagnostics; Easy Street rehabilitation program; eye bank; interim care; laboratory; long-term care (through Misericordia Place); Health Care for Lungs; occupational therapy; ophthalmology; pediatric dental surgery; Provincial Health Contact Centre; physiotherapy; recreation therapy; rehabilitation services; respiratory therapy; Sleep Disorder Centre; social work; spiritual & religious care; & support services.
Rosie Jacuzzi, President & CEO

WINNIPEG: Mount Carmel Clinic
Affiliated with: Winnipeg Regional Health Authority
886 Main St., Winnipeg, MB R2W 5L4

Tel: 204-582-2311 *Fax:* 204-582-6006
info@mountcarmel.ca
www.mountcarmel.ca

Year Founded: 1926
Note: Health services include: Aboriginal health & wellness; child; dental; general health; Hepatitis C clinic; homeless/harm reduction; immigrant/refugee; LGBT; mental health; pregnancy/parenting; reproductive/sexual health; & youth.
Bobbette Shoffner, Executive Director
204-582-0311, bshoffner@mountcarmel.ca
Al Shpeller, Director, Operations
ashpeller@mountcarmel.ca

WINNIPEG: NorWest Co-op Community Health
Affiliated with: Winnipeg Regional Health Authority
Also Known As: Inkster/Nor'west Co-op Community Health Centre
785 Keewatin St., Winnipeg, MB R2X 3B9

Tel: 204-938-5900 *Fax:* 204-938-5994
www.norwestcoop.ca
Social Media: www.facebook.com/193978229794;
twitter.com/NorWestCoop; www.youtube.com/user/NorwestCoop

Note: Programs & services include: primary health care; community development; counselling & support services; & early learning & childcare. This health centre is in the same location as ACCESS NorWest.
Ivan Sabesky, President & Board Chair

WINNIPEG: Point Douglas Community Health Centre
Affiliated with: Winnipeg Regional Health Authority
601 Aikins St., Winnipeg, MB R2W 4J5

Tel: 204-940-2025
www.wrha.mb.ca

Note: Provides services related to: healthy parenting & early childhood development; healthy children & youth; nutrition promotion; communicable disease prevention & management; immunization; & more.

WINNIPEG: Reh-Fit Centre
Affiliated with: Winnipeg Regional Health Authority
Former Name: Manitoba Cardiac Institute
1390 Taylor Ave., Winnipeg, MB R3M 3V8
Tel: 204-488-8023 *Fax:* 204-488-4819
reh-fit@reh-fit.com
www.reh-fit.com
Social Media: www.facebook.com/RehFit; twitter.com/RehFit
Year Founded: 1979
Note: A certified medical fitness facility specializing in cardiac rehabilitation.
Scott Bailey, Board Chair
Sue Boreskie, Chief Executive Officer
204-488-5850
Patrick Harrington, Director, Finance
204-488-5858, patrick.harrington@reh-fit.com
Janet Cranston, Director, Health & Fitness
204-488-5855, janet.cranston@reh-fit.com
Karyn Sinopoli, Director, Membership & Marketing
204-488-5857

WINNIPEG: River Heights Community Health Service Centre
Affiliated with: Winnipeg Regional Health Authority
1001 Corydon Ave., Winnipeg, MB R3M 0B6
Tel: 204-940-2005
www.wrha.mb.ca

WINNIPEG: River Heights Health & Social Services Centre
Affiliated with: Winnipeg Regional Health Authority
#6, 677 Stafford St., Winnipeg, MB R3M 2X7
Tel: 204-938-5500
www.wrha.mb.ca

Note: Provides services related to: healthy parenting & early childhood development; healthy children & youth; nutrition promotion; communicable disease prevention & management; immunization; & more.

WINNIPEG: St. Boniface Community Office
Affiliated with: Winnipeg Regional Health Authority
170 Goulet St., Winnipeg, MB R2H 0R7
Tel: 204-940-2035
www.wrha.mb.ca

Note: Provides services related to: healthy parenting & early childhood development; healthy children & youth; nutrition promotion; communicable disease prevention & management; immunization; & more.

WINNIPEG: St. Vital Community Office
Affiliated with: Winnipeg Regional Health Authority
St. Vital Square, #6, 845 Dakota St., Winnipeg, MB R2M 5M3
Tel: 204-940-2045
www.wrha.mb.ca

Note: Provides services related to: healthy parenting & early childhood development; healthy children & youth; nutrition promotion; communicable disease prevention & management; immunization; & more. This office is in the same location as the Youville Community Health Centre.

WINNIPEG: Seven Oaks General Hospital
Affiliated with: Winnipeg Regional Health Authority
2300 McPhillips St., Winnipeg, MB R2V 3M3
Tel: 204-632-7133
www.sogh.ca
Social Media: www.facebook.com/SevenOaksGeneralHospital; twitter.com/sevenoakswpg
Year Founded: 1981
Number of Beds: 304 beds
Note: Programs & services include: Aboriginal health; core rehabilitation; day hospital; diagnostic; family medicine; geriatric mental health; geriatric rehabilitation; health library; intensive care; kidney health; Koldonan Medical Centre; laboratory; mental health; oncology clinic; orthopedic clinic; pharmacy; Prairie Trail at the Oaks; respiratory therapy; surgery; Surgery Centre; Urology Centre; urgent care; & Wellness Institute.
Carrie Solmundson, President & COO
Dr. Ricardo Lobato de Faria, Chief Medical Officer

WINNIPEG: Seven Oaks Health & Social Services Centre
Affiliated with: Winnipeg Regional Health Authority
#3, 1050 Leila Ave., Winnipeg, MB R2P 1W6
Tel: 204-938-5600
www.wrha.mb.ca

Note: Provides services related to: healthy parenting & early childhood development; healthy children & youth; nutrition promotion; communicable disease prevention & management; immunization; & more.

WINNIPEG: Street Connections
Affiliated with: Winnipeg Regional Health Authority
496 Hargrave St., Winnipeg, MB R3A 0X7
Tel: 204-981-0742
outreach@wrha.mb.ca
www.streetconnections.ca

Note: Mobile harm reduction program specializing in harm reduction & free services to those in need. Programs & services include: general assistance (housing, addictions, food, legal, & more); counselling; nursing services; prenatal services; clean drug use supplies; needle exchange; & safe sex supplies.

WINNIPEG: Victoria General Hospital (VGH)
Affiliated with: Winnipeg Regional Health Authority
2340 Pembina Hwy., Winnipeg, MB R3T 2E8
Tel: 204-269-3570
info@vgh.mb.ca
www.vgh.mb.ca
Social Media: www.facebook.com/VanIslandHealth; twitter.com/Vanislandhealth
Year Founded: 1971
Number of Beds: 203 beds
Note: Programs & services include: allied health services; audiology; mental health; surgery; Mature Womens Centre; critical care; oncology; medicine/family medicine; & urgent care.

WINNIPEG: Win Gardner Place
Affiliated with: Winnipeg Regional Health Authority
Former Name: North End Wellness Centre
363 McGregor St., Winnipeg, MB R2W 4X4
Tel: 204-925-4486
www.wingardnerplace.ca
Social Media: www.facebook.com/WinGardnerPlace; twitter.com/WinGardnerPlace

Note: A collaborative effort among the following organizations: Ma Mawi Wi Chi Itata Centre, the YMCA-YWCA of Winnipeg, North End Community Renewal Corp., SPLASH Child Enrichment Centre & the Winnipeg Regional Health Authority.

WINNIPEG: Winnipeg Regional Health Authority (WRHA)
650 Main St., 4th Fl., Winnipeg, MB R3B 1E2
Tel: 204-926-7000 *Fax:* 204-926-7007
www.wrha.mb.ca
Social Media: www.youtube.com/user/WinnipegHealthRegion

Population Served: 700000
Number of Employees: 28000
Note: The WRHA provides services to residents of the City of Winnipeg as well as the surrounding Rural Municipalities of East & West St. Paul, & the Town of Churchill in northern Manitoba. The authority also provides support & referral services to Manitobans who live outside its boundaries, as well as to residents of northwestern Ontario & Nunavut.
Karen Dunlop, Board Chair
Milton Sussman, President & CEO
Dr. Brock Wright, Chief Medical Officer & Senior Vice-President, Clinical Services
Réal Cloutier, Chief Operating Officer & Vice-President
Glenn McLennan, Chief Financial Officer & Vice-President
Dave Leschasin, Chief Human Resources Officer & Acting Vice-President
Dr. Catherine Cook, Vice-President, Population & Aboriginal Health

WINNIPEG: Winnipeg West Integrated Health & Social Services
Affiliated with: Winnipeg Regional Health Authority
280 Booth Dr., Winnipeg, MB R3J 3R5
Tel: 204-940-2040
www.wrha.mb.ca

Note: This office is in the same location as ACCESS Winnipeg West.

WINNIPEG: Women's Health Clinic Inc. (WHC)
Affiliated with: Winnipeg Regional Health Authority
419 Graham Ave., #A, Winnipeg, MB R3C 0M3
Tel: 204-947-1517 *Fax:* 204-943-3844
Toll-Free: 866-947-1517
TTY: 204-956-0385
whc@womenshealthclinic.org
www.womenshealthclinic.org
Social Media: www.facebook.com/WHCwpg; twitter.com/whcwpg
Year Founded: 1981
Note: Services include: parenting support; mental health; eating
disorder workshops & support groups; reproductive & sexual health;
nutrition counselling; primary care; & health promotion.
Amy Tuckett, Specialist, Communications
  atuckett@womenshealthclinic.org

WINNIPEG: Youville Centre - Community Health Resource Centre
Affiliated with: Winnipeg Regional Health Authority
Also Known As: Youville Community Health Centre
St. Vital Square, #6, 845 Dakota St., Winnipeg, MB R2M 5M3
Tel: 204-255-4840 *Fax:* 204-255-4903
www.youville.ca

Year Founded: 1984
Note: Programs & services include: health care & wellness education;
counselling; & support. This Centre is in the same location as the
WRHA St. Vital Community Office.
Patrick Griffith, Executive Director

WINNIPEGOSIS: Winnipegosis Community Health
Affiliated with: Prairie Mountain Health
PO Box 280, 230 Bridge St., Winnipegosis, MB R0L 2G0
Tel: 204-656-4881
www.prairiemountainhealth.ca

Note: Services include: transitional care; palliative care; rehabilitation;
diagnostic; laboratory; emergency/ambulance; occupational therapy;
home care; mental health; long-term care; primary health care; public
health; Manitoba Telehealth; & Meals on Wheels

WINNIPEGOSIS: Winnipegosis Health Centre
Affiliated with: Prairie Mountain Health
Former Name: Winnipegosis General Hospital
Also Known As: Winnipegosis & District Health Centre
PO Box 280, 230 Bridge St., Winnipegosis, MB R0L 2G0
Tel: 204-656-4881 *Fax:* 204-629-3489
www.prairiemountainhealth.ca
Number of Beds: 15 acute care beds
Note: Programs & services include: acute medicine; outpatient;
palliative care; & 24-hour emergency services.
Michelle Quennelle, Executive Director

NEW BRUNSWICK

BAIE-SAINTE-ANNE: Baie-Ste-Anne Health Centre
Affiliated with: Horizon Health Network
13, rue de l'Église, Baie-Sainte-Anne, NB E9A 1A9
Tel: 506-228-2004 *Fax:* 506-228-2008
www.horizonnb.ca

Note: Patients may access the services of a physician who works 2
days per week, & a full time nurse on site; monthly public health clinic;
laboratory clinic twice a week.

BATHURST: Hôpital régional Chaleur
Affiliée à: Vitalité Health Network
Ancien nom: Centre hospitalier régional
1750, promenade Sunset, Bathurst, NB E2A 4L7
Tél: 506-544-3000 *Téléc:* 506-544-2533
info@vitalitenb.ca
www.vitalitenb.ca
Nombre de lits: 215 lits
Note: Services: diagnostiques; chirurgie; cliniques de soins

ambulatoires; mère et à l'enfant; specialises; spécialisés de
réadaptation; thérapeutiques; programme de suivi des porteurs
d'implants cochléaires du Nouveau-Brunswick; et Pavillon UCT.

BATHURST: NB Extra Mural Program
Bathurst Unit
Affiliated with: Vitalité Health Network
1745 Vallée-Lourdes Dr., Bathurst, NB E2A 4P8
Tel: 506-544-3030 *Fax:* 506-544-3029

BATHURST: Vitalité Health Network
Former Name: Restigouche Health Authority/Régie de la santé du
Restigouche
#600, 275 Main St., Bathurst, NB E2A 1A9
Tel: 506-544-2133 *Fax:* 506-544-2145
Toll-Free: 888-472-2220
info@vitalitenb.ca
www.vitalitenb.ca
Year Founded: 2008
Number of Beds: 965 beds; 60 veterans' beds; 172 Restigouche
Hospital Centre beds
Population Served: 239600
Number of Employees: 7400
Note: The Vitalité Health Network amalgamates Regional Health
Authority 4, the Restigouche Health Authority, the Acadie-Bathurst
Health Authority, & the Beauséjour Health Authority. The network is
comprised of 11 hospitals, 9 health centres, 5 clinics, 10 community
mental health centres, 4 addiction service centres, 2 veterans' centres,
11 public & sexual health offices & 12 extra-mural program offices.
Michelyne Paulin, Board Chair
Gilles Lanteigne, President & CEO
Dr. France Desrosiers, Vice-President, Medical Services, Training &
  Research
Gisèle Beaulieu, Vice-President, Performance, Quality & Corporate
  Services
Jacques Duclos, Vice-President, Community Services & Mental Health
Stéphane Legacy, Vice-President, Outpatient & Professional Services
Johanne Roy, Vice-President, Clinical Services

BELLEDUNE: Centre de santé de Jacquet River Health Centre
Affiliated with: Vitalité Health Network
41 Mack St., Belledune, NB E8G 2R3
Tel: 506-237-3222 *Fax:* 506-237-3224
www.vitalitenb.ca

BLACKS HARBOUR: Fundy Health Centre
Affiliated with: Horizon Health Network
34 Hospital St., Blacks Harbour, NB E5H 1K2
Tel: 506-456-4200 *Fax:* 506-456-4259
horizon@horizonnb.ca
www.horizonnb.ca

BLACKVILLE: Blackville Health Centre
Affiliated with: Horizon Health Network
2 Schafer Lane, Blackville, NB E9B 1P4
Tel: 506-843-2910 *Fax:* 506-843-2911
www.horizonnb.ca

Note: Services include: addictions & mental health; clinical;
diagnostics; & therapy.

BOIESTOWN: Boiestown Health Centre
Affiliated with: Horizon Health Network
#2, 6154 rte 8, Boiestown, NB E6A 1M4
Tel: 506-369-2700 *Fax:* 506-369-2702
horizonnb.ca

CAMPBELLTON: Campbellton Regional Hospital
Affiliated with: Vitalité Health Network
PO Box 880, 189 Lily Lake Rd., Campbellton, NB E3N 3H3
Tel: 506-789-5000
info@vitalitenb.ca
www.vitalitenb.ca
Year Founded: 1991
Number of Beds: 163 beds/lits
Number of Employees: 900
Note: Programs & services include: acute psychiatry; ambulatory care;
audiology; care for veterans; clinical nutrition; diagnostic imaging &
laboratory; emergency; ENT (ears, nose & throat); geriatrics; general
surgery; intensive care; medical; obstetrics/gynecology; occupational

therapy; orthopedics; palliative care; pediatrics; psychology; recreology; rehabilitation; social work; speech-language pathology; & urology.

CAMPOBELLO: NB Extra Mural Program
St Stephen Unit - Campobello Office
Affiliated with: Horizon Health Network
640, rte 774, Campobello, NB E5E 1A5

Tel: 506-752-4100

CARAQUET: Hôpital de l'Enfant-Jésus (RHSJT)
Affiliated with: Vitalité Health Network
Former Name: Hôpital de l'Enfant-Jésus RHSJ
1, boul St-Pierre ouest, Caraquet, NB E1W 1B6

Tel: 506-726-2100 *Fax:* 506-726-2188
info@vitalitenb.ca
www.vitalitenb.ca

Note: Services: clinique avec un infirmier praticien; clinique de phénylcétonurie (PCU); clinique de tests de Pap; clinique mère-enfant; cliniques et programmes multidisciplinaires; Lifeline; médecine / soins palliatifs; programme de réadaptation cardiaque; services diagnostiques; services thérapeutiques; soins ambulatoires; soins spirituels et religieux; télésanté; unité de formation médicale; et urgence.

CARAQUET: NB Extra Mural Program - Caraquet Unit
Affiliated with: Vitalité Health Network
390 St. Pierre Blvd. West, Caraquet, NB E1W 1B7

Tel: 506-726-2800

CHIPMAN: Chipman Health Centre
Affiliated with: Horizon Health Network
9 Civic Ct., Chipman, NB E4A 2H8

Tel: 506-339-7650 *Fax:* 506-339-7652
www.horizonnb.ca

Note: Offers clinical, diagnostics, mental health, & therapy services.

DALHOUSIE: Centre de santé communautaire St. Joseph
Affiliated with: Vitalité Health Network
#1, 280, rue Victoria, Dalhousie, NB E8C 2R6

Tel: 506-684-7000 *Fax:* 506-684-4751
www.vitalitenb.ca

Note: Le Réseau de santé Vitalité regroupe les huit anciennes régies régionales dans la province. Le Centre a pour mission d'améliorer l'accès aux soins de santé primaires, et l'état de santé des collectivités; promotion de la santé, prévention des maladies et blessures, et traitement des maladies chroniques; services diagnostiques; soins ambulatoires.

DALHOUSIE: NB Extra Mural Program - Restigouche Unit
Affiliated with: Vitalité Health Network
#2, 280 Victoria St., Dalhousie, NB E8C 2R6

Tel: 506-684-7060 *Fax:* 506-684-7334

DIEPPE: NB Extra Mural Program
Blanche-Bourgeois Unit
Affiliated with: Vitalité Health Network
30 Englehart St., #B, Dieppe, NB E1A 8H3

Tel: 506-862-4400

DOAKTOWN: Central Miramichi Community Health Centre (CMCHC)
Affiliated with: Horizon Health Network
Former Name: Upper Miramichi Health Services Centre - Doaktown
11 Prospect St., Doaktown, NB E9C 1C3

Tel: 506-365-6100 *Fax:* 506-365-6104
horizonnb.ca
Lorri Amos, Nurse Manager

EDMUNDSTON: Hôpital régional d'Edmundston
Affiliée à: Vitalité Health Network
275, boul Hébert, Edmundston, NB E3V 4E4

Tél: 506-739-2200 *Téléc:* 506-739-2231
info@vitalitenb.ca
www.vitalitenb.ca

Nombre de lits: 169 lits
Personnel: 1000
Note: Services: audiologie; bénévoles et soins spirituels et religieux; clinique de réadaptation cardiaque; clinique sur les maladies

pulmonaires; dialyse rénale; électrodiagnostic; ergothérapie; imagerie médicale; médecine; nutrition clinique; obstétrique; oncologie; orthophonie; pédiatrie; pharmacie; psychiatrie; psychologie; services diagnostiques; soins ambulatoires; soins intensifs; soins prolongés et soins palliatifs; thérapie respiratoire; travailleurs sociaux en milieu hospitalier; unités de chirurgie; et urgence.

EDMUNDSTON: NB Extra Mural Program
Edmundston Unit
180 Hebert Blvd., Edmundston, NB E3V 4N4

Tel: 506-739-2160 *Fax:* 506-739-2163

FAIRHAVEN: Deer Island Health Centre
Affiliated with: Horizon Health Network
999 Rte. 772, Fairhaven, NB E5V 1P2

Tel: 506-747-4150 *Fax:* 506-747-4151
www.horizonnb.ca

Note: Patients may access the services of a physician who works 1 day per week & a nurse practitioner who works 3 days per week.

FREDERICTON: Dr. Everett Chalmers Regional Hospital
Affiliated with: Horizon Health Network
PO Box 9000, 700 Priestman St., Fredericton, NB E3B 5N5

Tel: 506-452-5400 *Fax:* 506-452-5670
www.horizonnb.ca
Social Media: www.facebook.com/120963024660628;
twitter.com/HorizonHealthNB;
www.linkedin.com/company/horizon-health-network

Year Founded: 1976
Number of Beds: 315 beds
Note: Programs & services include: Addictions & Mental Health (community forensics, children & youth treatment programs); Clinical Services (day surgery, dermatology, dialysis, ear, nose & throat, emergency, family medicine, gastroenterology, general surgery, geriatrics, gynecology surgery, intensive care, internal medicine, minor surgery, neonatal intensive care, opthalmology surgery, orthopedic surgery, pediatrics, palliative care, plastic surgery, physiatry, psychiatry, obstetrics, thoracic surgery, urology surgery, vascular surgery & oncology); Diagnostics & Testing (blood & specimen, bone marrow, breathing function, bronchoscopy, CT scan, cystoscopy, endoscopy, ECG, fluoroscopy, holter monitoring, EEG, pathology, MRI, mammography, nuclear medicine, spirometry, ultrasound & x-ray); Public Health Programs (health emergency, health promotion, healthy learners, children & adolescents, immunization, communicable disease prevention, HIV testing & sexual health program); & Support & Therapy (audiology, clinical nutrition, occupational, physiotherapy, psychology, recreational, respiratory, speech-language pathology, spiritual care, social work & telehealth).
Nicole Tupper, Executive Director

FREDERICTON: NB Extra Mural Program
Fredericton Unit
Affiliated with: Horizon Health Network
PO Box 9000, 700 Priestman St., Fredericton, NB E3B 5N5

Tel: 506-452-5800 *Fax:* 506-452-5858
horizonnb.ca

FREDERICTON: NB Extra Mural Program
Sussex Unit
Affiliated with: Horizon Health Network
Health Services Complex, #4, 20 Kennedy Dr., Fredericton, NB E4E 2P1

Tel: 506-432-3280 *Fax:* 506-432-3250

FREDERICTON: NB Extra Mural Program
Fredericton Unit - Boiestown Office
Affiliated with: Horizon Health Network
PO Box 9000, 700 Priestman St., Fredericton, NB E3B 5N5

Tel: 506-452-5800 *Fax:* 506-452-5858

FREDERICTON: Stan Cassidy Centre for Rehabilitation
Affiliated with: Horizon Health Network
800 Priestman St., Fredericton, NB E3B 0C7

Tel: 506-452-5225 *Fax:* 506-452-5190

Number of Beds: 20 beds
Note: Rehabilitation centre specializing in the treatment of complex neurological conditions, including brain injury, stroke, spinal cord injury, & neuromuscular disorders, as well as complex forms of autism spectrum disorder.

Robert Leckey, Medical Director
Gillian Hoyt-Hallett, Administrative Director

FREDERICTON JUNCTION: Fredericton Junction Health Centre
Affiliated with: Horizon Health Network
233 Sunbury Dr., Fredericton Junction, NB E5L 1S1
Tel: 506-368-6501 *Fax:* 506-368-6502
www.horizonnb.ca

Note: Services include: addictions & mental health; clinical; diagnostics; & therapy.

GRAND MANAN: Grand Manan Hospital
Affiliated with: Horizon Health Network
196 Rte. 776, Grand Manan, NB E5G 1A3
Tel: 506-662-4060
horizon@horizonnb.ca
www.horizonnb.ca
Social Media: www.facebook.com/HorizonNB/
twitter.com/HorizonHealthNB
www.linkedin.com/company/horizon-health-network
Number of Beds: 10 beds
Population Served: 5000
Specialties: Chronic diseases & women's health issues
Note: Programs & services include: clinical services (emergency, family medicine & palliative care); diagnostics & testing (blood & specimen collection, ECG & x-ray); & support & therapy (physiotherapy & Telehealth).

GRAND MANAN: NB Extra Mural Program
Affiliated with: Horizon Health Network
582 rte 776, Grand Manan, NB E5G 2C9

GRAND-SAULT: Hôpital général de Grand-Sault inc.
Affiliée à: Vitalité Health Network
CP 7061, 625, boul Evérard H. Daigle, Grand-Sault, NB E3Z 2R9
Tél: 506-473-7555 *Téléc:* 506-473-7530
info@vitalitenb.ca
www.vitalitenb.ca
Fondée en: 1962
Nombre de lits: 20 lits
Population desservi: 15000
Note: Services: chirurgie mineure; clinique du diabète; clinique sur l'hypertension; dermatologie; électrocardiographie; endocrinologie; gastro-entérologie; gynécologie/obstétrique; imagerie médicale; inhalothérapie; laboratoire; médecine interne; nutrition; oncologie; ophtalmologie; orthopédie; oto-rhino-laryngologie; pédiatrie; physiothérapie; programme mère/enfant; réadaptation cardiaque; rhumatologie; services de traitement des dépendances; soins préanesthésiques; soins médicaux d'un jour; traitement anticoagulant; traitements mineurs; et urologie.
Nicole Labrie, Directrice d'établissement

GRAND-SAULT: Programme extra mural du NB - Unite de Grand-Sault
Affiliée à: Vitalité Health Network
532, ch Madawaska, Grand-Sault, NB E3Y 1A3
Tél: 506-473-7492 *Téléc:* 506-473-7476

HARVEY STATION: Harvey Health Centre
Affiliated with: Horizon Health Network
Former Name: Harvey Community Hospital Ltd.
2019 Rte. 3, Harvey Station, NB E6K 3E9
Tel: 506-366-6400 *Fax:* 506-366-6403
horizon@horizonnb.ca
www.horizonnb.ca

HARVEY STATION: Swanhaven Adult Residential Facility
1915, Rte. 3, Harvey Station, NB E6K 3K1
Tel: 506-366-2950
Number of Beds: 28 beds
Note: Specialty: Long-term care
Malcolm Cairns, Contact

KEDGWICK: NB Extra Mural Program
Kedgwick Unit
Affiliated with: Vitalité Health Network
156 Notre-Dame St., Kedgwick, NB E3Y 2A9
Tel: 506-284-3444

LAMÈQUE: Hôpital de Lamèque/Centre de santé communautaire de Lamèque
Affiliée à: Vitalité Health Network
Également connu sous le nom de: Hôpital et CSC de Lamèque
29, rue de l'Hôpital, Lamèque, NB E8T 1C5
Tél: 506-344-2261 *Téléc:* 506-344-3403
info@vitalitenb.ca
www.vitalitenb.ca
Nombre de lits: 12 lits
Note: Services: clinique de dépistage du cancer du col de l'utérus (test Pap); clinique de gériatrie; clinique de vaccination contre la grippe; clinique pour femmes enceintes; clinique pour les patients sans médecin de famille (suivi par les infirmières praticiennes); développement communautaire; électrodiagnostic cardiaque; ergothérapie; imagerie médicale; laboratoire; médecine; nutrition clinique; pharmacie; physiothérapie; programme d'abandon du tabac; programme Santé active; programme Mes choix, Ma santé; programme pour les endeuillés; soins des problèmes de santé chroniques; soutien à l'allaitement; télésanté; thérapie respiratoire (inhalothérapie); travail social; et unité de médecine familiale.

LAMÈQUE: NB Extra Mural Program - Lamèque Unit
Affiliated with: Vitalité Health Network
13 Principale St., Lamèque, NB E8P 1M9
Tel: 506-344-3000

MCADAM: McAdam Health Centre
Affiliated with: Vitalité Health Network
15 Saunders Rd., McAdam, NB E6J 1K9
Tel: 506-784-6300 *Fax:* 506-784-6306
horizonnb.ca

Note: Provides primary care & outpatient services.

MINTO: Queens North Community Health Centre
Affiliated with: Horizon Health Network
1100 Pleasant Dr., Minto, NB E4B 2V6
Tel: 506-327-7800 *Fax:* 506-327-7850
horizonnb.ca

Note: Services include: primary health care; illness & injury prevention; chronic disease management; & community development.
Isabel Camp, Manager

MIRAMICHI: Horizon Health Network
Former Name: Regional Health Authority B
155 Pleasant St., Miramichi, NB E1V 1Y3
Tel: 506-623-5500 *Fax:* 506-623-5533
horizon@horizonnb.ca
www.horizonnb.ca
Social Media: www.facebook.com/HorizonNB;
twitter.com/HorizonHealthNB;
www.linkedin.com/company/horizon-health-network
Year Founded: 2008
Number of Beds: 1,650 beds
Area Served: Provinces of New Brunswick, PEI, & northern Nova Scotia
Number of Employees: 12400
Note: Along with the Vitalité Health Network, the Horizon Health Network amalgamates the 8 former regional health authorities in New Brunswick. Horizon Health Network serves the Moncton, Saint John, Fredericton & Miramichi areas, as well as communities in Nova Scotia & Prince Edward Island.
Grace Losier, Board Chair
Karen McGrath, President & CEO
Andrea Seymour, Chief Operating Officer & Vice-President, Corporate
Jean Daigle, Vice-President, Community
Gary Foley, Vice-President, Professional Services
Geri Geldart, Vice-President, Clinical
Dr. Édouard Hendriks, Vice-President, Medical, Academic & Research Affairs
Margaret Melanson, Vice-President, Quality & Patient Centred Care

MIRAMICHI: Miramichi Regional Hospital
Affiliated with: Horizon Health Network
500 Water St., Miramichi, NB E1V 3G5
Tel: 506-623-3000 *Fax:* 506-623-3465
horizon@horizonnb.ca
www.horizonnb.ca
Social Media: www.facebook.com/HorizonNB;
twitter.com/HorizonHealthNB;
www.linkedin.com/company/horizon-health-network
Number of Beds: 150 beds
Note: Programs & services include: Addictions & Mental Health
(children & youth, gambling, inpatient acute care psychiatric unit,
inpatient addictions, individual family & group counseling, community
care, methadone treatment, substance abuse, smoking cessation
program & youth outpatient); Clinical Services (day surgery,
dermatology, ear, nose & throat, emergency, family medicine, general
surgery, gynecology surgery, geriatrics, intensive care, internal
medicine, minor surgery, obstetrics, pediatrics, palliative care,
psychiatry, oncology, ophthalmology surgery, orthopedic surgery,
rehabilitation & urology surgery); Diagnostics & Testing (blood &
specimen collection, breathing function lab, CT scan, cystoscopy,
endoscopy, ECG, fluoroscopy, holter monitoring, pathology, MRI,
mammography, ultrasound, x-rays & spirometry); Public Health
Programs (early childhood, health emergency & promotion, healthy
learners, immunization, communicable disease, HIV testing & sexual
health); & Support & Therapy (audiology, clinical nutrition, occupational,
physiotherapy, recreational, respiratory, speech-language pathology,
spiritual care, social work & telehealth).
Marilyn Underhill, Executive Director

MIRAMICHI: NB Extra Mural Program
Miramichi Unit
Affiliated with: Horizon Health Network
500 Water St., Miramichi, NB E1V 3G5
Tel: 506-623-6350 *Fax:* 506-623-6370

MIRAMICHI: NB Extra Mural Program
Miramichi Unit - Blackville Office
Affiliated with: Horizon Health Network
500 Water St., Miramichi, NB E1V 3G5
Tel: 506-623-6312 *Fax:* 506-623-6370

MIRAMICHI: NB Extra Mural Program
Miramichi Unit - Neguac Office
Affiliated with: Horizon Health Network
500 Water St., Miramichi, NB E1V 3G5
Tel: 506-623-6312 *Fax:* 506-623-6370

MONCTON: Le Centre hospitalier universitaire
Dr-Georges-L.-Dumont (CHUDGLD)
Affiliated with: Vitalité Health Network
330, av Université, Moncton, NB E1C 2Z3
Tel: 506-862-4000
info@vitalitenb.ca
www.vitalitenb.ca
Number of Beds: 302 lits
Note: Services: Appel Dumont Response; Auberge Mgr-Henri-Cormier;
audiologie; chirurgie; clinique d'obstétrique; clinique de
gynéco-oncologie; clinique de santé du sein; clinique de traitement;
clinique d'oncologie médicale et clinique de radio-oncologie; clinique
d'oncologie palliative; curiethérapie de la prostate; imagerie médicale;
laboratoire et prises de sang; médecine générale et médecine interne;
néphrologie; nutrition clinique; physiothérapie; physique médicale;
programme provincial de PCU et centre de coordination du dépistage
des troubles métaboliques; psychologie; service de travail social;
service d'ergothérapie; service d'orthophonie; soins ambulatoires;
soins spirituels et religieux; thérapie respiratoire; travail social; urgence;
service de radiothérapie; soins palliatifs; thérapie systémique
communautaire; unité 4D (unité d'oncologie); unité des naissances
(3B); et unité de pédiatrie (3D).
Richard Losier, Chef des opérations de la zone Beauséjour

MONCTON: The Moncton Hospital
Affiliated with: Horizon Health Network
135 MacBeath Ave., Moncton, NB E1C 6Z8
Tel: 506-857-5511 *Fax:* 506-857-5545
horizon@horizonnb.ca
www.horizonnb.ca
Social Media: www.facebook.com/HorizonNB;
twitter.com/HorizonHealthNB;
www.linkedin.com/company/horizon-health-network
Number of Beds: 381 beds
Specialties: Critical care & trauma cases
Note: Programs & services include: Addictions & Mental Health
(inpatient acute care psychiatric unit, inpatient addictions, individual
family & group counseling, community care, methadone treatment &
smoking cessation program); Clinical Services (day surgery,
dermatology, ear, nose & throat, emergency, family medicine, general
surgery, gynecology surgery, gastroenterology, geriatrics, intensive
care, internal medicine, neurology, neurosurgery, neonatal intensive
care, minor surgery, obstetrics, oncology, ophthalmology surgery,
orthopedic surgery, palliative care, plastic surgery, rehabilitation,
rheumatology, thoracic surgery, urology surgery & vascular surgery);
Diagnostics & Testing (blood & specimen, bone marrow, breathing
function, bronchoscopy, CT scan, cystoscopy, endoscopy, ECG,
fluoroscopy, holter monitoring, neuro electrodiagnostics, pathology,
MRI, mammography, nuclear medicine, spirometry, ultrasound & x-ray);
& Support & Therapy (audiology, clinical nutrition, occupational,
physiotherapy, psychology, recreational, respiratory, speech-language
pathology, spiritual care, social work & Telehealth).
Nancy Parker, Executive Director

MONCTON: NB Extra Mural Program
Driscoll Unit
Affiliated with: Horizon Health Network
#107, 1600 Main St., Moncton, NB E1E 1G5
Tel: 506-867-6500 *Fax:* 506-867-6509
horizonnb.ca

Note: Home healthcare program for eligible residents

NACKAWIC: Nackawic Community Health Centre
Affiliated with: Horizon Health Network
Nackawic Shopping Centre, Upper Floor, #201, 135 Otis Dr.,
Nackawic, NB E6G 1H1
Tel: 506-575-6600 *Fax:* 506-575-6603

NÉGUAC: Neguac Health Centre
Affiliated with: Horizon Health Network
38 Otho St., Néguac, NB E9G 4H3
Tel: 506-776-3876 *Fax:* 506-776-3877
www.horizonnb.ca

Note: Provides clinical, diagnostics, & support & therapy services.

OROMOCTO: NB Extra Mural Program
Oromocto Unit
Affiliated with: Horizon Health Network
275A Restigouche Rd., Oromocto, NB E2V 2H1
Tel: 506-357-4900 *Fax:* 506-357-4904

OROMOCTO: NB Extra Mural Program
Oromocto Unit - Minto Office
Affiliated with: Horizon Health Network
275A Restigouche Rd., Oromocto, NB E2V 2H1
Tel: 506-357-4900 *Fax:* 506-357-2675

OROMOCTO: Oromocto Public Hospital
Affiliated with: Horizon Health Network
103 Winnebago St., Oromocto, NB E2V 1C6
Tel: 506-357-4700
horizon@horizonnb.ca
www.horizonnb.ca
Social Media: www.facebook.com/HorizonNB;
twitter.com/HorizonHealthNB;
www.linkedin.com/company/horizon-health-network
Number of Beds: 45 beds
Note: Programs & services include: Clinical Services (day surgery, ear,
nose & throat, emergency, family medicine, general surgery,
gynecology surgery, gastroenterology, geriatrics, minor surgery,
opthalmology surgery, plastic surgery, palliative care, rehabilitation &
urology surgery); Diagnostics & Testing (blood & specimen collection,

bronchoscopy, cystoscopy, endoscopy, ECG, fluoroscopy, holter monitoring, mammography, spirometry, ultrasound & x-ray); & Support & Therapy (clinical nutrition, occupational therapy, physiotherapy, recreational therapy, respiratory therapy, speech-language pathology, spiritual care & social work).
Robyn Dean, Assistant to Facility Manager

PAQUETVILLE: Centre de santé de Paquetville
Affiliée à: Vitalité Health Network
1096, rue du Parc, Paquetville, NB E8R 1J4
Tél: 506-764-2424 *Téléc:* 506-764-2425

PERTH-ANDOVER: Hotel-Dieu of St. Joseph
Affiliated with: Horizon Health Network
10 Woodland Hill, Perth-Andover, NB E7H 5H5
Tel: 506-273-7100 *Fax:* 506-273-7200
horizon@horizonnb.ca
www.horizonnb.ca
Social Media: www.facebook.com/HorizonNB;
twitter.com/HorizonHealthNB;
www.linkedin.com/company/horizon-health-network
Number of Beds: 27 beds
Population Served: 6000
Note: Programs & services include: Addictions & Mental Health (smoking cessation program); Clinical Services (day surgery, emergency, general surgery, family medicine, minor surgery, pediatrics, palliative care, oncology, rehabilitation); Diagnostics & Testing (blood & specimen collection, endoscopy, ECG, fluoroscopy, Holter monitoring, mammography, spirometry, x-rays & ultrasound); & Support & Therapy (clinical nutrition, occupational therapy, physiotherapy, respiratory therapy, speech-language pathology, spiritual care, social work & Telehealth).
Karen O'Regan, Facility Manager

PERTH-ANDOVER: NB Extra Mural Program
Perth Unit
Affiliated with: Horizon Health Network
35F Tribe Rd., Perth-Andover, NB E7H 0A8
Tel: 506-273-7222 *Fax:* 506-273-7220
horizonnb.ca

PETIT-ROCHER: Services Résidentiels Nepisiguit Inc.
#312, 702, rue Principale, Petit-Rocher, NB E8J 1V1
Tél: 506-542-2404 *Téléc:* 506-542-2406
www.gnb.ca
Nombre de lits: 22 lits
Note: Service résidentiel à toutes les personnes ayant des handicaps de la région Nepisiguit
Luc DeRoche, Directeur général

PETITCODIAC: Petitcodiac Health Centre
Affiliated with: Horizon Health Network
2501, 32 Railway Ave., Petitcodiac, NB E4Z 6H4
Tel: 506-756-3400 *Fax:* 506-756-3406
www.horizonnb.ca

Note: Number of staff: 2 physicians. Offers clinical, mental health, diagnostics, & drop-in nursing services.

PLASTER ROCK: Tobique Valley Community Health Centre (TVCHC)
Affiliated with: Horizon Health Network
Former Name: Tobique Valley Hospital Inc.
120 Main St., Plaster Rock, NB E7G 2E5
Tel: 506-356-6600 *Fax:* 506-356-6618
horizon@horizonnb.ca
www.horizonnb.ca
Year Founded: 1957
Note: Services include: addictions & mental health (smoking cessation program); clinical services (family medicine); diagnostics & testing (blood & specimen collection, ECG, Holter monitoring, x-ray, & spirometry); & support & therapy (clinical nutrition, occupational therapy, physiotherapy, respiratory therapy, speech language pathology, social work, & Telehealth).

POINTE-VERTE: Centre de santé de Chaleur Health Centre
Affiliée à: Vitalité Health Network
Ancien nom: Centre de santé Pointe Verte
382, rue Principale, Pointe-Verte, NB E8J 2X6
Tél: 506-542-2434

QUISPAMSIS: NB Extra Mural Program
Kennebecasis Valley Unit
Affiliated with: Horizon Health Network
Quispamsis Village Centre, PO Box 21025, 175 Hampton Rd., Quispamsis, NB E2E 4Z4
Tel: 506-848-4600 *Fax:* 506-848-4620
horizonnb.ca

REXTON: Health Services Centre Rexton
Affiliated with: Horizon Health Network
33 Main St., Rexton, NB E4W 0E5
Tel: 506-523-7940 *Fax:* 506-523-7949
www.horizonnb.ca
Year Founded: 1974
Note: Drop-in services, clinics, immunization, nutrition & diabetes education

RIVERSIDE-ALBERT: Albert County Health & Wellness Centre
Affiliated with: Horizon Health Network
8 Forestdale Rd., Riverside-Albert, NB E4H 3Y7
Tel: 506-882-3100 *Fax:* 506-882-3101
horizonnb.ca
Year Founded: 1961
Note: Multidisciplinary, primary health care services, including clinical services, support, therapy, diagnostics & testing, & addictions & mental health programs.

ROGERSVILLE: Rogersville Health Centre
Affiliated with: Horizon Health Network
9, rue des Ormes, Rogersville, NB E4Y 1S6
Tel: 506-775-2030 *Fax:* 506-775-2025
www.horizonnb.ca
Note: Provides daily nursing services, physician services by appointment four days per week, & laboratory services one day per week.

SACKVILLE: NB Extra Mural Program
Tantramar Unit
Affiliated with: Horizon Health Network
8 Main St., Sackville, NB E4L 4A3
Tel: 506-364-4400 *Fax:* 506-364-4405
horizonnb.ca
Year Founded: 1979
Note: Home healthcare program for eligible residents

SACKVILLE: Sackville Memorial Hospital
Affiliated with: Horizon Health Network
8 Main St., Sackville, NB E4L 4A3
Tel: 506-364-4100 *Fax:* 506-536-1983
www.horizonnb.ca
Social Media: www.facebook.com/HorizonNB;
twitter.com/HorizonHealthNB;
www.linkedin.com/company/horizon-health-network
Number of Beds: 21 beds
Number of Employees: 105
Note: Programs & services include: Addictions & Mental Health (geriatrics, smoking cessation program); Clinical Services (day surgery, emergency, family medicine & geriatrics); Diagnostics & Testing (ECG, Holter monitoring & x-ray); & Support & Therapy (clinical nutrition, occupational therapy, physiotherapy, respiratory, speech-language pathology, spiritual care, social work & Telehealth).

SAINT JOHN: Hospice Greater Saint John
Affiliated with: Horizon Health Network
Former Name: Hospice Saint John & Sussex
385 Dufferin Row, Saint John, NB E2M 2J9
Tel: 506-632-5593 *Fax:* 506-632-5592
info@hospicesj.ca
www.hospicesj.ca
Year Founded: 1983
Number of Beds: 10 beds
Number of Employees: 7
Sandy Johnson, CEO
506-632-5723, sjohnson@hospicesj.ca

SAINT JOHN: NB Extra Mural Program
Saint John Unit
Affiliated with: Horizon Health Network
Meditrust Pharmacy Building, 1490 Manawagonish Rd., Saint John, NB E2M 3Y4
Tel: 506-649-2626 *Fax:* 506-649-2540
horizonnb.ca

Note: In-home support
Dawn Marie Buck, Director

SAINT JOHN: Saint John Regional Hospital
Affiliated with: Horizon Health Network
PO Box 2100, 400 University Ave., Saint John, NB E2L 4L4
Tel: 506-648-6000
horizon@horizonnb.ca
www.horizonnb.ca
Social Media: www.facebook.com/HorizonNB;
twitter.com/HorizonHealthNB;
www.linkedin.com/company/horizon-health-network
Number of Beds: 445 beds
Note: Teaching hospital affiliated with Dalhousie University, New Brunswick Community College, University of New Brunswick & Memorial University in St. John's Newfoundland.
Programs & services include: Addictions & Mental Health (emergency & inpatient acute care psychiatry); Clinical Services (cardiac surgery, day surgery, dermatology, dialysis, ear, nose & throat, emergency, family medicine, general surgery, gynecology surgery, gastroenterology, geriatrics, intensive care, internal medicine, neonatal intensive care, minor surgery, pediatrics, palliative care, physiatry, plastic & burns, psychiatry, neurology, neurosurgery, obstetrics, oncology, ophthalmology surgery, orthopedic surgery, plastic surgery, rehabilitation, rheumatology, sleep centre, thoracic surgery, urology surgery, & vascular surgery); Diagnostics & Testing (blood & specimen collection, bone marrow, breathing function, bronchoscopy, CT scan, cystoscopy, endoscopy, ECG, fluoroscopy, holter monitoring, neuro electrodiagnostics, pathology, MRI, mammography, positron emissions tomography, nuclear medicine, spirometry, ultrasound & x-ray); & Support & Therapy (audiology, clinical nutrition, occupational therapy, physiotherapy, psychology, recreational therapy, respiratory therapy, speech-language pathology, spiritual care, social work & Telehealth).

SAINT JOHN: St. Joseph's Community Health Centre
Affiliated with: Horizon Health Network
116 Coburg St., Saint John, NB E2L 3K1
Tel: 506-632-5537 *Fax:* 506-632-5539
en.horizonnb.ca

SAINT JOHN: St. Joseph's Hospital
Affiliated with: Horizon Health Network
130 Bayard Dr., Saint John, NB E2L 3L6
Tel: 506-632-5555 *Fax:* 506-632-5551
horizon@horizonnb.ca
www.horizonnb.ca
Social Media: www.facebook.com/HorizonNB;
twitter.com/HorizonHealthNB;
www.linkedin.com/company/horizon-health-network
Number of Beds: 103 beds
Note: Programs & services include: Addictions & Mental Health (methadone treatment program); Clinical Services (day surgery, ear, nose & throat, emergency, general surgery, gynecology surgery, gastroenterology, geriatrics, minor surgery, oncology, ophthalmology surgery, orthopedic surgery, palliative care, plastic surgery & urology surgery); Diagnostics & Testing (blood & specimen collection, CT scan, cystoscopy, endoscopy, ECG, fluoroscopy, holter monitoring, neuro electrodiagnostics, mammography, spirometry, ultrasound & x-ray); & Support & Therapy (clinical nutrition, occupational therapy, physiotherapy, recreational therapy, respiratory therapy, speech-language pathology, spiritual care, social work & Telehealth).
Heather Oakley, Facility Administrator

SAINT JOHN: WorkSafeNB Rehabilitation Centre
Affiliated with: Horizon Health Network
PO Box 160, 1 Portland St., Saint John, NB E2L 3X9
Tel: 506-738-8411 *Fax:* 888-629-4722
Toll-Free: 800-222-9775
worksafenb.ca

Year Founded: 1965
Note: Occupational rehabilitation

Gerard M. Adams, President & CEO
Shelly Dauphinee, Vice-President, WorkSafe Services

SAINT-QUENTIN: Hôtel-Dieu St-Joseph de Saint-Quentin
Affiliée à: Vitalité Health Network
21, rue Canada, Saint-Quentin, NB E8A 2P6
Tél: 506-235-2300 *Téléc:* 506-235-7201
info@vitalitenb.ca
www.vitalitenb.ca
Nombre de lits: 6 lits
Population desservi: 6000
Personnel: 80
Note: Services: anticoagulant; clinique du prédiabète; clinique pulmonaire; diabète; gastroentérologie; hypertension artérielle; imagerie médicale; laboratoire; médecine interne; mère-enfant; nutrition; obstétrique; oncologie; ophtalmologie; pédiatrie; physiothérapie; préanesthésie; santé mentale; soins médicaux d'un jour; traitement des dépendances; traitements mineurs; urologie; et urgence.

SAINTE-ANNE-DE-MADAWASKA: Centre de santé Ste-Anne
Affiliated with: Vitalité Health Network
1, rue de la Clinique, Sainte-Anne-de-Madawaska, NB E7E 1B9
Tel: 506-445-6200 *Fax:* 506-445-6201

SHEDIAC: Centre médical régional de Shédiac
Affiliated with: Vitalité Health Network
PO Box 1477, 419, rue Main, Shediac, NB E4P 2B8
Tel: 506-533-2700
www.vitalitenb.ca

SHEDIAC: NB Extra Mural Program
Shediac Unit
Affiliated with: Vitalité Health Network
423 Main St., Shediac, NB E4P 2B6
Tel: 506-533-2800

ST STEPHEN: Charlotte County Hospital
Affiliated with: Horizon Health Network
4 Garden St., St Stephen, NB E3L 2L9
Tel: 506-465-4444 *Fax:* 506-465-4418
horizon@horizonnb.ca
www.horizonnb.ca
Social Media: www.facebook.com/HorizonNB;
twitter.com/HorizonHealthNB;
www.linkedin.com/company/horizon-health-network
Number of Beds: 44 beds
Note: Programs & services include: Addictions & Mental Health (methadone treatment program); Clinical Services (dialysis, emergency, family medicine, geriatrics, intensive care, minor surgery & palliative care); Diagnostics & Testing (blood & specimen collection, endoscopy, ECG, holter monitoring, mammography, ultrasound, spirometry & x-ray); & Support & Therapy (clinical nutrition, occupational therapy, physiotherapy, respiratory therapy & speech-language pathology).

ST STEPHEN: NB Extra Mural Program
St Stephen Unit
Affiliated with: Horizon Health Network
#100, 73 Milltown Blvd., St Stephen, NB E3L 1G5
Tel: 506-465-4520 *Fax:* 506-465-4523
horizonnb.ca

ST. GEORGE: NB Extra Mural Program
Eastern Charlotte Unit
Affiliated with: Horizon Health Network
122 Main St., St. George, NB E5C 3J9
Tel: 506-755-4660 *Fax:* 506-755-4665
horizonnb.ca

STANLEY: Stanley Health Services Centre
Affiliated with: Horizon Health Network
PO Box 340, Stanley, NB E6B 2K5
Tel: 506-367-7730 *Fax:* 506-367-7738
www.horizonnb.ca

Note: Offers physician services by appointment.

STE-ANNE DE KENT: Programme extra mural du NB - Kent Unit
Affiliée à: Vitalité Health Network
Stella-Maris-de-Kent Hospital, 7717 route 134, Ste-Anne de Kent, NB E4S 1H5

Tél: 506-743-7800

STE-ANNE-DE-KENT: Hôpital Stella-Maris-de-Kent
Affiliée à: Vitalité Health Network
7714, rte 134, Ste-Anne-de-Kent, NB E4S 1H5

Tél: 506-743-7800
info@vitalitenb.ca
www.vitalitenb.ca

Nombre de lits: 20 lits
Note: Services: alimentation et nutrition / clinique de nutrition; clinique de santé; clinique de soins de la femme; clinique du diabète; cliniques externes avec spécialistes; électrocardiogramme; ergothérapie; imagerie diagnostique; laboratoire; liaison autochtone; orthophonie; pharmacie; physiothérapie; service de l'environnement; services spirituels et religieux; thérapie respiratoire; unité de médecine; et urgence.

SUSSEX: Sussex Health Centre
Affiliated with: Horizon Health Network
75 Leonard Dr., Sussex, NB E4E 2P7

Tel: 506-432-3100 *Fax:* 506-432-3106
horizon@horizonnb.ca
www.horizonnb.ca
Social Media: www.facebook.com/HorizonNB;
twitter.com/HorizonHealthNB;
www.linkedin.com/company/horizon-health-network

Number of Beds: 25 beds
Population Served: 30000
Note: Programs & services include: Clinical Services (day surgery, emergency, family medicine, general surgery, palliative care & rehabilitation); Diagnostics & Testing (blood & specimen collection, ECG, holter monitoring, mammography, spirometry, ultrasound & x-ray); & Support & Therapy (audiology, clinical nutrition, occupational therapy, physiotherapy, respiratory therapy, speech-language pathology & spiritual care).

TRACADIE: NB Extra Mural Program - Tracadie Unit
Affiliated with: Vitalité Health Network
3512-2 Principale St., Tracadie, NB E1X 1C9

Tel: 506-394-4100

TRACADIE-SHEILA: Hôpital de Tracadie-Sheila
Affiliée à: Vitalité Health Network
CP 3180 Stn. Main, 400, rue des Hospitalières, Tracadie-Sheila, NB E1X 1G5

Tél: 506-394-3000 *Téléc:* 506-394-3034
info@vitalitenb.ca
www.vitalitenb.ca

Fondée en: 1991
Note: Services: 2e nord et soins concentres; diététique; électrodiagnostic; ergothérapie; imagerie médicale; laboratoire; médecine et pédiatrie; orthophonie; physiothérapie; service alimentaire; service de psychologie; soins ambulatoires; travail social; services spirituels et religieux; thérapie respiratoire; traitement des dépendances; unité satellite de dialyse; et urgence.

WATERVILLE: NB Extra Mural Program - Woodstock Unit
Affiliated with: Horizon Health Network
11300 rte 130, Waterville, NB E7P 0A4

Tel: 506-375-2539 *Fax:* 506-375-2675

WATERVILLE: Upper River Valley Hospital
Affiliated with: Horizon Health Network
11300 Rte 130, Waterville, NB E7P 0A4

Tel: 506-375-5900
horizon@horizonnb.ca
www.horizonnb.ca
Social Media: www.facebook.com/HorizonNB;
twitter.com/HorizonHealthNB;
www.linkedin.com/company/horizon-health-network

Number of Beds: 52 beds
Population Served: 45000
Number of Employees: 800
Note: Programs & services include: Addictions & Mental Health (smoking cessation program); Clinical Services (day surgery, dialysis, emergency, family medicine, general surgery, gastroenterology, geriatrics, intensive care, internal medicine, minor surgery, pediatrics, palliative care, obstetrics, oncology, ophthalmology surgery, rehabilitation & urology surgery); Diagnostics & Testing (blood & specimen collection, bone marrow biopsies, breathing function lab, CT scan, endoscopy, ECG, fluoroscopy, Holter monitoring, MRI, mammography, spirometry, ultrasound & x-ray); Public Health Programs (health emergency & promotion, healthy learners program, children & adolescents, immunization, communicable disease prevention, HIV testing & sexual health); & Support & Therapy (audiology, clinical nutrition, occupational, physiotherapy, psychology, respiratory therapy, speech-language pathology, spiritual care, social work & Telehealth).

NEWFOUNDLAND & LABRADOR

BADGER'S QUAY: Brookfield/Bonnews Health Care Centre
Affiliated with: Central Regional Health Authority
PO Box 209, Badger's Quay, NL A0G 1B0

Tel: 709-536-2405 *Fax:* 709-536-2433
www.centralhealth.nl.ca

Year Founded: 1944
Number of Beds: 12 beds
Population Served: 3000

BAIE VERTE: Baie Verte Peninsula Health Centre
Affiliated with: Central Regional Health Authority
1 Columbus Dr., Baie Verte, NL A0K 1B0

Tel: 709-532-4281 *Fax:* 709-532-4939
Number of Beds: 18 long-term care beds; 1 respite bed; 6 acute care beds; 1 palliative care bed
Note: Acute & long term care; dental clinic; addiction treatment; rehabilitation services.
Craig Davis, Director, Health Services
craig.davis@centralhealth.nl.ca

BELL ISLAND: Dr. Walter Templeman Health Care Centre
Affiliated with: Eastern Regional Health Authority
PO Box 580, Wabana, Bell Island, NL A0A 4H0

Tel: 709-488-2821 *Fax:* 709-488-2600
Number of Beds: 20 beds
Note: Services include: addictions; blood collection; community health; diagnostic imaging; emergency; inpatient; long-term care; minor procedures; outpatient clinics; palliative care; public health; & social work.
Katherine Walters, Site Manager

BLACK TICKLE: Black Tickle Community Clinic
Affiliated with: Labrador-Grenfell Regional Health Authority
General Delivery, Black Tickle, NL A0K 1N0

Tel: 709-471-8872 *Fax:* 709-471-8893
www.lghealth.ca

Number of Beds: 1 holding bed
Note: Primary health care services

BONAVISTA: Bonavista Peninsula Health Centre
Affiliated with: Eastern Regional Health Authority
Former Name: Bonavista Community Health Centre
20-24 Hospital Rd., Bonavista, NL A0C 1B0

Tel: 709-468-7881
Number of Beds: 10 beds
Note: Services include: blood collection; diagnostic imaging; emergency; inpatient; laboratory; radiography; & outpatient clinics.

BOTWOOD: Dr. Hugh Twomey Health Care Centre
Affiliated with: Central Regional Health Authority
PO Box 250, Botwood, NL A0H 1E0

Tel: 709-257-5250
www.centralhealth.nl.ca/dr-hugh-twomey-health-centre
Number of Beds: 77 long-term care beds; 2 respite beds; 1 palliative care bed
Note: Services include: diagnostic imaging; dietitian; emergency; laboratory; long-term care; outpatient; palliative care; rehabilitation; & respite care.
Allison Champion, Manager, Client Care Services
allison.champion@centralhealth.nl.ca

BUCHANS: A.M. Guy Memorial Health Centre
Affiliated with: Central Regional Health Authority
PO Box 39, Buchans, NL A0H 1G0

Tel: 709-672-3304

Number of Beds: 18 long-term beds; 2 acute care beds; 1 holding bed; 1 palliative bed
Note: Services include: chemotherapy; diagnostic imaging; laboratory; outpatient & 24 hour emergency; physician & nurse practitioner clinics; public health; recreation; & rehabilitation.
Pamela Brace, Director, Health Services
  pamela.brace@centralhealth.nl.ca

BURGEO: Calder Health Care Centre
Affiliated with: Western Regional Health Authority
PO Box 190, Burgeo, NL A0N 2H0
  Tel: 709-886-2898
  westernhealth.nl.ca

Number of Beds: 3 acute care beds; 18 continuing care beds
Population Served: 1900
Note: Services include: diagnostic & laboratory services; recreational therapy; occupational & physiotherapy; Telehealth; & chemotherapy.
Laurie Porter, Director, Health Services
  laurieporter@westernhealth.nl.ca

BURIN: Burin Peninsula Health Care Centre
Affiliated with: Eastern Regional Health Authority
PO Box 340, #51, 85 Main St., Burin, NL A0E 1E0
  Tel: 709-891-1040
  www.easternhealth.ca

Note: Features an interim clinic staffed with three hospital physicians

CARBONEAR: Carbonear General Hospital
Affiliated with: Eastern Regional Health Authority
86 Highroad South, Carbonear, NL A1Y 1A4
  Tel: 709-945-5111 *Fax:* 709-945-5511
  client.relations@easternhealth.ca
  www.easternhealth.ca
  Social Media: www.facebook.com/EasternHealthNL;
  twitter.com/EasternHealthNL

Number of Beds: 80 beds
Note: Programs & services include: blood collection; diagnostic imaging; dialysis; emergency; inpatient services; laboratory; outpatient services; & surgery.
Tonya Somerton, Acute Care Manager, Surgical Services & Children's & Women's Health

CARTWRIGHT: Cartwright Community Clinic
Affiliated with: Labrador-Grenfell Regional Health Authority
General Delivery, Cartwright, NL A0K 1V0
  Tel: 709-938-7285

Number of Beds: 1 bed
Number of Employees: 9

CHARLOTTETOWN: Charlottetown Community Clinic
Affiliated with: Labrador-Grenfell Regional Health Authority
Former Name: Charlottetown Nursing Station
General Delivery, Charlottetown, NL A0K 5Y0
  Tel: 709-949-0259

Number of Beds: 3 beds
Number of Employees: 4

CHURCHILL FALLS: Churchill Falls Community Health Centre
Affiliated with: Labrador-Grenfell Regional Health Authority
General Delivery, Churchill Falls, NL A0R 1A0
  Tel: 709-925-3381
  www.lghealth.ca

Number of Beds: 2 holding beds
Note: Offers primary health care.
Tony Wakeham, Chief Executive Officer

CLARENVILLE: Dr. G.B. Cross Memorial Hospital
Affiliated with: Eastern Regional Health Authority
67 Manitoba Dr., Clarenville, NL A5A 1K3
  Tel: 709-466-3411
  client.relations@easternhealth.ca
  www.easternhealth.ca
  Social Media: www.facebook.com/EasternHealthNL;
  twitter.com/EasternHealthNL

Number of Beds: 56 beds (including basinets)
Note: Programs & services include: blood collection; diagnostic imaging; emergency; inpatient services; outpatient services; surgery; & x-ray.

CORNER BROOK: Western Memorial Regional Hospital
Affiliated with: Western Regional Health Authority
PO Box 2005, 1 Brookfield Ave., Corner Brook, NL A2H 6J7
  Tel: 709-637-5000
  www.westernhealth.nl.ca
  Social Media: twitter.com/WesternHealthNL;
  www.youtube.com/WesternHealthNL

Number of Beds: 217 beds
Population Served: 78000
Note: Programs & services include: cardiology; emergency; geriatrics; internal medicine & surgery; intensive care; laboratory; medical imaging; medical; nephrology; neurology; nursing; obstetrics/gynecology; ophthalmology; orthopedics; pediatrics; pharmacy; psychiatry; renal care; surgical services; & urology.
Cynthia Davis, Vice-President, Patient Services

CORNER BROOK: Western Regional Health Authority
Former Name: Western Regional Integrated Health Authority
Also Known As: Western Health
Western Memorial Hospital, PO Box 2005, 1 Brookfield Ave.,
Corner Brook, NL A2H 6J7
  Tel: 709-637-5245 *Fax:* 709-637-5159
  www.westernhealth.nl.ca
  Social Media: twitter.com/WesternHealthNL;
  www.youtube.com/WesternHealthNL

Number of Beds: 293 acute care beds; 464 long-term care beds; 40 enhanced assisted living beds
Population Served: 78000
Number of Employees: 3100
Note: Health facilities include two hospitals: Sir Thomas Roddick Hospital (Stephenville) & Western Memorial Regional Hospital (Corner Brook); four health centres: Dr. Charles L. LeGrow Health Centre (Port aux Basques), Bonne Bay Health Centre (Norris Point), Calder Health Centre (Burgeo) & Rufus Guinchard Health Centre (Port Saunders); & four long-term care centres: Corner Brook Long Term Care Centre (Corner Brook), Bay St. George Long Term Care Centre (Stephenville Crossing), Protective Community Residences (Corner Brook), & Emile Benoit House (Stephenville Crossing).
Tom O'Brien, Acting Board Chair
Dr. Susan Gillam, President & CEO
Catherine McDonald, Chief Nursing Officer & Vice-President, Professional Practice & Health Protection
Cynthia Davis, Vice-President, Patient Services
Devon Goulding, CFO & Vice-President, Finance & Support Services
Donna Hicks, Acting Vice-President, Information & Quality
Michelle House, Vice-President, Population Health & Human Resources
Kelli O'Brien, Vice-President, Long Term Care & Rural Health
Dr. Dennis Rashleigh, Vice-President, Medical Services
Tara Pye, Acting Regional Director, Communications

FLOWERS COVE: Strait of Belle Isle Health Centre
Affiliated with: Labrador-Grenfell Regional Health Authority
PO Box 59, Flowers Cove, NL A0K 2N0
  Tel: 709-456-2401

Number of Beds: 3 beds
Note: Specialties: Ambulatory care; Family medicine; Public health services; Pre-natal classes; Post-natal visiting; Preschool & baby assessments; Dental services; Rehabilitation services; Home care

FOGO: Fogo Island Health Centre
Affiliated with: Central Regional Health Authority
PO Box 9, Fogo, NL A0G 2B0
  Tel: 709-266-2221
  www.centralhealth.nl.ca

Year Founded: 2004
Note: Programs & services include: acute care; long-term care; emergency; laboratory; community health services; & x-ray.
Natasha Decker, Manager, Client Care Services
  natasha.decker@centralhealth.nl.ca

FORTEAU: Labrador South Health Centre
Affiliated with: Labrador-Grenfell Regional Health Authority
Forteau, NL A0K 2P0
  Tel: 709-931-2450 *Fax:* 709-931-2000

Number of Beds: 5 in-patient beds

GANDER: James Paton Memorial Regional Health Centre
Affiliated with: Central Regional Health Authority
125 TransCanada Hwy., Gander, NL A1V 1P7
Tel: 709-256-2500 *Fax:* 709-256-7800
www.centralhealth.nl.ca
Number of Beds: 106 beds
Note: Programs & services include: acute care; emergency; & specialized medical services.
Lori Hillyard, Chief Operating Officer
lori.hillyard@centralhealth.nl.ca

GRAND BANK: Grand Bank Community Health Centre
Affiliated with: Eastern Regional Health Authority
PO Box 310, 3 Grandview Blvd., Grand Bank, NL A0E 1W0
Tel: 709-832-2500 *Fax:* 709-832-1164

Note: Services include: 24-hour ambulance; dental clinic; home care; optometrist; & public health.

GRAND FALLS-WINDSOR: Central Newfoundland Regional Health Centre (CNRHC)
Affiliated with: Central Regional Health Authority
50 Union St., Grand Falls-Windsor, NL A2A 2E1
Tel: 709-292-2500
www.centralhealth.nl.ca
Number of Beds: 130 acute care beds
Note: Programs & services include: emergency; acute care; & specialized medical services.
Kelly Adams, Chief Operating Officer
kelly.adams@centralhealth.nl.ca

GRAND FALLS-WINDSOR: Central Regional Health Authority
Also Known As: Central Health
Regional Office, 21 Carmelite Rd., Grand Falls-Windsor, NL A2A 1Y4
Tel: 709-292-2138
www.centralhealth.nl.ca
Number of Beds: 510 long-term care; 247 acute care; 13 palliative care; 9 respite; 5 restorative; 3 residential; & 24 bassinets
Area Served: 177 communities; half the landmass of the island
Population Served: 94000
Number of Employees: 3184
John George, Board Chair
Rosemarie Goodyear, Chief Executive Officer
rosemarie.goodyear@centralhealth.nl.
Sherry Freake, Chief Operating Officer & Vice-President, Acute Care (Gander)
sherry.freake@centralhealth.nl.ca
Sean Tulk, Chief Operating Officer & Vice-President, Diagnostics & IM (Grand Falls-Windsor)
sean.tulk@centralhealth.nl.ca
Joanne Pelley, Chief Nursing Officer & Vice-President, Population Health
joanne.pelley@centralhealth.nl.ca
Heather Brown, Vice-President, Long Term Care, Community Supports & Rural Health
heather.brown@centralhealth.nl.ca
Dr. Jeff Cole, Vice-President, Medical Services
jeff.cole@centralhealth.nl.ca
Terry Ings, Vice-President, Human Resources & Support Services
terry.ings@centralhealth.nl.ca
John Kattenbusch, Vice-President, Finance & Infrastructure
john.kattenbusch@centralhealth.nl.ca

HAPPY VALLEY-GOOSE BAY: Labrador Health Centre
Affiliated with: Labrador-Grenfell Regional Health Authority
Former Name: Melville Hospital
PO Box 7000 Stn. C, Happy Valley-Goose Bay, NL A0P 1C0
Tel: 709-897-2000
www.lghealth.ca
Number of Beds: 25 beds
Note: Programs & services include: emergency; satellite dialysis; laboratory & diagnostic imaging; physiotherapy; occupational therapy; speech-language pathology; oncology/chemotherapy; respiratory therapy; dietitian; community health & home care nursing; mental health & addictions; & obstetrics/gynecology.
Roland Hewitt, Nursing Site Manager
roland.hewitt@lghealth.ca

HAPPY VALLEY-GOOSE BAY: Labrador-Grenfell Regional Health Authority
Former Name: Grenfell Regional Health Services; Health Labrador Corporation
Also Known As: Labrador-Grenfell Health
Administration Bldg., Labrador-Grenfell Health, PO Box 7000 Stn. C, Happy Valley-Goose Bay, NL A0P 1C0
Fax: 709-896-4032
Toll-Free: 855-897-2267
www.lghealth.ca
Year Founded: 2005
Area Served: North of Bartlett's Harbour on the Northern Peninsula, Labrador
Population Served: 37000
Number of Employees: 1505
Note: Labrador-Grenfell Health partners with the following to deliver services to Aboriginal communities: Nunatsiavut Department of Health & Social Development; 2 Innu Band Councils; NunatuKavut (formerly the Labrador Métis Nation); Health Canada; & private practitioners.
Tony Wakeham, Chief Executive Officer
Roger Snow, Chief Financial Officer
Barbara Blake, COO (South) & Vice-President, People & Information
Delia Connell, COO (Labrador East) & Vice-President, Community & Aboriginal Affairs
Ozette Simpson, COO, Labrador West & Quality Management
Donnie Sampson, Chief Nurse & Vice-President, Nursing
Dr. Gabe Woollam, Vice-President, Medical Services

HARBOUR BRETON: Connaigre Peninsula Health Centre
Affiliated with: Central Regional Health Authority
Former Name: Harbour Breton Health Centre
PO Box 70, 1 Alexander Ave., Harbour Breton, NL A0H 1P0
Tel: 709-885-2043 *Fax:* 709-885-2358
Number of Beds: 6 acute beds; 12 continuing care beds; 1 palliative bed; 1 respite bed
Wendy Pierce, Manager, Client Care Services
wendy.pierce@centralhealth.nl.ca

HOPEDALE: Hopedale Community Clinic
Affiliated with: Labrador-Grenfell Regional Health Authority
General Delivery, Hopedale, NL A0P 1G0
Tel: 709-933-3857 *Fax:* 709-933-3744
Number of Beds: 3 beds
Number of Employees: 7
Note: Provides primary health care services.

LABRADOR CITY: Labrador West Health Centre
Affiliated with: Labrador-Grenfell Regional Health Authority
Former Name: Captain William Jackman Memorial Hospital
1700 Nichols-Adam Hwy., Labrador City, NL A2V 0B2
Tel: 709-285-8100
www.lghealth.ca
Number of Beds: 28 beds (including 14 long-term care beds)
Note: Programs & services include: emergency; outpatient; surgery; satellite dialysis; maternity care; obstetrics/gynecology; laboratory & diagnostic imaging; physiotherapy; occupational therapy; speech-language pathology; audiology; respiratory therapy; EEG; EKG; oncology/chemotherapy; dietary; diabetes education; mental health & addictions; & population health.
Wanda Slade, Nursing Site Manager
wanda.slade@lghealth.ca

MARY'S HARBOUR: Mary's Harbour Community Clinic
Affiliated with: Labrador-Grenfell Regional Health Authority
Mary's Harbour, NL A0K 3P0
Tel: 709-921-6228 *Fax:* 709-921-6975
Number of Beds: 1 holding bed; 1 crib
Note: Number of Employees: 3 nurses + 1 personal care attendant + 1 maintenance person.

NAIN: Nain Community Clinic
Affiliated with: Labrador-Grenfell Regional Health Authority
General Delivery, Nain, NL A0P 1L0
Tel: 709-922-2912 *Fax:* 709-922-2103
Number of Beds: 4 holding beds
Number of Employees: 16
Note: Offers primary health care services.

SECTION II:
General Resources

NORRIS POINT: Bonne Bay Health Centre
Affiliated with: Western Regional Health Authority
PO Box 70, Norris Point, NL A0K 3V0
Tel: 709-458-2211 *Fax:* 709-458-2074
Number of Beds: 8 acute care beds; 14 continuing care beds
Note: Services include: clinical dietitian; diagnostic; emergency care; laboratory; medical; nursing; occupational therapy; outpatient; palliative care; physiotherapy; recreation therapy; social work; & specialty clinics.

NORTHWEST RIVER: Mani Ashini Health Clinic
Affiliated with: Labrador-Grenfell Regional Health Authority
PO Box 450, 289 Shenum St., Northwest River, NL A0P 1M0
Tel: 709-497-8331 *Fax:* 709-497-8521

OLD PERLICAN: Dr. A.A. Wilkinson Memorial Health Centre
Affiliated with: Eastern Regional Health Authority
PO Box 70, Old Perlican, NL A0A 3G0
Tel: 709-587-2200
Number of Beds: 4 beds
Note: Offers laboratory, diagnostic imaging, x-ray, & blood collection services.

PLACENTIA: Placentia Health Centre
Affiliated with: Eastern Regional Health Authority
PO Box 480, 1 Corrigan Pl., Placentia, NL A0B 2Y0
Tel: 709-227-2061 *Fax:* 709-227-5476
www.easternhealth.ca
Number of Beds: 10 inpatient beds; 75 long-term care beds
Note: Acute care & long term care (Lions Manor Nursing Home) on an in-patient & out-patient basis; services include chemotherapy, diabetes education, emergency care, & pastoral care.
Dr. Sandeep Mangat, Contact

PORT HOPE SIMPSON: Port Hope Simpson Community Clinic
Affiliated with: Labrador-Grenfell Regional Health Authority
General Delivery, Port Hope Simpson, NL A0K 4E0
Tel: 709-960-0271 *Fax:* 709-960-0392
www.lghealth.ca
Year Founded: 1975
Note: Specialties: Emergency room, basic trauma, cardiac monitoring & resuscitation, dental suite. Number of staff: 8

PORT SAUNDERS: Rufus Guinchard Health Care Centre
Affiliated with: Western Regional Health Authority
PO Box 40, Port Saunders, NL A0K 4H0
Tel: 709-861-3139 *Fax:* 709-861-3772
Number of Beds: 1 palliative care bed; 6 acute care beds; 22 long-term care beds
Note: Services include laboratory, diagnostics, therapy, pharmacy, dietitian, & social work.

PORT AUX BASQUES: Dr. Charles L. LeGrow Health Centre
Affiliated with: Western Regional Health Authority
PO Box 250, Port aux Basques, NL A0M 1C0
Tel: 709-695-2175 *Fax:* 709-695-3118
westernhealth.nl.ca
Number of Beds: 14 acute care beds; 30 long-term care beds
Population Served: 9000
Note: Services include pharmacy, dietitian, physiotherapy, laboratory, & diagnostics.
Kathy Organ, Director, Health Services

POSTVILLE: Postville Community Clinic
Affiliated with: Labrador-Grenfell Regional Health Authority
General Delivery, Postville, NL A0P 1N0
Tel: 709-479-9851
www.lghealth.ca
Number of Beds: 1 bed, 1 crib
Number of Employees: 3

RODDICKTON: White Bay Central Health Centre
Affiliated with: Labrador-Grenfell Regional Health Authority
General Delivery, Roddickton, NL A0K 4P0
Tel: 709-457-2215
Note: Programs & services include: ambulatory care; family medicine; emergency; palliative care; public health, mental health, & home care nursing; dental; diagnostic; & child, youth, & family services

SPRINGDALE: Green Bay Community Health Centre
Affiliated with: Central Regional Health Authority
PO Box 280, 275 Main St., Springdale, NL A0J 1T0
Tel: 709-673-4676 *Fax:* 709-673-2114
Number of Beds: 9 beds (2 convalescent; 1 palliative; 5 holding; 1 assessment)
Note: Services include: clinical dietitian; diabetic education; emergency; laboratory; medical clinic; outpatient; physiotherapy; Telehealth; & x-ray.
Wayne Wellman, Manager, Support Services
wayne.wellman@centralhealth.nl.ca

ST LAWRENCE: U.S. Memorial Health Centre
Affiliated with: Eastern Regional Health Authority
PO Box 398, 1 Memorial Dr., St Lawrence, NL A0E 2V0
Tel: 709-873-2330 *Fax:* 709-873-2390
www.easternhealth.ca
Number of Beds: 40 beds
Note: Long term & protective care units, ambulatory care clinic, nutritional services, pharmacy, visiting specialty clinics

ST. ANTHONY: Charles S. Curtis Memorial Hospital
Affiliated with: Labrador-Grenfell Regional Health Authority
Also Known As: Curtis Hospital
#178, 200 West St., St. Anthony, NL A0K 4S0
Tel: 709-454-3333
www.lghealth.ca
Number of Beds: 50 beds
Note: Programs & services include: acute care; anaesthesia; dentistry; family practice; general surgery; internal medicine; obstetrics/gynecology; ophthalmology; orthopedics; pathology; pediatrics; emergency; intensive care; oncology/chemotherapy; day surgery; satellite dialysis; laboratory & diagnostic imaging; physiotherapy; occupational therapy; speech-language pathology; respiratory therapy; EEG/ECG; pharmacy; audiology; clinical nutrition; diabetes education; social work; mental health & addictions; & psychology.

ST. JOHN'S: Eastern Regional Health Authority
Also Known As: Eastern Health
Health Sciences Centre, Prince Philip Dr., St. John's, NL A1B 3V6
Tel: 709-777-6500 *Toll-Free:* 877-444-1399
client.relations@easternhealth.ca
www.easternhealth.ca
Info Line: 811
Social Media: www.facebook.com/EasternHealthNL;
twitter.com/EasternHealthNL
Number of Beds: 1,696 long term care beds; 987 acute care beds; 9 observation beds
Area Served: Avalon, Burin & Bonavista Peninsulas; 21,000 sq km
Population Served: 300000
Number of Employees: 13000
Note: Area served includes 111 incorporated municipalities, 69 local service districts, & 66 unincorporated municipal units.
Leslie O'Reilly, Board Chair
David S. Diamond, President & CEO
Collette Smith, Vice-President
Katherine Chubbs, Chief Nursing Officer & Vice-President
George Butt, Vice-President & Chief Financial Officer
Ron Johnson, Vice-President & Chief Information Officer
Oscar Howell, Vice-President, Healthcare Technology & Data
    Management
Debbie Molloy, Vice-President, Human Resources
Lynette Oates, Chief Communications Officer

ST. JOHN'S: Health Sciences Centre - General Hospital
Affiliated with: Eastern Regional Health Authority
300 Prince Phillip Dr., St. John's, NL A1B 3V6
Tel: 709-777-6300
client.relations@easternhealth.ca
www.easternhealth.ca
Social Media: www.facebook.com/EasternHealthNL;
twitter.com/EasternHealthNL
Note: A tertiary acute care facility & teaching hospital affiliated with Memorial University Schools of Medicine, Nursing, & Pharmacy. Programs & services include: blood collection; diagnostic imaging; dialysis; emergency; inpatient services; laboratory; outpatient services; radiography; & surgery.

ST. JOHN'S: St. Clare's Mercy Hospital
Affiliated with: Eastern Regional Health Authority
154 LeMarchant Rd., St. John's, NL A1C 5B8

Tel: 709-777-5000
client.relations@easternhealth.ca
www.easternhealth.ca
Social Media: www.facebook.com/EasternHealthNL;
twitter.com/EasternHealthNL

Year Founded: 1922
Note: Tertiary hospital. Programs & services include: blood collection; diagnostic imaging; dialysis; emergency; inpatient services; laboratory; outpatient services; radiography; & surgery.

STEPHENVILLE: Sir Thomas Roddick Hospital
Affiliated with: Western Regional Health Authority
142 Minnesota Dr., Stephenville, NL A2N 2V6

Tel: 709-643-5111
www.westernhealth.nl.ca
Social Media: twitter.com/WesternHealthNL;
www.youtube.com/WesternHealthNL

Year Founded: 2003
Number of Beds: 44 acute care beds
Population Served: 24000
Note: Programs & services include: emergency; medical; nursing; obstetric/gynecaelogical; outpatient; pharmacy; renal care; specialty clinics; & surgical.
Karen Alexander, Site Manager

TWILLINGATE: Notre Dame Bay Memorial Health Centre
Affiliated with: Central Regional Health Authority
General Delivery, Twillingate, NL A0G 4M0

Tel: 709-884-2131 Fax: 709-884-2586
Number of Beds: 31 long-term care beds; 19 acute care beds
Note: Specialties: Outpatient services; Social work; Physiotherapy; Recreation therapy; Dietetics; Diabetes education; Health promotion & protection; Respite care, for children with special needs
Victor Shea, Director, Health Services
victor.shea@centralhealth.nl.ca

WHITBOURNE: Dr. W. H. Newhook Community Health Centre
Affiliated with: Eastern Regional Health Authority
PO Box 449, 7 Whitbourne Ave., Whitbourne, NL A0B 3K0

Tel: 709-759-2300 Fax: 709-759-2387

Note: Emergency centre; family physicians; laboratory & diagnostic services
Dr. Stephanie A. Squibb, Contact
stephanie.squibb@easternhealth.ca

NORTHWEST TERRITORIES

AKLAVIK: Susie Husky Health & Social Services Centre
Affiliated with: Northwest Territories Health & Social Services Authority
Former Name: Susie Husky Health Centre
PO Box 114, Aklavik, NT X0E 0A0

Tel: 867-978-2516 Fax: 867-978-2160
www.bdhssa.hss.gov.nt.ca

Note: Specialties: Clinics, such as chronic disease & well child, woman, & man clinics; School health program; Health promotion; Dental therapy; Home care; Immunization programs; Rehabilitative services; Child protection; Child & family services; Palliative care. Number of Employees: 1 nurse in charge + 3 community health nurses + 2 community social service workers; 1 dental therapist + 1 community health representative + 1 home support worker + 1 clerk + 1 caretaker

BEHCHOKO: Behchoko Health Centre
Affiliated with: Tlicho Community Services Agency
Former Name: Rae Health Centre
PO Box 5, Behchoko, NT X0E 0Y0

Tel: 867-392-6075 Fax: 867-392-6612
www.tlicho.ca
Rebecca Nash, Nurse-in-Charge

BEHCHOKO: Tlicho Community Services Agency
PO Box 5, Behchoko, NT X0E 0Y0

Tel: 867-392-3000 Fax: 867-392-3001
tcsa@tlicho.net
www.tlicho.ca

Note: A person can contact a member of the primary community care team in their home community & receive access to healthcare services in their own community, in the region &, as necessary, outside the NWT.
Kevin Armstrong, Chief Executive Officer
kevin_armstrong@tlicho.net

COLVILLE LAKE: Colville Lake Health Centre
Affiliated with: Northwest Territories Health & Social Services Authority
PO Box 50, Colville Lake, NT X0E 1L0

Tel: 867-709-2409 Fax: 867-709-2504

DELINE: Deline Health Centre
Affiliated with: Northwest Territories Health & Social Services Authority
PO Box 199, Deline, NT X0E 0G0

Tel: 867-589-3111 Fax: 867-589-5570

FORT GOOD HOPE: Fort Good Hope Health Centre
Affiliated with: Northwest Territories Health & Social Services Authority
PO Box 9, Fort Good Hope, NT X0E 0N0

Tel: 867-598-3333 Fax: 867-598-2605

Population Served: 585

FORT LIARD: Fort Liard Health Centre
Affiliated with: Northwest Territories Health & Social Services Authority
General Delivery, Fort Liard, NT X0E 0A0

Tel: 867-770-4301 Fax: 867-770-3235

FORT MCPHERSON: William Firth Health Centre
Affiliated with: Northwest Territories Health & Social Services Authority
PO Box 56, Fort McPherson, NT X0E 0J0

Tel: 867-952-2586 Fax: 867-952-2620

FORT PROVIDENCE: Fort Providence Health Centre
Affiliated with: Northwest Territories Health & Social Services Authority
PO Box 260, Fort Providence, NT X0E 0L0

Tel: 867-699-4311 Fax: 867-699-3811

FORT RESOLUTION: Fort Resolution Health Centre
Affiliated with: Northwest Territories Health & Social Services Authority
General Delivery, Fort Resolution, NT X0E 0M0

Tel: 867-394-4511 Fax: 867-394-3117
www.yhssa.hss.gov.nt.ca

FORT SIMPSON: Fort Simpson Health Centre
Affiliated with: Northwest Territories Health & Social Services Authority
PO Box 246, Fort Simpson, NT X0E 0N0

Tel: 867-695-7000 Fax: 867-695-7017

FORT SMITH: Fort Smith Health Centre
Affiliated with: Northwest Territories Health & Social Services Authority
c/o Fort Smith Health & Social Services, PO Box 1080, 41 Breynet St., Fort Smith, NT X0E 0P0

Tel: 867-872-6203 Fax: 867-872-6260
www.hss.gov.nt.ca
Number of Beds: 25 beds

FORT SMITH: Fort Smith Public Health Unit
Affiliated with: Northwest Territories Health & Social Services Authority
PO Box 1080, 41 Breynet St., Fort Smith, NT X0E 0P0

Tel: 867-872-6203 Fax: 867-872-6260

GAMETI: Gamèti Health Centre
Affiliated with: Tlicho Community Services Agency
General Delivery, Gameti, NT X0E 1R0

Tel: 867-997-3141 Fax: 867-997-3045
www.tlicho.ca

HAY RIVER: H.H. Williams Memorial Hospital
Affiliated with: Hay River Health & Social Service Authority
3 Gaetz Dr., Hay River, NT X0E 0R8
Tel: 867-874-7169 *Fax:* 867-874-2926
Number of Beds: 10 beds
Note: Provides physician & emergency services; also includes a long-term care facility.

HAY RIVER: Hay River Health & Social Services Authority (HRHSSA)
37911 Mackenzie Hwy., Hay River, NT X0E 0R6
Tel: 867-874-8000 *Fax:* 867-874-8016
www.hrhssa.org
Social Media: www.youtube.com/user/HSSCommunications
Number of Beds: 29 hospital beds; 15 long-term care beds
Area Served: Southern shore of Great Slave Lake, NWT, Enterprise & Hay River
Population Served: 3800
Number of Employees: 185
Note: Facilities: Hay River Emergency Group Home; Hay River Public Health Unit; Hay River Social Services Office; H.H. Williams Memorial Hospital; Hay River Medical Clinic; Woodland Manor; Hay River Reserve Health Station; Hay River Reserve Social Services; Enterprise Social Services. Area served includes six outlying communities with a total population of more than 6,000 people.
Erin Griffiths, Chief Executive Officer
  867-874-8160, erin_griffiths@gov.nt.ca
Merle Engel, Director, Finance
  867-874-7119, merle_engel@gov.nt.ca
Sheryl Courtoreille, Director, Client Services
  867-874-8020, sheryl_courtoreille@gov.nt.ca
Bonnie Kimble, Contact, Quality Improvement
  867-874-8150, hrhssa_clientrelations@gov.nt.ca

HAY RIVER: Hay River Public Health Unit
Affiliated with: Hay River Health & Social Service Authority
3 Gaetz Dr., Hay River, NT X0E 0R8
Tel: 867-874-7201 *Fax:* 867-874-7109
www.hrhssa.org

HAY RIVER RESERVE: Anne Buggins Wellness Centre
Affiliated with: Northwest Territories Health & Social Services Authority
Hay River Reserve, NT X0E 1G4
www.dhssa.hss.gov.nt.ca

INUVIK: Beaufort-Delta Health & Social Services
Affiliated with: Northwest Territories Health & Social Services Authority
285 - 289 Mackenzie Rd., Inuvik, NT X0E 0T0
Tel: 867-777-8000
bdhssa_info@gov.nt.ca
www.bdhssa.hss.gov.nt.ca

INUVIK: Inuvik Public Health Unit
Affiliated with: Northwest Territories Health & Social Services Authority
Bag 2, Inuvik, NT X0E 0T0
Tel: 867-777-7246 *Fax:* 867-777-3255
Barb Lennie, Nurse-in-Charge

INUVIK: Inuvik Regional Hospital
Affiliated with: Northwest Territories Health & Social Services Authority
Bag 2, Inuvik, NT X0E 0T0
Tel: 867-777-8000 *Fax:* 867-777-8054
www.bdhssa.hss.gov.nt.ca
Social Media: www.youtube.com/HSSCommunications
Number of Beds: 51 beds
Note: Location: #285, 289 Mackenzie Rd., Inuvik. Programs & services include: acute care; dermatology; diagnostic imaging; ear, nose & throat (ENT); emergency; gynecology; health promotion; internal medicine; laboratory; long term care; medical social work; neurology; nutrition; obstetrical care; ophthalmology; orthopedics; pediatrics; pharmacy; physician family clinics; psychiatry; regional mental health & addictions program; regional; social services; rehabilitation; surgery; telehealth; & visiting specialist clinics.

JEAN MARIE RIVER: Jean Marie River Health Cabin
Affiliated with: Northwest Territories Health & Social Services Authority
General Delivery, Jean Marie River, NT X0E 0N0
Tel: 867-809-2900

LUTSELK'E: Lutselk'e Health Centre
Affiliated with: Northwest Territories Health & Social Services Authority
PO Box 56, Lutselk'e, NT X0E 1A0
Tel: 867-370-3111 *Fax:* 867-370-3022
Note: Specialties: Public health programs; Counselling & crisis intervention & referrals

NAHANNI BUTTE: Nahanni Butte Health Cabin
Affiliated with: Northwest Territories Health & Social Services Authority
General Delivery, Nahanni Butte, NT X0E 0N0
Tel: 867-602-2203

NORMAN WELLS: Norman Wells Health Centre
Affiliated with: Northwest Territories Health & Social Services Authority
PO Box 8, Norman Wells, NT X0E 0V0
Tel: 867-587-3333 *Fax:* 867-587-2934

PAULATUK: Paulatuk Health Centre
Affiliated with: Northwest Territories Health & Social Services Authority
PO Box 114, Paulatuk, NT X0E 1N0
Tel: 867-580-3231 *Fax:* 867-580-3300
Number of Beds: 1 bed

SACHS HARBOUR: Sachs Harbour Health Centre
Affiliated with: Northwest Territories Health & Social Services Authority
PO Box 14, Sachs Harbour, NT X0E 0Z0
Tel: 867-690-4181 *Fax:* 867-690-3802
Note: Services include: chronic disease clinic; emergency; diagnostic; home care; health promotion; disease prevention; & immunization

TROUT LAKE: Trout Lake Health Centre
Affiliated with: Northwest Territories Health & Social Services Authority
Trout Lake Health Cabin, Trout Lake, NT X0E 1Z0
Tel: 867-206-2838

TUKTOYAKTUK: Rosie Ovayouk Health Centre
Affiliated with: Northwest Territories Health & Social Services Authority
PO Box 1000, Tuktoyaktuk, NT X0E 1C0
Tel: 867-977-2321 *Fax:* 867-977-2535
Note: Diagnosis; rehabilitation; home care.

TULITA: Tulita Health Centre
Affiliated with: Northwest Territories Health & Social Services Authority
PO Box 134, Tulita, NT X0E 0K0
Tel: 867-588-3333 *Fax:* 867-588-3000
www.shssa.hss.gov.nt.ca
Note: Specialties: Primary care; Health promotion & prevention.
Number of Employees: 3 nurses + 2 prevention & health promotion workers + 1 community social service worker + 1 mental health & addictions worker + 1 home support worker + support staff

ULUKHAKTOK: Emegak Health Centre
Affiliated with: Northwest Territories Health & Social Services Authority
PO Box 160, Ulukhaktok, NT X0E 0S0
Tel: 867-396-3111 *Fax:* 867-396-3221

ULUKHAKTOK: Ulukhaktok Health Services
Affiliated with: Northwest Territories Health & Social Services Authority
PO Box 160, Ulukhaktok, NT X0E 0S0
Tel: 867-396-3111 *Fax:* 867-396-3221
Note: Specialties: assessments; crisis intervention; therapeutic

counselling; education & awareness. Number of employees: 1 mental health & addictions counsellor; 1 community wellness worker

WEKWEÈTI: Wekweèti Health Centre
Affiliated with: Tlicho Community Services Agency
General Delivery, Wekweèti, NT X0E 1W0
Tel: 867-713-2904

WHATI: Whati Health Centre
Affiliated with: Tlicho Community Services Agency
General Delivery, Whati, NT X0E 1P0
Tel: 867-573-3261 Fax: 867-573-3701
www.tlicho.ca

WRIGLEY: Wrigley Health Centre
Affiliated with: Northwest Territories Health & Social Services Authority
General Delivery, Wrigley, NT X0E 1E0
Tel: 867-581-3441 Fax: 867-581-3200

Note: Services include: child & family services; diagnostic; emergency; palliative care; health promotion; disease prevention; home care; immunization; mental health; & rehabilitation

YELLOWKNIFE: Northwest Territories Health & Social Services Authority (NTHSSA)
Government of the Northwest Territories, PO Box 1320, Yellowknife, NT X1A 2L9
Tel: 867-767-9090
hss_transformation@gov.nt.ca
www.nthssa.ca

Note: Formed in Aug. 2016 as a result of the amalgamation of six regional health authorities: Beaufort-Delta Health & Social Services Authority, Dehcho Health & Social Services Authority, Fort Smith Health & Social Services Authority, Sahtu Health & Social Services Authority, Stanton Territorial Health Authority, & Yellowknife Health & Social Services Authority.
Damien Healy, Communications Manager, Health & Social Services
867-767-9052, damien_healy@gov.nt.ca

YELLOWKNIFE: Stanton Territorial Hospital
Affiliated with: Northwest Territories Health & Social Services Authority
PO Box 10, 550 Byrne Rd., Yellowknife, NT X1A 2N1
Tel: 867-669-4111
www.stha.hss.gov.nt.ca
Social Media: www.youtube.com/user/HSSCommunications

Note: Programs & services include: diagnostic imaging; emergency; intensive care; medical day care; medicine; obstetrics; pediatrics; psychiatry; surgery; & surgical day care.
Brenda Fitzgerald, Chief Executive Officer, Stanton Territorial Health Authority
Dr. Bing Guthrie, Medical Director, Stanton Territorial Health Authority
David Keselman, Director, Patient Care Services, Stanton Territorial Health Authority

YELLOWKNIFE: Yellowknife Public Health Unit
Affiliated with: Northwest Territories Health & Social Services Authority
Jan Stirling Bldg., 4702 Franklin Ave., Yellowknife, NT X1A 1N2
Tel: 867-920-6570 Fax: 867-873-0158
yhssa_phadmin@gov.nt.ca

Note: Services include: immunization; family services; services for children & adults

NOVA SCOTIA

ADVOCATE HARBOUR: Bayview Memorial Health Centre
Affiliated with: Nova Scotia Health Authority
3375 Hwy. 209, Advocate Harbour, NS B0M 1A0
Tel: 902-392-2859 Fax: 902-392-2625
www.cha.nshealth.ca
Year Founded: 1989
Number of Beds: 10 beds (including 8 long-term-care beds)
Note: Provides community health services & long-term care.

AMHERST: Cumberland Regional Health Care Centre (CRHCC)
Affiliated with: Nova Scotia Health Authority
19428 Hwy 2, RR #6, Amherst, NS B4H 1N6
Tel: 902-667-3361 Fax: 902-667-6306
www.nshealth.ca
Year Founded: 2002
Note: Programs & services include: ambulatory care; cancer patient navigation; diabetes education; diagnostic imaging; dietary/nutrition; emergency; intensive care unit; laboratory; maternal/child unit; medical inpatient unit; palliative care; pharmacy; rehabilitative services; respiratory therapy; social work; & surgery.

ANNAPOLIS ROYAL: Annapolis Community Health Centre
Affiliated with: Nova Scotia Health Authority
PO Box 426, 821 St. George St., Annapolis Royal, NS B0S 1A0
Tel: 902-532-2381 Fax: 902-532-2113

Note: Programs & services include: diagnostic imaging; emergency; laboratory; mental health & addictions; occupational therapy; palliative care; physiotherapy; & public health.

ANTIGONISH: St. Martha's Regional Hospital
Affiliated with: Nova Scotia Health Authority
25 Bay St., Antigonish, NS B2G 2G4
Tel: 902-867-4500 Fax: 902-867-1059
www.nshealth.ca
Year Founded: 1906
Number of Beds: 89 beds
Note: Programs & services include: anesthesia; bone densitometry; cancer & supportive care; cardio-respiratory; chemotherapy; chronic pain clinic; clinical nutrition; colposcopy clinic; cystometry clinic; diabetes education; diagnostic imaging; emergency; foot clinic; general medical/surgical; geriatric assessment & rehabilitation/clinic; gynecology/obstetrics/midwifery; heart health clinic; hospice & palliative care; internal medicine; laboratory services; mental health inpatient/outpatient; obstetrics; occupational therapy; Open Arms Clinic; ophthalmology; orthoptics clinic; ostomy clinic; otolaryngology; pediatrics; physiotherapy; plastic surgery; pre-surgical assessment clinic; social work; spiritual & religious care; & wound care clinic.
Martha Cooper, Facility Manager
martha.cooper@nshealth.ca

BADDECK: Victoria County Memorial Hospital
Affiliated with: Nova Scotia Health Authority
PO Box 220, 30 Old Margaree Rd., Baddeck, NS B0E 1B0
Tel: 902-295-2112
www.nshealth.ca
Year Founded: 1949
Number of Beds: 12 beds
Note: Services include: ambulatory care; diabetes education; diagnostic imaging; emergency care; general medicine; general & specialized clinical support services; laboratory; mental health & addiction; & palliative care.
Rose Surette, Facility Manager

BERWICK: Western Kings Memorial Health Centre
Affiliated with: Nova Scotia Health Authority
PO Box 490, 121 Orchard St., Berwick, NS B0P 1E0
Tel: 902-538-3111 Fax: 902-538-9590
www.avdha.nshealth.ca

Note: Services include outpatient department, laboratory, diagnostic imaging, physiotherapy, nutritional counselling, dialysis, mental health clinic, & Victorian Order of Nurses Adult Day Care program.

BRIDGEWATER: Nova Scotia Health Authority - Annapolis Valley, South Shore, & South West Regional Office
Affiliated with: Nova Scotia Health Authority
#109, 215 Dominion St., Bridgewater, NS B4V 2K7
Tel: 902-543-0850 Fax: 902-543-8024
Info Line: 811
Dr. Lynda Earle, Medical Officer of Health

BRIDGEWATER: South Shore Regional Hospital
Affiliated with: Nova Scotia Health Authority
Former Name: Health Services Association of the South Shore
90 Glen Allan Dr., Bridgewater, NS B4V 3S6
Tel: 902-543-4603
www.nshealth.ca

SECTION III:
General Resources

Number of Beds: 80 beds
Specialties: Trauma care
Note: Programs & services include: 24 hour emergency; ambulatory care; anesthesiology; cardiology; diagnostic imaging; EKG; gastroenterology; general medicine; intensive care; internal medicine; laboratory; mental health; obstetrics; pathology; pediatrics; radiology; rehabilitation; respiratory therapy; rheumatology; & surgery.
Lynn Farrell, Site Manager

CANSO: Eastern Memorial Hospital
Affiliated with: Nova Scotia Health Authority
PO Box 10, 1746 Union St., Canso, NS B0H 1H0
Tel: 902-366-2794 *Fax:* 902-366-2740
www.nshealth.ca
Year Founded: 1948
Number of Beds: 6 beds
Note: Programs & services include: acute care; adult day clinic; adult mental health & addiction prevention & treatment services; ambulatory care; clinical nutrition; continuing care; diagnostic imaging; laboratory; Meals on Wheels; nurse practitioner; occupational therapy; outpatient/emergency; palliative care; physiotherapy; public health; respite care; seniors mental health; social work; spiritual care; & Telehealth.
Elaine MacMaster, Facility Manager
elaine.macmaster@nshealth.ca

CHETICAMP: Sacred Heart Community Health Centre
Affiliated with: Nova Scotia Health Authority
Former Name: Sacred Heart Hospital
PO Box 129, 15102 Cabot Trail, Cheticamp, NS B0E 1H0
Tel: 902-224-4000
www.nshealth.ca
Year Founded: 1999
Number of Beds: 10 beds
Note: Programs & services include: ambulatory care; emergency care; general diagnostic imaging; general medicine; laboratory; mental health & addiction; & palliative care.

DARTMOUTH: Dartmouth General Hospital (DGH)
Affiliated with: Nova Scotia Health Authority
325 Pleasant St., Dartmouth, NS B2Y 4G8
Tel: 902-465-8300
www.nshealth.ca
Year Founded: 1976
Population Served: 120000
Note: Programs & services include: CT scanning; dentistry; ear, nose, & throat surgery; general surgery; gynaecology; inpatient medical, surgical care, & critical care; laboratory; mammography; oral maxillofacial surgery; orthopedic surgery; outpatient; plastic surgery; radiography; renal dialysis; & urology.
Dr. Ravi Parkash, Site Chief
Heather Francis, Director, Health Services

DARTMOUTH: Regional Residential Services Society (RRSS)
#LKD1, 202 Brownlow Ave., Dartmouth, NS B3B 1T5
Tel: 902-465-4022 *Fax:* 902-465-3124
www.rrss.ns.ca
Number of Beds: 185 beds
Note: Developmental residences & group homes, supported apartments, short & long term respite services, personal support planning, counseling, assessment. Number of staff: 400+
Carol Ann Brennan, Executive Director
902-465-2702, carolann.brennan@rrss.ns.ca

DIGBY: Digby General Hospital
Affiliated with: Nova Scotia Health Authority
75 Warwick St., Digby, NS B0V 1A0
Tel: 902-245-2501 *Fax:* 902-245-2803
www.nshealth.ca
Number of Beds: 11 acute beds; 13 restorative care beds; 9 transition beds
Population Served: 18992
Note: Programs & services include: cardiac/respiratory; continuing care; day surgery; diabetes education; diagnostic imaging; dietitian; emergency; laboratory; mental health & addiction; Nova Scotia Hearing & Speech Centre; nurse practitioner; nutrition; palliative care; pharmacy; public health; rehabilitation; restorative care; social work; & Telehealth.

Hubert d'Entremont, Site Manager
902-245-2502, hubert.dentremont@nshealth.ca

EVANSTON: Strait Richmond Hospital
Affiliated with: Nova Scotia Health Authority
138 Hospital Rd., Evanston, NS B0E 1J0
Tel: 902-625-3100 *Fax:* 902-625-3804
www.nshealth.ca
Year Founded: 1980
Number of Beds: 15 beds; 5 restorative care beds
Note: Programs & services include: chemotherapy; diabetes education; diagnostic imaging; dialysis (QEII Satellite Clinic); EKG; emergency; foot care; Holter monitors; internal medicine; laboratory; loop monitors; mental health outpatient services; nutrition & dietetic counselling; occupational therapy; palliative care; pediatrics; physiotherapy; Renal Clinic; rheumatology; social work; & Surgical Service Clinic.
Kathy Chisholm, Facility Manager
kathy.chisholm@nshealth.ca

GUYSBOROUGH: Guysborough Memorial Hospital
Affiliated with: Nova Scotia Health Authority
PO Box 170, 10560 Rte. 16, Guysborough, NS B0H 1H0
Tel: 902-533-3702 *Fax:* 902-533-4066
www.nshealth.ca
Number of Beds: 10 beds
Note: Programs & services include: diabetes education; diagnostic imaging; EKG; emergency; foot care clinic; laboratory; mental health outpatient; nutrition & dietetic counseling; physiotherapy; social work; & Well Men's Clinic (urology).
Elaine MacMaster, Facility Manager
elaine.macmaster@nshealth.ca

HALIFAX: IWK Health Centre
PO Box 9700, 5850/5980 University Ave., Halifax, NS B3K 6R8
Tel: 902-470-8888
feedback@iwk.nshealth.ca
www.iwk.nshealth.ca
Social Media: www.facebook.com/iwkhealthcentre; twitter.com/iwkhealthcentre; www.youtube.com/iwkhealthcentre

Number of Employees: 3600
Note: The IWK Health Centre provides care to women, children, youth and families in the Maritime provinces and beyond. In addition to providing highly specialized (tertiary) care, the IWK also provides primary care services.
Tracy Kitch, President/CEO
Jocelyn Vince, Chief Nurse Executive & Vice-President, Patient Care

HALIFAX: Nova Scotia Health Authority
#201, 90 Lovett Lake Ct., Halifax, NS B3S 0H6
Toll-Free: 1-844-491-5890
wearelistening@nshealth.ca
www.nshealth.ca
Info Line: 811
Social Media: www.facebook.com/NovaScotiaHealthAuthority; twitter.com/healthns

Year Founded: 2015
Number of Beds: 3,198
Area Served: Province of Nova Scotia
Number of Employees: 23400
Note: All former Nova Scotia health districts mergerd in 2015, forming the Nova Scotia Health Authority. The new organization will oversee 10 hospitals, 35 community health centres, 33 auxiliaries & 37 community health boards.
Janet Knox, President & CEO
Steven Parker, Chair
Allan Horsburgh, CFO & Vice-President, Stewardship & Accountability
Lindsay Peach, Vice-President, Integrated Health Services Community Support
Tricia Cochrane, Vice-President, Population Health
Tim Guest, Chief Nursing Officer & Vice-President, Integrated Health Services Program Care
Paula Bond, Vice-President, Integrated Health Services Program Care
Dr. Lynne Harrigan, Vice-President, Medicine & Integrated Health Services
Carmelle d'Entremont, Vice-President, People & Organizational Development

Patrick McGrath, Vice-President, Research, Innovation & Knowledge Translation

HALIFAX: Nova Scotia Health Authority - Halifax, Eastern Shore & West Hants Regional Office
Affiliated with: Nova Scotia Health Authority
#5, 7 Mellor Ave., Halifax, NS B3B 0E6
Tel: 902-481-5800 *Fax:* 902-481-5803
Dr. Trevor Arnason, Medical Officer of Health

HALIFAX: Queen Elizabeth II Health Sciences Centre (QEII)
Affiliated with: Nova Scotia Health Authority
1796 Summer St., Halifax, NS B3H 2A7
Tel: 902-473-2700
www.cdha.nshealth.ca
Social Media: www.facebook.com/CapitalHealth;
twitter.com/capital_health;
www.linkedin.com/company/capital-district-health-authority

Note: The largest teaching hospital in Atlantic Canada, made up of 10 buildings on 2 sites (the Halifax Infirmary site & the Victoria General site). The QEII provides general & specialized medical care, including mental health programs; cancer care; long-term care; geriatric assessment & restorative care.

INVERNESS: Inverness Consolidated Memorial Hospital
Affiliated with: Nova Scotia Health Authority
Former Name: Inverness Consolidated Hospital
PO Box 610, 39 James St., Inverness, NS B0E 1N0
Tel: 902-258-2100
www.nshealth.ca
Number of Beds: 48 beds
Note: Services include: ambulatory care; continuing care; diabetes education; emergency care; general medicine; general surgery; laboratory; mental health & addiction; palliative care; & renal dialysis.

KENTVILLE: Valley Regional Hospital
Affiliated with: Nova Scotia Health Authority
150 Exhibition St., Kentville, NS B4N 5E3
Tel: 902-678-7381 *Fax:* 902-679-1904
www.nshealth.ca
Year Founded: 1992
Number of Employees: 700
Note: Programs & services include: addiction services; anaesthesia; asthma care; chronic pain; diabetes; diagnostic imaging; emergency; laboratory; mental health; Nova Scotia Hearing & Speech Centre; organ & tissue donation; palliative care; pastoral care; pharmacy; residential mental health; seniors mental health; & surgery.

LIVERPOOL: Queens General Hospital
Affiliated with: Nova Scotia Health Authority
175 School St., Liverpool, NS B0T 1K0
Tel: 902-354-3436
www.nshealth.ca
Number of Beds: 14 beds
Note: Programs & services include: 24-hour outpatients/emergency; asthma; blood collection; diabetes education; diagnostic imaging; day surgery/ambulatory care; EKG; endoscopy; family medicine; geriatrics; gynecology; internal medicine; palliative care; pediatrics; psychiatry; rehabilitation; & renal dialysis.

LOWER SACKVILLE: Cobequid Community Health Centre (CCHC)
Affiliated with: Nova Scotia Health Authority
40 Freer Lane, Lower Sackville, NS B4C 0A2
Tel: 902-869-6100 *Fax:* 902-869-6148
www.capitalhealth.ca
Note: Ambulatory care facility
Dr. Mike Clory, Site Chief
Margaret Merlin-Wilson, Director, Health Services

LUNENBURG: Fishermen's Memorial Hospital
Affiliated with: Nova Scotia Health Authority
PO Box 1180, 14 High St., Lunenburg, NS B0J 2C0
Tel: 902-634-8801
www.nshealth.ca
Number of Beds: 23 veterans' care beds; 10 addiction services beds; 12 restorative care beds; 12 alternate level of care beds; 6 acute care beds; 2 observation beds
Note: Services include: 16-hour emergency; addiction; ambulatory

care; blood collection; diagnostic imaging; EKG; general medicine; palliative care; rehabilitation; restorative care; & veterans long term care.

MIDDLE MUSQUODOBOIT: Musquodoboit Valley Memorial Hospital
Affiliated with: Nova Scotia Health Authority
492 Archibald Brook Rd., Middle Musquodoboit, NS B0N 1X0
Tel: 902-384-2220
www.nshealth.ca
Number of Beds: 6 inpatient beds; palliative care room
Note: Programs & services include: acute home nursing care; clinical nutrition; diabetic clinic & Meals-on-Wheels; diagnostic services (including laboratory, EKG & radiology); emergency services; occupational therapy; outpatient services; palliative services; physiotherapy; public health; Shared Care Mental Health; social work; & The Musquodoboit Valley Family Practice.

MIDDLETON: Soldiers Memorial Hospital
Affiliated with: Nova Scotia Health Authority
PO Box 730, 462 Main St., Middleton, NS B0S 1P0
Tel: 902-825-3411 *Fax:* 902-825-0599
www.nshealth.ca
Population Served: 40000
Note: Programs & services include: adult mental health & addiction; cardiac investigation; continuing care; diabetes education; diagnostic imaging; emergency; enterostomal therapy; laboratory; Nova Scotia Hearing & Speech Centre; occupational therapy; palliative care; pharmacy; physiotherapy; public health; social work; ophthalmology day surgery; & transitional care.

MUSQUODOBOIT HARBOUR: Twin Oaks Memorial Hospital
Affiliated with: Nova Scotia Health Authority
7704 - 7 Hwy., Musquodoboit Harbour, NS B0J 2L0
Tel: 902-889-2200
www.nshealth.ca
Year Founded: 1976
Number of Beds: 14 beds
Note: Programs & services include: acute care; addiction; diabetic & foot care clinics; diagnostic imaging; emergency; family practice; Home Care Nova Scotia; laboratory; Meals on Wheels; Nova Scotia Hearing & Speech Clinic; nutrition counselling; occupational therapy; outpatient care; palliative & respite services; physiotherapy; & social services.

NEILS HARBOUR: Buchanan Memorial Community Health Centre
Affiliated with: Nova Scotia Health Authority
32610 Cabot Trail, Neils Harbour, NS B0C 1N0
Tel: 902-336-2200
www.nshealth.ca
Year Founded: 1943
Population Served: 4200
Note: Programs & services include: ambulatory care; ECG; emergency care; general & specialized clinical support services; general diagnostic imaging; general medicine; medical laboratory; mental health & addiction; palliative care; & public health.

NEW GLASGOW: Aberdeen Hospital
Affiliated with: Nova Scotia Health Authority
835 East River Rd., New Glasgow, NS B2H 3S6
Tel: 902-752-7600
www.nshealth.ca
Number of Beds: 104 beds
Population Served: 48000
Note: Services include: diagnostic imaging; emergency; general surgery; internal medicine; laboratory; obstetrics & gynecology; ophthalmology; orthopedics; pediatrics; psychiatry; & rehabilitation.

NORTH SYDNEY: Northside General Hospital
Affiliated with: Nova Scotia Health Authority
PO Box 399, 520 Purves St., North Sydney, NS B2A 3M4
Tel: 902-794-8521
www.nshealth.ca
Note: Programs & services include: ambulatory care; clinical support; continuing care; diabetes education; diagnostic imaging; emergency; general medicine; laboratory; mental health & addiction; orthoptics; pain clinic; palliative care; renal dialysis; surgery; Telehealth; & Well Women's Clinic.

PARRSBORO: South Cumberland Community Care Centre
Affiliated with: Nova Scotia Health Authority
50 Jenks Ave., Parrsboro, NS B0M 1S0
Tel: 902-254-2540 *Fax:* 902-254-2504
www.nshealth.ca

Year Founded: 1975
Number of Beds: 16 beds (14 long-term care; 2 swing/palliative care beds)
Note: Programs & services include: adult day care; Collaborative Emergency Centre; diagnostic imaging; long term care; outpatient; palliative care; primary health care clinic; & rehabilitation.
Ron McCormick, Site Manager

PICTOU: Sutherland Harris Memorial Hospital
Affiliated with: Nova Scotia Health Authority
PO Box 1059, 222 Haliburton Rd., Pictou, NS B0K 1H0
Tel: 902-485-4324
www.nshealth.ca

Year Founded: 1966
Number of Beds: 20 long-term beds for veterans; 12 restorative care beds
Note: Programs & services include: Diabetes Education Clinic; geriatric consultation service; Northumberland Veterans Unit; occupational therapy; physiotherapy; recreation; Restorative Care Unit; Satellite Hemodialysis Clinic; social work; & speech-language therapy.

PUGWASH: North Cumberland Memorial Hospital
Affiliated with: Nova Scotia Health Authority
260 Gulf Shore Rd., Pugwash, NS B0K 1L0
Tel: 902-243-2521 *Fax:* 902-243-2941
www.nshealth.ca

Year Founded: 1966
Note: Services include: Collaborative Emergency Centre; diagnostic imaging; laboratory collection; outpatient; primary health care clinic; rehabilitative services; & short stay & palliative care.

SHEET HARBOUR: Eastern Shore Memorial Hospital
Affiliated with: Nova Scotia Health Authority
22637 Hwy. #7, Sheet Harbour, NS B0J 3B0
Tel: 902-885-2554
www.nshealth.ca

Year Founded: 1976
Number of Beds: 16 beds
Note: Programs & services include: acute care; Adult Day Clinic; adult mental health & addiction prevention & treatment; clinical nutrition; community blood collection; continuing care; diabetes management; diagnostic imaging; Home Care Nova Scotia; laboratory; Meals on Wheels; NS Hearing & Speech; nurse practitioner; occupational therapy; outpatient/emergency; palliative care; physiotherapy; primary care physicians; public health; respite care; Sexual Health Center; social services; social work; spiritual care; & Telehealth.
Roberta Duchesne, Manager, Health Services
Tracy Manuge, Facility Secretary

SHELBURNE: Roseway Hospital
Affiliated with: Nova Scotia Health Authority
PO Box 610, 1606 Lake Rd., Shelburne, NS B0T 1W0
Tel: 902-875-3011 *Fax:* 902-875-1580
www.nshealth.ca

Number of Beds: 19 beds
Population Served: 15000
Note: Programs & services include: 24 hour emergency; addiction; audiology; cardiac stress testing; continuing care; diabetes education; diagnostic; internal medicine; mental health centre; nutrition counselling; obstetrics & gynecology; occupational therapy; otolaryngology; palliative care; physiotherapy; speech therapy; & surgery.
Jodi Ybarra, Site Manager
 jybarra@swndha.nshealth.ca

SHERBROOKE: St. Mary's Memorial Hospital
Affiliated with: Nova Scotia Health Authority
PO Box 299, 91 Hospital Rd., Sherbrooke, NS B0J 3C0
Tel: 902-522-2882 *Fax:* 902-522-2556
www.nshealth.ca

Year Founded: 1949
Number of Beds: 6 beds
Note: Programs & services include: diabetes education; diagnostic imaging; EKG; emergency; foot care clinic; hospice & palliative care;

laboratory; nutrition & dietetic counselling; physiotherapy; social work; & Telehealth.
Debbie MacIsaac, Facility Manager
 debbie.macisaac@nshealth.ca

SPRINGHILL: All Saints Springhill Hospital (ASSH)
Affiliated with: Nova Scotia Health Authority
Also Known As: All Saints Hospital
10 Princess St., Springhill, NS B0M 1X0
Tel: 902-597-3773 *Fax:* 902-597-3440
www.nshealth.ca

Year Founded: 1963
Number of Beds: 10 restorative care beds; 10 inpatient addictions treatment beds; 8 transitional care beds; 2 palliative care beds
Note: Programs & services include: Addiction Services In-Patient Unit; Collaborative Emergency Centre; diagnostic imaging; dialysis; laboratory; outpatient; palliative care; Primary Health Care Clinic; rehabilitative services; & restorative care.

SYDNEY: Cape Breton Regional Hospital
Affiliated with: Nova Scotia Health Authority
1482 George St., Sydney, NS B1P 1P3
Tel: 902-567-8000
www.nshealth.ca

Year Founded: 1995
Note: Programs & services include: Addictions Primary Unit; ambulatory care; bone densitometer; Cape Breton Cancer Centre; cardio/pulmonary/neuro services; clinical support; diabetes education; diagnostic imaging; emergency trauma care; laboratory; medicine; mental health & addiction; MRI; obstetrics; palliative care; pediatrics; renal dialysis; specialized intensive care; & surgery.

SYDNEY: Nova Scotia Health Authority - Cape Breton, Guysborough, & Antigonish Regional Office
Affiliated with: Nova Scotia Health Authority
235 Townsend St., 2nd Fl., Sydney, NS B1P 5E7
Tel: 902-563-2400

SYDNEY: Public Health Services
Affiliated with: Nova Scotia Health Authority
235 Townsend St., 2nd Fl., Sydney, NS B1P 5E7
Tel: 902-563-2400 *Fax:* 902-563-0508

TATAMAGOUCHE: Lillian Fraser Memorial Hospital
Affiliated with: Nova Scotia Health Authority
PO Box 40, 110 Blair Ave., Tatamagouche, NS B0K 1V0
Tel: 902-657-2382 *Fax:* 902-657-3745
www.nshealth.ca

Number of Beds: 10 beds
Note: Programs & services include: diabetes clinic; diagnostic imaging; emergency; food services; inpatient medical unit; laboratory; medical day unit; nutrition counselling; outpatient clinics; palliative care; perinatal & gynecology clinic; physiotherapy; primary care; rehabilitation; surgical clinic; & Telehealth.

TRURO: Colchester East Hants Health Centre
Affiliated with: Nova Scotia Health Authority
Former Name: Colchester Regional Hospital
600 Abenaki Rd., Truro, NS B2N 5A1
Tel: 902-893-5554 *Toll-Free:* 800-460-2110
www.nshealth.ca

Number of Beds: 98 beds
Note: Programs & services include: asthma care; blood/specimen collection; breast screening; cardiovascular; colpolscopy; coronary care; CT scan; dermatology; diabetes; diagnostic imaging; dialysis; dietary/nutrition; ECG; emergency; enterostomal therapy; general medicine; hearing & speech; intensive care; laboratory; medical day unit; mental health & addiction; occupational therapy; oncology; ophthalmology; ostomy clinic; outpatients; palliative care; perinatal; pharmacy; physiotherapy; pre-operative clinic; rehabilitation; respiratory; social work; surgery; Telehealth; water testing; women & children's health; & wound management.

TRURO: Nova Scotia Health Authority - Colchester-East Hants, Cumberland, & Pictou Regional Office
Affiliated with: Nova Scotia Health Authority
600 Abenaki Rd., Truro, NS B2N 5A1
Tel: 902-893-5820 *Fax:* 902-893-5839

WATERVILLE: Kings Regional Rehabilitation Centre
PO Box 128, 1349 County Home Rd., Waterville, NS B0P 1V0
Tel: 902-538-3103 *Fax:* 902-538-7022
info@krrc.ns.ca
www.krrc.ns.ca
Number of Beds: 199 beds
Number of Employees: 600
Note: Residential rehabilitation centre for clients with mental illness, brain injury, & physical & intellectual disabilities; offers medical, dental, social work, psychiatry, & therapy services
Joe Haverstock, Chief Executive Officer
Tracie Sarsfield-Turner, Director, Clinical Services
Kirk Fredericks, Director, Plant & Environmental Services

WINDSOR: Hants Community Hospital
Affiliated with: Nova Scotia Health Authority
89 Payzant Dr., Windsor, NS B0N 2T0
Tel: 902-792-2000
www.nshealth.ca
Number of Beds: 24 general beds; 14 transitional beds
Note: Programs & services include: acute medical; ambulatory day surgical care; ambulatory specialty consultation clinics; cardiac investigation; chronic pain clinic; community mental health & addictions; diagnostic imaging; laboratory; Nova Scotia Hearing & Speech Clinic; occupational therapy; physiotherapy; public health; respiratory; social work; & Well Womens Clinics.
Dr. Mike Clory, Site Chief
Sherri Parker, Director, Health Services

WOLFVILLE: Eastern Kings Memorial Community Health Centre
Affiliated with: Nova Scotia Health Authority
Former Name: Eastern Kings Community Health Centre
23 Earnscliffe Ave., Wolfville, NS B4P 1X4
Tel: 902-542-2266 *Fax:* 902-542-4619
www.nshealth.ca

YARMOUTH: Yarmouth Regional Hospital
Affiliated with: Nova Scotia Health Authority
60 Vancouver St., Yarmouth, NS B5A 2P5
Tel: 902-742-3541 *Fax:* 902-742-0369
www.nshealth.ca
Number of Beds: 124 beds
Population Served: 61000
Note: Programs & services include: addictions & withdrawal management services; ambulatory care; breast screening; Cancer Care Centre; cardiovascular program; chronic pain clinic; continuing care; diabetes education; diagnostic imaging; emergency; falls prevention; family wellness; kidney clinic; intensive care unit; laboratory; mental health; obstetrics; occupational therapy; palliative care; physiotherapy; pre-natal clinic; public health; recreational therapy; renal dialysis; respiratory therapy; stroke program; surgery; & Veterans Place.
Chris Newell, Site Manager

NUNAVUT

ARCTIC BAY: Arctic Bay Health Centre
PO Box 60, Arctic Bay, NU X0A 0A0
Tel: 867-439-8816 *Fax:* 867-439-8315

ARVIAT: Arviat Health Centre
PO Box 510, Arviat, NU X0C 0E0
Tel: 867-857-3100 *Fax:* 867-857-3149
Sandy Ranahan, Nurse Manager

BAKER LAKE: Baker Lake Health Centre
PO Box 120, Baker Lake, NU X0C 0A0
Tel: 867-793-2816 *Fax:* 867-793-2812

CAMBRIDGE BAY: Cambridge Bay Health Centre
PO Box 83, Cambridge Bay, NU X0B 0C0
Tel: 867-983-2531 *Fax:* 867-983-2262
www.cambridgebay.ca
Number of Beds: 2 beds

CAPE DORSET: Cape Dorset Health Centre
PO Box 180, Cape Dorset, NU X0A 0C0
Tel: 867-897-8820

CHESTERFIELD INLET: Chesterfield Inlet Health Centre
PO Box 9, Chesterfield Inlet, NU X0C 0B0
Tel: 867-898-9968 *Fax:* 867-898-9122

CLYDE RIVER: Clyde River Health Centre
PO Box 40, Clyde River, NU X0A 0E0
Tel: 867-924-6377 *Fax:* 867-924-6244

CORAL HARBOUR: Coral Harbour Health Centre
PO Box 120, Coral Harbour, NU X0C 0C0
Tel: 867-925-9916 *Fax:* 867-925-8380

GJOA HAVEN: Gjoa Haven Kativik Health Centre
General Delivery, Gjoa Haven, NU X0B 1J0
Tel: 867-360-7441 *Fax:* 867-360-6110

GRISE FJORD: Grise Fjord Health Centre
PO Box 81, Grise Fjord, NU X0A 0J0
Tel: 867-980-9923 *Fax:* 867-980-9067

HALL BEACH: Hall Beach Health Centre
General Delivery, Hall Beach, NU X0A 0K0
Tel: 867-928-8827 *Fax:* 867-928-8847

IGLOOLIK: Igloolik Health Centre
PO Box 240, Igloolik, NU X0A 0L0
Tel: 867-934-2100 *Fax:* 867-934-2149

IQALUIT: Iqaluit Public Health Clinic
PO Box 1000, Iqaluit, NU X0A 0H0
Tel: 867-979-5306

IQALUIT: Qikiqtani General Hospital
1 Ring Rd., Iqaluit, NU X0A 0H0
Tel: 867-975-8600
www.gov.nu.ca/health/information/qikiqtani-general-hospital
Number of Beds: 35 beds
Population Served: 16000
Note: Programs & services include: allergist; cardiology; dermatology; ENT (ear, nose & throat specialist); internal medicine; gynaecology; neurology; ophthalmology; orthopaedics; paediatric cardiology, orthopedics, neurology; respirology; rheumatology; & urology.

KIMMIRUT: Kimmirut Health Centre
PO Box 30, Kimmirut, NU X0A 0N0
Tel: 867-939-2217 *Fax:* 867-939-2068

KUGAARUK: St. Theresa Kugaaruk Health Centre
General Delivery, Kugaaruk, NU X0B 1K0
Tel: 867-769-6441 *Fax:* 867-769-6059

KUGLUKTUK: Kugluktuk Health Centre
PO Box 288, Kugluktuk, NU X0E 0E0
Tel: 867-982-4531 *Fax:* 867-982-3115

NAUJAAT: Naujaat Health Centre
General Delivery, Naujaat, NU X0C 0H0
Tel: 867-462-9916 *Fax:* 867-462-4212
Number of Beds: 2 beds
Population Served: 1082

PANGNIRTUNG: Pangnirtung Health Centre
PO Box 454, Pangnirtung, NU X0A 0R0
Tel: 867-473-8977 *Fax:* 867-473-8519
www.pangnirtung.ca/home
Note: Specialty: General health care by registered nurses; Individual counseling & referral; Massage therapy; Workshops for stress relief

POND INLET: Pond Inlet Health Centre
PO Box 280, Pond Inlet, NU X0A 0S0
Tel: 867-899-7500 *Fax:* 867-899-7538
Year Founded: 2004
Population Served: 1290
Note: Comprehensive health care. Number of employees: 20
Sherry Parks, Supervisor, Health Programs

QIKIQTARJUAQ: Qikiqtarjuaq Health Centre
PO Box 911, Qikiqtarjuaq, NU X0A 0B0
Tel: 867-927-8916 *Fax:* 867-927-8217

QIKIQTARJUAQ: Qikiqtarjuaq Health Centre
PO Box 911, Qikiqtarjuaq, NU X0A 0B0
Tel: 867-927-8916 *Fax:* 867-927-8217

RANKIN INLET: Rankin Inlet Health Centre
PO Box 008, Rankin Inlet, NU X0C 0G0
Tel: 867-645-8300 *Fax:* 867-645-8304

RESOLUTE: Resolute Bay Health Centre
PO Box 180, Resolute, NU X0A 0V0
Tel: 867-252-3844 *Fax:* 867-252-3601

SANIKILUAQ: Sanikiluaq Health Centre
PO Box 157, Sanikiluaq, NU X0A 0W0
Tel: 867-266-8965 *Fax:* 867-266-8802

Note: Provides general health care, counseling & referral. Services in Inuktitut & English

TALOYOAK: Taloyoak Judy Hill Memorial Health Centre
General Delivery, Taloyoak, NU X0E 1B0
Tel: 867-561-5111 *Fax:* 867-561-6906

Number of Employees: 5

WHALE COVE: Whale Cove Health Centre
PO Box 45, Whale Cove, NU X0C 1J0
Tel: 867-896-9916 *Fax:* 867-896-9115

ONTARIO

AJAX: Carea Community Health Centre - Ajax Office
Former Name: The Youth Centre; Barbara Black Centre for Youth Resources
#5, 360 Bayly St., Ajax, ON L1S 1P1
Tel: 905-428-1212 *Fax:* 905-428-9151
info@careachc.ca
www.careachc.ca
Social Media: www.facebook.com/CareaCHC; twitter.com/careachc

Note: Offers community health & wellness programs, as well as primary care, counselling, & chronic disease management services
Andrea Peckham, Chair

AJAX: Central East Local Health Integration Network
Also Known As: Central East LHIN
Harwood Plaza, #204A, 314 Harwood Ave. South, Ajax, ON L1S 2J1
Tel: 905-427-5497 *Fax:* 905-427-9659
Toll-Free: 866-804-5446
centraleast@lhins.on.ca
www.centraleastlhin.on.ca
Social Media: twitter.com/CentralEastLHIN

Year Founded: 2005
Area Served: From Victoria Park to Algonquin Park; 16,673 sq km
Population Served: 1400000
Louis O'Brien, Board Chair
Deborah Hammons, Chief Executive Officer
Stewart Sutley, Senior Director, System Finance & Performance Management

AJAX: Rouge Valley Ajax & Pickering
Lakeridge Health
Affiliated with: Central East Local Health Integration Network
580 Harwood Ave. South, Ajax, ON L1S 2J4
Tel: 905-683-2320
patientrelations@rougevalley.ca
www.rougevalley.ca
Social Media: www.facebook.com/rougevalleyhealthsystem;
twitter.com/RougeValley; www.youtube.com/RougeValleyHealthSys
Number of Beds: 172 beds
Note: Programs & services include: clinical nutrition; diabetes education; emergency; mental health; obstetrics; Ontario Breast Screening Program; paediatrics; physiotherapy; regional cardiac care; speech-language pathology; & surgery.
Andrée Robichaud, President & CEO, RVHS
Dr. Naresh Mohan, Chief of Staff, RVHS
Amelia McCutcheon, Chief Nursing Executive & Vice-President, Patient Services, RHVS
Leigh Duncan, Director, Government Relations & Communications, RHVS
647-294-8885, lduncan@rougevalley.ca

ALEXANDRIA: Glengarry Memorial Hospital (HGMH)/Hôpital Glengarry Memorial
Affiliated with: Champlain Local Health Integration Network
20260 County Road 43, Alexandria, ON K0C 1A0
Tel: 613-525-2222
www.hgmh.on.ca

Year Founded: 1965
Note: Programs & services include: chronic care; dermatology; diabetes; dietary; foot care; gastroenterology; internal medicine; laboratory; neurology; obstetrics/gynecology; orthopedic medicine/surgery; orthotics; physiotherapy; psychiatry; pulmonary function; radiology; rehabilitation; surgery; & urology.
Linda Morrow, Chief Executive Officer
Dr. N. Kucherepa, Chief of Staff
Shelley Coleman, Chief Nursing Officer & Vice-President, Clinical Services

ALLISTON: Stevenson Memorial Hospital (SMH)
Affiliated with: Central Local Health Integration Network
PO Box 4000, 200 Fletcher Cres., Alliston, ON L9R 1W7
Tel: 705-435-3377
www.smhosp.on.ca
Social Media: twitter.com/Stevenson_News;
www.youtube.com/channel/UC9yZ4YnEocvc48T35ptQPCw
Year Founded: 1928
Number of Beds: 32 acute beds
Note: Programs & services include: acute care; day surgery; diagnostic imaging; dialysis; emergency; laboratory; mental health; obstetrics & gynecology; outpatient clinics; pharmacy; & physiotherapy/occupational therapy.
Jody Levac, President & CEO
Dr. Oswaldo C. Ramirez, Chief of Staff

ALMONTE: Almonte General Hospital (AGH)
Affiliated with: Champlain Local Health Integration Network
75 Spring St., Almonte, ON K0A 1A0
Tel: 613-256-2500 *Fax:* 613-256-8549
tmclelland@agh-fvm.com
www.almontegeneral.com
Number of Beds: 52 beds (21 medical & surgical, 5 obstetrical, & 26 chronic care)
Population Served: 11000
Note: Programs & services include: acute care; cardiology; complex continuing care; day hospital; dental surgery; diabetic education; emergency; geriatric assessment; long-term care program; obstetrics; occupational therapy; outpatient service clinics; physiotherapy; rehabilitation; respite care/convalescent care; & sexual assault support/treatment.
Mary Wilson Trider, President & CEO
613-256-2514, mwilsontrider@agh-fvm.com
Dr. Melissa Forbes, Chief of Staff
613-256-2514, mforbes@agh-fvm.com
Heather Garnett, Chief Nursing Officer & Vice-President, Patient & Resident Services
613-256-2514, hgarnett@agh-fvm.com

ARMSTRONG: NorWest Community Health Centre - Armstrong Site
Affiliated with: North West Local Health Integration Network
PO Box 104, Armstrong, ON P0T 1A0
Tel: 807-583-1145 *Fax:* 807-583-1147
www.norwestchc.org/armstrong.htm
Social Media: www.facebook.com/NorWestCHC

Wendy Talbot, CEO

ARNPRIOR: Arnprior & District Memorial Hospital
Affiliated with: Arnprior Regional Health
350 John St. North, Arnprior, ON K7S 2P6
Tel: 613-623-3166 *Fax:* 613-623-4844
www.arnpriorhospital.com

Number of Beds: 105 beds
Population Served: 30000
Number of Employees: 300
Note: Hospital Specialties: Emergency services; Diagnostic imaging; Acute care; Ontario Breast Screening Program; Diabetes clinic; Physiotherapy; Speech therapy; Urotherapy; Palliative care
Eric Hanna, President & CEO
eric.hanna@arnpriorhealth.com

ARNPRIOR: Arnprior Regional Health (ARH)
350 John St. North, Arnprior, ON K7S 2P6
Tel: 613-623-3166
www.arnpriorregionalhealth.ca

Year Founded: 2005
Note: Acute, long-term & other healthcare services
Barbara Darlow, Board Chair
Eric Hanna, President & CEO
Dr. Christine Schriver, Chief of Staff
Susan Leach, Chief Nursing Executive & Vice-President,
  Patient/Resident Services
Ron Marcotte, Vice-President, Human Resources
Wendy Knechtel, Manager, Communications

ATIKOKAN: Atikokan General Hospital (AGH)
Affiliated with: North West Local Health Integration Network
PO Box 2490, 120 Dorothy St., Atikokan, ON P0T 1C0
Tel: 807-597-4215 *Fax:* 807-597-4305
www.aghospital.on.ca
Social Media: www.facebook.com/AtikokanGeneralHospital;
www.twitter.com/AtikokanHosp;
www.linkedin.com/company/atikokan-general-hospital
Number of Beds: 41 beds
Number of Employees: 100
Note: Programs & services include: emergency services; diagnostic services; acute care; cardiac care; rehabilitation services; counselling & addictions program; diabetic counselling; complex continuing care; long-term care
Doug Moynihan, Chief Executive Officer
  moynihand@aghospital.on.ca
Kim Cross, CFO & Vice-President, Corporate Services
  crossk@aghospital.on.ca
Esther Richards, Chief Nursing Officer
  richardse@aghospital.on.ca

BANCROFT: QHC North Hastings Hospital
Quinte Health Care
Affiliated with: South East Local Health Integration Network
Former Name: North Hastings District Hospital
PO Box 157, 1-H Manor Lane, Bancroft, ON K0L 1C0
Tel: 613-332-2825 *Fax:* 613-332-3847
www.qhc.on.ca
Social Media: www.facebook.com/173689537296;
twitter.com/QuinteHealth; www.youtube.com/QuinteHealthCare
Year Founded: 1927
Note: Part of the North Hastings Health Centre Campus, which includes: six-chair dialysis unit; 110-bed long-term care facility; Family Health Team; public health; Community Care Access Centre; & Community Care North Hastings.
Mary Clare Egberts, President & CEO, Quinte Health Care
Dr. Dick Zoutman, Chief of Staff, Quinte Health Care
Carol Smith Romeril, Chief Nursing Officer, Quinte Health Care

BARRIE: Barrie Community Health Centre
490 Huronia Rd., Barrie, ON L4N 6M2
Tel: 705-734-9690 *Fax:* 705-734-0239
www.bchc.ca

Note: Provides community-focused health promotion, illness prevention, & primary care services. Services provided by physicians, registered nurses, social workers, physiotherapists, & dietitians. North Innisfil office located at: 902 Lockhart Rd., 705-431-9245.
Christine Colcy, Executive Director

BARRIE: CCAC North Simcoe Muskoka
#100, 15 Sperling Dr., Barrie, ON L4M 6K9
Tel: 705-721-8010 *Toll-Free:* 888-721-2222 ex
healthcareathome.ca/nsm
Social Media: twitter.com/NSMCCAC; www.youtube.com/ccacnsm

Note: With offices in Barrie & Huntsville, provides health & personal support services for individuals living independently at home or making the transition to alternative care settings; information & referral, advocacy.

BARRIE: Royal Victoria Regional Health Centre (RVH)
Affiliated with: North Simcoe Muskoka Local Health Integration Network
Former Name: Royal Victoria Hospital
201 Georgian Dr., Barrie, ON L4M 6M2
Tel: 705-728-9802 *Fax:* 705-792-3324
TTY: 705-739-5618
www.rvh.on.ca

Year Founded: 1897
Number of Beds: 299 beds
Number of Employees: 2500
Note: Programs & services include: cardiac; cardio-respiratory; intensive care; chronic disease management; renal services; education; emergency; Home First; imaging; laboratory; medicine; mental health & addictions; internal medicine; pharmacy; rehabilitation & acute geriatrics; stroke program; surgery; telemedicine; & women's & children's program. Has 350 physicians on staff.
Janice Skot, President & CEO
  skotj@rvh.on.ca
Nancy Savage, Executive Vice-President, Patient & Family Experience
  savagen@rvh.on.ca
Dr. Chris Tebbutt, Vice-President, Academic & Medical Affairs
  tebbuttc@rvh.on.ca
Treva McCumber, Chief Nursing Executive & Vice-President, Patient Programs
  mccumbert@rvh.on.ca

BARRY'S BAY: St. Francis Memorial Hospital (SFMH)
Affiliated with: Champlain Local Health Integration Network
PO Box 129, 7 St. Francis Memorial Dr., Barry's Bay, ON K0J 1B0
Tel: 613-756-3044 *Fax:* 613-756-0168
www.sfmhosp.com
Year Founded: 1960
Number of Beds: 20 beds
Population Served: 10000
Note: Programs & services include: active care unit; addictions treatment; bone density; complex continuing care; diabetic clinic; diagnostic imaging; discharge planning; ear, nose & throat; emergency; foot care clinic; general surgery; hemodialysis & nephrology; holter monitor; internal medicine; Meals on Wheels; medical laboratories; OBSP/mammography; Ontario Breast Screening Program; orthotist; palliative care; pastoral care; physiotherapy; pre-op clinics; recreation; respiratory therapy; St. Francis Health Centre; Telemedicine; x-ray; & ultrasound.
Randy Penney, Chief Executive Officer
  613-432-4851
Gregory McLeod, Chief Operating Officer
  613-756-3044
Mary-Ellen Harris, Director, Patient Care Services
  613-756-3044

BEARSKIN LAKE: Bearskin Lake Nursing Station
Affiliated with: North West Local Health Integration Network
PO Box 56, Bearskin Lake, ON P0V 1E0
Tel: 807-363-2582 *Fax:* 807-363-1021

Note: Programs & services include: diabetes clinic; health awareness workshop; alcohol/drug abuse workshop; communicable diseases clinic.
Wesley Nothing, Director, Health

BELLEVILLE: CCAC South East - Belleville Branch Office
Bayview Mall, 470 Dundas St. East, Belleville, ON K8N 1G1
Tel: 613-966-3530 *Fax:* 613-966-0996
Toll-Free: 800-668-0901
healthcareathome.ca
Jacqueline Redmond, CEO

BELLEVILLE: QHC Belleville General Hospital
Quinte Health Care
Affiliated with: South East Local Health Integration Network
265 Dundas St. East, Belleville, ON K8N 5A9
Tel: 613-969-7400 *Fax:* 613-968-8234
Toll-Free: 800-483-2811
www.qhc.on.ca
Social Media: www.facebook.com/173689537296;
twitter.com/QuinteHealth; www.youtube.com/QuinteHealthCare
Year Founded: 1886
Number of Beds: 206 beds
Note: Programs & services include: cardiology; complex continuing care; children's treatment centre; clinical nutrition; diabetes education; emergency; intensive care; laboratory; maternal/child service; medical day clinic; medical service; oncology; outpatient clinics; orthopaedics; pharmacy; psychiatry/mental health; radiology/diagnostic services; rehabilitation; stroke (District Stroke Centre & stroke prevention clinic); surgery; & symptom management/palliative care.

SECTION II:
General Resources

Mary Clare Egberts, President & CEO, Quinte Health Care
Dr. Dick Zoutman, Chief of Staff, Quinte Health Care
Carol Smith Romeril, Chief Nursing Officer & Vice-President, Quinte
  Health Care

BELLEVILLE: South East Local Health Integration Network
Also Known As: South East LHIN
71 Adam St., Belleville, ON K8N 5K3
                    Tel: 613-967-0196 *Fax:* 613-967-1341
                              Toll-Free: 866-831-5446
                    southeast.communications@lhins.on.ca
                              www.southeastlhin.on.ca
              Social Media: twitter.com/SouthEastLHIN;
                    www.youtube.com/user/SouthEastLHIN

Year Founded: 2005
Area Served: South East region of Ontario
Population Served: 10000
Note: The South East Local Health Integration Network plans,
manages, & funds the health care system at the local & regional levels.
Includes 7 hospitals, 37 long-term care homes, 1 Community Care
Access Centre, 5 Community Health Centres, 4 Addictions & Mental
Health Agencies, & 22 Community Support Agencies. The South East
region extends from Brighton on the west to Prescott & Cardinal on the
east, north to Perth & Smith Falls, & back to Bancroft.
Donna Segal, Board Chair
Paul Huras, Chief Executive Officer
Sherry Kennedy, Chief Operating Officer
Steve Goetz, Director, Performance Optimization
Paula Heinemann, Controller & Director, Corporate Services
Larry Hofmeister, Director, HSP Funding & Allocations
Michael Spinks, Chief Knowledge Officer

BLIND RIVER: North Shore Health Network - Blind River Site
(BRDHC)/Pavillion Santé du District de Blind River
Affiliated with: North East Local Health Integration Network
Former Name: Blind River District Health Centre; Robb Hospital;
St. Joseph's General Hospital
PO Box 970, 525 Causley St., Blind River, ON P0R 1B0
                    Tel: 705-356-2265 *Fax:* 705-356-1220
                              www.nshn.care

Year Founded: 1928
Number of Beds: 16 acute care beds
Number of Employees: 185
Note: Programs & services include: acute care; community support
services; diabetes; diagnostic imaging; dietitian; emergency &
ambulatory care; exercise & falls prevention; laboratory; long-term care;
oncology; & pharmacy. Has 50 physicians on staff.
Connie Lee, Interim Chief Executive Officer
Dr. Mark Fowler, Chief of Staff
Jennifer Stanton Smith, Chief Financial Officer

BOWMANVILLE: Lakeridge Health - Bowmanville Site
Affiliated with: Central East Local Health Integration Network
47 Liberty St. South, Bowmanville, ON L1C 2N4
                    Tel: 905-623-3331
                    patientrelations@lakeridgehealth.on.ca
                              www.lakeridgehealth.on.ca
              Social Media: www.facebook.com/LakeridgeHealth;
              twitter.com/lakeridgehealth; www.youtube.com/lakeridgehealth

Note: Programs & services include: cancer care; diagnostic centre;
emergency; mental health; & senior's health.
Matthew Anderson, President & CEO, Lakeridge Health
  905-576-8711
Dr. Tony Stone, Chief of Staff, Lakeridge Health
  905-576-8711
Leslie Motz, Chief Nursing Executive, Lakeridge Health
  905-576-8711

BRACEBRIDGE: South Muskoka Memorial Hospital Site
Muskoka Algonquin Healthcare (MAHC)
Affiliated with: North Simcoe Muskoka Local Health Integration
Network
75 Ann St., Bracebridge, ON P1L 2E4
                    Tel: 705-645-4404 *Fax:* 705-645-4594
                              www.mahc.ca
Year Founded: 1949
Number of Beds: 43 acute care beds; 16 complex continuing care beds
Number of Employees: 645

Note: Programs & services include: cardio-respiratory; cancer
supportive care & infusion clinic; clinical nutrition; complex continuing
care; diabetes education; diagnostic imaging; discharge planning;
emergency; fracture clinic; general surgery/endoscopy; gynaecological
surgery; intensive care; laboratory; obstetrics; palliative care; paediatric
clinic; pharmacy; rehabilitation; seniors assessment; speech-language
pathology; spiritual care; telemedicine; & urology. Muskoka Algonquin
Healthcare employs around 85 physicians.
Natalie Bubela, Chief Executive Officer, MAHC
  705-789-0022
Dr. Biagio Iannantuono, Interim Chief of Staff, MAHC
  705-789-2311
Karen Fleming, Chief Quality & Nursing Executive, MAHC
  705-645-4404

BRAMPTON: Brampton Civic Hospital
William Osler Health System
Affiliated with: Central West Local Health Integration Network
Also Known As: William Osler Health Centre
2100 Bovaird Dr. East, Brampton, ON L6R 3J7
                    Tel: 905-494-2120
                              www.williamoslerhs.ca
              Social Media: www.facebook.com/WilliamOslerHealth;
              twitter.com/OslerHealth; www.youtube.com/WilliamOslerTV;
              www.linkedin.com/company/william-osler-health-system
Year Founded: 2007
Number of Beds: 608 beds
Note: Programs & services include: cancer care; cardiac care; complex
continuing care; critical care; diabetes care; diagnostic imaging;
emergency; general & internal medicine; kidney care; laboratories;
mental health & addictions; naturopathic care; palliative care;
rehabilitation services; respirology; seniors' care; surgical services; &
women's & children's services.
Joanne Flewwelling, Interim President & CEO, William Osler Health
  System

BRAMPTON: CCAC Central West
199 County Court Blvd., Brampton, ON L6W 4P3
                    Tel: 905-796-0040 *Fax:* 905-796-5620
                              Toll-Free: 888-733-1177
                              healthcareathome.ca

Cathy Hecimovich, CEO

BRAMPTON: Central West Local Health Integration Network
Also Known As: Central West LHIN
#300, 8 Nelson St. West, Brampton, ON L6X 4J2
                    Tel: 905-455-1281 *Fax:* 905-455-0427
                              Toll-Free: 866-370-5446
                    centralwest@lhins.on.ca
                              www.centralwestlhin.on.ca

Year Founded: 2005
Area Served: From northern Dufferin County to northern Peel Region
Population Served: 840000
Note: Fifty health service providers in central west Ontario including a
community care access centre, 2 community health centres, 14
community support services, 2 hospitals (three sites), 23 long-term
care homes, & 8 mental health & addiction agencies.
Maria Britto, Board Chair
Scott McLeod, Chief Executive Officer
  scott.mcleod@lhins.on.ca
Kim Delahunt, Senior Director, Health System Integration
  kim.delahunt@lhins.on.ca
Brock Hovey, Senior Director, Health System Performance
  brock.hovey@lhins.on.ca
Neil McIntosh, Director, Performance & Accountability
  neil.mcintosh@lhins.on.ca
Tom Miller, Director, Communications & Community Engagement
  tom.miller@lhins.on.ca
Elizabeth Salvaterra, Director, ER/ALC & Decision Support
  elizabeth.salvaterra@lhins.on.ca

BRANTFORD: Brantford General Hospital
Brant Community Healthcare System
Affiliated with: Hamilton Niagara Haldimand Brant Local Health
Integration Network
Also Known As: The Brantford General
200 Terrace Hill St., Brantford, ON N3R 1G9

Tel: 519-751-5544
www.bchsys.org
Social Media: www.facebook.com/bchsys; twitter.com/BCHSYS;
www.youtube.com/user/bchsys2011;
www.linkedin.com/company/brantford-general-hospital
Year Founded: 1885
Number of Beds: 265 beds
Number of Employees: 1200
Note: Programs & services include: acute care; Brant Community
Cancer Clinic; critical care; CT scan; emergency; gynaecology; mental
health; obstetrics; paediatrics; S.C. Johnson Dialysis Clinic; & surgery.
Has 175 physicians on staff. Brant Community Healthcare System is
affiliated with the Michael G. DeGroote School of Medicine, McMaster
University.
James Hornell, President & CEO, Brant Community Healthcare System
jim.hornell@bchsys.org
Dr. Christopher O'Brien, Chief of Staff, Brant Community Healthcare
System
christopher.obrien@bchsys.org
Lina Rinaldi, Chief Operating Officer & Chief Nursing Executive, Brant
Community Healthcare System
lina.rinaldi@bchsys.org
MaryLou Toop, Interim Chief Financial Officer, Brant Community
Healthcare System
marylou.toop@bchsys.org

BRANTFORD: CCAC Hamilton Niagara Haldimand Brant - Brant
Branch Office
Building 4, #4, 195 Henry St., Brantford, ON N3S 5C9
Tel: 519-759-7752 Fax: 519-759-7130
Toll-Free: 800-810-0000
healthcareathome.ca

Note: Head office for the region
Melody Miles, CEO

BROCKVILLE: Brockville General Hospital (BGH)
Affiliated with: South East Local Health Integration Network
75 Charles St., Brockville, ON K6V 1S8
Tel: 613-345-5649 Fax: 613-345-3529
www.bgh-on.ca
Social Media: www.facebook.com/brockvillegeneralhospital;
twitter.com/BrockvilleGener; www.linkedin.com/company/5091498
Year Founded: 1885
Number of Beds: 140+ beds
Population Served: 99000
Number of Employees: 830
Note: Programs & services include: cardiology diagnostics; children's
speech & language therapy; diagnostic imaging; early language;
emergency; gynecology; inpatient rehabilitation; infant & child
development program; mental health; Ontario Breast Screening
Program; Ontario Telehealth Network; outpatient paediatric
physiotherapy; pain management; & stroke prevention. BGH's Garden
Street Site provides palliative care services.
Jeanette Despatie, Acting Chief Executive Officer
desje@bgh-on.ca
Dr. David Goldstein, Chief of Staff
golda@bgh-on.ca
Julie Caffin, Chief Nursing Officer & Vice-President
cafju@bgh-on.ca

BURLINGTON: CCAC Hamilton Niagara Haldimand Brant -
Burlington Branch Office
440 Elizabeth St., 4th Fl., Burlington, ON L7R 2M1
Tel: 905-639-5228 Fax: 905-639-8704
Toll-Free: 800-810-0000
healthcareathome.ca

Melody Miles, CEO

BURLINGTON: Joseph Brant Hospital
Affiliated with: Hamilton Niagara Haldimand Brant Local Health
Integration Network
Former Name: Joseph Brant Memorial Hospital
1230 North Shore Blvd., Burlington, ON L7S 1W7
Tel: 905-632-3737 Fax: 905-336-6480
www.josephbranthospital.ca
Social Media: www.facebook.com/JosephBrantHospital;
twitter.com/Jo_Brant; www.linkedin.com/company/joseph-brant-hospital
Number of Beds: 245 beds
Number of Employees: 1400
Note: Programs & services include: community mental health;
emergency; maternal & child; outpatient clinics; paediatric & gestational
diabetes clinic; palliative care (outpatient); & Wellness House. Has
175+ physicians on staff.
Eric J. Vandewall, President & CEO
ceo@josephbranthospital.ca
Dr. Wes Stephen, Chief of Staff

CAMBRIDGE: Cambridge Memorial Hospital
Affiliated with: Waterloo Wellington Local Health Integration
Network
Former Name: South Waterloo Memorial Hospital
700 Coronation Blvd., Cambridge, ON N1R 3G2
Tel: 519-621-2330 Fax: 519-740-4938
TTY: 519-621-9180
information@cmh.org
www.cmh.org
Year Founded: 1953
Note: Programs & services include: clinical nutrition & diabetes
education; diagnostic imaging; emergency; infection control; inpatient
surgery & ambulatory surgical services; laboratory & CRU;
medicine/medical day care; mental health (inpatient & outpatient);
perioperative; pharmacy; rehabilitation, Allied Health, seniors & COPD;
& women's & children's health.
Patrick Gaskin, Chief Executive Officer
519-621-2330
Dr. Kunuk Rhee, Chief of Staff
519-621-2330
Mike Prociw, Chief Financial Officer
519-621-2330
Sandra Hett, Chief Nursing Executive & Vice-President, Clinical
Programs
519-621-2330

CAMBRIDGE: Langs Farm Village Association
1145 Concession Rd., Cambridge, ON N3H 4L5
Tel: 519-653-1470 Fax: 519-653-6277
info@langs.org
www.langs.org
William Davidson, Executive Director
519-653-1470 ext 236, billd@langs.org
Kerry-Lynn Wilkie, Director, Health Link
519-653-1470 ext 234, kerrylynnw@langs.org

CAMPBELLFORD: Campbellford Memorial Hospital (CMH)
Affiliated with: Central East Local Health Integration Network
146 Oliver Rd., Campbellford, ON K0L 1L0
Tel: 705-653-1140 Fax: 705-653-4371
info@cmh.ca
www.cmh.ca
Social Media: www.facebook.com/cmhospitalfoundation;
twitter.com/cmhfoundation; www.youtube.com/cmhfoundation
Number of Beds: 34 beds
Population Served: 30000
Note: Programs & services include: cardiac/diabetes education;
emergency; laboratory; mammography; mental health; nursing care;
palliative care; physiotherapy (inpatient); surgery; & x-ray, bone mineral
density & ultrasound.
Brad Hilker, President & CEO
705-653-1140, bhilker@cmh.ca
Jan Raine, Chief Nursing Officer
705-653-1140, jraine@cmh.ca

CARLETON PLACE: Carleton Place & District Memorial Hospital (CPDMH)
Affiliated with: Champlain Local Health Integration Network
211 Lake Ave. East, Carleton Place, ON K7C 1J4
Tel: 613-257-2200 *Fax:* 613-257-3026
info@carletonplacehosp.com
www.carletonplacehospital.ca

Year Founded: 1955
Population Served: 25000
Note: Programs & services include: inpatient services (pastoral care & palliative care); outpatient services (dietitian, laboratory, physiotherapy, sleep lab, speech & language therapy, surgery, & Telemedicine); diagnostic (cardiac diagnostics, loop monitoring, radiography, & ultrasound); & emergency.
Mary Wilson Trider, President & CEO
  mwilsontrider@cpdmh.ca
Dr. Scott Higham, Chief of Staff
  chiefofstaff@cpdmh.ca

CHAPLEAU: Chapleau Health Services (SSCHS)/Services de sante de Chapleau
Affiliated with: North East Local Health Integration Network
6 Broomhead Rd., Chapleau, ON P0M 1K0
Tel: 705-864-1520 *Fax:* 705-864-0449
chapleauhr@sschs.ca
www.sschs.ca

Number of Beds: 14 acute care beds at Chapleau General Hospital; 19 long term care beds, 4 chronic care beds, & 2 respite beds at the Bignucolo Residence
Note: Programs & services include: emergency services; acute care; occupational therapy; rehabilitation services; adult mental health services; counselling; services for the for the developmentally disabled; diabetes education; community services, such as Meals on Wheels, home support services & lifeline; operation of a nursing station in Foleyet; long term care; chronic care; & respite care.
Gail Bignucolo, Chief Executive Officer
  705-864-3050
Dr. Kendra Saari, Chief of Staff

CHATHAM: CCAC Erie St. Clair
PO Box 306, 712 Richmond St., Chatham, ON N7M 5K4
Tel: 519-436-2222 *Toll-Free:* 888-447-4468
healthcareathome.ca

Note: Head Office located at the Chatham-Kent branch, with other branch offices located in Sarnia & Windsor. Provides access to in-home health & personal support services to help individuals live independently at home, & assists with the transition to long term care when living at home is no longer possible
Cathy Kelly, Interim CEO

CHATHAM: Chatham-Kent Health Alliance (CKHA)
Affiliated with: Erie St. Clair Local Health Integration Network
PO Box 2030, 80 Grand Ave. West, Chatham, ON N7M 5L9
Tel: 519-352-6400
www.ckha.on.ca
Social Media: www.facebook.com/ckhamedia; twitter.com/ckhamedia; www.youtube.com/ckhamedia

Year Founded: 1998
Number of Beds: 200+ beds (total for both CKHA sites)
Number of Employees: 1350
Note: Programs & services include: adult & pediatric day surgery; ambulatory care; arthritis & stroke aquatic program; bone mineral densitometry; cardiac; chemotherapy/oncology; chiropody clinic; chronic disease management; continence clinic; coronary artery disease clinic; CT scan; diabetes education; dialysis; district stroke centre; echocardiography; emergency; EMG; endoscopy; fluoroscopy; general radiography; general surgery; gynaecology; health education; inpatient family medicine; inpatient surgical unit; integrated acute stroke unit; intensive care; mammography; mental health & addictions; MRI; nuclear medicine; nurse practitioner clinic; occupational therapy; Ontario Breast Screening Program; ophthalmology; oral surgery/dentistry; orthopedic surgery; orthotist/prosthetist; otolaryngology; outpatient hand clinic; parkinson's class; physiatry consultations/clinic; physiotherapy; progressive care; rehabilitation/complex continuing care; respiratory health; secondary stroke prevention clinic; sexual assault treatment centre; social work; speech-language pathology; supportive care & palliative care;

therapeutic recreation; transitional stroke program; ultrasound; urology; women & children's health; & wound, skin & ostomy consultations.
Affiliated with the Schulich School of Medicine - University of Western Ontario.
Lori Marshall, President & CEO
  lmarshall@ckha.on.ca
Jerome Quenneville, Chief Financial Officer
  jquenneville@ckha.on.ca
Lisa Northcott, Interim Chief Nursing Executive
  lnorthcott@ckha.on.ca

CHATHAM: Erie St. Clair Local Health Integration Network (ESC LHIN)/RLISS d'Érié St. Clair
Also Known As: Erie St. Clair LHIN
180 Riverview Dr., Chatham, ON N7M 5Z8
Tel: 519-351-5677 *Fax:* 519-351-9672
Toll-Free: 866-231-5446
www.eriestclairlhin.on.ca
Social Media: www.facebook.com/esclhin1; twitter.com/ESCLHIN; www.youtube.com/user/esclhin

Year Founded: 2006
Area Served: 7234 sq km
Population Served: 636020
Note: Serves the counties of Chatham-Kent, Sarnia/Lambton & Windsor/Essex
Martin Girash, Board Chair
Ralph Ganter, Acting Chief Executive Officer
  ralph.ganter@lhins.on.ca
Pete Crvenkovski, Director, Performance Quality & Knowledge Management
  pete.crvenkovski@lhins.on.ca
Shannon Sasseville, Director, Communications, Public Affairs & Organizational Development
  shannon.sasseville@lhins.on.ca
Jacquie Séguin, Coordinator, Performance & Finance
  jacquelin.seguin@lhins.on.ca
Julie Franchuk, Coordinator, Communications
  julie.franchuk@lhins.on.ca

CHESLEY: South Bruce Grey Health Centre - Chesley Site
Affiliated with: South West Local Health Integration Network
Former Name: Chesley & District Memorial Hospital
39 - 2nd St. SE, Chesley, ON N0G 1L0
Tel: 519-363-2340 *Fax:* 519-363-9871
info@sbghc.on.ca
www.sbghc.on.ca
Social Media: www.facebook.com/sbghc; twitter.com/SBG_HC
Year Founded: 1944
Number of Beds: 19 beds (9 acute care beds, 10 restorative care beds)
Note: Programs & services include: cardio-respiratory; diagnostic imaging; emergency department; emergency response system; inpatient medical beds; laboratory; nutrition services; outpatient clinics; palliative care; & restorative care.
Paul Rosebush, President & CEO, SBGHC
  prosebush@sbghc.on.ca
Maureen Rydall, Chief Nursing Officer, SBGHC
  mrydall@sbghc.on.ca

CLINTON: Clinton Public Hospital
Huron Perth Healthcare Alliance
Affiliated with: South West Local Health Integration Network
98 Shipley St., Clinton, ON N0M 1L0
Tel: 519-482-3440 *Toll-Free:* 888-275-1102
administration@hpha.ca
www.hpha.ca

Number of Beds: 20 acute care beds
Note: Programs & services include: ambulatory clinics; bone density; dietitian; emergency; laboratory; social work; speech language pathology; surgical daycare; ultrasound; & x-ray.
Andrew Williams, President & CEO, HPHA
  519-272-8202, andrew.williams@hpha.ca
Dr. Laurel Moore, Chief of Staff, HPHA
  519-272-8210, dr.laurel.moore@hpha.ca
Mary Cardinal, Site Administrator
  519-272-8206, mary.cardinal@hpha.ca

COBOURG: Northumberland Hills Hospital
Affiliated with: Central East Local Health Integration Network
Former Name: Northumberland Health Care Corp.
1000 DePalma Dr., Cobourg, ON K9A 5W6
Tel: 905-372-6811 *Fax:* 905-372-4243
info@nhh.ca
www.nhh.ca
Social Media: twitter.com/NorHillsHosp

Number of Beds: 137 beds
Population Served: 60000
Number of Employees: 600
Note: Programs & services include: acute care (emergency, intensive care, medical/surgical inpatient, maternal child care, & surgical); diagnostics (diagnostic imaging & women's health); outpatient care (ambulatory care, cancer & supportive care clinic, community mental health services, dialysis, & Telemedicine); & post-acute care (rehabilitation, restorative care, & palliative care).
Linda Davis, President & CEO
905-377-7755, ldavis@nhh.ca
Helen Brenner, Chief Nursing Executive & Vice-President, Patient Services
905-377-7756, hbrenner@nhh.ca
Jennifer Gillard, Director, Communications & Community Engagement
905-377-7757, jgillard@nhh.ca

COCHRANE: The Lady Minto Hospital
MICs Group of Health Services
Affiliated with: North East Local Health Integration Network
PO Box 4000, 241 - 8 St., Cochrane, ON P0L 1C0
Tel: 705-272-7200 *Fax:* 705-272-5486
www.micsgroup.com

Year Founded: 1915
Number of Beds: 25 acute care beds; 8 complex continuing care beds; 37 long-term care beds
Note: Programs & services include: clinical nutrition; complex continuing care; diabetes; diagnostic imaging; emergency; general surgery; laboratory; oncology; physiotherapy; respiratory therapy; telemedicine; & visiting specialty clinics. The Villa Minto chronic care wing houses a long-term care unit.
Paul Chatelain, Chief Executive Officer, MICs Group of Health Services
Karen Hill, Chief Nursing Officer, MICs Group of Health Services

COLLINGWOOD: Collingwood G&M Hospital
Affiliated with: North Simcoe Muskoka Local Health Integration Network
Former Name: Collingwood General & Marine Hospital
459 Hume St., Collingwood, ON L9Y 1W9
Tel: 705-445-2550
www.cgmh.on.ca
Social Media: www.facebook.com/CollingwoodGMHospital; twitter.com/CollingwoodHosp; www.youtube.com/user/CollingwoodGMHosp; www.linkedin.com/company/collingwood-general-and-marine-hospital
Year Founded: 1887
Number of Beds: 68 beds
Population Served: 60000
Note: Programs & services include: ambulatory care; cardio-respiratory; community mental health; diagnostic imaging; dialysis; emergency; general medicine; general surgery; intensive care; laboratory services; obstetrics/gynaecology; orthopaedic surgery; rehabilitation; & Telemedicine.
Guy Chartrand, President & CEO
705-445-2550
Dr. Michael Lisi, Chief of Staff
Michael Lacroix, CFO & Vice-President, Corporate Services

CORNWALL: CCAC North East - Cornwall Branch Office
709 Cotton Mill St., Cornwall, ON K6H 7K7
Tel: 310-2222 *Toll-Free:* 800-267-0852
healthcareathome.ca/champlain

CORNWALL: Centre de santé communautaire de l'Estrie
#6, 841, rue Sydney, Cornwall, ON K6H 3J7
Tél: 613-937-2683 *Téléc:* 613-937-2698
info@cscestrie.on.ca
www.cscestrie.on.ca
Média social: www.facebook.com/179209222111118; twitter.com/CSCE_

Note: Programmes: santé physique; santé mentale; santé communautaire; nutrition; programme d'éducation sur le diabète
Marc Bisson, Directeur général
m.bisson@cscestrie.on.ca

CORNWALL: Cornwall Community Hospital
Affiliated with: Champlain Local Health Integration Network
840 McConnell Ave., Cornwall, ON K6H 5S5
Tel: 613-938-4240 *Fax:* 613-930-4502
communications@cornwallhospital.ca
www.cornwallhospital.ca

Note: Programs & services include: addiction services; adult counselling & treatment; Arterial Blood Gas (ABG); assault & sexual abuse program; Assertive Community Treatment Team (ACTT); cardiac stress test; cardio-respiratory therapy; children's mental health; critical care; CT scan; day hospital; dentistry; diabetes education; dialysis; ECG/EEG; emergency; geriatrics; gynecology/obstetrics; inpatient psychiatric care unit; internal medicine; laboratory; MRI; mammography; mental health & addictions; neurology; nuclear medicine; ophthalmology; orthopedics; palliative care; pediatrics; psychiatry; psychogeriatric service; radiology; regional hip & knee replacement program; rehabilitation; sleep clinic; spiritual care; spirometry; stroke prevention; surgery; thrombosis; ultrasound; urology; women & children's health; & x-ray.
Jeanette Despatie, President & Chief Executive Officer
Dr. Lorne Scharf, Chief of Staff
Heather Arthur, Chief Nursing Officer & Vice-President, Patient Services

DEEP RIVER: Deep River & District Hospital (DRDH)
Affiliated with: Champlain Local Health Integration Network
117 Banting Dr., Deep River, ON K0J 1P0
Tel: 613-584-3333 *Fax:* 613-584-4920
Toll-Free: 866-571-8168
www.drdh.org
Year Founded: 1974
Note: Programs & services include: acute inpatient care; children's speech-language program; diabetes; diagnostic imaging; DRDH physiotherapy centre; emergency; laboratory; mental health; nutritional counselling; & Ontario Telemedicine.
Richard Bedard, President & CEO
Kate Kobbes, Chief Nursing Officer

DRYDEN: Dryden Regional Health Centre (DRHC)
Affiliated with: North West Local Health Integration Network
PO Box 3003, 58 Goodall St., Dryden, ON P8N 2Z6
Tel: 807-223-8201 *Fax:* 807-223-2370
TTY: 807-223-8295
www.drhc.on.ca
Year Founded: 1952
Number of Beds: 41 beds (31 acute beds & 10 chronic/rehab beds)
Note: Programs & services include: crisis response (807-223-8884); diabetes education (807-223-8208); diagnostic imaging; dietary; laboratory; mental health & addiction (807-223-6678); occupational therapy; oncology; physiotherapy; & sexual assault/domestic violence services (807-223-7427).
Dr. Stephen Viherjoki, Chief of Staff
Doreen Armstrong-Ross, Chief Nursing Executive

DUNNVILLE: Haldimand War Memorial Hospital
Affiliated with: Hamilton Niagara Haldimand Brant Local Health Integration Network
206 John St., Dunnville, ON N1A 2P7
Tel: 905-774-7431 *Fax:* 905-774-6776
kanger@hwmh.ca
www.hwmh.ca
Number of Beds: 22 acute care beds; 2 transitional beds; 4 day surgery beds; 4 assess & restore beds; 13 chronic care beds
Note: Specializes in diagnostic imaging for acute life-threatening injuries or severe illnesses, as well as treatment for non-life-threatening injuries or illnesses such as broken bones, cuts, earaches, eye injuries, fever, infections, minor burns, nose & throat issues & sprains & strains.
David Montgomery, President & CEO

DURHAM: South Bruce Grey Health Centre - Durham Site
Affiliated with: South West Local Health Integration Network
Former Name: Durham Memorial Hospital
PO Box 638, 320 College St., Durham, ON N0G 1R0
Tel: 519-369-2340 *Fax:* 519-369-6180
info@sbghc.on.ca
www.sbghc.on.ca
Social Media: www.facebook.com/sbghc; twitter.com/SBG_HC
Year Founded: 1946
Number of Beds: 10 beds
Note: Programs & services include: cardio-respiratory; diagnostic imaging; emergency department; emergency response system; inpatient medical beds; laboratory; nutrition services; outpatient clinics; palliative care; & spiritual care.
Paul Rosebush, President & CEO, SBGHC
prosebush@sbghc.on.ca
Maureen Rydall, Chief Nursing Officer, SBGHC
mrydall@sbghc.on.ca

EAR FALLS: Ear Falls Community Health Centre
Affiliated with: North West Local Health Integration Network
PO Box 250, 25 Spruce St., Ear Falls, ON P0V 1T0
Tel: 807-222-3728 *Fax:* 807-222-2053
earfallsfht@live.com

Note: Programs & services include: blood & lab work; Ministry of Transportation medical reviews; Northern Ontario Travel Grant Application.

ELLIOT LAKE: St. Joseph's General Hospital
Affiliated with: North East Local Health Integration Network
70 Spine Rd., Elliot Lake, ON P5A 1X2
Tel: 705-848-7182 *Fax:* 705-848-6239
www.sjghel.ca
Year Founded: 1958
Number of Beds: 58 beds
Note: Programs & services include: emergency; bone density; cardiology; chemotherapy; chiropody; clinical nutrition; diabetes education; ears, nose, & throat; electrocardiogram; endoscopy; gastroenterology; gerontology; intensive care; mental health; nephrology; obstetrics; ophthalmology; orthopedics; paediatrics; palliative care; pastoral care; physiotherapy; radiology; renal dialysis (as a satellite of Sudbury Regional Hospital); speech therapy; social work; surgery; urology; & ultrasound. The hospital corporation also manages St. Joseph's Manor long term care facility, & the Oaks Substance Abuse Treatment Centre.
Pierre Ozolins, Chief Executive Officer

EMO: Emo Health Centre
Riverside Health Care Facilities Inc.
Affiliated with: North West Local Health Integration Network
PO Box 390, 170 Front St., Emo, ON P0W 1E0
Tel: 807-274-3261 *Fax:* 807-482-2493
www.riversidehealthcare.ca
Number of Beds: 12 long-term, 3 acute care beds
Note: Programs & services include: physiotherapy; dietician; diagnostics; urgent care.
Wayne Woods

ENGLEHART: Englehart & District Hospital Inc.
Affiliated with: North East Local Health Integration Network
PO Box 69, 61 - 5th St., Englehart, ON P0J 1H0
Tel: 705-544-2301 *Fax:* 705-544-5222
www.edhospital.on.ca

Note: Programs & services include: acute care; cancer care; complex continuing care; diabetes; diagnostic imaging; emergency; foot care; laboratory; occupational therapy; palliative care; physiotherapy; respiratory therapy; & Telemedicine.
Gary Sims, Chief Executive Officer

ESPANOLA: Espanola Regional Hospital & Health Centre (ERHHC)/Hôpital régional et centre de santé d'espanola
Affiliated with: North East Local Health Integration Network
Former Name: Espanola General Hospital
825 McKinnon Dr., Espanola, ON P5E 1R4
Tel: 705-869-1420 *Fax:* 705-869-3091
info@esphosp.on.ca
www.espanolaregionalhospital.ca

Year Founded: 1949
Note: Programs & services include: diagnostic imaging; emergency/acute care; Espanola Nursing Home; family health team; laboratory; pharmacy; physiotherapy; Queensway Place; & sleep lab.
Nicole Haley, Chief Executive Officer
Jane Battistelli, Chief Nursing Officer
Kim Roy, Chief Financial Officer

EXETER: South Huron Hospital Association (SHHA)
Affiliated with: South West Local Health Integration Network
24 Huron St. West, Exeter, ON N0M 1S2
Tel: 519-235-2700 *Fax:* 519-235-3405
shha.administration@shha.on.ca
www.shha.on.ca
Year Founded: 1953
Number of Beds: 19 beds
Note: Programs & services include: clinical nutrition & counselling; diabetes education; diagnostic imaging; emergency; inpatient services; laboratory; nursing; palliative care; physiotherapy; social work; speech language pathology; & Telemedicine.
Todd Stepanuik, President & CEO

FERGUS: Groves Memorial Community Hospital (GMCH)
Affiliated with: Waterloo Wellington Local Health Integration Network
235 Union St. East, Fergus, ON N1M 1W3
Tel: 519-843-2010
info@gmch.fergus.net
www.gmch.ca
Number of Beds: 44 beds
Population Served: 34500
Number of Employees: 277
Note: Programs & services include: ambulatory care; chiropody; diabetes education; diagnostic imaging; emergency; geriatric emergency management; Hospital Elder Life Care Program; inpatient medicine; infection prevention & control; laboratory; nutritional services; obstetrics; Ontario Breast Screening Program; outpatient oncology unit; pastoral services; pharmacy; physiotherapy; respiratory therapy; speech-language pathology; & surgery.
Stephen Street, President & CEO
Dr. Rick Gergovich, Chief of Staff

FOREST: North Lambton Community Health Centre
Affiliated with: Erie St. Clair Local Health Integration Network
PO Box 1120, 3 - 59 King St. West, Forest, ON N0N 1J0
Tel: 519-786-4545 *Fax:* 519-786-6318
nlinfo@nlchc.com
www.nlchc.com
Social Media: www.facebook.com/NorthLambtonCHC

Note: Programs for children, seniors, healthy living, excercise & diabetes education.
Kathy Bresett, Executive Director
kbresett@nlchc.com

FORT ERIE: Douglas Memorial Hospital Site
Niagara Health System / Système de santé de Niagara
Affiliated with: Hamilton Niagara Haldimand Brant Local Health Integration Network
230 Bertie St., Fort Erie, ON L2A 1Z2
Tel: 905-378-4647
patientrelations@niagarahealth.on.ca
www.niagarahealth.on.ca
Social Media: twitter.com/niagarahealth; www.youtube.com/niagarahealthsystem
Year Founded: 1931
Number of Beds: 55 beds
Note: Programs & services include: complex care; diagnostic imaging; laboratory; Ontario Breast Screening Clinic; outpatient mental health; & urgent care.
Dr. Kevin Smith, Chief Executive Officer, Niagara Health System
kevin.smith@niagarahealth.on.ca
Dr. Suzanne Johnston, President, Niagara Health System
suzanne.johnston@niagarahealth.on.ca
Dr. Thomas Stewart, Chief of Staff
dr.thomas.stewart@niagarahealth.on.c

FORT FRANCES: Fort Frances Tribal Area Health Services
Affiliated with: North West Local Health Integration Network
PO Box 608, Fort Frances, ON P9A 3M9
Tel: 807-274-2042 *Fax:* 807-274-2050
www.fftahs.com

Note: Programs & services include: behavioural health services; chiropody & foot care services; diabetes education; home & community care.
Calvin Morrisseau, Executive Director

FORT FRANCES: Gizhewaadiziwin Health Access Centre
Affiliated with: North West Local Health Integration Network
PO Box 686, Fort Frances, ON P9A 3M9
Tel: 807-274-3131 *Fax:* 807-274-6280
www.gizhac.com

Note: Programs & services include: primary care; nutrition; traditional healing; mental health; diabetes education.

FORT FRANCES: Riverside Health Care Facilities Inc.
Affiliated with: North West Local Health Integration Network
110 Victoria Ave., Fort Frances, ON P9A 2B7
Tel: 807-274-3266 *Fax:* 807-274-2898
riverside@rhcf.on.ca
www.riversidehealthcare.ca

Year Founded: 1989
Number of Beds: 55 beds (Fort Frances); 12 beds (Emo); 24 beds (Rainy River)
Note: Operates the La Verendrye General Hospital (Fort Frances - acute care, continuing care, obstetrics & surgery); the Emo Health Centre (Emo - acute care, urgent care, long term care, diagnostic imaging, physiotherapy, dental clinic); & Rainy River Health Centre (Rainy River - acute care, long term care, diagnostic imaging, dental clinic).
Ted Scholten, President & CEO
t.scholten@rhcf.on.ca

FORT FRANCES: La Verendrye General Hospital
Riverside Health Care Facilities Inc.
Affiliated with: North West Local Health Integration Network
110 Victoria Ave., Fort Frances, ON P9A 2B7
Tel: 807-274-3261 *Fax:* 807-274-2898
Number of Beds: 30 acute care beds; 25 medical & surgical beds
Note: Programs & services include: acute care; intermediate care. The hospital hosts visiting specialists each year.

GEORGETOWN: Georgetown Hospital
Halton Healthcare Services
Affiliated with: Mississauga Halton Local Health Integration Network
Former Name: Georgetown & District Memorial Hospital
1 Princess Anne Dr., Georgetown, ON L7G 2B8
Tel: 905-873-0111
pr@haltonhealthcare.on.ca
www.haltonhealthcare.on.ca
Social Media: www.facebook.com/HaltonHealthcare; twitter.com/haltonhlthcare; www.linkedin.com/company/3186579
Year Founded: 1961
Number of Beds: 33 acute care beds; 20 continuing care beds
Population Served: 59000
Number of Employees: 326
Note: Programs & services include: complex continuing care; diagnostic imaging; emergency; general medicine; mammography; medical & surgical services; outpatient clinics & community programs; rehabilitation & geriatrics; smoking cessation program; & supportive housing program.
Denise Hardenne, President & CEO, Halton Healthcare
Dr. Lorne Martin, Chief of Staff, Halton Healthcare
Cindy McDonell, COO & Family Practice Program Leader, Georgetown Hospital

GERALDTON: Geraldton District Hospital
Affiliated with: North West Local Health Integration Network
PO Box 4, 500 Hogarth Ave., Geraldton, ON P0T 1M0
Tel: 807-854-1862 *Fax:* 807-854-1568
www.geraldtondh.com

Year Founded: 1963
Number of Beds: 23 acute care beds; 26 long term care beds

Note: Programs & services include: diagnostic imaging; laboratory; nursing; nutrition; rehabilitation; social work; & Telemedicine.
Lucy Bonanno, Chief Executive Officer
lbonanno@geraldtondh.com
Sylvie Duranceau, Chief of Clinical Services
sduranceau@geraldtondh.com
Laurie Heerema, Chief Nursing Executive
lheerema@geraldtondh.com

GODERICH: Alexandra Marine & General Hospital (AMGH)
Affiliated with: South West Local Health Integration Network
120 Napier St., Goderich, ON N7A 1W5
Tel: 519-524-8323 *Fax:* 519-524-8504
amgh.administration@amgh.ca
www.amgh.ca
Year Founded: 1901
Number of Beds: 54 beds
Note: Programs & services include: ambulatory care clinics; Diabetes Education Centre; diagnostic; dialysis; emergency; medicine; mental health; obstetrics; palliative care; pharmacy; physiotherapy; speech language therapy; support services; & surgery.
Bruce Quigley, President & CEO
bruce.quigley@amgh.ca
Samantha Marsh, Chief Nursing Executive
samantha.marsh@amgh.ca
Jimmy Trieu, Chief Information Officer
jimmy.trieu@amgh.ca

GRAND BEND: Grand Bend Area Community Health Centre
PO Box 1269, 69 Main St. East, Grand Bend, ON N0M 1T0
Tel: 519-238-2362 *Fax:* 519-238-6478
www.gbachc.ca
Area Served: Grand Bend, Hensall, Thedford
Note: Programs & services include: diabetes education; dietitian; occupational therapy; physiotherapy; primary care; & social work
Dr. Glenn Bartlett, Executive Director

GRIMSBY: Hamilton Niagara Haldimand Brant Local Health Integration Network (HNHB LHI)/RLISS de Hamilton Niagara Haldimand Brant
Also Known As: Hamilton Niagara Haldimand Brant LHIN
264 Main St. East, Grimsby, ON L3M 1P8
Tel: 905-945-4930 *Fax:* 905-945-1992
Toll-Free: 866-363-5446
hamiltonniagarahaldimandbrant@lhins.on.ca
www.hnhblhin.on.ca
Social Media: twitter.com/HNHB_LHINgage; www.youtube.com/user/hnhblhin
Year Founded: 2005
Area Served: Brant, Burlington, Haldimand, Hamilton, Niagara, Norfolk
Population Served: 1400000
Note: Facilities: 86 long term care homes; 9 hospitals (23 hospital sites); 7 community health centres (10 sites); 1 community care access centre. Programs: 54 community support services; 45 community mental health & addictions programs.
Laurie Ryan-Hill, Acting Board Chair
Donna Cripps, Chief Executive Officer
donna.cripps@lhins.on.ca
Derek Bodden, Director, Finance
derek.bodden@lhins.on.ca
Emily Christoffersen, Director, Quality & Risk Management
emily.christoffersen@lhins.on.ca
Linda Hunter, Director, Health Links & Strategic Initiatives
linda.hunter@lhins.on.ca
Steve Isaak, Director, Health System Transformation
steven.isaak@lhins.on.ca
Trish Nelson, Director, Communications, Community Engagement, & Corporate Services
trish.nelson@lhins.on.ca
Rosalind Tarrant, Director, Access to Care
rosalind.tarrant@lhins.on.ca
Jennifer Everson, Physician Lead, Clinical Health System Transformation
jennifer.everson@lhins.on.ca

GRIMSBY: West Lincoln Memorial Hospital
Hamilton Health Sciences
Affiliated with: Hamilton Niagara Haldimand Brant Local Health Integration Network
169 Main St. East, Grimsby, ON L3M 1P3
Tel: 905-945-2253 *Fax:* 905-945-5016
www.wlmh.on.ca
Social Media: twitter.com/hamhealthsc;
www.vimeo.com/hamiltonhealthsciences

Number of Beds: 60 beds
Population Served: 65000
Number of Employees: 391
Note: Programs & services include: complex continuing care; diagnostic imaging; emergency; general medical; geriatric assessment (inpatient & outpatient); intensive care; mental health; obstetrics; outpatient diagnostic & treatment services; palliative care; & surgery. Has 124 medical staff. Affiliated with Michael G. DeGroote School of Medicine, McMaster University.
Rob MacIsaac, President & CEO, Hamilton Health Sciences

GUELPH: Guelph General Hospital
Affiliated with: Waterloo Wellington Local Health Integration Network
115 Delhi St., Guelph, ON N1E 4J4
Tel: 519-822-5350 *Fax:* 519-837-6773
TTY: 519-837-6437
info@gghorg.ca
www.gghorg.ca
Social Media: www.facebook.com/162349190488511;
twitter.com/FdnofGGH

Year Founded: 1875
Number of Beds: 182 beds (including 22 intensive care & step down, 65 surgery, 8 paediatric, 68 medicine & 22 obstetric)
Number of Employees: 1300
Note: Programs & services include: ambulatory care; bariatric surgery; bariatric medical program; cardio respiratory; critical care unit; diagnostic imaging; dietetics/nutritional counselling; emergency; family birthing unit; laboratory; medical unit; paediatric care; pharmacy; rehabilitation therapies; sexual assault & domestic violence; sleep lab; support services; & surgical suite. Employs 300 professional staff.
Marianne Walker, President & CEO

GUELPH: Waterloo Wellington CCAC - Guelph Branch
Also Known As: WWCCAC
#201, 450 Speedvale Ave. West, Guelph, ON N1H 7G7
Tel: 519-823-2550
healthcareathome.ca/ww

Note: Long-term care placement services; information & referral to other community services; in-home health services; school health support services; access to long-term care facilities; access to adult day programs; mental health & palliative care services

HAGERSVILLE: West Haldimand General Hospital
Affiliated with: Hamilton Niagara Haldimand Brant Local Health Integration Network
75 Parkview Rd., Hagersville, ON N0A 1H0
Tel: 905-768-3311 *Fax:* 905-768-1820
webmaster@whgh.ca
www.whgh.ca

Year Founded: 1964
Number of Beds: 23 inpatient beds
Note: Programs & services include: acute care; day surgery; diagnostic imaging; emergency; Haldimand Norfolk diabetes services; laboratory; nutrition; outpatient clinics & laboratory services; pastoral care; & physiotherapy.
Kelly Isfan, President & CEO
905-768-3311, kelly.isfan@whgh.ca
Nancy Gabel, Chief of Staff
905-768-3311, ngabel@hotmail.com

HALIBURTON: Haliburton Highlands Health Services - Haliburton Site (HHHS)
Affiliated with: Central East Local Health Integration Network
PO Box 115, 7199 Gelert Rd., Haliburton, ON K0M 1S0
Tel: 705-457-1392 *Fax:* 705-457-2398
www.hhhs.ca

Year Founded: 2000
Number of Beds: 14 acute care beds; 30 long-term care beds

Note: Programs & services include: acute cate/emergency; diabetes education; diagnostic imaging; infection control; mental health; physiotherapy; & Telemedicine.
Carolyn Plummer, President & CEO
705-457-2527, cplummer@hhhs.ca
Michelle Douglas, Interim Chief Nurse Executive & Director, Care
705-457-1392, mdouglas@hhhs.ca
Kathy Newton, Chief Financial Officer & Director, Finance
kanewton@hhhs.ca

HAMILTON: CCAC Hamilton Niagara Haldimand Brant - Hamilton Branch Office
#1, 211 Pritchard Rd., Hamilton, ON L8J 0G5
Tel: 905-523-8600 *Fax:* 905-528-1883
Toll-Free: 800-810-0000
healthcareathome.ca

Melody Miles, CEO

HAMILTON: Centre de santé communautaire Hamilton/Niagara
1320, rue Barton est, Hamilton, ON L8H 2W1
Tél: 905-528-0163 *Téléc:* 905-528-9196
Ligne sans frais: 866-437-7606
cschn@cschn.ca
www.cschn.ca

Marcel Castonguay, Directeur général

HAMILTON: Hamilton General Hospital
Hamilton Health Sciences
Affiliated with: Hamilton Niagara Haldimand Brant Local Health Integration Network
237 Barton St. East, Hamilton, ON L8L 2X2
Tel: 905-521-2100
www.hamiltonhealthsciences.ca
Social Media: www.facebook.com/140084176009847;
twitter.com/hamhealthsc; www.vimeo.com/hamiltonhealthsciences
Year Founded: 1848
Number of Beds: 304 beds (91 inpatient beds)
Specialties: Cardiovascular care, neuosciences, trauma & burn treatment
Note: Major programs & services include: cardiac & vascular; neurosciences & trauma; & Population Health Institute. Others include: addictions & mental health; emergency; Hospital Elder Life Program; pain management centre; palliative care consultation; Regional Rehabilitation Centre; rehabilitation & seniors health program; seniors health; sexual assault & domestic violence care; & STD clinic.
Rob MacIsaac, President & CEO, Hamilton Health Sciences
Teresa Smith, Vice-President, Adult Regional Care

HAMILTON: Hamilton Urban Core Community Health Centre
71 Rebecca St., Hamilton, ON L8R 1B6
Tel: 905-522-3233 *Fax:* 905-522-3433
administration@hucchc.com
www.hucchc.com
Social Media:
www.facebook.com/HamiltonUrbanCoreCommunityHealthCentre;
twitter.com/hucchc

Denise Brooks, Executive Director
dbrooks@hucchc.com

HAMILTON: Juravinski Hospital
Hamilton Health Sciences
Affiliated with: Hamilton Niagara Haldimand Brant Local Health Integration Network
Former Name: Mount Hamilton Hospital
711 Concession St., Hamilton, ON L8V 1C3
Tel: 905-521-2100
www.hamiltonhealthsciences.ca
Social Media: www.facebook.com/140084176009847;
twitter.com/hamhealthsc; www.vimeo.com/hamiltonhealthsciences
Year Founded: 1917
Note: Programs & services include: diagnostic services & medical diagnostic unit; emergency hematology oncology medicine & JCC Ambulance Care; perioperative services; rehabilitation; & surgical oncology, orthopedics & critical care program.
Rob MacIsaac, President & CEO, Hamilton Health Services

HAMILTON: North Hamilton Community Health Centre
438 Hughson St. North, Hamilton, ON L8L 4N5
Tel: 905-523-6611 *Fax:* 905-523-5173
www.nhchc.ca

Year Founded: 1987
Note: Offers a variety of services & programs, including programs for men & women living with HIV/AIDS & programs for new immigrants/refugees
Elizabeth Beader, CEO
beader@nhchc.ca

HAMILTON: St. Joseph's Healthcare Hamilton - Charlton Campus
St. Joseph's Health System
Affiliated with: Hamilton Niagara Haldimand Brant Local Health Integration Network
50 Charlton Ave. East, Hamilton, ON L8N 4A6
Tel: 905-522-1155
www.stjosham.on.ca
Social Media: www.facebook.com/stjosehshealthcarefoundation; twitter.com/STJOESHAMILTON; www.youtube.com/Stjoesfoundation; www.linkedin.com/company/st-joseph's-healthcare-hamilton
Number of Beds: 786 across the system
Note: Programs & services include: Best Foot Forward; Brant seniors mental health outreach program; audiology; Brant Assertive Community Treatment Team (ACTT); continence care clinic; cleghorn early psychosis intervention program; community schizophrenia service; east region mental health services; geriatric assessment clinic; Niagara seniors mental health outreach program; relaxation group; & spiritual care. Affiliated with the Faculty of Health Sciences at McMaster University & Mohawk College.
Dr. David Higgins, President
Winnie Doyle, Chief Nursing Executive & Vice-President, Clinical Programs

HAMILTON: St. Joseph's Healthcare Hamilton - King Campus
St. Joseph's Health System
Affiliated with: Hamilton Niagara Haldimand Brant Local Health Integration Network
2757 King St. East, Hamilton, ON L8G 5E4
Tel: 905-522-1155
www.stjosham.on.ca
Social Media: www.facebook.com/stjosehshealthcarefoundation; twitter.com/STJOESHAMILTON; www.youtube.com/Stjoesfoundation; www.linkedin.com/company/st-joseph's-healthcare-hamilton

Note: Programs & services include: diabetes; east region mental health services; family practice; chiropody clinic; Health for Older Adults; women's health centre; continence care; family asthma education; & urgent care. Affiliated with the Faculty of Health Sciences at McMaster University & Mohawk College.
Dr. David Higgins, President
Winnie Doylens, Chief Nursing Executive & Vice-President, Clinical Programs

HANOVER: Hanover & District Hospital (HDH)
Affiliated with: South West Local Health Integration Network
90 - 7 Ave., Hanover, ON N4N 1N1
Tel: 519-364-2340 *Fax:* 519-364-3984
info@hdhospital.ca
www.hanoverhospital.on.ca
Social Media: www.facebook.com/HDHospital; twitter.com/HDHospital; www.linkedin.com/company/hanover-&-district-hospital
Year Founded: 1923
Number of Beds: 80 beds
Note: Programs & services include: auxiliary services; chaplaincy services; diagnostic imaging; diabetes education program; emergency; Family Centered Care Suites; Family Centered Birthing Unit; hemodialysis; infection control; intensive care unit; laboratory; medical/surgical; pet therapy; pharmacy; rehabilitation; restorative care; & specialty clinics.
Katrina Wilson, President & CEO
519-364-2341
Dana Howes, Chief Nursing Officer & Vice-President, Patient Care Services
519-364-2341
Marnie Ferguson, Vice-President, Finance & Operations
519-364-2341

Stacy Hogg, Vice-President, Human Resources
519-364-2341

HAWKESBURY: Hôpital Général de Hawkesbury & District General Hospital Inc.
Affiliated with: Champlain Local Health Integration Network
1111 Ghislain St., Hawkesbury, ON K6A 3G5
Tel: 613-632-1111 *Fax:* 613-636-6183
info@hgh.ca
www.hgh.ca
Year Founded: 1984
Number of Beds: 69 beds
Note: Programs & services include: diagnostic imaging; emergency; Ontario Breast Screening Program; mental health & addictions; geriatric psychiatry; & physiotherapy.
Marc LeBoutillier, Chief Executive Officer
Dr. Julie Maranda, Chief of Staff
Denise Picard-Stencer, Chief Nursing Executive & Vice-President, Acute Care
Marcel Leclair, Vice-President, Finance & Corporate Services

HEARST: Hôpital Nôtre-Dame Hospital
CP 8000, 1405 Edward St., Hearst, ON P0L 1N0
Tél: 705-362-4291 *Téléc:* 705-372-2923
www.ndh.on.ca
Nombre de lits: 44 lits
France Dallaire, CEO

HORNEPAYNE: Hornepayne Community Hospital
PO Box 190, 278 Front St., Hornepayne, ON P0M 1Z0
Tel: 807-868-2442 *Fax:* 807-868-2697
Number of Beds: 12 long-term care beds; 8 acute care beds
Note: Provides medical, inpatient, & outpatient care services.
Heather Jaremy-Berube, Chief Executive Officer
heather.jaremyberube@hornepaynehospi
Julie Roy-Ward, Chief Financial Officer
julie.royward@hornepaynehospital.ca

HUNTSVILLE: Huntsville District Memorial Hospital Site
Muskoka Algonquin Healthcare (MAHC)
Affiliated with: North Simcoe Muskoka Local Health Integration Network
100 Frank Miller Dr., Huntsville, ON P1H 1H7
Tel: 705-789-2311 *Fax:* 705-789-0557
www.mahc.ca
Number of Beds: 37 acute care beds
Number of Employees: 650
Note: Programs & services include: cardio respiratory; clinical nutrition; complex continuing care; diabetes education; diagnostic imaging; District Stroke Centre; emergency; food & nutrition; fracture clinic; general surgery; intensive care unit; laboratory; obstetrics; oncology; paediatric clinic; prenatal clinic; palliative care; rehabilitation; social work; & Telemedicine. Muskoka Algonquin Healthcare employs around 85 physicians.
Natalie Bubela, Chief Executive Officer, MAHC
705-789-2311
Dr. Biagio Iannantuono, Interim Chief of Medical Staff, MAHC
705-789-2311
Karen Fleming, Chief Quality & Nursing Executive, MAHC
705-645-4404

HUNTSVILLE: Muskoka Algonquin Healthcare
Huntsville District Memorial Hospital, 100 Frank Miller Dr., Huntsville, ON P1H 1H7
Tel: 705-789-2311 *Fax:* 705-789-0557
www.mahc.ca
Number of Beds: 99 beds
Number of Employees: 645
Note: Provides emergency health services & acute care.
Natalie Bubela, CEO
Dr. Jan Goossens, Chief of Medical Staff
Karen Fleming, Cheif Quality & Nursing Executive

IGNACE: Mary Berglund Community Health Centre (MBCHC)
PO Box 450, 1100 Main St., Ignace, ON P0T 1T0
Tel: 807-934-6719 *Fax:* 807-934-6552
mbchced@bellnet.ca
Social Media: www.facebook.com/867609549975894

Note: Specialties: Primary care; Public health nursing; Physiotherapy; Chronic disease follow-up; Health promotion; Men's & women's wellness clinics; Blood sugar & blood pressure screening programs; Chiropractic services; Massage therapy
Gloria Pronger, Executive Director

INGERSOLL: Alexandra Hospital
Affiliated with: South West Local Health Integration Network
29 Noxon St., Ingersoll, ON N5C 3V6
Tel: 519-485-1700 *Fax:* 519-485-9606
feedback@ah.tvh.ca
www.alexandrahospital.on.ca
Year Founded: 1909
Number of Beds: 26 beds
Note: Programs & services include: ambulatory clinics; complex continuing care; day surgery; Diabetes Education Centre; diagnostics; emergency department; inpatient unit; intensive care; nutrition; occupational therapy; Oxford County Cardiac Rehabilitation & Secondary Prevention Program; palliative care program; & physiotherapy.
Frank Deutsch, Chief Financial Officer & Integrated Vice-President
519-485-1700, frank.deutsch@ah.tvh.ca
Julie Ellery, Chief Nursing Executive & Integrated Vice-President
519-485-1700, julie.ellery@ah.tvh.ca

IROQUOIS FALLS: Anson General Hospital
MICs Group of Health Services
Affiliated with: North East Local Health Integration Network
58 Anson Dr., Iroquois Falls, ON P0K 1E0
Tel: 705-258-3911 *Fax:* 705-258-3221
www.micsgroup.com
Year Founded: 1955
Number of Beds: 19 acute care beds; 15 complex continuing care beds; 69 long-term care beds
Note: Programs & services include: clinical nutrition; complex continuing care; diabetes; diagnostic imaging; emergency; laboratory; physiotherapy; respiratory therapy; visiting specialty clinics; & Telemedicine.
Paul Chatelain, Chief Executive Officer, MICs Group of Health Services
Karen Hill, Chief Nursing Officer, MICs Group of Health Services
Gail Waghorn, Chief Financial Officer, MICs Group of Health Services

KAPUSKASING: Sensenbrenner Hospital
Affiliated with: North East Local Health Integration Network
101 Progress Cres., Kapuskasing, ON P5N 3H5
Tel: 705-337-6111 *Fax:* 705-337-4021
info@senhosp.ca
www.senhosp.ca
Number of Beds: 53 beds
Note: Programs & services include: active care; continuing care; diabetes education; diagnostic imaging; dietitian; ECG/respiratory therapy; emergency; infection control; laboratory; occupational therapy; physiotherapy; pharmacy; special care unit; specialty clinics; spiritual care; & surgical suite.
France Dallaire, Chief Executive Officer
Pauline Fréchette-Keating, Assistant Administrator, Nursing Services
Chantal Boyer-Brochu, Assistant Administrator, Finance & Hospital Services
Jessica Allarie, Director, Human Resources

KEMPTVILLE: Kemptville District Hospital
Affiliated with: Champlain Local Health Integration Network
PO Box 2007, 2675 Concession Rd., Kemptville, ON K0G 1J0
Tel: 613-258-6133 *Fax:* 613-258-4997
info@kdh.on.ca
www.kdh.on.ca
Social Media: www.facebook.com/KemptvilleDistrictHospital; twitter.com/KDHonline; www.youtube.com/user/KemptvilleHospital
Number of Beds: 18 inpatient beds; 4 interim long-term care beds; 8 convalescent care beds; 10 surgical beds
Note: Programs & services include: 24 hour emergency; convalescent care; diabetes education; diagnostic imaging; education; in-hospital care; long-term care; outpatient care; & surgery.
Frank Vassallo, Chief Executive Officer
613-258-6133
Dr. Greg Leonard, Chief of Staff
Cathy Burke, Vice-President, Nursing & Clinical Services

KENORA: CCAC North West - Kenora Branch Office
#3, 35 Wolsley St., Kenora, ON P9N 0H8
Tel: 807-467-4757 *Fax:* 807-468-1437
Toll-Free: 877-661-6621
healthcareathome.ca
Tuija Puiras, CEO
807-346-3273, Fax: 807-345-8868, tuija.puiras@nw.ccac-ont.ca

KENORA: Lake of the Woods District Hospital (LWDH)
Affiliated with: North West Local Health Integration Network
21 Sylvan St., Kenora, ON P9N 3W7
Tel: 807-468-9861 *Fax:* 807-468-3939
admin@lwdh.on.ca
www.lwdh.on.ca
Year Founded: 1897
Note: Programs & services include: emergency & ambulatory care; mental health programs; acute care; intensive & surgical care services; diagnostic imaging; mammography; sexual assult centre; physiotherapy; & palliative care.
Mark Balcaen, President & CEO

KINCARDINE: South Bruce Grey Health Centre - Kincardine Site
Affiliated with: South West Local Health Integration Network
Former Name: Kincardine & District General Hospital
1199 Queen St., Kincardine, ON N2Z 1G6
Tel: 519-396-3331 *Fax:* 519-396-3699
www.sbghc.on.ca
Social Media: www.facebook.com/sbghc; twitter.com/SBG_HC
Year Founded: 1908
Number of Beds: 25 beds
Note: Programs & services include: cardio-respiratory; family birthing centre; diagnostic imaging; emergency department; emergency response system; inpatient medical beds; laboratory; nutrition services; palliative care; & pastoral care.
Paul Rosebush, President & CEO, SBGHC
prosebush@sbghc.on.ca
Maureen Rydall, Chief Nursing Officer, SBGHC
mrydall@sbghc.on.ca

KINGSTON: CCAC South East - Kingston Head Office
#200, 1471 John Counter Blvd., Kingston, ON K7M 8S8
Tel: 613-544-7090 *Fax:* 613-544-1494
Toll-Free: 800-869-8828
healthcareathome.ca
Jacqueline Redmond, CEO

KINGSTON: Kingston Community Health Centres (KCHC)
263 Weller Ave., Kingston, ON K7K 2V4
Tel: 613-542-2949 *Fax:* 613-542-7657
info@kchc.ca
www.kchc.ca
Social Media: www.facebook.com/KingstonCHC; twitter.com/kingstonchc
Year Founded: 1988
Lisa Lund, Interim Manager
lisal@kchc.ca

KINGSTON: Kingston General Hospital (KGH)
Affiliated with: South East Local Health Integration Network
76 Stuart St., Kingston, ON K7L 2V7
Tel: 613-548-3232 *Toll-Free:* 800-567-5722
www.kgh.on.ca
Info Line: 613-549-6666
Year Founded: 1838
Number of Beds: 440 beds
Population Served: 500000
Note: Teaching & research hospital affiliated with Queen's University. Programs & services include: cancer; cardiac; critical care; emergency; endocrinology & metabolism; gastroenterology; imaging; infectious diseases; internal medicine; medical genetics; mental health; nephrology & dialysis; neurology; obstetrics & gynecology; pathology & molecular medicine; pediatrics; pharmacy; respirology; rheumatology; sexual assault & domestic violence; & surgical, perioperative & anesthesiology.
Dr. David Pichora, President & CEO
khscceo@hdh.kari.net
Dr. Michael Fitzpatrick, Chief of Staff & Vice-President, Medical Affairs
fitzpatm@kgh.kari.net

KINGSTON: The Religious Hospitaliers of Saint-Joseph of the Hotel Dieu of Kingston (HDH)
Affiliated with: South East Local Health Integration Network
Also Known As: Hotel Dieu Hospital
166 Brock St., Kingston, ON K7L 5G2
Tel: 613-544-3310 *Fax:* 613-544-4498
Toll-Free: 855-554-3400
www.hoteldieu.com
Social Media: www.facebook.com/HotelDieuHospital;
www.youtube.com/user/HDHKingston
Year Founded: 1845
Note: An ambulatory care teaching facility with programs & services including: audiology; cardiac rehabilitation; child development; Children's Outpatient Centre (COPC); day surgery; detox centre; diabetes education; ENT; eating disorders; eye clinic; Geaganano Residence; infant development; infection & immunology; mental health; & urgent care. It is affiliated with Queen's University & is partnered with Kingston's university hospitals.
Dr. David Pichora, President & CEO
613-544-3310, hdhceo@hdh.kari.net
Dr. Michael Fitzpatrick, Chief of Staff & Vice-President, Medical Affairs
Silvie Crawford, Chief Nursing Executive & Executive Vice-President

KIRKLAND LAKE: CCAC North East - Kirkland Lake Branch Office
53 Government Rd. West, Kirkland Lake, ON P2N 2E5
Tel: 705-567-2222 *Fax:* 705-567-9407
Toll-Free: 888-602-2222
healthcareathome.ca/northeast

KIRKLAND LAKE: Kirkland & District Hospital
145 Government Rd. East, Kirkland Lake, ON P2N 3P4
Tel: 705-567-5251 *Fax:* 705-568-2102
Year Founded: 1976
Number of Beds: 62 beds (6 intensive care; 41 medical/surgical; 15 continuing complex care)
Number of Employees: 260
Note: Services include diagnostic imaging, respiratory therapy, diabetic clinic, physiotherapy, pastoral care, telemedicine, & renal dialysis.
Gary Sims, President & CEO
Mark Spiller, Chief of Staff

KITCHENER: Grand River Hospital - Freeport Health Centre
Affiliated with: Waterloo Wellington Local Health Integration Network
PO Box 9056, 3570 King St. East, Kitchener, ON N2A 2W1
Tel: 519-742-3611
info@grhosp.on.ca
www.grhosp.on.ca
Number of Beds: 567 beds (including Kitchener-Waterloo Site)
Note: Programs & services offered across both hospital sites include: cancer care; childbirth; children (including neonatal intensive care); complex continuing care; critical care; emergency; laboratory; medical imaging; medical program & stroke centre; mental health & addictions; renal care; pharmacy; rehabilitation; & surgery.
Malcolm Maxwell, President & CEO
malcolm.maxwell@grhosp.on.ca
Dr. Peter Potts, Joint Chief of Staff

KITCHENER: Grand River Hospital - Kitchener-Waterloo Site
Affiliated with: Waterloo Wellington Local Health Integration Network
PO Box 9056, 835 King St. West, Kitchener, ON N2G 1G3
Tel: 519-742-3611
info@grhosp.on.ca
www.grhosp.on.ca
Number of Beds: 567 beds (including Freeport Health Centre site)
Note: Programs & services offered across both hospital sites include: cancer care; childbirth; children (including neonatal intensive care); complex continuing care; critical care; emergency; laboratory; medical imaging; medical program & stroke centre; mental health & addictions; renal care; pharmacy; rehabilitation; & surgery.
Malcolm Maxwell, President & CEO
Dr. Peter Potts, Joint Chief of Staff
Judy Linton, Chief Nursing Executive & Vice-President, Clinical Services

KITCHENER: Kitchener Downtown Community Health Centre
44 Francis St. South, Kitchener, ON N2G 2A2
Tel: 519-745-4404 *Fax:* 519-745-3709
mail@kdchc.org
www.kdchc.org
Eric Goldberg, Executive Director
519-745-4404, egoldberg@kdchc.org

KITCHENER: St. Mary's General Hospital
St. Joseph's Health System
Affiliated with: Waterloo Wellington Local Health Integration Network
911 Queen's Blvd., Kitchener, ON N2M 1B2
Tel: 519-744-3311 *Fax:* 519-749-6426
info@smgh.ca
www.smgh.ca
Year Founded: 1924
Number of Beds: 150 acute care beds
Number of Employees: 1200
Note: Catholic hospital, home to the Regional Cardiac Care Centre. Other programs & services include respiratory care, day surgery, general medicine, & emergency care.
Don Shilton, President
519-749-6544, dshilton@smgh.ca
Dr. Peter Potts, Chief of Staff
Angela Stanley, Chief Nursing Executive & Vice-President, Patient Services
astanley@smgh.ca

KITCHENER: Waterloo Wellington Local Health Integration Network (WWLHIN)/RLISS de Waterloo Wellington
Also Known As: Waterloo Wellington LHIN
East Bldg., #220, 50 Sportsworld Crossing Rd., Kitchener, ON N2P 0A4
Tel: 519-650-4472 *Fax:* 519-650-3155
Toll-Free: 866-306-5446
waterloowellington@lhins.on.ca
www.waterloowellingtonlhin.on.ca
Social Media: www.facebook.com/WWLHIN; twitter.com/WW_LHIN;
www.youtube.com/user/TheWWLHIN
Year Founded: 2005
Area Served: Waterloo, Wellington, Guelph & southern Grey County; 4,800 sq km
Population Served: 778676
Note: A crown agency of Ontario that works to plan, integrate, & fund local health services
Joan Fisk, Board Chair
Bruce Lauckner, Chief Executive Officer
Toni Lemon, Chief Strategy Officer
Zeynep Danis, Senior Director, Finance & Corporate Support
Gloria Cardoso, Senior Director, Health System Integration

LANARK: North Lanark County Community Health Centre
207 Robertson Dr., Lanark, ON K0G 1K0
Tel: 613-259-2182 *Fax:* 613-259-5235
Toll-Free: 866-762-0496
info@nlchc.on.ca
www.northlanarkchc.on.ca
Jane Coyle, Director, Health Services

LEAMINGTON: Leamington District Memorial Hospital (LDMH)
Affiliated with: Erie St. Clair Local Health Integration Network
194 Talbot St. West, Leamington, ON N8H 1N9
Tel: 519-326-2373
www.leamingtonhospital.com
Number of Beds: 58 beds
Note: Programs & services include: 24 hour emergency; ambulatory care; diagnostic services; gynecology; intensive care; medicine; obstetrics; palliative care; rehabilitation; & surgery.
Terry Shields, Chief Executive Officer
Susan Gibson, Chief Financial Officer
Dr. Ejaz Ghumman, Chief of Staff

LINDSAY: CCAC Central East - Lindsay Branch Office
370 Kent St. West, Lindsay, ON K9V 6G8
Tel: 705-324-9165 *Fax:* 855-352-2555
Toll-Free: 800-263-3877
healthcareathome.ca
Kathryn Ramsay, CEO

SECTION II:
General Resources

LINDSAY: Ross Memorial Hospital (RMH)
Affiliated with: Central East Local Health Integration Network
10 Angeline St. North, Lindsay, ON K9V 4M8
Tel: 705-324-6111 *Fax:* 705-328-6087
Toll-Free: 800-510-7365
publicrelations@rmh.org
www.rmh.org
Social Media: twitter.com/RossMemorial

Year Founded: 1902
Number of Beds: 175 beds
Population Served: 80000
Number of Employees: 820
Note: Programs & services include: continuing care; critical care; diagnostic imaging; dialysis; Health First (disease management); infection prevention & control; laboratory; medical program; mental health; radiation oncology consulation; spiritual; Ontario Telemedicine Network (OTN); pharmacy; surgery; therapy; & woman & child.

LIONS HEAD: Lion's Head Hospital
Grey Bruce Health Services
Affiliated with: South West Local Health Integration Network
22 Moore St., Lions Head, ON N0H 1W0
Tel: 519-793-3424 *Fax:* 519-793-4407
web@gbhs.on.ca
www.gbhs.on.ca
Social Media: twitter.com/greybrucehealth
Number of Beds: 4 acute care beds
Note: Programs & services include: acute care; ambulatory care; diagnostic imaging (general radiography); emergency; laboratory; physiotherapy; & spiritual care.
Lance Thurston, President & CEO, Grey Bruce Health Services
519-376-2121

LISTOWEL: Listowel Memorial Hospital
Listowel Wingham Hospitals Alliance
Affiliated with: South West Local Health Integration Network
255 Elizabeth St. East, Listowel, ON N4W 2P5
Tel: 519-291-3120 *Fax:* 519-291-5440
www.lwha.ca
Year Founded: 1919
Number of Beds: 50 beds
Note: Programs & services include: breast health centre; complex continuing care; diabetes education; diagnostic imaging; emergency; laboratory; maternal/newborn; medical unit; occupational therapy; outpatient clinics; palliative care; pastoral care; physiotherapy; speech-language pathology; & surgery.
Karl Ellis, President & CEO
519-291-3120, karl.ellis@lwha.ca

LITTLE CURRENT: Manitoulin Health Centre
PO Box 640, 11 Meredith St., Little Current, ON P0P 1K0
Tel: 705-368-2300 *Fax:* 705-368-3566
www.manitoulinhealthcentre.com
Number of Beds: 32 beds
Note: Services include: chemotherapy; chiropody clinic; day surgery; dialysis; emergency care; laboratory; medical/surgical; mental health; nutrition counselling; obstetrics; paediatrics; physiotherapy; radiology; & ultrasound.
Derek Graham, CEO
Dr. Mike Bedard, President, Medical Staff
Dr. Stephen Cooper, Chief of Staff

LONDON: CCAC South West - London Branch Office
356 Oxford St. West, London, ON N6H 1T3
Tel: 519-473-2222 *Fax:* 519-472-4045
Toll-Free: 800-811-5146
TTY: 519-473-9626
info-london@sw.ccac-ont.ca
healthcareathome.ca

Note: Head office for the South West CCAC & regional office for London & E. Middlesex
Sandra Coleman, CEO, South West CCAC

LONDON: London Health Sciences Centre - University Hospital Site
Affiliated with: South West Local Health Integration Network
339 Windermere Rd., London, ON N6A 5A5
Tel: 519-685-8500
www.lhsc.on.ca
Info Line: 519-685-8380
Social Media: www.facebook.com/LHSCCanada; twitter.com/LHSCCanada; www.youtube.com/LHSCCanada

Note: Programs & services include: carpal tunnel syndrome & mononeuropathy clinic; Clinical Neurological Sciences (CNS); cochlear implant program; Critical Care Outreach Team (CCOT); dentistry; diagnostic imaging; EEG; emergency; family medicine & palliative care; general surgery; general cardiology & cardiovascular surgery; intensive care; motor neuron disease clinic; movement disorder clinic; multi-organ transplant; multiple sclerosis clinic; occupational therapy; orthopaedics; pathology & laboratory medicine; physiotherapy; prescription centre pharmacy; psychological; renal care; social work; speech-language pathology; & surgery.
Murray Glendining, President & CEO

LONDON: London Health Sciences Centre - Victoria Hospital Site
Affiliated with: South West Local Health Integration Network
PO Box 5010, 800 Commissioners Rd. East, London, ON N6A 5W9
Tel: 519-685-8500
www.lhsc.on.ca
Info Line: 519-685-8380
Social Media: www.facebook.com/LHSCCanada; twitter.com/LHSCCanada; www.youtube.com/LHSCCanada
Year Founded: 1995
Note: Programs & services include: adult mental health care; bleeding disorders; blood conservation; cardiac care; Cardiac Fitness Institute of Southwestern Ontario; Critical Care Trauma Centre (CCTC); emergency; family medicine & palliative care; fertility clinic; maternal newborn care; medical genetics program of Southwestern Ontario; occupational therapy; pathology & laboratory medicine; pharmacy services; physiotherapy; renal care; sleep & apnea assessment unit; sleep medicine clinic; social work; speech-language pathology; surgical services; trauma program; urology; & women's health care.
Murray Glendining, President & CEO

LONDON: London InterCommunity Health Centre
659 Dundas St., London, ON N5W 2Z1
Tel: 519-660-0874 *Fax:* 519-642-1532
mail@lihc.on.ca
www.lihc.on.ca
Social Media: www.facebook.com/LondonInterCommunityHealthCentre; twitter.com/HealthCentre
Year Founded: 1989
Note: Specialties: Inclusive & equitable health & social services to persons who experience barriers to care; Mental health care; Diabetes program; Options clinic HIV anonymous testing; Health & youth outreach services. Number of employees: 70
Scott Courtice, Executive Director
scourtice@lihc.on.ca

LONDON: St. Joseph's Health Care, London
Affiliated with: South West Local Health Integration Network
268 Grosvenor St., London, ON N6A 4V2
Tel: 519-646-6100
comdept@sjhc.london.on.ca
www.sjhc.london.on.ca
Social Media: www.facebook.com/stjosephslondon; twitter.com/stjosephslondon; www.youtube.com/stjosephslondon
Number of Beds: 1,141 beds
Note: Includes St. Joseph's Hospital; Parkwood Institute; St. Joseph's Family Medical & Dental Centre; Mount Hope Centre for Long Term Care; & Southwest Centre for Forensic Mental Health Care. Affiliated with Western University & Fanshawe College.
Dr. Gillian Kernaghan, President & CEO, St. Joseph's Health Care London

LONDON: St. Joseph's Hospital
Affiliated with: St. Joseph's Health Care, London
PO Box 5777, 268 Grosvenor St., London, ON N6A 4V2
Tel: 519-646-6100
www.sjhc.london.on.ca

Number of Beds: 28 beds
Note: Programs & services include: arthritis; bone disease & osteoporosis; diabetes education; diagnostic imaging; gastroenterology; otolaryngology; respirology; rheumatology; & ultrasound.

LONDON: South West Local Health Integration Network
Also Known As: South West LHIN
#700, 201 Queens Ave., London, ON N6A 1J1
Tel: 519-672-0445 *Toll-Free:* 866-294-5446
southwest@lhins.on.ca
www.southwestlhin.on.ca
Social Media: www.facebook.com/SouthWestLHIN;
twitter.com/SouthWestLHIN; www.youtube.com/user/SouthWestLHIN;
linkedin.com/company/south-west-local-health-integration-network
Year Founded: 2005
Area Served: Area from Lake Erie to the Bruce Peninsula; 21,639 sq km
Number of Employees: 200
Note: The South West Local Health Integration Network (LHIN) is a crown agency responsible for the planning, integration & funding of nearly 200 health service providers including hospitals, long-term care homes, mental health & addictions agencies, community support services, community health centres, & the South West Community Care Access Centre.
Lori Van Opstal, Interim Board Chair
Michael Barrett, Chief Executive Officer
Mark Brintnell, Senior Director, Performance & Accountability
Kelly Gillis, Senior Director, System Design & Integration
Lorri Lowe, Controller & Manager, Corporate Services

LONGLAC: NorWest Community Health Centre - Longlac Site
Affiliated with: North West Local Health Integration Network
PO Box 910, 99 Skinner Ave., Longlac, ON P0T 1T0
Tel: 807-876-2271 *Fax:* 807-876-2473
www.norwestchc.org/longlac.htm
Social Media: www.facebook.com/NorWestCHC

Note: Primary care services; programs for children & seniors.
Wendy Talbot, CEO

MANITOUWADGE: Manitouwadge General Hospital
Affiliated with: North West Local Health Integration Network
1 Health Care Cres., Manitouwadge, ON P0T 2C0
Tel: 807-826-3251 *Fax:* 807-826-4216
infoserv@mh.on.ca
www.mh.on.ca

Number of Beds: 18 beds
Note: Programs & services include: chemotherapy; diabetes education; laboratory; physiotherapy; & diagnostic imaging.
Jocelyn Bourgoin, Chief Executive Officer
jbourgoin@mh.on.ca
Adenola Bodunde, Chief Financial Officer
abodunde@mh.on.ca

MARATHON: Wilson Memorial General Hospital
North of Superior Healthcare Group
Affiliated with: North West Local Health Integration Network
PO Box 780, 26 Peninsula Rd., Marathon, ON P0T 2E0
Tel: 807-229-1740 *Fax:* 807-229-1721
wilson@nosh.ca
www.nosh.ca

Year Founded: 1971
Number of Beds: 21 beds
Population Served: 7500
Note: Programs & services include: chemotherapy; rehabilitation; diabetes education; & eye & foot specialty treatment.
Adam Brown, CEO
807-229-1740
Janet Gobeil, Chief Nursing Officer
807-229-1740

MARKDALE: Markdale Hospital
Grey Bruce Health Services
Affiliated with: South West Local Health Integration Network
Also Known As: Centre Grey Hospital
PO Box 406, Markdale, ON N0C 1H0
Tel: 519-986-3040
web@gbhs.on.ca
www.gbhs.on.ca
Social Media: twitter.com/greybrucehealth
Number of Beds: 14 acute care beds
Note: Programs & services include: acute care; ambulatory care; Diabetes Grey Bruce; diagnostic imaging; emergency; laboratory; physiotherapy; spiritual care; & surgery.
Lance Thurston, President & CEO, Grey Bruce Health Services
519-376-2121

MARKHAM: Central Local Health Integration Network
Also Known As: Central LHIN
#300, 60 Renfrew Dr., Markham, ON L3R 0E1
Tel: 905-948-1872 *Fax:* 905-948-8011
Toll-Free: 866-392-5446
central@lhins.on.ca
www.centrallhin.on.ca
Social Media: www.youtube.com/user/TheCentralLHIN
Year Founded: 2005
Area Served: 2,730 sq km
Population Served: 1800000
Note: Areas served include parts of northern Toronto & Etobicoke, most of York Region, & South Simcoe County.
Warren Jestin, Board Chair
Kim Baker, Chief Executive Officer
kim.baker@lhins.on.ca
Karin Dschankilic, Chief Financial Officer & Senior Director, Performance, Contracts & Allocation
karin.dschankilic@lhins.on.ca
Chantell Tunney, Senior Director, Planning, Integration & Community Engagement
chantell.tunney@lhins.on.ca
Jennifer Scott, Director, Performance, Contract & Allocation
jennifer.scott@lhins.on.ca
Robert Del Vecchio, Director, Finance & Risk Management
robert.delvecchio@lhins.on.ca
Andrea Gates, Director, Enabling Technologies & Decision Support
andrea.gates@lhins.on.ca

MARKHAM: Markham Stouffville Hospital - Markham Site (MSH)
Affiliated with: Central Local Health Integration Network
PO Box 1800, 381 Church St., Markham, ON L3P 7P3
Tel: 905-472-7000
TTY: 905-472-7585
myhospital@msh.on.ca
www.msh.on.ca
Info Line: 905-472-7100
Social Media: www.facebook.com/MarkhamStouffvilleHospital;
twitter.com/MSHospital; www.youtube.com/MSHospital
Year Founded: 1990
Number of Beds: 245 beds
Note: Programs & services include: diabetes education; diagnostic & respiratory; emergency; ICU/NICU; laboratory; maternal child; medical; mental health; oncology; outpatient ambulatory care; palliative care; rehabilitation & transitional care; speech & language program; & surgery.
Jo-anne Marr, President & CEO
Dr. David Austin, Chief of Staff

MATHESON: Bingham Memorial Hospital
MICs Group of Health Services
Affiliated with: North East Local Health Integration Network
PO Box 70, 507 - 8th Ave., Matheson, ON P0K 1N0
Tel: 705-273-2424 *Fax:* 705-273-2515
www.micsgroup.com
Year Founded: 1955
Number of Beds: 11 acute care beds; 6 complex continuing care beds; 20 long-term care beds
Note: Programs & services include: clinical nutrition; diabetes; diagnostic imaging; emergency; laboratory; respiratory therapy; Telemedicine; & visiting specialty clinics.
Paul Chatelain, Chief Executive Officer, MICs Group of Health Services

Karen Hill, Chief Nursing Officer, MICs Group of Health Services

MATTAWA: Mattawa Hospital
PO Box 70, 217 Turcotte Park Rd., Mattawa, ON P0H 1V0
Tel: 705-744-5511 Fax: 705-744-6020
admin@mattawahospital.ca
www.mattawahospital.ca

Year Founded: 1878
Number of Beds: 19 beds
Note: Specialties: Primary care; Acute care; Ambulatory programs; Diabetic resource centre; Adult & children's mental health services; Paediatric, urology, psychiatry, & women's clinic; Physiotherapy services; Palliative care
Jeremy Stevenson, President & CEO

MEAFORD: Meaford Hospital
Grey Bruce Health Services
Affiliated with: South West Local Health Integration Network
229 Nelson St. West, Meaford, ON N4L 1A3
Tel: 519-538-1311 Fax: 519-538-5500
web@gbhs.on.ca
www.gbhs.on.ca
Social Media: twitter.com/greybrucehealth
Number of Beds: 15 acute care beds
Note: Programs & services include: acute care; ambulatory care; Diabetes Grey Bruce; diagnostic imaging; emergency; laboratory; physiotherapy; spiritual care; & surgery.
Lance Thurston, President & CEO, Grey Bruce Health Services
519-376-2121

MERRICKVILLE: Merrickville District Community Health Centre
PO Box 550, 354 Read St., Merrickville, ON K0G 1N0
Tel: 613-269-3400 Fax: 613-269-4958
info@rideauchs.ca
www.rvds.ca

Note: Specialties: Social work; Dietitian services; Health education; Individual & family counselling; Case management, such as asthma; Foot care services; Flu clinics; Immunizations
Peter McKenna, Executive Director
613-269-3400, pmckenna@rideauchs.ca

MIDLAND: Georgian Bay General Hospital - Midland Site
Affiliated with: North Simcoe Muskoka Local Health Integration Network
PO Box 760, 1112 St. Andrews Dr., Midland, ON L4R 4P4
Tel: 705-526-1300 Fax: 705-526-4491
www.gbgh.on.ca
Number of Beds: 69 acute care beds; 21 complex care beds; 15 rehabilitation beds; 6 ICU beds
Note: Programs & services include: acute & intensive care; emergency; inpatient & ambulatory care; obstetrics; regional complex continuing care; regional rehabiliation; & surgery.
John Kurvink, Interim President & CEO
Dr. Martin Veall, Chief of Medical Staff
Liliana Canadic, Chief Nursing Executive & Vice-President, Patient Services

MILTON: Milton District Hospital
Halton Healthcare Services
Affiliated with: Mississauga Halton Local Health Integration Network
7030 Derry Rd., Milton, ON L9T 7H6
Tel: 905-878-2383 Fax: 905-878-7047
TTY: 905-878-7202
mdhinfodesk@haltonhealthcare.on.ca
www.haltonhealthcare.on.ca
Social Media: www.facebook.com/HaltonHealthcare; twitter.com/haltonhlthcare; www.linkedin.com/company/3186579
Year Founded: 1959
Number of Beds: 43 acute care beds; 20 complex continuing care beds
Population Served: 100000
Number of Employees: 379
Note: Programs & services include: acute hand program; asthma education; audiology & hearing aid services; breastfeeding clinics, drop-ins & prenatal classes; cardiac rehabilitation program; complex continuing care; ConnectCARE; diagnostic imaging; emergency; Falls Prevention Clinic; Halton Diabetes Centre; inpatient rehabilitation; mammography; medical & surgical services; mental health urgent care

clinic; obstetrics; outpatient rehabilitation; respiratory rehabilitation program; smoking cessation program; speech-language pathology; & Work-Fit Total Therapy Centre.
Denise Hardenne, President & CEO, Halton Healthcare
Dr. Lorne Martin, Chief of Staff, Halton Healthcare

MINDEMOYA: Manitoulin Health Centre
Mindemoya Medical Clinic
PO Box 150, Mindemoya, ON P0P 1S0
Tel: 705-377-5371 Fax: 705-377-5372
www.manitoulinhealthcentre.com
Number of Beds: 14 beds
Note: Provides physician, nursing, social work, & dietitian services.

MINDEN: Haliburton Highlands Health Services - Minden Site (HHHS)
Affiliated with: Central East Local Health Integration Network
PO Box 30, 6 McPherson St., Minden, ON K0M 2K0
Tel: 705-286-2140 Fax: 705-286-6384
www.hhhs.ca

Note: Programs & services include: community programs; diabetes education; long-term care; mental health; physiotherapy; primary care; & ultrasound.
Carolyn Plummer, President & CEO
705-457-2527, cplummer@hhhs.ca

MISSISSAUGA: The Credit Valley Hospital
Trillium Health Partners
Affiliated with: Mississauga Halton Local Health Integration Network
2200 Eglinton Ave. West, Mississauga, ON L5M 2N1
Tel: 905-813-2200 Fax: 905-813-4444
Toll-Free: 877-292-4284
cvhpr@cvh.on.ca
trilliumhealthpartners.ca
Social Media: twitter.com/Trillium_Health; www.youtube.com/user/TrilliumHealth; www.linkedin.com/company/2949012
Year Founded: 1985
Number of Beds: 382 beds
Number of Employees: 3125
Note: Programs & services include: ambulatory care; asthma education; cardiac; diabetes education; diagnostic imaging; emergency; geriatric emergency; gynaecology; maternity; mental health; obstetrics; oncology; paediatrics; & renal services.
Michelle E. DiEmanuele, President & CEO, Trillium Health Partners
Dr. Dante Morra, Chief of Staff, Trillium Health Partners
Kathryn Hayward-Murray, Chief Nursing Executive & Senior Vice-President, Patient Care Services, Trillium Health Partners

MISSISSAUGA: Mississauga Hospital
Trillium Health Partners
Affiliated with: Mississauga Halton Local Health Integration Network
Former Name: Queensway General Hospital
100 Queensway West, Mississauga, ON L5B 1B8
Tel: 905-848-7100 Fax: 905-848-7140
patient.relationsmh@trilliumhealthpartners.ca
trilliumhealthpartners.ca
Social Media: twitter.com/Trillium_Health; www.youtube.com/user/TrilliumHealth; www.linkedin.com/company/2949012
Number of Beds: 751 beds
Note: Programs & services include: emergency care centre; birthing centre; critical care; neurosurgery; stroke & cardiac care; sexual assault & domestic violence services; & women's & children's health (Colonel Harland Sanders Family Care Centre).
Michelle E. DiEmanuele, President & CEO, Trillium Health Partners
Dr. Dante Morra, Chief of Staff, Trillium Health Partners
Kathryn Hayward-Murray, Chief Nursing Executive & Senior Vice-President, Patient Care Services, Trillium Health Partners

MOOSE FACTORY: Weeneebayko Area Health Authority/Weeneebayko General Hospital (WAHA)
Affiliated with: North East Local Health Integration Network
PO Box 664, 19 Hospital Dr., Moose Factory, ON P0L 1W0
Tel: 705-658-4544 Fax: 705-658-4917
www.waha.ca

Note: Programs & services include: emergency room; operating room; in-patient; & out-patient.
Bernie D. Schmidt, President & CEO
Dr. Gordon Green, Chief of Staff

MOUNT BRYDGES: Southwest Middlesex Health Centre
22262 Mill Rd., RR#5, Mount Brydges, ON N0L 1W0
Tel: 519-264-2800 *Fax:* 519-264-2742
www.smhc.net

Year Founded: 1974
Area Served: Mount Brydges & the surrounding area
Note: Appointments are necessary.
Gary Wood, Centre Administrator

MOUNT FOREST: Louise Marshall Hospital
North Wellington Health Care Corporation
Affiliated with: Waterloo Wellington Local Health Integration Network
630 Dublin St., Mount Forest, ON N0G 2L3
Tel: 519-323-2210 *Fax:* 519-323-3741
www.nwhealthcare.ca

Year Founded: 1923
Number of Beds: 15 inpatient beds
Population Served: 15000
Note: Programs & services include: anesthesiology; emergency; ENT; general surgery; gynecology; inpatient & outpatient care; internal medicine; neurology; obstetrics; pathology; pediatrics; radiology; specialist clinics; supportive diagnostic services; & urology.
Stephen Street, President & CEO, North Wellington Health Care

NAPANEE: Lennox & Addington County General Hospital
Affiliated with: South East Local Health Integration Network
8 Richmond Park Dr., Napanee, ON K7R 2Z4
Tel: 613-354-3301 *Fax:* 613-354-7157
www.lacgh.com

Number of Beds: 52 beds (24 active care, 2 palliative care, 4 special care, 22 long-term care)
Number of Employees: 270
Note: Programs & services include: bone mineral densitometry; cardiopulmonary; chemotherapy; day surgery; diabetes education; diagnostic imaging; emergency; inpatient; laboratory; mammography; nutrition; occupational therapy; pharmacy; physiotherapy; & respiratory therapy.
Wayne Coveyduck, President & CEO
Dr. Kim Morrison, Chief of Staff

NEW LISKEARD: Centre de santé communautaire du Témiskaming
CP 38, 20 May St. South, New Liskeard, ON P0J 1P0
Tél: 705-647-5775 *Téléc:* 705-647-6011
Ligne sans frais: 800-835-2728
www.csctim.on.ca

Jocelyne Maxwell, Directrice générale

NEW LISKEARD: Temiskaming Hospital
Affiliated with: North East Local Health Integration Network
421 Shepherdson Rd., New Liskeard, ON P0J 1P0
Tel: 705-647-8121 *Fax:* 705-647-5800
www.temiskaming-hospital.com

Year Founded: 1980
Number of Beds: 59 beds (40 acute, 11 chronic, 5 obstetric & 3 special care unit beds)
Population Served: 30000
Number of Employees: 257
Note: Programs & services include: emergency; cardiac rehabilitation; diagnostic imaging (CT scans); laboratory; nutrition services; occupational therapy; pastoral care; pharmacy; physiotherapy; respiratory therapy; speech language pathology; & telestroke program. Visiting specialists conduct services in neurology, nephrology, obstetrics & gynecology, orthotics, rehab/physical medicine, psychiatry, ophthalmology, & pediatrics.
Margaret Beatty, President & CEO
  705-647-1088, mbeatty@temiskaming-hospital.com
Kevin Duke, Chief Financial Officer & Director, Corporate Services
  705-647-1088, kduke@temiskaming-hospital.com
Erin Montgomery, Chief Nurse/Health Professions Officer & Director, Operations
  705-647-1088, emontgomery@temiskaming-hospital.com

NEWBURY: Four Counties Health Services (FCHS)
Middlesex Hospital Alliance
Affiliated with: South West Local Health Integration Network
1824 Concession Dr., RR#3, Newbury, ON N0L 1Z0
Tel: 519-693-4441
www.mhalliance.on.ca

Population Served: 23000
Note: Programs & services include: ambulatory care; community support; diabetes education; diagnostic imaging; emergency; medical surgical day services; & physiotherapy.
Todd Stepanuik, President & CEO, Middlesex Hospital Alliance
Dr. Gary Perkin, Chief of Staff, Middlesex Hospital Alliance

NEWMARKET: CCAC Central - Newmarket Head Office
Former Name: Etobicoke & York CCAC
#1, 1100 Gorham St., Newmarket, ON L3Y 8Y8
Tel: 905-895-1240 *Fax:* 905-952-2404
info@central.ccac-ont.ca
healthcareathome.ca

Megan Allen-Lamb, CEO

NEWMARKET: Southlake Regional Health Centre
Affiliated with: Central Local Health Integration Network
Former Name: York County Hospital
596 Davis Dr., Newmarket, ON L3Y 2P9
Tel: 905-895-4521
www.southlakeregional.org
Social Media: www.facebook.com/southlakeregionalhealthcentre; twitter.com/southlake_news; www.youtube.com/SouthlakeRHC

Year Founded: 1922
Number of Beds: 400 beds
Note: Programs & services include: chronic diseases clinics & programs; emergency; ethics; health information; maternal child; medicine; mental health; musculoskelatal; regional cancer program; regional cardiac care program; rehabilitation; surgery; & spiritual care.
Dr. Dave Williams, President & CEO
Dr. Steven Beatty, Chief of Staff
Helena Hutton, Chief Operating Officer
Annette Jones, Chief Nursing Officer & Vice-President, Patient Experiences

NIAGARA FALLS: Greater Niagara General Site
Niagara Health System / Système de santé de Niagara
Affiliated with: Hamilton Niagara Haldimand Brant Local Health Integration Network
5546 Portage Rd., Niagara Falls, ON L2E 6X2
Tel: 905-378-4647
patientrelations@niagarahealth.on.ca
www.niagarahealth.on.ca
Social Media: twitter.com/niagarahealth; www.youtube.com/niagarahealthsystem

Year Founded: 1907
Number of Beds: 180+ beds
Note: Programs & services include: cardiology; complex care; critical care; diagnostic imaging; emergency; laboratory; medicine; off-site dialysis centre; Ontario Breast Screening Clinic; outpatient clinics; outpatient mental health; regional geriatric assessment; regional stroke services; surgery; & pharmacy.
Dr. Kevin Smith, Chief Executive Officer, Niagara Health System
  kevin.smith@niagarahealth.on.ca
Dr. Suzanne Johnston, President, Niagara Health System
  suzanne.johnston@niagarahealth.on.ca
Derek McNally, Chief Nursing Executive, Niagara Health System
  derek.mcnally@niagarahealth.on.ca
Linda Boich, Executive Vice-President, Niagara Health System
  linda.boich@niagarahealth.on.ca

NIAGARA ON THE LAKE: Niagara-on-the-Lake Site
Niagara Health System / Système de santé de Niagara
Affiliated with: Hamilton Niagara Haldimand Brant Local Health Integration Network
176 Wellington St., Niagara on the Lake, ON L0S 1J0
Tel: 905-378-4647 *Fax:* 905-468-7690
patientrelations@niagarahealth.on.ca
www.niagarahealth.on.ca
Social Media: twitter.com/niagarahealth; www.youtube.com/niagarahealthsystem

Year Founded: 1921
Note: Programs & services include: complex care; diagnostic imaging; & laboratory.
Dr. Kevin Smith, Chief Executive Officer, Niagara Health System
kevin.smith@niagarahealth.on.ca
Dr. Suzanne Johnston, President, Niagara Health System
suzanne.johnston@niagarahealth.on.ca

NIPIGON: Nipigon District Memorial Hospital
Affiliated with: North West Local Health Integration Network
PO Box 37, 125 Hogan Rd., Nipigon, ON P0T 2J0
Tel: 807-887-3026 *Fax:* 807-887-2800
admin@ndmh.ca
www.ndmh.ca
Number of Beds: 37 beds
Note: Services include: acute & complex continuing care; emergency services; diagnostic imaging; physiotherapy; respite care; & Telehealth.
Dr. Rhonda Crocker Ellacott, Chief Executive Officer
807-887-3026
Dan Hill, Chief Financial Officer
Dot Allen, Chief Nursing Officer

NORTH BAY: CCAC North East - North Bay Branch Office
1164 Devonshire Ave., North Bay, ON P1B 6X7
Tel: 705-476-2222 *Fax:* 705-474-0080
TTY: 888-533-2222
healthcareathome.ca
Richard Joly, CEO

NORTH BAY: North Bay Regional Health Centre (NBRHC)/Centre régional de santé de North Bay
Former Name: North Bay General Hospital; Northeast Mental Health Centre
PO Box 2500, 50 College Dr., North Bay, ON P1B 5A4
Tel: 705-474-8600 *Fax:* 705-495-7956
pr@nbrhc.on.ca
www.nbrhc.on.ca
Social Media: www.facebook.com/nbrhc; twitter.com/nbrhc; www.youtube.com/thenbrhc
Number of Beds: 420 beds
Note: The North Bay Regional Health Centre is the result of an amalgamation of the North Bay General Hospital & the Northeast Mental Health Centre, which occurred in 2010. The facility now offers acute, specialist & mental health services to North Bay & the surrounding communities.
Paul Heinrich, President & CEO

NORTH BAY: North East Local Health Integration Network
Also Known As: North East LHIN
555 Oak St. East, 3rd Fl., North Bay, ON P1B 8E3
Tel: 705-840-2872 *Fax:* 705-840-0142
Toll-Free: 866-906-5446
www.nelhin.on.ca
Social Media: www.facebook.com/NorthEastLHIN;
twitter.com/NorthEastLHIN; www.youtube.com/user/LHIN101;
linkedin.com/company/north-east-local-health-integration-network
Year Founded: 2005
Area Served: 400,000 sq km
Population Served: 565000
Note: The North East LHIN brings 150 of the region's health care partners together - hospitals, community support services, mental health & addictions, community health centres, long-term care homes, & the Community Care Access Centre.
Rick Cooper, Interim Board Chair
Louise Paquette, Chief Executive Officer
Tamara Shewciw, Chief Information Officer, eHealth & Project Management Office
Kate Fyfe, Senior Director, System Performance
Terry Tilleczek, Senior Director, Policy & Health System Planning
Cynthia Stables, Director, Community Engagement, Communications, & Cultural Diversity

OAKVILLE: Mississauga Halton Local Health Integration Network (MH LHIN)/RLISS Mississauga Halton
Also Known As: Mississauga Halton LHIN
#500, 700 Dorval Dr., Oakville, ON L6K 3V3
Tel: 905-337-7131 *Fax:* 905-337-8330
Toll-Free: 866-371-5446
mississaugahalton@lhins.on.ca
www.mississaugahaltonlhin.on.ca
Social Media: www.youtube.com/user/mhlhin
Year Founded: 2005
Area Served: 900 sq km
Note: Includes the south-west portion of the City of Toronto, the south part of Peel Region, & all of Halton Region except for Burlington, which is part of the Hamilton Niagara Haldimand Brant LHIN; includes the municipalities of South Etobicoke, Mississauga, Halton Hills, Oakville, & Milton
Mary Davies, Acting Board Chair
Bill MacLeod, Chief Executive Officer
Andrew Hussain, Regional Chief Information Officer
Dale McGregor, Chief Financial Officer & Senior Director, Health System Performance & Information Management
Liane Fernandes, Chief Strategy Officer & Senior Director, Health System Development

OAKVILLE: Oakville-Trafalgar Memorial Hospital
Halton Healthcare Services
Affiliated with: Mississauga Halton Local Health Integration Network
3001 Hospital Gate, Oakville, ON L6M 0L8
Tel: 905-845-2571 *Fax:* 905-338-4636
TTY: 905-815-5111
infodesk@haltonhealthcare.on.ca
www.haltonhealthcare.on.ca
Social Media: www.facebook.com/HaltonHealthcare;
twitter.com/haltonhlthcare; www.linkedin.com/company/3186579
Number of Beds: 457 beds
Population Served: 183000
Number of Employees: 2127
Note: Programs & services include: ambulatory care; complex continuing care; critical care; diagnostics; emergency care; maternal & child care; mental health; rehabilitation; & surgery.
Denise Hardenne, President & CEO, Halton Healthcare
Dr. Lorne Martin, Chief of Staff, Halton Healthcare
Carole Moore, COO, Oakville-Trafalgar Memorial Hospital

ORANGEVILLE: Headwaters Health Care Centre
Affiliated with: Central West Local Health Integration Network
Former Name: Headwaters Orangeville
100 Rolling Hills Dr., Orangeville, ON L9W 4X9
Tel: 519-941-2410 *Fax:* 519-942-0483
www.headwatershealth.ca
Year Founded: 1997
Number of Beds: 87 beds
Note: Programs & services include: ambulatory care; cardiac care; chemotherapy; complex continuing care; diabetes care; diagnostic imaging; dialysis; domestic & sexual assault program; emergency; intensive care unit; laboratory; mental health; nutrition; obstetrics; occupational therapy; ophthalmology; paediatrics; palliative care; pharmacy; physiotherapy; respiratory therapy; speech-language pathology; spiritual care; surgery; & Telemedicine.
Stacey Daub, President & CEO
519-941-2702, sdaub@headwatershealth.ca
Dr. Somaiah Ahmed, Chief of Staff & Vice-President, Medical Affairs
519-941-2702, sahmed@headwatershealth.ca

ORILLIA: North Simcoe Muskoka Local Health Integration Network
Also Known As: North Simcoe Muskoka LHIN
#128, 210 Memorial Ave., Orillia, ON L3V 7V1
Tel: 705-326-7750 *Fax:* 705-326-1392
Toll-Free: 866-903-5446
northsimcoemuskoka@lhins.on.ca
www.nsmlhin.on.ca
Social Media: twitter.com/NSMLHIN
Year Founded: 2005
Population Served: 453710
Number of Employees: 35
Note: Encompasses the District of Muskoka, most of the County of Simcoe and a portion of Grey County. North Simcoe Muskoka is home

to four First Nations. Health service providers include: 7 hospitals, 26 long-term care homes, 1 community care access centre, 3 community health centre, 29 community support services & 9 community mental health providers.

Robert Morton, Board Chair

Jill Tettmann, Chief Executive Officer
jill.tettmann@lhins.on.ca

Neil Walker, Chief Operating Officer
neil.walker@lhins.on.ca

Archie Outar, Senior Manager, Finance
archie.outar@lhins.on.ca

Jessica Dolan, Associate, Communications & New Media
jessica.dolan@lhins.on.ca

ORILLIA: Orillia Soldiers' Memorial Hospital (OSMH)
Affiliated with: North Simcoe Muskoka Local Health Integration Network
170 Colborne St. West, Orillia, ON L3V 2Z3

Tel: 705-325-2201 Fax: 705-325-7394
TTY: 705-325-1231
info@osmh.on.ca
www.osmh.on.ca

Social Media: www.facebook.com/TheOrilliaSoldiersMemorialHospital;
twitter.com/OSMH_News; www.youtube.com/OSMHVideos;
www.linkedin.com/company/orillia-soldiers-memorial-hospital

Number of Beds: 230 inpatient beds
Number of Employees: 1200
Note: Programs & services include: cancer care; chronic disease management; clinical nutrition services; critical care; diagnostic imaging; emergency; infection prevention & control; laboratory; maternal, child & youth; mental health services; rehabilitation; regional kidney care program; surgical services; & Telemedicine. Has 300 physicians on staff.

Pat Campbell, President & CEO
ceo@osmh.on.ca

Dr. Nancy Merrow, Chief of Medical Staff & Vice-President, Medical Affairs

Cheryl Harrison, Vice-President, Regional Patient Programs

OSHAWA: Carea Community Health Centre - Oshawa Office
Former Name: Oshawa Community Health Centre
115 Grassmere Ave., Oshawa, ON L1H 3X7

Tel: 905-723-0036 Fax: 905-723-3391
info@careachc.ca
www.careachc.ca

Social Media: www.facebook.com/CareaCHC; twitter.com/careachc

Note: Specialties: Child development; Youth recreation; Women's wellness; Health promotion; Family community outreach; Education services, such as the diabetes education program; Counselling; Parenting groups; Regular check-ups; Rehabilitation

Lee Kierstead, CEO

OSHAWA: Lakeridge Health - Oshawa Site
Affiliated with: Central East Local Health Integration Network
Former Name: Oshawa General Hospital
1 Hospital Ct., Oshawa, ON L1G 2B9

Tel: 905-576-8711
www.lakeridgehealth.on.ca

Social Media: www.facebook.com/LakeridgeHealth;
twitter.com/lakeridgehealth; www.youtube.com/lakeridgehealth

Number of Beds: 363 beds
Note: Programs & services include: ambulatory & rehabilitation centre; Central East Regional Cardiac Care Program; child, youth & family program; community respiratory services; dialysis unit; eating disorders program; emergency department; GAIN geriatric clinic; interact treatment program; mental health day treatment program; Ontario Breast Screening Program; paediatric feeding/swallowing clinic; pain clinic; palliative care; Pinewood Centre (alcohol & addictions); & positive care clinic.

Matthew Anderson, President & CEO, Lakeridge Health
905-576-8711

Dr. Tony Stone, Chief of Staff, Lakeridge Health
905-576-8711

Leslie Motz, Chief Nursing Executive, Lakeridge Health
905-576-8711

OTTAWA: Bruyère Continuing Care
Affiliated with: Champlain Local Health Integration Network
Former Name: Sisters of Charity of Ottawa Health Service
43 Bruyère St., Ottawa, ON K1N 5C8

Tel: 613-562-6262 Fax: 613-562-6367
communications@bruyere.org
www.bruyere.org

Social Media: www.facebook.com/bruyerecare;
twitter.com/bruyerecare; www.linkedin.com/company/bruyerecare

Year Founded: 1993
Number of Beds: 706 beds
Number of Employees: 2045
Note: Specializes in complex continuing care, rehabilitation, palliative care, long-term care, & seniors housing; includes Saint-Vincent Hospital, Élisabeth Bruyère Hospital, Élisabeth Bruyère Residence, Saint-Louis Residence, & Bruyère Village.

Daniel Levac, President & CEO

Dr. Shaun McGuire, Chief of Staff

Debbie Gravelle, Chief Nursing Executive & Senior Vice-President, Clinical Programs

Marc Guèvremont, Chief Financial Officer & Vice-President, Corporate Services

Jean-François Brunelle, Vice-President, Human Resources & Organizational Development

Amy Porteous, Vice-President, Public Affairs & Planning

Dr. Carol Wiebe, Vice-President, Medical Affairs

Heidi Sveistrup, Vice-President, Research & Academic Affairs

Melissa Donskov, Executive Director, Long-Term Care

OTTAWA: Carlington Community & Health Services
900 Merivale Rd., Ottawa, ON K1Z 5Z8

Tel: 613-722-4000 Fax: 613-761-1805
info@carlington.ochc.org
www.carlington.ochc.org

Cameron MacLeod, Executive Director

OTTAWA: Centretown Community Health Centre
420 Cooper St., Ottawa, ON K2P 2N6

Tel: 613-233-4443 Fax: 613-233-3987
TTY: 613-233-0651
info@centretownchc.org
www.centretownchc.org

Social Media: www.facebook.com/CentretownCHC;
twitter.com/centretownchc

Cathy Doolan, President

OTTAWA: Champlain Community Care Access Centre (CCAC)/Centre d'accès aux soins communautaires
Former Name: Ottawa Community Care Access Centre
#100, 4200 Labelle St., Ottawa, ON K1J 1J8

Tel: 613-745-5525 Fax: 613-745-6984
Toll-Free: 800-538-0520
TTY: 613-745-0049
information@champlain.ccac-ont.ca
healthcareathome.ca/champlain

Note: Specialties: Home care; Coordination of community care; Information about long-term care options

Marc Sougavinski, CEO

OTTAWA: Champlain Local Health Integration Network
Also Known As: Champlain LHIN
#204, 1900 City Park Dr., Ottawa, ON K1J 1A3

Tel: 613-747-6784 Fax: 613-747-6519
Toll-Free: 866-902-5446
champlain@lhins.on.ca
www.champlainlhin.on.ca

Social Media: twitter.com/champlainlhin;
www.youtube.com/user/ChamplainLHIN

Year Founded: 2005
Population Served: 1200000
Note: Area Served: Renfrew County; City of Ottawa; Prescott & Russell; Stormont; Dundas & Glengarry; North Grenville; four parts of North Lanark

Jean-Pierre Boisclair, Board Chair

Chantale LeClerc, Chief Executive Officer

Cal Martell, Senior Director, Health System Performance

Eric Partington, Senior Director, Health System Performance
Elaine Medline, Director, Communications

OTTAWA: Hôpital Montfort
Affiliée à: Champlain Local Health Integration Network
713, ch Montréal, Ottawa, ON K1K 0T2

Tél: 613-746-4621 *Ligne sans frais:* 866-670-4621
montfort@montfort.on.ca
www.hopitalmontfort.com
Média social: www.facebook.com/hopital.montfort;
twitter.com/hopitalmontfort; www.youtube.com/user/telehopitalmontfort;
www.linkedin.com/company/hopital-montfort

Nombre de lits: 289 lits
Note: Services: centre familiale de naissance; medicine; programme de cancérologie; programme de santé mentale; services diagnostiques incluant imagerie diagnostique et laboratoire du sommeil; services de santé cardiovasculaire et pulmonaire; services thérapeutiques y inclus la physiothérapie et clinique pour les troubles de la communication; soins ambulatoires; soins aux malades en phase critique y inclus les soins intensive et soins d'urgence; et soins palliatifs.
Dr. Bernard Leduc, Président-directeur général
Dr. Guy Moreau, Médecin-chef
Suzanne Robichaud, Chef de la pratique infirmière et vice-présidente, Services cliniques

OTTAWA: The Ottawa Hospital - Civic Campus
Affiliated with: Champlain Local Health Integration Network
1053 Carling Ave., Ottawa, ON K1Y 4E9

Tel: 613-722-7000
TTY: 613-761-4024
www.ottawahospital.on.ca
Social Media: www.facebook.com/OttawaHospital;
twitter.com/OttawaHospital; www.youtube.com/user/TheOttawaHospital
Year Founded: 1845
Number of Beds: 1,122 beds across the system
Note: Programs & services include: cardiology; emergency; family health team; Mohs Surgery Clinic; neurosciences; Regional Geriatric Program for Eastern Ontario; spinal surgery; trauma services; University of Ottawa Skills & Simulation Centre (uOSSC); vascular surgery; weight management clinic - Bariatric Centre of Excellence; & women's breast health centre. Total physicians across hospital system: 1,300.
Dr. Jack Kitts, President & CEO
  613-761-4800, jbkitts@toh.ca
Dr. Jeffrey Turnbull, Chief of Staff
  613-737-8459, jeturnbull@toh.ca
Dr. Debra A. Bournes, Chief Nursing Executive & Vice-President, Clinical Programs
  613-737-8899, dbournes@toh.ca

OTTAWA: The Ottawa Hospital - General Campus
Affiliated with: Champlain Local Health Integration Network
501 Smyth Rd., Ottawa, ON K1H 8L6

Tel: 613-722-7000
TTY: 613-761-4024
www.ottawahospital.on.ca
Social Media: www.facebook.com/OttawaHospital;
twitter.com/OttawaHospital; www.youtube.com/user/TheOttawaHospital
Year Founded: 1845
Number of Beds: 1,122 beds across the system
Specialties: Cardiovascular
Note: Programs & services include: bone marrow transplant; chest diseases centre; emergency; regional cancer program; rehabilitation centre; robotic surgery; thoracic surgery; total joint replacement; & the University of Ottawa Eye Institute. Total physicians across hospital system: 1,300.
Dr. Jack Kitts, President & CEO
  613-761-4800, jbkitts@toh.ca
Dr. Jeffrey Turnbull, Chief of Staff
  613-737-8459, jeturnbull@toh.ca
Dr. Debra A. Bournes, Chief Nursing Executive & Vice-President, Clinical Programs
  613-737-8899, dbournes@toh.ca

OTTAWA: The Ottawa Hospital - Riverside Campus
Affiliated with: Champlain Local Health Integration Network
1967 Riverside Dr., Ottawa, ON K1H 7W9

Tel: 613-722-7000
TTY: 613-761-4024
www.ottawahospital.on.ca
Social Media: www.facebook.com/OttawaHospital;
twitter.com/OttawaHospital; www.youtube.com/user/TheOttawaHospital
Year Founded: 1845
Number of Beds: 1,122 beds across the system
Note: Programs & services include: arthritis centre; eye care centre; family health team; Foustanellas Endocrine & Diabetes Centre; nephrology; & Shirley E. Greenberg Women's Health Centre. Total physicians across hospital system: 1,300. Affiliated with the University of Ottawa.
Dr. Jack Kitts, President & CEO
  613-761-4800, jbkitts@toh.ca
Dr. Jeffrey Turnbull, Chief of Staff
  613-737-8459, jeturnbull@toh.ca
Dr. Debra A. Bournes, Chief Nursing Executive & Vice-President, Clinical Programs
  613-737-8899, dbournes@toh.ca

OTTAWA: Pinecrest-Queensway Health & Community Services (PQCHC)
1365 Richmond Rd., 2nd Fl., Ottawa, ON K2B 6R7

Tel: 613-820-4922 *Fax:* 613-288-3407
info@pqchc.com
www.pqchc.com
Social Media: www.facebook.com/PQCHC; twitter.com/PQCHC
Year Founded: 1979
Wanda MacDonald, Chief Executive Officer

OTTAWA: Queensway Carleton Hospital (QCH)
Affiliated with: Champlain Local Health Integration Network
3045 Baseline Rd., Ottawa, ON K2H 8P4

Tel: 613-721-2000 *Toll-Free:* 888-824-9111
www.qch.on.ca
Social Media: www.facebook.com/caregrowswest
Year Founded: 1976
Number of Beds: 264 beds
Population Served: 400000
Number of Employees: 1955
Note: Programs & services include: childbirth centre; emergency; geriatric services; medical & surgical services; mental health; & rehabilitation. Has 276 physicians & 8 midwives on staff.
Tom Schonberg, President & CEO
Dr. Andrew Falconer, Chief of Staff
Leah Levesque, Chief Nursing Officer & Vice-President, Patient Care

OTTAWA: Rehabilitation Centre (TRC)
The Ottawa Hospital
505 Smyth Rd., Ottawa, ON K1H 8M2

Tel: 613-737-7350
TTY: 613-526-1132
feedback@toh.ca
www.ottawahospital.on.ca

Note: Specialties: Rehabilitation of persons with a disabling physical illness or injury; Prosthetics & orthotics; Physiotherapy; Occupational therapy; Respiratory therapy; Speech-language pathology; Psychological services; Vocational rehabilitation counselling; Social work; Research
Dr. Jack Kitts, President & CEO

OTTAWA: Sandy Hill Community Health Centre
221 Nelson St., Ottawa, ON K1N 1C7

Tel: 613-789-1500 *Fax:* 613-789-7962
www.shchc.ca
Year Founded: 1973
Note: Provides a variety of health & social services in the Eastern Ottawa region
David Gibson, Executive Director

OTTAWA: Somerset West Community Health Centre
55 Eccles St., Ottawa, ON K1R 6S3

Tel: 613-238-8210 *Fax:* 613-238-7595
info@swchc.on.ca
www.swchc.on.ca

Note: Programs & services include: pulmonary rehabilitation; asthma program; mental health; obstetrical care; HIV testing; dental screening; foot care; primary care; & services for seniors
Naini Cloutier, Executive Director

OTTAWA: South-East Ottawa Community Health Centre
#600, 1355 Bank St., Ottawa, ON K1H 8K7
Tel: 613-737-5115 *Fax:* 613-739-8199
office@seochc.on.ca
www.seochc.on.ca
Info Line: 613-737-4809
Social Media: www.facebook.com/142007129166107;
twitter.com/SEOCHC

Note: Programs & services include: diabetes education; dental screening; HIV testing; foot care; & mental health
Leslie McDiarmid, Executive Director

OWEN SOUND: CCAC North Bruce & Grey Counties
#3009, 1415 - 1 Ave. West, Owen Sound, ON N4K 4K8
Fax: 519-371-5612
healthcareathome.ca

Sandra Coleman, CEO, South West CCAC

OWEN SOUND: Owen Sound Hospital
Grey Bruce Health Services
Affiliated with: South West Local Health Integration Network
1800 - 8th St. East, Owen Sound, ON N4K 6M9
Tel: 519-376-2121
web@gbhs.on.ca
www.gbhs.on.ca
Social Media: twitter.com/greybrucehealth

Number of Beds: 244 beds
Note: Regional referral centre for Grey & Bruce counties. Programs & services include: acute care; acute inpatient rehabilitation; ambulatory care; cardiac rehabilitation program; critical care; Diabetes Grey Bruce; diagnostic imaging; dialysis; electro diagnostics; emergency; Grey Bruce District Stroke Centre; health centre pharmacy; mental health; occupational therapy; physiotherapy; respiratory therapy; restorative care unit; sleep lab; social work; spiritual care; surgery; & women & child care.
Lance Thurston, President & CEO, Grey Bruce Health Services
519-376-2121
Dr. Michael Marriott, Chief of Staff, Grey Bruce Health Services
519-376-2121

PALMERSTON: Palmerston & District Hospital
North Wellington Health Care Corporation
Affiliated with: Waterloo Wellington Local Health Integration Network
500 Whites Rd., Palmerston, ON N0G 2P0
Tel: 519-343-2030 *Fax:* 519-343-3821
www.nwhealthcare.ca

Year Founded: 1908
Number of Beds: 15 inpatient beds
Population Served: 15000
Note: Programs & services include: anesthesiology; emergency; ENT; general surgery; gynecology; inpatient & outpatient care; internal medicine; obstetrics; pathology; radiology; specialist clinics; & supportive diagnostic services.
Stephen Street, President & CEO, North Wellington Health Care

PARIS: Willett Hospital
Brant Community Healthcare System
Affiliated with: Hamilton Niagara Haldimand Brant Local Health Integration Network
Also Known As: The Willett
238 Grand River St. North, Paris, ON N3L 2N7
Tel: 519-442-2251
www.bchsys.org
Social Media: www.facebook.com/bchsys; twitter.com/BCHSYS;
www.youtube.com/user/bchsys2011;
www.linkedin.com/company/brantford-general-hospital
Year Founded: 1922
Number of Beds: 260+ beds (including Brantford General Hospital)
Specialties: Urgent care
Note: Programs & services include: diagnostic imaging; fitness centres & programs; rehabilitation (outpatient); walk-in medical clinics & urgent

care. Brant Community Healthcare System is affiliated with the Michael G. DeGroote School of Medicine, McMaster University.
James Hornell, President & CEO, Brant Community Healthcare System
jim.hornell@bchsys.org
Dr. Christopher O'Brien, Chief of Staff, Brant Community Healthcare System
christopher.obrien@bchsys.org
Lina Rinaldi, Chief Operating Officer & Chief Nursing Executive, Brant Community Healthcare System
lina.rinaldi@bchsys.org
MaryLou Toop, Interim Chief Financial Officer, Brant Community Healthcare System
marylou.toop@bchsys.org

PARRY SOUND: West Parry Sound Health Centre (WPSHC)
Affiliated with: North East Local Health Integration Network
6 Albert St., Parry Sound, ON P2A 3A4
Tel: 705-746-9321 *Fax:* 705-746-7364
www.wpshc.com

Year Founded: 1995
Number of Beds: 90 beds
Note: Programs & services include: acute & complex continuing care; rehabilitation; on-site Lakeland Long Term Care Facility; Community Care Access Centre; emergency services; surgery; diagnostic imaging; chemotherapy; sleep disorder clinic; lab; telehealth; Base Hospital Program & nursing stations in Britt, Pointe au Baril, Rosseau, Whitestone, Argyle & Moosedeer; specialist clinics
Donald Sanderson, CEO

PEMBROKE: Pembroke Regional Hospital
Affiliated with: Champlain Local Health Integration Network
Former Name: Pembroke General Hospital
705 MacKay St., Pembroke, ON K8A 1G8
Tel: 613-732-2811 *Fax:* 613-732-9986
pr@prh.email
www.pemreghos.org
Info Line: 866-996-0991
Social Media: www.youtube.com/user/pembrokeregionalhosp
Number of Beds: 203 beds
Note: Programs & services include: acute mental health; ambulatory clinics; clinical ethics; community mental health; diabetes education & nutrition; diagnostic imaging; dialysis; emergency/ICU; infection prevention & control; laboratory; maternal & child care; medical; rehabilitation (inpatient & outpatient); respiratory therapy; social work; spiritual care; & surgery.
Pierre Noel, President & CEO
pierre.noel@prh.email
Dr. Tom Hurley, Chief of Staff
thomas.hurley@prh.email
Francois Lemaire, Chief Nursing Executive & Vice-President, Patient Services - Acute Care
francois.lemaire@prh.email

PENETANGUISHENE: Georgian Bay General Hospital -
Penetanguishene Site
Affiliated with: North Simcoe Muskoka Local Health Integration Network
25 Jeffery St., Penetanguishene, ON L9M 1K6
Tel: 705-526-1300 *Fax:* 705-526-4491
www.gbgh.on.ca

Note: Programs & services include: dialysis unit; Georgian Bay Cancer Support Centre; & Hospice Huronia. There is no emergency service at this location.
John Kurvink, Interim President & CEO
Dr. Martin Veall, Chief of Medical Staff
Liliana Canadic, Chief Nursing Executive & Vice-President, Patient Services

PENETANGUISHENE: Hôpital Privé Beechwood Private Hospital
58 Church St., Penetanguishene, ON L9M 1B3
Tel: 705-549-7473 *Fax:* 705-549-7194
bph@rogers.com
Number of Beds: 20 beds
Larry Bellisle, CEO

PERTH: Perth & Smiths Falls District Hospital - Perth Site
Also Known As: Great War Memorial Site
33 Drummond St. West, Perth, ON K7H 2K1
Tel: 613-267-1500 Fax: 613-264-0365
webinquiry@psfdh.on.ca
www.psfdh.on.ca

Number of Beds: 85 beds
Note: Programs & services include: assistive devices program; breast screening centre; clinics (obstetrical, pain, pediatric, respirology, orthopedics, general surgery & internal medicine); day hospital; diagnostic imaging; early language; emergency; general medicine; internal medicine; laboratory; sexual assault support & domestic violence program; oncology/palliative care; orthopedics; pharmacy; rehabilitation program; stroke prevention; & urology.
Beverley McFarlane, President & CEO
bmcfarlane@psfdh.on.ca

PETERBOROUGH: CCAC Central East - Peterborough Branch
Office
#202, 700 Clonsilla Ave., Peterborough, ON K9J 5Y3
Tel: 705-743-2212 Fax: 855-352-2555
Toll-Free: 800-263-3877
healthcareathome.ca
Kathryn Ramsay, CEO

PETERBOROUGH: Peterborough Regional Health Centre (PRHC)
Affiliated with: Central East Local Health Integration Network
1 Hospital Dr., Peterborough, ON K9J 7C6
Tel: 705-743-2121 Fax: 705-876-5120
TTY: 705-876-5141
info@prhc.on.ca
www.prhc.on.ca
Social Media: twitter.com/PRHC1;
www.youtube.com/user/PRHChospital;
www.linkedin.com/company/1357436

Number of Beds: 494 beds
Population Served: 300000
Number of Employees: 2200
Note: Programs & services include: diagnostic imaging; emergency; laboratory; medicine; mental health; nutrition; outpatient; rehabilitation; pharmacy; social work; surgery; & woman & child.
Dr. Peter McLaughlin, President & CEO
Dr. Nancy Martin-Ronson, CNE, CIO & Vice-President, Professional & Diagnostic Services

PETROLIA: Charlotte Eleanor Englehart Hospital (CEEH)
Bluewater Health
Affiliated with: Erie St. Clair Local Health Integration Network
Former Name: Charlotte Eleanor Englehart Hospital
450 Blanche St., Petrolia, ON N0N 1R0
Tel: 519-882-4325 Fax: 519-882-3711
www.bluewaterhealth.ca
Social Media: www.facebook.com/bluewaterhealth;
www.youtube.com/bluewaterhealth

Year Founded: 1911
Number of Beds: 326 beds (total for both Bluewater sites)
Note: Programs & services include: acute care; ambulatory care; continuing care; diagnostic imaging; emergency; inpatient medicine; laboratory services; & primary care.
Mike Lapaine, President & CEO, Bluewater Health
mlapaine@bluewaterhealth.ca

PICKLE LAKE: Pickle Lake Health Centre
Affiliated with: North West Local Health Integration Network
PO Box 302, Pickle Lake, ON P0V 3A0
Tel: 807-928-2047 Fax: 807-928-2584
picklelake.healthclinic@picklelake.org

Note: Programs & services include: chronic disease management; disease prevention; nutritional counselling.

PICTON: QHC Prince Edward County Memorial Hospital
Quinte Health Care
Affiliated with: South East Local Health Integration Network
PO Box 1900, 403 Main St. East, Picton, ON K0K 2T0
Tel: 613-476-1008 Fax: 613-476-8600
www.qhc.on.ca
Social Media: www.facebook.com/173689537296;
twitter.com/QuinteHealth; www.youtube.com/QuinteHealthCare

Year Founded: 1959
Number of Beds: 15 beds
Note: Programs & services include: emergency; endoscopy; hospice; laboratory; outpatient clinics; pharmacy; primary care medical inpatients; Prince Edward Family Health Team; & radiology.
Mary Clare Egberts, President & CEO, Quinte Health Care
Dr. Dick Zoutman, Chief of Staff, Quinte Health Care
Carol Smith Romeril, Chief Nursing Officer & Vice-President, Quinte Health Care

PORT COLBORNE: Port Colborne Site
Niagara Health System / Système de santé de Niagara
Affiliated with: Hamilton Niagara Haldimand Brant Local Health Integration Network
260 Sugarloaf St., Port Colborne, ON L3K 2N7
Tel: 905-378-4647
patientrelations@niagarahealth.on.ca
www.niagarahealth.on.ca
Social Media: twitter.com/niagarahealth;
www.youtube.com/niagarahealthsystem

Year Founded: 1951
Number of Beds: 46 beds inpatient beds for complex continuing care; 35 beds at the New Port Centre for addiction recovery
Note: Programs & services include: addictions services; complex care; diagnostic imaging; laboratory; Ontario Breast Screening Clinic; outpatient clinics; & urgent care.
Dr. Kevin Smith, Chief Executive Officer, Niagara Health System
kevin.smith@niagarahealth.on.ca
Dr. Suzanne Johnston, President, Niagara Health System
suzanne.johnston@niagarahealth.on.ca
Dr. Thomas Stewart, Chief of Staff, Niagara Health System
dr.thomas.stewart@niagarahealth.on.c

PORT PERRY: Lakeridge Health - Port Perry Site
Affiliated with: Central East Local Health Integration Network
451 Paxton St., Port Perry, ON L9L 1L9
Tel: 905-985-7321
www.lakeridgehealth.on.ca
Social Media: www.facebook.com/LakeridgeHealth;
twitter.com/lakeridgehealth; www.youtube.com/lakeridgehealth

Note: Programs & services include: ambulatory rehabilitation centres/musculoskeletal physiotherapy clinics; diabetes education; & emergency.
Matthew Anderson, President & CEO, Lakeridge Health
905-576-8711
Dr. Tony Stone, Chief of Staff, Lakeridge Health
905-576-8711
Leslie Motz, Chief Nursing Executive, Lakeridge Health
905-576-8711

PORTLAND: Country Roads Community Health Centre
PO Box 58, 4319 Cove Rd., Portland, ON K0G 1V0
Tel: 613-272-3302 Fax: 613-272-3024
Toll-Free: 888-998-9927
info@crchc.on.ca
www.crchc.on.ca

Note: Programs & services include: immunization; pre-natal care, post-natal care, & early childhood development programs; lung health; pharmacy; nutrition counselling; dental; & diabetes prevention
Marty Crapper, Executive Director

RAINY RIVER: Rainy River Health Centre
Riverside Health Care Facilities Inc.
Affiliated with: North West Local Health Integration Network
115 - 4th St., Rainy River, ON P0W 1L0
Tel: 807-274-3261 Fax: 807-852-3565
www.riversidehealthcare.ca

Number of Beds: 24 beds
Note: Programs & services include: emergency; diagnostic imaging; acute care; & long term care.
Tammy McNally, Manager

RED LAKE: Red Lake Margaret Cochenour Memorial Hospital
Affiliated with: North West Local Health Integration Network
Also Known As: Red Lake Hospital
PO Box 5005, 51 Hwy. 105, Red Lake, ON P0V 2M0
Tel: 807-727-2066 *Fax:* 807-727-2923
www.redlakehospital.ca
Year Founded: 1973
Number of Beds: 12 acute care beds; 4 chronic care beds; 2 obstetrics beds
Note: Services include: emergency; laboratory; nursing; diagnostic imaging; physiotherapy; support services; & Family Health Team.
Angela Bishop, President & CEO
807-727-3800, ceo@redlakehospital.ca
Rebecca Ross, Chief Nursing Executive
Alex McAuley, Chief Financial Officer

RENFREW: Renfrew Victoria Hospital
Affiliated with: Champlain Local Health Integration Network
Also Known As: RVH
499 Raglan St. North, Renfrew, ON K7V 1P6
Tel: 613-432-4851 *Fax:* 613-432-8649
www.renfrewhosp.com
Social Media: www.facebook.com/renfrewvictoriahospital
Year Founded: 1897
Number of Beds: 101 beds
Number of Employees: 450
Note: Programs & services include: ambulatory; counselling; diagnostic; emergency; inpatient; outreach programs; & rehabilitation. Affiliated with Algonquin College & Cambrian College.
Randy Penney, President & CEO
613-432-4851
Christine Ferguson, Vice-President, Patient Care Services
613-432-4851

RICHARDS LANDING: North Shore Health Network - Richards Landing Site
Affiliated with: North East Local Health Integration Network
PO Box 188, 1180 Richards St., Richards Landing, ON P0R 1J0
Tel: 705-246-2570 *Fax:* 705-246-2569
www.nshn.care

Note: Services include emergency & diagnostics.
Connie Lee, Chief Nursing Officer & Director, Clinical Services
Dr. Lenka Snajdrova, Chief of Staff

RICHMOND HILL: CCAC Central - Richmond Hill Site
Former Name: York Region CCAC
#400, 9050 Yonge St., Richmond Hill, ON L4C 9S6
Tel: 905-763-9928 *Fax:* 905-952-2404
info@central.ccac-ont.ca
healthcareathome.ca
Megan Allen-Lamb, CEO

RICHMOND HILL: Mackenzie Richmond Hill Hospital
Mackenzie Health
Affiliated with: Central Local Health Integration Network
Former Name: York Central Hospital
10 Trench St., Richmond Hill, ON L4C 4Z3
Tel: 905-883-1212 *Fax:* 905-883-2455
mackenziehealth.ca
Social Media: www.facebook.com/MackenzieHealth;
twitter.com/mackenziehealth;
www.youtube.com/user/MackenzieHealthVideo;
www.linkedin.com/company/mackenzie-health
Number of Beds: 241 acute care beds; 168 long-term care beds; 84 complex continuing care beds; 22 integrated stroke beds (all Mackenzie Health sites)
Number of Employees: 2641
Note: Has 465 physicians on staff.
Altaf Stationwala, President & CEO, Mackenzie Health
Dr. Steven Jackson, Chief of Staff, Mackenzie Health

SARNIA: Bluewater Health
Affiliated with: Erie St. Clair Local Health Integration Network
Former Name: Charlotte Eleanor Englehart Hospital; Sarnia General Hospital; St. Joseph's Health
Norman Site, 89 Norman St., Sarnia, ON N7T 6S3
Tel: 519-464-4400 *Fax:* 519-464-4407
www.bluewaterhealth.ca
Social Media: www.facebook.com/bluewaterhealth;
www.youtube.com/bluewaterhealth
Year Founded: 2002
Number of Beds: 326 beds (total for both Bluewater sites)
Number of Employees: 2500
Note: Programs & services include: ambulatory care; bone density; Cancer Care Assessment & Treatment Centre; cancer clinic; cardiology; communication disorders; CT scan; day hospital; day surgery; diabetes & clinical nutrition; diagnostic imaging; dialysis; district stroke centre; eating disorders; emergency; endoscopy; infection prevention & control; inpatient medicine, rehabilitation, & surgery; intensive care; laboratory; mammography; maternal/infant/child; mental health & addiction; MRI; nuclear medicine; nutrition & food services; occupational therapy; outpatient rehabilitation; palliative care; Pat Mailloux Eye Centre; physiotherapy; prostate cancer clinic; respiratory therapy; rural health; sexual/domestic assault treatment centre; social work; spiritual care; surgery; Telemedicine; ultrasound; withdrawal management; & x-ray.
Mike Lapine, President & CEO
519-464-4400, mlapaine@bluewaterhealth.ca
Dr. Michel Haddad, Chief of Professional Staff
519-464-4400, mhaddad@bluewaterhealth.ca
Shannon Landry, Chief Nursing Executive
519-464-4400, slandry@bluewaterhealth.ca
Julia Oosterman, Chief, Communications & Public Affairs
519-464-4400, joosterman@bluewaterhealth.ca
Laurie Zimmer, Vice-President, Operations
519-464-4400, lzimmer@bluewaterhealth.ca
Samer Abou-Sweid, Vice-President, Operations
519-464-4400, sabousweid@bluewaterhealth.ca

SAULT STE MARIE: Community Care Access Centre
390 Bay St., Sault Ste Marie, ON P6A 1X2
Tel: 705-949-1808 *Fax:* 705-949-1663
Toll-Free: 800-668-7705
healthcareathome.ca

Note: Provides long term care in home.
Richard Joly, CEO

SAULT STE MARIE: Group Health Centre Sault Ste. Marie
240 McNabb St., Sault Ste Marie, ON P6B 1Y5
Tel: 705-759-1234 *Fax:* 705-759-7469
Toll-Free: 800-461-2407
inquiries@ghc.on.ca
www.ghc.on.ca

Note: GHC is a consumer-sponsored health care facility, built by private funds donated by local union members. A partnership of the Sault Ste. Marie & District Group Health Association & the Algoma District Medical Group. Number of staff: 300+
Alex Lambert, President & CEO
705-759-5606

SAULT STE MARIE: Sault Area Hospital (SAH)
Affiliated with: North East Local Health Integration Network
750 Great Northern Rd., Sault Ste Marie, ON P6B 0A8
Tel: 705-759-3434 *Fax:* 705-541-7810
publicaffairs@sah.on.ca
www.sah.on.ca
Number of Beds: 293 beds
Population Served: 115000
Number of Employees: 1850
Note: Programs & services include: emergency & critical care; medicine; surgery; obstetrics, maternity & pediatrics; mental health & addiction; complex continuing care; & rehabilitation.
Ron Gagnon, President & CEO
Dr. Heather O'Brien, Chief of Staff
Elizabeth Ferguson, Chief Nursing Officer & Vice-President, Clinical Operations

SEAFORTH: CCAC South West - Seaforth Branch
PO Box 580, 32 Centennial Dr., Seaforth, ON N0K 1W0
Tel: 519-527-0000 *Fax:* 519-527-1255
Toll-Free: 800-267-0535
healthcareathome.ca

Sandra Coleman, CEO, South West CCAC

SEAFORTH: Seaforth Community Hospital
Huron Perth Healthcare Alliance
Affiliated with: South West Local Health Integration Network
24 Centennial Dr., Seaforth, ON N0K 1W0
Tel: 519-527-1650 *Fax:* 519-527-8414
Toll-Free: 888-275-1102
www.hpha.ca

Year Founded: 1965
Number of Beds: 20 beds
Note: Programs & services include: adult speech therapy services; ambulatory clinics; community stroke rehabilitation team; complex continuing care; emergency; imaging; Huron Perth Diabetes Education Program; laboratory; medicine; occupational therapy; physiotherapy; & social work.
Andrew Williams, President & CEO, HPHA
519-272-8202, andrew.williams@hpha.ca
Dr. Laurel Moore, Chief of Staff, HPHA
519-272-8210, dr.laurel.moore@hpha.ca
Anne Campbell, Site Administrator
519-272-8210, anne.campbell@hpha.ca

SIMCOE: CCAC Hamilton Niagara Haldimand Brant -
Haldimand-Norfolk Branch Office
76 Victoria St., Simcoe, ON N3Y 1L5
Tel: 519-426-7400 *Fax:* 519-426-4384
Toll-Free: 800-810-0000
healthcareathome.ca

Melody Miles, CEO

SIMCOE: Norfolk General Hospital
Affiliated with: Hamilton Niagara Haldimand Brant Local Health
Integration Network
365 West St., Simcoe, ON N3Y 1T7
Tel: 519-426-0130 *Fax:* 519-429-6998
www.ngh.on.ca
Social Media: www.facebook.com/NGHSimcoe;
twitter.com/NorfolkGeneralH
Number of Beds: 106 beds (including 45 chronic beds)
Note: Programs & services include: breast screening; complex care; continence care; detox (Holmes House); diabetes; diagnostic imaging; emergency; ICU; infection control; laboratory; obesity & metabolic surgery; obstetrics; palliative care; rehabilitation; respiratory; social work; stroke clinic; surgery; & surgical day care & endoscopy.
Kelly Isfan, President & CEO
519-426-0130, Fax: 519-429-6998
Heather Riddell, Vice-President, Patient Care
519-426-0130

SIOUX LOOKOUT: Sioux Lookout Meno Ya Win Health Centre
(SLMHC)
Affiliated with: North West Local Health Integration Network
PO Box 909, 1 Meno Ya Win Way, Sioux Lookout, ON P8T 1B4
Tel: 807-737-3030
info@slmhc.on.ca
www.slmhc.on.ca
Number of Beds: 60 beds
Note: Primary health care services including a broad range of basic & some specialist hospital services, specialized community based programs & services responding to population health needs (withdrawal management, suicide, TB, etc.), long term care, & integrated traditional & modern medicine. Serves Nishnawbe-Aski communities north of Sioux Lookout, the Treaty #3 community of Lac Seul First Nation, as well as residents of Pickle Lake & Savant Lake.
Heather Lee, Chief Nursing Executive & Vice-President, Health
Services
Dr. Teresa O'Driscoll, Chief of Staff
Dean Osmond, Chief Operating Officer & Vice-President, Corporate
Services
Jennifer Lawrance, Vice-President, Quality & Support Services

SMITHS FALLS: CCAC South East - Smiths Falls Branch Office
#1, 52 Abbott St. North, Smiths Falls, ON K7A 1W3
Tel: 613-283-8012 *Fax:* 613-283-0308
Toll-Free: 800-267-6041
healthcareathome.ca

Jacqueline Redmond, CEO

SMITHS FALLS: Perth & Smiths Falls District Hospital - Smiths
Falls Site
Affiliated with: South East Local Health Integration Network
60 Cornelia St. West, Smiths Falls, ON K7A 2H9
Tel: 613-283-2330 *Fax:* 613-283-8990
webinquiry@psfdh.on.ca
www.psfdh.on.ca

Year Founded: 1995
Number of Beds: 97 beds
Population Served: 44000
Note: Programs & services include: assistive devices program; clinics; dialysis; diagnostic imaging; emergency; general medicine; general surgery; internal medicine; laboratory; obstetrics/gynaecology; oncology/palliative care; orthopedics; pharmacy; sexual assault support & domestic violence program; & urology.
Beverley McFarlane, President & CEO
613-283-2330, bmcfarlane@psfdh.on.ca
Dr. Peter Roney, Chief of Staff

SMOOTH ROCK FALLS: Hôpital de Smooth Rock Falls Hospital
(HSRFH)
Affiliated with: North East Local Health Integration Network
Also Known As: SRF Hospital
107 Kelly Rd., Smooth Rock Falls, ON P0L 2B0
Tel: 705-338-2781 *Fax:* 705-338-4410
info@srfhosp.ca
www.srfhosp.ca

Number of Beds: 14 acute care beds; 23 long term care beds
Number of Employees: 85
Note: Programs & services include: acute care; long term care; emergency services; laboratory; physiotheraphy; & diagnostic imaging.
Fabien Hébert, Chief Executive Officer
705-338-3212, fhebert@srfhosp.ca
Steven Blier, Chief Financial Officer
705-362-2906, sblier@ndh.on.ca
Chantal Tessier, Chief Nursing Officer
705-338-3215, ctessier@srfhosp.ca

SOUTHAMPTON: Southampton Hospital
Grey Bruce Health Services
Affiliated with: South West Local Health Integration Network
340 High St., Southampton, ON N0H 2L0
Tel: 519-797-3230
web@gbhs.on.ca
www.gbhs.on.ca
Social Media: twitter.com/greybrucehealth
Number of Beds: 16 acute care beds
Note: Programs & services include: acute care; ambulatory care; Diabetes Grey Bruce; diagnostic imaging; emergency; laboratory; physiotherapy; spiritual care; & surgery.
Lance Thurston, President & CEO, Grey Bruce Health Services
519-376-2121

ST CATHARINES: CCAC Hamilton Niagara Haldimand Brant -
Niagara Branch Office
149 Hartzel Rd., St Catharines, ON L2P 1N6
Tel: 905-684-9441 *Fax:* 905-684-8463
Toll-Free: 800-810-0000
healthcareathome.ca

Melody Miles, CEO

ST CATHARINES: Hôtel Dieu Shaver Health & Rehabilitation
Centre
Affiliated with: Hamilton Niagara Haldimand Brant Local Health
Integration Network
Former Name: Hôtel-Dieu Health Sciences Hospital - Niagara
541 Glenridge Ave., St Catharines, ON L2T 4C2
Tel: 905-685-1381 *Fax:* 905-687-4871
www.hoteldieushaver.org

Number of Beds: 134 beds
Number of Employees: 400
Note: Complex continuing care, rehabilitation, & palliative care.

Jane Rufrano, CEO & CFO
  jane.rufrano@hoteldieushaver.org
Dr. Jack Luce, Chief of Staff
  dr.johnthomas.luce@hoteldieushaver.o
Jennifer Hansen, Chief Nursing Officer & Director, Nursing
  jennifer.hansen@hoteldieushaver.org
David Ceglie, Vice-President, Clinical Services
  david.ceglie@hoteldieushaver.org
Lynne Pay, Vice-President, Corporate Services
  lynne.pay@hoteldieushaver.org
Mary Jane Johnson, Director, Commmunications
  maryjane.johnson@hoteldieushaver.org

ST CATHARINES: St. Catharines General Site
Niagara Health System / Système de santé de Niagara
Affiliated with: Hamilton Niagara Haldimand Brant Local Health
Integration Network
1200 Fourth Ave., St Catharines, ON L2S 0A9

Tel: 905-378-4647
patientrelations@niagarahealth.on.ca
www.niagarahealth.on.ca
Social Media: twitter.com/niagarahealth;
www.youtube.com/niagarahealthsystem

Year Founded: 1865
Number of Beds: 375 beds
Note: Programs & services include: cardiology; children's health; critical care; diagnostic imaging; emergency & urgent care; kidney care; laboratory; medicine; mental health & addictions; Ontario Breast Screening Clinic; outpatient services; pharmacy; surgery; Walker Family Cancer Centre; women's & babies health.
Dr. Kevin Smith, Chief Executive Officer, Niagara Health System
  kevin.smith@niagarahealth.on.ca
Dr. Suzanne Johnston, President, Niagara Health System
  suzanne.johnston@niagarahealth.on.ca
Derek McNally, Chief Nursing Executive, Niagara Health System
  derek.mcNally@niagarahealth.on.ca

ST JACOBS: Woolwich Community Health Centre
PO Box 370, 10 Parkside Dr., St Jacobs, ON N0B 2N0

Tel: 519-664-3794 *Fax:* 519-664-2182
genmail@wchc.on.ca
www.wchc.on.ca

Year Founded: 1985
Note: Focuses on primary health care, illness prevention, & health promotion services.
Denise Squire, Executive Director

ST MARYS: St. Marys Memorial Hospital
Huron Perth Healthcare Alliance
Affiliated with: South West Local Health Integration Network
267 Queen St. West, St Marys, ON N4X 1B6

Tel: 519-284-1332 *Fax:* 519-284-8324
Toll-Free: 888-275-1102
administration@hpha.ca
www.hpha.ca

Year Founded: 1950
Number of Beds: 20 beds
Note: Programs & services include: ambulatory clinics; complex continuing care; emergency; Huron Perth Diabetes Education Program; laboratory; medicine unit; occupational therapy; physiotherapy; social work; & spiritual care.
Andrew Williams, President & CEO, HPHA
  519-272-8202, andrew.williams@hpha.ca
Dr. Laurel Moore, Chief Of Staff, HPHA
  519-272-8210, dr.laurel.moore@hpha.ca
Marie Ormerod, Site Administrator
  519-272-8210, marie.ormerod@hpha.ca

ST THOMAS: CCAC St. Thomas
#70, 1063 Talbot St., St Thomas, ON N5P 1G4

Tel: 519-631-9907 *Fax:* 519-631-2236
info-stthomas@sw.ccac-ont.ca
healthcareathome.ca

Sandra Coleman, CEO, South West CCAC

ST THOMAS: St. Thomas-Elgin General Hospital
Affiliated with: South West Local Health Integration Network
189 Elm St., St Thomas, ON N5R 5C4

Tel: 519-631-2030 *Fax:* 519-631-1825
TTY: 519-631-7789
publicrelations@stegh.on.ca
www.stegh.on.ca
Social Media: www.facebook.com/804890622863889;
twitter.com/stegh_cares

Year Founded: 1954
Number of Beds: 158 beds
Number of Employees: 850
Note: Programs & services include: acute medical unit; cardiac intensive care; clinical nutrition; continuing care; diagnostic imaging; education programs; emergency; laboratory; mental health care; pastoral care; surgery; & women & children's program.
Dr. Nancy Whitmore, President & CEO
Karen Davies, Chief Nursing Executive
Mary Stewart, Vice-President

STRATFORD: CCAC South West - Stratford Branch Office
Former Name: Perth County Community Care Access Centre
65 Lorne Ave. East, Stratford, ON N5A 6S4

Tel: 519-273-2222 *Fax:* 519-273-2847
Toll-Free: 800-269-3683
healthcareathome.ca

Sandra Coleman, CEO, South West CCAC

STRATFORD: Stratford General Hospital
Huron Perth Healthcare Alliance
Affiliated with: South West Local Health Integration Network
46 General Hospital Dr., Stratford, ON N5A 2Y6

Tel: 519-272-8210 *Fax:* 519-271-7137
Toll-Free: 888-275-1102
administration@hpha.ca
www.hpha.ca

Year Founded: 1896
Number of Beds: 135 beds
Note: Programs & services include: ambulatory clinics; cardio respiratory; chemotherapy; complex continuing care & rehabilitation; critical care (ICU & telemetry); dialysis; emergency; Huron Perth Diabetes Education Program; Huron Perth District Stroke Centre; imaging; inpatient mental health services; laboratory services; maternal child unit; medicine; social work; spiritual care; & surgery.
Andrew Williams, President & CEO, HPHA
  519-272-8202, andrew.williams@hpha.ca
Dr. Laurel Moore, Chief of Staff, HPHA
  519-272-8210, dr.laurel.moore@hpha.ca
Ken Haworth, Site Administrator
  519-272-8210, ken.haworth@hpha.ca

STRATHROY: Strathroy Middlesex General Hospital
Middlesex Hospital Alliance
Affiliated with: South West Local Health Integration Network
395 Carrie St., Strathroy, ON N7G 3J4

Tel: 519-245-5295 *Fax:* 519-245-0366
admin@mha.tvh.ca
www.mhalliance.on.ca

Year Founded: 1914
Number of Beds: 54 beds
Population Served: 35000
Number of Employees: 300
Note: Programs & services include: ambulatory care clinics; diabetes education program; diagnostic imaging; emergency; intensive care; medical inpatient unit; medical surgical inpatient unit; obstetrics inpatient unit; occupational therapy; physiotherapy; speech-language pathology; & surgery.
Todd Stepanuik, President & CEO, Middlesex Hospital Alliance
Dr. Gary Perkin, Chief of Staff, Middlesex Hospital Alliance

STURGEON FALLS: The West Nipissing General Hospital
(WNGH)/L'Hôpital général de Nipissing Ouest
Affiliated with: North East Local Health Integration Network
725 Coursol Rd., Sturgeon Falls, ON P2B 2Y6

Tel: 705-753-3110 *Fax:* 705-753-0210
administration@wngh.ca
www.wngh.ca

Year Founded: 1977
Number of Beds: 98 beds

Note: Programs & services include: diagnostic & therapeutic; dietitian; emergency; inpatient services; outpatient services; pharmacy; physiotherapy; & Telemedicine.
Cynthia Désormiers, Chief Executive Officer
Dr. Klère Bourgault, Chief of Staff
Jo-Ann Lennon Labelle, Chief Nursing Officer

SUDBURY: CCAC North-East - Sudbury Branch Office
Rainbow Centre, #41-C, 40 Elm St., Sudbury, ON P3C 1S8
Tel: 705-522-3461 *Fax:* 705-522-3855
Toll-Free: 800-461-2919
healthcareathome.ca

Richard Joly, CEO

SUDBURY: Centre de santé communautaire du Grand Sudbury
19, ch Frood, Sudbury, ON P3C 4Y9
Tél: 705-670-2274 *Téléc:* 705-670-2277
www.santesudbury.ca
Média social: www.facebook.com/ajeunesse

Lynne Dupuis, Présidente

SUDBURY: Health Sciences North (HSN)
Affiliated with: North East Local Health Integration Network
41 Ramsey Lake Rd., Sudbury, ON P3E 5J1
Tel: 705-523-7100 *Fax:* 705-523-7112
Toll-Free: 866-469-0822
communications@hsnsudbury.ca
www.hsnsudbury.ca
Social Media: www.facebook.com/HSNSudbury;
twitter.com/HSN_Sudbury;
www.youtube.com/user/healthsciencesnorth;
www.linkedin.com/company/health-sciences-north
Number of Beds: 454 beds
Number of Employees: 3900
Note: Programs & services include: cancer care; domestic violence & sexual assault treatment; mental health & addiction services; & transitional & rehabilitative care.
Dr. Denis-Richard Roy, President & CEO
Dr. Chris Bourdon, Chief of Staff
David McNeil, Chief Nursing Executive

SUDBURY: Ramsey Lake Health Centre
Affiliated with: Health Sciences North
Former Name: Sudbury Regional Hospital - Laurentian Site
41 Ramsey Lake Rd., Sudbury, ON P3E 5J1
Tel: 705-523-7100 *Fax:* 705-523-7112
Toll-Free: 866-469-0822
www.hsnsudbury.ca

Note: Programs & services include critical care, palliative care, emergency care, medical imaging, rehabilitation, & mental health services.

SUDBURY: Sudbury & District Health Unit (SDHU)
1300 Paris St., Sudbury, ON P3E 3A3
Tel: 705-522-9200 *Fax:* 705-522-5182
Toll-Free: 866-522-9200
www.sdhu.com
Social Media: twitter.com/SD_PublicHealth

Number of Employees: 250+
Penny Sutcliffe, Medical Officer of Health & CEO

SUDBURY: Sudbury Outpatient Centre
Affiliated with: Health Sciences North
865 Regent St. South, Sudbury, ON P3E 3Y9
Tel: 705-523-7100 *Toll-Free:* 866-469-0822
www.hsnsudbury.ca
Number of Beds: 189 beds
Dr. Denis-Richard Roy, President & CEO, Health Sciences North

TERRACE BAY: The McCausland Hospital
North of Superior Healthcare Group
Affiliated with: North West Local Health Integration Network
PO Box 370, 20B Cartier Rd., Terrace Bay, ON P0T 2W0
Tel: 807-825-3273 *Fax:* 807-825-9623
www.nosh.ca
Year Founded: 1980
Number of Beds: 45 beds (23 community beds, 22 long-term beds)

Population Served: 4000
Note: Services include: emergency; cancer care; diabetes program; diagnostic imaging (ECG, Holter monitors, radiology, ultrasound); laboratory; obstetrics & gynecology; physiotherapy; seniors drop-in program; & surgery.
Adam Brown, CEO
807-825-3273

THESSALON: North Shore Health Network - Thessalon Site
Affiliated with: North East Local Health Integration Network
135 Dawson St., Thessalon, ON P0R 1L0
Tel: 705-842-2014
www.nshn.care

Note: Programs & services include: diagnostic imaging; emergency; & surgery.
Connie Lee, Interim Chief Executive Officer

THORNHILL: Shouldice Hospital Ltd.
Affiliated with: Central Local Health Integration Network
7750 Bayview Ave., Thornhill, ON L3T 4A3
Tel: 905-889-1125 *Fax:* 905-889-4216
Toll-Free: 800-291-7750
postoffice@shouldice.com
www.shouldice.com
Year Founded: 1945
Number of Beds: 89 beds
Specialties: Hernia repair
Note: Has 10 surgeons on staff.
John Hughes, Chief Administrative Officer

THUNDER BAY: Anishnawbe Mushkiki Thunder Bay Aboriginal Health Centre
Affiliated with: North West Local Health Integration Network
29 Royston Ct., Thunder Bay, ON P7A 4Y7
Tel: 807-343-4843 *Fax:* 807-343-4728
info@mushkiki.com
mushkiki.com

Note: Programs & services include: clinic care; culture; education; intervention; prevention.

THUNDER BAY: Hogarth Riverview Manor
St. Joseph's Care Group
300 Lillie St. North, Thunder Bay, ON P7C 4Y7
Tel: 807-625-1110 *Fax:* 807-623-4520
www.sjcg.net
Number of Beds: 96 beds
Note: Long-term care home
Tracy Buckler, President & CEO, St. Joseph's Care Group

THUNDER BAY: North West Local Health Integration Network
Also Known As: North West LHIN
#201, 975 Alloy Dr., Thunder Bay, ON P7B 5Z8
Tel: 807-684-9425 *Fax:* 807-684-9533
Toll-Free: 866-907-5446
northwest@lhins.on.ca
www.northwestlhin.on.ca
Social Media: www.facebook.com/nwlhin; twitter.com/NorthWestLHIN
Year Founded: 2005
Population Served: 235900
Note: The North West LHIN is responsible for planning, integrating & funding local health services, including hospitals, the Community Care Access Centre, community health centres, long-term care homes, community support service agencies & community mental health & addiction services. The North West LHIN extends from just west of White River to the Manitoba border & from Hudson Bay in the north down to the United States border.
Gil Labine, Board Chair
Laura Kokocinski, Chief Executive Officer
Brian Ktytor, Acting Chief Operating Officer
Susan Pilatzke, Senior Director, Health System Transformation
Chris Wcislo, Controller & Manager, Corporate Services

THUNDER BAY: NorWest Community Health Centre - Thunder Bay Site
Affiliated with: North West Local Health Integration Network
525 Simpson St., Thunder Bay, ON P7C 3J6
Tel: 807-622-8235 *Fax:* 807-622-7637
Toll-Free: 866-357-5454
www.norwestchc.org/thunder_bay.htm
Social Media: www.facebook.com/NorWestCHC

Wendy Talbot, CEO

THUNDER BAY: St. Joseph's Hospital
St. Joseph's Care Group
Affiliated with: North West Local Health Integration Network
PO Box 3251, 35 Algoma St. North, Thunder Bay, ON P7B 5G7
Tel: 807-343-2431 *Fax:* 807-343-0144
sjcg@tbh.net
www.sjcg.net

Note: Programs & services include: ambulatory care clinics; chiropody & foot care; day hospital; general rehabilitation; geriatric assessment & rehabilitative care; hospice/palliative care; orthopedic physiotherapy & occupational therapy; outpatient neurology rehabilitation; pulmonary rehabilitation; rheumatic disease; & transition.
Tracy Buckler, President & CEO, St. Joseph's Care Group

THUNDER BAY: Thunder Bay Regional Health Sciences Centre
Affiliated with: North West Local Health Integration Network
980 Oliver Rd., Thunder Bay, ON P7B 6V4
Tel: 807-684-6000
tbrhsc@tbh.net
www.tbrhsc.net
Year Founded: 2004
Number of Beds: 375 acute care beds (28 beds for anesthetic recovery, 40 beds for day surgery recovery)
Number of Employees: 2800
Note: A comprehensive, multi-disciplinary, acute care facility with services incuding ambulatory care, cardio respiratory services, critical care, diagnostic assessment, diagnostic imaging, emergency, laboratory services, palliative care, prevention & screening, rehabilitation, supportive care, surgery, & Telemedicine. The TBRHSC amalgamates the former Port Arthur & McKellar sites of the Thunder Bay Regional Hospital.
Jean Bartkowiak, President & CEO
Dr. Gordon Porter, Chief of Staff
Dr. Rhonda Crocker Ellacott, Chief Nursing Executive
Dr. Mark Henderson, Executive Vice-President, Patient Services

TILLSONBURG: Tillsonburg District Memorial Hospital (TDMH)
Affiliated with: South West Local Health Integration Network
167 Rolph St., Tillsonburg, ON N4G 3Y9
Tel: 519-842-3611 *Fax:* 519-688-1031
mail@tdmh.on.ca
www.tillsonburghospital.on.ca
Number of Beds: 51 beds
Note: Programs & services include: ambulatory care; complex continuing care; diabetes education; diagnostic & treatment; dialysis; emergency; intensive coronary care; medical/surgical unit; palliative care; rehabilitation; & surgery.
Dr. Mohamed Abdalla, Chief of Staff
Julie Ellery, Integrated Vice-President, Nursing

TIMMINS: Misiway Milopemahtesewin Community Health Centre
130 Wilson Ave., Timmins, ON P4N 2S9
Tel: 705-264-2200 *Fax:* 705-264-2243
www.misiway.ca

Note: Clinic services; traditional healing services; diabetes education program.
Rachel Cull, Executive Director

TIMMINS: North East Community Care Access Centre - Timmins Branch Office
#101, 330 - 2nd Ave., Timmins, ON P4N 8A4
Tel: 705-267-7766 *Fax:* 705-267-7795
Toll-Free: 888-668-2222
healthcareathome.ca/northeast

Richard Joly, CEO

TIMMINS: Timmins & District Hospital (TADH)/L'Hôpital de Timmins et du district
Affiliated with: North East Local Health Integration Network
700 Ross Ave. East, Timmins, ON P4N 8P2
Tel: 705-267-2131 *Fax:* 705-267-6311
generalinquiries@tadh.com
www.tadh.com
Year Founded: 1993
Number of Beds: 134 beds
Number of Employees: 920
Note: Programs & services include: cardiopulmonary; complex continuing care; critical care; emergency; maternal child; medical; medical imaging; mental health; nephrology; oncology; palliative care; rehabilitation; sleep centre; surgery; & Telemedicine.
Blaise MacNeil, President & CEO
Dr. Harry Voogjarv, Chief of Staff
Joan Ludwig, Chief Nursing Officer

TOBERMORY: Tobermory Clinic
PO Box 220, 7275 Hwy. 6, Tobermory, ON N0H 2R0
Tel: 519-596-2305 *Fax:* 519-596-2979

Note: Specialties: Family health; Community care; Minor day surgery; Mental health counselling. Number of Employees: 4 physicians + 1 nurse practitioner + 1 social worker + several clinic nurses
Pamela Loughlean, Executive Director

TORONTO: Access Alliance Multicultural Community Health Centre
#500, 340 College St., Toronto, ON M5T 3A9
Tel: 416-324-8677 *Fax:* 416-324-9074
mail@accessalliance.ca
www.accessalliance.ca
Social Media: www.facebook.com/AccessAlliance;
twitter.com/accessalliance

Note: Provides community health services to refugees & immigrants
Erik Landriault, Board Chair

TORONTO: Anishnawbe Health Toronto
225 Queen St. East, Toronto, ON M5A 1S4
Tel: 416-360-0486 *Fax:* 416-365-1083
www.aht.ca
Year Founded: 1984
Note: An accredited community health centre, utilizing traditional healing approaches. A range of services is available, including fetal alcohol spectrum disorder services, diabetic care, HIV testing, mental health services & psychiatry, counselling, naturopathy, chiropody, women's services, massage therapy, & dental services. Other centres located at: 179 Gerrard St. East, 416-920-2605; & 22 Vaughan Rd., 416-657-0379. Mental Health Crisis Management Service: 416-891-8606.
Joe Hester, Executive Director

TORONTO: Anne Johnston Health Station
2398 Yonge St., Toronto, ON M4P 2H4
Tel: 416-486-8666 *Fax:* 416-486-8660
info@ajhs.ca
www.ajhs.ca
Social Media: www.facebook.com/theannejohnstonhealthstation;
twitter.com/ajhealthstation

Note: Programs & services include: chiropody; counselling; occupational therapy; nutrition; physiotherapy; Seniors Home Health Program; & youth health clinic
Brenda McNeill, Executive Director

TORONTO: Bernard Betel Centre for Creative Living
1003 Steeles Ave. West, Toronto, ON M2R 3T6
Tel: 416-225-2112 *Fax:* 416-225-2097
reception@betelcentre.org
www.betelcentre.org

Note: Provides education, recreation, arts, fitness & health services
Gail Gould, Executive Director

TORONTO: Black Creek Community Health Centre
#5, 2202 Jane St., Toronto, ON M3M 1A4
Tel: 416-249-8000 *Fax:* 416-249-4594
www.bcchc.com
Social Media: twitter.com/BlackCreekCHC

Note: Programs & services include: clinical services; counselling; dietitian; & diabetes education
Cheryl Prescod, Executive Director

TORONTO: Bridgepoint Active Healthcare
Sinai Health System
Affiliated with: Toronto Central Local Health Integration Network
Former Name: The Riverdale Hospital
Also Known As: Bridgepoint Hospital
1 Bridgepoint Dr., Toronto, ON M4M 2B5
Tel: 416-461-8252 *Fax:* 416-461-5696
www.bridgepointhealth.ca
Social Media: www.facebook.com/BridgepointHealth;
twitter.com/BridgepointTO; www.youtube.com/bridgepointhospital;
www.linkedin.com/company/bridgepoint-health
Number of Beds: 404 beds
Specialties: Complex continuing care & rehabilitation
Note: Programs & services include: ambulatory care; diabetes education; dialysis; endocrinology; general internal medicine; geriatric psychiatry; neurological care; orthopedic care; pain management; palliative care; physiatry; therapeutic recreation; & urgent care.
Dr. Gary Newton, President & CEO, Sinai Health System
Jane Merkley, Chief Nurse Executive & Executive Vice-President, Patient Care & Quality
Joan Sproul, Chief Administrative Officer & Executive Vice-President, Finance
Dr. Maureen Shandling, Executive Vice-President, Academic & Medical Affairs

TORONTO: Casey House Hospice
9 Huntley St., Toronto, ON M4Y 2K8
Tel: 416-962-7600 *Fax:* 416-962-5147
heart@caseyhouse.on.ca
www.caseyhouse.com
Social Media:
www.facebook.com/pages/Casey-House-Toronto/111871308199;
twitter.com/caseyhouseTO; www.youtube.com/caseyhousetv;
www.linkedin.com/company/casey-house-foundation
Year Founded: 1988
Number of Beds: 13 beds
Note: Hospice; home care office
Stephanie Karapita, CEO
Dr. Ann Stewart, MD, MSc, CCFP, Medical Director
416-962-7660

TORONTO: CCAC Central - Sheppard Site
#700, 45 Sheppard Ave. East, Toronto, ON M2N 5W9
Tel: 416-222-2241 *Fax:* 416-222-6517
info@central.ccac-ont.ca
healthcareathome.ca

Megan Allen-Lamb, CEO

TORONTO: CCAC Central East - Scarborough Branch Office
#801, 100 Consilium Pl., Toronto, ON M1H 3E3
Tel: 416-750-2444 *Fax:* 855-352-2555
Toll-Free: 800-263-3877
healthcareathome.ca
Kathryn Ramsay, CEO

TORONTO: CCAC Toronto Central
#305, 250 Dundas St. West, Toronto, ON M5T 2Z5
Tel: 416-506-9888 *Fax:* 416-506-0374
Toll-Free: 866-243-0061
TTY: 416-506-1512
feedback@toronto.ccac-ont.ca
healthcareathome.ca
Bill Tottle, CEO

TORONTO: CCAC Toronto Central - East Site
Former Name: East York Access Centre
2494 Danforth Ave., Toronto, ON M4C 1L1
Tel: 416-506-9888
feedback@toronto.ccac-ont.ca
healthcareathome.ca
Bill Tottle, CEO

TORONTO: Central Toronto Community Health Centres
Queen West Community Health Centre
168 Bathurst St., Toronto, ON M5V 2R4
Tel: 416-703-8482 *Fax:* 416-703-8479
info@ctchc.com
www.ctchc.com

Note: Medical services (with specialized services for the homeless), psychiatric & mental health services, individual & group counselling, harm reduction program (safer sex, safer drug use, Hepatitis C & HIV prevention), needle exchange, diabetes education program, chiropody, perinatal nursing, dental clinic.
Angela Robertson, Executive Director
arobertson@ctchc.com

TORONTO: Central Toronto Community Health Centres
Shout Clinic
168 Bathurst St., Toronto, ON M5V 2R4
Tel: 416-703-8482
info@ctchc.com
www.ctchc.com

Year Founded: 1992
Note: Walk-in medical clinic providing comprehensive health care services to homeless & street involved youth, 16-24 years of age.
Anne Marie DiCenso, Director, Community Health & Development
adicenso@ctchc.com

TORONTO: Centre francophone de Toronto
Ancien nom: Centre médico-social communautaire
#303, 555, rue Richmond ouest, Toronto, ON M5V 3B1
Tél: 416-922-2672 *Téléc:* 416-922-6624
infos@centrefranco.org
www.centrefranco.org
Média social: www.facebook.com/Centre.francophone.de.Toronto;
twitter.com/CentrefrancoT; www.linkedin.com/company/659599

Lise Marie Baudry, Directrice générale

TORONTO: Davenport Perth Neighbourhood Centre (DPNCHC)
1900 Davenport Rd., Toronto, ON M6N 1B7
Tel: 416-656-8025 *Fax:* 416-656-1264
info@dpnchc.ca
www.dpnchc.ca
Social Media: twitter.com/DPNCHC

Note: Offers primary health care, health promotion, disease prevention, & mental health services
Kim Fraser, Executive Director
kfraser@dpnchc.ca

TORONTO: Don Mills Surgical Unit Inc. (DMSU)
Centric Health Surgical
Affiliated with: Central Local Health Integration Network
#208, 20 Wynford Dr., Toronto, ON M3C 1J4
Tel: 416-441-2111 *Fax:* 416-441-2114
www.centrichealthepcn.ca/facilities/don-mills-surgical-unit
Year Founded: 1960
Note: Surgical services & procedures offered include: general, orthopaedic, ophthalmology, plastic surgery, upper & lower extremity, cosmetics, dental & ENT. Has 20 surgeons on staff.

TORONTO: East End Community Health Centre
1619 Queen St. East, Toronto, ON M4L 1G4
Tel: 416-778-5858 *Fax:* 416-778-5855
www.eastendchc.on.ca

Note: Services include counselling, physiotherapy, nutrition, & medical.
Joyce Kalsen, Executive Director

TORONTO: Etobicoke General Hospital (EGH)
William Osler Health System
Affiliated with: Central West Local Health Integration Network
Also Known As: William Osler Health Centre
101 Humber College Blvd., Toronto, ON M9V 1R8
Tel: 416-747-2120
www.williamoslerhs.ca
Social Media: www.facebook.com/WilliamOslerHealth;
twitter.com/OslerHealth; www.youtube.com/WilliamOslerTV;
www.linkedin.com/company/william-osler-health-system
Number of Beds: 262 beds
Note: Programs & services include: cancer care; cardiac care; complex
continuing care; critical care; diabetes care; diagnostic imaging;
emergency; general & internal medicine; joint assessment centre;
kidney care; laboratories; mental health & addictions; naturopathic
care; palliative care; rehabilitation services; respirology; seniors' care;
surgical services; & women's & children's services.
Matthew Anderson, President & CEO, William Osler Health System

TORONTO: Family Health Centre
Michael Garron Hospital
840 Coxwell Ave., Toronto, ON M4C 5T2
Tel: 416-469-6464 Fax: 416-469-6164
ptrep@tegh.on.ca (Patients); community@tegh.on.ca (Community)
www.tegh.on.ca
Year Founded: 2002
Note: Specialties: Low-risk obstetrics; Psychotherapy; Telephone
health advisory service

TORONTO: Flemingdon Health Centre
10 Gateway Blvd., Toronto, ON M3C 3A1
Tel: 416-429-4991 Fax: 416-422-3573
fhcinfo@fhc-chc.com
www.fhc-chc.com

Note: Programs & services include: medical care; health education;
immunization; obstetrical care; nutrition counselling; chiropody; social
services; health promotion; & diabetes prevention programs
John Elliott, Executive Director

TORONTO: Four Villages Community Health Centre
1700 Bloor St. West, Toronto, ON M6P 4C3
Tel: 416-604-0640
info@4villages.on.ca
www.4villageschc.ca

Note: Programs & services include: chronic disease & pain
management; nutrition; & mental health
Tariq Asmi, Chief Executive Officer

TORONTO: Humber River Regional Hospital - Finch St. Site
2111 Finch Ave. West, Toronto, ON M3N 1N1
Tel: 416-744-2500
www.hrrh.on.ca

Note: Affiliated with the University of Toronto & Queen's University.

TORONTO: Humber River Regional Hospital - Wilson Ave. Site
Affiliated with: Toronto Central Local Health Integration Network
1235 Wilson Ave., Toronto, ON M3M 0B2
Tel: 416-242-1000
www.hrh.ca
Social Media: www.youtube.com/humberriverhospital
Year Founded: 2015
Number of Beds: 656 beds (all sites)
Number of Employees: 3300
Note: Programs & services include: acute care; adult day treatment;
assessment program; child & adolescent mental health inpatient unit;
child & adolescent outpatient services; community treatment program;
early intervention in psychosis program; elective inpatient withdrawal
management program; general psychiatry unit; geriatric psychiatry
outpatient clinic services; geriatric psychiatry outreach team; Humber
River Hospital funded clinic; Humber River Rehabilitation Centre;
intensive day treatment; internal geriatric psychiatry consultation teams;
outpatient services; psychogeriatric outreach & consultation team; &
transition child & adolescent program. Affiliated with the University of
Toronto & Queen's University.
Barb Collins, President & CEO
Dr. Narenda Singh, Chief of Staff

Marg Czaus, Chief Nursing Officer

TORONTO: Lawrence Heights Community Health Centre
12 Flemington Rd., Toronto, ON M6A 2N4
Tel: 416-787-1661 Fax: 416-787-3761
www.unisonhcs.org
Social Media: www.facebook.com/UnisonHCS; twitter.com/unisonhcs

Note: Programs & services include: medical care; counselling; diabetes
management; dietitian; dental; footcare; & seniors health care
Michelle Joseph, Chief Executive Officer

TORONTO: Michael Garron Hospital - Toronto East Health Network
Affiliated with: Toronto Central Local Health Integration Network
Former Name: Toronto East General Hospital
825 Coxwell Ave., Toronto, ON M4C 3E7
Tel: 416-461-8272 Fax: 416-469-6106
community@tegh.on.ca
www.tegh.on.ca
Info Line: 416-469-6487
Social Media: www.facebook.com/TorontoEastGeneral;
twitter.com/EastGeneral; www.youtube.com/user/TorontoEastGeneral;
www.linkedin.com/company/toronto-east-general-hospital
Year Founded: 1929
Population Served: 400000
Number of Employees: 2500
Note: Affiliated with the University of Toronto. Programs & services
include: acute care; breastfeeding centre for families; complex
continuing care; inpatient rehabilitation; alternate level of care; cancer
care; cardiology; child development centre; DEC NET (Diabetes
Education Community Network of East Toronto); diabetes care;
diagnostic imaging; East Toronto postpartum adjustment program;
emergency; family health centre; geriatric assessment; hematology;
mental health outpatient programs; neonatal care; nephrology;
obstetrics; palliative care; pediatrics; prolonged-ventilation weaning
centre; psychiatry; respiratory diseases; & surgery.
Sarah Downey, President & CEO
Dr. Ian Fraser, Chief of Staff
Irene Andress, Chief Nursing Executive & Program Director,
ER/Medicine/Nursing Resource Team

TORONTO: Mount Sinai Hospital
Affiliated with: Toronto Central Local Health Integration Network
600 University Ave., Toronto, ON M5G 1X5
Tel: 416-596-4200
TTY: 416-586-8275
communicationsandmarketing@mtsinai.on.ca
www.mountsinai.on.ca
Social Media: www.facebook.com/MountSinaiHospital;
twitter.com/MountSinai; www.youtube.com/user/MountSinaiHospital;
www.linkedin.com/company/mount-sinai-hospital-toronto
Year Founded: 1923
Number of Beds: 442 beds
Number of Employees: 4528
Note: Teaching & research Hospital, affiliated with the University of
Toronto. Home to six Centres of Excellence: Frances Bloomberg
Centre for Women's & Infants' Health; Christopher Sharp Centre for
Surgical Oncology; The Daryl A. Katz Centre for Urgent & Critical Care;
The Centre for Inflammatory Bowel Disease; Centre for
Musculoskeletal Disease; & The Lunenfeld-Tanenbaum Research
Institute.
Hospital programs & services include: acute care; Alzheimer's support
& training centre; arthritis & autoimmune diseases; asthma; audiology;
cancer (breast, colon & sarcoma); cardiology; Chinese outreach
program; clinic for HIV related concerns; day surgery; dental clinic;
diabetes education; digestive diseases; eye clinic; family medicine
centre; geriatric psychiatry; nutrition counselling; Ontario Breast
Screening Program; orthopedics; pain management; palliative care;
psychiatric unit; rehabilitation; speech disorders; sports medicine;
urology; & women's & infants' health programs.
Carey Lucki, Interim President & Vice-President, Client Services
Samir Sinha, Chief Clinical Advisor

TORONTO: North York General Hospital - Branson Ambulatory Care Centre
Affiliated with: Toronto Central Local Health Integration Network
555 Finch Ave. West, Toronto, ON M2R 1N5

Tel: 416-633-9420
www.nygh.on.ca
Social Media: www.facebook.com/NorthYorkGeneralHospital;
twitter.com/NYGH_News; www.youtube.com/user/NYGHNews
Number of Beds: 419 acute beds (all sites); 192 long-term care beds (all sites)
Note: Programs & services include: adolescent eating disorder program; cataract high volume centre; diabetes education centre; Gale & Graham Wright Prostate Centre; laboratory medicine; medical imaging; mental health; pharmacy; Total Joint Assessment Centre (TJAC); & Urgent Care Centre (UCC).
Dr. Tim Rutledge, President & CEO
Dr. Everton Gooden, Chief of Staff
Karyn Popovich, Chief Nursing Executive & Vice-President, Clinical Programs, Quality & Risk

TORONTO: North York General Hospital - General Site
Affiliated with: Toronto Central Local Health Integration Network
4001 Leslie St., Toronto, ON M2K 1E1

Tel: 416-756-6000
www.nygh.on.ca
Social Media: www.facebook.com/NorthYorkGeneralHospital;
twitter.com/NYGH_News; www.youtube.com/user/NYGHNews
Number of Beds: 419 acute beds (all sites); 192 long-term care beds (all sites)
Note: Community teaching hospital affiliated with the University of Toronto. Programs & services include: cancer care; child & teen; diagnostic imaging; emergency & urgent care; genetics; family & community medicine; laboratory; maternal newborn care; medicine & elder care; mental health; pharmacy; & surgery.
Dr. Tim Rutledge, President & CEO
Everton Gooden, Chief of Staff
Karyn Popovich, Chief Nursing Executive & Vice-President, Clinical Programs, Quality & Risk

TORONTO: Parkdale Community Health Centre
1229 Queen St. West, Toronto, ON M6K 1L2

Tel: 416-537-2455 *Fax:* 416-537-5133
www.pchc.on.ca
Social Media: twitter.com/ParkdaleCHC
Year Founded: 1984
Note: Specialties: Service in several languages; Primary care; Educational programs, such as pre- & post-natal classes; Support groups; Counselling; Mental health support; HIV testing
Shirley Roberts, Interim Executive Director

TORONTO: Princess Margaret Hospital
University Health Network
Affiliated with: Toronto Central Local Health Integration Network
Also Known As: Princess Margaret Cancer Centre
610 University Ave., Toronto, ON M5G 2M9

Tel: 416-946-2000
www.theprincessmargaret.ca
Social Media: www.facebook.com/UniversityHealthNetwork;
twitter.com/UHN_News; www.youtube.com/UHNToronto;
www.linkedin.com/company/university-health-network
Year Founded: 1952
Number of Beds: 202 beds
Number of Employees: 3000
Note: A teaching hospital of the University of Toronto, & a top cancer treatment & research centre. Programs & services include: allied health; dental oncology, ocular & maxillofacial prosthetics; laboratory medicine; medical imaging; medical oncology & hematology; oncology nursing; patient education & survivorship; pharmacy; psychosocial oncology & palliative care; radiation medicine; & surgical oncology. The Ontario Cancer Institute comprises the research wing of the hospital.

TORONTO: Queensway Health Centre
Trillium Health Partners
Affiliated with: Mississauga Halton Local Health Integration Network
150 Sherway Dr., Toronto, ON M9C 1A5

Tel: 416-259-6671
Patient.RelationsMH@trilliumhealthpartners.ca
trilliumhealthpartners.ca
Social Media: twitter.com/Trillium_Health;
www.youtube.com/user/TrilliumHealth;
www.linkedin.com/company/2949012
Note: An ambulatory care facility with services including urgent care centre, day surgery, diabetes management centre, cardiac wellness & rehabilitation, Kingsway Financial Spine Centre, & The Betty Wallace Women's Health Centre (focusing on osteoporosis & breast disease). There is no emergency centre here; it is located at the Mississauga branch.
Michelle E. DiEmanuele, President & CEO, Trillium Health Partners
Dr. Dante Morra, Chief of Staff, Trillium Health Partners
Kathryn Haywood-Murray, Chief Nursing Executive & Senior Vice-President, Patient Care Services, Trillium Health Partners

TORONTO: Regent Park Community Health Centre
465 Dundas St. East, Toronto, ON M5A 2B2

Tel: 416-364-2261 *Fax:* 416-364-0822
www.regentparkchc.org
Year Founded: 1973
Note: Emphasis on an integrated approach: health promotion, disease prevention, social services. A community-founded & operated facility, with a focus on comprehensive, accessible care. Services in English, Cantonese, Mandarin, Vietnamese, Somali & Spanish. The Pathways to Education Program for youth at risk, created & first implemented in Regent Park, has been adopted by communities across Canada
Greg Webster, Board President

TORONTO: Rouge Valley Centenary
Scarborough & Rouge Hospital
Affiliated with: Central East Local Health Integration Network
2867 Ellesmere Rd., Toronto, ON M1E 4B9

Tel: 416-284-8131
patientrelations@rougevalley.ca
www.rougevalley.ca
Social Media: www.facebook.com/rougevalleyhealthsystem;
twitter.com/RougeValley; www.youtube.com/RougeValleyHealthSys
Year Founded: 1967
Number of Beds: 307 beds
Note: Programs & services include: acute care; cancer care; cardiac care; continuing care; critical care; diabetes education; diagnostic imaging; emergency; geriatric assessment; maternal newborn care; mental health; paediatrics; palliative care; respiratory therapy; & surgical care.
Andrée Robichaud, Interim President & CEO, Scarborough & Rouge Hospital
Dr. Naresh Mohan, Interim Chief Medical Officer
Linda Calhoun, Chief Nursing Executive, Scarborough & Rouge Hospital
Cara Flemming, Chief Financial Officer, Scarborough & Rouge Hospital

TORONTO: Runnymede Healthcare Centre
Affiliated with: Toronto Central Local Health Integration Network
625 Runnymede Rd., Toronto, ON M6S 3A3

Tel: 416-762-7316 *Fax:* 416-762-3836
communications@runnymedehc.ca
www.runnymedehc.ca
Social Media: www.facebook.com/RunnymedeHC;
twitter.com/RunnymedeHC; www.youtube.com/RunnymedeHC;
www.linkedin.com/company/runnymedehc
Year Founded: 1945
Note: Complex continuing care hospital with rehabilitation, speech therapy, dental care, & foot care services.
Connie Dejak, President & CEO
Raj Sewda, Chief Nursing Executive & Chief Privacy Officer
Stewart Boecker, Chief Financial Officer & Vice-President, Finance
Sharleen Ahmed, Vice-President, Strategy, Quality & Clinical Programs
Richard Mendonca, Vice-President, Human Resources & Organizational Development

SECTION II:
General Resources

TORONTO: St. Joseph's Health Centre Toronto
Affiliated with: Toronto Central Local Health Integration Network
30 The Queensway, Toronto, ON M6R 1B5

Tel: 416-530-6000
TTY: 416-530-6820
www.stjoe.on.ca

Social Media: www.facebook.com/MySt.Joes; twitter.com/mystjoes;
www.youtube.com/user/StJoesHealthCentre;
www.linkedin.com/company/st.-joseph's-health-centre-toronto

Year Founded: 1921
Number of Beds: 381 beds
Number of Employees: 2550
Note: Programs & services include: acute care; cardiology; cancer care; diabetes; diagnostic imaging; dialysis; ear, nose & throat (ENT); elderly community health services; family medicine centre; geriatric emergency & outpatient services; gynecology; Lifeline; mental health programs; obstetrics; ophthalmology; orthopedics; pediatrics; pre & postnatal care; psychiatric unit; respiratory care; sleep lab; speech disorders; surgery; & urology. This teaching hospital was founded by the Sisters of St. Joseph. Has 400 physicians on staff.
Elizabeth Buller, President & CEO
Dr. Ted Rogovein, Chief of Staff
Jenni Glad-Timmons, Chief Nursing Executive & Director,
    Interprofessional Practice

TORONTO: St. Michael's Hospital
Affiliated with: Toronto Central Local Health Integration Network
30 Bond St., Toronto, ON M5B 1W8

Tel: 416-360-4000
www.stmichaelshospital.com
Social Media: www.facebook.com/116986731666237;
twitter.com/StMikesHospital;
www.youtube.com/user/StMichaelsHospital;
www.linkedin.com/company/st.-michael's-hospital

Number of Beds: 463 inpatient beds
Number of Employees: 6066
Note: Catholic hospital with a focus on teaching & research, affiliated with the University of Toronto. Programs & services include: acute care; addiction; arthritis; breast centre; cancer care; cardiology; chiropody; critical care; diabetes clinic; dialysis; fracture clinic; general internal medicine; geriatrics; gynecology; hemophilia; HIV/AIDS; inner city health program; inpatient oncology; mental health; mobility; multiple sclerosis; neo-natal intensive care; neurosurgery; obstetrics; Ontario Breast Screening Program; ophthalmology; osteoporosis; outpatient services; palliative care; pediatrics; services for seniors; stroke centre; respirology; sleep laboratory; specialized complex care; trauma centre; urology; & vascular disease.
Robert Howard, President & CEO
Dr. Douglas Sinclair, Executive Vice-President & Chief Medical Officer
Sonya Canzian, Chief Nursing Executive, Chief Health Disciplines
    Exec., & Executive Vice-President, Programs

TORONTO: The Salvation Army Toronto Grace Health Centre (TGHC)
Affiliated with: Toronto Central Local Health Integration Network
Also Known As: Toronto Grace Hospital
47 Austin Terrace, Toronto, ON M5R 1Y8

Tel: 416-925-2251 Fax: 416-925-3211
www.torontograce.org
Social Media: www.facebook.com/torontogracehealthcentre;
twitter.com/torontogracehc;
www.linkedin.com/company/toronto-grace-health-centre

Year Founded: 1905
Number of Beds: 119 beds
Note: Complex continuing care facility providing services such as foot clinic/chiropody, palliative care & slow-paced rehabilitation.
Marilyn Rook, President & CEO
Dr. John Ruth, Medical Director
Janet Harris, Chief Nursing Executive
Ralph Anstey, Chief Financial Officer

TORONTO: Scarborough Centre for Healthy Communities
Former Name: West Hill Community Services
2660 Eglinton Ave. East, Toronto, ON M1K 2S3

Tel: 416-642-9445
www.schcontario.ca
Info Line: 416-847-4173

Year Founded: 1977
Number of Employees: 130
Note: Offers 38 integrated services across 11 sites. They provide medical assistance through their clinics, are involved in a youth program, & have other social support programs including a food bank.
Jeanie Joaquin, CEO

TORONTO: The Scarborough Hospital - Birchmount Campus
Scarborough & Rouge Hospital
Affiliated with: Central East Local Health Integration Network
Former Name: The Scarborough Hospital - Grace Campus
3030 Birchmount Rd., Toronto, ON M1W 3W3

Tel: 416-495-2400
www.tsh.to
Social Media: www.facebook.com/ScarboroughHospital;
twitter.com/ScarboroughHosp;
www.youtube.com/user/TSHCommunications;
www.linkedin.com/company/the-scarborough-hospital

Number of Beds: 215 beds
Number of Employees: 3105
Note: A health facility with emphasis on emergency outpatient psychiatric concerns, notably its Regional Crisis Program, an emergency response team to acute psychiatric crises. Affiliated with the University of Toronto.
Robert Biron, President & CEO
Dr. Tom Chan, Chief of Medical Staff
Linda Calhoun, Chief Nursing Executive & Vice-President, Integrated
    Care & Patient Experience

TORONTO: The Scarborough Hospital - General Campus
Scarborough & Rouge Hospital
Affiliated with: Central East Local Health Integration Network
3050 Lawrence Ave. East, Toronto, ON M1P 2V5

Tel: 416-438-2911
www.tsh.to
Social Media: www.facebook.com/ScarboroughHospital;
twitter.com/ScarboroughHosp;
www.youtube.com/user/TSHCommunications;
www.linkedin.com/company/the-scarborough-hospital

Year Founded: 1956
Number of Beds: 277 beds
Number of Employees: 3105
Note: Programs & services include: adult mental health; diabetes education; Dorif Lawrence Breast Clinic; emergency; family & community medicine; maternal/newborn; medical; Ontario Breast Screening Program; outpatient services; paediatrics; prenatal classes; & surgery. Affiliated with the University of Toronto.
Robert Biron, President & CEO
Dr. Tom Chan, Chief of Medical Staff
Linda Calhoun, Chief Nursing Executive & Vice-President, Integrated
    Care & Patient Experience

TORONTO: South Riverdale Community Health Centre
955 Queen St. East, Toronto, ON M4M 3P3

Tel: 416-461-1925
www.srchc.ca

Note: Programs & services include: counselling; diabetes education; environmental health; nutrition; chiropody; health care clinic; physiotherapy; & Teleophthalmology
Lynne Raskin, Chief Executive Officer

TORONTO: Stonegate Community Health Centre
150 Berry Rd., Toronto, ON M8Y 1W3

Tel: 416-231-7070 Fax: 416-231-2663
info@stonegatechc.org
www.stonegatechc.org
Social Media: www.facebook.com/318730301566322;
twitter.com/StonegateCHC

Note: Specialties: asthma education; chiropody; counselling; dental; diabetes education; dietitian; medical; & smoking cessation
Bev Leaver, Executive Director

TORONTO: Sunnybrook Health Sciences Centre - Bayview Campus
Affiliated with: Toronto Central Local Health Integration Network
2075 Bayview Ave., Toronto, ON M4N 3M5

Tel: 416-480-6100
www.sunnybrook.ca
Social Media: www.facebook.com/SunnybrookHSC;
twitter.com/Sunnybrook; www.youtube.com/SunnybrookMedia
Year Founded: 1948
Number of Beds: 1,325 beds (including bassinet beds)
Note: A comprehensive health facility with a focus on cancer care (Odette Cancer Centre), cardiac care (Schulich Heart Centre), musculoskeletal care (Holland Musculoskeletal Program), brain science program (stroke, dementias, mood disorders), women's health, infertility, perinatal care, pediatrics, emergency services, trauma & critical care, veterans' care & residence, research & education.
Barry McLellan, President & CEO
Malcolm Moffat, Executive Vice-President, Programs
Andy Smith, Chief Medical Executive & Executive Vice-President, Programs
Michael Young, Chief Admin. Executive & Executive Vice-President

TORONTO: Toronto Central Local Health Integration Network (TC LHIN)/RLISS du Centre-Toronto
Also Known As: Toronto Central LHIN
#201, 425 Bloor St. East, Toronto, ON M4W 3R4

Tel: 416-921-7453 *Fax:* 416-921-0117
Toll-Free: 866-383-5446
torontocentral@lhins.on.ca
www.torontocentrallhin.on.ca
Social Media: twitter.com/tc_lhin;
www.youtube.com/user/TorontoCentralLHIN
Year Founded: 2005
Area Served: City of Toronto, Scarborough, North York & Etobicoke
Population Served: 1200000
Note: 170 health service providers including hospitals, the Toronto Central Community Care Access Centre, community support services, community health centres, mental health & addictions agencies & long-term care homes are funded through the TC LHIN.
Dr. Vivek Goel, Board Chair
Susan Fitzpatrick, Chief Executive Officer
Sophia Ikura, Senior Director, Strategy, Community Engagement & Population Health
Raj Krishnapillai, Senior Director, Finance, Corporate & Shared Services
William B. Manson, Senior Director, Performance Management & Health Analytics

TORONTO: Toronto General Hospital (TGH)
University Health Network
Affiliated with: Toronto Central Local Health Integration Network
200 Elizabeth St., Toronto, ON M5G 2C4

Tel: 416-340-3111
www.uhn.ca/corporate/AboutUHN/OurHospitals/TGH
Social Media: www.facebook.com/UniversityHealthNetwork;
twitter.com/UHN_News; www.youtube.com/UHNToronto;
www.linkedin.com/company/university-health-network
Year Founded: 1829
Number of Beds: 457 beds
Note: A comprehensive health care & teaching facility, its specialties include cardiac care (Peter Munk Cardiac Centre), transplantation, kidney diseases & care, tropical disease, eating disorders, nephrology, psychiatry, HIV/AIDS care, & telemedicine. It is home to the MaRS Discovery District, a not-for-profit research corporation with funding from both private & public sectors. Affiliated with the University of Toronto.

TORONTO: Toronto Rehabilitation Institute
University Health Network
Affiliated with: Toronto Central Local Health Integration Network
Also Known As: Toronto Rehab
550 University Ave., Toronto, ON M5G 2A2

Tel: 416-597-3422 *Fax:* 416-597-1977
www.uhn.ca/torontorehab
Social Media: www.facebook.com/UniversityHealthNetwork;
twitter.com/UHN_News; www.youtube.com/UHNToronto;
www.linkedin.com/company/university-health-network

Note: Rehabilitation & complex continuing care; includes Lakeside Long-Term Care Centre; Lyndhurst Centre; E.W. Bickle Centre; Rumsey Centre, & University Centre
Dr. Peter Pisters, President & CEO

TORONTO: Toronto Western Hospital
University Health Network
Affiliated with: Toronto Central Local Health Integration Network
399 Bathurst St., Toronto, ON M5T 2S8

Tel: 416-603-2581
www.uhn.ca/corporate/AboutUHN/OurHospitals/TWH
Social Media: www.facebook.com/UniversityHealthNetwork;
twitter.com/UHN_News; www.youtube.com/UHNToronto;
www.linkedin.com/company/university-health-network
Year Founded: 1905
Number of Beds: 280 beds
Note: Primary areas of focus are neural & sensory sciences, community & population health & musculoskeletal health & arthritis. Programs & services include: acquired brain injury clinic; aneurysm clinic; artists health centre; asthma; cardiac & pulmonary rehab; diabetes education; eye clinic; memory clinic; mental health & addictions; movement disorders clinic; sleep clinic; stroke clinic; Tourette's Clinic; & tuberculosis clinic. Affiliated with the University of Toronto.

TORONTO: University Health Network (UHN)
Affiliated with: Toronto Central Local Health Integration Network
R. Fraser Elliot Building, 1st Fl., 190 Elizabeth St., Toronto, ON M5G 2C4

Tel: 416-340-4800
www.uhn.ca
Social Media: www.facebook.com/UniversityHealthNetwork;
twitter.com/UHN_News; www.youtube.com/UHNToronto;
www.linkedin.com/company/university-health-network
Number of Beds: 1,295 beds (total, all sites)
Number of Employees: 14318
Note: Comprised of Princess Margaret Hospital, Toronto General Hospital, Toronto Western Hospital & Toronto Rehab, UHN is a comprehensive health care, research & teaching facility with fields of focus including cancer care, cardiac care, musculoskeletal health & arthritis, neuroscience, ophthalmology, surgical & critical care, transplantation. The network is affiliated with the University of Toronto, Faculty of Medicine.
Dr. Peter Pisters, President & CEO
Michael Nader, Executive Vice-President, Clinical Operations
Dr. Charles Chan, Executive Vice-President, Clinical Programs Quality & Safety

TORONTO: West Park Healthcare Centre
Affiliated with: Toronto Central Local Health Integration Network
Former Name: West Park Hospital
82 Buttonwood Ave., Toronto, ON M6M 2J5

Tel: 416-243-3600 *Fax:* 416-243-8947
feedback@westpark.org
www.westpark.org
Social Media: www.facebook.com/WestParkHealthcareCentre;
twitter.com/westparkhcc; www.youtube.com/WestParkhealthcare;
www.linkedin.com/company/218953
Year Founded: 1904
Number of Beds: 200 long-term care beds; 140 complex continung care beds; 130 rehab beds
Number of Employees: 932
Note: Rehabilitation & chronic care facility
Anne-Marie Malek, President & CEO
Dr. Nora Cullen, Chief of Staff
Jay Cooper, CFO & Vice-President, Corporate Services
Jan Walker, CIO & Vice-President, Strategy & Innovation
Barbara Bell, Chief Nurse & Health Professions Officer
Liliana Catapano, Chief Human Resource Officer
Shelley Ditty, Vice-President, Planning & Development
Donna Renzetti, Vice-President, Programs

TORONTO: Women's College Hospital (WCH)
Affiliated with: Toronto Central Local Health Integration Network
76 Grenville St., Toronto, ON M5S 1B2

Tel: 416-323-6400
info@wchospital.ca
www.womenscollegehospital.ca
Social Media: www.facebook.com/wchospital; twitter.com/wchospital;
www.youtube.com/wchospital
Year Founded: 1928
Note: Programs & services include: asthma; breastfeeding support;
breast screening; cardiac rehabilitation for women; child & family
psychiatry; chronic pain; complex care; Crossroads Refugee Health
Clinic; day surgery; diabetes education (TRIDEC); environmental
health; gynecology; headache clinic; infertility; mental health programs;
osteoporosis; prenatal & postnatal support; Ricky Kanee Schacter
Dermatology Centre; sexual assault & domestic violence care centre;
WISE program; & Women's Health Matters (online resource). The
hospital was renovated in 2016, offering updated access to diagnostic
imaging services & additional operating rooms.
Marilyn Emery, President & CEO
Dr. Danielle Martin, Vice-President, Medical Affairs & Health System
   Solutions

TORONTO: Women's Health in Women's Hands
#500, 2 Carlton St., Toronto, ON M5B 1J3

Tel: 416-593-7655 *Fax:* 416-593-5867
info@whiwh.com
www.whiwh.com
Year Founded: 1993
Number of Employees: 33
Note: Provides mental & physical health services for women ages 16 &
above.
Notisha Massaquoi, Executive Director
   notisha@whiwh.com

TRENTON: QHC Trenton Memorial Hospital
Quinte Health Care
Affiliated with: South East Local Health Integration Network
242 King St., Trenton, ON K8V 5S6

Tel: 613-392-2540 *Fax:* 613-392-3749
www.qhc.on.ca
Social Media: www.facebook.com/173689537296;
twitter.com/QuinteHealth; www.youtube.com/QuinteHealthCare
Year Founded: 1951
Number of Beds: 31 beds
Note: Programs & services include: cardiology; clinical nutrition;
diabetes education; emergency services; laboratory; medical services;
Nursing Home Ready Unit; outpatient clinics; pharmacy;
psychiatry/mental health crisis clinic; radiology/diagnostic services;
surgery; & symptom management/palliative care.
Mary Clare Egberts, President & CEO, Quinte Health Care
Dr. Dick Zoutman, Chief of Staff, Quinte Health Care
Carol Smith Romeril, Chief Nursing Officer & Vice-President, Quinte
   Health Care

TWEED: Gateway Community Health Centre
PO Box 99, 41 McClellan St., Tweed, ON K0K 3J0

Tel: 613-478-1211 *Fax:* 613-478-6692
Toll-Free: 855-478-1211
www.gatewaychc.org
Year Founded: 1991
Note: Programs & services include: primary care; chronic disease
management; nutritional counselling; mental health; & health promotion
Lyn Linton, Executive Director

UXBRIDGE: Markham Stouffville Hospital - Uxbridge Site (MSH)
Affiliated with: Central Local Health Integration Network
Also Known As: Uxbridge Cottage Hospital
PO Box 5003, 4 Campbell Dr., Uxbridge, ON L9P 1S4

Tel: 905-852-9771
myhospital@msh.on.ca
www.msh.on.ca
Social Media: www.facebook.com/MarkhamStouffvilleHospital;
twitter.com/MSHospital; www.youtube.com/MSHospital
Year Founded: 1959
Number of Beds: 20 beds
Note: Programs & services include: day surgery; diagnostic imaging;
emergency; laboratory; & physiotherapy.

Jo-anne Marr, President & CEO
Dr. David Austin, Chief of Staff

WALKERTON: South Bruce Grey Health Centre - Walkerton Site
Affiliated with: South West Local Health Integration Network
Former Name: County of Bruce General Hospital
PO Box 1300, 21 McGivern St. West, Walkerton, ON N0G 2V0

Tel: 519-881-1220 *Fax:* 519-881-0452
info@sbghc.on.ca
www.sbghc.on.ca
Social Media: www.facebook.com/sbghc; twitter.com/SBG_HC
Year Founded: 1900
Number of Beds: 31 beds (25 acute care beds, 6 obstetric beds)
Note: Programs & services include: cardio-respiratory; family birthing
centre; diagnostic imaging; emergency department; emergency;
inpatient medical beds; laboratory; nutrition services; outpatient clinics;
palliative care; & pastoral care.
Paul Rosebush, President & CEO, SBGHC
   prosebush@sbghc.on.ca
Maureen Rydall, Chief Nursing Officer, SBGHC
   mrydall@sbghc.on.ca

WALLACEBURG: Chatham-Kent Health Alliance - Sydenham
Campus (CKHA)
Affiliated with: Erie St. Clair Local Health Integration Network
PO Box 2030, 325 Margaret Ave., Wallaceburg, ON N8A 2A7

Tel: 519-352-6400
www.ckha.on.ca
Social Media: www.facebook.com/ckhamedia; twitter.com/ckhamedia;
www.youtube.com/ckhamedia
Year Founded: 1952
Number of Beds: 200+ beds (total for both CKHA sites)
Note: Programs & services include: ambulatory care; diagnostic
imaging; emergency; inpatient medicine unit; laboratory; rehabilitation
therapy; & respiratory services.
Lori Marshall, President & CEO, CKHA
   lmarshall@ckha.on.ca

WATERLOO: CCAC Waterloo Wellington
141 Weber St. South, Waterloo, ON N2J 2A9

Tel: 519-748-2222 *Fax:* 519-883-5555
Toll-Free: 888-883-3313
information@ww.ccac-ont.ca
healthcareathome.ca

Note: Head office for the region
Dale Clement, CEO

WAWA: Lady Dunn Health Centre
PO Box 179, 17 Government Rd., Wawa, ON P0S 1K0

Tel: 705-856-2335 *Fax:* 705-856-7533
Toll-Free: 866-832-3321
www.ldhc.com
Number of Beds: 16 long-term care beds; 10 acute care beds; 2 respite
beds
Population Served: 4352
Note: Programs & services include: 24 hour emergency; acute care;
diagnostic; long-term care; obstetrics; oncology; & physiotherapy.
Kadean Ogilvie-Pinter, Chief Executive Officer & Director, Patient Care
   Services
   kogilvie@ldhc.com
Geraldine Dumont, Chief Financial Officer
   gdumont@ldhc.com
Dr. Mike Cotterill, Chief of Staff

WELLAND: Welland Hospital Site
Niagara Health System / Système de santé de Niagara
Affiliated with: Hamilton Niagara Haldimand Brant Local Health
Integration Network
65 - 3rd St., Welland, ON L3B 4W6

Tel: 905-378-4647
patientrelations@niagarahealth.on.ca
www.niagarahealth.on.ca
Social Media: twitter.com/niagarahealth;
www.youtube.com/niagarahealthsystem
Year Founded: 1908
Number of Beds: 155 beds (including 15 nephrology beds)
Note: Programs & services include: ambulatory clinics; complex care;
critical care; diabetes education; diagnostic imaging; emergency;

laboratory; long-term care; medicine; Ontario Breast Screening Clinic; ophthalmology; satellite dialysis centre; & surgery.
Dr. Kevin Smith, Chief Executive Officer, Niagara Health System
    kevin.smith@niagarahealth.on.ca
Dr. Suzanne Johnston, President, Niagara Health System
    suzanne.johnston@niagarahealth.on.ca
Derek McNally, Chief Nursing Executive, Niagara Health System
    derek.mcnally@niagarahealth.on.ca

WEST LORNE: West Elgin Community Health Centre
153 Main St., West Lorne, ON N0L 2P0
Tel: 519-768-1715 Fax: 519-768-2548
info@wechc.on.ca
www.wechc.on.ca

Note: Provides health services & community programs to residents of the western Elgin area
Andy Kroeker, Executive Director
    akroeker@wechc.on.ca

WHITBY: CCAC Central East - Whitby Head Office
Former Name: Durham Access to Care
920 Champlain Ct., Whitby, ON L1N 6K9
Tel: 905-430-3308 Fax: 905-430-0645
Toll-Free: 800-263-3877
healthcareathome.ca

Kathryn Ramsay, CEO

WHITBY: Lakeridge Health - Whitby Site
Affiliated with: Central East Local Health Integration Network
300 Gordon St., Whitby, ON L1N 5T2
Tel: 905-668-6831
www.lakeridgehealth.on.ca
Social Media: www.facebook.com/LakeridgeHealth;
twitter.com/lakeridgehealth; www.youtube.com/lakeridgehealth
Number of Beds: 42+ beds
Note: Programs & services include: ambulatory rehabilitation centres/musculoskeletal physiotherapy clinics; diabetes education; & respiratory rehabilitation.
Matthew Anderson, President & CEO, Lakeridge Health
    905-576-8711
Dr. Tony Stone, Chief of Staff, Lakeridge Health
    905-576-8711
Leslie Motz, Chief Nursing Executive, Lakeridge Health
    905-576-8711

WIARTON: Wiarton Hospital
Grey Bruce Health Services
Affiliated with: South West Local Health Integration Network
369 Mary St., Wiarton, ON N0H 2T0
Tel: 519-534-1260 Fax: 519-534-5159
web@gbhs.on.ca
www.gbhs.on.ca
Social Media: twitter.com/greybrucehealth
Number of Beds: 22 beds
Note: Programs & services include: acute care; ambulatory care; complex continuing care; Diabetes Grey Bruce; diagnostic imaging; emergency; laboratory; North Bruce Community Mental Health Team; physiotherapy; spiritual care; & surgery.
Lance Thurston, President & CEO, Grey Bruce Health Services
    519-376-2121

WINCHESTER: Winchester District Memorial Hospital (WDMH)
Affiliated with: Champlain Local Health Integration Network
566 Louise St., Winchester, ON K0C 2K0
Tel: 613-774-2420 Fax: 613-774-0453
www.wdmh.on.ca
Number of Beds: 70 beds
Number of Employees: 320
Note: Programs & services include: clinics; complex continuing care; diabetes education; diagnostic imaging; emergency; enhanced care; inpatient laboratory; maternity; medical day care; medical/surgical; occupational therapy; Ontario breast screening program; physiotherapy; Robillard Hearing Centre; sleep lab; & surgical day care. Has 135 physicians, dentists & midwives on staff. Affiliated with approximately 20 college & university programs.
Cholly Boland, Chief Executive Officer
    cboland@wdmh.on.ca

Lynn Hall, Chief Nursing Executive & Senior Vice-President, Clinical Services & Professional Practice Leader
    lhall@wdmh.on.ca

WINDSOR: CCAC Erie St. Clair - Windsor Branch
5415 Tecumseh Rd. East, 2nd Fl., Windsor, ON N8T 1C5
Tel: 519-258-8211 Fax: 519-351-5842
Toll-Free: 888-447-4468
healthcareathome.ca/eriestclair

WINDSOR: Hôtel-Dieu Grace Healthcare
Affiliated with: Erie St. Clair Local Health Integration Network
1453 Prince Rd., Windsor, ON N9C 3Z4
Tel: 519-257-5111
www.hdgh.org
Social Media: www.facebook.com/HDGHF; twitter.com/HDGHWindsor;
www.youtube.com/user/HOTELDIEUGRACE

Note: Programs & services include: acquired brain injury; addiction & mental health; adult day program; bariatric assessment & treatment; cardiac; chiropody; community crisis centre; complex continuing care; concurrent disorder program; dual diagnosis; stabilization; geriatrics; mood & anxiety treatment; palliative program; pharmacy; Regional Children's Centre; rehabiliation; remedial measures; residential rehabilitation; wellness program for extended psychosis; & withdrawal management services.
Janice Kaffer, President & CEO
Marie Campagna, Chief Financial Officer & Vice-President, Corporate Services & New Business Development
Ester Lipnicki, Chief Nursing Officer & Vice-President, Restorative Care
Dr. Andrea Steen, Vice-President, Medical Affairs

WINDSOR: Sandwich Community Health Centre
Affiliated with: Windsor Essex Community Health Centre
3320 College Ave., Windsor, ON N9C 0E1
Tel: 519-258-6002 Fax: 519-258-3693
www.wechc.org
Year Founded: 1982
Note: Focuses on providing primary health care & counselling.
Glenn Bartlett, Executive Director

WINDSOR: Windsor Regional Hospital - Metropolitan Campus
Affiliated with: Erie St. Clair Local Health Integration Network
1995 Lens Ave., Windsor, ON N8W 1L9
Tel: 519-254-5577 Fax: 519-254-2317
www.wrh.on.ca
Social Media: www.facebook.com/WindsorRegionalHospital;
twitter.com/WRHospital; www.youtube.com/user/WRHWeCare
Year Founded: 1928
Number of Beds: 483+ beds (total of all WRH sites)
Population Served: 400000
Note: Programs & services on both campuses include: cardiac care; complex trauma; emergency services; intensive care; medicine; neonatal intensive care; paediatric services; regional cancer services; renal dialysis; stroke & neurosurgery; & surgery.
David Musyj, President & CEO

WINDSOR: Windsor Regional Hospital - Ouellette Campus
Affiliated with: Erie St. Clair Local Health Integration Network
1030 Ouellette Ave., Windsor, ON N9A 1E1
Tel: 519-973-4411
www.wrh.on.ca
Social Media: www.facebook.com/WindsorRegionalHospital;
twitter.com/WRHospital; www.youtube.com/user/WRHWeCare
Year Founded: 1888
Number of Beds: 469 beds (total of all WRH sites)
Population Served: 400000
Note: Acquired by Windsor Regional Hospital in 2013; renovations in 2008 expanded emergency services, operating rooms & diagnostic imaging departments. Programs & services on both campuses include: cardiac care; complex trauma; emergency services; family birthing centre; intensive care; medicine; neonatal intensive care; paediatric services; regional cancer services; renal dialysis; stroke & neurosurgery; & surgery.
David Musyj, President & CEO

WINGHAM: Wingham & District Hospital
Listowel Wingham Hospitals Alliance
Affiliated with: South West Local Health Integration Network
270 Carling Terrace, Wingham, ON N0G 2W0
Tel: 519-357-3210 *Fax:* 519-357-2931
www.lwha.ca

Number of Beds: 36 beds
Note: Programs & services include: breast health; diabetes education; diagnostic imaging; emergency; inpatient/medical; laboratory; maternal/newborn; nutrition; oncology; outpatient clinics; surgical; & therapy.
Karl Ellis, President & CEO
519-357-3210, karl.ellis@lwha.ca

WOODSTOCK: CCAC South West - Woodstock Branch Office
1147 Dundas St., Woodstock, ON N4S 8W3
Tel: 519-539-1284 *Fax:* 519-539-0065
Toll-Free: 800-561-5490
info-woodstock@sw.ccac-ont.ca
healthcareathome.ca

Sandra Coleman, CEO, South West CCAC

WOODSTOCK: Woodstock General Hospital
Affiliated with: South West Local Health Integration Network
310 Juliana Dr., Woodstock, ON N4V 0A4
Tel: 519-421-4211 *Fax:* 519-421-4247
info@wgh.on.ca
www.wgh.on.ca

Number of Beds: 178 beds
Note: Programs & services include: ambulatory care; complex continuing care; critical care; diagnostic imaging; inpatient rehabilitation; intensive rehabilitation outpatient program; maternal child services; medical/surgical unit; mental health; surgery; & urology.
Natasa Veljovic, President & CEO
Dr. Malcolm MacLeod, Chief of Staff
Jayne Menard, Chief Nursing Officer & Vice-President, Patient Care

WOODSTOCK: Woodstock Private Hospital
Affiliated with: South West Local Health Integration Network
369 Huron St., Woodstock, ON N4S 7A5
Tel: 519-537-8162 *Fax:* 519-537-7204

Number of Beds: 16 beds
Note: Chronic care hospital
Lisa Figg, Administrator

PRINCE EDWARD ISLAND

ALBERTON: Western Hospital
Affiliated with: Health PEI
PO Box 10, 148 Poplar St., Alberton, PE C0B 1B0
Tel: 902-853-8650 *Fax:* 902-853-8658
www.healthpei.ca/westernhospital

Number of Beds: 27 beds (25 medical, 2 palliative)
Population Served: 8000
Note: Services include: addiction; diagnostic imaging; dialysis; laboratory; pharmacy; physiotherapy; & nutrition counselling.

CHARLOTTETOWN: Euston Street Group Home
Affiliated with: Health PEI
190 Euston St., Charlottetown, PE C1A 1W8
Tel: 902-566-2964

Note: Respite care is available for adolescents who are in the care of the Director of Child Welfare.

CHARLOTTETOWN: Health PEI
PO Box 2000, 16 Garfield St., Charlottetown, PE C1A 7N8
Tel: 902-368-6130 *Fax:* 902-368-6136
healthpei@gov.pe.ca
www.healthpei.ca
Info Line: 811
Social Media: twitter.com/health_pei

Year Founded: 2010
Number of Beds: 595 long-term care beds
Area Served: Province-wide
Population Served: 148649
Number of Employees: 5000
Note: Health PEI is responsible for the operation & delivery of publicly funded health services & long term care in Prince Edward Island.

Phyllis Horne, Board Chair
phorne@gov.pe.ca
Dr. Michael Mayne, Chief Executive Officer
Andrew MacDougall, Director, Long Term Care
asmacdougall@gov.pe.ca
Calvin Joudrie, Subsidization Manager, Long Term Care
ccjoudrie@gov.pe.ca
Shelley MacCallum, Gerontological Clinical Nurse Coordinator
slmaccallum@ihis.org

CHARLOTTETOWN: Home Care Support - Hillsborough Hospital
Affiliated with: Health PEI
Hillsborough Hospital Annex, 115 Deacon Grove Lane, Charlottetown, PE C1A 7N5
Tel: 902-368-4790

CHARLOTTETOWN: Queen Elizabeth Hospital Inc. (QEH)
Affiliated with: Health PEI
PO Box 6600, 60 Riverside Dr., Charlottetown, PE C1A 8T5
Tel: 902-894-2111
TTY: 902-894-2204
www.healthpei.ca/qeh

Year Founded: 1982
Number of Beds: 243 beds
Note: Acute care hospital, with burn care services; coronary care; psychiatry; physiotherapy; occupational therapy; orthpedic & specialized gynecological surgery; eye surgery; plastic surgery; neonatal intensive care; cancer care; diagnostic imaging
Dr. Michael Mayne, Chief Executive Officer, Health PEI

MONTAGUE: Home Care Support - Health PEI Montague
Affiliated with: Health PEI
PO Box 490, 6 Harmony Lane, Montague, PE C0A 1R0
Tel: 902-838-0786

MONTAGUE: King's County Memorial Hospital
Affiliated with: Health PEI
PO Box 490, 409 MacIntyre Ave., Montague, PE C0A 1R0
Tel: 902-838-0777 *Fax:* 902-838-0770
www.healthpei.ca/kcmh

Number of Beds: 30 beds
Note: Services include: emergency; inpatient; & ambulatory care.

O'LEARY: Community Hospital O'Leary
Affiliated with: Health PEI
PO Box 160, 14 MacKinnon Dr., O'Leary, PE C0B 1V0
Tel: 902-859-8700 *Fax:* 902-859-8774
www.healthpei.ca/cho

Year Founded: 1957
Number of Beds: 13 extended care beds
Note: Services include: diagnostic imaging; laboratory; pharmacy; physiotherapy; & nutrition counselling.

O'LEARY: Home Care Support - Community Hospital
Affiliated with: Health PEI
PO Box 160, 14 MacKinnon Dr., O'Leary, PE C0B 1V0
Tel: 902-859-8730

SOURIS: Souris Hospital
Affiliated with: Health PEI
PO Box 640, 17 Knights Ave., Souris, PE C0A 2B0
Tel: 902-687-7150 *Fax:* 902-687-7175
www.healthpei.ca

Number of Beds: 17 beds
Population Served: 7000
Note: Acute care rural facility. Services include: addiction; ambulatory; diabetes program; diagnostic imaging; extended care; home care; mental health; palliative care; renal program; & public health nursing.

SUMMERSIDE: Prince County Hospital (PCH)
Affiliated with: Health PEI
PO Box 3000, 65 Roy Boates Ave., Summerside, PE C1N 2A9
Tel: 902-438-4200 *Fax:* 902-438-4511
www.healthpei.ca/pch

Number of Beds: 110 beds
Note: Services include: ambulatory care; emergency; hemodialysis; inpatient mental health; intensive care; obstetrics; & pediatrics.
Arlene Gallant-Bernard, Chief Administrative Officer

TYNE VALLEY: Stewart Memorial Hospital
Affiliated with: Health PEI
PO Box 10, 6926 rte 12, Tyne Valley, PE C0B 2C0
Tel: 902-831-7900 *Fax:* 902-831-7901
www.healthpei.ca/smh

Number of Beds: 23 beds
Note: Services include: nursing; medical; dental care; nutrition; podiatry; occupational therapy; & physiotherapy.

QUÉBEC

ALMA: CSSS de Lac-Saint-Jean-Est
Affiliée à: CIUSSS du Saguenay-Lac-Saint-Jean
CP 1300, 300, boul Champlain Sud, Alma, QC G8B 5W3
Tél: 418-669-2000 *Téléc:* 418-668-9695
www.santealma.qc.ca

Note: Les Installations (Services de CH, CHSLD, et CLSC): Hôpital d'Alma; CLSC Secteur-Centre (Alma); CLSC Secteur-Nord (L'Ascension-de-Notre-Seigneur); CLSC Secteur-Sud (Métabetchouan-Lac-à-la-Croix); Centre d'hébergement Isidore-Gauthier; Centre d'hébergement Métabetchouan-Lac-à-la-Croix; Centre d'hébergement Le normandie

AMOS: CRDI Abitibi-Témiscamingue Clair-Foyer
Affiliée à: CISSS de l'Abitibi-Témiscamingue
841, 3e rue Ouest, Amos, QC J9T 2T4
Tél: 819-732-6511 *Téléc:* 819-732-0922
www.cisss-at.gouv.qc.ca

Nombre de lits: 31 lits
Note: Centre de réadaptation (déficience intellectuelle); services de support.

AMOS: CSSS Les Eskers de l'Abitibi (CSSSEA)
Affiliée à: CISSS de l'Abitibi-Témiscamingue
622, 4e rue ouest, Amos, QC J9T 2S2
Tél: 819-732-3341 *Téléc:* 819-732-7054
www.cisss-at.gouv.qc.ca

Nombre de lits: 96 lits de courte durée; 103 lits d'hébergement; 24 lits en ressources intermédiaires
Région desservi: MRC d'Abitibi (19 municipalités)
Population desservi: 25000
Personnel: 900
Note: Les Installations (Services de CH, CHSLD, et CLSC): Hôpital Hôtel-Dieu d'Amos (819-732-3341); Centre d'hébergement Harricana (819-732-6521); CLSC Les Eskers (Amos, Barraute, Berry, Guyenne, La Corne, La Motte, Landrienne, Launay, Preissac, Rochebaucourt, Saint-Dominique-du-Rosaire, Saint-Félix-de-Dalquier, Saint-Marc-de-Figuery, Saint-Mathieu-d'Harricana, Sainte-Gertrude-Manneville, Trécesson - secteur La Ferme, Trécesson - secteur Villemontel).
Le Territoire desservi: 17 municipalités, deux territoires non organisés (TNO) et la communauté algonquine de Pikogan, MRC d'Abitibi

AMOS: Hôpital Hôtel-Dieu d'Amos
Affiliée à: CISSS de l'Abitibi-Témiscamingue
622, 4e rue Ouest, Amos, QC J9T 2S2
Tél: 819-732-3341

Note: Services diagnostiques; urgence et traumatologie; othopédie; rhumatologie; ophtalmologie; chirurgie plastique/reconstructive/maxillo-faciale; gynécologie; obstétrique; gériatrie; physiothérapie; réadaptation cardio-respiratoire.

AMQUI: CSSS de la Matapédia
135, av Gaétan-Archambeault, Amqui, QC G5J 2K5
Tél: 418-629-2211
www.csssmatapedia.qc.ca

Personnel: 502
Note: Services à la population: Services hospitaliers et urgence; Services diagnostiques; Services de réadaptation; Services ambulatoires; Services de pastorale; Services offerts en CLSC; Services de soutien à domicile; Services d'hébergement de longue durée; Services gériatriques

AMQUI: Hôpital d'Amqui
Affiliée à: CISSS du Bas-St-Laurent
135, av Gaétan-Archambault, Amqui, QC G5J 2K5
Tél: 418-629-2211
www.cisss-bsl.gouv.qc.ca

Population desservi: 21000

AUPALUK: Dispensaire d'Aupaluk
Aupaluk, QC J0M 1X0
Tél: 819-491-9090

Nombre de lits: 1 lit

BAIE-COMEAU: Centre de protection et de réadaptation de la Côte-Nord
Affiliée à: CISSS de la Côte-Nord
835, boul Joliet, Baie-Comeau, QC G5C 1P5
Tél: 418-589-9927 *Téléc:* 418-589-4304
www.cisss-cotenord.gouv.qc.ca

Nombre de lits: 225 lits

BAIE-COMEAU: Centre intégré de santé et de services sociaux de la Côte-Nord
835, boul Jolliet, Baie-Comeau, QC G5C 1P5
Tél: 418-589-9845 *Téléc:* 418-589-8574
Ligne sans frais: 800-463-5142
www.cisss-cotenord.gouv.qc.ca
Info Line: 811
Média social: www.facebook.com/cisss.cotenord
Région desservi: Tadoussac à Blanc-Sablon, 1,300 km
Population desservi: 95000
Marc Fortin, Président-directeur général

BAIE-COMEAU: Hôpital Le Royer
Affiliée à: CISSS de la Côte-Nord
635, boul Jolliet, Baie-Comeau, QC G5C 1P1
Tél: 418-589-3701 *Téléc:* 418-589-9654
Fondée en: 1951
Nombre de lits: 85 lits de santé physique; 21 lits de psychiatrie
Note: Pprogrammes et services comprennent: chirurgie; médecine nucléaire; pédopsychiatrie; radiologie; urologie

BAIE-SAINT-PAUL: Hôpital de Baie-Saint-Paul
Affiliée à: CIUSSS de la Capitale-Nationale
74, rue Ambroise-Fafard, Baie-Saint-Paul, QC G3Z 2J6
Tél: 418-435-5150

Nombre de lits: 40 lits hospitaliers; 56 lits de soins de longue durée
Note: Services: anesthésiologie, chirurgie gériatrie, psychiatrie, radiologie, ophtalmologie, urologie; soins généraux et spécialisés; urgence.

BASSIN: CLSC de Bassin
Affiliée à: CISSS des Iles
599, ch du Bassin, Bassin, QC G4T 0C8
Tél: 418-937-2572 *Téléc:* 418-937-5381

BEDFORD: CLSC de Bedford
Affiliée à: CISSS de la Montérégie-Ouest
34, rue St-Joseph, Bedford, QC J0J 1A0
Tél: 450-248-4321 *Téléc:* 450-248-7435
www.santemonteregie.qc.ca/lapommeraie

BELOEIL: CLSC des Patriotes
Affiliée à: CISSS de la Montérégie-Est
300, rue Serge-Pepin, Beloeil, QC J3G 0B8
Tél: 450-536-2572 *Téléc:* 450-536-6367
www.santemonteregie.qc.ca/richelieu-yamaska
Fondée en: 1985
Région desservi: MRC de la Vallée-du-Richelieu
Spécialités: Cliniques de vaccination; Clinique du diabète; Programmes en périnatalité; Services à domicile aux personnes en perte d'autonomie

BONAVENTURE: Centre de réadaptation de la Gaspésie
MRC de Bonaventure
238, av Port-Royal, Bonaventure, QC G0C 1E0
Tél: 418-534-4243 *Téléc:* 418-534-2411

BOUCHERVILLE: CLSC des Seigneuries de Boucherville
Affiliée à: CISSS de la Montérégie-Est
160, boul De Montarville, Boucherville, QC J4B 6S2
Tél: 450-468-3530 *Téléc:* 450-468-8530
www.santemonteregie.qc.ca

BROSSARD: CHSLD Vigi Brossard
Affiliée à: Vigi Santé Ltée
5955, boul Grande-Allée, Brossard, QC J4Z 3G4
Tél: 450-656-8500 *Téléc:* 450-656-8586
www.vigisante.com
Nombre de lits: 66 lits
Note: Agence/région administrative: Agence de la santé et des services sociaux de Montérégie.

CANDIAC: CLSC Kateri
Affiliée à: CISSS de la Montérégie-Ouest
90, boul Marie-Victorin, Candiac, QC J5R 1C1
Tél: 450-659-7661 *Téléc:* 450-444-6260
Nombre de lits: 340 lits

CANTLEY: CLSC Cantley
Affiliated with: CISSS de l'Outaouais
850, Montée de la Source, Cantley, QC J8V 3H4
Tel: 819-459-1112 *Fax:* 819-827-5818
Toll-Free: 877-459-1112

CAP-CHAT: CLSC de Cap-Chat
Affiliée à: CISSS de la Gaspésie
CP 415, 49, rue Notre-Dame, Cap-Chat, QC G0J 1E0
Tél: 418-786-5594 *Téléc:* 418-786-2638
www.cisss-gaspesie.gouv.qc.ca

CAP-AUX-MEULES: Centre intégré de santé et de services sociaux des Îles
430, ch Principal, Cap-aux-Meules, QC G4T 1R9
Tél: 418-986-2121
www.cisssdesiles.com
Info Line: 811
Média social: www.facebook.com/151244821567542

Population desservi: 80353
Yvette Fortier, Présidente-directrice générale

CAP-AUX-MEULES: CLSC de Cap-aux-Meules
Affiliée à: CISSS des Îles
420, ch Principal, Cap-aux-Meules, QC G4T 1R9
Tél: 418-986-2572 *Téléc:* 418-986-4911

CAP-AUX-MEULES: Hôpital de l'Archipel
Affiliée à: CISSS des Îles
430, ch Principal, Cap-aux-Meules, QC G4T 1R9
Tél: 418-986-2121
Nombre de lits: 105 lits

CAPLAN: CLSC de Caplan
Affiliée à: CISSS de la Gaspésie
96, boul Perron ouest, Caplan, QC G0C 1H0
Tél: 418-388-2572 *Téléc:* 418-388-5646

CARLETON: Point de service - Réadaptation Carleton-sur-Mer
314, boul Perron ouest, Carleton, QC G0C 1J0
Tél: 418-364-6037

CHANDLER: CLSC de Chandler
Affiliée à: CISSS de la Gaspésie
CP 1090, 633, av Daigneault, Chandler, QC G0C 1K0
Tél: 418-689-2572 *Téléc:* 418-689-4707
Nombre de lits: 62 lits
Chantal Duguay, Directrice générale

CHANDLER: CSSS du Rocher-Percé
Affiliée à: CISSS la Gaspésie
451, rue Monseigneur Ross est, Chandler, QC G0C 1K0
Tél: 418-689-2261 *Téléc:* 418-689-5551
www.csssrocherperce.com
Nombre de lits: 52 lits en soins de courte durée; 36 lits en soins de longue durée; 62 lits en hébergement de longue durée; 5 lits en psychiatrie
Région desservi: MRC du Rocher-Percé
Note: Les Installations (Services de CH, CHSLD, et CLSC): Hôpital de Chandler (418-689-2261); Centre d'hébergement Villa-Pabos

(418-689-6621); CLSC Chandler (418-689-2572); CLSC Percé (418-782-2572); CLSC Gascons (418-396-2572)

CHANDLER: Hôpital de Chandler
Affiliée à: CISSS de la Gaspésie
451, rue Mgr Ross Est, Chandler, QC G0C 1K0
Tél: 418-689-2261
www.cisss-gaspesie.gouv.qc.ca
Nombre de lits: 155 lits
Note: Soins hospitaliers; soins de longue durée; a fusionné avec le CLSC-CHSLD Pabok en 2004.

CHANDLER: Point de service - Réadaptation Rocher-Percé
Affiliée à: CISSS de la Gaspésie
#102, 328, boul René-Lévesque ouest, Chandler, QC G0C 1K0
Tél: 418-689-4286

CHÂTEAUGUAY: Centre intégré de santé et de services sociaux de la Montérégie-Ouest
200, boul Brisebois, Châteauguay, QC J6K 4W8
Tél: 450-699-2425
www.santemo.quebec
Info Line: 811

Population desservi: 430000
Personnel: 8700
Yves Masse, Président-directeur général
Claude Jolin, Président, Conseil d'administration

CHÂTEAUGUAY: CLSC Châteauguay
Affiliée à: CISSS de la Montérégie-Ouest
95, ave de la Verdure, Châteauguay, QC J6K 0E8
Tél: 450-699-3333 *Téléc:* 450-691-6202

CHÂTEAUGUAY: CSSS Jardins-Roussillon
Affiliée à: CISSS de la Montérégie-Ouest
200, boul Brisebois, Châteauguay, QC J6K 4W8
Tél: 450-699-2425
www.santemonteregie.qc.ca/jardins-roussillon

Population desservi: 189000
Note: Les Installations (Services de CH, CHSLD, et CLSC): Hôpital Anna-Laberge (450-699-2425); Centre d'hébergement de Châteauguay (450-692-8231); Centre d'hébergement de La Prairie (450-659-9148); Centre d'hébergement de Saint-Rémi (450-454-4694); Centre de services Lauzon (450-699-7901); CLSC Châteauguay (450-699-3333); CLSC Jardin-du-Québec, Napierville (450-245-3336); CLSC Jardin-du-Québec, Saint-Rémi (450-454-4671); CLSC Kateri (450-659-7661); Centre d'hébergement Champlain Châteauguay (450-632-4451, poste 313); Centre d'hébergement Champlain Jean-Louis-Lapierre (450-632-4451, poste 313); Centre hospitalier Kateri Memorial (450-638-3930).
Le Territoire desservi: Candiac, Châteauguay, Delson, Hemmingford Canton et Village, La Prairie, Léry, Mercier, Napierville, Saint-Bernard-de-Lacolle, Saint-Constant, Saint-Cyprien de Napierville, Sainte-Catherine, Sainte-Clotilde, Saint-Édouard, Sainte-Martine, Saint-Isidore, Saint-Jacques-le-Mineur, Saint-Mathieu, Saint-Michel, Saint-Patrice-de-Sherrington, Saint-Philippe, Saint-Rémi, Saint-Urbain-Premier

CHÂTEAUGUAY: Hôpital Anna-Laberge
Affiliée à: CISSS de la Montérégie-Ouest
200, boul Brisebois, Châteauguay, QC J6K 4W8
Tél: 450-699-2425
www.santemonteregie.qc.ca
Fondée en: 1988
Nombre de lits: 226 lits hospitaliers
Yves Masse, Directeur général, CISSS de la Montérégie-Ouest

CHERTSEY: CLSC de Chertsey
Affiliée à: CISSS de Lanaudière
485, rue Dupuis, Chertsey, QC J0K 3K0
Tél: 450-882-2488

CHIBOUGAMAU: Centre régional de santé et services sociaux de la Baie-James (CRSSSBJ)
Également connu sous le nom de: CRSSS de la Baie-James
312, 3e rue, Chibougamau, QC G8P 1N5
Tél: 418-748-3575 *Téléc:* 418-748-6391
Ligne sans frais: 866-748-2676
info.crsssbj@ssss.gouv.qc.ca
www.crsssbaiejames.gouv.qc.ca
Média social: www.facebook.com/CRSSSBJ

Fondée en: 1996
Région desservi: Nord-du-Québec
Note: Centres de santé (CS): Centre de santé René-Ricard; Centre de santé de Chibougamau; Centre de santé Lebel; Centre de santé Isle-Dieu; Centre de santé de Radisson
Nathalie Boisvert, Présidente-directrice générale
Dr. Éric Goyer, Directeur, Santé publique
Jean-Luc Imbeault, Directeur, ressources financières, techniques et informationnelles
Jean Lemoyne, Directeur, services professionnels, et des services multidisciplinaires
Luc Néron, Directeur, soins infirmiers
Jean-Pierre Savary, Directeur, Ressources humaines

CHICOUTIMI: Centre intégré universitaire de santé et de services sociaux du Saguenay-Lac-St-Jean
Également connu sous le nom de: CIUSSS Saguenay-Lac-St-Jean
930, rue Jacques-Cartier est, Chicoutimi, QC G7H 7K9
Tél: 418-545-4980 *Téléc:* 418-545-8791
Ligne sans frais: 800-370-4980
info@santesaglac.gouv.qc.ca
santesaglac.com
Info Line: 811
Média social: www.facebook.com/SanteSagLac; twitter.com/CIUSSS_SLSJ

Population desservi: 278560
Personnel: 10000
Martine Couture, Présidente-directrice générale
Gilles Gagnon, Président-directeur général adjoint
Michel Martel, Directeur, Ressources financières
Donald Aubin, Directeur, Santé publique

CHICOUTIMI: CSSS de Chicoutimi
Affiliée à: CIUSSS du Saguenay-Lac-Saint-Jean
CP 5006, 305, rue Saint-Vallier, Chicoutimi, QC G7H 5H6
Tél: 418-541-1000 *Téléc:* 418-541-1144
www.csss-chicoutimi.qc.ca

Note: Les Installations (Services de CH, CHSLD, et CLSC): Hôpital de Chicoutimi (418-541-1000); Centre d'hébergement Beaumanoir (418-698-3900); Centre d'hébergement Mgr-Victor-Tremblay (418-698-3907); Centre d'hébergement de la Colline (418-549-5474); CLSC de Chicoutimi (418-543-2221); CLSC Maintien à domicile (418-693-3924). Médecins: 300

CHICOUTIMI: Hôpital de Chicoutimi
Affiliée à: CIUSSS du Saguenay-Lac-St-Jean
305, rue Saint-Vallier, Chicoutimi, QC G7H 5H6
Tél: 418-541-1000 *Téléc:* 418-541-1144
Ligne sans frais: 866-404-7468

CHISASIBI: Conseil Cri de la santé et des services sociaux de la Baie James (CCSSSBJ)/Cree Board of Health & Social Services of James Bay
PO Box 250, Chisasibi, QC J0M 1E0
Tel: 819-855-2744 *Fax:* 819-855-2098
cbhssjb-ccsssbj@ssss.gouv.qc.ca
www.creehealth.org
Social Media: www.facebook.com/creehealth; twitter.com/creehealth; www.youtube.com/creehealth

Year Founded: 1978
Area Served: Terres-Cries-de-la-Baie-James
Bella M. Petawabano, Président/représentant de l'Autorité regional des cris

CHISASIBI: Hôpital de Chisasibi
Affiliée à: Conseil Cri de la santé et des services sociaux de la Baie James
21, rue Maamuu, Chisasibi, QC J0M 1E0
Tél: 819-855-2844 *Téléc:* 819-855-9060
www.creehealth.org/services/chisasibi-hospital
Nombre de lits: 17 servent aux soins actifs (5 en pédiatrie); 9 aux malades chroniques; 3 aux soins respiratoires; 9 hémodialyse
Personnel: 34
Philippe Lubino, Directeur

COATICOOK: Centre hospitalier de Coaticook
Affiliée à: CIUSSS de l'Estrie
138, rue Jeanne-Mance, Coaticook, QC J1A 1W3
Tél: 819-849-9102
www.santeestrie.qc.ca

COATICOOK: CSSS de la MRC de Coaticook
Affiliée à: CIUSSS de l'Estrie
163, rue Jeanne-Mance, Coaticook, QC J1A 1W3
Tél: 819-849-9102
www.santeestrie.qc.ca

Fondée en: 2005
Région desservi: MRC de Coaticook (12 municipalités)
Personnel: 300
Note: Les Installations (Services de CH, CHSLD, et CLSC): Centre hospitalier de Coaticook (819-849-9102); CLSC (1 point de service); 1 centre d'hébergement en soins de longue durée (92 lits); Clinique médicale GMF des Frontières (819-849-4808)

COWANSVILLE: CSSS la Pommeraie
Affiliée à: CIUSSS de l'Estrie
950, rue Principale, Cowansville, QC J2K 1K3
Tél: 450-266-4342 *Téléc:* 450-263-8669

Fondée en: 2004
Nombre de lits: 279 lits
Population desservi: 52000
Personnel: 1382
Note: Les Installations (Services de CH, CHSLD, et CLSC): Hôpital Brome-Missisquoi-Perkins (450-266-4342, option 5); Centre d'accueil de Cowansville (450-266-4342, option 3); CHSLD de Bedford (450-248-4304); Foyer Sutton (450-538-3332); Les Foyers Farnham (450-293-3167); CLSC de Bedford (450-248-4321 poste 0); CLSC de Cowansville (450-266-4342, option 4); CLSC de Farnham (450-293-3622); CLSC de Sutton (450-266-4342, option 4); CLSC de VIlle de Lac-Brome (450-242-2001); Service de soutien à domicile (450-266-4342, option 2).
Le Territoire desservi: La MRC de Brome-Missisquoi en plus des municipalités de Sainte-Brigide-d'Iberville et de l'Ange-Gardien

DIXVILLE: Centre d'accueil Dixville inc.
CRDITED Estrie
301, rue Saint-Alexandre, Dixville, QC J0B 1P0
Tél: 819-346-8471 *Téléc:* 819-849-6673
info.crditedestrie@ssss.gouv.qc.ca
www.crditedestrie.qc.ca

Fondée en: 1958
Note: Le centre de réadaptation en déficience intellectuelle et troubles envahissants du développement Estre (CRDITED Estrie) est composé de deux établissements du réseau de la santé et des services sociaux du Québec, soit le Centre d'accueil Dixville inc. et le Centre Notre-Dame de l'Enfant (Sherbrooke) inc.
Gaétan Duford, Président, Conseil d'administration
Danielle Lareau, Directrice générale, et secrétaire, conseil d'administration

DOLBEAU-MISTASSINI: CSSS Maria-Chapdelaine
Affiliée à: CIUSSS du Saguenay-Lac-Saint-Jean
L'Hôpital, 2000, boul Sacré-Coeur, Dolbeau-Mistassini, QC G8L 2R5
Tél: 418-276-1234 *Téléc:* 418-276-4355
Nombre de lits: 292 lits
Population desservi: 28285
Personnel: 750
Note: Les Installations (Services de CH, CHSLD, et CLSC): L'Hôpital, Dolbeau-Mistassini; L'Oasis, Dolbeau-Mistassini; Les Jardins du Monastère, Dolbeau-Mistassini; Centre de Normandin, Normandin

DOLBEAU-MISTASSINI: Hôpital de Dolbeau-Mistassini
Affiliée à: CIUSSS du Saguenay-Lac-Saint-Jean
2000, boul Sacré-Coeur, Dolbeau-Mistassini, QC G8L 2R5
Tél: 418-276-1234 *Téléc:* 418-276-4355

DONNACONA: CSSS de Portneuf
Affiliée à: CIUSSS de la Capitale-Nationale
250, boul Gaudreau, Donnacona, QC G3M 1L7
Tél: 418-285-3025
www.ciusss-capitalenationale.gouv.qc.ca
Fondée en: 1999
Note: Les Installations (Services de CH, CHSLD, et CLSC): Hôpital
régional de Portneuf (418-337-4611); Centre d'hébergement
Donnacona (418-285-3025); Centre d'hébergement Pont-Rouge
(418-873-4661); Centre d'hébergement Saint-Casimir (418-339-2861);
Centre d'hébergement Saint-Marc-des-Carrières (418-268-3511);
Centre d'hébergement Saint-Raymond (418-337-4661); CLSC
Donnacona (418-285-2626); CLSC Pont-Rouge (418-873-6062); CLSC
Rivière-à-Pierre (418-323-2253); CLSC Saint-Marc-des-Carrières
(418-268-3571); CLSC Saint-Raymond (418-337-4611); CLSC
Saint-Ubalde (418-277-2256). Médecins: 45

DRUMMONDVILLE: CLSC Drummond
Affiliée à: CIUSSS de la Mauricie-et-du-Centre-du-Québec
350, rue Saint-Jean, Drummondville, QC J2B 5L4
Tél: 819-474-2572
www.ciusssmcq.ca

DRUMMONDVILLE: Hôpital Sainte-Croix
Affiliée à: CIUSSS de la santé Mauricie-et-du-Centre-du-Québec
570, rue Heriot, Drummondville, QC J2B 1C1
Tél: 819-478-6464
ciusssmcq.ca

Note: Anatomopathologie, chirurgie générale, gynécologie-obstétrique,
pédiatrie, médecine familiale/interne/nucléaire, ophtalmologie,
orthopédie, psychiatrie, radiologie, urologie.

FORESTVILLE: Pavillon Forestville
Affiliée à: CISSS de la Côte-Nord
CP 790, 2, 7e rue, Forestville, QC G0T 1E0
Tél: 418-587-2212 *Téléc:* 418-587-2865
Nombre de lits: 20 lits
Marc Fortin, Directeur général

**GASPÉ: Centre intégré de santé et de services sociaux de la
Gaspésie**
215, boul de York ouest, Gaspé, QC G4X 2W2
Tél: 418-368-3301 *Téléc:* 418-368-6850
www.cisss-gaspesie.gouv.qc.ca
Info Line: 811
Fondée en: 2015
Population desservi: 80238
Chantal Duguay, Présidente-directrice générale

GASPÉ: CLSC de Gaspé
Affiliée à: CISSS de la Gaspésie
CP 6397, 205, boul de York ouest, 2e étage, Gaspé, QC G4X 2V7
Tél: 418-368-2572
Note: CSSS Côte-de-Gaspé.

GASPÉ: CLSC de Rivière-au-Renard
Affiliée à: CISSS de la Gaspésie
154, boul Renard Est, Gaspé, QC G4X 5R5
Tél: 418-269-2572
Nombre de lits: 3 lits

GASPÉ: CSSS de La Côte-de-Gaspé
Affiliée à: CISSS de la Gaspésie
215, boul de York Ouest, Gaspé, QC G4X 2W2
Tél: 418-368-3301 *Ligne sans frais:* 877-666-8766
www.cisss-gaspesie.gouv.qc.ca

Note: Les Installations (Services de CH, CHSLD, et CLSC): Hôpital
Hotel-Dieu de Gaspé (418-368-3301); Centre d'hébergement Mgr-Ross
(418-368-3301); CLSC de Barachois (418-645-2572); CLSC de Gaspé
(418-368-2572); CLSC de Grande-Vallée (418-393-2572); CLSC de
Murdochville (418-784-2572); CLSC de Rivière-au-Renard
(418-269-2572); Unité de médecine familiale (418-368-6663)

GASPÉ: Hôpital de Gaspé
Affiliée à: CISSS de la Gaspésie
215, boul de York Ouest, Gaspé, QC G4X 2W2
Tél: 418-368-3301

GASPÉ: Point de service - Réadaptation Gaspé
Affiliée à: CISSS de la Gaspésie
150, rue Mgr Ross, Gaspé, QC G4X 2S7
Tél: 418-368-2306

**GATINEAU: Centre intégré de santé et de services sociaux de
l'Outaouais**
80, av Gatineau, Gatineau, QC J8T 4J3
Tél: 819-966-6000 *Téléc:* 819-966-6570
Ligne sans frais: 800-267-2325
relationaveclacommunauteagence07@ssss.gouv.qc.ca
cisss-outaouais.gouv.qc.ca
Info Line: 811

Population desservi: 389496
Note: Centres de santé et de services sociaux (CSSS): CSSS du
Pontiac; CSSS de la Vallée-de-la-Gatineau; CSSS des Collines;
CSSS de Gatineau; CSSS de Papineau
Jean Hébert, Président-directeur général

GATINEAU: CLSC de Gatineau - Point de service de la Gappe
Affiliée à: CISSS de l'Outaouais
777, boul de la Gappe, Gatineau, QC J8T 8R2
Tél: 819-966-6550

Note: Services généraux santé; soins infirmiers et ambulatoires;
consulation médicale pour les clientèles vulnérables.

GATINEAU: CLSC de Gatineau - Point de service Gatineau
Affiliée à: CISSS de l'Outaouais
80, av Gatineau, Gatineau, QC J8T 4J3
Tél: 819-966-6590 *Téléc:* 819-966-6572

Note: Centre local de services communautaires.

GATINEAU: CLSC de Gatineau - Point de service LeGuerrier
Affiliée à: CISSS de l'Outaouais
425, rue LeGuerrier, Gatineau, QC J9H 6N8
Tél: 819-966-6540 *Téléc:* 819-966-6541

GATINEAU: CLSC Vallée-de-la-Lièvre
Affiliée à: CISSS de l'Outaouais
578, rue Maclaren est, Gatineau, QC J8L 2W1
Tél: 819-986-3359 *Téléc:* 819-986-5671

GATINEAU: CSSS de Gatineau
Affiliée à: CISSS de l'Outaouais
777, boul de la Gappe, Gatineau, QC J8T 8R2
Tél: 819-966-6550 *Téléc:* 819-966-6565
www.csssgatineau.qc.ca
Média social: twitter.com/csssgatineau
Fondée en: 2004
Population desservi: 230000
Personnel: 5500
Note: Les Installations (Services de CH, CHSLD, et CLSC): Hôpital de
Gatineau (819-966-6100); Hôpital de Hull (819-966-6200); Hôpital de
jour gériatrique (819-664-2060); Hôpital Pierre-Janet (819-771-7761);
Centre d'hébergement - Foyer du Bonheur (819-966-6410); Centre
d'hébergement - La Pietà (819-966-6420); Centre d'hébergement - Bon
séjour (819-966-6450); Centre d'hébergement - Renaissance
(819-966-6440); CLSC de Gatineau - boul de la Gappe
(819-966-6550); CLSC de Gatineau - av Gatineau (819-966-6550);
CLSC de Gatineau - rue Saint-Rédempteur (819-966-6510); CLSC de
Gatineau - boul du Mont-Bleu (819-966-6530); CLSC de Gatineau -
boul Saint-Raymond (819-966-6525); CLSC de Gatineau - rue
LeGuerrier (819-966-6540); CLSC de Gatineau - Maison Bruyère
(819-966-6540); CLSC de Gatineau - boul Alexandre-Taché
(819-966-6580); Unité de médecine familiale (819-966-6380); Maison
de naissance de l'Outaouais (819-966-6585); Pavillon Marcel D'amour
(819-776-8093); Résidence de Hull (819-770-2992); Équipe de
réadaptation (819-772-9777, poste 7221); Résidence Corbeil
(819-777-2042); Résidence de Gatineau (819-568-3349)

GATINEAU: CSSS de Papineau
Affiliée à: CISSS de l'Outaouais
578, rue MacLaren Est, Gatineau, QC J8L 2W1
Tél: 819-986-3359
csss_papineau@ssss.gouv.qc.ca
www.cssspapineau.qc.ca

Note: Les Installations (Services de CH, CHSLD, et CLSC): Hôpital de Papineau (819-986-3341); Centre d'hébergement Vallée-de-la-Lièvre (819-986-4115); CLSC et Centre d'hébergement Petite-Nation (819-983-7341); CLSC Vallée-de-la-Lièvre (rue Maclaren est, Gatineau; av Buckingham, Gatineau; Val-des-Bois)

GATINEAU: Hôpital de Gatineau
Affiliée à: CISSS de l'Outaouais
909, boul La Vérendrye ouest, Gatineau, QC J8P 7H2
Tél: 819-966-6100

GATINEAU: Hôpital de Hull
Affiliée à: CISSS de l'Outaouais
116, boul Lionel-Émond, Gatineau, QC J8Y 1W7
Tél: 819-966-6200

GATINEAU: Hôpital de Papineau
Affiliée à: CISSS de l'Outaouais
155, rue Maclaren est, Gatineau, QC J8L 0C2
Tél: 819-986-3341

Nombre de lits: 63 lits hospitaliers

GATINEAU: Hôpital Pierre-Janet
Affiliée à: CISSS de l'Outaouais
20, rue Pharand, Gatineau, QC J9A 1K7
Tél: 819-771-7761 Téléc: 819-771-2908
www.chpj.ca
Fondée en: 1965
Nombre de lits: 87 lits

GATINEAU: Pavillon du Parc inc.
Affiliée à: CISSS de l'Outaouais
124, rue Lois, Gatineau, QC J8Y 3R7
Tél: 819-770-1022 Téléc: 819-770-1023
www.pavillonduparc.qc.ca
Nombre de lits: 92 lits
Note: Centre de réadaptation
Jean Dansereau, Directeur général

GRANDE-VALLéE: CLSC de Grande-Vallée
Affiliée à: CISSS de la Gaspésie
CP 190, 71, rue St-François-Xavier ouest, Grande-Vallée, QC G0E 1K0
Tél: 418-393-2001

Note: CSSS Côte-de-Gaspé.

GREENFIELD PARK: Centre intégré de santé et de services sociaux de la Montérégie-Centre
3120, boul Taschereau, Greenfield Park, QC J4V 2H1
Tél: 450-466-5000 Téléc: 450-466-8887
www.santemc.quebec
Info Line: 811

Population desservi: 383000
Personnel: 8900
Richard Deschamps, Président-directeur général

GREENFIELD PARK: CSSS Champlain - Charles-Le Moyne (CSSSCCLM)
Affiliée à: CISSS de la Montérégie-Centre
3120, boul Taschereau, Greenfield Park, QC J4V 2H1
Tél: 450-466-5000
www.santemonteregie.qc.ca/champlain
Nombre de lits: 473 lits d'hospitalisation et 195 en hébergement
Population desservi: 210000
Personnel: 4700
Note: Les Installations (Services de CH, CHSLD, et CLSC): Hôpital Charles-Le Moyne (450-466-5000); Centre d'hébergement Champlain (450-672-3320); Centre d'hébergement Henriette-Céré (450-672-3320); CLSC Saint-Hubert (450-443-7400); CLSC Samuel-de-Champlain (450-445-4452); Centre Saint-Lambert (450-672-3320); Centre de recherche appliquée (450-466-5433); Centre de recherche clinique (450-466-5024); Centre de prêt d'équipements Panama

(450-462-5193); Centre externe de néphrologie Greenfield Park (450-466-5000, poste 3645); Centre externe de néphrologie Saint-Lambert (450-466-5000, poste 3646); Clinique externe de pédopsychiatrie (450-466-5000, poste 2414); Hôpital de jour pour adolescents (450-466-5000, poste 2008); Clinique externe de psychiatrie pour adultes (450-466-5620); Clinique externe de psychiatrie pour adultes (450-466-5453); Centre de jour, Clinique Labonté (450-466-5455); Maison Brodeur (450-448-4763); Suivi intensif dans la communauté (450-466-5605); Groupe de médecine familiale de l'Unité de médecine familiale Charles-Le Moyne (450-466-5630).
Le Territoire desservi: Arrondissements de Greenfield Park, du Vieux-Longueuil et de Saint-Hubert. Affilié à l'Université de Sherbrooke.

GREENFIELD PARK: Hôpital Charles LeMoyne
Affiliée à: CISSS de la Montérégie-Centre
3120, boul Taschereau, Greenfield Park, QC J4V 2H1
Tél: 450-466-5000

Note: L'Hôpital est le centre hospitalier régional et universitaire de la Montérégie; affilié à l'Université de Sherbrooke; soins et services de court durée en santé physique, santé mentale, réadaptation; recherche; enseignement universitaire.

GROSSE-ILE: CLSC de l'Est
Affiliée à: CISSS des Iles
773, ch Principal, Grosse-Ile, QC G4T 6B5
Tél: 418-985-2572 Téléc: 418-985-2862

HUNTINGDON: CLSC Huntingdon
Affiliée à: CISSS de la Montérégie-Ouest
10, rue King, Huntingdon, QC J0S 1H0
Tél: 450-829-2321 Téléc: 450-264-6801
www.santemonteregie.qc.ca/haut-saint-laurent

Spécialités: Services médicaux; Santé mentale adulte et jeunesse; Santé publique; Clinique de vaccination; Soutien à domicile

ILE D'ENTRÉE: CLSC de l'Ile d'Entrée
Affiliée à: CISSS des Iles
Ile d'Entrée, QC G4T 1Z1
Tél: 418-986-4299 Téléc: 418-986-4094

JOLIETTE: Centre d'hébergement de Saint-Eusèbe
Affiliée à: CISSS de Lanaudière
585, boul Manseau, Joliette, QC J6E 3E5
Tél: 450-759-1662
www.csssnl.qc.ca
Nombre de lits: 159 lits

JOLIETTE: Centre de réadaptation La Myriade
Affiliée à: CISSS de Lanaudière
339, boul Base-de-Roc, Joliette, QC J6E 5P3
Tél: 450-753-9600 Téléc: 450-753-1930
www.crlamyriade.qc.ca
Nombre de lits: 38 lits
Daniel Castonguay, Président-directeur général, CISSS de Lanaudière

JOLIETTE: Centre intégré de santé et de services sociaux de Lanaudière
260, rue Lavaltrie Sud, Joliette, QC J6E 5X7
Tél: 450-759-1157 Téléc: 450-756-1157
Ligne sans frais: 800-668-9229
santelanaudiere@ssss.gouv.qc.ca
www.santelanaudiere.qc.ca
Info Line: 811

Population desservi: 502846
Note: Centres de santé et de services sociaux (CSSS): CSSS du Sud de Lanaudière; CSSS du Nord de Lanaudière
Daniel Castonguay, Président-directeur général
Jacques Perreault, Président, Conseil d'administration

JOLIETTE: CSSS du Sud de Lanaudière
Affiliée à: CISSS de Lanaudière
Centre administratif, 260, rue Lavaltrie Sud, Joliette, QC J6E 5X7
Tél: 450-759-1157 Téléc: 450-756-0598
Ligne sans frais: 800-668-9229
www.csss.sudlanaudiere.ca

Note: Les Installations (Services de CH, CHSLD, et CLSC): Hôpital Pierre-Le Gardeur; CLSC Lamater; CLSC Meilleur; Centres d'hébergement; Centre de jour L'Escale; Hôpital de jour de psychiatrie de la MRC Les Moulins; Hôpital de jour de psychiatrie de la MRC de L'Assomption; Clinique externe de psychiatrie de Charlemagne; SIME (Suivi Intensif dans le Milieu en Équipe); Clinique externe de psychiatrie de L'Assomption

JONQUIÈRE: CLSC de Jonquière
Affiliée à: CIUSSS du Saguenay-Lac-St-Jean
3667, boul Harvey, Jonquière, QC G7X 3A9
Tél: 418-695-2572

JONQUIÈRE: CSSS de Jonquière
Affiliée à: CIUSSS du Saguenay-Lac-Saint-Jean
Centre administratif et hospitalier, CP 1200, 2230, rue de l'Hôpital, Jonquière, QC G7X 7X2
Tél: 418-695-7700
www.csssjonquiere.qc.ca
Nombre de lits: 294 lits d'hébergement; 5 lits d'hébergement temporaire; 70 lits d'hospitalisation; 15 lits en Unité de réadaptation fonctionnelle intensive
Personnel: 1500
Note: Les Installations (Services de CH, CHSLD, et CLSC): Centre administratif et hospitalier; CLSC Jonquière (St-Ambroise); Centre de réadaptation en déficience physique; Centre de réadaptation en dépendance; Centre d'hébergement Des Chênes; Centre d'hébergement Georges-Hébert; Centre d'hébergement Ste-Marie; Centre d'hébergement des Années d'Or

JONQUIÈRE: Hôpital de Jonquière
Affiliée à: CIUSSS du Saguenay-Lac-St-Jean
2230, rue de l'Hôpital, Jonquière, QC G7X 7X2
Tél: 418-695-7700 *Téléc:* 418-695-7729

KAHNAWAKE: Kateri Memorial Hospital Centre
Affiliated with: CISSS de la Montérégie-Ouest
Also Known As: Tehsakotitsén:tha
PO Box 10, Kahnawake, QC J0L 1B0
Tel: 450-638-3930 *Fax:* 450-638-4634
www.kmhc.ca
Number of Beds: 43 beds/lits
Note: Services include family medicine, home care, community health, infection prevention & control, nutrition services, occupational therapy, physiotherapy, speech therapy, & social services.
Susan Horne, Executive Director
Lynda Delisle, Director, Operations
Dr. Suzanne Jones, Director, Professional Services
Valerie Diabo, Director, Nursing

KAWAWACHIKAMACH: CLSC Naskapi
Affiliée à: CISSS de la Côte-Nord
CP 5154, Kawawachikamach, QC G0G 2Z0
Tél: 418-585-2897 *Téléc:* 418-585-3126
Région desservi: La communauté autochtone de Kawawachikamach

KIPAWA: Kebaowek Health Centre
Ancien nom: Health Centre of Eagle Village
3 Omiga St., Kipawa, QC J0Z 2H0
Tél: 819-627-9060 *Téléc:* 819-627-1885
www.kebaowek.ca

KUUJJUAQ: Centre de santé Tulattavik de l'Ungava
Affiliée à: Régie régionale de la santé et des services sociaux Nunavik
CP 149, Kuujjuaq, QC J0M 1C0
Tél: 819-964-2905
Nombre de lits: 15 lits hospitaliers; 10 lits de soins de longue durée
Note: Urgence; soins médicaux; soins infirmiers; maternité; radiologie; pharmacie; électrocardiographie; laboratoire; physiothérapie.

KUUJJUAQ: Centre de santé Tulattavik de l'Ungava
CP 149, Kuujjuaq, QC J0M 1C0
Tél: 819-964-2905
Nombre de lits: 23 lits

KUUJJUAQ: Régie régionale de la santé et des services sociaux Nunavik (RRSSSN)/Nunavik Regional Board of Health & Social Services
PO Box 900, Kuujjuaq, QC J0M 1C0
Tel: 819-964-2222 *Fax:* 819-964-2888
Toll-Free: 844-964-2244
info@sante-services-sociaux.ca
www.nrbhss.gouv.qc.ca
Social Media: www.facebook.com/perspectivenunavik;
twitter.com/PNunavik; vimeo.com/user21609307;
www.linkedin.com/company/3480026
Number of Beds: 50 lits; 12 lits (personnes en perte d'autonomie); 14 lits (direction régionale de la réadaptation)
Area Served: Nunavik; 14 communautés; sous-régions: Hudson et Ungava
Number of Employees: 65

LA BAIE: CSSS Cléophas-Claveau
Affiliée à: CIUSSS du Saguenay-Lac-Saint-Jean
Centre hospitalier, 1000, rue Docteur-Desgagné, La Baie, QC G7B 2Y6
Tél: 418-544-3381 *Téléc:* 418-544-0770
www.cssscleophasclaveau.qc.ca

Note: Les Installations (Services de CH, CHSLD, et CLSC): Centre hospitalier; Centre d'hébergement Bagotville; Centre d'hébergement St-Joseph; CLSC de La Baie; CLSC L'Anse-Saint-Jean

LA BAIE: Hôpital de La Baie
Affiliée à: CIUSSS du Saguenay-Lac-St-Jean
CP 38, 1000, rue Docteur-Desgagné, La Baie, QC G7B 3P9
Tél: 418-544-3381 *Téléc:* 416-544-0770

LA MALBAIE: CLSC de La Malbaie
Affiliée à: CIUSSS de la Capitale-Nationale
535, boul de Comporté, La Malbaie, QC G5A 1S8
Tél: 418-665-6413
www.ciusss-capitalenationale.gouv.qc.ca

LA MALBAIE: Hôpital de La Malbaie
Affiliée à: CIUSSS de la Capitale-Nationale
303, rue St-Étienne, La Malbaie, QC G5A 1T1
Tél: 418-665-1700

LA POCATIÈRE: L'Hôpital Notre-Dame-de-Fatima
Affiliée à: CISSS du Bas-St-Laurent
1201, 6e av Pilote, La Pocatière, QC G0R 1Z0
Tél: 418-856-7000 *Téléc:* 418-856-4737
Nombre de lits: 49 lits

LA SARRE: Centre hospitalier de La Sarre
Affiliée à: CISSS de l'Abitibi-Témiscamingue
679, 2e rue Est, La Sarre, QC J9Z 2X7
Tél: 819-333-2311

LA SARRE: CSSS des Aurores-Boréales (CSSSAB)
Affiliée à: CISSS de l'Abitibi-Témiscamingue
679, 2e rue Est, La Sarre, QC J9Z 2X7
Tél: 819-333-2311 *Téléc:* 819-333-4316
www.cisss-at.gouv.qc.ca

Population desservi: 21308
Note: Les Installations (Services de CH, CHSLD, et CLSC): Centre de soins de courte durée (Centre hospitalier et siège social, 819-333-2311); Centre d'hébergement de soins de longue durée de Macamic (819-782-4661); Centre d'hébergement de soins de longue durée de La Sarre (819-333-5525); Centre d'hébergement de soins de longue durée de Palmarolle (819-787-2612); CLSC (Beaucanton, Duparquet, Dupuy, Gallichan, La Sarre, Macamic, Normétal, Palmarolle, Taschereau)

LA TUQUE: CSSS du Haut-Saint-Maurice (CSSSHSM)
Affiliée à: CIUSSS de la Mauricie et du Centre-du-Québec
885, boul Ducharme, La Tuque, QC G9X 3C1
Tél: 819-523-4581
www.ciusssmcq.ca

Note: Le Territoire desservi: Les régions du Centre-du-Québec, de Lanaudière, des Laurentides, de l'Abitibi-Témiscamingue, de la Baie-James, de Québec et du Saguenay-Lac Saint-Jean

LASALLE: CLSC de LaSalle
Affiliée à: CIUSSS de l'Ouest-de-l'Ile-de-Montréal
8550, boul Newman, LaSalle, QC H8N 1Y5
                    Tél: 514-364-2572 *Téléc:* 514-364-6365
                    www.ciusss-ouestmtl.gouv.qc.ca

LASALLE: CSSS de Dorval-Lachine-LaSalle (CSSS DLL)
Affiliée à: CIUSSS de l'Ouest-de-l'Ile-de-Montréal
8585, Terrasse Champlain, LaSalle, QC H8P 1C1
                    Tél: 514-639-0660
                    www.csssdll.qc.ca

Personnel: 2000
Note: Les Installations (Services de CH, CHSLD, et CLSC): Hôpital de LaSalle / Longue durée de l'hôpital de LaSalle (514-362-8000); CLSC de LaSalle (514-364-2572); CLSC de Dorval-Lachine (514-639-0650); Centre d'hébergement de Dorval (514-631-9094); Centre d'hébergement de Lachine (514-634-7161); Centre d'hébergement de LaSalle (514-364-6700); Centre d'hébergement Nazaire-Piché (514-637-2326).
Le Territoire desservi: Les arrondissements montréalais de LaSalle et Lachine; La municipalité de Dorval

LASALLE: Hôpital de LaSalle
Affiliée à: CIUSSS de l'Ouest-de-l'Ile-de-Montréal
8585, Terrasse Champlain, LaSalle, QC H8P 1C1
                    Tél: 514-362-8000
                    www.ciusss-ouestmtl.gouv.qc.ca

LAC-MÉGANTIC: CSSS du Granit
Affiliée à: CIUSSS de l'Estrie
3569, rue Laval, Lac-Mégantic, QC G6B 1A5
                    Tél: 819-583-0330 *Téléc:* 819-583-5239
                    Ligne sans frais: 800-827-2572

Note: Les Installations (Services de CH, CHSLD, et CLSC): CHSLD - Centre de jour (Point de service Lac-Mégantic); CLSC-CHSLD - Centre de jour (Point de service Lambton); CLSC (Point de chute Saint-Ludger); CLSC (Point de chute Notre-Dame des Bois)

LACHINE: CLSC de Dorval-Lachine
Affiliée à: CIUSSS de l'Ouest-de-l'Ile-de-Montréal
1900, rue Notre-Dame, Lachine, QC H8S 2G2
                    Tél: 514-639-0650 *Téléc:* 514-639-0666
                    www.csssdll.qc.ca

Note: Services de santé; services sociaux curatifs et préventifs.

LAVAL: Centre intégré de santé et de services sociaux de Laval
Également connu sous le nom de: CISSS de Laval
1755, boul René-Laennec, Laval, QC H7M 3L9
                    Tél: 450-978-8608
            communications.cisssslaval@ssss.gouv.qc.ca
                    www.lavalensante.com
                    Info Line: 811
Média social: www.facebook.com/cissslaval; twitter.com/cissslaval; www.youtube.com/csssdelaval

Fondée en: 2015
Population desservi: 429430
Note: Centres de santé et de services sociaux (CSSS): CSSS de Laval
Caroline Barbir, Présidente-directrice générale
Yves Carignan, Président, Conseil d'administration

LAVAL: CLSC des Mille-Iles
Affiliée à: CISSS de Laval
4731, boul Levesque Est, Laval, QC H7C 1M9
                    Tél: 450-661-2572 *Téléc:* 450-661-6177

Note: Les autres points de service CLSC: Marigot (2 sites), Mille-Iles (304, boul Cartier ouest), Ruisseau-Papineau (2 sites), et Sainte-Rose.

LAVAL: CRDI Normand-Laramée
304, boul Cartier Ouest, Laval, QC H7N 2J2
                    Tél: 450-972-2099
                    crdinl@ssss.gouv.qc.ca
                    www.crdinl.qc.ca

Note: Le CRDI Normand-Laramée est membre actif du Consortium national de recherche sur l'intégration sociale.
Julie Vaillancourt, Directrice générale

Isabelle Portelance, Responsable, direction des services à la clientèle

LAVAL: CSSS de Laval
Affiliée à: CISSS de Laval
1515, boul Chomedey, Laval, QC H7V 3Y7
                    Tél: 450-978-8300
                    www.cssslaval.qc.ca
                Média social: www.youtube.com/csssdelaval

Fondée en: 2004
Nombre de lits: 751 lits d'hébergement longue durée; 512 lits d'hospitalisation courte durée; 489 lits au permis d'hospitalisation de courte durée
Note: Les Installations (Services de CH, CHSLD, et CLSC): Hôpital de la Cité-de-la-Santé, avec centre de prélèvements, UMF et CICL (450-668-1010); Centre ambulatoire (450-978-8300); Centre d'hébergement Fernand-Larocque (450-661-5440); Centre d'hébergement Idola-Saint-Jean (450-668-6750); Centre d'hébergement de La Pinière (450-661-3305); Centre d'hébergement Rose-de-Lima (450-622-6996); Centre d'hébergement de Sainte-Dorothée (450-689-0933); Centre intégré de services de première ligne de l'ouest de l'Ile (450-627-2530); CLSC du Marigot (450-668-1803); CLSC des Mille-Iles (450-661-2572, 450 972-6808); CLSC du Ruisseau-Papineau (450-687-5690); CLSC de Sainte-Rose (450-622-5110)

LAVAL: Hôpital de la Cité-de-la-Santé
Affiliée à: CISSS de Laval
1755, boul René-Laennec, Laval, QC H7M 3L9
                    Tél: 450-668-1010

LAVAL: Jewish Rehabilitation Hospital (JRH)/Hôpital juif de réadaptation
Affiliée à: CISSS de Laval
3205, Place Alton-Goldbloom, Laval, QC H7V 1R2
                    Tél: 450-688-9550
                    www.hjr-jrh.qc.ca

Fondée en: 1962
Nombre de lits: 132 lits
Personnel: 550

LES ILES-DE-LA-MADELEINE: Centre de réadapation en déficience physique des Iles-de-la-Madeleine
Affiliée à: CISSS de la Gaspésie
695, ch des Caps, Les Iles-de-la-Madeleine, QC G4T 2S9
                    Tél: 418-986-4870 *Téléc:* 418-986-2623
                    www.cisss-gaspesie.gouv.qc.ca

Note: Déficience physique.

LÉVIS: Centre de réadaptation en déficience intellectuelle de Chaudière-Appalaches
Affiliée à: CISSS de Chaudière-Appalaches
55, rue du Mont-Marie, Lévis, QC G6V 0B8
                    Tél: 418-833-3218 *Téléc:* 418-833-9849
                    Ligne sans frais: 866-333-3218
                    www.cisss-ca.gouv.qc.ca
Nombre de lits: 674 lits

LÉVIS: Centre de réadaptation en déficience physique de Charny
Affiliée à: CISSS de Chaudière-Appalaches
9500, boul. du Centre-Hospitalier, Lévis, QC G6X 0A1
                    Tél: 418-380-2064 *Téléc:* 418-380-2096
                    www.cisss-ca.gouv.qc.ca
Nombre de lits: 48 lits
Note: Programmes: Déficience auditive, Déficience du langage, Déficience motrice (enfant, adulte), Clinique de sclérose en plaques, Programme d'évaluation & de réadaptation en conduite automobile, Neurotraumatisme, Dépistage du traumatisme craniocérébral léger, Programme intensif de gestion autonome de la douleur, et Programme de suppléance à la communication.

LÉVIS: Hôtel-Dieu de Lévis
Affiliée à: CISSS de Chaudière-Appalache
143, rue Wolfe, Lévis, QC G6V 3Z1
                    Tél: 418-835-7121 *Ligne sans frais:* 888-835-7105

Note: Associé à l'Université Laval.

LONGUEUIL: Centre de réadaptation en déficience intellectuelle Montérégie-est (CRDITED)
1255, rue Beauregard, Longueuil, QC J4K 2M3
Tél: 450-679-6511 *Téléc:* 450-928-3315
www.crditedme.ca

Nombre de lits: 1157 lits
Yves Masse, Président-directeur général

LONGUEUIL: CLSC de Longueuil-Ouest
Affiliée à: CISSS de la Montérégie-Est
201, boul Curé-Poirier Ouest, Longueuil, QC J4J 2G4
Tél: 450-651-9830 *Téléc:* 450-651-4606
www.santemonteregie.qc.ca

LONGUEUIL: CLSC Simonne-Monet-Chartrand
Affiliée à: CISSS de la Montérégie-Est
1303, boul Jacques-Cartier est, Longueuil, QC J4M 2Y8
Tél: 450-463-2850 *Téléc:* 450-646-7552
www.santemonteregie.qc.ca

LONGUEUIL: CSSS Pierre-Boucher
Affiliée à: CISSS de la Montérégie-Est
1333, boul Jacques-Cartier Est, Longueuil, QC J4M 2A5
Tél: 450-468-8111
www.santemonteregie.qc.ca/cssspierreboucher

Fondée en: 2004
Population desservi: 250000
Personnel: 4400
Note: Les Installations (Services de CH, CHSLD, et CLSC): Hôpital Pierre-Boucher (450-468-8111); Centre d'hébergement de Contrecoeur (450-468-8410); Centre d'hébergement de Lajemmerais (450-463-2995); Centre d'hébergement de Mgr-Coderre (450-448-3111); Centre d'hébergement du Chevalier-De Lévis (450-670-5110); Centre d'hébergement du Manoir-Trinité (450-674-4948); Centre d'hébergement Jeanne-Crevier (450-641-0590); Centre d'hébergement René-Lévesque (450-651-2210); CLSC de Longueuil-Ouest (450-651-9830); CLSC des Seigneuries de Boucherville (450-655-3630; CLSC des Seigneuries de Contrecoeur (450-468-8413; CLSC des Seigneuries de Saint-Amable (450-468-5250); CLSC des Seigneuries de Sainte-Julie (450-468-3670); CLSC des Seigneuries de Varennes (450-677-2917); CLSC des Seigneuries de Verchères (450-448-3700); CLSC Simonne-Monet-Chartrand (450-463-2850); Centre d'accueil Saint-Laurent inc. (450-670-5480).
Le Territoire desservi: Arrondissement du Vieux-Longueuil, Boucherville, Calixa-Lavallée, Contrecoeur, Saint-Amable, Sainte-Julie, Varennes et Verchères

LONGUEUIL: Hôpital Pierre-Boucher
Affiliée à: CISSS de la Montérégie-Est
1333, boul Jacques-Cartier Est, Longueuil, QC J4M 2A5
Tél: 450-468-8111

Note: Services comprennent: urgence; soins intensifs; soins palliatifs; services médicaux; chirurgie; psychiatrie.

LOW: CLSC de Low
Affiliée à: CISSS de l'Outaouais
CP 130, 334, rte 105, Low, QC J0X 2C0
Tél: 819-422-3548 *Téléc:* 819-422-3568

MAGOG: CSSS de Memphrémagog
Affiliée à: CIUSSS de l'Estrie
50, rue Saint-Patrice Est, Magog, QC J1X 3X3
Tél: 819-843-2572 *Ligne sans frais:* 800-268-2572
www.santeestrie.qc.ca

Note: Les Installations (Services de CH, CHSLD, et CLSC): Hôpital de Memphrémagog; Point de service de Mansonville (450-292-3376); Point de service de Stanstead (819-876-7521)

MANIWAKI: CSSS de la Vallée-de-la-Gatineau (CSSSVG)
Affiliée à: CISSS de l'Outaouais
309, boul Desjardins, Maniwaki, QC J9E 2E7
Tél: 819-449-4690 *Téléc:* 819-449-7330
www.csssvg.qc.ca

Population desservi: 20000
Note: Les Installations (Services de CH, CHSLD, et CLSC): L'hôpital de Maniwaki; Le Foyer Père Guinard de Maniwaki; Le Foyer d'accueil de Gracefield; Les CLSC de Low, Gracefield, et Maniwaki
Natalie Jobin, Direction santé physique
nathaliejobin@ssss.gouv.qc.ca

MANIWAKI: Hôpital de Maniwaki
Affiliée à: CISSS de l'Outaouais
309, boul Desjardins, Maniwaki, QC J9E 2E7
Tél: 819-449-4690

Fondée en: 1998
Nombre de lits: 36 lits de courte durée; 4 lits soins intermédiaires

MANSFIELD-ET-PONTEFRACT: CSSS du Pontiac
Affiliée à: CISSS de l'Outaouais
CP 430, 160, ch de la Chute, Mansfield-et-Pontefract, QC J0X 1R0
Tél: 819-683-3000 *Téléc:* 819-683-3682
Ligne sans frais: 800-567-9625
www.santepontiac.qc.ca
Média social: www.facebook.com/213024748134

Fondée en: 1996
Population desservi: 20000
Note: Les Installations (Services de CH, CHSLD, et CLSC): Centre Hospitalier du Pontiac; Pavillon Centre d'accueil Pontiac; Pavillon Manoir Sacré Cour; CLSC Bryson; CLSC Chapeau; CLSC de Mansfield-et-Pontefract, Fort-Coulonge; CLSC Otter-Lake; CLSC Quyon; CLSC Rapides-des-Joachims
Jean-Guy Patenaude, Président, Conseil d'administration
Richard Grimard, Directeur général

MARIA: CSSS de la Baie-des-Chaleurs (CSSSBC)
Affiliée à: CISSS de la Gaspésie
Centre administratif, 419, boul Perron, Maria, QC G0C 1Y0
Tél: 418-759-3443 *Téléc:* 418-759-5063
www.cisss-gaspesie.gouv.qc.ca

Fondée en: 2004
Nombre de lits: 77 lits
Région desservi: MRC d'Avignon; MRC de Bonaventure
Population desservi: 32591
Personnel: 1100
Note: Les Installations (Services de CH, CHSLD, et CLSC): Hôpital de Maria (418-759-3443); Centre d'hébergement de Maria (418-759-3458); Centre d'hébergement de Matapédia (418-865-2221); Centre d'hébergement de New Carlisle (418-752-3386); CLSC Malauze de Matapédia (418-865-2221); CLSC de Pointe-à-la-Croix (418-788-5454); CLSC de Saint-Omer (418-364-7064); CLSC de Caplan (418-388-2572); CLSC de Paspébiac (418-752-2572); Unité de médecine familiale Baie-des-Chaleurs (418-759-1336, poste 2811).
Médecins: 67

MARIA: Hôpital de Maria
Affiliée à: CISSS de la Gaspésie
419, boul Perron, Maria, QC G0C 1Y0
Tél: 418-759-3443
www.cisss-gaspesie.gouv.qc.ca

Nombre de lits: 77 lits
Note: Unité de médecine familiale: 418-759-1336.
Chantal Duguay, Présidente-directrice générale, CISSS de la Gaspésie

MARSOUI: CLSC de Marsoui
Affiliée à: CISSS de la Gaspésie
CP 415, 8, rte Principale Est, Marsoui, QC G0E 1S0
Tél: 418-288-5511 *Téléc:* 418-288-2572
www.cisss-gaspesie.gouv.qc.ca

MASHAM: CLSC des Collines
Affiliée à: Centre de santé et de services sociaux des Collines
9, ch Passe-Partout, Masham, QC J0X 2W0
Tél: 819-459-1112 *Téléc:* 819-456-4531
Ligne sans frais: 877-459-1112
www.santedescollines.qc.ca

Nombre de lits: Centre d'hébergement La Pêche: 32 lits.
Note: Y compris le Centre d'hébergement La Pêche et le CLSC Masham.
André Désilets, Directeur général

MATANE: CSSS de Matane
Affiliée à: CISSS du Bas-St-Laurent
Centre Administratif, Hôpital de Matane, 333, rue Thibault, Matane,
QC G4W 2W5

Tél: 418-562-3135 *Téléc:* 418-562-9374
www.csssmatane.com

Population desservi: 22057
Note: Les Installations (Services de CH, CHSLD, et CLSC): Hôpital de Matane (45 lits); Centre d'hébergement de Matane (106 lits); CLSC de Matane (Les Méchins, Baie-des-Sables)

MATANE: Hôpital de Matane
Affiliée à: CISSS du Bas-St-Laurent
333, rue Thibault, Matane, QC G4W 2W5
Tél: 418-562-3135 *Téléc:* 418-562-9374

Population desservi: 21000

MATAPÉDIA : CLSC Malauze de Matapédia
Affiliée à: CISSS de la Gaspésie
CP 190, 14, boul Perron, Matapédia, QC G0J 1V0
Tél: 418-865-2221 *Téléc:* 418-865-2317

Note: Services sociaux; programme petite enfance; clinique de vaccination et dépistage; programme de santé mentale; services aux personnes handicapées; soutien à domicile; service dentaire. Le centre d'hébergement est situé au deuxième étage du CLSC.

MÉTABETCHOUAN-LAC-A-LA-CROIX: CLSC Secteur-Sud
Affiliée à: Centre de santé et de services sociaux de
Lac-Saint-Jean-Est
1895, rte 169, Métabetchouan-Lac-a-la-Croix, QC G8G 1B4
Tél: 418-669-2000
Nombre de lits: 168 lits

MONT-LAURIER: Hôpital de Mont-Laurier
Affiliée à: CISSS des Laurentides
2561, ch de la Lièvre sud, Mont-Laurier, QC J9L 3G3
Tél: 819-623-1234 *Téléc:* 819-440-4299

MONT-LOUIS: CLSC de Mont-Louis
Affiliée à: CISSS de la Gaspésie
CP 100, 19, 1e av Ouest, Mont-Louis, QC G0E 1T0
Tél: 418-797-2744 *Téléc:* 418-797-5173
www.cisss-gaspesie.gouv.qc.ca

MONTMAGNY: Hôpital de Montmagny
Affiliée à: CISSS de Chaudière-Appalaches
350, boul Taché Ouest, Montmagny, QC G5V 3R8
Tél: 418-248-0630

Nombre de lits: 101 lits
Note: Services: anesthésiologie; chirurgie; ergothérapie; gériatrie; gynécologie-obstétrique; hémodialyse; inhalothérapie; laboratoires; médecine d'urgence; nutrition; oncologie; orthopédie; oto-rhino-laryngologie et ophtalmologie; pédiatrie; pédopsychiatrie et psychiatrie; pharmacie; physiothérapie; radiologie

MONTRÉAL: Atelier le Fil d'Ariane inc.
#100, 4837, rue Boyer, Montréal, QC H2J 3E6
Tél: 514-842-5592 *Téléc:* 514-842-8343
atelier.bureau.ariane@ssss.gouv.qc.ca
www.atelierlefildariane.org
Média social: www.facebook.com/www.atelierlefildariane.org
Nombre de lits: 20 places
Note: Un atelier de travail pour des adultes ayant des limitations fonctionnelles sur le plan intellectuel; l'atelier favorise l'intégration sociale & communautaire & l'autonomie personnelle & professionnelle des artisans.
Gaétan Gagné, Directeur général

MONTRÉAL: Brassard Plasticien
Ancien nom: Centre métropolitain de Chirurgie Plastique Inc.
995, rue de Salaberry, Montréal, QC H3L 1L2
Tél: 514-288-2097 *Téléc:* 514-288-3547
www.drbrassard.com

Nombre de lits: 17 lits
Dr. Pierre Brassard, Directeur général

MONTRÉAL: Centre d'accueil le programme de Portage inc.
Également connu sous le nom de: Portage
885, square Richmond, Montréal, QC H3J 1V8
Tél: 514-939-0202
info@portage.ca
www.portage.ca
Média social: www.facebook.com/PortageCanada;
twitter.com/PortageCanada
Fondée en: 1970
Note: Portage operates drug addiction treatment centres in the Québec cities of Montréal, Québec, Beaconsfield, Prévost, & Saint-Malachie. Centres in Atlantic Canada, Ontario, & British Columbia assist adolescents.

MONTRÉAL: Centre de réadaptation Constance-Lethbridge
Affiliée à: CIUSSS du Centre-Ouest-de-l'Ile-de-Montréal
7005, boul de Maisonneuve Ouest, Montréal, QC H4B 1T3
Tél: 514-487-1770 *Ligne sans frais:* 866-487-1891
www.constance-lethbridge.qc.ca
Média social: www.facebook.com/ConstanceLethbridge

Note: Déficience motrice

MONTRÉAL: Centre de réadaptation en dépendance de Montréal -
Institut universitaire
Ancien nom: Centre Dollard-Cormier
950, rue de Louvain est, Montréal, QC H2M 2E8
Tél: 514-385-1232
www.ciusss-centresudmtl.gouv.qc.ca
Nombre de lits: 55 lits
M. Jacques Couillard, Directeur général

MONTRÉAL: Centre hospitalier de l'Université de Montréal
Affiliée à: CIUSSS du Centre-Sud-de-l'Ile-de-Montréal
3840, rue St-Urbain, Montréal, QC H2W 1T8
Tél: 514-890-8000
www.chumontreal.qc.ca
Média social: www.facebook.com/chum.montreal;
twitter.com/chumontreal; www.youtube.com/user/chumontreal
Nombre de lits: 1217 lits hospitaliers, 170 lits longue durée
Fabrice Brunet, Président-Directeur général

MONTRÉAL: Centre hospitalier de St. Mary
Affiliée à: CIUSSS de l'Ouest-de-l'Ile-de-Montréal
3830, av Lacombe, Montréal, QC H3T 1M5
Tél: 514-345-3511
www.smhc.qc.ca
Nombre de lits: 271 lits hospitaliers
Ralph Dadoun, Directeur général

MONTRÉAL: Centre hospitalier universitaire Sainte-Justine
Affiliée à: CIUSSS du Centre-Ouest-de-l'Ile-de-Montréal
3175, ch de la Côte-Sainte-Catherine, Montréal, QC H3T 1C5
Tél: 514-345-4931
www.chusj.org
Média social: www.facebook.com/ChuSteJustine;
twitter.com/ChuSteJustine
Nombre de lits: 55 lits
Fabrice Brunet, Président-directeur général

MONTRÉAL: Centre intégré universitaire de santé et de services
sociaux de l'Ouest-de-l'Ile-de-Montréal
Institut universitaire en santé mentale Douglas, 6875, boul Lasalle,
Pavillon Dobell, Montréal, QC H4H 1R3
Tél: 514-630-2123 *Téléc:* 514-888-4462
informations.comtl@ssss.gouv.qc.ca
www.ciusss-ouestmtl.gouv.qc.ca
Info Line: 811
Population desservi: 368740
Benoît Morin, Président-directeur général

MONTRÉAL: Centre intégré universitaire de santé et de services
sociaux du Centre-Ouest-de-l'Ile-de-Montréal
3755, ch de la Côte Sainte-Catherine, #B, Montréal, QC H3T 1E3
Tél: 514-340-8222
www.ciusss-centreouestmtl.gouv.qc.ca
Info Line: 811

Population desservi: 341700

Lawrence Rosenberg, Président-directeur général

MONTRÉAL: Centre intégré universitaire de santé et de services sociaux du Centre-Sud-de-l'Île-de-Montréal
6161, rue Laurendeau, Montréal, QC H4E 3X6
Tél: 514-362-1000 *Téléc:* 514-732-5107
www.ciusss-centresudmtl.gouv.qc.ca
Média social: www.facebook.com/ciusss_csmtl;
twitter.com/ciusss_csmtl;
www.linkedin.com/company/ciusss-centre-sud-de-l'île-de-montréal

Population desservi: 300000
Personnel: 15000
Sonia Bélanger, Présidente-directrice générale

MONTRÉAL: Centre intégré universitaire de santé et de services sociaux du Nord-de-l'Île-de-Montréal
555, boul Gouin ouest, Montréal, QC H4J 1C8
Tél: 514-336-6673
ciusss-nordmtl.gouv.qc.ca
Média social: www.facebook.com/CIUSSSnmtl

Population desservi: 411000
Pierre Gfeller, Président-directeur général

MONTRÉAL: Centre intégré universitaire de santé et de services sociaux de l'Est-de-l'île-de-Montréal
5415, boul de l'Assomption, Montréal, QC H1T 2M4
Tél: 514-251-4000
www.ciusss-estmtl.gouv.qc.ca
Nombre de lits: 1279 lits de courte durée; 2502 lits d'hébergement de longue durée
Population desservi: 527000
Yvan Gendron, Président-directeur général

MONTRÉAL: Centre Miriam
Affiliée à: CIUSSS du Centre-Ouest-de-l'Île-de-Montréal
8160, ch Royden, Montréal, QC H4P 2T2
Tél: 514-345-0210 *Téléc:* 514-345-8965
mircea.bruj.miriam@ssss.gouv.qc.ca
www.centremiriam.ca
Fondée en: 1960
Note: Soutient les personnes ayant une déficience intellectuelle.
Dr. Abraham Fuks, M.D., Président, Conseil d'administration
Daniel Amar, Directeur général

MONTRÉAL: Clinique communautaire de Pointe St-Charles
500, av Ash, Montréal, QC H3K 2R4
Tél: 514-937-9251 *Téléc:* 514-937-3492
ccpsc.qc.ca
Marie-Claude Rose, Présidente
Luc Leblanc, Coordonnateur général de la Clinique

MONTRÉAL: CLSC d'Ahuntsic
Affiliée à: CIUSSS du Nord-de-l'Île-de-Montréal
1165, boul Henri-Bourassa Est, Montréal, QC H2C 3K2
Tél: 514-384-2000
www.csssamn.ca

Spécialités: Prélèvements; Services sociaux courants; Réadaptation; Information sur les vaccins

MONTRÉAL: CLSC de Benny Farm
Affiliée à: CIUSSS du Centre-Ouest-de-l'Île-de-Montréal
6484, av Monkland, Montréal, QC H4B 1H3
Tél: 514-484-7878 *Téléc:* 514-485-6406
www.cssscavendish.qc.ca

Note: Les Services: Centre de prélèvements; Clinique d'hypertension artérielle du CSSS Cavendish (514-484-7878, poste 3098); Maladie pulmonaire obstructive chronique (514-484-7878); Centre d'abandon du tabagisme (514 484-7878, poste 3068); Clinique de la santé des femmes (514-484-7878, poste 3067)

MONTRÉAL: CLSC de Bordeaux-Cartierville
Affiliée à: CIUSSS du Nord-de-l'Île-de-Montréal
11822, av du Bois-de-Boulogne, Montréal, QC H3M 2X6
Tél: 514-331-2572
www.csssbcstl.qc.ca

MONTRÉAL: CLSC de Côte-des-Neiges
Affiliée à: CIUSSS du Centre-Ouest-de-l'Île-de-Montréal
5700, ch de la Côte-des-Neiges, Montréal, QC H3T 2A8
Tél: 514-731-8531 *Téléc:* 514-731-9600
www.csssdelamontagne.qc.ca

MONTRÉAL: CLSC de Hochelaga-Maisonneuve
Affiliée à: CIUSSS de l'Est-de-l'Île-de-Montréal
4201, rue Ontario Est, Montréal, QC H1V 1K2
Tél: 514-253-2181
www.cssslucilleteasdale.qc.ca

Spécialités: Les services de santé; Les services sociaux

MONTRÉAL: CLSC de Mercier-Est — Anjou
Affiliée à: CIUSSS de l'Est-de-l'Île-de-Montréal
9503, rue Sherbooke Est, Montréal, QC H1L 6P2
Tél: 514-356-2572
www.cssspointe.ca

Note: Les Services: Sevices de prélèvement; Services pour les futurs parents, nourrissons, enfant âgés de moins de 5 ans et leurs parents; Clinique des jeunes (jeunes âgés de 12 à 18 ans); Santé mentale; Radiologie

MONTRÉAL: CLSC de Montréal-Nord
Affiliée à: CIUSSS du Nord-de-l'Île-de-Montréal
11441, boul Lacordaire, Montréal, QC H1G 4J9
Tél: 514-384-2000
www.csssamn.ca

Spécialités: Clinique des adultes; Clinique des jeunes; Informations et counselling; Clinique d'avortement; Pose de dispositifs intra-utérins (DIU)

MONTRÉAL: CLSC de Parc Extension
Affiliée à: CIUSSS du Centre-Ouest-de-l'Île-de-Montréal
7085, rue Hutchison, Montréal, QC H3N 1Y9
Tél: 514-273-9591
www.csssdelamontagne.qc.ca

Spécialités: Soins infirmiers et médicaux; Services psychosociaux; Réadaptation; Aide domestique; Assistance personnelle

MONTRÉAL: CLSC de Rivière-des-Prairies
Affiliée à: CIUSSS de l'Est-de-l'Île-de-Montréal
8655, boul Perras, Montréal, QC H1E 4M7
Tél: 514-494-4924

Spécialités: Les services de santé; Les services sociaux

MONTRÉAL: CLSC de Rosemont
Affiliée à: CIUSSS de l'Est-de-l'Île-de-Montréal
Centre administratif, 2909, rue Rachel Est, Montréal, QC H1W 0A9
Tél: 514-524-3541
www.cssslucilleteasdale.qc.ca

Spécialités: Services de santé; Services psychosociaux; Services sociaux scolaires; Services de maintien à domicile; Service de santé dentaire

MONTRÉAL: CLSC de Saint-Henri
Affiliée à: CIUSSS du Centre-Sud-de-l'Île-de-Montréal
3833, rue Notre-Dame ouest, Montréal, QC H4C 1P8
Tél: 514-933-7541
www.sov.qc.ca

MONTRÉAL: CLSC de Saint-Michel
Affiliée à: CIUSSS de l'Est-de-l'Île-de-Montréal
3355, rue Jarry est, Montréal, QC H1Z 2E5
Tél: 514-722-3000
www.csss-stleonardstmichel.qc.ca

Spécialités: Clinique médicale; Prélèvements; Vaccination (514-374-8223); Soutien à domicile

MONTRÉAL: CLSC de Villeray
Affiliée à: CIUSSS du Nord-de-l'Île-de-Montréal
1425, rue Jarry est, Montréal, QC H2E 1A7
Tél: 514-376-4141
www.cssscoeurdelile.ca

Fondée en: 1985
Spécialités: Promotion de la santé; Intervention psychosociale; Services thérapeutiques; Vaccination des enfants; Support à l'allaitement; Soutien à domicile

MONTRÉAL: CLSC des Faubourgs - Visitation
Affiliée à: CIUSSS du Centre-Sud-de-l'Ile-de-Montréal
1705, rue de la Visitation, Montréal, QC H2L 3C3
Tél: 514-527-2361 *Téléc:* 514-598-7754
www.ciusss-centresudmtl.gouv.qc.ca

MONTRÉAL: CLSC du Plateau Mont-Royal
Affiliée à: CIUSSS du Centre-Sud-de-l'Ile-de-Montréal
4625, av de Lorimier, Montréal, QC H2H 2B4
Tél: 514-521-7663
www.csssjeannemance.ca

Spécialités: Services psychosociaux; Services médicaux courants; Service en nutrition; Service d'échange de seringues pour personnes toxicomanes; Réadaptation

MONTRÉAL: CLSC Métro
Affiliée à: CIUSSS du Centre-Ouest-de-l'ile-de-Montréal
1801, boul de Maisonneuve Ouest, Montréal, QC H3H 1J9
Tél: 514-934-0354
www.csssdelamontagne.qc.ca

Spécialités: Clinique médicale; Services sociaux; Programmes de santé pour les écoles et les garderies; Thérapie familiale et de couple

MONTRÉAL: CLSC Olivier-Guimond
Affiliée à: CIUSSS de l'Est-de-l'Ile-de-Montréal
5810, rue Sherbrooke Est, Montréal, QC H1N 1B2
Tél: 514-255-2365
www.cssslucilleteasdale.qc.ca

Spécialités: Maladies infectieuses; Santé mentale; Violence conjugale et familiale; Santé dentaire; Nutrition; Réadaptation

MONTRÉAL: CLSC Pointe-aux-Trembles - Montréal-Est
Affiliée à: CIUSSS de l'Est-de-l'Ile-de-Montréal
13926, rue Notre-Dame est, Montréal, QC H1A 1T5
Tél: 514-642-4050
www.cssspointe.ca

Spécialités: Services sociaux; Réadaptation; Aide domestique; Vaccination

MONTRÉAL: CLSC Saint-Louis-du-Parc
Affiliée à: CIUSSS du Centre-Sud-de-l'Ile-de-Montréal
#100, 15, av du Mont-Royal Ouest, Montréal, QC H2T 2R9
Tél: 514-286-9657 *Téléc:* 514-286-9706
www.ciusss-centresudmtl.gouv.qc.ca

MONTRÉAL: La Corporation du centre de réadaptation Lucie-Bruneau
Affiliée à: CIUSSS du Centre-Sud-de-l'Ile-de-Montréal
2275, av Laurier est, Montréal, QC H2H 2N8
Tél: 514-527-4527 *Téléc:* 514-527-0979
www.ciusss-centresudmtl.gouv.qc.ca

Nombre de lits: 50 lits
Note: Centre de réadaptation (déficience motrice)
Pierre Paul Milette, Directeur général adjoint santé physique générale, CIUSSS du Centre-Sud-de-l'Ile-de-Montréal

MONTRÉAL: CSSS Cavendish
Affiliée à: CIUSSS du Centre-Ouest-de-l'Ile-de-Montréal
Centre administratif, 5425, av Bessborough, Montréal, QC H4V 2S7
Tél: 514-484-7878 *Téléc:* 514-483-4596
www.cssscavendish.qc.ca

Fondée en: 2004
Population desservi: 121900
Personnel: 1400
Note: Les Installations (Services de CH, CHSLD, et CLSC): Hôpital Richardson (514-484-7878); CLSC René-Cassin (514-484-7878); CLSC de Notre-Dame-de-Grâce - Montréal-Ouest (514-484-7878); Centre d'hébergement Henri-Bradet (514-484-7878); Centre d'hébergement St-Andrew (514-932-3630); Centre d'hébergement Father-Dowd (514-932-3630); Centre d'hébergement St-Margaret (514-932-3630)

MONTRÉAL: CSSS d'Ahuntsic et Montréal-Nord (CSSSAM-N)
Affiliée à: CIUSSS du Nord-de-l'Ile-de-Montréal
1725, boul Gouin est, Montréal, QC H2C 3H6
Tél: 514-384-2000
www.csssamn.ca

Population desservi: 170000
Note: Les Installations (Services de CH, CHSLD, et CLSC): Hôpital Fleury; Centre d'hébergement de Louvain; Centre d'hébergement Laurendeau; Centre d'hébergement Légaré; Centre d'hébergement Paul-Lizotte; CLSC d'Ahuntsic; CLSC de Montréal-Nord

MONTRÉAL: CSSS de l'Ouest-de-l'Ile
Affiliée à: CIUSSS de l'Ouest-de-l'Ile-de-Montréal
160, av Stillview, Montréal, QC H9R 2Y2
Tél: 514-630-2225
www.csssouestdelile.qc.ca

Nombre de lits: 227 lits d'hospitalisation de courte durée; 155 lits d'hébergement de longue durée
Population desservi: 220000
Personnel: 2125
Note: Les Installations (Services de CH, CHSLD, et CLSC): Hôpital général du Lakeshore (514-630-2225); CLSC de Pierrefonds (514-626-2572); CLSC du Lac-Saint-Louis (514-697-4110); Centre d'hébergement Denis-Benjamin-Viger (514-620-6310).
Le Territoire desservi: Les arrondissments de de Pierrefonds-Roxboro et de L'Ile-Bizard-Sainte-Geneviève; Les villes de Baie d'Urfé, Beaconsfield, Dollard-des-Ormeaux, Kirkland, Pointe-Claire, Sainte-Anne-de-Bellevue, et Senneville

MONTRÉAL: CSSS de la Montagne
Affiliée à: CIUSSS du Centre-Ouest-de-l'Ile-de-Montréal
1980, rue Sherbrooke Ouest, Montréal, QC H3H 1E8
Tél: 514-731-8531
www.csssdelamontagne.qc.ca
Média social: www.facebook.com/CSSSdelaMontagne

Note: Les Installations (Services de CH, CHSLD, et CLSC): CLSC de Côte-des-Neiges, Montréal (514-731-8531); CLSC de Côte-des-Neiges, Point de service Outremont; CLSC Métro (514-934-0354); CLSC de Parc-Extension (514-273-9591); Maison de naissance Côte-des-Neiges (514-736-2323); Programme régional d'accueil et d'intégration des demandeurs d'asile (PRAIDA).
Le Territoire desservi: Le quartier Côte-des-Neiges de l'arrondissement Côte-des-Neiges / Notre-Dame-de-Grâce; L'arrondissement Outremont; Le quartier Parc-Extension de l'arrondissement Villeray-Saint-Michel-Parc-Extension; Le district Peter-McGill de l'arrondissement Ville-Marie; Une partie de l'arrondissement Plateau Mont-Royal; Les villes de Mont-Royal et Westmount
Denis Sirois, Président, Conseil d'administration
Marc Sougavinski, Directeur général

MONTRÉAL: CSSS de la Pointe-de-l'Ile
Affiliée à: CIUSSS de l'Est-de-l'Ile-de-Montréal
9503, rue Sherbrooke Est, Montréal, QC H1L 6P2
Tél: 514-356-2572
www.cssspointe.ca

Population desservi: 191980
Note: Les Installations (Services de CH, CHSLD, et CLSC): Centre d'hébergement Biermans (514-351-9891); Centre d'hébergement François-Séguenot (514-642-4050); Centre d'hébergement Judith-Jasmin (514-354-5990); Centre d'hébergement Pierre-Joseph-Triest (514-353-1227); CLSC de Mercier-Est-Anjou (514-356-2572); CLSC de Pointe-aux-Trembles-Montréal-Est (514-642-4050); CLSC de Rivière-des-Prairies (514-494-4924); Manoir Claudette Barré (514-351-0200); Ressource intermédiaire Claudette Barré (514-351-0200); Ressource intermédiaire Limoges (514-852-3898)

MONTRÉAL: Hôpital Catherine Booth de l'Armée du Salut
Affiliée à: CIUSSS du Centre-Ouest-de-l'Ile-de-Montréal
4375, av Montclair, Montréal, QC H4B 2J5
Tél: 514-484-7878

Note: Réadaptation

MONTRÉAL: Hôpital de réadaptation Lindsay
6363, ch Hudson, Montréal, QC H3S 1M9

Tél: 514-737-3661
www.irglm.qc.ca

Fondée en: 1914
Note: Hôpital spécialisé de courte-durée

MONTRÉAL: Hôpital de réadaptation Villa Medica
225, rue Sherbrooke est, Montréal, QC H2X 1C9

Tél: 514-288-8201
info@villamedica.ca
www.villamedica.ca

Nombre de lits: 150 lits
Note: Centre hospitalier de réadaptation
Anne Beauchamp, Directrice générale

MONTRÉAL: Hôpital de Verdun
Affiliée à: CIUSSS du Centre-Sud-de-l'Ile-de-Montréal
4000, boul LaSalle, Montréal, QC H4G 2A3

Tél: 514-362-1000
www.ciusss-centresudmtl.gouv.qc.ca

MONTRÉAL: Hôpital du Sacré-Coeur de Montréal
Affiliée à: CIUSSS du Nord-de-l'Ile-de-Montréal
5400, boul Gouin ouest, Montréal, QC H4J 1C5

Tél: 514-338-2222
www.hscm.ca

Nombre de lits: 554 lits hospitaliers
Note: outpatient services & trauma centre

MONTRÉAL: Hôpital Fleury
Affiliée à: CIUSSS du Nord-de-l'Ile-de-Montréal
2180, rue Fleury Est, Montréal, QC H2B 1K3

Tél: 514-384-2000
ciusss-nordmtl.gouv.qc.ca

Nombre de lits: 174 lits
Région desservi: Le territoire d'Ahuntsic et de Montréal-Nord, QC
Spécialités: Prélèvements; Urgence psychiatrique

MONTRÉAL: Hôpital général de Montréal
1650, av Cedar, Montréal, QC H3G 1A4

Tél: 514-934-1934
www.muhc.ca

Fondée en: 1821
Nombre de lits: 533 beds
Normand Rinfret, Directeur général, MUHC

MONTRÉAL: Hôpital général juif Sir Mortimer B. Davis
Affiliée à: CIUSSS du Centre-Ouest-de-l'Ile-de-Montréal
3755, ch Côte Ste-Catherine, Montréal, QC H3T 1E2

Tél: 514-340-8222 *Téléc:* 514-340-7510
jgh.ca

Nombre de lits: 637 lits hospitaliers
Personnel: 4869
Lawrence Rosenberg, Président-directeur général
Georges Bendavid, Directeur, Services techniques par intérim

MONTRÉAL: Hôpital Jean-Talon
Affiliée à: CIUSSS du Nord-de-l'Ile-de-Montréal
1385, rue Jean-Talon Est, Montréal, QC H2E 1S6

Tél: 514-495-6767
www.cssscoeurdelile.ca

MONTRÉAL: Hôpital Maisonneuve-Rosemont
Affiliée à: CIUSSS de l'Est-de-l'Ile-de-Montréal
5415, boul de l'Assomption, Montréal, QC H1T 2M4

Tél: 514-252-3400
www.maisonneuve-rosemont.org
Média social: www.facebook.com/351488907544;
www.youtube.com/user/HMRmontreal

MONTRÉAL: Hôpital Marie-Clarac
3530, boul Gouin est, Montréal, QC H1H 1B7

Tél: 514-321-8800 *Téléc:* 514-321-9626
ressourceshumaines.macl@ssss.gouv.qc.ca
www.hopitalmarie-clarac.qc.ca

Nombre de lits: 204 lits
Sr. Pierre-Anne Mandato, Directrice générale

MONTRÉAL: Hôpital Mont-Sinai
Affiliée à: CIUSSS du Centre-Ouest-de-l'Ile-de-Montréal
5690, boul Cavendish, Montréal, QC H4W 1S7

Tél: 514-369-2222 *Téléc:* 514-369-2225
www.sinaimontreal.ca

Fondée en: 1909
Nombre de lits: 107 lits
Note: Services comprennent: soins respiratoires; soins palliatifs; soins long-terme; services de soutien. Affilié avec McGill University
Barbara Gold, Responsable

MONTRÉAL: Hôpital Richardson
Affiliée à: CIUSSS du Centre-Ouest-de-l'Ile-de-Montréal
5425, rue Bessborough, Montréal, QC H4V 2S7

Tél: 514-484-7878 *Téléc:* 514-483-4596
www.cssscavendish.qc.ca

Anna Maria Malorni, Personne ressource
514-484-7878, annamaria.malorni.cvd@ssss.gouv.qc.c

MONTRÉAL: Hôpital Santa Cabrini
Affiliée à: CIUSSS de l'Est-de-l'Ile-de-Montréal
5655, rue St-Zotique est, Montréal, QC H1T 1P7

Tél: 514-252-6000
www.santacabrini.qc.ca

Nombre de lits: 472 lits hospitaliers
Jean-Fançois Foisy, Directeur général

MONTRÉAL: Institut de réadaptation
Gingras-Lindsay-de-Montréal
Affiliée à: CIUSSS du Centre-Sud-de-l'Ile-de-Montréal
Ancien nom: Institut de réadaptation de Montréal
6300, av Darlington, Montréal, QC H3S 2J4

Tél: 514-340-2085 *Téléc:* 514-340-2091
www.irglm.qc.ca
Média social: www.youtube.com/user/IRGLM

Fondée en: 1949
Nombre de lits: 200 lits
Note: Centre de réadaptation
Dany Lavallée, Coordonnateur par intérim, Services des bénévoles

MONTRÉAL: Institut Philippe Pinel de Montréal
10905, boul Henri-Bourassa est, Montréal, QC H1C 1H1

Tél: 514-648-8461
www.pinel.qc.ca

Fondée en: 1927
Nombre de lits: 292 lits
Personnel: 700
Dre Renée Fugère, Preésidente-Directrice générale
Anne Côté, Directrice, Services techniques

MONTRÉAL: Institut universitaire en santé mentale Douglas
Ancien nom: Hôpital Douglas
6875, boul LaSalle, Montréal, QC H4H 1R3

Tél: 514-761-6131 *Téléc:* 514-761-6131
www.douglas.qc.ca
Média social: www.facebook.com/institutdouglas;
twitter.com/institutdouglas; www.youtube.com/douglasinstitute

Nombre de lits: 266 lits
Note: Mental hospital affiliated with McGill University; also community services, outpatient services, housing, social rehabilitation, specialized services (eating disorders, alcoholism & drug abuse, schizophrenia, aging, dementia & Alzheimer dementia)
Lynne McVey, Directrice générale

MONTRÉAL: Maison Elisabeth
2131, av de Marlowe, Montréal, QC H4A 3L4

Tél: 514-482-2488 *Téléc:* 514-482-9467
info@maisonelizabeth.ca
www.maisonelizabethhouse.com

Nombre de lits: 18 lits
Linda Schachtler, Directrice générale

MONTRÉAL: Santé au travail
6600, Côte-des-neiges, Montréal, QC H3S 2A9

Tél: 514-858-2460 *Téléc:* 514-858-6568

MONTRÉAL-NORD: Château Beaurivage
Affiliée à: Résidences Azur
6880, boul Gouin Est, Montréal-Nord, QC H1G 6L8
Tél: 514-323-7222 *Téléc:* 514-328-8987
chateaubeaurivage@residencesazur.com
www.residencesazur.com/39-residence-chateau-beaurivage.html
Média social: www.facebook.com/792621820777770

Julie Dagenais, Directrice générale

MURDOCHVILLE: CLSC de Murdochville
Affiliée à: CISSS de la Gaspésie
600, rue William-May, Murdochville, QC G0E 1W0
Tél: 418-784-2572 *Téléc:* 418-784-3629

Note: CSSS Côte-de-Gaspé.

NICOLET: CSSS de Bécancour-Nicolet-Yamaska (CSSSBNY)
Affiliée à: CIUSSS de la Mauricie et du Centre-du-Québec
Centre administratif, Centre Christ-Roi, 675, rue St-Jean-Baptiste, Nicolet, QC J3T 1S4
Tél: 819-293-2071 *Téléc:* 819-293-6160
Ligne sans frais: 800-263-2572
www.ciusssmcq.ca
Info Line: 811

Population desservi: 44000
Personnel: 1000
Note: Les Installations (Services de CH, CHSLD, et CLSC): Centre Christ-Roi (819-293-2071); Centre Filles de la Sagesse (819-293-8337); Centre Fortierville (819-287-4442); Centre d'hébergement Deschaillons (819-292-2262); Centre d'hébergement Fortierville (819-287-4686); Centre d'hébergement Lucien-Shooner (450-568-2712); Centre d'hébergement Romain-Becquet (819-263-2245); Centre d'hébergement Saint-Célestin (819-229-3617); Point de service Gentilly (819-298-2144); Point de service Saint-Grégoire (819-233-2719); Point de service Saint-Léonard-d'Aston (819-399-3666)

NOTRE-DAME-DU-LAC: CSSS de Témiscouata
Affiliée à: CISSS du Bas-St-Laurent
58, rue de l'Église, Notre-Dame-du-Lac, QC G0L 1X0
Tél: 418-899-6751
www.cisss-bsl.gouv.qc.ca

Note: Les Installations (Services de CH, CHSLD, et CLSC): Hôpital de Notre-Dame-du-Lac; CLSC de Cabano; CLSC de Dégelis; CLSC de Lac-des-Aigles; CLSC de Pohénégamook; Clinique médicale de Squatec; Centre d'hébergement Squatec; Centre d'hébergement St-Louis; Centre d'hébergement Rivière-Bleue; La Maison du Lac; La Villa Saint-Louis; Résidence Dégelico; Les Habitations Jules Edouard; R.I. Véronique Lavoie; Le Manoir de l'Érable Argenté

NOTRE-DAME-DU-LAC: Hôpital de Notre-Dame-du-Lac
Affiliée à: CISSS du Bas-St-Laurent
58, rue de l'Église, Notre-Dame-du-Lac, QC G0L 1X0
Tél: 418-899-6751 *Téléc:* 418-899-2809
Ligne sans frais: 855-899-2424
Nombre de lits: 35 lits

ORMSTOWN: CSSS du Haut-Saint-Laurent (CSSSHSL)
Affiliée à: CISSS de la Montérégie-Ouest
28, rue Gale, Ormstown, QC J0S 1K0
Tél: 450-829-2321
www.santemonteregie.qc.ca/haut-saint-laurent
Nombre de lits: 125 lits (longue durée); 49 lits (courte durée); 9 lits (hébergement temporaire)
Note: Les Installations (Services de CH, CHSLD, et CLSC): Hôpital Barrie Memorial (450-829-2321); Centre d'hébergement d'Ormstown (450-829-2321); Centre d'hébergement du comté de Huntingdon (450-829-2321); CLSC Huntingdon (450-829-2321); Point de service du CLSC Huntingdon (450-829-2321).
Le Territoire desservi: La MRC du Haut Saint-Laurent (Dundee, Elgin, Franklin, Godmanchester, Havelock, Hinchinbrooke, Howick, Huntingdon, Ormstown, Saint-Anicet, Saint-Chrysostome, Sainte-Barbe, Très-Saint-Sacrement)

ORMSTOWN: Hôpital Barrie Memorial
Affiliée à: CISSS de la Montérégie-Ouest
28, rue Gale, Ormstown, QC J0S 1K0
Tél: 450-829-2321 *Téléc:* 450-829-3582
www.santemonteregie.qc.ca/haut-saint-laurent
Fondée en: 2006
Note: Affilié à l'université McGill.

PASPÉBIAC: CLSC de Paspébiac
Affiliée à: CISSS de la Gaspésie
273, boul Gérard-D.-Lévesque, Paspébiac, QC G0C 2K0
Tél: 418-752-2572

PERCÉ: CLSC de Barachois
Affiliée à: CISSS de la Gaspésie
1070, rte 132 Est, Percé, QC G0C 1A0
Tél: 418-645-2572 *Téléc:* 418-645-2106

Note: CSSS Côte-de-Gaspé.

PERCÉ: CLSC de Percé
Affiliée à: CISSS de la Gaspésie
CP 269, 98, rte 132 ouest, Percé, QC G0C 2L0
Tél: 418-782-2572

Note: CSSS du Rocher-Percé.

PLESSISVILLE: CLSC-CHSLD de l'Érable
Affiliée à: CIUSSS de la Mauricie-et-du-Centre-du-Québec
1331, rue Saint-Calixte, Plessisville, QC G6L 1P4
Tél: 819-362-6301 *Téléc:* 819-362-6812
fondation_erable@ssss.gouv.qc.ca
www.cssssae.qc.ca
Nombre de lits: 40 lits de soins de longue durée
Note: CLSC de l'Érable, et l'Unité de soins longue durée de l'Érable.

POHÉNÉGAMOOK: CLSC de Pohénégamook
Affiliée à: CISSS du Bas-St-Laurent
1922, rue St-Vallier, Pohénégamook, QC G0L 1J0
Tél: 418-859-2450 *Téléc:* 418-859-1285

POINTE-CLAIRE: CLSC du Lac-Saint-Louis
Affiliée à: CIUSSS de l'Ouest-de-l'Île-de-Montréal
180, av Cartier, Pointe-Claire, QC H9S 4S1
Tél: 514-697-4110
www.csssouestdelile.qc.ca

Note: Les Services: Santé sexuelle (514-697-4110, poste 1313); Suivis post-natals (514-697-4110, poste 1346); Soutien à l'allaitement (514-697-4110, poste 1346); Suivi diététique (514-697-4110, poste 1346); Vaccination (514-697-4110); Suivis intensifs et continus pour la clientèle vulnérable (514-697-4110, poste 1346); Clinique des jeunes (514-697-4110, poste 1313); Services psychosociaux (514-697-4110, poste 1334); Santé dentaire (514-697-4110)

POINTE-CLAIRE: Hôpital général du Lakeshore
Affiliée à: CIUSSS de l'Ouest-de-l'Île-de-Montréal
160, av Stillview, Pointe-Claire, QC H9R 2Y2
Tél: 514-630-2225
www.ciusss-ouestmtl.gouv.qc.ca
Nombre de lits: 227 lits hospitaliers

POINTE-À-LA-CROIX: CLSC de Pointe-à-la-Croix
Affiliée à: CISSS de la Gaspésie
CP 389, 48, boul Interprovincial, Pointe-à-la-Croix, QC G0C 1L0
Tél: 418-788-5454 *Téléc:* 418-788-2510

PORT-DANIEL-GASCONS: CLSC Gascons
Affiliée à: CISSS de la Gaspésie
CP 28, 63, rte 132, Port-Daniel-Gascons, QC G0C 1P0
Tél: 418-396-2572 *Téléc:* 418-396-2367

Note: CSSS du Rocher-Percé.

PUVIRNITUQ: Centre de santé Inuulitsivik
Affiliated with: Régie régionale de la santé et des services sociaux Nunavik
ch Baie D'Hudson, Puvirnituq, QC J0M 1P0
Tel: 819-988-2957
recruitment.csi@ssss.gouv.qc.ca
www.inuulitsivik.ca

Number of Beds: 17 lits hospitaliers; 8 lits de soins de longue durée
Note: Soins médicaux, soins dentaires; sages-femmes; services en santé mentale; télémedicine; laboratoire; points de service: Akulivik, Inukjuak, Ivujivik, Kuujjuarapik, Puvirnituq, Salluit et Umiujuaq.
Jane Beaudoin, Directrice générale
  jane.beaudoin.csi@ssss.gouv.qc.ca

PUVIRNITUQ: Centre de santé Inuulitsivik
ch Baie d'Hudson, Puvirnituq, QC J0M 1P0

Tél: 819-988-2957
recrutement.csi@ssss.gouv.qc.ca
www.inuulitsivik.ca

Nombre de lits: 8 lits
Jane Beaudoin, Directrice générale

QUÉBEC: Centre d'hébergement Christ-Roi
Affiliée à: CIUSSS de la Capitale-Nationale
900, boul Wilfrid-Hamel, Québec, QC G1M 2R9

Tél: 418-682-1711

Nombre de lits: 142 lits
Note: Hébergement permanent/soins de longue durée, hôpital de jour, hébergement temporaire, consultations externes

QUÉBEC: Centre de réadaptation en déficience intellectuelle de Québec (CRDIQ)
Affiliée à: CIUSSS de la Capitale-Nationale
7843, rue des Santolines, Québec, QC G1G 0G3

Tél: 418-683-2511 *Téléc:* 418-683-9735
www.crdiq.qc.ca

Fondée en: 2001
Nombre de lits: 530 lits
Catherine Chagnon, Agente d'information, CIUSSS de la
  Capitale-Nationale

QUÉBEC: Centre de réadaptation Ubald-Villeneuve
2525, ch de la Canardière, Québec, QC G1J 2G3

Tél: 418-663-5008 *Téléc:* 418-663-6575
communication@cruv.qc.ca
www.cruv.qc.ca

Andrée Deschênes, Directrice générale

QUÉBEC: Centre hospitalier de l'Université Laval (CHUL)
Centre hospitalier universitaire de Québec
Affiliée à: CIUSSS de la Capitale-Nationale
2705, boul Laurier, Québec, QC G1V 4G2

Tél: 418-525-4444 *Téléc:* 418-654-2762
www.chudequebec.ca

Note: Affilié à l'Université Laval.
Gertrude Bourdon, Présidente-directrice générale

QUÉBEC: Centre hospitalier universitaire de Québec (CHUQ)
11, côte du Palais, Québec, QC G1R 2J6

Tél: 418-525-4444
www.chuq.qc.ca
Média social: www.facebook.com/chudequebec;
twitter.com/chudequebec; www.youtube.com/user/chudequebec;
linkedin.com/company/centre-hospitalier-universitaire-de-qu-bec

Personnel: 13500
Gertrude Bourdon, Présidente-Directrice générale

QUÉBEC: Centre intégré universitaire de santé et de services sociaux de la Capitale-Nationale
Également connu sous le nom de: CIUSSS de la Capitale-Nationale
2915, av du Bourg-Royal, Québec, QC G1C 3S2

Tél: 418-266-1019 *Téléc:* 418-661-2845
www.ciusss-capitalenationale.gouv.qc.ca
Info Line: 811
Média social: www.facebook.com/538181276359816;
twitter.com/CIUSSS_CN

Fondée en: 2015
Région desservi: Les territoires de Charlevoix et de Portneuf (69 municipalités)
Population desservi: 737787
Note: Le CIUSSS de la Capitale-Nationale est la fusion des Agence de la santé et des services sociaux de la Capitale-Nationale, Centre de réadaptation en déficience intellectuelle de Québec (CDRIQ), Centre de réadaptation en dépendance de Québec, CSSS de Charlevoix,

CSSS de la Vieille-Capitale, CSSS de Portneuf, CSSS de Québec-Nord, Centre jeunesse de Québec-Institut universitaire, Institut de réadaptation en déficience physique de Québec (IRDPQ), Institut universitaire en santé mentale de Québec (IUSMQ) et Hôpital Jeffrey Hale-Saint Brigid's (établissement regroupé).
Michel Delamarre, Président-directeur général
Simon Lemay, Président, Conseil d'administration

QUÉBEC: CLSC de la Basse-Ville
Affiliée à: CIUSSS de la Capitale-National
50, rue Saint-Joseph, Québec, QC G1K 3A5

Tél: 418-529-2572 *Téléc:* 418-524-3234

QUÉBEC: CLSC de la Haute-Ville
Affiliée à: CIUSSS de la Capitale-Nationale
55, ch Ste-Foy, Québec, QC G1R 1S9

Tél: 418-641-2572
www.csssvc.qc.ca

Note: Services: Consultations médicales (418-682-75940);
Consultations psychosociales (418-641-2572); Clinique jeunesse (418-682-7594); Contraception orale d'urgence (418-682-7594); Cours prénataux (418-641-2572); Vaccination (418-682-7594); Soutien à domicile (418-651-3888)

QUÉBEC: CLSC de la Jacques-Cartier (Loretteville)
Affiliée à: CIUSSS de la Capitale-Nationale
11999A, rue de l'Hôpital, Québec, QC G2A 2T7

Tél: 418-843-2572 *Téléc:* 418-843-3880
www.csssqn.qc.ca

Spécialités: Clinique prénatale (418-661-7195); Soutien à domicile; Services infirmiers

QUÉBEC: CSSS de la Vieille-Capitale
Affiliée à: CIUSSS de la Capitale-Nationale
1, av du Sacré-Coeur, Québec, QC G1N 2W1

Tél: 418-529-4777
www.ciusss-capitalenationale.gouv.qc.ca

Fondée en: 2004
Note: Les Installations (Services de CH, CHSLD, et CLSC): CLSC de Cap-Rouge-Saint-Augustin; CLSC de la Basse-Ville; CLSC de la Haute-Ville; CLSC de la Haute-Ville, édifice Courchesne; CLSC de Limoilou; CLSC de L'Ancienne-Lorette; CLSC de Sainte-Foy-Sillery; CLSC de Sainte-Foy-Sillery, Pavillon Marguerite-D'Youville; CLSC des Rivières; Centre d'hébergement Christ-Roi; Centre d'hébergement de Limoilou; Centre d'hébergement Hôpital général de Québec; Centre d'hébergement Le Faubourg; Centre d'hébergement Louis-Hébert; Centre d'hébergement Notre-Dame-de-Lourdes; Centre d'hébergement Sacré-Cour; Centre d'hébergement Saint-Antoine; Unité de médecine familiale de la Haute-Ville; Unité de médecine familiale Laurier; Unité de médecine familiale Laval; Unité de médecine familiale Saint-François d'Assise

QUÉBEC: CSSS Québec-Nord
Affiliée à: CIUSSS de la Capitale-Nationale
Centre administratif, 2915, av du Bourg-Royal, Québec, QC G1C 3S2

Tél: 418-266-1019
www.ciusss-capitalenationale.gouv.qc.ca

Fondée en: 2004
Nombre de lits: 900+ lits
Population desservi: 300000
Personnel: 3000
Note: Les Installations (Services de CH, CHSLD, et CLSC): Hôpital Ste-Anne-de-Beaupré; Hôpital Chauveau; Centre d'hébergement du Fargy; Centre d'hébergement Saint-Augustin; Centre d'hébergement Yvonne-Sylvain; Centre d'hébergement Roy-Rousseau; Centre d'hébergement Charlesbourg; Centre d'hébergement Alphonse-Bonenfant; Centre d'hébergement Loretteville; CLSC de la Jacques-Cartier (Loretteville, Sainte-Catherine-de-la-Jacques-Cartier); CLSC La Source Sud; CLSC La Source Nord; CLSC La Source La Maisonnée; CLSC Orléans (Beauport, Ile d'Orléans, Beaupré, Maizerets, Montmorency); Unité de médecine familiale

QUÉBEC: Hôpital Chauveau
Affiliée à: CIUSSS de la Capitale-Nationale
11999, rue de l'Hôpital, Québec, QC G2A 2T7
Tél: 418-842-3651 *Téléc:* 418-842-8660
www.csssqn.qc.ca

Note: Services: anesthésie, chirurgie, gériatrie, psychiatrie, radiologie, ophtalmologie, urologie; soins généraux et spécialisés; urgence.
Dr. Gilles Caron, Chef du service de l'urgence

QUÉBEC: Hôpital de l'Enfant-Jésus
Affiliée à: CIUSSS de la Capitale-Nationale
1401, 18e rue, Québec, QC G1J 1Z4
Tél: 418-649-0252
www.cha.quebec.qc.ca

Note: Affilié à l'Université Laval et Université de Québec.
Marie Girard, Directrice générale

QUÉBEC: Hôpital du Saint-Sacrement
Centre hospitalier affilié universitaire de Québec
Affiliée à: CIUSSS de la Capitale-Nationale
1050, ch Sainte-Foy, Québec, QC G1S 4L8
Tél: 418-682-7511
www.cha.quebec.qc.ca

Note: Affilié à l'Université Laval et Université de Québec.
Marie Girard, Directrice générale

QUÉBEC: Hôpital Jeffery Hale
Affiliée à: CIUSSS de la Capitale-Nationale
1250, ch Ste-Foy, Québec, QC G1S 2M6
Tél: 418-684-5333 *Ligne sans frais:* 888-984-5333
www.jhsb.ca
Nombre de lits: 99 lits de soins de longue durée

QUÉBEC: Hôpital Sainte-Anne-de-Beaupré
Affiliée à: CIUSSS de la Capitale-Nationale
11000, rue des Montagnards, Québec, QC G0A 1E0
Tél: 418-827-3726
Nombre de lits: 158 lits d'hébergement et de soins de longue durée; 9 lits UTRF; 3 lits de soins palliatifs; 2 lits de transition
Note: Services infirmiers, médicaux, et psychosociaux.

QUÉBEC: Hôpital Saint-François d'Assise
Centre hospitalier universitaire de Québec
Affiliée à: CIUSSS de la Capitale-Nationale
10, rue de l'Espinay, Québec, QC G1L 3L5
Tél: 418-525-4444 *Téléc:* 418-525-6338
www.chudequebec.ca

Note: Affilié à l'Université Laval.

QUÉBEC: L'Hôtel-Dieu de Québec
Centre hospitalier universitaire de Québec
Affiliée à: CIUSSS de la Capitale-Nationale
11, côte du Palais, Québec, QC G1R 2J6
Tél: 418-525-4444 *Téléc:* 418-691-5205
www.chudequebec.ca

Note: Affilié à l'Université Laval.

QUÉBEC: Institut de réadaptation en déficience physique de Québec
Affiliée à: CIUSSS de la Capitale-Nationale
525, boul Wilfrid Hamel, Québec, QC G1M 2S8
Tél: 418-529-9141 *Téléc:* 418-529-7318
TTY: 418-649-3733
www.irdpq.qc.ca
Média social: www.youtube.com/user/VideosIRDPQ
Nombre de lits: 165 lits
Note: Centre de réadaptation (déficience physique)

QUÉBEC: La Maison Michel Sarrazin
Affiliée à: CIUSSS de la Capitale-Nationale
2101, ch St-Louis, Québec, QC G1T 2P5
Tél: 418-688-0878 *Téléc:* 418-681-8636
info@michel-sarrazin.ca
www.michel-sarrazin.ca

Nombre de lits: 15 lits
Alain-Philippe Lemieux, Directeur général

RICHELIEU: CLSC du Richelieu
Affiliée à: CISSS de la Montérégie-Centre
300, ch de Marieville, Richelieu, QC J3L 3V8
Tél: 450-658-7561 *Téléc:* 450-658-4390
www.santemonteregie.qc.ca/haut-richelieu-rouville

Spécialités: Rencontres prénatales; Clinique de la petite enfance
(450-658-7561, poste 4164)

RICHMOND: CLSC de Richmond
Affiliée à: CIUSSS de l'Estrie
110, rue Barlow, Richmond, QC J0B 2H0
Tél: 819-542-2777
www.santeestrie.qc.ca

RIMOUSKI: Centre de réadaptation en déficience intellectuelle du Bas St-Laurent (CRDITED)
Affiliée à: CISSS du Bas-St-Laurent
Ancien nom: Centre de réadaptation intellectuelle du Bas St-Laurent
325, rue Saint-Jean-Baptiste est, Rimouski, QC G5L 1Y8
Tél: 418-723-4425 *Téléc:* 418-723-3196
info.crditedbsl@ssss.gouv.qc.ca
www.crditedbsl.ca
Louise Brassard, Conseillère, Communication et à la gestion de la qualité
louise.brassard.crditedbsl@ssss.gouv

RIMOUSKI: Centre intégré de santé et de services sociaux du Bas-St-Laurent
Également connu sous le nom de: CISSS Bas-St-Laurent
355, boul Saint-Germain ouest, Rimouski, QC G5L 3N2
Tél: 418-724-3000
www.cisss-bsl.gouv.qc.ca
Info Line: 811

Nombre de lits: 476 lits de courte durée
Population desservi: 200880
Personnel: 8000
Isabelle Malo, Présidente-directrice générale
Hugues St-Pierre, Président, Conseil d'administration

RIMOUSKI: CLSC Rimouski
Affiliée à: CISSS du Bas-St-Laurent
165, rue des Gouverneurs, Rimouski, QC G5L 7R2
Tél: 418-727-5493
www.cisss-bsl.gouv.qc.ca

Personnel: 2200
Note: 3 autres points de service: Saint-Fabien, Saint-Marcellin, et Saint-Narcisse

RIMOUSKI: Hôpital régional de Rimouski
Affiliée à: CISSS du Bas-St-Laurent
150, av Rouleau, Rimouski, QC G5L 5T1
Tél: 418-724-3000
Nombre de lits: 255 lits

RIVIÉRE-ROUGE: Centre de services de Rivière-Rouge
Affiliée à: CISSS des Laurentides
1525, rue L'Annonciation nord, Rivière-Rouge, QC J0T 1T0
Tél: 819-275-2118
www.santelaurentides.qc.ca

RIVIÉRE-DU-LOUP: Le Centre hospitalier régional du Grand-Portage (CHRGP)
Affiliée à: CISSS du Bas-St-Laurent
75, rue Saint-Henri, Rivière-du-Loup, QC G5R 2A4
Tél: 418-868-1000 *Téléc:* 418-868-1032
Nombre de lits: 145 lits

RIVIÉRE-DU-LOUP: CLSC de Rivière-du-Loup
22, rue Saint-Laurent, Rivière-du-Loup, QC G5R 4W5
Tél: 418-867-2642 *Téléc:* 418-867-4713
www.cisss-bsl.gouv.qc.ca

RIVIÉRE-DU-LOUP: CSSS de Rivière-du-Loup
Le Centre hospitalier régional de Grand-Portage, 75, rue St-Henri, Rivière-du-Loup, QC G5R 2A4
Tél: 418-868-1010 *Téléc:* 418-868-1032
www.csssriviereduloup.qc.ca

Personnel: 1500
Note: Les Installations (Services de CH, CHSLD, et CLSC): Centre hospitalier régional de Grand-Portage ((CHRGP); Centre d'hébergement Saint-Joseph; Centre d'hébergement Saint-Antonin; Centre d'hébergement St-Cyprien; CLSC Rivière et Marées; L'Estran Centre de réadaptation en alcoolisme et toxicomanie du Bas-Saint-Laurent
Doris Laliberté-Kirouac, Présidente, Conseil d'administration
Daniel Lévesque, Directeur général et secrétaire

ROBERVAL: Centre de réadaptation en déficience intellectuelle du Saguenay-Lac-Saint-Jean
Affiliée à: CIUSSS du Saguenay-Lac-Saint-Jean
835, rue Roland, Roberval, QC G8H 3J5
Tél: 418-275-1360 *Téléc:* 418-275-6595
www.crdited02.qc.ca
Média social: www.facebook.com/CRDITEDduSLSJ

Personnel: 600
Note: Centre de réadaptation pour personnes présentant une déficience intellectuelle
Johanne Houde, Directrice générale

ROBERVAL: CSSS Domaine-du-Roy
Affiliée à: CIUSSS du Saguenay-Lac-Saint-Jean
Édifice Hôtel-Dieu de Roberval, 450, rue Brassard, Roberval, QC G8H 1B9
Tél: 418-275-0110 *Téléc:* 418-275-6202
www.santesaglac.com

Note: Les Installations (Services de CH, CHSLD, et CLSC): Hôtel-Dieu de Roberval; Centre d'hébergement Roberval; Centre d'hébergement Saint-Félicien; CLSC Saint-Félicien; CLSC Roberval; Mission de Centre de réadaptation en alcoolisme et autres toxicomanies (CRAT); Centre de réadaptation pour alcooliques et autres toxicomanes Saint-Antoine

ROBERVAL: Hôtel-Dieu de Roberval
Affiliée à: CIUSSS du Saguenay-Lac-Saint-Jean
450, rue Brassard, Roberval, QC G8H 1B9
Tél: 418-275-0110
Nombre de lits: 135 lits
Note: L'hôpital offre service d'urgence, médecine générale/interne/nucléaire, ophtalmologie, obstétrique, orthopédie, pédiatrie, chirurgie, psychiatrie, urologie, réadaptation physique.

ROUYN-NORANDA: Centre de réadaptation La Maison
Affiliée à: CISSS de l'Abitibi-Témiscamingue
100, ch Docteur-Lemay, Rouyn-Noranda, QC J9X 5T2
Tél: 819-762-6592 *Téléc:* 819-762-2049
www.cisss-at.gouv.qc.ca
Nombre de lits: 55 lits
Note: Centre de réadaptation (déficience physique, troubles envahissants du développement).
Line St-Amour, Directrice générale
line_st-amour@ssss.gouv.qc.ca

ROUYN-NORANDA: Centre intégré de santé et de services sociaux de l'Abitibi-Témiscamingue
1, 9e rue, Rouyn-Noranda, QC J9X 2A9
Tél: 819-764-3264 *Téléc:* 819-764-2948
info_sante-abitibi-temiscamingue@ssss.gouv.qc.ca
www.cisss-at.gouv.qc.ca
Info Line: 811
Fondée en: 2015
Région desservi: La région de l'Abitibi-Témiscamingue (65 municipalités)
Population desservi: 147700
Note: Centres de santé et de services sociaux (CSSS): CSSS des Aurores-Boréales; CSSS les Eskers de l'Abitibi; CSSS de Rouyn-Noranda; CSSS de la Vallée-de-l'Or; CSSS du Témiscamingue
Jacques Boissonneault, Président-directeur général
Claude Morin, Président, Conseil d'administration

ROUYN-NORANDA: CLSC de Rouyn-Noranda
Affiliée à: CISSS de l'Abitibi-Témiscamingue
1, 9e rue, Rouyn-Noranda, QC J9X 2A9
Tél: 819-762-5599
www.cisss-at.gouv.qc.ca
Note: Point de service CLSC, et consultations externes CHSGS.

ROUYN-NORANDA: CSSS de Rouyn-Noranda (CSSSRN)
Affiliée à: CIUSSS de l'Abitibi-Témiscamingue
4, 9e rue, Rouyn-Noranda, QC J9X 2B2
Tél: 819-764-5131 *Téléc:* 819-764-2948
www.cisss-at.gouv.qc.ca
Fondée en: 2004
Population desservi: 39615
Personnel: 1200
Note: Les Installations (Services de CH, CHSLD, et CLSC): Hôpital, Rouyn-Noranda (819-764-5131); Centre d'hébergement, Rouyn-Noranda (819-762-0908); CLSC, Rouyn-Noranda (819-762-8144) (Beaudry-Cloutier, Cadillac, Cléricy-Mont-Brun, Montbeillard-Rollet, Destor)

ROUYN-NORANDA: Hôpital de Rouyn-Noranda
Affiliée à: CISSS de l'Abitibi-Témiscamingue
4, 9e rue, Rouyn-Noranda, QC J9X 2B2
Tél: 819-764-5131

SAINT-CHARLES-BORROMÉE: Centre hospitalier régional de Lanaudière (CHRDL)
Affiliée à: CISSS de Lanaudière
1000, boul Sainte-Anne, Saint-Charles-Borromée, QC J6E 6J2
Tél: 450-759-8222

SAINT-CHARLES-BORROMÉE: CSSS du Nord de Lanaudière
Affiliée à: CIUSSS de Lanaudière
1000, boul Sainte-Anne, Saint-Charles-Borromée, QC J6E 6J2
Tél: 450-759-8222
www.csssnl.qc.ca
Région desservi: MRC de D'Autray, de Joliette, de Matawinie, et de Montcalm
Population desservi: 200000
Personnel: 4700
Note: Les Installations (Services de CH, CHSLD, et CLSC): Centre hospitalier régional De Lanaudière; Centre d'hébergement Alphonse-Rondeau; Centre d'hébergement Desy; Centre d'hébergement Sainte-Élisabeth; Centre d'hébergement Parphilia-Ferland; Centre d'hébergement Saint-Eusèbe; Centre d'hébergement du Piedmont; Centre d'hébergement Saint-Donat; Centre d'hébergement Brassard; Centre d'hébergement Saint-Antoine de Padoue; Centre d'hébergement Saint-Jacques; Centre d'hébergement Saint-Liguori; CLSC de Berthier; CLSC de Lavaltrie; CLSC de Saint-Gabriel; CLSC de Joliette; CLSC de Chertsey; CLSC de Saint-Jean-de-Matha; CLSC de Saint-Donat; CLSC de Saint-Michel-des-Saints; CLSC de Saint-Esprit; Centre de réadaptation en dépendances Le Tremplin de Saint-Charles-Borromée; Centre de réadaptation en dépendances Le Tremplin de Repentigny; Centre de réadaptation en dépendances Le Tremplin de Terrebonne; Services externes psychiatriques intégrés pour adultes de Rawdon; Services psychiatriques pour enfants et adolescents; Unité de médecine familiale du Nord de Lanaudière.
Nombre de médecins, dentistes, et de pharmaciens: 350
Daniel Castonguay, Directeur général

SAINT-EUSTACHE: CSSS du Lac-des-Deux-Montagnes
Affiliée à: CISSS des Laurentides
Direction générale, 520, boul Arthur-Sauvé, Saint-Eustache, QC J7R 5B1
Tél: 450-473-6811 *Téléc:* 450-473-6966
Ligne sans frais: 888-234-3837
www.moncsss.com
Média social: twitter.com/CSSS2Montagnes
Fondée en: 2004
Note: Les Installations (Services de CH, CHSLD, et CLSC): Hôpital de Saint-Eustache (450-473-6811); Centre d'hébergement de Saint-Eustache (450-472-0013); Centre d'hébergement de Saint-Benoît (450-258-2481); CLSC Jean-Olivier-Chénier (450-491-1233); CLSC Mirabel (450-475-7938); Clinique externe de psychiatrie (450-473-1533

SAINT-EUSTACHE: Hôpital de Saint-Eustache
Affiliée à: CISSS des Laurentides
520, boul Arthur-Sauvé, Saint-Eustache, QC J7R 5B1
Tél: 450-473-6811 Téléc: 450-473-6966
Ligne sans frais: 888-234-3837
Nombre de lits: 261 lits

SAINT-FÉLICIEN: CLSC Saint-Félicien - Édifice Bon-Conseil
Affiliée à: CIUSSS du Saguenay-Lac-St-Jean
CP 10, 1228, boul Sacré-Coeur, Saint-Félicien, QC G8K 2P8
Tél: 418-679-5270 Téléc: 418-679-1748

SAINT-FÉLICIEN: CLSC Saint-Félicien - Édifice Hôtel de Ville
Affiliée à: CIUSSS du Saguenay-Lac-St-Jean
CP 10, 1209, boul Sacré-Coeur, Saint-Félicien, QC G8K 2P8
Tél: 418-679-5270 Téléc: 418-679-3510

SAINT-GEORGES: Hôpital de Saint-Georges
Affiliée à: CISSS de Chaudière-Appalaches
1515, 17e rue Ouest, Saint-Georges, QC G5Y 4T8
Tél: 418-228-2031 Téléc: 418-227-3825
Nombre de lits: 142 lits
Note: Services: chirurgie générale; gynécologie-obstétrique; psychiatrie; radiologie

SAINT-HUBERT: CLSC Saint-Hubert
Affiliée à: CISSS de la Montérégie-Centre
6800, boul Cousineau, Saint-Hubert, QC J3Y 8Z4
Tél: 450-443-7400
www.santemonteregie.qc.ca/champlain
Région desservi: L'arrondissement Saint-Hubert de la Ville de Longueuil
Spécialités: Rencontres prénatales (450-443-7400, option 6); Consultations psychosociales (450-443-7400, poste 7318)

SAINT-HYACINTHE: Centre intégré de santé et de services sociaux de la Montérégie-Est
2750, boul Laframboise, Saint-Hyacinthe, QC J2S 4Y8
Tél: 450-771-3333
santeme.quebec
Fondée en: 2015
Population desservi: 510000
Personnel: 11800
Louise Potvin, Présidente-directrice générale

SAINT-HYACINTHE: Hôpital Honoré-Mercier
Affiliée à: CISSS de la Montérégie-Est
2750, boul Laframboise, Saint-Hyacinthe, QC J2S 4Y8
Tél: 450-771-3333
Nombre de lits: 213 lits en soins aigus; 35 lits de psychiatrie courte durée; 25 lits en hébergement santé mentale
Note: Services comprennent: centre mère-enfant-famille; Pédiatrie; Soins intensifs; Chirurgie.

SAINT-JEAN-SUR-RICHELIEU: CLSC de la Vallée-des-Forts
Affiliée à: CISSS de la Montérégie-Centre
978, boul du Séminaire nord, Saint-Jean-sur-Richelieu, QC J3A 1E5
Tél: 450-358-2572 Téléc: 450-349-0724

SAINT-JEAN-SUR-RICHELIEU: CSSS Haut-Richelieu - Rouville
Affiliée à: CISSS de la Montérégie-Centre
978, boul du Séminaire Nord, Saint-Jean-sur-Richelieu, QC J3A 1E5
Tél: 450-358-2572
www.santemonteregie.qc.ca/haut-richelieu-rouville
Fondée en: 2004
Population desservi: 182000
Personnel: 4000
Note: Les Installations (Services de CH, CHSLD, et CLSC): Hôpital du Haut-Richelieu, Saint-Jean-sur-Richelieu (450-359-5000); Centre d'hébergement Champagnat, Saint-Jean-sur-Richelieu (450-347-3769); Centre d'hébergement Georges-Phaneuf, Saint-Jean-sur-Richelieu (450-346-1133); Centre d'hébergement Gertrude-Lafrance, Saint-Jean-sur-Richelieu (450-359-5555); Centre d'hébergement Sainte-Croix, Marieville (450-460-4475); Centre d'hébergement Saint-Joseph, Chambly (450-658-6271); Centre d'hébergement Val-Joli, Saint-Césaire (450-469-3194); CLSC de Henryville (450-299-2828); CLSC de la Vallée-des-Forts, Saint-Jean-sur-Richelieu (450-358-2572); CLSC de Saint-Césaire (450-469-0269); CLSC du Richelieu (450-658-7561); Manoir Soleil, Chambly (450-658-4441);

Clinique jeunesse 12-21 ans, Saint-Jean-sur-Richelieu (450-358-2572); Clinique jeunesse du Bassin de Chambly 12-24 ans, Chambly (450-658-2016); Point de chute de Lacolle (450-299-2828); Services de consultation externe - psychiatrie, réadaptation pédiatrique, clinique d'évaluation TED (450-346-2222).
Médecins: 300.
Le Territoire desservi: MRC de Rouville, MRC du Haut-Richelieu et MRC de la Vallée-du-Richelieu (21 municipalités)

SAINT-JEAN-SUR-RICHELIEU: Hôpital du Haut-Richelieu
Affiliée à: CISSS de la Montérégie-Centre
920, boul du Séminaire Nord, Saint-Jean-sur-Richelieu, QC J3A 1B7
Tél: 450-359-5000 Téléc: 450-359-5251
Ligne sans frais: 866-967-4825
Nombre de lits: 307 lits
Personnel: 1500

SAINT-JEAN-SUR-RICHELIEU: Les services de réadaptation du Sud-Ouest et du Renfort
Affiliée à: CISSS de la Montérégie-Ouest
#105, 315, rue MacDonald, Saint-Jean-sur-Richelieu, QC J3B 8J3
Tél: 450-348-6121 Téléc: 450-348-8440
www.srsor.qc.ca
Nombre de lits: 581 lits
Gilles Bertrand, Directeur général
Lisa Charest, Agente administrative
lisa.charest@rrsss16.gouv.qc.ca

SAINT-JÉRÔME: Centre intégré de santé et de services sociaux des Laurentides
290, rue Montigny, Saint-Jérôme, QC J7Z 5T3
Tél: 450-432-2777 Ligne sans frais: 866-963-2777
www.santelaurentides.gouv.qc.ca
Info Line: 811
Fondée en: 2015
Population desservi: 595202
Personnel: 13500
Jean-François Foisy, Président-directeur général
André Poirier, Président, Conseil d'administration

SAINT-JÉRÔME: CSSS de Saint-Jérôme
Affiliée à: CISSS des Laurentides
290, rue de Montigny, Saint-Jérôme, QC J7Z 5T3
Tél: 450-432-2777 Ligne sans frais: 866-963-2777
www.cdsj.org
Nombre de lits: 405 lits de courte durée dont 85 en psychiatrie; 305 lits répartis en trois centres d'hébergement
Note: Les Installations (Services de CH, CHSLD, et CLSC): Hôpital régional de Saint-Jérôme (450-432-2777); Centre d'hébergement Youville (450-432-2777, poste 26761); Centre d'hébergement L'Auberge (450-432-2777, poste 23621); Centre d'hébergement Lucien-G.-Rolland (450-432-2777, poste 23221); CLSC de Saint-Jérôme, famille, enfance, jeunesse, services à la collectivité (450-432-2777, poste 25000); CLSC de Saint-Jérôme, soutien à domicile (450-432-2777, poste 26221); CLSC de Saint-Jérôme, santé mentale et services psychosociaux (450-432-2777, poste 26500); Clinique de développement (450-432-2777, poste 23600); Maison de naissance du Boisé (450-432-2777, poste 23660); Centre de prélèvements (450-432-2777, poste 22197).
Médecins: 350

SAINT-JÉRÔME: Hôpital régional de Saint-Jérôme
Affiliée à: CISSS des Laurentides
290, rue de Montigny, Saint-Jérôme, QC J7Z 5T3
Tél: 450-432-2777 Ligne sans frais: 866-963-2777

SAINT-LÉONARD: CLSC de Saint-Léonard
Affiliée à: CIUSSS de l'Est-de-l'Île-de-Montréal
5540, rue Jarry Est, Saint-Léonard, QC H1P 1T9
Tél: 514-722-3000
www.csss-stleonardstmichel.qc.ca

SAINT-LUDGER: CLSC Saint-Ludger
Affiliée à: CIUSSS de l'Estrie
210-A, rue La Salle, Saint-Ludger, QC G0M 1W0
Tél: 819-583-2572
www.santeestrie.qc.ca

SAINT-OMER: CLSC de Saint-Omer
Affiliée à: CISSS de la Gaspésie
CP 10, 102, boul Perron, Saint-Omer, QC G0C 2Z0
Tél: 418-364-7064 *Téléc:* 418-364-7119

SAINT-PASCAL: CSSS de Kamouraska
Affiliée à: CISSS du Bas-St-Laurent
575, av Martin, Saint-Pascal, QC G0L 3Y0
Tél: 418-856-7000
www.cisss-bsl.gouv.qc.ca

Note: Les Installations (Services de CH, CHSLD, et CLSC): Hôpital Notre-Dame-de-Fatima (49 lits); Centre d'hébergement D'Anjou, Saint-Pacôme (53 lits); Centre d'hébergement Thérèse-Martin, Rivière-Ouelle (46 lits); Centre d'hébergement Villa Maria, Saint-Alexandre (52 lits); CLSC, Saint-Pascal; CLSC, La Pocatière; CLSC, Saint-André

SAINT-PAULIN: CLSC de St-Paulin
Affiliée à: CIUSSS de la Mauricie-et-du-Centre-du-Québec
2841, rue Laflèche, Saint-Paulin, QC J0K 3G0
Tél: 819-268-2572
www.csssm.qc.ca

Spécialités: Services infirmiers courants; Vaccination

SAINT-RAYMOND: Hôpital régional de Portneuf
Affiliée à: CIUSSS de la Capitale-Nationale
700, rue Saint-Cyrille, Saint-Raymond, QC G3L 1W1
Tél: 418-337-4611

SAINT-RÉMI: CLSC Jardin-du-Québec
Affiliée à: CISSS de la Montérégie-Ouest
2, rue Sainte-Famille, Saint-Rémi, QC J0L 2L0
Tél: 450-454-4671 *Téléc:* 450-454-4538

SAINT-SIMÉON: CLSC de Saint-Siméon
Affiliée à: CIUSSS de la Capitale-Nationale
371, rue Saint-Laurent, Saint-Siméon, QC G0T 1X0
Tél: 418-638-2369
www.ciusss-capitalenationale.gouv.qc.ca
Nombre de lits: 18 lits
Note: Centre local de services communautaires (418-638-2369); centre d'hébergement et centre de jour.

SAINTE-AGATHE-DES-MONTS: CSSS des Sommets
Affiliée à: CISSS des Laurentides
Pavillon administratif Jacques-Duquette, 234, rue Saint-Vincent, Sainte-Agathe-des-Monts, QC J8C 2B8
Tél: 819-324-4000 *Ligne sans frais:* 855-766-6387
www.csss-sommets.com
Nombre de lits: 217 lits de longue durée; 104 lits de courte durée
Région desservi: MRC des Laurentides et des environs
Population desservi: 46517
Personnel: 1500
Note: Les Installations (Services de CH, CHSLD, et CLSC): Hôpital Laurentien (819-324-4000); Pavillon Philippe-Lapointe (819-324-4000); Centre d'hébergement de Mont-Tremblant (819-425-2793); Centre d'hébergement de Labelle (819-686-2372); CLSC de Sainte-Agathe-des-Monts (819-326-3111); CLSC de Mont-Tremblant (819-425-3771); CLSC de Labelle (819-686-2117)

SAINTE-AGATHE-DES-MONTS: Hôpital Laurentien
Affiliée à: CISSS des Laurentides
234, rue Saint-Vincent, Sainte-Agathe-des-Monts, QC J8C 2B8
Tél: 819-324-4000

SAINTE-ANNE-DE-BELLEVUE: Hôpital Sainte-Anne
Affiliée à: CIUSSS de l'Ouest-de-l'Île-de-Montréal
305, boul des Anciens-Combattants, Sainte-Anne-de-Bellevue, QC H9X 1Y9
Tél: 514-457-3440 *Ligne sans frais:* 800-361-9287
ifnormations.comtl@ssss.gouv.qc.ca
www.ciusss-ouestmtl.gouv.qc.ca
Nombre de lits: 590 lits
Rachel Corneille-Gravel, Directrice générale

SAINTE-ANNE-DES-MONTS: Point de service - Réadaptation Route du Parc
Affiliée à: CISSS de la Gaspésie
230, rte du Parc, Sainte-Anne-des-Monts, QC G4V 2C4
Tél: 418-763-3325

SAINTE-MARIE: Centre intégré de santé et de services sociaux de Chaudière-Appalaches
363, rte Cameron, Sainte-Marie, QC G6E 3E2
Tél: 418-386-3363 *Téléc:* 418-386-3361
reception.cisss-ca@ssss.gouv.qc.ca
www.cisss-ca.gouv.qc.ca
Info Line: 811

Population desservi: 424856
Daniel Paré, Président-directeur général
Brigitte Busque, Présidente, Conseil d'administration

SALABERRY-DE-VALLEYFIELD: CSSS du Suroît
Affiliée à: CISSS de la Montérégie-Ouest
150, rue Saint-Thomas, Salaberry-de-Valleyfield, QC J6T 6C1
Tél: 450-371-9920 *Ligne sans frais:* 800-694-9920
www.santemonteregie.qc.ca
Région desservi: Salaberry-de-Valleyfield; Beauharnois; Vaudreuil-Dorion
Note: Les Installations (Services de CH, CHSLD, et CLSC): Hôpital du Suroît (450-371-9920); Centre d'hébergement Cécile-Godin (450-429-6403); Centre d'hébergement Docteur-Aimé-Leduc (450-373-4818); CLSC de Beauharnois (450-429-6455); CLSC de Salaberry-de-Valleyfield (450-371-0143); Centre de jour pour adultes, Salaberry-de-Valleyfield (450-373-7321); Clinique externe pour adultes, Salaberry-de-Valleyfield (450-373-6252); Clinique externe pour jeunes, Salaberry-de-Valleyfield (450-373-5705); Clinique externe pour adultes, Vaudreuil-Dorion (450-455-7967); Clinique externe pour jeunes, Vaudreuil-Dorion (450-455-3356)

SALABERRY-DE-VALLEYFIELD: Hôpital du Suroît
Affiliée à: CISSS de la Montérégie-Ouest
150, rue Saint-Thomas, Salaberry-de-Valleyfield, QC J6T 6C1
Tél: 450-371-9920

SEPT-ILES: Hôpital de Sept-Iles
Affiliée à: CISSS de la Côte-Nord
45, rue du Père-Divet, Sept-Iles, QC G4R 3N7
Tél: 418-962-9761 *Téléc:* 418-962-7604

Note: Services: cardiologie; chirurgie générale; médecine nucléaire; obstétrique gynécologie; radiologie diagnostique

SHAWINIGAN: CSSS de l'Énergie
Affiliée à: CIUSSS de la Mauricie et du Centre-du-Québec
Centre administratif, 243, 1e rue de la Pointe, Shawinigan, QC G9N 1K2
Tél: 819-536-7500
info@cssse.qc.ca
www.etrehumain.ca

Note: Les Installations (Services de CH, CHSLD, et CLSC): Hôpital du Centre-de-la-Mauricie (819-536-7500); Centre d'hébergement Joseph-Garceau (819-537-5173); Centre d'hébergement Laflèche (819-533-2500); Centre d'hébergement Saint-Maurice (819-536-0071); CLSC du Centre-de-la-Mauricie (819-539-8371); CIC de Shawinigan (819-537-6647); Centre régional de santé mentale (819-536-7500)

SHAWINIGAN: Hôpital du Centre-de-la-Mauricie
Affiliée à: CIUSSS de la Mauricie-et-du-Centre-du-Québec
50, 119e rue, Shawinigan, QC G9P 5K1
Tél: 819-536-7500
www.ciusssmcq.ca

SHAWVILLE: Hôpital du Pontiac
Affiliée à: CISSS de l'Outaouais
200, rue Argue, Shawville, QC J0X 2Y0
Tél: 819-647-2211

SHERBROOKE: Centre de réadaptation Estrie (CRE)
Affiliée à: CIUSSS de l'Estrie
#200, 300, rue King est, Sherbrooke, QC J1G 1B1
Tél: 819-346-8411 *Téléc:* 819-346-4580
www.santeestrie.qc.ca
Média social: www.youtube.com/user/readaptationestrie

Spécialités: Réadaptation fonctionnelle intensive; Ressources résidentielles et d'hébergement

SHERBROOKE: Centre hospitalier universitaire de Sherbrooke - Édifice Murray (CHUS)
Affiliée à: CIUSSS de l'Estrie
500, rue Murray, Sherbrooke, QC J1G 2K6
Tél: 819-346-1110 *Ligne sans frais:* 866-638-2601
www.santeestrie.qc.ca
Média social: www.youtube.com/user/CHUSSherbrooke
Fondée en: 1995
Nombre de lits: 677 lits
Région desservi: Sherbrooke; Haut-St-François; Val-St-François; MRC de Coaticook
Personnel: 6244
Note: Programmes et services comprennent: chimiothérapie cérébrale; neurochirurgie par scalpel-gamma; neurochirurgie assistée par IRM 3D avancé; dépistage du cancer colorectal; production de radioisotopes par cyclotron (au Centre de recherche). Associé à l'Université de Sherbrooke.
Patricia Gauthier, Présidente-directrice générale, CIUSSS de l'Estrie

SHERBROOKE: Centre hospitalier universitaire de Sherbrooke - Fleurimont (CHUS)
Affiliée à: CIUSSS de l'Estrie
3001, 12e av Nord, Sherbrooke, QC J1H 5N4
Tél: 819-346-1110 *Ligne sans frais:* 866-638-2601
www.santeestrie.qc.ca
Fondée en: 1995
Nombre de lits: 677 lits
Région desservi: Sherbrooke; Haut-St-François; Val-St-François; MRC de Coaticook
Personnel: 6244
Note: Programmes et services comprennent: chimiothérapie cérébrale; neurochirurgie par scalpel-gamma; neurochirurgie assistée par IRM 3D avancé; dépistage du cancer colorectal; production de radioisotopes par cyclotron (au Centre de recherche). Associé à l'Université de Sherbrooke.

SHERBROOKE: Centre hospitalier universitaire de Sherbrooke - Hôtel-Dieu (CHUS)
Affiliée à: CIUSSS de l'Estrie
580, rue Bowen Sud, Sherbrooke, QC J1G 2E8
Tél: 819-346-1110 *Ligne sans frais:* 866-638-2601
www.santeestrie.qc.ca
Fondée en: 1995
Nombre de lits: 677 lits
Région desservi: Sherbrooke; Haut-St-François; Val-St-François; MRC de Coaticook
Personnel: 6244
Note: Programmes et services comprennent: chimiothérapie cérébrale; neurochirurgie par scalpel-gamma; neurochirurgie assistée par IRM 3D avancé; dépistage du cancer colorectal; production de radioisotopes par cyclotron (au Centre de recherche). Associé à l'Université de Sherbrooke.

SHERBROOKE: Centre intégré universitaire de santé et de services sociaux de l'Estrie
Également connu sous le nom de: CIUSSS de l'Estrie
375, rue Argyll, Sherbrooke, QC J1J 3H5
Tél: 819-780-2222
www.santeestrie.qc.ca
Info Line: 811
Média social: www.facebook.com/SanteEstrie;
twitter.com/CIUSSE_CHUS; www.linkedin.com/company/2789705
Région desservi: Lac-Mégantic à Granby, environ 13,000 km2
Population desservi: 500000
Personnel: 17000
Patricia Gauthier, Présidente-directrice générale

SHERBROOKE: Centre Jean-Patrice Chiasson/Maison St-Georges
1930, rue King ouest, Sherbrooke, QC J1J 2E2
Tél: 819-821-2500
Nombre de lits: 40 places
Note: Centre de réadaptation des drogues
Murray McDonald, Directeur général

SHERBROOKE: CLSC de Sherbrooke - Point de service 50 rue Camirand
Affiliée à: CIUSSS de l'Estrie
50, rue Camirand, Sherbrooke, QC J1H 4J5
Tél: 819-780-2220
www.santeestrie.qc.ca
Note: Autres points de service: 1200, rue King est et 8, rue Speid.

SHERBROOKE: Hôpital et centre d'hébergement Argyll
Affiliée à: CIUSSS de l'Estrie
375, rue Argyll, Sherbrooke, QC J1J 3H5
Tél: 819-780-2222
Note: Programmes et services comprennent: centre d'hébergement; centre de prélèvements; cliniques ambulatoires gériatriques; unité de courte durée gériatrique.

SHERBROOKE: Hôpital et centre d'hébergement D'Youville
Affiliée à: CIUSSS de l'Estrie
1036, rue Belvédère Sud, Sherbrooke, QC J1H 4C4
Tél: 819-780-2222
Note: Programmes et services comprennent: centre d'hébergement; hôpital de jour; unité de réadaptation; centre de recherche sur le vieillissement.

SHERBROOKE: Villa Marie-Claire inc.
470, rue Victoria, Sherbrooke, QC J1H 3J2
Tél: 819-563-1622 *Téléc:* 819-563-6990

SOREL-TRACY: CLSC Gaston-Bélanger
Affiliée à: CISSS de la Montérégie-Est
Également connu sous le nom de: CLSC du Havre
30, rue Ferland, Sorel-Tracy, QC J3P 3C7
Tél: 450-746-4545
Nombre de lits: 18 lits

SOREL-TRACY: CSSS Pierre-De Saurel
Affiliée à: CISSS de la Montérégie-Est
400, av Hôtel-Dieu, Sorel-Tracy, QC J3P 1N5
Tél: 450-746-6000
www.santemonteregie.qc.ca/sorel-tracy
Fondée en: 2004
Note: Les Installations (Services de CH, CHSLD, et CLSC): Hôtel-Dieu de Sorel (450-746-6000); Centre d'hébergement Élisabeth-Lafrance (450-746-5555); Centre d'hébergement de Tracy (450-743-4924); Centre d'hébergement J.-Arsène-Parenteau (450-742-5936); CLSC Gaston-Bélanger (450-746-4545); Résidence Sorel-Tracy inc. (450-742-9428); Centre de jour, Sorel-Tracy (450-743-5569); Hôpital de jour, Sorel-Tracy (450-743-5569).
Le Territoire desservi: Massueville; Saint-Gérard-de-Majella; Saint-Roch-de-Richelieu; Saint-Aimé; Saint-Joseph-de-Sorel; Sorel-Tracy; Saint-David; Sainte-Anne-de-Sorel; Saint-Ours; Yamaska; Sainte-Victoire-de-Sorel; Saint-Robert

SOREL-TRACY: Hôtel-Dieu de Sorel
Affiliée à: CISSS de la Montérégie-Est
400, av de l'Hôtel-Dieu, Sorel-Tracy, QC J3P 1N5
Tél: 450-746-6000

STE-ANNE-DES-MONTS: Centre de réadaptation de la Gaspésie
Affiliée à: CISSS de la Gaspésie
230, rte du Parc, Ste-Anne-des-Monts, QC G4V 2C4
Tél: 418-763-3325
Nombre de lits: 131 lits

STE-ANNE-DES-MONTS: CLSC de Sainte-Anne-des-Monts
Affiliée à: CISSS de la Gaspésie
50, rue Belvédère, Ste-Anne-des-Monts, QC G4V 1X4
Tél: 418-763-7771 *Téléc:* 418-763-7176
www.cisss-gaspesie.gouv.qc.ca

STE-CATHERINE-DE-LA-J-CARTIER: CLSC de la Jacques-Cartier (Sainte-Catherine-de-la- Jacques-Cartier)
Affiliée à: CIUSSS de la Capitale-Nationale
4570, rte de Fossambault, Ste-Catherine-de-la-J-Cartier, QC G3N 2T6
Tél: 418-843-2572 *Téléc:* 418-843-3880
www.csssqn.qc.ca

Spécialités: Soutien à domicile; Services infirmiers

TERREBONNE: CLSC Lamater - boul des Seigneurs
Affiliée à: CISSS de Lanaudière
2099, boul des Seigneurs, Terrebonne, QC J6X 4A7

Tél: 450-471-2881 *Téléc:* 450-471-8235
www.csss.sudlanaudiere.ca

Spécialités: Clinique médicale; Services sociaux scolaires; Service en santé mentale; Services dentaires préventifs; Clinique des jeunes; Vaccination

TERREBONNE: Hôpital Pierre-Le Gardeur
Affiliée à: CISSS de Lanaudière
911, montée des Pionniers, Terrebonne, QC J6V 2H2

Tél: 450-654-7525 *Ligne sans frais:* 888-654-7525

Note: Programmes et services comprennent chirurgies, cliniques spécialisées, suppléance rénale, centre d'oncologie et soins en santé psychiatrique.

THETFORD MINES: Hôpital de Thetford Mines
Affiliée à: CISSS de Chaudière-Appalaches
1717, rue Notre-Dame Est, Thetford Mines, QC G6G 2V4

Tél: 418-338-7777

Nombre de lits: 130 lits
Note: Services: chirurgie générale; gynécologie-obstétrique; médecine nucléaire; pédiatrie; psychiatrie; radiologie; urologie

TROIS-PISTOLES: Centre hospitalier Trois-Pistoles
Affiliée à: CISSS du Bas-St-Laurent
550, rue Notre-Dame Est, Trois-Pistoles, QC G0L 4K0

Tél: 418-851-1111 *Téléc:* 418-851-2944

TROIS-PISTOLES: CSSS des Basques
550, rue Notre-Dame est, Trois-Pistoles, QC G0L 4K0

Tél: 418-851-1111
www.csssbasques.qc.ca

Personnel: 210

TROIS-RIVIÈRES: Centre de réadaptation Interval
Affiliée à: CIUSSS de la Mauricie-et-du-Centre-du-Québec
1775, rue Nicolas-Perrot, Trois-Rivières, QC G9A 1C5

Tél: 819-378-4083 *Téléc:* 819-693-0237
www.centreinterval.qc.ca

Note: Centre de réadaptation (déficience motrice)
Bruno Landry, Directeur général

TROIS-RIVIÈRES: Centre de service Laviolette
Affiliée à: CIUSSS de la Mauricie-et-du-Centre-du-Québec
1274, rue Laviolette, Trois-Rivières, QC G9A 1W4

Tél: 819-379-5650
www.cssstr.qc.ca

Spécialités: Soutien à domicile

TROIS-RIVIÈRES: Centre hospitalier affilié universitaire régional
Affiliée à: CIUSSS de la Mauricie-et-du-Centre-du-Québec
1991, boul du Carmel, Trois-Rivières, QC G8Z 3R9

Tél: 819-697-3333

Note: Affilié à l'Université de Montréal en Mauricie.

TROIS-RIVIÈRES: Centre intégré universitaire de santé et de services sociaux de la Mauricie-et-du-Centre-du-Québec
858, terrasse Turcotte, Trois-Rivières, QC G9A 5C5

Tél: 819-375-3111
www.ciusssmcq.ca
Info Line: 811

Fondée en: 2015
Population desservi: 510163
Note: Fournit des services dans les domaines suivants: Arthabaska-et-de-l'Érable, Bécancour-Nicolet-Yamaska, Drummond, De l'Énergie (Shawinigan et les environs), Haut-Saint-Maurice, Maskinongé, Trois-Rivières et Vallée-de-la-Batiscan.
Martin Beaumont, Président-directeur général
Richard Desrochers, Président du conseil d'administration

TROIS-RIVIÈRES: Centre St-Joseph
Affiliée à: CIUSSS de la Mauricie-et-du-Centre-du-Québec
731, rue Sainte-Julie, Trois-Rivières, QC G9A 1Y1

Tél: 819-370-2100
www.ciusssmcq.ca

Nombre de lits: 198 lits hospitaliers; 100 lits de soins de longue durée
Note: Centre St-Joseph: services hospitaliers; Centre d'hébergement pour personnes âgées

TROIS-RIVIÈRES: CRDITED de la Mauricie et du Centre-du-Québec
3255, rue Foucher, Trois-Rivières, QC G8Z 1M6

Tél: 819-379-6868 *Téléc:* 819-379-5155
Ligne sans frais: 888-379-7732
www.crditedmcq.qc.ca
Média social: www.facebook.com/crditedmcq.iu;
twitter.com/crditedmcqiu;
www.youtube.com/channel/UCv3p3-3l6FoqZSX5sCDEGxQ

Région desservi: La région sociosanitaire de la Mauricie et du Centre-du-Québec
Note: Le Centre de réadaptation en déficience intellectuelle et en troubles envahissants du développement de la Mauricie et du Centre-du-Québec (CRDITED MCQ) est affilié à l'Université du Québec à Trois-Rivières (UQTR).
Sylvie Dupras, Directrice générale

TROIS-RIVIÈRES: CSSS de Trois-Rivières
Affiliée à: CIUSSS de la Mauricie et du Centre-du-Québec
731, rue Ste-Julie, Trois-Rivières, QC G9A 1Y1

Tél: 819-370-2100
www.cssstr.qc.ca
Média social: www.facebook.com/csss.trois.rivieres;
www.youtube.com/cssstr

Note: Les Installations (Services de CH, CHSLD, et CLSC): Centre hospitalier affilié universitaire régional (819-697-3333); Centre Cloutier-du Rivage (819-370-2100); Centre St-Joseph (819-370-2100); Centre d'hébergement Cooke (819-370-2100); Centre d'hébergement Louis-Denoncourt (819-376-2566); Centre d'hébergement Roland-Leclerc (819-370-2100); Centre de services Les Forges (819-379-5650); Centre Ste-Geneviève (819-370-2200, poste 46101); Centre de l'Horloge (819-370-2100); Centre Arc-en-Ciel (pédopsychiatrie, 819-374-6291); Centre de prêt d'équipement (819-370-2100)

TROIS-RIVIÈRES: Domremy Mauricie-Centre-du-Québec
440, rue des Forges, Trois-Rivières, QC G9A 2H5

Tél: 819-374-4744
DomremyMCQ@ssss.gouv.qc.ca
www.domremymcq.ca

Fondée en: 1958
Note: Centre de réadaptation des drogues
Nathalie Magnan, Directrice générale

VAL-D'OR: CSSS de la Vallée-de-l'Or (CSSSVO)
Affiliée à: CISSS de l'Abitibi-Témiscamingue
Pavillon Germain-Bigué, 725, 6e rue, Val-d'Or, QC J9P 3Y1

Tél: 819-825-5858 *Téléc:* 819-825-7873
www.cisss-at.gouv.qc.ca
Média social: www.facebook.com/189290301107018

Fondée en: 2004
Nombre de lits: 88 lits (CH); 183 lits (CHSLD)
Population desservi: 43000
Personnel: 1300
Note: Les Installations (Services de CH, CHSLD, et CLSC): Hôpital de Val-d'Or (819-825-5858); Hôpital psychiatrique de Malartic (819-825-5858); Centre d'hébergement de Val-d'Or (819-825-5858); Centre d'hébergement Saint-Martin de Malartic (819-825-5858); CLSC de Val-d'Or (819-825-5858); CLSC de Senneterre (819-825-5858); CLSC de Malartic (819-825-5858); Unité de médecine familiale de la Vallée-de-l'Or (819-825-5858, poste 3549); Clinique externe de psychiatrie (819-825-5858)

VAL-D'OR: Hôpital de Val-d'Or
Affiliée à: CISSS de l'Abitibi-Témiscamingue
725, 6e rue, Val-d'Or, QC J9P 3Y1

Tél: 819-825-5858

Note: Programmes et services comprennent: audiologie; biochimie;

chirurgie générale; gastro-entérologie; médecine nucléaire; néphrologie; pneumologie; réadaptation physique; santé mentale

VERDUN: Centre d'hébergement du Manoir-de-Verdun
Affiliée à: CIUSSS du Centre-Sud-de-l'Ile-de-Montréal
Ancien nom: CHSLD Champlain - Manoir de Verdun
5500, boul Lasalle, Verdun, QC H4H 1N9
Tél: 514-769-8801
www.ciusss-centresudmtl.gouv.qc.ca
Nombre de lits: 225 lits

VICTORIAVILLE: CLSC Suzor-Côté
Affiliée à: CIUSSS de la Mauricie-et-du-Centre-du-Québec
100, rue de l'Ermitage, Victoriaville, QC G6P 9N2
Tél: 819-758-7281 Téléc: 819-758-5009
www.ciusssmcq.ca
Fondée en: 1981

VICTORIAVILLE: CSSS d'Arthabaska-et-de-l'Érable
Affiliée à: CIUSSS de la Mauricie et du Centre-du-Québec
Centre administratif, 5, rue des Hospitalières, Victoriaville, QC G6P 6N2
Tél: 819-357-2030
www.csssae.qc.ca

Note: Les Installations (Services de CH, CHSLD, et CLSC): Hôtel-Dieu d'Arthabaska; CLSC Suzor-Coté; CLSC des Bois-Francs; CLSC de l'Érable; CLSC Saint-Louis; Centre d'hébergement du Chêne; Centre d'hébergement du Roseau; Centre d'hébergement des Étoiles-d'Or; Centre d'hébergement du Sacré-Coeur; Centre d'hébergement des Quatre-Vents; Centre d'hébergement des Bois-Francs; Centre d'hébergement de Saint-Eusèbe; Centre d'hébergement du Tilleul

VICTORIAVILLE: Hôtel-Dieu d'Arthabaska
Affiliée à: CIUSSS de la Mauricie-et-du-Centre-du-Québec
5, rue des Hospitalières, Victoriaville, QC G6P 6N2
Tél: 819-357-2030
www.ciusssmcq.ca
Nombre de lits: 178 lits de santé physique; 21 lits de psychiatrie

VILLE-MARIE: CSSS du Témiscamingue (CSSST)
Affiliée à: CISSS de l'Abitibi-Témiscamingue
Ancien nom: CSSS du Lac-Témiscamingue; CSSS de Témiscaming-et-de-Kipawa
Services administratifs, 22, rue Notre-Dame Nord, Ville-Marie, QC J9V 1W8
Tél: 819-629-2420 Téléc: 819-629-3257
www.cisss-at.gouv.qc.ca
Fondée en: 2011
Population desservi: 17000
Personnel: 600
Note: Les Installations (Services de CH, CHSLD, et CLSC): Pavillon Sainte-Famille (CH et CLSC); Pavillon Témiscaming-Kipawa (CH, CLSC, et CHSLD); Pavillon Duhamel (CHSLD). Points de services: Angliers; Laforce; Latulipe; Moffet; Nédélec; Notre-Dame-du-Nord; Rémigny

VILLE-MARIE: Hôpital de Ville-Marie
Affiliée à: CISSS de l'Abitibi-Témiscamingue
22, rue Notre-Dame Nord, Ville-Marie, QC J9V 1W8
Tél: 819-629-2420

WAKEFIELD: CSSS des Collines
Affiliée à: CISSS de l'Outaouais
101, ch Burnside, Wakefield, QC J0X 3G0
Tél: 819-459-1112 Téléc: 819-459-1894
www.santedescollines.qc.ca

Note: Les Installations (Services de CH, CHSLD, et CLSC): L'Hôpital Mémorial de Wakefield; Le Centre d'hébergement La Pêche; Le CLSC des Collines (Cantley, Chelsea, Masham, Val-des-Monts). Les Municipalités: Cantley; Chelsea; La Pêche; Val-des-Monts (excluant le secteur Poltimore)
André Désilets, Directeur général

WAKEFIELD: Hôpital Mémorial de Wakefield
Affiliée à: CISSS de l'Outaouais
101, ch Burnside, Wakefield, QC J0X 3G0
Tél: 819-459-1112 Téléc: 819-459-1894
Ligne sans frais: 877-459-1112
Nombre de lits: 16 lits

WEEDON: CSSS du Haut-Saint-François
Affiliée à: CIUSSS de l'Estrie
460, 2e av, Weedon, QC J0B 3J0
Tél: 819-821-4000 Téléc: 819-877-3714
www.santeestrie.qc.ca
Région desservi: MRC du Haut-Saint-François (14 municipalités)
Note: Les Installations (Services de CH, CHSLD, et CLSC): Centre d'hébergement d'East Angus (819-832-2487); Centre d'hébergement de Weedon (819-877-2500); CLSC de Weedon (819-877-3434); CLSC de Cookshire (819-875-3373); CLSC de La Patrie (819-888-2811); CLSC d'East Angus (819-832-4961)

WINDSOR: CSSS du Val-Saint-François
Affiliée à: CIUSSS de l'Estrie
Centre administratif, 79, rue Allen, Windsor, QC J1S 2P8
Tél: 819-542-2777
www.santeestrie.qc.ca
Média social: twitter.com/csssvsf; www.linkedin.com/company/1149395

Note: Les Installations (Services de CH, CHSLD, et CLSC): CLSC - Urgence mineure de Windsor; CLSC de Richmond; CLSC de Valcourt; Centre d'hébergement de Windsor; Centre d'hébergement de Richmond; Centre d'hébergement de Valcourt

SASKATCHEWAN

ARBORFIELD: Arborfield & District Health Care Centre
Affiliated with: Kelsey Trail Regional Health Authority
PO Box 160, 5 Ave., Arborfield, SK S0E 0A0
Tel: 306-769-4200 Fax: 306-769-8759
Number of Beds: 36 beds
Note: Programs & services include: clinic; laboratory; day care; health care.

ARCOLA: Arcola Health Centre
Affiliated with: Sun Country Health Region
PO Box 419, 607 Prairie Ave., Arcola, SK S0C 0G0
Tel: 306-455-2771
www.suncountry.sk.ca
Number of Beds: 12 acute care beds
Note: Programs & services include: Telehealth; palliative care; mental health services; & acute care services.
Enoch Pambour, Contact

ASSINIBOIA: Assiniboia Union Hospital
Affiliated with: Five Hills Health Region
501 - 6 Ave., Assiniboia, SK S0H 0B0
Tel: 306-642-9400
Info Line: 306-642-9444
Number of Beds: 22 long term care beds; 12 acute care beds; 4 respite/palliative care beds
Note: Programs & services include: emergency services; acute care; laboratory; respite care; & palliative care.

BALCARRES: Balcarres Integrated Care Centre
Affiliated with: Regina Qu'Appelle Health Region
PO Box 340, 100 South Elgin St., Balcarres, SK S0G 0C0
Tel: 306-334-6260 Fax: 306-334-2865
Year Founded: 1999
Number of Beds: 44 beds
Note: Programs & services include: addictions counselling; dietitian; electrocardiogram; laboratory; long-term care; mental health therapist; outpatient/ambulatory care; physical therapy; physician & nurse practitioner; & x-ray.

BEAUVAL: Beauval Health Centre
Affiliated with: Keewatin Yatthé Regional Health Authority
PO Box 68, Beauval, SK S0M 0G0
Tel: 306-288-4800 Fax: 306-288-2225
Toll-Free: 866-848-8022

Note: Addiction treatments; mental health; dentistry; ambulance.

BEECHY: Beechy Health Centre
Affiliated with: Heartland Regional Health Authority
PO Box 68, 226 - 1st Ave. North, Beechy, SK S0L 0C0
Tel: 306-859-2118 Fax: 306-859-2206

Note: Programs & services include: primary health care; lab/radiology services; visiting community health services: public health, counselling, occupational health, nutrition.

BENGOUGH: Bengough Health Centre
Affiliated with: Sun Country Health Region
PO Box 399, 400 - 2 St. West, Bengough, SK S0C 0K0
Tel: 306-268-2048

Note: Programs & services include: diabetes; home care; palliative care.

BIG RIVER: Big River Health Centre
Affiliated with: Prince Albert Parkland Regional Health Authority
220 - 1st Ave. North, Big River, SK S0J 0E0
Tel: 306-469-2220 *Fax:* 303-469-2193
Number of Beds: 34 long-term care beds; 1 interim bed
Note: Programs & services include: chronic disease management; home care; laboratory; mental health; primary health care clinic; public health nursing; special care home; & x-ray.

BIGGAR: Biggar & District Health Centre
Affiliated with: Heartland Regional Health Authority
PO Box 130, 501 - 1 Ave. West, Biggar, SK S0K 0M0
Tel: 306-948-3323
Number of Beds: 53 long term care beds; 13 acute care beds
Note: Services include: acute care; diagnostics; emergency; home care; laboratory; long term care; outpatient; physicians; Telehealth; & x-ray.

BIGGAR: Biggar Home Care Office
Affiliated with: Heartland Regional Health Authority
PO Box 130, Biggar, SK S0K 0M0
Tel: 306-948-3323 *Fax:* 306-948-2011

BIGGAR: Eatonia Home Care Office
Affiliated with: Heartland Regional Health Authority
PO Box 400, 205 - 2 Ave. West, Biggar, SK S0L 0Y0
Tel: 306-967-2985 *Fax:* 306-967-2373

BIRCH HILLS: Birch Hills Health Centre
Affiliated with: Prince Albert Parkland Regional Health Authority
PO Box 578, 3 Wilson St., Birch Hills, SK S0J 0G0
Tel: 306-749-3331 *Fax:* 306-749-2440

BLACK LAKE: Athabasca Health Authority (AHA)
PO Box 124, Black Lake, SK S0J 0H0
Tel: 306-439-2200 *Fax:* 306-439-2212
www.athabascahealth.ca
Info Line: 811

Population Served: 4500
Number of Employees: 82
Note: Provides health care services to the First Nations communities of Black Lake, Fond du Lac, Stony Rapids, Uranium City, Camsell Portage & Hatchet Lake.
Jennifer Conley, Chief Executive Officer
jconley@athabascahealth.ca

BLACK LAKE: Athabasca Health Facility
Affiliated with: Athabasca Health Authority
PO Box 124, 224 Chicken Indian Reserve, Black Lake, SK S0J 0H0
Tel: 306-439-2200 *Fax:* 306-439-2211

Year Founded: 2003
Note: Programs & services include: acute care, birthing services, long term care, emergency & ambulatory care, public health, mental health, addictions therapy, traditional healing, radiology & lab services.

BLACK LAKE: Black Lake Denesuline Health Centre/Nursing Station
Affiliated with: Athabasca Health Authority
PO Box 135, Black Lake, SK S0J 0H0
Tel: 306-284-2020 *Fax:* 306-284-2090

BORDEN: Borden Primary Health Centre
Affiliated with: Saskatoon Health Region
Former Name: Borden Community Health Centre
PO Box 90, 308 Shepard St., Borden, SK S0K 0N0
Tel: 306-997-2110 *Fax:* 306-997-2114

BROADVIEW: Broadview Hospital
Affiliated with: Regina Qu'Appelle Health Region
PO Box 100, 901 Nina St., Broadview, SK S0G 0K0
Tel: 306-696-5500 *Fax:* 306-696-2611

Note: Programs & services include: ambulatory care; emergency; inpatient; laboratory; Native liaison worker; outpatient; palliative care; perinatal/delivery; & x-ray.
Zachary Phillips, Manager

BUFFALO NARROWS: Buffalo Narrows Health Centre
Affiliated with: Keewatin Yatthé Regional Health Authority
PO Box 40, Buffalo Narrows, SK S0M 0J0
Tel: 306-235-5800 *Fax:* 306-235-4500
Toll-Free: 866-848-8011

Note: Programs & services include: pharmacy; mental & public health; long term care; acute care; laboratory.

BUFFALO NARROWS: Keewatin Yatthé Regional Health Authority (KYRHA)
Metis Society Bldg., PO Box 40, Buffalo Narrows, SK S0M 0J0
Tel: 306-235-2220 *Fax:* 306-235-4604
www.kyrha.ca
Info Line: 811
Social Media: www.facebook.com/KeewatinYatthe; twitter.com/KYHealthRegion
Area Served: Northwest Saskatchewan; 1/4 of the province
Number of Employees: 350
Note: In 2017, it was announced that Keewatin Yatthé Regional Health Authority, along with 11 other Saskatchewan health regions, will consolidate to form one provincial health authority.
Tina Rasmussen, Board Chair
Jean-Marc Desmeules, Chief Executive Officer
Edward Harding, Executive Director, Finance & Infrastructure

CABRI: Prairie Health Care Centre
Affiliated with: Cypress Regional Health Authority
PO Box 79, 517 - 1 St. North, Cabri, SK S0N 0J0
Tel: 306-587-2623
Number of Beds: 17 long term care beds; 3 multipurpose beds
Note: Programs & services include: outpatient procedures; lab/x-ray; physiotherapy; respite; speech language pathology

CANOE NARROWS: Canoe Narrows/Lake Health Centre & Nursing Station
Affiliated with: Keewatin Yatthé Regional Health Authority
PO Box 229, Canoe Narrows, SK S0M 0K0
Tel: 306-829-2140 *Fax:* 306-829-4450

CANORA: Canora Hospital
Affiliated with: Sunrise Regional Health Authority
PO Box 749, 1219 Main St., Canora, SK S0A 0L0
Tel: 306-563-5621 *Fax:* 306-563-5571

Year Founded: 1968
Number of Beds: 16 acute care beds
Note: Programs & services include: 24 hour emergency; cardiac; laboratory; medicine; occupational therapy; outpatient; pharmacy; physical therapy; & x-ray.
Jennifer Richardson, Manager, Health Services

CARLYLE: Carlyle Community Health
Affiliated with: Sun Country Health Region
PO Box 670, 206 Railway Ave. East, Carlyle, SK S0C 0R0
Tel: 306-453-6131 *Fax:* 306-453-6799

CARLYLE: Carlyle Medical Clinic
Affiliated with: Sun Country Health Region
PO Box 1090, 214 Main St., Carlyle, SK S0C 0R0
Tel: 306-453-6795 *Fax:* 306-453-6796

Liette Hrabia, Contact

CARROT RIVER: Carrot River Health Centre
Affiliated with: Kelsey Trail Regional Health Authority
PO Box 250, 4101 - 1 Ave. West, Carrot River, SK S0E 0L0
Tel: 306-768-3100 *Fax:* 306-768-3233
Number of Beds: 36 beds(35 long term care bed, 1 respite bed)
Bessie Lefebvre, Director, Health Services

CENTRAL BUTTE: Central Butte Regency Hospital
Affiliated with: Five Hills Health Region
PO Box 40, 601 Canada St., Central Butte, SK S0H 0T0
Tel: 306-796-2190
Number of Beds: 22 long term care beds; 5 alternate level of care beds
Note: Programs & services include acute care & special care home.

CHRISTOPHER LAKE: Little Red Health Centre
Affiliated with: Prince Albert Parkland Health Region
PO Box 330, Christopher Lake, SK S0J 0N0
Tel: 306-982-4294 Fax: 306-982-3672

CLEARWATER RIVER: Clearwater River Dene First Nation Health Centre
Affiliated with: Keewatin Yatthé Regional Health Authority
PO Box 5040, Clearwater River, SK S0M 3H0
Tel: 306-822-2378 Fax: 306-822-2297

CLIMAX: Border Health Centre
Affiliated with: Cypress Regional Health Authority
PO Box 60, 301 - 1 St. West, Climax, SK S0N 0N0
Tel: 306-293-2222
Number of Beds: 4 beds

CORONACH: Coronach Health Centre
Affiliated with: Sun Country Health Region
PO Box 150, 240 South Ave. East, Coronach, SK S0H 0Z0
Tel: 306-267-2022

Note: Programs & services include: diabetes program; dietitian services; home care; palliative care; rehabilitation services; respite care; telehealth; mental health services
Dawn Gold, Contact

CREIGHTON: Creighton Health Centre
Affiliated with: Mamawetan Churchill River Health Region
PO Box 219, 298 - 1st St. East, Creighton, SK S0P 0A0
Tel: 306-688-8620 Fax: 306-688-8629

CUMBERLAND HOUSE: Cumberland House Health Centre
Affiliated with: Kelsey Trail Regional Health Authority
PO Box 8, 2nd Ave., Cumberland House, SK S0E 0S0
Tel: 306-888-2244 Fax: 306-884-2269

CUPAR: Cupar Health Clinic
Affiliated with: Regina Qu'Appelle Health Region
PO Box 100, 217 Stanley St., Cupar, SK S0G 0Y0
Tel: 306-723-4300 Fax: 306-723-4416

Note: Programs & services offered include: lab and x-ray services; system wide admission/discharge department (SWADD).

CUT KNIFE: Cut Knife Health Complex
Affiliated with: Prairie North Health Region
PO Box 220, 102 Dion Ave., Cut Knife, SK S0M 0N0
Tel: 306-398-4718 Fax: 306-398-2206
www.pnrha.ca
Number of Beds: 28 long-term care beds; 2 respite beds; 1 palliative care bed; 2 observation beds
Note: attached Special Care Home

DAVIDSON: Davidson Health Centre
Affiliated with: Heartland Regional Health Authority
PO Box 758, 900 Government Rd., Davidson, SK S0G 1A0
Tel: 306-567-2801 Fax: 306-567-2073
Number of Beds: 38 beds
Number of Employees: 70
Note: Services include: acute care; diagnostics; emergency; home care; laboratory; long-term care; outpatient; physicians; public health nurse; Telehealth; & x-ray.

DAVIDSON: Davidson Home Care Office
Affiliated with: Heartland Regional Health Authority
PO Box 669, Davidson, SK S0G 1A0
Tel: 306-567-2302 Fax: 306-567-2073

DEBDEN: Big River First Nation Health Centre
Affiliated with: Prince Albert Parkland Health Region
PO Box 160, Debden, SK S0J 0S0
Tel: 306-724-4664 Fax: 306-724-4555

DELISLE: Delisle Primary Health Centre
Affiliated with: Saskatoon Health Region
PO Box 119, 305 - 1 St. West, Delisle, SK S0L 0P0
Tel: 306-493-2810 Fax: 306-493-2812

DILLON: Buffalo River Health Centre
Affiliated with: Keewatin Yatthé Regional Health Authority
PO Box 130, Dillon, SK S0M 0S0
Tel: 306-282-2132 Fax: 306-282-2117

DINSMORE: Dinsmore Health Care Centre
Affiliated with: Heartland Regional Health Authority
PO Box 219, 207 - 1st St. East, Dinsmore, SK S0L 0T0
Tel: 306-846-2222 Fax: 306-846-2225

Population Served: 375
Note: Programs & services include: long term care; visiting care services include physiotherapy, occupational therapy, mental health consultation, nutrition, child health.

DODSLAND: Dodsland Clinic
Former Name: Dodsland Health Centre
4 Ave., Dodsland, SK S0L 0V0
Tel: 306-356-2104

Note: Community-owned clinic

EASTEND: Eastend Wolf Willow Health Centre
Affiliated with: Cypress Regional Health Authority
PO Box 490, 555 Redcoat Dr., Eastend, SK S0N 0T0
Tel: 306-295-3534
Number of Beds: 25 beds (23 long term care, 2 multipurpose)
Note: Programs & services include: lab/x-ray; mental health programs; physiotherapy; long term care; palliative beds; respite care.

EATONIA: Eatonia Health Centre
Affiliated with: Heartland Regional Health Authority
PO Box 400, 205 - 2nd Ave. West, Eatonia, SK S0L 0Y0
Tel: 306-967-2591 Fax: 306-967-2373

Note: Programs & services include: physician services; wellness program; lab/radiology; home care services; emergency services; occupational therapy; pharmacy deliveries.

EDAM: Lady Minto Health Care Centre
Affiliated with: Prairie North Health Region
PO Box 330, Edam, SK S0M 0V0
Tel: 306-397-5560 Fax: 306-397-2225
Number of Beds: 14 long-term care beds; 3 respite beds; 2 convalescent beds; 1 palliative bed
Note: Programs & services include: laboratory/diagnostic imaging; home care; addictions; family counseling; occupational therapy.

ELROSE: Elrose Health Centre
Affiliated with: Heartland Regional Health Authority
PO Box 100, 505 Main St., Elrose, SK S0L 0Z0
Tel: 306-378-2882 Fax: 306-378-2812

Note: Programs & services include: long term care; respite/palliative & convalescent.

ESTERHAZY: Esterhazy Home Care Office
Affiliated with: Sunrise Regional Health Authority
PO Box 1570, 216 Ancona St., Esterhazy, SK S0A 0X0
Tel: 306-745-6700 Fax: 306-745-3206

ESTERHAZY: Esterhazy Public Health Office
Affiliated with: Sunrise Regional Health Authority
PO Box 849, 216 Ancona St., Esterhazy, SK S0A 0X0
Tel: 306-745-3200 Fax: 306-745-3207

ESTERHAZY: St. Anthony's Hospital
Affiliated with: Sunrise Regional Health Authority
PO Box 280, 216 Ancona St., Esterhazy, SK S0A 0X0
Tel: 306-745-3973 Fax: 306-745-3245
Year Founded: 1940
Number of Beds: 14 acute care beds
Note: Services include: 24 hour emergency; dietitian; laboratory; medicine; outpatient; pastoral care; & x-ray.

ESTEVAN: St. Joseph's Hospital
Affiliated with: Sun Country Health Region
1176 Nicholson Rd., Estevan, SK S4A 0H3
Tel: 306-637-2400
stjosephsestevan.ca

Note: Programs & services include: adult day program; diagnostic; dialysis; emergency; endoscopy; intensive care; laboratory; long term care; medical unit; & pharmacy.
Greg Hoffort, Executive Director
  greg.hoffort@schr.sk.ca

ESTON: Eston Health Centre
Affiliated with: Heartland Regional Health Authority
PO Box 667, 800 Main St., Eston, SK S0L 1A0
Tel: 306-962-3667 Fax: 306-962-3900

ESTON: Eston Home Care Office
Affiliated with: Heartland Regional Health Authority
PO Box 667, 822 Main St., Eston, SK S0L 1A0
Tel: 306-962-3215

FILLMORE: Fillmore Health Centre
Affiliated with: Sun Country Health Region
PO Box 246, 100 Main St., Fillmore, SK S0G 1N0
Tel: 306-722-3315

Note: Programs & services include: ambulartory servicing; diabetes program; home care; palliative care; public health inspection
Linda Wilson, Contact

FOAM LAKE: Foam Lake Health Centre
Affiliated with: Sunrise Regional Health Authority
PO Box 190, 715 Saskatchewan Ave. East, Foam Lake, SK S0A 1A0
Tel: 306-272-3325 Fax: 306-272-4449

FOND DU LAC: Fond du Lac Denesuline Health Centre/Nursing Station
Affiliated with: Athabasca Health Authority
PO Box 213, Fond du Lac, SK S0J 0W0
Tel: 306-686-2003 Fax: 306-686-2145

FORT QU'APPELLE: All Nations' Healing Hospital (ANHH)
Affiliated with: Regina Qu'Appelle Health Region
PO Box 300, 450 - 8th St., Fort Qu'Appelle, SK S0G 1S0
Tel: 306-332-5611 Fax: 306-332-5033
www.rqhealth.ca

Number of Beds: 14 acute care beds
Population Served: 2500
Note: Hospital Specialties: First Nations health services; acute care; emergency services; women's health; palliative care; laboratory; & radiology.
Lorna Breitkreuz, Director, Client Services

FORT QU'APPELLE: Fort Qu'Appelle Community Health Services Centre
Affiliated with: Regina Qu'Appelle Health Region
178 Boundary Ave. North, Fort Qu'Appelle, SK S0G 1S0
Tel: 306-332-3300

GAINSBOROUGH: Gainsborough & Area Health Centre
Affiliated with: Sun Country Health Region
PO Box 420, 312 Stephens St., Gainsborough, SK S0C 0Z0
Tel: 306-685-2277

Note: Programs & services include: telehealth; palliative care; respite care; long term care; home care; diabetes edcation program; convalescent care
Donna Davis, Contact

GOODSOIL: L. Gervais Memorial Health Centre
Affiliated with: Prairie North Health Region
PO Box 100, Main St., Goodsoil, SK S0M 1A0
Tel: 306-238-2100 Fax: 306-238-4449
www.pnrha.ca

Number of Beds: 12 long-term care beds; 2 respite beds; 4 convalescent/palliative beds
Note: Health centre with a nursing home & attached special care home. Services include diagonistic imaging/laboratory; ambulatory services; home care; occupational therapy

GRAVELBOURG: St. Joseph's Hospital/Foyer d'Youville
Affiliated with: Five Hills Health Region
PO Box 810, 216 Bettez St., Gravelbourg, SK S0H 1X0
Tel: 306-648-3185 Fax: 306-648-3440
Number of Beds: 9 acute care beds; 49 long term care beds; 1 respite/palliative/convalescent bed
Number of Employees: 110
Note: Services include: acute care; diagnostics; emergency; long term care; palliative/respite care; occupational therapy; & physiotherapy.
Patricia MacEwan, CEO

GREEN LAKE: Green Lake Health Centre
Affiliated with: Keewatin Yatthé Regional Health Authority
PO Box 29, Green Lake, SK S0M 1B0
Tel: 306-832-6257 Toll-Free: 877-800-0002

GRENFELL: Grenfell Health Centre
Affiliated with: Regina Qu'Appelle Health Region
PO Box 243, 721 Stella St., Grenfell, SK S0G 2B0
Tel: 306-697-2853 Fax: 306-697-3459

Note: Programs & services include: laboratory and x-ray services; public and mental health programs; addiction; nutrition; community therapy

GULL LAKE: Gull Lake Special Care Centre
Affiliated with: Cypress Regional Health Authority
PO Box 539, 751 Grey St., Gull Lake, SK S0N 1A0
Tel: 306-672-4700

Number of Beds: 36 beds
Note: Programs & services include lab/x-ray; child and youth counselling; dietitian; physiotherapy; day program; home care; palliative care; respite care.

HAFFORD: Hafford Special Care Centre
Affiliated with: Prince Albert Parkland Regional Health Authority
PO Box 130, 213 South Ave. East, Hafford, SK S0J 1A0
Tel: 306-549-2108 Fax: 306-549-2104
Number of Beds: 22 long-term care beds; 2 interim beds
Note: Services include: day programs; respite care; & rehabilitation services.
Doreen Madwid, Facility Manager
  dmadwid@paphr.sk.ca

HERBERT: Herbert & District Integrated Health Facility
Affiliated with: Cypress Regional Health Authority
PO Box 520, 405 Herbert Ave., Herbert, SK S0H 2A0
Tel: 306-784-2466
Number of Beds: 36 long term care beds; 6 acute care beds; 2 multipurpose beds
Note: Programs & services include: acute care; addictions; child & youth counsellor; dietitian; emergency; home care; laboratory; long-term care; mental health; outpatient procedures; palliative care; physiotherapy; public health nurse; respite care; speech language pathology; & x-ray.

HODGEVILLE: Hodgeville Health Centre
Affiliated with: Cypress Regional Health Authority
PO Box 232, 105 Main St., Hodgeville, SK S0H 2B0
Tel: 306-677-2292

HUDSON BAY: Hudson Bay Health Care Facility
Affiliated with: Kelsey Trail Regional Health Authority
PO Box 940, 614 Prince St., Hudson Bay, SK S0E 0Y0
Tel: 306-865-5600 Fax: 306-865-2429
Number of Beds: 20 long term care beds; 2 respite care beds
Note: Programs & services include: 24 hour emergency outpatient care; ambulance; acute care; day care; laboratory; mental health; palliative care; primary health care; radiology; & Telehealth.

HUMBOLDT: Humboldt District Health Complex (HDHC)
Affiliated with: Saskatoon Health Region
Former Name: St. Elizabeth's Hospital
PO Box 10, 515 - 14th Ave., Humboldt, SK S0K 2A0
Tel: 306-682-2603
www.saskatoonhealthregion.ca

Year Founded: 2011
Note: Programs & services include: home care; mental health; addiction services; laboratory/x-ray; & therapy.

HUMBOLDT: Humboldt Public Health Office
Affiliated with: Saskatoon Health Region
PO Box 1930, 515 - 14th Ave., Humboldt, SK S0K 2A0
Tel: 306-682-2626 *Toll-Free:* 855-613-8205

ILE-A-LA-CROSSE: St. Joseph's Hospital
Affiliated with: Keewatin Yatthé Regional Health Authority
PO Box 500, Ile-a-la-Crosse, SK S0M 1C0
Tel: 306-833-2016 *Fax:* 306-833-2556

Note: Services include: acute care; dental therapy; emergency care; home care; inpatient social detox; laboratory; long-term care; mental health; physical therapy; physician; public health clinic; & x-ray.

IMPERIAL: Long Lake Valley Integrated Facility
Affiliated with: Regina Qu'Appelle Health Region
PO Box 180, Imperial, SK S0G 2J0
Tel: 306-963-2210 *Fax:* 306-963-2518
Year Founded: 1992
Number of Beds: 15 long term care beds; 3 respite or palliative beds
Note: Programs & services include: short-term & long-term care; Respite & day care services; well baby clinics; foot care clinics; outreach programs; education programs

INDIAN HEAD: Indian Head Union Hospital
Affiliated with: Regina Qu'Appelle Health Region
PO Box 340, 300 Hospital St., Indian Head, SK S0G 2K0
Tel: 306-695-4000 *Fax:* 306-695-4002

Note: Services include: ambulatory care; emergency; inpatient services; & outpatient services.

INVERMAY: Invermay Health Centre
Affiliated with: Sunrise Regional Health Authority
PO Box 160, 303 - 4 Ave. North, Invermay, SK S0A 1M0
Tel: 306-593-2133 *Fax:* 306-593-4566
www.sunrisehealthregion.sk.ca
Number of Beds: 26 beds (24 long term care beds, 2 respite beds)
Note: Programs & services include child and youth worker; drug and alcohol programs; visiting occupational therapy; behaviour management; public health office; adult day wellness program

ITUNA: Ituna Home Care Office
Affiliated with: Sunrise Regional Health Authority
PO Box 130, 320 - 5 Ave. NE, Ituna, SK S0A 1N0
Tel: 306-795-2911 *Fax:* 306-795-3592

ITUNA: Ituna Pioneer Health Care Centre
Affiliated with: Sunrise Regional Health Authority
PO Box 130, 320 - 5 Ave. East, Ituna, SK S0A 1N0
Tel: 306-795-2471 *Fax:* 306-795-3592
Number of Beds: 38 beds (35 long term care beds, 2 respite beds, 1 transition bed)
Note: Programs & services include adult day programs.

JAMES SMITH: James Smith Health Centre
Affiliated with: Prince Albert Parkland Health Region
PO Box 506, James Smith, SK S0J 1H0
Tel: 306-864-2454 *Fax:* 306-864-2536

KAMSACK: Kamsack Home Care Office
Affiliated with: Sunrise Regional Health Authority
PO Box 1053, 341 Stewart St., Kamsack, SK S0A 1S0
Tel: 306-542-2212 *Fax:* 306-542-3902

KAMSACK: Kamsack Hospital/Kamsack Nursing Home
Affiliated with: Sunrise Regional Health Authority
PO Box 429, 341 Stewart St., Kamsack, SK S0A 1S0
Tel: 306-542-2635 *Fax:* 306-542-4360
Number of Beds: 20 acute care beds; 61 long-term care beds; 2 respite beds
Note: Services include: 24 hour emergency; cardiac services; intensive care; laboratory; medicine; outpatient services; pediatrics; pharmacy; physiotherapy; & x-ray.

KAMSACK: Kamsack Public Health Office
Affiliated with: Sunrise Regional Health Authority
PO Box 218, 359 Queen Elizabeth Blvd., Kamsack, SK S0A 1S0
Tel: 306-542-4295 *Fax:* 306-542-2995

KELVINGTON: Kelvington & Area Hospital
Affiliated with: Kelsey Trail Regional Health Authority
PO Box 70, 701 - 6th Ave. West, Kelvington, SK S0A 1W0
Tel: 306-327-5500 *Fax:* 306-327-5115
www.kelseytrailhealth.ca

Note: Services include: 24 hour emergency outpatient care; inpatient acute care; laboratory; palliative care; radiology; & Telehealth.
Karri Franklin, Facility Administrator

KERROBERT: Kerrobert Health Centre
Affiliated with: Heartland Regional Health Authority
PO Box 350, 365 Alberta Ave., Kerrobert, SK S0L 1R0
Tel: 306-834-2646 *Fax:* 306-834-1004
Year Founded: 1959
Number of Beds: 47 beds

KERROBERT: Kerrobert Home Care Office
Affiliated with: Heartland Regional Health Authority
PO Box 320, 365 Alberta Ave., Kerrobert, SK S0L 1R0
Tel: 306-834-2646 *Fax:* 306-834-1007

KINCAID: Kincaid Wellness Centre
Affiliated with: Five Hills Regional Health Authority
PO Box 179, Kincaid, SK S0H 2J0
Tel: 306-264-3233 *Fax:* 306-264-3878
www.fhhr.ca/Kincaid.htm

KINDERSLEY: Kindersley & District Health Centre
Affiliated with: Heartland Regional Health Authority
1003 - 1 St. West, Kindersley, SK S0L 1S2
Tel: 306-463-1000
Number of Beds: 21 acute care beds; 77 long-term care beds; 7 alternate level of care beds
Note: Long term care; acute care.

KINDERSLEY: Kindersley Home Care Office
Affiliated with: Heartland Regional Health Authority
1003 - 1 St. West, Kindersley, SK S0L 1S2
Tel: 306-463-1000 *Fax:* 306-463-4550

KINISTINO: Kinistino Medical Clinic
Affiliated with: Prince Albert Parkland Regional Health Authority
PO Box 100, 401 Meyers Ave., Kinistino, SK S0J 1H0
Tel: 306-864-2212 *Fax:* 306-864-3220

KIPLING: Kipling Community Health
Affiliated with: Sun Country Health Region
PO Box 480, 602 Main St., Kipling, SK S0G 2S0
Tel: 306-736-2522 *Fax:* 306-736-2300

KIPLING: Kipling Integrated Health Centre
Affiliated with: Sun Country Health Region
PO Box 420, 906 Industrial Dr., Kipling, SK S0G 2S0
Tel: 306-736-2552
Number of Beds: 32 long-term care beds; 12 acute care beds; 1 respite bed
Note: Programs & services include: diabetes program; dietitian services; respite care; rehabilitation; palliative care; & Telehealth.
Kelly Beattie, Contact

KYLE: Kyle & District Health Centre
Affiliated with: Heartland Regional Health Authority
PO Box 70, 208 - 3 Ave. East, Kyle, SK S0L 1T0
Tel: 306-375-2251 *Fax:* 306-375-2422

KYLE: Kyle Home Care Office
Affiliated with: Heartland Regional Health Authority
PO Box 68, Kyle, SK S0L 1T0
Tel: 306-375-2400 *Fax:* 306-375-2422

LA LOCHE: La Loche Health Centre
Affiliated with: Keewatin Yatthé Regional Health Authority
Bag Service 1, La Loche, SK S0M 1G0
Tel: 306-822-3200 *Fax:* 306-822-2274
Toll-Free: 888-688-7087

Note: Services include: acute care; dental therapy; emergency; home care; inpatient social detox; laboratory; long-term care; medical health clinic; mental health & addictions; physical therapy; physician; public health clinic; & x-ray.

LA RONGE: Mamawetan Churchill River Health Region
PO Box 6000, La Ronge, SK S0J 1L0
Tel: 306-425-2422 *Fax:* 306-425-5513
www.mcrhealth.ca
Info Line: 811
Social Media: www.facebook.com/MCRHealth;
twitter.com/MCR_Health

Year Founded: 2002
Area Served: Northeastern Saskatchewan; 25% of the province
Population Served: 24442
Number of Employees: 300
Note: Operates facilities in the following communities: Creighton, La Ronge, Pinehouse, Sandy Bay & Weyakwin. In 2017, it was announced that Mamawetan Churchill River Health Region, along with 11 other Saskatchewan health regions, will consolidate to form one provincial health authority.
Ron Woytowich, Board Chair
Andrew McLetchie, Chief Executive Officer

LA RONGE: La Ronge Health Centre
Affiliated with: Mamawetan Churchill River Health Region
PO Box 6000, 227 Backlund St., La Ronge, SK S0J 1L0
Tel: 306-425-2422 *Fax:* 306-425-5513

LAFLECHE: LaFleche & District Health Centre
Affiliated with: Five Hills Regional Health Authority
PO Box 159, 315 Main St., Lafleche, SK S0H 2K0
Tel: 306-472-5230
www.fhhr.ca/Lafleche.htm

Number of Beds: 16 beds

LAMPMAN: Lampman Community Health Centre
Affiliated with: Sun Country Health Region
PO Box 100, 309 - 2 Ave. East, Lampman, SK S0C 1N0
Tel: 306-487-2561

Note: Programs & services include: dietitian services; ambulartory services; home care; meergency medical services; palliative care; respite care
Cyndee Hoium, Contact

LANGENBURG: Langenburg Health Care Complex
Affiliated with: Sunrise Regional Health Authority
PO Box 370, 200 Heritage Dr., Langenburg, SK S0A 2A0
Tel: 306-743-2661 *Fax:* 306-743-5025

LANGENBURG: Langenburg Home Care Office
Affiliated with: Sunrise Regional Health Authority
PO Box 370, 200 Heritage Dr., Langenburg, SK S0A 2A0
Tel: 306-743-5005 *Fax:* 306-743-2844

LANGENBURG: Langenburg Public Health Office
Affiliated with: Sunrise Regional Health Authority
PO Box 160, 200 Heritage Dr., Langenburg, SK S0A 2A0
Tel: 306-743-2801 *Fax:* 306-743-2899

LANIGAN: Lanigan Hospital
Affiliated with: Saskatoon Health Region
PO Box 609, 36 Downing St. East, Lanigan, SK S0K 2M0
Tel: 306-365-1400 *Fax:* 306-365-3354
www.saskatoonhealthregion.ca

Year Founded: 1968
Number of Beds: 4 acute care beds; 6 long-term care beds
Number of Employees: 88
Note: Services include: acute care; home care; laboratory; long-term care; mental health & addiction; occupational therapy; physiotherapy; public health; & x-ray.

LEADER: Leader Hospital
Affiliated with: Cypress Regional Health Authority
PO Box 129, 423 Main St., Leader, SK S0N 1H0
Tel: 306-628-3845

Number of Beds: 10 acute/multipurpose beds
Note: Services include: acute care; addictions; dietitian; emergency; home care; laboratory; mental health; outpatient; pharmacy; physiotherapy; podiatry; psychiatry; public health nurse; & x-ray.

LEADER: Leader Primary Health Care Site
Affiliated with: Cypress Regional Health Authority
PO Box 638, 519 Main St. East, Leader, SK S0N 1H0
Tel: 306-628-4584

LEASK: Mistawasis Health Centre
Affiliated with: Prince Albert Parkland Health Region
PO Box 148, Leask, SK S0J 1M0
Tel: 306-466-4507 *Fax:* 306-466-2220

LEOVILLE: Evergreen Health Centre
Affiliated with: Prince Albert Parkland Regional Health Authority
PO Box 160, Leoville, SK S0J 1N0
Tel: 306-984-2136 *Fax:* 306-984-2046

LEOVILLE: Pelican Lake (Chitek) Health Centre
Affiliated with: Prince Albert Parkland Health Region
PO Box 361, Leoville, SK S0J 1N0
Tel: 306-984-4716 *Fax:* 306-984-4728

LEROY: Leroy Community Health & Social Centre
Affiliated with: Saskatoon Health Region
PO Box 7, 211 - 1 Ave. NE, Leroy, SK S0K 2P0
Tel: 306-286-3347 *Fax:* 306-286-3888
www.saskatoonhealthregion.ca

LESTOCK: St. Joseph's Integrated Care Centre
Affiliated with: Regina Qu'Appelle Health Region
PO Box 280, 508 Westmoor St., Lestock, SK S0A 2G0
Tel: 306-274-2300 *Fax:* 306-274-2301

Number of Beds: 10 beds
Note: Services include: adult day care; long-term care; & respite care.

LLOYDMINSTER: Lloydminster & Area Home Care Services
Affiliated with: Prairie North Health Region
3830 - 43 Ave., Lloydminster, SK S9V 1Y3
Tel: 306-820-6200 *Fax:* 306-825-3666

LLOYDMINSTER: Lloydminster & District Co-operative Health Services Ltd.
4808 - 50 St., Lloydminster, SK S9V 0M8
Tel: 306-825-6536

LLOYDMINSTER: Lloydminster Hospital
Affiliated with: Prairie North Health Region
3820 - 43 Ave., Lloydminster, SK S9V 1Y5
Tel: 306-820-6000 *Fax:* 306-825-6516

Note: Services include: community cancer centre; hemodialysis; magnetic resonance imaging; obstetrics; occupational therapy; palliative care; & physical therapy.

LOON LAKE: Loon Lake Health Centre & Special Care Home
Affiliated with: Prairie North Health Region
PO Box 69, 510 - 2nd St., Loon Lake, SK S0M 1L0
Tel: 306-837-2114 *Fax:* 306-837-2268
Number of Beds: 12 long-term care beds; 4 short-term beds; 1 respite bed; 1 palliative bed
Note: Services include: addictions; diagnostic imaging; dietitian; home care; laboratory; medical clinic; occupational therapy; & public health.

LUCKY LAKE: Lucky Lake Health Centre
Affiliated with: Heartland Regional Health Authority
PO Box 250, 1 Ave., Lucky Lake, SK S0L 1Z0
Tel: 306-858-2133 *Fax:* 306-858-2312

MACKLIN: Macklin Home Care Office
Affiliated with: Heartland Regional Health Authority
PO Box 190, Macklin, SK S0L 2C0
Tel: 306-753-3202 *Fax:* 306-753-2181

MACKLIN: St. Joseph's Health Centre
Affiliated with: Heartland Regional Health Authority
PO Box 190, Hwy. 31 North, Macklin, SK S0L 2C0
Tel: 306-753-2115 *Fax:* 306-753-2181

MAIDSTONE: Maidstone Health Complex
Affiliated with: Prairie North Health Region
PO Box 160, 214 - 5th Ave. East, Maidstone, SK S0M 1M0
Tel: 306-893-2622 *Fax:* 306-893-2922
Number of Beds: 11 acute beds; 24 long-term care beds; 2 respite beds
Note: Services include: addictions; ambulance; Collaborative Emergency Centre; diagnostic imaging; dietitian; home care; laboratory; medical clinic; occupational therapy; physiotherapy; & public health.

MARCELIN: Muskeg Lake Health Centre
Affiliated with: Prince Albert Parkland Health Region
PO Box 224, Marcelin, SK S0J 1R0
Tel: 306-466-4914 *Fax:* 306-466-4919

MARYFIELD: Maryfield Health Centre
Affiliated with: Sun Country Health Region
PO Box 164, 233 Main St., Maryfield, SK S0G 3K0
Tel: 306-646-2133

Note: Programs & services include: diabetes program; mental health services; primary health care; palliative care.
Nikki Ford, Contact

MEADOW LAKE: Meadow Lake Community Services
Affiliated with: Prairie North Health Region
#9, 711 Centre St., Meadow Lake, SK S9X 1E6
Tel: 306-236-1570 *Fax:* 306-236-4974

MEADOW LAKE: Meadow Lake Hospital
Affiliated with: Prairie North Health Region
#2, 711 Centre St., Meadow Lake, SK S9X 1E6
Tel: 306-236-1500 *Fax:* 306-236-3244

Note: Services include: acute care; home care; mental health; palliative care; & therapy.

MEADOW LAKE: Northwest Health Facility
Affiliated with: Prairie North Health Region
Also Known As: Meadow Lake Hospital
#2, 711 Centre St., Meadow Lake, SK S9X 1E6
Tel: 306-236-1500 *Fax:* 306-236-3244

Note: Specialty: Acute care; Diagnostic imaging

MELFORT: Melfort Home Care Office
Affiliated with: Kelsey Trail Regional Health Authority
PO Box 1480, 401 Burns Ave. East, Melfort, SK S0E 1A0
Tel: 306-752-1780 *Fax:* 306-752-1786

MELFORT: Melfort Hospital
Affiliated with: Kelsey Trail Regional Health Authority
PO Box 1480, 510 Broadway Ave., Melfort, SK S0E 1A0
Tel: 306-752-8700 *Fax:* 306-752-8711

Note: Programs & services include: 24 hour emergency outpatient care; chemotherapy; endoscopy; general surgery; inpatient acute care; laboratory; labour & delivery; palliative care; radiology; & Telehealth.
Nadine Mevel-Degerness, Facility Administrator

MELFORT: Melfort Public Health Office
Affiliated with: Kelsey Trail Regional Health Authority
PO Box 6500, 107 Crawford Ave. East, Melfort, SK S0E 1A0
Tel: 306-752-6310 *Fax:* 306-752-6353

MELVILLE: Melville Public Health Office
Affiliated with: Sunrise Regional Health Authority
PO Box 62, 200 Heritage Dr., Melville, SK S0A 2P0
Tel: 306-728-7310 *Fax:* 306-728-4925

MELVILLE: Melville/Ituna Home Care Office
Affiliated with: Sunrise Regional Health Authority
PO Box 2348, 200 Heritage Dr., Melville, SK S0A 2P0
Tel: 306-728-7300 *Fax:* 306-728-4925

MELVILLE: St. Peter's Hospital
Affiliated with: Sunrise Regional Health Authority
PO Box 1810, 200 Heritage Dr., Melville, SK S0A 2P0
Tel: 306-728-5407 *Fax:* 306-728-4870

Year Founded: 1942
Number of Beds: 30 acute care beds
Number of Employees: 87
Note: Programs & services include: 24 hour emergency; chemotherapy outreach program; dietitian; endoscopy; laboratory; medicine; outpatient; pastoral care; pharmacy; physiotherapy; social work; & x-ray.
Lisa Alspach, Facility Manager

MELVILLE: Saul Cohen Family Resource Centre
Affiliated with: Sunrise Regional Health Authority
PO Box 164, 200 Heritage Dr., Melville, SK S0A 2P0
Tel: 306-728-7320 *Fax:* 306-728-4925

Note: Outpatient counseling & support individuals & families affected by addictions
Sherry Shumay

MIDALE: Mainprize Manor & Health Centre
Affiliated with: Sun Country Health Region
PO Box 239, 206 South St., Midale, SK S0C 1S0
Tel: 306-458-2300

Note: Programs & service offered: Doctor clinics; Outpatient service; Day respite care; Long-term care
Cyndee Hoium, Contact

MONT NEBO: Ahtahkakoop Health Centre
Affiliated with: Prince Albert Parkland Health Regionty
PO Box 64, Mont Nebo, SK S0J 1X0
Tel: 306-468-2747 *Fax:* 306-468-2967

MONTMARTRE: Montmartre Health Centre
Affiliated with: Regina Qu'Appelle Health Region
PO Box 206, 237 - 2 Ave. East, Montmartre, SK S0G 3M0
Tel: 306-424-2222 *Fax:* 306-424-2227

MOOSE JAW: Crescent View Clinic
Affiliated with: Five Hills Health Region
131A - 1st Ave. NE, Moose Jaw, SK S6H 0Y8
Tel: 306-691-2040

MOOSE JAW: Dr. F.H. Wigmore Regional Hospital
Affiliated with: Five Hills Health Region
55 Diefenbaker Dr., Moose Jaw, SK S6J 0C2
Tel: 306-694-0200
www.fhhr.ca/MooseJawHospital.htm
Number of Beds: 115 beds
Note: Services include: emergency; diagnostics; dialysis; laboratory; mental health outpatient services; patient education; surgery; & therapy.

MOOSE JAW: Five Hills Health Region
55 Diefenbaker Dr., Moose Jaw, SK S6J 0C2
Tel: 306-694-0296 *Fax:* 306-694-0282
Toll-Free: 888-425-1111
inquiries@fhhr.ca
www.fhhr.ca
Info Line: 811

Area Served: South-central Saskatchewan
Population Served: 54000
Number of Employees: 1200
Note: Five Hills Health Region is home to 14 acute care, long term care, wellness, & health facilities. In 2017, it was announced that Five Hills Health Region, along with 11 other Saskatchewan health regions, will consolidate to form one provincial health authority.
Betty Collicott, Board Chair
Cheryl Craig, President & CEO
Dr. Fred Wigmore, Senior Medical Officer
Dr. Mark Vooght, Medical Health Officer
Georgia Hutchinson, Interim Vice-President, Continuing Care
Laurie Albinet, Vice-President, Clinical Services
Jim Allen, Vice-President, Environmental Services
Terry Hutchinson, Vice-President, Community Health Services
Kyle Matthies, Vice-President, People & Quality

MOOSOMIN: Southeast Integrated Care Centre - Moosomin
Affiliated with: Regina Qu'Appelle Health Region
Former Name: Moosomin Union Hospital
601 Wright Rd., Moosomin, SK S0G 3N0
Tel: 306-435-3303 *Fax:* 306-435-3211
Number of Beds: 27 acute care beds; 58 long-term care beds
Note: Services include: acute care; diagnostics; emergency; home care; laboratory; long-term care; mental health; outpatient; physiotherapy; & public health.

MOSSBANK: Mossbank Health Centre
Affiliated with: Five Hills Regional Health Authority
PO Box 322, Mossbank, SK S0H 3G0
Tel: 306-354-2300 *Fax:* 306-354-2819
www.fhhr.ca/Mossbank.htm

MUSKODAY: Muskoday Health Centre
Affiliated with: Prince Albert Parkland Health Region
PO Box 40, Muskoday, SK S0J 3H0
Tel: 306-764-6737 *Fax:* 306-764-4664

NAICAM: Naicam Home Care Office
Affiliated with: Kelsey Trail Regional Health Authority
305 - 1 St. South, Naicam, SK S0K 2Z0
Tel: 306-874-2276

NEILBURG: Manitou Health Centre
Affiliated with: Prairie North Health Region
PO Box 190, 105 - 2nd Ave. West, Neilburg, SK S0M 2C0
Tel: 306-823-4262 *Fax:* 306-823-4590

Note: Programs & services include: laboratory/diagnostic imaging; home care; public health; addictions

NEUDORF: Neudorf Health & Social Centre
410 Main St., Neudorf, SK S0A 2T0
Tel: 306-748-2878

NIPAWIN: Nipawin Hospital
Affiliated with: Kelsey Trail Regional Health Authority
PO Box 389, 800 - 6 St. East, Nipawin, SK S0E 1E0
Tel: 306-862-6100 *Fax:* 306-862-9310
www.kelseytrailhealth.ca

Note: Programs & services include: 24 hour emergency outpatient care; chemotherapy; endoscopy; general surgery; inpatient acute care; laboratory; labour & delivery; palliative care; pediatrician; radiology; & Telehealth.
Linda Brothwell, Facility Administrator

NIPAWIN: Nipawin Public Health Office
Affiliated with: Kelsey Trail Regional Health Authority
PO Box 389, 210 - 2 St. West, Nipawin, SK S0E 1E0
Tel: 306-862-7230 *Fax:* 306-862-0763

NOKOMIS: Nokomis Health Centre
Affiliated with: Saskatoon Health Region
PO Box 98, 103 - 2 Ave. East, Nokomis, SK S0G 3R0
Tel: 306-528-2114 *Fax:* 306-528-4445
Number of Beds: 14 beds

NORQUAY: Norquay Health Centre
Affiliated with: Sunrise Regional Health Authority
PO Box 190, Norquay, SK S0A 2V0
Tel: 306-594-2133 *Fax:* 306-594-2488
Number of Beds: 30 long term care beds; 2 respite beds
Note: Programs & services include: laboratory/diagnostic imaging; home care; public health; addictions. Palliative care beds provided as needed.

NORQUAY: Norquay Home Care Office
Affiliated with: Sunrise Regional Health Authority
PO Box 535, 355 East Rd. Allowance South, Norquay, SK S0A 2V0
Tel: 306-594-2277 *Fax:* 306-594-2220

NORTH BATTLEFORD: Battlefords Union Hospital
Affiliated with: Prairie North Health Region
1092 - 107 St., North Battleford, SK S9A 1Z1
Tel: 306-446-6600 *Fax:* 306-446-6561

Note: Services include: acute care; diagnostic imaging; dialysis; & laboratory.

NORTH BATTLEFORD: Prairie North Health Region (PNHR)
Battlefords Union Hospital, 1092 - 107 St., North Battleford, SK S9A 1Z1
Tel: 306-446-6606
www.pnrha.ca
Info Line: 811

Area Served: Northwest part of central Saskatchewan
Population Served: 82499
Number of Employees: 3300
Note: In 2017, it was announced that Prairie North Health Region, along with 11 other Saskatchewan health regions, will consolidate to form one provincial health authority.
Bonnie O'Grady, Chair
David Fan, Chief Executive Officer

Derek Miller, Vice-President, Finance & Operations
Irene Denis, Vice-President, People, Strategy & Performance
Gloria King, Vice-President, Integrated Health Services
Vikki Smart, Vice-President, Primary Health Services
Dr. Kevin Govender, Co-Senior Medical Officer
Dr. Wilhelm Retief, Co-Senior Medical Officer
Dr. Gavin Van de Venter, Co-Senior Medical Officer

NORTH BATTLEFORD: Saskatchewan Hospital
Affiliated with: Prairie North Health Region
PO Box 39, North Battleford, SK S9A 2X8
Tel: 306-446-6800 *Fax:* 306-445-5392

Note: psychiatric rehabilitation hospital

OUTLOOK: Outlook & District Health Centre
Affiliated with: Heartland Regional Health Authority
PO Box 369, 500 Semple St., Outlook, SK S0L 2N0
Tel: 306-867-8676

Year Founded: 2008
Number of Beds: 10 acute care beds; 42 long-term care beds; 6 alternate level of care beds
Note: Programs & services include: acute care; diagnostics; dietitian; emergency; foot care; home care; laboratory; long term care; mental health counselling; occupational therapy; outpatient; physicians; physiotherapy; public health; & Telehealth.

OUTLOOK: Outlook Home Care Office
Affiliated with: Heartland Regional Health Authority
PO Box 1100, Outlook, SK S0L 2N0
Tel: 306-867-8676 *Fax:* 306-867-2069

OXBOW: Galloway Health Centre
Affiliated with: Sun Country Health Region
PO Box 268, 917 Tupper St., Oxbow, SK S0C 2B0
Tel: 306-483-2956

Note: Programs & services include: convalescent care; respite care; telehealth.
Caroline Hill, Contact

PANGMAN: Pangman Health Centre
Affiliated with: Sun Country Health Region
PO Box 90, 211 Keeler St., Pangman, SK S0C 2C0
Tel: 306-442-2044

Note: Programs & services include: rehabilitation services; public health inspection; mental health services; diabetes program; ambulance services; home care; palliative care

PARADISE HILL: Paradise Hill Health Centre
Affiliated with: Prairie North Health Region
PO Box 179, Paradise Hill, SK S0M 2G0
Tel: 306-344-2255 *Fax:* 306-344-2277
Number of Beds: No patient/resident care beds
Note: Programs & services include: laboratory; clinic; dietician; addiction treatment.

PATUANAK: English River Health Services
Affiliated with: Keewatin Yatthé Regional Health Authority
PO Box 60, Patuanak, SK S0M 2H0
Tel: 306-396-2072 *Fax:* 306-396-2177

PINEHOUSE: Pinehouse Health Centre
Affiliated with: Mamawetan Churchill River Health Region
PO Box 70, Pinehouse, SK S0J 2B0
Tel: 306-884-5670 *Fax:* 306-884-5699

Note: Programs & services include: public health; health education; primary care; addiction services; mental health services; home care services

PONTEIX: Ponteix Health Centre
Affiliated with: Cypress Regional Health Authority
PO Box 600, 428 - 2 Ave., Ponteix, SK S0N 1Z0
Tel: 306-625-3382 *Fax:* 306-625-3764

Note: Programs & services include: Radiology, Laboratory Services, Home Care, Nutrition, Mental Health, Baby Clinic, Public Health, Foyer St. Joseph Nursing Home, Ambulance Service.

PORCUPINE PLAIN: Porcupine Carragana Hospital
Affiliated with: Kelsey Trail Regional Health Authority
PO Box 70, Windsor Ave., Porcupine Plain, SK S0E 1H0
Tel: 306-278-6262 *Fax:* 306-278-3088
Number of Beds: 3 respite beds
Note: Programs & services include: 24 hour emergency outpatient care; ambulance; home care; inpatient acute care; laboratory; palliative care; radiology; & Telehealth.
Chris Pohl, Facility Administrator

PREECEVILLE: Preeceville & District Health Centre
Affiliated with: Sunrise Regional Health Authority
Former Name: Preeceville Hospital; Preeceville & District Integrated Health Care Facility
PO Box 469, 712 - 7 St. NE, Preeceville, SK S0A 3B0
Tel: 306-547-2102 *Fax:* 306-547-2223
www.sunrisehealthregion.sk.ca
Number of Beds: 10 acute care beds; 38 long-term care beds; 2 respite beds
Note: Programs & services include: dietitian; emergency; laboratory; mental health & addictions; outpatient; pharmacy; physician; physiotherapy; primary health care; Telehealth; & x-ray.
Monica Dutchak, Manager

PREECEVILLE: Preeceville Home Care Office
Affiliated with: Sunrise Regional Health Authority
PO Box 407, 712 - 7 Ave. NW, Preeceville, SK S0A 3B0
Tel: 306-547-4441 *Fax:* 306-547-5514

PREECEVILLE: Preeceville Public Health & Physiotherapy Office
Affiliated with: Sunrise Regional Health Authority
PO Box 466, 239 Highway Ave. East, Preeceville, SK S0A 3B0
Tel: 306-547-2815 *Fax:* 306-547-2092

PRINCE ALBERT: Associate Medical Clinic
Affiliated with: Prince Albert Parkland Health Region
#400, 20 - 14 St. West, Prince Albert, SK S6V 3K8
Tel: 306-764-1513 *Fax:* 306-764-3091

PRINCE ALBERT: Crescent Heights Family Medical Centre
Affiliated with: Prince Albert Parkland Health Region
#114, 2805 - 6 Ave. East, Prince Albert, SK S6V 6Z6
Tel: 306-763-2681 *Fax:* 306-953-1024

PRINCE ALBERT: First Nations & Inuit Health North Service Centre
Affiliated with: Prince Albert Parkland Health Region
PO Box 5000, 3601 - 5 Ave. East, Prince Albert, SK S6V 7V6
Tel: 306-953-8600 *Fax:* 306-953-8566

PRINCE ALBERT: Prince Albert Co-Operative Health Centre
Affiliated with: Prince Albert Parkland Regional Health Authority
110 - 8th St. East, Prince Albert, SK S6V 0V7
Tel: 306-763-6464 *Fax:* 306-763-2101
www.coophealth.com
Year Founded: 1962
Frank Regel, Board Chair
Renee Danylczuk, Executive Director

PRINCE ALBERT: Prince Albert Medical Clinic
Affiliated with: Prince Albert Parkland Health Region
681 - 15th St. West, Prince Albert, SK S6V 7H9
Tel: 306-764-1505 *Fax:* 306-764-7751

PRINCE ALBERT: Prince Albert Parkland Regional Health Authority (PAPHR)
1521 - 6th Ave. West, Prince Albert, SK S6V 5K1
Tel: 306-765-6400 *Fax:* 306-765-6401
www.paphr.ca
Info Line: 811
Social Media: www.facebook.com/paphr; twitter.com/PAParkHealth
Area Served: North central Saskatchewan
Population Served: 82578
Note: In 2017, it was announced that Prince Albert Parkland Regional Health Authority, along with 11 other Saskatchewan health regions, will consolidate to form one provincial health authority.
Brenda Abrametz, Board Chair
Cecile Hunt, President & CEO
Brett Enns, Vice-President, Primary Health Services
Don McKay, Vice-President, Human Resources
Cheryl Elliott, Vice-President, Finance & Corporate Support Services
Carol Gregoryk, Vice-President, Integrated Health Services

Pat Stuart, Vice-President, Clinical Support Services & Quality Performance
Dr. Randy Friesen, Co-Senior Medical Officer
Dr. Cecil Hammond, Co-Senior Medical Officer

PRINCE ALBERT: South Hill Family Practice
Affiliated with: Prince Albert Parkland Health Region
2685 - 2nd Ave. West, Prince Albert, SK S6V 5E3
Tel: 306-922-9570 *Fax:* 306-922-2464

PRINCE ALBERT: Victoria Hospital
Affiliated with: Prince Albert Parkland Regional Health Authority
1200 - 24 St. West, Prince Albert, SK S6V 5T4
Tel: 306-765-6000 *Fax:* 306-763-2871

Note: Services include: ambulatory care; anesthesiology; diagnostic imaging; dialysis; emergency; day surgery; general surgery; inpatient; intensive care; internal medicine; laboratory; obstetrics & gynecology; orthopedics; pediatrics; & psychiatry.

PRINCE ALBERT: West Hill Medical Clinic
Affiliated with: Prince Albert Parkland Health Region
#1A, 2995 - 2nd Ave. West, Prince Albert, SK S6V 5V5
Tel: 306-765-8500 *Fax:* 306-765-8501

QUILL LAKE: Quill Lake Community Health & Social Centre
Affiliated with: Saskatoon Health Region
PO Box 126, Quill Lake, SK S0A 3E0
Tel: 306-383-2266

RADVILLE: Radville Marian Health Centre
Affiliated with: Sun Country Health Region
PO Box 310, 840 Conrad Ave., Radville, SK S0C 0G0
Tel: 306-869-2224
Number of Beds: 25 beds
Note: Programs & services include: palliative care; home care; diabetes program; acute care services.

RADVILLE: Radville Public Health Office
Affiliated with: Sun Country Health Region
PO Box 683, 840 Conrad Ave., Radville, SK S0C 2G0
Tel: 306-869-2555 *Fax:* 306-369-3118
Judy DeRoose, Contact

RAYMORE: Raymore Community Health & Social Centre
Affiliated with: Regina Qu'Appelle Health Region
PO Box 134, 806 - 2 Ave., Raymore, SK S0A 3J0
Tel: 306-746-2231 *Fax:* 306-746-4639
Year Founded: 1981

REDVERS: Redvers Health Centre
Affiliated with: Sun Country Health Region
PO Box 30, 18 Eichhorst St., Redvers, SK S0C 2H0
Tel: 306-452-4004
Number of Beds: 7 acute care beds; 23 long-term care beds; 1 respite/multipurpose bed
Note: Programs & services include: inpatient care; long-term care; & emergency outpatient services.
Polly Godenir, Contact

REGINA: Al Ritchie Health Action Centre
Affiliated with: Regina Qu'Appelle Health Region
325 Victoria Ave., Regina, SK S4N 0P5
Tel: 306-766-7660

Note: Programs & services include: GED exam support services; skills registry; job search support; prenatal nutrition advice; community computer; Dad's Group; family crafts; quit smoking program; seniors' potluck lunch; community kitchen; foot care; primary care nurse (by appt); food bank referrals; video lending library.

REGINA: Four Directions Community Health Centre
Affiliated with: Regina Qu'Appelle Health Region
3510 - 5 Ave., Regina, SK S4T 0M2
Tel: 306-766-7540

REGINA: Meadow Primary Health Care Centre
Affiliated with: Regina Qu'Appelle Health Region
4006 Dewdney Ave., Regina, SK S4T 1A2
Tel: 306-766-6399 *Toll-Free:* 855-766-6399

REGINA: Pasqua Hospital
Affiliated with: Regina Qu'Appelle Health Region
4101 Dewdney Ave., Regina, SK S4T 1A5
Tel: 306-766-2222
www.rqhealth.ca/facilities/pasqua-hospital

REGINA: Regina General Hospital
Affiliated with: Regina Qu'Appelle Health Region
Former Name: Victoria Hospital
1440 - 14 Ave., Regina, SK S4P 0W5
Tel: 306-766-4444
www.rqhealth.ca/facilities/regina-general-hospital
Year Founded: 1901
Note: Offers full-range acute care services; home to the Wasakaw Pisim Native Health Centre, Sleep Disorders Centre, and 50-bed mental health facility

REGINA: Regina Qu'Appelle Health Region (RQHR)
2180 - 23 Ave., Regina, SK S4S 0A5
Tel: 306-766-5100 *Fax:* 306-766-5414
www.rqhealth.ca
Info Line: 811
Social Media: www.facebook.com/ReginaQuAppelleHealthRegion;
twitter.com/rqhealth; www.youtube.com/user/rqhr;
www.linkedin.com/company/regina-qu'appelle-health-region
Area Served: 26,663 sq km
Population Served: 289362
Number of Employees: 11000
Note: In 2017, it was announced that Regina Qu'Appelle Health Region, along with 11 other Saskatchewan health regions, will consolidate to form one provincial health authority.
Dick Carter, Board Chair
Keith Dewar, President & CEO
  keith.dewar@rqhealth.ca
Dr. George Carson, Senior Medical Officer
  george.carson@rqhealth.ca

REGINA BEACH: Regina Beach Primary Health Care Centre
Affiliated with: Regina Qu'Appelle Health Region
410 Centre St., Regina Beach, SK S0G 4C0
Tel: 306-729-3395 *Fax:* 306-729-3395
Toll-Free: 855-766-6399

ROCKGLEN: Grasslands Health Centre
Affiliated with: Five Hills Regional Health Authority
PO Box 219, 1006 Hwy. 2, Rockglen, SK S0H 3R0
Tel: 306-476-2030
www.fhhr.ca
Number of Beds: 17 beds

ROSE VALLEY: Rose Valley Health Centre
Affiliated with: Kelsey Trail Regional Health Authority
PO Box 310, 119 McCallum St., Rose Valley, SK S0E 1M0
Tel: 306-322-2115 *Fax:* 306-322-2037

ROSETOWN: Heartland Regional Health Authority
Also Known As: Heartland Health Region
PO Box 2110, 301 Centennial Dr., Rosetown, SK S0L 2V0
Tel: 306-882-4111 *Fax:* 306-882-1389
Toll-Free: 800-631-7686
heartland@hrha.sk.ca
www.hrha.sk.ca
Info Line: 811
Number of Beds: 481 long term care beds; 82 acute care; 58 program beds
Area Served: West-central Saskatchewan; 41,770 sq km
Population Served: 44256
Note: Facilities in 16 communities, including a district hospital in Kindersley. Services include primary & acute health care, emergency services, telehealth, public health, dental health, counselling, addictions services, occupation therapy, speech & language therapy, nutrition. In 2017, it was announced that Heartland Regional Health Authority, along with 11 other Saskatchewan health regions, will consolidate to form one provincial health authority.
Gayle Riendeau, Interim President & CEO
Stacey Bosch, Vice-President, Corporate Services
Jeannie Munro, Vice-President, Primary Health & Quality Services
Sheila Pajunen, Vice-President, Human Resources
Sheila Pajunen, Vice-President, Human Resources
Dr. Lyle Williams, Senior Medical Officer

Wayne Pierrepont, Director, Environmental Services/Capital Projects

ROSETOWN: Rosetown & District Health Centre
Affiliated with: Heartland Regional Health Authority
PO Box 850, Hwy. 4 North, Rosetown, SK S0L 2V0
Tel: 306-882-2672 *Fax:* 306-882-3335
Year Founded: 1964
Gail Adamowski, Facility Manager

ROSETOWN: Rosetown Home Care Office
Affiliated with: Heartland Regional Health Authority
PO Box 624, Rosetown, SK S0L 2V0
Tel: 306-882-4100 *Fax:* 306-882-4251

ROSTHERN: Rosthern Hospital
Affiliated with: Saskatoon Health Region
2016 - 2 St., Rosthern, SK S0K 3R0
Tel: 306-232-4811
www.saskatoonhealthregion.ca
Year Founded: 1950
Number of Beds: 30 beds
Number of Employees: 60
Note: Acute care facility with six physicians on-staff.

ROSTHERN: Rosthern Public Health Office
Affiliated with: Saskatoon Health Region
PO Box 216, 2014 - 6th St., Rosthern, SK S0K 3R0
Tel: 306-232-6001 *Toll-Free:* 888-301-4636

SANDY BAY: Sandy Bay Health Centre
Affiliated with: Mamawetan Churchill River Health Region
PO Box 210, Sandy Bay, SK S0P 0G0
Tel: 306-754-5400 *Fax:* 306-754-5429
Note: Programs & services include: primary care; public health; health education; telehealth; home care services

SASKATOON: 20th & Q Pediatric Specialists & Family Walk-In
Affiliated with: Saskatoon Health Region
1631 - 20th St. West, Saskatoon, SK S7M 0Z9
Tel: 306-384-9888

SASKATOON: Blairmore Medical Clinic
Affiliated with: Saskatoon Health Region
225 Betts Ave., Saskatoon, SK S7M 1L2
Tel: 306-652-6400

SASKATOON: Children's Hospital of Saskatchewan
Affiliated with: Saskatoon Health Region
c/o Saskatoon Health Region - Royal Univ. Hospital, 103 Hospital Dr., 3rd Fl., Saskatoon, SK S7N 0W8
Tel: 306-655-2293
childrenshospitalsask@saskatoonhealthregion.ca
Social Media: www.facebook.com/childrenhospSK;
twitter.com/childrenhospSK; www.pinterest.com/childrenshospsk
Note: Programs & services include: maternal services; children's sleep lab; children's Hemodialysis

SASKATOON: Idylwyld Centre Public Health Office
Affiliated with: Saskatoon Health Region
#101, 310 Idylwyld Dr. North, Saskatoon, SK S7L 0Z2
Tel: 306-655-4620

SASKATOON: Lakeside Medical Clinic
Affiliated with: Saskatoon Health Region
3919 - 8th St. East, Saskatoon, SK S7H 5M7
Tel: 306-374-6884 *Fax:* 306-374-2552
www.lakeside.ca
Social Media: twitter.com/LMCSaskatoon

SASKATOON: Lenore Medical Clinic
Affiliated with: Saskatoon Health Region
#4, 123 Lenore Dr., Saskatoon, SK S7K 7H9
Tel: 306-242-6700

SASKATOON: MediClinic
Affiliated with: Saskatoon Health Region
#101, 3333 - 8th St. East, Saskatoon, SK S7H 4K1
Tel: 306-955-1530
www.mediclinic-sk.com
Social Media: twitter.com/Mediclinicon8th

Year Founded: 1982

SASKATOON: North East Public Health Office
Affiliated with: Saskatoon Health Region
#108, 407 Ludlow St., Saskatoon, SK S7S 1P3
Tel: 306-655-4700

SASKATOON: Our Neighbourhood Health Centre
Affiliated with: Saskatoon Health Region
1120 - 20th St. West, Saskatoon, SK S7M 0Y8
Tel: 306-655-3250

SASKATOON: Primary Health Centre South East - Scott-Forget Towers
Affiliated with: Saskatoon Health Region
#100, 2501 Louise St., Saskatoon, SK S7J 3M1
Tel: 306-655-4550

SASKATOON: Royal University Hospital
Affiliated with: Saskatoon Health Region
103 Hospital Dr., Saskatoon, SK S7N 0W8
Tel: 306-655-1000
www.saskatoonhealthregion.ca
Year Founded: 1955
Note: Affiliated with the University of Saskatchewan.

SASKATOON: St. Paul's Hospital
Saskatchewan Catholic Health Corporation
Affiliated with: Saskatoon Health Region
1702 - 20 St., Saskatoon, SK S7M 0Z9
Tel: 306-655-5000 *Fax:* 306-655-5900
info@stpaulshospital.org
www.stpaulshospital.org
Jean Morrison, President & CEO

SASKATOON: Saskatoon City Hospital
Affiliated with: Saskatoon Health Region
701 Queen St., Saskatoon, SK S7K 0M7
Tel: 306-655-8000
www.saskatoonhealthregion.ca
Year Founded: 1909

SASKATOON: Saskatoon Community Clinic
Affiliated with: Saskatoon Health Region
455 - 2nd Ave. North, Saskatoon, SK S7K 2C2
Tel: 306-652-0300 *Fax:* 306-664-4120
member.relations@communityclinic.sk.ca
www.saskatooncommunityclinic.ca
Year Founded: 1962
Note: Health services are offered at the Downtown Clinic & the Westside Clinic.
Anne Doucette, President, Board of Directors

SASKATOON: Saskatoon Health Region (SRHA)
Saskatoon City Hospital, Level 1 Administration, 701 Queen St., Saskatoon, SK S7K 0M7
Tel: 306-655-7500
general.inquiries@saskatoonhealthregion.ca
www.saskatoonhealthregion.ca
Info Line: 811
Social Media: www.facebook.com/SaskatoonHealthRegion;
twitter.com/SaskatoonHealth;
www.youtube.com/user/SaskatoonHealthReg
Area Served: 34,120 sq km
Population Served: 350000
Note: The health region serves over 100 regional municipalities, cities, towns, villages, & First Nation communities in Saskatchewan. Facilities include hospitals, long term care facilities, primary health care sites, public health centres, mental health & addictions centres & community-based sites. In 2017, it was announced that Saskatoon Health Region, along with 11 other Saskatchewan health regions, will consolidate to form one provincial health authority.
Mike Stensrud, Board Chair
Dan Florizone, President & CEO
Dr. Cory Neudorf, Chief Medical Health Officer
Jackie Mann, Vice-President, Integrated Health Services
Diane Shendruk, Vice-President, Integrated Health Services
Petrina McGrath, Vice-President, People, Practice & Quality
Nilesh Kavia, Vice-President, Finance & Corporate Services
Dr. George Pylypchuk, Vice-President, Practitioner Staff Affairs

SASKATOON: Saskatoon Minor Emergency Clinic
Affiliated with: Saskatoon Health Region
3110 Laurier Dr., Saskatoon, SK S7L 5J7
Tel: 306-978-2200

SASKATOON: South East Public Health Office
Affiliated with: Saskatoon Health Region
3006 Taylor St. East, Saskatoon, SK S7H 4J2
Tel: 306-655-4730 *Toll-Free:* 855-613-8216

SHAUNAVON: Shaunavon Hospital & Care Centre
Affiliated with: Cypress Regional Health Authority
PO Box 789, 660 - 4 St. East, Shaunavon, SK S0N 2M0
Tel: 306-297-2644 *Fax:* 306-297-1949
Number of Beds: 41 long term care beds; 10 acute/multidisciplinary beds; 3 multipurpose beds
Note: Programs & services include: acute care; addictions program; child & youth counsellor; day program; dietitian; emergency; home care; laboratory; long-term care; mental health; physiotherapy; podiatry; public health nurse; respite care; speech language pathology; & x-ray.

SHELLBROOK: Parkland Integrated Health Centre
Affiliated with: Prince Albert Parkland Regional Health Authority
#100, Dr. J.L. Spencer Dr., Shellbrook, SK S0J 2E0
Tel: 306-747-2603 *Fax:* 306-747-3004
Number of Beds: 20 acute care beds; 34 long-term care beds
Note: Services include: home care; laboratory; mental health; public health; therapy; & x-ray.

SHELLBROOK: Shellbrook Doctors Office
Affiliated with: Prince Albert Parkland Health Region
PO Box 1030, 206 - 2nd Ave. West, Shellbrook, SK S0J 2E0
Tel: 306-747-2552 *Fax:* 306-747-2141

SHELLBROOK: Shellbrook Home Care
Affiliated with: Prince Albert Parkland Health Region
PO Box 70, 211 - 2 Ave. West, Shellbrook, SK S0J 2E0
Tel: 306-747-4266 *Fax:* 306-747-3004

SHELLBROOK: Shellbrook Medical Clinic
Affiliated with: Prince Albert Parkland Health Region
PO Box 504, 208 - 2nd Ave. West, Shellbrook, SK S0J 2E0
Tel: 306-747-2171 *Fax:* 306-747-2173

SMEATON: Smeaton Health Centre
Affiliated with: Kelsey Trail Regional Health Authority
PO Box 158, 2nd Ave. West, Smeaton, SK S0J 2J0
Tel: 306-426-2051 *Fax:* 306-426-2299

SOUTHEY: Southey Health Action Centre
Affiliated with: Regina Qu'Appelle Health Region
PO Box 519, 280 Burns Ave., Southey, SK S0G 4P0
Tel: 306-726-2239 *Fax:* 306-726-4472
Year Founded: 1995

SPALDING: Spalding Community Health Centre
Affiliated with: Saskatoon Health Region
PO Box 220, Spalding, SK S0K 4C0
Tel: 306-872-2011

SPIRITWOOD: Spiritwood & District Health Complex
Affiliated with: Prince Albert Parkland Regional Health Authority
400 1st St. East, Spiritwood, SK S0J 2M0
Tel: 306-883-2133 *Fax:* 306-883-4440
Number of Beds: 43 long-term care beds; 3 respite beds
Note: Services include: addiction services; Collaborative Emergency Centre; home care; laboratory; mental health; primary health care clinic; public health; therapy; & x-ray.

SPIRITWOOD: Spiritwood Home Care
Affiliated with: Prince Albert Parkland Health Region
PO Box 69, 400 - 1 St. East, Spiritwood, SK S0J 2M0
Tel: 306-883-4266 *Fax:* 306-883-4440

SPIRITWOOD: Spiritwood Indian Health Services
Affiliated with: Prince Albert Parkland Health Region
PO Box 579, 100 Railroad Ave. West, Spiritwood, SK S0J 2M0
Tel: 306-883-2905 *Fax:* 306-883-2535

SPIRITWOOD: Spiritwood Medical Clinic
Affiliated with: Prince Albert Parkland Health Region
PO Box 668, Spiritwood, SK S0J 2M0
Tel: 306-883-2140 *Fax:* 306-883-3211

SPIRITWOOD: Witchekan Lake Health Centre
Affiliated with: Prince Albert Parkland Health Region
PO Box 359, Spiritwood, SK S0J 2M0
Tel: 306-883-2552 *Fax:* 306-883-2578

ST WALBURG: St. Walburg Health Complex
Affiliated with: Prairie North Health Region
PO Box 339, 410 - 3rd Ave. West, St Walburg, SK S0M 2T0
Tel: 306-248-6719 *Fax:* 306-248-3413
Number of Beds: 31 beds (28 long term care bed, 1 respite, 1 palliative, 1 convalescent)
Note: Attached special care home. Programs offered include diagnostic imaging; medical clinic services; dietitian; family counseling; mental health programs; physiotherapy; occupational therapy

STRASBOURG: Strasbourg & District Health Centre
Affiliated with: Saskatoon Health Region
303 Edward St., Strasbourg, SK S0G 4V0
Tel: 306-725-3220
Year Founded: 1974
Note: Specialties: Physiotherapy; Counselling; Public health services

STURGEON LAKE: Sturgeon Lake Health Centre
Affiliated with: Prince Albert Parkland Health Region
Comp 5, Site 12, RR#1, Sturgeon Lake, SK S0J 2E0
Tel: 306-764-9352 *Fax:* 306-763-0767

SWIFT CURRENT: Cypress Health Region's Community Health Services
Affiliated with: Cypress Regional Health Authority
350 Cheadle St. West, Swift Current, SK S9H 4G3
Tel: 306-778-5280

SWIFT CURRENT: Cypress Regional Health Authority
Also Known As: Cypress Health Region
429 - 4th Ave. NE, Swift Current, SK S9H 2J9
Tel: 306-778-5100 *Fax:* 306-773-9513
Toll-Free: 888-461-7443
info@cypressrha.ca
www.cypresshealth.ca
Info Line: 811
Social Media: www.facebook.com/cypresshealth;
twitter.com/cypresshealth; www.youtube.com/user/cypresshealthsk
Year Founded: 2002
Area Served: Western Saskatchewan; 44,000 sq km
Population Served: 45394
Number of Employees: 1700
Note: In 2017, it was announced that Cypress Regional Health Authority, along with 11 other Saskatchewan health regions, will consolidate to form one provincial health authority.
Lyle Quintin, Board Chair
Beth Vachon, Chief Executive Officer
Dr. Ivo Radevski, Senior Medical Officer
Beth Adashynski, Vice-President, Performance & Quality
Larry Allsen, CFO & Vice-President, Corporate Services
Bryce Martin, Vice-President, Primary Health Care
Brenda Schwan, Vice-President, Continuing Care
Kim Kruse, Director, Executive & Board Support

SWIFT CURRENT: Cypress Regional Hospital
Affiliated with: Cypress Regional Health Authority
Former Name: Swift Current Regional Hospital
2004 Saskatchewan Dr., Swift Current, SK S9H 5M8
Tel: 306-778-9400
cypresshealth.ca
Year Founded: 1951
Number of Beds: 91 acute care beds
Note: Programs & services include: emergency; general surgery; intensive care; internal medicine; obstetrics & gynecology; pathology; pediatrics; psychiatry; & radiology.

THEODORE: Theodore Health Centre
Affiliated with: Sunrise Regional Health Authority
PO Box 70, 615 Anderson Ave., Theodore, SK S0A 4C0
Tel: 306-647-2115 *Fax:* 306-647-2238
Number of Beds: 19 beds (18 long term care beds, 1 respite/palliative care bed)
Note: Specialties: Long-term care; Nursing services; Phlebotomy service; Respite care; Palliative care

THEODORE: Theodore Public Health Office
Affiliated with: Sunrise Regional Health Authority
PO Box 292, 615 Anderson Ave., Theodore, SK S0A 4C0
Tel: 306-647-2353 *Fax:* 306-647-2238

TISDALE: Kelsey Trail Regional Health Authority
PO Box 1780, Tisdale, SK S0E 1T0
Tel: 306-873-6600 *Fax:* 306-873-2372
tdemarsh@kthr.sk.ca
www.kelseytrailhealth.ca
Info Line: 811
Social Media: www.facebook.com/123342694465;
twitter.com/kelseytrail;
www.linkedin.com/company/kelsey-trail-health-region
Area Served: 44,369.62 sq km
Population Served: 42650
Number of Employees: 1683
Note: In 2017, it was announced that Kelsey Trail Regional Health Authority, along with 11 other Saskatchewan health regions, will consolidate to form one provincial health authority.
Rennie Harper, Board Chair
Shane Merriman, Chief Executive Officer

TISDALE: Tisdale Hospital
Affiliated with: Kelsey Trail Regional Health Authority
PO Box 1630, 2010 - 110th Ave. West, Tisdale, SK S0E 1T0
Tel: 306-873-6500 *Fax:* 306-873-5994
www.kelseytrailhealth.ca

Note: Services include: 24 hour emergency outpatient care; chemotherapy; inpatient acute care; laboratory; labour & delivery; palliative care; radiology; sigmiodoscopy; & Telehealth.
Tracey Farber, Administrator

TISDALE: Tisdale Public Health Office
Affiliated with: Kelsey Trail Regional Health Authority
PO Box 1297, 800 - 1 St. East, Tisdale, SK S0E 1T0
Tel: 306-873-8282 *Fax:* 306-873-2168

TURTLEFORD: Riverside Health Complex
Affiliated with: Prairie North Health Region
PO Box 10, Turtleford, SK S0M 2Y0
Tel: 306-845-2195 *Fax:* 306-845-2772
Number of Beds: 29 beds
Note: Attached special care home

UNITY: Unity & District Health Centre
Affiliated with: Heartland Regional Health Authority
Former Name: Unity Hospital
PO Box 741, Airport Rd., Unity, SK S0K 4L0
Tel: 306-228-2666 *Fax:* 306-228-2292
Year Founded: 2001
Note: Programs & services include: acute care; diagnostic services; maternity services; community health services; public health nursing; mental health services; counselling; physiotherapy; occupational therapy; home care; long-term care; respite care; palliative care
Kim Halter, Facility Manager
Randy Scherr, Supervisor, Plant Maintenance

UNITY: Unity Home Care Office
Affiliated with: Heartland Regional Health Authority
PO Box 1538, Unity, SK S0K 4L0
Tel: 306-228-2666 *Fax:* 306-228-2292

URANIUM CITY: Uranium City Health Centre
Affiliated with: Athabasca Health Authority
PO Box 360, Uranium City, SK S0J 2W0
Tel: 306-498-2412 *Fax:* 306-498-2577

VANGUARD: Vanguard Health Centre
Affiliated with: Cypress Regional Health Authority
PO Box 190, Division St., Vanguard, SK S0N 2V0
Tel: 306-582-2044

WADENA: Wadena Hospital
Affiliated with: Saskatoon Health Region
PO Box 10, 533 - 5 St. NE, Wadena, SK S0A 4J0
Tel: 306-338-2515
www.saskatoonhealthregion.ca
Year Founded: 1967
Number of Beds: 52 beds

Number of Employees: 107
Note: Provides acute, respite, & long-term care services.

WADENA: Wadena Primary Health Team
Affiliated with: Saskatoon Health Region
533 - 5th St. NE, Wadena, SK S0A 4J0
Tel: 306-338-2597

WADENA: Wadena Public Health Office
Affiliated with: Saskatoon Health Region
PO Box 10, 533 - 5 St. NE, Wadena, SK S0A 4J0
Tel: 306-338-2538 *Toll-Free:* 855-338-9994

WAHPETON: Wahpeton Health Centre
Affiliated with: Prince Albert Parkland Health Region
PO Box 128, Wahpeton, SK S6V 5R4
Tel: 306-922-6772 *Fax:* 306-922-6774

WAKAW: Wakaw Health Centre
Affiliated with: Saskatoon Health Region
Former Name: Wakaw Hospital
PO Box 309, 301 - 1 St. North, Wakaw, SK S0K 4P0
Tel: 306-233-4611

Year Founded: 1956
Note: Services include: acute care; diagnostic imaging; home care; laboratory; mental health; & palliative care.

WATROUS: Watrous Hospital
Affiliated with: Saskatoon Health Region
PO Box 130, 702 - 4 St. East, Watrous, SK S0K 4T0
Tel: 306-946-1200
www.saskatoonhealthregion.ca

Note: Services include: acute care; diagnostic imaging; laboratory; public health; & therapy.

WATROUS: Watrous Primary Health Centre
Affiliated with: Saskatoon Health Region
403 Main St., Watrous, SK S0K 4T0
Tel: 306-946-2075

WATROUS: Watrous Public Health Office
Affiliated with: Saskatoon Health Region
PO Box 130, 704 - 4th Ave., Watrous, SK S0K 4T0
Tel: 306-946-2102 *Toll-Free:* 877-817-9336

WATSON: Watson Community Health Centre
Affiliated with: Saskatoon Health Region
PO Box 220, Watson, SK S0K 4V0
Tel: 306-287-3791

WAWOTA: Wawota Memorial Health Centre
Affiliated with: Sun Country Health Region
PO Box 60, 609 Choo Foo Cres., Wawota, SK S0G 5A0
Tel: 306-739-5200
Number of Beds: 29 long-term care beds; 3 respite/multipurpose beds
Note: Programs & services include: child speech language pathology; diabetes program; dietitian; emergency medical services; mental health; occupational therapy; palliative care; & Telehealth.
Holly Hodgson, Contact

WEYAKWIN: Weyakwin Health Centre
Affiliated with: Mamawetan Churchill River Health Region
PO Box 8, Weyakwin, SK S0J 1W0
Tel: 306-663-6100 *Fax:* 306-663-6165

WEYBURN: Sun Country Health Region (SCHR)
808 Souris Valley Rd., Weyburn, SK S4H 2Z9
Tel: 306-842-8339
info@schr.sk.ca
www.suncountry.sk.ca
Info Line: 811

Year Founded: 2002
Area Served: Southeast portion of Saskatchewan; 33,239 sq km
Population Served: 59690
Note: In 2017, it was announced that Sun Country Health Region, along with 11 other Saskatchewan health regions, will consolidate to form one provincial health authority.
Marilyn Charlton, Board Chair
Marga Cugnet, President & CEO
306-842-8718

Dean Biesenthal, Vice-President, Human Resources
306-842-8724
Janice Giroux, Vice-President, Community Health
306-842-8652
Murray Goeres, Interim Vice-President, Health Facilities
306-842-8706
John Knoch, Vice-President, Corporate & Finance
306-842-8714
Dr. Dimitri Louvish, Vice-President, Medical
306-842-8651

WEYBURN: Weyburn Community Health Services
Affiliated with: Sun Country Health Region
PO Box 2003, 900 Saskatchewan Dr., Weyburn, SK S4H 2Z9
Tel: 306-842-8618 *Fax:* 306-842-8637

Note: Programs & services include: mental health services; telehealth.
Janice Giroux, Contact

WEYBURN: Weyburn General Hospital
Affiliated with: Sun Country Health Region
201 - 1 Ave. NE, Weyburn, SK S4H 0N1
Tel: 306-842-8400
Number of Beds: 40 acute care beds
Note: Programs & services include: acute care; addiction services; diabetes education program; mental health services; occupational therapy; palliative care; rehabilitation; & spiritual care.
James Anderson, Contact

WEYBURN: Weyburn Primary Health Care Clinic
Affiliated with: Sun Country Health Region
#204, 117 - 3 St., Weyburn, SK S4H 0W3
Tel: 306-842-8790

WHITEWOOD: Whitewood Community Health Centre
Affiliated with: Regina Qu'Appelle Health Region
PO Box 669, 921 Gambetta St., Whitewood, SK S0G 5C0
Tel: 306-735-2688 *Fax:* 306-735-2512

Specialties: Outpatient / ambulatory care services
Note: Programs & services: public health (306-435-6279); parenting plus (306-697-4048); mental health services for children (306-697-4021); mental health services for adults (306-697-4023); nutrition services (306-697-4037); home care services (306-696-2500).

WILKIE: Wilkie Health Centre
Affiliated with: Heartland Regional Health Authority
PO Box 459, 304 - 7 Ave. East, Wilkie, SK S0K 4W0
Tel: 306-843-2644 *Fax:* 306-843-3222

WILKIE: Wilkie Home Care Office
Affiliated with: Heartland Regional Health Authority
PO Box 459, 304 - 7 St. East, Wilkie, SK S0K 4W0
Tel: 306-843-2644 *Fax:* 306-843-3222

WILLOW BUNCH: Willow Bunch Health Centre
Affiliated with: Five Hills Regional Health Authority
PO Box 6, Willow Bunch, SK S0H 4K0
Tel: 306-473-2310 *Fax:* 306-473-2677
www.fhhr.ca/WillowBunch.htm

WOLSELEY: Wolseley Memorial Integrated Health Centre
Affiliated with: Regina Qu'Appelle Health Region
PO Box 458, 801 Ouimet St., Wolseley, SK S0G 5H0
Tel: 306-698-4440 *Fax:* 306-698-4434

Note: Services include: ambulatory care; laboratory; outpatient; palliative care; & x-ray.

WYNYARD: Wynyard & District Community Health Centre
Affiliated with: Saskatoon Health Region
PO Box 1539, 210 Ave. B East, Wynyard, SK S0A 4T0
Tel: 306-554-3363
Paul Lendzyk, Executive Director

WYNYARD: Wynyard Integrated Facility
Affiliated with: Saskatoon Health Region
PO Box 670, 300 - 10 St. East, Wynyard, SK S0A 4T0
Tel: 306-554-2586
www.saskatoonhealthregion.ca

Number of Beds: 59 beds
Number of Employees: 100
Note: Acute care; long-term care; respite care.
Cheryl Sinclair, Manager, Client Services

YORKTON: Sunrise Health & Wellness Centre
Affiliated with: Sunrise Regional Health Authority
#25, 259 Hamilton Rd., Yorkton, SK S3N 4C6
Tel: 306-786-6363 Fax: 306-786-6364

YORKTON: Sunrise Regional Health Authority
270 Bradbrooke Dr., Yorkton, SK S3N 2K6
Tel: 306-786-0100 Fax: 306-786-0122
Toll-Free: 800-505-9220
www.sunrisehealthregion.sk.ca
Info Line: 811
Social Media: www.facebook.com/sunrisehealthreg;
twitter.com/SunriseRegion

Number of Employees: 2900
Note: Sunrise Health Region stretches from the Qu'Appelle Valley to the northern boreal forest, & from the parklands of the Manitoba border into the Saskatchewan prairie farmlands. In 2017, it was announced that Sunrise Regional Health Authority, along with 11 other Saskatchewan health regions, will consolidate to form one provincial health authority.
Don Rae, Board Chair
Suann Laurent, President & CEO
Dr. Phillip Fourie, Senior Medical Officer & Vice-President, Medical Services
Christina Denysek, Vice-President, Strategy & Partnerships
Lorelei Stusek, Vice-President, Corporate Services

YORKTON: Yorkton Home Care Office
Affiliated with: Sunrise Regional Health Authority
PO Box 5016, 270 Bradbrooke Dr., Yorkton, SK S3N 3Z4
Tel: 306-786-0711 Fax: 306-786-0707

YORKTON: Yorkton Public Health Office
Affiliated with: Sunrise Regional Health Authority
150 Independent St., Yorkton, SK S3N 0S7
Tel: 306-786-0600 Fax: 306-786-0620

YORKTON: Yorkton Regional Health Centre
Affiliated with: Sunrise Regional Health Authority
270 Bradbrooke Dr., Yorkton, SK S3N 2K6
Tel: 306-782-2401 Fax: 306-786-6295
Number of Beds: 87 acute care beds
Note: Services include: 24 hour emergency; diagnostic laboratory; hemodialysis; intensive care; medical imaging; obstetrics; outpatient; pediatrics; pharmacy; respiratory therapy; & social work.

YUKON TERRITORY

BEAVER CREEK: Beaver Creek Health Centre
PO Box 3, Beaver Creek, YT Y0B 1A0
Tel: 867-862-4444 Fax: 867-862-7909

CARMACKS: Carmacks Health Centre
PO Box 230, Carmacks, YT Y0B 1C0
Tel: 867-863-4444 Fax: 867-863-6612
Number of Beds: 2 beds

DAWSON: Dawson City Community Hospital
Yukon Hospital Corporation
Former Name: Dawson City Health Centre
PO Box 870, 501 - 6th Ave., Dawson, YT Y0B 1G0
Tel: 867-993-4444 Fax: 867-993-4317
yukonhospitals.ca/dawson-city-hospital
Number of Beds: 6 beds
Number of Employees: 28
Note: Services offered by the Dawson Community Health Centre & Dawson Medical Clinic are now located within this facility. Programs & services include: ambulatory care; basic diagnostic & lab tests; communicable disease screening; diagnostic imaging; emergency; healthy lifestyle support; hearing services; house calls; immunizations; infant & preschool health exams; inpatient care; mental health services; palliative care; pharmacy; physiotherapy; pre & post-natal education; school health program; third party medical assessments; & travel health education & immunizations.
Jason Bilsky, Chief Executive Officer, Yukon Hospital Corporation

DESTRUCTION BAY: Destruction Bay Health Centre
General Delivery, Destruction Bay, YT Y0B 1H0
Tel: 867-841-4444 Fax: 867-841-5274

FARO: Faro Health Centre
PO Box 99, Faro, YT Y0B 1K0
Tel: 867-994-4444 Fax: 867-994-3457

HAINES JUNCTION: Haines Junction Health Centre
PO Box 5369, Haines Junction, YT Y0B 1L0
Tel: 867-634-4444 Fax: 867-634-2733

MAYO: Mayo Health Centre
PO Box 98, 21 Centre St., Mayo, YT Y0B 1M0
Tel: 867-996-4444 Fax: 867-996-2018

Note: Specialties: Public health services; Health promotion services; Home care services. Number of Employees: 1 doctor + 3 community nurse practitioners

OLD CROW: Old Crow Health Centre
PO Box 92, Old Crow, YT Y0B 1N0
Tel: 867-996-4444 Fax: 867-966-3614
www.oldcrow.ca/nursing
Year Founded: 1960
Number of Employees: 4
Note: Specialties: Nursing care; Health promotion; Home & community care

PELLY CROSSING: Pelly Crossing Health Centre
PO Box 20, Pelly Crossing, YT Y0B 1P0
Tel: 867-537-4444 Fax: 867-537-3611

ROSS RIVER: Ross River Health Centre
General Delivery, Ross River, YT Y0B 1S0
Tel: 867-969-4444 Fax: 867-969-2014

TESLIN: Teslin Health Centre
PO Box 70, Teslin, YT Y0B 1B0
Tel: 867-390-4444 Fax: 867-390-2217

Note: Specialties: Public health services; Health promotion; Clinical care by community nurses; Home care

WATSON LAKE: Watson Lake Health Centre
PO Box 500, Watson Lake, YT Y0A 1C0
Tel: 867-536-5255 Fax: 867-536-5258

WATSON LAKE: Watson Lake Hospital
Yukon Hospital Corporation
817 Ravenhill Dr., Watson Lake, YT Y0A 1C0
Tel: 867-536-4444
yukonhospitals.ca/yukonhospitalsfacilities/watsonlake
Number of Beds: 6 beds
Number of Employees: 32
Note: Programs & services include: ambulatory care; convalescent care; diagnostic services (laboratory & medical imaging); emergency; First Nations health program; inpatient care; respite care; & stabilization, observation & monitoring.
Carol Chiasson, Facility Administrator
Jason Bilsky, Chief Executive Officer, Yukon Hospital Corporation

WHITEHORSE: Whitehorse General Hospital (WGH)
Yukon Hospital Corporation
5 Hospital Rd., Whitehorse, YT Y1A 3H7
Tel: 867-393-8700
www.whitehorsehospital.ca
Year Founded: 1902
Number of Beds: 55 beds
Number of Employees: 486
Specialties: Medical imaging services; Laboratory services; Diabetes Education Centre; Nutrition services; First Nations health programs; Therapy services
Note: Programs & services include: First Nations health programs; cancer care; cardiac stress testing; diabetes education; emergency; environmental; intensive care; laboratory; maternity; medical; medical imaging (CT scanning, digital mammography, MRI & ultrasound); nutrition; pediatrics; pharmacy; social work; specialists clinic; surgery; therapy; & pastoral care.
Dr. Sherillynne Himmelsbach, Medical Staff, Yukon Hospital Corporation

Charitable Foundations

National Associations

Achilles Canada
119 Snowden Ave., Toronto ON M4N 2A8
Tel: 416-485-6451; *Fax:* 416-485-0823
www.achillescanada.ca
Previous Name: Achilles Track Club Canada
Overview: A medium-sized national charitable organization founded in 1999
Mission: To encourage & assist all persons with disabilities (visual disability, cerebral palsy, paraplegia, arthritis, epilepsy, multiple sclerosis, amputation, cystic fibrosis, stroke, cancer, traumatic head injury, & many others) to enjoy running for health in a social environment
Chief Officer(s):
Brian McLean, Contact
bmclean@achillescanada.ca

Acupuncture Canada
Tower II, #109, 895 Don Mills Rd., Toronto ON M3C 1W3
Tel: 416-752-3988; *Fax:* 416-752-4398
www.acupuncturecanada.org
Previous Name: Acupuncture Foundation of Canada Institute
Overview: A medium-sized national organization founded in 1995
Mission: To define & maintain the highest professional standards for the use of acupuncture; To gain recognition of acupuncture's legitimate place in western medicine as a safe, efficient complement to conventional medical treatment; To design educational training programs for physicians, physiotherapists, RNs, dentists, chiropractors & naturopaths in the methodology & practice of acupuncture
Affliation(s): World Federation of Acupuncture Societies; Pan Pacific Medical Acupuncture Forum
Chief Officer(s):
Jacek Brachaniec, President
Cathy Donald, Treasurer
Ronda Kellington, Executive Director
rkellington@acupuncturecanada.org
Ann Eldemire, Administrative Coordinator
aeldemire@acupuncturecanada.org
Sheila Williams, Director, Education Administration
Christina Rogoza, Director, Education Curriculum

Air Canada Foundation
Montréal QC
e-mail: foundation-fondation@aircanada.ca
www.aircanada.com/en/about/community/foundation
Overview: A medium-sized national charitable organization founded in 2012
Mission: To help connect sick children to the medical care they need; to help alleviate child poverty

L'Arche Foundation
#300, 10271 Yonge St., Richmond Hill ON L4C 3B5
Tel: 905-770-7696; *Fax:* 905-884-4819
Toll-Free: 800-571-0212
e-mail: info@larchefoundation.ca
www.larchefoundation.ca
www.facebook.com/larchecanadafoundation
www.twitter.com/LArcheCanadaF1
Overview: A medium-sized national charitable organization overseen by L'Arche Canada
Mission: To raise money to support the activities of L'Arche Canada
Member of: L'Arche International
Chief Officer(s):
Gary Sim, President & CEO

The Belinda Stronach Foundation (TBSF)
Toronto ON
www.tbsf.ca
www.youtube.com/user/TheTBSFChannel
Overview: A small national charitable organization founded in 2008
Mission: Assists girls and women and Aboriginal youth in Canada and youth in developing nations to achieve a better life through the provision of programs that enhance basic health and education, improve economic and political independence and that promote civic involvement.

Chief Officer(s):
Belinda Stronach, President & CEO

Best Buddies Canada (BBC) / Vrais Copains
#907, 1243 Islington Ave., Toronto ON M8X 1Y9
Tel: 416-531-0003; *Fax:* 416-531-0325
Toll-Free: 888-779-0061
e-mail: info@bestbuddies.ca
www.bestbuddies.ca
www.facebook.com/BestBuddiesCanada
twitter.com/BestBuddiesCND
www.youtube.com/user/bestbuddiescanada
Overview: A medium-sized national charitable organization founded in 1995
Mission: To enhance communities by offering one-to-one friendships & leadership development opportunities for people with intellectual & developmental disabilities
Member of: Best Buddies International
Chief Officer(s):
Stephen Pinnock, Executive Director
sp@bestbuddies.ca
Ethel Maamo, Manager, Programs
ethelm@bestbuddies.ca

Canadian Abilities Foundation
#803, 255 Duncan Mill Rd., Toronto ON M3B 3H9
Tel: 416-421-7944; *Fax:* 416-421-8418
e-mail: abilities@bcsgroup.com
www.abilities.ca
twitter.com/abilitiescanada
Overview: A small national charitable organization founded in 1988
Mission: To provide information, inspiration & opportunity to Canadians with disabilities
Chief Officer(s):
Caroline Tapp-McDougall, Executive Director & Managing Editor
Publications:
• Abilities
Type: Magazine; *Frequency:* Quarterly; *Accepts Advertising*
Profile: For people with disabilities, their families, friends, & professionals

Canadian Association of Medical Teams Abroad (CAMTA)
103 Laurier Dr., Edmonton AB T5R 5P6
Tel: 780-486-7161; *Fax:* 403-223-9020
e-mail: info@camta.com
camta.com
www.facebook.com/237638586268756
twitter.com/camta
Overview: A small national charitable organization founded in 2001
Mission: CAMTA provides orthopedic surgeries to pediatric and adult patients in Ecuador.
Chief Officer(s):
Marc Moreau, President
Francisco Gallardo, Secretary
Veronica Kong, Executive Director

Canadian Digestive Health Foundation (CDHF) / Fondation canadienne for la promotion de la santé digestive
#455, 2525 Old Bronte Rd., Oakville ON L6M 4J2
Tel: 905-847-2002
www.cdhf.ca
www.linkedin.com/company/649009
www.facebook.com/CDHFdn
twitter.com/TheCDHF
www.youtube.com/user/CDHFtube
Overview: A medium-sized national charitable organization founded in 1994 overseen by Canadian Association of Gastroenterology
Mission: To raise funds for the protection, promotion, & improvement of digestive health
Chief Officer(s):
Richard Fedorak, President
Catherine Mulvale, Executive Director
Publications:
• Canadian Digestive Health Foundation Newsletter
Type: Newsletter
Profile: Current information from digestive health experts across Canada

Canadian Foundation for Healthcare Improvement (CFHI) / Fondation canadienne pour l'amélioration des services de santé (FCASS)

#700, 1565 Carling Ave., Ottawa ON K1Z 8R1

Tel: 613-728-2238; *Fax:* 613-728-3527
Other Communication: registration@cfhi-fcass.ca
e-mail: info@cfhi-fcass.ca
www.cfhi-fcass.ca
www.linkedin.com/company/canadian-foundation-for-healthcare-improv
emen
www.facebook.com/107329739320566
twitter.com/cfhi_fcass
www.youtube.com/user/CHSRF

Previous Name: Canadian Health Services Research Foundation
Overview: A large national organization founded in 1996
Mission: To funds management & policy research in health services; To support applied health services & nursing researchers; To support the synthesis & dissemination of research results; To support the use of research results by decision makers in the health system
Chief Officer(s):
R. Lynn Stevenson, Chair
Maureen O'Neil, President, 613-728-2238 Ext. 237
  maureen.oneil@cfhi-fcass.ca
Nancy Quattrocchi, Vice-President, Corporate Services
  nancy.quattrocchi@cfhi.fcass.ca
Stephen Samis, Vice-President, Programs
  stephen.samis@cfhi-fcass.ca
Publications:
• @CFHI-FCASS [Canadian Foundation for Healthcare Improvement] Bulletin
Type: Newsletter; *Frequency:* Monthly
Profile: Current reports & activities from the Canadian Foundation for Healthcare Improvement
• Canadian Foundation for Healthcare Improvement Annual Report
Type: Yearbook; *Frequency:* Annually
Profile: Organizational highlights from the past year
• CFHI [Canadian Foundation for Healthcare Improvement] Strategic Directions 2009-2013
Profile: An outline of activities & initiatives
• Pass it on! [a series of publications from the Canadian Foundation for Healthcare Improvement]
Profile: Innovative approaches to successful changes in healthcare

Canadian Foundation for Pharmacy (CFP) / Fondation canadienne pour la pharmacie

5809 Fieldon Rd., Mississauga ON L5M 5K1

Tel: 905-997-3238; *Fax:* 905-997-4264
www.cfpnet.ca
www.linkedin.com/groups/Canadian-Foundation-Pharmacy-7473036

Previous Name: Canadian Foundation for the Advancement of Pharmacy
Overview: A medium-sized national charitable organization founded in 1945
Mission: To provide programs for the advancement of the pharmacy profession in Canada
Affiliation(s): Canadian Phamacists Association
Chief Officer(s):
Marshall Moleschi, President
Dayle Acorn, Executive Director
  dacorn@cfpnet.ca

Canadian Foundation for Physically Disabled Persons (CFPDP)

#265, 6 Garamond Ct., Toronto ON M3C 1Z5

Tel: 416-760-7351; *Fax:* 416-760-9405
e-mail: info@cfpdp.com
www.cfpdp.com
www.facebook.com/cffpdp
twitter.com/cffpdp

Overview: A small national charitable organization founded in 1984
Mission: To provide financial assistance to organizations sharing concern for physically disabled adults; To help create awareness in the public & business communities, & in government of the needs of physically disabled adults in the areas of housing, employment, education, accessibility, sports & recreation, & research
Chief Officer(s):
Vim Kochhar, Chair
  vimkochhar@sympatico.ca

Dorothy Price, Executive Director
  dorothyprice@sympatico.ca

Canadian Magen David Adom for Israel (CMDA) / Magen David Adom canadien pour Israël

#3155, 6900, boul Decarie, Montréal QC H3X 2T8

Tel: 514-731-4400; *Fax:* 514-731-2490
Toll-Free: 800-731-2848
e-mail: info@cmdai.org
www.cmdai.org
www.linkedin.com/company/10863533
www.facebook.com/CanadianMagenDavidAdom
twitter.com/CanadianMDA
www.youtube.com/user/CanadianMDA

Overview: A small international charitable organization founded in 1976
Mission: To raise funds to purchase medical supplies to be sent to Israel
Member of: International Red Cross
Affiliation(s): Magen David Adom, Israel
Chief Officer(s):
Sidney Benizri, National Executive Director
  sbenizri@cmdai.org

Canadian Medical Foundation (CMF) / La Fondation médicale canadienne

1870 Alta Vista Dr., Ottawa ON K1G 6R7

Fax: 613-526-7555
Toll-Free: 866-530-4979
e-mail: info@cmf.ca
www.medicalfoundation.ca
twitter.com/CdnMedicalFound
www.youtube.com/CdnMedicalFoundation

Overview: A large national charitable organization founded in 1987
Mission: Physicians striving for excellence in health care through charitable action together & in partnership with others; organized, guided & funded by physicians CMF makes decisive, targeted funding decisions in areas physicians feel will provide the best impact
Chief Officer(s):
Ruth Collins-Nakai, Chair
Lee Gould, President & CEO
Publications:
• Best Practice
Type: Newsletter; *Frequency:* Quarterly

Canadian MedicAlert Foundation / Fondation canadienne MedicAlert

Morneau Shepell Centre II, #600, 895 Don Mills Rd, Toronto ON M3C 1W3

Tel: 416-696-0267; *Fax:* 800-392-8422
Toll-Free: 800-668-1507
e-mail: customerservice@medicalert.ca
www.medicalert.ca
www.facebook.com/medicalertcanada
twitter.com/medicalertCA
www.youtube.com/medicalertCA

Also Known As: MedicAlert
Overview: A large national charitable organization founded in 1961
Mission: To provide lifelong access to personal & medical information in order to protect & save the lives of its members; MedicAlert is a non-profit organization that provides all Canadians with medical protection in an emergency situation
Affiliation(s): MedicAlert Foundation International
Chief Officer(s):
Robert Ridge, MBA, President & CEO
Dorothy Griesbach, CPA, Director & CPO, Finance & Corporate Affairs

Canadian Melanoma Foundation (CMF)

c/o Div. of Dermatology, Univ. of British Columbia, 835 - 10th Ave. West, Vancouver BC V5Z 4E8

Tel: 604-875-4747; *Fax:* 604-873-9919
www.derm.ubc.ca/division/cmf/cmf1.htm

Overview: A small national organization
Mission: A non-profit organization dedicated to improving cancer prevention and cure.

Canadian National Autism Foundation (CNAF)
PO Box 66512, 38 King St. East, Stoney Creek ON L8G 5E5
Tel: 905-930-8682; *Fax:* 905-930-9744
e-mail: info@cnaf.net
www.cnaf.net
Overview: A small national charitable organization founded in 2000
Mission: To increase autism awareness; To assist families; To raise funds to support Canadian-based autism research
Chief Officer(s):
Tina Fougere, President & Founder

Canadian Tinnitus Foundation
#404, 1688 - 152 St., Surrey BC V4A 4N2
Tel: 604-317-2952
e-mail: info@findthecurenow.org
www.findthecurenow.org
www.facebook.com/CanadianTinnitusFoundation
Overview: A medium-sized national organization
Mission: A not-for-profit organization working to expand awareness & generate funding for tinnitus research
Chief Officer(s):
Nathan Nowak, President
John Jabat, Vice-President
Brian Cassidy, Treasurer
Elizabeth Eayrs, Secretary

Children's Wish Foundation of Canada / Fondation canadienne rêves d'enfants
#350, 1101 Kingston Rd., Pickering ON L1V 1B5
Tel: 905-839-8882; *Fax:* 905-839-3745
Toll-Free: 800-700-4437
e-mail: nat@childrenswish.ca
www.childrenswish.ca
www.linkedin.com/company/children's-wish-foundation-of-canada
www.facebook.com/ChildrensWish
twitter.com/Childrens_wish
www.instagram.com/childrenswishfoundation
Overview: A large national charitable organization founded in 1984
Mission: The Foundation grants wishes to children suffering from a high risk, life-threatening illnesses
Chief Officer(s):
Chris Kotsopoulos, CEO
chris.kotsopoulos@childrenswish.ca
Sandra Hancox, National Director, Chapter Relations
sandra.hancox@childrenswish.ca
Sandy Watt, National Director, Marketing
sandy.watt@childrenswish.ca

Alberta & N.W.T. Chapter - Calgary
#270, 2323 - 32 Ave. NE, Calgary AB T2E 6Z3
Tel: 403-265-9039; *Fax:* 403-265-1704
Toll-Free: 800-267-9474
e-mail: ab@childrenswish.ca
www.facebook.com/ChildrensWishAB
twitter.com/ChildrensWishAB
Chief Officer(s):
Kyla Martin, Provincial Director
kyla.martin@childrenswish.ca

Alberta & N.W.T. Chapter - Edmonton
#200, 9750 - 51 Ave. NW, Edmonton AB T6E 0A6
Tel: 780-340-9039; *Fax:* 587-881-0064
Toll-Free: 800-267-9474
e-mail: ab@childrenswish.ca
www.facebook.com/ChildrensWishAB
twitter.com/ChildrensWishAB
Chief Officer(s):
Kyla Martin, Provincial Director
kyla.martin@childrenswish.ca

British Columbia & Yukon Chapter
#450, 319 West Pender St., Vancouver BC V6B 1T3
Tel: 604-299-2241; *Fax:* 604-299-1228
Toll-Free: 800-267-9474
e-mail: bc@childrenswish.ca
www.facebook.com/ChildrensWishBC
twitter.com/cwfbc
Chief Officer(s):

Jennifer Petersen, Provincial Director
jennifer.petersen@childrenswish.ca
Bureau de Montréal
#904, 4200, boul St. Laurent, Montréal QC H2W 2R2
Tél: 514-289-1777; *Téléc:* 514-298-8504
Ligne sans frais: 800-267-9474
Courriel: qo@revesdenfants.ca
www.facebook.com/revesenfants
twitter.com/Reves_denfants
Chief Officer(s):
Juli Meilleur, Directrice générale
juli.meilleur@childrenswish.ca

Bureau de Québec
Halles Fleur de Lys, #904, 245, rue Soumande, Québec QC G1M 3H6
Tél: 418-650-2111; *Téléc:* 418-650-3466
Ligne sans frais: 800-267-9474
Courriel: qe@revesdenfants.ca
www.facebook.com/revesenfants
twitter.com/Reves_denfants
Chief Officer(s):
Pierre-Luc Berthiaume, Directeur régional, Est-du-Québec
pierre-luc.berthiaume@revesdenfants.ca

Manitoba & Nunavut Chapter
350 St. Mary Ave., Winnipeg MB R3C 3J2
Tel: 204-945-9474; *Fax:* 204-945-9479
Toll-Free: 800-267-9474
e-mail: mb@childrenswish.ca
www.facebook.com/ChildrensWishMB
twitter.com/ChildrensWishMB
Chief Officer(s):
Maria Toscano, Provincial Director
maria.toscano@childrenswish.ca

National Capital Region
#206, 1800 Bank St., Ottawa ON K1V 0W3
Tel: 613-221-9474; *Fax:* 613-221-9441
Toll-Free: 800-267-9474
e-mail: ncr@childrenswish.ca
www.facebook.com/ChildrensWishNatCap
twitter.com/ChildrensWishNC
Chief Officer(s):
Leanne Brown, Regional Director
Leanne.Brown@childrenswish.ca

New Brunswick Chapter
#C202, 600 Main St., Saint John NB E2K 1J5
Tel: 506-632-0099; *Fax:* 506-635-6924
Toll-Free: 800-267-9474
e-mail: nb@childrenswish.ca
www.facebook.com/ChildrensWishFoundationNB
twitter.com/NBChildrensWish
Chief Officer(s):
Kelly Hare, Chapter Director
kelly.hare@childrenswish.ca

Newfoundland & Labrador Chapter
#211 - 31 Peet St., St. John's NL A1B 3W8
Tel: 709-739-9474; *Fax:* 709- 72-6947
Toll-Free: 800-267-9474
e-mail: nl@childrenswish.ca
www.facebook.com/ChildrensWishNL
twitter.com/cwfnl
Chief Officer(s):
Edie Newton, Provincial Director
edie.newton@childrenswish.ca

Nova Scotia Chapter
#105, 238 Brownlow Ave., Dartmouth NS B3B 2B4
Tel: 902-492-1984; *Fax:* 902-492-1908
Toll-Free: 800-267-9474
e-mail: ns@childrenswish.ca
www.facebook.com/ChildrensWishNS
twitter.com/ChildrensWishNS
Chief Officer(s):
Cheryl Matthews, Provincial Director
cheryl.matthews@childrenswish.ca

Ontario Chapter
#360, 1101 Kingston Rd., Pickering ON L1V 1B5

Tel: 905-427-5353; *Fax:* 905-427-0536
Toll-Free: 800-267-9474
e-mail: on@childrenswish.ca
www.facebook.com/ChildrensWishON
twitter.com/ChildrensWishON

Chief Officer(s):
Tiffany MacDonald, Provincial Director
tiffany.macdonald@childrenswish.ca

Prince Edward Island Chapter
Midtown Plaza, #7, 375 University Ave., Charlottetown PE C1A 2S2

Tel: 902-566-5526; *Fax:* 902-894-8412
Toll-Free: 800-267-9474
e-mail: pei@childrenswish.ca
www.facebook.com/ChildrensWishPE
twitter.com/ChildrensWishPE

Chief Officer(s):
Beth Corney Gauthier, Provincial Director
beth.corneygauthier@childrenswish.ca

Saskatchewan Chapter
3602 Millar Ave., Saskatoon SK S7K 3L3

Tel: 306-955-0511; *Fax:* 306-653-9474
Toll-Free: 800-267-9474
e-mail: sk@childrenswish.ca

Chief Officer(s):
Gay Anderson, Provincial Director
gay.anderson@childrenswish.ca

Doctors without Borders Canada (MSF) / Médecins sans frontières Canada (MSF-C)
#402, 720 Spadina Ave., Toronto ON M5S 2T9

Tel: 416-964-0619; *Fax:* 416-963-8707
Toll-Free: 800-982-7903
e-mail: msfcan@msf.ca
www.msf.ca
www.linkedin.com/company/6952
www.facebook.com/msf.english
twitter.com/MSF_Canada
www.youtube.com/user/MSFCanada

Also Known As: MSF Canada
Overview: A small national charitable organization founded in 1991
Mission: To offer assistance to populations in distress, to victims of natural or man-made disasters & to victims of armed conflict, without discrimination & irrespective of race, religion, creed or political affiliation.
Chief Officer(s):
Heather Culbert, President
Stephen Cornish, Executive Director

Québec Office
#220, 1470, rue Peel, Montréal QC H3A 1T1

Tél: 514-845-5621; *Téléc:* 514-845-3707
Ligne sans frais: 866-878-5621
Courriel: msfqc@msf.ca

Dreams Take Flight
PO Box 7000, Stn. Airport, Dorval QC H4Y 1J2

Tel: 204-479-5267
e-mail: canada@dreamstakeflight.ca
www.dreamstakeflight.ca
www.facebook.com/DreamsTakeFlightCanada
twitter.com/DreamsTakeFlight

Overview: A small national charitable organization founded in 1989
Mission: To provide Disney vacations to children with mental & physical disabilities
Chief Officer(s):
Bev Watson, President
ntl.president@dreamstakeflight.ca

Easter Seals Canada / Timbres de Pâques Canada
#401, 40 Holly St., Toronto ON M4S 3C3

Tel: 416-932-8382; *Fax:* 416-932-9844
Toll-Free: 877-376-6362
e-mail: info@easterseals.ca
www.easterseals.ca
www.facebook.com/eastersealscanada
twitter.com/easterseals

Also Known As: Canadian Rehabilitation Council for the Disabled
Previous Name: Easter Seals/March of Dimes National Council
Overview: A medium-sized national charitable organization founded in 1962
Mission: To enhance the quality of life, self-esteem, & self-determination of Canadians with physical disabilities; To support the social & economic integration of people with disabilities
Member of: Imagine Canada's Ethical Code Program
Chief Officer(s):
Dave Starrett, Chief Executive Officer, 416-932-8382 Ext. 250
Alex Krievins, National Director, Programs & Development, 416-932-8382 Ext. 228
Frank Williamson, Director, Finance, 416-932-8382 Ext. 222
Publications:
• Easter Seals Canada Annual Report
Type: Yearbook; *Frequency:* Annually
Profile: Messages from the Chair of the Board & the Chief Executive Officer, information about the organization's programs & fundraising efforts, & the treasurer's report

Fondation Diane Hébert Inc
132, rue Blainville Est, Sainte-Thérèse-de-Blainville QC J7E 1M2

Tél: 450-971-1112; *Téléc:* 450-971-1818
Ligne sans frais: 877-971-1110
Courriel: fdh@macten.net

Aperçu: *Dimension:* moyenne; *Envergure:* nationale; Organisme sans but lucratif; fondée en 1987
Mission: Services directs offerts aux patients en attente de greffes, aux greffés et à leur famille autant sur le plan moral, physique ou financier; prêt d'équipements médicaux tels que chaises roulantes électriques; la Fondation vise aussi à sensibiliser la population au don d'organes
Membre de: Info Don D'Organes; Québec Transplant; Canadian Transplant Association

Fragile X Research Foundation of Canada (FXRFC)
167 Queen St. West, Brampton ON L6Y 1M5

Tel: 905-453-9366
e-mail: info@fragilexcanada.ca
www.fragilexcanada.ca

Overview: A small national charitable organization founded in 1997
Mission: To raise public awareness of Fragile X; to raise money for Fragile X research & support services; to establish a support system for those with & affected by Fragile X
Chief Officer(s):
Carlo Paribello, President / Medical Director
medical@fragilexcanada.ca

The Gairdner Foundation
MaRS Centre, South Tower, #407, 101 College St., Toronto ON M5G 1L7

Tel: 416-596-9996; *Fax:* 416-596-9992
e-mail: thegairdner@gairdner.org
www.gairdner.org
www.facebook.com/263607420316593
twitter.com/GairdnerAwards
www.youtube.com/user/CanadaGairdnerAwards

Overview: A small national charitable organization founded in 1957
Mission: To recognize researchers who have made signifcant contributions to the medical science field
Chief Officer(s):
Janet Rossant, President & Scientific Director
janet.rossant@gairdner.org
Penny Balberman, Financial Director
penny@gairdner.org
Nora Cox, Office Manager
nora@gairdner.org

Guillain-Barré Syndrome Foundation of Canada (GBSFCI)
PO Box 80060, Stn. Rossland Garden, 3100 Garden St., Whitby ON
L1R 0H1

Tel: 647-560-6842
Toll-Free: 866-224-3301
www.gbs-cidp.org/canada
www.facebook.com/gbscidp

Overview: A medium-sized national charitable organization founded in 1985
Mission: To provide information about GBS & CIDP; To provide education, research, & support to individuals, families & friends affected by GBS, CIDP & related disorders
Affliation(s): Guillain-Barré Syndrome Foundation International
Chief Officer(s):
Donna Hartlen, Executive Director

Health Charities Coalition of Canada (HCCC) / Coalition canadienne des organismes bénévoles en santé
41 Empress Ave., Annex D, Ottawa ON K1R 7E9

Tel: 613-232-7266
www.healthcharities.ca

Overview: A small national organization founded in 2000
Mission: To provide health policy leadership for the health of all people of Canada; To act as a collective authoritative voice of national health charities in public policy & health research issues that affect the lives of the people of Canada
Chief Officer(s):
Connie Côté, Executive Director

Help Fill a Dream Foundation of Canada
4085 Quadra St., #D, Victoria BC V8X 1K5

Tel: 250-382-3135; *Fax:* 250-382-2711
Toll-Free: 866-382-2711
e-mail: contact@helpfilladream.com
helpfilladream.com
www.facebook.com/helpfilladream
twitter.com/helpfilladream

Overview: A small national charitable organization founded in 1986
Mission: To fill the dreams of children under 19 years of age who have life-threatening illness in BC
Chief Officer(s):
Craig Smith, Executive Director

Hospital for Sick Children Foundation (HSCF)
525 University Ave., 14th Fl., Toronto ON M5G 2L3

Tel: 416-813-6166; *Fax:* 416-813-5024
Toll-Free: 800-661-1083
www.sickkidsfoundation.com
www.facebook.com/sickkidsfoundation
twitter.com/sickkids
www.youtube.com/sickkidsfoundation

Overview: A medium-sized national charitable organization founded in 1972
Mission: To invest contributions in paediatric care, research & education to help children at The Hospital for Sick Children, throughout Canada, & around the world
Chief Officer(s):
Ted Garrard, President/CEO
Kathleen Taylor, Chair
L. Robin Cardozo, Chief Operating Officer, 416-813-2937
  robin.cardozo@sickkidsfoundation.com
Josee Bertrand, Director, Finance
  josee.bertrand@sickkidsfoundation.com
Noelle de la Mothe, Director, Direct Marketing
  noelle.delamothe@sickkidsfoundation.com
Nora Paradis, Director, Human Resources
  nora.paradis@sickkidsfoundation.com

Jacob's Ladder - The Canadian Foundation for Control of Neurodegenerative Disease
#400, 505 Consumers Rd., Toronto ON M2J 4V8

Tel: 416-485-0078; *Fax:* 800-611-2449
e-mail: info@jacobsladder.ca
www.jacobsladder.ca
www.facebook.com/154447297910994
twitter.com/JacobsLadder_

Overview: A medium-sized national charitable organization founded in 1998

Mission: To raise awareness of neurodegenerative disease; To lower occurrences of neurodegenerative disease in the future
Chief Officer(s):
Jeff Schwartz, Co-Founder
Ellen Schwartz, Co-Founder

JMJ Children's Fund of Canada Inc
PO Box 20051, 390 Rideau St. East, Ottawa ON K1N 9N5

e-mail: amdg3@rogers.com
www.jmjchildren.ca

Overview: A small national organization founded in 1972
Mission: To assist children in need of food, medication & schooling; to provide physiotherapy for the physically disabled

Kids Help Phone (KHP) / Jeunesse j'écoute
#300, 439 University Ave., Toronto ON M5G 1Y8

Tel: 416-586-5437
Toll-Free: 800-668-6868
e-mail: info@kidshelpphone.ca
kidshelpphone.ca
www.linkedin.com/company/kids-help-phone
www.facebook.com/KidsHelpPhone
twitter.com/kidshelpphone
www.youtube.com/user/KidsHelpPhone

Overview: A medium-sized national charitable organization founded in 1989
Mission: To provide a national, bilingual, 24-hours a day, 365 days of the year, toll-free, professionally staffed, confidential counselling service to young people; To help young people deal with concerns large or small; To contribute to awareness of children's issues & the development of policies & practices to help Canadian children
Member of: Child Helpline International; Alliance of Information & Referral Systems
Chief Officer(s):
Sharon Wood, President & CEO

Alberta/Northwest Territories
4331 Manhattan Rd. SE, Calgary AB T2G 4B1

Tel: 403-476-0385
Toll-Free: 866-297-4101
e-mail: alberta@kidshelpphone.ca

Atlantic Region
#301, 1600 Bedford Hwy., Bedford NS B4A 1E8

Tel: 902-457-4779
Toll-Free: 888-470-8880
e-mail: atlantic@kidshelpphone.ca

British Columbia/Yukon
#1100, 1200 West 73 Ave., Vancouver BC V6P 6G5

Tel: 604-267-7057
Toll-Free: 877-267-7057
e-mail: bc@kidshelpphone.ca

Manitoba
#320, 145 Pacific Ave., Winnipeg MB R3B 2Z6

Tel: 204-770-8053
e-mail: manitoba@kidshelpphone.ca

Ontario
#300, 439 University Ave., Toronto ON M5G 1Y8

Tel: 416-586-5437
Toll-Free: 800-268-3062
e-mail: ontario@kidshelpphone.ca

Québec
#303, 5605, av de Gaspé, Montréal QC H2T 2A4

Tel: 514-273-7007
Toll-Free: 866-814-1010
e-mail: quebec@kidshelpphone.ca

Saskatchewan
#120, 2150 Scarth St., Regina SK S4P 2H7

Tel: 306-780-9492
Toll-Free: 866-321-4125
e-mail: saskatchewan@kidshelpphone.ca

Make-A-Wish Canada / Fais-Un-Voeu Canada
#520, 4211 Yonge St., Toronto ON M2P 2A9

Tel: 416-224-9474; *Fax:* 416-224-8795
Toll-Free: 888-822-9474
e-mail: nationaloffice@makeawish.ca
makeawish.ca
www.linkedin.com/company/422218
www.facebook.com/makeawish.ca
twitter.com/MakeAWishCA
www.youtube.com/user/makeawishcanada

Overview: A large national charitable organization founded in 1980
Mission: The Foundation grants wishes to children suffering from a high risk, life-threatening illnesses
Chief Officer(s):
Jennifer Klotz-Ritter, President & Chief Executive Officer Ext. 6112
   jennifer.ritter@makeawish.ca

March of Dimes Canada (MODC) / Mars de dix sous du Canada
10 Overlea Blvd., Toronto ON M4H 1A4

Tel: 416-425-3463; *Fax:* 416-425-1920
Toll-Free: 800-263-3463
www.marchofdimes.ca
www.facebook.com/marchofdimescanada
twitter.com/modcanada
www.youtube.com/user/marchofdimescda

Also Known As: Rehabilitation Foundation for Disabled Persons, Canada
Overview: A large national charitable organization founded in 2001
Mission: To provide support services to people with disabilities, their families & caregivers across Canada
Affliation(s): Ontario March of Dimes; Ontario March of Dimes Non-Profit Housing Corporation (NPHC); OMOD Independence Non-Profit Corporation; Rehabilitation Foundation for Disabled Persons Inc., U.S.; Polio Canada; Stroke Recovery Canada
Chief Officer(s):
Jenelle Ross, Chair
Andria Spindel, President & CEO
Zullfikar Chaggan, Chief Financial Officer
Chris Harrison, Chief Administrative Officer
Jerry Lucas, Chief Operating Officer

March of Dimes Non-Profit Housing Corporation (NPHC)
March of Dimes Canada Head Office, 10 Overlea Blvd., Toronto ON M4H 1A4

Tel: 416-425-3463; *Fax:* 416-425-1920
Toll-Free: 800-263-3463
e-mail: nphc@marchofdimes.ca
www.marchofdimes.ca/nphc

Overview: A small national charitable organization founded in 1992
Mission: To develop & promote affordable supportive housing for people with physical disabilities
Affliation(s): March of Dimes Canada
Chief Officer(s):
Cameron Whale, Chair
Publications:
• Ontario March of Dimes Non-Profit Housing Corporation Annual Report
Type: Yearbook; *Frequency:* Annually

Meningitis Research Foundation of Canada
PO Box 28015, Stn. Parkdale, Waterloo ON N2L 6J8

Tel: 519-664-0244
Toll-Free: 800-643-1303
e-mail: fund@meningitis.ca
www.meningitis.ca
www.facebook.com/meningitisca
twitter.com/meningitisCA

Overview: A small national charitable organization
Mission: To raise funds to promote education & research in order to prevent death & disability from meningitis & other infections of the central nervous system; To provide support & education to patients & their families affected by meningitis; To increase public awareness of meningitis; To promote better understanding of the disease among healthcare professionals; To provide funds for research into improved diagnosis, treatment, & prevention of meningitis
Chief Officer(s):
Kathryn Blain, Chair

The Paterson Foundation
1918 Yonge St., Thunder Bay ON P7E 6T9

www.patersonfoundation.ca
Overview: A small national charitable organization founded in 1970
Mission: To assist educational, religious & cultural, charitable, non-profit registered organizations with particular interest in health care & relief work
Chief Officer(s):
Donald C. Paterson, President

Phoenix Community Works Foundation (PCWF)
330 Bloor St. West, Toronto ON M5S 3A7

Tel: 416-964-3388
e-mail: info@pcwf.ca
www.pcwf.ca

Overview: A medium-sized national charitable organization founded in 1973
Mission: To assist in the development of a healthy community by encouraging creativity; To promote educational programs relating to the emotional, intellectual & physical well-being of individuals & society; To foster studies & experimental projects related to the physical & social environments; To promote studies & programs in area of emotional health
Chief Officer(s):
Larry Rooney, Executive Director

Right to Play
Thomson Bldg., PO Box 64, #1900, 65 Queen St. West, Toronto ON M5H 2M5

Tel: 416-498-1922; *Fax:* 416-498-1942
e-mail: info@righttoplay.com
www.righttoplay.com
www.linkedin.com/company/right-to-play
www.facebook.com/RightToPlayCAN
twitter.com/RighttoPlayCAN
www.youtube.com/user/RightToPlayCan

Previous Name: Olympic Aid
Overview: A medium-sized international charitable organization founded in 2002
Mission: Educating and empowering children and youth to use sport and play to overcome the effects of poverty, conflict and disease in disadvantaged communities.
Chief Officer(s):
Johann Koss, President & CEO

Ronald McDonald House Charities of Canada (RMHC) / Oeuvres pour enfants Ronald McDonald du Canada
1 McDonald's Place, Toronto ON M3C 3L4

Tel: 416-446-3493; *Fax:* 416-446-3588
Toll-Free: 800-387-8808
e-mail: rmhc@ca.mcd.com
www.rmhccanada.ca
www.facebook.com/RMHCCanada

Previous Name: Ronald McDonald Children's Charities of Canada
Overview: A medium-sized national charitable organization founded in 1982
Mission: To help children in need by improving the physical & emotional quality of life for children with serious illnesses, disabilities &/or chronic conditions, allowing them to lead happier, healthier & more productive lives
Chief Officer(s):
Cathy Loblaw, President & CEO
   cathy.loblaw@ca.mcd.com
Roxanna Kassam-Kara, Director, Marketing & Communications
   roxanna.kassamkara@ca.mcd.com
Kelly Glover, Coordinator
   kelly.glover@ca.mcd.com

Scottish Rite Charitable Foundation of Canada
4 Queen St. South, Hamilton ON L8P 3R3

Tel: 905-522-0033; *Fax:* 905-522-3716
e-mail: info@srcf.ca
www.srcf.ca

Overview: A medium-sized national charitable organization founded in 1964
Mission: To provide assistance through major grants in the physical/biological & socio/economic areas; To support research into the causes & treatment of intellectual impairment
Chief Officer(s):

Gareth Taylor, President
James E. Ford, Secretary
Publications:
• Clarion [a publication of The Scottish Rite Charitable Foundation of Canada]
Type: Magazine
• The Foundation Newsletter [a publication of The Scottish Rite Charitable Foundation of Canada]
Type: Newsletter
• The Scottish Rite Charitable Foundation of Canada Annual Report
Type: Report

Starlight Children's Foundation Canada
#105, 1375 Transcanada Hwy., Dorval QC H9P 2W8
Toll-Free: 888-782-7947
e-mail: info@starlightcanada.org
www.starlightcanada.org
www.linkedin.com/groups?gid=1414967
www.facebook.com/starlightcanada
twitter.com/StarlightCanada
www.youtube.com/CanadaStarlight
Overview: A medium-sized national charitable organization
Mission: To brighten the lives of seriously ill children & their families by providing both in-hospital & out-patient programs to enhance their ability to cope with the stress of illness
Chief Officer(s):
Brian J.H. Bringolf, Executive Director
brian.bringolf@starlightcanada.ca
Trevor Dicaire, Vice-President
trevor.dicaire@starlightcanada.org
Jeannie O'Regan, Vice-President, Special Events & Operations
jeannie.oregan@starlightcanada.org
Michele Vantrepote, Manager, Communications
Palermo Coronado, Coordinator, Finance

British Columbia Chapter
Odd Fellows' Hall, 1443 West 8th Ave., Vancouver BC V6H 1C9
Tel: 604-742-0272; *Fax:* 604-742-0274
e-mail: infovancouver@starlightcanada.org
Chief Officer(s):
Heather Burnett, Regional Coordinator
heather@starlightcanada.org

Calgary Chapter
8 Mount Norquay Gate SE, Calgary AB T2Z 2L3
Tel: 403-457-0344; *Fax:* 403-457-0384
Toll-Free: 800-880-1004
e-mail: infocalgary@starlightcanada.org
Chief Officer(s):
Laura Stow, Regional Coordinator
laura.stow@starlightcanada.org

Montréal Chapter
105, 1375, rte Transcanadienne, Dorval QC H9P 2W8
Tel: 514-288-9474; *Fax:* 514-287-0635
Toll-Free: 888-782-7947
e-mail: starlight@starlightquebec.org
www.starlightquebec.org
Chief Officer(s):
Brian J.H. Bringolf, Executive Director
brian@starlightquebec.org

Sunshine Dreams for Kids / Rayons de Soleil pour enfants
#100, 300 Wellington St., London ON N6B 2L5
Tel: 519-642-0990; *Fax:* 519-642-1201
Toll-Free: 800-461-7935
e-mail: info@sunshine.ca
www.sunshine.ca
www.linkedin.com/company/sunshine-foundation-of-canada
www.facebook.com/SunshineFound
twitter.com/SunshineFound
www.youtube.com/user/SunshineFound
Also Known As: The Sunshine Foundation of Canada
Overview: A medium-sized national charitable organization founded in 1987
Mission: To fulfill the dreams of children between the ages of three & nineteen who are challenged by a severe physical disability or life-threatening illness
Chief Officer(s):

Ed Holder, President

The Terry Fox Foundation / La Fondation Terry Fox
#150, 8960 University High St., Burnaby BC V5A 4Y6
Tel: 604-200-0541; *Fax:* 604-701-0247
Toll-Free: 888-836-9786
Other Communication: contact@terryfoxrun.org;
international@terryfox.org
e-mail: national@terryfoxrun.org
www.terryfoxrun.org
www.facebook.com/TheTerryFoxFoundation
twitter.com/TerryFoxCanada
www.youtube.com/terryfoxcanada
Also Known As: Terry Fox Run
Overview: A large national charitable organization founded in 1980
Mission: To maintain the vision & principles of Terry Fox while raising money for cancer research through the annual Terry Fox Run, memoriam donations & planned gifts. All money raised by the Foundation is distributed through the National Cancer Institute of Canada
Chief Officer(s):
Bill Pristanski, Chair
Judith Fox, International Director, 604-239-8576
international@terryfoxrun.org

Alberta/NWT/Nunavut Office
#D10, 6115 - 3rd St. SE, Calgary AB T2H 2L2
Tel: 403-212-1336; *Fax:* 403-212-1343
Toll-Free: 888-836-9786
Chief Officer(s):
Wendy Kennelly, Provincial Director
wendy.kennelly@terryfoxrun.org

British Columbia/Yukon Office
2669 Shaughnessy St., Port Coquitlam BC V3C 3G7
Tel: 604-464-2666; *Fax:* 604-464-2664
Toll-Free: 888-836-9786
e-mail: bcyukon@terryfoxrun.org
Chief Officer(s):
Donna White, Provincial Director

International
#150, 8960 University High St., Burnaby BC V5A 4Y6
e-mail: international@terryfoxrun.org
Chief Officer(s):
Rhonda Risenrough, International Director
Rhonda.risebrough@terryfox.org

Manitoba Office
1214 Chevrier Blvd., #A, Winnipeg MB R3T 1Y3
Tel: 204-231-5282; *Fax:* 204-321-5365
Toll-Free: 888-836-9786
e-mail: mb@terryfoxrun.org
Chief Officer(s):
Tammy Ferrante, Provincial Director

New Brunswick/PEI Office
#493, 605 Prospect St., Fredericton NB E3B 6B8
Tel: 506-458-2618; *Fax:* 506-459-4572
Toll-Free: 888-836-9786
e-mail: nbpei@terryfoxrun.org
Chief Officer(s):
Gwen Smith-Walsh, Provincial Director

Newfoundland & Labrador
#202, 835 Topsail Rd., Mount Pearl NL A1N 3J6
Tel: 709-576-8428; *Fax:* 709-747-7277
Toll-Free: 888-836-9786
e-mail: nl@terryfoxrun.org
Chief Officer(s):
Heather Strong, Provincial Director

Nova Scotia Office
#203, 3600 Kempt Rd., Halifax NS B3K 4X8
Tel: 902-423-8131; *Fax:* 902-492-3639
Toll-Free: 888-836-9786
e-mail: ns@terryfoxrun.org
Chief Officer(s):
Barbara Pate, Provincial Director

Ontario Office

#900, 1200 Eglinton Ave. Wast, Toronto ON M3C 1H9
Tel: 416-924-8252; *Fax:* 416-924-6597
Toll-Free: 888-836-9786
e-mail: ontario@terryfoxrun.org

Chief Officer(s):
Martha McClew, Provincial Director

Québec Office
#207, 10 Churchill Blvd., Greenfield Park QC J4V 2L7
Tel: 450-923-9747; *Fax:* 450-923-8468
Toll-Free: 888-836-9786
e-mail: qc@terryfoxrun.org

Chief Officer(s):
Peter Sheremeta, Provincial Director

Saskatchewan Office
1812 - 9th Ave. North, Regina SK S4R 7T4
Tel: 306-757-1662; *Fax:* 306-757-7422
Toll-Free: 888-836-9786

Chief Officer(s):
Heather Mackenzie, Provincial Director
heather.mackenzie@terryfoxrun.org

United Way of Canada - Centraide Canada
#900, 116 Albert St., Ottawa ON K1P 5G3
Tel: 613-236-7041; *Fax:* 613-236-3087
Toll-Free: 800-267-8221
e-mail: info@unitedway.ca
www.unitedway.ca
ca.linkedin.com/company/united-way-centraide-canada
www.facebook.com/UnitedWayCentraide
twitter.com/UnitedWayCanada
www.youtube.com/UnitedWayofCanada

Also Known As: Centraide Canada - United Way of Canada
Overview: A large national charitable organization
Mission: To create opportunities for a better life for all; To inspire Canadians to make a lasting difference in their communities
Affiliation(s): United Way International
Chief Officer(s):
Jacline A. Nyman, President/CEO

YMCA Canada
#601, 1867 Younge St., Toronto ON M4S 1Y5
Tel: 416-967-9622; *Fax:* 416-967-9618
www.ymca.ca
www.facebook.com/YMCACanada
twitter.com/YMCA_Canada

Also Known As: The National Council of Young Men's Christian Associations of Canada
Overview: A large national charitable organization founded in 1851
Mission: Dedicated to the growth of all persons in spirit, mind & body, & in a sense of responsibility to each other & the global community; fosters & stimulates the development of strong member associations & advocates on their behalf regionally, nationally & internationally
Affiliation(s): Canadian Centre for Philanthropy; Canadian Child Care Federation; Canadian Coalition for the Rights of Children; Canadian Council for International Cooperation; Canadian Council on Children & Youth; Canadian Recreational Canoeing Association; Coalition on National Voluntary Organizations; Conference Board of Canada; Huronia Tourism Association; National Fitness Leadership Advisory Committee; National Life Guard Service; National Voluntary Health Agencies; National Youth Serving Agencies; Partnership Africa Canada; Resorts Ontario; Royal Life Saving Society; Voluntary Sector Round Table
Chief Officer(s):
Scott Haldane, President/CEO
Bahadur Madhani, Chair

Brockville & Area YMCA-YWCA
345 Park St., Brockville ON K6V 5Y7
Tel: 613-342-7961; *Fax:* 613-342-8223
e-mail: ymca@brockvilley.com
www.brockvilley.com
www.facebook.com/163865009971
twitter.com/YMCABrockville

Chief Officer(s):
Kim Charteris, Interim CEO
kcharteris@brockvilley.com

Family YMCA of Windsor - Essex County

500 Victoria Ave., Windsor ON N9A 4M8
Tel: 519-258-9622; *Fax:* 519-258-9629
e-mail: windsor@ymca.ca
ymcawo.ca/windsor-essex-contact
www.facebook.com/12860181433

Chief Officer(s):
Giles Denis, Contact, 519-258-9622 Ext. 225
dgiles@ymcawo.ca

National Capital Region YMCA - YWCA de la région de la capitale nationale
180 Argyle Ave., Ottawa ON K2P 1B7
Tel: 613-237-1320; *Fax:* 613-788-5052
www.ymcaywca.ca
www.facebook.com/ymcaywca
twitter.com/YMCAYWCA_Ottawa
www.youtube.com/user/ymcaywcaottawa

Chief Officer(s):
Deirdre Speers, President & CEO

Northern Alberta YMCA
#300, 10030 - 102A Ave., Edmonton AB T5J 0G5
Tel: 780-425-9622; *Fax:* 780-428-9469
edmonton.ymca.ca
www.facebook.com/82802289395

Chief Officer(s):
Nick Parkinson, President & CEO
nparkinson@edmonton.ymca.ca

Owen Sound Family YMCA
700 10th Street East, Owen Sound ON N4K 0C6
Tel: 519-376-0484; *Fax:* 519-376-0487
Toll-Free: 800-265-3711
e-mail: membership@ymcaowensound.on.ca
www.ymcaowensound.on.ca

Chief Officer(s):
Gayle Graham, CEO, 519-376-0484 Ext. 204
ggraham@ymcaowensound.on.ca

Timmins Family YMCA
376 Poplar Ave., Timmins ON P4N 4S4
Tel: 705-360-4381; *Fax:* 705-360-4382
e-mail: info@timminsymca.org
www.timminsymca.org

Chief Officer(s):
Wayne Bozzer, Executive Director
wbozzer@timminsymca.org

YMCA - YWCA of Brantford
143 Wellington St., Brantford ON N3S 3Y8
Tel: 519-752-6568; *Fax:* 519-759-8431
e-mail: brantford_membership@ymca.ca
www.ymcahbb.ca
www.facebook.com/ymcahamiltonburlingtonbrantford
twitter.com/ymcahbb

Chief Officer(s):
Jim Commerford, President & Chief Executive Officer, 905-317-4919
jim_commerford@ymca.ca

YMCA - YWCA of Moose Jaw
220 Fairford St. East, Moose Jaw SK S6H 6H2
Tel: 306-692-0688; *Fax:* 306-694-5034
www.moosejawymca.ca
www.facebook.com/mjymca

Chief Officer(s):
Jana Bollinger, President

YMCA - YWCA of Saint John
130 Broadview Ave., Saint John NB E2L 5C5
Tel: 506-634-4860; *Fax:* 506-634-0783
e-mail: admin@saintjohny.com
www.saintjohny.com
www.facebook.com/SaintJohnY
twitter.com/Y_SaintJohn

Chief Officer(s):
Jill Keliher, Director

YMCA - YWCA of the Central Okanagan

375 Hartman Rd., Kelowna BC V1X 2M9
Tel: 250-491-9622; *Fax:* 250-765-7962
e-mail: info@ymca-ywca.com
www.ymcaokanagan.ca

Chief Officer(s):
Sharon Peterson, CEO
speterson@ymca-ywca.com

YMCA - YWCA of Winnipeg
3550 Portage Ave., Winnipeg MB R3K 0Z8
Tel: 204-832-7002; *Fax:* 204-889-9002
e-mail: info@ymcaywca.mb.ca
www.ywinnipeg.ca
www.facebook.com/ywinnipeg
twitter.com/YWinnipeg
www.youtube.com/user/YWinnipeg

Chief Officer(s):
Kent Paterson, President & CEO

YMCA of Barrie
22 Grove St. West, Barrie ON L4N 1M7
Tel: 705-726-6421; *Fax:* 705-726-0508
e-mail: barrie@ymcaofsimcoemuskoka.ca

YMCA of Belleville & Quinte
433 Victoria Ave., Belleville ON K8N 2G1
Tel: 613-966-9622; *Fax:* 613-962-9247
e-mail: info@bellevilleymca.ca
www.bellevilleymca.ca

Chief Officer(s):
Robert J. Gallagher, CEO

YMCA of Brandon
231 - 8th St., Brandon MB R7A 3X2
Tel: 204-727-5456; *Fax:* 204-726-0995
e-mail: info@ymcabrandon.com
www.ymcabrandon.com

Chief Officer(s):
Lon Culling, CEO

YMCA of Calgary
101 - 3 St. SW, 2nd Fl., Calgary AB T2P 4G6
Tel: 403-237-9622; *Fax:* 403-269-4661
e-mail: nkaminer@calgary.ymca.ca
www.ymcacalgary.org
www.facebook.com/146637995640

Chief Officer(s):
Helene Weir, President & CEO, 403-781-1670
hweir@calgary.ymca.ca

YMCA of Cape Breton
399 Charlotte St., Sydney NS B1P 1E3
Tel: 902-562-9622; *Fax:* 902-564-2063
e-mail: info@cbymca.com
www.cbymca.com
www.facebook.com/YMCAcapebreton

Chief Officer(s):
Andre Gallant, CEO

YMCA of Chatham-Kent
101 Courthouse Lane, Chatham ON N7L 0B5
Tel: 519-360-9622; *Fax:* 519-360-9629
www.ymcaswo.ca/membership_branches-ymca_of_chathamkent.php
Chief Officer(s):
Amy Wadsworth, General Manager, 519-360-9622 Ext. 103

YMCA of Chilliwack
45844 Hocking Ave., Chilliwack BC V2P 1B4
Tel: 604-792-3371; *Fax:* 604-792-7298
e-mail: chilliwack@gv.ymca.cag
www.vanymca.org/centres/chilliwack
twitter.com/ChilliwackYMCA

Chief Officer(s):
Yvonne Comfort, General Manager

YMCA of Collingwood & District
PO Box 592, 200 Hume St., Collingwood ON L9Y 4E8
Tel: 705-445-5705; *Fax:* 705-445-7732
ymcaofsimcoemuskoka.ca/health_fitness_recreation/collingwood.html
Chief Officer(s):
Rob Armstrong, CEO, 705-726-9622 Ext. 437

YMCA of Cumberland
PO Box 552, 92 Church St., Amherst NS B4H 4A1
Tel: 902-667-9112; *Fax:* 902-661-4692
e-mail: info@cumberland.ymca.ca
www.ymcaofcumberland.com
www.facebook.com/29565029610

Chief Officer(s):
Trina Clarke, CEO
tclarke@ymcaofcumberland.com

YMCA of Exploits Valley
13 Prices Ave., Grand Falls-Windsor NL A2B 1C9
Tel: 709-489-9622; *Fax:* 709-489-8404
e-mail: shaunette_skinner@exploitsvalley.ymca.ca
www.exploitsvalleyymca.ca
www.facebook.com/2263448125

Chief Officer(s):
Shaunette Skinner, Contact

YMCA of Fort Erie
1555 Garrison Rd., Fort Erie ON L2A 1P8
Tel: 905-871-9622; *Fax:* 905-871-9228
www.ymcaofniagara.org/membership_branches-fort_erie.php

YMCA of Fredericton
570 York St., Fredericton NB E3B 3R2
Tel: 506-462-3000; *Fax:* 506-462-3007
www.ymcafredericton.nb.ca
www.facebook.com/260446094448
twitter.com/FrederictonYMCA

Chief Officer(s):
Barb Ramsay, CEO
barb.ramsay@ymcafredericton.org
Ruth Claybourn, Manager, Family Services
Ruth.Claybourn@ymcafredericton.org
Lisa Hanson-Ouellette, Manager, Member Services
Lisa.Hanson-Ouellette@ymcafredericton.org

YMCA of Greater Halifax/Dartmouth
#306, 5670 Spring Garden Road, Halifax NS B3J 1H6
Tel: 902-423-4261
www.ymcahrm.ns.ca

Chief Officer(s):
Bette Watson-Borg, CEO
bette_watson-borg@ymca.ca

YMCA of Greater Moncton
30 War Veterans Ave., Moncton NB E1C 0B3
Tel: 506-857-0606; *Fax:* 506-859-8198
e-mail: info@ymcamoncton.com
www.ymcamoncton.ca
www.facebook.com/107599097472

Chief Officer(s):
Zane Korytko, CEO
zane.korytko@ymcamoncton.com

YMCA of Greater Montréal
1435, rue Drummond, 4e étage, Montréal QC H3G 1W3
Tel: 514-849-5331; *Fax:* 514-849-5863
ymcamontreal.qc.ca/centres_en.htm

Chief Officer(s):
Stéphanie Vaillancourt, CEO

YMCA of Greater Toronto
#300, 2200 Yonge St., Toronto ON M4S 2C6
Tel: 416-928-9622; *Fax:* 416-928-2030
e-mail: memberservices@ymcagta.org
www.ymcagta.org
www.facebook.com/YMCAGTA
twitter.com/ymcagta
www.youtube.com/user/ymcagta

Chief Officer(s):
Medhat Mahdy, President & CEO

YMCA of Greater Vancouver
100 - 5055 Joyce Street, Vancouver BC V5R 6B2
Tel: 604-681-9622; *Fax:* 604-688-0220
e-mail: info@gv.ymca.cag
www.vanymca.org

Chief Officer(s):
Stephen Butz, President & CEO

YMCA of Greater Victoria
851 Broughton St., Victoria BC V8W 1E5
Tel: 250-386-7511; *Fax:* 250-380-1933
e-mail: memberservices@victoriay.com
www.victoriay.com
www.facebook.com/13153669353503
Chief Officer(s):
Jennie Edgecombe, CEO
jedgecombe@victoriay.com

YMCA of Hamilton/Burlington/Brantford
79 James St. South, Hamilton ON L8P 2Z1
Tel: 905-529-7102; *Fax:* 905-529-6682
e-mail: hamilton_downtown@ymca.ca
www.ymcahbb.ca
Chief Officer(s):
Jim Commerford, CEO, 905-317-4919
jim_commerford@ymca.ca

YMCA of Humber Community
PO Box 836, 2 Herald Ave., Corner Brook NL A2H 6H6
Tel: 709-639-9676; *Fax:* 709-634-9622
www.humbercommunityymca.ca
Chief Officer(s):
Christine Young, CEO

YMCA of Kingston
100 Wright Cres., Kingston ON K7L 4T9
Tel: 613-546-2647; *Fax:* 613-549-0654
e-mail: contact@kingston.ymca.ca
www.kingston.ymca.ca
Chief Officer(s):
Mary Kloosterman, CEO
mary_kloosterman@kingston.ymca.ca

YMCA of Lethbridge
515 Stafford Dr. South, Lethbridge AB T1J 2L3
Tel: 403-327-9622; *Fax:* 403-320-6475
e-mail: ymca@lethbridgeymca.org
www.lethbridgeymca.org
Chief Officer(s):
Jennifer Petracek-Kolb, CEO
jennifer@lethbridgeymca.org

YMCA of London
382 Waterloo St., London ON N6B 2N8
Tel: 519-667-3300; *Fax:* 519-433-8527
www.ymcawo.ca
Chief Officer(s):
Shaun Elliott, CEO
selliott@ymcawo.ca

YMCA of Lunenburg County
75 High St., Bridgewater NS B4V 1V8
Tel: 902-543-9622; *Fax:* 902-543-6545
e-mail: jill_sutherland@ymca.ca
www.ymcalunenburgcounty.org
Chief Officer(s):
Yvonne Smith, CEO
yvonne_smith@ymca.ca

YMCA of Medicine Hat
150 Ash Ave. SE, Medicine Hat AB T1A 3A9
Tel: 403-527-4426; *Fax:* 403-529-5702
www.medicinehatymca.ca
www.facebook.com/YMCAMH
twitter.com/MedicineHatYMCA
www.youtube.com/channel/UC96Lsbg-f7NaDDx3DW_VDIw
Chief Officer(s):
Sharon Hayward, CEO
sharon@medicinehatymca.ca

YMCA of Midland
Little Lake Park, PO Box 488, 560 Little Lake Park Rd., Midland ON L4R 4L3
Tel: 705-526-7828; *Fax:* 705-526-8735
www.ymcaofsimcoemuskoka.ca/health_fitness_recreation/midland.html

YMCA of Niagara

43 Church Street, St Catharines ON L2R 7E1
Tel: 905-646-9622; *Fax:* 905-646-4213
www.ymcaofniagara.org
Chief Officer(s):
Stephen Butz, CEO

YMCA of North Bay
186 Chippewa St. West, North Bay ON P1B 6G2
Tel: 705-497-9622; *Fax:* 705-474-5116
www.ymcanorthbay.com
www.facebook.com/ymcanorthbay
Chief Officer(s):
Kim Kanmacher, CEO

YMCA of Northumberland
339 Elgin St. West, Cobourg ON K9A 4X5
Tel: 905-372-0161; *Fax:* 905-377-8940
www.ymcanorthumberland.com
www.facebook.com/93308676120
Chief Officer(s):
Eunice Kirkpatrick, CEO, 905-372-4318 Ext. 310
ekirkpatrick@ymcanorthumberland.com

YMCA of Oakville
410 Rebecca St., Oakville ON L6K 1K7
Tel: 905-845-3417; *Fax:* 905-842-6792
e-mail: customerservice@oakville.ymca.ca
www.ymcaofoakville.com
www.linkedin.com/company/ymca-of-oakville
www.facebook.com/YMCAOakville
twitter.com/YMCAOakville
Chief Officer(s):
Kyle Barber, President & CEO

YMCA of Orillia
300 Peter St. North, Orillia ON L3V 5A2
Tel: 705-325-6168; *Fax:* 705-325-0243
e-mail: orillia@ymcaofsimcoemuskoka.ca
www.ymcaofsimcoemuskoka.ca
Chief Officer(s):
Gilda Evely, General Manager
gilda_evely@ymca.ca

YMCA of Peterborough
123 Aylmer St. South, Peterborough ON K9J 3H8
Tel: 705-748-9622; *Fax:* 705-741-3719
e-mail: kelly_wilson@ymca.ca
www.peterboroughymca.org
twitter.com/YMCA_of_Ptbo
Chief Officer(s):
Robert Gallagher, CEO
bob_gallagher@ymca.ca

YMCA of Pictou County
RR #3, 2756 Westville Rd., New Glasgow NS B2H 5C6
Tel: 902-752-0202; *Fax:* 902-755-3446
e-mail: frontdesk@pcymca.ca
www.pcymca.ca
www.facebook.com/YMCAPictouCounty
Chief Officer(s):
Dave MacIntyre, General Manager

YMCA of Prince George
PO Box 1808, 2020 Massey Dr., Prince George BC V2L 4V7
Tel: 250-562-9341; *Fax:* 250-564-2474
e-mail: info@pgymca.bc.ca
www.pgymca.bc.ca
www.facebook.com/NBCYMCA
twitter.com/NBCY
www.youtube.com/user/PGYMCA
Chief Officer(s):
Amanda Alexander, CEO, 250-562-9341 Ext. 116

YMCA of Regina
2400 - 13th Ave., Regina SK S4P 0V9
Tel: 306-757-9622; *Fax:* 306-525-5508
ymcaregina.squarespace.com
www.facebook.com/YMCARegina
Chief Officer(s):
Randy Klassen, CEO
rklassen@regina.ymca.ca

YMCA of St. John's
PO Box 21291, 84 Elizabeth Ave., St. John's NL A1A 5G6
Tel: 709-726-9622; *Fax:* 709-576-0410
www.ynortheastavalon.com
www.linkedin.com/groups/YMCA-Northeast-Avalon-1903327
www.facebook.com/348363604436
twitter.com/@YMCAofNEA
Chief Officer(s):
Jason Brown, President & CEO
jbrown@ynortheastavalon.com

YMCA of St Thomas - Elgin
20 High St., St Thomas ON N5R 5V2
Tel: 519-631-2418; *Fax:* 519-631-4131
www.ymcawo.ca
Chief Officer(s):
Katie Payler, General Manager, 519-631-2418 Ext. 226
kpayler@ymcawo.ca

YMCA of Sarnia - Lambton
1015 Finch Dr., Sarnia ON N7S 8G5
Tel: 519-336-9622; *Fax:* 519-336-7818
Chief Officer(s):
Ian Foss, General Manager

YMCA of Saskatoon
25 - 22nd St. East, Saskatoon SK S7K 0C7
Tel: 306-652-7515; *Fax:* 306-652-2828
e-mail: ymca@ymcasaskatoon.org
www.ymcasaskatoon.org
Chief Officer(s):
Dean Dodge, CEO

YMCA of Sault Ste Marie
235 McNabb St., Sault Ste Marie ON P6B 1Y3
Tel: 705-949-3133; *Fax:* 705-949-3344
e-mail: info@ssmymca.ca
www.sault.ymca.ca
Chief Officer(s):
Kim Caruso, CEO
kim.caruso@ssmymca.ca

YMCA of Stratford - Perth
204 Downie St. South, Stratford ON N5A 1X4
Tel: 519-271-0480; *Fax:* 519-271-0489
e-mail: cathy_clay@ymca.ca
www.stratfordperthymca.com
Chief Officer(s):
Mimi Price, CEO
mimi_price@ymca.ca

YMCA of Sudbury
140 Durham St., Sudbury ON P3E 3M7
Tel: 705-673-9136; *Fax:* 705-675-8777
e-mail: memberservices@sudbury.ymca.ca
www.sudbury.ymca.ca
www.facebook.com/YMCASudbury
Chief Officer(s):
Kim Kanmacher, CEO

YMCA of Summerside
212 Green St., Summerside PE C1N 1Y4
Tel: 902-436-3446; *Fax:* 902-436-4935
e-mail: mail@ymcapei.ca
www.ymcapei.ca
Chief Officer(s):
Ron Perry, President

YMCA of ville de Québec/Québec City
650, Wilfrid-Laurier, Québec QC G1R 2L4
Tel: 418-522-0800
e-mail: ymca02@globetrotter.net
Chief Officer(s):
Claude Gagné, CEO

YMCA of Wood Buffalo

Westwood Centre, 221 Tundra Dr., Fort McMurray AB T9H 4Z7
Tel: 780-790-9622; *Fax:* 780-743-4045
e-mail: nahanni_alma@ymca.ca
www.ymca.woodbuffalo.org
www.facebook.com/FortMcMurrayYmcaWoodbuffalo
twitter.com/YMCAWoodBuffalo
instagram.com/ymcawoodbuffalo
Chief Officer(s):
Nahanni Alma, Senior Director, Membership Sales & Service,
780-790-9622 Ext. 226

YMCA of Yarmouth
PO Box 86, 275 Main St., Yarmouth NS B5A 4B1
Tel: 902-742-7181; *Fax:* 902-742-7676
e-mail: denise_reid@ymca.ca
www.ymcayarmouth.net
www.facebook.com/YmcaYarmouth
Chief Officer(s):
Yvonne Smith, CEO
Yvonne_Smith@ymca.ca

YMCAs of Cambridge & Kitchener-Waterloo
#203, 460 Frederick Street, Kitchener ON N2H 2P5
Tel: 519-584-7479
e-mail: ymcacambridge@ymca.ca
www.ymcacambridgekw.ca
Chief Officer(s):
John Haddock, CEO, 519-584-7479 Ext. 200

YMCA-YWCA of Guelph
130 Woodland Glen Dr., Guelph ON N1G 4M3
Tel: 519-824-5150; *Fax:* 519-824-4729
e-mail: contact@guelphy.org
www.guelphy.org
Chief Officer(s):
Bonk Jim, CEO

YMCA-YWCA of Kamloops
400 Battle St., Kamloops BC V2C 2L7
Tel: 250-372-7725; *Fax:* 250-372-3023
e-mail: dharris@kamloopsy.org
www.kamloopsy.org
Chief Officer(s):
Colin Reid, CEO, 250-372-7725 Ext. 202
creid@kamloopsy.org

Provincial Associations

ALBERTA

Alberta Cancer Foundation (ACF)
#710, 10123 - 99 St. NW, Edmonton AB T5J 3H1
Tel: 780-643-4400; *Fax:* 780-643-4398
Toll-Free: 866-412-4222
e-mail: acfonline@albertacancer.ca
albertacancer.ca
www.facebook.com/albertacancerfoundation
twitter.com/albertacancer
www.youtube.com/user/ABCancerFoundation
Overview: A small provincial charitable organization founded in 1984
Mission: To raise funds to support & enhance the programs &
treatment facilities of the Alberta Cancer Board
Member of: Alberta Cancer Board
Chief Officer(s):
Myka Osinchuk, CEO

Alberta Children's Hospital Foundation
2888 Shaganappi Trail NW, Calgary AB T3B 6A8
Tel: 403-955-8818; *Fax:* 403-955-8840
Toll-Free: 877-715-5437
e-mail: kids@achf.com
www.childrenshospital.ab.ca
www.facebook.com/AlbertaChildrensHospitalFoundation
www.youtube.com/user/ACHF1
Overview: A small provincial charitable organization founded in 1957
Mission: To raise money on behalf of the Alberta Children's Hospital in
order to improve the services provided to patients & to fund research
Chief Officer(s):
Saifa Koonar, President & CEO

Alberta Easter Seals Society
#103, 811 Manning Rd. NE, Calgary AB T2E 7L4
Tel: 403-235-5662; *Fax:* 403-248-1716
Toll-Free: 877-732-7837
e-mail: calgary@easterseals.ab.ca
www.easterseals.ab.ca
www.facebook.com/EasterSealsAlberta
twitter.com/easterseals AB
pinterest.com/clienttell
Previous Name: Alberta Rehabilitation Council for the Disabled
Overview: A medium-sized provincial charitable organization founded in 1951 overseen by Easter Seals Canada
Mission: To represent interests of all people with disabilities in Alberta; to promote change at all policy-making levels through public awareness campaigns, projects, seminars; to provide mobility equipment; to conduct public awareness programs; to provide recreational activities through summer camp - Camp Horizon; to provide a residential home program - Easter Seals McQueen Residence
Chief Officer(s):
Susan Boivin, Chief Executive Officer, 403-325-5662 Ext. 212
   susan@easterseals.ab.ca

Kids Cancer Care Foundation of Alberta
#302, 609 - 14 St. NW, Calgary AB T2N 2A1
Tel: 403-216-9210; *Fax:* 403-216-9215
Toll-Free: 888-554-2267
e-mail: staff@kidscancercare.ab.ca
www.kidscancercare.ab.ca
www.facebook.com/KCCFA
twitter.com/KidsCancerCare
instagram.com/kidscancercare
Overview: A small provincial charitable organization
Mission: To help improve the lives of children who are suffering from cancer
Chief Officer(s):
Christine McIver, Founder & CEO

The Rainbow Society of Alberta
6604 - 82nd Ave., Edmonton AB T6B 0E7
Tel: 780-469-3306; *Fax:* 780-469-2935
www.rainbowsociety.ab.ca
www.facebook.com/pages/Rainbow-Society-of-Alberta/317391988337
twitter.com/RainbowSociety
Overview: A small provincial charitable organization founded in 1986
Mission: To grant the wishes of Alberta children between the ages of three years & eighteen who have been diagnosed with a chronic or life-threatening illness
Member of: Volunteer Centre of Edmonton & Calgary
Affiliation(s): The Rainbow Society Inc.
Chief Officer(s):
Craig Hawkins, Executive Director

   Calgary
   PO Box 1153, Stn. M, Calgary AB T2P 2K9
   Tel: 403-252-3891; *Fax:* 403-254-5183
   Chief Officer(s):
   Sharon Francis, Fund Development Manager
   sharonf@rainbowsociety.ab.ca

Sickle Cell Foundation of Alberta
PO Box 55041, Stn. New Knottwood, 1704 Millwoods Rd. SW, Edmonton AB T6K 3N0
Tel: 780-450-4943
e-mail: scfoa@telus.ca
www.sicklecellfoundationofalberta.org
Overview: A small provincial organization
Mission: To promote awareness about sickle cell disorder in Alberta
Chief Officer(s):
Ekua Yorke, Founder & Coordinator

BRITISH COLUMBIA

British Columbia Lions Society for Children with Disabilities (BCLS)
3981 Oak St., Vancouver BC V6H 4H5
Tel: 604-873-1865; *Fax:* 604-873-0166
Toll-Free: 800-818-4483
e-mail: info@lionsbc.ca
www.lionsbc.ca
www.facebook.com/125279254193295
twitter.com/LionsBC
Also Known As: Lions Society of BC; Easter Seals; BC Lions Foundation for Children with Disabilities
Overview: A large provincial charitable organization founded in 1952
Mission: To provide as many services as possible to children with disabilities; to enhance the lives of children with special needs; to continue building, not only specialized services & facilities, but challenging young hearts & minds as well; giving children with disabilities self-esteem, self-confidence & a sense of independence
Member of: Easter Seals Canada
Affiliation(s): Easter Seal House Society; 24 HR Relay Society

   Victoria Office
   2095 Granite St., Victoria BC V8S 3G5
   Tel: 250-370-0518; *Fax:* 250-370-5098
   Toll-Free: 888-868-2822
   e-mail: info@forthekidsbc.org

British Columbia's Children's Hospital Foundation (BCCHF)
938 West 28th Ave., Vancouver BC V5Z 4H4
Tel: 604-875-2444; *Fax:* 604-875-2596
Toll-Free: 888-663-3033
e-mail: info@bcchf.ca
www.bcchf.ca
www.facebook.com/BCChildrens
twitter.com/BCCHF
www.youtube.com/user/bcchf
Overview: A small provincial charitable organization
Mission: To make positive differences in the lives of children by raising funds to support British Columbia's Children's Hospital & its related health partners
Member of: Children's & Women's Health Centre of British Columbia
Chief Officer(s):
Don Lindsay, Chair
Teri Nicholas, President & CEO
Hitesh Kothary, Chief Financial Officer
Debora Sweeney, Chief Strategy Officer
Maria Faccio, Chief Philanthropy Offier
Lillian Hum, Chief Philanthropy Offier

Kinsmen Foundation of British Columbia & Yukon (KRF)
c/o David Owen, #3, 33361 Wren Cres., Abbotsford BC V2S 5V9
Tel: 604-852-4501; *Fax:* 604-852-4501
e-mail: kinsmenfoundationofbc@shaw.ca
www.kinsmenfoundationofbc.ca
Overview: A medium-sized provincial charitable organization founded in 1952 overseen by Easter Seals Canada
Mission: Committed to providing funding for services & technologies empowering British Columbians with physical disabilities to live more independently
Chief Officer(s):
David Owen, Volunteer Chief Administrative Officer

Variety - The Children's Charity of BC
4300 Still Creek Dr., Burnaby BC V5C 6C6
Tel: 604-320-0505
Toll-Free: 800-310-5437
e-mail: info@variety.bc.ca
www.variety.bc.ca
www.facebook.com/variety.bc.ca
twitter.com/VarietyBC
www.youtube.com/user/VarietyBC
Also Known As: Variety Club
Overview: A medium-sized provincial charitable organization founded in 1965
Mission: To raise funds throughout the province of B.C. for the benefit of B.C.'s children with special needs; To provide funds for capital costs; To create new centres or improve existing facilities & purchase

specialized equipment
Member of: Variety Clubs International
Chief Officer(s):
Kristy Gill, Executive Director
  kristy.gill@variety.bc.ca

MANITOBA

Children's Hospital Foundation of Manitoba
#CE501, 840 Sherbrook St., Winnipeg MB R3A 1S1
Tel: 204-787-4000; *Fax:* 204-787-4114
Toll-Free: 866-953-5437
Other Communication: Donations 204-953-5437
goodbear.mb.ca
www.facebook.com/childrenshospitalfoundation
twitter.com/chfmanitoba
www.youtube.com/user/DRGoodbear1
Overview: A large provincial charitable organization founded in 1971
Mission: To help raise funds for the Winnipeg Children's Hospital & the Manitoba Institute of Child Health in order to provide patients with improved health care services & to fund research
Chief Officer(s):
Lawrence Prout, President & CEO
  lprout@hsc.mb.ca

The Dream Factory
#303, 1 Wesley Ave., Winnipeg MB R3C 4C6
Tel: 204-989-4010; *Fax:* 204-944-9549
Toll-Free: 866-989-4010
e-mail: dream@thedreamfactory.ca
www.thedreamfactory.ca
www.facebook.com/TheDreamFactoryMB
twitter.com/DreamFactoryMB
www.youtube.com/user/TheDreamFactoryMB
Previous Name: The Rainbow Society
Overview: A small provincial charitable organization founded in 1983
Mission: To provide the opportunity for children (ages 3 to 18) who are suffering from life-threatening illness to fulfill their dreams
Affiliation(s): Rainbow Society of Alberta
Chief Officer(s):
Leilani Kagan, President
Howard Koks, Executive Director
  howard@thedreamfactory.ca
Alyssa Slike, Officer, Development
  alyssa@thedreamfactory.ca
Cindy Titus, Coordinator, Communications & Fundraising
  cindy@thedreamfactory.ca
Isaura Clark, Coordinator, Volunteer
  isaura@thedreamfactory.ca

Manitoba Medical Service Foundation Inc. (MMSF)
PO Box 1046, Stn. Main, Winnipeg MB R3G 3P3
Tel: 204-788-6801; *Fax:* 204-774-1761
e-mail: info@mmsf.ca
www.mmsf.ca
Overview: A medium-sized provincial organization founded in 1971
Mission: To consider the provision of funds for the advancement of scientific, educational, & other activities to maintain & improve the health & welfare of the citizens of Manitoba
Affiliation(s): Manitoba Blue Cross
Chief Officer(s):
Greg Hammond, Executive Director
Lindsay Du Val, Chair

Variety - The Children's Charity of Manitoba, Tent 58 Inc.
#2, 1313 Border St., Winnipeg MB R3H 0X4
Tel: 204-982-1050; *Fax:* 204-475-3198
e-mail: admin@varietymanitoba.com
www.varietymanitoba.com
www.facebook.com/varietymanitoba
twitter.com/Varietymanitoba
www.youtube.com/user/varietymanitoba
Overview: A medium-sized provincial charitable organization founded in 1979
Member of: Variety International - The Children's Charity
Chief Officer(s):
Jerry Maslowsky, Chief Executive Officer

NEW BRUNSWICK

Easter Seals New Brunswick (ESNB) / Les Timbres de Pâques N.-B.
65 Brunswick St., Fredericton NB E3B 1G5
Tel: 506-458-8739; *Fax:* 506-457-2863
e-mail: info@easterseals.nb.ca
www.easterseals.nb.ca
www.facebook.com/246795441998452
twitter.com/EasterSealsNB
Also Known As: Canadian Rehabilitation Council for the Disabled (New Brunswick)
Overview: A medium-sized provincial charitable organization founded in 1966 overseen by Easter Seals Canada
Mission: To provide rehabilitation services & programs to persons with disabilities in New Brunswick; To improve public attitudes towards disabled persons; To provide disabled persons with new opportunities; to provide orthopedic appliances, rehabilitative equipment, technical aids & computers; To advocate on behalf of disabled persons; To serve as information resource centre for disabled persons, students, the public & health professionals; To hold the franchise for the Easter Seals campaign; To provide interprovincial transportation assistance to treatment & diagnostic centres
Chief Officer(s):
Julia Latham, Executive Director
Publications:
• Easter Seals New Brunswick Annual Report
Type: Report; *Frequency:* Annually

NEWFOUNDLAND AND LABRADOR

Easter Seals Newfoundland & Labrador
Husky Energy Easter Seals House, 206 Mount Scio Rd., St. John's NL A1B 4L5
Tel: 709-754-1399; *Fax:* 709-754-1398
e-mail: info@easterseals.nf.ca
www.easterseals.nf.ca
www.linkedin.com/company/easter-seals-newfoundland-and-labrador
www.facebook.com/EasterSealsNL
twitter.com/eastersealsnl
Previous Name: Newfoundland Society for the Physically Disabled Inc.
Overview: A medium-sized provincial organization founded in 1950 overseen by Easter Seals Canada
Mission: To maximize the abilities & enhancing the lives of children & youth with physical disabilities through recreational, social & other therapeutic programs, direct assistance, education & advocacy
Chief Officer(s):
Mark Bradbury, Chief Executive Officer, 709-754-1399 Ext. 222
  markb@eastersealsnl.ca

The International Grenfell Association (IGA)
PO Box 75, 430 Topsail Rd., St. John's NL A1E 4N1
Tel: 709-745-6162; *Fax:* 709-745-6163
e-mail: iga@nfld.net
www.grenfellassociation.org
Overview: A small provincial charitable organization founded in 1914
Mission: To provide funds in support of initiatives that benefit the health, education, social & cultural well-being of the people of Northern Newfoundland & Coastal Labrador, working in partnership with government & other agencies
Chief Officer(s):
Paul Canning, Administrator

NOVA SCOTIA

Easter Seals Nova Scotia (AFNS)
3670 Kempt Rd., Halifax NS B3K 4X8
Tel: 902-453-6000
e-mail: mailing@easterseals.ns.ca
www.easterseals.ns.ca
www.facebook.com/ESnovascotia
twitter.com/Eastersealsns
www.youtube.com/user/eastersealsns
Previous Name: Abilities Foundation of Nova Scotia
Overview: A medium-sized provincial charitable organization founded in 1931 overseen by Easter Seals Canada
Mission: To enable Nova Scotians with physical disabilities to enhance their quality of life by realizing their individual potential

Chief Officer(s):
Henk van Leeuwen, President & CEO, 902-453-6000 Ext. 222
  henk@easterseals.ns.ca
Publications:
• Easter Seals Nova Scotia Annual Report
Type: Report; *Frequency:* Annually

ONTARIO

The Easter Seal Society (Ontario) (TESS) / Société du timbre de Pâques de l'Ontario
#700, 1 Concorde Gate, Toronto ON M3C 3C6
Tel: 416-421-8377; *Fax:* 416-696-1035
Toll-Free: 800-668-6252
e-mail: info@easterseals.org
www.easterseals.org
www.linkedin.com/company/107859
www.facebook.com/MoneyMart24HourRelay
twitter.com/eastersealsont
www.youtube.com/user/Eastersealsont
Overview: A large provincial charitable organization founded in 1922 overseen by Easter Seals Canada
Mission: To help children with physical disabilities achieve their full individual potential & future independence
Member of: National Society of Fundraising Executives; Canadian Centre for Philanthropy; Ontario Association for Children's Treatment Centres
Affiliation(s): BC Lions Society for Children with Disabilities; Newfoundland Society for the Physically Disabled; Québec Easter Seal Society; Easter Seal Ability Council - Alberta; Saskatchewan Abilities Council; Society for Manitobans with Disabilities; Rotary Club of Charlottetown; Abilities Foundation of Nova Scotia; CRCD New Brunswick branch; National Easter Seal Society, USA
Chief Officer(s):
Duncan Hawthorne, Chair
Carol Lloyd, President & CEO

Eastern Region - Kingston
#111, 993 Princess St., Kingston ON K7L 1H3
Tel: 613-547-4126
Toll-Free: 888-667-0043

Eastern Region - Ottawa
#350, 1101 Prince of Wales Dr., Ottawa ON K2C 3W7
Tel: 613-226-3051
Toll-Free: 800-561-4313

Northern Region - Sault Ste. Marie
364 Queen St. East, Sault Ste Marie ON P6A 1Z1
Tel: 705-945-1279
Chief Officer(s):
Carolyn O'Connor, Contact
  coconnor@easterseals.org

Northern Region - Sudbury
887 Notre Dame Ave., #F, Sudbury ON P3A 2T2
Tel: 705-566-8858
Toll-Free: 800-316-5730
Chief Officer(s):
Carmen Bazinet, Contact
  cbazinet@easterseals.org

Northern Region - Thunder Bay
#201, 91 Cumberland St. South, Thunder Bay ON P7B 6A7
Tel: 807-345-7622
Toll-Free: 800-267-3778

Western Region - Burlington / Mississauga / Oakville
PO Box 209, 4035 Fairview St., Burlington ON L7L 6E8
Tel: 289-208-1040
Chief Officer(s):
Susan Smith, Regional Manager
  ssmith@easterseals.org

Western Region - Windsor / Sarnia
2117 Pelissier St., Windsor ON N8X 1N3
Tel: 519-944-0044
Toll-Free: 888-535-5623

Lupus Foundation of Ontario (LFO)
PO Box 687, 294 Ridge Rd. North, Ridgeway ON L0S 1N0
Tel: 905-894-4611; *Fax:* 905-894-4616
Toll-Free: 800-368-8377
e-mail: lupusont@vaxxine.com
www.vaxxine.com/lupus
Overview: A medium-sized provincial charitable organization founded in 1977 overseen by Lupus Canada
Mission: To serve the lupus patient community as a charitable organization
Chief Officer(s):
Laurie Kroeker, President

Ontario Foundation for Visually Impaired Children Inc. (OFVIC)
PO Box 1116, Stn. D, Toronto ON M6P 3K2
Tel: 416-767-5977; *Fax:* 416-767-5530
e-mail: ofvic@look.ca
Overview: A small provincial organization
Chief Officer(s):
April Cornell, Executive Director

Ontario March of Dimes (OMOD) / Marche des dix sous de l'Ontario
10 Overlea Blvd., Toronto ON M4H 1A4
Tel: 416-425-3463; *Fax:* 416-425-1920
Toll-Free: 800-263-3463
www.marchofdimes.ca
www.facebook.com/marchofdimescanada
twitter.com/modcanada
www.youtube.com/user/marchofdimescda
Also Known As: Rehabilitation Foundation for the Disabled
Overview: A large provincial charitable organization founded in 1951
Mission: To maximize the independence, personal empowerment & community participation of people with physical disabilities
Affiliation(s): March of Dimes Canada; Ontario March of Dimes Non-Profit Housing Corporation (NPHC); OMOD Independence Non-Profit Corporation; Rehabilitation Foundatation for Disabled Persons Inc., U.S.; Polio Canada; Stroke Recovery Canada
Chief Officer(s):
Andria Spindel, President & CEO
Jerry Lucas, Vice-President & COO

Reach for the Rainbow
20 Torlake Cres., Toronto ON M8Z 1B3
Tel: 416-503-0088; *Fax:* 416-503-0485
e-mail: info@reachfortherainbow.ca
www.reachfortherainbow.ca
www.facebook.com/ReachForTheRainbow
twitter.com/RFTRCharity
www.youtube.com/RFTRCharity
Overview: A small provincial charitable organization founded in 1983
Mission: To offer integrated recreational & respite programs for disabled children within the province of Ontario
Chief Officer(s):
David Neal, Executive Director
  dneal@reachfortherainbow.ca
Lisa Carty, Chair

Variety - The Children's Charity (Ontario)
3701 Danforth Ave., Toronto ON M1N 2G2
Tel: 416-699-7167; *Fax:* 416-699-5752; *TTY:* 416-699-8147
e-mail: info@varietyvillage.on.ca
www.varietyvillage.ca
Previous Name: Variety Club of Ontario, Tent 28
Overview: A medium-sized provincial organization founded in 1945
Mission: To improve the quality of life for children with disabilities & to promote their integration into society
Member of: Variety Clubs International
Affiliation(s): Variety Village; Variety Ability Systems Inc.
Chief Officer(s):
Karen Stintz, President & CEO
  kstintz@varietyvillage.on.ca

Villa Charities Inc. (Toronto District)
901 Lawrence Ave. West, Toronto ON M6A 1C3
Tel: 416-789-7011; *Fax:* 416-789-3951
www.villacharities.com
Previous Name: Italian Canadian Benevolent Corporation (Toronto District)

Overview: A medium-sized provincial charitable organization founded in 1971
Mission: To develop social programs that enhace the lives of their senior members & promote Italian heritage
Affliation(s): Villa Colombo Services for Seniors; Columbus Centre; VITA Community Living Services; Caboto Terrace; Casa DelZotto; Casa Abruzzo; Villa Colombo Vaughan Di Poce Centre
Chief Officer(s):
Aldo Cundari, Chair
Frank Chiarotto, Vice-Chair
Joseph Arcuri, Treasurer

Wellspring Cancer Support Foundation / Fondation Wellspring pour les personnes atteintes de cancer
4 Charles St. East, Toronto ON M4Y 1T1
Tel: 416-961-1928; *Fax:* 416-961-3721
Toll-Free: 877-499-9904
www.wellspring.ca
wwww.facebook.com/WellspringCAN
twitter.com/wellspringCAN
www.youtube.com/user/WellspringCancer
Overview: A medium-sized provincial charitable organization
Chief Officer(s):
John Philp, Chair
Christina Smith, CEO

QUÉBEC

Bechtel Foundation of Canada
#350, 1981 McGill College Ave., Montréal QC H3A 3A8
Tel: 514-871-1711; *Fax:* 514-871-1392
www.bechtel.com
Overview: A small provincial organization founded in 1949
Mission: To finance educational activities in engineering & the support of community & national health, welfare & cultural organizations
Chief Officer(s):
John McVey, General Manager
jmcvey@bechtel.com

The Farha Foundation / La Fondation Farha
#100, 576, rue Sainte-Catherine Est, Montréal QC H2L 2E1
Tel: 514-270-4900; *Fax:* 514-270-5363
e-mail: farha@farha.qc.ca
www.farha.qc.ca
www.facebook.com/FondationFARHAFoundation
twitter.com/FarhaFoundation
www.youtube.com/user/farhafondation
Overview: A medium-sized provincial charitable organization founded in 1992
Mission: To raise funds to improve the quality of life for persons living with HIV & AIDS throughout Québec
Chief Officer(s):
Nancy Farha, Executive Director Ext. 223
n.farha@farha.qc.ca

Fondation Marie-Éve Saulnier
#102, 3925, Grande-Allée, Saint-Hubert QC J4T 2V8
Tél: 450-926-9000; *Téléc:* 450-766-8843
www.fondationmarieevesaulnier.qc.ca
www.facebook.com/Fondation.Marie.Eve.Saulnier2014
twitter.com/FondationMES
www.youtube.com/channel/UCKSL9-vwaPFPiHGDYXjLs_g
Aperçu: *Dimension:* petite; *Envergure:* provinciale; fondée en 1997
Mission: La Fondation Marie-Éve Saulnier améliore au jour le jour la qualité de vie des enfents atteints de cancer.
Membre(s) du bureau directeur:
Linda Langlois Saulnier, Directrice générale

Fondation pour la recherche sur la moelle épinière
#400, 6020 rue Jean-Talon Est, Montréal QC H1S 3B1
Tél: 514-341-7272; *Téléc:* 514-341-8884
Ligne sans frais: 877-341-7272
Courriel: info@moelleepiniere.com
www.moelleepiniere.com
www.facebook.com/MEMOQuebec
twitter.com/MEMOQuebec
Nom précédent: Fondation André Sénécal pour la recherche sur la moelle épinière
Aperçu: *Dimension:* moyenne; *Envergure:* provinciale; fondée en 1994

Mission: A pour but de récolter des fonds pour financer, principalement, la recherche scientifique et médicale sur les lésions médullaires
Membre(s) du bureau directeur:
Walter Zelaya, Directeur général
wzelaya@moelleepiniere.com

Fondation québécoise de la maladie coeliaque (FQMC) / Québec Celiac Foundation
#230, 4837, rue Boyer, Montréal QC H2J 3E6
Tél: 514-529-8806; *Téléc:* 514-529-2046
Courriel: info@fqmc.org
www.fqmc.org
Aperçu: *Dimension:* petite; *Envergure:* provinciale; Organisme sans but lucratif; fondée en 1983
Mission: Diffuser de l'information sur la maladie et le régime sans gluten; faciliter l'approvisionnement; encourager les initiatives des membres; supporter les membres et défendre leurs droits; favoriser la recherche; soliciter des fonds pour réaliser ses mandats
Membre(s) du bureau directeur:
Suzanne Laurencelle, Directrice Générale

Société pour les enfants handicapés du Québec (SEHQ) / Quebec Society for Disabled Children
2300, boul René-Lévesque ouest, Montréal QC H3H 2R5
Tél: 514-937-6171; *Téléc:* 514-937-0082
Ligne sans frais: 877-937-6171
Courriel: sehq@enfantshandicapes.com
www.enfantshandicapes.com
www.facebook.com/enfantshandicapes
twitter.com/SEHQ
Aperçu: *Dimension:* moyenne; *Envergure:* provinciale; Organisme sans but lucratif; fondée en 1930 surveillé par Easter Seals Canada
Mission: Voué au bien-être des enfants handicapés et de leur famille; grâce aux contributions publiques qui lui sont versées et aux efforts conjugués de bénévoles et des permanents, la société offre des services directs et professionnels qui favorisent le développement personnel des enfants et leur intégration dans la communauté
Membre(s) du bureau directeur:
Ronald Davidson, Directeur général, 877-937-6171 Ext. 210
rdavidson@enfantshandicapes.com
Carolle Desjardins, Directrice, Financement, 877-937-6171 Ext. 232
cdesjardins@enfantshandicapes.com
Nicole Amzallag, Séjours de groupes et classes nature, 877-937-6171 Ext. 212
namzallag@enfantshandicapes.com

SASKATCHEWAN

Children's Hospital Foundation of Saskatchewan
#1, 345 - 3 Ave. South, Saskatoon SK S7K 1M6
Tel: 306-931-4887
Toll-Free: 888-808-5437
e-mail: info@chfsask.ca
www.childrenshospitalsask.ca
www.facebook.com/CHFSask
twitter.com/childhospitalsk
www.youtube.com/user/ChildHospitalSK
Overview: A small provincial charitable organization
Mission: To help raise funds for the Children's Hospital of Saskatchewan in order to provide patients with improved health care services & to fund research
Chief Officer(s):
Brynn Boback-Lane, President & CEO

YUKON TERRITORY

Yukon Foundation
PO Box 31622, Whitehorse YT Y1A 6L2
Tel: 867-393-2454
e-mail: yukonfoundation@klondiker.com
www.yukonfoundation.com
Overview: A small provincial organization founded in 1980
Mission: To promote educational advancement and scientific or medical research for the enhancement of human knowledge; provide support intended to contribute to the mental, cultural and physical well-being of residents of Yukon; and promote the cultural heritage of Yukon.
Chief Officer(s):

Sophie Partridge, Executive Director

Local Associations
ALBERTA

Calgary Children's Foundation
c/o CHQR FM, #170, 200 Barclay Parade SW, Calgary AB T2P 4R5
Tel: 403-444-4337
Overview: A small local organization
Mission: To promote the mental & physical health & welfare of children & certain adults who are disadvantaged & reside within Alberta
Chief Officer(s):
Betty Jo Kaiser, Administrator
  bettyjo.kaiser@corusent.com

Chinook Regional Hospital Foundation (CRHF)
960 - 19th St. South, Lethbridge AB T1J 1W5
Tel: 403-388-6001; *Fax:* 403-388-6604
e-mail: info@crhfoundation.com
www.crhfoundation.ca
www.facebook.com/crhfoundation.ca
twitter.com/crh_foundation
Also Known As: CRH Foundation
Overview: A small local charitable organization
Mission: To raise, receive & distribute funds for equipment & programs in order to enhance patient services at Chinook Regional Hospital; Primarily fund the purchase & maintenance of equipment that will enhance care & attract medical specialists
Chief Officer(s):
Jason Vanden Hoek, Executive Director

Kids Kottage Foundation
10107 - 134 Ave., Edmonton AB T5E 1J2
Tel: 780-448-1752; *Crisis Hot-Line:* 780-944-2888
e-mail: info@kidskottage.org
www.kidskottage.org
www.facebook.com/kidskottageYEG
twitter.com/KidsKottageEDM
Previous Name: Canadian Foundation for the Love of Children
Overview: A medium-sized local charitable organization founded in 1987
Mission: To promote the health & well-being of children & their families; To prevent child abuse & neglect by supporting families in crisis
Chief Officer(s):
Lori Reiter, Executive Director
Dianne Petersen, Program Manager

Lo-Se-Ca Foundation
#215, 1 Carnegie Dr., St Albert AB T8N 5B1
Tel: 780-460-1400
www.loseca.ca
www.facebook.com/115663645142959
twitter.com/losecafdn
Overview: A small local charitable organization founded in 1988
Mission: To promote the quality of life of families & individuals by providing services within a Christian environment; to enhance human well-being, worth & dignity of life for all persons with disabilities
Member of: Alberta Association of Rehabilitation Centres; Persons with Developmental Disabilities
Chief Officer(s):
Marie Renaud, Executive Director
  mrenaud@loseca.ca

BRITISH COLUMBIA

David Foster Foundation
212 Henry St., Victoria BC V9A 3H9
Tel: 250-475-1223; *Fax:* 250-475-1193
Toll-Free: 877-777-7675
e-mail: info@davidfosterfoundation.com
www.davidfosterfoundation.com
www.linkedin.com/company/david-foster-foundation
www.facebook.com/DavidFosterFoundation
twitter.com/davidfosterfdn
Overview: A small local charitable organization founded in 1986

Mission: To provide financial assistance to families of children undergoing transplant surgery; To raise public awareness regarding organ donation
Chief Officer(s):
Michael Ravenhill, CEO
  mravenhill@davidfosterfoundation.com

Lions Gate Hospital Foundation
231 East 15th St., North Vancouver BC V7L 2L7
Tel: 604-984-5785; *Fax:* 604-984-5786
e-mail: info@lghfoundation.com
www.lghfoundation.com
www.facebook.com/lghfoundation
twitter.com/LGHFoundation
instagram.com/lghfoundation
Overview: A small local charitable organization
Mission: To help raise money on behalf of 10 health care centres to fund research & improve patient care
Chief Officer(s):
Judy Savage, President
  judy.savage@vch.ca

Portuguese Canadian Seniors Foundation
5455 Imperial St., Burnaby BC V5J 1E5
Tel: 604-873-2979; *Fax:* 604-873-2974
www.pcsf.ca
www.youtube.com/user/THEPCSF
Overview: A small local organization founded in 1987
Chief Officer(s):
Maria Viegas Guerreiro, President

Vernon Jubilee Hospital Foundation
2101 - 32nd St., Vernon BC V1T 5L2
Tel: 250-558-1362; *Fax:* 250-558-4133
e-mail: info@vjhfoundation.org
www.vjhfoundation.org
www.facebook.com/VJHFoundation
Overview: A small local charitable organization founded in 1981
Mission: To support & raise funds for Vernon Jubilee Hospital, as well as residential care facilities & community care programs
Chief Officer(s):
Sue Beaudry, Director, Development, 250-558-1200 Ext. 1405

Victoria Hospitals Foundation (VHF)
1952 Bay St., Victoria BC V8R 1J8
Tel: 250-519-1750; *Fax:* 250-519-1751
e-mail: vhf@viha.ca
www.victoriahf.ca
www.facebook.com/VictoriaHF
twitter.com/ourvichospitals
Previous Name: Greater Victoria Hospitals Foundation
Overview: A small local charitable organization founded in 1989
Mission: To raise funds for Victoria's major hospitals: Victoria General & Royal Jubilee, which also serve the entire Vancouver Island
Affiliation(s): Vancouver Island Health Authority
Chief Officer(s):
Melanie Mahlman, President & CEO
Publications:
• InTouch [a publication of Victoria Hospitals Foundation]
Type: Newsletter; *Frequency:* Quarterly
Profile: Relays news about funding activities & priorities at the hospitals

West Vancouver Community Foundation
775 - 15th St., West Vancouver BC V7T 2S9
Tel: 604-925-8153; *Fax:* 604-925-8154
e-mail: westvanfoundation@telus.net
www.westvanfoundation.com
www.facebook.com/westvanfoundation
Overview: A small local charitable organization founded in 1979
Mission: To improve the quality of life in West Vancouver; to assist organizations & people through grants & awards, with special emphasis on health, education, the arts, social services & West Vancouver's physical environment
Member of: Community Foundations of Canada
Chief Officer(s):
Geoff Jopson, Chair
Delaina Bell, Executive Director

NEW BRUNSWICK

Cerebral Palsy Foundation (St. John) Inc.
PO Box 2152, Saint John NB E2L 3V1

Tel: 506-648-0322
e-mail: mail@cpfsj.ca
www.cpfsj.ca

Overview: A small local organization

Chipman Community Care Inc.
PO Box 435, Chipman NB E4A 3N4

Tel: 506-339-5565; *Fax:* 506-339-6823
e-mail: communitycareinc@hotmail.com

Overview: A small local charitable organization founded in 1987
Mission: To promote total community wellness among youth to seniors
Member of: Association of Food Banks & C.V.A.'s for New Brunswick; Atlantic Alliance of Food Banks & C.V.A.'s
Chief Officer(s):
Mary West, President

Fondation CHU Dumont Foundation
330 University Ave., Moncton NB E1C 2Z3

Tel: 506-862-4285; *Fax:* 506-862-4474
Toll-Free: 800-862-6775
e-mail: info@fondationdumont.ca
www.chudumont.ca
www.facebook.com/ChuDumont

Overview: A small local charitable organization
Mission: To raise money on behalf of the Dr. Georges L. Dumont Hospital to improve the services offered to patients & to fund research
Chief Officer(s):
Jacques B. LeBlanc, President & CEO

Friends of The Moncton Hospital Foundation
135 MacBeath Ave., Moncton NB E1C 6Z8

Tel: 506-857-5488; *Fax:* 506-857-5753
e-mail: friends@horizonnb.ca
www.friendsfoundation.ca
www.facebook.com/FriendsofTMH
twitter.com/FriendsofTMH
www.youtube.com/user/FriendsofTMH

Overview: A small local charitable organization founded in 1965
Mission: To raise money on behalf of the Moncton Hospital in order to improve the services offered to patients & fund research
Chief Officer(s):
Linda Saunders, President & CEO
linda.saunders@horizonnb.ca

NEWFOUNDLAND AND LABRADOR

Dr. H. Bliss Murphy Cancer Care Foundation
Dr. H. Bliss Murphy Cancer Centre, 300 Prince Philip Dr., St. John's NL A1B 3V6

Tel: 709-777-7589; *Fax:* 709-777-2372
cancercarefoundation.nl.ca
www.facebook.com/cancercarefoundation
twitter.com/Cancercarefdn
www.youtube.com/user/Cstarz76

Overview: A small local charitable organization
Mission: To raise money on behalf of the Dr. H. Bliss Murphy Cancer Centre in order to improve the services offered to patients & to fund research
Chief Officer(s):
Lynette Hillier, Executive Director, 709-777-7590, Fax: 797-772-372
lynette.hillier@easternhealth.ca

Janeway Children's Hospital Foundation
300 Prince Philip Dr., St. John's NL A1B 3V6

Tel: 709-777-4640; *Fax:* 709-777-4489
e-mail: janewayfoundation@easternhealth.ca
www.janewayfoundation.nf.ca
www.facebook.com/JanewayNL
twitter.com/JanewayNL
www.youtube.com/user/janewayfoundation

Overview: A small local charitable organization
Mission: To raise money on behalf of the Janeway Childnren's Hospital that helps fund research & improve patient care
Chief Officer(s):
Lynn Sparkes, Executive Director

NOVA SCOTIA

Cape Breton Regional Hospital Foundation
#209, 45 Weatherbee Rd., Sydney NS B1M 0A1

Tel: 902-567-7752
e-mail: foundation@cbdha.nshealth.ca
www.becauseyoucare.ca
www.facebook.com/CapeBretonCares
twitter.com/BecauseUCare
instagram.com/becauseucare

Overview: A small local charitable organization
Mission: To raise money on behalf of the Cape Breton Regional Hospital in order to improve the services provided to patients & to fund research
Chief Officer(s):
Brad Jacobs, CEO, 902-567-8186
brad.jacobs@nshealth.ca

IWK Health Centre Foundation (IWKF)
#B220, 5855 Spring Garden Rd., Halifax NS B3H 4S2

Tel: 902-470-8085
Toll-Free: 800-595-2266
e-mail: foundationmail@iwk.nshealth.ca
iwkfoundation.org
www.facebook.com/iwkfoundation
twitter.com/IWKFoundation
www.instagram.com/iwkfoundation

Overview: A small local charitable organization
Mission: To raise money on behalf of the IWK Health Centre that helps fund research & improve patient care
Chief Officer(s):
Jennifer Gillivan, ICD.D, President & CEO
jennifer.gillivan@iwk.nshealth.ca

Regional Occupation Centre Foundation
Regional Occupation Centre, 3 MacQuarrie Dr. Ext., Port Hawkesbury NS B9A 3A3

Tel: 902-625-0132; *Fax:* 902-625-5344
www.rocsociety.ca/Foundation

Also Known As: ROC Foundation
Overview: A small local charitable organization founded in 2009
Mission: To raise funds to support the mission & objectives of the Regional Occupation Centre Society

ONTARIO

Acclaim Health
2370 Speers Rd., Oakville ON L6L 5M2

Tel: 905-827-8800; *Fax:* 905-827-3390
Toll-Free: 800-387-7127
www.acclaimhealth.ca
ca.linkedin.com/company/acclaim-health
www.facebook.com/acclaimhealth
twitter.com/AcclaimHealth

Overview: A small local charitable organization founded in 1971
Mission: To provide elderly patients with home health care solutions; to help improve their patients' quality of life through volunteer visitors
Chief Officer(s):
Angelia Brewer, RN, MBA, CEO
abrewer@acclaimhealth.ca

Alva Foundation
c/o Graham Hallward, 199 Albertus Ave., Toronto ON M4R 1J6

e-mail: info@alva.ca
www.alva.ca

Previous Name: Southam Foundation
Overview: A medium-sized local charitable organization founded in 1965
Mission: To fund research into risk factors in early childhood development (pre-natal to 3 years of age); To fund pilot programs on demonstrations of new therapies serving the constituency described above
Chief Officer(s):
Christopher Kerrigan, President
Graham F. Hallward, Chair, Donations Committee

Baycrest Foundation
3560 Bathurst St., 2nd Fl., Toronto ON M6A 2E1
Tel: 416-785-2875; *Fax:* 416-785-4296
e-mail: donations@baycrest.org
www.baycrest.org/give
Overview: A small local charitable organization founded in 1979
Mission: To raise money on behalf of the Baycrest Centre, which helps funds research for age related diseases
Chief Officer(s):
Josh Cooper, President & CEO, 416-785-2500 Ext. 2415
jcooper@baycrest.org

Bob Rumball Foundation for the Deaf
2395 Bayview Ave., Toronto ON M2L 1A2
Tel: 416-449-9651; *TTY:* 416-449-2728
Other Communication: 416-640-0723
e-mail: fundraising@bobrumball.org
www.bobrumball.org
www.facebook.com/86097284911
twitter.com/BobRumball
www.instagram.com/bobrumball
Previous Name: Ontario Mission of the Deaf
Overview: A small local organization founded in 1872
Mission: To meet the social, recreational, educational & spiritual needs of the deaf community & raise funds for The Bob Rumball Centre for the Deaf in Toronto, The Bob Rumball Associations for the Deaf in Milton, The Bob Rumball Long Term Care Home for the Deaf in Barrie & The Bob Rumball Camp for the Deaf in Parry Sound.
Chief Officer(s):
Derek Rumball, Executive Director

CAMH Foundation
Bell Gateway Building, 100 Stokes St., 5th Fl., Toronto ON M6J 1H4
Tel: 416-979-6909; *Fax:* 416-979-6910
Toll-Free: 800-414-0471
e-mail: foundation@camh.ca
www.supportcamh.ca
ca.linkedin.com/company/camh-foundation
www.facebook.com/end.stigma
twitter.com/endstigma
www.instagram.com/camhfoundation
Also Known As: Centre for Addiction & Mental Health Foundation
Overview: A small local charitable organization
Mission: To raise money on behalf of CAMH in order to improve the services provided to patients & to fund research
Chief Officer(s):
Darrell Gregersen, President & CEO
Darrell.Gregersen@camh.ca

Catholic Charities of The Archdiocese of Toronto
#400, 1155 Yonge St., Toronto ON M4T 1W2
Tel: 416-934-3401; *Fax:* 416-934-3402
e-mail: info@catholiccharitiestor.org
www.catholiccharitiestor.org
twitter.com/charitiescares
Previous Name: Council of Catholic Charities
Overview: A medium-sized local licensing charitable organization founded in 1913
Mission: To ensure the provision of health & social sciences; To provide leadership & advocacy on behalf of member agencies & those in need; To serve people living & working throughout the Greater Toronto Area, as well as in Simcoe, Durham, Peel, & York
Affiliation(s): Catholic Family Services of Toronto & 26 member agencies
Chief Officer(s):
Thomas Cardinal Collins, Chair
Carmela Pallotto, President
Michael Fullan, Executive Director

C.G. Jung Foundation of Ontario
14 Elm St., Toronto ON M5G 1S7
Tel: 416-961-9767; *Fax:* 416-961-6659
e-mail: info@cgjungontario.com
www.cgjungontario.com
Also Known As: Ontario Association of Jungian Analysts
Overview: A small local charitable organization founded in 1971
Mission: To disseminate information about the psychological teachings of Carl Gustav Jung through lectures, seminars, workshops, a library &

a bookstore; a list of Jungian analysts is available for referral
Member of: International Association of Jungian Analysts
Chief Officer(s):
Catherine Johnson, Administrator
Publications:
• Chiron [a publication of the C.G. Jung Foundation of Ontario]
Type: Newsletter; *Editor:* Robert Black; *ISSN:* 1918-6142

Chai-Tikvah The Life & Hope Foundation
#313, 4600 Bathurst St., Toronto ON M2R 3V2
Tel: 416-634-3050
e-mail: info@lifeandhope.ca
www.lifeandhope.ca
Overview: A small local charitable organization
Mission: To support individuals with mental illness by providing secure housing options & services, & promoting their inclusion in society
Chief Officer(s):
David Drutz, Chair
Rochelle Goldman-Brown, Executive Director

The Children's Aid Foundation of York Region
#19, 201 Millway Ave., Vaughan ON L4K 5K8
Tel: 905-738-8675
www.cafyr.org
www.facebook.com/184207384932619
Overview: A small local organization
Mission: To improve the lives of abused children through enrichment, education, & prevention; To raise funds to support the children & families served by Children's Aid Societies
Chief Officer(s):
Attilio Lio, President

Children's Aid Society of Toronto (CASMT)
30 Isabella St., Toronto ON M4Y 1N1
Tel: 416-924-4640
www.torontocas.ca
www.youtube.com/channel/UCY5JSHV7wnG5mB5OLTLIn6Q
Previous Name: Children's Aid Society of Metropolitan Toronto
Overview: A large local organization founded in 1891
Mission: To protect children from emotional, sexual & physical harm by working with individual children & their families; to provide a high standard & continuity of substitute parental care for those children who cannot remain at home; to develop prevention programs
Member of: Ontario Association of Children's Aid Societies; Child Welfare League of Canada; Child Welfare League of America
Chief Officer(s):
Anthony Fralick, Chair
David Rivard, CEO
Publications:
• Communicate [a publication of the Children's Aid Society of Toronto]
Type: Newspaper

Children's Health Foundations
345 Westminster Ave., London ON N6C 4V3
Tel: 519-432-8564; *Fax:* 519-432-5907
Toll-Free: 888-834-2696
e-mail: info@childhealth.ca
childhealth.ca
www.facebook.com/CHFHope
twitter.com/CHFHope
www.youtube.com/user/ChildrensRaisingHope
Overview: A small local charitable organization founded in 1922
Mission: To help raise funds for children's hospitals in order to provide patients with improved health care services & to fund research
Chief Officer(s):
Sherri Bocchini, Chief Development Officer
sbocchini@childhealth.ca
Tracy Loosemore, Chief Operating Officer
tloosemore@childhealth.ca

Children's Hospital of Eastern Ontario Foundation
415 Smyth Rd., Ottawa ON K1H 8M8
Tel: 613-737-2780; *Fax:* 613-738-4818
Toll-Free: 800-561-5638
www.cheofoundation.com
www.facebook.com/CHEOkids
twitter.com/cheohospital
www.youtube.com/user/CHEOvideos
Also Known As: Children's Hospital Foundation

Overview: A medium-sized local charitable organization founded in 1974
Mission: To advance the physical, mental, & social well-being of children & their families in Eastern Ontario & Western Quebec by raising, managing, & disbursing funds; To support the Children's Hospital of Eastern Ontario
Member of: Children's Miracle Network Telethon
Chief Officer(s):
Mahesh Mani, Chair
Len Hanes, Director, Communications
  lhanes@cheofoundation.com

Community One Foundation
PO Box 760, Stn. F, Toronto ON M4Y 2N6

Tel: 416-920-5422
e-mail: info@communityone.ca
www.communityone.ca
www.facebook.com/CommunityOneFoundation
twitter.com/C1Foundation
instagram.com/c1foundation

Previous Name: Lesbian & Gay Community Appeal Foundation
Overview: A medium-sized local charitable organization founded in 1980
Mission: To raise & disburse funds for the advancement of lesbian, gay, bisexual & transgender projects, artists & organizations; To fund projects in the areas of health & social services, arts & culture, research & education, political & legal
Member of: Canadian Centre for Philanthropy
Chief Officer(s):
Terrance Greene, Co-Chair
Kevin Ormsby, Co-Chair

Hamilton Community Foundation (HCF)
#700, 120 King St. West, Hamilton ON L8P 4V2

Tel: 905-523-5600; *Fax:* 905-523-0741
e-mail: info@hamiltoncommunityfoundation.ca
hamiltoncommunityfoundation.ca
www.facebook.com/HamCommFdn
twitter.com/HamCommFdn

Overview: A small local charitable organization founded in 1954
Mission: To distribute grants in perpetuity to those of Hamilton/Wentworth & Burlington region. Grants in the past have been for adult basic education, theatre arts, residential redevelopment, environment, poverty reduction, youth activities, preschool, sexual assualt centre, community healthcare.
Member of: Canadian Centre for Philanthropy; Council on Foundations; Community Foundations of Canada
Chief Officer(s):
Brent J. Foreman, Chair
Terry Cooke, President & CEO Ext. 224
  terry.cooke@hamiltoncommunityfoundation.ca

London Health Sciences Foundation (LHSF)
747 Base Line Rd. East, London ON N6C 2R6

Tel: 519-685-8409; *Fax:* 519-685-8265
e-mail: foundation@lhsc.on.ca
www.lhsf.ca
www.facebook.com/lhsf.ca
twitter.com/LHSFCanada
www.youtube.com/LHSFCanada

Overview: A small local charitable organization
Mission: To help raise money on behalf of the London Health Sciences Centre to fund research & improve patient care
Chief Officer(s):
John H. MacFarlane, President, 519-685-8409 Ext. 58482

Markham Stouffville Hospital Foundation
PO Box 1800, 381 Church St., Markham ON L3P 7P3

Tel: 905-472-7059; *Fax:* 905-472-7018
e-mail: mshfoundation@msh.on.ca
www.mshf.on.ca
www.facebook.com/markhamstouffvillehospital
twitter.com/mshospital
www.youtube.com/mshospital

Also Known As: MSH Foundation
Overview: A small local charitable organization
Mission: To raise money on behalf of the Markham Stouffville Hospital in order to fund research & improve patient care

Chief Officer(s):
Suzette Strong, Chief Executive Officer, 905-472-7396
  suzette@msh.on.ca

Mon Sheong Foundation
11211 Yonge St., Richmond Hill ON L4S 0E9

Tel: 905-883-9288; *Fax:* 905-883-9855
Toll-Free: 866-708-0002
e-mail: msf@monsheong.org
www.monsheong.org
twitter.com/MonSheong
instagram.com/monsheong

Overview: A medium-sized local organization founded in 1964
Mission: To recognize the Chinese language & philosophy through caring for the elderly & edifying the young; To provide programs & services which respond to the needs of communities
Member of: Ontario Association of Nonprofit Homes & Services for Seniors
Affliation(s): Ontario Hospital Association
Chief Officer(s):
Stephanie Wong, CEO

Mount Sinai Hospital Foundation
#1001, 522 University Ave., Toronto ON M5G 1W7

Tel: 416-586-8203; *Fax:* 416-586-8639
Toll-Free: 877-565-8555
e-mail: foundation@mtsinai.on.ca
www.mshfoundation.ca
www.youtube.com/user/MountSinaiFoundation

Overview: A small local charitable organization founded in 1923
Mission: The Foundation raises & stewards funds to support the Mount Sinai Hospital's patient care, research & education. In 2008, more than $344 million has been raised to fund The Best Medicine Campaign, to support research, innovative programs, improved facilities & technology. Mount Sinai Hospital's Centres of Excellence include: the Samuel Lunenfeld Research Institute, Women's & Infants' Health, Oncology, Acute & Chronic Medicine, & Laboratory Medicine & Infection Control
Chief Officer(s):
Brent S. Belzberg, Chair
Kevin Goldthorp, President
Publications:
• The Best Medicine Matters [a publication of the Mount Sinai Hospital Foundation]
Type: Newsletter; *Frequency:* q.

North York General Foundation
4001 Leslie St., Toronto ON M2K 1E1

Tel: 416-756-6944; *Fax:* 416-756-9047
e-mail: foundation@nygh.on.ca
www.nyghfoundation.ca
www.linkedin.com/company/north-york-general-foundation
www.facebook.com/NYGHFoundation
twitter.com/NYGHFoundation
www.youtube.com/NYGHFoundation

Overview: A small local charitable organization
Mission: To raise money on behalf of North York General Hospital in order to fund research & improve patient care
Chief Officer(s):
Terry Pursell, President & CEO

Princess Margaret Cancer Foundation
700 University Ave., 10th Fl., Toronto ON M5G 1Z5

Tel: 416-946-6560; *Fax:* 416-946-6563
Toll-Free: 866-224-6560
e-mail: info@thepmcf.ca
www.thepmcf.ca
www.facebook.com/thePMCF
twitter.com/thePMCF
www.youtube.com/user/PrincessMargaretHF

Overview: A small local charitable organization
Mission: To raise funds to support cancer research at the Princess Margaret Cancer Centre
Chief Officer(s):
Tom Ehrlich, Chair
Paul Alofs, President & CEO
Kenzie Broddy, Manager, Communications
  kenzie.broddy@thepmcf.ca

St. Joseph's Healthcare Foundation
224 James St. South, Hamilton ON L8P 3A9

Tel: 905-521-6036; *Fax:* 905-577-0860
Toll-Free: 866-478-5037
e-mail: info@stjoesfoundation.ca
www.stjoesfoundation.ca
www.facebook.com/stjosephshealthcarefoundation
twitter.com/stjoeshamilton
www.instagram.com/stjoeshamilton

Overview: A small local charitable organization founded in 1970
Mission: To raise money for St. Joseph's Healthcare Hamilton
Chief Officer(s):
Sera Filice-Armenio, President & CEO

Simcoe Muskoka Family Connexions
#7, 60 Bell Farm Rd., Barrie ON L4M 5G6

Tel: 705-726-6587; *Fax:* 705-726-9788
Toll-Free: 800-461-4236
www.simcoecas.com

Merged from: Children's Aid Society of Simcoe County; Family, Youth & Child Services of Muskoka
Overview: A medium-sized local organization
Mission: To provide guidance & counseling to families & protection for children
Chief Officer(s):
Susan Carmichael, Executive Director

Sudbury Manitoulin Children's Foundation
PO Box 1264, Stn. B, 296 Larch St., Sudbury ON P3E 4S7

Tel: 705-673-2227; *Fax:* 705-673-8798
www.smcf.com
www.facebook.com/SudburyManitoulinChildrensFoundationSMCF
twitter.com/SMCF_1976

Overview: A small local charitable organization
Mission: To develop programs designed to assist children & families from the Sudbury-Manitoulin area
Chief Officer(s):
Anne Salter Dorland, Executive Director
anne@smcf.com

Toronto General & Western Hospital Foundation
R. Fraser Elliot Bldg., #5S-801, 190 Elizabeth St., Toronto ON M5G 2C4

Tel: 416-340-3935; *Fax:* 416-340-4864
Toll-Free: 877-846-4483
e-mail: foundation@uhn.ca
www.tgwhf.ca
www.facebook.com/tgwhf
www.twitter.com/tgwhf
www.youtube.com/user/TGWHFoundation

Previous Name: Toronto Hospital Foundation
Overview: A small local charitable organization
Mission: To raise funds for research, education & the enhancement of patient care at University Health Network.
Chief Officer(s):
Tennys J.M. Hanson, President & CEO

Trillium Health Partners Foundation
Clinical & Administrative Bldg., 100 Queensway West, 5th Fl., Mississauga ON L5B 1B8

Tel: 905-848-7575; *Fax:* 905-804-7927
e-mail: foundation@thp.ca
trilliumgiving.ca
www.facebook.com/TrilliumHealthPartnersFoundation
twitter.com/trilliumhealth
www.youtube.com/user/TrilliumHeroes

Merged from: Trillium Health Centre Foundation; Credit Valley Hospital Foundation
Overview: A small local charitable organization founded in 2013
Mission: To help raise funds for the Credit Valley Hospital, the Mississauga Hospital & the Queensway Health Centre in order to provide patients with improved health care services & to fund research
Chief Officer(s):
Steve Hoscheit, President & CEO
Steve.Hoscheit@thp.ca

Prince County Hospital Foundation (PCHF)
PO Box 3000, 65 Roy Boates Ave., Summerside PE C1N 2A9

Tel: 902-432-2547; *Fax:* 902-432-2551
e-mail: info@pchcare.com
www.pchcare.com
www.facebook.com/PCHFoundation
twitter.com/PCHFoundation

Overview: A medium-sized local charitable organization
Mission: To raise money for Prince County Hospital in order to keep up with medical equipment needs
Chief Officer(s):
Heather Matheson, Managing Director
hematheson@ihis.org
Bevan Woodacre, Officer, Communications
bdwoodacre@ihis.org
Lisa Schurman-Smith, Manager, Finance & Administration
leschurman@ihis.org
Kelly Arsenault, Administrator, Database
kmarsenault@ihis.org

Queen Elizabeth Hospital Foundation
PO Box 6600, 60 Riverside Dr., Charlottetown PE C1A 8T5

Tel: 902-894-2425; *Fax:* 902-894-2433
e-mail: info@qehfoundation.pe.ca
www.qehfoundation.pe.ca
www.facebook.com/QEHFoundation
twitter.com/QEHFoundation

Also Known As: QEH Foundation
Overview: A small local charitable organization
Mission: To receive donations on behalf of the Queen Elizabeth Hospital & utilize those funds in order to improve the quality of care at the Queen Elizabeth Hospital
Chief Officer(s):
Tracey Comeau, Chief Executive Officer
tacomeau@qehfoundation.pe.ca

Birks Family Foundation / Fondation de la famille Birks
#1200, 615, boul René-Lévesque Ouest, Montréal QC H3B 1P5

e-mail: secretarytreasurer@birksfamilyfoundation.ca
www.birksfamilyfoundation.ca

Overview: A small local charitable organization founded in 1961

The EJLB Foundation
#1050, 1350, rue Sherbrooke Ouest, Montréal QC H3G 1J1

Fax: 514-843-4080
e-mail: general@fondationecho.ca
www.ejlb.qc.ca

Overview: A small local organization founded in 1983
Mission: Provides grants to organizations with areas of interest in mental health and the environment
Chief Officer(s):
Kevin Leonard, Executive Director

Eldee Foundation
c/o Bloomfield & Associates, #1720, 1080, Côte du Beaver Hill, Montréal QC H2Z 1S8

Tel: 514-871-9571; *Fax:* 514-397-0816
www.eldeefoundation.ca

Overview: A small local charitable organization founded in 1961
Mission: To provides grants mostly for education & medical research to organizations primarily for the benefit of persons of the Jewish faith
Chief Officer(s):
Harry J.F. Bloomfield, President

Fondation Cardio-Montérégienne (FOCAM)
#230, 1750, boul Marie-Victorin, Longueuil QC J4G 1A5

Tél: 450-468-3333; *Téléc:* 450-468-3334
www.fondationcardio-monteregienne.ca

Aperçu: *Dimension:* petite; *Envergure:* locale
Mission: Encourager et soutenir l'avancement de la science médicale au moyen de dons permettant l'acquisition d'équipements reliés à la médecine cardiaque.

Fondation Centre de cancérologie Charles-Bruneau
4515, rue de Rouen, Montréal QC H1V 1H1
Tél: 514-256-0404; *Téléc:* 514-256-2116
Ligne sans frais: 877-256-0404
Courriel: fondation@charlesbruneau.qc.ca
charlesbruneau.qc.ca
www.facebook.com/fcharlesbruneau
twitter.com/fcharlesbruneau
www.youtube.com/fcharlesbruneau
Aperçu: *Dimension:* petite; *Envergure:* locale; Organisme sans but lucratif
Mission: Pour amasser des fonds qui finance la recherche sur le cancer pédiatrique
Membre(s) du bureau directeur:
Rébecca Dumont, Directrice générale
rdumont@charlesbruneau.qc.ca

Fondation CHU de Québec
Hôpital Saint-François d'Assise, #E1-152, 10, rue de l'Espinay, Québec QC G1L 3L5
Tél: 418-525-4385; *Téléc:* 418-525-4393
Courriel: fondation.chuq@chuq.qc.ca
www.fondationduchuq.org
twitter.com/FCHUQ
Aperçu: *Dimension:* petite; *Envergure:* locale; Organisme sans but lucratif
Mission: Pour augmenter des fonds sur le compte de 5 hôpitaux pour améliorer les services offerts aux patients et à financer la recherche
Membre(s) du bureau directeur:
Marie-Claude Paré, Présidente et chef de la direction
marie-claude.pare@chudequebec.ca

Fondation CHU Sainte-Justine
#335, 5757, av Decelles, Montréal QC H3S 2C3
Tél: 514-345-4710; *Téléc:* 514-345-4718
Ligne sans frais: 888-235-3667
Courriel: fondation@sainte-justine.org
www.fondation-sainte-justine.org
www.facebook.com/fondationsaintejustine
twitter.com/fondstejustine
www.youtube.com/user/FondationHSJ
Aperçu: *Dimension:* petite; *Envergure:* locale; Organisme sans but lucratif; fondée en 1987
Mission: Pour amasser des fonds pour le compte de le CHU Sainte-Justine que aident à améliorer les services offerts aux patients et à financer la recherche
Membre(s) du bureau directeur:
Maud Cohen, Présidente et directrice générale

Fondation de l'Hôpital de Montréal pour enfants / Montréal Children's Hospital Foundation
1, Place Alexis Nihon, #1420, 3400, boul de Maisonneuve Ouest, Montréal QC H3Z 3B8
Tel: 514-934-4846; *Fax:* 514-939-3551
Toll-Free: 866-934-4846
e-mail: info@fhme.com
fondationduchildren.com
www.facebook.com/lechildren
twitter.com/hopitalchildren
www.youtube.com/montrealchildrens
Overview: A small local charitable organization
Mission: Pour amasser des fonds au nom de l'Hôpital de Montréal pour enfants afin de financer la recherche et améliorer les soins aux patients
Chief Officer(s):
Marie-Josée Gariépy, Présidente
mgar@fhme.com

Fondation de l'Hôpital du Sacré-Coeur de Montréal
5400, boul Gouin Ouest, Montréal QC H4J 1C5
Tél: 514-338-2303; *Téléc:* 514-338-3153
Ligne sans frais: 866-453-3666
Courriel: fondation.hsc@ssss.gouv.qc.ca
www.fhscm.com
www.linkedin.com/company/5323549
www.facebook.com/FondationHopitalSacreCoeur
twitter.com/fhscm
www.youtube.com/user/HSCM2009

Aperçu: *Dimension:* petite; *Envergure:* locale; Organisme sans but lucratif; fondée en 1976
Mission: Pour amasser des fonds au nom du Hôpital du Sacré-Coeur de Montréal afin de financer la recherche et améliorer les soins aux patients
Membre(s) du bureau directeur:
Paul Bergeron, Directeur général
paul.bergeron.cnmtl@ssss.gouv.qc.ca

Fondation de l'Hôpital Général de Montréal / Montréal General Hospital Foundation
#E6-129, 1650, av Cedar, Montréal QC H3G 1A4
Tel: 514-934-8230; *Fax:* 514-937-7683
e-mail: info@mghfoundation.com
www.mghfoundation.com
Overview: A small local charitable organization founded in 1973
Mission: Pour amasser des fonds au nom de l'Hôpital Général de Montréal afin de financer la recherche et améliorer les soins aux patients
Chief Officer(s):
Jean-Guy Gourdeau, Président & directeur exécutif
jggourdeau@mghfoundation.com

Fondation de l'Hôpital Maisonneuve-Rosemont
#270, 5345, boul de L'Assomption, Montréal QC H1T 4B3
Tél: 514-252-3435; *Téléc:* 514-252-3943
Courriel: info@fondationhmr.ca
fondationhmr.ca
www.linkedin.com/company-beta/10080977
www.facebook.com/fondationhmr
twitter.com/fondationhmr
www.youtube.com/user/FondationHMR
Aperçu: *Dimension:* petite; *Envergure:* locale; Organisme sans but lucratif
Mission: Pour amasser des fonds pour le compte de l'Hôpital Maisonneuve-Rosemont que contribuent à améliorer les services offerts aux patients et à financer la recherche
Membre(s) du bureau directeur:
Lucie Drapeau, Directrice générale

Fondation du CHUM
#800, 465, rue McGill, Montréal QC H2Y 2H1
Tél: 514-890-8077; *Téléc:* 514-412-7393
Ligne sans frais: 877-570-0797
Courriel: info@fondationduchum.com
fondationduchum.com
www.linkedin.com/company/fondation-du-chum
www.facebook.com/FondationCHUM
twitter.com/FondationCHUM
www.youtube.com/user/fondationduchum
Aperçu: *Dimension:* petite; *Envergure:* locale; Organisme sans but lucratif
Mission: Pour amasser des fonds pour le compte de le Centre hospitalier de l'Université de Montréal pour améliorer les services offerts aux patients et à financer la recherche
Membre(s) du bureau directeur:
Luce Moreau, Présidente-directrice générale

Fondation Hôpital Charles-LeMoyne (FHCLM)
3120, boul Taschereau, Greenfield Park QC J4V 2H1
Tél: 450-466-5487; *Téléc:* 450-672-1716
www.fhclm.ca
www.facebook.com/FondationCharlesLeMoyne
Nom précédent: Fondation Charles LeMoyne
Aperçu: *Dimension:* petite; *Envergure:* locale; Organisme sans but lucratif; fondée en 1964
Mission: S'occuper de réunir les fonds pour que l'Hôpital Charles LeMoyne puisse acheter et remplacer de l'équipement spécialisé et pour permettre la recherche médicale
Membre(s) du bureau directeur:
Danièle J. Martin, Directrice générale

Fondation Institut de Cardiologie de Montréal / Montréal Heart Institute Foundation
4100, rue Molson, Montréal QC N1Y 3N1

Tel: 514-593-2525; *Fax:* 514-376-5400
Toll-Free: 877-518-2525
e-mail: ficmdon@icm-mhi.org
www.icm-mhi.org/fr/fondation
www.facebook.com/institutcardiologiemontreal
twitter.com/ICMtl
www.youtube.com/user/InstituteCardioMtl

Overview: A small local charitable organization founded in 1977
Mission: Pour amasser des fonds au nom de l'Institut de Cardiologie de Montréal afin de financer la recherche
Chief Officer(s):
Mélanie La Couture, Directrice générale
melanie.lacouture@icm-mhi.org

Fondation Santé Gatineau
Pavillon Desjardins, #B-202, 116, boul Lionel-Émond, Gatineau QC J8Y 1W7

Tél: 819-966-6108; *Téléc:* 819-966-6012
Courriel: csssgatineau_info_fondation@ssss.gouv.qc.ca
www.fondationsantegatineau.ca
www.facebook.com/FondationSanteGatineau
twitter.com/FondSanteGat

Aperçu: *Dimension:* petite; *Envergure:* locale; Organisme sans but lucratif
Mission: Pour augmenter des fonds sur le compte du CSSS de Gatineau pour améliorer les services offerts aux patients et à financer la recherche
Membre(s) du bureau directeur:
Jean Pigeon, Directeur général

Jewish General Hospital Foundation (JGHF) / Hôpital général juif fondation (HGJF)
#A107, 3755 Côte-Sainte-Catherine Rd., Montréal QC H3T 1E2

Tel: 514-340-8251; *Fax:* 514-340-8220
e-mail: info@jghfoundation.org
www.jghfoundation.org
www.facebook.com/FHGJ.JGHF

Overview: A small local charitable organization founded in 1969
Mission: To raise money on behalf of the Jewish General Hospital in order to fund research & improve patient care
Chief Officer(s):
Myer Bick, President & CEO
mbick@fon.jgh.mcgill.ca

McGill University Health Centre Foundation
#900, 2155, rue Guy, Montréal QC H3H 2R9

Tel: 514-931-5656; *Fax:* 514-931-5696
www.muhcfoundation.com

Also Known As: MUHC Foundation
Overview: A small local charitable organization
Mission: To raise money on behalf of the McGill University Health Centre in order to fund research & improve patient care
Chief Officer(s):
Julie Quenneville, President
julie.quenneville@muhc.mcgill.ca
Lorraine Balleine, Director, Finance & Administration
lorraine.balleine@muhc.mcgill.ca

SASKATCHEWAN

Lloydminster Region Health Foundation (LRHF)
#116, 4910 - 50 St., Lloydminster SK S9V 0Y5

Tel: 306-820-6161; *Fax:* 306-825-3680
lrhf.ca
www.facebook.com/LloydRHF

Overview: A small local charitable organization founded in 1983
Mission: To help raise money on behalf of 4 health care centres to fund research & improve patient care
Chief Officer(s):
Wendy Plandowski, CEO
wendy.plandowski@lrhf.ca

Royal University Hospital Foundation (RUHF)
#1626, 103 Hospital Dr., Saskatoon SK S7N 0W8

Tel: 306-655-1984
e-mail: info@ruhf.org
www.ruhf.org
www.facebook.com/RoyalUniversityHospitalFoundation
twitter.com/RUHFoundation
www.youtube.com/channel/UCUu4nSywH8WtF7lQHZVgFTQ

Overview: A small local charitable organization founded in 1983
Mission: To help provide additional funds for the Royal University Hospital, a university teaching hospital
Chief Officer(s):
Arla Gustafson, CEO

Telemiracle/Kinsmen Foundation Inc.
2217C Hanselman Ct., Saskatoon SK S7L 6A8

Tel: 306-244-6400; *Fax:* 306-653-5730
www.telemiracle.com
www.facebook.com/Telemiracle
twitter.com/Telemiracle

Overview: A small local charitable organization
Mission: To provide special needs equipment & medical assistance to people in Saskatchewan
Chief Officer(s):
Cindy Xavier, Executive Director

International Associations

African Medical & Research Foundation Canada (AMREF Canada)
#403, 489 College St., Toronto ON M6G 1A5

Tel: 416-961-6981; *Fax:* 416-961-6984
Toll-Free: 888-318-4442
e-mail: info@amrefcanada.org
www.amrefcanada.org
www.facebook.com/amrefcanada
twitter.com/amrefcanada
www.youtube.com/amrefcanada

Also Known As: Flying Doctors
Overview: A medium-sized international charitable organization founded in 1957
Mission: Development agency working to enhance community health in East & Southern Africa; headquartered in Nairobi, Kenya; eleven national offices in both Europe & America; acts as support office in raising private & public funds for overseas health programs & also plays active role in maintaining working relations with Canadian International Development Agency (CIDA)
Member of: Canadian Council for International Cooperation
Affliation(s): African Medical & Research Foundations Nairobi; Canadian Centre for Philanthropy; Ontario Council for International Cooperation; Canadian Council for International Cooperation; Canadian Society of International Health
Chief Officer(s):
Anne-Marie Kamanye, Executive Director

Aga Khan Foundation Canada (AKFC)
The Delegation of the Ismaili Imamat, 199 Sussex Dr., Ottawa ON K1N 1K6

Tel: 613-237-2532; *Fax:* 613-567-2532
Toll-Free: 800-267-2532
e-mail: info@akfc.ca
www.akfc.ca

Overview: A medium-sized international charitable organization founded in 1980
Mission: To support cost-effective development projects in Asia & Africa in the fields of primary health care, education & rural development, with special attention paid to the needs of women. Major initiatives include: The Pakistan-Canada Social Institutions Development Program; the Tajikistan Institutional Support Program and the Non-Formal Education Program of the Bangladesh Rural Advancement Committee.
Chief Officer(s):
Khalil Z. Shariff, CEO

Association for Healthcare Philanthropy (AHP)
#400, 313 Park Ave., Falls Church VA 22046 USA

Tel: 703-532-6243; *Fax:* 703-532-7170
e-mail: ahp@ahp.org
www.ahp.org
www.linkedin.com/groups/Association-Healthcare-Philanthropy-114275
7
www.facebook.com/AHPIntl
twitter.com/AHPIntl

Overview: A small international organization founded in 1967
Mission: Educational organization and advocacy body for health care fundraising professionals in Canada & the United States.
Member of: Association for Healthcare Philathropy
Chief Officer(s):
David L. Flood, Chair
Steven W. Churchill, President & CEO

Canada India Village Aid Association (CIVA)
1822 West 2nd Ave., Vancouver BC V6J 1H9

e-mail: projects@civaid.ca
www.civaid.ca

Overview: A small international charitable organization founded in 1981
Mission: To raise funds to support anti-poverty projects benefiting the peoples of rural India; to foster self-help & self-reliance, particularly through sustainable development & women's empowerment, collaborating with Indian non-profit agencies & organizations in various fields of development, education, health care, & environmental concern.
Chief Officer(s):
Ashok Kotwal, Contact

Canadian Feed The Children (CFTC)
#123, 6 Lansing Sq., Toronto ON M2J 1T5

Tel: 416-757-1220; *Fax:* 416-757-3318
Toll-Free: 800-387-1221
e-mail: contact@canadianfeedthechildren.ca
www.canadianfeedthechildren.ca
www.linkedin.com/company/canadian-feed-the-children
www.facebook.com/CanadianFeedTheChildren
twitter.com/cdnfeedchildren
www.youtube.com/user/canadianfeed

Overview: A medium-sized international charitable organization founded in 1986
Mission: To alleviate the impact of poverty on children; To work with local partners overseas & in Canada to enhance the well-being of children & the self-sufficiency of their families & communities
Member of: Canadian Council for International Cooperation
Chief Officer(s):
Debra Kerby, President & CEO
Anne Marshall, Chief Financial Officer
Peter Timmerman, Vice-President, Programs
Gail Black, Vice-President, Development
Jennifer Watson, Vice-President, Communications

Canadian Friends of Bikur Cholim Hospital
329 Joicey Blvd., Toronto ON M5N 2V8

Tel: 416-781-6960

Overview: A small international organization
Mission: To support & raise funds for Bakir Cholim Hospital in Jerusalem
Chief Officer(s):
David Kleiner, Secretary-Treasurer
dkleiner@danatrading.com

Christian Children's Fund of Canada (CCFC)
1200 Denison St., Markham ON L3R 8G6

Tel: 905-754-1001; *Fax:* 905-754-1002
Toll-Free: 800-263-5437
Other Communication: media@ccfcanada.ca
e-mail: donor-relations@ccfcanada.ca
www.ccfcanada.ca
www.facebook.com/CCFC
twitter.com/CCFCanada
www.youtube.com/c/ccfcanada

Overview: A large international charitable organization founded in 1960

Mission: To focus upon community development ministry, starting with basic assistance & leading to programs stressing self-help & eventual independence; To work with colleagues & partners in developing countries; To reach out to children & families of all faiths
Member of: Canadian Council of Christian Charities; Better Business Bureau; ChildFund Alliance; Imagine Canada
Affiliation(s): Canadian Marketing Association; Association of Fundraising Professionals
Chief Officer(s):
Douglas Ellenor, Chair
Terrance M Slobodian, Vice-President, Fund Development & Communications
Jim Carrie, Vice-President, Global Operations
Jeff Hogan, CPA; CA; CSR-P, Vice-President, Finance & Corporate Services
Publications:
• Child Essentials Newsletter
Type: Newsletter; *Frequency:* monthly
• ChildVoice
Type: Magazine; *Frequency:* s-a.; *Editor:* Vicki Quigley
Profile: Magazine for donors featuring stories of sponsored children

Coffin-Lowry Syndrome Foundation (CLSF)
675 Kalima Pl. NW, Issaquah WA 98027 USA

Tel: 425-427-0939
e-mail: coffinlowry@gmail.com
clsf.info

Overview: A small international organization founded in 1991
Mission: To serve as a clearinghouse of information on the syndrome, a support group for parents with CLS children & a general forum for exchanging experiences, advice & information with other CLS families; to seek to become a visible group in the medical, scientific, educational & professional communities in order to facilitate referrals of newly diagnosed individuals, & to encourage medical & behavioural research in order to improve methods of social integration of CLS individuals
Chief Officer(s):
Mary C. Hoffman, Chairperson

Compassion Canada
PO Box 5591, London ON N6A 5G8

Tel: 519-668-0224; *Fax:* 866-685-1107
Toll-Free: 800-563-5437
e-mail: info@compassion.ca
www.compassion.ca

Overview: A medium-sized international charitable organization founded in 1963
Mission: To provide sponsors for children in Third World countries; To aid community development projects in cooperation with Canadian International Development Agency; To be an advocate for children, to release them from their spiritual, economic, social & physical poverty & to enable them to become responsible & fulfilled Christian adults
Member of: Better Business Bureau; Canadian Council of Christian Charities; Association of Evangelical Relief & Development Organizations; Evangelical Fellowship of Canada
Chief Officer(s):
Barry Slauenwhite, President & CEO
Jim Bartholomew, Vice-President, Strategy & Marketing
Tim DeWeerd, Vice-President, Business Services
Deb Wilkins, Vice-President, Engagement

Dystonia Medical Research Foundation Canada / Fondation de recherches médicales sur la dystonie
#305, 121 Richmond St. West, Toronto ON M5H 2K1

Tel: 416-488-6974; *Fax:* 416-488-5878
Toll-Free: 800-361-8061
e-mail: info@dystoniacanada.org
www.dystoniacanada.org
www.facebook.com/DMRFC

Also Known As: DMRF Canada
Overview: A small international charitable organization founded in 1976
Mission: To advance & support research relating to dystonia; To build awareness about the illness in order to educate both medical & lay communities; To sponsor patient & family support groups & programs
Member of: Dystonia Medical Research Foundation
Chief Officer(s):

SECTION III: Appendices

Stefanie Ince, Executive Director
stefanieince@dystoniacanada.org

Alberta - Calgary Support Group
c/o Developmental Disabilities Resource Centre, 4631
Richardson Way SW, Calgary AB T3E 7B7
Toll-Free: 800-361-8061
Chief Officer(s):
Margaret Roy, Contact, 403-271-4438
roymg@telusplanet.net

British Columbia - Kelowna Area Support Group
Kelowna BC
Tel: 250-763-7739
Chief Officer(s):
Anne Skomedal, Contact
rskomedal@shaw.ca

Manitoba - Winnipeg Support Group
Winnipeg MB

New Brunswick - Moncton Support Group
Moncton NB
Chief Officer(s):
Shirley Sharkey, Contact, 506-204-2722
j.s.sharkey@rogers.com

Nova Scotia - Port Hawesbury Area Contact
Port Hawkesbury NS
Chief Officer(s):
Marcellin Chiasson, Contact, 902-625-1811
marcellin.chiasson@ns.sympatico.ca

Nunavut - Iqaluit Area Contact
Iqaluit NU
Tel: 867-979-3791
e-mail: info@dystoniacanada.org
Chief Officer(s):
Sharon Gee, Contact
sharon_gee@hotmail.com

Ontario - Golden Triangle Support Group
c/o Judy Harsch, #808, 7 Christopher Ct., Guelph ON N1G 4V6
Chief Officer(s):
Judy Harsch, Contact, 519-767-9721
jjmarie@rogers.com

Ontario - Hamilton Support Group
Hamilton ON
Chief Officer(s):
Laurie Bell, Contact, 905-774-4111
landbell@rogers.com

Ontario - London Support Group
London ON
Chief Officer(s):
Michelle & Bruce Goodhue, Contacts, 519-455-7457
bgood137@sympatico.ca

Ontario - Ottawa Support Group
Ottawa ON
Tel: 613-224-6888
Toll-Free: 800-361-8061
Chief Officer(s):
John Heney, Contact
jjheney@netrover.com

Ontario - Sudbury Support Group
Sudbury ON
Chief Officer(s):
Mary Guy, Contact, 705-524-0606
maryguy@personainternet.com

Ontario - Toronto Support Group
Toronto ON
Chief Officer(s):
Wendy Paul, Contact, Membership co-ordinator & support,
416-789-0154
dmrft@rogers.com

Québec - Montréal Support Group
Montréal QC
Chief Officer(s):
Chloe Belisle, Contact, 514-696-0949

Saskatchewan - Saskatoon Support Group
SK
Chief Officer(s):
Diane Haugen, Contact, 306-477-0577
dystonia@sasktel.net

Ethiopiaid
#900, 275 Slater St., Ottawa ON K1P 5H9
Tel: 613-238-4481
e-mail: info@ethiopiaid.ca
www.ethiopiaid.ca
www.facebook.com/EthiopiaidCanada
twitter.com/EthiopiaidCAN
Overview: A medium-sized international charitable organization founded in 1989
Mission: To create lasting & positive change in Ethiopia by tackling the problems of poverty, ill health & poor education; To donate to local community projects in Ethiopia
Chief Officer(s):
Olivier Bonnet, Executive Director
Jennifer Naidoo, Officer, Development & Communications

Joubert Syndrome & Related Disoarders Foundation (JSRDF)
c/o Pete Asman, Treasurer, 1415 West Ave., Cincinnati OH 45215
USA
Tel: 614-864-1362
e-mail: president@jsrdf.org
www.jsrdf.org
www.facebook.com/180691234440
twitter.com/jsrdf
Overview: A small international charitable organization founded in 1992
Mission: To serve as an international network of parents who share knowledge, experience & emotional support; to educate physicians & their support teams; to increase awareness & understanding of Joubert Syndrome; to provide support to families who have loved ones diagnosed with Joubert Syndrome
Chief Officer(s):
Karen Tompkins, President
president@jsrdf.org

Samaritan's Purse Canada (SPC)
20 Hopewell Way NE, Calgary AB T3J 5H5
Tel: 403-250-6565; *Fax:* 403-250-6567
Toll-Free: 800-663-6500
e-mail: info@samaritan.ca
www.samaritanspurse.ca
www.facebook.com/samaritanspurse.ca
twitter.com/spcanada
www.youtube.com/user/samaritanspursecan; pinterest.com/spcanada
Also Known As: Operation Christmas Child
Overview: A large international charitable organization founded in 1973
Mission: To meet both physical & spiritual needs of people who are victims of war, poverty, natural disasters, disease & famine; To provide emergency relief & development programs, & medical projects
Member of: Canadian Council of Christian Charities
Affliation: Samaritan's Purse USA
Chief Officer(s):
Franklin Graham, President & CEO
Fred Weiss, Executive Director

Save a Family Plan (SAFP)
PO Box 3622, London ON N6A 4L4
Tel: 519-672-1115; *Fax:* 519-672-6379
e-mail: safpinfo@safp.org
www.safp.org
www.facebook.com/pages/Save-A-Family-Plan/117934038235594
twitter.com/SaveaFamilyPlan
Overview: A large international charitable organization founded in 1965
Mission: Implements sustainable family & community development programs in 5 states in India, with 41 social service societies, 26 homes of health, approximately 10,550 grass roots community organiziations & 15,000 poor families; programs are developed through needs assessments; within all aspects of programming, environmental & gender impact assessments are undertaken. Offices in Canada, the

U.S. & India
Member of: Coalition for the Right of Children
Chief Officer(s):
Lesley Tordoff, Executive Director
Lois Côté, President
Publications:
• Ektha (Unity)
Type: Newsletter

Seva Canada Society
#100, 2000 West 12th Ave., Vancouver BC V6J 2G2
Tel: 604-713-6622; *Fax:* 604-733-4292
Toll-Free: 877-460-6622
www.seva.ca
www.facebook.com/sevacanada
twitter.com/sevacanada
www.instagram.com/sevacanada
Previous Name: Seva Service Society
Overview: A small international charitable organization founded in 1982
Mission: To prevent blindness in developing countries through the implementation of local eye care programs
Member of: British Columbia Council for International Cooperation
Chief Officer(s):
Penny Lyons, Executive Director
Ken Bassett, Director, Program
Deanne Berman, Director, Marketing & Communications
Christine Smith, Director, Development
Lisa Demers, Manager, Operations & Program

Teamwork Children's Services International
5983 Ladyburn Cres., Mississauga ON L5M 4V9
Tel: 905-542-1047
www.teamworkchildrenservices.com
Overview: A small international charitable organization
Mission: To provide a safe environment for disadvantaged children in rural areas of Africa; To help children become productive citizens through the provision of physical & mental care, education, & vocational training
Chief Officer(s):
Joel Chacha, Executive Director
jchacha@teamworkchildrenservices.com

United Mitochondrial Disease Foundation (UMDF)
#201, 8085 Saltsburg Rd., Pittsburgh PA 15239 USA
Tel: 412-793-8077; *Fax:* 412-793-6477
Toll-Free: 888-317-8633
e-mail: info@umdf.org
www.umdf.org
Overview: A small international organization founded in 1995
Mission: To promote research & education for the diagnosis, treatment & cure of mitochondrial disorders & to provide support to affected individuals & families
Chief Officer(s):
Charles A. Mohan, CEO/Executive Director
chuckm@umdf.org
Charles A. Mohan, Jr., CEO

Death and Bereavement

National Associations

Canadian Hospice Palliative Care Association (CHPCA) / Association canadienne de soins palliatifs (ACSP)
Annex D, Saint-Vincent Hospital, 60 Cambridge St. North, Ottawa ON K1R 7A5
Tel: 613-241-3663; *Fax:* 613-241-3986
Toll-Free: 800-668-2785
Other Communication: Info Line: 1-877-203-4636
www.chpca.net
www.facebook.com/CanadianHospicePalliativeCare
twitter.com/CanadianHPCAssn
Overview: A large national charitable organization founded in 1991
Mission: CHPCA provides leadership in the pursuit of excellence in the care of people approaching death in Canada, in order to lessen suffering, loneliness, & grief. The national association works to develop national standards of practice for hospice palliative care.

Member of: Quality End of Life Care Coalition; HEAL; Canadian Care Giver Coalition; Health Charities Council of Canada
Chief Officer(s):
Laurie Anne O'Brien, President
Jeff Christiansen, Secretary-Treasurer
Sharon Baxter, Executive Director
Publications:
• AVISO
Type: Newsletter; *Frequency:* Quarterly
• Canadian Hospice Palliative Care Association National Office Update
Type: Newsletter; *Frequency:* Monthly
Profile: Events, research news, awards, policy news, & resources
• Directory of Hospice Palliative Care Services
Type: Directory
Profile: Information on the availability of hospice palliative care services across Canada, featuring listings of programs & services, contact information, population served, & area of care

Canadian Society of Palliative Care Physicians (CSPCP) / Société canadienne des médecins de soins palliatifs (SCMSP)
c/o Fraser Health Authority, #400, 13450 - 102 Ave., Surrey BC V3T 0H1
Tel: 604-341-3174; *Fax:* 604-587-4644
e-mail: office@cspcp.ca
www.cspcp.ca
Overview: A medium-sized national organization
Mission: The CSPCP is a membership organization for patients and their families, though the advancement and improvement of palliative medicine and training.
Chief Officer(s):
Susan MacDonald, President
Kim Taylor, Executive Director

Council on Palliative Care / Conseil des Soins Palliatifs
3605, rue de la Montagne, Montréal QC H3G 2M1
Tel: 514-845-0795
e-mail: fmpa202@gmail.com
www.mcgill.ca/council-on-palliative-care
www.facebook.com/CouncilOnPalliativeCare
twitter.com/PalliativeCares
Overview: A small national organization founded in 1994
Mission: To work in association with McGill University to raise public awareness & support of palliative care; To increase the availability of palliative care
Chief Officer(s):
Suzanne O'Brien, Co-Chair
John Sanford, Co-Chair
Publications:
• Council on Palliative Care Newsletter
Type: Newsletter
Profile: Council news, articles about palliative care, meeting highlights, & upcoming events

Cryonics Society of Canada (CSC)
PO Box 11514, 600 The East Mall, Toronto ON M9B 4B0
e-mail: csc4@cryocdn.org
www.cryocdn.org
Overview: A small national organization founded in 1988
Mission: To promote & provide information to the public about cryonics; To assist individuals in making cryonic suspension arrangements; To encourage research in cryonics & other life-extension sciences

Dying with Dignity (DWD) / Mourir dans la dignité
#802, 55 Eglinton Ave. East, Toronto ON M4P 1G8
Tel: 416-486-3998; *Fax:* 416-486-5562
Toll-Free: 800-495-6156
www.dyingwithdignity.ca
www.facebook.com/DWDCanada
twitter.com/DWDCanada
www.youtube.com/user/DWDCanada
Overview: A medium-sized national charitable organization founded in 1980
Mission: To improve the quality of dying for all Canadians in accordance with their own wishes, values & beliefs
Affliation(s): World Federation of Right to Die Societies
Chief Officer(s):
Shanaaz Gokool, Chief Executive Officer
Valerie Fernandes, Director, Operations & Programs

Anya Colangelo, Coordinator, Membership & Office
Kelsey Goforth, Coordinator, National Volunteer & Events
Cory Ruf, Coordinator, Communications
Nino Sekopet, Manager, Personal Support & Advocacy

Last Post Fund (LPF) / Fonds du Souvenir
#401, 505, boul René-Lévesque ouest, Montréal QC H2Z 1Y7
Tel: 514-866-2727; *Fax:* 514-866-1471
Toll-Free: 800-465-7113
e-mail: info@lastpost.ca
www.lastpostfund.ca
Overview: A medium-sized national charitable organization founded in 1909
Mission: To ensure that no war veterans, or certain other persons who meet the wartime service eligibility criteria, are denied a funeral & burial due to lack of funds
Chief Officer(s):
Barry Keeler, President
Raymond Mikkola, Vice-President, West
Derek Sullivan, Vice-President, East
Jean-Pierre Goyer, Executive Director

Alberta Branch
Canada Place, #1130, 9700 Jasper Ave., Edmonton AB T5J 4C3
Tel: 780-495-3766; *Fax:* 780-495-6960
Toll-Free: 888-495-3766

British Columbia Branch
#307, 7337 - 137th St., Surrey BC V3W 1A4
Tel: 604-572-3242; *Fax:* 604-572-3306
Toll-Free: 800-268-0248

Newfoundland-Labrador Branch
Prudential Bldg., 49 Elizabeth Ave., St. John's NL A1A 1W9
Tel: 709-579-4288; *Fax:* 709-579-0966
Toll-Free: 888-579-4288

Nova Scotia Branch
Chebucto Place, #200A, 7105 Chebucto Rd., Halifax NS B3L 4W8
Tel: 902-455-5283; *Fax:* 902-455-4058
Toll-Free: 800-565-4777

Ontario Branch
#905, 55 St. Clair Ave. East, Toronto ON M4T 1M2
Tel: 416-923-1608; *Fax:* 416-923-3695
Toll-Free: 800-563-2508

Saskatchewan Branch
Princeton Towers, #400, 123 - 2e Ave. South, Saskatoon SK S7K 736
Tel: 306-975-6045; *Fax:* 306-975-4306
Toll-Free: 800-667-3668
e-mail: lastpost@sasktel.net

United Kingdom Representative
High Commission of Canada, Canada House, Trafalgar Sq., London SW1Y 5BJ United Kingdom
Tel: 44 (0) 207 004 6075
Chief Officer(s):
Suzanne Happe, Veterans Affairs Officer
suzanne.happe@international.gc.ca

The Right to Die Society of Canada (RTDSC) / Société Canadienne pour le Droit de Mourir (SCDM)
145 Macdonell Ave., Toronto ON M6R 2A4
Tel: 416-535-0690
Toll-Free: 866-535-0690
e-mail: info@righttodie.ca
www.righttodie.ca
Previous Name: The Right to Die Network of Canada
Overview: A small national organization founded in 1991
Mission: To work with legislators, policy makers & the public to expand the range of humane options for people who are suffering intolerably from incurable conditions & who want a self-directed dying; to work with sufferers to expand their awareness of the options that are legal & may be appropriate for them
Chief Officer(s):
Ruth von Fuchs, President & Secretary

Provincial Associations

ALBERTA

Alberta Hospice Palliative Care Association (AHPCA)
#1245, 70 Ave. SE, Calgary AB T2H 2X8
Tel: 403-206-9938; *Fax:* 403-206-9958
e-mail: director@ahpca.ca
www.ahpca.ca
www.facebook.com/AlbertaHospicePalliativeCare
twitter.com/AHPCA
www.youtube.com/watch?v=6Z3044hPlrl
Previous Name: Palliative Care Association of Alberta
Overview: A medium-sized provincial charitable organization
Mission: To engage in actions & strategies that result in comprehensive, equitable & quality end of life care for Albertans
Member of: Canadian Palliative Care Association
Chief Officer(s):
Pansy Angevine, Chair
Leslie Penny, Treasurer
Jennifer Elliott, Executive Director
Theresa Bellows, Road Show Coordinator
Reilly Bellows, Social Media
Publications:
• Alberta Hospice Palliative Care Association Newsletter
Type: Newsletter
Profile: Association highlights, including membership information & courses
• Alberta Hospice Palliative Care Association Volunteer Training Manual
Type: Manual
Profile: Information based upon the CHPCA Norms of Practice

BRITISH COLUMBIA

British Columbia Hospice Palliative Care Association (BCHPCA)
#1100, 1200 West 73rd Ave., Vancouver BC V6P 6G5
Tel: 604-267-7024; *Fax:* 604-267-7026
Toll-Free: 877-410-6297
e-mail: office@bchpca.org
www.bchpca.org
Overview: A medium-sized provincial charitable organization
Mission: To ensure the quality of life for all British Columbians affected by life-limiting illness, death, & bereavement; To act as a collective voice in British Columbia, advocating for hospice palliative care at all levels
Member of: Canadian Hospice Palliative Care Association
Chief Officer(s):
Lorraine Gerard, Executive Director
ed@bchpca.org

MANITOBA

Palliative Manitoba (HPCM)
2109 Portage Ave., Winnipeg MB R3J 0L3
Tel: 204-889-8525; *Fax:* 204-888-8874
Toll-Free: 800-539-0295
e-mail: info@manitobahospice.mb.ca
palliativemanitoba.ca
www.facebook.com/pages/Palliative-Manitoba/1397723373824559
twitter.com/PalliativeMB
Previous Name: Hospice & Palliative Care Manitoba
Overview: A medium-sized provincial charitable organization founded in 1983
Mission: To champion the development of hospice palliative care for the people of Manitoba through education, information, advocacy & support to service delivery
Member of: Canadian Hospice Palliative Care Association
Chief Officer(s):
Mary Williams, Executive Director
mwilliams@manitobahospice.mb.ca
Lynda Wolf, President
Bob Brennan, Treasurer
Kelly Morris, Vice-President
Publications:
• Hospice & Palliative Care Manitoba Annual Report
Type: Yearbook; *Frequency:* Annually
Profile: Highlights of the year plus financial statements

• The Hospice Companion
Type: Newsletter; *Frequency:* Semiannually; *Price:* Free with
membership in Hospice & Palliative Care Manitoba
Profile: Information about volunteering, upcoming events, news from
regions, & membership news

NEW BRUNSWICK

New Brunswick Hospice Palliative Care Association
Fredericton Medical Clinic, #302, 1015 Regent St., Fredericton NB
E3B 6H5
       e-mail: info@nbhpca-aspnb.ca
       www.nbhpca-aspnb.ca
       www.facebook.com/763652390348798
Previous Name: New Brunswick Palliative Care Association
Overview: A small provincial organization
Mission: To promote principles & standards for hospice palliative care
in New Brunswick
Member of: Canadian Palliative Care Association
Chief Officer(s):
Renée Turcotte, President
  president@nbhpca-aspnb.ca

NEWFOUNDLAND AND LABRADOR

Newfoundland & Labrador Palliative Care Association (NLPCA)
PO Box 39023, 390 Topsail Rd., St. John's NL A1E 5Y7
       www.nlpalliativecareassociation.com
Overview: A medium-sized provincial charitable organization founded
in 1993
Mission: To strive for excellence in the care of persons near death; To
lessen the suffering & loneliness of people approaching the end of life
Member of: Canadian Hospice Palliative Care Association (CHPCA)
Chief Officer(s):
Debbie Squires, President
Daphne Crane-Burt, Secretary

NOVA SCOTIA

Nova Scotia Hospice Palliative Care Association (NSHPCA)
PO Box 103, Lakeside NS B3T 1M6
       Tel: 902-818-9139
       e-mail: info@nshpca.ca
       www.nshpca.ca
Overview: A medium-sized provincial charitable organization founded
in 1995
Mission: To strive towards achieving comfort & peace for persons
living & dying with a life-threatening illness throughout Nova Scotia; to
promote the philosophy & principles of palliative care through
networking, public & professional education, advocacy & research; to
educate & improve public awareness of the needs of those with a
life-threatening illness; thus enabling & empowering communities to
recognize the values, needs & wishes of all persons across all stages
of life
Member of: Canadian Palliative Care Association
Chief Officer(s):
Carolyn Marshall, President

ONTARIO

Bereavement Ontario Network (BON)
174 Oxford St., Woodstock ON N4S 6B1
       Tel: 519-290-0219
       e-mail: info@bereavementontarionetwork.ca
       www.bereavementontarionetwork.ca
Overview: A medium-sized provincial charitable organization
Mission: To connect organizations & individuals throughout the
province that work in the field of grief, bereavement, & mourning as
professionals & volunteers
Chief Officer(s):
Susan McCoy, Chair
  smccoy2140@rogers.com

Hospice Palliative Care Ontario (HPCO)
#707, 2 Carlton St., Toronto ON M5B 1J3
       Tel: 416-304-1477; *Fax:* 416-304-1479
       Toll-Free: 800-349-3111
       e-mail: info@hpco.ca
       www.hpco.ca
       twitter.com/hpcontario
       www.youtube.com/user/hpcotube
Merged from: Hospice Association of Ontario; Ontario Palliative
Care Association
Overview: A medium-sized provincial charitable organization founded
in 2011
Mission: To act as a voice on issues related to the provision of quality
end-of-life care for Ontarians; To advance palliative care standards of
practice; To advocate for the development of hospice palliative care
services in Ontario
Member of: Canadian Hospice Palliative Care Association (CHPCA)
Chief Officer(s):
Rick Firth, President & CEO, 416-304-1477 Ext. 24
  rfirth@hpco.ca
Paula Neil, Director, Operations
  pneil@hpco.ca
Michelle Colero, Manager, Development
  mcolero@hpco.ca
Publications:
• Hospice Palliative Care Ontario Newsletter
Type: Newsletter
Profile: Association reports, conferences, & articles
• Ontario Palliative Care Association Annual Report
Type: Yearbook; *Frequency:* Annually

PRINCE EDWARD ISLAND

Hospice Palliative Care Association of Prince Edward Island
c/o Hospice PEI, 5 Brighton Rd., Charlottetown PE C1A 8T6
       Tel: 902-368-4498
       e-mail: hpca@hospicepei.ca
       www.hospicepei.ca
       www.facebook.com/253154211534608
Previous Name: Island Hospice Association
Overview: A medium-sized provincial organization founded in 1985
Mission: To provide care & support to the terminally ill & their families
& to those who are bereaved
Member of: Canadian Hospice Palliative Care Association
Chief Officer(s):
Linda Callard, Chair

QUÉBEC

Réseau des soins palliatifs du Québec
CP 321, Succ. Chef, Granby QC J2G 8E5
       Tél: 514-826-9400; *Téléc:* 438-238-1336
       Courriel: info@aqsp.org
       www.aqsp.org
       twitter.com/PalliatifQc
Aperçu: *Dimension:* moyenne; *Envergure:* provinciale; fondée en 1990
Mission: Offrir aux intervenants de différentes disciplines de soins et
de services, un organisme de référence et d'échange en soins
palliatifs; favoriser le perfectionnement par la formation, le raffinement
des soins et la recherche, pour assurer une meilleure qualité de vie aux
malades atteints de maladie à issue fatale
Membre(s) du bureau directeur:
Alberte Déry, Présidente, Conseil d'administration
Marlène Côté, Vice-présidente, Conseil d'administration
Francine Lamarche, Coordonnatrice

SASKATCHEWAN

Saskatchewan Palliative Care Association
PO Box 37053, Regina SK S4S 7K3
       Tel: 306-522-3232
       Toll-Free: 888-614-8016
       e-mail: info@saskpalliativecare.org
       www.saskpalliativecare.org
Overview: A medium-sized provincial charitable organization founded
in 1991
Mission: To promote the philosophy & principles of palliative care
through networking, education, advocacy & research; to improve quality

of life for the dying
Member of: Canadian Palliative Care Association
Chief Officer(s):
Jeff Christiansen, President
  JChristiansen@speersfuneralchapel.com

Local Associations

BRITISH COLUMBIA

North Shore Hospice Society
231 East 15th St., North Vancouver BC V7L 2L7
Tel: 604-984-5785
www.northshorehospicepalliative.com
Previous Name: Lions Gate Hospice Society
Overview: A small local charitable organization founded in 1982
Mission: To support hospice/palliative care for people at the end of their lives & to support their family & friends in the North Vancouver area
Chief Officer(s):
Jo-Ann Wood, Chair

ONTARIO

Hospice of Waterloo Region
298 Lawrence Ave., Kitchener ON N2M 1Y4
Tel: 519-743-4114; *Fax:* 519-743-7021
e-mail: hospice@hospicewaterloo.ca
www.hospicewaterloo.ca
www.facebook.com/hospicewaterloo
twitter.com/hospicewaterloo
www.youtube.com/channel/UCUd8GumvtdxvoGo0WGT2Fog
Overview: A small local charitable organization
Mission: To provide comfort, care & support to people affected by life-threatening illness; To offer services in hospitals, long-term care facilities or in the home
Chief Officer(s):
Judy Nairn, Executive Director
  judy@hospicewaterloo.ca

Homeopathic Medicine

National Associations

Alliance for Chiropractic (AFC)
#126, 17A - 218 Silvercreek Pkwy. North, Guelph ON N1H 8E8
Tel: 519-822-1879; *Fax:* 519-822-1239
Toll-Free: 877-997-9927
www.allianceforchiropractic.com
Previous Name: Chiropractic Awareness Council
Overview: A small national organization founded in 1998
Mission: To promote public awareness of chiropractic life principles by promoting an awareness of the devastating effects of vertebral subluxation complex on the expression of human health potential; To educate the public with the conviction that chiropractic care is an integral aspect of health for people of all ages & to society in general
Member of: Chiropractic Coalition
Chief Officer(s):
Craig Hazel, Chair

American Association of Naturopathic Physicians (AANP)
#250, 818 - 18th St., NW, Washington DC 20006 USA
Tel: 202-237-8150; *Fax:* 202-237-8152
Toll-Free: 866-538-2267
e-mail: member.services@naturopathic.org
www.naturopathic.org
www.linkedin.com/groups/1213117
www.facebook.com/theAANP
twitter.com/AANP
Overview: A small international organization
Mission: Represents licensed or licensable naturopathic physicians who are graduates of four-year, residential graduates programs
Affiliation(s): Canadian Association of Naturopathic Doctors; College of Naturopathic Doctors of Alberta; British Columbia Naturopathic Association; Manitoba Naturopathic Association; New Brunswick Association of Naturopathic Doctors; Newfoundland and Labrador Association of Naturopathic Doctors; Nova Scotia Association of Naturopathic Doctors; Ontario Association of Naturopathic Doctors;

Prince Edward Island Association of Naturopathic Doctors; Quebec Association of Naturopathic Medicine; Saskatchewan Association of Naturopathic Practitioners; Yukon Naturopathic Association
Chief Officer(s):
Dennis Reynolds, Interim Executive Director, 202-849-6306
  dennis.reynolds@naturopathic.org

Canadian Association for Integrative & Energy Therapies (CAIET)
Tel: 416-221-5639; *Fax:* 416-221-7126
www.caiet.org
www.facebook.com/epccanada
twitter.com/CEPConference
Overview: A small national organization
Mission: A Canadian nonprofit organization of licensed mental health professionals and related energy and integrative health practitioners promoting knowledge and understanding of Energy Psychology and related fields.
Chief Officer(s):
Sharon Cass-Toole, President & Executive Director

Canadian Association of Acupuncture & Traditional Chinese Medicine (CAACTM)
c/o Chinese Medicine & Acupuncture Clinic of Toronto, 3195 Sheppard Ave. East, 2nd Fl., Toronto ON M1T 3K1
Tel: 416-493-8447; *Fax:* 416-493-9450
Toll-Free: 888-299-9799
e-mail: info@caatcm.com
www.caatcm.com
Overview: A small national organization founded in 1994
Mission: To promote & improve the practice of traditional Chinese medicine & acupuncture in the prevention & treatment of diseases, & the restoration & maintenance of health; To implement acceptable standards of practice within the profession

The Canadian Association of Naturopathic Doctors (CAND) / Association canadienne des docteurs en naturopathie
#200, 20 Holly St., Toronto ON M2S 3B1
Tel: 416-496-8633; *Fax:* 416-496-8634
Toll-Free: 800-551-4381
www.cand.ca
www.facebook.com/NaturopathicDrs
twitter.com/naturopathicdrs
Previous Name: Canadian Naturopathic Association
Overview: A medium-sized national organization founded in 1955
Mission: CAND is a not-for-profit professional organization that promotes naturopathic medicine to the public, insurance companies & corporations. CAND encourages professional, educational & networking activities among its members, & standardization of educational requirements for practitioners
Chief Officer(s):
Shawn O'Reilly, Executive Director
Alex McKenna, Marketing Director

Canadian Chiropractic Association (CCA) / Association chiropratique canadienne (ACC)
#6, 186 Spadina Ave., Toronto ON M5T 3B2
Tel: 416-585-7902; *Fax:* 416-585-2970
Toll-Free: 877-222-9303
e-mail: info@chiropractic.ca
www.chiropracticcanada.ca
www.linkedin.com/company/canadian-chiropractic-association
www.facebook.com/canadianchiropracticassociation
twitter.com/CanChiroAssoc
www.youtube.com/CanChiroAssoc
Overview: A large national organization founded in 1953
Mission: To see every Canadian have full & equitable access to chiropractic care; To promote the integration of chiropractic into the Canadian health care system
Affiliation(s): Canadian Chiropractic Examining Board; Canadian Federation of Chiropractic Regulatory & Educational Accrediting Boards; Canadian Chiropractic Historical Association; Canadian Memorial Chiropractic College; Université du Québec á Trois-Rivières Programme de Doctorat en Chiropratique; Canadian Chiropractic Protective Association; Canadian Chiropractic Research Foundation; World Federation of Chiropractic
Chief Officer(s):
Alison Dantas, CEO, 416-585-7902 Ext. 226
  adantas@chiropractic.ca

Publications:
• Canadian Chiropractic Association Membership Directory [a publication of the Canadian Chiropractic Association]
Type: Directory; *Price:* Free with CCA membership
Profile: A listing of all associate members
• Canadian Chiropractic Association Update
Type: Newsletter
• The CCA [Canadian Chiropractic Association] Report
Type: Newsletter; *Price:* Free with CCA membership
• Journal of the Canadian Chiropractic Association (JCCA)
Frequency: Quarterly; *Accepts Advertising; Editor:* Dr. Allan Gotlib;
ISSN: 1715-6181; *Price:* Free with CCA membership; $30
Canadiannon-members; $74 foreign
Profile: Peer-reviewed research & communication between the CCA &
its members

**Canadian Chiropractic Examining Board (CCEB) / Conseil
canadien des examens chiropratiques**
#230, 1209 - 59th Ave. SE, Calgary AB T2H 2P6
Fax: 403-230-3321
e-mail: exams@cceb.ca
www.cceb.ca

Overview: A small national organization founded in 1962
Mission: To provide high quality exams for licensure
Member of: National Certification Commission

**Canadian Chiropractic Research Foundation (CCRF) / La
Fondation canadienne pour la recherche en chiropratique**
#6, 186 Spadina Ave., Toronto ON M5T 3B2
Tel: 416-585-7902; *Fax:* 416-585-2970
Toll-Free: 877-222-9303
www.canadianchiropracticresearchfoundation.com
Previous Name: Chiropractic Foundation for Spinal Research
Overview: A small national charitable organization founded in 1976
Mission: To fund & facilitate health services & research related to the
practice of chiropractic
Affliation(s): Canadian Chiropractic Association; Canadian Institute for
Health Research
Chief Officer(s):
Drew Potter, President
dpotter@chiropractic.ca

The Canadian College of Naturopathic Medicine (CCNM)
1255 Sheppard Ave. East, Toronto ON M2K 1E2
Tel: 416-498-1255
Toll-Free: 866-241-2266
www.ccnm.edu
www.linkedin.com/in/ccnmalumni
www.facebook.com/myccnm
twitter.com/myccnm
www.youtube.com/myccnm
Overview: A medium-sized national licensing organization
Mission: To promote naturopathic medicine; To educate its students &
expand members' knowledge about naturopathic medicine
Chief Officer(s):
Colleen McQuarrie, Chair

**Canadian Federation of Aromatherapists / La fédération
canadienne d'aromathérapistes**
124 Sweet Water Cres., Richmond Hill ON L4S 2B4
Tel: 519-746-1594; *Fax:* 519-746-9493
e-mail: cfamanager@cfacanada.com
www.cfacanada.com
www.facebook.com/CanadianAromatherapy
twitter.com/cfaaromatherapy
Overview: A medium-sized national organization founded in 1993
Mission: To maintain a register of aromatherapy practitioners, schools,
& instructors who meet established minimum standards; To act as a
unified voice of the profession; To maintain the highest ethical
standards of the profession
Chief Officer(s):
Danielle Sade, President
daniellesade@hotmail.ca

**Canadian Federation of Chiropractic Regulatory & Educational
Accrediting Boards (CFCREAB)**
#2301, 30 Gloucester St., Toronto ON M4Y 1L6
Tel: 416-697-7458
www.chirofed.ca

Previous Name: Canadian Federation of Chiropractic Regulatory
Boards
Overview: A medium-sized national organization founded in 1978
Mission: To promote unified standards for the operations of all
licensing & regulatory boards; To aid in problems confronting individual
boards; To promote & aid cooperation between chiropractic learning
boards & regulatory boards
Chief Officer(s):
H. James Duncan, Chief Executive Officer

**Canadian Holistic Nurses Association (CHNA) / Association
canadienne des infirmières en soins holistiques**
www.chna.ca
www.facebook.com/CHNA.ca
Overview: A small national organization founded in 1986
Mission: To further the development of holistic nursing practice; To
promote CHNA standards of practice
Affiliation(s): Canadian Nurses Association
Chief Officer(s):
Linda Turner, President
lturner@langara.bc.ca
Jane Aitken-Herring, Secretary
djherring@pei.sympatico.ca
Susan Morris, Acting Contact, Membership
sbmorrisis@shaw.ca
Publications:
• Canadian Holistic Nurses Association Member Directory
Type: Directory
• Canadian Holistic Nurses Association Newsletter
Type: Newsletter; *Editor:* Wendy Snefjella

Canadian Horticultural Therapy Association (CHTA)
PO Box 74628, 2768 West Broadway, Vancouver BC V6K 4P4
e-mail: admin@chta.ca
www.chta.ca
www.facebook.com/119374542077
Overview: A small national organization
Mission: To promote the use & awareness of horticulture as a
therapeutic modality; horticultural therapy is a process which uses
plants, horticultural activities, & the natural world to promote
awareness & well-being by improving the body, mind, & spirit
Chief Officer(s):
Christina Klein, Chair
chair@chta.ca

Canadian Hypnosis Association (CHA)
121 Wallis St., Parksville BC V9P 1K7
Tel: 250-248-0480
www.canadianhypnosisassociation.ca
Previous Name: Canadian Hypnotherapy Association
Overview: A small national organization founded in 1977
Mission: To determine standards for hypnotherapy in Canada & to
promote the therapeutic value of hypnosis
Chief Officer(s):
Joe Friede, President

Canadian Institute of Iridology
PO Box 13576, Stn. Best Buy, Mississauga ON L5N 8G5
Tel: 416-231-6298; *Fax:* 905-824-0063
e-mail: iridologyplus@hotmail.com
www.cdninstiridology.com
Overview: A small national organization founded in 1989
Mission: To provide a professional teaching forum in the field of
iridology
Affiliation(s): The Iridologists' Association of Canada (Ir.A.C.)

**Canadian Massage Therapist Alliance (CMTA) / Alliance
Canadienne de Massothérapeutes**
#16, 1724 Quebec Ave., Saskatoon SK S7K 1V9
Tel: 306-384-7077
e-mail: info@crmta.ca
www.crmta.ca
www.facebook.com/CRMTA
Overview: A medium-sized national organization founded in 1991
Mission: To foster & advance the art, science & philosophy of
massage therapy through nationwide cooperation in a professional,
ethical & practical manner for the betterment of health care in Canada

Canadian Memorial Chiropractic College (CMCC)
6100 Leslie St., Toronto ON M2H 3J1
Tel: 416-482-2340; *Fax:* 416-646-1114
Toll-Free: 800-463-2923
e-mail: communications@cmcc.ca
www.cmcc.ca
Overview: A medium-sized national organization founded in 1945
Mission: To advance the art, science & philosophy of chiropractic; To educate chiropractors; To further the development of the chiropractic profession; To improve the health of society
Member of: Canadian Chiropractic Association
Chief Officer(s):
David Gryfe, Chair
Rahim Karim, Vice-Chair
Publications:
• CMCC [Canadian Memorial Chiropractic College] Annual Report
Type: Yearbook; *Frequency:* Annually
• CMCC [Canadian Memorial Chiropractic College] Academic Calendar
Frequency: Annually
Profile: Academic programs & course descriptions
• CMCC [Canadian Memorial Chiropractic College] Research Report
Frequency: Irregular
Profile: A summary of research activities undertaken at CMCC
• Primary Contact: A Magazine for Canadian Chiropractors
Type: Magazine; *Frequency:* 3 pa; *Editor:* Shannon Clark
Profile: Articles, continuing education, CMCC events, & members

Canadian Natural Health Association (CNHA)
#105, 5 Wakunda Pl., Toronto ON M4A 1A2
Tel: 416-686-7056
Previous Name: Canadian Natural Hygiene Society
Overview: A medium-sized national charitable organization founded in 1960
Mission: To establish leadership in healthy, natural lifestyle education & support services; to assist by providing resources to help make people healthier

Canadian Reiki Association (CRA)
#24, 2350 New St., Burlington ON L7R 4P8
Toll-Free: 800-835-7525
e-mail: reiki@reiki.ca
www.reiki.ca
www.facebook.com/groups/6813158154
twitter.com/reikicanada
www.pinterest.com/canadianreikias
Overview: A small national organization founded in 1997
Mission: Provides members with a national voice; encourages high educational standards; promotes ethical practices & teaching; assists the public with referrals to practitioners & teachers; committed to enlightening & educating communites about Reiki
Member of: Volunteer Canada
Chief Officer(s):
Bonnie Smith, President
bonnie@reiki.ca

Canadian Society of Chinese Medicine & Acupuncture (CSCMA)
#402, 245 Fairview Mall Dr., Toronto ON M2J 4T1
Tel: 416-597-6769; *Fax:* 416-597-9928
e-mail: office@tcmcanada.org
www.tcmcanada.org
Overview: A small national organization founded in 1994
Mission: To unite traditional Chinese medicine (TCM) & acupuncture practitioners, & to advocate for legal recognition & regulation of TCM in Canada
Chief Officer(s):
Zhao Cheng, President
Gengmin Tang, Secretary General
Publications:
• The Canadian Society of Chiense Medicine & Acupuncture Publication
Type: Journal

Chinese Canadian Chiropractic Society (CCCS)
c/o Federation of Chinese Canadian Professionals, 55 Glenn Hawthorne Blvd., Mississauga ON L5R 3S6
Tel: 905-890-3235; *Fax:* 905-568-5293
fccpontario.com/professional-sections/chiropractic
Overview: A small national organization founded in 2001

Mission: Created in order to educate the Chinese community about the benefits of chiropractic care
Chief Officer(s):
Frank Nhan, Representative

Chinese Medicine & Acupuncture Association of Canada (CMAAC)
154 Wellington St., London ON N6B 2K8
Tel: 519-642-1970; *Fax:* 519-642-2932
e-mail: headoffice@cmaac.ca
www.cmaac.ca
Overview: A medium-sized national organization founded in 1983
Mission: To unite practitioners of Eastern & Western Medicine; To develop & establish high standards of education & training for practitioners; To promote & attend international conferences; To assist in the exchange of scientific research; To act as an educational vehicle for the public
Member of: World Federation of Acupuncture
Affliation(s): World Wildlife Fund Canada; Canadian Health Care Anti-Fraud Association
Chief Officer(s):
Cedric Cheung, President

Alberta Chapter
414 Lee Ridge Rd., Edmonton AB T6K 0N7
Tel: 780-497-4610; *Fax:* 780-461-6366
Chief Officer(s):
King Sang Wong, President

Manitoba Chapter
1036 Portage Ave., Winnipeg MB R3G 0S2
Tel: 204-284-4047; *Fax:* 204-284-5755
Chief Officer(s):
Lin Liu, President
liulin1036@hotmail.com

New Brunswick Chapter
NB
Tel: 506-382-1288
Chief Officer(s):
Hui Zhang, President
zhanghuiacu@hotmail.com

Newfoundland Chapter
16 Dan's Rd., Portugal Cove-St. Philips NL A1M 1H3
Tel: 709-895-2907; *Fax:* 709-754-5802
Chief Officer(s):
Michelle Collett, President
collettmichele@hotmail.com

Nova Scotia Chapter
6066 Quinpool Rd., Halifax NS B3L 1A1
Tel: 902-832-0688; *Fax:* 902-835-3298
e-mail: acup@eastlink.ca
Chief Officer(s):
Diana Tong Li, President

Ontario Office
117 King St. East, Oshawa ON L1H 1B9
Tel: 905-721-4917; *Fax:* 905-721-4336
Chief Officer(s):
Jane Cheung, Chair, TCM Policy Development & Communications Committee

Québec Chapter
1312, rue Jean-Charles Catin, Cap Rouge ON G1Y 2X3
Tel: 613-569-8947; *Fax:* 613-569-8947
Chief Officer(s):
Gasan Askerow, President
askerow@bell.net

Saskatchewan Chapter
3829B Albert St. South, Regina SK S4S 3R4
Tel: 306-584-9888; *Fax:* 306-584-9888
e-mail: saskatchewanacupuncture@gmail.com
Chief Officer(s):
Diana Dong Yue Zhang, President

Corporation des praticiens en médecine douce du Canada (CPMDQ)
CP 51071, 101, boul Cardinal-Léger, Pincourt QC J7V 9T3

Téléc: 514-221-3740
Ligne sans frais: 800-624-6627
Courriel: info@cpmdq.com
www.cpmdq.com

Aperçu: Dimension: petite; *Envergure:* nationale; fondée en 1991
Mission: De contribuer à l'essor d'une société où les individus, leurs familles et leurs communautés seraient responsables et capables d'assurer le développement et l'amélioration de leur santé physique, psychologique, spirituelle et sociale, grâce à des solutions globales, novatrices et durables.

Homeopathic College of Canada (HCC)

e-mail: info@homeopathy.edu
www.homeopathy.edu

Also Known As: International Academy of Homeopathy
Overview: A small national organization founded in 1995
Mission: To maintain the highest professional standards of homeopathy; To provide international leadership in the fields of homeopathy & complementary medicine; To promote homeopathy as an alternative & complement within the health care system; To provide treatment effectively & economically within the health care system
Member of: Ontario Homeopathic Association; Homeopathic Medical Council of Canada
Chief Officer(s):
John Crellin, M.D., Ph.D., Dean
Idoia Ania, Contact, Student Affairs

Homeopathic Medical Association Of Canada (HMAC)
2649 Islington Ave., Toronto ON M9V 2X6

e-mail: info@hmac.ca
www.hmac.ca

Overview: A small national organization
Mission: To serve homeopathic practitioners across Canada; To uphold the code of ethics
Chief Officer(s):
Gangadhar Hanchate, President, 647-668-3567
  grao_hanchate@yahoo.com
Publications:
• Homeopathic Medical Council of Canada Journal
Type: Journal
Profile: Featuring a list of homeopathic doctors who are members of the council

National United Professional Association of Trained Homeopaths (NUPATH)
#102, 2680 Matheson Blvd., Mississauga ON L4W 0A5

Tel: 905-267-8539; *Fax:* 905-267-3401
e-mail: info@nupath.org
www.nupath.org

Overview: A medium-sized national organization founded in 1993
Mission: To represent homeopathic practitioners in Canada
Chief Officer(s):
Sushila Lalsingh, President

Natural Health Practitioners of Canada (NHP)
10339 - 124 St., 6th Fl, Edmonton AB T5N 3W1

Tel: 780-484-2010; *Fax:* 780-484-3605
Toll-Free: 888-711-7701
e-mail: growingtogether@nhpcanada.org
www.nhpcanada.org
www.linkedin.com/companies/nhpcanada
www.facebook.com/nhpcanada
twitter.com/NHPCANADA
www.youtube.com/nhpcanada

Previous Name: Association of Massage Therapists & Wholistic Practitioners
Overview: A medium-sized national organization founded in 1988
Mission: To maintain professional standards of practitioners practising in massage therapy & wholistic practice in order to benefit services to clients
Chief Officer(s):
Kelly Sloan, Executive Director

Natural Health Practitioners of Canada Association (NHPCA) / Association des Praticiens de la santé naturelle du Canada (PSNC)
10339 - 124 St. NW, 6th Fl, Edmonton AB T5N 3W1

Tel: 780-484-2010; *Fax:* 780-484-3605
Toll-Free: 888-711-7701
e-mail: growingtogether@nhpcanada.org
www.nhpcanada.org
www.linkedin.com/companies/nhpcanada
www.facebook.com/nhpcanada
twitter.com/NHPCANADA
www.youtube.com/nhpcanada

Overview: A medium-sized national organization founded in 1988
Mission: To provide programs, services and products for members in the service of public wellness and to serve the public by promoting and advocating the wellness professions.
Chief Officer(s):
Kelly Sloan, Executive Director
Publications:
• Connections [a publication of the Natural Health Practitioners of Canada]
Type: Magazine; *Frequency:* Quarterly

Reflexology Association of Canada (RAC) / Association canadienne de réflexologie
#304, 414 Graham Ave., Winnipeg MB R3C 0L8

Tel: 204-477-4909; *Fax:* 204-477-4955
Toll-Free: 877-722-3338
e-mail: memberservices@reflexolog.org
www.reflexologycanada.ca

Overview: A medium-sized national organization founded in 1976
Mission: To set & maintain high standards among practising reflexologists; To advance quality training; To develop an effective referral system across Canada
Chief Officer(s):
Judy Carey, Executive Director
Mary Jardine, President

Tara Canada Network Association
PO Box 15270, Vancouver BC V6B 5B1

Toll-Free: 888-278-8272
e-mail: information@share-international.ca
www.taracanada.org/pp3
www.facebook.com/ShareInternationalCanada

Overview: A small national charitable organization
Mission: To provide information on the emergence of Maitreya, the World Teacher, & on transmission meditation, a specialized form of group meditation
Affiliation(s): Share International Canada

Trager Canada
PO Box 28079, 1795 Henderson Hwy., Winnipeg MB R2G 4E9

Tel: 204-396-4747
Toll-Free: 888-724-3788
e-mail: admin@trager.ca
www.trager.ca

Previous Name: Trager Practitioners of S. Central Ontario
Overview: A small national licensing organization founded in 1981
Mission: To support & encourage the expanding practice of the Trager Approach & Mentastics movement re-education in Canada
Member of: Trager International

Provincial Associations

ALBERTA

Alberta College & Association of Chiropractors (ACAC)
Manulife Place, 11203 - 70 St. NW, Edmonton AB T5B 1T1

Tel: 780-420-0932; *Fax:* 780-425-6583
Other Communication: Blog: www.everydaychiropractic.com
e-mail: office@albertachiro.com
www.albertachiro.com
www.facebook.com/AlbertaChiropractors
twitter.com/AlbertaChiro
www.youtube.com/user/albertachiro

Previous Name: College of Chiropractors of Alberta; Alberta Chiropractic Association
Overview: A medium-sized provincial licensing organization founded in 1986 overseen by Canadian Chiropractic Association

Mission: To ensure quality chiropractic care that enhances the well-being & protects the rights of the people of Alberta; To promote the art, science, & philosophy of chiropractic & its value in the health care community
Chief Officer(s):
Deb Manz, Chief Executive Officer
 dmanz@albertachiro.com

Alberta College of Acupuncture & Traditional Chinese Medicine (ACATCM)
Main Lobby, 4935 - 40 Ave. NW, Calgary AB T3A 2N1

Tel: 403-286-8788
Toll-Free: 888-789-9984
e-mail: info@acatcm.com
www.acatcm.com

Overview: A medium-sized provincial organization founded in 1997
Mission: To maintain & strengthen leadership in Acupuncture & Traditional Chinese Medical education; To provide quality education in Acupuncture & TCM; To provide continuing education programs to health care professionals seeking to enhance their skills; To help graduates achieve success as primary health care providers using the principles of Traditional Chinese Medicine
Affiliation(s): Beijing University of Chinese Medicine
Chief Officer(s):
Dennis Lee, Co-President
Colton Oswald, Co-President

College of Naturopathic Doctors of Alberta (CNDA)
813 - 14th St. NW, Calgary AB T2N 2A4

Tel: 403-266-2446; *Fax:* 403-226-2433
e-mail: secretary@cnda.net
www.cnda.net
twitter.com/CollegeNDAB

Previous Name: Alberta Association of Naturopathic Practitioners
Overview: A small provincial organization overseen by The Canadian Association of Naturopathic Doctors
Mission: To maintain a high standard of practice among naturopathic doctors.
Chief Officer(s):
Alissa Gaul, President

Massage Therapist Association of Alberta (MTAA)
#2, 7429 - 49 St., Red Deer AB T4P 1N2

Tel: 403-340-1913; *Fax:* 403-346-2269
e-mail: info@mtaalberta.com
www.mtaalberta.com
www.facebook.com/MTAAlberta

Overview: A small provincial organization founded in 1953
Mission: To promote massage therapy through member services, education, professional standards & advocacy
Member of: Canadian Massage Therapist Alliance

BRITISH COLUMBIA

Association of Complementary & Integrative Physicians of BC (ACIPBC)
PO Box 526, #185, 911 Yates St., Victoria BC V8V 4Y9

www.acpbc.org

Overview: A small provincial organization founded in 1995
Mission: To ensure the delivery of quality holistic patient care through education, information, research, & the professional development of physicians
Affiliation(s): Canadian Complementary Medical Association
Chief Officer(s):
Bill Code, President
Publications:
• ACIPBC [Association of Complementary & Integrative Physicians of BC] Newsletter
Type: Newsletter; *Frequency:* Quarterly

British Columbia Chiropractic Association (BCCA)
#125, 3751 Shell Rd., Richmond BC V6X 2W2

Tel: 604-270-1332; *Fax:* 604-278-0093
Toll-Free: 866-256-1474
www.bcchiro.com
www.facebook.com/bcchiro
twitter.com/bcchiro
www.youtube.com/bcchiropractic

Overview: A medium-sized provincial organization founded in 1934 overseen by Canadian Chiropractic Association
Mission: To represent BC chiropractors in matters relating to health policy, public relations & health authorities
Chief Officer(s):
Jay Robinson, President

British Columbia Naturopathic Association (BCNA)
2238 Pine St., Vancouver BC V6J 5G4

Tel: 604-736-6646; *Fax:* 604-736-6048
Toll-Free: 800-277-1128
e-mail: bcna@bcna.ca
www.bcna.ca
www.facebook.com/BCNaturopathicAssociation
twitter.com/BCnaturopath
www.youtube.com/user/BCNaturopathicAssoc

Overview: A small provincial organization founded in 1993 overseen by The Canadian Association of Naturopathic Doctors
Mission: To act on behalf of the naturopathic profession in British Columbia; To advance the welfare of members of the profession
Affiliation(s): Canadian Association of Naturopathic Doctors
Publications:
• Your Health
Type: Newsletter; *Frequency:* Quarterly
Profile: Research & articles

Canadian Shiatsu Society of British Columbia (CSSBC)
123 Carrie Cates Ct., North Vancouver BC V7M 3K7

Tel: 604-349-8508
e-mail: info@shiatsupractor.org
www.shiatsupractor.org

Overview: A small provincial organization
Mission: To set high educational & professional standards for Shiatsu Therapy in British Columbia; To provide the Shiatsupractor (SPR) certification

College of Chiropractors of British Columbia (CCBC)
#125, 3751 Shell Rd., Richmond BC V6X 2W2

Tel: 604-270-1332; *Fax:* 604-278-0093
Toll-Free: 866-256-1474
www.chirobc.com

Previous Name: British Columbia College of Chiropractors
Overview: A medium-sized provincial organization
Mission: To deal with concerns from the public or practitioners regarding BC chiropractic doctors
Affiliation(s): British Columbia Chiropractic Association
Chief Officer(s):
David Olson, Chair
Avtar Jassal, Vice-Chair
Publications:
• College of Chriopractors of British Columbia Annual Report
Type: Yearbook; *Frequency:* Annually
Profile: Reports from the chair, the registrar, & committee chairs
• College of Chriopractors of British Columbia Professional Conduct Handbook
Type: Handbook; *Number of Pages:* 36
Profile: Contents include the code of ethics plus the standards, limits, & conditions of practice

College of Naturopathic Physicians of British Columbia (CNPBC)
#840, 605 Robson St., Vancouver BC V6B 5J3

Tel: 604-688-8236; *Fax:* 604-688-8476
Toll-Free: 877-611-8236
e-mail: office@cnpbc.bc.ca
www.cnpbc.bc.ca

Previous Name: Association of Naturopathic Physicians of British Columbia
Overview: A small provincial licensing organization founded in 1936
Mission: To set standards of professional practice amongst naturopathic physicians in BC.
Chief Officer(s):
Howard Greenstein, CEO & Registrar
 registrar@cnpbc.bc.ca

College of Traditional Chinese Medicine Practitioners & Acupuncturists of British Columbia (CTCMABC)
1664 - West 8th Ave., Vancouver BC V6J 1V4
Tel: 604-738-7100; *Fax:* 604-738-7171
e-mail: info@ctcma.bc.ca
www.ctcma.bc.ca
Overview: A small provincial organization founded in 1996
Mission: To protect the public by establishing a system of mandatory registration in which practitioners have to meet & maintain standards in TCM & acupuncture care established by the College
Chief Officer(s):
Mary S. Watterson, Registrar & CEO
Publications:
• Balance [a publication of the College of Traditional Chinese Medicine Practitioners & Acupuncturists of British Columbia]
Type: Newsletter; *Frequency:* 4 pa

International College of Traditional Chinese Medicine of Vancouver (ICTCMV)
#201, 1508 West Broadway, Vancouver BC V6J 1W8
Tel: 604-731-2926; *Fax:* 604-731-2964
e-mail: info@tcmcollege.com
www.tcmcollege.com
www.facebook.com/tcmcollegevan
Overview: A medium-sized provincial organization founded in 1986
Mission: To provide TCM training to foster effective & ethical TCM doctors; To raise awareness of TCM; To promote medical ethics; To support TCM research
Chief Officer(s):
Laina Ho, President

MANITOBA

Manitoba Association of Asian Physicians (MAAP)
c/o Dr. Rajat Kumar, President, 675 McDermot Ave., Winnipeg MB R3E 0V9
www.maap.ca
Overview: A small provincial organization founded in 1985

Manitoba Chiropractors' Association (MCA)
#610, 1445 Portage Ave., Winnipeg MB R3G 3P4
Tel: 204-942-3000; *Fax:* 204-942-3010
www.mbchiro.org
Overview: A medium-sized provincial licensing organization founded in 1945 overseen by Canadian Chiropractic Association
Mission: To act as both a regulatory body & a professional association to serve the public & the chiropractors of Manitoba; To foster high standards of chiropractic health care for Manitobans; To ensure that safe, ethical, & competent servicew are provided by Manitoba chiropractors
Chief Officer(s):
Taras Luchak, Executive Director
Ernie Miron, Registrar

Manitoba Naturopathic Association (MNA)
PO Box 434, 971 Corydon Ave., Winnipeg MB R3M 0Y0
Tel: 204-947-0381
e-mail: info@mbnd.ca
www.mbnd.ca
Overview: A small provincial licensing organization founded in 1946 overseen by The Canadian Association of Naturopathic Doctors
Mission: To act as a regulatory body for the profession of naturopathy, in accordance with The Naturopathic Act of Manitoba
Chief Officer(s):
Lesley Phimister, Executive Director & Registrar

Massage Therapy Association of Manitoba Inc. (MTAM)
#304, 428 Portage Ave., Winnipeg MB R3C 0E2
Tel: 204-927-7979; *Fax:* 204-927-7978
Toll-Free: 866-605-1433
e-mail: info@mtam.mb.ca
www.mtam.mb.ca
www.linkedin.com/company/2511272
www.facebook.com/MTAManitoba
twitter.com/MTAManitoba
Overview: A small provincial organization founded in 1973
Mission: To promote & enhance massage therapy in Manitoba; To ensure safe & ethical massage therapy practice; To represent members & support their professional growth

Chief Officer(s):
Sheila Molloy, Executive Director

NEW BRUNSWICK

New Brunswick Association of Naturopathic Doctors (NBAND)
c/o Crystal Charest, 2278 King George Hwy., Miramichi NB E1V 6N6
Tel: 506-773-3700; *Fax:* 506-773-3704
www.nband.ca
twitter.com/NewBrunswickNDs
Overview: A small provincial organization overseen by The Canadian Association of Naturopathic Doctors
Mission: To educate the public on the philosophies and values of Naturopathic Medicine and to promote the profession within the province.
Chief Officer(s):
Crystal Charest, Contact

New Brunswick Chiropractors' Association (NBCA) / Association des chiropraticiens du Nouveau-Brunswick
#206, 944 Prospect St., Fredericton NB E3B 9M6
Tel: 506-455-6800; *Fax:* 506-455-4430
e-mail: comments@nbchiropractic.ca
www.nbchiropractic.ca
Overview: A medium-sized provincial licensing organization founded in 1958 overseen by Canadian Chiropractic Association
Mission: To regulate the practice of chiropractic medicine & govern its members in accordance with the Act & the by-laws, in order to serve & protect the public interests; To establish, maintain, develop & enforce standards of qualification for the practice of chiropractic, including the required knowledge, skill & efficiency; To establish, maintain, develop & enforce standards of professional ethics; To promote public awareness of the role of the Association & the work of chiropractic, & to communicate & cooperate with other professional organizations for the advancement of the best interests of the Association, including the publication of books, papers & journals; To encourage studies in chiropractic & provide assistance & facilities for special studies & research
Chief Officer(s):
Mohamed El-Bayoumi, Chief Executive Officer

New Brunswick Massotherapy Association (NBMA) / Association des massothérapeutes du Nouveau-Brunswick (AMNB)
10, rue des Oiseaux, Pointe-Verte NB E8J 2V6
Toll-Free: 855-642-2662
e-mail: info@nbma-amnb.ca
www.nbma-amnb.ca
Overview: A small provincial organization

NEWFOUNDLAND AND LABRADOR

Newfoundland & Labrador Chiropractic Association
#285W, 120 Torbay Rd., St. John's NL A1A 2G8
Tel: 709-739-7762; *Fax:* 709-739-7703
www.nlchiropractic.ca
Overview: A medium-sized provincial organization overseen by Canadian Chiropractic Association

NOVA SCOTIA

Nova Scotia Association of Naturopathic Doctors (NSAND)
PO Box 245, Lower Sackville NS B4C 2S9
Tel: 902-431-8001
e-mail: info@nsand.ca
www.nsand.ca
www.facebook.com/novascotiaassociationofNDs
twitter.com/NSAND_
Overview: A small provincial organization founded in 1995 overseen by The Canadian Association of Naturopathic Doctors
Mission: To be a resource for its members & to inform the public about naturopathic medicine.
Chief Officer(s):
Bryan Rade, President
Florence Woolaver, Administrator

Nova Scotia College of Chiropractors (NSCC)
Park Lane Terraces, PO Box 142, #502, 5657 Spring Garden Rd.,
Halifax NS B3J 3R4

Tel: 902-407-4255; *Fax:* 902-425-2441
e-mail: inquiries@chiropractors.ns.ca
www.chiropractors.ns.ca

Overview: A small provincial organization founded in 1953 overseen
by Canadian Chiropractic Association
Mission: To promote & improve the proficiency of chiropractors in all
matters relating to the practice of chiropractic; To protect the public
from untrained & unqualified persons acting as chiropractors; To
advance the chiropractic profession
Chief Officer(s):
John K. Sutherland, Executive Director

ONTARIO

College of Chiropractors of Ontario
#902, 130 Bloor St. West, Toronto ON M5S 1N5
Tel: 416-922-6355; *Fax:* 416-925-9610
Toll-Free: 877-577-4772
e-mail: cco.info@cco.on.ca
www.cco.on.ca

Overview: A small provincial organization
Mission: To develop admission, conduct, & practice standards
Chief Officer(s):
Jo-Ann Willson, Registrar
jpwillson@cco.on.ca

The College of Naturopaths of Ontario
150 John St., 10th Fl., Toronto ON M5V 3E3
Tel: 416-583-6010; *Fax:* 416-583-6011
e-mail: info@collegeofnaturopaths.on.ca
www.collegeofnaturopaths.on.ca

Previous Name: Board of Directors of Drugless Therapy, Naturopathy
(Ontario)
Overview: A small provincial licensing organization founded in 1925
Mission: To register & regulate naturopathic doctors in Ontario; To
investigate complaints from patients & the public
Member of: Federation of Health Regulatory Colleges of Ontario
Affiliation(s): North American Board of Naturopathic Examiners;
Ontario Association of Naturopathic Doctors
Chief Officer(s):
Andrew Parr, Registrar & CEO
registrar@collegeofnaturopaths.on.ca
Syed Mehdi, Officer, Finance & Administration
Erica Laugalys, Manager, Examinations & Entry to Practise
Anna Jeremian, Manager, Membership

**Ontario Association of Acupuncture & Traditional Chinese
Medicine (OAATCM)**
370B Dupont St., Toronto ON M5R 3G3
Tel: 416-944-2265

Overview: A small provincial organization
Mission: To encourage the standardization of educational
requirements for all practitioners of traditional Chinese medicine (TCM);
To support high standards of professional training, competency &
qualifications of TCM practitioners

Ontario Association of Naturopathic Doctors (OAND)
#603, 789 Don Mills Rd., Toronto ON M3C 1T5
Tel: 416-233-2001; *Fax:* 416-233-2924
Toll-Free: 877-628-7284
e-mail: info@oand.org
www.oand.org
www.facebook.com/ndontario
twitter.com/OANDorg

Previous Name: Ontario Naturopathic Association
Overview: A medium-sized provincial organization founded in 1950
overseen by The Canadian Association of Naturopathic Doctors
Mission: To act as a voice for naturopathic doctors in Ontario
Affiliation(s): Canadian Association of Naturopathic Doctors
Chief Officer(s):
Chrystine Langille, CEO
clangille@oand.org
Alfred Hauk, Chair
Angeli Chitale, Secretary

**Ontario Chiropractic Association (OCA) / Association
chiropratique de l'Ontario**
#200, 20 Victoria St., Toronto ON M5C 2N8
Tel: 416-860-0070; *Fax:* 416-860-0857
Toll-Free: 877-327-2273
e-mail: oca@chiropractic.on.ca
www.chiropractic.on.ca
www.facebook.com/ontariochiropracticassociation
twitter.com/ON_Chiropractic

Overview: A medium-sized provincial organization founded in 1929
overseen by Canadian Chiropractic Association
Mission: To serve its members by promoting the philosophy, art, &
science of chiropractic & thereby enhance the health & well-being of
the citizens of Ontario
Chief Officer(s):
Kristina Peterson, President

Ontario College of Reflexology (OCR)
PO Box 220, New Liskeard ON P0J 1P0
Tel: 705-647-5354; *Fax:* 705-995-3415
Toll-Free: 888-627-3338
Other Communication: info@ocr.edu; membership@ocr.edu;
referral@ocr.edu
e-mail: ocr@ocr.edu
www.ocr.edu
www.facebook.com/ontarioreflexology
twitter.com/profbisson
plus.google.com/+OcrEdu

Overview: A small provincial organization
Mission: To provide accreditation for reflexologists in the province of
Ontario, where required & as permitted by applicable statues of
Ontario; To improve & maintain the qualifications & standards of the
reflexology profession; To promote reflexology in the province
Chief Officer(s):
Donald A. Bisson, Chair
Publications:
• OCR [Ontario College of Reflexology] Foot Notes
Type: Newsletter; *Frequency:* Quarterly

Ontario Herbalists Association (OHA)
PO Box 123, Stn. D, Toronto ON M9A 4X2
Tel: 416-236-0090
Toll-Free: 877-642-4372
e-mail: info@herbalists.on.ca
www.herbalists.on.ca
www.facebook.com/herbalists.on.ca
twitter.com/Ontarioherbs

Overview: A medium-sized provincial organization founded in 1979
Mission: To bring together people with interest in & knowledge about
herbs; To facilitate a sharing of information & research; To promote
advancement of understanding of medicinal plants; To serve as liaison
between herbalists & other healing professionals & to work actively for
recognition & promotion of herbal therapy
Member of: British Herbal Medicine Association
Chief Officer(s):
Diane Kent, President

Ontario Homeopathic Association (OHA)
#801, 60 Pleasant Bldv., Toronto ON M4T 1K1
Tel: 416-516-6109; *Fax:* 416-516-7725
e-mail: info@ontariohomeopath.com
www.ontariohomeopath.com
www.linkedin.com/pub/ontario-homeopathic-association/5a/614/581
www.facebook.com/OntarioHomeopathicAssociation
twitter.com/OntHomeopath

Overview: A medium-sized provincial organization founded in 1992
Mission: To promote homeopathy; to educate physicians in the areas
of homeopathy

Registered Massage Therapists' Association of Ontario (RMTAO)
#704, 1243 Islington Ave., Toronto ON M8X 1Y9
Tel: 416-979-2010; *Fax:* 416-979-1144
Toll-Free: 800-668-2022
e-mail: info@rmtao.com
www.rmtao.com
twitter.com/RMTAO

Previous Name: Ontario Massage Therapist Association
Overview: A medium-sized provincial organization founded in 1936

Mission: To advocate on behalf of all masssage therapists in Ontario; To ensure public access to the services of massage therapists; To encourage high standards for massage therapists
Chief Officer(s):
Andrew Lewarne, Exec. Director and Chief Exec. Officer, 416-979-2010 Ext. 301
andrew@rmtao.com
Jill Haig, Manager, Operations, 416-979-2010 Ext. 303
jill@rmtao.com
Laura Fixman, Contact, Communications & Member Services, 416-979-2010 Ext. 100
laura@rmtao.com

Shiatsu Therapy Association of Ontario (STAO)
#1056, 7B Pleasant Blvd., Toronto ON M4T 1K2
Tel: 416-923-7826
Toll-Free: 877-923-7826
e-mail: info@shiatsuassociation.com
www.shiatsuassociation.com
Overview: A small provincial organization founded in 1983
Mission: To promote awareness of Shiatsu to the public, health care professionals, government agencies & insurance companies; to protect the integrity of the profession with high educational standards & dedication to safeguarding the welfare of the public through strict adherence by its members to the STAO code of conduct
Chief Officer(s):
Carolyn Kozole, Administrator, 416-719-4590

PRINCE EDWARD ISLAND

Prince Edward Island Chiropractic Association (PEICA)
#280, 119 Kent St., Charlottetown PE C1A 1N3
Tel: 902-892-4454; *Fax:* 902-892-4454
e-mail: dtownchiro@pei.aibn.com
Overview: A small provincial organization overseen by Canadian Chiropractic Association
Mission: To represent the chiropractic profession in Prince Edward Island; To advance the chiropractic profession in the province; To encourage high standards of service; To protect the residents of Prince Edward Island from unqualified individuals acting as chiropractors
Chief Officer(s):
Christopher McCarthy, Registrar

Prince Edward Island Massage Therapy Association
PO Box 1882, Charlottetown PE C1A 7N5
Fax: 902-368-7281
Toll-Free: 866-566-1955
www.peimta.com
Overview: A medium-sized provincial organization
Mission: To raise the awareness of all Islanders on the benefits of therapeutic massage
Chief Officer(s):
Jennifer White, President
president@peimta.com

QUÉBEC

Académie de Réflexologie du Québec
1285, rue de la Visitation, Sainte-Foy QC G1W 3K5
Tél: 418-651-8575
Ligne sans frais: 800-701-8575
www.academiereflexologie.ca
Aperçu: *Dimension:* petite; *Envergure:* provinciale; fondée en 1984
Mission: Faire connaître la remarquable efficacité des thérapies réflexes pour améliorer rapidement de beaucoup la santé; grâce à de meilleures connaissances en biochimie cellulaire et en neurobiologie, l'Académie de Réflexologie du Québec a développé depuis de nombreuses années des nouvelles techniques très performantes (massage articulaire ou massage intégral) qui agissent simultanément pour détecter (prévenir), détendre (relaxer) et qui ont un effet thérapeutique profond pour résoudre d'innombrables problèmes de santé; de ses recherches est née la carrière de Thérapeute Réflexe; toute personne certifiée est assujettie à un code de déontologie et appartient à son regroupement professionnel de même formation; le maître massothérapeute travaille avec les bases majeures du corps humain, dont les réflexes des différents méchanismes du système nerveux autonome
Membre de: Association des maîtres massothérapeutes

Alliance des massothérapeutes du Québec (AMQ)
147, boul Laurier, Saint-Basile-le-Grand QC J3N 1A9
Tél: 450-441-1117; *Téléc:* 450-441-1157
Ligne sans frais: 888-687-1786
Courriel: info@massotherapeutes.qc.ca
www.massotherapeutes.qc.ca
www.facebook.com/1471162382012847
twitter.com/AllianceMasso
Aperçu: *Dimension:* petite; *Envergure:* provinciale; Organisme sans but lucratif; fondée en 1999
Mission: Vérifier les qualifications des massothérapeutes et offrir un service de formation afin que membres demeurent à l'avant-garde de la profession et des besoins du public
Membre(s) du bureau directeur:
Marie-Josée Poisson, Présidente

Association des Acupuncteurs du Québec (L'AAQ)
#203, 1453, rue Beaubien Est, Montréal QC H2G 3C6
Tél: 514-564-5115
Ligne sans frais: 844-564-5115
Courriel: info@acupuncture-quebec.com
www.acupuncture-quebec.com
fr-ca.facebook.com/128162563939912
Nom précédent: Association d'Acupuncture du Québec
Aperçu: *Dimension:* petite; *Envergure:* provinciale; Organisme sans but lucratif; fondée en 2000
Mission: Promouvoir la médecine traditionnelle chinoise et l'acupuncture; défendre les intêrets de ses membres
Affliation(s): Ordre des acupuncteurs du Québec; Département d'acupuncture: Collège de Rosemont; Distributeurs de l'AAQ
Membre(s) du bureau directeur:
Mélanie Lévesque, Présidente

Association des chiropraticiens du Québec
7960, boul Métropolitain Est, Montréal QC H1K 1A1
Tél: 514-355-0557; *Téléc:* 514-355-0070
Ligne sans frais: 866-292-4476
Courriel: acq@chiropratique.com
www.chiropratique.com
www.facebook.com/AssoDesChirosQc
twitter.com/AssoChiroQc
www.youtube.com/user/AssoDesChirosQc
Aperçu: *Dimension:* moyenne; *Envergure:* provinciale; fondée en 1967 surveillé par Canadian Chiropractic Association
Mission: Défendre les intérêts professionnels, sociaux et économiques de ses membres

Association des herboristes de la province de Québec
CP 80, 7, av 70e ouest, Blainville QC J7C 1R7
Tél: 450-435-2979
Courriel: herbesunivers@bellnet.ca
Aperçu: *Dimension:* petite; *Envergure:* provinciale

Association des massologues et techniciens en massage du Canada - Association des massothérapeutes professionnels du Québec
#200, 5967, rue Jean-Talon est, Saint-Léonard QC H1S 1M5
Téléc: 514-727-6555
Ligne sans frais: 888-434-6914
Aperçu: *Dimension:* moyenne; *Envergure:* provinciale; Organisme sans but lucratif; fondée en 1984

Association des naturopathes professionnels du Québec (ANPQ)
192 Saint-Joseph, Terrebonne QC J6W 2Y7
Tél: 450-824-3550; *Téléc:* 450-824-1887
Ligne sans frais: 888-268-2516
Courriel: anm.anpq@videotron.ca
www.anpq.qc.ca
Aperçu: *Dimension:* petite; *Envergure:* provinciale; fondée en 1971
Mission: Association à but non lucratif et à charte provinciale qui regroupe des praticiens en naturopathie dûment qualifiés
Membre(s) du bureau directeur:
Yves Dussault, Président

Association québécoise des phytothérapeutes (AQP)
3805, rue Bélair, Montréal QC H2A 2C1
Tél: 514-722-8888; *Téléc:* 514-722-5164
Ligne sans frais: 800-268-5878
Courriel: associatio1@bellnet.ca
www.aqp-annspq.ca

Également appelé: Association des naturopathes et naturothérapeutes spécialisés en phytothérapie
Aperçu: *Dimension:* moyenne; *Envergure:* provinciale; fondée en 1969
Mission: Regrouper les phytothérapeutes; favoriser l'atteinte d'un niveau de compétence supérieure; assurer la protection du public; contribuer à l'avancement de la phytothérapie

Fédération québécoise des massothérapeutes (FQM)
#400, 4428, boul St-Laurent, Montréal QC H2W 1Z5
Tél: 514-597-0505; *Téléc:* 514-597-0141
Ligne sans frais: 800-363-9609
Courriel: administration@fqm.qc.ca
www.fqm.qc.ca
www.facebook.com/massotherapie.FQM
twitter.com/FederationFQM
www.youtube.com/user/FQMmassotherapie
Aperçu: *Dimension:* moyenne; *Envergure:* provinciale; Organisme sans but lucratif; Organisme de réglementation; fondée en 1979
Mission: Regrouper les massothérapeutes afin de promouvoir la massothérapie sous l'intérêt public et de valoriser la profession de la massothérapie
Membre(s) du bureau directeur:
Sylvie Bédard, Présidente directrice générale
sylvie.bedard@fqm.qc.ca

Mon Réseau Plus, Association professionnelle des massothérapeutes spécialisés du Québec inc.
2285, rue St-Pierre, Drummondville QC J2C 5A7
Téléc: 819-472-2900
Ligne sans frais: 800-461-1312
Courriel: info@monreseauplus.com
www.monreseauplus.com
www.linkedin.com/company/mon-r-seau-plus
www.facebook.com/MonReseauPlus.Massotherapie
twitter.com/MonReseauPlus
Également appelé: Mon Réseau +
Merged from: AMOC; CMA; CMAPPAC
Aperçu: *Dimension:* petite; *Envergure:* provinciale; fondée en 2008
Mission: Représenter les activités professionnelles de ses membres
Membre(s) du bureau directeur:
Martin Vallée, Président-directeur général
mvallee@monreseauplus.com

Ordre des acupuncteurs de Québec (OAQ)
#1106, 505, boul René-Lévesque ouest, Montréal QC H2Z 1Y7
Tél: 514-523-2882; *Téléc:* 514-523-9669
Ligne sans frais: 800-474-5914
Courriel: info@o-a-q.org
www.o-a-q.org
Aperçu: *Dimension:* petite; *Envergure:* provinciale
Mission: Réglementer et de surveiller des activités professionnelles qui comportent des risques de préjudices pour le public
Membre(s) du bureau directeur:
Raymond Bourret, President
president@o-a-q.org

Québec Association of Naturopathic Medicine (QANM) / Association de medecine naturapathique du Québec (AMNQ)
1173 boul du Mont Royal ouest, Montréal QC H2V 2H6
Tel: 514-755-6629
e-mail: info@qanm.org
qanm.org
www.linkedin.com/groups/AMNQ-QANM-4267434
www.facebook.com/amnq.qanm
twitter.com/amnq_qanm
Overview: A small provincial organization founded in 1995
Affliation(s): Canadian Association of Naturopathic Doctors
Chief Officer(s):
André Saine, DC, ND, President

Syndicat professionnel des homéopathes du Québec (SPHQ)
#106, 1600, av de Lorimier, Montréal QC H2K 3W5
Tél: 514-525-2037
Ligne sans frais: 800-465-5788
Courriel: accueil@sphq.org
www.sphq.org
Aperçu: *Dimension:* petite; *Envergure:* provinciale; Organisme sans but lucratif; fondée en 1989

Affliation(s): Fédération des professionnèles; Confédération des Syndicats Nationaux; Bureau fédéral des médecines alternatives; L'International Council for Homeopathy; Homéopathes de Terre Sans Frontières

SASKATCHEWAN

Chiropractors' Association of Saskatchewan (CAS)
3420A Hill Ave., Regina SK S4S 0W9
Tel: 306-585-1411; *Fax:* 306-585-0685
e-mail: admin@saskchiropractic.ca
www.saskchiropractic.ca
www.youtube.com/user/SaskChiro
Overview: A medium-sized provincial organization founded in 1943 overseen by Canadian Chiropractic Association
Mission: To standardize & elevate chiropractic methods
Chief Officer(s):
Kevin Henbid, President
Denise Gerein, Registrar
dgerein@saskchiropractic.ca

Massage Therapist Association of Saskatchewan (MTAS)
#16, 1724 Quebec Ave., Saskatoon SK S7K 1V9
Tel: 306-384-7077; *Fax:* 306-384-7175
e-mail: mtas@sasktel.net
www.saskmassagetherapy.com
www.linkedin.com/company/massage-therapist-association-of-saskatchewan
www.facebook.com/145260445598968
twitter.com/SaskMassage
Overview: A small provincial licensing organization founded in 1997
Mission: To encourage the science & practice of massage therapy
Member of: Canadian Massage Therapist Alliance; Saskatchewan Chamber of Commerce
Chief Officer(s):
Lori Green, Executive Director
lorigreen@saskmassagetherapy.com
Jayne Little, Manager, Member Services

Saskatchewan Association of Naturopathic Practitioners (SANP)
2706 13th Ave., Regina SK S4T 1N7
Tel: 306-543-4325; *Fax:* 306-543-4330
e-mail: info@sanp.ca
www.sanp.ca
www.facebook.com/SaskNDs
Overview: A small provincial licensing organization overseen by The Canadian Association of Naturopathic Doctors
Mission: To act as the governing body for naturopathic doctors in Saskatchewan; To license & regulate naturopathic physicians in the province; To ensure members are educated & trained according to strict standards
Chief Officer(s):
Laura Stark, President
president@sanp.ca
Wendy Presant-Jahn, Vice-President
vicepresident@sanp.ca
Kathleen Fyffe, Secretary
secretary@sanp.ca
Jacqui Fleury, Treasurer, 306-373-5209
treasurer@sanp.ca
Vanessa DiCicco, Registrar
registrar@sanp.ca

Local Associations

NOVA SCOTIA

Atlantic Therapeutic Touch Network (ATTN) / Le réseau Toucher Thérapeutique de l'Atlantique
PO Box 24073, 21 MicMac Blvd., Dartmouth NS B3A 4T4
e-mail: info@atlanticttn.com
www.atlanticttn.com
www.facebook.com/725635027565929
Overview: A small local organization founded in 1996
Chief Officer(s):
Judy Donovan-Whitty, Coordinator & Secretary

QUÉBEC

Réseau Tara Canada (Québec)
CP 156, Succ. Ahuntsic, Montréal QC H3L 3N7

Ligne sans frais: 888-886-8272
Courriel: medias@taraquebec.org
www.taraquebec.org
www.facebook.com/ShareInternationalCanada

Également appelé: Réseau Tara; Tara Québec
Aperçu: *Dimension:* petite; *Envergure:* locale; Organisme sans but lucratif; fondée en 1985
Mission: Répandre le message de l'Enseignant universel Maitreya, le Christ, dirigeant de la Hiérarchie spirituelle de la planète
Membre de: Tara Canada
Affliation(s): Partage International Canada; Tara Canada Network Association

International Associations

Sivananda Ashram Yoga Camp
673 - 8 Ave., Val Morin QC J0T 2R0

Tel: 819-322-3226
Toll-Free: 800-263-9642
e-mail: hq@sivananda.org
www.sivananda.org
www.facebook.com/SivanandaYogaCamp
twitter.com/sivanandacamp

Previous Name: Yoga Vedanta Centre
Overview: A small international charitable organization founded in 1963
Mission: To practice classical Indian yoga
Member of: International Sivananda Yoga Vedanta Centres

Centre Sivananda de Yoga Vedanta de Montréal
5178, boul St-Laurent, Montréal QC H2T 1R8

Tél: 514-279-3545
Courriel: montreal@sivananda.org
www.sivananda.org/montreal
www.facebook.com/sivanandayogamontreal

Sivananda Yoga Vedanta Centre
77 Harbord St., Toronto ON M5S 1G4

Tel: 416-966-9642
e-mail: toronto@sivananda.org
www.sivananda.org/toronto
www.facebook.com/sivanandatoronto
twitter.com/sivanandatoronto

World Federation of Chiropractic (WFC) / La Fédération mondiale de chiropratique
#601, 160 Eglinton Ave. East, Toronto ON M4P 3B5

Tel: 416-484-9978; *Fax:* 416-484-9665
e-mail: info@wfc.org
www.wfc.org
www.facebook.com/WorldFederationofChiropractic

Overview: A medium-sized international organization founded in 1988
Mission: To increase awareness of & access to chiropractic
Member of: Council of International Organizations of Medical Sciences (CIOMS)
Affliation(s): World Health Organization (WHO)
Chief Officer(s):
Richard Brown, Secretary-General

Yasodhara Ashram Society
PO Box 9, Kootenay Bay BC V0B 1X0

Tel: 250-227-9224; *Fax:* 250-227-9494
Toll-Free: 800-661-8711
e-mail: info@yasodhara.org
www.yasodhara.org

Overview: A small international charitable organization founded in 1963
Mission: To maintain a centre for adults engaged in a life of spiritual intent; to provide instruction in & opportunities for religious & spiritual practice
Chief Officer(s):
Swami Lalitananda, President

National Publications

Alive
Owned By: Alive Publishing Group
#100, 12751 Vulcan Way, Richmond, BC V6V 3C8

Fax: 800-663-6597
Toll-Free: 800-663-6580
Social Media: plus.google.com/+aliveHealthMag
twitter.com/alivehealth
www.faceboo k.com/alive.health.wellness

Circulation: 200,000 *Frequency:* Monthly
Topics include health, wellness, natural health.
Ryan Benn, Publisher

Canadian Chiropractor
Owned By: Annex Publishing & Printing Inc.
PO Box 530, 105 Donly Dr. South, Simcoe, ON N3Y 4N5

Fax: 519-429-3094
Toll-Free: 888-599-2228

Circulation: 5,800 *Frequency:* 8 times a year
Mari-Len De Guzman, Editor, mdeguzman@annexweb.com
Martin McAnulty, Publisher, mmcanulty@annexweb.com

Massage Therapy Canada
Owned By: Annex Publishing & Printing Inc.
PO Box 530, 105 Donly Dr. South, Simcoe, ON N3Y 4N5

Fax: 519-429-3094
Toll-Free: 888-599-2228
Social Media: twitter.com/MTCanadaMag
www.facebook.com/MassageTherapyCanada

Circulation: 5,800 *Frequency:* 4 times a year
Mari-Len De Guzman, Editor, 905-726-4659,
mdeguzman@annexweb.com

Provincial/Local Publications

Mosaic Mind, Body & Spirit Magazine
PO Box 80588 Bellerose, St. Albert, AB T8N 7C3

Tel: 780-572-5880; *Fax:* 780-939-0588
mosaicmagazine@shaw.ca
Social Media: www.facebook.com/218630024830514

Circulation: 100,000 *Frequency:* Quarterly
Holistic medicine.
Connie Brisson, Publisher/Editor

WHOLifE Journal
PO Box 278, Kamsack, SK S0A 1S0

Tel: 306-542-3616; *Fax:* 306-542-3619
editor@wholife.com

Circulation: 17,000 *Frequency:* 6 times a year
Covers natural health & wellness for body, mind & spirirt, plus environmental issues
Melva Armstrong, Publisher/Editor

National Schools

ONTARIO

***Ottawa:* International Academy Health Education Centre**
380 Forest St., Ottawa, ON K2B 8E6, Canada

Tel: 613-820-0318; *Fax:* 613-820-7478
Toll-Free: 800-267-8732
info@intlacademy.com
www.intlacademy.com
www.facebook.com/internationalacademyhealtheducation
www.youtube.com/channel/UCCzjnU6PgSoZwvIKjIC1hhg

Note: Nutrition; herbs; iridology; reflexology; aromatherapy; homeopathy; shiatsu/accupressure; massage
Dorothy Marshall, Ph.D., N.D., C.H.H.P., N., Executive Director

***Ottawa:* International Academy of Natural Health Sciences**
380 Forest St., Ottawa, ON K2B 8E6, Canada

Tel: 613-820-0318; *Fax:* 613-820-7478
Toll-Free: 1-800-267-8732
naturalhealth@intlacademy.com
www.intlacademy.com

Note: Nutrition; herbs; iridology; reflexology
Paul Raven, Principal
Tanya Sparkes, Program Director

Toronto: **The Canadian College of Naturopathic Medicine**
1255 Sheppard Ave. East, Toronto, ON M2K 1E2, Canada
Tel: 416-498-1255; *Toll-Free:* 1-866-241-2266
www.ccnm.edu
www.facebook.com/myccnm
twitter.com/myccnm
www.youtube.com/myccnm

Enrollment: 600
Number of Employees: 100 full time; 100 part time *Note:* Naturopathic medical education, research & clinical practice; 4,500+ hours of classroom & clinical training
Nicholas De Groot, Dean
Bob Bernhardt, President & CEO

Local Schools

Edmonton: **Grant MacEwan University**
Also known as: MacEwan University
P.O. Box 1796
Edmonton, AB T5J 2P2, Canada
Toll-Free: 888-497-4622
info@macewan.ca
www.macewan.ca
www.facebook.com/MacEwanUniversity
twitter.com/macewanu
www.linkedin.com/edu/school?id=21055
www.youtube.com/macewanchannel
Deborah Saucier, President

National Libraries

Canadian Memorial Chiropractic College
6100 Leslie St., Toronto, ON M2H 3J1
Tel: 416-482-2340; *Fax:* 416-482-4816
www.cmcc.ca/Page.aspx?pid=377

Collection: Chiropractic History
Margaret Butkovic, Library Director
416-482-2340 ext. 159
Kent Murnaghan, Reference Librarian
416-482-2340 ext. 205
Steve Zoltai, Collection Development Librarian
Todd Vasey, Library Technician (Cataloguing)
Deanne Collier, Library Technician
Shabana Siddiqui, Library Technician (Serials)

Indigenous Health Issues

National Associations

The Belinda Stronach Foundation (TBSF)
Toronto ON
www.tbsf.ca
www.youtube.com/user/TheTBSFChannel
Overview: A small national charitable organization founded in 2008
Mission: Assists girls and women and Aboriginal youth in Canada and youth in developing nations to achieve a better life through the provision of programs that enhance basic health and education, improve economic and political independence and that promote civic involvement.
Chief Officer(s):
Belinda Stronach, President & CEO

Canadian Aboriginal AIDS Network (CAAN)
6520 Salish Dr., Vancouver BC V6N 2C7
Tel: 604-266-7616; *Fax:* 604-266-7612
www.caan.ca
www.facebook.com/CAAN.ca
twitter.com/caan_says

Overview: A medium-sized national organization
Mission: To provide support & advocacy for Aboriginal people living with or affected by HIV/AIDS, TB, aging, mental illness, or other co-morbidity issues
Chief Officer(s):
Emma Palmantier, Chair
Ken Clement, Chief Executive Officer, 604-266-7616 Ext. 227
Merv Thomas, Manager, National Programs Communications, 604-266-7616 Ext. 226

Publications:
• Canadian Journal of Aboriginal Community-Based HIV/AIDS Research (CJACBR)
Type: Journal; *Frequency:* Annually; *Editor:* Renee Masching et al.
Profile: A peer-reviewed journal directed toward Aboriginal HIV/AIDS service organizations, Aboriginal people living with HIV/AIDS, community leaders, policy & decision-makers, & anyone with an interest in HIV/AIDS

Canadian Indigenous Nurses Association (CINA)
50 Driveway, Ottawa ON K2P 1E2
Tel: 613-724-4677
e-mail: info@anac.on.ca
www.indigenousnurses.ca
twitter.com/aboriginalnurse
Previous Name: Aboriginal Nurses Association of Canada; Indian & Inuit Nurses of Canada
Overview: A large national charitable organization founded in 1974
Mission: To work with & on behalf of Aboriginal nurses to promote the development & practice of Aboriginal nursing in order to improve the health of Aboriginal people
Member of: Canadian Nurses Association
Affiliation(s): Health Canada; Canadian Nurses Association
Chief Officer(s):
Lisa Bourque-Bearskin, President
Ada Roberts, Vice-President
Publications:
• The Aboriginal Nurse [a publication of the Canadian Indigenous Nurses Association]
Type: Newsletter; *Frequency:* 3 pa; *Accepts Advertising; Editor:* Connie Toulouse; *Price:* Free with membership in the Aboriginal Nurses Association of Canada

First Nations Breast Cancer Society
#309, 1333 East 7th Ave., Vancouver BC V5N 1R6
Tel: 604-872-4390; *Fax:* 604-875-0779
e-mail: echoes@fnbreastcancer.bc.ca
www.fnbreastcancer.bc.ca
Overview: A small national organization founded in 1995
Mission: Offers breast cancer education and support to First Nations women.
Chief Officer(s):
Jacqueline Davis, President
jdavis@fnbreastcancer.bc.ca

Indigenous Physicians Association of Canada (IPAC)
#305, 323 Portage Ave., Winnipeg MB R3B 2C1
e-mail: info@ipac-amic.org
www.ipac-amic.org
Overview: A small national organization
Mission: To serve the interests of Indigenous physicians, medical students & the health related interests of Indigenous people in Canada
Chief Officer(s):
Darlene Kitty, President

Ki-Low-Na Friendship Society (KFS)
442 Leon Ave., Kelowna BC V1Y 6J3
Tel: 250-763-4905; *Fax:* 250-861-5514
e-mail: reception@kfs.bc.ca
www.kfs.bc.ca
Previous Name: Central Okanagan Indian Friendship Society
Overview: A small national charitable organization founded in 1974
Mission: To promote total well-being for Native people in all human dimensions: physical, spiritual, mental & emotional
Member of: United Way
Chief Officer(s):
Edna Terbasket, Executive Director

National Association of Friendship Centres (NAFC) / Association nationale des centres d'amitié
275 MacLaren St., Ottawa ON K2P 0L9
Tel: 613-563-4844; *Fax:* 613-594-3428
Toll-Free: 877-563-4844
e-mail: nafcgen@nafc.ca
nafc.ca
www.linkedin.com/company/national-association-of-friendship-centres
www.facebook.com/TheNAFC
twitter.com/NAFC_ANCA
Overview: A medium-sized national organization founded in 1971

Mission: To assist friendship centres in communication, funding & training
Chief Officer(s):
Erin Corston, Executive Director
  ecorston@nafc.ca

National Native Addictions Partnership Foundation (NNAPF) / Fondation autochtone nationale de partenariat pour la lutte contre les dépendances
PO Box 183, Muskoday SK S0J 3H0
Tel: 306-763-4714; Fax: 306-763-5993
Toll-Free: 866-763-4714
e-mail: info@nnapf.org
www.nnapf.org
www.facebook.com/423836911040446
twitter.com/NNAPF
Overview: A small national organization founded in 1998
Mission: To advocate, develop, facilitate, & monitor strategies designed to continuously upgrade & enhance the quality of ideas, information, program methodologies, financial allocations & skills of service providers comprising the program
Chief Officer(s):
Austin Bear, President
Janice Nicotine, Vice-President

Native Women's Association of Canada (NWAC) / L'Association des femmes autochtones du Canada (AFAC)
#4, 155 International Rd., Akwesasne ON K6H 5R7
Tel: 613-722-3033
Toll-Free: 800-461-4043
e-mail: reception@nwac.ca
www.nwac.ca
www.facebook.com/NWAC.AFAC
twitter.com/NWAC_CA
Overview: A medium-sized national organization founded in 1974
Mission: To enhance, promote & foster the social, economic, cultural & political well-being of First Nations & Métis women with First Nations & Canadian societies; To help empower women by being involved in developing & changing legislation which affects them, & by involving them in the development & delivery of programs promoting equal opportunity for Aboriginal women. Satellite office located at 1 Nicholas St., 9th Fl., Ottawa.
Member of: Indigenous Survival International
Chief Officer(s):
Francyne Joe, Interim President

Red Road HIV/AIDS Network (RRHAN)
#61-1959 Marine Dr., North Vancouver BC V7P 3G1
Tel: 778-340-3388; Fax: 778-340-3328
e-mail: info@red-road.org
www.red-road.org
twitter.com/RRHAN
Overview: A small national organization founded in 1999
Mission: The Red Road HIV/AIDS Network works to reduce or prevent the spread of HIV/AIDS; improve the health and wellness of Aboriginal people living with HIV/AIDS; and increase awareness about HIV/AIDS and establish a network which supports the development and delivery of culturally appropriate, innovative, coordinated, accessible, inclusive and accountable HIV/AIDS programs and services
Chief Officer(s):
Kim Louie, Executive Director
  klouie@red-road.org
Heidi Standeven, Provincial Coordinator
  hstandeven@red-road.org
Publications:
• Bloodlines Magazine
Type: Magazine
Profile: a forum in which Aboriginal Persons Living with HIV/AIDS can share their personal experiences, discuss issues affecting them, offer advice and suggestions to their peers.
• Red Road Aboriginal HIV/AIDS Resource Directory
Type: Directory; Frequency: Semi-Annually

Regroupement des centres d'amitié autochtone du Québec (RCAAQ)
#100, 85, boul Maurice-Bastien, Wendake QC G0A 4V0
Tél: 418-842-6354; Téléc: 418-842-9795
Ligne sans frais: 877-842-6354
Courriel: infos@rcaaq.info
www.rcaaq.info
www.facebook.com/RCAAQ
twitter.com/rcaaq
www.youtube.com/rcaaq
Aperçu: Dimension: moyenne; Envergure: nationale; Organisme sans but lucratif; fondée en 1976 surveillé par National Association of Friendship Centres
Mission: Etre la voix provinciale des centres existants ou en voie de développement et de leurs communautés; appuyer ses membres dans l'atteinte de leurs objectifs; favoriser leur concertation et les représenter collectivement pour qu'ils remplissent au mieux leur mandat
Membre(s) du bureau directeur:
Tanya Sirois, Directrice générale

2-Spirited People of the First Nations (TPFN)
#105, 145 Front St. East, Toronto ON M5A 1E3
Tel: 416-944-9300; Fax: 416-944-8381
www.2spirits.com
www.facebook.com/2spiritsTO
www.instagram.com/2spirits_com
Previous Name: Gays & Lesbians of the First Nations
Overview: A medium-sized national charitable organization founded in 1989
Mission: To create a place where Aboriginal 2-Spirited people can grow & learn together as a community, fostering a positive, self-sufficient image, honouring our past & building a future; to work together toward bridging the gap between the 2-Spirited, Lesbian, Gay, Bisexual & Transgendered community & our Aboriginal identity
Member of: Ontario AIDS Network; Toronto Aboriginal Social Services Association; Canadian Aboriginal AIDS Network
Chief Officer(s):
Art Zoccole, Executive Director Ext. 222
  art@2spirits.com

Provincial Associations

ALBERTA

Alberta Aboriginal Women's Society
PO Box 5168, Stn. Main, Peace River AB T8S 1R8
Tel: 780-624-3416; Fax: 780-624-3409
e-mail: aaws@telusplanet.net
Overview: A medium-sized provincial organization overseen by Native Women's Association of Canada
Chief Officer(s):
Ruth Kidder, President

Alberta Native Friendship Centres Association (ANFCA)
10336 - 121 St., Edmonton AB T5N 1K8
Tel: 780-423-3138; Fax: 780-425-6277
www.anfca.com
Overview: A medium-sized provincial organization founded in 1970 overseen by National Association of Friendship Centres
Mission: To assist friendship centres in communication, funding & training
Chief Officer(s):
Nelson Mayer, Executive Director
  anfca.director@telus.net

Napi Friendship Association
PO Box 657, 622 Charlotte St., Pincher Creek AB T0K 1K0
Tel: 403-627-4224; Fax: 403-627-2564
e-mail: napiyouthcoordinator@gmail.com
www.okinapi.com
www.facebook.com/napiyouthprograms
Overview: A small provincial charitable organization overseen by Alberta Native Friendship Centres Association
Mission: To create better communication & understanding between the residents of Pincher Creek & the Peigan Nation
Member of: Alberta Native Friendship Centres Association

BRITISH COLUMBIA

Association of BC First Nations Treatment Programs
PO Box 325, Invermere BC V0A 1K0
Tel: 778-526-2501; *Fax:* 778-526-2505
Overview: A small provincial organization
Mission: To provide a forum that promotes culturally relevant practices to enhance & advance the continuum of care in addressing addictions among First Nations peoples

British Columbia Aboriginal Network on Disability Society (BCANDS)
1179 Kosapsum Cres., Victoria BC V9A 7K7
Tel: 250-381-7303; *Fax:* 250-381-7312
Toll-Free: 888-815-5511; *TTY:* 888-815-5511
e-mail: bcands@bcands.bc.ca
www.bcands.bc.ca
www.linkedin.com/company/3252163
www.facebook.com/386847191382585
twitter.com/bcands1
Overview: A small provincial charitable organization founded in 1991
Mission: To promote the betterment of Aboriginal people with disabilities
Chief Officer(s):
Stephen Lytton, President
Ruby Reid, Secretary-Treasurer
Neil Belanger, Executive Director

British Columbia Association of Aboriginal Friendship Centres (BCAAFC)
551 Chatham St., Victoria BC V8T 1E1
Tel: 250-388-5522; *Fax:* 250-388-5502
Toll-Free: 800-990-2432
e-mail: frontdesk@bcaafc.com
www.bcaafc.com
www.facebook.com/pages/BC-Friendship-Centres/160027657353593
Overview: A medium-sized provincial organization overseen by National Association of Friendship Centres
Mission: To promote the betterment of Aboriginal Friendship Centres in British Columbia by acting as a unifying body for the Centres; To establish & maintain communications between Aboriginal Friendship Centres, other associations, & government
Chief Officer(s):
Paul Lacerte, Executive Director
Publications:
• BC Association of Aboriginal Friendship Centres Annual Report
Type: Report; *Frequency:* Annually

British Columbia Native Women's Association
144 Briar Ave., Kamloops BC V2B 1C1
Tel: 250-554-4556; *Fax:* 250-554-4573
www.facebook.com/bc.nativewomensassociation
Overview: A medium-sized provincial organization overseen by Native Women's Association of Canada

Native Brotherhood of British Columbia (NBBC) / Fraternité des Indiens de la Colombie-Britannique
#110, 100 Park Royal South, West Vancouver BC V7T 1A2
Tel: 604-913-2997; *Fax:* 604-913-2995
nativebrotherhood.ca
Overview: A medium-sized provincial organization founded in 1931
Mission: To improve the social, spiritual, economic & physical conditions of its members, including education, health & living; To cooperate with other organizations which are involved with the advancement of Indian welfare; To focus on capacity building, particularly resources with economic potential

Union of British Columbia Indian Chiefs
#500, 342 Water St., Vancouver BC V6B 1B6
Tel: 604-684-0231; *Fax:* 604-684-5726
Toll-Free: 800-793-9701
e-mail: ubcic@ubcic.bc.ca
www.ubcic.bc.ca
www.facebook.com/UBCIC
twitter.com/UBCIC
www.youtube.com/UBCIC
Overview: A medium-sized provincial organization founded in 1969
Mission: To settle land claims & Aboriginal rights in BC; To improve the social, economic, health, & education of Aboriginal people in BC; To provide a political voice for Aboriginal people in BC

Member of: Assembly of First Nations; World Council of Indigenous Peoples
Chief Officer(s):
Stewart Phillip, President

MANITOBA

Manitoba Association of Friendship Centres (MAC)
#102, 150 Henry Ave., Winnipeg MB R3B 0J7
Tel: 204-942-6299
www.friendshipcentres.ca
www.facebook.com/FriendshipCentres
Overview: A medium-sized provincial charitable organization founded in 1971 overseen by National Association of Friendship Centres
Mission: To assist friendship centres in communication, funding & training
Chief Officer(s):
Adam Blanchard, Executive Director

Mother of Red Nations Women's Council of Manitoba (MORN)
#300, 141 Bannatyne Ave., Winnipeg MB R3B 0R3
Tel: 204-942-6676
morn.cimnet.ca/cim/92C270_397T18346.dhtm
Previous Name: Aboriginal Women of Manitoba
Overview: A small provincial organization overseen by Native Women's Association of Canada
Mission: To represent Aboriginal women in Manitoba & serve as their primary political & advocacy organization; To promote, protect & support the spiritual, emotional, physical & mental well-being of all Aboriginal women & children in the province
Affiliation(s): Native Woman's Association of Canada

Native Addictions Council of Manitoba (NACM)
160 Salter St., Winnipeg MB R2W 4K1
Tel: 204-586-8395; *Fax:* 204-589-3921
e-mail: info@nacm.ca
www.mts.net/~nacm/
Also Known As: Pritchard House
Overview: A small provincial charitable organization founded in 1972
Mission: To provide traditional holistic healing services to First Peoples through treatment of addictions; each member of First Peoples has the right to wellness.

NEW BRUNSWICK

New Brunswick Aboriginal Women's Council
29 Big Cove Rd., Elsipogtog NB E4W 2S5
Tel: 506-523-9518; *Fax:* 506-523-8350
e-mail: nbawca@nb.aibn.com
Previous Name: New Brunswick Native Indian Women's Council
Overview: A medium-sized provincial organization overseen by Native Women's Association of Canada
Chief Officer(s):
Sarah Rose, President

NEWFOUNDLAND AND LABRADOR

Labrador Native Women's Association
PO Box 542, Stn. B, Happy Valley-Goose Bay NL A0P 1S0
Tel: 709-896-5071; *Fax:* 709-896-5071
www.exec.gov.nl.ca/exec/wpo/aboriginalwomen
Overview: A small provincial organization

Newfoundland Native Women's Association
PO Box 22, Benoits Cove NL A0L 1A0
Tel: 709-789-3430; *Fax:* 709-789-2207
e-mail: nf.nativewomen@nf.aibn.com
Overview: A small provincial organization overseen by Native Women's Association of Canada
Mission: To enhance, promote & foster the social, economic, cultural and political well-being of First Nations and Métis women within First Nation, Métis and Canadian societies.

NORTHWEST TERRITORIES

Northwest Territories/Nunavut Council of Friendship Centres
PO Box 2285, #209, 4817 - 49th St., Yellowknife NT X1A 2P6
Tel: 867-669-7063; *Fax:* 867-669-7064
ntnucfc.wildapricot.org
Overview: A small provincial organization overseen by National Association of Friendship Centres

Mission: To assist friendship centres in the Northwest Territories & Nunavut

NOVA SCOTIA

Nova Scotia Native Women's Society (NSNWA)
PO Box 805, Truro NS B2N 5E8
Tel: 902-893-7402; *Fax:* 902-897-7162
www.facebook.com/nsnwa
Overview: A medium-sized provincial organization founded in 1972 overseen by Native Women's Association of Canada
Member of: Native Women's Association of Canada (NWAC)

ONTARIO

Métis National Council (MNC) / Ralliement national des Métis
#4, 340 MacLaren St., Ottawa ON K2P 0M6
Tel: 613-232-3216; *Fax:* 613-232-4262
Toll-Free: 800-928-6330
e-mail: info@metisnation.ca
www.metisnation.ca
www.facebook.com/186735084697421
twitter.com/MNC_tweets
www.youtube.com/user/MetisNationalCouncil
Overview: A medium-sized provincial organization founded in 1983
Mission: To represent the Métis both nationally & internationally; To secure a healthy space for the Métis Nation's existence within Canada
Chief Officer(s):
Clément Chartier, President

Ontario Federation of Indian Friendship Centres (OFIFC)
219 Front St. East, Toronto ON M5A 1E8
Tel: 416-956-7575; *Fax:* 416-956-7577
Toll-Free: 800-772-9291
e-mail: ofifc@ofifc.org
www.ofifc.org
www.facebook.com/TheOFIFC
twitter.com/theofifc
Also Known As: Ontario Federation of Friendship Centres
Overview: A medium-sized provincial organization founded in 1971 overseen by National Association of Friendship Centres
Mission: To represent the collective interests of Ontario's friendship centres; To administer programs delivered by friendship centres, such as justice, health, employment, & family support; To improve the quality of life for Aboriginal people for equal access & participation in Canadian society
Chief Officer(s):
Sheila McMahon, President

Ontario Native Women's Association (ONWA)
PO Box 15-684, 150 City Rd., Fort William First Nation ON P7J 1J7
Tel: 807-577-1492; *Fax:* 807-623-1104
Toll-Free: 800-667-0816
www.onwa.ca
www.facebook.com/onwa7
twitter.com/_onwa_
Overview: A medium-sized provincial organization founded in 1972 overseen by Native Women's Association of Canada
Mission: To foster & promote the economic, social, cultural, & political well-being of First Nations & Métis women in Ontario; To represent Native women on issues that affect their lives
Chief Officer(s):
Dawn Harvard, President

PRINCE EDWARD ISLAND

Aboriginal Women's Association of Prince Edward Island
PO Box 145, 312 Sweetgrass Trail, Lennox Island PE C0B 1P0
Tel: 902-831-3059; *Fax:* 902-831-3027
e-mail: info@awapei.org
www.awapei.org
www.facebook.com/193334154037222
twitter.com/awapei1
Overview: A small provincial organization founded in 1975 overseen by Native Women's Association of Canada
Mission: To address issues of concern to off-reserve Aboriginal women; To improve the educational, social & economic conditions surrounding Aboriginal women
Chief Officer(s):

Judith Clark, President

QUÉBEC

Femmes autochtones du Québec inc. (FAQ) / Québec Native Women Inc.
CP 1989, Kahnawake QC J0L 1B0
Tél: 450-632-0088; *Téléc:* 450-632-9280
Courriel: info@faq-qnw.org
www.faq-qnw.org
www.facebook.com/FAQQNW
twitter.com/FAQQNW
vimeo.com/user14258370
Aperçu: *Dimension:* moyenne; *Envergure:* provinciale; Organisme sans but lucratif; fondée en 1974 surveillé par Native Women's Association of Canada
Mission: Appuyer les efforts des femmes autochtones pour l'amélioration de leurs conditions de vie par la promotion de la non-violence, de la justice et de l'égalité des droits et de les soutenir dans leur engagement au sein de leur communauté
Membre(s) du bureau directeur:
Viviane Michel, Présidente

SASKATCHEWAN

Aboriginal Friendship Centres of Saskatchewan
115 Wall St., Saskatoon SK S7K 6C2
Tel: 306-955-0762; *Fax:* 306-955-0972
www.afcs.ca
www.facebook.com/192129454182112
twitter.com/afcsk
www.youtube.com/user/theAFCS
Overview: A medium-sized provincial organization founded in 1963 overseen by National Association of Friendship Centres
Mission: The objectives of the Aboriginal Friendship Centres (AFC) of Sask. are: the promotion of the goals and objectives of its member Friendship Centres; the facilitation of communication and cooperation amongst all Centres w/in SK,.; the providing of information regarding the operation and dvlp. of AFCs to the public; negotiation with all tiers of gov't on matters of concern to the member Centres; assistance in Program Dvlp.; and assistance to all members in terms of funding information, debt recovery plans, financial negotiation, and networking.
Chief Officer(s):
Gwen Bear, Executive Director

Saskatchewan Aboriginal Women's Circle Corporation
PO Box 1174, Yorkton SK S3N 2X3
Tel: 306-783-1228; *Fax:* 306-783-1771
e-mail: sawcc@hotmail.com
Previous Name: Saskatchewan Native Women's Association
Overview: A small provincial organization founded in 1972 overseen by Native Women's Association of Canada
Mission: To walk in balance with guidance by the creator; to unite people together as healthy nations to ensure a better life for future generations

YUKON TERRITORY

Yukon Aboriginal Women's Council
#202, 307 Jarvis St., Whitehorse YT Y1A 2H3
Tel: 867-667-6162; *Fax:* 867-668-7539
e-mail: yawc@northwestel.net
Overview: A small provincial organization founded in 1983 overseen by Native Women's Association of Canada
Mission: To create equal opportunities for Aboriginal women by implementing programs aimed to improving their quality of life

Local Associations

ALBERTA

Aboriginal Friendship Centre of Calgary
#101, 427 - 51 Ave. SE, Calgary AB T2H 0M8
Tel: 403-270-7379
e-mail: info@afccalgary.org
www.afccalgary.org
www.facebook.com/AboriginalFriendshipCentreOfCalgary
www.twitter.com/AbYouthCouncil
Overview: A small local organization overseen by Alberta Native Friendship Centres Association

Member of: Alberta Native Friendship Centres Association
Chief Officer(s):
Sandra Sutter, President

Athabasca Native Friendship Centre Society
4919 - 53 St., Athabasca AB T9S 1L1
Tel: 780-675-3086; Fax: 780-675-3063
e-mail: anfcs@telusplanet.net
anfca.com/friendship-centres/athabasca
Overview: A small local organization founded in 1988 overseen by Alberta Native Friendship Centres Association
Mission: The Society is a non-profit, social services agency administering programs & services to meet the needs of all Aboriginal people of the region, both transient & resident.
Member of: Alberta Native Friendship Centres Association (ANFCA)
Chief Officer(s):
Laureen Houle, Executive Director

Bonnyville Canadian Native Friendship Centre
PO Box 5399, 4711 - 50 Ave., Bonnyville AB T9N 2G5
Tel: 780-826-3374; Fax: 780-826-2540
e-mail: bcnfced@incentre.net
www.facebook.com/bonnyvillefriendshipcentre
Overview: A small local organization founded in 1971 overseen by Alberta Native Friendship Centres Association
Mission: To create a healthy, productive community through innovative & cultural services
Member of: Alberta Native Friendship Centres Association

Canadian Native Friendship Centre (CNFC)
11728 - 95 St., Edmonton AB T5G 1L9
Tel: 780-760-1900; Fax: 780-760-1900
www.cnfc.ca
www.facebook.com/CNFCEdmonton
Also Known As: CNFC Edmonton
Overview: A small local charitable organization founded in 1962 overseen by Alberta Native Friendship Centres Association
Mission: To improve the quality of life of Aboriginal Peoples in an urban environment by supporting self-determined activities encouraging equal access to & participation in Canadian society while respecting Aboriginal cultural distinctiveness
Member of: National Association of Friendship Centres; Alberta Native Friendship Centres Association
Chief Officer(s):
Ron Walker, Executive Director

Cold Lake Native Friendship Centre
PO Box 1978, 5015 - 55 St., Cold Lake AB T9M 1P4
Tel: 780-594-7526; Fax: 780-594-1599
e-mail: cold1@telus.net
clnfc.ca/index.php/home/cold-lake-friendship-centre
www.facebook.com/ColdLakeFriendshipCentre
Previous Name: Grand Centre Canadian Native Friendship Centre
Overview: A small local charitable organization overseen by Alberta Native Friendship Centres Association
Mission: The Centre aims to facilitate the advancement of cultural, social, recreation between Natives & non-Native people of Cold Lake area.
Member of: Alberta Native Friendship Centres Association (ANFCA)
Chief Officer(s):
Agnes Gendron, Executive Director

Edmonton Aboriginal Senior Centre (NSC)
Cottage E, 10107 - 134 Ave., Edmonton AB T5E 1J2
Tel: 780-476-6595
e-mail: manager@easc.ca
www.easc.ca
Previous Name: Métis Women's Council of Edmonton
Overview: A small local charitable organization founded in 1986
Mission: To promote welfare, education & interests of Aboriginal seniors within the Edmonton area

Edson Friendship Centre
#13, 5023 - 3rd Ave., Edson AB T7E 1X7
Tel: 780-723-5494; Fax: 780-723-4359
e-mail: efc99@telus.net
www.facebook.com/110865509072047
Overview: A small local charitable organization founded in 1986 overseen by Alberta Native Friendship Centres Association

Member of: National Association of Friendship Centre; Alberta Native Friendship Centres Association

Grande Prairie Friendship Centre
10507 - 98 Ave., Grande Prairie AB T8V 4L1
Tel: 780-532-5722; Fax: 780-539-5121
e-mail: gpfriend@telusplanet.net
gpfriendshipcenter.wordpress.com
Overview: A small local organization overseen by Alberta Native Friendship Centres Association
Member of: Alberta Native Friendship Centres Association
Chief Officer(s):
Miranda Laroche, Executive Director

High Level Native Friendship Centre
PO Box 1735, 11000 - 95 St., High Level AB T0H 1Z0
Tel: 780-926-3355; Fax: 780-926-2038
e-mail: hlnfcs.ed@gmail.com
anfca.com/friendship-centres/high-level
Overview: A small local organization overseen by Alberta Native Friendship Centres Association
Member of: Alberta Native Friendship Centres Association
Chief Officer(s):
Barb Adekat, Executive Director

High Prairie Native Friendship Centre
PO Box 1448, 4919 - 51 Ave., High Prairie AB T0G 1E0
Tel: 780-523-4511; Fax: 780-523-3055
e-mail: edhpnfc@gmail.com
www.facebook.com/260735773965759
Overview: A small local organization founded in 1975 overseen by Alberta Native Friendship Centres Association
Mission: To improve the quality of life for Aboriginal people in urban areas by supporting self-determined activities that encourage: the development of human and community resources; the improvement of socio-economic and physical conditions; better understanding and relationships between Aboriginal and non-Aboriginal citizens; and the enhancement of Aboriginal culture among Aboriginal people and the communities they reside in.
Member of: Alberta Native Friendship Centres Association

Hinton Friendship Centre
PO Box 6720, Stn. Main, 965 Switzer Dr., Hinton AB T7V 1X6
Tel: 780-865-5189; Fax: 780-865-1756
e-mail: main@fchinton.com
www.hintonfriendshipcentre.ca
Overview: A small local organization founded in 1995 overseen by Alberta Native Friendship Centres Association
Member of: Alberta Native Friendship Centres Association
Chief Officer(s):
Yvonne Oshanyk, Executive Director

Lac La Biche Canadian Native Friendship Centre
PO Box 2338, 10105 Churchill Dr., Lac La Biche AB T0A 2C0
Tel: 780-623-3249; Fax: 780-623-1846
www.llb-cnfc.com
www.facebook.com/llbcnfc
twitter.com/LLBCNFC
Overview: A small local organization overseen by Alberta Native Friendship Centres Association
Mission: Dedicated to providing culturally-based programs and services that respond to the distinct needs of urban Aboriginal people in their communities and bridging the gaps that occur between Aboriginal and non-Aboriginal peoples in urban areas.
Member of: Alberta Native Friendship Centres Association
Chief Officer(s):
Donna Webster, Executive Director
donna@llb-cnfc.com

Mannawanis Native Friendship Centre
PO Box 1358, 4901 - 50 St., St Paul AB T0A 3A0
Tel: 780-645-4630; Fax: 780-645-1980
Other Communication: Alt. E-mail: mannawanis@hotmail.com
e-mail: mannatfc@mcsnet.ca
Overview: A small local charitable organization overseen by Alberta Native Friendship Centres Association
Mission: To co-exist in a safe & unified environment that supports the development of healthy aboriginal families, providers & members of the community

Member of: Alberta Native Friendship Centres Association
Affiliation(s): Alberta Food Bank Association; Canadian Food Bank Association

Métis Child & Family Services Society (Edmonton) (MCFS)
10437 - 123rd St., Edmonton AB T5N 1N8
Tel: 780-452-6100; *Fax:* 780-452-8944
e-mail: reception@metischild.com
www.metischild.com
Overview: A small local organization founded in 1984
Mission: To promote the health & well-being of Aboriginal children & families by building the capacity of the Métis community through the provision of culturally sensitive & appropriate services & programs
Chief Officer(s):
Don Langford, Executive Director
ed1@metischild.com

Nistawoyou Association Friendship Centre
8310 Manning Ave., Fort McMurray AB T9H 1W1
Tel: 780-743-8555; *Fax:* 780-750-0527
e-mail: nistawoyou@gmail.com
Overview: A small local organization founded in 1964 overseen by Alberta Native Friendship Centres Association
Mission: To develop social & recreational activities in the Aboriginal communities in & around Fort McMurray
Member of: Alberta Native Friendship Centres Association
Affiliation(s): Fort McMurray United Way
Chief Officer(s):
Theresa Nahwegahbow, Executive Director

Red Deer Native Friendship Society
4808-51 Ave., Red Deer AB T4N 4H3
Tel: 403-340-0020; *Fax:* 403-324-1610
anfca.com/friendship-centres/red-deer
Overview: A small local organization founded in 1984 overseen by Alberta Native Friendship Centres Association
Mission: To inform the community of the problems experiences by Aboriginal people living in urban areas, & to work with the community to resolve these problems where possible; To provide a medium for the development of Aboriginal Leadership in the community; To promote friendship & understanding between Aboriginal & Non-Aboriginal people; To preserve & promote Aboriginal Culture & Heritage within the community; To assist Aboriginal people to use & derive advantages from services & facilities & to improve generally the lives of Aboriginal people; To establish organizational leadership, management effectiveness & responsive program planning & delivery in addressing the issues facing the Native community
Member of: Alberta Native Friendship Centres Association
Chief Officer(s):
Lianne Hazell, Executive Director
lhazell@rdnfs.com

Rocky Native Friendship Society
PO Box 1927, 4917 - 52 St., Rocky Mountain House AB T4T 1B4
Tel: 403-845-2788; *Fax:* 403-845-3093
www.friendshipcentre.shawbiz.ca
www.facebook.com/147332261987888
Overview: A small local organization founded in 1975 overseen by Alberta Native Friendship Centres Association
Mission: To create a healthy & supportive community to empower Aboriginal people in the Rocky Mountain House area; To strengthen Aboriginal cultural awareness
Member of: Alberta Native Friendship Centres Association
Affiliation(s): Alberta Native Friendship Centres Association
Chief Officer(s):
Helge Nome, President
Douglas Bonaise, Vice-President
Tani Amarook, Treasurer
Merle White, Executive Director

Sagitawa Friendship Centre / Where the Rivers Meet
PO Box 5083, 10108 - 100 Ave., Peace River AB T8S 1R7
Tel: 780-624-2443; *Fax:* 780-624-2728
e-mail: tracy-sagitawa@telus.net
anfca.com/friendship-centres/peace-river
Overview: A small local organization founded in 1964 overseen by Alberta Native Friendship Centres Association

Mission: To encourage respect & acceptance of all people; To enhance the quality of life of Aboriginal people in the Peace River area
Member of: Alberta Native Friendship Centres Association
Chief Officer(s):
Tracy Zweifel, Executive Director

Sik-ooh-kotoki Friendship Society
1709 - 2nd Ave. South, Lethbridge AB T1J 0E8
Tel: 403-328-2414; *Fax:* 403-327-0087
e-mail: sikooh@telusplanet.net
anfca.com/friendship-centres/lethbridge
Also Known As: Lethbridge Friendship Centre
Overview: A small local organization founded in 1969 overseen by Alberta Native Friendship Centres Association
Mission: To improve the quality of life for Aboriginal peoples in an urban environment by supporting self-determined activities which encourage equal access to, & participation in Canadian society & which respect & strengthen the increasing emphasis on Aboriginal cultural distinctiveness
Member of: Alberta Native Friendship Centres Association
Chief Officer(s):
Yolande Weasel Head, Executive Director
yolande.ywh@shaw.ca

Slave Lake Native Friendship Centre
416 - 6 Ave., Slave Lake AB T0G 2A2
Tel: 780-849-3039; *Fax:* 780-849-2402
Other Communication: Alt. E-mail: slnfced@gmail.com
e-mail: slnfc2@gmail.com
anfca.com/friendship-centres/slave-lake
Overview: A small local organization founded in 1972 overseen by Alberta Native Friendship Centres Association
Mission: To be a leader in the community by implementing new programs/services that will serve the needs of the Aboriginal people in order to improve their self-reliance & well being
Member of: Alberta Native Friendship Centres Association
Chief Officer(s):
Jamie Linington, Executive Director

BRITISH COLUMBIA

Cariboo Friendship Society
99 South 3rd Ave., Williams Lake BC V2G 1J1
Tel: 250-398-6831; *Fax:* 250-398-6115
e-mail: admin@cfswl.ca
www.cariboofriendshipsociety.ca
Overview: A small local organization founded in 1969
Mission: To promote healthy lifestyles, & fostering fellowship & understanding between people by providing holistic programs & services to all.
Chief Officer(s):
Rosanna McGregor, Executive Director
rmcgregor@cfswl.ca

Dze L K'ant Friendship Centre Society
PO Box 2920, 1188 Main St., Smithers BC V0J 2N0
Tel: 250-847-5211; *Fax:* 250-847-5144
e-mail: dzelkant@gmail.com
www.dzelkant.com
Previous Name: Dze L K'ant Indian Friendship Centre Society
Overview: A small local charitable organization founded in 1974 overseen by British Columbia Association of Aboriginal Friendship Centres
Mission: The Centre is a community-based organization providing programs & services to enhance self-reliance, self-efficiency & self-awareness among Aboriginal people.
Member of: BC Association of Aboriginal Friendship Centres
Chief Officer(s):
Annette Morgan, Executive Director
Genevieve Poirier, Program Director

Dease Lake Location
PO Box 328, 71 Stikine, Dease Lake BC V0C 1L0
Tel: 250-771-3147
e-mail: deasepop@gmail.com

Houston Location
3383 - 11 St., Houston BC V0J 1Z0
Tel: 250-845-2131; *Fax:* 250-845-2136
e-mail: aecdhouston@gmail.com

First Nations Friendship Centre (FNFC)
2904 - 29th Ave., Vernon BC V1T 1Y7
Tel: 250-542-1247; *Fax:* 205-542-3707
e-mail: fnfc@shawcable.com
Also Known As: First Nations Friendship Centre Society
Overview: A small local charitable organization founded in 1975
Mission: To improve the quality of life for Native People in a welcome environment, by supporting self-determined activities which encourage equal access to & participation in Canadian society & which respect Native cultural distinctiveness

Friendship House Association of Prince Rupert
744 Fraser St., Prince Rupert BC V8J 1P9
Tel: 250-627-1717; *Fax:* 250-627-7533
e-mail: reception@friendshiphouse.ca
www.friendshiphouse.ca
www.facebook.com/235609558272
Overview: A small local organization founded in 1958
Mission: To provide educational & cultural programs to the First Nations community in Prince Rupert

Healing Our Spirit BC Aboriginal HIV/AIDS Society
137 East 4 Ave., Vancouver BC V5T 1G4
Tel: 604-879-8884; *Fax:* 604-879-9926
Toll-Free: 866-745-8884
e-mail: info@healingourspirit.org
www.healingourspirit.org
Overview: A medium-sized local charitable organization founded in 1992
Mission: To prevent & reduce the spread of HIV infection in First Nation communities & to support those affected by HIV/AIDS.
Member of: Canadian Aboriginal AIDS Network
Affliation(s): Red Road HIV/AIDS Network; BC Aboriginal AIDS Awareness Program; AIDS Vancouver; BC Persons with AIDS
Chief Officer(s):
Winston Thompson, Executive Director
winston@healingourspirit.org
Leonard George, President

Mission Indian Friendship Centre (MIFC)
33150A - 1st Ave., Mission BC V2V 1G4
Tel: 604-826-1281; *Fax:* 604-826-4956
www.mifcs.bc.ca/programs.html
www.facebook.com/missionfriendshipcentresociety
Overview: A small local charitable organization founded in 1973
Mission: To provide acceptable assistance & services to the community, without prejudice from an aboriginal perspective
Affliation(s): all First Nations organizations

Nawican Friendship Centre
1320 - 102 Ave., Dawson Creek BC V1G 2C6
Tel: 250-782-5202; *Fax:* 250-782-8411
e-mail: community@nawican.ca
Overview: A small local organization founded in 1971

Pacific Association of First Nations' Women
2017 Dundas St., Vancouver BC V5L 1J5
Tel: 604-872-1849; *Fax:* 604-872-1845
pafnw.ca
Also Known As: Pacific Association of First Nations' Women
Previous Name: Association of First Nations' Women; West Coast Professional Native Women's Association
Overview: A small local organization founded in 1981
Mission: To assist Aboriginal women & their families with health, education & social services issues
Member of: Council of Aboriginal Women of BC
Affliation(s): Vancouver Aboriginal Council
Chief Officer(s):
Joy Chalmers, Contact, Community Homecare Services Program
joy_bc@hotmail.com

Positive Living North: No kheyoh t'sih'en t'sehena Society (PLN)
#1, 1563 - 2nd Ave., Prince George BC V2L 3B8
Tel: 250-562-1172; *Fax:* 250-562-3317
Toll-Free: 888-438-2437
www.positivelivingnorth.ca
www.facebook.com/103410213083441
Previous Name: Prince George AIDS Prevention Program; AIDS Prince George; Prince George AIDS Society

Overview: A small local organization founded in 1992 overseen by Canadian AIDS Society
Mission: To provide services to people live with HIV & their families; 75 per cent of PLN's clients are of Aboriginal descent
Chief Officer(s):
Vanessa West, Executive Director
Publications:
• Common Threads [a publication of Positive Living North]
Type: Newsletter; *Frequency:* Quarterly

Prince George Native Friendship Centre
1600 - 3rd Ave., Prince George BC V2L 3G6
Tel: 250-564-3568; *Fax:* 250-563-0924
e-mail: info@pgnfc.com
www.pgnfc.com
Overview: A small local organization founded in 1969
Mission: To serve the needs of Aboriginal people residing in the urban area; To improve the quality of life in the community as a whole
Chief Officer(s):
Emma Palmantier, President
Joan Sutherland, Treasurer

Quesnel Tillicum Society Friendship Centre
319 North Fraser Dr., Quesnel BC V2J 1Y9
Tel: 250-992-8347; *Fax:* 250-992-5708
www.quesnel-friendship.org
www.facebook.com/QuesnelTillicum
twitter.com/QuesnelTillicum
Overview: A small local charitable organization founded in 1971
Mission: To improve the quality of life & to meet the needs of First Nations & other people who are faced with adjusting to the social, economic & cultural lifestyle of the community
Member of: National Association of Friendship Centres
Chief Officer(s):
Tony Goulet, Executive Director
tony.goulet@qnfc.bc.ca

Tansi Friendship Centre Society
PO Box 418, 5301 South Access Rd., Chetwynd BC V0C 1J0
Tel: 250-788-2996; *Fax:* 250-788-2353
e-mail: reception@tansifcs.com
www.facebook.com/groups/181117091978465
Overview: A small local organization overseen by Food Banks British Columbia
Member of: Food Banks British Columbia

Tillicum Lelum Aboriginal Friendship Centre
774B Centre St., Nanaimo BC V9R 4Z6
Tel: 250-753-4417; *Fax:* 250-753-8122
www.tillicumlelum.ca
Overview: A small local organization
Mission: To provide programs & services designed to improve the quality of life for Aboriginal people
Chief Officer(s):
Grace Elliott-Nielsen, Executive Director

Vancouver Aboriginal Friendship Centre Society (VAFCS)
1607 East Hastings St., Vancouver BC V5L 1S7
Tel: 604-251-4844; *Fax:* 604-251-1986
e-mail: info@vafcs.org
www.vafcs.org
www.facebook.com/354262331330400
Overview: A small local charitable organization founded in 1963
Mission: To assist Aboriginal people making a transition to the urban community by providing social, cultural & recreational programs & services
Chief Officer(s):
John Webster, Chair

Victoria Native Friendship Centre (VNFC)
231 Regina Ave., Victoria BC V8Z 1J6
Tel: 250-384-3211; *Fax:* 250-384-1586
www.vnfc.ca
www.facebook.com/150790278331058
twitter.com/VNFCTWEET
Overview: A small local organization founded in 1969
Mission: To meet the needs of Native people in the greater Victoria area by providing them with services & information designed to enhance their traditional values

Member of: United Way; Association of Aboriginal Post-Secondary Institutions
Chief Officer(s):
Bruce Parisian, Executive Director

MANITOBA

Brandon Friendship Centre
836 Lorne Ave., Brandon MB R7A 0T8
Tel: 204-727-1407; Fax: 204-726-0902
e-mail: bfcinc@mts.net
Overview: A small local charitable organization
Mission: To provide services to the community with an emphasis on Aboriginal culture.

Dauphin Friendship Centre (DFC)
210 - 1st Ave. NE, Dauphin MB R7N 1A7
Tel: 204-638-5707; Fax: 204-638-4799
e-mail: dfcexec@mts.net
www.dauphinfriendshipcentre.com
www.facebook.com/DauphinFriendshipCenter
Overview: A small local charitable organization founded in 1974
Mission: To enhance the quality of life for Aboriginal and Non-Aboriginal people in the community by working together to provide services and programs to meet the needs of its membership and community.
Affliation(s): Manitoba Association of Friendship Centres; National Association of Friendship Centres

Elbert Chartrand Friendship Centre
PO Box 1448, 1413 Main St. East, Swan River MB R0L 1Z0
Tel: 204-734-9301; Fax: 204-734-3090
Overview: A small local organization
Mission: To promote continuous public relations aimed at creating and developing mutual understanding and to improve relations between people of Indian descent and others

Flin Flon Aboriginal Friendship Association Inc.
57 Church St., Flin Flon MB R8A 1K8
Tel: 204-687-3900
e-mail: p.e.c@mymts.net
flinflonfriendshipcentre.ca
Previous Name: Flin Flon Indian & Metis Friendship Centre; Flin Flon Indian-Metis Friendship Association Inc.
Overview: A small local organization founded in 1966
Mission: To encourage active participation of Aboriginal people in Canadian society, promoting awareness of Aboriginal cultural; to provide culturally sensitive programs & services to members of the community.

Indian & Metis Friendship Centre of Winnipeg Inc. (IMFC)
45 Robinson St., Winnipeg MB R2W 5H5
Tel: 204-586-8441; Fax: 204-582-8261
imfcentre.net
twitter.com/IMFC_BINGO
Overview: A small local organization founded in 1959
Chief Officer(s):
Jim Sinclair, Executive Director

Lynn Lake Friendship Centre
625 Gordon Ave., Lynn Lake MB R0B 0W0
Tel: 204-356-2407
Overview: A small local organization
Mission: Provides programs and services to meet the needs of the Aboriginal and Non Aboriginal people in Lynn Lake and surrounding area.

Ma-Mow-We-Tak Friendship Centre Inc. / The Gathering Place
4 Nelson Rd., Thompson MB R8N 0B4
Tel: 204-677-0950
www.mamowwetak.com
Overview: A small local organization founded in 1976
Mission: To support Aboriginal people making the transition from life on the reserve or isolated communities to urban life in Thompson, Manitoba; To operate as a non-sectarian, non-political, non-profit, charitable organization, geared to meeting the needs of Aboriginal people in Thompson and the surrounding area
Chief Officer(s):
Anita Campbell, Executive Director

The Pas Friendship Centre Inc.
PO Box 2638, The Pas MB R9A 1M3
Tel: 204-627-7500; Fax: 204-623-4268
e-mail: tpfc@mts.net
Overview: A small local organization
Chief Officer(s):
Ron Chief, Executive Director

Portage Friendship Centre Inc. (PFC)
20 - 3rd St. NE, Portage la Prairie MB R1N 1N4
Tel: 204-239-6333; Fax: 204-856-2470
e-mail: info@ptgfc.org
www.ptgfc.org
www.facebook.com/PortageFriendshipCentre
Previous Name: Portage La Prairie Friendship Centre
Overview: A small local organization founded in 1966
Chief Officer(s):
Jacqueline Stasiuk, President
Shirley Bernard, Executive Director
s_bernard@ptgfc.org

Riverton & District Friendship Centre
PO Box 359, 53 Laura Ave., Riverton MB R0C 2R0
Tel: 204-378-2800; Fax: 204-378-5705
e-mail: rdfc@mymts.net
www.rivertonfc.com
Overview: A small local charitable organization founded in 1981
Mission: To provide a meeting place for individuals & community groups of different cultures; To create fellowship between the native members of the Riverton area
Member of: Manitoba Association of Friendship Centres
Affliation(s): National Association of Friendship Centres; National Aboriginal Health Organization
Chief Officer(s):
Tanis Grimolfson, Executive Director

Selkirk Friendship Centre (SFC)
425 Eveline St., Selkirk MB R1A 2J5
Tel: 204-482-7525; Fax: 204-785-8124
www.facebook.com/144548738915132
Overview: A small local organization founded in 1968
Mission: Promotes the progress in the educational, social, ecomonic, social, athletic & cultural life of both Aboriginal & Non-Aboriginal peoples

NEWFOUNDLAND AND LABRADOR

Labrador Friendship Centre
PO Box 767, Stn. B, 49 Grenfell St., Happy Valley-Goose Bay NL A0P 1E0
Tel: 709-896-8302; Fax: 709-896-8731
www.lfchvgb.ca
Overview: A small local organization
Mission: To meet the needs of Aboriginal people in Labrador through the provision of programs & services
Chief Officer(s):
Jennifer Hefler-Elson, Executive Director
jhefler-elson@lfchvgb.ca

St. John's Native Friendship Centre
716 Water St., St. John's NL A1E 1C1
Tel: 709-726-5902; Fax: 709-722-0874
www.sjnfc.com
twitter.com/St_Johns_NFC
Overview: A small local organization
Mission: To provide programs & services for Aboriginal people
Member of: National Association of Friendship Centres
Chief Officer(s):
Christopher Sheppard, Executive Director

NORTHWEST TERRITORIES

Soaring Eagle Friendship Centre
PO Box 396, #2, 8 Gagnier St., Hay River NT X0E 1G1
Tel: 867-874-6581; Fax: 867-874-3362
e-mail: soaringeaglefc@northwestel.net
www.facebook.com/SoaringEagleFriendshipCentre
Overview: A small local organization

Zhahti Koe Friendship Centre
PO Box 209, Fort Providence NT X0E 0L0
Tel: 867-699-3801; *Fax:* 867-699-4355
Overview: A small local organization

NOVA SCOTIA

Healing Our Nations (HON)
31 Gloster Ct., Dartmouth NS B3B 1X9
Tel: 902-492-4255
e-mail: ea@accesswave.ca
www.hon93.ca
www.facebook.com/Healing.Our.Nations
Also Known As: Atlantic First Nations AIDS Task Force
Overview: A small local organization founded in 1991 overseen by Canadian AIDS Society
Mission: To educate First Nation people about HIV/AIDS; to improve the community by elimiating family violence, substance abuse, mental & spiritual malaise leading to depression & suicide.
Member of: Canadian HIV/AIDS Legal Network
Affiliation(s): Union of NS Indians; Union of NB Indians; Atlantic Policy Congress; Mawiw Council; Confederacy of Mainland Mi'Kmaq
Chief Officer(s):
Julie Thomas, Program Manager

Mi'kmaq Native Friendship Centre
2158 Gottingen St., Halifax NS B3K 3B4
Tel: 902-420-1576; *Fax:* 902-423-6130
www.mymnfc.com
www.facebook.com/121366117945828
Overview: A small local charitable organization founded in 1973 overseen by National Association of Friendship Centres
Mission: To promote the educational & cultural advancement of native people in & about the Halifax/Dartmouth area; to assist people of native descent who have newly arrived in the area to settle in; to strive to create & improve mutual understanding between people of native descent & others.
Chief Officer(s):
Tony Thomas, Chair

NUNAVUT

Pulaarvik Kablu Friendship Centre
PO Box 429, Rankin Inlet NU X0C 0G0
Tel: 867-645-2600; *Fax:* 867-645-2538
e-mail: recept_pkfcmain@qiniq.com
www.pulaarvik.ca
Previous Name: Sappujijijit Friendship Centre
Overview: A small local organization founded in 1973
Member of: National Association of Friendship Centres
Chief Officer(s):
Marianne Taparti, Chair
George Dunkerley, Executive Director

ONTARIO

Atikokan Native Friendship Centre (ANFC)
PO Box 1510, #307, 309 Main St., Atikokan ON P0T 1C0
Tel: 807-597-1213; *Fax:* 807-597-1473
atikokaninfo.com/business/atikokan-native-friendship-centre
Overview: A small local charitable organization founded in 1983
Mission: To serve as a meeting place for urban, Aboriginal people and also community members regardless of nationality; to provide an Aboriginal Family Support program for families with children up to 6 years old (includes parent relief/ mom/dads & tots, prenatal and postnatal support); to provide health outreach services, healing & wellness services, family violence initiatives, crisis intervention services, seniors care support services, cultural events, educational assistance, food bank, resource library, community support &d assistance for newcomers & community referral services.
Member of: Ontario Federation of Indian Friendship Centres
Chief Officer(s):
Sarah Laurich, Contact
sarahlaurich@gmail.com

Barrie Native Friendship Centre (BNFC)
175 Bayfield St., Barrie ON L4M 3B4
Tel: 705-721-7689; *Fax:* 705-721-7418
Overview: A small local charitable organization founded in 1987

Mission: To promote social activities, community awareness, culture-language, information/resources, employment/education/staffing, children's programs; to assist urban Natives; to work in cooperation with non-Native community
Member of: Ontario Federation of Indian Friendship Centres
Chief Officer(s):
Samantha Kinoshameg, Executive Director
executivedirector@bnfc.ca

CanAm Indian Friendship Centre of Windsor (CAIFC)
2929 Howard Ave., Windsor ON N8X 4W4
Tel: 519-253-3243; *Fax:* 519-253-7876
e-mail: admin@caifc.ca
www.caifc.ca
Overview: A small local charitable organization founded in 1981
Mission: To advocate on behalf of Aboriginal people in Windsor; To improve the quality of life of community members
Affliation(s): Ontario Federation of Indian Friendship Centres

Dryden Native Friendship Centre (DNFC)
74 Queen St., Dryden ON P8N 1A4
Tel: 807-223-4180; *Fax:* 807-223-6275
e-mail: dnfc@drytel.net
www.ofifc.org/centre/dryden-native-friendship-centre
www.facebook.com/Apatisiwin
Overview: A small local organization founded in 1984
Member of: Ontario Federation of Indian Friendship Centres

Fort Erie Native Friendship Centre
796 Buffalo Rd., Fort Erie ON L2A 5H2
Tel: 905-871-8931
e-mail: reception@fenfc.org
www.fenfc.org
www.facebook.com/FortErieNFC
Overview: A small local organization
Mission: To enhance all aspects of Native life through such programs as day care services & the distribution of business attire & advice to those seeking employment.

Georgian Bay Native Friendship Centre (GBNFC)
175 Yonge St., Midland ON L4R 2A7
Tel: 705-526-5589; *Fax:* 705-526-7662
e-mail: gbnfc@gbnfc.com
www.gbnfc.com
Overview: A small local charitable organization founded in 1984
Mission: To provide youth activities & programs, to create opportunities for them to have a voice & participate in the community.
Member of: Ontario Federation of Indian Friendship Centres
Chief Officer(s):
Compton Khan, Executive Director
edirector@gbnfc.com

Indian Friendship Centre in Sault Ste Marie
122 East St., Sault Ste Marie ON P6A 3C7
Tel: 705-256-5634; *Fax:* 705-942-3227
e-mail: info@ssmifc.ca
www.ssmifc.com
www.facebook.com/ssm.ifc
twitter.com/ssmifc
Overview: A small local organization founded in 1972
Mission: To provide a comprehensive range of social programs to improve the overall well-being of its community; to nurture Indian self-expression & leadership, & it encourages the study of Indian needs, the planning of services from both public & private agencies.
2nd location: 29 Welington St., East, Sault Ste. Marie.
Member of: Ontario Federation of Indian Friendship Centres
Affiliation(s): National Association of Friendship Centres
Chief Officer(s):
Cathy Syrette, Executive Director
director@ssmifc.ca

Ininew Friendship Centre
PO Box 1499, 190 - 3rd Ave., Cochrane ON P0L 1C0
Tel: 705-272-4497; *Fax:* 705-272-3597
e-mail: reception@ininewfriendshipcentre.ca
www.ininewfriendshipcentre.ca
www.facebook.com/pages/ininew-friendship-centre/115600240820
Overview: A small local organization

Mission: To improve the quality of life for everyone in the community by offering a wide variety of programs, covering health management, social work, sports & other communal activities.
Chief Officer(s):
Desmond O'Connor, President
  president@ininewfriendshipcentre.ca
Jack Solomon, Executive Director
  executive@ininewfriendshipcentre.ca

James Bay Association for Community Living
PO Box 460, #18, 4 St., Moosonee ON P0L 1Y0
                  Tel: 705-336-2378; *Fax:* 705-336-2694
                  www.jbacl.org
Previous Name: Moosonee-Moose Factory Association for Community Living
Overview: A small local charitable organization
Mission: To address the residential requirements of individuals with developmental disabilities; To integrate developmentally disabled people into their home communities; To work towards supported employment & independent living (area covers west coast of James Bay) so that all persons live in a state of dignity, share in all elements of living in the community & have the opportunity to participate effectively
Member of: Community Living Ontario
Chief Officer(s):
Weena Saunders, President
Mark Storey, Executive Director
  mark.storey@jbacl.org

Kapuskasing Friendship Centre (KFC)
41 Murdock St., Kapuskasing ON P5N 1H9
                  Tel: 705-337-1935; *Fax:* 705-335-6789
                  e-mail: kifc@ntl.sympatico.ca
           www.ofifc.org/centre/kapuskasing-friendship-centre
Previous Name: Kapuskasing Indian Friendship Centre
Overview: A small local organization founded in 1985
Mission: To help improve the lives of the Aboriginal community in the Kapuskasing area through participation in Canadian society which values Native culture
Member of: Ontario Federation of Indian Friendship Centres

Moosonee Native Friendship Centre
PO Box 478, Moosonee ON P0L 1Y0
                  Tel: 705-336-2808; *Fax:* 705-336-2929
                  www.onlink.net/~mcap
Overview: A small local organization founded in 1982
Mission: To assist the Aboriginal population of Moosonee with establishing a better quality of life, spiritually, culturally, socially & economically
Member of: Ontario Federation of Indian Friendship Centres

N'Amerind (London) Friendship Centre
260 Colbourne St., London ON N6B 2S6
                  Tel: 519-672-0131; *Fax:* 519-672-0717
                  www.namerind.on.ca
                  www.facebook.com/namerindfc
Overview: A small local organization founded in 1967
Mission: To promote the intellectual, spiritual & physical well being of Native people, with a focus on Urban Natives
Member of: Ontario Federation of Indian Friendship Centres
Chief Officer(s):
Donna Phillips, President
Al Day, Executive Director
  aday@namerind.on.ca

N'swakamok Native Friendship Centre
110 Elm St., Sudbury ON P3C 1T5
                  Tel: 705-674-2128; *Fax:* 705-671-3539
                  e-mail: nnfcadmin@on.aibn.com
                  www.nfcsudbury.org
Overview: A small local organization founded in 1967
Mission: To provide social programs & services to the Native population
Chief Officer(s):
Marie Meawasige, Executive Director

Native Child & Family Services of Toronto (NCFST)
30 College St., Toronto ON M5G 1K2
                  Tel: 416-969-8510; *Fax:* 416-928-0706
  Other Communication: After Hours Emergency Service: 416-924-4646
                  e-mail: info@nativechild.org
                  www.nativechild.org
                  twitter.com/ncfst
Overview: A medium-sized local charitable organization founded in 1986
Mission: To provide caring, well-being, quality of life, & healing to children in need in Toronto's Native community
Chief Officer(s):
Kenn Richard, Executive Director

Ne'Chee Friendship Centre
PO Box 241, 1301 Railway St., Kenora ON P9N 3X3
                  Tel: 807-468-5440; *Fax:* 807-468-5340
                  e-mail: reception@nechee.org
                  www.nechee.org
Overview: A small local charitable organization founded in 1976
Member of: Ontario Federation of Indian Friendship Centres; National Association of Friendship Centres
Chief Officer(s):
Patti Fairfield, Executive Director
  aces@nechee.org

Nishnawbe - Gamik Friendship Centre
52 King St., Sioux Lookout ON P8T 1B8
                  Tel: 807-737-1909; *Fax:* 807-737-1805
                  Toll-Free: 800-619-9519
                  e-mail: ches@ngfc.net
                  www.ngfc.net
Overview: A small local organization founded in 1971
Mission: To provide a meeting place for people of Aboriginal ancestry & others in the Sioux Lookout, Ontario region to exchange ideas & to develop mutual understanding & appreciation; To advance native language & culture
Member of: Ontario Federation of Indian Friendship Centres
Chief Officer(s):
Che September, Exeuctive Director
Kelly Anderson, President

North Bay Indian Friendship Centre (NBIFC)
980 Cassells St., North Bay ON P1B 4A6
                  Tel: 705-472-2811
                  e-mail: info@nbifc.org
                  www.nbifc.org
                  www.facebook.com/197057837005772
Overview: A small local organization founded in 1974
Mission: To improve the quality of life for First Nation, Metis, & Inuit people in North Bay, Ontario
Member of: Ontario Federation of Indian Friendship Centres

Odawa Native Friendship Centre
250 City Centre Ave., Ottawa ON K1R 6K7
                  Tel: 613-722-3811; *Fax:* 613-722-4667
                  e-mail: info@odawa.on.ca
                  www.odawa.on.ca
                  www.facebook.com/Odawa.Friendship
Overview: A small local charitable organization
Affliation(s): Ontario Federation of Indian Friendship Centres
Chief Officer(s):
Neal Freeland, President
  president@odawa.on.ca
Morgan Hare, Executive Director, 613-722-3811 Ext. 246
  executive.director@odawa.on.ca

Parry Sound Friendship Centre
13 Bowes St., Parry Sound ON P2A 2K7
                  Tel: 705-746-5970; *Fax:* 705-746-2612
             e-mail: postmaster@parrysoundfriendshipcentre.com
                  www.parrysoundfriendshipcentre.com
Overview: A medium-sized local organization founded in 1966
Member of: National Association of Friendship Centres; Ontario Federation of Indian Friendship Centres
Chief Officer(s):
Gail Hall, Executive Director

Red Lake Indian Friendship Centre (RLIFC)
PO Box 244, Red Lake ON P0V 2M0
Tel: 807-727-2847; *Fax:* 807-727-3253
www.rlifc.ca
Previous Name: District Indian Youth Club
Overview: A small local charitable organization founded in 1964
Mission: To provide a gathering place for the Aboriginal community in the Red Lake, Ontario region; To promote economic development for Aboriginal people
Member of: Ontario Federation of Indian Friendship Centres

Thunder Bay Indian Friendship Centre (TBIFC)
401 North Cumberland St., Thunder Bay ON P7A 4P7
Tel: 807-345-5840; *Fax:* 807-344-8945
e-mail: TBIFC@shawcable.com
www.tbifc.ca
Overview: A small local organization founded in 1964
Mission: To serve as a meeting place for the Native community in Thunder Bay, Ontario; To address issues that affect the lives of Native people
Member of: Ontario Federation of Indian Friendship Centres
Chief Officer(s):
Debbie Sault, President
Whitney Knott, Secretary
Audrey Fisher, Treasurer

Thunderbird Friendship Centre
PO Box 430, 301 Beamish Ave. West, Geraldton ON P0T 1M0
Tel: 807-854-1060; *Fax:* 807-854-0861
Toll-Free: 888-854-1060
e-mail: reception@thunderbirdfriendshipcentre.ca
Overview: A small local organization founded in 1971
Mission: To provide a meeting place for the Aboriginal & non-Aboriginal people of the Geraldton, Ontario area
Member of: Ontario Federation of Indian Friendship Centres
Chief Officer(s):
Karen Stephenson, Executive Director
karen.stephenson@thunderbirdfriendshipcentre.ca

Timmins Native Friendship Centre
179 Kirby Ave., Timmins ON P4N 1K1
Tel: 705-268-6262; *Fax:* 705-268-6266
e-mail: reception@tnfc.ca
www.tnfc.ca
www.facebook.com/TimminsNativeFriendshipCentre
Overview: A small local organization
Mission: To provide a culturally sensitive, helpful environment for Aboriginal & non-Aboriginal people in Timmins, Ontario; To improve the quality of life for Aboriginal & non-Aboriginal people in the Timmins community
Member of: Ontario Federation of Indian Friendship Centres
Chief Officer(s):
Veronica Nicholson, Executive Director
vnicholson@tnfc.ca
Roseanne Ross, Director, Finance

United Native Friendship Centre (UNFC)
PO Box 752, Fort Frances ON P9A 3N1
Tel: 807-274-8541; *Fax:* 807-274-4110
Toll-Free: 877-496-9034
Other Communication: Aboriginal Headstart Phone: 807-274-7244
e-mail: inquiry@unfc.org
www.unfc.org
Overview: A small local charitable organization founded in 1973
Mission: To enhance the lives of Native & non-Native peoples; to serve Aboriginal people with special services in the fields of social, educational, & cultural development while at the same time building a bridge of understanding between Native & non-Native people
Member of: Ontario Federation of Indian Friendship Centres
Chief Officer(s):
Sheila McMahon, Executive Director
smcmahon@unfc.org
Publications:
• UNFC [United Native Friendship Centre] Newsletter
Type: Newsletter
Profile: Features centre updates & event dates

Circle of Life Centre

616 Mowat Ave., Fort Frances ON P9A 3N1

QUÉBEC

Native Friendship Centre of Montréal Inc. (NFCM) / Centre d'amitié autochtone de Montréal Inc.
2001 St. Laurent Blvd., Montréal QC H2X 2T3
Tel: 514-499-1854; *Fax:* 514-499-9436
Toll-Free: 855-499-1854
e-mail: info@nfcm.org
www.nfcm.org
Overview: A medium-sized local charitable organization founded in 1974
Mission: To promote, develop & enhance the quality of life of the urban Aboriginal community of Montréal
Member of: National Association of Friendship Centres
Chief Officer(s):
Brett W. Pineau, Executive Director

SASKATCHEWAN

Battlefords Indian & Métis Friendship Centre
960 - 103 St., North Battleford SK S9A 1K2
Tel: 306-445-8216
e-mail: nbimfc@sasktel.net
www.afcs.ca/battleford-friendship-centre.html
www.facebook.com/366725376804735
Also Known As: Battlefords Friendship Centre
Overview: A small local charitable organization founded in 1969
Member of: Aboriginal Friendship Centres of Saskatchewan

Buffalo Narrows Friendship Centre
PO Box 189, 351 Buffalo St., Buffalo Narrows SK S0M 0J0
Tel: 306-235-4633; *Fax:* 306-235-4544
e-mail: bnfc@sasktel.net
www.afcs.ca/buffalo-narrows.html
Overview: A small local organization
Chief Officer(s):
Brenda Chartier, Executive Director

Ile-a-la-Crosse Friendship Centre Inc.
PO Box 160, Lajeunesse Ave., Ile-a-la-Crosse SK S0M 1C0
Tel: 306-833-2313; *Fax:* 306-833-2216
e-mail: ilx.friendctr.inc@sasktel.net
ilealacrossefc.weebly.com
www.facebook.com/4925553507971
Overview: A small local organization founded in 1980
Mission: The Centre provides referrals, information, social, cultural, health awareness & sports & recreational programs to help ensure a better quality of life for the community & area.
Member of: Aboriginal Friendship Centres of Saskatchewan; National Association of Friendship Centres
Chief Officer(s):
Myra Malboeuf, Executive Director

Indian & Metis Friendship Centre of Prince Albert (IMFCPA)
1409 - 1st Ave. East, Prince Albert SK S6V 1G2
Tel: 306-764-3431; *Fax:* 306-763-3205
e-mail: paimfc.reception@sasktel.net
www.facebook.com/IMFCPA
Previous Name: Prince Albert Indian & Métis Friendship Centre
Overview: A small local organization founded in 1963
Mission: To promote understanding, cooperation, & trust; To recognize the social, cultural, & recreational needs of aboriginal people in Prince Albert & the surrounding area
Affliation(s): Aboriginal Friendship Centres of Saskatchewan
Chief Officer(s):
Connie Farber, Executive Director
Publications:
• Prince Albert Indian & Métis Friendship Centre Newsletter
Type: Newsletter; *Frequency:* Monthly

Kikinahk Friendship Centre
PO Box 254, 320 Boardman St., La Ronge SK S0J 1L0
Tel: 306-425-2051
www.facebook.com/141174299305567
Previous Name: Neginuk Friendship Centre
Overview: A small local organization founded in 1977
Mission: To provide a cultural centre for Indian, Métis & non-status Indian persons

Chief Officer(s):
Ron Woytowich, Executive Director

Lloydminster Native Friendship Centre (LNFC)
PO Box 1364, 4602 - 49 Ave., Lloydminster SK S9V 1K4
Tel: 306-825-6558; *Fax:* 306-825-6565
e-mail: reception@LNFC.org
www.lnfc.org

Overview: A small local charitable organization founded in 1982 overseen by Alberta Native Friendship Centres Association
Mission: To provide services to residents from SK & AB, within an approximate 11 km radius; to promote better understanding & relations between the different cultures within our community; to develop wellness, education, cultural & social programs & activities for children & their families; to promote the well-being & enhancement of quality of life for all people within the community through partnership with community & government agencies; to seek avenues of financial security to ensure viable & sustainable operation
Member of: Alberta Native Friendship Centres Association
Chief Officer(s):
Audrey Parke, President & Secretary
Bonnie Start, Executive Director

Moose Mountain Friendship Centre
PO Box 207, 112 Main St., Carlyle SK S0M OJO
Tel: 306-453-2425; *Fax:* 306-453-6777
Overview: A small local organization

Qu'Appelle Valley Friendship Centre (QVFC)
PO Box 240, Fort Qu'Appelle SK S0G 1S0
Tel: 306-332-5616; *Fax:* 306-332-5091
e-mail: admin@qvfc.ca
www.qvfc.ca

Overview: A small local charitable organization founded in 1980
Mission: To provide support & direct services to the Aboriginal community; To strive to bridge the gap between Aboriginial people & society at large, through assisting in the process of social interaction, sharing of cultures & the educating of harmonious working relationships between all communities & cultures
Affiliation(s): Friendship Centres of Saskatachewant; National Friendship Centre
Chief Officer(s):
Rob Donison, Executive Director
rdonison@qvfc.ca

Saskatoon Indian & Métis Friendship Centre
168 Wall St., Saskatoon SK S7K 1N4
Tel: 306-244-0174; *Fax:* 306-664-2536
e-mail: reception_SIMFC@shaw.ca
www.simfc.ca
www.facebook.com/groups/SIMFCUpcomingEvents
Overview: A small local organization
Mission: To improve the quality of life for Aboriginal people in the City of Saskatoon.
Member of: Charities; donations; corporate sponsorship; government
Chief Officer(s):
Bill Mintram, Executive Director

Yorkton Friendship Centre
139 Dominion Ave., Yorkton SK S3N 1S3
Tel: 306-782-2822; *Fax:* 306-782-6662
Overview: A small local organization

YUKON TERRITORY

Skookum Jim Friendship Centre
3159 - 3rd Ave., Whitehorse YT Y1A 1G1
Tel: 867-633-7680; *Fax:* 867-668-4460
e-mail: sjfcfriends@northwestel.net
www.skookumjim.com
www.facebook.com/skookumjimfriendshipcentre
vimeo.com/user5226474
Overview: A small local organization founded in 1962 overseen by National Association of Friendship Centres
Mission: Committed to a vision of bettering the spiritual, emotional, mental & physical well being of First Nations peoples, fostering the way of Friendship & understanding between people
Chief Officer(s):
Marney Paradis, Executive Director, 867-633-7687
sjfcexecutive@northwestel.net

National Libraries

First Nations & Inuit Health Branch (Health Canada)
Tunney's Pasture, 200 Eglantine Driveway, Ottawa, ON K1A 0K9
Fax: 613-952-5770
Toll-Free: 866-225-0709
TTY: 800-465-773
www.hc-sc.gc.ca/fniah-spnia/pubs/index-eng.php

Health Canada/ Santé Canada
70 Colombine Driveway, Ottawa, ON K1A 0K9
Tel: 613-957-2991; *Fax:* 613-941-5366
Toll-Free: 866-225-0709
info@hc-sc.gc.ca
www.hc-sc.gc.ca

Profile: The library serves the information needs of employees at Health Canada & the Public Health Agency of Canada. The print collection is located in closed stacks at the National Research Council's facility in Ottawa, & access is administered by Infotrieve Canada Inc. **Collection:** Print materials; extensive electronic collections of ejournals, ebooks, & databases (available by intranet only)
Lynda Gamble, Portfolio Manager
Kathryn Jackson, Portfolio Manager

Pauktuutit Inuit Women of Canada
#520, 1 Nicholas St., Ottawa, ON K1N 7B7
Tel: 613-238-3977; *Fax:* 613-238-1787
Toll-Free: 800-667-0749
info@pauktuutit.ca
www.pauktuutit.ca
Social Media: www.youtube.com/pauktuutit; twitter.com/Pauktuutit; www.facebook.com/pauktuutit
Tracy O'Hearn, Executive Director
tohearn@pauktuutit.ca
Irina Appa, Executive Assistant
iappa@pauktuutit.ca

Provincial Libraries

BC Aboriginal Network on Disability Society
1179 Kosapsum Cres., Victoria, BC V9A 7K7
Tel: 250-381-7303; *Fax:* 250-381-7312
Toll-Free: 888-815-5511
bcands@bcands.bc.ca
www.bcands.bc.ca
Neil Belanger, Executive Director
exdir@bcands.bc.ca

Healing Our Nations
31 Gloster Ct., Dartmouth, NS B3B 1X9
Tel: 902-492-4255
ea@accesswave.ca
www.hon93.ca

National Government

Health Canada / Santé Canada
Tunney's Pasture, Ottawa, ON K1A 0K9
Tel: 613-957-2991
Fax: 613-941-5366
Toll-Free: 866-225-0709
TTY: 800-465-7735
info@hc-sc.gc.ca
www.hc-sc.gc.ca
Other Communication: Information on Medical Marijuana:
1-866-337-7705; omc-bcm@hc-sc.gc.ca
twitter.com/healthcanada
www.facebook.com/HealthyCdns
www.youtube.com/user/healthcanada
In partnership with provincial & territorial governments, Health Canada (HC) develops health policy, enforces health regulations, promotes disease prevention, & enhances healthy living for all Canadians. HC ensures that health services are available & accessible to First Nations & Inuit communities. It works closely with other federal departments, agencies & health stakeholders to reduce health & safety risks to Canadians. Through its Health Intelligence Network, HC works with other levels of government & the health care system in the surveillance,

prevention, control & research of disease outbreaks across Canada & around the world. It also monitors health & safety risks related to the sale & use of drugs, food, chemicals, pesticides, medical devices & certain consumer products. HC negotiates agreements regarding hazardous materials in the workplace, performs medical assessments for pilots & air traffic controllers, & conducts environmental health assessments. As of April 1, 2013, Health Canada assumed the responsibilities & functions under the Hazardous Materials Information Review Act, formerly carried out by the Hazardous Materials Information Review Commission.

Minister, Health, Hon. Jane Philpott, P.C.
Tel: 613-992-3640
Fax: 613-992-3642
Jane.Philpott@parl.gc.ca

Deputy Minister, Simon Kennedy
Tel: 613-957-0212

Director, Parliamentary Affairs, Peter Cleary
Tel: 613-957-0200

Director, Communications, David Clements
Tel: 613-957-0200

Director, Policy, Caroline Pitfield
Tel: 613-957-0200

Press Secretary, Andrew MacKendrick
Tel: 613-957-0200

Departmental Liaison (PHAC & CIHR), Marianne DeVito
Tel: 613-957-0200

First Nations & Inuit Health Branch (FNIHB) / Direction générale de la santé des Premières nations et des Inuits (DGSPNI)

Assists First Nations & Inuit communities & people to address health inequalities & diseases threats through health surveillance & population health interventions. Ensures the availability of, or access to, health services for First Nations & Inuit people. Devolves control & management of community-based health services to First Nations & Inuit communities & organizations. The Environmental Health Division addresses conditions in the environment that could affect the health of community members, such as drinking water quality, mould, food safety, facilities inspections, transportation of dangerous goods. The Environmental Research Division conducts, coordinates & funds contaminants-related research, coordinates the replacement or upgrading of diesel-fuel tanks & remediation of fuel oil-contaminated sites, lab services for testing of PCBs & mercury, drinking water-related research & testing.

Senior Assistant Deputy Minister, Sony Perron
Tel: 613-957-7701
Assistant Deputy Minister, Regional Operations, Valerie Gideon
Tel: 613-946-1722
Chief Medical Officer of Health & Executive Director, Population & Public Health, Tom Wong
Tel: 613-952-9616
Director General, Non-Insured Health Benefits Directorate, Scott Doidge
Tel: 613-954-8825
Director General, Strategic Policy, Planning & Information, Mary-Luisa Kapelus
Tel: 613-954-2445
Director General, Delivery, Active Response & Coordination, Aruna Sadana
Tel: 613-954-0765
Director General, Branch, Anthony Sangster
Tel: 613-818-1243
Executive Director, Primary Health Care, Robin Buckland
Tel: 613-957-6359
Executive Director, Operational Services & Systems Division, Jean Pruneau
Tel: 613-960-3656
Executive Director, Internal Client Services Directorate, Susan Russell
Tel: 613-952-3151

Acting Executive Director, Policy & Partnerships, Tasha Stefanis
Tel: 613-941-1606
Director, Environmental Public Health Division, Ivy Chan
Tel: 613-948-7773
Director, Primary Health Care Systems, Leila Gillis
Tel: 613-952-7492
Director, Communicable Disease Control, Erin E. Henry
Tel: 613-957-1151
Director, Home, Community & Preventative Care Division, Jacques Néron
Tel: 613-948-5445

Local Hospitals & Health Centres

ALBERTA

CALGARY: Sunrise Native Addictions Services Society
Affiliated with: Alberta Health Services
Former Name: Native Addictions Services
Also Known As: SUNRISE
1231 - 34 Ave. NE, Calgary, AB T2E 6N4
Tel: 403-261-7921 *Fax:* 403-261-7945
nasgeneral@nass.ca
www.nass.ca

Year Founded: 1974
Number of Beds: 36
Area Served: Calgary & area
Number of Employees: 32
Note: Offers 12-step & Aboriginal-based addiction programming. Only treatment centre in Calgary that uses Aboriginal Spiritual Teachings as a core part of the program. Serves people 18 & over, of all nationalities.
Leslie Big Bull, Director, Operations
403-261-7921, lbigbull@nass.ca
Bryan Flack, Program Director
403-261-7921, bflack@nass.ca
Deborah Axworthy, Manager, Administration
403-261-7921, daxworthy@nass.ca

EDMONTON: Poundmaker's Lodge Treatment Centres (PMLTC)
Affiliated with: Alberta Health Services
PO Box 34007 Stn. Kingsway Mall, Edmonton, AB T5G 3G4
Tel: 780-458-1884 *Fax:* 780-459-1876
Toll-Free: 866-458-1884
info@poundmaker.org
www.poundmakerslodge.ca
Social Media: www.facebook.com/poundmakers.lodge;
twitter.com/pmltc14

Year Founded: 1973
Number of Beds: 64 beds
Number of Employees: 58
Specialties: Alcohol & drug treatment
Note: Aboriginal addiction treatment centre near Edmonton, Alberta. Provides holistic addiction treatment using concepts based in traditional First Nations, Metis, & Inuit beliefs as well as 12-step, abstinence based recovery. Serves adults aged 18 years & over from all walks of life.
Lacey Kaskamin, Coordinator, Community Engagement
780-458-1884, lacey-kaskamin@poundmaker.org
Linden Jessome, Executive Assistant
780-458-1884, linden-jessome@poundmaker.org
Darlene Marchuk, Clinical Manager
780-458-1884, darlene-marchuk@poundmaker.org

MANITOBA

WINNIPEG: Aboriginal Health & Wellness Centre
Affiliated with: Winnipeg Regional Health Authority
#215, 181 Higgins Ave., Winnipeg, MB R3B 3G1
Tel: 204-925-3700 *Fax:* 204-925-3709
www.wrha.mb.ca

Note: Programs & services include: traditional medicine; diabetes education; children's health; & health promotion.
Holly MacLean, Director, Wellness

WINNIPEG: Native Addictions Council of Manitoba (NACM)
Affiliated with: Winnipeg Regional Health Authority
160 Salter St., Winnipeg, MB R2W 4K1

Tel: 204-586-8395 *Fax:* 204-589-3921
www.nacm.ca

Year Founded: 1971
Note: Provides holistic treatment of addictions

QUÉBEC

WEMOTACI: Conseil de la Nation Atikamekw
Wemotaci, QC G0X 3R0

Tél: 819-523-6153 *Téléc:* 819-523-8706

Nombre de lits: 9
Constant Awashish, Président

Sports for the Disabled

National Associations

Achilles Canada
119 Snowden Ave., Toronto ON M4N 2A8

Tel: 416-485-6451; *Fax:* 416-485-0823
www.achillescanada.ca

Previous Name: Achilles Track Club Canada
Overview: A medium-sized national charitable organization founded in 1999
Mission: To encourage & assist all persons with disabilities (visual disability, cerebral palsy, paraplegia, arthritis, epilepsy, multiple sclerosis, amputation, cystic fibrosis, stroke, cancer, traumatic head injury, & many others) to enjoy running for health in a social environment
Chief Officer(s):
Brian McLean, Contact
bmclean@achillescanada.ca

Canadian Amputee Golf Association (CAGA)
PO Box 6091, Stn. A, Calgary AB T2H 2L4

e-mail: canamps@caga.ca
www.caga.ca

Overview: A small national organization founded in 2000
Mission: To provide support for amputees both before & after amputation; To raise awareness to the general population on the effects of amputation; To offer rehabilitation, through teaching amputees golf; To run amputee golf tournaments
Chief Officer(s):
Gwen Davies, President

Canadian Amputee Sports Association (CASA) / Association canadienne des sports pour amputés
Toronto ON

www.canadianamputeesports.ca
Overview: A medium-sized national charitable organization founded in 1977
Mission: To promote & organize amateur sport competitions in Canada for persons who are without a limb or part of a limb; To promote research in prosthetic devices for sport activities; To select a Canadian national team for participation in international sports events for amputees
Affliation(s): Canadian Paralympic Committee; Hockey Canada

Canadian Association for Disabled Skiing (CADS) / Association canadienne pour les skieurs handicapés (ACSH)
791 Strathcona Dr. SW, Calgary AB T3H 1N8

Tel: 587-315-5870; *Fax:* 866-531-9644
disabledskiing.ca
Overview: A medium-sized national charitable organization founded in 1976
Mission: To assist individuals with a disability to participate in recreational & competitive snow skiing & snowboarding
Chief Officer(s):
Maureen O'Hara-Leman, Executive Director
executive.director@disabledskiing.ca
Publications:
• The Perspective: CADS National Newsletter
Type: Newsletter; *Editor:* Karen Elliott
Profile: Reports from the Canadian Association for Disabled Skiing, plus programming & forthcoming events

Canadian Deaf Curling Association (CDCA) / Association de Curling des Sourdes du Canada
Vancouver BC

Tel: 604-734-2250; *Fax:* 604-734-2254; *TTY:* 250-539-3264
www.deafcurlcanada.org
Also Known As: Deaf Curl Canada
Overview: A small national organization overseen by Canadian Deaf Sports Association
Mission: To provide deaf & hard of hearing curlers with opportunities across Canada
Member of: Canadian Deaf Sports Association; Canadian Curling Association
Affliation(s): British Columbia Deaf Sports Federation; Alberta Deaf Curling Association; Saskatchewan Deaf Sports Association; Manitoba Deaf Curling Association; Ontario Deaf Curling Assocation; Association de Curling des Sourds du Quebec; Nova Scotia Deaf Curling Association
Chief Officer(s):
Bradford Bentley, President
president@deafcurlcanada.org
Allard Thomas, Vice-President
Susanne Beriault, Secretary
cdca-secretary@gmail.com
David Pickard, Treasurer
dpickard@telus.net
Dean Sutton, Chief Technical Director
curlingtd@shaw.ca

Canadian Deaf Golf Association (CDGA) / Association Canadienne de Golf des Sourds
#20, 51 Sholto Drive, London ON N6G 2E9

cdga1993.wixsite.com/cdga
Overview: A small national organization overseen by Canadian Deaf Sports Association
Mission: To aid in the development of leadership & golfing skills among deaf golfers across Canada
Member of: Canadian Deaf Sports Association
Chief Officer(s):
Dana McCarthy, President
cdgapresident@gmail.com
Peter Mitchell, Vice-President
pmitchell25@rogers.com
Paul Landry, Secretary
pauljlandry@shaw.ca
Adam Redmond, Treasurer
cdgatreasurer@gmail.com
Aurele Bourgeois, Director
abourgeois10@cogeco.ca

Canadian Electric Wheelchair Hockey Association (CEWHA)
#920, 200 Yorkland Blvd., Toronto ON M2J 5C1

Tel: 416-757-8544; *Fax:* 416-490-9334
e-mail: info@cewha.ca
www.cewha.ca
www.facebook.com/cewha
twitter.com/canadianewha
www.youtube.com/cewhanational
Overview: A small national charitable organization founded in 1980
Mission: To provide a hockey program for persons with disabilities who have limited upper body strength & mobility
Chief Officer(s):
John Blackburn, Executive Director

Canadian Paralympic Committee (CPC) / Comité paralympique canadien
#100, 85 Plymouth St., Ottawa ON K1S 3E2

Tel: 613-569-4333; *Fax:* 613-569-2777
www.paralympic.ca
www.facebook.com/CDNParalympics
twitter.com/CDNParalympics
www.youtube.com/user/CDNParalympics
Previous Name: Canadian Federation of Sport Organizations for the Disabled
Overview: A medium-sized national charitable organization founded in 1982
Mission: To support disabled athletes through the establishment of a sustainable Paralymic sport system; To inspire all disabled Canadians

to participate in sports
Affliation(s): International Paralympic Committee
Chief Officer(s):
Karen O'Neill, Chief Executive Officer, 613-569-4333 Ext. 223
koneill@paralympic.ca
Gaétan Tardif, President
Laurie Cairns, Executive Director, Corporate Services
lcairns@paralympic.ca
François Robert, Executive Director, Partnerships
frobert@paralympic.ca
Martin Richard, Executive Director, Communications & Marketing
mrichard@paralympic.ca
Catherine Gosselin-Després, Executive Director, Sport
cgosselin-despres@paralympic.ca

Canadian Society for Psychomotor Learning & Sport Psychology (CSPLSP) / Société canadienne d'apprentissage psychomoteur et de psychologie du sport (SCAPPS)
#360, 125 University Private, Ottawa ON K1N 6N5
www.scapps.org

Overview: A small national organization founded in 1977
Mission: To promote the study of motor development, motor learning, motor control, & sport psychology
Chief Officer(s):
Chris Shields, President
Erin Cressman, Secretary, Communications
Publications:
• Journal of Exercise, Movement, and Sport [a publication of the Canadian Society for Psychomotor Learning & Sport Psychology]
Type: Journal; *Editor:* Joel Barnes

Canadian Therapeutic Riding Association / Association canadienne d'équitation thérapeutique
5420 Hwy. 6 North, RR#5, Guelph ON N1H 6J2
Tel: 519-767-0700; *Fax:* 519-767-0435
e-mail: ctra@golden.net
www.cantra.ca
twitter.com/CanTRA_ACET

Also Known As: CanTRA
Overview: A large national charitable organization founded in 1980
Mission: To foster therapeutic riding for persons with disabilities by establishing riding standards in collaboration with the medical profession; To accredit programs, certify instructors & promote research; To promote equestan sport & competition for persons with disabilities
Member of: Riding for Disabled International; Canadian Paralympic Committee; Canadian Equestrian Federation
Chief Officer(s):
Eliane Trempe, President
Publications:
• CanTRA [Canadian Therapeutic Riding Association] Caller / L'Appel ACET
Type: Newsletter; *Frequency:* q.; *Price:* free with membership
Profile: CanTRA conferences, articles, events, bylaws changes, & clinics
• Communiqué [a publication of the Canadian Therapeutic Riding Association]
Type: Newsletter; *Price:* free with membership
Profile: Information for CanTRA members, published between CanTRA Caller newsletters

Canadian Wheelchair Basketball Association (CWBA) / Association canadienne de basketball en fauteuil roulant (ACBFR)
#8, 6 Antares Dr., Phase 1, Ottawa ON K2E 8A9
Tel: 613-260-1296; *Fax:* 613-260-1456
Toll-Free: 877-843-2922
e-mail: info@wheelchairbasketball.ca
www.wheelchairbasketball.ca
www.facebook.com/wheelchairbasketball
twitter.com/WCBballCanada
www.youtube.com/WheelchairBball
Also Known As: Wheelchair Basketball Canada
Overview: A medium-sized national charitable organization founded in 1994
Mission: To act as the governing body for wheelchair basketball in Canada
Member of: Canadian Paralympic Committee; International Wheelchair

Basketball Federation
Affliation(s): Canada Basketball
Chief Officer(s):
Wendy Gittens, Executive Director
wgittens@wheelchairbasketball.ca
Jeff Dunbrack, Director, High Performance
jdunbrack@wheelchairbasketball.ca
Courtney Pollock, Manager, Communications & Marketing
cpollock@wheelchairbasketball.ca
Ryan Lauzon, Coordinator, Programs
rlauzon@wheelchairbasketball.ca
Lindsay Crone, Coordinator, Communications
lcrone@wheelchairbasketball.ca
Cori Droogh, Coordinator, Special Projects
cdroogh@wheelchairbasketball.ca
Publications:
• Around The Rim [a publication of the Canadian Wheelchair Basketball Association]
Type: Newsletter
• CWBA [Canadian Wheelchair Basketball Association] Annual Report
Type: Yearbook; *Frequency:* Annually

Canadian Wheelchair Sports Association (CWSA) / Association canadienne des sports en fauteuil roulant (ACSFR)
#108, 2255 St. Laurent Blvd., Ottawa ON K1G 4K3
Tel: 613-523-0004; *Fax:* 613-523-0149
e-mail: info@cwsa.ca
www.cwsa.ca
www.facebook.com/wheelchairrugbycanada
twitter.com/wcrugbycanada
www.youtube.com/wheelsportscanada
Overview: A large national charitable organization founded in 1967
Mission: To promote excellence & develop opportunities for Canadians in wheelchair sport
Affliation(s): International Stoke Mandeville Wheelchair Sports Federation
Chief Officer(s):
Donald Royer, President
Cathy Cadieux, Executive Director
ccadieux@cwsa.ca
Duncan Campbell, Director, National Development, 604-333-3539, Fax: 604-333-3450
duncancampbell@cwsa.ca
Andy Van Neutegem, Director, High Performance, Fax: 250-220-2501
andy@cwsa.ca
Nancy Wong, Program Coordinator, 604-333-3539, Fax: 604-333-3450
nancywong@cwsa.ca
Marnie McRoberts, Lead Medical Officer, 416-529-7731
marnie@cwsa.ca

Special Olympics Canada (SOC) / Olympiques spéciaux Canada
#600, 21 St. Clair Ave. East, Toronto ON M4T 1L9
Tel: 416-927-9050; *Fax:* 416-927-8475
Toll-Free: 888-888-0608
e-mail: info@specialolympics.ca
www.specialolympics.ca
www.facebook.com/SpecialOCanada
twitter.com/SpecialOCanada
www.youtube.com/specialocanada
Previous Name: Canadian Special Olympics Inc.
Overview: A large national organization founded in 1969
Mission: To provide sport training & competition for people with an intellectual disability, at local, regional, provincial, national & international levels, year round
Affliation(s): Special Olympics International; The Order of United Commercial Travelers of America; The Sandbox Project
Chief Officer(s):
Sharon Bollenbach, Chief Executive Officer, 416-927-9050 Ext. 4389
sbollenbach@specialolympics.ca

Provincial Associations

ALBERTA

Alberta Amputee Sports & Recreation Association (AASRA)
PO Box 86093, Stn. Marda Loop, Calgary AB T2T 6B7
Tel: 403-201-0507
e-mail: info@aasra.ab.ca
www.aasra.ab.ca
www.facebook.com/495810413773520
Overview: A small provincial charitable organization founded in 1977
Mission: To support & provide opportunities for amputees in recreational & sporting activities, in events for both the disabled & able-bodied; To provide moral support to new amputees & family
Chief Officer(s):
Rachael Pasay, President

Alberta Cerebral Palsy Sport Association (ACPSA)
Percy Page Centre, 11759 Groat Rd., Edmonton AB T5M 3K6
Tel: 780-422-2904; *Fax:* 780-422-2663
e-mail: contact@acpsa.ca
www.acpsa.ca
www.facebook.com/165504436855126
twitter.com/AlbertaCPSports
instagram.com/powerchair_sports
Also Known As: Sportability Alberta
Overview: A small provincial charitable organization founded in 1984 overseen by Canadian Cerebral Palsy Sports Association
Mission: To promote recreational & competitive sporting opportunities for persons with cerebral palsy, brain injury & related conditions
Member of: Canadian Cerebral Palsy Sports Association

Alberta Deaf Sports Association (ADSA)
#205, 11404 - 142 St., Edmonton AB T5M 1V1
e-mail: info@albertadeafsports.ca
www.albertadeafsports.ca
www.facebook.com/AlbertaDeafSports
Also Known As: Federation of Silent Sports of Alberta
Overview: A medium-sized provincial charitable organization founded in 1974 overseen by Canadian Deaf Sports Association
Mission: To coordinate sport & recreation activities for deaf people in Alberta; To promote competition at the local, provincial, regional, & national levels; To select Alberta athletes to compete in national championships for the World Games of the Deaf
Member of: Canadian Deaf Sports Association
Chief Officer(s):
Grant Underschultz, President
Brenda Hillcox, Secretary
Publications:
• Alberta Deaf Sports Newsletter
Type: Newsletter
Profile: Highlights of past events & notice of future events

Alberta Northern Lights Wheelchair Basketball Society
Saville Community Sports Centre, #2-209, 11610 - 65 Ave., Edmonton AB T6G 2E1
e-mail: info@albertanorthernlights.com
www.albertanorthernlights.com
www.facebook.com/172864392765380
Overview: A medium-sized provincial charitable organization founded in 1976
Mission: To develop health, fitness, & sport for men, women, & children with physical disabilities
Chief Officer(s):
Neil Feser, Manager, Program

Alberta Therapeutic Recreation Association (ATRA)
8038 Fairmount Dr. SE, Calgary AB T2H 0Y1
Tel: 403-258-2520; *Fax:* 403-255-2234
Toll-Free: 888-258-2520
e-mail: atra@alberta-tr.org
www.alberta-tr.org
Overview: A small provincial organization founded in 1985
Mission: To offer mentorships, continuing education, bursaries, & awards
Chief Officer(s):
Kari Medd, President
president@alberta-tr.org

Canadian Association for Disabled Skiing - Alberta (CADS Alberta)
11759 Groat Rd., Edmonton AB T5M 3K6
Tel: 780-427-8104; *Fax:* 780-422-2663
e-mail: info@cadsalberta.ca
www.cadsalberta.ca
www.facebook.com/CADSAB
twitter.com/CADSAlberta
Overview: A small provincial charitable organization founded in 1961 overseen by Canadian Association for Disabled Skiing
Mission: CADS Alberta is a volunteer-based organization assisting individuals with a disability to lead fuller lives through active participation in recreational & competitive snow skiing & snowboarding. It is a registered charity, BN: 133967406RR0001.
Member of: Canadian Association for Disabled Skiing
Affliation(s): Canadian Ski Instructors' Alliance (CSIA), Canadian Association of Snowboard Instructors (CASI)
Chief Officer(s):
Edward Shaw, President
president@cadsalberta.ca
Sharon Veeneman, Executive Coordinator

Calgary Zone
CADS Calgary, Canada Olympic Park, 88 Canada Olympic Rd. SW, Calgary AB T3B 5R5
Tel: 403-286-8050
e-mail: info@cadscalgary.ca
www.cadscalgary.ca
twitter.com/CADSCalgary
Chief Officer(s):
John Bowman, Chair
chair@cadscalgary.ca

Edmonton Zone
CADS Edmonton, PO Box 35073, 10818 Jasper Ave., Edmonton AB T5J 0B7
Tel: 780-669-3856
e-mail: info@cadsedmonton.ca
www.cadsedmonton.ca
www.facebook.com/150695641627414
twitter.com/CADSEdmonton
Chief Officer(s):
Dale Loyer, President

Rocky Mountain Zone
Rocky Mountain Adaptive Sports Centre, #2, 201 Carey, Canmore AB T1W 2R7
Tel: 403-431-1354
e-mail: info@rockymountainadaptive.com
www.rockymountainadaptive.com
Chief Officer(s):
Jamie McCulloch, Executive Director, 403-431-1154
jamie@rockymountainadaptive.com

Paralympic Sports Association (Alberta) (PSA)
#305, 11010 101 St., Edmonton AB T5H 4B9
Tel: 780-439-8687; *Fax:* 780-432-0486
e-mail: info@parasports.net
www.parasports.net
www.linkedin.com/company/paralympic-sports-association
www.facebook.com/PSASports
twitter.com/Sports_PSA
Overview: A medium-sized provincial charitable organization founded in 1965
Mission: To provide sports & recreation programs for people with physical disabilities
Affliation(s): Wheelchair Sports Alberta
Chief Officer(s):
Amy MacKinnon, Executive Director
executivedirector@parasports.net
Amy Hayward, Coordinator, Programs
programs@parasports.net

Special Olympics Alberta (SOA)
Percy Page Centre, 11759 Groat Rd., Edmonton AB T5M 3K6
Tel: 780-415-0719; *Fax:* 780-415-1306
Toll-Free: 800-444-2883
e-mail: info@specialolympics.ab.ca
www.specialolympics.ab.ca
www.facebook.com/specialolympicsalberta
twitter.com/SpecialOAlberta
Previous Name: Alberta Special Olympics Inc.
Overview: A medium-sized provincial charitable organization founded in 1980 overseen by Special Olympics Canada
Mission: To enrich the lives of Albertans with an intellectual disability, through sport
Chief Officer(s):
John Byrne, President & CEO
jbyrne@specialolympics.ab.ca

Wheelchair Sports Alberta
11759 Groat Rd., Edmonton AB T5M 3K6
Tel: 780-427-8699
Toll-Free: 888-453-6770
e-mail: wsa1@telus.net
www.abwheelchairsport.ca
www.facebook.com/WheelchairSportsAlberta
twitter.com/WSA_Alberta
Overview: A small provincial organization
Mission: To develop wheelchair sports throughout Alberta
Member of: Canadian Wheelchair Sports Association
Chief Officer(s):
Sharleen Edwards, Executive Director

BRITISH COLUMBIA

BC Adaptive Snowsports (BCAS)
780 Marine Dr. SW, Vancouver BC V6P 5Y7
Tel: 604-333-3630
e-mail: info@bcadaptive.com
www.bcadaptive.com
linkedin.com/company/the-disabled-skiers-association-of-bc
www.facebook.com/bcadaptive
twitter.com/BC_adaptive
Previous Name: Disabled Skiers Association of BC
Overview: A medium-sized provincial charitable organization founded in 1973 overseen by Canadian Association for Disabled Skiing
Mission: To promote adaptive skiing, snowboarding, & mountain accessbility as a form of rehabiliation for participants with physical disabilities; To contribute to an inclusive & healthy lifestyle for residents of British Columbia
Member of: BC Disability Sports; Canadian Association for Disabled Skiing
Chief Officer(s):
Wayne Leslie, Executive Director, 604-333-3631
wayne@bcadaptive.com

British Columbia Therapeutic Recreation Association (BCTRA)
PO Box 93597, Stn. Nelson Park, Vancouver BC V6E 4L7
Other Communication: membership@bctra.org
e-mail: info@bctra.org
www.bctra.org
Overview: A small provincial organization founded in 1991
Mission: To represent Therapeutic Recreation Professionals & their practice within BC
Chief Officer(s):
Brenda Kinch, President
president@bctra.org

British Columbia Therapeutic Riding Association (BCTRA)
3885B - 96th St., Delta BC V4K 3N3
Tel: 604-590-0897
e-mail: ponypalstra@yahoo.ca
www.vcn.bc.ca/bctra
Overview: A small provincial charitable organization founded in 1986
Mission: To adhance the quality of life of people with disabilities
Member of: Canadian Therapeutic Riding Association; Horse Council of British Columbia
Affliation(s): Horse Council BC; Sports & Fitness Council for the Disabled
Chief Officer(s):
Candice Miller, President

British Columbia Wheelchair Sports Association (BCWSA)
780 Southwest Marine Dr., Vancouver BC V6P 5Y7
Tel: 604-333-3520; *Fax:* 604-333-3450
Toll-Free: 877-737-3090
e-mail: info@bcwheelchairsports.com
www.bcwheelchairsports.com
www.facebook.com/BCWSA
twitter.com/BCWSA
www.youtube.com/user/BCWheelchairSports
Overview: A medium-sized provincial charitable organization
Mission: To promote & develop wheelchair sport opportunities for British Columbians who identify with physical disabilities
Member of: Canadian Wheelchair Sports Association
Chief Officer(s):
Gail Hamamoto, Executive Director, 604-333-3520 Ext. 201
gail@bcwheelchairsports.com

Disabled Sailing Association of BC (DSA)
#318, 425 Carrall St., Vancouver BC V6B 6E3
Tel: 604-688-6464; *Fax:* 604-688-6463
e-mail: dsa@disabilityfoundation.org
www.disabledsailingbc.org
www.facebook.com/DisabledSailingAssociation
twitter.com/DisabilityFdn
Overview: A small provincial charitable organization founded in 1989
Mission: To help people with disabilities live independent lives
Affliation(s): BC Sport & Fitness Council for the Disabled; Sam Sullivan Disability Foundation

Special Olympics BC (SOBC)
#210, 3701 East Hastings St., Burnaby BC V5C 2H6
Tel: 604-737-3078; *Fax:* 604-737-3080
Toll-Free: 888-854-2276
e-mail: info@specialolympics.bc.ca
www.specialolympics.bc.ca
www.facebook.com/specialolympicsbc
twitter.com/sobcsociety
Previous Name: British Columbia Special Olympics
Overview: A medium-sized provincial charitable organization founded in 1980 overseen by Special Olympics Canada
Mission: To provide individuals with intellectual disabilities the opportunity to participate in sporting events at the regional, provincial, national, or international levels
Member of: Special Olympics Canada
Affliation(s): Special Olympics International
Chief Officer(s):
Dan Howe, President & CEO, 604-737-3079
dhowe@specialolympics.bc.ca
Christina Hadley, Vice-President, Fund Development & Communications
chadley@specialolympics.bc.ca
Lois McNary, Vice-President, Sport
lmcnary@specialolympics.bc.ca
Josh Pasnak, Manager, Finance & Administration
jpasnak@specialolympics.bc.ca
Lauren Openshaw, Office Administrator
lopenshaw@specialolympics.bc.ca

Victoria
PO Box 31121, Stn. University Heights, Victoria BC V8N 6J3
Tel: 250-213-5467
www.victoriaspecialolympics.com
Chief Officer(s):
Kim Perkins, Coordinator, Public Relations
kim@kimperkins.ca
Kristina D'Sa, Secretary
specialo.kristinadsa@gmail.com

MANITOBA

Manitoba Cerebral Palsy Sports Association (MCPSA)
MB
Overview: A small provincial organization overseen by Canadian Cerebral Palsy Sports Association
Mission: To assist in the development of sport for the disabled in Manitoba by providing an opportunity for a wider participation for persons with cerebral palsy & other neuromuscular disorders
Member of: Canadian Cerebral Palsy Sports Association

Manitoba Deaf Sports Association Inc. (MDSA)
c/o Sport Manitoba, 145 Pacific Ave., Winnipeg MB R3B 2Z6
www.mdsaassoc.com
Overview: A small provincial organization overseen by Canadian Deaf
Sports Association
Mission: To provide sporting opportunities for deaf people in Manitoba
Member of: Canadian Deaf Sports Association
Chief Officer(s):
Brenda Comte, President
 mdsapresident72@gmail.com
Shawna Joynt, Vice-President
Kenneth Anderson, Treasurer
Joseph Comte, Technical Director

Manitoba Riding for the Disabled Association Inc. (MRDA)
145 Pacific Ave., Winnipeg MB R3B 2Z6
Tel: 204-925-5905; *Fax:* 204-925-5792
e-mail: exedir@mrda.cc
www.mrda.cc
www.facebook.com/105010909544565
Overview: A small provincial charitable organization founded in 1977
Mission: To provide a therapeutic horseback riding program for
children with disabilities.
Member of: Canadian Therapeutic Riding Association
Chief Officer(s):
Peter Manastyrsky, Executive Director

Manitoba Wheelchair Sports Association
145 Pacific Ave., Winnipeg MB R3B 2Z6
Tel: 204-925-5790; *Fax:* 204-925-5792
e-mail: mwsa@sportmanitoba.ca
www.mwsa.ca
www.facebook.com/manitobawheelchairsports
Overview: A small provincial organization founded in 1962
Mission: Committed to leadership in the promotion of well being and a
healthy lifestyle through the development of sport and fitness related
opportunities for physically disabled Manitobans.
Member of: Canadian Wheelchair Sports Association
Chief Officer(s):
Samuel Unrau, Interim Executive Director

Special Olympics Manitoba (SOM)
#304, 145 Pacific Ave., Winnipeg MB R3B 2Z6
Tel: 204-925-5628; *Fax:* 204-925-5635
Toll-Free: 888-333-9179
e-mail: som@specialolympics.mb.ca
www.specialolympics.mb.ca
www.facebook.com/SpecOManitoba
twitter.com/SpecOManitoba
www.instagram.com/specomanitoba
Previous Name: Manitoba Special Olympics
Overview: A small provincial charitable organization founded in 1980
overseen by Special Olympics Canada
Mission: To enrich the lives of Manitobans with an intellectual
disability, through active participation in sport
Member of: Special Olympics Inc.
Chief Officer(s):
Jennifer Campbell, President & CEO, 204-925-5632
 jcampbell@specialolympics.mb.ca

NEW BRUNSWICK

Canadian Association for Disabled Skiing - New Brunswick
c/o Lloyd Gagnon, 59 rue Carrier, Edmundston NB E3V EY2
Tel: 506-739-9662
Overview: A medium-sized provincial charitable organization overseen
by Canadian Association for Disabled Skiing
Mission: To provide skiing opportunities for individuals with disabilities
Member of: Canadian Association for Disabled Skiing
Chief Officer(s):
Lloyd Gagnon, President
 lloyd@disabledskiing.ca
Jim Bowland, Technical Coordinator
 jimbowland.cadsnb@nb.sympatico.ca

Special Olympics New Brunswick
#103, 411 St. Mary's St., Fredericton NB E3B 8H4
Tel: 506-455-0404; *Fax:* 506-455-0410
e-mail: infosonb@specialolympics.ca
www.specialolympicsnb.ca
www.facebook.com/specialolympicsnb
twitter.com/specialonb
Previous Name: New Brunswick Special Olympics
Overview: A small provincial charitable organization founded in 1979
overseen by Special Olympics Canada
Mission: To offer athletic programs to people with intellectual
disabilites in New Brunswick
Chief Officer(s):
Josh Astle, Executive Director

NEWFOUNDLAND AND LABRADOR

Canadian Association for Disabled Skiing - Newfoundland &
Labrador Division
6 Albany Pl., St. John's NL A1E 1Y2
Tel: 709-753-3625; *Fax:* 709-777-4884
disabledskiing.ca/?page_id=123
Also Known As: CADS Newfoundland/Labrador
Overview: A small provincial organization overseen by Canadian
Association for Disabled Skiing
Member of: Canadian Association for Disabled Skiing
Chief Officer(s):
Marg Tibbo, Representative
 margaret.tibbo@easternhealth.ca

Newfoundland & Labrador Deaf Sports Association (NLDSA)
58 First St., Mount Pearl NL A1N 1Y3
Overview: A small provincial organization overseen by Canadian Deaf
Sports Association
Mission: To govern fitness, amateur sports & recreation for deaf
people in Newfoundland & Labrador
Member of: Canadian Deaf Sports Association
Chief Officer(s):
Bryan Johnson, Acting President
 bryan.johnson@nf.sympatico.ca

Special Olympics Newfoundland & Labrador
87 Elizabeth Ave., St. John's NL A1B 1R6
Tel: 709-738-1923; *Fax:* 709-738-0119
Toll-Free: 877-738-1913
e-mail: sonl@sonl.ca
www.sonl.ca
www.facebook.com/TeamSONL
twitter.com/SpecialONL
Previous Name: Newfoundland-Labrador Special Olympics
Overview: A small provincial charitable organization founded in 1986
overseen by Special Olympics Canada
Mission: To provide sport, fitness & recreation programs for individuals
with an intellectual disability
Chief Officer(s):
Trish Williams, Executive Director
 trishw@sonl.ca

Wheelchair Sports Association of Newfoundland & Labrador
(WSANL)
NL
Overview: A small provincial organization
Member of: Canadian Wheelchair Sports Association

NORTHWEST TERRITORIES

Special Olympics Northwest Territories (SONWT)
PO Box 1691, Yellowknife NT X1A 2N1
Tel: 867-446-2873
www.sonwt.ca
Previous Name: Northwest Territories Special Olympics
Overview: A small provincial organization founded in 1989 overseen
by Special Olympics Canada
Mission: Special Olympics N.W.T. is the territorial sport governing
body responsible for the delivery of sport for people with intellectual
disabilities in the Northwest Territories.
Member of: Sport North; Special Olympics Canada
Chief Officer(s):
Lynn Elkin, Executive Director
 lynn@sonwt.ca

NOVA SCOTIA

Canadian Association for Disabled Skiing - Nova Scotia
c/o Alpine Ski Nova Scotia, 5516 Spring Garden Rd., 4th Fl., Halifax
NS B3J 1G6

Tel: 902-425-5450; *Fax:* 902-425-5606
e-mail: alpinens@sportnovascotia.ca
disabledskiing.ca/provincial-programs/nova-scotia
Also Known As: CADS Nova Scotia
Overview: A medium-sized provincial organization overseen by
Canadian Association for Disabled Skiing
Member of: Alpine Canada Alpin; Canadian Association for Disabled
Skiing
Chief Officer(s):
Lorraine Burch, Executive Director

Nova Scotia Deaf Sports Association (NSDSA)
5516 Spring Garden Rd., 4th Fl., Halifax NS B3J 1G6
Overview: A small provincial organization overseen by Canadian Deaf
Sports Association
Mission: To govern fitness, amateur sports & recreation for deaf
people in Nova Scotia.
Member of: Canadian Deaf Sports Association
Chief Officer(s):
Matt Ayyash, President

Nova Scotia Recreation Professionals in Health (NSRPH)
c/o MacGillivray Guest Home, 25 Xavier Dr., Sydney NS B1S 2R9
Tel: 902-539-6110; *Fax:* 902-567-0437
www.nsrph.com
www.facebook.com/NSRPH
Overview: A small provincial organization founded in 1994
Mission: To allow for recreation professionals to communicate,
network, & share concerns & ideas; To advocate for the necessity &
benefits of recreation in the health care system
Chief Officer(s):
Shelly Luddington, President
shelly.luddington@theadmiralltc.com
Dawn MacDonald, Vice-President, Communications
Dawn.MacDonald@nscc.ca

Special Olympics Nova Scotia (SONS)
#201, 5516 Spring Garden Rd., Halifax NS B3J 1G6
Tel: 902-429-2266; *Fax:* 902-425-5606
Toll-Free: 866-299-2019
www.sons.ca
www.facebook.com/SpecialONS
twitter.com/SpecialONS
instagram.com/SpecialONS
Previous Name: Nova Scotia Special Olympics
Overview: A small provincial charitable organization founded in 1978
overseen by Special Olympics Canada
Mission: Special Olympics is a non-profit organization dedicated to
providing year-round sports training and athletic competition in a variety
of Olympic-type sports for children and adults with an intellectual
disability.
Chief Officer(s):
Mike Greek, President & CEO
greekmr@sportnovascotia.ca

ONTARIO

**Canadian Association for Disabled Skiing - National Capital
Division (CADS-NCD)**
1216 Bordeau Grove, Ottawa ON K1C 2M7

Tel: 819-827-4378
www.cads-ncd.ca
Overview: A medium-sized provincial charitable organization overseen
by Canadian Association for Disabled Skiing
Mission: To provide disabled individuals with skiing opportunities
Member of: Canadian Association for Disabled Skiing
Chief Officer(s):
Bernie Simpson, President
berniesimpson@outlook.com

Canadian Association for Disabled Skiing - Ontario
145 Dew St., King City ON L7B 1L1

Tel: 647-280-1307
www.disabledskiingontario.com
www.facebook.com/cads.ontario
twitter.com/cads_ontario
www.flickr.com/photos/cadsontario
Also Known As: CADS Ontario
Overview: A medium-sized provincial organization overseen by
Canadian Association for Disabled Skiing
Mission: To provide a skiing program for people with disabilities
Member of: Canadian Association for Disabled Skiing
Chief Officer(s):
Gwen Binsfeld, President

Ontario Amputee & Les Autres Sports Association (OALASA)
c/o Rodney Reimer, 15 Tanner Dr., London ON N5W 6B4

oalasa.webs.com
Previous Name: Ontario Amputee Sports Association
Overview: A small provincial organization founded in 1976
Member of: Sport for Disabled Ontario; Canadian Amputee Sports
Association
Chief Officer(s):
Rodney Reimer, President, 519-659-7452
rodreimer@rogers.com

Ontario Cerebral Palsy Sports Association (OCPSA)
PO Box 60082, Ottawa ON K1T 0K9
Tel: 613-723-1806; *Fax:* 613-723-6742
Toll-Free: 866-286-2772
ocpsa.com
Overview: A small provincial organization overseen by Canadian
Cerebral Palsy Sports Association
Mission: To provide, promote & coordinate competitive opportunities
for persons with with cerebral palsy & other neuromuscular disorders in
Ontario.
Member of: Canadian Cerebral Palsy Sports Association
Affliation(s): Canadian Sport Institute - Ontario; Coaches Association
of Ontario; ParaSport Ontario
Chief Officer(s):
Don Sinclair, President

**Ontario Therapeutic Riding Association (OnTRA) / Association
ontarienne d'équitation thérapeutique**
47 Fairlane Rd., London ON N6K 3E3

e-mail: president@ontra.ca
www.ontra.ca
Overview: A small provincial charitable organization founded in 1983
Mission: The Ontario Therapeutic Riding Association (OnTRA)
promotes horseback riding as a form of therapy and sport for children
and adults living with physical, cognitive, emotional, and/or behavioural
challenges. OnTRA provides volunteers and therapeutic riding
professionals with on-going information and training to ensure riders
with disabilities receive the best possible therapy.
Member of: Canadian Therapeutic Riding Association; Ontario
Equestrian Federation

Ontario Track 3 Ski Association for the Disabled
#4, 61 Advance Rd., Toronto ON M8Z 2S6
Tel: 416-233-3872; *Fax:* 416-233-7862
Toll-Free: 877-308-7225
e-mail: track3@track3.org
www.track3.org
www.facebook.com/OntarioTrack3
twitter.com/OntarioTrack3
Also Known As: Track 3
Overview: A small provincial charitable organization founded in 1972
Mission: To discover ability through the magic of snow sports.
Chief Officer(s):
Naomi Schafler, Executive Director
Publications:
• On Track
Type: Newsletter; *Frequency:* Quarterly; *Accepts Advertising*

Ontario Wheelchair Sports Association (OWSA)
#101, 100 Sunrise Ave., Toronto ON M4A 1B3
e-mail: info@owsa.ca
www.owsa.ca
www.facebook.com/WheelchairSportsON
twitter.com/WSA_Ontario
Overview: A medium-sized provincial organization founded in 1972
Mission: To provide sporting & recreational opportunities for athletes who compete in wheelchairs
Member of: Canadian Wheelchair Sports Association
Affliation(s): Canadian Wheelchair Sports Association
Chief Officer(s):
Ken Thom, President
kenthom@rogers.com
Laura Wilson, Executive Director
laura@owsa.ca

ParaSport Ontario
#104, 3 Concorde Gate, Toronto ON M3C 3N7
Tel: 416-426-7187; *Fax:* 416-426-7361
Toll-Free: 800-265-1539
e-mail: info@parasportontario.ca
www.parasportontario.ca
twitter.com/parasport_ont
www.instagram.com/parasportontario
Previous Name: Sport for Disabled - Ontario; Paralympics Ontario
Overview: A medium-sized provincial charitable organization founded in 1981
Mission: To provide leadership, resources, & opportunities to ensure a strong community for disabled persons in the Ontario sport & recreation community
Affliation(s): Ontario Amputee & Les Autres Sports Association; Ontario Blind Sports Association; Ontario Cerebral Palsy Sports Association; Ontario Wheelchair Sports Association
Chief Officer(s):
Alan Trivett, Executive Director, 416-426-7186
alan@parasportontario.ca

Special Olympics Ontario (SOO)
#200, 65 Overlea Blvd., Toronto ON M4H 1P1
Tel: 416-447-8326; *Fax:* 416-447-6336
Toll-Free: 888-333-5515
www.specialolympicsontario.com
www.facebook.com/specialolympicsontario
twitter.com/soontario
www.youtube.com/specialolympicson
Previous Name: Ontario Special Olympics
Overview: A medium-sized provincial charitable organization founded in 1979 overseen by Special Olympics Canada
Mission: To provide sports training & competition for people with an intellectual disability through community-based programs
Member of: Special Olympics Canada
Chief Officer(s):
Glenn MacDonell, President & Chief Executive Officer, 416-447-8326 Ext. 225
glennm@specialolympicsontario.com
Linda Ashe, Vice-President, 416-447-8326 Ext. 220
lindaa@specialolympicsontario.com
Willie E, Manager, Accounting Services, 416-447-8326 Ext. 223
williee@specialolympicsontario.com
Lynn Miller, Manager, Marketing Services, 416-447-8326 Ext. 226
lynnm@specialolympicsontario.com
James Noronha, Manager, Program Services, 416-447-8326 Ext. 240
jamesn@specialolympicsontario.com

PRINCE EDWARD ISLAND

ParaSport & Recreation PEI
Royalty Center House Of Sport, #123, 40 Enman Cres., Charlottetown PE C1E 1E6
Tel: 902-368-4540; *Fax:* 902-368-4548
e-mail: info@parasportpei.ca
www.parasportpei.ca
www.facebook.com/141822665843254
twitter.com/ParaSportPEI
Previous Name: Paralympics PEI Inc.
Overview: A small provincial charitable organization founded in 1974

Mission: To ensure the ample provision of sport & recreation opportunities for persons who are physically challenged
Member of: Canadian Blind Sport Association; Canadian Association for Disabled Skiing; Canadian Wheelchair Sports Association
Affliation(s): The JoyRiders Therapeutic Riding Association of PEI Inc.; The Canadian Council of the Blind - Prince County and Queensland Chapters; The Abegweit Club of Summerside; G.E.A.R. (Getting Everyone Accessibly Riding)
Chief Officer(s):
Tracy Stevenson, Executive Director
tracy@parasportpei.ca

Special Olympics Prince Edward Island (SOPEI)
PO Box 822, #240, 40 Enman Cres., Charlottetown PE C1A 7L9
Tel: 902-368-8919
Toll-Free: 800-287-1196
e-mail: sopei@sopei.com
www.sopei.com
www.facebook.com/Specialopei
twitter.com/Specialopei
www.youtube.com/channel/UCqsAGVtPqgIJeQRN_GeNOtw
Previous Name: PEI Special Olympics
Overview: A small provincial charitable organization founded in 1987 overseen by Special Olympics Canada
Mission: To provide sport, recreation & fitness for the intellectually disabled in PEI; To provide competititve opportunities for its members
Chief Officer(s):
Charity Sheehan, Executive Director
csheehan@sopei.com

QUÉBEC

Association québécoise de sports pour paralytiques cérébraux (AQSPC)
4545, av Pierre-de Coubertin, Montréal QC H1V 0B2
Tél: 514-252-3143; *Téléc:* 514-254-1069
www.sportpc.qc.ca
www.facebook.com/189413534433667
Aperçu: *Dimension:* petite; *Envergure:* provinciale surveillé par Canadian Cerebral Palsy Sports Association
Membre de: Canadian Cerebral Palsy Sports Association
Membre(s) du bureau directeur:
José Malo, Directrice générale, 514-252-3143 Ext. 3742
jmalo@sportpc.qc.ca

Jeux Olympiques Spéciaux du Québec Inc. (OSQ) / Québec Special Olympics
#200, 1274, rue Jean-Talon est, Montréal QC H2R 1W3
Tél: 514-843-8778; *Téléc:* 514-843-8223
Ligne sans frais: 877-743-8778
www.olympiquesspeciaux.qc.ca
www.facebook.com/olympiquesspeciauxquebec
twitter.com/athletesOSQ
Aperçu: *Dimension:* petite; *Envergure:* provinciale; fondée en 1981 surveillé par Special Olympics Canada
Mission: Les Olympiques spéciaux, actifs dans plus de 170 pays, ont pour mission d'enrichir, par le sport, la vie des personnes présentant une déficience intellectuelle. Plus de 3.7 millions d'athlètes spéciaux, de tous âges, sont inscrits dans le monde dont plus de 31,000 au Canada et 4,850 aux programmes récréatifs scolaire ou compétitifs offerts dans toutes les régions du Québec. Les 14 sports officiels sont pratiqués à l'intérieur d'un réseau de compétitions annuelles, comptant plus de 80 événements conçus pour tous les niveaux d'habiletés.
Membre de: Special Olympics Canada
Membre(s) du bureau directeur:
Daniel Granger, Président

SASKATCHEWAN

Regina Therapeutic Riding Association (RTRA)
PO Box 474, Regina SK S4P 3A2
Tel: 306-530-0794
e-mail: ReginaTRA@sasktel.net
rtra.ca
www.facebook.com/reginatherapeuticridingassociation
Overview: A small provincial charitable organization founded in 1992
Mission: To provide medically supervised horseback riding lessons for individuals with special needs.
Chief Officer(s):

SECTION III: Appendices

John Van Knoll, Chair

Saskatchewan Ski Association - Skiing for Disabled (SASKI)
1860 Lorne St., Saskatoon SK S4P 2L7

Tel: 306-780-9236; *Fax:* 306-781-6021
www.saski.ca

Also Known As: SASKI - Skiing for Disabled
Overview: A medium-sized provincial organization founded in 1982
overseen by Canadian Association for Disabled Skiing
Mission: To promote all aspects of winter skiing in Saskatchewan,
including alpine, biathlon, cross country & skiing for disabled, & to
provide assistance to clubs & individual athletes, instruction & training,
adaptive equipment, & a resource library
Member of: Canadian Association for Disabled Skiing
Chief Officer(s):
Pat Prokopchuk, Contact
prokr@sasktel.net

Saskatchewan Wheelchair Sports Association (SWSA)
510 Cynthia St., Saskatoon SK S7L 7K7

Tel: 306-975-0824
e-mail: info@swsa.ca
www.swsa.ca
www.facebook.com/182080694193
twitter.com/skwcsports
www.youtube.com/user/SKWheelchairSports

Overview: A small provincial organization founded in 1977
Mission: Dedicated to developing & supporting opportunities for
children, teens & adults with disabilities to participate in the
Association's sport, recreation & leisure time activities to the best of
their abilities.
Member of: Canadian Wheelchair Sports Association

Special Olympics Saskatchewan
353 Broad St., Regina SK S4R 1X2

Tel: 306-780-9247; *Fax:* 306-780-9441
Toll-Free: 888-307-6226
e-mail: sos@specialolympics.sk.ca
www.specialolympics.sk.ca
www.facebook.com/SOSaskatchewan
twitter.com/SpecialOSask
www.youtube.com/user/SpecialOSk

Previous Name: Saskatchewan Special Olympics Society
Overview: A small provincial organization overseen by Special
Olympics Canada
Mission: To enhance the lives of persons with intellectual disabilities
through sport
Chief Officer(s):
Faye Matt, Chief Executive Officer, 306-780-9277
fmatt@specialolympics.sk.ca

YUKON TERRITORY

Special Olympics Yukon (SOY) / Les Jeux Olympiques Spéciaux du Yukon
4061 4th Ave., Whitehorse YT Y1A 1H1

Tel: 867-668-6511; *Fax:* 867-667-4237
e-mail: info@specialolympicsyukon.ca
www.specialolympicsyukon.ca
www.facebook.com/191453284318177
twitter.com/SpecialOYukon

Previous Name: Yukon Special Olympics
Overview: A medium-sized provincial charitable organization founded
in 1981 overseen by Special Olympics Canada
Mission: To provide a full continuum of sport apportunities for
Yukoners with a mental disability
Affliation(s): Special Olympics International
Chief Officer(s):
Serge Michaud, Executive Director
smichaud@specialolympicsyukon.ca
Brettanie Deal-Porter, Program Director
bdealporter@specialolympicsyukon.ca
Sylvia Anderson, Coordinator, Marketing & Development
sanderson@specialolympicsyukon.ca

Local Associations
ALBERTA

Lethbridge Therapeutic Riding Association (LTRA)
RR#8-24-6, Lethbridge AB T1J 4P4

Tel: 403-328-2165; *Fax:* 403-317-0235
e-mail: info@ltra.ca
www.ltra.ca

Also Known As: Rainbow Riding Centre
Overview: A small local charitable organization founded in 1977
Mission: To provide the opportunity for improved physical & emotional
well-being for people of all ages & abilities who participate in
therapeutic, recreational, educational & competitive riding programs at
Rainbow Riding Centre
Member of: Canadian Therapeutic Riding Association
Chief Officer(s):
Rick Austin, Executive Director
raustin@ltra.ca

Little Bits Therapeutic Riding Association
PO Box 29016, Stn. Pleasantview, Edmonton AB T6H 5Z6

Tel: 780-476-1233; *Fax:* 780-476-7252
Other Communication: Volunteering Inquiries, E-mail:
volunteers@littlebits.ca
e-mail: info@littlebits.ca
www.littlebits.ca
www.facebook.com/LittleBitsVolunteers

Overview: A small local charitable organization founded in 1978
Mission: To provide recreational riding programs that have therapeutic
benefits for disabled children & adults in Edmonton & surrounding area.
Physical address: Whitemud Equine Learning Centre Asociation,
12504 Fox Dr. NW, Edmonton, AB T6G 2L6
Member of: Central Canadian Therapeutic Riding Association; North
American Riding for the Handicapped Association
Chief Officer(s):
Linda Rault, Riding Administrator
Publications:
• Little Bits Therapeutic Riding Association e-Newsletter
Type: Newsletter

Mount View Special Riding Association (MVSRA)
PO Box 1637, Didsbury AB T0M 0W0

Tel: 403-335-9146; *Fax:* 403-556-6480
www.mountviewriding.com

Previous Name: Mountview Handicapped Riding Association
Overview: A small local charitable organization founded in 1983
Mission: To provide recreational & therapeutic riding to specially abled
adults & children with mental &/or physical disabilities
Member of: Canadian Therapeutic Riding Association
Chief Officer(s):
Karla Brautigam, President
Karla@asc-mva.ab.ca

Peace Area Riding for the Disabled (PARDS)
8202 - 84 St., Grande Prairie AB T8X 0L6

Tel: 780-538-3211; *Fax:* 780-538-3683
e-mail: info@pards.ca
www.pards.ca

Overview: A small local charitable organization founded in 1984
Mission: To enhance the lives of individuals with disabilities through
"equine assisted therapy"; To promoten physical, emotional, intellectual
& social growth for individuals with disabilities through therapeutic
riding services; To build a community that embraces differences &
supports growth & success for all of its members
Member of: Canadian Therapeutic Riding Association
Chief Officer(s):
Jennifer Douglas, Executive Director

Quest Support Services Inc.
PO Box 1201, Stn. Main, Lethbridge AB T1J 4A4

Tel: 403-381-9515; *Fax:* 403-320-6555
www.questsupport.com
twitter.com/QuestLethbridge

Previous Name: Quest Residential & Support Services
Overview: A small local organization founded in 1993
Mission: To provide services for people with developmental
disabilities, community based agencies
Chief Officer(s):

Michael Tamura, Owner

BRITISH COLUMBIA

Comox Valley Therapeutic Riding Society (CVTRS)
PO Box 3666, Courtenay BC V9N 7P1
Tel: 250-338-1968; *Fax:* 250-338-4137
e-mail: cvtrs@telus.net
www.cvtrs.com

Also Known As: Therapeutic Riding
Overview: A small local charitable organization founded in 1986
Mission: To provide a therapeutic riding program for physically, mentally & emotionally disabled, hearing & visually impaired children & adults
Member of: Canadian Therapeutic Riding Association
Affliation(s): North American Handicapped Riding Association
Chief Officer(s):
Nancy King, Executive Director

Cowichan Therapeutic Riding Association (CRTA)
c/o Providence Farm, 1843 Tzouhalem Rd., Duncan BC V9L 5L6
Tel: 250-746-1028; *Fax:* 250-746-1033
e-mail: info@ctra.ca
www.ctra.ca
www.facebook.com/cowichantherapeuticridingassociation
instagram.com/cowichantherapeuticriding
Overview: A small local charitable organization founded in 1985
Mission: To use horses to help persons with various disabilities in the Cowichan area of British Columbia achieve physical & mental health, behavioral, communication, cognitive, & social goals; To provide therapeutic or sporting activities in a safe environment with qualified instruction in order to improve the quality of life for persons with disabilities
Publications:
• The Leading Rein
Type: Newsletter; *Accepts Advertising*
Profile: Updates from the association, including a calendar of events, & information on upcoming riding programs

Errington Therapeutic Riding Association (ETRA)
Pyramid Stables, PO Box 462, 7581 Harby Rd., Lantzville, Parksville BC V9P 2G6
e-mail: etrainfo@shaw.ca
www.etra.ca
www.facebook.com/ETRAPledgeRide2016
Overview: A small local organization founded in 1989
Mission: ETRA is an independent, non-profit association that gives people with disabilities the chance to ride a horse, to improve their physical and/or mental well-being, & enhance their sense of achievement & self-worth.
Member of: CanTRA; B.C. Therapeutic Riding Association
Affliation(s): BC Therapeutic Riding Association; Canadian Therapeutic Riding Association
Chief Officer(s):
Regine Eder, President
regine.eder@shaw.ca

Pacific Riding for Developing Abilities (PRDA)
1088 - 208 St., Langley BC V2Z 1T4
Tel: 604-530-8717; *Fax:* 604-530-8617
www.prda.ca
www.facebook.com/PRDALangley
Previous Name: Pacific Riding for Disabled Association
Overview: A small local charitable organization founded in 1973
Mission: To enhance the quality of life for people with a range of disabilities, providing therapeutic equestrian activities & educational opportunities.
Member of: Canadian Therapeutic Riding Association; Langley Chamber of Commerce; North American Riding for the Handicapped Association
Affliation(s): Ishtar Transition Housing Society; Burnaby Association for Community Inclusion
Chief Officer(s):
Michelle Ingall, Executive Director

Chilliwack Branch
47240 Greenhill Rd., Chilliwack BC V2R 4T2
Tel: 604-858-2149

Vancouver Branch

c/o Southlands Riding Club, 7025 Macdonald St., Vancouver BC V6N 1G2
Tel: 604-263-4817; *Fax:* 604-263-1281

Victoria Therapeutic Riding Association (VTRA)
PO Box 412, Brentwood Bay BC V8M 1R3
Tel: 778-426-0506
vtra.ca
www.facebook.com/VictoriaTherapeuticRidingAssociation
twitter.com/VicTherapeutic
instagram.com/victherapeutic
Previous Name: Victoria Riding for Disabled Association
Overview: A small local charitable organization founded in 1982
Mission: To provide a therapeutic riding program for children & adults with disabilities to promote their physical, psychological, & social well-being
Member of: Canadian Therapeutic Riding Association
Affliation(s): B.C. Therapeutic Riding Association; Horse Council of British Columbia; Volunteer Victoria; Canadian Therapeutic Riding Association's; Association of Fundraising Professionals
Chief Officer(s):
Annie Brothwell, President
Audrey Cooper, Executive Director
Publications:
• The Stable Voice [a publication of Victoria Therapeutic Riding Association]
Type: Newsletter; *Frequency:* q.

NEW BRUNSWICK

Cavalier Riding Club Ltd. (CRC)
705 Pine Glen Rd., Pine Glen NB E1J 1S1
Tel: 506-386-7652
cavalierridingclub.weebly.com
Also Known As: Greater Moncton Riding for the Disabled; CRC Therapeutic Horseback Riding for the Disabled
Overview: A small local organization
Mission: To use hippotherapy in order to treat certain physical and emotional conditions of individuals with a disability
Member of: Canadian Therapeutic Riding Association

NOVA SCOTIA

Antigonish Therapeutic Riding Association
1216 Ohio East Rd., Antigonish NS B2G 2K8
Tel: 902-863-4853
www.facebook.com/399942843470547
Overview: A small local charitable organization founded in 1987
Mission: To provide a therapeutic and recreational horseback riding program for physically, mentally, and emotionally handicapped people, and to promote public awareness of such a program

Halifax Area Leisure & Therapeutic Riding Association
196 Moss Close, Lawrencetown NS B2Z 1S5
Tel: 902-435-9344
e-mail: haltr2@live.ca
www.bengallancers.com/special-needs-haltr
www.facebook.com/HalifaxJrBengalLancers
twitter.com/Bengal_Lancers
instagram.com/hfxjrbengallancers
Previous Name: Lancer Rehab Riders
Overview: A small local charitable organization
Mission: HALTR is a volunteer-run group that provides horse-riding & driving programs for people with special needs. It is a registered charity, BN: 890783947RR0001.
Member of: Equine Canada; Canadian Therapeutic Riding Association
Affliation(s): Sport Canada
Chief Officer(s):
Sallie Murphy, Program Manager

ONTARIO

Central Ontario Developmental Riding Program (CODRP)
Pride Stables, 584 Pioneer Tower Rd., Kitchener ON N2P 2H9
Tel: 519-653-4686; *Fax:* 519-653-5565
e-mail: info@pridestables.com
www.pridestables.com
www.facebook.com/PrideStables
Also Known As: Pride Stables

Overview: A small local charitable organization founded in 1973
Mission: To provide a safe, high-quality riding program for persons with disabilities; to foster personal growth & improvement through the use of horses as a medium for development & therapy with the assistance of volunteers
Member of: Ontario Equestrian Federation; Association of Riding Establishments of Ontario
Affiliation(s): Ontario Therapeutic Riding Association (ONTRA)
Chief Officer(s):
Heather Mackneson, Executive Director

CharterAbility
PO Box 60024, Oakville ON L6J 6G4
Tel: 905-466-2016
e-mail: info@charterability.com
www.charterability.com
Overview: A small local organization
Mission: To promote accessible boating & provide a barrier-free, fully accessible, charter boat service on Lake Ontario for groups of people of all ages with disabilities or mobility impairments
Chief Officer(s):
Stephen Cull, Founder & President

Community Association for Riding for the Disabled (CARD)
4777 Dufferin St., Toronto ON M3H 5T3
Tel: 416-667-8600; *Fax:* 416-739-7520
e-mail: info@card.ca
www.card.ca
Overview: A medium-sized local charitable organization founded in 1969
Mission: To improve the lives of children & adults with disabilities through therapeutic riding programs
Member of: Canadian Therapeutic Riding Association
Affiliation(s): Ontario Therapeutic Riding Association
Chief Officer(s):
Penny Smith, Executive Director
  penny@card.ca
Seana Waldon, Director, Therapeutic Riding Services
  seana@card.ca
Judy Wanless, Director, Volunteer Services
  judy@card.ca
Bonnie Hartley, Coordinator, Fundraising & Events
  bonnie@card.ca

Equestrian Association for the Disabled
8360 Leeming Rd., RR#3, Mount Hope ON L0R 1W0
Tel: 905-679-8323; *Fax:* 905-679-1705
e-mail: info@tead.on.ca
www.tead.on.ca
www.facebook.com/TEADStables
Also Known As: TEAD
Overview: A small local charitable organization founded in 1978
Mission: To enhance the life of children & adults with physical, mental, & emotional handicaps, through equestrian therapy
Chief Officer(s):
Hilary Webb, Manager, Programs, 905-679-8323 Ext. 224
  hilary@tead.on.ca
Helen Clayton, Manager, Farm, 905-679-8323 Ext. 230
  helen@tead.on.ca

Lanark County Therapeutic Riding Program (LCTRP)
30 Bennett St., Carleton Place ON K7C 4J9
Tel: 613-257-7121; *Fax:* 613-257-2675
e-mail: info@therapeuticriding.ca
www.therapeuticriding.ca
Overview: A small local charitable organization founded in 1986
Mission: To provide individuals a holistic approach to therapy, rehabilitation & recreation; the opportunity to experience freedom & movement astride a horse
Member of: Canadian Therapeutic Riding Association; Ontario Therapeutic Riding Association; Lanark Health & Community Services
Chief Officer(s):
Maria Hofbauer, Head Instructor

Mirabel Morgan Special Riding Centre
1201 - 2nd Line South, Bailieboro ON K0L 1B0
Tel: 705-939-6485
e-mail: mirabelmf@gmail.com
Overview: A small local organization

Mission: Year round program for anyone who wishes to ride who has medical, physical, or emotional needs; for those who enjoy the outdoors & animals, want to improve flexibility, balance, joint, muscle & nerve stimulation; designed to meet unique needs, limitations & abilities of the rider
Member of: Canadian Therapeutic Riding Association

PARD Therapeutic Riding (PARD)
PO Box 1654, Peterborough ON K9J 5S4
Tel: 705-742-6441
e-mail: pardtherapeuticriding@gmail.com
www.pard.ca
www.facebook.com/PARDTherapeuticRiding
Previous Name: Peterborough Association for Riding for the Disabled
Overview: A small local charitable organization
Mission: Provides the benefits of riding to people with disabilities.
Member of: Canadian Therapeutic Riding Association; Ontario Therapeutic Riding Association
Chief Officer(s):
Kathy Carruthers, Program Coordinator

Quinte Therapeutic Riding Association (QUINTRA)
173 McGee Rd., RR#2, Stirling ON K0K 3E0
Tel: 613-395-4472
www.quintra.org
Overview: A small local charitable organization founded in 1985
Mission: To offer therapeutic horseback-riding sessions to disabled children & young adults to maximize the disabled person's physical & mental capabilities; To improve disabled young people's self-confidence & the ability to cope with everyday living
Member of: Canadian Therapeutic Riding Association; Ontario Therapeutic Riding Association
Affiliation(s): United Way of Quinte
Chief Officer(s):
Barb Davis, Contact, 613-395-2990
  barbara.davis@sympatico.ca

SARI Therapeutic Riding
12659 Medway Rd., RR#1, Arva ON N0M 1C0
Tel: 519-666-1123; *Fax:* 519-666-1971
e-mail: office@sari.ca
www.sari.ca
www.facebook.com/SARITherapeuticRiding
twitter.com/SARITherapeutic
www.youtube.com/channel/UCWEQ6cSSY89McQFCwwTxLow
Also Known As: Special Ability Riding Institute
Previous Name: SARI Riding for Disabled
Overview: A medium-sized local charitable organization founded in 1978
Mission: To provide opportunities for people with special needs to move towards greater independence & freedom by providing therapeutic riding & driving programs which meet individual needs; To balance safety & challenge to maximize opportunities for growth; To support contributions of participants, parents, volunteers & staff
Member of: Canadian Therapeutic Riding Association
Affiliation(s): Ontario Therapeutic Riding Association
Chief Officer(s):
Diane Blackall, Executive Director

Sunrise Therapeutic Riding & Learning Centre
6920 Concession 1, RR#2, Puslinch ON N0B 2J0
Tel: 519-837-0558; *Fax:* 519-837-1233
Other Communication: Barn office phone: 519-827-0558, ext. 30
e-mail: info@sunrise-therapeutic.ca
www.sunrise-therapeutic.ca
www.facebook.com/224072694372280
Also Known As: Sunrise
Previous Name: Sunrise Equestrian & Recreation Centre for the Disabled
Overview: A small local charitable organization founded in 1982
Mission: To develop the full potential of children & adults with disabilites & lead them closer to independence through therapy, recreation, horse riding, life skills & farm related activity programme
Member of: Canadian Therapeutic Riding Association; Ontario Therapeutic Riding Association
Affiliation(s): Ontario's Promise
Chief Officer(s):

Rob Vandebelt, Chief Executive Officer, 519-837-0558 Ext. 32
   rob@sunrise-therapeutic.ca
Nikki Duffield, Program Director & Head Instructor, 519-837-0558 Ext.
   29
   nikkid@sunrise-therapeutic.ca
Lynne O'Brien, Manager, Operations & Volunteer, 519-837-0558 Ext.
   31
   lynne@sunrise-therapeutic.ca
Publications:
• Pony Express [a publication of the Sunrise Therapeutic Riding &
Learning Centre]
Type: Newsletter; *Frequency:* Irregular
Profile: News & profiles on members

Therapeutic Ride Algoma
2627 Second Line West, Sault Ste Marie ON P6A 6K4
                               Tel: 705-759-9282
              e-mail: therapeuticridealgoma@hotmail.ca
                              www.ridealgoma.com

Overview: A small local organization
Member of: Canadian Therapeutic Riding Association
Chief Officer(s):
Bob Trainor, President

Windsor-Essex Therapeutic Riding Association (WETRA) /
Association d'équitation thérapeutique Windsor-Essex
3323 North Maklen Rd., RR#2, Essex ON N8M 2X6
              Tel: 519-726-7682; *Fax:* 519-726-4403
                              e-mail: info@wetra.ca
                                   www.wetra.ca
                    www.facebook.com/525824287490852
                              twitter.com/WETRA_

Overview: A small local charitable organization founded in 1969
Mission: To improve the quality of life of physically, emotionally,
mentally challenged persons through equine related therapy
Member of: Canadian Therapeutic Riding Association
Affliation(s): Ontario Therapeutic Riding Association
Chief Officer(s):
Becky Mills, Managing Director

QUÉBEC

Association des sports pour aveugles de Montréal (ASAM)
4545, av Pierre-de Coubertin, Montréal QC H1V 0B2
                               Tél: 514-252-3178
              Courriel: infoasaq@sportsaveugles.qc.ca
                     www.sportsaveugles.qc.ca/asam
                     www.facebook.com/ASAMONTREAL

Aperçu: *Dimension:* petite; *Envergure:* locale; Organisme sans but
lucratif; fondée en 1983
Mission: Promouvoir l'accessibilité et la pratique des sports et loisirs
aux personnes handicapées visuelles; organiser et structurer les
différentes activités sportives; recruter et former des bénévoles
accompagnateurs
Affliation(s): Association sportive des aveugles du Québec
Membre(s) du bureau directeur:

Nathalie Chartrand, Directrice générale
   nchartrand@sportsaveugles.qc.ca

SASKATCHEWAN

Regina Therapeutic Recreation Association (RTRA)
c/o Sandra Procyk, 1150 Broadway Ave., Regina SK S4P 4V3
                  e-mail: regina_tra@hotmail.com
                       nonprofits.accesscomm.ca/rtra

Overview: A small local organization
Mission: To provide professional development, education, & support to
recreation practitioners & students in any vocational setting in Regina &
surrounding area
Chief Officer(s):
Angela Strelioff, Chair
   rec.mutchmor@sasktel.net

International Associations

International Committee of Sports for the Deaf (ICSD) / Comité
international des Sports des Sourds (CISS)
Maison du Sport International, Av. de Rhondanie 54, Lausanne
CH-1007 Switzerland
              Tel: 41 78 733 35 67; *Fax:* 7 (499) 255 04 36
                              e-mail: office@ciss.org
                                   www.ciss.org

Also Known As: International Deaflympics
Overview: A medium-sized international charitable organization
founded in 1924
Mission: To organize sporting events for deaf & hard of hearing
athletes
Member of: International Olympic Committee; General Assembly of
International Sports Federations
Affliation(s): Canadian Deaf Sports Association
Chief Officer(s):
Valery Rukhledev, President
   president@ciss.org

Professional Association of Therapeutic Horsemanship
International (PATH)
PO Box 33150, Denver CO 80233 USA
                  Tel: 303-452-1212; *Fax:* 303-252-4610
                          Toll-Free: 800-369-7433
                                   www.pathintl.org

Previous Name: North American Riding for the Handicapped
Association
Overview: A medium-sized international charitable organization
founded in 1969
Mission: Promotes the benefit of the horse riding for individuals with
physical, emotional & learning disabilities
Chief Officer(s):
Kathy Alm, Chief Executive Officer
   kalm@pathintl.org

This statistics section starts with tables of health topics that include geographic regions (Canada and its provinces) and age-standardized rates. Topics include overall health and mental health, life stress, specific conditions such as diabetes and cancer, injuries in the last 12 months, leisure-time physical activity, exposure to second-hand smoke at home, and sense of community well being, among others. Most topics break down into sub-categories-such as Both Sexes, Males, and Females-for a total of 158 tables. They include data for up to eleven years, from 2003 to 2014.

Following the health trends tables is a section of graphs on wait times-referral to appointment, appointment to treatment, referral to treatment-by province. The data includes statistics for the years 1993/1994 and 2016 for easy comparison.

AGE-STANDARDIZED RATES, PERCEIVED HEALTH, VERY GOOD OR EXCELLENT (%), [6] BOTH SEXES, CANADA, PROVINCES AND TERRITORIES

Geography	2003	2005	2007	2008	2009	2010	2011	2012	2013	2014
Canada	59.7	61.5	61.2	60.6	62.2	61.9	61.6	61.9	61.3	60.9
Newfoundland and Labrador	67.4	65.6	64.0	63.5	59.3	65.4	62.2	61.1	63.6	61.7
Prince Edward Island	66.2	60.2	59.3	63.2	62.9	67.0	59.7	60.6	59.7	62.0
Nova Scotia	60.0	60.1	59.5	58.6	62.1	60.8	61.1	60.7	60.9	60.2
New Brunswick	52.1	56.8	58.1	57.6	58.4	57.1	56.6	57.8	57.7	55.7
Quebec	58.6	61.2	61.6	61.3	63.3	61.5	61.7	61.7	60.9	60.8
Ontario	58.3	62.0	61.2	60.9	62.8	62.6	61.7	62.5	62.0	61.0
Manitoba	62.4	60.7	61.5	55.9	61.8	58.4	58.0	60.3	60.3	61.0
Saskatchewan	61.6	59.7	58.4	56.6	61.0	59.7	58.7	59.0	60.1	62.4
Alberta	63.7	62.4	62.6	63.4	61.8	62.4	62.7	62.9	62.5	63.5
British Columbia	61.6	61.0	60.5	58.7	60.6	62.6	62.7	61.4	60.4	59.2
Yukon [4]	54.3	57.4	55.8	61.6	60.8	57.8	60.1	57.1	59.7	58.7
Northwest Territories [4]	54.4	60.5	50.7	47.9	49.6	45.4	46.9	52.0	53.7	50.9
Nunavut [4,5]	52.1	46.8	54.4	42.9	41.6	45.9	42.7	42.2	35.7	34.7

Source: Statistics Canada. *Table 105-0503 - Health indicator profile, age-standardized rate, annual estimates, by sex, Canada, provinces and territories, occasional,* CANSIM (database). (accessed: March 1, 2017)

Please see footnotes [30], [31], [57], [58], [59], [60], [61], [62], [64] for characteristics of the age-standardized rate.

AGE-STANDARDIZED RATES, PERCEIVED HEALTH, VERY GOOD OR EXCELLENT (%), [6] MALES, CANADA, PROVINCES AND TERRITORIES

Geography	2003	2005	2007	2008	2009	2010	2011	2012	2013	2014
Canada	60.8	61.9	61.8	60.9	62.7	61.7	61.9	62.2	62.1	60.6
Newfoundland and Labrador	64.6	64.7	62.8	59.9	57.9	66.5	63.0	56.6	63.3	60.9
Prince Edward Island	69.3	56.3	56.3	65.3	61.9	64.2	56.3	62.8	62.8	58.9
Nova Scotia	57.5	59.0	57.9	59.7	63.9	58.8	60.7	59.8	58.7	60.3
New Brunswick	51.1	56.6	56.1	56.8	60.4	56.8	57.3	56.6	57.5	54.4
Quebec	60.3	61.8	62.4	61.4	64.7	60.2	60.9	63.4	61.1	60.1
Ontario	59.5	62.7	62.4	60.8	63.1	63.2	62.3	62.7	63.9	61.0
Manitoba	63.0	62.0	61.7	57.2	58.9	61.2	59.9	56.5	62.8	59.5
Saskatchewan	61.4	60.2	59.3	55.7	58.9	58.9	59.3	60.3	59.1	64.7
Alberta	66.0	62.0	60.4	65.3	60.3	61.2	61.2	61.7	63.2	62.5
British Columbia	62.5	61.8	62.1	60.0	62.4	62.1	65.5	63.6	59.6	59.6
Yukon [4]	59.4	56.9	56.7	61.9	59.3	57.0	59.5	54.6	57.6	56.9
Northwest Territories [4]	58.2	61.3	49.9	48.9	52.9	43.2	49.5	53.9	49.4	47.5
Nunavut [4, 5]	54.5	44.8	60.3	49.5	40.5	49.7	46.5	41.7	31.8E	36.5

Symbol Legend:
E   Use with caution

Source: Statistics Canada. *Table 105-0503 - Health indicator profile, age-standardized rate, annual estimates, by sex, Canada, provinces and territories, occasional,* CANSIM (database). (accessed: March 1, 2017)

Please see footnotes 30, 31, 57, 58, 59, 60, 61, 62, 64 for characteristics of the age-standardized rate.

AGE-STANDARDIZED RATES, PERCEIVED HEALTH, VERY GOOD OR EXCELLENT (%), [6] FEMALES, CANADA, PROVINCES AND TERRITORIES

Geography	2003	2005	2007	2008	2009	2010	2011	2012	2013	2014
Canada	58.6	61.0	60.6	60.2	61.8	62.2	61.3	61.5	60.6	61.1
Newfoundland and Labrador	70.1	66.4	65.1	66.8	60.6	64.5	61.5	65.4	63.9	62.6
Prince Edward Island	63.2	63.7	62.1	61.3	63.8	69.5	63.0	58.6	56.9	64.9
Nova Scotia	62.2	61.2	61.0	57.6	60.4	62.6	61.5	61.5	62.9	60.1
New Brunswick	53.0	56.9	60.0	58.4	56.6	57.4	55.9	58.9	58.0	57.0
Quebec	56.9	60.6	60.9	61.2	61.9	62.8	62.5	60.1	60.6	61.5
Ontario	57.2	61.3	59.9	61.0	62.6	62.0	61.2	62.4	60.1	61.0
Manitoba	61.7	59.4	61.3	54.6	64.7	55.6	56.1	64.1	57.8	62.4
Saskatchewan	61.8	59.3	57.5	57.5	63.1	60.6	58.1	57.7	61.1	60.1
Alberta	61.3	62.8	64.9	61.3	63.4	63.7	64.3	64.3	61.9	64.4
British Columbia	60.8	60.2	58.9	57.4	58.8	63.2	60.1	59.3	61.3	58.7
Yukon [4]	49.3	58.0	54.9	61.3	62.3	58.6	60.8	59.6	61.7	60.5
Northwest Territories [4]	50.3	59.7	51.6	46.8	46.4	47.8	44.3	50.1	58.4	54.5
Nunavut [4][5]	49.9	49.1	48.7	36.2	42.6	42.0	38.2E	42.8	39.6	32.6

Symbol Legend:
E   Use with caution

Source: Statistics Canada. *Table 105-0503 - Health indicator profile, age-standardized rate, annual estimates, by sex, Canada, provinces and territories, occasional,* CANSIM (database). (accessed: March 1, 2017)

Please see footnotes 30, 31, 57, 58, 59, 60, 61, 62, 64 for characteristics of the age-standardized rate.

AGE-STANDARDIZED RATES, PERCEIVED HEALTH, FAIR OR POOR (%), [6] BOTH SEXES, CANADA, PROVINCES AND TERRITORIES

Geography	2003	2005	2007	2008	2009	2010	2011	2012	2013	2014
Canada	10.6	10.3	10.4	10.3	9.9	10.3	10.3	9.7	9.7	10.2
Newfoundland and Labrador	10.0	10.6	9.8	10.6	11.6	11.3	11.0	11.5	9.8	9.8
Prince Edward Island	9.2	12.6	11.1	12.5	12.1	9.1	11.1	9.8	10.2	8.6
Nova Scotia	12.2	12.6	12.5	13.1	10.1	12.3	11.6	11.4	12.1	11.9
New Brunswick	15.1	12.8	13.5	13.2	11.4	14.6	12.5	13.0	12.1	12.8
Quebec	9.8	9.2	8.6	8.7	8.3	8.6	8.8	8.4	9.4	9.3
Ontario	11.1	10.3	10.7	11.0	10.3	11.1	10.6	9.6	9.6	11.0
Manitoba	10.1	10.3	10.6	11.3	9.9	11.2	11.8	8.8	8.9	9.1
Saskatchewan	10.7	11.5	11.1	11.3	10.3	10.0	10.8	11.9	9.7	9.0
Alberta	9.3	10.5	10.3	8.9	10.4	10.0	11.0	10.4	9.1	9.0
British Columbia	10.3	10.6	11.4	10.7	10.9	9.7	10.5	10.7	10.0	10.4
Yukon [4]	11.6	9.8	11.0	9.6E	10.5E	11.9	11.5	10.9	10.0	11.6
Northwest Territories [4]	12.4	14.3	12.9	13.1	13.4	15.3	15.6	10.6	10.8	13.1
Nunavut [4, 5]	12.8	15.9	10.7E	18.8	11.7E	12.7E	16.8	17.8	17.5	F

Symbol Legend:
E   Use with caution
F   Too unreliable to be published

Source: Statistics Canada. *Table 105-0503 - Health indicator profile, age-standardized rate, annual estimates, by sex, Canada, provinces and territories, occasional,* CANSIM (database). (accessed: March 1, 2017)

Please see footnotes 30, 31, 57, 58, 59, 60, 61, 62, 64 for characteristics of the age-standardized rate.

AGE-STANDARDIZED RATES, PERCEIVED HEALTH, FAIR OR POOR (%), [6] MALES, CANADA, PROVINCES AND TERRITORIES

Geography	2003	2005	2007	2008	2009	2010	2011	2012	2013	2014
Canada	9.5	9.8	10.0	10.1	9.6	10.2	9.8	9.4	9.6	10.2
Newfoundland and Labrador	10.7	10.5	11.1	12.0	11.9	11.8	9.0	14.7	10.5	10.8
Prince Edward Island	8.2	13.2	11.6	11.8	13.0	10.5	12.7E	9.0E	10.1	8.9E
Nova Scotia	11.7	12.9	13.3	13.8	10.5	12.8	13.3	12.2	13.1	10.1
New Brunswick	15.5	12.0	13.8	13.9	11.3	14.2	11.7	13.4	11.5	12.6
Quebec	8.6	8.7	8.2	8.9	8.2	9.5	8.1	7.9	9.6	9.5
Ontario	9.8	9.8	9.8	10.3	9.9	10.7	9.9	8.9	9.0	10.8
Manitoba	9.6	10.3	9.2	9.4	10.8	9.8	11.3	8.8	8.3	9.6
Saskatchewan	10.1	10.7	12.0	10.4	10.3	9.1	9.7	11.4	9.8	8.9
Alberta	8.3	10.1	10.7	8.9	10.5	9.3	11.7	11.0	9.1	9.3
British Columbia	9.4	9.9	11.1	10.8	9.2	10.1	9.4	9.7	10.9	10.5
Yukon [4]	10.9	13.6E	9.4E	6.8E	8.0E	14.5E	12.6E	13.4E	9.6E	12.4E
Northwest Territories [4]	9.7E	13.4E	12.7	14.0E	10.9E	13.6E	13.1	9.5E	11.1	15.5
Nunavut [4,5]	8.0E	19.4	10.5E	16.2E	13.4E	F	14.2E	18.1E	23.7E	F

Symbol Legend:
E   Use with caution
F   Too unreliable to be published

Source: Statistics Canada. *Table 105-0503 - Health indicator profile, age-standardized rate, annual estimates, by sex, Canada, provinces and territories, occasional,* CANSIM (database). (accessed: March 1, 2017)

Please see footnotes 30, 31, 57, 58, 59, 60, 61, 62, 64 for characteristics of the age-standardized rate.

AGE-STANDARDIZED RATES, PERCEIVED HEALTH, FAIR OR POOR (%), [6] FEMALES, CANADA, PROVINCES AND TERRITORIES

Geography	2003	2005	2007	2008	2009	2010	2011	2012	2013	2014
Canada	11.6	10.8	10.8	10.6	10.3	10.3	10.9	10.1	9.7	10.2
Newfoundland and Labrador	9.3	10.7	8.7	9.3	11.3	10.8	12.9	8.4	9.2	8.9
Prince Edward Island	10.2	12.0	10.6	13.1	11.4	7.9	9.7[E]	10.5	10.4	8.4[E]
Nova Scotia	12.6	12.4	11.7	12.3	9.8	11.8	10.0	10.7	11.1	13.6
New Brunswick	14.6	13.6	13.3	12.6	11.4	14.9	13.3	12.6	12.6	13.0
Quebec	11.0	9.8	9.0	8.6	8.3	7.7	9.5	8.8	9.2	9.2
Ontario	12.4	10.7	11.5	11.7	10.7	11.4	11.2	10.2	10.2	11.1
Manitoba	10.7	10.3	11.9	13.2	8.9	12.5	12.4	8.9	9.4	8.6
Saskatchewan	11.3	12.3	10.2	12.3	10.3	10.9	11.9	12.4	9.6	9.0
Alberta	10.3	11.0	9.9	8.9	10.2	10.8	10.3	9.7	9.1	8.7
British Columbia	11.2	11.3	11.7	10.5	12.5	9.3	11.6	11.7	9.1	10.3
Yukon [4]	12.3[E]	6.2[E]	12.7[E]	12.5[E]	13.0[E]	9.3[E]	10.4[E]	8.5[E]	10.5[E]	10.8[E]
Northwest Territories [4]	15.4	15.3[E]	13.0[E]	12.1[E]	15.7[E]	17.0	18.2[E]	11.8[E]	10.6[E]	10.6[E]
Nunavut [4, 5]	17.6[E]	11.8[E]	10.9[E]	21.4[E]	10.1[E]	13.5[E]	19.8[E]	17.5[E]	11.1[E]	F

Symbol Legend:
E   Use with caution
F   Too unreliable to be published

Source: Statistics Canada. *Table 105-0503 - Health indicator profile, age-standardized rate, annual estimates, by sex, Canada, provinces and territories, occasional,* CANSIM (database). (accessed: March 27, 2017)

Please see footnotes 30, 31, 57, 58, 59, 60, 61, 62, 64 for characteristics of the age-standardized rate.

AGE-STANDARDIZED RATES, PERCEIVED MENTAL HEALTH, VERY GOOD OR EXCELLENT (%), [7]
BOTH SEXES, CANADA, PROVINCES AND TERRITORIES

Geography	2003	2005	2007	2008	2009	2010	2011	2012	2013	2014
Canada	73.8	74.8	75.2	75.0	74.4	74.4	73.1	72.2	71.6	71.5
Newfoundland and Labrador	76.8	77.9	77.9	78.2	75.9	76.8	73.4	73.7	74.5	72.5
Prince Edward Island	77.1	77.0	74.3	75.8	73.6	77.4	72.4	72.7	68.4	69.8
Nova Scotia	75.4	73.7	73.8	72.7	75.9	73.5	72.7	71.0	68.4	69.9
New Brunswick	68.8	71.2	71.4	72.8	69.3	70.3	69.9	70.8	68.4	64.8
Quebec	76.8	76.6	77.4	77.6	77.2	75.9	75.4	75.1	73.9	74.2
Ontario	72.9	74.9	74.9	75.3	74.6	75.0	73.2	72.6	71.4	70.8
Manitoba	75.0	72.5	73.9	72.2	71.9	70.9	67.8	69.8	71.5	69.0
Saskatchewan	73.9	73.3	74.0	72.8	72.8	72.7	69.1	67.7	71.6	68.8
Alberta	73.8	74.6	76.1	74.3	74.1	73.9	74.9	71.6	72.9	72.5
British Columbia	71.2	73.1	72.4	71.9	71.1	72.3	70.7	68.3	67.8	70.4
Yukon [4]	74.7	75.5	72.8	73.5	75.5	72.1	66.1	70.9	66.4	63.2
Northwest Territories [4]	69.4	74.1	67.2	60.2	63.4	56.6	60.0	63.2	65.3	59.2
Nunavut [4, 5]	68.5	63.2	67.6	65.0	70.3	70.2	50.9	57.6	55.0	56.0

Source: Statistics Canada. *Table 105-0503 - Health indicator profile, age-standardized rate, annual estimates, by sex, Canada, provinces and territories, occasional,* CANSIM (database). (accessed: March 9, 2017)

Please see footnotes 30, 31, 57, 58, 59, 60, 61, 62, 64 for characteristics of the age-standardized rate.

AGE-STANDARDIZED RATES, PERCEIVED MENTAL HEALTH, VERY GOOD OR EXCELLENT (%), [7] MALES, CANADA, PROVINCES AND TERRITORIES

Geography	2003	2005	2007	2008	2009	2010	2011	2012	2013	2014
Canada	74.0	75.3	75.9	76.0	75.2	75.1	73.9	73.3	72.6	72.8
Newfoundland and Labrador	76.4	77.6	76.9	79.7	78.2	78.2	73.5	74.8	75.6	74.7
Prince Edward Island	77.4	75.6	72.2	77.3	70.5	76.4	73.3	76.2	72.3	68.8
Nova Scotia	73.3	73.8	73.3	73.9	76.6	72.4	72.5	71.0	69.5	75.1
New Brunswick	67.8	71.4	73.7	72.0	68.9	71.6	71.3	72.2	68.2	65.6
Quebec	77.1	76.8	79.0	77.7	78.4	76.3	76.2	77.0	75.1	74.2
Ontario	73.4	75.6	76.1	77.3	74.9	76.7	73.7	73.6	73.3	72.5
Manitoba	74.4	73.5	73.4	74.2	70.1	70.0	68.0	69.1	72.2	70.1
Saskatchewan	73.8	73.2	74.1	72.9	72.7	74.2	68.6	67.9	71.9	70.8
Alberta	74.5	75.1	76.3	75.6	73.7	73.9	75.6	73.3	72.3	74.2
British Columbia	70.6	73.8	71.6	71.0	73.6	71.9	73.1	68.4	67.5	71.8
Yukon [4]	80.3	75.4	69.6	71.4	71.7	71.8	64.7	71.3	65.5	63.3
Northwest Territories [4]	74.1	78.6	70.0	60.7	67.6	56.9	67.1	64.3	64.4	58.2
Nunavut [4, 5]	69.2	63.2	68.4	64.8	74.7	73.1	54.3	56.8	61.3	61.6

Source: Statistics Canada. *Table 105-0503 - Health indicator profile, age-standardized rate, annual estimates, by sex, Canada, provinces and territories, occasional,* CANSIM (database). (accessed: March 27, 2017)

Please see footnotes 30, 31, 57, 58, 59, 60, 61, 62, 64 for characteristics of the age-standardized rate.

AGE-STANDARDIZED RATES, PERCEIVED MENTAL HEALTH, VERY GOOD OR EXCELLENT (%), [7] FEMALES, CANADA, PROVINCES AND TERRITORIES

Geography	2003	2005	2007	2008	2009	2010	2011	2012	2013	2014
Canada	73.7	74.3	74.4	74.1	73.7	73.7	72.3	71.1	70.6	70.2
Newfoundland and Labrador	77.1	78.2	78.8	76.8	73.8	75.5	73.2	72.7	73.4	70.5
Prince Edward Island	76.8	78.3	76.2	74.4	76.2	78.3	71.6	69.6	64.8	70.7
Nova Scotia	77.3	73.6	74.2	71.6	75.3	74.5	73.0	71.0	67.4	64.9
New Brunswick	69.7	71.0	69.2	73.5	69.7	69.0	68.7	69.5	68.5	64.1
Quebec	76.6	76.3	75.8	77.4	75.9	75.5	74.6	73.3	72.7	74.3
Ontario	72.4	74.2	73.8	73.4	74.2	73.3	72.8	71.6	69.6	69.2
Manitoba	75.6	71.5	74.2	70.3	73.7	71.7	67.7	70.6	70.8	68.0
Saskatchewan	74.1	73.4	73.9	72.6	72.8	71.2	69.7	67.5	71.2	66.7
Alberta	73.1	74.1	75.8	72.9	74.4	73.9	74.0	69.9	73.5	70.7
British Columbia	71.7	72.3	73.2	72.8	68.7	72.7	68.3	68.2	68.2	69.0
Yukon [4]	69.5	75.6	76.1	75.6	79.2	72.4	67.5	70.6	67.3	63.0
Northwest Territories [4]	64.4	69.3	64.3	59.7	59.3	56.3	52.6	61.9	66.4	60.2
Nunavut [4,5]	67.9	63.2	66.8	65.1	66.3	67.2	47.1E	58.5	48.5	49.8

Symbol Legend:
E   Use with caution

Source: Statistics Canada. *Table 105-0503 - Health indicator profile, age-standardized rate, annual estimates, by sex, Canada, provinces and territories, occasional,* CANSIM (database). (accessed: March 27, 2017)

Please see footnotes 30, 31, 57, 58, 59, 60, 61, 62, 64 for characteristics of the age-standardized rate.

AGE-STANDARDIZED RATES, PERCEIVED MENTAL HEALTH, FAIR OR POOR (%), [7] BOTH SEXES, CANADA, PROVINCES AND TERRITORIES

Geography	2003	2005	2007	2008	2009	2010	2011	2012	2013	2014
Canada	4.5	4.7	4.6	4.9	4.9	5.1	5.4	5.6	6.1	6.3
Newfoundland and Labrador	3.2	3.3	3.5	3.4	3.0	3.3	3.3[E]	6.3	4.9	5.3
Prince Edward Island	4.5	4.5	4.3[E]	4.0[E]	4.9[E]	4.7[E]	4.0[E]	6.1	6.7	6.8[E]
Nova Scotia	4.1	4.6	5.4	5.4	3.9	6.1	5.9	6.5	8.0	7.7
New Brunswick	6.3	5.3	5.4	4.8	5.8	6.5	5.4	6.0	5.7	7.2
Quebec	3.5	3.6	3.2	3.4	3.5	4.3	4.0	3.6	4.7	4.2
Ontario	4.7	4.9	4.8	5.5	5.4	5.5	5.8	6.1	6.4	7.2
Manitoba	3.9	4.7	5.2	5.4	5.4	5.2	7.5	6.8	5.2	6.9
Saskatchewan	4.9	4.9	4.2	5.5	5.4	5.0	6.7	7.4	7.4	5.2
Alberta	4.6	5.4	4.8	4.5	4.7	4.8	4.9	5.3	5.7	5.8
British Columbia	5.9	5.8	5.8	6.2	5.8	5.8	6.6	6.6	7.8	7.3
Yukon [4]	3.9[E]	4.0[E]	3.1[E]	7.2[E]	5.5[E]	6.3[E]	6.5[E]	4.7[E]	6.8	7.8[E]
Northwest Territories [4]	3.6[E]	4.7	4.5[E]	4.0[E]	6.1[E]	8.1	6.4[E]	7.4[E]	8.6[E]	9.0[E]
Nunavut [4, 5]	5.2[E]	8.4[E]	3.8[E]	5.5[E]	6.9[E]	F	4.2[E]	12.3[E]	5.1[E]	F

Symbol Legend:
E   Use with caution
F   Too unreliable to be published

Source: Statistics Canada. *Table 105-0503 - Health indicator profile, age-standardized rate, annual estimates, by sex, Canada, provinces and territories, occasional,* CANSIM (database). (accessed: March 27, 2017)

Please see footnotes 30, 31, 57, 58, 59, 60, 61, 62, 64 for characteristics of the age-standardized rate.

AGE-STANDARDIZED RATES, PERCEIVED MENTAL HEALTH, FAIR OR POOR (%), [7] MALES, CANADA, PROVINCES AND TERRITORIES

Geography	2003	2005	2007	2008	2009	2010	2011	2012	2013	2014
Canada	4.2	4.3	4.5	4.5	4.6	4.8	5.0	5.0	5.7	5.4
Newfoundland and Labrador	3.6	2.8	4.2[E]	3.5[E]	2.2[E]	3.1[E]	3.4[E]	8.2[E]	5.0[E]	6.2[E]
Prince Edward Island	3.7[E]	4.8[E]	4.3[E]	4.3[E]	5.5[E]	6.7[E]	F	5.7[E]	6.5[E]	6.6[E]
Nova Scotia	4.4	4.8	4.4[E]	5.0[E]	3.5[E]	5.8[E]	5.7[E]	5.8[E]	7.2	4.0[E]
New Brunswick	6.4	5.0	4.8[E]	5.1	6.6[E]	7.6	3.6[E]	5.6[E]	5.4[E]	5.7[E]
Quebec	3.4	3.3	3.4	3.8	3.2	4.6	3.6	3.4	4.3	3.6
Ontario	4.1	4.6	4.8	4.6	5.4	4.6	5.3	5.1	6.0	6.2
Manitoba	3.4	4.4	4.6[E]	3.0[E]	5.7[E]	4.8[E]	7.3[E]	7.4[E]	4.5	6.5
Saskatchewan	4.4	5.0	4.4	5.5	5.7	3.9[E]	6.6[E]	6.9[E]	7.1	4.8
Alberta	3.9	4.8	4.0	4.3	4.3	3.9	5.2	4.5	5.4	4.7
British Columbia	5.5	4.9	6.3	5.6	4.9	6.4	5.8	6.4	7.5	7.0
Yukon [4]	F	4.8[E]	F	7.8[E]	5.8[E]	4.3[E]	4.8[E]	F	5.1[E]	4.9[E]
Northwest Territories [4]	3.5[E]	4.7[E]	4.1[E]	F	F	6.8[E]	4.2[E]	9.0[E]	7.9[E]	10.6[E]
Nunavut [4,5]	F	7.7[E]	F	5.5[E]	F	F	F	F	F	5.0[E]

Symbol Legend:
E   Use with caution
F   Too unreliable to be published

Source: Statistics Canada. *Table 105-0503 - Health indicator profile, age-standardized rate, annual estimates, by sex, Canada, provinces and territories, occasional,* CANSIM (database). (accessed: March 27, 2017)

Please see footnotes 30, 31, 57, 58, 59, 60, 61, 62, 64 for characteristics of the age-standardized rate.

AGE-STANDARDIZED RATES, PERCEIVED MENTAL HEALTH, FAIR OR POOR (%), [Z] FEMALES, CANADA, PROVINCES AND TERRITORIES

Geography	2003	2005	2007	2008	2009	2010	2011	2012	2013	2014
Canada	4.9	5.1	4.6	5.3	5.1	5.4	5.9	6.1	6.5	7.1
Newfoundland and Labrador	2.8	3.8	2.9E	3.3E	3.8E	3.5E	3.2E	4.5E	4.8E	4.5E
Prince Edward Island	5.2E	4.2	4.4E	3.7E	4.3E	3.0E	F	6.5E	6.8E	7.0E
Nova Scotia	3.9	4.5	6.2	5.9	4.3	6.4	6.1E	7.2E	8.7	11.3
New Brunswick	6.3	5.7	6.0	4.5	4.9	5.5	7.1	6.3	6.0	8.6
Quebec	3.6	3.9	3.0	2.9	3.8	4.0	4.4	3.9	5.1	4.8
Ontario	5.3	5.2	4.9	6.4	5.5	6.3	6.4	7.0	6.7	8.1
Manitoba	4.3	5.0	5.8	7.8	5.0	5.7	7.7	6.2	5.9	7.2
Saskatchewan	5.5	4.8	4.0	5.5	5.2	6.1	6.7	7.9E	7.7	5.6
Alberta	5.3	6.0	5.6	4.7	5.1	5.6	4.6	6.1	5.9	6.9
British Columbia	6.2	6.6	5.4	6.8	6.6	5.3	7.5	6.7	8.1	7.5
Yukon [4]	4.7E	3.3E	5.3E	F	F	8.3E	8.2E	6.0E	8.4E	10.8E
Northwest Territories [4]	3.7E	4.6E	4.9E	4.7E	6.8E	9.6E	8.7E	5.7E	9.2E	7.4E
Nunavut [4, 5]	F	9.1E	5.1E	F	4.9E	F	F	16.3E	F	F

Symbol Legend:
E   Use with caution
F   Too unreliable to be published

Source: Statistics Canada. *Table 105-0503 - Health indicator profile, age-standardized rate, annual estimates, by sex, Canada, provinces and territories, occasional,* CANSIM (database). (accessed: March 27, 2017)

Please see footnotes 30, 31, 57, 58, 59, 60, 61, 62, 64 for characteristics of the age-standardized rate.

AGE-STANDARDIZED RATES, PERCEIVED LIFE STRESS, QUITE A LOT (15 YEARS AND OVER) (%), [10], [11] BOTH SEXES, CANADA, PROVINCES AND TERRITORIES

Geography	2003	2005	2007	2008	2009	2010	2011	2012	2013	2014
Canada	24.1	22.9	22.6	22.2	23.3	23.5	23.9	23.0	23.3	23.5
Newfoundland and Labrador	14.6	14.6	12.6	11.4	13.1	15.5	13.2	13.5	15.4	16.9
Prince Edward Island	14.9	17.1	14.0	16.1	14.1	13.7	18.3	16.1	19.6	17.6
Nova Scotia	18.5	21.0	18.7	18.8	19.1	18.9	20.4	17.1	20.4	20.0
New Brunswick	24.5	19.5	20.7	18.6	21.8	20.6	19.3	18.6	19.7	21.1
Quebec	28.9	26.2	27.5	26.7	26.9	27.7	29.4	27.9	27.0	27.6
Ontario	24.3	22.7	21.9	21.8	24.0	23.3	23.2	22.3	23.5	22.4
Manitoba	20.4	20.0	19.8	19.1	20.4	19.7	22.9	20.6	19.6	22.3
Saskatchewan	21.0	21.0	18.8	20.0	19.2	19.7	18.8	20.3	20.0	20.8
Alberta	22.3	21.4	21.4	21.1	22.3	21.8	24.3	22.3	20.5	21.6
British Columbia	21.0	22.4	21.0	20.8	20.2	22.6	20.1	21.4	22.4	23.9
Yukon [4]	16.8	21.8	20.9	21.4	19.9	17.4	20.9	21.1	21.0	25.3
Northwest Territories [4]	19.3	17.6	19.0	11.1	17.6	18.0	17.9	18.7	16.8E	20.1
Nunavut [4], [5]	21.7E	18.4	15.4E	18.4	17.7	16.7E	23.4	19.2	16.5E	17.7

Symbol Legend:
E   Use with caution

Source: Statistics Canada. *Table 105-0503 - Health indicator profile, age-standardized rate, annual estimates, by sex, Canada, provinces and territories, occasional,* CANSIM (database). (accessed: March 27, 2017)

Please see footnotes 30, 31, 57, 58, 59, 60, 61, 62, 64 for characteristics of the age-standardized rate.

AGE-STANDARDIZED RATES, PERCEIVED LIFE STRESS, QUITE A LOT (15 YEARS AND OVER) (%), [10, 11] MALES, CANADA, PROVINCES AND TERRITORIES

Geography	2003	2005	2007	2008	2009	2010	2011	2012	2013	2014
Canada	23.3	22.0	21.6	21.0	21.6	21.9	22.3	21.2	21.4	22.6
Newfoundland and Labrador	15.0	13.2	10.4	13.0	12.1	17.0	12.7	13.3	13.9	17.8
Prince Edward Island	12.5	14.8	13.3	16.4	10.8E	12.8E	19.1E	16.2E	14.1E	14.4E
Nova Scotia	17.5	18.1	19.8	19.7	20.1	16.9	22.7	13.7	19.1	18.8
New Brunswick	24.8	18.1	20.9	19.7	20.8	18.4	17.8	15.5	18.7	20.2
Quebec	27.7	25.9	26.9	25.8	24.9	24.5	27.3	27.4	25.1	26.9
Ontario	23.5	21.6	20.2	20.0	21.9	21.9	21.8	19.6	21.2	20.9
Manitoba	19.3	18.1	18.5	16.1	19.5	17.4	22.1	22.0	18.6	19.4
Saskatchewan	19.9	20.3	18.3	18.8	19.2	19.9	17.5	18.3	19.6	18.7
Alberta	21.5	21.7	20.1	19.7	21.2	20.7	23.1	20.3	17.7	22.3
British Columbia	20.3	20.4	21.4	19.9	18.2	22.7	17.5	19.9	21.6	23.9
Yukon [4]	12.4E	21.7	17.3E	22.3	18.9	15.8E	18.3	17.3E	17.0	24.6
Northwest Territories [4]	21.1	17.6	19.3E	8.5E	18.3	15.4	13.2E	15.4E	12.7E	18.0
Nunavut [4, 5]	17.8E	16.3E	14.3E	20.6E	15.0E	17.5E	26.8E	16.9E	11.4E	16.1E

Symbol Legend:
E   Use with caution

Source: Statistics Canada. *Table 105-0503 - Health indicator profile, age-standardized rate, annual estimates, by sex, Canada, provinces and territories, occasional,* CANSIM (database). (accessed: March 27, 2017)

Please see footnotes 30, 31, 57, 58, 59, 60, 61, 62, 64 for characteristics of the age-standardized rate.

AGE-STANDARDIZED RATES, PERCEIVED LIFE STRESS, QUITE A LOT (15 YEARS AND OVER) (%), [10, 11] FEMALES, CANADA, PROVINCES AND TERRITORIES

Geography	2003	2005	2007	2008	2009	2010	2011	2012	2013	2014
Canada	25.0	23.9	23.6	23.4	25.0	25.1	25.4	24.7	25.2	24.3
Newfoundland and Labrador	14.2	15.9	14.8	10.0	14.1	14.0	13.7	13.7	16.9	16.1
Prince Edward Island	17.3	19.2	14.7	15.8	17.1	14.4	17.4	15.9	24.7	20.4
Nova Scotia	19.4	23.7	17.6	18.1	18.2	20.7	18.3	20.3	21.6	21.1
New Brunswick	24.1	20.8	20.5	17.6	22.7	22.7	20.7	21.5	20.7	22.0
Quebec	30.1	26.5	28.1	27.5	28.8	30.9	31.5	28.5	28.8	28.2
Ontario	25.0	23.8	23.6	23.6	26.1	24.8	24.5	24.9	25.8	23.9
Manitoba	21.5	21.8	21.0	22.0	21.3	21.9	23.6	19.1	20.7	25.0
Saskatchewan	22.1	21.7	19.4	21.3	19.2	19.6	20.2	22.4	20.3	23.0
Alberta	23.1	21.2	22.7	22.4	23.3	23.0	25.6	24.3	23.4	20.9
British Columbia	21.7	24.2	20.7	21.6	22.1	22.5	22.6	23.0	23.2	23.9
Yukon [4]	21.0	21.9	24.7	20.5	20.9E	18.9	23.6	25.0	24.9	25.9
Northwest Territories [4]	17.5	17.7	18.8	14.0E	16.8E	20.8E	22.7	22.2	21.3	22.2
Nunavut [4, 5]	25.4E	21.0E	16.4E	16.1E	20.0E	16.0E	19.5E	21.9E	21.7E	19.6E

Symbol Legend:
E   Use with caution

Source: Statistics Canada. *Table 105-0503 - Health indicator profile, age-standardized rate, annual estimates, by sex, Canada, provinces and territories, occasional,* CANSIM (database). (accessed: March 27, 2017)

Please see footnotes 30, 31, 57, 58, 59, 60, 61, 62, 64 for characteristics of the age-standardized rate.

AGE-STANDARDIZED RATES, OVERWEIGHT OR OBESE, ADULT (18 YEARS AND OVER) (%), [38], [39], [40], [41] BOTH SEXES, CANADA, PROVINCES AND TERRITORIES

Geography	2003	2005	2007	2008	2009	2010	2011	2012	2013	2014
Canada	48.1	48.6	49.2	49.6	49.8	50.6	50.4	50.7	51.7	52.1
Newfoundland and Labrador	59.3	61.6	61.1	61.2	62.2	61.6	68.5	61.1	66.8	66.9
Prince Edward Island	59.1	59.5	59.0	57.7	57.1	54.9	54.0	60.9	60.5	59.5
Nova Scotia	54.2	56.4	55.9	62.1	57.9	58.3	58.2	58.4	59.2	60.5
New Brunswick	56.2	59.0	58.2	59.2	61.5	61.0	56.9	57.7	62.5	61.1
Quebec	46.0	45.4	46.2	46.3	46.9	49.7	47.9	48.2	51.3	49.0
Ontario	48.2	48.4	49.9	49.9	49.6	50.9	50.7	51.4	51.0	52.6
Manitoba	54.1	53.6	54.2	53.6	56.4	59.7	58.0	55.8	55.6	60.1
Saskatchewan	55.8	57.3	55.2	59.2	57.1	59.3	58.4	57.8	60.0	57.1
Alberta	50.6	51.2	52.5	52.0	54.4	50.8	51.5	52.2	53.9	53.8
British Columbia	42.3	44.6	42.7	43.5	43.3	42.1	44.6	44.8	45.0	46.2
Yukon [4]	51.6	49.5	52.3	49.5	51.1	47.1	54.2	48.4	62.1	54.8
Northwest Territories [4]	54.5	58.9	58.5	61.9	61.2	54.2	58.5	61.5	57.1	63.3
Nunavut [4] [5]	52.9	61.3	53.0	63.7	56.5	63.1	63.6	52.7	60.0	50.8

Source: Statistics Canada. *Table 105-0503 - Health indicator profile, age-standardized rate, annual estimates, by sex, Canada, provinces and territories, occasional,* CANSIM (database). (accessed: March 27, 2017)

Please see footnotes [30], [31], [57], [58], [59], [60], [61], [62], [64] for characteristics of the age-standardized rate.

AGE-STANDARDIZED RATES, OVERWEIGHT OR OBESE, ADULT (18 YEARS AND OVER) (%), [38], [39], [40], [41] MALES, CANADA, PROVINCES AND TERRITORIES

Geography	2003	2005	2007	2008	2009	2010	2011	2012	2013	2014
Canada	56.2	56.9	57.5	57.2	57.4	59.1	58.2	58.5	60.4	60.1
Newfoundland and Labrador	66.5	68.5	64.0	67.7	74.6	66.4	75.7	71.3	72.4	71.6
Prince Edward Island	69.1	65.8	68.5	66.4	66.7	64.3	63.8	71.3	63.6	61.7
Nova Scotia	63.4	65.2	63.5	65.8	65.1	66.5	65.5	68.0	61.6	66.1
New Brunswick	62.3	65.8	65.1	67.6	66.4	63.7	59.9	67.2	66.9	67.3
Quebec	54.3	53.7	53.9	54.3	54.1	58.7	56.0	55.6	59.8	57.6
Ontario	56.1	56.7	58.1	57.9	56.9	59.4	58.0	59.4	59.8	60.4
Manitoba	62.6	61.4	62.0	59.9	64.0	66.9	64.1	66.1	63.5	67.5
Saskatchewan	62.9	66.3	64.7	67.1	62.9	69.1	65.5	67.6	68.8	62.5
Alberta	58.3	59.2	60.4	59.9	62.9	59.2	60.8	57.8	63.6	62.4
British Columbia	50.9	53.2	52.9	50.3	52.5	52.1	53.5	52.3	55.3	55.4
Yukon [4]	56.9	53.4	60.1	52.7	54.8	50.8	59.2	57.2	66.7	57.8
Northwest Territories [4]	58.3	63.1	62.2	61.2	62.8	61.5	62.9	61.1	59.2	68.9
Nunavut [4], [5]	56.9	65.3	50.0	72.4	51.7	61.1	69.2	50.7	56.4	48.3

Source: Statistics Canada. *Table 105-0503 - Health indicator profile, age-standardized rate, annual estimates, by sex, Canada, provinces and territories, occasional,* CANSIM (database). (accessed: March 27, 2017)

Please see footnotes 30, 31, 57, 58, 59, 60, 61, 62, 64 for characteristics of the age-standardized rate.

AGE-STANDARDIZED RATES, OVERWEIGHT OR OBESE, ADULT (18 YEARS AND OVER) (%), [38], [39], [40], [41] FEMALES, CANADA, PROVINCES AND TERRITORIES

Geography	2003	2005	2007	2008	2009	2010	2011	2012	2013	2014
Canada	39.9	40.2	41.0	41.9	42.0	41.8	42.5	42.8	42.9	43.9
Newfoundland and Labrador	52.0	54.6	58.2	55.1	50.5	57.0	61.2	50.9	61.3	62.2
Prince Edward Island	48.5	53.4	50.0	49.4	48.7	45.4	44.0	51.2	57.5	57.6
Nova Scotia	45.1	47.8	48.6	58.6	51.0	50.8	51.4	49.4	57.0	55.2
New Brunswick	50.0	52.1	51.7	50.7	56.8	58.5	53.9	48.8	58.1	55.1
Quebec	37.5	36.9	38.5	38.1	39.5	40.4	39.5	40.6	42.5	40.1
Ontario	40.2	40.0	41.8	42.0	42.2	42.4	43.5	43.4	42.1	44.7
Manitoba	45.3	45.6	46.2	47.1	48.4	52.5	51.6	44.8	47.3	52.6
Saskatchewan	48.2	47.7	45.8	50.9	50.8	49.1	50.8	47.4	50.6	51.1
Alberta	42.2	42.5	43.9	43.4	45.0	41.6	41.4	46.1	43.5	44.6
British Columbia	33.3	35.9	32.8	36.6	34.1	31.8	35.5	37.3	34.4	36.6
Yukon [4]	46.1	45.6	44.5	46.2	47.2	43.2	48.7	39.7	57.2	51.6
Northwest Territories [4]	50.1	53.8	54.4	62.8	59.5	46.3	53.2	62.0	54.8	57.0
Nunavut [4],[5]	48.7	56.3	56.5	52.6	61.0	65.6	56.6	55.5	64.1	54.0

Source: Statistics Canada. *Table 105-0503 - Health indicator profile, age-standardized rate, annual estimates, by sex, Canada, provinces and territories, occasional,* CANSIM (database). (accessed: March 27, 2017)

Please see footnotes [30], [31], [57], [58], [59], [60], [61], [62], [64] for characteristics of the age-standardized rate.

AGE-STANDARDIZED RATES, OVERWEIGHT, ADULT (18 YEARS AND OVER) (%), [38], [39], [40], [41] BOTH SEXES, CANADA, PROVINCES AND TERRITORIES

Geography	2003	2005	2007	2008	2009	2010	2011	2012	2013	2014
Canada	33.2	33.3	33.0	32.8	32.6	33.1	32.8	33.1	33.6	32.5
Newfoundland and Labrador	38.8	37.7	38.8	34.6	36.2	33.4	39.9	35.5	37.7	36.8
Prince Edward Island	38.2	36.5	37.0	35.6	34.4	36.1	31.5	34.8	34.4	36.3
Nova Scotia	34.4	35.6	34.8	37.0	34.9	33.4	36.5	32.8	33.3	33.0
New Brunswick	36.1	36.5	37.4	36.0	33.3	34.2	32.9	31.8	37.0	36.4
Quebec	32.4	31.5	31.2	31.3	30.9	34.3	31.8	32.1	33.5	31.6
Ontario	33.4	33.5	33.6	33.4	32.9	32.9	33.1	34.0	34.0	32.8
Manitoba	35.4	35.5	35.6	33.4	34.4	35.6	36.6	35.8	32.1	36.0
Saskatchewan	35.5	36.2	34.1	34.2	35.6	37.9	37.2	33.1	35.0	32.7
Alberta	34.8	35.3	33.7	34.0	35.7	32.6	32.8	33.8	34.9	32.9
British Columbia	30.6	31.7	30.9	30.7	30.4	29.7	30.2	31.2	30.7	30.8
Yukon [4]	31.6	30.9	26.3	32.1	30.4	30.7	36.8	31.5	42.9	33.2
Northwest Territories [4]	31.7	33.6	35.7	37.0	35.0	30.9	32.8	35.2	32.7	29.6
Nunavut [4, 5]	32.2	34.7	33.5	32.5	30.7		35.8	30.8	33.1	26.6E

Symbol Legend:
E   Use with caution

Source: Statistics Canada. *Table 105-0503 - Health indicator profile, age-standardized rate, annual estimates, by sex, Canada, provinces and territories, occasional,* CANSIM (database). (accessed: March 27, 2017)

Please see footnotes 30, 31, 57, 58, 59, 60, 61, 62, 64 for characteristics of the age-standardized rate.

AGE-STANDARDIZED RATES, OVERWEIGHT, ADULT (18 YEARS AND OVER) (%), [38],[39],[40],[41] MALES, CANADA, PROVINCES AND TERRITORIES

Geography	2003	2005	2007	2008	2009	2010	2011	2012	2013	2014
Canada	40.5	40.5	40.1	39.4	39.1	40.1	39.3	40.5	40.8	38.9
Newfoundland and Labrador	46.0	43.4	40.6	38.9	45.0	37.4	44.6	43.3	45.1	40.0
Prince Edward Island	46.9	41.9	46.7	46.7	42.2	44.1	39.4	43.3	37.0	37.5
Nova Scotia	41.8	44.8	41.4	44.3	41.2	38.4	41.9	42.8	36.8	38.7
New Brunswick	42.6	43.4	45.4	44.2	38.6	35.7	36.1	40.6	43.1	41.9
Quebec	40.3	38.4	37.6	38.3	37.2	42.0	38.7	39.4	39.2	38.7
Ontario	40.4	40.8	40.9	40.0	38.9	39.9	39.1	41.9	42.1	38.8
Manitoba	42.9	42.1	41.7	39.0	40.5	44.8	42.2	45.9	37.8	41.4
Saskatchewan	40.6	43.0	41.8	40.1	40.5	46.4	43.2	40.0	42.6	37.2
Alberta	41.8	42.0	40.2	40.8	42.9	39.3	39.7	39.4	43.0	39.6
British Columbia	37.8	39.4	40.1	36.6	38.0	36.6	38.1	37.1	38.4	38.0
Yukon [4]	38.3	37.8	30.4	37.7	34.5	31.7	40.0	38.6	43.3	37.8
Northwest Territories [4]	35.4	37.5	41.5	35.8	39.1	36.4	38.4	38.8	35.2	34.2
Nunavut [4],[5]	36.4	40.8	33.4	36.2	25.7E	37.9E	46.1	33.3	36.2E	25.8E

Symbol Legend:
E Use with caution

Source: Statistics Canada. *Table 105-0503 - Health indicator profile, age-standardized rate, annual estimates, by sex, Canada, provinces and territories, occasional,* CANSIM (database). (accessed: March 27, 2017)

Please see footnotes [30], [31], [57], [58], [59], [60], [61], [62], [64] for characteristics of the age-standardized rate.

AGE-STANDARDIZED RATES, OVERWEIGHT, ADULT (18 YEARS AND OVER) (%), [38], [39], [40], [41] FEMALES, CANADA, PROVINCES AND TERRITORIES

Geography	2003	2005	2007	2008	2009	2010	2011	2012	2013	2014
Canada	25.8	26.0	25.8	26.1	26.0	25.9	26.1	25.6	26.2	26.0
Newfoundland and Labrador	31.5	32.1	37.0	30.6	28.0	29.6	35.2	27.8	30.3	33.4
Prince Edward Island	28.9	31.3	27.9	25.1	27.5	28.0	23.5	27.0	31.8	35.3
Nova Scotia	27.1	26.7	28.4	30.0	28.7	28.8	31.4	23.4	30.1	27.5
New Brunswick	29.4	29.4	29.8	27.8	28.4	32.8	29.7	23.4	30.9	31.0
Quebec	24.3	24.5	24.8	24.2	24.5	26.3	24.6	24.6	27.6	24.2
Ontario	26.3	26.1	26.4	26.8	26.8	25.8	27.1	26.1	25.7	26.8
Manitoba	27.5	28.8	29.3	27.6	28.0	26.3	30.7	25.0	26.2	30.5
Saskatchewan	30.1	28.9	26.3	27.9	30.3	28.9	30.8	25.8	26.8	27.7
Alberta	27.4	28.1	26.7	26.7	27.6	25.2	25.2	27.7	26.0	25.9
British Columbia	23.1	23.9	21.9	24.8	22.7	22.6	22.1	25.2	22.8	23.4
Yukon [4]	24.7	24.1	22.1	26.2	26.3	29.7	33.3	24.3E	42.4	28.3
Northwest Territories [4]	27.6	29.0	29.2	38.4	31.0	25.0	26.3	31.0	29.9	24.3E
Nunavut [4], [5]	27.9	26.9	33.6E	27.7E	35.4E	43.2E	22.9E	27.3E	29.3E	27.6E

Symbol Legend:
E   Use with caution

Source: Statistics Canada. *Table 105-0503 - Health indicator profile, age-standardized rate, annual estimates, by sex, Canada, provinces and territories, occasional,* CANSIM (database). (accessed: March 27, 2017)

Please see footnotes [30], [31], [57], [58], [59], [60], [61], [62], [64] for characteristics of the age-standardized rate.

AGE-STANDARDIZED RATES, OBESE, ADULT (18 YEARS AND OVER) (%), [38], [39], [40], [41] BOTH SEXES, CANADA, PROVINCES AND TERRITORIES

Geography	2003	2005	2007	2008	2009	2010	2011	2012	2013	2014
Canada	14.9	15.3	16.3	16.7	17.2	17.5	17.7	17.6	18.2	19.5
Newfoundland and Labrador	20.5	23.8	22.3	26.6	25.9	28.2	28.5	25.6	29.1	30.2
Prince Edward Island	20.9	23.0	22.0	22.1	22.7	18.8	22.4	26.1	26.1	23.2
Nova Scotia	19.8	20.8	21.1	25.1	23.1	24.9	21.7	25.6	25.9	27.5
New Brunswick	20.1	22.5	20.8	23.2	28.1	26.8	24.0	26.0	25.5	24.8
Quebec	13.6	13.8	15.1	14.9	16.0	15.4	16.1	16.2	17.8	17.4
Ontario	14.8	14.9	16.3	16.5	16.7	18.0	17.6	17.4	17.0	19.7
Manitoba	18.8	18.1	18.6	20.2	22.0	24.1	21.4	20.0	23.5	24.2
Saskatchewan	20.3	21.1	21.2	25.0	21.5	21.5	21.2	24.7	25.1	24.4
Alberta	15.7	15.9	18.8	17.9	18.8	18.2	18.7	18.4	19.1	20.9
British Columbia	11.7	12.9	11.8	12.7	12.9	12.4	14.4	13.6	14.3	15.3
Yukon [4]	19.9	18.6	26.0	17.4	20.6	16.4	17.3	17.0	19.2	21.6
Northwest Territories [4]	22.7	25.2	22.9	24.9	26.1	23.3	25.6	26.3	24.4	33.7
Nunavut [4], [5]	20.7	26.6	19.5	31.2	25.8	22.9E	27.8	22.0	26.9	24.2

Symbol Legend:
E   Use with caution

Source: Statistics Canada. *Table 105-0503 - Health indicator profile, age-standardized rate, annual estimates, by sex, Canada, provinces and territories, occasional,* CANSIM (database). (accessed: March 27, 2017)

Please see footnotes [30], [31], [57], [58], [59], [60], [61], [62], [64] for characteristics of the age-standardized rate.

AGE-STANDARDIZED RATES, OBESE, ADULT (18 YEARS AND OVER) (%), [38], [39], [40], [41] MALES, CANADA, PROVINCES AND TERRITORIES

Geography	2003	2005	2007	2008	2009	2010	2011	2012	2013	2014
Canada	15.8	16.4	17.4	17.8	18.4	19.1	18.9	18.0	19.6	21.2
Newfoundland and Labrador	20.5	25.1	23.4	28.8	29.6	29.0	31.1	28.0	27.3	31.6
Prince Edward Island	22.1	23.9	21.8	19.7	24.5	20.2	24.4	28.0	26.6	24.3
Nova Scotia	21.7	20.4	22.1	21.5	23.9	28.1	23.6	25.2	24.8	27.3
New Brunswick	19.7	22.3	19.7	23.4	27.8	28.0	23.8	26.5	23.8	25.4
Quebec	14.0	15.3	16.4	16.0	17.0	16.7	17.3	16.3	20.6	18.9
Ontario	15.7	15.9	17.2	17.9	17.9	19.4	18.9	17.6	17.7	21.6
Manitoba	19.7	19.3	20.4	20.9	23.5	22.0	21.9	20.1	25.7	26.1
Saskatchewan	22.4	23.3	22.9	26.9	22.5	22.7	22.3	27.6	26.2	25.3
Alberta	16.5	17.2	20.3	19.1	20.0	20.0	21.1	18.4	20.5	22.8
British Columbia	13.1	13.8	12.8	13.7	14.4	15.5	15.4	15.1	16.9	17.4
Yukon [4]	18.6	15.5E	29.7	15.0E	20.4	19.1E	19.2	18.6E	23.4	20.0
Northwest Territories [4]	22.9	25.7	20.7	25.3	23.8E	25.2E	24.6	22.3	23.9	34.7
Nunavut [4], [5]	20.5	24.4	16.6E	36.2E	26.0E	23.3E	23.1E	17.4E	20.2E	22.5E

Symbol Legend:
E   Use with caution

Source: Statistics Canada. *Table 105-0503 - Health indicator profile, age-standardized rate, annual estimates, by sex, Canada, provinces and territories, occasional,* CANSIM (database). (accessed: March 27, 2017)

Please see footnotes 30, 31, 57, 58, 59, 60, 61, 62, 64 for characteristics of the age-standardized rate.

AGE-STANDARDIZED RATES, OBESE, ADULT (18 YEARS AND OVER) (%), [38], [39], [40], [41] FEMALES, CANADA, PROVINCES AND TERRITORIES

Geography	2003	2005	2007	2008	2009	2010	2011	2012	2013	2014
Canada	14.0	14.2	15.2	15.7	15.9	15.9	16.4	17.2	16.7	17.8
Newfoundland and Labrador	20.4	22.6	21.2	24.6	22.4	27.3	26.0	23.2	31.0	28.8
Prince Edward Island	19.6	22.0	22.1	24.3	21.2	17.4	20.5	24.3	25.7	22.3
Nova Scotia	18.0	21.2	20.2	28.6	22.3	21.9	20.0	26.0	26.9	27.7
New Brunswick	20.6	22.7	21.9	22.9	28.4	25.7	24.2	25.5	27.2	24.2
Quebec	13.2	12.4	13.8	13.8	15.1	14.0	14.9	16.1	14.9	15.9
Ontario	13.9	13.9	15.5	15.2	15.4	16.6	16.4	17.3	16.4	17.9
Manitoba	17.8	16.9	16.9	19.5	20.4	26.2	20.9	19.8	21.1	22.1
Saskatchewan	18.1	18.8	19.4	23.0	20.5	20.1	20.0	21.6	23.8	23.4
Alberta	14.8	14.4	17.2	16.7	17.4	16.4	16.2	18.4	17.4	18.8
British Columbia	10.3	12.1	10.9	11.8	11.3	9.2	13.4	12.1	11.6	13.2
Yukon [4]	21.3	21.6	22.4	19.9	20.9	13.4E	15.3	15.4	14.8E	23.3
Northwest Territories [4]	22.6	24.8	25.3	24.3E	28.5	21.3	26.9	31.0	24.9	32.7
Nunavut [4, 5]	20.8	29.4	22.9E	24.9E	25.5	22.4E	33.7E	28.1E	34.8E	26.4E

Symbol Legend:
E   Use with caution

Source: Statistics Canada. *Table 105-0503 - Health indicator profile, age-standardized rate, annual estimates, by sex, Canada, provinces and territories, occasional,* CANSIM (database). (accessed: March 27, 2017)

Please see footnotes [30], [31], [57], [58], [59], [60], [61], [62], [64] for characteristics of the age-standardized rate.

AGE-STANDARDIZED RATES, ARTHRITIS (%), [12], [13] BOTH SEXES, CANADA, PROVINCES AND TERRITORIES

Geography	2003	2005	2007	2008	2009	2010	2011	2012	2013	2014
Canada	16.1	15.3	13.8	13.9	13.2	13.6	14.2	12.7	13.0	13.3
Newfoundland and Labrador	19.3	18.8	17.4	17.1	17.5	18.2	16.1	17.9	16.1	18.7
Prince Edward Island	19.1	18.2	16.5	15.8	15.7	13.8	16.8	14.7	16.4	14.8
Nova Scotia	22.4	20.3	20.0	18.3	19.7	21.7	17.4	16.8	17.6	17.9
New Brunswick	19.2	18.2	15.8	17.3	14.3	15.8	15.0	14.1	15.5	19.0
Quebec	12.9	12.8	9.8	9.7	8.9	9.4	13.0	8.5	7.8	8.5
Ontario	16.9	16.2	15.2	15.5	14.6	14.8	15.1	13.7	14.6	15.0
Manitoba	17.1	17.0	14.2	16.0	14.9	16.1	16.0	14.6	16.2	15.2
Saskatchewan	17.7	17.1	14.8	16.1	15.6	15.6	15.3	14.7	13.6	14.1
Alberta	17.5	15.6	14.6	14.6	14.4	14.8	13.9	13.8	14.8	14.8
British Columbia	15.0	14.1	13.5	13.0	12.2	12.8	12.1	13.1	12.9	12.5
Yukon [4]	19.0	16.5	15.4	12.5	14.6	15.5	14.1	12.6	17.8	16.8
Northwest Territories [4]	16.4	17.0	12.8	13.1	16.8	16.3	13.7E	17.6	14.1	17.7
Nunavut [4], [5]	11.8E	12.8E	11.3	18.1	11.5E	16.5E	12.1E	14.8E	14.0E	16.6E

Symbol Legend:
E   Use with caution

Source: Statistics Canada. *Table 105-0503 - Health indicator profile, age-standardized rate, annual estimates, by sex, Canada, provinces and territories, occasional,* CANSIM (database). (accessed: March 27, 2017)

Please see footnotes 30, 31, 57, 58, 59, 60, 61, 62, 64 for characteristics of the age-standardized rate.

AGE-STANDARDIZED RATES, ARTHRITIS (%), [12], [13] MALES, CANADA, PROVINCES AND TERRITORIES

Geography	2003	2005	2007	2008	2009	2010	2011	2012	2013	2014
Canada	12.2	11.8	10.7	10.9	10.1	10.6	10.6	9.9	10.1	10.6
Newfoundland and Labrador	16.4	14.2	14.9	14.6	12.8	15.9	14.9	16.4	11.8	14.8
Prince Edward Island	15.6	15.2	14.2	12.4	11.8	13.1	12.9	12.5	14.1	12.2
Nova Scotia	19.3	17.0	17.1	15.4	15.9	17.7	13.5	11.7	14.9	14.5
New Brunswick	15.0	13.7	13.8	14.2	11.7	11.7	11.7	12.6	11.6	16.9
Quebec	8.6	9.4	7.2	7.1	6.3	6.8	8.5	5.9	5.2	6.4
Ontario	12.8	12.4	11.7	12.2	11.0	11.4	11.6	10.8	11.4	11.9
Manitoba	14.5	14.4	10.7	10.1	11.9	11.6	13.1	12.1	15.0	13.2
Saskatchewan	15.1	14.2	12.0	13.2	13.1	12.8	13.3	12.0	10.8	12.0
Alberta	13.0	12.1	11.8	12.2	11.2	11.6	10.8	10.9	11.9	12.3
British Columbia	12.1	10.8	10.6	10.5	9.8	10.9	8.8	10.8	10.6	9.3
Yukon [4]	16.3	13.7	12.1E	9.9E	10.1E	15.4E	11.7	11.0E	14.9E	12.3
Northwest Territories [4]	13.7	14.6	11.0E	12.2E	13.3E	12.1E	8.5E	19.3	12.9E	17.7
Nunavut [4], [5]	3.8E	13.2	6.6E	17.9E	F	13.8E	12.0E	13.3E	F	F

Symbol Legend:

E Use with caution

F Too unreliable to be published

Source: Statistics Canada. *Table 105-0503 - Health indicator profile, age-standardized rate, annual estimates, by sex, Canada, provinces and territories, occasional,* CANSIM (database). (accessed: March 27, 2017)

Please see footnotes 30, 31, 57, 58, 59, 60, 61, 62, 64 for characteristics of the age-standardized rate.

AGE-STANDARDIZED RATES, ARTHRITIS (%), [12], [13] FEMALES, CANADA, PROVINCES AND TERRITORIES

Geography	2003	2005	2007	2008	2009	2010	2011	2012	2013	2014
Canada	19.8	18.8	16.7	16.8	16.2	16.5	17.6	15.4	15.8	16.0
Newfoundland and Labrador	22.1	23.2	19.8	19.4	21.9	20.4	17.2	19.3	20.0	22.5
Prince Edward Island	22.5	20.9	18.5	19.0	19.1	14.4	20.6	16.9	18.5	17.3
Nova Scotia	25.4	23.4	22.9	21.0	23.3	25.4	21.0	21.6	20.1	21.2
New Brunswick	23.3	22.5	17.8	20.3	16.7	19.8	18.1	15.6	19.4	20.9
Quebec	17.1	16.1	12.2	12.3	11.5	12.0	17.4	11.1	10.4	10.6
Ontario	20.9	19.9	18.6	18.7	18.0	18.0	18.4	16.6	17.7	17.9
Manitoba	19.6	19.5	17.5	21.9	17.8	20.5	19.0	17.0	17.4	17.1
Saskatchewan	20.3	19.9	17.5	19.1	18.0	18.5	17.3	17.4	16.5	16.2
Alberta	21.9	19.1	17.4	17.1	17.8	18.1	17.1	16.7	17.8	17.3
British Columbia	17.8	17.2	16.3	15.4	14.4	14.8	15.2	15.4	15.1	15.7
Yukon [4]	21.6	19.3	18.7	15.1	19.1	15.7	16.6	14.4	20.7	21.3
Northwest Territories [4]	19.3	19.7	14.7	14.1E	20.3	20.9	19.0E	15.7	15.4E	17.7
Nunavut [4], [5]	19.5E	F	16.0E	18.2E	12.5E	F	12.2E	16.5E	15.6E	23.7E

Symbol Legend:
E   Use with caution
F   Too unreliable to be published

Source: Statistics Canada. *Table 105-0503 - Health indicator profile, age-standardized rate, annual estimates, by sex, Canada, provinces and territories, occasional,* CANSIM (database). (accessed: March 27, 2017)

Please see footnotes 30, 31, 57, 58, 59, 60, 61, 62, 64 for characteristics of the age-standardized rate.

AGE-STANDARDIZED RATES, DIABETES (%), [14], [15] BOTH SEXES, CANADA, PROVINCES AND TERRITORIES

Geography	2003	2005	2007	2008	2009	2010	2011	2012	2013	2014
Canada	4.2	4.3	5.1	5.0	5.1	5.4	5.1	5.2	5.3	5.2
Newfoundland and Labrador	5.7	5.9	7.5	7.5	6.7	6.5	8.6	5.7	6.2	6.5
Prince Edward Island	4.7	5.5	5.1	6.2	5.1	7.3	5.5	5.9	6.3	5.6
Nova Scotia	4.8	5.7	5.6	5.6	5.9	6.5	6.6	6.6	5.7	6.0
New Brunswick	4.8	4.9	6.0	6.2	5.4	6.0	6.7	5.6	5.5	5.7
Quebec	4.0	4.4	4.8	4.9	4.7	4.4	4.6	4.9	5.5	5.0
Ontario	4.2	4.4	5.4	5.2	5.4	6.2	5.5	5.5	5.5	5.8
Manitoba	4.7	3.9	4.4	4.4	5.0	5.0	5.5	5.1	5.7	4.2
Saskatchewan	4.3	4.3	4.8	5.5	4.9	6.1	4.9	5.5	5.9	5.3
Alberta	3.7	3.9	4.5	4.6	4.7	5.2	4.5	5.7	5.0	4.7
British Columbia	4.1	4.0	4.8	4.2	4.5	4.3	4.1	4.5	4.2	4.1
Yukon [4]	5.2E	4.9E	5.3	2.3E	4.2E	5.4E	4.2E	6.9E	4.7E	7.3
Northwest Territories [4]	6.1	4.7E	5.1E	4.6E	5.9E	3.6E	4.4E	4.7E	5.3E	8.7E
Nunavut [4], [5]	F	F	F	F	5.4E	F	F	F	F	F

Symbol Legend:

E   Use with caution

F   Too unreliable to be published

Source: Statistics Canada. *Table 105-0503 - Health indicator profile, age-standardized rate, annual estimates, by sex, Canada, provinces and territories, occasional,* CANSIM (database). (accessed: March 27, 2017)

Please see footnotes 30, 31, 57, 58, 59, 60, 61, 62, 64 for characteristics of the age-standardized rate.

AGE-STANDARDIZED RATES, DIABETES (%), [14], [15] MALES, CANADA, PROVINCES AND TERRITORIES

Geography	2003	2005	2007	2008	2009	2010	2011	2012	2013	2014
Canada	4.4	4.7	5.6	5.3	5.6	6.2	5.5	5.6	5.7	5.9
Newfoundland and Labrador	6.4	6.1	7.1	7.7	6.8	5.8	7.8	5.0	6.4	5.4
Prince Edward Island	6.0	6.4	6.1[E]	7.3[E]	6.6[E]	9.1[E]	6.4[E]	6.2	6.7[E]	6.6[E]
Nova Scotia	5.1	5.4	6.9	6.0	6.2	7.5	6.6	6.8	6.6	6.4
New Brunswick	4.9	4.6	6.7	5.9	5.5	7.0	7.9	7.2	4.9	6.3
Quebec	4.1	4.6	5.4	5.2	5.5	5.0	5.0	5.1	6.1	5.5
Ontario	4.4	5.0	5.9	5.6	5.8	7.4	6.1	5.5	5.6	6.6
Manitoba	5.7	4.6	4.9	4.7	6.0	5.1	5.8[E]	7.5	6.2	4.6
Saskatchewan	4.3	5.0	5.2	5.9	5.1	5.4	5.2	5.9	6.7	5.5
Alberta	4.1	4.1	4.4	4.7	5.5	6.1	5.0	6.2	5.8	5.7
British Columbia	4.7	4.2	5.6	4.6	5.1	5.1	4.2	4.9	4.7	4.8
Yukon [4]	5.6[E]	3.2[E]	4.1[E]	2.7[E]	F	6.8[E]	3.8[E]	8.4[E]	4.0[E]	7.0[E]
Northwest Territories [4]	6.5[E]	4.3[E]	F	6.0[E]	F	2.7[E]	4.1[E]	4.1[E]	5.6[E]	F
Nunavut [4], [5]	F	F	F	F	F	F	F	F	F	F

Symbol Legend:
E   Use with caution
F   Too unreliable to be published

Source: Statistics Canada. *Table 105-0503 - Health indicator profile, age-standardized rate, annual estimates, by sex, Canada, provinces and territories, occasional,* CANSIM (database). (accessed: March 27, 2017)

Please see footnotes 30, 31, 57, 58, 59, 60, 61, 62, 64 for characteristics of the age-standardized rate.

AGE-STANDARDIZED RATES, DIABETES (%), [14], [15] FEMALES, CANADA, PROVINCES AND TERRITORIES

Geography	2003	2005	2007	2008	2009	2010	2011	2012	2013	2014
Canada	3.9	4.0	4.6	4.7	4.5	4.6	4.7	4.9	4.9	4.6
Newfoundland and Labrador	5.1	5.7	7.9	7.3	6.7	7.2	9.3	6.4	6.1	7.5
Prince Edward Island	3.4	4.7	4.3E	5.2E	3.9E	5.6E	4.7E	5.6E	6.0	4.7
Nova Scotia	4.4	6.0	4.4	5.3	5.6	5.6	6.7	6.4	4.8	5.7
New Brunswick	4.6	5.3	5.3	6.6	5.3	5.1	5.5	4.1	6.0	5.1
Quebec	3.9	4.2	4.2	4.5	4.0	3.8	4.2	4.6	4.8	4.6
Ontario	4.1	3.7	4.9	4.9	5.0	5.0	5.0	5.4	5.3	5.1
Manitoba	3.7	3.3	4.0	4.1	4.0	4.9	5.3	2.7	5.2	3.9
Saskatchewan	4.3	3.7	4.4	5.1	4.7	6.8	4.5	5.0	5.1E	5.1
Alberta	3.3	3.6	4.6	4.5	3.8	4.3	4.0	5.1	4.2	3.7
British Columbia	3.4	3.8	4.1	3.7	4.0	3.6	4.1	4.2	3.7	3.5
Yukon [4]	4.7E	6.6E	6.4E	F	5.7E	4.1E	4.6E	5.3E	5.4E	7.5E
Northwest Territories [4]	5.6E	5.3E	5.2E	F	F	F	4.6E	5.3E	5.0E	7.7E
Nunavut [4], [5]	F	F	F	F	F	F	F	F	F	F

Symbol Legend:
E   Use with caution
F   Too unreliable to be published

Source: Statistics Canada. *Table 105-0503 - Health indicator profile, age-standardized rate, annual estimates, by sex, Canada, provinces and territories, occasional,* CANSIM (database). (accessed: March 27, 2017)

Please see footnotes 30, 31, 57, 58, 59, 60, 61, 62, 64 for characteristics of the age-standardized rate.

AGE-STANDARDIZED RATES, ASTHMA (%), [16] BOTH SEXES, CANADA, PROVINCES AND TERRITORIES

Geography	2003	2005	2007	2008	2009	2010	2011	2012	2013	2014
Canada	8.5	8.4	8.1	8.6	8.3	8.6	8.8	8.3	8.1	8.2
Newfoundland and Labrador	9.0	9.6	5.5	8.4	9.5	8.5	9.3	8.8	8.3	8.7
Prince Edward Island	9.1	8.6	9.1	7.5	7.6	11.2	11.8E	8.9E	8.3	8.8
Nova Scotia	9.4	9.9	11.3	10.4	10.0	10.0	10.3	10.4	9.5	10.2
New Brunswick	9.2	8.8	9.0	9.4	7.9	8.6	10.2	9.7	10.1	7.7
Quebec	8.7	8.7	8.2	9.0	7.6	8.8	9.5	8.3	8.5	9.1
Ontario	8.4	8.1	8.1	8.4	8.4	8.4	7.9	8.1	7.6	7.7
Manitoba	9.0	7.9	7.5	11.0	11.2	9.4	11.6	7.5	9.4	9.2
Saskatchewan	8.1	8.8	8.8	8.6	9.1	8.6	8.9	10.7	7.3	8.3
Alberta	9.3	8.6	8.9	8.0	8.8	9.4	9.1	7.9	8.8	8.3
British Columbia	7.5	8.4	6.9	7.5	7.6	7.9	8.4	8.0	7.3	7.5
Yukon [4]	8.2	8.9	8.5	8.0E	10.2	9.6	9.9E	9.8	8.4	6.6
Northwest Territories [4]	8.1	8.4	5.3E	6.3E	6.7E	7.0	6.6E	6.7E	5.3E	8.7E
Nunavut [4] [5]	4.6E	5.2E	F	F	5.7E	F	6.3E	3.5E	8.5E	6.7E

Symbol Legend:
E   Use with caution
F   Too unreliable to be published

Source: Statistics Canada. *Table 105-0503 - Health indicator profile, age-standardized rate, annual estimates, by sex, Canada, provinces and territories, occasional,* CANSIM (database). (accessed: March 29, 2017)

Please see footnotes 30, 31, 57, 58, 59, 60, 61, 62, 64 for characteristics of the age-standardized rate.

AGE-STANDARDIZED RATES, ASTHMA (%), [16] MALES, CANADA, PROVINCES AND TERRITORIES

Geography	2003	2005	2007	2008	2009	2010	2011	2012	2013	2014
Canada	7.3	7.1	6.8	7.4	7.0	7.4	7.6	7.1	7.2	7.1
Newfoundland and Labrador	8.9	8.2	4.8E	7.6	9.1	7.1E	7.5	8.8E	4.8E	8.4E
Prince Edward Island	7.5	7.0	7.7E	7.0E	7.9E	10.1E	11.1E	6.5E	8.2E	8.8E
Nova Scotia	8.0	8.4	8.6	8.2E	8.3E	9.2E	9.1	8.4E	9.3	7.4E
New Brunswick	7.6	8.2	6.5	8.0	6.1	7.7	7.3E	8.6	8.5E	7.4E
Quebec	7.4	6.7	7.0	7.6	7.4	6.9	8.3	7.2	7.2	8.3
Ontario	7.0	6.8	6.6	7.3	7.0	7.3	6.9	7.0	6.8	6.5
Manitoba	7.7	7.7	6.1	8.9	8.5	7.7	10.3E	6.4E	10.4	7.7
Saskatchewan	6.9	8.2	8.6	8.8	8.9	8.1	8.3	8.2	5.9	7.2
Alberta	8.2	7.4	7.3	6.8	6.7	8.9	8.3	7.4	8.1	7.2
British Columbia	6.9	7.0	6.4	6.8	5.6	7.0	6.8	6.2	6.9	6.6
Yukon [4]	6.0E	6.7E	6.8E	5.7E	6.9E	6.3E	6.9E	9.6E	6.8E	F
Northwest Territories [4]	8.0E	5.4E	F	4.6E	5.3E	4.5E	5.9E	4.9E	4.2E	7.3E
Nunavut [4, 5]	F	F	F	F	5.4E	F	F	F	8.1E	8.7E

Symbol Legend:

E Use with caution

F Too unreliable to be published

Source: Statistics Canada. *Table 105-0503 - Health indicator profile, age-standardized rate, annual estimates, by sex, Canada, provinces and territories, occasional,* CANSIM (database). (accessed: March 29, 2017)

Please see footnotes 30, 31, 57, 58, 59, 60, 61, 62, 64 for characteristics of the age-standardized rate.

AGE-STANDARDIZED RATES, ASTHMA (%), [16] FEMALES, CANADA, PROVINCES AND TERRITORIES

Geography	2003	2005	2007	2008	2009	2010	2011	2012	2013	2014
Canada	9.7	9.8	9.4	9.7	9.6	9.8	9.9	9.5	9.0	9.3
Newfoundland and Labrador	9.2	11.0	6.2	9.1	9.9	9.8	11.0	8.9	11.7	9.0
Prince Edward Island	10.6	10.1	10.4	8.0E	7.4E	12.3	12.5E	11.2E	8.3E	8.7E
Nova Scotia	10.8	11.3	13.8	12.5	11.7	10.7	11.5	12.2	9.7	12.9
New Brunswick	10.7	9.4	11.4	10.7	9.7	9.5	12.9	10.7	11.7	8.0
Quebec	10.0	10.6	9.4	10.3	7.8	10.6	10.7	9.4	9.8	9.9
Ontario	9.8	9.3	9.6	9.5	9.7	9.6	8.8	9.2	8.5	9.0
Manitoba	10.2	8.1	8.9	13.0	13.8	11.1	12.8	8.5	8.4	10.6
Saskatchewan	9.2	9.3	9.0	8.4	9.2	9.0	9.5	13.2	8.7	9.5
Alberta	10.5	9.7	10.4	9.2	10.9	10.0	9.8	8.5	9.6	9.4
British Columbia	8.2	9.7	7.4	8.3	9.6	8.8	9.9	9.8	7.6	8.4
Yukon [4]	10.3	10.9	10.2E	10.3E	13.5E	13.0E	13.0E	9.9E	10.0E	9.0E
Northwest Territories [4]	8.3E	11.7	8.4E	F	F	9.8E	7.4E	8.6E	6.5E	10.2E
Nunavut [4, 5]	F	F	F	F	F	F	8.4E	F	F	F

Symbol Legend:
E   Use with caution
F   Too unreliable to be published

Source: Statistics Canada. *Table 105-0503 - Health indicator profile, age-standardized rate, annual estimates, by sex, Canada, provinces and territories, occasional,* CANSIM (database). (accessed: March 29, 2017)

Please see footnotes 30, 31, 57, 58, 59, 60, 61, 62, 64 for characteristics of the age-standardized rate.

AGE-STANDARDIZED RATES, HIGH BLOOD PRESSURE (%), [17] BOTH SEXES, CANADA, PROVINCES AND TERRITORIES

Geography	2003	2005	2007	2008	2009	2010	2011	2012	2013	2014
Canada	13.0	13.2	13.8	14.0	14.2	14.2	14.4	14.0	14.1	13.9
Newfoundland and Labrador	15.0	16.3	17.3	16.5	16.8	18.7	17.0	16.7	17.0	18.5
Prince Edward Island	13.4	13.2	14.3	15.5	14.8	15.1	15.9	15.1	16.9	15.5
Nova Scotia	15.6	15.0	15.7	16.0	16.6	15.9	17.4	17.1	14.6	14.3
New Brunswick	14.3	16.4	15.9	15.5	16.1	17.2	16.5	17.2	17.0	16.4
Quebec	12.6	12.7	13.0	13.3	13.8	13.4	13.1	13.3	13.1	12.9
Ontario	13.4	13.8	14.6	14.4	14.8	14.8	15.0	13.9	15.1	14.6
Manitoba	12.8	13.5	13.8	15.6	14.3	14.0	15.7	13.6	15.9	15.1
Saskatchewan	12.9	13.5	14.5	15.4	15.0	14.8	14.9	15.5	14.4	13.2
Alberta	12.5	12.9	14.0	14.3	14.1	14.3	14.2	15.2	13.9	14.2
British Columbia	11.8	11.3	11.9	12.3	12.1	12.2	13.1	12.7	11.9	11.7
Yukon [4]	12.5	13.1	15.7	10.8	14.1	12.1	13.2	12.7	14.1	12.9
Northwest Territories [4]	14.4	10.9	13.8	13.2	15.3E	13.5	10.5E	9.5	15.7	13.5
Nunavut [4,5]	9.9E	9.6E	7.3E	10.0E	18.4E	10.0E	19.6	17.7	16.6E	12.6E

Symbol Legend:
E Use with caution

Source: Statistics Canada. *Table 105-0503 - Health indicator profile, age-standardized rate, annual estimates, by sex, Canada, provinces and territories, occasional,* CANSIM (database). (accessed: March 29, 2017)

Please see footnotes 30, 31, 57, 58, 59, 60, 61, 62, 64 for characteristics of the age-standardized rate.

AGE-STANDARDIZED RATES, HIGH BLOOD PRESSURE (%), [17] MALES, CANADA, PROVINCES AND TERRITORIES

Geography	2003	2005	2007	2008	2009	2010	2011	2012	2013	2014
Canada	12.0	12.5	13.1	13.6	13.8	14.1	14.3	13.9	14.7	14.5
Newfoundland and Labrador	13.5	14.9	15.2	14.9	14.7	20.1	15.1	17.8	15.8	19.0
Prince Edward Island	11.9	12.7	15.3	15.7	14.7	16.1	16.9	17.9	16.5	16.2
Nova Scotia	14.7	13.5	14.9	15.4	15.3	15.7	17.2	17.0	15.4	14.1
New Brunswick	13.3	16.0	14.7	14.6	14.4	16.4	16.2	17.1	17.1	18.1
Quebec	10.4	11.4	12.3	12.3	12.7	12.8	12.4	12.6	12.9	13.0
Ontario	13.1	13.4	13.8	14.1	14.7	14.9	15.4	14.2	16.0	15.5
Manitoba	11.6	12.9	13.9	15.3	15.0	14.5	15.2	14.3	16.5	16.9
Saskatchewan	12.2	12.6	13.3	14.7	14.7	14.2	14.3	16.4	16.0	12.5
Alberta	11.8	12.9	12.8	14.4	14.3	13.3	14.0	14.9	13.8	14.7
British Columbia	11.2	10.8	11.7	12.3	12.0	13.0	13.5	12.5	13.1	12.7
Yukon [4]	12.0E	11.1E	18.4	11.5E	13.9E	12.1E	13.5E	17.4	13.6	10.7E
Northwest Territories [4]	14.1	10.5	15.3E	17.0	12.5E	14.2	8.8E	8.1E	15.3	19.1
Nunavut [4,5]	F	11.8E	8.2E	F	18.6E	8.5E	26.4E	19.1E	11.7E	F

Symbol Legend:

E   Use with caution

F   Too unreliable to be published

Source: Statistics Canada. *Table 105-0503 - Health indicator profile, age-standardized rate, annual estimates, by sex, Canada, provinces and territories, occasional,* CANSIM (database). (accessed: March 29, 2017)

Please see footnotes 30, 31, 57, 58, 59, 60, 61, 62, 64 for characteristics of the age-standardized rate.

AGE-STANDARDIZED RATES, HIGH BLOOD PRESSURE (%), [17] FEMALES, CANADA, PROVINCES AND TERRITORIES

Geography	2003	2005	2007	2008	2009	2010	2011	2012	2013	2014
Canada	13.9	13.9	14.5	14.4	14.6	14.3	14.5	14.1	13.6	13.2
Newfoundland and Labrador	16.3	17.6	19.4	18.1	18.7	17.3	18.9	15.8	18.2	18.0
Prince Edward Island	14.8	13.7	13.4	15.4	14.9	14.1	14.9	12.6	17.4	14.8
Nova Scotia	16.6	16.3	16.5	16.5	17.8	16.1	17.6	17.1	14.0	14.6
New Brunswick	15.3	16.8	17.0	16.3	17.8	18.0	16.7	17.4	16.9	14.7
Quebec	14.7	14.0	13.6	14.3	14.9	14.1	13.9	14.0	13.2	12.9
Ontario	13.7	14.2	15.3	14.7	14.9	14.7	14.7	13.7	14.2	13.7
Manitoba	14.0	14.1	13.7	16.0	13.6	13.5	16.2	13.0	15.3	13.4
Saskatchewan	13.6	14.5	15.7	16.0	15.4	15.4	15.4	14.5	12.8	13.9
Alberta	13.2	12.9	15.2	14.2	13.9	15.3	14.4	15.6	14.0	13.6
British Columbia	12.5	11.8	12.1	12.3	12.2	11.5	12.8	12.9	10.8	10.7
Yukon [4]	12.9E	15.0	12.9	10.1E	14.4E	12.1	13.0	8.0E	14.6	15.1
Northwest Territories [4]	14.7	11.3	12.2E	9.1E	18.0E	12.8	12.2E	11.0E	16.2	7.8E
Nunavut [4, 5]	F	7.2E	6.5E	15.4E	18.2E	F	11.7E	16.2E	21.7E	15.7E

Symbol Legend:
E   Use with caution
F   Too unreliable to be published

Source: Statistics Canada. *Table 105-0503 - Health indicator profile, age-standardized rate, annual estimates, by sex, Canada, provinces and territories, occasional,* CANSIM (database). (accessed: March 29, 2017)

Please see footnotes 30, 31, 57, 58, 59, 60, 61, 62, 64 for characteristics of the age-standardized rate.

AGE-STANDARDIZED RATES, MOOD DISORDER (%), [53] BOTH SEXES, CANADA, PROVINCES AND TERRITORIES

Geography	2003	2005	2007	2008	2009	2010	2011	2012	2013	2014
Canada	5.1	5.5	6.2	6.6	6.1	6.4	6.8	6.9	7.5	7.6
Newfoundland and Labrador	4.0	4.3	4.6	5.0	4.2	6.1	6.5	8.0	6.7	6.9
Prince Edward Island	4.5	3.9	6.3	6.5E	5.7E	8.0	7.0E	8.2E	10.7	9.9
Nova Scotia	6.0	7.6	7.7	8.1	7.8	9.1	9.3	9.2	10.8	11.4
New Brunswick	7.0	5.3	8.9	5.8	6.3	7.5	7.8	8.0	7.5	11.0
Quebec	3.7	3.9	4.5	4.5	4.5	5.1	4.7	5.0	5.2	4.8
Ontario	5.4	5.9	6.6	7.3	6.6	6.5	7.4	7.2	8.1	8.2
Manitoba	4.5	5.8	6.4	8.2	6.1	6.4	8.3	8.8	7.1	7.4
Saskatchewan	5.1	5.5	6.6	7.6	7.0	6.5	8.4	7.5	7.8	8.1
Alberta	5.9	6.0	6.0	6.7	6.5	7.4	6.5	7.5	6.8	8.5
British Columbia	6.2	6.4	7.8	7.5	7.1	6.9	7.6	7.7	9.4	8.6
Yukon [4]	3.9E	6.1	7.2E	8.3E	9.9E	10.8	10.1E	5.2E	7.6	8.5
Northwest Territories [4]	4.7	5.9E	4.3E	3.7E	6.1E	7.0E	6.8E	4.9E	7.9E	6.8E
Nunavut [4,5]	F	4.0E	F	F	4.3E	5.7E	F	5.8E	F	F

Symbol Legend:

E   Use with caution

F   Too unreliable to be published

Source: Statistics Canada. *Table 105-0503 - Health indicator profile, age-standardized rate, annual estimates, by sex, Canada, provinces and territories, occasional,* CANSIM (database). (accessed: March 29, 2017)

Please see footnotes 30, 31, 57, 58, 59, 60, 61, 62, 64 for characteristics of the age-standardized rate.

AGE-STANDARDIZED RATES, MOOD DISORDER (%), [53] MALES, CANADA, PROVINCES AND TERRITORIES

Geography	2003	2005	2007	2008	2009	2010	2011	2012	2013	2014
Canada	3.6	3.8	4.4	4.8	4.4	4.9	4.8	5.2	6.1	5.7
Newfoundland and Labrador	3.0E	2.6	3.5E	4.5E	2.5E	5.3E	3.8E	6.6E	5.2E	4.9E
Prince Edward Island	3.3E	3.3E	6.1E	6.1E	3.8E	7.4E	6.2E	F	8.0E	5.7E
Nova Scotia	4.2	5.1	5.6E	6.0E	5.6E	8.0E	5.3E	7.0E	8.3	6.5E
New Brunswick	4.8	4.2	7.5	4.4E	5.1E	5.1E	4.9E	7.0E	6.2E	7.4E
Quebec	3.0	3.1	3.6	3.8	3.2	4.4	3.7	4.0	4.0	3.8
Ontario	3.8	4.0	4.3	5.3	4.8	4.6	5.5	5.6	6.3	6.3
Manitoba	3.5	3.5	4.1E	4.9E	4.5E	4.3E	5.6E	6.6E	3.8E	5.5
Saskatchewan	3.8	3.9	4.5	6.3	5.3	5.0E	6.5E	6.1E	6.5	4.6
Alberta	3.3	3.6	3.9	4.3	4.3	4.7	4.5	4.9	5.1	5.9
British Columbia	4.4	4.3	5.6	5.2	4.9	5.8	4.7	5.1	9.8	7.1
Yukon [4]	F	5.2E	F	F	7.6E	11.3E	6.7E	5.0E	F	6.1E
Northwest Territories [4]	3.0E	4.3E	F	F	F	F	F	F	5.4E	5.9E
Nunavut [4, 5]	F	F	F	F	F	F	F	F	F	F

Symbol Legend:
E Use with caution
F Too unreliable to be published

Source: Statistics Canada. *Table 105-0503 - Health indicator profile, age-standardized rate, annual estimates, by sex, Canada, provinces and territories, occasional,* CANSIM (database). (accessed: March 29, 2017)

Please see footnotes 30, 31, 57, 58, 59, 60, 61, 62, 64 for characteristics of the age-standardized rate.

SECTION IV:
Statistics

AGE-STANDARDIZED RATES, MOOD DISORDER (%), [53] FEMALES, CANADA, PROVINCES AND TERRITORIES

Geography	2003	2005	2007	2008	2009	2010	2011	2012	2013	2014
Canada	6.6	7.1	8.0	8.3	7.9	7.9	8.7	8.7	8.8	9.5
Newfoundland and Labrador	4.9	5.8	5.7	5.4E	5.8E	6.8E	9.0	9.4	8.1	8.7
Prince Edward Island	5.6	4.4	6.5E	6.8E	7.4E	8.6E	7.7E	11.5E	13.2	13.8E
Nova Scotia	7.7	10.0	9.7	10.0	9.9	10.2	12.8	11.2	13.0	16.3
New Brunswick	9.0	6.4	10.4	7.3	7.4	9.9	10.5	9.0	8.9	14.4
Quebec	4.3	4.7	5.3	5.1	5.8	5.7	5.7	5.9	6.3	5.7
Ontario	7.0	7.6	8.8	9.3	8.3	8.3	9.2	8.8	9.8	10.0
Manitoba	5.4	8.0	8.5	11.4	7.6	8.3	11.0	10.9	10.3	9.3
Saskatchewan	6.4	7.1	8.6	9.0	8.7	8.0	10.3	8.9	9.0	11.7
Alberta	8.6	8.5	8.1	9.2	8.8	10.2	8.7	10.2	8.6	11.3
British Columbia	7.9	8.5	9.9	9.7	9.2	8.0	10.4	10.4	9.0	10.2
Yukon [4]	6.2E	6.9E	9.7E	10.8E	12.2E	10.2	13.5E	5.3E	12.3	11.0E
Northwest Territories [4]	6.5E	7.6E	4.1E	F	F	10.2E	11.4E	7.8E	10.7E	7.7E
Nunavut [4,5]	F	6.0E	F	F	5.2E	F	F	7.8E	F	F

Symbol Legend:
E   Use with caution
F   Too unreliable to be published

Source: Statistics Canada. *Table 105-0503 - Health indicator profile, age-standardized rate, annual estimates, by sex, Canada, provinces and territories, occasional,* CANSIM (database). (accessed: March 29, 2017)

Please see footnotes 30, 31, 57, 58, 59, 60, 61, 62, 64 for characteristics of the age-standardized rate.

AGE-STANDARDIZED RATES, PAIN OR DISCOMFORT, MODERATE OR SEVERE (%), [18, 19] BOTH SEXES, CANADA, PROVINCES AND TERRITORIES

Geography	2003	2005	2007	2008	2009	2010	2011	2012	2013	2014
Canada	9.6	9.8	10.2	11.0	10.6	10.6	12.6	12.7	12.2	12.4
Newfoundland and Labrador	9.5	10.7	9.9	11.8	9.7	9.8	13.7	14.0	11.2	10.9
Prince Edward Island	10.7	11.2	12.1	10.2	7.8	10.4	15.9	15.0	14.5	12.9
Nova Scotia	9.4	12.5	11.5	12.7	11.7	13.9	14.5	14.6	15.0	13.3
New Brunswick	12.4	12.3	11.4	11.8	13.3	10.9	13.8	13.1	13.1	13.8
Quebec	10.7	9.9	9.8	10.0	10.6	10.8	12.6	13.8	12.5	12.2
Ontario	8.9	9.6	10.6	11.4	10.6	10.6	13.1	12.4	12.1	12.6
Manitoba	8.4	10.7	9.3	12.1	10.5	11.1	12.4	11.9	13.2	11.5
Saskatchewan	8.5	10.0	9.1	8.0	9.9	10.0	13.3	11.3	10.5	9.4
Alberta	9.3	8.9	8.8	10.8	10.8	10.7	11.4	12.1	12.2	12.2
British Columbia	9.7	9.2	10.4	11.5	10.2	9.8	11.5	12.3	11.4	12.7
Yukon [4]	11.0	10.9	11.9	9.5E	10.6	12.0	12.2	16.8	14.7	12.0
Northwest Territories [4]	9.0	11.2	6.4E	7.3	8.2E	8.9	10.3E	11.6	9.7	9.6E
Nunavut [4, 5]	8.4E	8.2	7.5	9.8E	8.3E	9.1E	7.6E	15.7	10.3E	12.8

Symbol Legend:
E   Use with caution

Source: Statistics Canada. *Table 105-0503 - Health indicator profile, age-standardized rate, annual estimates, by sex, Canada, provinces and territories, occasional,* CANSIM (database). (accessed: March 29, 2017)

Please see footnotes 30, 31, 57, 58, 59, 60, 61, 62, 64 for characteristics of the age-standardized rate.

AGE-STANDARDIZED RATES, PAIN OR DISCOMFORT, MODERATE OR SEVERE (%),[18, 19] MALES, CANADA, PROVINCES AND TERRITORIES

Geography	2003	2005	2007	2008	2009	2010	2011	2012	2013	2014
Canada	7.4	8.3	8.2	9.1	9.0	9.3	10.6	10.3	9.8	10.7
Newfoundland and Labrador	9.0	9.7	8.0	10.9	7.4	9.0	9.6E	13.6	9.6	8.7
Prince Edward Island	7.8	9.9	11.3	6.5E	5.7E	12.7E	13.6E	12.7	14.2	11.5E
Nova Scotia	7.2	12.3	10.2	10.5	11.6	12.5	14.1	11.8	12.7	10.5
New Brunswick	11.9	12.2	10.0	10.4	11.4	8.6	12.1	10.7	9.4	13.8
Quebec	8.5	7.7	7.5	8.5	8.6	9.7	10.2	11.1	9.5	10.5
Ontario	6.7	8.1	8.4	9.4	8.9	8.9	10.8	9.4	9.9	10.7
Manitoba	6.1	9.1	7.9	9.1	11.0	9.5	10.0	11.1	11.1	10.6
Saskatchewan	8.4	9.1	6.7	5.3	8.4	9.2	11.7	9.4	9.2	9.0
Alberta	6.9	7.3	7.7	9.0	10.0	9.1	10.5	9.4	10.2	9.9
British Columbia	6.9	8.1	8.9	9.3	7.9	9.4	9.8	11.3	9.0	12.3
Yukon [4]	9.8E	9.4E	7.5E	8.5E	8.2E	11.9E	12.1E	18.2E	12.9E	11.2E
Northwest Territories [4]	8.1	9.4E	5.7E	5.7E	6.2E	F	6.8E	10.9E	6.5E	8.6E
Nunavut [4, 5]	F	8.2E	7.4E	7.1E	9.9E	F	F	17.9E	12.8	12.5E

Symbol Legend:
E Use with caution
F Too unreliable to be published

Source: Statistics Canada. *Table 105-0503 - Health indicator profile, age-standardized rate, annual estimates, by sex, Canada, provinces and territories, occasional,* CANSIM (database). (accessed: March 29, 2017)

Please see footnotes 30, 31, 57, 58, 59, 60, 61, 62, 64 for characteristics of the age-standardized rate.

AGE-STANDARDIZED RATES, PAIN OR DISCOMFORT, MODERATE OR SEVERE (%), [18, 19] FEMALES, CANADA, PROVINCES AND TERRITORIES

Geography	2003	2005	2007	2008	2009	2010	2011	2012	2013	2014
Canada	11.7	11.2	12.1	12.8	12.2	11.9	14.7	15.1	14.5	13.9
Newfoundland and Labrador	10.0	11.7	11.8	12.6	11.9	10.7	17.7	14.4	12.7	13.1
Prince Edward Island	13.4	12.4	12.9	13.7	9.7	8.2	18.2	17.1	14.7	14.1
Nova Scotia	11.4	12.7	12.6	14.7	11.8	15.2	14.8	17.2	17.1	16.0
New Brunswick	12.9	12.5	12.7	13.2	15.1	13.1	15.3	15.3	16.8	13.9
Quebec	12.8	12.0	12.1	11.4	12.6	11.9	15.1	16.4	15.5	13.9
Ontario	11.1	10.9	12.7	13.3	12.2	12.2	15.3	15.2	14.2	14.4
Manitoba	10.7	12.2	10.6	14.9	9.9	12.7	14.9	12.7	15.3	12.3
Saskatchewan	8.6	10.8	11.5	10.7	11.5	10.8	15.0	13.2	11.8	9.7
Alberta	11.7	10.6	10.0	12.7	11.5	12.4	12.3	14.9	14.3	14.5
British Columbia	12.4	10.3	11.9	13.5	12.5	10.1	13.3	13.2	13.8	13.2
Yukon [4]	12.3E	12.3	16.3	10.5E	13.0E	12.2E	12.3E	15.4	16.5	12.8
Northwest Territories [4]	9.9	13.3	7.2E	9.1E	10.2E	12.6	14.0E	12.5E	13.3	10.8E
Nunavut [4, 5]	14.6E	8.1E	7.5E	12.6E	6.8E	F	11.2E	13.1E	F	13.2E

Symbol Legend:
E   Use with caution
F   Too unreliable to be published

Source: Statistics Canada. *Table 105-0503 - Health indicator profile, age-standardized rate, annual estimates, by sex, Canada, provinces and territories, occasional,* CANSIM (database). (accessed: March 29, 2017)

Please see footnotes [30], [31], [57], [58], [59], [60], [61], [62], [64] for characteristics of the age-standardized rate.

AGE-STANDARDIZED RATES, PAIN OR DISCOMFORT THAT PREVENTS ACTIVITIES (%), [19], [20] BOTH SEXES, CANADA, PROVINCES AND TERRITORIES

Geography	2003	2005	2007	2008	2009	2010	2011	2012	2013	2014
Canada	10.0	10.3	10.9	11.4	11.2	11.4	13.3	13.4	13.2	13.4
Newfoundland and Labrador	9.9	10.3	10.5	11.5	10.4	10.5	12.5	15.4	10.8	12.3
Prince Edward Island	11.3	11.7	12.1	10.0	8.7	11.0	16.5	14.7	16.7	12.7
Nova Scotia	10.8	11.2	12.7	12.7	11.0	14.8	14.1	14.6	16.2	15.5
New Brunswick	12.6	12.0	11.4	12.0	12.6	12.2	14.6	12.4	13.7	15.3
Quebec	9.1	8.0	8.2	8.9	9.2	9.5	10.5	12.1	10.9	11.4
Ontario	9.9	10.8	12.0	12.2	12.1	12.2	14.6	13.8	13.9	13.8
Manitoba	9.5	11.7	10.4	13.3	11.9	12.9	16.2	14.0	15.0	13.6
Saskatchewan	10.0	11.4	10.3	9.2	12.0	10.6	14.0	11.6	11.7	11.0
Alberta	10.4	10.4	10.5	12.0	11.6	11.1	12.0	14.3	13.7	13.4
British Columbia	11.3	11.3	12.5	12.7	11.6	11.8	14.1	13.8	13.6	15.1
Yukon [4]	12.2E	15.5	13.9	12.2	12.7	13.7	15.9	15.9	18.2	18.3
Northwest Territories [4]	11.0	12.0	8.8	9.2E	8.9E	11.3	10.8E	13.1	15.4	12.7
Nunavut [4],[5]	8.2E	10.2	10.3E	11.6	8.7E	11.7	12.1E	19.4	11.5E	17.0E

Symbol Legend:
E   Use with caution

Source: Statistics Canada. *Table 105-0503 - Health indicator profile, age-standardized rate, annual estimates, by sex, Canada, provinces and territories, occasional,* CANSIM (database). (accessed: March 29, 2017)

Please see footnotes 30, 31, 57, 58, 59, 60, 61, 62, 64 for characteristics of the age-standardized rate.

AGE-STANDARDIZED RATES, PAIN OR DISCOMFORT THAT PREVENTS ACTIVITIES (%), [19], [20] MALES, CANADA, PROVINCES AND TERRITORIES

Geography	2003	2005	2007	2008	2009	2010	2011	2012	2013	2014
Canada	7.7	8.4	8.7	9.2	9.4	9.7	11.3	11.1	10.7	11.3
Newfoundland and Labrador	9.5	8.7	8.1	10.6	8.1	9.4	8.3E	14.8E	7.9	8.7
Prince Edward Island	8.2	10.1	12.2	6.6E	6.9E	11.6E	14.2E	13.5E	13.9E	10.0E
Nova Scotia	7.3	10.6	11.4	10.0	10.8	12.4	13.4	11.8	14.0	11.2
New Brunswick	13.3	11.6	10.0	10.4	10.7	10.1	11.5	10.4	10.9	14.7
Quebec	7.1	5.7	6.5	7.6	7.5	8.5	8.5	10.0	8.0	9.4
Ontario	7.3	9.0	9.1	9.8	9.9	9.9	12.4	11.1	11.5	11.4
Manitoba	7.0	9.5	9.2	8.8	11.7	10.4	14.9	12.7	12.4	13.5
Saskatchewan	10.1	10.8	6.5	6.8	10.7	10.0	12.1	9.3	10.3	10.6
Alberta	7.5	7.9	9.5	10.0	10.6	9.1	11.0	12.0	11.9	11.4
British Columbia	8.3	10.1	10.2	10.0	9.3	10.9	11.9	11.3	11.2	13.7
Yukon [4]	11.5E	14.0E	8.8E	9.0E	10.4E	13.1	15.5E	16.0E	14.8	16.6
Northwest Territories [4]	9.9	7.5E	5.6E	8.2E	F	8.3E	7.0E	12.5E	14.8E	12.4E
Nunavut [4],[5]	F	10.4E	8.2E	9.6E	10.4E	11.6E	F	16.4E	16.2E	16.5E

Symbol Legend:
E Use with caution
F Too unreliable to be published

Source: Statistics Canada. *Table 105-0503 - Health indicator profile, age-standardized rate, annual estimates, by sex, Canada, provinces and territories, occasional,* CANSIM (database). (accessed: March 29, 2017)

Please see footnotes 30, 31, 57, 58, 59, 60, 61, 62, 64 for characteristics of the age-standardized rate.

AGE-STANDARDIZED RATES, PAIN OR DISCOMFORT THAT PREVENTS ACTIVITIES (%), [19, 20] FEMALES, CANADA, PROVINCES AND TERRITORIES

Geography	2003	2005	2007	2008	2009	2010	2011	2012	2013	2014
Canada	12.3	12.0	13.0	13.5	12.9	13.1	15.3	15.7	15.6	15.4
Newfoundland and Labrador	10.4	12.0	12.8	12.3	12.5	11.6	16.6	15.9	13.7	15.7
Prince Edward Island	14.2	13.2	11.9	13.1	10.4	10.5	18.7	15.8	19.2	15.1
Nova Scotia	14.1	11.7	13.9	15.2	11.2	17.0	14.7	17.1	18.3	19.7
New Brunswick	11.9	12.5	12.8	13.5	14.3	14.2	17.5	14.3	16.5	15.9
Quebec	11.1	10.3	9.8	10.2	10.9	10.5	12.5	14.1	13.9	13.4
Ontario	12.4	12.6	14.7	14.5	14.1	14.4	16.8	16.4	16.3	16.2
Manitoba	12.0	13.8	11.6	17.7	12.0	15.3	17.5	15.3	17.5	13.6
Saskatchewan	9.8	12.0	14.0	11.7	13.3	11.2	15.8	13.9	13.1	11.3
Alberta	13.3	12.9	11.5	14.0	12.6	13.1	13.0	16.6	15.6	15.6
British Columbia	14.3	12.4	14.8	15.3	13.9	12.6	16.3	16.1	15.9	16.4
Yukon [4]	12.9E	16.9E	18.9	15.5	15.0E	14.4	16.3	15.8	21.7	20.2
Northwest Territories [4]	12.3E	16.9	12.3E	10.3E	11.2E	14.5	14.7E	13.8	16.1E	12.9E
Nunavut [4, 5]	14.6E	9.9E	12.4E	13.7E	7.1E	11.7E	18.7E	22.7E	F	17.5E

Symbol Legend:
E   Use with caution
F   Too unreliable to be published

Source: Statistics Canada. *Table 105-0503 - Health indicator profile, age-standardized rate, annual estimates, by sex, Canada, provinces and territories, occasional,* CANSIM (database). (accessed: March 29, 2017)

Please see footnotes 30, 31, 57, 58, 59, 60, 61, 62, 64 for characteristics of the age-standardized rate.

PROPORTION OF BIRTHS WITH LOW BIRTH WEIGHT (%), BOTH SEXES, CANADA, PROVINCES AND TERRITORIES [1, 3, 4, 5, 6, 7, 8, 9, 10, 18, 19]

Geography	2003	2004	2005	2006	2007	2008	2009	2010	2011	2012
Canada [11, 12]	5.9	5.9	6.0	6.1	6.0	6.0	6.1	6.2	6.1	6.1
Newfoundland and Labrador [11, 12]	5.6	5.8	5.9	5.6	5.4	6.1	5.5	6.7	5.9	5.3
Prince Edward Island	4.2	5.5	5.4	4.9	5.8	5.1	6.5	5.3	4.5	5.6
Nova Scotia	5.7	5.9	6.3	6.4	5.7	5.9	5.8	6.2	6.0	6.4
New Brunswick	5.1	5.6	5.9	5.8	4.9	5.2	6.1	5.6	5.9	6.0
Quebec	5.7	5.9	5.7	5.8	5.7	5.6	5.8	5.7	5.7	5.6
Ontario	6.1	5.9	6.2	6.2	6.2	6.3	6.4	6.6	6.5	6.4
Manitoba	5.5	5.6	5.4	5.9	5.6	5.5	5.5	5.8	5.8	6.0
Saskatchewan	5.6	5.5	5.7	5.6	5.5	5.4	5.7	5.6	5.7	5.8
Alberta	6.3	6.4	6.6	6.9	6.6	6.8	6.9	6.8	6.6	7.0
British Columbia	5.4	5.7	5.7	5.6	5.8	5.5	5.4	5.5	5.6	5.8
Yukon [14]	5.1	4.7	3.8	5.5	6.4	4.3	6.8	6.3	4.9	4.4
Northwest Territories [14, 15, 16]	5.9	5.6	5.1	3.8	4.3	6.0	4.8	3.7	5.2	5.5
Nunavut [13, 14, 16]	8.0	6.9	8.4	8.5	6.2	8.2	8.4	7.6	7.7	7.7

Source: Statistics Canada. *Table 102-4005 - Low birth weight (less than 2,500 grams) and borderline viable birth weight-adjusted low birth weight (500 to less than 2,500 grams), by sex, Canada, provinces and territories, annual,* CANSIM (database). (accessed: March 29, 2017)

PROPORTION OF BIRTHS WITH LOW BIRTH WEIGHT (%), MALES, CANADA, PROVINCES AND TERRITORIES [1, 3, 4, 5, 6, 7, 8, 9, 10, 18, 19]

Geography	2003	2004	2005	2006	2007	2008	2009	2010	2011	2012
Canada [11, 12]	5.4	5.6	5.6	5.7	5.6	5.6	5.7	5.7	5.7	5.7
Newfoundland and Labrador [11, 12]	5.4	5.4	5.9	4.9	4.7	5.6	5.4	5.5	5.1	5.2
Prince Edward Island	4.4	5.2	6.0	4.4	6.1	4.4	6.8	5.8	4.4	5.5
Nova Scotia	5.6	5.3	5.8	5.7	5.4	5.3	5.6	5.8	5.6	5.9
New Brunswick	5.0	5.6	5.8	5.6	4.6	5.0	5.6	5.2	5.4	5.9
Quebec	5.2	5.4	5.2	5.4	5.3	5.0	5.3	5.2	5.3	5.1
Ontario	5.5	5.6	5.8	5.8	5.9	6.0	6.0	6.0	6.1	6.0
Manitoba	5.3	5.4	5.1	5.7	5.2	5.4	5.3	5.3	5.6	5.7
Saskatchewan	5.2	5.2	5.5	5.4	5.2	5.2	5.3	5.3	5.5	5.1
Alberta	6.1	5.9	6.4	6.4	6.1	6.3	6.4	6.5	6.2	6.4
British Columbia	4.9	5.4	5.2	5.1	5.5	5.3	5.2	5.2	5.3	5.5
Yukon [14]	6.3	2.8	0.6	4.0	7.5	4.8	6.8	4.6	3.9	2.6
Northwest Territories [14, 15, 16]	6.7	5.9	5.8	3.7	4.1	5.3	4.3	3.6	4.3	5.0
Nunavut [13, 14, 16]	6.7	9.1	8.9	6.0	5.3	8.8	9.0	6.3	7.6	8.6

Source: Statistics Canada. *Table 102-4005 - Low birth weight (less than 2,500 grams) and borderline viable birth weight-adjusted low birth weight (500 to less than 2,500 grams), by sex, Canada, provinces and territories, annual,* CANSIM (database). (accessed: March 29, 2017)

PROPORTION OF BIRTHS WITH LOW BIRTH WEIGHT (%), FEMALES, CANADA, PROVINCES AND TERRITORIES [1, 3, 4, 5, 6, 7, 8, 9, 10, 18, 19]

Geography	2003	2004	2005	2006	2007	2008	2009	2010	2011	2012
Canada [11, 12]	6.3	6.3	6.4	6.5	6.4	6.4	6.5	6.7	6.5	6.6
Newfoundland and Labrador [11, 12]	5.9	6.2	5.9	6.3	6.1	6.6	5.6	8.0	6.7	5.5
Prince Edward Island	4.0	5.9	4.7	5.5	5.6	5.8	6.2	4.9	4.6	5.6
Nova Scotia	5.8	6.5	6.8	7.1	6.1	6.5	6.0	6.7	6.4	6.8
New Brunswick	5.3	5.6	6.1	6.0	5.2	5.5	6.5	6.0	6.4	6.1
Quebec	6.2	6.4	6.2	6.2	6.2	6.2	6.3	6.3	6.2	6.1
Ontario	6.7	6.2	6.7	6.6	6.6	6.7	6.8	7.2	6.9	6.8
Manitoba	5.7	5.7	5.7	6.0	6.0	5.7	5.7	6.3	6.0	6.4
Saskatchewan	5.9	6.0	6.0	5.9	5.8	5.7	6.1	5.8	6.0	6.4
Alberta	6.5	6.9	6.8	7.5	7.2	7.2	7.4	7.2	7.1	7.6
British Columbia	5.9	5.9	6.1	6.1	6.1	5.7	5.7	5.8	5.9	6.1
Yukon [14]	3.8	6.4	7.0	7.1	5.2	3.7	6.7	8.1	6.0	6.2
Northwest Territories [14, 15, 16]	5.1	5.4	4.2	3.9	4.5	6.6	5.4	3.8	6.2	6.1
Nunavut [13, 14, 16]	9.3	4.4	8.0	11.6	7.0	7.5	7.9	8.8	7.7	6.9

Source: Statistics Canada. *Table 102-4005 - Low birth weight (less than 2,500 grams) and borderline viable birth weight-adjusted low birth weight (500 to less than 2,500 grams), by sex, Canada, provinces and territories, annual,* CANSIM (database). (accessed: March 29, 2017)

AGE-STANDARDIZED RATES, CHRONIC OBSTRUCTIVE PULMONARY DISEASE (COPD) (%), [56] BOTH SEXES, CANADA, PROVINCES AND TERRITORIES

Geography	2003	2005	2007	2008	2009	2010	2011	2012	2013	2014
Canada	4.3	4.3	..	4.5	4.1	4.1	3.8	3.9	4.0	3.6
Newfoundland and Labrador	4.2	5.1	..	5.0	4.4	4.8	3.3E	4.1	4.3E	3.4
Prince Edward Island	5.1	5.5	..	4.3E	3.0E	3.9E	6.1E	5.6E	4.5E	4.7E
Nova Scotia	5.7	6.5	..	5.6	6.6	5.2	5.8	4.8	3.9	4.8
New Brunswick	5.5	4.9	..	4.7	4.9	4.9	5.9	5.1	4.2	4.5
Quebec	4.5	4.3	..	4.2	4.7	4.0	4.3	4.1	4.1	4.0
Ontario	4.3	4.3	..	4.5	3.9	4.2	3.4	3.7	4.0	3.4
Manitoba	2.9	4.1	..	5.3	3.7	4.5	4.0E	4.2E	2.9	3.1E
Saskatchewan	3.0	4.3	..	4.4	3.9	4.6E	4.2	4.3	2.8	4.2
Alberta	3.7	4.1	..	4.8	3.5	3.7	3.9	3.7	4.2	3.8
British Columbia	4.1	3.7	..	4.2	3.6	3.6	3.4	3.8	4.0	3.2
Yukon [4]	4.5E	5.4E	..	4.4E	F	6.2E	4.3E	3.6E	3.5E	5.4E
Northwest Territories [4]	F	3.7E	..	F	F	F	F	3.6E	F	F
Nunavut [4,5]	F	F	..	F	F	F	F	F	F	F

Symbol Legend:
.. Not Available
E Use with caution
F Too unreliable to be published

Source: Statistics Canada. *Table 105-0503 - Health indicator profile, age-standardized rate, annual estimates, by sex, Canada, provinces and territories, occasional,* CANSIM (database). (accessed: March 29, 2017)

Please see footnotes 30, 31, 57, 58, 59, 60, 61, 62, 64 for characteristics of the age-standardized rate.

AGE-STANDARDIZED RATES, CHRONIC OBSTRUCTIVE PULMONARY DISEASE (COPD) (%), [56] MALES, CANADA, PROVINCES AND TERRITORIES

Geography	2003	2005	2007	2008	2009	2010	2011	2012	2013	2014
Canada	3.6	3.9	..	4.2	3.9	3.7	3.3	3.5	3.6	3.3
Newfoundland and Labrador	3.2E	4.3	..	4.4E	3.9E	4.0E	3.6E	5.2E	3.3E	2.8E
Prince Edward Island	4.1E	5.8E	..	3.7E	3.1E	3.8E	F	5.3E	F	5.2E
Nova Scotia	4.7	5.5	..	5.6E	5.1E	4.2E	5.2	5.1E	3.4E	4.3E
New Brunswick	6.3	4.9	..	4.0E	2.5E	3.9E	4.3E	4.8E	4.0E	4.9E
Quebec	3.7	3.5	..	3.2	5.0	3.4	3.9	4.0	3.7	3.4
Ontario	3.7	4.0	..	4.4	3.6	3.9	2.5	3.2	3.5	2.9
Manitoba	2.5	4.3	..	5.5E	3.3E	3.3E	3.7E	3.0E	2.1E	2.6E
Saskatchewan	2.9E	3.6	..	6.0E	3.4E	5.0E	4.1E	3.3E	2.7E	4.2E
Alberta	2.8	4.2	..	5.3E	3.4E	3.2	3.9	3.4	4.2	3.4E
British Columbia	3.5	3.3	..	4.0	3.6	3.5E	3.1	2.9	3.7	3.8E
Yukon [4]	5.2E	F	..	F	F	F	6.3E	F	F	F
Northwest Territories [4]	F	F	..	F	F	F	F	F	F	F
Nunavut [4] [5]	F	F	..	F	F	F	F	F	F	F

Symbol Legend:
.. Not Available
E Use with caution
F Too unreliable to be published

Source: Statistics Canada. *Table 105-0503 - Health indicator profile, age-standardized rate, annual estimates, by sex, Canada, provinces and territories, occasional,* CANSIM (database). (accessed: March 29, 2017)

Please see footnotes 30, 31, 57, 58, 59, 60, 61, 62, 64 for characteristics of the age-standardized rate.

AGE-STANDARDIZED RATES, CHRONIC OBSTRUCTIVE PULMONARY DISEASE (COPD) (%), [56] FEMALES, CANADA, PROVINCES AND TERRITORIES

Geography	2003	2005	2007	2008	2009	2010	2011	2012	2013	2014
Canada	4.9	4.7	..	4.7	4.3	4.5	4.4	4.3	4.3	4.0
Newfoundland and Labrador	5.1[E]	5.8	..	5.6[E]	4.9[E]	5.5[E]	3.0[E]	3.0[E]	5.1[E]	3.9[E]
Prince Edward Island	6.0[E]	5.1[E]	..	4.9[E]	F	4.1[E]	8.1[E]	F	4.6[E]	4.3[E]
Nova Scotia	6.7	7.5	..	5.7	7.9	6.0	6.3	4.6[E]	4.4	5.4
New Brunswick	4.7	4.9	..	5.3	7.2[E]	5.8	7.2[E]	5.4[E]	4.5	4.1[E]
Quebec	5.3	5.1	..	5.2	4.5	4.6	4.7	4.3	4.6	4.6
Ontario	4.9	4.6	..	4.6	4.2	4.5	4.2	4.2	4.4	3.9
Manitoba	3.3	3.9	..	5.1	4.1[E]	5.6[E]	4.3[E]	5.3[E]	3.7[E]	3.5[E]
Saskatchewan	3.1	5.0	..	2.9	4.4	4.1[E]	4.4[E]	5.4[E]	2.8[E]	4.3[E]
Alberta	4.5	4.1	..	4.3	3.6	4.2	3.9	4.0	4.3[E]	4.1
British Columbia	4.6	4.0	..	4.3	3.7	3.6	3.8	4.5	4.3	2.6
Yukon [4]	3.8[E]	F	..	F	F	F	F	4.8[E]	4.4[E]	F
Northwest Territories [4]	F	F	..	F	F	F	F	F	F	F
Nunavut [4, 5]	F	F	..	F	F	F	F	F	F	F

Symbol Legend:
.. Not Available
E Use with caution
F Too unreliable to be published

Source: Statistics Canada. *Table 105-0503 - Health indicator profile, age-standardized rate, annual estimates, by sex, Canada, provinces and territories, occasional,* CANSIM (database). (accessed: March 29, 2017)

Please see footnotes 30, 31, 57, 58, 59, 60, 61, 62, 64 for characteristics of the age-standardized rate.

AGE-STANDARDIZED RATES, INJURIES WITHIN THE PAST 12 MONTHS CAUSING LIMITATION OF NORMAL ACTIVITIES (%), [54, 55, 65] BOTH SEXES, CANADA, PROVINCES AND TERRITORIES

Geography	2003	2005	2007	2008	2009	2010	2011	2012	2013	2014
Canada	13.5	14.1	..	..	15.1	15.7	..	..	16.9	16.4
Newfoundland and Labrador	13.4	12.4	..	..	14.1	15.3			17.0	16.7
Prince Edward Island	12.9	13.0	..	..	11.6	13.0	..	..	17.7	16.9
Nova Scotia	14.9	15.9	..	..	15.6	16.3	..		18.1	18.9
New Brunswick	13.6	12.2	..	..	14.7	15.7	..	..	14.9	17.2
Quebec	11.9	12.3	..	..	14.8	14.5	..	..	16.2	15.4
Ontario	13.1	14.2	..	..	14.1	15.2	..	..	15.5	14.7
Manitoba	15.7	14.0	..	..	17.5	16.9	..	..	20.3	19.9
Saskatchewan	14.2	15.0	..	..	15.9	17.6	..		20.2	18.9
Alberta	15.4	14.8	..	..	16.6	17.0	18.1	19.2	17.3	17.6
British Columbia	15.4	16.8	..	..	17.1	17.0	..	..	20.1	19.9
Yukon [4]	17.8	15.7	..	..	15.6	18.2	..	..	25.7	26.4
Northwest Territories [4]	11.5	16.6	..	..	13.9	13.3	15.0	17.4	15.9	20.6
Nunavut [4, 5]	14.1E	10.1	..	..	16.4	18.6E	..	..	12.9	9.2E

Symbol Legend:
.. Not Available
E Use with caution

Source: Statistics Canada. *Table 105-0503 - Health indicator profile, age-standardized rate, annual estimates, by sex, Canada, provinces and territories, occasional,* CANSIM (database). (accessed: March 29, 2017)

Please see footnotes 30, 31, 57, 58, 59, 60, 61, 62, 64 for characteristics of the age-standardized rate.

AGE-STANDARDIZED RATES, INJURIES WITHIN THE PAST 12 MONTHS CAUSING LIMITATION OF NORMAL ACTIVITIES (%), [54], [55], [65] MALES, CANADA, PROVINCES AND TERRITORIES

Geography	2003	2005	2007	2008	2009	2010	2011	2012	2013	2014
Canada	15.9	17.0	..	..	17.6	18.2	..	..	19.1	18.1
Newfoundland and Labrador	16.1	13.7	..	..	16.5	18.5	..	..	16.4	20.2
Prince Edward Island	16.1	16.5	..	..	12.9E	12.7E	..	..	17.5	21.3
Nova Scotia	16.7	19.7	..	..	15.3	19.9	..	..	21.7	21.1
New Brunswick	16.3	14.8	..	..	17.3	16.2	..	..	15.9	19.6
Quebec	14.3	14.7	..	..	18.4	17.3	..	..	17.8	17.5
Ontario	15.3	16.9	..	..	16.3	17.8	..	..	17.3	15.6
Manitoba	17.3	16.6	..	..	20.3	17.9	..	..	18.9	21.4
Saskatchewan	16.6	17.6	..	..	18.1	18.4	..	..	25.9	20.1
Alberta	17.8	18.1	..	..	18.2	19.3	20.8	22.0	19.7	20.2
British Columbia	18.0	20.4	..	..	19.6	19.9	..	..	24.7	21.7
Yukon [4]	22.1	17.4	..	..	20.5	17.9	..	..	26.1	29.9
Northwest Territories [4]	14.0	18.0	..	..	16.2E	12.6	17.0E	21.1	15.7	24.0
Nunavut [4], [5]	17.4E	13.4	..	..	22.8E	17.8E	..	..	16.7	F

Symbol Legend:
.. Not Available
E Use with caution
F Too unreliable to be published

Source: Statistics Canada. *Table 105-0503 - Health indicator profile, age-standardized rate, annual estimates, by sex, Canada, provinces and territories, occasional,* CANSIM (database). (accessed: March 31, 2017)

Please see footnotes [30], [31], [57], [58], [59], [60], [61], [62], [64] for characteristics of the age-standardized rate.

AGE-STANDARDIZED RATES, INJURIES WITHIN THE PAST 12 MONTHS CAUSING LIMITATION OF NORMAL ACTIVITIES (%), [54, 55, 65] FEMALES, CANADA, PROVINCES AND TERRITORIES

Geography	2003	2005	2007	2008	2009	2010	2011	2012	2013	2014
Canada	11.3	11.4	..	..	12.7	13.2	..	..	14.7	14.7
Newfoundland and Labrador	10.8	11.1	..	..	11.8	12.1	..	..	17.6	13.5
Prince Edward Island	9.8	9.8	..	..	10.4	13.3	..	..	18.0	12.9E
Nova Scotia	13.1	12.3	..	..	16.0	13.1	..	..	14.7	16.7
New Brunswick	10.9	9.8	..	..	12.2	15.2	..	..	14.0	15.0
Quebec	9.5	9.9	..	..	11.3	11.7	..	..	14.7	13.2
Ontario	11.0	11.6	..	..	11.9	12.8	..	..	13.7	13.8
Manitoba	14.1	11.5	..	..	14.7	16.0	..	..	21.7	18.4
Saskatchewan	11.9	12.4	..	..	13.7	16.9	..	..	14.5	17.7
Alberta	13.0	11.5	..	..	15.0	14.6	15.2	16.3	14.8	14.9
British Columbia	12.9	13.4	..	..	14.7	14.2	..	..	15.5	18.0
Yukon [4]	13.7E	14.1	..	..	10.7E	18.4	..	..	25.3	22.9
Northwest Territories [4]	8.9	15.0	..	..	11.7E	14.0E	12.8E	13.5E	16.0	17.0
Nunavut [4, 5]	10.9E	6.1E	..	..	10.8E	19.5E	..	..	9.0E	F

Symbol Legend:
.. Not Available
E Use with caution
F Too unreliable to be published

Source: Statistics Canada. *Table 105-0503 - Health indicator profile, age-standardized rate, annual estimates, by sex, Canada, provinces and territories, occasional,* CANSIM (database). (accessed: March 31, 2017)

Please see footnotes 30, 31, 57, 58, 59, 60, 61, 62, 64 for characteristics of the age-standardized rate.

AGE-STANDARDIZED RATES, INJURIES WITHIN THE PAST 12 MONTHS, SOUGHT MEDICAL ATTENTION (%), [54], [55], [65] BOTH SEXES, CANADA, PROVINCES AND TERRITORIES

Geography	2003	2005	2007	2008	2009	2010	2011	2012	2013	2014
Canada	8.3	8.6	..	..	8.4	8.2	..	..	8.7	8.5
Newfoundland and Labrador	9.1	8.1	..	..	8.5	9.3			8.3	9.6
Prince Edward Island	7.6	8.2	..	..	8.1	7.3			9.1	9.6
Nova Scotia	8.6	9.0	..	..	8.8	9.5	..		10.4	9.3
New Brunswick	8.2	6.9	..	..	8.1	8.3	..		7.6	8.8
Quebec	7.3	7.4	..	..	8.1	7.0	..	..	8.3	8.0
Ontario	7.9	8.4	..	..	7.6	8.0	..		8.0	7.5
Manitoba	10.1	8.5	..	..	9.9	7.7	..		10.1	11.3
Saskatchewan	8.8	10.0	..	..	9.5	9.0	..		9.1	9.0
Alberta	9.8	9.3	..	..	10.2	9.2	9.5	9.1	8.0	9.0
British Columbia	9.2	10.5	..	..	8.9	9.5	..		11.1	10.5
Yukon [4]	10.4	8.9	..	..	10.4	12.8	..		14.0	15.3
Northwest Territories [4]	6.8E	9.2	..	..	5.7E	6.3	7.8E	9.7	8.2E	8.4
Nunavut [4], [5]	8.9E	6.8	..	..	9.8E	14.8E	..		7.2E	F

Symbol Legend:
.. Not Available
E Use with caution
F Too unreliable to be published

Source: Statistics Canada. *Table 105-0503 - Health indicator profile, age-standardized rate, annual estimates, by sex, Canada, provinces and territories, occasional,* CANSIM (database). (accessed: March 31, 2017)

Please see footnotes [30], [31], [57], [58], [59], [60], [61], [62], [64] for characteristics of the age-standardized rate.

AGE-STANDARDIZED RATES, INJURIES WITHIN THE PAST 12 MONTHS, SOUGHT MEDICAL ATTENTION (%), [54, 55, 65] MALES, CANADA, PROVINCES AND TERRITORIES

Geography	2003	2005	2007	2008	2009	2010	2011	2012	2013	2014
Canada	9.7	10.0	..	..	9.5	9.3	..	..	9.6	9.2
Newfoundland and Labrador	11.0	8.8	..	..	10.4	10.7	..	..	8.4	10.1
Prince Edward Island	8.6	9.8	..	..	9.6E	6.1E	..	..	8.3E	10.7E
Nova Scotia	9.9	10.2	..	..	8.4	10.6	..	..	12.3	9.3
New Brunswick	9.7	7.8	..	..	8.6	8.7	..	..	9.0	10.7
Quebec	8.9	8.6	..	..	10.3	8.4	..	..	9.3	8.8
Ontario	9.2	9.8	..	..	8.5	9.2	..	..	8.6	7.7
Manitoba	10.5	9.5	..	..	11.2	8.3	..	..	8.8	12.7
Saskatchewan	10.3	11.7	..	..	11.5	9.2	..	..	11.1	11.1
Alberta	11.4	10.7	..	..	10.3	9.9	10.4	9.6	8.9	10.5
British Columbia	11.0	12.6	..	..	9.7	11.1	..	..	13.1	11.3
Yukon [4]	14.9E	10.5	..	..	14.7	12.5E	..	..	14.3E	18.6E
Northwest Territories [4]	8.4E	9.5	..	..	6.6E	6.2E	9.7E	12.0E	5.9E	8.9E
Nunavut [4, 5]	13.4E	9.1	..	..	13.3E	F	..	..	8.4E	F

Symbol Legend:
.. Not Available
E Use with caution
F Too unreliable to be published

Source: Statistics Canada. *Table 105-0503 - Health indicator profile, age-standardized rate, annual estimates, by sex, Canada, provinces and territories, occasional,* CANSIM (database). (accessed: March 31, 2017)

Please see footnotes 30, 31, 57, 58, 59, 60, 61, 62, 64 for characteristics of the age-standardized rate.

AGE-STANDARDIZED RATES, INJURIES WITHIN THE PAST 12 MONTHS, SOUGHT MEDICAL ATTENTION (%), [54], [55], [65] FEMALES, CANADA, PROVINCES AND TERRITORIES

Geography	2003	2005	2007	2008	2009	2010	2011	2012	2013	2014
Canada	6.8	7.2	..	..	7.2	7.1	..	..	7.7	7.8
Newfoundland and Labrador	7.2	7.4	..	..	6.8	8.0			8.3E	9.2
Prince Edward Island	6.6	6.9	..	..	6.7E	8.5E	..		9.9	8.5E
Nova Scotia	7.3	7.9	..	..	9.2	8.5			8.6	9.4
New Brunswick	6.7	6.1	..	..	7.5	8.0	..		6.2	7.0
Quebec	5.7	6.3	..	..	6.0	5.5	..	..	7.4	7.3
Ontario	6.7	7.1	..	..	6.7	7.0	..		7.4	7.3
Manitoba	9.8	7.4	..	..	8.6	7.1E	..		11.5	9.8
Saskatchewan	7.3	8.4	..	..	7.5	8.9			7.2	6.9
Alberta	8.2	7.9	..	..	10.0	8.5	8.6	8.6	7.1	7.5
British Columbia	7.5	8.5	..	..	8.1	7.9	..		9.0	9.8
Yukon [4]	5.9E	7.4E	..	..	6.0E	13.1E	..		13.8E	11.9E
Northwest Territories [4]	5.1E	8.9	..	..	F	6.4E	5.7E	7.3E	10.7E	8.0E
Nunavut [4], [5]	4.6E	F	..	..	F	F	..		F	F

Symbol Legend:
.. Not Available
E Use with caution
F Too unreliable to be published

Source: Statistics Canada. *Table 105-0503 - Health indicator profile, age-standardized rate, annual estimates, by sex, Canada, provinces and territories, occasional,* CANSIM (database). (accessed: March 31, 2017)

Please see footnotes [30], [31], [57], [58], [59], [60], [61], [62], [64] for characteristics of the age-standardized rate.

AGE-STANDARDIZED RATES, CANCER INCIDENCE (PER 100,000 POPULATION), BOTH SEXES, CANADA, PROVINCES AND TERRITORIES

Geography	2003	2004	2005	2006	2007	2008	2009	2010	2011	2012	2013
Canada	518.2	523.4	526.9	527.9	533.0	522.3	522.8	514.0	517.2	505.3	513.6
Newfoundland and Labrador [4, 18]	448.4	453.0	469.8	556.4	567.6	579.9	574.3	568.2	572.1	550.5	556.6
Prince Edward Island	613.7	578.5	566.2	564.7	604.6	569.5	561.4	535.1	555.2	551.4	526.9
Nova Scotia	563.1	578.1	580.8	615.9	594.5	564.6	550.0	571.9	549.0	563.1	554.6
New Brunswick	535.0	537.1	572.3	580.1	580.7	581.4	566.4	549.4	541.8	529.8	538.1
Quebec [4, 18, 20]	546.7	551.2	553.4	546.5	547.0	553.2	551.5	531.6	531.6	531.6	531.6
Ontario [4, 18, 21]	503.3	515.1	524.3	524.5	529.4	504.1	507.2	506.7	509.4	488.0	516.9
Manitoba	520.7	541.1	521.9	518.6	534.2	533.3	540.7	530.0	534.7	512.7	509.7
Saskatchewan	522.1	534.8	524.6	508.1	531.4	531.6	520.7	503.2	511.0	504.0	500.7
Alberta	543.3	530.5	515.2	520.5	514.3	514.9	511.9	502.3	513.6	498.4	485.4
British Columbia	484.2	477.6	483.4	484.7	502.7	491.6	497.2	482.7	493.3	489.0	480.4
Yukon	450.8	543.1	549.1	390.7	488.8	367.4	480.6	444.1	438.1	396.0	429.8
Northwest Territories [5]	645.3	575.3	571.7	458.3	613.5	495.2	558.1	512.1	504.5	570.9	454.9
Nunavut [5]	897.0	465.8	874.3	680.6	512.2	426.4	554.1	449.4	450.7	429.2	411.6

Source: Statistics Canada. *Table 103-0554 - New cases and 2011 age-standardized rate for primary cancer (based on the July 2016 CCR tabulation file), by cancer type and sex, Canada, provinces and territories, annual (number unless otherwise noted),* CANSIM (database). (accessed: March 31, 2017)

Primary types of cancer (ICD-O-3) 2, 3, 6 = Total, all primary sites of cancer
Census population structure = 2011 Census population structure 13
Characteristics 14, 15, 16 = New cancer cases (age-standardized rate per 100,000 population) 17

Also see footnotes 1, 2, 3, 19

AGE-STANDARDIZED RATES, CANCER INCIDENCE (PER 100,000 POPULATION), MALES, CANADA, PROVINCES AND TERRITORIES

Geography	2003	2004	2005	2006	2007	2008	2009	2010	2011	2012	2013
Canada	609.0	615.7	614.7	616.1	618.9	601.9	594.3	577.5	581.0	557.7	568.3
Newfoundland and Labrador [4, 18]	511.5	532.6	544.5	689.6	675.4	685.2	707.0	677.8	655.9	594.8	615.2
Prince Edward Island	744.7	708.0	674.3	734.6	741.3	670.6	715.3	613.3	684.2	650.9	609.2
Nova Scotia	687.8	707.8	690.4	747.6	708.5	656.8	645.3	652.3	623.8	634.5	634.8
New Brunswick	651.0	664.1	700.5	703.8	708.7	721.8	668.1	652.8	626.7	613.7	613.5
Quebec [4, 18, 20]	658.2	666.7	659.9	646.0	638.6	643.1	637.8	602.5	602.5	602.5	602.5
Ontario [4, 18, 21]	583.4	599.4	608.3	608.4	610.0	573.5	565.5	565.1	568.6	525.1	565.7
Manitoba	608.1	622.4	587.6	596.0	620.4	597.5	601.5	591.9	591.0	555.0	548.1
Saskatchewan	617.8	656.8	631.6	574.6	614.5	624.0	592.7	552.1	570.4	569.9	546.0
Alberta	643.3	616.3	597.3	607.4	594.1	599.8	593.7	569.9	585.9	562.3	539.9
British Columbia	562.8	547.4	553.2	559.8	588.5	568.2	562.4	539.1	551.4	541.0	528.6
Yukon	588.6	619.4	578.0	372.0	516.0	346.8	524.6	419.2	477.2	408.8	443.5
Northwest Territories [5]	673.9	718.4	750.2	545.0	684.4	440.1	633.0	540.1	519.0	561.9	543.6
Nunavut [5]	1,015.2	477.3	951.3	657.4	480.6	475.5	605.2	456.2	385.0	397.0	401.6

Source: Statistics Canada. *Table 103-0554 - New cases and 2011 age-standardized rate for primary cancer (based on the July 2016 CCR tabulation file), by cancer type and sex, Canada, provinces and territories, annual (number unless otherwise noted)*, CANSIM (database). (accessed: March 31, 2017)

Primary types of cancer (ICD-O-3) [2], [3], [6] = Total, all primary sites of cancer
Census population structure = 2011 Census population structure [13]
Characteristics [14], [15], [16] = New cancer cases (age-standardized rate per 100,000 population) [17]

Also see footnotes [1], [2], [3], [19]

AGE-STANDARDIZED RATES, CANCER INCIDENCE (PER 100,000 POPULATION), FEMALES, CANADA, PROVINCES AND TERRITORIES

Geography	2003	2004	2005	2006	2007	2008	2009	2010	2011	2012	2013
Canada	455.2	458.3	465.7	465.7	471.4	466.0	472.1	470.3	472.8	469.9	476.9
Newfoundland and Labrador [4, 18]	397.5	388.2	413.6	449.5	480.9	492.8	463.9	482.6	503.5	516.9	506.0
Prince Edward Island	520.1	472.8	473.1	430.4	490.4	491.7	439.6	474.3	450.9	476.5	468.6
Nova Scotia	470.8	481.3	498.8	517.3	508.6	495.7	478.0	514.3	492.0	509.9	495.3
New Brunswick	450.6	446.4	480.0	484.6	480.1	471.1	484.7	465.7	475.0	465.9	480.0
Quebec [4, 18, 20]	478.8	479.4	488.7	486.0	490.3	499.5	500.2	492.0	492.0	492.0	492.0
Ontario [4, 18, 21]	448.2	455.3	464.6	464.4	471.2	454.5	465.9	465.8	468.1	464.3	484.6
Manitoba	462.8	486.9	482.5	468.7	472.4	490.1	503.0	487.2	497.9	485.9	486.3
Saskatchewan	448.9	437.8	440.6	459.2	465.5	461.0	465.2	468.0	467.1	454.8	467.4
Alberta	466.7	466.4	454.5	455.2	456.5	449.7	448.5	451.0	459.2	449.6	447.0
British Columbia	425.0	423.9	431.0	427.6	434.7	431.9	445.7	438.9	446.0	447.3	442.2
Yukon	390.5	454.5	527.6	408.2	453.2	383.5	455.3	468.7	382.8	384.0	416.9
Northwest Territories [5]	707.7	480.0	428.4	380.5	561.6	530.6	509.8	484.6	474.4	588.2	373.6
Nunavut [5]	961.9	445.7	774.2	693.4	538.8	381.5	488.2	444.7	507.2	448.0	410.8

Source: Statistics Canada. *Table 103-0554 - New cases and 2011 age-standardized rate for primary cancer (based on the July 2016 CCR tabulation file), by cancer type and sex, Canada, provinces and territories, annual (number unless otherwise noted),* CANSIM (database). (accessed: March 31, 2017)

Primary types of cancer (ICD-O-3) 2, 3, 6 = Total, all primary sites of cancer
Census population structure = 2011 Census population structure 13
Characteristics 14, 15, 16 = New cancer cases (age-standardized rate per 100,000 population) 17

Also see footnotes 1, 2, 3, 19

SECTION IV: Statistics

AGE-STANDARDIZED RATES, COLON CANCER INCIDENCE (PER 100,000 POPULATION), BOTH SEXES, CANADA, PROVINCES AND TERRITORIES

Geography	2003	2004	2005	2006	2007	2008	2009	2010	2011	2012	2013
Canada	45.2	45.9	45.9	44.9	45.2	44.8	43.7	42.5	42.4	41.7	41.6
Newfoundland and Labrador [4, 18]	65.4	63.6	62.6	69.6	69.5	62.9	59.5	63.3	66.4	65.7	64.2
Prince Edward Island	43.8	53.9	57.9	44.5	42.6	57.8	49.3	42.5	58.3	44.8	54.5
Nova Scotia	55.6	55.6	53.2	54.9	55.4	58.5	47.0	56.1	51.9	53.5	47.9
New Brunswick	45.4	38.8	44.1	40.7	42.6	43.3	44.3	42.6	41.4	43.3	45.8
Quebec [4, 18, 20]	48.1	48.4	49.0	46.6	46.9	47.5	47.4	45.7	45.7	45.7	45.7
Ontario [4, 18, 21]	44.3	46.5	46.1	45.2	45.7	44.2	42.7	39.5	39.5	38.0	37.7
Manitoba	45.0	46.5	44.7	45.1	47.5	46.2	47.6	47.9	47.8	40.7	41.7
Saskatchewan	45.4	46.6	45.3	41.3	44.0	44.4	43.1	45.1	44.6	47.2	51.4
Alberta	41.9	40.1	39.6	40.4	38.7	37.9	39.2	40.6	39.9	36.4	36.2
British Columbia	39.2	39.9	40.9	39.8	39.8	40.1	38.7	38.3	38.6	41.4	41.9
Yukon	36.4	63.5	66.2	51.1	38.7	40.2	29.2	37.9	19.7	52.7	32.8
Northwest Territories [5]	69.7	98.1	30.6	60.5	80.4	67.1	58.3	65.6	62.4	83.6	32.0
Nunavut [5]	120.3	38.8	128.1	145.1	91.3	27.0	34.1	53.0	87.8	47.2	93.4

Source: Statistics Canada. *Table 103-0554 - New cases and 2011 age-standardized rate for primary cancer (based on the July 2016 CCR tabulation file), by cancer type and sex, Canada, provinces and territories, annual (number unless otherwise noted)*, CANSIM (database). (accessed: March 31, 2017)

Primary types of cancer (ICD-O-3) [2], [3], [6] = Colon excluding rectum [C18.0-C18.9, C26.0] [7]
Census population structure = 2011 Census population structure [13]
Characteristics [14], [15], [16] = New cancer cases (age-standardized rate per 100,000 population) [17]

Also see footnotes [1], [2], [3], [19]

AGE-STANDARDIZED RATES, COLON CANCER INCIDENCE (PER 100,000 POPULATION), MALES, CANADA, PROVINCES AND TERRITORIES

Geography	2003	2004	2005	2006	2007	2008	2009	2010	2011	2012	2013
Canada	51.9	52.1	52.6	51.8	52.3	51.6	50.6	47.6	48.0	46.8	47.2
Newfoundland and Labrador [4, 18]	72.2	76.1	68.8	81.2	81.1	69.5	74.8	66.9	71.4	73.3	69.9
Prince Edward Island	47.9	54.3	56.7	48.4	54.7	57.0	51.9	52.6	72.6	41.4	70.1
Nova Scotia	67.8	59.3	59.5	57.9	66.1	66.4	53.7	64.5	51.3	58.2	54.7
New Brunswick	50.4	41.9	51.4	47.9	49.7	51.5	49.9	44.7	45.1	50.0	50.6
Quebec [4, 18, 20]	55.9	55.2	56.6	55.9	55.2	55.5	55.0	52.9	52.9	52.9	52.9
Ontario [4, 18, 21]	50.3	53.1	53.0	52.2	52.6	50.8	49.0	44.4	44.9	41.2	43.4
Manitoba	56.0	54.8	51.9	52.6	54.9	55.4	55.9	52.7	53.8	51.4	43.4
Saskatchewan	52.4	52.7	52.1	47.2	49.9	54.8	49.8	47.6	51.1	54.9	63.0
Alberta	48.5	46.4	44.6	47.2	44.0	44.3	46.7	44.4	46.9	42.3	39.3
British Columbia	44.8	43.9	46.9	43.8	46.4	45.2	45.2	42.4	43.3	45.7	45.9
Yukon	50.0	85.1	31.2	63.2	43.7	28.5	x	30.1	x	55.8	38.5
Northwest Territories [5]	151.7	141.3	x	82.7	78.7	50.6	65.4	49.8	75.2	60.4	x
Nunavut [5]	104.7	x	122.7	145.7	106.8	x	32.0	36.7	128.7	41.3	58.7

Symbol Legend:
X   Suppressed to meet the confidentiality requirements of the Statistics Act

Source: Statistics Canada. *Table 103-0554 - New cases and 2011 age-standardized rate for primary cancer (based on the July 2016 CCR tabulation file), by cancer type and sex, Canada, provinces and territories, annual (number unless otherwise noted),* CANSIM (database). (accessed: March 31, 2017)

Primary types of cancer (ICD-O-3) 2, 3, 6 = Colon excluding rectum [C18.0-C18.9, C26.0] 7
Census population structure = 2011 Census population structure 13
Characteristics 14, 15, 16 = New cancer cases (age-standardized rate per 100,000 population) 17

Also see footnotes 1, 2, 3, 19

AGE-STANDARDIZED RATES, COLON CANCER INCIDENCE (PER 100,000 POPULATION), FEMALES, CANADA, PROVINCES AND TERRITORIES

Geography	2003	2004	2005	2006	2007	2008	2009	2010	2011	2012	2013
Canada	39.8	41.0	40.6	39.3	39.5	39.3	38.2	38.2	37.8	37.5	37.0
Newfoundland and Labrador [4, 18]	60.8	53.9	56.7	61.0	59.4	56.6	47.3	60.0	62.4	58.7	59.0
Prince Edward Island	41.2	50.9	58.0	41.0	33.5	57.3	49.3	34.3	46.4	46.7	42.6
Nova Scotia	46.4	53.1	47.1	53.2	48.1	52.7	42.3	49.6	52.5	50.7	41.6
New Brunswick	41.4	36.2	38.6	34.7	36.7	37.4	38.9	39.8	37.9	37.0	41.3
Quebec [4, 18, 20]	42.1	43.4	43.3	39.9	40.9	42.1	41.5	40.1	40.1	40.1	40.1
Ontario [4, 18, 21]	39.6	40.9	40.4	39.3	40.1	38.5	37.8	35.5	35.2	35.3	33.1
Manitoba	36.6	39.9	39.7	39.3	41.2	39.4	41.1	43.5	43.1	32.1	39.8
Saskatchewan	39.0	41.3	39.8	36.2	38.5	35.6	37.3	42.8	38.7	40.8	41.1
Alberta	36.4	35.2	35.2	34.5	34.0	32.1	32.7	37.4	34.5	31.5	34.1
British Columbia	34.4	36.8	35.8	36.6	34.4	36.0	33.5	34.6	34.4	37.4	38.3
Yukon	x	38.4	90.0	37.3	30.5	53.3	x	46.3	x	52.2	x
Northwest Territories [5]	57.3	47.4	35.2	x	77.6	84.0	52.0	78.4	43.1	105.2	35.6
Nunavut [5]	146.7	23.0	x	141.9	69.1	x	36.9	x	x	56.4	128.6

Symbol Legend:
X Suppressed to meet the confidentiality requirements of the Statistics Act

Source: Statistics Canada. *Table 103-0554 - New cases and 2011 age-standardized rate for primary cancer (based on the July 2016 CCR tabulation file), by cancer type and sex, Canada, provinces and territories, annual (number unless otherwise noted),* CANSIM (database). (accessed: March 31, 2017)

Primary types of cancer (ICD-O-3) 2, 3, 6 = Colon excluding rectum [C18.0-C18.9, C26.0] 7
Census population structure = 2011 Census population structure 13
Characteristics 14, 15, 16 = New cancer cases (age-standardized rate per 100,000 population) 17

Also see footnotes 1, 2, 3, 19

AGE-STANDARDIZED RATES, LUNG CANCER INCIDENCE (PER 100,000 POPULATION), BOTH SEXES, CANADA, PROVINCES AND TERRITORIES

Geography	2003	2004	2005	2006	2007	2008	2009	2010	2011	2012	2013
Canada	75.4	76.0	76.4	75.7	75.8	74.3	73.6	70.9	69.6	70.1	69.3
Newfoundland and Labrador [4, 18]	55.8	53.8	61.8	80.9	73.3	73.2	82.2	76.7	69.8	73.2	75.0
Prince Edward Island	80.1	89.0	83.6	79.8	84.6	82.3	95.2	82.6	71.7	77.6	66.8
Nova Scotia	88.2	87.4	90.6	91.2	91.3	85.3	85.1	86.2	83.4	90.8	81.2
New Brunswick	89.4	88.8	91.8	94.6	91.3	93.6	89.0	81.5	76.9	80.1	85.5
Quebec [4, 18, 20]	96.4	97.4	95.9	94.5	95.2	96.2	92.5	86.8	86.8	86.8	86.8
Ontario [4, 18, 21]	64.6	65.8	68.0	66.8	65.8	62.7	63.2	62.7	61.9	62.5	61.9
Manitoba	78.5	79.9	81.0	73.8	75.3	77.7	77.6	73.3	71.9	70.0	68.8
Saskatchewan	69.3	68.4	71.1	72.5	72.3	71.8	67.4	73.6	74.7	67.5	71.1
Alberta	71.7	68.1	66.7	68.8	66.8	68.0	68.2	64.0	62.8	62.3	61.3
British Columbia	66.8	68.4	66.1	64.2	68.5	64.5	64.6	61.5	59.2	61.7	59.5
Yukon	73.1	77.9	88.9	50.7	73.7	57.8	92.1	70.9	54.3	72.5	75.0
Northwest Territories [5]	80.9	108.5	97.3	83.2	97.9	99.4	78.1	65.6	84.1	102.1	68.1
Nunavut [5]	439.5	210.8	312.4	276.1	194.4	163.0	232.5	217.0	150.2	153.7	144.9

Source: Statistics Canada. *Table 103-0554 - New cases and 2011 age-standardized rate for primary cancer (based on the July 2016 CCR tabulation file), by cancer type and sex, Canada, provinces and territories, annual (number unless otherwise noted),* CANSIM (database). (accessed: March 31, 2017)

Primary types of cancer (ICD-O-3) 2, 3, 6 = Lung and bronchus [C34.0-C34.9] 7
Census population structure = 2011 Census population structure 13
Characteristics 14, 15, 16 = New cancer cases (age-standardized rate per 100,000 population) 17

Also see footnotes 1, 2, 3, 19

AGE-STANDARDIZED RATES, LUNG CANCER INCIDENCE (PER 100,000 POPULATION), MALES, CANADA, PROVINCES AND TERRITORIES

Geography	2003	2004	2005	2006	2007	2008	2009	2010	2011	2012	2013
Canada	96.3	96.4	94.9	93.0	92.6	88.8	87.4	83.5	81.3	81.1	79.4
Newfoundland and Labrador [4, 18]	79.2	75.2	78.7	104.2	96.8	102.7	115.7	100.1	94.8	93.1	87.8
Prince Edward Island	106.6	110.8	102.0	92.5	96.3	115.1	126.7	111.7	92.0	102.1	82.2
Nova Scotia	114.7	116.1	117.7	114.8	109.1	98.7	104.2	99.1	98.0	103.4	94.3
New Brunswick	127.4	119.8	117.0	114.1	123.2	116.0	113.9	105.5	97.3	100.1	105.5
Quebec [4, 18, 20]	133.6	134.5	130.4	126.1	124.5	123.3	115.9	108.0	108.0	108.0	108.0
Ontario [4, 18, 21]	80.7	81.2	82.3	81.2	78.4	72.8	73.6	73.5	71.1	71.2	69.4
Manitoba	89.2	95.1	94.6	86.3	92.8	91.0	86.6	79.6	78.9	72.4	76.1
Saskatchewan	84.9	83.3	85.2	79.1	83.6	80.6	75.9	80.1	80.3	75.1	74.0
Alberta	87.5	79.9	77.0	81.2	77.7	76.2	81.0	71.1	68.3	67.1	66.1
British Columbia	78.1	79.4	75.2	72.4	77.8	73.2	70.8	68.0	65.4	66.9	64.1
Yukon	77.1	66.8	149.1	28.9	74.1	34.3	85.8	59.6	61.7	95.8	61.8
Northwest Territories [5]	35.3	98.5	138.1	104.5	122.5	95.7	61.5	78.0	81.4	142.5	104.3
Nunavut [5]	406.0	215.7	369.1	251.8	236.3	185.2	252.1	258.1	59.3	142.8	163.2

Source: Statistics Canada. *Table 103-0554 - New cases and 2011 age-standardized rate for primary cancer (based on the July 2016 CCR tabulation file), by cancer type and sex, Canada, provinces and territories, annual (number unless otherwise noted)*, CANSIM (database). (accessed: March 31, 2017)

Primary types of cancer (ICD-O-3) [2], [3], [6] = Lung and bronchus [C34.0-C34.9] [7]
Census population structure = 2011 Census population structure [13]
Characteristics [14], [15], [16] = New cancer cases (age-standardized rate per 100,000 population) [17]

Also see footnotes [1], [2], [3], [19]

AGE-STANDARDIZED RATES, LUNG CANCER INCIDENCE (PER 100,000 POPULATION), FEMALES, CANADA, PROVINCES AND TERRITORIES

Geography	2003	2004	2005	2006	2007	2008	2009	2010	2011	2012	2013
Canada	60.4	61.3	63.1	63.5	63.8	63.9	63.7	61.7	61.4	62.4	62.1
Newfoundland and Labrador [4, 18]	35.5	34.8	47.8	61.8	53.5	49.7	56.6	58.1	49.6	57.1	65.1
Prince Edward Island	62.3	76.0	67.5	72.7	75.1	53.8	70.8	59.4	54.3	60.4	55.9
Nova Scotia	67.9	66.5	71.6	74.4	79.1	75.9	70.4	77.8	72.5	82.5	72.4
New Brunswick	61.0	67.8	74.4	80.5	68.6	76.8	70.4	63.5	61.6	66.2	70.8
Quebec [4, 18, 20]	72.1	72.0	72.7	74.0	75.4	78.3	77.6	73.1	73.1	73.1	73.1
Ontario [4, 18, 21]	52.9	54.5	57.8	56.3	56.7	55.3	55.6	54.5	55.4	56.2	56.5
Manitoba	70.7	69.0	71.1	65.6	63.0	68.7	73.7	69.2	67.3	68.9	63.9
Saskatchewan	58.0	57.4	61.1	68.2	64.3	65.7	61.5	68.5	70.8	62.1	69.8
Alberta	59.9	59.3	59.5	60.4	59.5	62.7	58.7	58.9	59.1	59.4	58.3
British Columbia	59.1	60.6	58.9	59.1	61.4	57.9	60.0	56.6	54.5	58.0	56.3
Yukon	66.2	89.9	x	75.5	79.1	80.9	99.1	82.4	40.8	45.9	90.7
Northwest Territories [5]	131.2	124.8	60.9	62.7	75.6	94.3	95.2	49.6	83.6	66.4	29.5
Nunavut [5]	512.3	204.0	237.8	295.2	147.7	139.3	200.7	175.8	224.9	158.6	124.2

Symbol Legend:
X   Suppressed to meet the confidentiality requirements of the Statistics Act

Source: Statistics Canada. *Table 103-0554 - New cases and 2011 age-standardized rate for primary cancer (based on the July 2016 CCR tabulation file), by cancer type and sex, Canada, provinces and territories, annual (number unless otherwise noted),* CANSIM (database). (accessed: March 31, 2017)

Primary types of cancer (ICD-O-3) [2], [3], [6] = Lung and bronchus [C34.0-C34.9] [7]
Census population structure = 2011 Census population structure [13]
Characteristics [14], [15], [16] = New cancer cases (age-standardized rate per 100,000 population) [17]

Also see footnotes [1], [2], [3], [19]

AGE-STANDARDIZED RATES, BREAST CANCER INCIDENCE (PER 100,000 POPULATION), BOTH SEXES, CANADA, PROVINCES AND TERRITORIES

Geography	2003	2004	2005	2006	2007	2008	2009	2010	2011	2012	2013
Canada	67.7	67.8	68.1	67.9	68.1	66.5	67.9	68.2	68.4	66.4	66.4
Newfoundland and Labrador [4, 18]	60.2	59.4	63.3	59.0	60.6	66.6	60.2	62.1	64.9	64.5	69.4
Prince Edward Island	87.0	75.6	61.0	57.5	58.3	72.2	60.4	82.8	64.1	72.2	73.9
Nova Scotia	66.3	67.2	72.8	75.1	66.9	71.8	68.0	72.5	68.0	69.7	61.7
New Brunswick	69.7	61.7	70.3	65.6	66.9	65.2	67.8	66.1	66.8	61.4	63.7
Quebec [4, 18, 20]	70.6	71.1	70.7	71.0	71.0	70.4	71.1	69.4	69.4	69.4	69.4
Ontario [4, 18, 21]	67.1	67.9	68.1	68.5	68.9	65.6	67.5	68.3	68.4	66.4	66.6
Manitoba	70.2	71.3	69.7	69.0	69.1	69.9	69.3	68.7	72.2	68.3	65.3
Saskatchewan	66.5	65.0	65.3	67.2	67.6	65.1	69.5	65.5	66.3	64.3	68.3
Alberta	68.8	69.5	63.9	64.6	65.4	62.5	65.3	66.9	65.7	65.1	62.9
British Columbia	62.8	63.0	65.4	63.2	64.7	64.0	65.7	67.0	69.2	62.7	64.5
Yukon	48.4	78.2	89.1	76.2	46.2	45.0	59.8	59.9	69.6	75.5	76.4
Northwest Territories [5]	125.2	54.4	46.4	51.0	61.0	51.5	64.1	71.4	61.2	69.1	60.2
Nunavut [5]	9.7	27.4	77.4	51.2	x	37.6	x	34.8	33.4	37.3	10.7

Symbol Legend:
X Suppressed to meet the confidentiality requirements of the Statistics Act

Source: Statistics Canada. *Table 103-0554 - New cases and 2011 age-standardized rate for primary cancer (based on the July 2016 CCR tabulation file), by cancer type and sex, Canada, provinces and territories, annual (number unless otherwise noted),* CANSIM (database). (accessed: March 31, 2017)

Primary types of cancer (ICD-O-3) [2], [3], [6] = Breast [C50.0-C50.9] [7]
Census population structure = 2011 Census population structure [13]
Characteristics [14], [15], [16] = New cancer cases (age-standardized rate per 100,000 population) [17]

Also see footnotes [1], [2], [3], [19]

AGE-STANDARDIZED RATES, BREAST CANCER INCIDENCE (PER 100,000 POPULATION), MALES, CANADA, PROVINCES AND TERRITORIES

Geography	2003	2004	2005	2006	2007	2008	2009	2010	2011	2012	2013
Canada	1.4	1.2	1.2	1.1	1.2	1.2	1.3	1.4	1.2	1.3	1.2
Newfoundland and Labrador [4, 18]	x	x	x	0.5	x	x	1.5	1.2	x	1.6	1.2
Prince Edward Island	3.5	x	x	x	x	x	x	2.9	x	x	x
Nova Scotia	2.0	x	3.4	1.6	1.8	1.5	1.1	2.9	2.4	1.6	1.1
New Brunswick	2.0	x	0.3	1.2	1.9	x	1.4	0.9	x	2.7	2.2
Quebec [4, 18, 20]	1.1	1.2	1.4	1.0	1.1	1.7	1.3	1.4	1.4	1.4	1.4
Ontario [4, 18, 21]	1.7	1.5	1.3	1.3	1.3	1.1	1.4	1.4	1.5	1.2	1.2
Manitoba	1.4	1.3	x	0.6	1.0	1.3	1.0	1.7	x	1.3	0.7
Saskatchewan	x	1.1	0.7	1.3	x	0.8	1.3	1.7	1.2	1.0	1.2
Alberta	1.3	1.1	1.2	0.9	1.2	0.9	1.2	0.6	0.8	0.9	0.6
British Columbia	1.2	0.9	0.6	0.9	1.1	1.0	1.2	1.3	0.7	1.3	1.1
Yukon	x	x	x	x	x	x	x	x	x	x	x
Northwest Territories [5]	x	x	x	x	x	x	x	x	4.6	x	x
Nunavut [5]	x	x	x	x	x	x	x	x	x	x	x

Symbol Legend:
X   Suppressed to meet the confidentiality requirements of the Statistics Act

Source: Statistics Canada. *Table 103-0554 - New cases and 2011 age-standardized rate for primary cancer (based on the July 2016 CCR tabulation file), by cancer type and sex, Canada, provinces and territories, annual (number unless otherwise noted),* CANSIM (database). (accessed: March 31, 2017)

Primary types of cancer (ICD-O-3) 2, 3, 6 = Breast [C50.0-C50.9] 7
Census population structure = 2011 Census population structure 13
Characteristics 14, 15, 16 = New cancer cases (age-standardized rate per 100,000 population) 17

Also see footnotes 1, 2, 3, 19

AGE-STANDARDIZED RATES, BREAST CANCER INCIDENCE (PER 100,000 POPULATION), FEMALES, CANADA, PROVINCES AND TERRITORIES

Geography	2003	2004	2005	2006	2007	2008	2009	2010	2011	2012	2013
Canada	126.5	127.0	127.8	127.8	128.4	125.7	128.4	129.4	130.0	126.3	126.4
Newfoundland and Labrador [4, 18]	115.0	112.3	120.9	112.5	115.1	125.9	112.7	117.2	123.4	123.0	131.8
Prince Edward Island	162.8	141.6	113.4	108.1	109.8	136.6	112.4	153.4	120.7	135.5	137.2
Nova Scotia	121.5	124.5	133.2	139.6	122.9	133.9	127.4	134.4	126.7	130.8	115.3
New Brunswick	128.8	115.3	131.6	121.8	124.5	122.0	127.1	124.7	126.3	115.3	119.6
Quebec [4, 18, 20]	130.6	131.4	131.2	132.6	132.8	131.9	133.6	131.3	131.3	131.3	131.3
Ontario [4, 18, 21]	124.9	126.6	127.7	128.5	129.2	123.5	126.9	128.6	128.7	125.4	126.0
Manitoba	131.5	134.1	131.1	130.1	130.4	131.5	131.4	130.5	138.1	130.0	125.2
Saskatchewan	126.2	122.9	124.3	127.7	129.4	124.5	132.4	124.5	126.6	123.9	132.1
Alberta	131.3	133.1	121.8	123.8	125.6	120.2	125.9	130.1	127.7	126.9	123.3
British Columbia	119.4	119.7	124.7	120.2	123.2	122.3	126.2	128.7	133.5	120.3	123.8
Yukon	92.2	158.4	164.8	147.5	94.6	92.9	128.2	125.3	145.2	142.3	155.8
Northwest Territories [5]	275.2	115.4	94.8	113.4	126.8	107.8	138.0	154.4	118.8	141.8	119.8
Nunavut [5]	20.3	58.2	171.2	106.4	x	83.9	x	74.2	71.3	x	x

Symbol Legend:
X   Suppressed to meet the confidentiality requirements of the Statistics Act

Source: Statistics Canada. *Table 103-0554 - New cases and 2011 age-standardized rate for primary cancer (based on the July 2016 CCR tabulation file), by cancer type and sex, Canada, provinces and territories, annual (number unless otherwise noted),* CANSIM (database). (accessed: March 31, 2017)

Primary types of cancer (ICD-O-3) 2, 3, 6 = Breast [C50.0-C50.9] 7
Census population structure = 2011 Census population structure 13
Characteristics 14, 15, 16 = New cancer cases (age-standardized rate per 100,000 population) 17

Also see footnotes 1, 2, 3, 19

AGE-STANDARDIZED RATES, CURRENT SMOKER, DAILY OR OCCASIONAL (%), [22], [23], [24], [25], [26], [28] BOTH SEXES, CANADA, PROVINCES AND TERRITORIES

Geography	2003	2005	2007	2008	2009	2010	2011	2012	2013	2014
Canada	23.4	22.2	22.6	21.9	20.5	21.1	20.4	20.6	19.6	18.5
Newfoundland and Labrador	25.1	24.1	26.6	25.2	24.3	24.1	22.1	27.1	21.0	22.4
Prince Edward Island	24.6	22.8	22.9	20.8	21.2	24.5	23.9	24.2	20.4	21.9
Nova Scotia	24.5	23.8	25.7	24.1	24.8	23.2	22.0	23.9	22.2	23.5
New Brunswick	26.0	23.6	24.4	24.3	23.1	23.9	22.4	24.6	22.3	21.9
Quebec	26.4	24.8	25.6	24.0	23.1	23.8	21.9	24.4	21.9	20.3
Ontario	22.6	21.3	21.2	20.3	18.9	19.5	19.9	19.2	18.1	17.8
Manitoba	23.5	21.5	23.6	25.1	21.7	19.4	21.5	20.5	20.0	16.4
Saskatchewan	25.3	25.0	27.2	25.5	22.7	23.4	24.2	20.2	23.9	20.5
Alberta	22.9	22.9	22.0	22.6	22.8	22.4	21.4	21.2	20.4	18.5
British Columbia	19.2	18.4	18.4	19.1	16.3	18.1	15.9	15.3	16.9	15.1
Yukon [4]	28.2	29.9	36.1	30.4	35.3	26.9	28.2	29.2	25.2	24.9
Northwest Territories [4]	36.0	36.6	37.0	33.8	37.1	38.8	36.5	35.0	33.3	32.5
Nunavut [4, 5]	63.8	51.1	56.9	51.6	57.0	51.9	55.2	51.5	57.1	58.1

Source: Statistics Canada. *Table 105-0503 - Health indicator profile, age-standardized rate, annual estimates, by sex, Canada, provinces and territories, occasional,* CANSIM (database). (accessed: March 31, 2017)

Please see footnotes [30], [31], [57], [58], [59], [60], [61], [62], [64] for characteristics of the age-standardized rate.

AGE-STANDARDIZED RATES, CURRENT SMOKER, DAILY OR OCCASIONAL (%), [22], [23], [24], [25], [26], [28] MALES, CANADA, PROVINCES AND TERRITORIES

Geography	2003	2005	2007	2008	2009	2010	2011	2012	2013	2014
Canada	25.6	24.4	25.5	25.0	23.1	24.7	23.0	23.5	22.7	22.0
Newfoundland and Labrador	28.7	24.7	31.7	27.4	29.7	25.6	25.5	30.0	23.1	26.4
Prince Edward Island	27.7	26.3	27.4	24.3	23.1	28.1	26.7	26.7	27.5	28.0
Nova Scotia	26.2	25.2	27.3	27.2	26.3	24.3	22.7	27.4	25.7	25.0
New Brunswick	26.8	26.2	28.6	24.3	23.7	27.1	21.8	28.8	27.0	23.7
Quebec	27.8	25.8	28.1	26.4	24.7	27.3	23.1	28.2	24.3	23.2
Ontario	25.6	24.3	24.5	24.2	22.2	23.5	24.4	22.1	21.2	22.4
Manitoba	24.1	23.0	26.8	28.3	23.8	21.7	22.7	21.3	21.3	20.5
Saskatchewan	26.4	26.1	28.1	28.5	24.2	25.7	25.6	20.0	26.1	20.8
Alberta	24.7	25.8	25.2	25.3	26.0	26.1	23.5	25.5	24.7	21.4
British Columbia	21.8	20.3	21.1	22.1	18.1	21.9	17.2	16.4	20.2	18.3
Yukon [4]	27.9	31.4	37.2	31.8	38.3	27.5	30.9	30.4	23.8	27.9
Northwest Territories [4]	37.2	35.1	39.6	37.1	37.6	38.5	41.6	36.0	32.7	37.2
Nunavut [4, 5]	63.7	52.5	58.0	50.6	63.0	45.8	53.1	53.7	47.6	54.5

Source: Statistics Canada. *Table 105-0503 - Health indicator profile, age-standardized rate, annual estimates, by sex, Canada, provinces and territories, occasional,* CANSIM (database). (accessed: March 31, 2017)

Please see footnotes 30, 31, 57, 58, 59, 60, 61, 62, 64 for characteristics of the age-standardized rate.

AGE-STANDARDIZED RATES, CURRENT SMOKER, DAILY OR OCCASIONAL (%), [22], [23], [24], [25], [26], [28] FEMALES, CANADA, PROVINCES AND TERRITORIES

Geography	2003	2005	2007	2008	2009	2010	2011	2012	2013	2014
Canada	21.3	20.1	19.7	18.9	18.0	17.6	17.9	17.8	16.6	15.1
Newfoundland and Labrador	21.8	23.5	21.8	23.0	19.2	22.6	18.9	24.3	18.9	18.6
Prince Edward Island	21.6	19.6	18.8	17.4	19.5	21.2	21.3	22.0	13.9	16.3
Nova Scotia	22.8	22.5	24.3	21.3	23.4	22.2	21.3	20.7	18.9	22.1
New Brunswick	25.3	21.1	20.3	24.4	22.6	20.8	22.9	20.7	17.7	20.3
Quebec	25.1	23.9	23.1	21.6	21.4	20.3	20.6	20.5	19.5	17.4
Ontario	19.6	18.3	18.1	16.7	15.6	15.6	15.7	16.5	15.2	13.3
Manitoba	22.9	20.0	20.6	22.0	19.5	17.1	20.3	19.6	18.8	12.5
Saskatchewan	24.2	24.0	26.3	22.6	21.1	21.1	22.8	20.5	21.7	20.2
Alberta	21.1	19.9	18.7	19.9	19.6	18.7	19.2	16.8	16.1	15.6
British Columbia	16.5	16.5	15.8	16.2	14.4	14.4	14.7	14.3	13.5	11.9
Yukon [4]	28.5	28.4	35.1	29.0	32.3	26.3	25.4	28.1	26.7	21.8
Northwest Territories [4]	34.6	38.1	34.3	30.2	36.5	39.1	31.4	33.9	33.9	27.6
Nunavut [4], [5]	63.8	49.6	55.9	52.5	51.5	58.3	57.7	49.0	66.9	62.2

Source: Statistics Canada. *Table 105-0503 - Health indicator profile, age-standardized rate, annual estimates, by sex, Canada, provinces and territories, occasional,* CANSIM (database). (accessed: March 31, 2017)

Please see footnotes [30], [31], [57], [58], [59], [60], [61], [62], [64] for characteristics of the age-standardized rate.

AGE-STANDARDIZED RATES, CURRENT SMOKER, DAILY (%), [22], [23], [24], [26], [28] BOTH SEXES, CANADA, PROVINCES AND TERRITORIES

Geography	2003	2005	2007	2008	2009	2010	2011	2012	2013	2014
Canada	17.9	16.7	17.5	16.9	15.6	15.5	15.1	15.4	14.2	13.4
Newfoundland and Labrador	20.7	19.4	20.7	19.4	18.9	18.9	18.2	21.8	15.6	17.2
Prince Edward Island	21.1	17.9	17.9	16.4	15.5	19.6	20.8	20.0	17.2	18.1
Nova Scotia	20.3	18.7	20.4	19.7	19.9	19.2	17.8	17.7	17.1	16.7
New Brunswick	22.2	18.9	20.5	20.5	18.3	19.3	17.7	18.5	17.9	16.0
Quebec	20.7	18.6	19.9	18.7	17.3	17.0	16.3	18.3	15.7	14.6
Ontario	16.8	15.9	16.5	15.5	14.3	14.6	14.6	14.2	13.1	13.3
Manitoba	18.4	16.8	19.6	19.2	14.6	14.9	15.0	15.2	15.7	11.1
Saskatchewan	19.5	19.6	22.1	20.6	17.8	19.1	18.6	15.2	17.4	15.3
Alberta	17.5	17.6	17.2	17.5	17.3	16.2	16.3	16.3	15.0	13.9
British Columbia	13.9	12.8	13.2	14.2	12.3	12.5	11.2	11.0	11.5	9.4
Yukon [4]	21.7	24.9	31.4	24.9	25.3	22.1	23.7	22.5	18.9	18.4
Northwest Territories [4]	29.5	28.6	27.1	26.7	30.7	30.4	27.3	28.3	25.3	24.7
Nunavut [4] [5]	57.2	45.7	50.9	47.5	52.4	48.8	47.2	47.1	47.8	52.2

Source: Statistics Canada. *Table 105-0503 - Health indicator profile, age-standardized rate, annual estimates, by sex, Canada, provinces and territories, occasional,* CANSIM (database). (accessed: March 31, 2017)

Please see footnotes 30, 31, 57, 58, 59, 60, 61, 62, 64 for characteristics of the age-standardized rate.

AGE-STANDARDIZED RATES, CURRENT SMOKER, DAILY (%), [22], [23], [24], [26], [28] MALES, CANADA, PROVINCES AND TERRITORIES

Geography	2003	2005	2007	2008	2009	2010	2011	2012	2013	2014
Canada	19.6	18.5	19.7	19.4	17.5	18.1	16.8	17.8	16.3	15.8
Newfoundland and Labrador	23.6	20.4	25.1	22.2	22.5	19.9	19.8	24.6	16.6	20.9
Prince Edward Island	24.0	22.0	21.7	18.4	16.2E	20.9	23.8	21.0	24.5	21.7
Nova Scotia	21.6	19.4	20.9	22.5	21.1	21.8	17.5	19.7	19.6	16.8
New Brunswick	23.3	20.6	23.7	20.4	19.4	22.0	16.9	22.3	21.1	16.6
Quebec	22.0	19.8	22.3	21.1	18.3	19.3	17.6	21.1	17.4	16.0
Ontario	18.8	18.3	18.8	18.5	16.7	17.7	17.4	16.8	15.0	16.7
Manitoba	18.3	17.6	21.2	21.2	16.7	16.7	15.0	14.9	16.3	14.7
Saskatchewan	20.4	20.4	22.9	22.5	19.1	19.9	19.4	14.1	18.3	16.0
Alberta	19.2	20.1	19.2	19.2	19.9	19.0	18.0	20.3	18.3	16.0
British Columbia	16.0	14.2	15.2	16.6	14.2	14.3	11.7	12.4	13.9	11.2
Yukon [4]	22.1	26.6	32.0	24.6	27.2	24.3	27.6	23.2	17.9	21.2
Northwest Territories [4]	30.5	28.4	27.1	30.9	31.4	30.8	32.8	28.1	25.3	28.6
Nunavut [4],[5]	56.3	47.6	50.7	46.0	58.1	42.1	42.8	47.1	40.0E	49.8

Symbol Legend:
E   Use with caution

Source: Statistics Canada. *Table 105-0503 - Health indicator profile, age-standardized rate, annual estimates, by sex, Canada, provinces and territories, occasional,* CANSIM (database). (accessed: March 31, 2017)

Please see footnotes [30], [31], [57], [58], [59], [60], [61], [62], [64] for characteristics of the age-standardized rate.

AGE-STANDARDIZED RATES, CURRENT SMOKER, DAILY (%), [22], [23], [24], [26], [28] FEMALES, CANADA, PROVINCES AND TERRITORIES

Geography	2003	2005	2007	2008	2009	2010	2011	2012	2013	2014
Canada	16.3	14.9	15.4	14.5	13.7	13.0	13.5	13.0	12.2	11.1
Newfoundland and Labrador	18.0	18.5	16.4	16.7	15.6	18.0	16.6	19.1	14.7	13.7
Prince Edward Island	18.3	14.2	14.5	14.5	14.8	18.3	17.9	19.1	10.5	14.7E
Nova Scotia	19.0	18.1	19.8	17.0	18.8	16.8	18.1	15.9	14.8	16.6
New Brunswick	21.0	17.2	17.3	20.6	17.3	16.7	18.4	15.0	14.9	15.5
Quebec	19.5	17.5	17.6	16.3	16.3	14.7	15.0	15.5	13.9	13.1
Ontario	14.8	13.5	14.3	12.6	12.0	11.5	11.9	11.6	11.2	10.1
Manitoba	18.5	16.1	18.1	17.3	12.6	13.2	15.0	15.5	15.0	7.5
Saskatchewan	18.7	18.9	21.4	18.6	16.6	18.3	17.8	16.3	16.5	14.6
Alberta	15.7	15.0	15.3	15.7	14.7	13.4	14.6	12.2	11.6	11.7
British Columbia	12.0	11.4	11.3	12.0	10.5	10.7	10.7	9.7	9.1	7.7
Yukon [4]	21.3	23.3	30.9	25.3	23.5	19.8	19.6	21.8	20.0	15.6E
Northwest Territories [4]	28.5	28.9	27.0	22.1	30.0	30.0	21.6	28.7	25.3	20.7
Nunavut [4,5]	58.1	43.6	51.1	49.0	47.2	55.7	52.2	47.1	56.0	54.9

Symbol Legend:
E Use with caution

Source: Statistics Canada. *Table 105-0503 - Health indicator profile, age-standardized rate, annual estimates, by sex, Canada, provinces and territories, occasional,* CANSIM (database). (accessed: March 31, 2017)

Please see footnotes 30, 31, 57, 58, 59, 60, 61, 62, 64 for characteristics of the age-standardized rate.

AGE-STANDARDIZED RATES, PHYSICAL ACTIVITY DURING LEISURE-TIME, MODERATELY ACTIVE OR ACTIVE (%), [36, 37] BOTH SEXES, CANADA, PROVINCES AND TERRITORIES

Geography	2003	2005	2007	2008	2009	2010	2011	2012	2013	2014
Canada	52.3	52.7	51.0	51.3	53.2	53.1	54.8	54.7	56.3	54.6
Newfoundland and Labrador	45.3	46.6	49.0	45.5	48.8	49.5	51.3	53.8	49.6	49.6
Prince Edward Island	45.7	45.6	49.9	49.1	52.0	52.3	50.5	55.8	49.8	52.2
Nova Scotia	50.1	50.2	49.8	49.4	53.4	55.8	56.0	56.2	58.6	54.5
New Brunswick	46.9	47.6	45.4	50.2	51.0	54.1	53.3	55.3	52.5	51.8
Quebec	48.9	49.2	47.5	48.4	50.4	50.6	51.8	49.7	52.9	51.7
Ontario	51.8	53.4	50.5	50.1	51.4	51.3	54.6	54.7	55.4	53.6
Manitoba	52.2	49.0	53.8	53.8	55.0	55.0	55.1	55.3	57.9	54.4
Saskatchewan	51.9	51.3	48.5	50.0	53.5	52.1	55.1	54.4	55.5	53.0
Alberta	55.4	54.4	54.7	53.7	57.0	56.4	56.0	55.2	57.3	57.8
British Columbia	60.5	59.6	57.4	59.1	60.9	59.3	60.3	62.3	64.9	61.9
Yukon [4]	60.5	57.4	56.0	52.8	55.1	62.4	61.5	67.5	66.7	64.8
Northwest Territories [4]	51.9	49.0	48.9	39.7	40.6	48.4	50.6	55.2	56.4	57.0
Nunavut [4, 5]	32.9	41.6	38.3	43.3	42.6	44.2	33.2	47.5	43.5	36.9

Source: Statistics Canada. *Table 105-0503 - Health indicator profile, age-standardized rate, annual estimates, by sex, Canada, provinces and territories, occasional,* CANSIM (database). (accessed: March 31, 2017)

Please see footnotes 30, 31, 57, 58, 59, 60, 61, 62, 64 for characteristics of the age-standardized rate.

AGE-STANDARDIZED RATES, PHYSICAL ACTIVITY DURING LEISURE-TIME, MODERATELY ACTIVE OR ACTIVE (%), [36], [37] MALES, CANADA, PROVINCES AND TERRITORIES

Geography	2003	2005	2007	2008	2009	2010	2011	2012	2013	2014
Canada	55.9	55.4	54.2	55.3	57.3	56.1	57.5	57.2	58.9	57.7
Newfoundland and Labrador	52.1	51.5	56.4	48.8	54.3	51.4	57.0	55.3	51.6	55.8
Prince Edward Island	48.0	46.7	52.5	50.5	54.8	55.2	51.9	58.6	51.7	54.2
Nova Scotia	53.8	52.1	53.6	54.6	56.8	58.1	59.4	59.4	62.3	59.0
New Brunswick	51.1	50.9	47.8	52.8	58.2	56.4	58.8	53.5	56.5	58.9
Quebec	53.0	53.1	51.8	54.3	55.9	54.6	55.7	52.4	55.5	54.6
Ontario	55.7	57.0	54.1	55.1	55.7	55.2	57.2	57.9	58.4	56.4
Manitoba	55.7	51.8	55.5	54.6	58.1	59.3	58.3	55.9	62.2	56.4
Saskatchewan	52.9	52.4	51.9	52.9	56.7	53.4	57.9	55.3	55.7	56.7
Alberta	56.9	53.5	54.5	54.9	58.8	57.9	56.1	56.0	58.8	61.4
British Columbia	63.5	60.3	59.5	60.0	63.5	59.8	62.0	65.4	66.9	64.2
Yukon [4]	61.9	62.0	57.5	55.3	59.4	62.1	62.7	73.5	70.8	66.4
Northwest Territories [4]	53.8	51.6	50.4	38.9	50.3	49.6	53.5	57.4	60.0	54.2
Nunavut [4,5]	34.9	41.8	44.9	47.2	49.0	42.8	33.1	57.0	52.5	43.1

Source: Statistics Canada. *Table 105-0503 - Health indicator profile, age-standardized rate, annual estimates, by sex, Canada, provinces and territories, occasional,* CANSIM (database). (accessed: March 31, 2017)

Please see footnotes [30], [31], [57], [58], [59], [60], [61], [62], [64] for characteristics of the age-standardized rate.

AGE-STANDARDIZED RATES, PHYSICAL ACTIVITY DURING LEISURE-TIME, MODERATELY ACTIVE OR ACTIVE (%), [36], [37] FEMALES, CANADA, PROVINCES AND TERRITORIES

Geography	2003	2005	2007	2008	2009	2010	2011	2012	2013	2014
Canada	48.9	50.1	47.9	47.4	49.2	50.1	52.3	52.3	53.8	51.7
Newfoundland and Labrador	38.9	41.9	42.2	42.5	43.7	47.6	46.0	52.3	47.7	43.8
Prince Edward Island	43.5	44.5	47.6	47.9	49.6	49.7	49.2	53.2	48.1	50.4
Nova Scotia	46.7	48.3	46.4	44.5	50.2	53.7	52.9	53.3	55.2	50.3
New Brunswick	43.1	44.6	43.1	47.9	44.4	51.9	48.2	57.0	48.7	45.1
Quebec	44.9	45.5	43.3	42.5	45.1	46.6	48.0	47.1	50.4	48.8
Ontario	48.2	49.9	46.9	45.3	47.2	47.6	52.1	51.7	52.5	51.0
Manitoba	48.8	46.4	52.1	53.0	51.9	50.9	52.0	54.7	53.8	52.4
Saskatchewan	50.9	50.3	45.3	47.2	50.3	50.9	52.3	53.6	55.3	49.3
Alberta	54.0	55.3	54.8	52.6	55.2	54.9	55.9	54.4	55.8	54.1
British Columbia	57.5	59.0	55.5	58.2	58.5	58.9	58.7	59.2	62.9	59.5
Yukon [4]	59.1	53.0	54.4	50.3	51.0	62.8	60.4	61.8	62.7	63.1
Northwest Territories [4]	50.0	46.1	47.4	40.6	31.0	47.2	47.5	52.7	52.6	60.0
Nunavut [4], [5]	30.9	41.3	31.8	39.5	36.9	45.7E	33.3	36.5	34.1E	29.9E

Symbol Legend:
E   Use with caution

Source: Statistics Canada. *Table 105-0503 - Health indicator profile, age-standardized rate, annual estimates, by sex, Canada, provinces and territories, occasional,* CANSIM (database). (accessed: March 31, 2017)

Please see footnotes [30], [31], [57], [58], [59], [60], [61], [62], [64] for characteristics of the age-standardized rate.

AGE-STANDARDIZED RATES, PHYSICAL ACTIVITY DURING LEISURE-TIME, INACTIVE (%), [36], [37] BOTH SEXES, CANADA, PROVINCES AND TERRITORIES

Geography	2003	2005	2007	2008	2009	2010	2011	2012	2013	2014
Canada	47.7	47.3	49.0	48.7	46.8	46.9	45.2	45.3	43.7	45.4
Newfoundland and Labrador	54.7	53.4	51.0	54.5	51.2	50.5	48.7	46.2	50.4	50.4
Prince Edward Island	54.3	54.4	50.1	50.9	48.0	47.7	49.5	44.2	50.2	47.8
Nova Scotia	49.9	49.8	50.2	50.6	46.6	44.2	44.0	43.8	41.4	45.5
New Brunswick	53.1	52.4	54.6	49.8	49.0	45.9	46.7	44.7	47.5	48.2
Quebec	51.1	50.8	52.5	51.6	49.6	49.4	48.2	50.3	47.1	48.3
Ontario	48.2	46.6	49.5	49.9	48.6	48.7	45.4	45.3	44.6	46.4
Manitoba	47.8	51.0	46.2	46.2	45.0	45.0	44.9	44.7	42.1	45.6
Saskatchewan	48.1	48.7	51.5	50.0	46.5	47.9	44.9	45.6	44.5	47.0
Alberta	44.6	45.6	45.3	46.3	43.0	43.6	44.0	44.8	42.7	42.2
British Columbia	39.5	40.4	42.6	40.9	39.1	40.7	39.7	37.7	35.1	38.1
Yukon [4]	39.5	42.6	44.0	47.2	44.9	37.6	38.5	32.5	33.3	35.2
Northwest Territories [4]	48.1	51.0	51.1	60.3	59.4	51.6	49.4	44.8	43.6	43.0
Nunavut [4], [5]	67.1	58.4	61.7	56.7	57.4	55.8	66.8	52.5	56.5	63.1

Source: Statistics Canada. *Table 105-0503 - Health indicator profile, age-standardized rate, annual estimates, by sex, Canada, provinces and territories, occasional,* CANSIM (database). (accessed: March 31, 2017)

Please see footnotes 30, 31, 57, 58, 59, 60, 61, 62, 64 for characteristics of the age-standardized rate.

AGE-STANDARDIZED RATES, PHYSICAL ACTIVITY DURING LEISURE-TIME, INACTIVE (%), [36, 37] MALES, CANADA, PROVINCES AND TERRITORIES

Geography	2003	2005	2007	2008	2009	2010	2011	2012	2013	2014
Canada	44.1	44.6	45.8	44.7	42.7	43.9	42.5	42.8	41.1	42.3
Newfoundland and Labrador	47.9	48.5	43.6	51.2	45.7	48.6	43.0	44.7	48.4	44.2
Prince Edward Island	52.0	53.3	47.5	49.5	45.2	44.8	48.1	41.4	48.3	45.8
Nova Scotia	46.2	47.9	46.4	45.4	43.2	41.9	40.6	40.6	37.7	41.0
New Brunswick	48.9	49.1	52.2	47.2	41.8	43.6	41.2	46.5	43.5	41.1
Quebec	47.0	46.9	48.2	45.7	44.1	45.4	44.3	47.6	44.5	45.4
Ontario	44.3	43.0	45.9	44.9	44.3	44.8	42.8	42.1	41.6	43.6
Manitoba	44.3	48.2	44.5	45.4	41.9	40.7	41.7	44.1	37.8	43.6
Saskatchewan	47.1	47.6	48.1	47.1	43.3	46.6	42.1	44.7	44.3	43.3
Alberta	43.1	46.5	45.5	45.1	41.2	42.1	43.9	44.0	41.2	38.6
British Columbia	36.5	39.7	40.5	40.0	36.5	40.2	38.0	34.6	33.1	35.8
Yukon [4]	38.1	38.0	42.5	44.7	40.6	37.9	37.3	26.5	29.2	33.6
Northwest Territories [4]	46.2	48.4	49.6	61.1	49.7	50.4	46.5	42.6	40.0	45.8
Nunavut [4, 5]	65.1	58.2	55.1	52.8	51.0	57.2	66.9	43.0	47.5	56.9

Source: Statistics Canada. *Table 105-0503 - Health indicator profile, age-standardized rate, annual estimates, by sex, Canada, provinces and territories, occasional,* CANSIM (database). (accessed: March 31, 2017)

Please see footnotes 30, 31, 57, 58, 59, 60, 61, 62, 64 for characteristics of the age-standardized rate.

AGE-STANDARDIZED RATES, PHYSICAL ACTIVITY DURING LEISURE-TIME, INACTIVE (%), [36], [37] FEMALES, CANADA, PROVINCES AND TERRITORIES

Geography	2003	2005	2007	2008	2009	2010	2011	2012	2013	2014
Canada	51.1	49.9	52.1	52.6	50.8	49.9	47.7	47.7	46.2	48.3
Newfoundland and Labrador	61.1	58.1	57.8	57.5	56.3	52.4	54.0	47.7	52.3	56.2
Prince Edward Island	56.5	55.5	52.4	52.1	50.4	50.3	50.8	46.8	51.9	49.6
Nova Scotia	53.3	51.7	53.6	55.5	49.8	46.3	47.1	46.7	44.8	49.7
New Brunswick	56.9	55.4	56.9	52.1	55.6	48.1	51.8	43.0	51.3	54.9
Quebec	55.1	54.5	56.7	57.5	54.9	53.4	52.0	52.9	49.6	51.2
Ontario	51.8	50.1	53.1	54.7	52.8	52.4	47.9	48.3	47.5	49.0
Manitoba	51.2	53.6	47.9	47.0	48.1	49.1	48.0	45.3	46.2	47.6
Saskatchewan	49.1	49.7	54.7	52.8	49.7	49.1	47.7	46.4	44.7	50.7
Alberta	46.0	44.7	45.2	47.4	44.8	45.1	44.1	45.6	44.2	45.9
British Columbia	42.5	41.0	44.5	41.8	41.5	41.1	41.3	40.8	37.1	40.5
Yukon [4]	40.9	47.0	45.6	49.7	49.0	37.2	39.6	38.2	37.3	36.9
Northwest Territories [4]	50.0	53.9	52.6	59.4	69.0	52.8	52.5	47.3	47.4	40.0
Nunavut [4] [5]	69.1	58.7	68.2	60.5	63.1	54.3	66.7	63.5	65.9	70.1

Source: Statistics Canada. *Table 105-0503 - Health indicator profile, age-standardized rate, annual estimates, by sex, Canada, provinces and territories, occasional,* CANSIM (database). (accessed: March 31, 2017)

Please see footnotes 30, 31, 57, 58, 59, 60, 61, 62, 64 for characteristics of the age-standardized rate.

AGE-STANDARDIZED RATES, FRUIT AND VEGETABLE CONSUMPTION, 5 TIMES OR MORE PER DAY (%), [34], [35] BOTH SEXES, CANADA, PROVINCES AND TERRITORIES

Geography	2003	2005	2007	2008	2009	2010	2011	2012	2013	2014
Canada	41.3	43.8	43.9	43.9	45.7	43.6	40.7	40.9	41.1	39.8
Newfoundland and Labrador	26.3	22.9	29.0	33.4	30.3	29.3	28.9	25.6	25.3	26.6
Prince Edward Island	31.1	33.1	38.7	34.8	37.4	35.5	30.8	33.3	30.9	31.4
Nova Scotia	32.5	34.1	34.2	36.5	37.1	35.9	35.8	33.5	33.3	32.1
New Brunswick	34.0	36.8	38.2	38.7	40.4	38.0	36.1	32.1	37.0	35.6
Quebec	45.4	52.9	52.7	54.1	54.4	51.1	47.3	47.8	47.8	47.2
Ontario	41.9	42.8	42.0	40.6	44.1	42.9	38.9	39.6	39.4	38.0
Manitoba	36.3	34.5	36.8	34.0	38.5	34.9	37.0	36.0	32.2	31.1
Saskatchewan	36.6	36.2	36.6	39.9	40.1	37.4	33.3	37.7	38.0	35.8
Alberta	39.3	39.1	41.7	45.2	43.2	41.1	41.9	37.5	42.7	39.5
British Columbia	41.9	44.0	44.4	42.3	45.6	42.3	40.0	42.0	40.6	39.5
Yukon [4]	44.8	45.6	39.7	37.1	46.0	54.1	41.2	40.2	32.6	42.8
Northwest Territories [4]	33.3	28.2	26.6	21.3	25.5	26.0	27.6	37.5	37.7	32.5
Nunavut [4],[5]	28.7	25.0	25.8	22.5E	29.7	22.2	19.4	25.8	22.8	22.8

Symbol Legend:
E   Use with caution

Source: Statistics Canada. *Table 105-0503 - Health indicator profile, age-standardized rate, annual estimates, by sex, Canada, provinces and territories, occasional,* CANSIM (database). (accessed: March 31, 2017)

Please see footnotes [30], [31], [57], [58], [59], [60], [61], [62], [64] for characteristics of the age-standardized rate.

AGE-STANDARDIZED RATES, FRUIT AND VEGETABLE CONSUMPTION, 5 TIMES OR MORE PER DAY (%), [34], [35] MALES, CANADA, PROVINCES AND TERRITORIES

Geography	2003	2005	2007	2008	2009	2010	2011	2012	2013	2014
Canada	34.6	36.4	36.9	37.4	40.2	36.9	34.3	34.6	34.7	32.7
Newfoundland and Labrador	23.4	18.1	25.8	29.6	24.8	22.3	26.0	21.1	21.9	21.4
Prince Edward Island	25.1	25.2	30.1	28.6	31.0	30.8	24.1	24.9	21.6	25.0
Nova Scotia	26.4	30.0	27.2	31.9	32.5	29.7	29.9	27.9	29.5	26.5
New Brunswick	27.6	29.4	30.9	30.7	33.6	32.2	29.2	21.8	30.5	29.5
Quebec	37.2	44.6	44.3	47.2	47.9	41.9	40.3	40.2	39.1	38.3
Ontario	36.0	35.1	36.0	34.3	39.0	37.8	32.4	34.9	34.1	30.8
Manitoba	30.4	28.1	29.1	28.6	31.5	29.7	27.1	26.1	27.6	25.0
Saskatchewan	27.4	29.7	27.1	31.7	33.6	30.4	27.0	29.9	31.5	28.6
Alberta	30.7	33.4	33.2	37.6	36.7	33.5	33.9	30.6	35.6	34.2
British Columbia	35.8	36.8	38.2	36.1	41.5	36.0	35.8	35.1	34.4	32.9
Yukon [4]	41.2	42.6	40.1	33.4	40.3	49.8	34.3	30.0	27.2	34.5
Northwest Territories [4]	27.8	23.9	19.9	16.8E	24.3	22.6	24.5	34.8	34.3	24.4
Nunavut [4],[5]	25.1	24.6	16.0E	22.9E	23.1E	18.0E	16.2E	20.4E	20.7E	18.0E

Symbol Legend:
E   Use with caution

Source: Statistics Canada. *Table 105-0503 - Health indicator profile, age-standardized rate, annual estimates, by sex, Canada, provinces and territories, occasional,* CANSIM (database). (accessed: March 31, 2017)

Please see footnotes 30, 31, 57, 58, 59, 60, 61, 62, 64 for characteristics of the age-standardized rate.

AGE-STANDARDIZED RATES, FRUIT AND VEGETABLE CONSUMPTION, 5 TIMES OR MORE PER DAY (%), [34], [35] FEMALES, CANADA, PROVINCES AND TERRITORIES

Geography	2003	2005	2007	2008	2009	2010	2011	2012	2013	2014
Canada	47.9	50.8	50.6	50.2	51.1	50.0	47.0	47.0	47.4	46.8
Newfoundland and Labrador	29.1	27.5	32.0	36.8	35.3	35.9	31.7	29.9	28.5	31.5
Prince Edward Island	36.7	40.2	46.4	40.6	42.8	39.8	37.3	40.9	39.5	37.1
Nova Scotia	38.1	38.0	40.6	40.7	41.4	41.5	41.0	38.5	36.7	37.5
New Brunswick	39.8	43.7	44.8	46.3	46.7	43.4	42.5	41.5	43.0	41.4
Quebec	53.3	60.9	60.7	60.9	60.8	60.2	54.1	55.2	56.4	55.9
Ontario	47.5	50.2	47.6	46.5	49.0	47.8	45.0	44.1	44.6	45.0
Manitoba	42.1	40.6	44.1	39.3	45.1	39.9	47.2	46.0	36.6	36.9
Saskatchewan	45.4	42.6	45.8	47.8	46.3	44.3	39.4	45.6	44.5	43.0
Alberta	47.9	44.7	50.3	52.9	50.0	49.0	50.0	44.4	50.0	45.1
British Columbia	47.8	50.8	50.3	48.3	49.4	48.4	44.0	48.6	46.8	45.9
Yukon [4]	48.0	48.6	39.4	40.7	51.4	58.3	48.1	50.2	37.8	51.3
Northwest Territories [4]	39.0	32.9	33.5	26.3	26.7	29.6	30.7	40.5	41.3	40.7
Nunavut [4],[5]	32.2	25.5E	35.7	22.2E	35.7E	26.4E	23.0E	32.0E	24.9E	27.9

Symbol Legend:
E   Use with caution

Source: Statistics Canada. *Table 105-0503 - Health indicator profile, age-standardized rate, annual estimates, by sex, Canada, provinces and territories, occasional,* CANSIM (database). (accessed: March 31, 2017)

Please see footnotes [30], [31], [57], [58], [59], [60], [61], [62], [64] for characteristics of the age-standardized rate.

AGE-STANDARDIZED RATES, BREASTFEEDING INITIATION (%), [49], [50], [65] FEMALES, CANADA, PROVINCES AND TERRITORIES

Geography	2003	2005	2007	2008	2009	2010	2011	2012	2013	2014
Canada	84.6	86.9	87.0	88.5	87.2	87.1	88.2	90.3	..	..
Newfoundland and Labrador	63.8	61.3	68.5	70.3	60.7	64.0	54.7	56.9	..	..
Prince Edward Island	77.6	72.0	77.0	71.5	72.6	75.2	91.3	64.5	..	..
Nova Scotia	76.9	74.1	74.7	74.6	76.7	78.9	80.3	86.5	85.5	89.1
New Brunswick	64.5	77.1	75.2	75.0	83.4	79.1	70.3	78.4	81.3	76.7
Quebec	76.5	82.7	82.3	86.7	81.7	83.7	88.6	89.8	89.8	87.1
Ontario	87.0	87.8	88.5	89.8	87.7	89.7	87.0	90.8	91.8	89.8
Manitoba	88.6	89.7	86.6	82.1	86.4	91.0	94.2	91.2	..	..
Saskatchewan	87.3	88.8	82.9	92.2	90.0	89.7	85.1	86.3	..	..
Alberta	91.3	92.7	92.5	91.7	92.4	89.6	93.5	91.6	95.0	95.0
British Columbia	93.3	93.4	95.2	94.8	97.3	88.5	94.4	97.0	..	..
Yukon [4]	90.8	99.1	98.1	97.6	100.0	93.2	93.1	99.3	..	..
Northwest Territories [4]	75.0	92.9	88.0	88.0	87.4	92.6	97.5	92.8	87.2	90.0
Nunavut [4] [5]	75.5	75.0	70.1	69.0	75.4	61.3E	79.7	83.5	70.2	77.4

Symbol Legend:
.. Not available
E Use with caution

Source: Statistics Canada. *Table 105-0503 - Health indicator profile, age-standardized rate, annual estimates, by sex, Canada, provinces and territories, occasional,* CANSIM (database). (accessed: March 31, 2017)

Please see footnotes [30], [31], [57], [58], [59], [60], [61], [62], [64] for characteristics of the age-standardized rate.

AGE-STANDARDIZED RATES, EXCLUSIVE BREASTFEEDING, AT LEAST 6 MONTHS (%), [49], [51], [52], [65], [66] FEMALES, CANADA, PROVINCES AND TERRITORIES

Geography	2003	2005	2007	2008	2009	2010	2011	2012	2013	2014
Canada	16.8	20.1	20.9	25.1	24.2	27.9	28.0	24.4	..	..
Newfoundland and Labrador	8.2E	12.1E	10.6E	F	16.3E	17.7E	F	17.6E	..	..
Prince Edward Island	11.9E	11.9E	16.4E	F	21.5E	16.5E	F	F	..	..
Nova Scotia	14.2E	15.2E	14.4E	18.0E	13.7E	23.6E	25.3E	20.7E	35.9E	31.0E
New Brunswick	8.4E	15.1E	12.0E	17.6E	15.7E	21.2E	20.4E	27.2E	23.1E	16.1E
Quebec	9.6	14.0	14.2	18.3	18.7	21.7	22.5	15.9	22.8	23.1
Ontario	17.3	19.6	21.4	25.6	22.9	29.4	27.8	22.7	33.1	27.5
Manitoba	18.4E	25.0	19.5E	27.0	32.7E	28.5E	36.2	22.6E	..	..
Saskatchewan	18.6	22.2	27.6	26.8	33.1	34.3	26.3	36.6	..	..
Alberta	21.9	22.4	17.6	31.2	29.7	30.4	26.9E	27.7	32.6	30.9
British Columbia	27.1	31.2	39.8	35.7	33.4	35.1	41.9	41.4	..	..
Yukon [4]	F	42.1E	35.9E	41.3E	33.2E	44.4E	F	41.7E	..	..
Northwest Territories [4]	23.9E	26.1E	28.0E	F	38.1E	34.4E	F	F	35.2E	36.8E
Nunavut [4], [5]	32.9E	31.1E	16.7E	31.8E	29.6E	F	34.4E	F	31.2E	F

Symbol Legend:
.. Not available
E Use with caution
F Too unreliable to be published

Source: Statistics Canada. *Table 105-0503 - Health indicator profile, age-standardized rate, annual estimates, by sex, Canada, provinces and territories, occasional,* CANSIM (database). (accessed: March 31, 2017)

Please see footnotes [30], [31], [57], [58], [59], [60], [61], [62], [64] for characteristics of the age-standardized rate.

AGE-STANDARDIZED RATES, CONTACT WITH A MEDICAL DOCTOR IN THE PAST 12 MONTHS (%), [45], [46], [65] BOTH SEXES, CANADA, PROVINCES AND TERRITORIES

Geography	2003	2005	2007	2008	2009	2010	2011	2012	2013	2014
Canada	80.0	80.1	78.2	78.5	79.4	79.3	..	77.1	76.9	77.1
Newfoundland and Labrador	83.0	83.2	79.0	80.4	77.3	82.0	..	81.1	80.6	78.3
Prince Edward Island	84.7	83.6	81.4	80.6	82.2	81.2	..	77.9	79.0	77.4
Nova Scotia	85.0	85.1	81.9	81.1	79.5	84.4	..	79.9	78.7	79.4
New Brunswick	81.8	80.8	78.9	75.1	78.9	78.6	..	76.6	76.3	76.8
Quebec	74.8	74.7	73.7	74.8	75.4	75.3	..	73.8	73.8	74.8
Ontario	81.2	81.4	80.5	80.8	82.2	80.6	..	78.4	77.9	78.9
Manitoba	79.1	80.3	75.3	77.3	80.1	79.7	78.1	79.6	79.4	72.9
Saskatchewan	81.5	82.4	78.8	78.0	80.1	80.2	..	77.0	76.8	74.3
Alberta	81.5	81.0	76.6	76.3	77.3	79.4	..	74.9	76.3	74.7
British Columbia	82.4	82.9	80.3	80.0	79.9	80.6	..	79.4	78.8	79.2
Yukon [4]	83.8	79.2	75.5	79.6	80.7	84.1	..	78.0	82.6	75.6
Northwest Territories [4]	71.2	77.2	68.5	67.6	69.9	66.9	..	71.3	68.8	70.0
Nunavut [4], [5]	56.2	61.4	51.8	55.1	60.9	55.5	..	63.5	54.0	49.2

Symbol Legend:
.. Not available

Source: Statistics Canada. *Table 105-0503 - Health indicator profile, age-standardized rate, annual estimates, by sex, Canada, provinces and territories, occasional,* CANSIM (database). (accessed: March 31, 2017)

Please see footnotes [30], [31], [57], [58], [59], [60], [61], [62], [64] for characteristics of the age-standardized rate.

AGE-STANDARDIZED RATES, CONTACT WITH A MEDICAL DOCTOR IN THE PAST 12 MONTHS (%), [45], [46], [65] MALES, CANADA, PROVINCES AND TERRITORIES

Geography	2003	2005	2007	2008	2009	2010	2011	2012	2013	2014
Canada	73.6	73.9	71.4	71.2	72.7	72.6	..	70.3	70.4	70.5
Newfoundland and Labrador	75.9	75.6	72.6	76.4	68.7	74.1	..	77.9	71.9	70.4
Prince Edward Island	76.6	77.1	74.0	75.8	76.8	75.4	..	70.9	72.9	71.9
Nova Scotia	78.7	77.9	75.1	73.7	74.0	79.0	..	71.6	74.2	71.3
New Brunswick	75.2	73.8	72.2	67.9	73.1	68.9	..	67.9	69.1	68.9
Quebec	66.8	67.0	65.4	64.7	66.1	67.1	..	65.2	64.8	65.1
Ontario	75.4	75.9	74.8	74.9	77.2	75.3	..	71.7	71.9	73.0
Manitoba	73.0	74.7	67.5	70.8	74.3	73.0	71.2	75.3	75.0	64.4
Saskatchewan	76.5	76.9	72.6	71.1	73.3	73.9	..	70.7	70.1	69.1
Alberta	74.9	75.1	68.9	68.4	69.2	71.9	..	68.3	71.2	69.9
British Columbia	77.1	78.0	74.3	73.6	73.7	74.3	..	74.5	73.3	75.2
Yukon [4]	77.1	68.7	69.0	73.8	76.2	77.7	..	77.7	80.7	65.2
Northwest Territories [4]	62.7	69.6	61.3	62.6	61.8	64.4	..	65.5	62.6	67.6
Nunavut [4], [5]	49.2	58.6	48.9	49.4	52.7	52.6	..	56.7	51.4	52.2

Symbol Legend:
.. Not available

Source: Statistics Canada. *Table 105-0503 - Health indicator profile, age-standardized rate, annual estimates, by sex, Canada, provinces and territories, occasional,* CANSIM (database). (accessed: March 31, 2017)

Please see footnotes 30, 31, 57, 58, 59, 60, 61, 62, 64 for characteristics of the age-standardized rate.

AGE-STANDARDIZED RATES, CONTACT WITH A MEDICAL DOCTOR IN THE PAST 12 MONTHS (%), [45], [46], [65] FEMALES, CANADA, PROVINCES AND TERRITORIES

Geography	2003	2005	2007	2008	2009	2010	2011	2012	2013	2014
Canada	86.2	86.0	84.8	85.6	86.0	85.7	..	83.8	83.4	83.6
Newfoundland and Labrador	89.8	90.5	85.1	84.2	85.3	89.6	..	84.2	89.0	85.8
Prince Edward Island	92.5	89.6	88.1	85.1	87.1	86.6	..	84.5	84.8	82.6
Nova Scotia	90.9	91.9	88.3	88.0	84.8	89.2	..	87.6	82.9	87.3
New Brunswick	88.2	87.5	85.4	82.1	84.6	87.9	..	84.8	83.2	84.4
Quebec	82.6	82.1	81.9	84.8	84.5	83.4	..	82.3	82.8	84.4
Ontario	86.8	86.8	86.0	86.5	87.2	85.8	..	84.9	83.8	84.6
Manitoba	85.1	85.9	83.0	83.8	85.9	86.2	85.0	83.8	83.7	81.3
Saskatchewan	86.5	87.9	84.9	84.8	86.7	86.5	..	83.4	83.6	79.6
Alberta	88.2	87.0	84.4	84.5	85.7	87.3	..	81.7	81.5	79.7
British Columbia	87.6	87.7	86.2	86.2	86.0	86.9	..	84.1	84.4	83.1
Yukon [4]	90.4	89.4	82.0	85.4	85.2	90.7	..	78.3	84.5	86.3
Northwest Territories [4]	80.5	85.5	76.2	73.2	78.0	69.6	..	77.6	75.5	72.4
Nunavut [4], [5]	63.0	64.8	54.8	60.9	68.0	58.5	..	71.3	56.7	45.8

Symbol Legend:
.. Not available

Source: Statistics Canada. *Table 105-0503 - Health indicator profile, age-standardized rate, annual estimates, by sex, Canada, provinces and territories, occasional,* CANSIM (database). (accessed: March 31, 2017)

Please see footnotes 30, 31, 57, 58, 59, 60, 61, 62, 64 for characteristics of the age-standardized rate.

AGE-STANDARDIZED RATES, PARTICIPATION AND ACTIVITY LIMITATION, SOMETIMES OR OFTEN (%), [21, 65] BOTH SEXES, CANADA, PROVINCES AND TERRITORIES

Geography	2003	2005	2007	2008	2009	2010	2011	2012	2013	2014
Canada	30.1	28.3	29.6	27.1	25.6	26.1	..	30.9	29.2	29.9
Newfoundland and Labrador	29.2	31.7	32.2	30.3	27.6	28.9	..	37.5	34.3	29.2
Prince Edward Island	28.5	29.2	32.9	30.1	23.8	26.2	..	32.4	35.4	32.2
Nova Scotia	36.1	36.1	35.8	35.5	29.9	34.0	..	38.1	40.0	37.3
New Brunswick	31.5	31.1	29.8	29.3	31.4	28.9	..	35.0	29.7	33.8
Quebec	27.2	25.6	23.0	20.8	22.7	24.2	..	30.1	25.1	26.8
Ontario	30.6	28.1	31.5	27.6	25.8	26.1	..	29.3	28.7	29.5
Manitoba	30.5	29.5	33.4	35.2	28.9	31.1	..	33.8	32.6	32.3
Saskatchewan	29.4	30.8	33.0	29.7	27.8	26.6	..	33.6	29.1	32.1
Alberta	32.3	29.3	32.8	30.9	27.4	27.5	..	29.9	32.1	31.9
British Columbia	30.6	29.1	30.2	28.5	25.1	24.7	..	33.4	31.1	31.9
Yukon [4]	35.7	28.8	29.5	26.8	29.7	27.9	34.4	39.1	40.8	44.4
Northwest Territories [4]	31.4	29.0	29.0	24.8	26.8	24.3	28.3	38.9	37.6	41.1
Nunavut [4, 5]	35.8	35.9	29.3	34.5	27.5	30.1	24.2	41.7	26.3	32.7

Symbol Legend:
.. Not available

Source: Statistics Canada. *Table 105-0503 - Health indicator profile, age-standardized rate, annual estimates, by sex, Canada, provinces and territories, occasional,* CANSIM (database). (accessed: March 31, 2017)

Please see footnotes 30, 31, 57, 58, 59, 60, 61, 62, 64 for characteristics of the age-standardized rate.

AGE-STANDARDIZED RATES, PARTICIPATION AND ACTIVITY LIMITATION, SOMETIMES OR OFTEN (%), [21], [65] MALES, CANADA, PROVINCES AND TERRITORIES

Geography	2003	2005	2007	2008	2009	2010	2011	2012	2013	2014
Canada	28.3	27.1	28.0	26.0	23.7	24.8	..	29.5	27.3	27.9
Newfoundland and Labrador	29.8	32.0	30.7	30.3	25.0	28.1	..	41.6	31.2	26.5
Prince Edward Island	27.0	28.0	34.2	30.0	22.7	27.9	..	31.4	35.0	30.0
Nova Scotia	35.9	35.1	35.1	34.9	28.9	31.9	..	35.5	37.7	29.2
New Brunswick	30.8	29.8	28.8	29.3	30.5	27.9	..	36.5	28.0	31.6
Quebec	24.8	24.3	21.3	19.9	21.2	23.9	..	28.6	23.6	25.6
Ontario	28.5	27.3	29.7	26.6	24.0	24.1	..	27.4	26.5	27.1
Manitoba	29.3	28.0	32.7	32.4	28.2	28.6	..	32.1	30.0	31.3
Saskatchewan	30.3	30.5	32.8	29.2	25.2	25.1	..	33.3	29.4	29.4
Alberta	29.4	28.1	31.2	29.5	25.2	26.3	..	29.6	31.3	29.9
British Columbia	30.4	27.3	28.4	26.6	22.1	23.7	..	31.6	28.8	30.6
Yukon [4]	35.1	28.0	24.6	26.2	30.0	32.6	35.2	42.1	41.1	41.0
Northwest Territories [4]	30.2	26.5	28.1	26.7	24.9	19.8	24.9	36.7	38.3	38.0
Nunavut [4,5]	35.2	44.0	27.9	34.9	34.3E	35.8E	22.9E	42.3	31.7	31.5

Symbol Legend:
.. Not available
E Use with caution

Source: Statistics Canada. *Table 105-0503 - Health indicator profile, age-standardized rate, annual estimates, by sex, Canada, provinces and territories, occasional,* CANSIM (database). (accessed: March 31, 2017)

Please see footnotes 30, 31, 57, 58, 59, 60, 61, 62, 64 for characteristics of the age-standardized rate.

AGE-STANDARDIZED RATES, PARTICIPATION AND ACTIVITY LIMITATION, SOMETIMES OR OFTEN (%), [21, 65] FEMALES, CANADA, PROVINCES AND TERRITORIES

Geography	2003	2005	2007	2008	2009	2010	2011	2012	2013	2014
Canada	31.8	29.4	31.2	28.2	27.4	27.4	..	32.3	31.0	31.9
Newfoundland and Labrador	28.7	31.4	33.5	30.3	30.0	29.8	..	33.5	37.2	31.8
Prince Edward Island	29.8	30.3	31.8	30.2	24.7	24.7	..	33.2	35.7	34.2
Nova Scotia	36.3	37.0	36.5	36.0	30.8	36.0	..	40.5	42.1	45.0
New Brunswick	32.2	32.4	30.8	29.3	32.2	29.9	..	33.6	31.3	35.9
Quebec	29.5	26.8	24.6	21.7	24.2	24.4	..	31.5	26.6	28.0
Ontario	32.7	28.9	33.1	28.6	27.6	28.0	..	31.1	30.8	31.7
Manitoba	31.7	31.0	34.1	38.0	29.6	33.5	..	35.4	35.2	33.3
Saskatchewan	28.6	31.0	33.1	30.2	30.3	28.0	..	33.9	28.7	34.8
Alberta	35.3	30.6	34.3	32.3	29.7	28.8	..	30.3	33.0	34.0
British Columbia	30.8	30.9	32.0	30.4	27.9	25.6	..	35.3	33.5	33.2
Yukon [4]	36.3	29.6	34.3	27.5	29.5	23.1	33.5	36.1	40.6	47.8
Northwest Territories [4]	32.7	31.7	30.0	22.6	28.7	29.2	31.7	41.3	36.8	44.3
Nunavut [4, 5]	36.3	26.5	30.7	34.0	21.4E	24.2E	25.6E	41.1	20.8E	34.1E

Symbol Legend:
.. Not available
E Use with caution

Source: Statistics Canada. *Table 105-0503 - Health indicator profile, age-standardized rate, annual estimates, by sex, Canada, provinces and territories, occasional,* CANSIM (database). (accessed: March 31, 2017)

Please see footnotes 30, 31, 57, 58, 59, 60, 61, 62, 64 for characteristics of the age-standardized rate.

AGE-STANDARDIZED RATES, INFLUENZA IMMUNIZATION, LESS THAN ONE YEAR AGO (%), [47], [48] BOTH SEXES, CANADA, PROVINCES AND TERRITORIES

Geography	2003	2005	2007	2008	2009	2010	2011	2012	2013	2014
Canada	26.1	32.0	29.8	29.8	30.3	23.5	27.9	26.4	26.6	29.5
Newfoundland and Labrador	15.1	20.3	21.5	23.7	27.0	18.2	26.0	20.4	23.2	25.6
Prince Edward Island	21.6	28.2	28.8	26.6	29.9	22.8	28.2	28.5	27.7	34.8
Nova Scotia	28.5	36.0	36.8	36.9	37.2	40.4	47.0	38.5	39.5	43.5
New Brunswick	20.7	25.3	24.9	28.9	27.8	30.9	32.8	32.4	33.7	34.8
Quebec	18.2	23.0	23.3	24.2	25.8	12.6	20.2	18.9	20.8	20.6
Ontario	33.7	40.6	35.1	34.5	33.2	25.1	30.6	28.7	28.4	32.4
Manitoba	18.1	26.1	24.6	25.0	27.6	27.1	24.7	25.8	25.3	26.9
Saskatchewan	20.9	25.6	24.1	27.8	28.6	24.2	29.1	28.4	23.4	33.9
Alberta	23.7	28.1	27.8	27.7	30.6	29.0	30.8	27.0	28.1	32.5
British Columbia	25.1	30.6	29.8	27.9	29.3	28.1	26.6	28.7	27.5	30.7
Yukon [4]	22.2	34.0	30.6	31.1	33.9	46.3	32.5	28.2	27.9	30.6
Northwest Territories [4]	27.5	41.0	37.0	39.0	37.8	35.3	40.4	38.9	35.5	36.7
Nunavut [4, 5]	30.5	47.6	38.8	45.1	40.1	52.7	45.6	31.2	33.4	39.6

Source: Statistics Canada. *Table 105-0503 - Health indicator profile, age-standardized rate, annual estimates, by sex, Canada, provinces and territories, occasional,* CANSIM (database). (accessed: March 31, 2017)

Please see footnotes [30], [31], [57], [58], [59], [60], [61], [62], [64] for characteristics of the age-standardized rate.

AGE-STANDARDIZED RATES, INFLUENZA IMMUNIZATION, LESS THAN ONE YEAR AGO (%), [47], [48] MALES, CANADA, PROVINCES AND TERRITORIES

Geography	2003	2005	2007	2008	2009	2010	2011	2012	2013	2014
Canada	23.3	29.1	26.5	26.3	27.2	20.7	24.8	22.8	23.8	25.7
Newfoundland and Labrador	14.0	18.5	17.9	19.8	26.7	16.1	21.9	18.9	20.6	22.8
Prince Edward Island	18.6	25.4	25.9	23.1	25.7	20.9	21.2	21.7	25.1	27.5
Nova Scotia	26.0	31.6	34.4	30.3	30.3	33.3	44.9	32.7	34.6	35.4
New Brunswick	18.6	23.2	19.3	26.3	24.0	25.5	27.4	28.5	30.5	29.2
Quebec	16.4	20.8	20.3	20.8	22.0	9.8	17.1	16.2	18.0	17.2
Ontario	30.1	37.4	31.8	31.5	31.2	23.5	28.2	24.7	25.6	30.1
Manitoba	15.2	23.6	21.2	21.5	24.7	25.7	22.3	22.9	24.5	22.4
Saskatchewan	17.4	22.7	20.0	21.9	23.2	20.1	25.1	21.2	18.2	29.3
Alberta	21.0	24.8	24.3	23.6	26.3	23.2	26.6	24.8	25.3	26.3
British Columbia	22.7	28.1	27.4	25.2	26.6	25.8	23.3	25.0	25.4	25.3
Yukon [4]	21.9	26.1	27.4	28.4	26.0	42.0	29.2	29.4	23.5	25.8
Northwest Territories [4]	24.1	35.8	36.3	37.8	37.8	34.7	34.4	33.2	27.8	33.8
Nunavut [4], [5]	28.2	47.3	40.4	39.3	31.3	53.0	46.3	31.5	33.9	44.7

Source: Statistics Canada. *Table 105-0503 - Health indicator profile, age-standardized rate, annual estimates, by sex, Canada, provinces and territories, occasional,* CANSIM (database). (accessed: March 31, 2017)

Please see footnotes 30, 31, 57, 58, 59, 60, 61, 62, 64 for characteristics of the age-standardized rate.

AGE-STANDARDIZED RATES, INFLUENZA IMMUNIZATION, LESS THAN ONE YEAR AGO (%), [47, 48] FEMALES, CANADA, PROVINCES AND TERRITORIES

Geography	2003	2005	2007	2008	2009	2010	2011	2012	2013	2014
Canada	28.8	34.8	32.9	33.0	33.2	26.2	30.8	29.8	29.3	33.2
Newfoundland and Labrador	16.1	21.9	24.8	27.3	27.3	20.2	30.0	21.8	25.6	28.2
Prince Edward Island	24.4	30.7	31.5	29.8	33.5	24.4	34.9	34.6	30.1	41.3
Nova Scotia	30.7	40.0	39.0	43.1	43.5	46.7	48.9	43.9	44.1	51.3
New Brunswick	22.7	27.3	30.1	31.3	31.3	35.9	37.8	36.1	36.7	40.0
Quebec	20.0	25.2	26.2	27.6	29.5	15.3	23.3	21.5	23.5	23.9
Ontario	37.2	43.7	38.3	37.3	35.2	26.6	32.8	32.4	31.0	34.5
Manitoba	20.8	28.5	27.8	28.5	30.5	28.4	27.0	28.7	26.0	31.3
Saskatchewan	24.2	28.5	27.9	33.4	33.8	28.3	33.1	35.7	28.5	38.6
Alberta	26.4	31.4	31.4	31.9	34.9	35.0	35.2	29.3	31.0	38.8
British Columbia	27.4	33.0	32.2	30.5	31.8	30.4	29.7	32.3	29.6	35.9
Yukon [4]	22.5	41.7	33.7	33.7	41.6	50.8	35.6	26.9	32.1	35.4
Northwest Territories [4]	31.0	46.7	37.6	40.3	37.9	35.9	46.5	45.1	43.6	39.8
Nunavut [4, 5]	32.8	48.0	37.1	50.8	47.7	52.5	44.8	30.8	32.9	33.9E

Symbol Legend:
E   Use with caution

Source: Statistics Canada. *Table 105-0503 - Health indicator profile, age-standardized rate, annual estimates, by sex, Canada, provinces and territories, occasional,* CANSIM (database). (accessed: March 31, 2017)

Please see footnotes 30, 31, 57, 58, 59, 60, 61, 62, 64 for characteristics of the age-standardized rate.

AGE-STANDARDIZED RATES, REGULAR MEDICAL DOCTOR (%), [44] BOTH SEXES, CANADA, PROVINCES AND TERRITORIES

Geography	2003	2005	2007	2008	2009	2010	2011	2012	2013	2014
Canada	84.9	84.6	83.5	83.2	83.4	83.1	83.1	83.5	82.8	83.3
Newfoundland and Labrador	85.0	86.5	87.2	86.6	85.6	88.4	90.1	90.5	86.9	88.6
Prince Edward Island	92.2	88.9	87.3	85.6	89.8	90.3	85.4	87.9	86.9	89.5
Nova Scotia	94.5	94.0	93.5	93.1	92.2	92.4	91.9	89.8	89.0	87.8
New Brunswick	92.0	92.8	91.1	89.6	90.8	91.5	91.2	92.1	90.7	93.3
Quebec	72.0	72.7	70.7	70.0	70.1	71.2	71.1	71.9	71.6	71.6
Ontario	91.2	90.6	89.7	90.3	90.6	89.9	90.1	90.3	90.2	91.6
Manitoba	82.7	82.8	83.1	81.8	84.2	84.6	84.9	82.6	81.7	81.8
Saskatchewan	84.6	83.0	83.1	80.9	82.1	82.7	78.7	81.3	78.8	78.9
Alberta	83.6	82.1	81.5	80.4	79.9	78.6	78.9	80.4	79.4	79.1
British Columbia	88.3	87.9	86.8	85.5	85.5	84.1	84.1	84.0	82.6	82.4
Yukon [4]	81.7	73.7	76.7	76.9	77.0	76.8	78.9	70.4	72.4	72.2
Northwest Territories [4]	45.2	49.3	41.4	39.6	37.8	41.5	34.5	38.3	41.6	42.5
Nunavut [4,5]	29.4E	17.0E	15.6	12.1E	12.9E	16.6E	21.0	18.8	15.7E	20.1

Symbol Legend:
E   Use with caution

Source: Statistics Canada. *Table 105-0503 - Health indicator profile, age-standardized rate, annual estimates, by sex, Canada, provinces and territories, occasional,* CANSIM (database). (accessed: March 31, 2017)

Please see footnotes 30, 31, 57, 58, 59, 60, 61, 62, 64 for characteristics of the age-standardized rate.

AGE-STANDARDIZED RATES, REGULAR MEDICAL DOCTOR (%), [44] MALES, CANADA, PROVINCES AND TERRITORIES

Geography	2003	2005	2007	2008	2009	2010	2011	2012	2013	2014
Canada	80.4	80.3	78.6	78.6	78.9	78.3	78.5	78.8	78.5	79.4
Newfoundland and Labrador	80.5	82.4	84.5	83.6	80.2	83.9	86.2	87.3	81.9	83.9
Prince Edward Island	90.6	85.6	85.2	84.0	88.2	89.2	83.6	88.9	82.0	90.8
Nova Scotia	92.7	91.3	90.4	90.0	88.7	89.1	89.8	85.3	85.4	84.9
New Brunswick	89.7	90.6	88.3	84.9	90.8	89.0	88.7	89.5	88.0	90.7
Quebec	64.4	65.5	61.2	62.5	61.5	63.5	64.2	64.8	64.7	65.3
Ontario	88.4	88.2	87.2	87.7	88.2	86.9	87.7	87.6	87.5	89.5
Manitoba	77.9	78.2	77.2	76.0	80.0	80.8	77.4	77.7	75.8	76.2
Saskatchewan	79.5	77.1	75.9	76.2	77.3	78.7	72.8	74.4	74.3	71.6
Alberta	77.5	75.7	74.8	74.4	74.4	72.2	71.3	73.9	75.1	74.6
British Columbia	85.1	84.8	83.8	81.5	82.4	79.5	80.7	79.9	79.0	78.9
Yukon [4]	77.6	66.0	73.9	69.7	70.8	75.0	71.0	69.2	73.8	67.6
Northwest Territories [4]	37.1	41.8	39.5	34.1	37.1	36.3	31.1	34.1	33.9	40.4
Nunavut [4,5]	F	18.2E	13.2E	F	F	17.9E	16.6E	15.7E	17.5E	23.8

Symbol Legend:
E   Use with caution
F   Too unreliable to be published

Source: Statistics Canada. *Table 105-0503 - Health indicator profile, age-standardized rate, annual estimates, by sex, Canada, provinces and territories, occasional,* CANSIM (database). (accessed: March 31, 2017)

Please see footnotes 30, 31, 57, 58, 59, 60, 61, 62, 64 for characteristics of the age-standardized rate.

AGE-STANDARDIZED RATES, REGULAR MEDICAL DOCTOR (%), 44 FEMALES, CANADA, PROVINCES AND TERRITORIES

Geography	2003	2005	2007	2008	2009	2010	2011	2012	2013	2014
Canada	89.2	88.8	88.4	87.7	87.8	87.8	87.6	88.0	87.0	87.2
Newfoundland and Labrador	89.4	90.5	89.8	89.3	90.6	92.7	93.8	93.5	91.7	93.0
Prince Edward Island	93.8	91.8	89.3	87.1	91.3	91.2	87.2	87.0	91.5	88.3
Nova Scotia	96.1	96.6	96.3	96.0	95.5	95.4	93.8	93.9	92.3	90.6
New Brunswick	94.3	95.0	93.7	94.2	90.9	93.8	93.6	94.6	93.4	95.8
Quebec	79.4	79.7	80.0	77.5	78.5	78.7	78.1	79.0	78.4	77.8
Ontario	93.8	92.8	92.1	92.8	93.0	92.7	92.5	92.9	92.8	93.6
Manitoba	87.4	87.2	88.8	87.5	88.3	88.2	92.5	87.5	87.4	87.4
Saskatchewan	89.7	88.9	90.1	85.5	86.8	86.7	84.7	88.2	83.4	86.3
Alberta	89.7	88.6	88.3	86.5	85.7	85.2	86.7	87.1	83.8	83.6
British Columbia	91.4	91.0	89.7	89.4	88.5	88.6	87.5	88.0	86.1	85.9
Yukon 4	85.8	81.1	79.5	84.2	83.2	78.7	86.9	71.7	71.1	77.0
Northwest Territories 4	53.9	57.6	43.6E	45.8	38.5	47.1	38.2	42.6	49.9	44.6
Nunavut 4, 5	28.4E	15.5	17.9E	14.3E	16.7E	15.2E	26.1	22.3E	F	15.9E

Symbol Legend:
E   Use with caution
F   Too unreliable to be published

Source: Statistics Canada. *Table 105-0503 - Health indicator profile, age-standardized rate, annual estimates, by sex, Canada, provinces and territories, occasional,* CANSIM (database). (accessed: March 31, 2017)

Please see footnotes 30, 31, 57, 58, 59, 60, 61, 62, 64 for characteristics of the age-standardized rate.

AGE-STANDARDIZED RATES, EXPOSURE TO SECOND-HAND SMOKE AT HOME (%), [27] BOTH SEXES, CANADA, PROVINCES AND TERRITORIES

Geography	2003	2005	2007	2008	2009	2010	2011	2012	2013	2014
Canada	10.7	8.9	7.5	6.8	6.4	6.0	5.7	4.8	4.6	4.0
Newfoundland and Labrador	14.0	11.8	9.4	8.2	8.2	6.8	5.8	4.8E	4.6	4.7E
Prince Edward Island	12.0	13.5	8.3	8.2	6.9E	5.2E	8.5	8.2E	5.0E	4.3E
Nova Scotia	12.5	10.6	7.7	7.1	7.4	8.5	5.1	7.0	8.5	5.1
New Brunswick	13.2	12.5	8.9	9.0	7.9	6.8	7.4	6.4	5.8	4.6
Quebec	16.1	13.5	12.1	9.9	9.7	8.9	9.1	6.9	6.9	6.0
Ontario	9.4	7.4	5.8	6.0	5.4	5.4	4.9	4.2	4.0	3.4
Manitoba	10.9	8.6	9.2	6.9	6.0	5.7	4.4	5.0	4.1	3.3
Saskatchewan	10.6	7.6	8.5	7.9	6.9	6.2	4.9	5.7	5.3	3.7
Alberta	9.0	7.9	6.2	5.6	5.8	5.9	5.3	4.8	3.5	4.4
British Columbia	5.8	5.0	4.7	3.8	3.6	2.9	2.6	2.6	2.5	2.1
Yukon [4]	13.0	7.8E	11.9E	6.9E	12.1E	7.7E	5.2E	F	5.8E	3.1E
Northwest Territories [4]	13.9	16.7	12.0E	5.2E	8.4E	7.5E	8.6E	4.7E	6.3E	5.1E
Nunavut [4, 5]	11.2E	13.2E	11.0E	11.4E	F	F	F	9.3E	5.5E	F

Symbol Legend:
E Use with caution
F Too unreliable to be published

Source: Statistics Canada. *Table 105-0503 - Health indicator profile, age-standardized rate, annual estimates, by sex, Canada, provinces and territories, occasional,* CANSIM (database). (accessed: March 31, 2017)

Please see footnotes 30, 31, 57, 58, 59, 60, 61, 62, 64 for characteristics of the age-standardized rate.

AGE-STANDARDIZED RATES, EXPOSURE TO SECOND-HAND SMOKE AT HOME (%), [27] MALES, CANADA, PROVINCES AND TERRITORIES

Geography	2003	2005	2007	2008	2009	2010	2011	2012	2013	2014
Canada	11.6	9.6	8.3	7.5	7.0	6.8	6.2	4.9	4.3	4.4
Newfoundland and Labrador	14.8	12.6	12.8	11.1E	10.5	8.6E	6.3E	7.3E	4.9E	4.4E
Prince Edward Island	12.1	15.7	8.8E	8.7E	9.8E	5.7E	10.9E	10.3E	5.4E	F
Nova Scotia	14.9	11.5	6.7	7.9	7.0E	8.5E	5.6E	6.2E	9.7E	6.8E
New Brunswick	14.4	12.8	9.8	8.9	7.2E	7.7	8.8E	8.3E	6.3E	4.4E
Quebec	17.1	14.7	14.3	10.6	10.4	9.7	9.8	7.4	6.4	6.7
Ontario	9.9	7.9	6.1	6.7	6.3	6.0	5.0	4.2	3.7	3.4
Manitoba	13.0	8.5	8.4	8.7	7.3E	5.9E	5.7E	5.6E	3.5E	3.2E
Saskatchewan	11.5	8.4	10.1	7.5	6.7E	6.6	4.3	5.7E	4.0E	3.7E
Alberta	10.0	8.6	6.8	6.7	6.8	7.4	6.7	4.1	2.8E	5.4
British Columbia	6.0	5.0	5.0	4.0	3.4	3.4	2.8	2.3E	2.4E	2.1E
Yukon [4]	16.7E	8.9E	16.0E	9.8E	13.4E	9.7E	F	F	6.9E	F
Northwest Territories [4]	15.8	19.8	15.9E	F	11.2E	F	11.1E	F	7.2E	7.1E
Nunavut [4, 5]	14.0E	14.3E	11.2E	F	F	F	F	F	F	F

Symbol Legend:
E Use with caution
F Too unreliable to be published

Source: Statistics Canada. *Table 105-0503 - Health indicator profile, age-standardized rate, annual estimates, by sex, Canada, provinces and territories, occasional,* CANSIM (database). (accessed: March 31, 2017)

Please see footnotes 30, 31, 57, 58, 59, 60, 61, 62, 64 for characteristics of the age-standardized rate.

AGE-STANDARDIZED RATES, EXPOSURE TO SECOND-HAND SMOKE AT HOME (%), [27] FEMALES, CANADA, PROVINCES AND TERRITORIES

Geography	2003	2005	2007	2008	2009	2010	2011	2012	2013	2014
Canada	10.0	8.3	6.8	6.1	5.8	5.4	5.2	4.8	4.8	3.7
Newfoundland and Labrador	13.3	11.1	6.6	5.7E	6.3E	5.1E	5.4E	2.5E	4.2E	5.0E
Prince Edward Island	11.9	11.7	7.8E	7.8E	4.4E	4.8E	6.3E	6.4E	4.6E	F
Nova Scotia	10.4	9.8	8.6	6.5	7.7	8.6E	4.6E	7.7E	7.5E	3.6E
New Brunswick	12.0	12.2	8.2	9.1	8.5	6.0	6.1E	4.9E	5.4E	4.8E
Quebec	15.1	12.3	10.1	9.2	9.1	8.2	8.5	6.4	7.3	5.4
Ontario	8.9	7.0	5.4	5.4	4.6	4.8	4.8	4.2	4.2	3.3
Manitoba	8.9	8.6	10.0	5.2E	4.9	5.5E	3.1E	4.3E	4.6E	3.4E
Saskatchewan	9.7	6.8	6.9	8.3	7.2	5.9	5.6	5.6E	6.5E	3.6E
Alberta	8.0	7.2	5.7	4.5	4.8	4.5	4.0	5.5	4.1E	3.3
British Columbia	5.5	4.9	4.5	3.7	3.9	2.4E	2.3E	2.8E	2.6E	2.1E
Yukon [4]	9.4E	6.8E	8.0E	F	10.8E	5.7E	7.7E	F	F	F
Northwest Territories [4]	11.9E	13.1	8.1E	5.0E	F	F	F	F	5.4E	F
Nunavut [4,5]	8.3E	12.0E	10.9E	F	F	F	F	F	F	F

Symbol Legend:
E   Use with caution
F   Too unreliable to be published

Source: Statistics Canada. *Table 105-0503 - Health indicator profile, age-standardized rate, annual estimates, by sex, Canada, provinces and territories, occasional,* CANSIM (database). (accessed: March 31, 2017)

Please see footnotes 30, 31, 57, 58, 59, 60, 61, 62, 64 for characteristics of the age-standardized rate.

AGE-STANDARDIZED RATES, EXPOSURE TO SECOND-HAND SMOKE IN THE PAST MONTH, IN VEHICLES AND/OR PUBLIC PLACES (%), [29] BOTH SEXES, CANADA, PROVINCES AND TERRITORIES

Geography	2003	2005	2007	2008	2009	2010	2011	2012	2013	2014
Canada	25.1	19.8	17.2	15.4	15.5	15.8	17.8	17.6	17.2	18.1
Newfoundland and Labrador	23.8	17.9	18.6	16.3	14.5	15.0	19.3	15.6	15.3	16.2
Prince Edward Island	23.2	15.0	14.8	13.8	11.3	11.3	19.3	14.7	14.8	15.7
Nova Scotia	24.3	16.1	19.1	18.0	15.9	16.1	18.5	14.6	16.3	17.9
New Brunswick	25.7	16.4	17.5	15.9	17.0	15.3	18.7	17.8	16.4	17.4
Quebec	32.2	27.2	17.6	14.5	15.1	14.8	19.4	17.9	16.8	17.0
Ontario	23.3	18.0	17.2	16.1	15.8	17.2	17.5	17.7	17.7	19.3
Manitoba	25.2	12.9	14.5	14.9	15.6	17.5	19.0	20.1	18.4	19.9
Saskatchewan	28.8	16.6	15.7	14.7	13.9	13.8	15.2	14.0	19.2	16.6
Alberta	25.9	22.5	20.2	15.8	15.3	14.9	17.3	18.9	16.8	20.0
British Columbia	16.7	14.9	15.3	14.5	15.5	14.7	16.3	16.8	16.7	15.6
Yukon [4]	30.6	12.9	10.0E	6.9E	8.4E	7.7E	11.0	10.8E	14.1	8.9
Northwest Territories [4]	38.3	19.0	12.2	7.1E	11.9E	13.1	15.1	19.4E	26.2	21.8
Nunavut [4,5]	24.8E	13.1E	13.4E	15.0E	F	F	F	30.4E	17.8E	14.9E

Symbol Legend:
E Use with caution
F Too unreliable to be published

Source: Statistics Canada. *Table 105-0503 - Health indicator profile, age-standardized rate, annual estimates, by sex, Canada, provinces and territories, occasional,* CANSIM (database). (accessed: March 31, 2017)

Please see footnotes 30, 31, 57, 58, 59, 60, 61, 62, 64 for characteristics of the age-standardized rate.

AGE-STANDARDIZED RATES, EXPOSURE TO SECOND-HAND SMOKE IN THE PAST MONTH, IN VEHICLES AND/OR PUBLIC PLACES (%), [29] MALES, CANADA, PROVINCES AND TERRITORIES

Geography	2003	2005	2007	2008	2009	2010	2011	2012	2013	2014
Canada	28.1	22.2	18.7	16.5	17.1	17.1	19.6	18.6	17.8	19.6
Newfoundland and Labrador	27.8	20.5	22.1	19.9	16.7	20.0	21.2	17.6	13.7	15.7
Prince Edward Island	27.5	17.4	15.8	18.6	15.0E	11.6E	19.3	17.0E	17.6E	21.1E
Nova Scotia	28.7	18.2	18.0	20.3	16.1	17.3	18.8	17.4	18.8	19.9
New Brunswick	28.5	18.3	17.9	18.7	17.8	20.0	19.9	20.2	17.0	19.9
Quebec	35.8	30.6	19.3	15.1	16.2	15.8	20.9	20.1	17.8	18.5
Ontario	26.1	19.9	18.3	17.1	17.5	18.3	19.5	17.8	17.6	20.8
Manitoba	27.8	14.3	14.2	17.8	19.5	18.8	21.3	21.1	19.7	20.7
Saskatchewan	32.5	19.7	20.3	15.6	14.3	14.6	16.8	15.5	21.1	18.4
Alberta	29.7	25.6	23.3	17.1	18.2	17.1	20.0	19.3	17.5	21.5
British Columbia	18.5	16.2	16.0	14.9	16.8	15.3	17.4	18.3	18.0	17.0
Yukon [4]	33.0	13.4E	9.3E	7.4E	10.4E	F	11.5E	12.9E	13.5E	10.0E
Northwest Territories [4]	41.7	18.4	13.8E	F	13.1E	12.9E	17.7	16.3E	28.6	23.3
Nunavut [4,5]	29.7	16.5E	F	19.0E	F	F	F	F	13.4E	F

Symbol Legend:
E Use with caution
F Too unreliable to be published

Source: Statistics Canada. *Table 105-0503 - Health indicator profile, age-standardized rate, annual estimates, by sex, Canada, provinces and territories, occasional,* CANSIM (database). (accessed: March 31, 2017)

Please see footnotes 30, 31, 57, 58, 59, 60, 61, 62, 64 for characteristics of the age-standardized rate.

AGE-STANDARDIZED RATES, EXPOSURE TO SECOND-HAND SMOKE IN THE PAST MONTH, IN VEHICLES AND/OR PUBLIC PLACES (%), [29] FEMALES, CANADA, PROVINCES AND TERRITORIES

Geography	2003	2005	2007	2008	2009	2010	2011	2012	2013	2014
Canada	22.3	17.6	16.0	14.5	14.0	14.7	16.2	16.7	16.7	16.8
Newfoundland and Labrador	20.2	15.4	15.7	13.1	12.7	10.3	17.7	13.8	16.7	16.7
Prince Edward Island	19.4	13.1	14.0	9.8E	8.1E	11.0E	19.2	12.7	12.6E	11.5E
Nova Scotia	20.3	14.2	20.0	16.0	15.7	15.2	18.3	12.3	14.2	16.0
New Brunswick	23.1	14.6	17.2	13.3	16.3	11.1	17.5	15.8	15.9	15.0
Quebec	28.9	23.9	16.1	13.9	14.0	14.0	18.0	15.9	15.9	15.6
Ontario	20.9	16.2	16.2	15.3	14.4	16.1	15.8	17.6	17.8	18.0
Manitoba	22.8	11.7	14.7	12.2	11.9	16.3	16.7	19.1	17.1	19.1
Saskatchewan	25.2	13.5	11.3	13.8	13.5	13.1	13.6	12.4	17.3	14.8
Alberta	22.3	19.6	17.2	14.6	12.7	12.9	14.7	18.6	16.2	18.5
British Columbia	15.1	13.6	14.6	14.2	14.2	14.2	15.3	15.4	15.5	14.4
Yukon [4]	28.3	12.4E	10.6E	F	F	8.9E	10.5E	F	14.7E	7.9E
Northwest Territories [4]	34.8	19.7	10.5E	10.2E	10.7E	13.4E	12.7E	22.6E	23.5E	20.5
Nunavut [4, 5]	20.0E	F	F	10.7E	F	F	F	F	25.1E	F

Symbol Legend:
E   Use with caution
F   Too unreliable to be published

Source: Statistics Canada. *Table 105-0503 - Health indicator profile, age-standardized rate, annual estimates, by sex, Canada, provinces and territories, occasional,* CANSIM (database). (accessed: March 31, 2017)

Please see footnotes 30, 31, 57, 58, 59, 60, 61, 62, 64 for characteristics of the age-standardized rate.

AGE-STANDARDIZED RATES, EXPOSURE TO SECOND-HAND SMOKE IN THE PAST MONTH, IN VEHICLES (%), [29] BOTH SEXES, CANADA, PROVINCES AND TERRITORIES

Geography	2003	2005	2007	2008	2009	2010	2011	2012	2013	2014
Canada	10.5	8.5	8.9	7.7	7.6	7.3	7.1	6.8	6.2	6.4
Newfoundland and Labrador	15.2	10.6	13.4	12.3	10.5	10.6	9.7	8.4	8.3	8.6
Prince Edward Island	13.8	12.2	9.6	9.4	7.0E	6.8E	10.9	7.5	10.1E	5.3E
Nova Scotia	13.7	9.6	12.9	11.7	9.8	9.1	9.4	6.7	7.2	8.5
New Brunswick	13.6	11.4	11.8	10.2	9.8	10.1	11.0	8.2	8.3	9.1
Quebec	12.3	9.5	10.1	8.1	9.2	8.0	8.3	8.3	7.2	7.4
Ontario	10.0	8.2	8.6	7.1	6.7	6.9	6.4	5.8	5.1	6.3
Manitoba	11.4	8.7	7.9	8.8	9.2	9.7	7.4	8.7	8.4	5.5
Saskatchewan	11.6	9.6	10.4	9.3	9.2	7.5	8.5	6.9	9.2	7.0
Alberta	10.1	9.2	8.8	8.6	7.5	7.2	7.8	7.9	6.2	6.9
British Columbia	7.1	6.0	6.3	5.7	6.0	5.3	4.8	5.4	5.5	3.7
Yukon [4]	14.1	7.2	7.8E	1.9E	5.9E	4.5E	7.4E	F	9.7	4.5E
Northwest Territories [4]	18.9	9.6	8.2	5.2E	9.0E	7.8E	9.1E	11.7E	14.7	11.9
Nunavut [4, 5]	15.0E	6.7E	F	F	F	F	F	F	F	F

Symbol Legend:
E   Use with caution
F   Too unreliable to be published

Source: Statistics Canada. *Table 105-0503 - Health indicator profile, age-standardized rate, annual estimates, by sex, Canada, provinces and territories, occasional,* CANSIM (database). (accessed: March 31, 2017)

Please see footnotes 30, 31, 57, 58, 59, 60, 61, 62, 64 for characteristics of the age-standardized rate.

AGE-STANDARDIZED RATES, EXPOSURE TO SECOND-HAND SMOKE IN THE PAST MONTH, IN VEHICLES (%), [29] MALES, CANADA, PROVINCES AND TERRITORIES

Geography	2003	2005	2007	2008	2009	2010	2011	2012	2013	2014
Canada	11.8	9.6	9.7	8.5	8.7	8.2	7.8	7.6	6.6	7.5
Newfoundland and Labrador	18.1	11.9	16.0	16.2	11.2	14.6	11.4	9.9E	8.4	9.0E
Prince Edward Island	16.4	14.2	10.5E	12.9E	8.2E	7.4E	9.6E	7.6E	12.9E	7.5E
Nova Scotia	16.2	10.7	11.6	12.9	9.2	10.0E	9.4E	8.4E	9.3E	9.9E
New Brunswick	15.5	11.9	11.5	11.7	9.9	13.4	13.0	10.6E	8.2E	10.4
Quebec	13.3	11.0	11.3	8.4	10.0	8.8	8.8	9.8	6.9	8.6
Ontario	11.3	8.8	9.3	8.1	7.8	7.9	6.7	6.3	5.4	7.4
Manitoba	13.4	9.4	6.7	10.9	12.9	8.8	9.4	11.2	8.8E	5.7E
Saskatchewan	12.0	12.5	12.9	9.8	8.7	7.6	10.3E	8.3	10.6	7.8
Alberta	11.6	10.6	10.2	9.2	9.2	8.4	9.4	6.6	7.2	7.9
British Columbia	8.2	7.0	6.8	6.0	7.3	6.0	5.0	6.9	6.4	5.2
Yukon [4]	14.7E	6.7E	6.7E	3.3E	6.9E	F	8.1E	F	11.1E	F
Northwest Territories [4]	20.6	9.8E	10.2E	F	11.6E	F	11.0E	11.3E	16.6	14.6E
Nunavut [4, 5]	18.4E	F	F	F	F	F	F	F	F	F

Symbol Legend:
E Use with caution
F Too unreliable to be published

Source: Statistics Canada. *Table 105-0503 - Health indicator profile, age-standardized rate, annual estimates, by sex, Canada, provinces and territories, occasional,* CANSIM (database). (accessed: March 31, 2017)

Please see footnotes 30, 31, 57, 58, 59, 60, 61, 62, 64 for characteristics of the age-standardized rate.

AGE-STANDARDIZED RATES, EXPOSURE TO SECOND-HAND SMOKE IN THE PAST MONTH, IN VEHICLES (%), [29] FEMALES, CANADA, PROVINCES AND TERRITORIES

Geography	2003	2005	2007	2008	2009	2010	2011	2012	2013	2014
Canada	9.4	7.6	8.1	6.9	6.7	6.4	6.5	6.0	5.8	5.4
Newfoundland and Labrador	12.7	9.4	11.3	8.8E	9.9E	6.8	8.2E	7.1E	8.2E	8.3E
Prince Edward Island	11.5	10.5	8.9E	6.4E	5.9E	6.3E	12.1E	7.3E	7.9E	F
Nova Scotia	11.6	8.6	14.0	10.7	10.3	8.4E	9.4	5.3E	5.4E	7.2E
New Brunswick	11.8	11.0	12.0	8.8	9.6	7.2	9.2	6.2E	8.4	7.9E
Quebec	11.3	8.1	9.0	7.8	8.5	7.3	7.9	6.9	7.4	6.3
Ontario	8.9	7.6	7.9	6.2	5.8	6.1	6.0	5.3	4.9	5.4
Manitoba	9.4	8.1	8.9	7.0	5.8E	10.4E	5.6	6.3E	8.1E	5.3E
Saskatchewan	11.2	6.9	8.1	8.8	9.6	7.3	6.7E	5.6	7.8	6.3E
Alberta	8.6	7.8	7.4	7.9	5.9	6.1	6.2	9.2	5.3	5.9
British Columbia	6.1	5.1	5.8	5.5	4.8	4.7	4.7	4.0	4.6	2.4E
Yukon [4]	13.5E	7.6E	8.8E	F	F	5.3E	6.8E	F	8.3E	F
Northwest Territories [4]	17.1E	9.4E	6.3E	8.1E	F	6.5E	F	12.1E	12.6E	9.5E
Nunavut [4, 5]	F	F	F	4.5E	F	F	F	F	F	F

Symbol Legend:
E   Use with caution
F   Too unreliable to be published

Source: Statistics Canada. *Table 105-0503 - Health indicator profile, age-standardized rate, annual estimates, by sex, Canada, provinces and territories, occasional,* CANSIM (database). (accessed: March 31, 2017)

Please see footnotes 30, 31, 57, 58, 59, 60, 61, 62, 64 for characteristics of the age-standardized rate.

AGE-STANDARDIZED RATES, EXPOSURE TO SECOND-HAND SMOKE IN THE PAST MONTH, IN PUBLIC PLACES (%), [29] BOTH SEXES, CANADA, PROVINCES AND TERRITORIES

Geography	2003	2005	2007	2008	2009	2010	2011	2012	2013	2014
Canada	20.4	15.4	11.6	10.5	10.5	11.6	13.5	13.6	13.6	14.7
Newfoundland and Labrador	14.6	10.9	9.4	7.1	6.0	6.7	13.1	9.0	10.4	11.0
Prince Edward Island	13.5	6.0	7.0	6.4E	5.9E	6.3E	12.0	9.4	8.2	11.6
Nova Scotia	16.3	9.7	10.7	9.1	8.4	9.2	13.0	10.3	12.3	13.2
New Brunswick	20.1	7.3	8.6	8.1	8.9	7.3	11.5	11.3	11.0	11.1
Quebec	28.1	23.9	10.7	8.9	8.6	9.8	13.9	12.9	12.7	13.1
Ontario	18.5	13.5	12.1	11.8	11.8	13.6	13.9	14.3	14.9	16.1
Manitoba	20.4	6.1	9.0	8.9	9.1	11.3	14.1	16.1	13.2	16.9
Saskatchewan	24.6	10.0	8.1	7.6	7.4	8.3	9.7	9.6	13.5	11.8
Alberta	21.3	18.3	15.0	10.3	10.6	10.1	12.3	14.4	12.4	16.2
British Columbia	13.1	11.2	11.5	11.3	12.1	12.4	13.7	13.5	13.2	13.7
Yukon [4]	23.6	7.8E	4.5E	5.1E	F	F	4.3E	7.2E	7.7E	6.7E
Northwest Territories [4]	30.5	13.0	5.5E	3.1E	4.2E	7.3E	9.8	14.1E	15.7	14.2
Nunavut [4, 5]	18.3E	F	F	F	F	F	F	F	16.3E	12.9E

Symbol Legend:
E   Use with caution
F   Too unreliable to be published

Source: Statistics Canada. *Table 105-0503 - Health indicator profile, age-standardized rate, annual estimates, by sex, Canada, provinces and territories, occasional,* CANSIM (database). (accessed: March 31, 2017)

Please see footnotes 30, 31, 57, 58, 59, 60, 61, 62, 64 for characteristics of the age-standardized rate.

AGE-STANDARDIZED RATES, EXPOSURE TO SECOND-HAND SMOKE IN THE PAST MONTH, IN PUBLIC PLACES (%), [29] MALES, CANADA, PROVINCES AND TERRITORIES

Geography	2003	2005	2007	2008	2009	2010	2011	2012	2013	2014
Canada	23.2	17.4	12.4	10.9	11.7	12.4	14.9	13.7	13.9	15.6
Newfoundland and Labrador	16.7	12.5	11.8	8.5E	7.2	8.4E	15.0	9.9E	8.9	12.5E
Prince Edward Island	15.4	7.6E	7.6E	8.9E	8.5E	7.1E	13.7E	11.7E	9.0E	15.7E
Nova Scotia	19.0	10.6	10.3	9.9	9.2	9.4E	13.3	10.9E	14.7	14.4
New Brunswick	22.8	9.2	9.0	9.9	9.5	9.4E	11.6	10.8	12.5E	13.0
Quebec	32.0	27.1	11.2	9.5	9.5	10.2	15.6	13.9	13.7	13.8
Ontario	21.0	15.3	12.8	12.3	13.1	14.5	15.6	13.7	14.8	17.1
Manitoba	22.5	6.9	9.3	10.7	11.2	13.4	14.9	15.5	13.9	17.9
Saskatchewan	28.1	11.4	11.3	8.3	8.0	9.1	10.0	9.4	14.5	13.1
Alberta	24.7	20.8	17.3	10.4	12.3	11.7	14.4	15.5	12.3	17.5
British Columbia	14.7	11.9	12.0	11.3	13.3	12.6	14.0	13.9	13.5	13.8
Yukon [4]	25.7	7.7E	F	F	F	F	F	10.5E	5.5E	7.1E
Northwest Territories [4]	35.1	12.0	F	F	F	6.4E	12.4E	F	16.6	13.7E
Nunavut [4] [5]	21.7E	10.1E	F	F	F	F	F	F	12.6E	F

Symbol Legend:
E   Use with caution
F   Too unreliable to be published

Source: Statistics Canada. *Table 105-0503 - Health indicator profile, age-standardized rate, annual estimates, by sex, Canada, provinces and territories, occasional,* CANSIM (database). (accessed: March 31, 2017)

Please see footnotes 30, 31, 57, 58, 59, 60, 61, 62, 64 for characteristics of the age-standardized rate.

AGE-STANDARDIZED RATES, EXPOSURE TO SECOND-HAND SMOKE IN THE PAST MONTH, IN PUBLIC PLACES (%), [29] FEMALES, CANADA, PROVINCES AND TERRITORIES

Geography	2003	2005	2007	2008	2009	2010	2011	2012	2013	2014
Canada	17.7	13.5	10.9	10.0	9.4	10.8	12.2	13.4	13.3	13.9
Newfoundland and Labrador	12.8	9.3	7.4E	5.8E	5.1E	5.1E	11.3	8.2	11.8	9.7
Prince Edward Island	11.9	4.6E	6.6E	4.4E	3.7E	5.7E	10.4E	7.4E	7.5E	8.4E
Nova Scotia	13.8	8.9	11.0	8.5	7.7E	8.9E	12.6	9.9	10.3	12.1
New Brunswick	17.6	5.5	8.3	6.4	8.3	5.5E	11.4	11.7	9.7	9.3
Quebec	24.4	20.9	10.3	8.3	7.8	9.4	12.3	12.0	11.9	12.4
Ontario	16.2	11.9	11.5	11.5	10.7	12.8	12.4	14.8	15.0	15.2
Manitoba	18.4	5.3	8.7	7.2E	7.2E	9.3	13.4	16.6	12.5	16.1
Saskatchewan	21.2	8.7	5.0	7.0	6.7	7.6	9.4	9.9	12.6	10.5
Alberta	18.1	15.9	12.8	10.2	8.9	8.6	10.3	13.4	12.4	15.0
British Columbia	11.6	10.6	11.0	11.3	11.1	12.2	13.4	13.2	13.0	13.6
Yukon [4]	21.5E	8.0E	F	F	F	F	4.9E	4.1E	9.9E	6.3E
Northwest Territories [4]	25.8	14.1E	F	F	6.4E	8.3E	7.5E	18.6E	14.7E	14.6E
Nunavut [4] [5]	15.0E	F	F	F	F	F	F	F	22.4E	F

Symbol Legend:
E   Use with caution
F   Too unreliable to be published

Source: Statistics Canada. *Table 105-0503 - Health indicator profile, age-standardized rate, annual estimates, by sex, Canada, provinces and territories, occasional,* CANSIM (database). (accessed: March 31, 2017)

Please see footnotes 30, 31, 57, 58, 59, 60, 61, 62, 64 for characteristics of the age-standardized rate.

AGE-STANDARDIZED RATES, INFANT MORTALITY RATE (PER 1,000 LIVE BIRTHS), BOTH SEXES, CANADA, PROVINCES AND TERRITORIES

Geography	2003	2004	2005	2006	2007	2008	2009	2010	2011	2012	2013
Canada [11, 12]	5.3	5.3	5.4	5.0	5.1	5.0	4.9	5.0	4.8	4.8	5.0
Newfoundland and Labrador [11, 12]	5.0	5.1	6.2	5.3	7.5	5.1	6.3	5.3	6.3	5.7	6.4
Prince Edward Island	4.9	4.3	2.2	2.1	5.0	2.0	3.4	3.6	4.2	3.8	2.1
Nova Scotia	5.7	4.6	4.0	4.0	3.3	3.5	3.4	4.6	4.9	4.6	3.4
New Brunswick	4.1	4.3	4.1	4.0	4.3	3.2	5.8	3.4	3.5	5.7	4.7
Quebec	4.4	4.6	4.6	5.1	4.5	4.3	4.4	5.0	4.3	5.0	4.9
Ontario	5.3	5.5	5.6	5.0	5.2	5.3	5.0	5.0	4.6	4.8	4.9
Manitoba	8.0	7.0	6.6	6.0	7.3	6.5	6.3	6.7	7.7	5.6	5.6
Saskatchewan	6.3	6.2	8.3	6.1	5.8	6.2	6.7	5.9	6.7	5.4	7.5
Alberta	6.6	5.8	6.8	5.3	6.0	6.2	5.5	5.9	5.3	4.2	5.3
British Columbia	4.2	4.3	4.5	4.1	4.0	3.7	3.6	3.8	3.8	3.8	3.7
Yukon [14]	6.0	11.0	0.0	8.2	8.4	5.3	7.8	5.2	0.0	2.3	2.5
Northwest Territories [14, 15, 16]	5.7	0.0	4.2	10.2	4.1	9.7	15.5	1.4	7.2	4.4	7.5
Nunavut [13, 14, 16]	19.8	16.1	10.0	13.4	15.1	16.1	14.8	14.5	26.3	21.4	16.4

Source: Statistics Canada. *Table 102-0030 - Infant mortality, by sex and birth weight, Canada, provinces and territories, annual,* CANSIM (database). (accessed: March 31, 2017)

Sex [5], [6] = Both sexes
Birth weight [3], [6], [19] = All birth weights [7], [8]
Characteristics [2], [17], [18] = Infant mortality rate per 1,000 live births [3], [4], [8], [10]

Also see footnotes [1], [5], [9]

AGE-STANDARDIZED RATES, INFANT MORTALITY RATE (PER 1,000 LIVE BIRTHS), MALES, CANADA, PROVINCES AND TERRITORIES

Geography	2003	2004	2005	2006	2007	2008	2009	2010	2011	2012	2013
Canada [11, 12]	5.7	5.5	5.9	5.4	5.5	5.4	5.1	5.5	5.3	5.0	5.3
Newfoundland and Labrador [11, 12]	6.4	5.2	5.6	6.7	6.5	5.2	7.4	6.0	6.2	8.4	6.0
Prince Edward Island	4.2	5.6	2.9	2.7	7.4	2.6	5.5	5.5	4.0	1.5	2.8
Nova Scotia	7.6	5.5	3.8	3.7	3.3	2.8	3.4	4.6	5.8	4.2	3.2
New Brunswick	3.9	5.1	4.0	4.4	5.7	4.2	5.9	4.9	4.4	6.1	5.3
Quebec	4.3	4.6	5.4	5.3	4.8	4.4	4.5	5.3	4.7	5.0	5.2
Ontario	5.5	5.8	5.7	5.6	5.7	5.9	5.3	5.4	5.1	5.1	5.4
Manitoba	9.8	7.2	6.6	6.3	8.1	6.2	6.7	8.0	8.5	5.2	6.9
Saskatchewan	7.5	7.1	9.3	6.6	4.7	7.8	6.8	6.0	7.9	5.3	8.4
Alberta	7.7	6.3	7.6	5.7	6.2	6.3	5.6	6.3	5.2	4.6	5.2
British Columbia	4.7	4.1	5.2	4.2	4.8	4.1	3.3	4.0	4.4	4.2	3.6
Yukon [14]	11.4	5.6	0.0	5.1	16.0	10.7	14.6	5.1	0.0	4.4	0.0
Northwest Territories [14, 15, 16]	8.6	0.0	8.0	8.4	5.4	19.6	10.7	2.8	5.7	5.8	8.7
Nunavut [13, 14, 16]	20.6	24.9	5.9	14.4	25.4	23.1	18.3	20.3	35.8	32.3	14.8

Source: Statistics Canada. *Table 102-0030 - Infant mortality, by sex and birth weight, Canada, provinces and territories, annual,* CANSIM (database). (accessed: March 31, 2017)

Sex 5, 6 = Both sexes
Birth weight 3, 6, 19 = All birth weights 7, 8
Characteristics 2, 17, 18 = Infant mortality rate per 1,000 live births 3, 4, 8, 10

Also see footnotes 1, 5, 9

AGE-STANDARDIZED RATES, INFANT MORTALITY RATE (PER 1,000 LIVE BIRTHS), FEMALES, CANADA, PROVINCES AND TERRITORIES

Geography	2003	2004	2005	2006	2007	2008	2009	2010	2011	2012	2013
Canada [11], [12]	4.8	5.0	5.0	4.6	4.7	4.6	4.7	4.6	4.3	4.5	4.6
Newfoundland and Labrador [11], [12]	3.5	5.1	6.8	3.7	8.5	5.0	5.1	4.6	6.4	2.8	6.8
Prince Edward Island	5.7	3.0	1.5	1.5	2.8	1.4	1.4	1.5	4.3	6.1	1.5
Nova Scotia	3.6	3.6	4.1	4.4	3.3	4.2	3.5	4.6	3.9	4.9	3.7
New Brunswick	4.2	3.5	4.1	3.5	2.9	2.2	5.7	1.9	2.6	5.2	4.1
Quebec	4.4	4.7	3.8	4.8	4.1	4.2	4.3	4.6	3.9	4.9	4.7
Ontario	5.1	5.3	5.4	4.3	4.7	4.7	4.7	4.5	4.1	4.6	4.3
Manitoba	6.0	6.9	6.7	5.7	6.4	6.8	5.9	5.3	6.9	6.0	4.4
Saskatchewan	5.1	5.2	7.2	5.6	6.9	4.6	6.7	5.8	5.3	5.5	6.5
Alberta	5.4	5.3	5.9	4.8	5.9	6.1	5.3	5.4	5.3	3.9	5.4
British Columbia	3.7	4.5	3.7	4.0	3.2	3.4	3.9	3.5	3.3	3.4	3.8
Yukon [14]	0.0	16.0	0.0	11.9	0.0	0.0	0.0	5.4	0.0	0.0	5.6
Northwest Territories [14], [15], [16]	2.8	0.0	0.0	12.1	2.8	0.0	20.8	0.0	8.9	2.9	6.2
Nunavut [13], [14], [16]	19.0	5.8	13.9	12.1	5.0	8.1	11.3	9.2	15.4	9.8	18.1

Source: Statistics Canada. *Table 102-0030 - Infant mortality, by sex and birth weight, Canada, provinces and territories, annual,* CANSIM (database). (accessed: March 31, 2017)

Sex [5], [6] = Both sexes
Birth weight [3], [6], [19] = All birth weights [7], [8]
Characteristics [2], [17], [18] = Infant mortality rate per 1,000 live births [3], [4], [8], [10]

Also see footnotes [1], [5], [9]

AGE-STANDARDIZED RATES, LIFE EXPECTANCY AT BIRTH (YEARS),[18, 19, 20, 22] BOTH SEXES, CANADA, PROVINCES AND TERRITORIES

Geography [7, 8]	2000-2002	2005-2007	2006-2008	2007-2009
Canada [0]	79.6	80.7	80.9	81.1
Newfoundland and Labrador [10]	77.9	78.3	78.5	78.9
Prince Edward Island [11] [9]	78.6	80.2	80.2	80.2
Nova Scotia [12] [10]	78.9	79.7	79.9	80.1
New Brunswick [13] [11]	79.0	80.0	80.2	80.2
Quebec [24]	79.3	80.7	81.0	81.2
Ontario by Local Health Integration Network [35] [12]	79.8	81.0	81.3	81.5
Ontario by Health Unit [35] [12]	79.8	81.0	81.3	81.5
Manitoba [46] [14]	78.5	79.3	79.5	79.5
Saskatchewan [47] [14]	79.0	79.5	79.5	79.6
Alberta [48] [17]	79.6	80.5	80.6	80.7
British Columbia [59]	80.4	81.2	81.4	81.7
Yukon [60]	77.2	77.0	76.7	76.7
Northwest Territories [61]	78.0	78.0	77.1	77.4
Nunavut [62]	73.0	72.0	72.2	71.6

Source: Statistics Canada. *Table 102-4307 - Life expectancy, at birth and at age 65, by sex, three-year average, Canada, provinces, territories, health regions and peer groups, occasional (years unless otherwise noted)*, CANSIM (database). (accessed: March 31, 2017)

AGE-STANDARDIZED RATES, LIFE EXPECTANCY AT BIRTH (YEARS),[18, 19, 20, 22] MALES, CANADA, PROVINCES AND TERRITORIES

Geography [7, 8]	2000-2002	2005-2007	2006-2008	2007-2009
Canada [0]	77.0	78.3	78.5	78.8
Newfoundland and Labrador [10]	75.3	75.8	76.2	76.5
Prince Edward Island [11] [9]	75.4	77.6	77.5	77.5
Nova Scotia [12] [10]	76.3	77.1	77.4	77.7
New Brunswick [13] [11]	76.1	77.4	77.6	77.5
Quebec [24]	76.4	78.2	78.6	78.8
Ontario by Local Health Integration Network [35] [12]	77.4	78.8	79.0	79.2
Ontario by Health Unit [35] [12]	77.4	78.8	79.0	79.2
Manitoba [46] [14]	75.7	76.8	76.9	77.0
Saskatchewan [47] [14]	76.2	76.9	76.9	77.0
Alberta [48] [17]	77.1	78.1	78.3	78.5
British Columbia [59]	78.0	78.9	79.2	79.5
Yukon [60]	74.9	74.6	74.3E	74.2E
Northwest Territories [61]	75.6	75.3	74.6E	75.1E
Nunavut [62]	70.8	68.9	69.2E	68.8E

Symbol Legend:
E   Use with caution

Source: Statistics Canada. *Table 102-4307 - Life expectancy, at birth and at age 65, by sex, three-year average, Canada, provinces, territories, health regions and peer groups, occasional (years unless otherwise noted),* CANSIM (database). (accessed: March 31, 2017)

AGE-STANDARDIZED RATES, LIFE EXPECTANCY AT BIRTH (YEARS),[18, 19, 20, 22] FEMALES, CANADA, PROVINCES AND TERRITORIES

Geography [7, 8]	2000-2002	2005-2007	2006-2008	2007-2009
Canada [0]	82.0	83.0	83.1	83.3
Newfoundland and Labrador [10]	80.6	80.8	80.9	81.2
Prince Edward Island [11] [9]	81.7	82.7	82.9	82.8
Nova Scotia [12] [10]	81.4	82.2	82.3	82.4
New Brunswick [13] [11]	81.9	82.5	82.7	82.8
Quebec [24]	82.0	83.1	83.3	83.4
Ontario by Local Health Integration Network [35] [12]	82.1	83.1	83.4	83.6
Ontario by Health Unit [35] [12]	82.1	83.1	83.4	83.6
Manitoba [46] [14]	81.2	81.8	82.0	81.9
Saskatchewan [47] [14]	81.8	82.0	82.1	82.1
Alberta [48] [17]	82.1	82.9	83.0	83.0
British Columbia [59]	82.8	83.5	83.6	83.9
Yukon [60]	79.7	79.8	79.4E	79.1E
Northwest Territories [61]	80.8	81.3	80.0E	80.1E
Nunavut [62]	74.3	76.0	76.2E	75.2E

Symbol Legend:
E   Use with caution

Source: Statistics Canada. *Table 102-4307 - Life expectancy, at birth and at age 65, by sex, three-year average, Canada, provinces, territories, health regions and peer groups, occasional (years unless otherwise noted),* CANSIM (database). (accessed: March 31, 2017)

AGE-STANDARDIZED RATES, LIFE EXPECTANCY AT AGE 65 (YEARS),[18], [19], [20], [22] BOTH SEXES, CANADA, PROVINCES AND TERRITORIES

Geography [L] [8]	2000-2002	2005-2007	2006-2008	2007-2009
Canada [0]	18.9	19.8	20.0	20.2
Newfoundland and Labrador [10]	17.3	17.9	18.0	18.2
Prince Edward Island [11] [9]	18.2	19.4	19.4	19.3
Nova Scotia [12] [10]	18.3	18.9	19.1	19.3
New Brunswick [13] [11]	18.4	19.3	19.4	19.5
Quebec [24]	18.7	19.8	20.0	20.1
Ontario by Local Health Integration Network [35] [12]	18.9	19.9	20.2	20.3
Ontario by Health Unit [35] [12]	18.9	19.9	20.2	20.3
Manitoba [46] [14]	18.7	19.4	19.5	19.6
Saskatchewan [47] [14]	19.0	19.6	19.6	19.7
Alberta [48] [17]	19.3	20.0	20.1	20.2
British Columbia [59]	19.6	20.4	20.5	20.7
Yukon [60]	17.5	17.3	17.0	17.0
Northwest Territories [61]	17.6	18.2	17.6	18.0
Nunavut [62]	15.1	14.4	15.2	15.2

Source: Statistics Canada. *Table 102-4307 - Life expectancy, at birth and at age 65, by sex, three-year average, Canada, provinces, territories, health regions and peer groups, occasional (years unless otherwise noted),* CANSIM (database). (accessed: March 31, 2017)

AGE-STANDARDIZED RATES, LIFE EXPECTANCY AT AGE 65 (YEARS),[18, 19, 20, 22] MALES, CANADA, PROVINCES AND TERRITORIES

Geography [7, 8]	2000-2002	2005-2007	2006-2008	2007-2009
Canada [0]	17.0	18.1	18.3	18.5
Newfoundland and Labrador [10]	15.4	16.2	16.5	16.6
Prince Edward Island [11] [9]	16.0	17.5	17.6	17.6
Nova Scotia [12] [10]	16.4	17.1	17.4	17.5
New Brunswick [13] [11]	16.3	17.5	17.7	17.7
Quebec [24]	16.5	18.0	18.2	18.3
Ontario by Local Health Integration Network [35] [12]	17.2	18.3	18.5	18.7
Ontario by Health Unit [35] [12]	17.2	18.3	18.5	18.7
Manitoba [46] [14]	16.7	17.5	17.6	17.7
Saskatchewan [47] [14]	16.9	17.8	17.8	17.9
Alberta [48] [17]	17.4	18.3	18.4	18.5
British Columbia [59]	18.0	18.9	19.0	19.2
Yukon [60]	16.4	15.8	15.7E	15.8E
Northwest Territories [61]	16.3	16.1	15.9E	16.6E
Nunavut [62]	15.4	13.3	14.2E	13.9E

Symbol Legend:
E   Use with caution

Source: Statistics Canada. *Table 102-4307 - Life expectancy, at birth and at age 65, by sex, three-year average, Canada, provinces, territories, health regions and peer groups, occasional (years unless otherwise noted),* CANSIM (database). (accessed: March 31, 2017)

AGE-STANDARDIZED RATES, LIFE EXPECTANCY AT AGE 65 (YEARS),[18, 19, 20, 22] FEMALES, CANADA, PROVINCES AND TERRITORIES

Geography [7, 8]	2000-2002	2005-2007	2006-2008	2007-2009
Canada [0]	20.5	21.3	21.5	21.6
Newfoundland and Labrador [10]	19.2	19.5	19.4	19.7
Prince Edward Island [11] [9]	20.1	20.9	21.0	20.7
Nova Scotia [12] [10]	19.8	20.5	20.7	20.9
New Brunswick [13] [11]	20.2	20.9	20.9	21.1
Quebec [24]	20.5	21.3	21.5	21.6
Ontario by Local Health Integration Network [35] [12]	20.4	21.3	21.6	21.7
Ontario by Health Unit [35] [12]	20.4	21.3	21.6	21.7
Manitoba [46] [14]	20.4	20.9	21.1	21.2
Saskatchewan [47] [14]	20.8	21.2	21.2	21.3
Alberta [48] [17]	20.9	21.5	21.6	21.6
British Columbia [59]	21.1	21.7	21.8	22.0
Yukon [60]	18.8	19.1	18.6E	18.4E
Northwest Territories [61]	19.2	20.9	19.6E	19.7E
Nunavut [62]	14.3	16.3	16.8E	17.0E

Symbol Legend:
E   Use with caution

Source: Statistics Canada. *Table 102-4307 - Life expectancy, at birth and at age 65, by sex, three-year average, Canada, provinces, territories, health regions and peer groups, occasional (years unless otherwise noted),* CANSIM (database). (accessed: March 31, 2017)

AGE-STANDARDIZED RATES, TOTAL, ALL CAUSES OF DEATH (PER 100,000 POPULATION), BOTH SEXES, CANADA, PROVINCES AND TERRITORIES

Geography, place of residence [3], [4]	2003	2004	2005	2006	2007	2008	2009	2010	2011	2012	2013
Canada, place of residence	825.6	805.0	792.5	760.2	759.7	748.6	725.2	706.0	693.3	693.7	686.2
Newfoundland and Labrador, place of residence	975.7	968.9	983.0	962.8	945.8	938.7	884.7	881.4	863.7	850.6	873.5
Prince Edward Island, place of residence	898.6	907.4	811.1	847.8	795.4	812.1	846.4	731.5	802.2	765.4	775.7
Nova Scotia, place of residence	888.7	893.6	876.8	843.4	842.0	814.2	795.6	781.8	786.5	778.7	796.9
New Brunswick, place of residence	881.5	861.4	833.0	799.4	810.7	808.3	781.5	751.1	745.2	748.5	746.9
Quebec, place of residence	829.6	818.1	794.5	744.8	759.2	742.4	726.4	715.2	700.5	697.2	680.1
Ontario, place of residence	821.7	787.1	785.3	747.7	743.1	727.2	706.4	687.7	669.5	666.1	659.8
Manitoba, place of residence	876.1	870.7	850.1	832.4	823.3	819.3	796.1	777.1	780.8	778.8	764.1
Saskatchewan, place of residence	852.9	831.7	822.0	827.4	812.8	822.4	790.8	795.5	784.3	778.8	779.4
Alberta, place of residence	817.9	795.7	787.7	768.4	756.2	764.9	739.2	705.6	698.2	709.9	709.3
British Columbia, place of residence	765.0	757.0	737.9	723.7	722.4	718.0	679.4	652.6	642.2	657.6	649.6
Yukon, place of residence	871.6	1,070.1	1,012.0	1,110.2	1,042.9	1,148.0	1,045.9	1,095.8	1,079.1	892.3	884.4
Northwest Territories, place of residence	1,351.3	874.6	909.0	1,086.7	973.0	1,047.2	932.6	890.4	834.2	968.7	945.1
Nunavut, place of residence	1,406.7	1,211.2	1,282.4	1,438.5	1,296.2	1,314.7	1,548.4	1,097.4	1,541.3	1,233.9	1,590.3

Source: Statistics Canada. Table 102-0553 - Deaths and mortality rate (age standardization using 2011 population), by selected grouped causes and sex, Canada, provinces and territories, annual, CANSIM (database). (accessed: March 31, 2017)

Cause of death (ICD-10) [6], [7], [8] = Total, all causes of death [A00-Y89]
Characteristics [14], [15], [16], [17], [18], [19], [21] = Age-standardized mortality rate per 100,000 population

Also see footnotes [1], [2], [5], [13], [22], [23], [24], [25], [26], [27]

AGE-STANDARDIZED RATES, TOTAL, ALL CAUSES OF DEATH (PER 100,000 POPULATION), MALES, CANADA, PROVINCES AND TERRITORIES

Geography, place of residence [3] [4]	2003	2004	2005	2006	2007	2008	2009	2010	2011	2012	2013
Canada, place of residence	1,026.2	993.7	974.3	933.1	930.1	916.0	883.1	853.7	834.5	843.4	829.6
Newfoundland and Labrador, place of residence	1,221.1	1,245.5	1,255.1	1,192.8	1,175.7	1,152.9	1,094.2	1,078.9	1,039.7	1,054.8	1,029.2
Prince Edward Island, place of residence	1,147.5	1,140.7	980.5	1,086.6	1,005.7	1,018.5	1,031.7	927.5	948.9	916.9	1,006.0
Nova Scotia, place of residence	1,104.1	1,113.8	1,104.8	1,050.1	1,039.8	1,007.5	982.1	963.9	947.9	949.7	983.7
New Brunswick, place of residence	1,128.2	1,074.8	1,054.2	968.0	1,021.7	1,008.5	959.9	923.7	920.7	924.8	897.4
Quebec, place of residence	1,055.5	1,036.9	1,003.7	934.6	937.4	916.9	886.6	864.2	843.5	853.4	822.1
Ontario, place of residence	1,013.3	961.7	944.6	911.2	904.6	887.5	860.7	832.1	807.0	809.3	800.9
Manitoba, place of residence	1,108.4	1,082.6	1,046.2	1,029.0	1,022.9	1,015.4	974.6	935.0	940.6	946.1	937.2
Saskatchewan, place of residence	1,078.7	1,043.6	1,031.5	1,023.3	996.0	1,029.0	978.6	967.7	951.7	960.3	944.0
Alberta, place of residence	1,008.3	972.5	973.7	943.3	922.8	927.9	897.7	855.9	838.2	866.2	858.2
British Columbia, place of residence	921.7	911.6	895.9	867.3	875.4	860.8	815.4	780.6	768.9	785.5	775.2
Yukon, place of residence	1,032.3	1,300.5	1,260.3	1,569.5	1,212.8	1,383.7	1,334.9	1,308.0	1,480.9	1,131.3	980.5
Northwest Territories, place of residence	1,470.1	984.6	1,230.9	1,378.5	1,084.3	1,256.5	1,109.3	1,034.8	885.3	1,130.2	1,110.0
Nunavut, place of residence	1,396.8	1,382.5	1,524.3	1,568.9	1,533.5	1,669.0	1,901.5	1,033.0	1,351.8	1,343.6	1,742.5

Source: Statistics Canada. *Table 102-0553 - Deaths and mortality rate (age standardization using 2011 population), by selected grouped causes and sex, Canada, provinces and territories, annual,* CANSIM (database). (accessed: March 31, 2017)

Cause of death (ICD-10) [6], [7], [8] = Total, all causes of death [A00-Y89]
Characteristics [14], [15], [16], [17], [18], [19], [21] = Age-standardized mortality rate per 100,000 population

Also see footnotes [1], [2], [5], [13], [22], [23], [24], [25], [26], [27]

AGE-STANDARDIZED RATES, TOTAL, ALL CAUSES OF DEATH (PER 100,000 POPULATION), FEMALES, CANADA, PROVINCES AND TERRITORIES

Geography, place of residence 3, 4	2003	2004	2005	2006	2007	2008	2009	2010	2011	2012	2013
Canada, place of residence	680.0	666.4	658.1	631.6	631.3	623.0	604.8	591.3	582.2	580.3	575.6
Newfoundland and Labrador, place of residence	791.3	772.8	786.3	787.8	780.9	782.9	719.4	726.9	726.7	695.3	749.9
Prince Edward Island, place of residence	735.2	752.2	686.2	683.6	630.6	659.9	704.2	579.1	685.4	651.8	601.9
Nova Scotia, place of residence	731.9	730.9	714.1	686.6	699.2	672.7	653.9	646.9	664.8	655.0	657.1
New Brunswick, place of residence	704.0	706.3	674.2	672.7	658.1	659.5	645.4	621.7	608.4	615.1	631.6
Quebec, place of residence	674.2	669.3	650.9	614.6	630.7	618.4	609.2	603.8	591.8	585.8	576.5
Ontario, place of residence	683.1	658.5	665.9	626.2	621.3	608.0	590.3	576.6	562.9	557.7	552.0
Manitoba, place of residence	714.0	715.7	708.0	687.2	674.1	673.2	663.5	654.6	653.5	652.4	630.1
Saskatchewan, place of residence	680.8	669.7	661.5	675.0	671.3	660.2	644.2	654.9	650.6	636.4	648.5
Alberta, place of residence	676.1	660.4	645.1	634.2	626.5	637.0	612.9	582.8	584.0	589.4	592.4
British Columbia, place of residence	641.6	634.0	612.8	606.3	599.1	602.0	568.6	548.9	536.4	553.0	544.0
Yukon, place of residence	702.1	915.7	785.9	916.0	846.9	916.7	871.7	915.2	780.3	674.3	785.0
Northwest Territories, place of residence	1,290.5	736.7	646.1	807.6	847.8	840.2	739.3	736.1	755.9	838.4	793.7
Nunavut, place of residence	1,528.5	1,044.9	962.2	1,259.2	994.9	946.8	1,295.2	1,094.3	1,695.0	1,073.0	1,474.3

Source: Statistics Canada. *Table 102-0553 - Deaths and mortality rate (age standardization using 2011 population), by selected grouped causes and sex, Canada, provinces and territories, annual,* CANSIM (database). (accessed: March 31, 2017)

Cause of death (ICD-10) 6, 7, 8 = Total, all causes of death [A00-Y89]
Characteristics 14, 15, 16, 17, 18, 19, 21 = Age-standardized mortality rate per 100,000 population

Also see footnotes 1, 2, 5, 13, 22, 23, 24, 25, 26, 27

AGE-STANDARDIZED RATES, ALL MALIGNANT NEOPLASMS, DEATHS (PER 100,000 POPULATION), BOTH SEXES, CANADA, PROVINCES AND TERRITORIES

Geography, place of residence [3], [4]	2003	2004	2005	2006	2007	2008	2009	2010	2011	2012	2013
Canada, place of residence	237.6	234.8	230.3	225.5	224.6	221.5	217.1	213.2	209.8	210.0	205.5
Newfoundland and Labrador, place of residence	257.1	242.6	264.7	261.2	266.8	247.6	264.6	244.6	241.6	237.4	249.7
Prince Edward Island, place of residence	270.8	252.8	222.3	235.1	214.4	229.4	246.3	204.6	223.5	227.4	225.8
Nova Scotia, place of residence	270.2	266.5	259.8	258.2	251.2	247.3	240.7	239.3	243.2	237.0	234.4
New Brunswick, place of residence	256.8	237.6	244.8	232.4	233.3	239.4	238.2	217.0	210.7	213.8	214.8
Quebec, place of residence	254.3	254.6	248.8	243.8	245.9	243.8	237.5	234.4	231.3	231.9	223.0
Ontario, place of residence	233.8	228.6	225.5	219.5	215.6	213.7	208.7	206.7	204.0	202.0	196.9
Manitoba, place of residence	237.2	248.3	234.6	235.3	232.2	226.5	224.5	220.6	214.1	217.1	212.9
Saskatchewan, place of residence	230.1	225.3	222.3	222.6	218.1	214.8	209.3	214.8	207.7	205.9	206.4
Alberta, place of residence	225.3	222.1	215.7	211.5	209.6	207.0	204.8	194.6	189.1	193.2	192.5
British Columbia, place of residence	212.2	213.6	206.6	202.1	207.2	200.1	195.7	193.1	187.9	191.8	190.5
Yukon, place of residence	316.5	276.9	326.2	360.5	338.2	332.3	285.8	366.3	284.8	259.6	281.1
Northwest Territories, place of residence	393.9	243.6	266.8	236.9	195.4	310.3	222.3	325.1	244.8	258.3	231.0
Nunavut, place of residence	376.4	445.3	484.9	586.7	451.6	409.5	517.4	233.7	507.4	434.1	468.2

Source: Statistics Canada. *Table 102-0553 - Deaths and mortality rate (age standardization using 2011 population), by selected grouped causes and sex, Canada, provinces and territories, annual,* CANSIM (database). (accessed: March 31, 2017)

Cause of death (ICD-10) [6], [7], [8] = Malignant neoplasms [C00-C97]
Characteristics [14], [15], [16], [17], [18], [19], [21] = Age-standardized mortality rate per 100,000 population

Also see footnotes [1], [2], [5], [13], [22], [23], [24], [25], [26], [27]

AGE-STANDARDIZED RATES, ALL MALIGNANT NEOPLASMS, DEATHS (PER 100,000 POPULATION), MALES, CANADA, PROVINCES AND TERRITORIES

Geography, place of residence [3] [4]	2003	2004	2005	2006	2007	2008	2009	2010	2011	2012	2013
Canada, place of residence	294.3	289.4	283.9	276.7	273.8	270.0	263.6	255.6	251.6	253.5	246.2
Newfoundland and Labrador, place of residence	322.7	314.7	341.7	358.9	331.9	319.4	333.3	301.0	295.5	295.6	287.9
Prince Edward Island, place of residence	317.6	315.1	249.5	285.3	272.9	266.9	288.9	237.5	270.2	285.5	304.1
Nova Scotia, place of residence	327.1	335.5	333.4	331.1	310.0	314.1	292.4	287.0	288.0	288.4	284.7
New Brunswick, place of residence	338.4	310.8	315.3	285.8	293.8	315.5	290.4	258.4	257.8	271.9	257.4
Quebec, place of residence	328.2	328.3	317.6	307.5	306.2	301.0	292.0	287.1	282.0	284.8	269.7
Ontario, place of residence	287.5	278.4	271.3	269.3	259.9	258.9	253.7	248.4	245.9	244.1	236.9
Manitoba, place of residence	294.4	299.4	291.1	283.7	287.7	272.2	266.7	259.2	257.7	261.5	252.4
Saskatchewan, place of residence	289.3	280.9	268.7	269.9	266.8	266.8	254.3	248.8	239.6	248.8	243.8
Alberta, place of residence	270.5	265.0	267.1	253.1	253.6	245.2	248.3	231.4	224.8	233.0	229.9
British Columbia, place of residence	251.0	252.0	250.8	237.5	248.4	240.1	234.4	225.0	220.2	221.2	223.9
Yukon, place of residence	401.4	290.7	419.9	407.6	402.4	345.4	329.1	410.3	310.8	326.5	360.0
Northwest Territories, place of residence	411.4	298.5	386.2	249.5	203.9	332.1	224.4	361.7	219.7	326.2	262.3
Nunavut, place of residence	373.9	397.4	493.8	600.2	533.1	480.0	483.1	322.3	491.9	430.2	515.2

Source: Statistics Canada. *Table 102-0553 - Deaths and mortality rate (age standardization using 2011 population), by selected grouped causes and sex, Canada, provinces and territories, annual,* CANSIM (database). (accessed: March 31, 2017)

Cause of death (ICD-10) [6], [7], [8] = Malignant neoplasms [C00-C97]
Characteristics [14], [15], [16], [17], [18], [19], [21] = Age-standardized mortality rate per 100,000 population

Also see footnotes [1], [2], [5], [13], [22], [23], [24], [25], [26], [27]

AGE-STANDARDIZED RATES, ALL MALIGNANT NEOPLASMS, DEATHS (PER 100,000 POPULATION), FEMALES, CANADA, PROVINCES AND TERRITORIES

Geography, place of residence [3] [4]	2003	2004	2005	2006	2007	2008	2009	2010	2011	2012	2013
Canada, place of residence	200.2	198.6	194.1	191.3	190.6	188.7	184.7	183.3	180.3	180.1	177.3
Newfoundland and Labrador, place of residence	207.7	194.5	209.9	193.8	220.8	199.9	214.1	205.5	204.6	194.1	222.9
Prince Edward Island, place of residence	246.1	212.4	206.5	203.5	169.3	206.6	220.7	178.8	191.5	185.0	169.6
Nova Scotia, place of residence	231.0	218.5	208.7	205.5	212.6	203.0	205.2	206.5	213.2	203.8	198.6
New Brunswick, place of residence	204.7	188.9	195.7	196.3	194.6	185.0	203.7	187.8	177.3	174.2	187.4
Quebec, place of residence	207.4	208.9	205.3	204.3	206.9	206.9	201.4	198.6	197.6	198.2	192.8
Ontario, place of residence	198.6	195.7	194.7	186.3	184.4	183.3	177.5	177.5	174.5	173.0	168.9
Manitoba, place of residence	201.4	216.2	199.0	203.2	193.9	197.8	198.8	194.0	182.1	186.3	187.2
Saskatchewan, place of residence	190.0	186.9	190.2	191.3	185.8	177.4	176.2	190.2	186.3	177.3	179.3
Alberta, place of residence	196.1	193.0	179.3	183.8	179.7	180.1	173.7	167.2	163.8	165.4	166.3
British Columbia, place of residence	185.4	186.5	174.6	176.9	176.2	171.5	166.8	170.0	162.9	170.3	165.3
Yukon, place of residence	219.3	295.7	228.7	353.8	270.8	303.4	289.1	326.8	258.1	190.6	228.0
Northwest Territories, place of residence	416.4	188.0	210.6	227.7	192.1	281.3	210.5	278.7	262.7	204.3	194.9
Nunavut, place of residence	352.9	494.2	415.9	540.5	334.7	320.4	555.8	148.7	488.4	418.5	452.2

Source: Statistics Canada. *Table 102-0553 - Deaths and mortality rate (age standardization using 2011 population), by selected grouped causes and sex, Canada, provinces and territories, annual,* CANSIM (database). (accessed: March 31, 2017)

Cause of death (ICD-10) 6, 7, 8 = Malignant neoplasms [C00-C97]
Characteristics 14, 15, 16, 17, 18, 19, 21 = Age-standardized mortality rate per 100,000 population

Also see footnotes 1, 2, 5, 13, 22, 23, 24, 25, 26, 27

AGE-STANDARDIZED RATES, DISEASES OF THE HEART, DEATHS (PER 100,000 POPULATION), BOTH SEXES, CANADA, PROVINCES AND TERRITORIES

Geography, place of residence [3] [4]	2003	2004	2005	2006	2007	2008	2009	2010	2011	2012	2013
Canada, place of residence	196.6	187.6	179.9	167.8	164.1	159.8	150.1	143.0	135.6	136.4	134.8
Newfoundland and Labrador, place of residence	257.1	263.4	243.9	246.2	232.0	214.9	201.6	190.7	180.5	178.0	182.8
Prince Edward Island, place of residence	242.3	244.3	229.3	249.2	216.6	187.9	202.7	179.2	177.2	156.7	167.6
Nova Scotia, place of residence	216.0	200.8	205.3	184.9	178.8	166.2	160.3	154.9	147.3	144.8	156.0
New Brunswick, place of residence	221.5	223.4	189.0	171.7	170.4	165.7	158.6	154.4	150.3	148.2	148.2
Quebec, place of residence	184.5	174.7	163.0	150.3	152.6	145.9	138.5	136.1	124.8	126.0	120.2
Ontario, place of residence	201.4	188.3	184.6	169.4	162.2	156.5	148.2	138.4	131.7	131.5	130.7
Manitoba, place of residence	201.2	210.8	196.3	186.0	182.2	184.5	162.7	160.7	159.1	162.1	158.3
Saskatchewan, place of residence	203.2	200.5	194.9	196.4	185.0	185.7	172.5	172.0	162.8	167.0	164.4
Alberta, place of residence	211.0	206.8	197.5	185.2	182.1	183.2	178.8	167.5	163.5	165.6	166.2
British Columbia, place of residence	175.8	167.0	160.4	155.0	153.9	156.8	138.7	130.8	123.5	127.4	126.8
Yukon, place of residence	202.3	229.1	200.6	153.6	267.9	186.9	170.1	205.0	187.0	153.3	144.4
Northwest Territories, place of residence	330.2	203.7	108.8	222.0	227.8	187.7	211.4	183.4	171.0	160.9	182.0
Nunavut, place of residence	248.8	238.2	235.2	164.3	196.7	109.7	172.9	171.5	122.7	177.9	214.8

Source: Statistics Canada. *Table 102-0553 - Deaths and mortality rate (age standardization using 2011 population), by selected grouped causes and sex, Canada, provinces and territories, annual,* CANSIM (database). (accessed: March 31, 2017)

Cause of death (ICD-10) [6], [7], [8] = Diseases of heart [I00-I09, I11, I13, I20-I51]
Characteristics [14], [15], [16], [17], [18], [19], [21] = Age-standardized mortality rate per 100,000 population

Also see footnotes [1], [2], [5], [13], [22], [23], [24], [25], [26], [27]

AGE-STANDARDIZED RATES, DISEASES OF THE HEART, DEATHS (PER 100,000 POPULATION), MALES, CANADA, PROVINCES AND TERRITORIES

Geography, place of residence [3] [4]	2003	2004	2005	2006	2007	2008	2009	2010	2011	2012	2013
Canada, place of residence	260.0	245.2	233.9	219.0	213.8	209.4	195.9	186.1	175.8	179.6	176.2
Newfoundland and Labrador, place of residence	342.3	346.2	317.1	295.1	294.8	264.8	255.2	243.6	225.8	228.4	228.6
Prince Edward Island, place of residence	318.2	358.4	297.1	353.3	310.5	264.4	249.8	268.1	217.7	197.8	222.6
Nova Scotia, place of residence	292.0	265.8	272.7	239.8	233.7	225.0	216.1	215.0	201.3	197.0	224.2
New Brunswick, place of residence	294.1	286.4	249.7	229.3	227.1	214.0	207.5	205.5	197.7	202.2	190.5
Quebec, place of residence	244.9	233.5	215.8	200.2	197.3	190.9	179.9	172.6	159.4	164.3	153.7
Ontario, place of residence	264.6	244.6	236.0	219.9	211.3	206.9	194.5	181.3	171.3	174.9	171.4
Manitoba, place of residence	276.8	282.5	261.2	245.7	252.4	258.2	220.4	215.2	209.0	218.7	214.0
Saskatchewan, place of residence	277.4	269.5	264.7	264.5	236.5	248.9	231.5	227.7	215.9	219.1	221.2
Alberta, place of residence	274.4	262.7	259.2	244.8	232.6	233.1	231.5	216.2	210.8	215.2	218.0
British Columbia, place of residence	228.3	211.6	202.6	193.9	199.0	196.7	174.7	168.0	158.5	163.1	161.5
Yukon, place of residence	129.6	272.6	268.0	116.9	374.5	271.2	248.8	250.5	350.6	310.6	206.6
Northwest Territories, place of residence	309.0	249.6	136.5	222.9	263.4	297.8	315.4	181.2	228.0	244.9	253.5
Nunavut, place of residence	313.5	394.5	337.9	222.2	291.1	190.4	314.0	210.3	128.7	311.1	252.1

Source: Statistics Canada. *Table 102-0553 - Deaths and mortality rate (age standardization using 2011 population), by selected grouped causes and sex, Canada, provinces and territories, annual,* CANSIM (database). (accessed: March 31, 2017)

Cause of death (ICD-10) 6, 7, 8 = Diseases of heart [I00-I09, I11, I13, I20-I51]
Characteristics 14, 15, 16, 17, 18, 19, 21 = Age-standardized mortality rate per 100,000 population

Also see footnotes 1, 2, 5, 13, 22, 23, 24, 25, 26, 27

AGE-STANDARDIZED RATES, DISEASES OF THE HEART, DEATHS (PER 100,000 POPULATION), FEMALES, CANADA, PROVINCES AND TERRITORIES

Geography, place of residence [3] [4]	2003	2004	2005	2006	2007	2008	2009	2010	2011	2012	2013
Canada, place of residence	149.3	144.2	139.2	128.7	125.7	121.6	114.3	109.2	103.3	103.2	102.0
Newfoundland and Labrador, place of residence	192.5	198.9	185.7	203.0	184.6	173.8	157.0	146.3	140.5	139.7	141.8
Prince Edward Island, place of residence	183.6	173.3	173.0	174.1	142.6	131.8	157.4	115.4	143.8	124.1	128.4
Nova Scotia, place of residence	161.3	152.4	157.8	141.4	136.7	122.0	119.0	111.1	105.0	105.9	105.8
New Brunswick, place of residence	164.3	173.7	144.6	127.7	128.3	129.9	117.3	116.0	112.7	108.0	114.3
Quebec, place of residence	140.9	133.9	125.2	114.7	118.0	112.2	107.0	107.6	97.4	97.1	94.0
Ontario, place of residence	154.0	145.2	145.5	130.6	124.3	118.1	112.1	105.2	100.2	98.6	98.6
Manitoba, place of residence	147.2	156.4	144.5	142.4	128.6	127.2	116.5	117.5	119.9	117.1	112.2
Saskatchewan, place of residence	146.0	146.3	141.1	142.7	141.6	136.3	126.2	127.0	119.5	124.9	119.1
Alberta, place of residence	161.3	160.6	150.3	137.9	141.7	142.0	137.4	127.2	124.2	126.0	124.7
British Columbia, place of residence	134.7	132.3	127.4	122.8	118.4	123.3	109.0	100.4	93.8	98.3	97.4
Yukon, place of residence	252.8	198.8	141.4	172.8	170.2	121.5	117.0	161.3	70.3	27.6	82.6
Northwest Territories, place of residence	315.8	141.3	78.6	230.5	173.2	96.9	113.6	184.0	105.2	95.7	123.2
Nunavut, place of residence	142.3	14.0	129.3	98.7	57.3	15.8	63.6	103.5	143.0	56.2	157.2

Source: Statistics Canada. *Table 102-0553 - Deaths and mortality rate (age standardization using 2011 population), by selected grouped causes and sex, Canada, provinces and territories, annual,* CANSIM (database). (accessed: March 31, 2017)

Cause of death (ICD-10) 6, 7, 8 = Diseases of heart [I00-I09, I11, I13, I20-I51]
Characteristics 14, 15, 16, 17, 18, 19, 21 = Age-standardized mortality rate per 100,000 population

Also see footnotes 1, 2, 5, 13, 22, 23, 24, 25, 26, 27

AGE-STANDARDIZED RATES, CEREBROVASCULAR DISEASES, DEATHS (PER 100,000 POPULATION), BOTH SEXES, CANADA, PROVINCES AND TERRITORIES

Geography, place of residence [3, 4]	2003	2004	2005	2006	2007	2008	2009	2010	2011	2012	2013
Canada, place of residence	57.2	53.0	49.1	46.4	45.4	43.7	42.9	40.1	37.6	36.9	36.1
Newfoundland and Labrador, place of residence	72.1	71.6	74.7	68.9	63.8	68.4	64.1	59.0	52.0	49.0	54.6
Prince Edward Island, place of residence	69.7	75.0	53.6	40.8	46.5	48.3	52.8	45.9	51.5	40.3	38.7
Nova Scotia, place of residence	59.8	63.1	54.3	51.2	52.7	52.4	48.3	45.0	44.6	45.3	41.8
New Brunswick, place of residence	58.1	51.9	48.8	46.4	46.3	45.4	43.0	39.5	39.6	43.3	40.0
Quebec, place of residence	44.6	40.7	38.7	38.4	37.2	35.5	35.2	33.7	31.4	30.3	31.8
Ontario, place of residence	59.4	55.5	51.1	47.4	45.9	43.1	43.6	40.7	36.6	35.9	34.5
Manitoba, place of residence	61.0	57.1	52.3	51.3	49.9	48.1	50.9	48.7	43.8	45.8	44.6
Saskatchewan, place of residence	61.9	52.4	50.6	47.0	50.1	46.6	44.2	39.4	44.6	41.5	39.3
Alberta, place of residence	63.9	57.2	53.4	50.0	43.6	44.5	43.1	38.7	38.8	37.8	36.2
British Columbia, place of residence	63.3	58.3	53.7	50.6	52.7	51.3	47.8	44.8	42.8	42.7	41.3
Yukon, place of residence	95.4	66.1	61.1	74.0	54.4	91.4	59.5	65.2	79.6	41.8	34.0
Northwest Territories, place of residence	54.9	73.6	25.1	25.0	39.7	38.5	54.4	27.2	75.0	71.0	34.9
Nunavut, place of residence	118.8	80.9	87.4	35.8	26.9	93.9	4.4	29.9	85.8	35.0	35.2

Source: Statistics Canada. *Table 102-0553 - Deaths and mortality rate (age standardization using 2011 population), by selected grouped causes and sex, Canada, provinces and territories, annual,* CANSIM (database). (accessed: March 31, 2017)

Cause of death (ICD-10) 6, 7, 8 = Cerebrovascular diseases [I60-I69]
Characteristics 14, 15, 16, 17, 18, 19, 21 = Age-standardized mortality rate per 100,000 population

Also see footnotes 1, 2, 5, 13, 22, 23, 24, 25, 26, 27

AGE-STANDARDIZED RATES, CEREBROVASCULAR DISEASES, DEATHS (PER 100,000 POPULATION), MALES, CANADA, PROVINCES AND TERRITORIES

Geography, place of residence [3] [4]	2003	2004	2005	2006	2007	2008	2009	2010	2011	2012	2013
Canada, place of residence	62.6	56.6	52.5	50.0	48.2	46.0	45.6	42.2	39.7	40.0	38.2
Newfoundland and Labrador, place of residence	85.3	79.7	85.3	67.2	75.9	66.8	73.5	66.2	61.1	55.9	59.9
Prince Edward Island, place of residence	87.5	79.2	54.2	34.3	39.6	53.4	59.1	44.6	58.2	44.8	40.8
Nova Scotia, place of residence	66.6	61.0	57.9	52.7	58.1	51.8	50.9	45.9	49.6	49.2	43.2
New Brunswick, place of residence	53.5	53.6	52.8	45.7	46.5	47.0	46.1	35.6	40.0	46.3	43.1
Quebec, place of residence	50.1	44.5	42.0	42.3	39.9	35.6	38.3	35.3	31.9	34.5	32.7
Ontario, place of residence	65.5	59.0	53.4	50.7	49.1	46.2	44.9	43.6	39.1	37.9	37.1
Manitoba, place of residence	63.6	63.5	55.3	55.7	46.7	55.6	57.1	51.1	45.8	46.6	46.0
Saskatchewan, place of residence	67.9	49.3	62.3	52.4	52.3	52.0	48.0	39.3	50.9	49.7	41.0
Alberta, place of residence	69.9	64.8	58.1	52.0	47.2	47.5	45.3	40.2	40.4	39.7	36.4
British Columbia, place of residence	64.7	60.1	55.0	54.9	54.2	52.0	50.5	46.6	43.7	45.5	44.0
Yukon, place of residence	127.4	63.3	71.9	149.3	53.6	91.1	27.8	67.7	76.4	47.7	13.8
Northwest Territories, place of residence	63.0	45.8	67.9	30.7	32.4	42.4	70.5	37.8	64.9	82.2	54.7
Nunavut, place of residence	125.6	128.4	37.0	60.0	26.0	222.7	3.1	24.3	94.5	50.3	26.9

Source: Statistics Canada. *Table 102-0553 - Deaths and mortality rate (age standardization using 2011 population), by selected grouped causes and sex, Canada, provinces and territories, annual,* CANSIM (database). (accessed: March 31, 2017)

Cause of death (ICD-10) 6, 7, 8 = Cerebrovascular diseases [I60-I69]
Characteristics 14, 15, 16, 17, 18, 19, 21 = Age-standardized mortality rate per 100,000 population

Also see footnotes 1, 2, 5, 13, 22, 23, 24, 25, 26, 27

AGE-STANDARDIZED RATES, CEREBROVASCULAR DISEASES, DEATHS (PER 100,000 POPULATION), FEMALES, CANADA, PROVINCES AND TERRITORIES

Geography, place of residence [3] [4]	2003	2004	2005	2006	2007	2008	2009	2010	2011	2012	2013
Canada, place of residence	53.2	49.9	46.1	43.4	42.9	41.4	40.5	37.9	35.5	34.3	34.2
Newfoundland and Labrador, place of residence	61.8	65.9	66.5	67.7	55.2	67.2	55.6	51.3	44.9	43.6	49.9
Prince Edward Island, place of residence	63.1	70.2	50.0	43.0	50.2	43.7	45.8	46.6	47.7	39.8	38.0
Nova Scotia, place of residence	53.8	62.1	50.2	49.8	48.5	51.8	45.6	43.0	40.8	42.2	39.3
New Brunswick, place of residence	58.8	49.9	45.8	46.1	45.1	44.3	40.7	41.4	37.6	40.1	36.9
Quebec, place of residence	41.0	37.6	36.0	35.3	35.0	34.3	32.8	32.1	30.2	27.5	30.5
Ontario, place of residence	54.9	52.5	48.8	44.4	43.3	40.5	42.1	38.0	34.4	33.9	32.5
Manitoba, place of residence	58.3	51.6	49.1	47.8	50.6	42.3	45.7	45.6	41.1	44.9	42.9
Saskatchewan, place of residence	57.2	53.7	41.5	43.0	47.4	43.0	41.7	38.3	39.8	35.5	37.9
Alberta, place of residence	59.8	51.5	49.9	47.8	40.3	42.5	40.6	36.2	37.0	35.9	35.6
British Columbia, place of residence	61.2	56.1	51.9	47.2	50.4	49.9	45.0	42.8	41.6	39.8	38.6
Yukon, place of residence	80.7	67.4	43.1	37.7	47.2	68.5	84.9	58.1	87.9	35.6	52.9
Northwest Territories, place of residence	85.4	97.5	0.0	17.8	44.1	34.0	30.7	16.2	80.4	56.2	15.5
Nunavut, place of residence	118.9	5.6	199.3	0.0	25.4	10.1	6.0	36.4	78.4	16.8	42.0

Source: Statistics Canada. *Table 102-0553 - Deaths and mortality rate (age standardization using 2011 population), by selected grouped causes and sex, Canada, provinces and territories, annual,* CANSIM (database). (accessed: March 31, 2017)

Cause of death (ICD-10) [6], [7], [8] = Cerebrovascular diseases [I60-I69]
Characteristics [14], [15], [16], [17], [18], [19], [21] = Age-standardized mortality rate per 100,000 population

Also see footnotes [1], [2], [5], [13], [22], [23], [24], [25], [26], [27]

AGE-STANDARDIZED RATES, CHRONIC LOWER RESPIRATORY DISEASES, DEATHS (PER 100,000 POPULATION), BOTH SEXES, CANADA, PROVINCES AND TERRITORIES

Geography, place of residence [3] [4]	2003	2004	2005	2006	2007	2008	2009	2010	2011	2012	2013
Canada, place of residence	37.2	35.7	36.3	32.7	34.5	34.3	33.1	31.6	32.0	31.3	32.5
Newfoundland and Labrador, place of residence	46.5	41.0	41.4	38.9	40.9	49.9	44.6	44.7	42.0	47.6	41.4
Prince Edward Island, place of residence	36.8	32.4	25.5	27.7	36.7	29.8	33.9	36.9	38.0	44.7	37.6
Nova Scotia, place of residence	42.1	50.1	44.7	43.0	47.2	41.5	43.8	47.8	48.0	44.7	49.0
New Brunswick, place of residence	42.1	37.1	35.9	39.7	39.7	41.9	42.1	38.0	40.8	35.0	38.5
Quebec, place of residence	42.1	43.4	42.8	35.8	38.8	35.9	35.6	33.1	32.6	33.0	35.1
Ontario, place of residence	34.5	31.1	33.0	28.8	30.8	30.2	29.7	28.3	28.5	27.9	28.4
Manitoba, place of residence	36.8	33.3	36.0	32.5	30.7	35.3	32.6	32.6	33.0	32.5	33.1
Saskatchewan, place of residence	34.7	34.1	32.6	34.9	36.4	37.4	31.8	34.4	34.8	31.8	34.9
Alberta, place of residence	36.3	34.9	36.3	35.9	35.9	37.7	34.2	32.6	35.8	34.4	35.6
British Columbia, place of residence	34.1	32.8	33.0	31.4	32.0	34.8	32.3	30.3	30.7	28.6	30.4
Yukon, place of residence	22.4	45.9	74.2	50.5	54.0	93.9	76.5	65.4	69.4	54.1	37.5
Northwest Territories, place of residence	92.7	29.6	95.0	55.7	65.5	59.7	68.4	55.7	34.3	58.0	111.4
Nunavut, place of residence	220.3	105.7	131.1	266.6	199.3	305.8	148.0	259.1	318.5	140.1	171.4

Source: Statistics Canada. *Table 102-0553 - Deaths and mortality rate (age standardization using 2011 population), by selected grouped causes and sex, Canada, provinces and territories, annual,* CANSIM (database). (accessed: March 31, 2017)

Cause of death (ICD-10) [6], [7], [8] = Chronic lower respiratory diseases [J40-J47]
Characteristics [14], [15], [16], [17], [18], [19], [21] = Age-standardized mortality rate per 100,000 population

Also see footnotes [1], [2], [5], [13], [22], [23], [24], [25], [26], [27]

AGE-STANDARDIZED RATES, CHRONIC LOWER RESPIRATORY DISEASES, DEATHS (PER 100,000 POPULATION), MALES, CANADA, PROVINCES AND TERRITORIES

Geography, place of residence [3], [4]	2003	2004	2005	2006	2007	2008	2009	2010	2011	2012	2013
Canada, place of residence	53.3	49.7	50.3	44.5	46.7	46.5	42.9	40.9	39.9	40.3	40.8
Newfoundland and Labrador, place of residence	76.5	70.0	71.1	46.0	74.2	79.2	61.2	65.0	53.4	67.6	58.5
Prince Edward Island, place of residence	58.6	52.1	36.1	40.6	49.1	40.9	45.6	63.1	46.8	60.6	52.0
Nova Scotia, place of residence	62.5	73.0	63.6	59.1	61.0	60.7	59.6	59.0	57.8	60.3	69.6
New Brunswick, place of residence	62.4	56.3	52.5	53.9	59.3	57.1	59.9	56.8	56.4	46.5	50.4
Quebec, place of residence	66.8	66.3	64.3	52.8	55.7	49.7	47.9	45.1	41.2	42.8	46.6
Ontario, place of residence	47.1	41.7	44.5	38.1	40.8	40.5	37.9	35.6	35.2	35.8	35.2
Manitoba, place of residence	54.4	47.0	50.9	47.7	40.6	47.3	42.7	41.6	41.8	41.3	42.4
Saskatchewan, place of residence	47.6	52.3	45.0	47.5	51.8	50.4	39.9	46.0	45.3	42.7	44.6
Alberta, place of residence	51.4	45.8	49.4	49.2	46.9	51.6	45.1	42.4	44.9	42.5	42.0
British Columbia, place of residence	45.3	40.1	41.7	39.7	41.2	44.8	38.9	36.5	37.4	37.1	34.7
Yukon, place of residence	46.3	40.0	116.3	48.0	56.6	131.2	117.4	108.4	102.3	77.8	49.0
Northwest Territories, place of residence	140.6	43.5	110.6	99.1	86.5	52.2	137.5	26.7	45.7	102.0	99.2
Nunavut, place of residence	0.0	61.3	121.6	281.9	186.8	297.5	93.5	81.4	292.8	94.2	242.1

Source: Statistics Canada. *Table 102-0553 - Deaths and mortality rate (age standardization using 2011 population), by selected grouped causes and sex, Canada, provinces and territories, annual,* CANSIM (database). (accessed: March 31, 2017)

Cause of death (ICD-10) [6], [7], [8] = Chronic lower respiratory diseases [J40-J47]
Characteristics [14], [15], [16], [17], [18], [19], [21] = Age-standardized mortality rate per 100,000 population

Also see footnotes [1], [2], [5], [13], [22], [23], [24], [25], [26], [27]

AGE-STANDARDIZED RATES, CHRONIC LOWER RESPIRATORY DISEASES, DEATHS (PER 100,000 POPULATION), FEMALES, CANADA, PROVINCES AND TERRITORIES

Geography, place of residence 3, 4	2003	2004	2005	2006	2007	2008	2009	2010	2011	2012	2013
Canada, place of residence	28.4	27.7	28.3	26.0	27.5	27.2	27.3	26.2	27.2	25.9	27.3
Newfoundland and Labrador, place of residence	28.4	25.3	23.3	34.6	23.1	32.5	33.1	32.1	35.3	37.2	31.3
Prince Edward Island, place of residence	26.3	21.6	21.4	20.7	30.7	20.6	25.9	19.7	31.8	34.5	27.6
Nova Scotia, place of residence	31.1	37.4	34.1	35.1	39.6	31.3	34.4	41.5	42.4	35.4	35.5
New Brunswick, place of residence	31.2	26.2	27.4	32.1	29.0	32.9	31.8	27.6	31.8	28.3	31.7
Quebec, place of residence	29.9	31.7	32.5	27.3	30.3	28.7	29.0	26.9	28.0	27.9	28.9
Ontario, place of residence	27.6	25.2	26.1	23.4	25.1	24.0	24.8	23.9	24.4	23.2	24.0
Manitoba, place of residence	27.3	26.0	28.6	23.9	26.0	27.3	26.6	27.5	27.6	27.5	27.7
Saskatchewan, place of residence	27.7	22.6	24.4	27.2	27.2	29.5	27.7	26.8	28.3	25.0	29.1
Alberta, place of residence	27.9	28.4	27.8	27.7	29.0	30.0	27.6	26.1	30.0	29.9	32.0
British Columbia, place of residence	27.5	27.7	27.7	25.9	26.0	28.1	28.0	26.3	26.0	22.7	27.1
Yukon, place of residence	0.0	45.4	58.3	61.4	49.1	58.5	66.2	22.2	45.5	39.0	24.3
Northwest Territories, place of residence	68.2	16.4	81.6	12.7	47.6	73.2	12.7	85.8	22.9	29.6	111.2
Nunavut, place of residence	722.4	185.1	137.7	240.6	221.6	314.3	178.3	424.3	350.4	181.5	95.2

Source: Statistics Canada. *Table 102-0553 - Deaths and mortality rate (age standardization using 2011 population), by selected grouped causes and sex, Canada, provinces and territories, annual,* CANSIM (database). (accessed: March 31, 2017)

Cause of death (ICD-10) 6, 7, 8 = Chronic lower respiratory diseases [J40-J47]
Characteristics 14, 15, 16, 17, 18, 19, 21 = Age-standardized mortality rate per 100,000 population

Also see footnotes 1, 2, 5, 13, 22, 23, 24, 25, 26, 27

AGE-STANDARDIZED RATES, UNINTENTIONAL INJURIES, DEATHS (PER 100,000 POPULATION), BOTH SEXES, CANADA, PROVINCES AND TERRITORIES

Geography, place of residence [3, 4]	2003	2004	2005	2006	2007	2008	2009	2010	2011	2012	2013
Canada, place of residence	31.2	30.4	31.3	31.0	31.3	31.5	30.8	31.8	31.2	32.0	31.6
Newfoundland and Labrador, place of residence	27.0	27.2	29.1	28.3	21.4	31.3	29.3	31.2	29.6	27.8	30.1
Prince Edward Island, place of residence	34.4	53.7	23.8	42.9	35.1	42.8	43.6	33.5	39.1	29.3	37.8
Nova Scotia, place of residence	30.5	35.3	36.7	37.6	45.1	44.7	43.1	38.2	39.9	42.9	45.2
New Brunswick, place of residence	41.3	35.2	36.6	37.2	40.3	36.8	35.2	38.3	35.8	35.0	33.6
Quebec, place of residence	29.3	29.5	30.1	28.8	26.3	26.9	25.8	27.0	26.6	25.7	26.6
Ontario, place of residence	29.5	29.6	30.2	31.1	31.5	31.1	30.6	32.6	31.4	33.0	32.8
Manitoba, place of residence	34.1	38.8	37.0	39.7	39.7	41.0	42.1	40.1	41.7	42.0	39.5
Saskatchewan, place of residence	44.5	38.2	39.9	41.3	40.0	48.9	45.3	48.3	46.5	46.6	41.7
Alberta, place of residence	30.8	28.4	31.1	28.6	32.0	30.7	27.8	27.6	25.9	27.5	28.2
British Columbia, place of residence	34.0	28.9	31.3	27.6	30.1	30.2	31.1	31.5	33.1	33.7	31.2
Yukon, place of residence	78.8	105.2	94.1	98.4	70.1	64.4	111.7	67.6	44.1	39.0	42.2
Northwest Territories, place of residence	112.9	37.6	58.2	111.3	63.1	41.9	66.1	41.4	30.6	53.8	68.0
Nunavut, place of residence	56.6	66.9	69.7	39.6	38.9	76.1	124.5	46.0	63.7	74.0	54.5

Source: Statistics Canada. *Table 102-0553 - Deaths and mortality rate (age standardization using 2011 population), by selected grouped causes and sex, Canada, provinces and territories, annual,* CANSIM (database). (accessed: March 31, 2017)

Cause of death (ICD-10) [6], [7], [8] = Accidents (unintentional injuries) [V01-X59, Y85-Y86]
Characteristics [14], [15], [16], [17], [18], [19], [21] = Age-standardized mortality rate per 100,000 population

Also see footnotes [1], [2], [5], [13], [22], [23], [24], [25], [26], [27]

AGE-STANDARDIZED RATES, UNINTENTIONAL INJURIES, DEATHS (PER 100,000 POPULATION), MALES, CANADA, PROVINCES AND TERRITORIES

Geography, place of residence [3], [4]	2003	2004	2005	2006	2007	2008	2009	2010	2011	2012	2013
Canada, place of residence	42.0	40.6	42.7	41.3	42.1	42.3	41.1	42.2	41.7	42.0	41.4
Newfoundland and Labrador, place of residence	37.2	41.2	43.6	38.5	28.4	40.9	46.6	43.6	39.6	38.2	34.8
Prince Edward Island, place of residence	56.1	75.0	29.5	41.5	41.0	59.8	65.7	44.5	53.0	40.4	54.8
Nova Scotia, place of residence	41.6	47.0	49.7	50.8	61.5	58.0	57.8	51.6	55.1	53.4	58.6
New Brunswick, place of residence	57.8	49.8	49.9	48.4	57.7	49.5	47.5	50.3	51.6	49.3	44.0
Quebec, place of residence	39.1	39.1	40.9	39.1	36.0	36.9	33.8	34.8	37.2	33.5	35.3
Ontario, place of residence	38.3	37.6	40.5	40.8	40.5	40.4	40.6	43.1	39.7	42.6	42.5
Manitoba, place of residence	45.6	51.6	50.1	50.0	54.4	53.8	53.7	51.2	53.6	53.8	52.3
Saskatchewan, place of residence	63.9	53.9	53.9	56.9	55.0	64.1	62.4	64.5	62.9	63.2	55.4
Alberta, place of residence	43.5	40.7	43.2	39.0	46.2	44.9	38.9	39.7	37.2	39.6	39.7
British Columbia, place of residence	46.2	40.6	43.0	38.4	42.4	41.9	41.6	42.3	45.2	44.4	40.6
Yukon, place of residence	103.2	120.5	144.4	81.0	47.9	95.5	166.8	79.9	65.3	35.9	47.5
Northwest Territories, place of residence	154.5	45.2	78.9	151.3	61.8	70.2	63.9	48.1	39.6	50.1	101.1
Nunavut, place of residence	80.1	81.5	123.1	72.5	54.7	136.1	282.0	82.3	57.9	112.5	62.7

Source: Statistics Canada. *Table 102-0553 - Deaths and mortality rate (age standardization using 2011 population), by selected grouped causes and sex, Canada, provinces and territories, annual,* CANSIM (database). (accessed: March 31, 2017)

Cause of death (ICD-10) [6], [7], [8] = Accidents (unintentional injuries) [V01-X59, Y85-Y86]
Characteristics [14], [15], [16], [17], [18], [19], [21] = Age-standardized mortality rate per 100,000 population

Also see footnotes [1], [2], [5], [13], [22], [23], [24], [25], [26], [27]

AGE-STANDARDIZED RATES, UNINTENTIONAL INJURIES, DEATHS (PER 100,000 POPULATION), FEMALES, CANADA, PROVINCES AND TERRITORIES

Geography, place of residence [3, 4]	2003	2004	2005	2006	2007	2008	2009	2010	2011	2012	2013
Canada, place of residence	21.7	21.0	21.3	21.8	21.5	21.9	21.6	22.4	21.9	23.1	22.8
Newfoundland and Labrador, place of residence	16.7	14.9	17.4	19.2	14.3	21.7	16.4	19.5	19.7	16.3	23.5
Prince Edward Island, place of residence	16.4	35.3	18.7	41.8	27.2	25.7	25.9	23.7	27.7	19.2	22.5
Nova Scotia, place of residence	21.0	25.0	26.2	24.9	31.1	32.6	30.0	27.2	26.7	33.2	32.5
New Brunswick, place of residence	26.0	21.8	24.7	26.1	25.7	24.5	23.2	27.4	21.3	23.0	23.3
Quebec, place of residence	20.7	20.5	20.4	20.1	17.4	18.0	18.2	19.5	17.5	18.8	19.1
Ontario, place of residence	21.9	22.3	21.4	22.9	23.3	23.5	22.2	23.6	24.0	24.8	24.4
Manitoba, place of residence	24.9	27.4	26.2	30.6	27.3	28.6	31.9	30.1	30.5	31.8	28.8
Saskatchewan, place of residence	26.9	24.5	27.2	26.0	25.5	35.1	30.2	32.8	31.1	31.1	28.8
Alberta, place of residence	19.5	17.0	19.3	19.0	19.4	17.6	17.7	16.6	15.2	16.7	18.2
British Columbia, place of residence	22.4	18.0	20.7	17.2	19.2	19.3	20.9	21.7	22.2	24.0	22.1
Yukon, place of residence	51.7	89.9	40.2	108.1	85.9	33.8	70.5	50.5	19.6	42.4	37.3
Northwest Territories, place of residence	76.0	31.9	27.1	70.3	58.9	14.3	64.0	28.7	22.9	55.9	41.3
Nunavut, place of residence	29.0	62.9	0.0	5.1	21.5	15.3	52.7	4.7	60.1	29.8	41.0

Source: Statistics Canada. *Table 102-0553 - Deaths and mortality rate (age standardization using 2011 population), by selected grouped causes and sex, Canada, provinces and territories, annual,* CANSIM (database). (accessed: March 31, 2017)

Cause of death (ICD-10) 6, 7, 8 = Accidents (unintentional injuries) [V01-X59, Y85-Y86]
Characteristics 14, 15, 16, 17, 18, 19, 21 = Age-standardized mortality rate per 100,000 population

Also see footnotes 1, 2, 5, 13, 22, 23, 24, 25, 26, 27

AGE-STANDARDIZED RATES, DIABETES MELLITUS, DEATHS (PER 100,000 POPULATION), BOTH SEXES, CANADA, PROVINCES AND TERRITORIES

Geography, place of residence [3] [4]	2003	2004	2005	2006	2007	2008	2009	2010	2011	2012	2013
Canada, place of residence	29.1	27.8	27.2	24.2	23.9	23.6	21.1	20.5	20.7	19.7	19.2
Newfoundland and Labrador, place of residence	58.1	57.9	49.6	44.5	48.8	51.4	40.5	35.9	38.6	38.4	36.2
Prince Edward Island, place of residence	14.3	20.8	24.5	17.5	21.4	17.7	11.4	14.9	20.5	15.9	22.0
Nova Scotia, place of residence	31.8	28.6	28.4	28.4	24.6	26.2	21.5	24.9	22.4	23.2	21.4
New Brunswick, place of residence	36.9	37.9	36.5	26.3	27.4	24.9	23.4	21.5	23.7	24.3	23.9
Quebec, place of residence	25.7	24.2	22.6	21.4	19.9	19.7	17.7	17.0	17.0	15.1	15.2
Ontario, place of residence	32.0	29.6	29.5	25.7	25.6	25.9	22.9	22.2	21.7	20.4	19.1
Manitoba, place of residence	37.3	40.0	38.2	34.2	32.9	32.1	29.1	27.3	32.0	25.6	26.3
Saskatchewan, place of residence	32.4	31.9	29.7	29.8	29.4	26.8	29.1	24.5	25.1	27.2	30.0
Alberta, place of residence	20.8	19.2	19.9	16.9	17.9	16.8	14.7	13.4	16.6	15.6	15.4
British Columbia, place of residence	24.3	25.2	25.2	22.4	23.0	22.1	19.8	20.8	20.7	21.7	21.5
Yukon, place of residence	10.5	48.6	12.6	32.4	27.2	11.0	42.5	42.5	55.4	14.6	15.7
Northwest Territories, place of residence	16.0	33.5	20.5	30.3	12.2	13.2	6.5	15.6	8.8	12.0	4.4
Nunavut, place of residence	0.0	0.0	9.3	0.0	0.0	10.5	0.0	7.5	4.5	16.7	18.1

Source: Statistics Canada. *Table 102-0553 - Deaths and mortality rate (age standardization using 2011 population), by selected grouped causes and sex, Canada, provinces and territories, annual,* CANSIM (database). (accessed: March 31, 2017)

Cause of death (ICD-10) [6], [7], [8] = Diabetes mellitus [E10-E14]
Characteristics [14], [15], [16], [17], [18], [19], [21] = Age-standardized mortality rate per 100,000 population

Also see footnotes [1], [2], [5], [13], [22], [23], [24], [25], [26], [27]

AGE-STANDARDIZED RATES, DIABETES MELLITUS, DEATHS (PER 100,000 POPULATION), MALES, CANADA, PROVINCES AND TERRITORIES

Geography, place of residence [3] [4]	2003	2004	2005	2006	2007	2008	2009	2010	2011	2012	2013
Canada, place of residence	35.6	35.1	33.4	30.5	30.5	29.3	26.4	26.1	26.3	24.7	24.4
Newfoundland and Labrador, place of residence	55.8	67.6	50.4	47.3	53.3	46.4	49.3	38.3	47.7	47.7	43.7
Prince Edward Island, place of residence	18.4	25.2	38.7	20.2	27.3	23.2	18.8	21.2	25.2	19.7	23.9
Nova Scotia, place of residence	39.0	37.2	34.8	38.4	32.0	32.2	27.7	32.2	29.8	27.4	26.7
New Brunswick, place of residence	51.0	45.6	46.9	33.1	37.9	30.4	28.6	25.8	27.8	28.5	30.1
Quebec, place of residence	31.7	28.8	28.0	27.3	24.9	24.2	21.9	22.3	20.9	18.4	19.5
Ontario, place of residence	39.7	37.3	35.9	31.7	32.5	32.9	28.9	28.2	27.5	25.3	24.2
Manitoba, place of residence	41.8	53.4	40.0	43.3	45.6	40.4	33.3	32.8	42.4	30.3	32.1
Saskatchewan, place of residence	39.6	42.7	38.5	38.7	37.6	33.9	37.9	34.3	31.6	36.4	41.6
Alberta, place of residence	24.6	24.1	26.1	19.3	23.4	20.0	18.3	17.1	21.2	20.2	19.4
British Columbia, place of residence	30.4	33.4	31.8	29.8	29.1	28.2	24.8	26.5	26.7	28.5	27.4
Yukon, place of residence	0.0	32.0	22.5	85.9	32.6	0.0	26.2	70.9	116.6	14.9	4.9
Northwest Territories, place of residence	0.0	39.2	10.6	57.6	23.3	25.3	5.0	12.9	0.0	6.3	4.2
Nunavut, place of residence	0.0	0.0	17.8	0.0	0.0	0.0	0.0	14.1	0.0	4.1	41.7

Source: Statistics Canada. *Table 102-0553 - Deaths and mortality rate (age standardization using 2011 population), by selected grouped causes and sex, Canada, provinces and territories, annual,* CANSIM (database). (accessed: March 31, 2017)

Cause of death (ICD-10) 6, 7, 8 = Diabetes mellitus [E10-E14]
Characteristics 14, 15, 16, 17, 18, 19, 21 = Age-standardized mortality rate per 100,000 population

Also see footnotes 1, 2, 5, 13, 22, 23, 24, 25, 26, 27

AGE-STANDARDIZED RATES, DIABETES MELLITUS, DEATHS (PER 100,000 POPULATION), FEMALES, CANADA, PROVINCES AND TERRITORIES

Geography, place of residence [3] [4]	2003	2004	2005	2006	2007	2008	2009	2010	2011	2012	2013
Canada, place of residence	24.2	22.6	22.4	19.4	18.9	19.2	17.0	16.1	16.4	15.7	15.0
Newfoundland and Labrador, place of residence	58.3	50.4	47.0	41.1	46.0	53.3	36.7	33.1	33.5	31.2	30.4
Prince Edward Island, place of residence	10.7	19.2	14.0	15.8	16.7	12.1	5.8	8.9	17.8	12.9	19.7
Nova Scotia, place of residence	26.4	22.8	23.7	20.8	18.4	21.8	17.1	19.8	17.6	19.6	17.3
New Brunswick, place of residence	27.3	32.6	30.1	21.5	19.3	21.6	19.0	18.6	20.3	20.9	20.4
Quebec, place of residence	21.4	20.5	18.6	17.1	16.0	16.1	14.7	13.4	13.7	12.3	11.8
Ontario, place of residence	26.2	24.1	24.4	20.9	20.4	20.5	18.1	17.3	17.1	16.4	15.0
Manitoba, place of residence	33.9	30.9	36.3	27.3	24.2	25.4	25.3	22.8	24.1	21.7	21.2
Saskatchewan, place of residence	26.0	23.7	23.1	23.3	23.7	20.9	22.7	16.9	19.6	20.2	21.2
Alberta, place of residence	18.0	15.8	15.6	14.8	13.8	14.2	11.9	10.3	13.0	12.2	12.5
British Columbia, place of residence	19.3	19.4	20.2	16.5	18.2	17.2	15.5	16.0	15.8	16.3	16.4
Yukon, place of residence	23.9	45.2	0.0	8.8	17.8	22.4	50.6	22.4	19.7	12.1	21.3
Northwest Territories, place of residence	30.9	25.4	21.7	0.0	0.0	0.0	9.2	20.4	14.8	17.0	4.7
Nunavut, place of residence	0.0	0.0	0.0	0.0	0.0	21.5	0.0	0.0	10.0	32.6	0.0

Source: Statistics Canada. *Table 102-0553 - Deaths and mortality rate (age standardization using 2011 population), by selected grouped causes and sex, Canada, provinces and territories, annual,* CANSIM (database). (accessed: March 31, 2017)

Cause of death (ICD-10) 6, 7, 8 = Diabetes mellitus [E10-E14]
Characteristics 14, 15, 16, 17, 18, 19, 21 = Age-standardized mortality rate per 100,000 population

Also see footnotes 1, 2, 5, 13, 22, 23, 24, 25, 26, 27

AGE-STANDARDIZED RATES, ALZHEIMER'S DISEASE, DEATHS (PER 100,000 POPULATION), BOTH SEXES, CANADA, PROVINCES AND TERRITORIES

Geography, place of residence [3], [4]	2003	2004	2005	2006	2007	2008	2009	2010	2011	2012	2013
Canada, place of residence	21.1	20.5	20.4	19.3	19.3	20.8	19.1	18.7	17.7	17.5	17.0
Newfoundland and Labrador, place of residence	30.0	31.9	23.1	28.6	26.0	25.9	19.4	22.9	18.5	15.6	17.1
Prince Edward Island, place of residence	21.1	21.1	11.7	19.2	17.4	20.6	20.7	18.6	16.6	22.4	17.2
Nova Scotia, place of residence	23.0	23.2	25.4	20.9	25.7	27.3	25.8	28.3	25.3	25.9	23.7
New Brunswick, place of residence	23.3	27.7	20.1	21.6	24.9	20.9	19.5	19.2	19.0	19.4	20.9
Quebec, place of residence	28.7	27.3	29.2	26.8	27.5	27.9	26.6	26.7	25.8	25.7	25.3
Ontario, place of residence	20.1	19.3	19.7	17.8	17.6	19.4	17.5	17.2	15.6	15.6	14.6
Manitoba, place of residence	12.8	14.4	14.5	13.9	12.8	12.7	11.6	11.5	11.8	9.4	9.9
Saskatchewan, place of residence	19.6	18.5	18.5	18.3	17.4	19.2	14.5	12.0	13.8	10.8	10.4
Alberta, place of residence	16.8	16.1	15.0	15.8	13.9	17.5	15.0	13.9	12.7	11.9	10.8
British Columbia, place of residence	15.1	14.5	12.9	13.2	13.1	15.6	15.2	13.7	13.8	14.0	13.9
Yukon, place of residence	13.4	15.7	33.0	32.5	15.8	30.5	22.7	17.8	29.9	17.0	19.0
Northwest Territories, place of residence	14.6	11.3	0.0	13.5	10.4	30.3	0.0	0.0	9.1	6.3	17.0
Nunavut, place of residence	0.0	0.0	0.0	0.0	0.0	39.4	0.0	0.0	24.6	0.0	0.0

Source: Statistics Canada. *Table 102-0553 - Deaths and mortality rate (age standardization using 2011 population), by selected grouped causes and sex, Canada, provinces and territories, annual,* CANSIM (database). (accessed: March 31, 2017)

Cause of death (ICD-10) [6], [7], [8] = Alzheimer's disease [G30]
Characteristics [14], [15], [16], [17], [18], [19], [21] = Age-standardized mortality rate per 100,000 population

Also see footnotes [1], [2], [5], [13], [22], [23], [24], [25], [26], [27]

AGE-STANDARDIZED RATES, ALZHEIMER'S DISEASE, DEATHS (PER 100,000 POPULATION), MALES, CANADA, PROVINCES AND TERRITORIES

Geography, place of residence [3], [4]	2003	2004	2005	2006	2007	2008	2009	2010	2011	2012	2013
Canada, place of residence	17.8	16.7	16.9	16.0	16.0	17.4	16.2	15.7	15.3	14.6	14.5
Newfoundland and Labrador, place of residence	27.0	25.3	13.9	19.6	20.3	23.0	13.3	19.2	19.0	12.0	15.8
Prince Edward Island, place of residence	17.5	9.4	3.2	9.9	8.5	16.0	17.6	9.2	12.6	10.6	15.4
Nova Scotia, place of residence	20.6	19.7	22.5	17.3	23.7	22.3	20.8	26.1	22.7	19.4	20.9
New Brunswick, place of residence	23.2	22.6	14.0	16.8	19.8	19.0	17.7	16.9	20.5	15.0	15.3
Quebec, place of residence	22.7	21.1	23.9	21.8	21.7	22.9	22.5	20.8	21.1	20.0	21.6
Ontario, place of residence	16.7	16.5	16.7	15.2	15.7	16.2	15.3	14.7	13.2	13.9	12.4
Manitoba, place of residence	11.0	12.9	11.4	11.2	10.3	11.6	9.8	8.7	11.9	9.1	8.1
Saskatchewan, place of residence	19.7	17.0	16.0	13.9	16.4	18.8	13.5	11.3	13.5	11.3	10.7
Alberta, place of residence	16.0	11.3	12.9	15.6	11.1	15.3	13.7	12.8	10.4	10.7	9.4
British Columbia, place of residence	13.4	12.7	12.1	11.3	10.4	13.0	12.3	12.7	13.5	12.2	12.5
Yukon, place of residence	36.5	51.8	54.0	92.3	11.8	35.0	50.4	19.4	0.0	19.7	9.8
Northwest Territories, place of residence	0.0	0.0	0.0	23.0	0.0	31.5	0.0	0.0	18.5	13.1	23.9
Nunavut, place of residence	0.0	0.0	0.0	0.0	0.0	0.0	0.0	0.0	0.0	0.0	0.0

Source: Statistics Canada. *Table 102-0553 - Deaths and mortality rate (age standardization using 2011 population), by selected grouped causes and sex, Canada, provinces and territories, annual,* CANSIM (database). (accessed: March 31, 2017)

Cause of death (ICD-10) [6], [7], [8] = Alzheimer's disease [G30]
Characteristics [14], [15], [16], [17], [18], [19], [21] = Age-standardized mortality rate per 100,000 population

Also see footnotes [1], [2], [5], [13], [22], [23], [24], [25], [26], [27]

AGE-STANDARDIZED RATES, ALZHEIMER'S DISEASE, DEATHS (PER 100,000 POPULATION), FEMALES, CANADA, PROVINCES AND TERRITORIES

Geography, place of residence [3], [4]	2003	2004	2005	2006	2007	2008	2009	2010	2011	2012	2013
Canada, place of residence	22.5	22.2	22.0	20.8	20.9	22.4	20.4	20.2	19.0	18.9	18.2
Newfoundland and Labrador, place of residence	32.6	35.5	27.8	32.9	29.5	28.0	22.2	24.2	18.6	17.5	17.4
Prince Edward Island, place of residence	22.9	25.9	15.0	22.6	21.5	23.3	23.5	23.4	17.9	28.3	16.1
Nova Scotia, place of residence	24.7	24.9	27.0	22.7	26.6	29.2	28.0	28.9	26.7	28.9	24.6
New Brunswick, place of residence	23.6	30.7	22.9	24.2	27.3	21.7	19.7	20.4	18.4	21.3	23.7
Quebec, place of residence	31.1	29.6	31.2	28.7	30.2	30.1	28.5	29.3	28.2	28.1	27.1
Ontario, place of residence	21.5	20.5	20.9	19.0	18.4	20.8	18.4	18.5	16.7	16.3	15.7
Manitoba, place of residence	13.9	15.0	16.1	15.4	13.8	13.5	12.7	13.2	11.5	9.7	10.7
Saskatchewan, place of residence	19.3	19.4	19.7	20.6	18.0	18.9	15.1	12.1	14.0	10.4	10.3
Alberta, place of residence	17.2	18.4	16.1	15.9	15.3	18.6	15.5	14.4	14.0	12.6	11.9
British Columbia, place of residence	15.7	15.4	13.3	13.9	14.5	17.1	16.7	14.3	13.8	14.9	14.6
Yukon, place of residence	0.0	0.0	39.3	13.3	15.7	35.1	0.0	16.5	46.9	15.0	25.1
Northwest Territories, place of residence	19.1	22.7	0.0	0.0	18.3	32.6	0.0	0.0	0.0	0.0	11.9
Nunavut, place of residence	0.0	0.0	0.0	0.0	0.0	57.3	0.0	0.0	40.0	0.0	0.0

Source: Statistics Canada. *Table 102-0553 - Deaths and mortality rate (age standardization using 2011 population), by selected grouped causes and sex, Canada, provinces and territories, annual,* CANSIM (database). (accessed: March 31, 2017)

Cause of death (ICD-10) [6], [7], [8] = Alzheimer's disease [G30]
Characteristics [14], [15], [16], [17], [18], [19], [21] = Age-standardized mortality rate per 100,000 population

Also see footnotes [1], [2], [5], [13], [22], [23], [24], [25], [26], [27]

AGE-STANDARDIZED RATES, INFLUENZA AND PNEUMONIA, DEATHS (PER 100,000 POPULATION), BOTH SEXES, CANADA, PROVINCES AND TERRITORIES

Geography, place of residence [3] [4]	2003	2004	2005	2006	2007	2008	2009	2010	2011	2012	2013
Canada, place of residence	18.9	21.2	20.6	17.4	17.8	17.0	17.7	14.9	16.2	15.9	17.5
Newfoundland and Labrador, place of residence	20.0	19.9	20.9	16.2	16.0	16.5	15.9	11.8	16.5	14.0	21.5
Prince Edward Island, place of residence	38.8	48.2	28.4	40.0	40.4	40.0	31.8	22.1	40.0	21.2	24.0
Nova Scotia, place of residence	23.4	22.0	22.6	21.4	21.9	18.7	17.4	15.5	18.9	15.6	15.8
New Brunswick, place of residence	19.1	18.0	21.5	16.4	16.4	15.2	13.7	12.4	18.3	12.3	14.2
Quebec, place of residence	12.3	17.3	18.6	13.3	14.9	15.7	18.1	15.4	17.4	18.5	21.9
Ontario, place of residence	20.4	19.3	21.1	16.5	17.6	15.9	17.1	14.3	15.4	14.8	15.9
Manitoba, place of residence	21.5	19.1	22.7	20.4	18.3	18.2	16.8	15.4	15.9	17.3	17.0
Saskatchewan, place of residence	24.0	24.8	23.2	22.7	20.0	20.5	20.3	18.0	18.8	16.8	21.3
Alberta, place of residence	17.0	18.9	18.4	19.7	18.5	18.2	16.7	12.6	13.7	15.0	15.1
British Columbia, place of residence	22.4	32.6	21.9	21.3	20.6	19.3	19.2	16.3	15.1	14.6	15.3
Yukon, place of residence	3.2	26.4	12.4	25.5	4.8	17.4	10.9	29.9	8.5	26.7	31.0
Northwest Territories, place of residence	68.6	31.3	46.1	80.4	39.8	62.8	26.0	8.8	19.6	13.3	27.9
Nunavut, place of residence	1.5	94.5	16.8	8.6	30.3	4.6	85.6	0.0	8.8	0.0	75.9

Source: Statistics Canada. *Table 102-0553 - Deaths and mortality rate (age standardization using 2011 population), by selected grouped causes and sex, Canada, provinces and territories, annual,* CANSIM (database). (accessed: March 31, 2017)

Cause of death (ICD-10) 6, 7, 8 = Influenza and pneumonia [J09-J18]
Characteristics 14, 15, 16, 17, 18, 19, 21 = Age-standardized mortality rate per 100,000 population

Also see footnotes 1, 2, 5, 13, 22, 23, 24, 25, 26, 27

AGE-STANDARDIZED RATES, INFLUENZA AND PNEUMONIA, DEATHS (PER 100,000 POPULATION), MALES, CANADA, PROVINCES AND TERRITORIES

Geography, place of residence [3] [4]	2003	2004	2005	2006	2007	2008	2009	2010	2011	2012	2013
Canada, place of residence	23.7	26.9	24.7	21.7	22.1	21.4	21.8	18.5	19.7	19.6	21.7
Newfoundland and Labrador, place of residence	23.5	30.8	29.8	26.4	22.7	20.1	15.9	13.1	18.6	18.2	29.3
Prince Edward Island, place of residence	46.4	46.3	37.0	45.6	55.1	45.5	23.8	21.1	42.9	18.0	34.9
Nova Scotia, place of residence	27.0	29.2	27.1	22.4	26.8	24.5	22.8	19.8	21.9	20.6	19.1
New Brunswick, place of residence	26.9	20.4	29.6	16.5	21.8	18.8	16.8	18.4	26.1	13.0	18.4
Quebec, place of residence	16.3	22.3	23.1	17.1	18.7	20.8	22.2	19.5	20.9	22.5	26.7
Ontario, place of residence	25.4	24.7	24.1	20.2	21.3	19.2	22.1	17.6	18.7	18.6	20.1
Manitoba, place of residence	28.6	24.9	28.7	25.4	22.5	22.7	22.1	20.7	18.6	22.7	22.6
Saskatchewan, place of residence	25.7	32.9	30.5	31.0	25.6	28.1	23.9	20.7	23.8	18.1	24.5
Alberta, place of residence	22.1	23.0	22.5	26.7	22.3	23.0	19.9	15.8	16.8	19.0	19.0
British Columbia, place of residence	26.9	38.5	25.1	24.4	24.6	23.6	22.1	19.4	19.4	18.1	18.6
Yukon, place of residence	5.9	6.3	0.0	92.3	8.3	19.7	11.3	76.3	18.1	39.2	0.0
Northwest Territories, place of residence	115.9	27.0	71.3	101.9	87.0	69.5	29.0	17.9	30.3	21.9	49.5
Nunavut, place of residence	0.0	111.5	27.1	0.0	0.0	0.0	89.8	0.0	18.0	0.0	48.6

Source: Statistics Canada. *Table 102-0553 - Deaths and mortality rate (age standardization using 2011 population), by selected grouped causes and sex, Canada, provinces and territories, annual,* CANSIM (database). (accessed: March 31, 2017)

Cause of death (ICD-10) [6], [7], [8] = Influenza and pneumonia [J09-J18]
Characteristics [14], [15], [16], [17], [18], [19], [21] = Age-standardized mortality rate per 100,000 population

Also see footnotes [1], [2], [5], [13], [22], [23], [24], [25], [26], [27]

AGE-STANDARDIZED RATES, INFLUENZA AND PNEUMONIA, DEATHS (PER 100,000 POPULATION), FEMALES, CANADA, PROVINCES AND TERRITORIES

Geography, place of residence [3, 4]	2003	2004	2005	2006	2007	2008	2009	2010	2011	2012	2013
Canada, place of residence	16.3	18.0	18.2	14.9	15.3	14.5	15.2	12.7	13.9	13.6	15.1
Newfoundland and Labrador, place of residence	17.6	14.5	17.0	11.1	12.6	14.1	15.4	10.7	14.4	11.7	17.7
Prince Edward Island, place of residence	36.9	52.9	23.8	36.7	32.1	37.7	36.6	22.7	35.9	23.0	16.0
Nova Scotia, place of residence	20.5	18.3	19.7	20.6	19.5	16.1	14.4	13.1	17.7	12.7	14.4
New Brunswick, place of residence	14.4	16.6	16.6	16.4	13.1	12.4	11.7	8.9	14.1	11.4	11.7
Quebec, place of residence	10.5	14.5	16.2	11.2	12.5	12.9	15.7	13.1	15.5	16.0	19.3
Ontario, place of residence	17.9	16.4	19.2	14.2	15.4	13.7	14.0	12.2	13.2	12.5	13.4
Manitoba, place of residence	17.1	15.6	19.8	17.0	16.6	15.6	13.5	12.1	14.1	13.6	13.3
Saskatchewan, place of residence	22.6	19.7	18.1	17.0	17.0	16.1	17.4	16.1	15.1	16.2	19.6
Alberta, place of residence	14.3	16.3	16.2	15.7	16.0	15.8	14.5	10.7	11.8	12.5	12.8
British Columbia, place of residence	19.8	28.9	19.7	19.3	17.8	16.7	17.3	14.3	12.2	12.5	13.2
Yukon, place of residence	0.0	37.1	24.7	0.0	0.0	15.2	11.5	4.8	0.0	19.1	55.1
Northwest Territories, place of residence	46.5	32.3	21.0	47.8	3.4	52.3	24.4	0.0	11.5	4.9	15.3
Nunavut, place of residence	3.3	107.5	0.0	18.2	72.3	9.9	64.3	0.0	0.0	0.0	124.3

Source: Statistics Canada. *Table 102-0553 - Deaths and mortality rate (age standardization using 2011 population), by selected grouped causes and sex, Canada, provinces and territories, annual,* CANSIM (database). (accessed: March 31, 2017)

Cause of death (ICD-10) 6, 7, 8 = Influenza and pneumonia [J09-J18]
Characteristics 14, 15, 16, 17, 18, 19, 21 = Age-standardized mortality rate per 100,000 population

Also see footnotes 1, 2, 5, 13, 22, 23, 24, 25, 26, 27

AGE-STANDARDIZED RATES, INTENTIONAL SELF-HARM, DEATHS (PER 100,000 POPULATION), BOTH SEXES, CANADA, PROVINCES AND TERRITORIES

Geography, place of residence [3], [4]	2003	2004	2005	2006	2007	2008	2009	2010	2011	2012	2013
Canada, place of residence	12.1	11.4	11.6	10.8	11.0	11.1	11.5	11.6	11.3	11.3	11.5
Newfoundland and Labrador, place of residence	8.9	10.0	10.4	10.5	10.5	8.4	9.1	12.5	10.7	8.3	10.7
Prince Edward Island, place of residence	10.1	6.0	9.5	5.8	10.0	8.9	11.2	9.0	8.6	7.3	10.8
Nova Scotia, place of residence	10.6	9.4	9.2	11.4	9.4	10.1	13.8	10.4	11.4	12.2	12.3
New Brunswick, place of residence	12.1	11.8	13.0	12.1	10.6	14.0	11.1	14.0	13.7	15.1	10.9
Quebec, place of residence	16.7	15.1	16.0	14.8	14.0	14.7	13.7	14.1	14.0	13.3	13.9
Ontario, place of residence	8.8	8.4	9.0	8.5	8.6	8.0	9.2	9.1	9.0	9.2	9.3
Manitoba, place of residence	14.6	11.7	14.2	12.1	10.7	13.3	14.8	12.0	11.9	13.7	12.8
Saskatchewan, place of residence	11.7	11.1	12.0	11.1	12.9	13.0	15.6	12.8	13.3	12.0	12.6
Alberta, place of residence	14.3	14.4	12.8	12.0	13.5	13.6	13.4	14.3	13.0	13.2	13.6
British Columbia, place of residence	10.9	11.2	9.6	8.8	10.1	10.4	10.8	11.1	10.6	10.5	10.5
Yukon, place of residence	20.6	24.0	12.9	8.9	5.8	7.3	5.7	10.1	14.6	18.7	17.7
Northwest Territories, place of residence	22.1	22.0	9.0	11.1	17.5	20.2	13.4	15.5	11.7	17.8	18.7
Nunavut, place of residence	89.0	61.9	45.8	49.7	51.5	50.5	53.4	58.8	58.9	58.2	108.5

Source: Statistics Canada. *Table 102-0553 - Deaths and mortality rate (age standardization using 2011 population), by selected grouped causes and sex, Canada, provinces and territories, annual,* CANSIM (database). (accessed: March 31, 2017)

Cause of death (ICD-10) [6], [7], [8] = Intentional self-harm (suicide) [X60-X84, Y87.0]
Characteristics [14], [15], [16], [17], [18], [19], [21] = Age-standardized mortality rate per 100,000 population

Also see footnotes [1], [2], [5], [13], [22], [23], [24], [25], [26], [27]

AGE-STANDARDIZED RATES, INTENTIONAL SELF-HARM, DEATHS (PER 100,000 POPULATION), MALES, CANADA, PROVINCES AND TERRITORIES

Geography, place of residence [3] [4]	2003	2004	2005	2006	2007	2008	2009	2010	2011	2012	2013
Canada, place of residence	19.0	17.6	18.1	17.0	16.9	17.0	18.1	17.8	17.1	17.4	17.6
Newfoundland and Labrador, place of residence	14.2	16.2	17.0	18.0	20.4	14.9	17.1	21.4	16.8	13.0	15.0
Prince Edward Island, place of residence	17.6	7.7	17.8	10.4	18.9	15.6	22.2	14.3	13.4	9.2	20.7
Nova Scotia, place of residence	17.1	15.8	16.5	19.2	14.7	16.9	21.6	18.1	18.3	17.7	19.0
New Brunswick, place of residence	20.2	19.3	20.9	21.1	16.3	22.8	19.0	23.0	21.4	24.7	18.4
Quebec, place of residence	26.4	22.9	25.4	23.2	22.2	22.5	21.4	21.8	21.7	20.7	21.7
Ontario, place of residence	13.9	12.9	13.8	13.2	13.5	12.3	14.2	13.4	13.4	14.3	14.5
Manitoba, place of residence	23.1	16.9	23.0	18.6	15.7	17.6	21.3	16.9	15.0	18.5	17.7
Saskatchewan, place of residence	19.3	18.2	18.4	17.3	18.8	18.1	24.7	19.7	20.3	18.7	17.8
Alberta, place of residence	21.5	22.2	18.9	18.4	19.0	20.8	20.9	21.4	19.3	19.8	20.2
British Columbia, place of residence	16.8	17.4	14.6	14.2	14.9	15.8	17.2	18.0	16.1	16.1	15.6
Yukon, place of residence	40.2	47.1	21.0	12.2	11.7	13.3	11.3	5.0	26.9	31.5	30.4
Northwest Territories, place of residence	42.8	34.4	17.3	17.4	26.2	31.5	18.8	25.6	22.7	30.6	19.5
Nunavut, place of residence	128.3	99.5	74.1	81.0	77.9	79.3	89.0	84.6	93.7	88.2	160.8

Source: Statistics Canada. Table 102-0553 - Deaths and mortality rate (age standardization using 2011 population), by selected grouped causes and sex, Canada, provinces and territories, annual, CANSIM (database). (accessed: March 31, 2017)

Cause of death (ICD-10) 6, 7, 8 = Intentional self-harm (suicide) [X60-X84, Y87.0]
Characteristics 14, 15, 16, 17, 18, 19, 21 = Age-standardized mortality rate per 100,000 population

Also see footnotes 1, 2, 5, 13, 22, 23, 24, 25, 26, 27

AGE-STANDARDIZED RATES, INTENTIONAL SELF-HARM, DEATHS (PER 100,000 POPULATION), FEMALES, CANADA, PROVINCES AND TERRITORIES

Geography, place of residence [3] [4]	2003	2004	2005	2006	2007	2008	2009	2010	2011	2012	2013
Canada, place of residence	5.5	5.5	5.4	5.0	5.3	5.5	5.3	5.7	5.7	5.5	5.7
Newfoundland and Labrador, place of residence	3.8	4.2	4.1	3.0	1.2	2.1	1.5	3.8	4.7	3.7	6.4
Prince Edward Island, place of residence	2.9	4.4	1.5	1.3	1.4	2.8	1.4	4.0	4.0	5.5	1.3
Nova Scotia, place of residence	4.2	3.4	2.2	3.9	4.7	3.7	6.6	3.0	5.2	7.0	5.8
New Brunswick, place of residence	4.2	4.6	5.4	4.0	5.0	5.6	3.5	5.5	6.5	5.7	3.7
Quebec, place of residence	7.3	7.7	7.1	6.8	6.0	7.2	6.2	6.7	6.4	6.1	6.3
Ontario, place of residence	4.3	4.2	4.5	4.2	4.2	4.0	4.5	5.0	4.7	4.4	4.5
Manitoba, place of residence	6.2	6.7	5.5	5.5	5.6	9.3	8.9	7.4	8.7	9.2	8.0
Saskatchewan, place of residence	4.2	4.2	5.7	4.9	7.5	8.2	6.8	5.9	6.3	5.2	7.5
Alberta, place of residence	7.3	6.7	6.7	6.1	8.0	6.5	5.7	7.2	6.7	6.5	7.2
British Columbia, place of residence	5.2	5.1	4.8	3.7	5.5	5.3	4.7	4.4	5.4	5.2	5.6
Yukon, place of residence	0.0	0.0	5.1	4.9	0.0	0.0	0.0	15.9	0.0	5.2	5.2
Northwest Territories, place of residence	0.0	9.0	0.0	3.8	8.5	8.3	7.2	3.6	0.0	3.7	16.8
Nunavut, place of residence	47.0	22.2	16.5	17.2	23.3	19.8	15.0	31.1	20.7	25.3	52.0

Source: Statistics Canada. *Table 102-0553 - Deaths and mortality rate (age standardization using 2011 population), by selected grouped causes and sex, Canada, provinces and territories, annual,* CANSIM (database). (accessed: March 31, 2017)

Cause of death (ICD-10) [6], [7], [8] = Intentional self-harm (suicide) [X60-X84, Y87.0]
Characteristics [14], [15], [16], [17], [18], [19], [21] = Age-standardized mortality rate per 100,000 population

Also see footnotes [1], [2], [5], [13], [22], [23], [24], [25], [26], [27]

AGE-STANDARDIZED RATES, NEPHRITIS, NEPHROTIC SYNDROME AND NEPHROSIS, DEATHS (PER 100,000 POPULATION), BOTH SEXES, CANADA, PROVINCES AND TERRITORIES

Geography, place of residence [3] [4]	2003	2004	2005	2006	2007	2008	2009	2010	2011	2012	2013
Canada, place of residence	13.1	12.8	12.7	12.4	12.4	12.1	11.0	11.3	9.3	9.3	8.0
Newfoundland and Labrador, place of residence	21.1	21.2	23.5	23.8	21.5	18.8	20.1	24.2	17.4	20.2	16.4
Prince Edward Island, place of residence	14.5	14.9	21.3	18.9	14.3	18.7	15.3	14.5	14.1	17.7	10.1
Nova Scotia, place of residence	13.6	15.5	16.8	12.7	12.9	13.1	13.4	11.5	9.5	10.2	8.4
New Brunswick, place of residence	17.0	16.2	15.4	15.3	15.8	15.2	12.4	15.5	14.4	12.8	11.9
Quebec, place of residence	14.3	13.2	13.6	12.6	12.6	13.6	12.5	12.7	11.5	11.9	9.2
Ontario, place of residence	12.4	12.4	11.6	11.8	11.6	11.0	9.9	10.3	8.1	8.0	7.5
Manitoba, place of residence	15.8	14.5	14.5	13.9	12.6	12.9	11.9	12.8	11.3	10.7	8.8
Saskatchewan, place of residence	14.7	16.9	16.6	17.8	18.2	15.9	16.0	16.8	14.4	14.3	13.8
Alberta, place of residence	11.1	11.4	11.9	10.7	11.6	12.7	11.2	10.6	8.8	8.0	8.0
British Columbia, place of residence	10.7	10.5	10.2	10.9	11.0	9.5	7.9	8.4	5.2	5.6	4.3
Yukon, place of residence	14.9	4.6	3.3	37.7	3.1	19.6	5.6	8.9	5.0	13.1	16.2
Northwest Territories, place of residence	15.1	0.0	12.4	13.5	45.0	20.9	12.6	32.9	5.5	17.7	15.1
Nunavut, place of residence	31.0	0.0	10.9	0.0	54.0	20.4	101.6	50.5	0.0	29.3	49.0

Source: Statistics Canada. *Table 102-0553 - Deaths and mortality rate (age standardization using 2011 population), by selected grouped causes and sex, Canada, provinces and territories, annual,* CANSIM (database). (accessed: April 4, 2017)

Cause of death (ICD-10) 6, 7, 8 = Nephritis, nephrotic syndrome and nephrosis [N00-N07, N17-N19, N25-N27]
Characteristics 14, 15, 16, 17, 18, 19, 21 = Age-standardized mortality rate per 100,000 population

Also see footnotes 1, 2, 5, 13, 22, 23, 24, 25, 26, 27

SECTION IV: Statistics

AGE-STANDARDIZED RATES, NEPHRITIS, NEPHROTIC SYNDROME AND NEPHROSIS, DEATHS (PER 100,000 POPULATION), MALES, CANADA, PROVINCES AND TERRITORIES

Geography, place of residence [3] [4]	2003	2004	2005	2006	2007	2008	2009	2010	2011	2012	2013
Canada, place of residence	17.3	18.1	17.4	16.7	16.2	16.1	14.2	14.0	12.2	11.8	10.2
Newfoundland and Labrador, place of residence	26.8	26.2	30.0	37.3	29.2	30.0	22.5	31.7	19.9	29.1	22.2
Prince Edward Island, place of residence	21.7	18.0	33.7	30.8	25.8	30.9	18.4	10.9	22.9	25.3	12.1
Nova Scotia, place of residence	16.2	24.6	21.6	17.5	17.8	16.2	18.6	14.1	14.5	13.5	11.6
New Brunswick, place of residence	23.3	21.3	19.4	21.2	21.1	16.8	15.8	21.0	18.8	12.9	12.4
Quebec, place of residence	19.7	19.9	19.6	17.2	16.9	19.5	15.4	15.7	14.9	15.9	10.7
Ontario, place of residence	17.0	17.2	15.4	15.7	14.9	14.4	13.2	12.9	10.9	10.0	10.4
Manitoba, place of residence	21.0	20.9	20.3	17.4	16.2	15.8	18.1	16.0	15.0	13.7	11.1
Saskatchewan, place of residence	19.2	24.2	22.4	23.7	20.6	21.9	21.2	21.2	18.6	18.3	18.7
Alberta, place of residence	13.9	16.1	17.3	13.9	16.3	16.5	13.6	12.0	11.4	10.2	9.4
British Columbia, place of residence	13.1	13.7	13.7	14.1	14.9	11.5	10.5	10.5	6.7	6.2	5.2
Yukon, place of residence	16.9	0.0	0.0	107.3	6.0	57.9	11.3	0.0	0.0	7.4	0.0
Northwest Territories, place of residence	29.9	0.0	26.7	23.0	52.8	25.5	0.0	45.2	11.5	48.6	0.0
Nunavut, place of residence	49.9	0.0	20.4	0.0	0.0	11.7	188.6	32.6	0.0	53.0	27.0

Source: Statistics Canada. *Table 102-0553 - Deaths and mortality rate (age standardization using 2011 population), by selected grouped causes and sex, Canada, provinces and territories, annual,* CANSIM (database). (accessed: April 4, 2017)

Cause of death (ICD-10) [6], [7], [8] = Nephritis, nephrotic syndrome and nephrosis [N00-N07, N17-N19, N25-N27]
Characteristics [14], [15], [16], [17], [18], [19], [21] = Age-standardized mortality rate per 100,000 population

Also see footnotes [1], [2], [5], [13], [22], [23], [24], [25], [26], [27]

AGE-STANDARDIZED RATES, NEPHRITIS, NEPHROTIC SYNDROME AND NEPHROSIS, DEATHS (PER 100,000 POPULATION), FEMALES, CANADA, PROVINCES AND TERRITORIES

Geography, place of residence [3], [4]	2003	2004	2005	2006	2007	2008	2009	2010	2011	2012	2013
Canada, place of residence	10.6	10.0	10.0	9.9	10.0	9.7	9.0	9.6	7.5	7.7	6.7
Newfoundland and Labrador, place of residence	18.4	18.3	20.1	16.8	17.4	11.9	17.2	20.2	16.7	14.3	12.4
Prince Edward Island, place of residence	10.1	13.7	12.8	12.7	9.2	11.9	12.3	16.9	8.6	13.3	8.6
Nova Scotia, place of residence	12.3	11.2	14.1	10.0	9.7	11.2	10.9	9.8	6.8	8.3	6.9
New Brunswick, place of residence	13.8	13.3	12.0	12.3	12.8	14.4	10.3	11.8	11.1	12.5	11.2
Quebec, place of residence	11.1	9.9	10.1	9.8	10.3	10.4	10.8	10.9	9.4	9.4	8.1
Ontario, place of residence	10.0	9.7	9.6	9.5	9.6	8.8	8.0	8.6	6.4	6.6	5.8
Manitoba, place of residence	13.1	10.9	11.3	11.7	10.4	11.5	8.0	11.2	9.2	9.3	7.4
Saskatchewan, place of residence	11.8	12.6	13.0	14.5	16.2	11.6	12.6	13.8	11.6	11.5	10.4
Alberta, place of residence	9.1	8.9	8.6	8.8	8.5	10.5	9.7	9.5	7.2	6.9	7.0
British Columbia, place of residence	9.2	8.4	8.0	8.7	8.6	8.2	6.4	7.1	4.2	5.1	3.7
Yukon, place of residence	13.5	10.9	7.2	0.0	0.0	0.0	0.0	16.5	9.3	13.4	26.1
Northwest Territories, place of residence	0.0	0.0	0.0	0.0	44.9	16.3	20.3	19.1	0.0	0.0	26.4
Nunavut, place of residence	0.0	0.0	0.0	0.0	138.1	33.3	57.3	52.5	0.0	0.0	68.1

Source: Statistics Canada. *Table 102-0553 - Deaths and mortality rate (age standardization using 2011 population), by selected grouped causes and sex, Canada, provinces and territories, annual,* CANSIM (database). (accessed: April 4, 2017)

Cause of death (ICD-10) [6], [7], [8] = Nephritis, nephrotic syndrome and nephrosis [N00-N07, N17-N19, N25-N27]
Characteristics [14], [15], [16], [17], [18], [19], [21] = Age-standardized mortality rate per 100,000 population

Also see footnotes [1], [2], [5], [13], [22], [23], [24], [25], [26], [27]

AGE-STANDARDIZED RATES, SENSE OF COMMUNITY BELONGING, SOMEWHAT STRONG OR VERY STRONG (%), [43] BOTH SEXES, CANADA, PROVINCES AND TERRITORIES

Geography	2003	2005	2007	2008	2009	2010	2011	2012	2013	2014
Canada	63.2	63.6	64.1	64.2	64.7	64.9	64.3	65.5	65.2	65.6
Newfoundland and Labrador	79.1	78.2	78.1	79.3	79.7	77.4	75.9	75.3	74.8	74.9
Prince Edward Island	73.4	73.6	68.8	75.3	70.7	71.3	72.2	73.2	72.0	74.6
Nova Scotia	69.9	70.8	68.3	71.9	69.8	71.5	69.9	69.6	70.4	72.3
New Brunswick	71.6	72.5	66.5	70.3	72.7	70.5	69.9	70.1	69.7	69.5
Quebec	55.0	54.1	58.4	56.9	56.3	56.7	55.1	59.2	56.9	57.3
Ontario	63.7	64.7	64.7	66.5	66.3	67.3	66.3	67.4	67.1	67.5
Manitoba	68.1	67.6	67.2	67.6	68.4	64.6	67.0	67.9	69.5	68.1
Saskatchewan	71.7	70.9	68.8	69.0	70.2	71.1	72.7	73.1	70.8	73.8
Alberta	64.0	64.2	62.7	60.5	64.8	62.0	63.9	64.6	63.8	66.8
British Columbia	67.0	68.8	68.3	66.4	68.0	68.8	68.4	65.9	69.5	67.4
Yukon [4]	70.1	69.1	71.0	72.7	71.1	81.1	78.9	73.5	72.2	72.4
Northwest Territories [4]	79.2	74.3	78.6	82.2	82.0	77.2	80.5	80.6	79.3	80.5
Nunavut [4, 5]	81.2	81.7	79.6	87.0	84.1	88.4	83.5	85.5	86.1	86.4

Source: Statistics Canada. *Table 105-0503 - Health indicator profile, age-standardized rate, annual estimates, by sex, Canada, provinces and territories, occasional,* CANSIM (database). (accessed: April 4, 2017)

Please see footnotes 30, 31, 57, 58, 59, 60, 61, 62, 64 for characteristics of the age-standardized rate.

AGE-STANDARDIZED RATES, SENSE OF COMMUNITY BELONGING, SOMEWHAT STRONG OR VERY STRONG (%), [43] MALES, CANADA, PROVINCES AND TERRITORIES

Geography	2003	2005	2007	2008	2009	2010	2011	2012	2013	2014
Canada	62.7	63.1	63.1	64.2	63.8	64.0	62.3	64.7	64.0	64.8
Newfoundland and Labrador	79.1	77.8	77.5	79.0	78.7	77.9	75.2	75.5	73.2	75.1
Prince Edward Island	78.5	72.7	70.5	80.0	72.0	74.7	74.5	72.5	72.5	76.9
Nova Scotia	70.5	71.1	68.2	74.7	71.3	71.6	71.5	67.0	71.4	73.3
New Brunswick	73.0	73.2	64.7	69.9	75.5	69.8	69.6	73.7	67.6	68.0
Quebec	54.9	55.3	58.1	56.7	55.2	57.0	53.4	58.1	56.1	55.7
Ontario	63.0	63.5	63.4	66.9	64.8	65.9	64.9	66.6	66.1	67.4
Manitoba	67.2	68.4	66.8	66.8	66.1	62.6	63.4	71.4	69.9	67.2
Saskatchewan	70.9	71.2	67.4	68.5	69.0	72.0	74.4	71.5	69.2	72.7
Alberta	62.9	62.5	61.1	59.6	64.6	61.6	60.1	65.4	61.3	66.6
British Columbia	66.1	67.6	67.8	66.5	67.7	66.2	64.6	63.7	67.7	65.6
Yukon [4]	71.5	68.8	69.9	72.3	71.8	81.6	75.3	73.3	73.0	72.0
Northwest Territories [4]	78.6	74.4	76.2	82.4	83.6	78.0	81.0	82.4	77.5	78.1
Nunavut [4, 5]	80.8	79.5	76.6	87.7	85.3	86.9	81.7	85.6	82.6	87.6

Source: Statistics Canada. *Table 105-0503 - Health indicator profile, age-standardized rate, annual estimates, by sex, Canada, provinces and territories, occasional,* CANSIM (database). (accessed: April 4, 2017)

Please see footnotes 30, 31, 57, 58, 59, 60, 61, 62, 64 for characteristics of the age-standardized rate.

AGE-STANDARDIZED RATES, SENSE OF COMMUNITY BELONGING, SOMEWHAT STRONG OR VERY STRONG (%), [43] FEMALES, CANADA, PROVINCES AND TERRITORIES

Geography	2003	2005	2007	2008	2009	2010	2011	2012	2013	2014
Canada	63.7	64.1	65.0	64.2	65.7	65.8	66.2	66.2	66.4	66.4
Newfoundland and Labrador	79.2	78.5	78.6	79.6	80.6	77.0	76.5	75.2	76.2	74.7
Prince Edward Island	68.7	74.3	67.2	71.0	69.6	68.1	70.0	73.8	71.7	72.6
Nova Scotia	69.3	70.5	68.5	69.2	68.4	71.4	68.6	71.9	69.5	71.4
New Brunswick	70.3	71.8	68.1	70.7	70.1	71.2	70.1	66.7	71.6	71.0
Quebec	55.2	53.0	58.7	57.2	57.5	56.4	56.7	60.4	57.7	58.9
Ontario	64.2	65.8	65.9	66.1	67.7	68.6	67.6	68.2	68.1	67.7
Manitoba	69.1	66.9	67.5	68.4	70.7	66.5	70.6	64.3	69.1	69.0
Saskatchewan	72.4	70.7	70.2	69.5	71.4	70.2	71.1	74.6	72.4	75.0
Alberta	65.1	66.0	64.4	61.3	65.1	62.5	67.9	63.7	66.4	66.9
British Columbia	67.9	69.9	68.8	66.2	68.2	71.4	72.1	68.1	71.3	69.2
Yukon [4]	68.8	69.3	72.0	73.0	70.4	80.6	82.4	73.7	71.4	72.8
Northwest Territories [4]	79.7	74.3	81.2	82.0	80.5	76.2	79.9	78.6	81.3	83.0
Nunavut [4,5]	81.6	84.3	82.6	86.3	83.0	90.0	85.6	85.3	89.8	85.0

Source: Statistics Canada. *Table 105-0503 - Health indicator profile, age-standardized rate, annual estimates, by sex, Canada, provinces and territories, occasional,* CANSIM (database). (accessed: April 4, 2017)

Please see footnotes 30, 31, 57, 58, 59, 60, 61, 62, 64 for characteristics of the age-standardized rate.

AGE-STANDARDIZED RATES, LIFE SATISFACTION, SATISFIED OR VERY SATISFIED (%), [8, 9] BOTH SEXES, CANADA, PROVINCES AND TERRITORIES

Geography	2003	2005	2007	2008	2009	2010	2011	2012	2013	2014
Canada	91.4	91.9	92.1	91.7	92.5	92.6	92.9	93.0	92.4	92.8
Newfoundland and Labrador	94.0	93.8	93.7	94.1	92.8	92.7	93.3	93.3	93.5	94.5
Prince Edward Island	94.2	93.8	94.6	94.2	94.6	95.3	94.2	94.6	94.1	95.0
Nova Scotia	92.9	92.0	92.3	92.4	91.9	92.8	93.7	94.1	92.5	91.8
New Brunswick	91.9	93.0	93.4	93.2	92.4	92.8	94.2	94.5	93.2	92.7
Quebec	91.9	93.0	93.0	92.7	94.5	94.4	94.7	94.1	93.8	94.1
Ontario	90.6	91.2	91.1	90.8	91.9	91.9	91.8	93.1	91.4	91.9
Manitoba	92.4	91.8	92.7	91.8	92.1	91.8	91.5	91.4	93.0	93.6
Saskatchewan	92.6	92.9	92.8	92.3	93.8	93.3	93.3	92.6	93.7	94.8
Alberta	92.5	92.1	92.9	92.3	91.5	91.3	92.8	92.9	92.3	93.0
British Columbia	90.6	90.8	92.1	90.8	91.5	92.2	92.5	90.8	92.3	92.4
Yukon [4]	88.4	91.0	91.3	89.2	90.6	93.4	95.0	92.6	90.9	91.7
Northwest Territories [4]	91.0	93.2	93.0	94.2	93.4	88.9	90.5	88.7	90.7	88.9
Nunavut [4, 5]	87.8	90.3	94.6	91.9	86.7	92.2	91.3	84.1	87.1	87.2

Source: Statistics Canada. *Table 105-0503 - Health indicator profile, age-standardized rate, annual estimates, by sex, Canada, provinces and territories, occasional,* CANSIM (database). (accessed: April 4, 2017)

Please see footnotes 30, 31, 57, 58, 59, 60, 61, 62, 64 for characteristics of the age-standardized rate.

AGE-STANDARDIZED RATES, LIFE SATISFACTION, SATISFIED OR VERY SATISFIED (%), [8, 9] MALES, CANADA, PROVINCES AND TERRITORIES

Geography	2003	2005	2007	2008	2009	2010	2011	2012	2013	2014
Canada	91.3	91.9	92.2	91.8	92.6	92.6	92.9	92.8	92.6	93.1
Newfoundland and Labrador	93.5	94.2	94.2	92.8	92.7	92.8	94.5	93.6	93.5	93.8
Prince Edward Island	94.8	93.8	93.6	94.1	94.1	96.4	93.5	94.4	96.1	93.7
Nova Scotia	92.9	92.4	93.4	93.5	91.2	93.5	94.1	94.3	93.3	94.3
New Brunswick	92.0	92.7	93.1	92.8	92.2	91.2	94.6	94.3	94.0	94.6
Quebec	91.9	93.0	93.0	91.8	94.3	94.3	94.4	94.1	94.0	93.6
Ontario	90.5	91.4	91.1	91.5	91.9	92.4	92.0	92.8	91.6	92.4
Manitoba	92.2	91.9	93.1	92.7	91.8	92.0	92.6	90.0	94.7	93.5
Saskatchewan	92.4	92.8	92.7	92.0	93.3	93.9	94.4	92.8	95.4	95.1
Alberta	92.8	91.4	93.2	92.2	91.9	91.3	92.0	92.7	91.3	93.9
British Columbia	90.4	91.0	91.7	91.0	92.9	91.1	92.8	91.1	92.2	92.9
Yukon [4]	88.5	89.5	94.2	90.4	90.9	92.8	95.7	96.1	94.2	89.2
Northwest Territories [4]	92.8	93.5	92.8	93.0	94.6	87.6	95.0	90.0	91.7	90.0
Nunavut [4, 5]	88.2	88.2	94.2	94.5	87.5	93.2	94.7	85.8	87.7	89.1

Source: Statistics Canada. *Table 105-0503 - Health indicator profile, age-standardized rate, annual estimates, by sex, Canada, provinces and territories, occasional,* CANSIM (database). (accessed: April 4, 2017)

Please see footnotes 30, 31, 57, 58, 59, 60, 61, 62, 64 for characteristics of the age-standardized rate.

AGE-STANDARDIZED RATES, LIFE SATISFACTION, SATISFIED OR VERY SATISFIED (%), [8], [9] FEMALES, CANADA, PROVINCES AND TERRITORIES

Geography	2003	2005	2007	2008	2009	2010	2011	2012	2013	2014
Canada	91.4	91.8	92.1	91.5	92.4	92.6	92.8	93.1	92.3	92.5
Newfoundland and Labrador	94.5	93.4	93.3	95.3	92.8	92.7	92.1	93.0	93.5	95.1
Prince Edward Island	93.5	93.9	95.5	94.4	95.0	94.2	94.8	94.9	92.4	96.1
Nova Scotia	92.8	91.6	91.3	91.4	92.6	92.1	93.3	93.9	91.7	89.5
New Brunswick	91.7	93.3	93.6	93.7	92.6	94.2	93.9	94.7	92.5	90.9
Quebec	92.0	93.1	93.0	93.5	94.8	94.6	95.1	94.1	93.6	94.5
Ontario	90.6	90.9	91.0	90.1	91.9	91.5	91.5	93.4	91.2	91.5
Manitoba	92.6	91.7	92.3	90.8	92.5	91.6	90.5	92.9	91.3	93.7
Saskatchewan	92.7	93.1	92.9	92.5	94.2	92.7	92.3	92.4	92.0	94.5
Alberta	92.3	92.8	92.7	92.4	91.0	91.3	93.7	93.0	93.3	92.1
British Columbia	90.8	90.7	92.5	90.7	90.1	93.2	92.2	90.6	92.5	92.0
Yukon [4]	88.4	92.3	88.4	88.0	90.3	94.0	94.4	89.2	87.7	94.2
Northwest Territories [4]	89.2	92.8	93.2	95.4	92.2	90.4	85.8	87.4	89.7	87.7
Nunavut [4], [5]	87.4	92.9	95.0	89.3	85.9	91.1	87.5	82.0	86.6	85.1

Source: Statistics Canada. *Table 105-0503 - Health indicator profile, age-standardized rate, annual estimates, by sex, Canada, provinces and territories, occasional,* CANSIM (database). (accessed: April 4, 2017)

Please see footnotes [30], [31], [57], [58], [59], [60], [61], [62], [64] for characteristics of the age-standardized rate.

Footnotes

CANSIM Table 105-0503 - Health indicator profile, age-standardized rate, annual estimates, by sex, Canada, provinces and territories

Source: Statistics Canada, Canadian Community Health Survey (CCHS)

Since 2009, all rates in this table are calculated excluding non-response categories ("refusal", "don't know", and "not stated") in the denominator.

4. Beginning with the 2008 and 2007/2008 reference period, weighting controls on the proportion of Aboriginal and non-Aboriginal as well as capital and non-capital have been put in place for Yukon and the Northwest Territories. Similar controls for Inuit and non-Inuit have also been put in place for Nunavut for the same reference periods. This may affect some of the comparability to previous reference periods where no such controls were in place.

5. In Nunavut, starting in 2013, the coverage was expanded to represent 92% of the targeted population. Before 2013, the coverage was 71% since the survey covered only the 10 largest communities.

6. Population aged 12 and over who reported perceiving their own health status as being either excellent or very good or fair or poor, depending on the indicator. Perceived health refers to the perception of a person's health in general, either by the person himself or herself, or, in the case of proxy response, by the person responding. Health means not only the absence of disease or injury but also physical, mental and social well being.

7. Population aged 12 and over who reported perceiving their own mental health status as being excellent or very good or fair or poor, depending on the indicator. Perceived mental health refers to the perception of a person's mental health in general. Perceived mental health provides a general indication of the population suffering from some form of mental disorder, mental or emotional problems, or distress, not necessarily reflected in perceived health.

8. Population aged 12 and over who reported being satisfied or very satisfied with their life in general.

9. In 2009, the question on life satisfaction was changed from a five-point answer category to an eleven-point scale. A grouped variable was developed to provide a concordance between the two scales and is now the basis for this indicator. Please see the variable GENGSWL in the derived variables documentation.

10. Data for this indicator are collected from population aged 15 years and over only.

11. Population aged 15 and over who reported perceiving that most days in their life were quite a bit or extremely stressful. Perceived life stress refers to the amount of stress in the person's life, on most days, as perceived by the person or, in the case of proxy response, by the person responding.

12. Population aged 15 and over who reported that they have been diagnosed by a health professional as having arthritis.

13. Arthritis includes rheumatoid arthritis and osteoarthritis, but excludes fibromyalgia. In the 2011 French questionnaire, the word "arthrose" was added to the arthritis question as respondents tend to associate the word "arthrite" with rheumatoid arthritis and "arthrose" with degenerative arthritis. This lead to an increase in reported arthritis for 2011. However, the word "arthrose" was then omitted from the question in 2012, leading to a decrease in the reported arthritis estimates for the province of Quebec and subsequently at the national level. Therefore, the data for the arthritis indicator in 2011 should be used with caution.

14. Population aged 12 and over who reported that they have been diagnosed by a health professional as having Type 1 or Type 2 diabetes.

15. Diabetes includes females 15 and over who reported that they have been diagnosed with gestational diabetes.

16. Population aged 12 and over who reported that they have been diagnosed by a health professional as having asthma.

17. Population aged 12 and over who reported that they have been diagnosed by a health professional as having high blood pressure.

18. Population aged 12 and over who reported that they usually have pain or discomfort.

19. Canada and provincial estimates are based on sub-sample weights for 2005 and 2003 data.

20. Population aged 15 and over who reported having pain or discomfort that prevents activities.

21. Population aged 12 and over who reported being limited in selected activities (home, school, work and other activities) because of a physical condition, mental condition or health problem which has lasted or is expected to last 6 months or longer.

22. Population aged 12 and over who reported being a current smoker.

23. Daily smoker refers to those who reported smoking cigarettes every day.

24. Does not take into account the number of cigarettes smoked.

25. Occasional smoker refers to those who reported smoking cigarettes occasionally. This includes former daily smokers who now smoke occasionally.

26. Statistics Canada has two main surveys that produce National and Provincial smoking rates. The Canadian Community Health Survey (CCHS), and the Canadian Tobacco, Alcohol and Drugs Survey (CTADS), which replaces the Canadian Tobacco Use Monitoring Survey (CTUMS) beginning in 2013. Users should be aware of a number of differences between CCHS and CTADS. CCHS collects information from respondents aged 12 and over, CTADS collects information from respondents aged 15 and over; the two surveys use different sampling frames; the annual sample for CTADS is 20,000 compared to 65,000 for CCHS; in CCHS, smoking questions are asked in the context of a wide range of health-related behaviours whereas in CTADS, all questions are related to the use of multiple products and substances with addictive properties. Although these factors can influence the estimates produced at a single point in time, the trends produced by the two surveys have been noted to be very consistent over time. Rather than comparing smoking rates produced from the two surveys, Statistics Canada advises users to choose a single source, based on their objectives, and to use that source consistently.

27. Non-smoking population aged 12 and over who reported that at least one person smoked inside their home every day or almost every day. Smoking inside the home excludes smoking inside the garage, whether attached or detached.

28. Data collected for this indicator is based on the question referring to smoking of cigarettes only. Note that data on smoking alternative tobacco products is captured in a different module (TAL).

29. Non-smoking population aged 12 and over who reported being exposed to second-hand smoke in private vehicles and/or public places on every day or almost every day in the past month.

30. The coefficient of variation characteristic (CV) is no longer available in this table. Data quality flags ('E' use with caution and 'F' too unreliable to be published), which are based on CVs, are still applied to counts and percentages when appropriate.

31. Percentages are rounded to the nearest tenth. Numbers are rounded to the nearest unit.

32. Population aged 12 and over who reported having 5 or more drinks on one occasion, at least once a month in the past year.

33. Starting in 2009, the denominator includes all respondents aged 12 and over. This change applies to rates from all years in this table. In data released before 2009, the denominator included only those respondents who reported having had at least one drink in the past 12 months. Increasing the population in the denominator reduces the estimate rates. This change was implemented to produce more comparable rates over time and is more consistent with methods used in calculating other indicators in this table.

34. Indicates the usual number of times (frequency) per day a person reported eating fruits and vegetables. Measure does not take into account the amount consumed.

35. Canada and provincial estimates are based on sub-sample weights for 2005 data.

36. Population aged 12 and over who reported the nature, frequency and duration of their participation in leisure-time physical activity.

37. Respondents are classified as active, moderately active or inactive based on an index of average daily physical activity over the past 3 months. For each leisure time physical activity the respondent is engaged in, an average daily energy expenditure is calculated by multiplying the number of times the activity was performed by the average duration of the activity by the energy cost (kilocalories per kilogram of body weight per hour) of the activity. The index is calculated as the sum of the average daily energy expenditures of all activities. Respondents are classified as follows: 3.0 kcal/kg/day or more = physically active; 1.5 to 2.9 kcal/kg/day = moderately active; less than 1.5 kcal/kg/day = inactive.

38. Body mass index (BMI) is a method of classifying body weight according to health risk. According to the World Health Organization (WHO) and Health Canada guidelines, health risk levels are associated with each of the following BMI categories: normal weight = least health risk; underweight and overweight = increased health risk; obese, class I = high health risk; obese, class II = very high health risk; obese, class III = extremely high health risk.

39. Body mass index (BMI) is calculated by dividing the respondent's body weight (in kilograms) by their height (in metres) squared.

40. A definition change was implemented in 2004 to conform with the World Health Organization (WHO) and Health Canada guidelines for body weight classification. The index is calculated for the population aged 18 and over, excluding pregnant females and persons less than 3 feet (0.914 metres) tall or greater than 6 feet 11 inches (2.108 metres).

41. According to the World Health Organization (WHO) and Health Canada guidelines, the index for body weight classification is: less than 18.50 (underweight); 18.50 to 24.99 (normal weight); 25.00 to 29.99 (overweight); 30.00 to 34.99 (obese, class I); 35.00 to 39.99 (obese, class II); 40.00 or greater (obese, class III).

42. A definition change was implemented in 2013 to conform with the World Health Organization (WHO) and Health Canada guidelines for Heavy drinking. Heavy drinking refers to males who reported having 5 or more drinks, or women who reported having 4 or more drinks, on one occasion, at least once a month in the past year. While this indicator remains comparable for males to the 5 or more drinks indicator published in previous years, it is no longer comparable for females.

43. Population aged 12 and over who reported their sense of belonging to their local community as being very strong or somewhat strong. Research shows a high correlation of sense of community-belonging with physical and mental health.

44. Population aged 12 and over who reported that they have a regular medical doctor. In 2005 and 2003, the indicator in French only included "médecin de famille". Starting in 2007, this concept was widened to "médecin régulier", which includes "médecin de famille".

45. Population aged 12 and over who reported having consulted with a medical doctor in the past 12 months.

46. Medical doctor includes family or general practitioners as well as specialists such as surgeons, allergists, orthopaedists, gynaecologists or psychiatrists. For population aged 12 to 17, includes pediatricians.

47. Population aged 12 and over who reported when they had their last influenza immunization (flu shot).

48. The 2009 data on flu shots may include H1N1 vaccines received in the Fall of 2009. In 2010, the word "seasonal" was added to the questions in order to collect the two types of vaccines separately. After 2010, the separate module on H1N1 vaccines is not asked as the H1N1 flu shot is now given in combination with the seasonal flu vaccine.

49. Based on information provided by females aged 15 to 55 who had a baby in the last 5 years.

50. Initiated breastfeeding refers to mothers who breastfed or tried to breastfeed their last child even if only for a short time.

51. Exclusive breastfeeding refers to an infant receiving only breast milk, without any additional liquid (even water) or solid food.

52. The numerator includes mothers who have exclusively breastfed for at least 6 months and who may or may not be still breastfeeding. The denominator includes all mothers who had a baby in the past 5 years but excludes mothers who were still breastfeeding and who had not introduced any other liquids or solid foods to the baby's feeds. Previously, this indicator included in the numerator, only mothers who had stopped breastfeeding and for whom we knew they had introduced other liquids or solid foods to the baby's feeds when the baby was 6 months or more. The denominator included mothers who had stopped breastfeeding and for whom we knew when they had introduced other liquids or solid foods to the baby's feeds. This modification will produce lower rates of 6 months exclusive breastfeeding as mothers who have had a baby in the past 5 years and have not breastfed are now included in the denominator. This change was implemented to produce more comparable rates over time and is more consistent with methods used in calculating other indicators.

53. Population aged 12 and over who reported that they have been diagnosed by a health professional as having a mood disorder, such as depression, bipolar disorder, mania or dysthymia.

54. Population aged 12 and over who sustained injuries in the past 12 months and who sought medical attention from a health professional in the 48 hours following the injury.

55. Respondents aged 12 and over who sustained injuries in the past 12 months which were serious enough to limit normal activities. For those with more than one injury in the past 12 months, refers to "the most serious injury", as identified by the respondent. Repetitive strain injuries are not included.

56. Population aged 35 and over who reported being diagnosed by a health professional with chronic bronchitis, emphysema or chronic obstructive pulmonary disease (COPD).

57. Age-standardized (age-adjusted) rates have been calculated using the direct method, and the 1991 Canadian Census population structure. The use of a standard population results in more meaningful rate comparisons, as it adjusts for variations in population age distributions over time and across different geographic areas.

58. The confidence interval illustrates the degree of variability associated with a rate. Wide confidence intervals indicate high variability, thus, these rates should be interpreted with due caution. When comparing estimates, it is important to use confidence intervals to determine if differences between values are statistically significant.

59. Bootstrapping techniques were used to produce the 95% confidence intervals (CIs).

60. Data with a coefficient of variation (CV) from 16.6% to 33.3% are identified as follows: (E) use with caution.

61. Data with a coefficient of variation (CV) greater than 33.3% were suppressed due to extreme sampling variability and are identified as follows: (F) too unreliable to be published.

62. The following standard symbols are used in this Statistics Canada table: (..) for figures not available for a specific reference period and (...) for figures not applicable.

63. This variable provides direction and statistical significance of the difference between estimates (p < 0.05). A value of +1 means the difference observed is significantly higher, -1 means the difference is significantly lower and 0 means the difference is not statistically significant.

64. Starting with the 2010 and 2009/2010 Canadian Community Health Survey (CCHS) datasets, the 2006 Census population counts have been used to produce the population projection counts. These counts are used to ensure that the CCHS survey weights and resulting estimates included in this CANSIM table are consistent with known population totals. Prior to 2010, 2001 Census population counts were used. Evaluation studies have confirmed that the impact of this change on CCHS estimates should be minimal.

65. This indicator is derived from data collected from an optional content module. Only provincial and sub-provincial estimates are available for years when the module was selected by a given province. National estimates are not available unless the module became part of biennial or quadrennial common content blocks in a given survey year. Please refer to the document "CCHS content overview" available for the survey under the documentation section of the Definitions, data sources and methods page on the Statistics Canada website.

66. In the 2011 questionnaire, in order to improve the quality of the data, the question measuring when other liquids or solids were introduced to the baby's feeds was split into two separate questions. One addresses the addition of other liquids and the other addresses the addition of other solids to the baby's feeds.

Source: Statistics Canada. *Table 105-0503 - Health indicator profile, age-standardized rate, annual estimates, by sex, Canada, provinces and territories, occasional,* CANSIM (database). (accessed: April 11, 2017)

CANSIM Table 102-4005 - Low birth weight (less than 2,500 grams) and borderline viable birth weight-adjusted low birth weight (500 to less than 2,500 grams), by sex, Canada, provinces and territories

1. Source: Statistics Canada, Canadian Vital Statistics, Birth Database

3. Over time, there has been increased registration of live births with birth weight less than 500 grams. To improve comparability of this indicator over an extended time period, low birth weight birth counts and low birth weight birth rates are calculated two ways, including and excluding live births with birth weight under 500 grams.

4. Counts and rates in this table exclude: live births to mothers not resident in Canada; live births to mothers resident in Canada, province or territory of residence unknown; live births with unknown birth weight.

5. Rates in this table are based on place of residence for indicators derived from birth events.

6. Missing data on sex of infant were imputed based on birth registration number.

7. Standard low birth weight birth counts in this table include all live births with birth weight less than 2,500 grams.

8. Standard low birth weight birth rates are calculated as follows: low birth weight birth counts in a given year divided by live birth counts for the same year with known birth weight.

9. Borderline viable birth weight-adjusted low birth weight counts in this table are calculated by subtracting the number of live births with a birth

weight of less than 500 grams from the standard low birth weight counts in the same year.

10. Borderline viable birth weight-adjusted low birth weight birth rates in this table are calculated as follows: (subtract the number of live births with a birth weight of less than 500 grams from the standard low birth weight birth counts in the same year) and divide by (live birth counts for the same year with a known birth weight greater than 499 grams).

11. Live births for the years 1979 to 1981 and 1985 to 1990 to mothers resident in Newfoundland and Labrador were adjusted to correct for undercounts.

12. No data on birth weight are available for 1979 to 1990 live births to mothers resident in Newfoundland and Labrador.

13. Live births for the years 1979 to 1990 to mothers resident in Nunavut are included with live births to mothers resident in the Northwest Territories.

14. Number and proportion of low birth weight births for Yukon, the Northwest Territories and Nunavut should be interpreted with caution due to a small underlying count.

15. Northwest Territories excluding Nunavut.

16. Nunavut and the Northwest Territories (excluding Nunavut) came into existence on April 1, 1999. Data for these two territories are shown combined and separated for years 1991 to 1999 and separated from 2000 on. Historical data prior to 1991 are shown for the two territories combined as the "Northwest Territories including Nunavut" series; it was terminated in 1999. The vital statistics data that pertain to these territories for 1999 were previously published on the basis of the legal definition of each territory, as per the date of the event. Vital events for Nunavut that occurred before April 1, 1999 were tabulated with those of the Northwest Territories; only those events that occurred from April 1, 1999 on were tabulated separately. See the paper versions of the following publications for data year 1999: catalogue numbers 84F0001XPB, 84F0210XPB, 84F0211XPB, 84F0208XPB and 84F0209XPB.

17. The following standard symbols are used in this Statistics Canada table: (..) for figures not available for a specific reference period, (...) for figures not applicable and (x) for figures suppressed to meet the confidentiality requirements of the Statistics Act.

18. Live birth is the complete expulsion or extraction from its mother of a product of conception, irrespective of the duration of the pregnancy, which, after such separation, breathes or shows any other evidence of life, such as beating of the heart, pulsation of the umbilical cord, or definite movement of voluntary muscles, whether or not the umbilical cord has been cut or the placenta is attached.

19. Birth weight is the first weight of the newborn obtained immediately after birth, expressed in grams.

Source: Statistics Canada. *Table 102-4005 - Low birth weight (less than 2,500 grams) and borderline viable birth weight-adjusted low birth weight (500 to less than 2,500 grams), by sex, Canada, provinces and territories, annual,* CANSIM (database). (accessed: April 11, 2017)

CANSIM Table 103-0554 - New cases and 2011 age-standardized rate for primary cancer (based on the July 2016 CCR tabulation file), by cancer type and sex, Canada, provinces and territories

1. Data sources include Statistics Canada's Canadian Cancer Registry Database and Demography Division Population estimates as of July 1st 2016, released September 27th, 2016. Statistics Canada maintains the CCR which is comprised of data supplied by the provinces and territories whose cooperation is gratefully acknowledged.

2. World Health Organization, International Classification of Diseases for Oncology, Third Edition (ICD-O-3) and the International Agency for Research on Cancer (IARC) rules for determining multiple primary types (source: International Agency for Research on Cancer, World

Health Organization, International Association of Cancer Registries, and European Network of Cancer Registries. International Rules for Multiple Primary Cancers, ICD-O Third Edition, Internal Report No.2004/02. Lyon: International Agency for Research on Cancer, 2004).

3. Cancer incidence refers to new primary sites of malignant neoplasms. The Canadian Cancer Registry (CCR) is a dynamic database that can be updated with new records or changes to previous records, therefore, the incidence counts may vary from one release to the next. In particular, data for the most recent years often represent an undercount of total cases due to a delay in the reporting of new cancer cases to the Canadian Cancer Registry. These missing cases are added to their appropriate diagnosed year with the reporting of a new reference year.

4. Although the Canadian Cancer Registry (CCR) strives to achieve national uniformity, reporting procedures and completeness still vary across the country. Specific issues follow: a) Because Quebec relies primarily on hospital data (i.e., hospitalizations or day surgeries) for cancers diagnosed until the end of 2010, the number of cases of some cancers are underestimated (source: Brisson J, Major D, Pelletier E. Evaluation of the completeness of the Fichier des tumeurs du Québec. Institut national de la santé publique du Québec; 2003). Also, Quebec does not participate in national duplicate resolution process and in the national linkage between the CCR and the Canadian Vital Statistics Death Database. These processes reduce duplicate person and tumour records, identify cases missed by provincial/territorial registries, and enhance the accuracy of vital status information. b) There may be under-reporting of cancer cases in Newfoundland and Labrador due to incomplete linkage of cancer data with death data. c) Differences may exist between the content of the CCR and the provincial/territorial cancer registries because of incomplete updating of the CCR by the provinces and territories.

5. Nunavut became a territory in April 1999 and historical data are provided for comparison purposes. Current and historical cancer data are presented for the current boundaries of the Northwest Territories and Nunavut.

6. Cancer types are defined using the Surveillance, Epidemiology and End Results (SEER) program, based on International Classification of Diseases for Oncology, Third Edition (ICD-O-3). Included are all invasive types and in situ for bladder.

7. Excluding morphology types M-9050 to M-9055; M-9140; M-9590 to M-9992.

8. Other non-epithelial skin, excluding morphology types M-8000 to M-8005, M-8010 to M-8046, M-8050 to M-8084, M-8090 to M-8110, M-8720 to M-8790, M-9050 to M-9055, M-9140, M-9590 to M-9992.

9. Brain, excluding morphology types M-9050 to M-9055; M-9140; M-9530 to M-9539; M-9590 to M-9992.

10. Non-Hodgkin lymphoma, M-9590 to M-9597, M-9670 to M-9729, M-9735 to M-9738; M-9811 to M-9818, all sites except C42.0, C42.1, C42.4; M-9823, all sites except C42.0, C42.1, C42.4; M-9827, all sites except C42.0, C42.1, C42.4; M-9837, all sites except C42.0, C42.1, C42.4.

11. Other leukemia, M-9733, M-9742, M-9800, M-9801, M-9805,M-9806 to M-9809, M-9820, M-9831, M-9832 to M-9834, M-9860, M-9870, M-9891, M-9930, M-9931, M-9940, M-9948, M-9963, M-9964; C42.0, M-9827; C42.1, M-9827; C42.4, M-9827.

12. Other, ill-defined and unknown sites, M-9740, M-9741, M-9750 to M-9769, M-9950, M-9960 to M-9962, M-9965 to M-9967, M-9970, M-9971, M-9975, M-9980, M-9982 to M-9987, M-9989, M-9991, M-9992; C42.0 to C42.4, excluding M-9050 to M-9055, M-9140, M-9590 to M-9992; C76.0 to C76.8, excluding M-9050 to M-9055, M-9140, M-9590 to M-9992; C77.0 to C77.9, excluding M-9050 to M-9055, M-9140, M-9590 to M-9992; C80.9, excluding M-9050 to M-9055, M-9140, M-9590 to M-9992.

13. Cancer incidence rates are age-standardized using the direct method and the final 2011 Canadian postcensal population structure (Age standardization).

14. Confidence intervals convey the degree of precision associated with a rate. Wide confidence intervals convey imprecision (i.e., high variability) and should be interpreted and compared cautiously. Two-sided 95% confidence intervals for age-standardized incidence rates are calculated according to Fay and Feuer (1997) (source: Fay MP, Feuer EJ. Confidence intervals for directly standardized rates: a method based on the gamma distribution. Statistics in Medicine 1997, 16: 791-801).

15. To prevent inappropriate disclosure of health-related information, the actual number of cases of a specific cancer is randomly rounded to a lower or higher multiple of 5; true zeros and actual counts evenly divisible by 5 are not affected. Random rounding is applied to each cell count independently. Specifically, an unbiased random rounding procedure is applied such that numbers ending in 0 or 5 are not rounded; numbers ending in a 1 or 6 are rounded up with a probability of 0.20 and down with a probability of 0.80; numbers ending in 2 or 7 are rounded up and down with probabilities of 0.40 and 0.60, respectively; numbers ending in 3 or 8 are rounded up and down with probabilities of 0.60 and 0.40, respectively; and, numbers ending in 4 or 9 are rounded up and down with probabilities of 0.80 and 0.20, respectively. Consequently, columns and rows will sum to totals only by chance. By design, differences between the rounded and actual counts will never exceed 4 and actual counts are more likely to be rounded to the nearest multiple of 5. The randomly rounded number of cases is used to calculate the incidence rate and 95% confidence limits. The age-standardized incidence rate and 95% confidence interval, however, are calculated using the actual number of cases in the age-specific strata. When the rounded total number of cases is zero, the actual age-standardized incidence rate and 95% confidence interval are suppressed to maintain the ambiguity of zeros. Otherwise, users could decipher when the actual value is zero rather than a one to four.

16. The following standard symbols are used in this Statistics Canada table: (..) for figures not available for a specific reference period, (...) for figures not applicable and (x) for figures suppressed to meet the confidentiality requirements of the Statistics Act.

17. The use of a standard population results in more meaningful incidence rate comparisons, because it adjusts for variations in population age distributions over time and across geographic areas.

18. Death certificate only (DCO) cases: Ontario has no DCO cases reported from 2008 to 2014 (just over 1,000 DCO cases were reported in 2007); Quebec has no DCO cases reported for 2010 (just under 1,400 DCO cases were reported in 2009).

19. To reduce the number of duplicate cases, a national duplicate resolution process was completed up to December 31, 2014 for all provinces and territories, except Quebec. A similar process was completed up to December 31, 2008 for Quebec records only. A death clearance linkage was completed up to December 31, 2008 for all provinces and territories, except Quebec. Death clearance was performed by linking cancer records to the Canadian Vital Statistics Death Database (excluding Quebec deaths).

20. Cancer incidence data for Quebec are not available for the 2011, 2012, 2013 and 2014 diagnosis years in the Canadian Cancer Registry. For CANSIM tables 103-0550 and 103-0554, annual count and rate data for Quebec for 2011 to 2013 have been copied using the 2010 data. This assumes that annual cancer incidence and population counts in Quebec for 2011 to 2013 have been unchanged since 2010. Data for Canada for 2011 to 2013 include the copied data for Quebec and this should be considered in any interpretation of the data. CANSIM tables 103-0555 and 103-0556 do not contain Quebec.

21. As of October 2014 Ontario has implemented a new cancer reporting system, the Ontario Cancer Registry. The first year Ontario reported to the CCR using the new system is the 2013 diagnosis year.

The adoption of the new rules may have contributed to the increase in the incidence number of certain types of cancer reported by Ontario.

Source: Statistics Canada. *Table 103-0554 - New cases and 2011 age-standardized rate for primary cancer (based on the July 2016 CCR tabulation file), by cancer type and sex, Canada, provinces and territories, annual (number unless otherwise noted)*, CANSIM (database). (accessed: April 11, 2017)

CANSIM Table 102-0030 - Infant mortality, by sex and birth weight, Canada, provinces and territories

1. Sources: Statistics Canada, Canadian Vital Statistics, Birth and Death Databases

2. Infant mortality corresponds to the death of a child under one year of age.

3. Counts and rates in this table exclude: live births to mothers not resident in Canada; live births to mothers resident in Canada, province or territory of residence unknown; deaths of infants not resident in Canada; and deaths of infants resident in Canada, province or territory of residence unknown.

4. Rates in this table are based on place of residence for indicators derived from birth and death events.

5. Missing data on sex of infant were imputed based on birth or death registration number.

6. Over time, there has been increased registration of live births with birth weight less than 500 grams. To improve comparability of this indicator over an extended time period, infant death counts and infant mortality rates are calculated two ways, including and excluding live births with birth weight under 500 grams.

7. Standard infant death counts in this table include all infant deaths regardless of birth weight.

8. Standard infant mortality rates are calculated as follows: infant death counts in a given year divided by live birth counts for the same year, regardless of birth weight.

9. Borderline viable birth weight-adjusted infant death counts in this table are calculated by subtracting the number of live births with a birth weight of less than 500 grams from the standard infant death counts in the same year.

10. Borderline viable birth weight-adjusted infant mortality rates in this table are calculated as follows: (subtract the number of live births with a birth weight of less than 500 grams from the standard infant death counts in the same year) and divide by (live birth counts for the same year with a known birth weight greater than 499 grams). Occasionally, this method will result in an estimate of infant mortality rate that is higher than the standard infant mortality rate. This happens when there are no live births under 500 grams but there are live births with unknown birth weight. This method creates an incongruous measure of infant mortality whenever all infant deaths occur in one sex and all births under 500 grams occur in the opposite sex, as occurred in Yukon in 2000. In that case, subtraction of the one female birth under 500 grams from the one male infant death generated a value of 0 for both sexes.

11. Live births for the years 1979 to 1981 and 1985 to 1990 to mothers resident in Newfoundland and Labrador were adjusted to correct for undercounts.

12. No data on birth weight are available for 1979 to 1990 live births to mothers resident in Newfoundland and Labrador.

13. Live births for the years 1979 to 1990 to mothers resident in Nunavut are included with live births to mothers resident in the Northwest Territories.

14. Infant mortality rates for Yukon, the Northwest Territories and Nunavut should be interpreted with caution due to a small underlying count.

15. Northwest Territories excluding Nunavut.

16. Nunavut and the Northwest Territories (excluding Nunavut) came into existence on April 1, 1999. Data for these two territories are shown combined and separated for years 1991 to 1999 and separated from 2000 on. Historical data prior to 1991 are shown for the two territories combined as the "Northwest Territories including Nunavut" series; it was terminated in 1999. The vital statistics data that pertain to these territories for 1999 were previously published on the basis of the legal definition of each territory, as per the date of the event. Vital events for Nunavut that occurred before April 1, 1999 were tabulated with those of the Northwest Territories; only those events that occurred from April 1, 1999 on were tabulated separately. See the paper versions of the following publications for data year 1999: catalogue numbers 84F0001XPB, 84F0210XPB, 84F0211XPB, 84F0208XPB and 84F0209XPB.

17. The following standard symbols are used in this Statistics Canada table: (..) for figures not available for a specific reference period, (...) for figures not applicable and (x) for figures suppressed to meet the confidentiality requirements of the Statistics Act.

18. Death refers to the permanent disappearance of all evidence of life at any time after a live birth has taken place. Stillbirths are excluded.

19. Live birth is the complete expulsion or extraction from its mother of a product of conception, irrespective of the duration of the pregnancy, which, after such separation, breathes or shows any other evidence of life, such as beating of the heart, pulsation of the umbilical cord, or definite movement of voluntary muscles, whether or not the umbilical cord has been cut or the placenta is attached.

20. Birth weight is the first weight of the newborn obtained immediately after birth, expressed in grams.

Source: Statistics Canada. *Table 102-0030 - Infant mortality, by sex and birth weight, Canada, provinces and territories, annual*, CANSIM (database). (accessed: April 11, 2017)

CANSIM Table 102-4307 - Life expectancy, at birth and at age 65, by sex, three-year average, Canada, provinces, territories, health regions and peer groups

1. Sources: Statistics Canada, Canadian Vital Statistics, Death Database and Demography Division (population estimates). The CANSIM table 102-4307 is an update of CANSIM table 102-0218.

2. Life expectancy is the number of years a person would be expected to live, starting from birth (for life expectancy at birth) and similarly for other age groups, if the age- and sex-specific mortality rates for a given observation period (such as a calendar year) were held constant over the estimated life span.

3. In this table, the calculation of life expectancy is based on three consecutive years of death data and population estimates.

4. Life expectancy is calculated with Greville's method for abridged life tables (Greville, TNE., "United States Life Tables and Actuarial Tables, 1939-1941", Public Health Service, Washington, 1946).

5. Rates used in this table for the calculation of life expectancy are calculated with data that exclude: births to mothers not resident in Canada; births to mothers resident in Canada, province or territory of residence unknown; deaths of non-residents of Canada; deaths of residents of Canada whose province or territory of residence was unknown; deaths for which age or sex of decedent was unknown.

6. Rates used for the calculation of life expectancy in this table are based on data tabulated by place of residence.

7. Health regions are administrative areas defined by provincial ministries of health according to provincial legislation. The health

regions presented in this table are based on boundaries and names in effect as of October 2011. For complete Canadian coverage, each northern territory represents a health region.

8. Peer groups are aggregations of health regions that share similar socio-economic and demographic characteristics, based on 2006 Census data. These are useful in the analysis of health regions, where important differences may be detected by comparing health regions within a peer group. The ten peer groups are identified by the letters A through J, which are appended to the health region 4-digit code. Caution should be taken when comparing data for the peer groups over time due to changes in the peer groups. For more information on the peer groups classification, consult Statistics Canada's publication "Health Indicators" (catalogue number 82-221-XWE).

9. Prince Edward Island restructured and collapsed the four administrative areas into one in November 2005. As of May 2012, data for Prince Edward Island are disseminated at the provincial level only.

10. Minor name changes have been made to Nova Scotia health regions. For example, Zone 1 is now called South Shore/South West Nova while DHA 9 is now referred to as the Capital District Health Authority. For more information consult Statistics Canada's publication Health Regions: Boundaries and Correspondence with Census Geography" (catalogue number 82-402-XWE).

11. The province of New Brunswick has made minor name changes to its health regions. 'Regions' are now referred to as 'Zones'. In addition, a descriptive name for each Zone has been added. For example, Zone 1 will now be referred to as 'Zone 1 (Moncton)'. In February 2006 a small boundary change in New Brunswick occurred: Cambridge-Narrows village (population 717) was reassigned from Region 2 to Region 3. For more information consult Statistics Canada's publication "Health Regions: Boundaries and Correspondence with Census Geography" (catalogue number 82-402-XWE).

12. In Ontario, Public Health Units (PHU) administer health promotion and disease prevention programs. Local Health Integration Networks (LHIN) are responsible for planning, funding and administering health care programs and services across the province. Data are provided for both PHUs and LHINs. However, since the weights for the Canadian Community Health Survey sample are primarily based on PHUs, only estimates for rates (percentages) are available by LHIN in the profile. Special LHIN weights are available upon request. These weights will allow for more precise estimation at the LHIN level including the estimation of totals.

14. In Manitoba and Saskatchewan, health regions are referred to as Health Authorities (HA) or Regional Health Authorities (RHA).

15. To avoid data suppression, northern regions in Manitoba have been grouped with neighbouring regions, as follows: Churchill Regional Health Authority (4690) is combined with Burntwood Regional Health Authority (4680) and referred to as Burntwood/Churchill (4685).

16. To avoid data suppression, northern regions in Saskatchewan have been grouped with neighbouring regions, as follows: Athabasca Health Authority (4713) is combined with Mamawetan Churchill River Regional Health Authority (4711) and Keewatin Yatthé Regional Health Authority (4712) and referred to as Mamawetan/Keewatin/Athabasca (4714).

17. As of Fall 2011, Alberta data are disseminated at five new Zone levels. They were approved for use in November 2010 in Alberta by the Joint Alberta Health Services - Alberta Health and Wellness Geographies Committee and are aggregations of the previous nine Regional Health Authorities. For more information consult Statistics Canada's publication 'Health Regions: Boundaries and Correspondence with Census Geography' (catalogue number 82-402-XWE).

18. The 95% confidence interval (CI) illustrates the degree of variability associated with a number.

19. Wide confidence intervals (CIs) indicate high variability, thus, these numbers or rates should be interpreted and compared with due caution.

20. The following standard symbols are used in this Statistics Canada table: (..) for figures not available for a specific reference period, (...) for figures not applicable and (x) for figures suppressed to meet the confidentiality requirements of the Statistics Act.

21. This variable provides direction and statistical significance of the difference between estimates (p < 0.05). A value of +1 means the difference observed is significantly higher, -1 means the difference is significantly lower and 0 means the difference is not statistically significant.

22. For small populations (less than 25,000), life expectancy is shown with an 'E' (use with caution) to indicate that the quality of the estimates are more affected by the imputation method used when there are no deaths for a given age group.

Source: Statistics Canada. *Table 102-4307 - Life expectancy, at birth and at age 65, by sex, three-year average, Canada, provinces, territories, health regions and peer groups, occasional (years unless otherwise noted),* CANSIM (database). (accessed: April 11, 2017)

CANSIM Table 102-0553 - Deaths and mortality rate (age standardization using 2011 population), by selected grouped causes and sex, Canada, provinces and territories

1. Sources: Statistics Canada, Canadian Vital Statistics, Birth and Death Databases and Appendix II of the publication "Mortality Summary List of Causes" (catalogue number 84F0209XIE)

2. Death refers to the permanent disappearance of all evidence of life at any time after a live birth has taken place. Stillbirths are excluded.

3. The geographic distribution of deaths in this table is based on the deceased's usual place of residence.

4. Counts in this table exclude deaths of non-residents of Canada.

5. For data year 2000 to 2009, missing data on sex of the deceased were imputed based on death registration number. Starting with 2010 data year, missing data on sex of the deceased were imputed based on the cause of death information and a logistic regression.

6. The cause of death tabulated is the underlying cause of death. This is defined as (a) the disease or injury which initiated the train of events leading directly to death, or (b) the circumstances of the accident or violence which produced the fatal injury. The underlying cause is selected from the conditions listed on the medical certificate of cause of death.

7. World Health Organization (WHO), International Statistical Classification of Diseases and Related Health Problems, Tenth Revision (ICD-10)

8. National Center for Health Statistics, United States. "B" list in "Instruction Manual; Part 9; ICD-10 Cause-of-Death Lists for Tabulating Mortality Statistics".

9. Other and unspecified infectious and parasitic diseases and their sequelae A00, A05, A20 to A36, A42 to A44, A48 to A49, A54 to A79, A81 to A82, A85.0 to A85.1, A85.8, A86 to B04, B06 to B09, B25 to B49, B55 to B99.

10. All other diseases (residual) D65 to E07, E15 to E34, E65 to F99, G04 to G14, G23 to G25, G31 to H93, K00 to K22, K29 to K31, K50 to K66, K71 to K72, K75 to K76, K83 to M99, N13.0 to N13.5, N13.7 to N13.9, N14, N15.0, N15.8 to N15.9, N20 to N23, N28 to N39, N41 to N64, N80 to N98. As of 2003, also includes U04.

11. Motor vehicle accidents V02 to V04, V09.0, V09.2, V12 to V14, V19.0 to V19.2, V19.4 to V19.6, V20 to V79, V80.3 to V80.5, V81.0 to V81.1, V82.0 to V82.1, V83 to V86, V87.0 to V87.8, V88.0 to V88.8, V89.0, V89.2.

12. Other land transport accidents V01, V05 to V06, V09.1, V09.3 to V09.9, V10 to V11, V15 to V18, V19.3, V19.8 to V19.9, V80.0 to V80.2,

V80.6 to V80.9, V81.2 to V81.9, V82.2 to V82.9, V87.9, V88.9, V89.1, V89.3, V89.9.

13. The following standard symbols are used in this Statistics Canada table: (..) for figures not available for a specific reference period and (...) for figures not applicable.

14. The population estimates used for the 2000 mortality rate calculations are July 1, 2000 updated postcensal estimates, adjusted for net census undercoverage and include non-permanent residents. These population estimates appear in the publication "Annual Demographic Statistics, 2001" (catalogue number 91-213-XIB/XPB).

15. The population estimates used for the 2001 mortality rate calculations are July 1, 2001 updated postcensal estimates, adjusted for net census undercoverage and include non-permanent residents. These population estimates appear in the publication "Annual Demographic Statistics, 2002" (catalogue number 91-213-XIB/XPB).

16. The population estimates used for the 2002 mortality rate calculations are July 1, 2002 updated postcensal estimates, adjusted for net census undercoverage and include non-permanent residents. These population estimates appear in the publication "Annual Demographic Statistics, 2003" (catalogue number 91-213-XIB/XPB).

17. The population estimates used for the 2003 mortality rate calculations are July 1, 2003 updated postcensal estimates, adjusted for net census undercoverage and include non-permanent residents. These population estimates appear in the publication "Annual Demographic Statistics, 2004" (catalogue number 91-213-XIB/XPB).

18. The population estimates used for the 2004 mortality rate calculations are July 1, 2004 updated postcensal estimates, adjusted for net census undercoverage and include non-permanent residents. These population estimates appear in the publication "Annual Demographic Statistics, 2005" (catalogue number 91-213-XIB/XPB).

19. For data year 2005 to 2009, the population estimates used to calculate the mortality rates are presented in the Appendix II of the publication "Mortality Summary List of Causes" (catalogue number 84F0209XIE).

20. The category "Unknown province or territory" refers to deaths of residents of Canada with province or territory of residence unknown. Starting with the 2010 data year, province or territory of residence is imputed where unknown.

21. Starting with the 2010 data year, information regarding the population estimates used for the mortality rate calculations is found in the "Data sources" entry for survey number 3233.

22. The totals (all causes of death) by age group and/ or sex presented in this table may not reflect those given in CANSIM tables 102-0501 to 102-0510, 102-0030 due to the correction of age or sex information that was inconsistent with the underlying cause of death.

23. For reference years 2000 to 2009, the crude and age-standardized mortality rates for the category "Both sexes" have been corrected. The correction affects only the rates for the following 9 sex-specific grouped causes of death: Malignant neoplasm of cervix uteri [C53], Malignant neoplasms of corpus uteri and uterus, part unspecified [C54-C55], Malignant neoplasm of ovary [C56], Malignant neoplasm of prostate [C61], Hyperplasia of prostate [N40], Inflammatory diseases of female pelvic organs [N70-N76], Pregnancy, childbirth and the puerperium [O00-O99], Pregnancy with abortive outcome [O00-O07] and Other complications of pregnancy, childbirth and the puerperium [O10-O99]. Prior to the correction, the rates for these 9 groups were calculated using either the male or female population; the corrected values use the combined male-female population, making them consistent with the 2010 and 2011 rates.

24. During the production of each year's birth/death/stillbirth statistics, data from previous years may be revised to reflect any updates or changes that have been received from the provincial and territorial vital statistics registrars.

25. Starting with the 2013 reference year, information regarding new and terminated cause of death codes, as well as any changes to the cause of death descriptions, are available upon request; please contact Statistics Canada's Statistical Information Service (toll-free 1-800-263-1136; 514-283-8300; STATCAN.infostats-infostats.STATCAN@Canada.ca).

26. The 2011 Canadian population is used as the standard population for the calculation of the age-standardized mortality rates presented in this table. Age-standardization removes the effects of differences in the age structure of populations among areas and over time. Age-standardized mortality rates show the number of deaths per 1,000 population (or 100,000 population) that would have occurred in a given area if the age structure of the population of that area was the same as the age structure of a specified standard population. For age-standardized mortality rates using the 1991 Canadian Census of Population, see CANSIM table 102-0552. Further information on age-standardized mortality rates can be found in Vital Statistics Death Database - Glossary (http://www23.statcan.gc.ca/imdb-bmdi/document/3233_D4_T9_V1-eng.htm).

27. Starting with the 2013 reference year, a new coding system was used to select the underlying cause of death. For more information or to obtain documentation regarding the impact of this change, please contact Statistics Canada's Statistical Information Service (toll-free 1-800-263-1136; 514-283-8300; STATCAN.infostats-infostats.STATCAN@Canada.ca).

Source: Statistics Canada. *Table 102-0553 - Deaths and mortality rate (age standardization using 2011 population), by selected grouped causes and sex, Canada, provinces and territories, annual,* CANSIM (database). (accessed: April 11, 2017)

Graph 1: Median wait between referral by GP and appointment with specialist, by province, 1993 and 2016

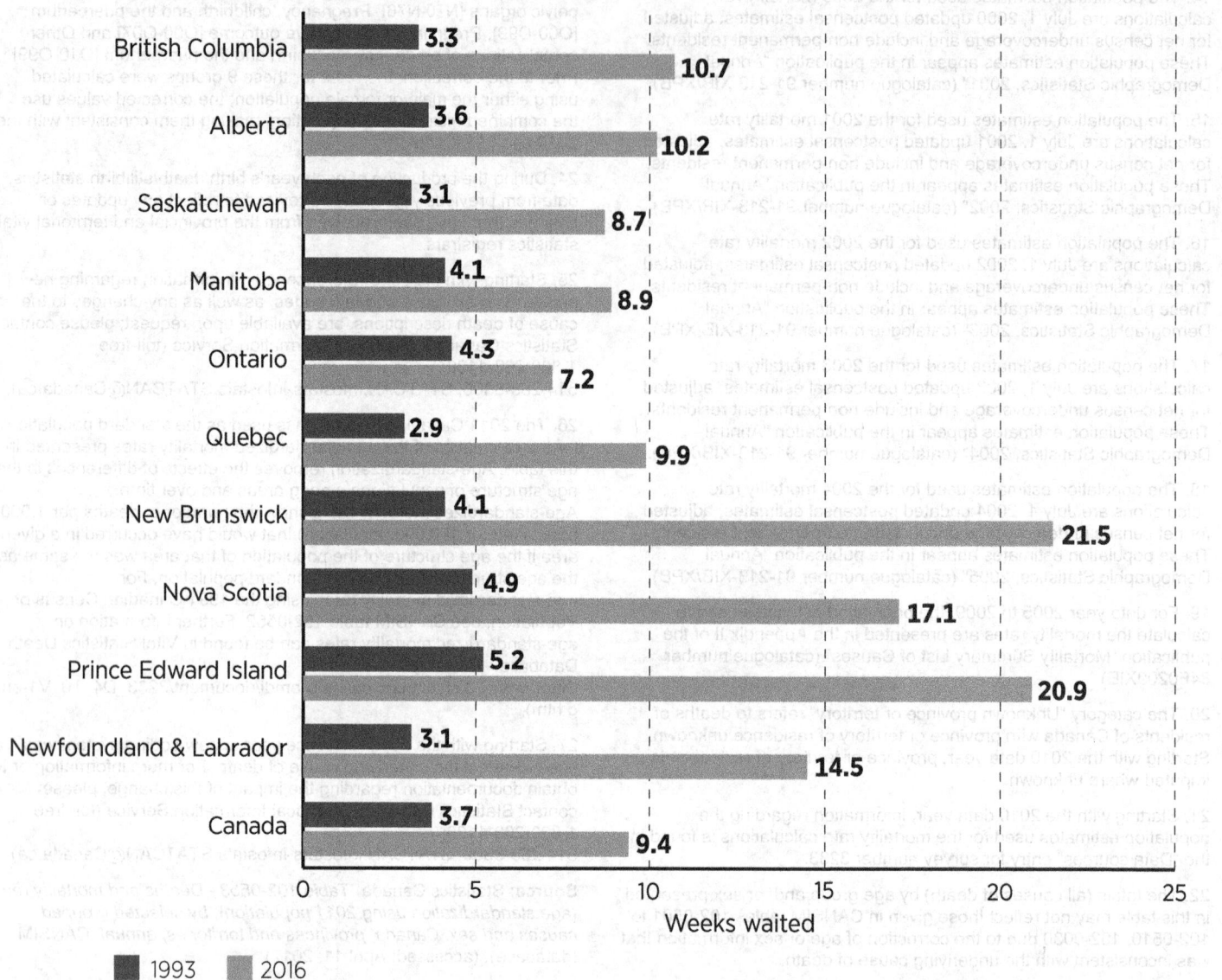

Province	1993	2016
British Columbia	3.3	10.7
Alberta	3.6	10.2
Saskatchewan	3.1	8.7
Manitoba	4.1	8.9
Ontario	4.3	7.2
Quebec	2.9	9.9
New Brunswick	4.1	21.5
Nova Scotia	4.9	17.1
Prince Edward Island	5.2	20.9
Newfoundland & Labrador	3.1	14.5
Canada	3.7	9.4

Weeks waited

■ 1993 ■ 2016

Source: The Fraser Institute's national waiting list survey, 2016; *Waiting Your Turn, 1997.*

Graph 2: Median wait between referral by GP and appointment with specialist, by specialty, 1993 and 2016

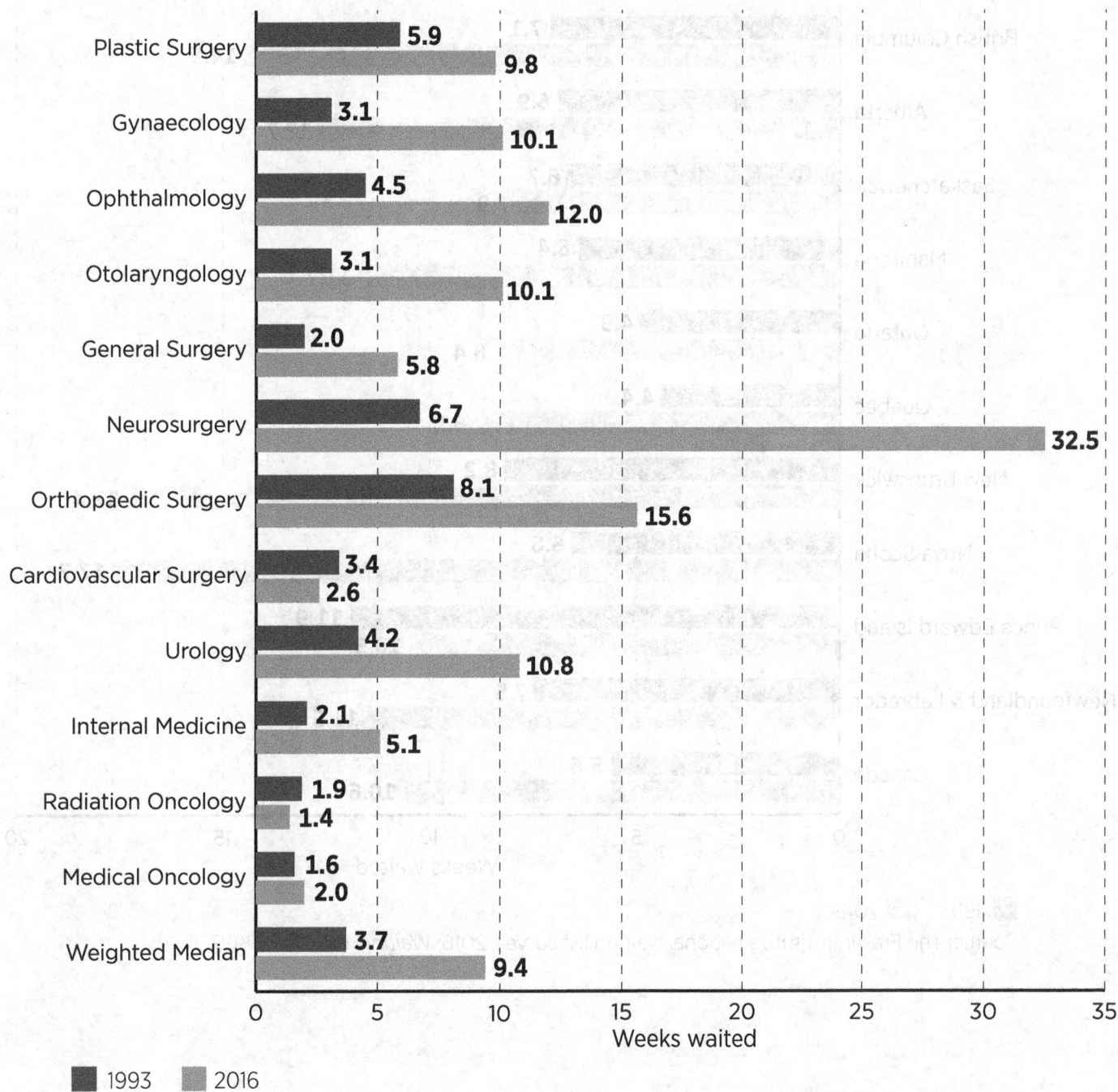

Plastic Surgery
- 5.9
- 9.8

Gynaecology
- 3.1
- 10.1

Ophthalmology
- 4.5
- 12.0

Otolaryngology
- 3.1
- 10.1

General Surgery
- 2.0
- 5.8

Neurosurgery
- 6.7
- 32.5

Orthopaedic Surgery
- 8.1
- 15.6

Cardiovascular Surgery
- 3.4
- 2.6

Urology
- 4.2
- 10.8

Internal Medicine
- 2.1
- 5.1

Radiation Oncology
- 1.9
- 1.4

Medical Oncology
- 1.6
- 2.0

Weighted Median
- 3.7
- 9.4

Weeks waited (0, 5, 10, 15, 20, 25, 30, 35)

■ 1993 ■ 2016

Source: The Fraser Institute's national waiting list survey, 2016; *Waiting Your Turn, 1997.*

Graph 3: Median wait between appointment with specialist and treatment, by province, 1993 and 2016

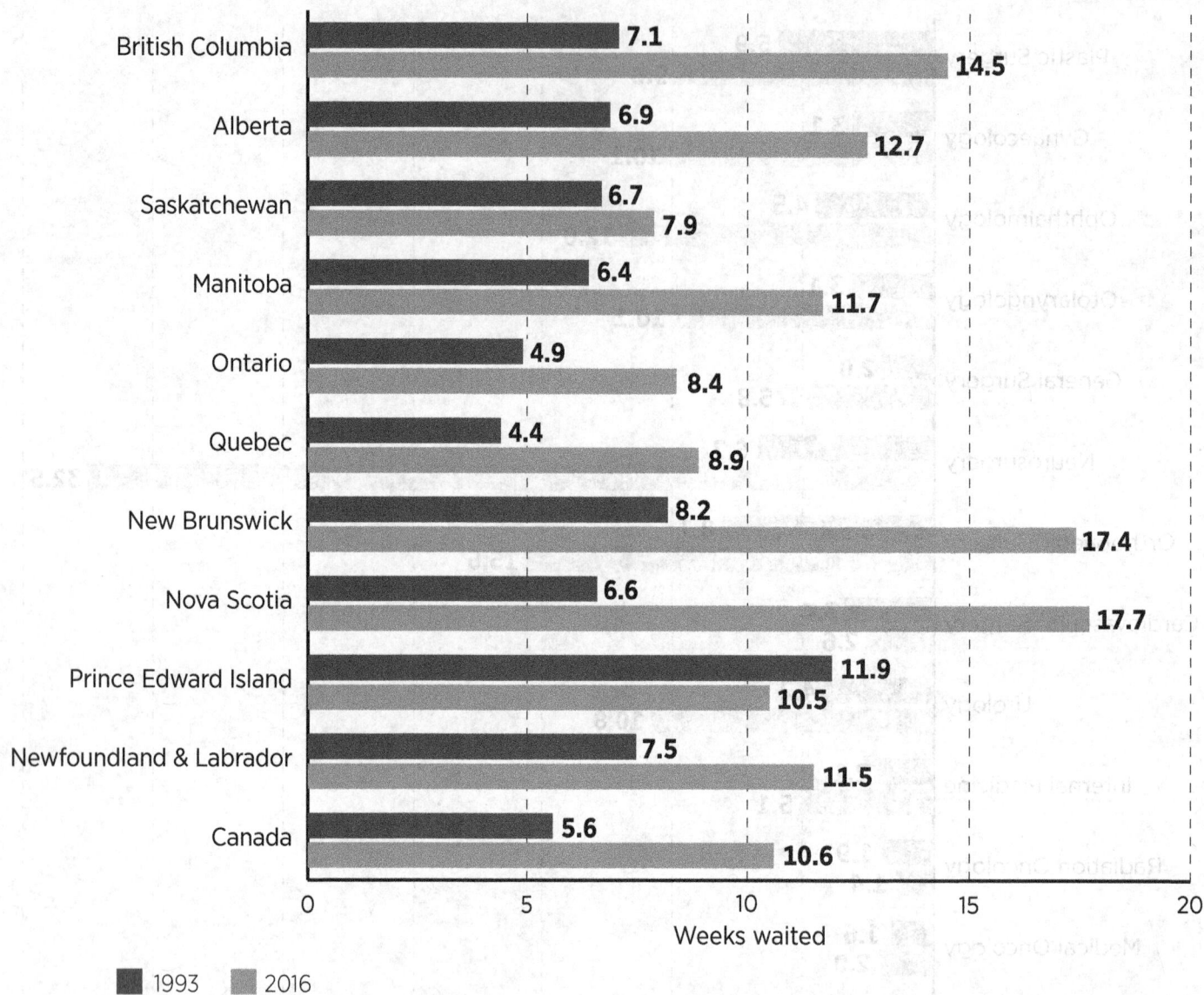

Province	1993	2016
British Columbia	7.1	14.5
Alberta	6.9	12.7
Saskatchewan	6.7	7.9
Manitoba	6.4	11.7
Ontario	4.9	8.4
Quebec	4.4	8.9
New Brunswick	8.2	17.4
Nova Scotia	6.6	17.7
Prince Edward Island	11.9	10.5
Newfoundland & Labrador	7.5	11.5
Canada	5.6	10.6

Weeks waited

■ 1993 ■ 2016

Source: The Fraser Institute's national waiting list survey, 2016; *Waiting Your Turn, 1997*.

Source: © Bacchus Barua and Feixue Ren (2016). Waiting Your Turn: Wait Times for Health Care in Canada, 2016 Report. *Fraser Institute.* https://www.fraserinstitute.org/studies/waiting-your-turn-wait-times-for-health-care-in-canada-2016. *Accessed March 2, 2017.*

Graph 4: Median wait between appointment with specialist and treatment, by specialty, 1993 and 2016

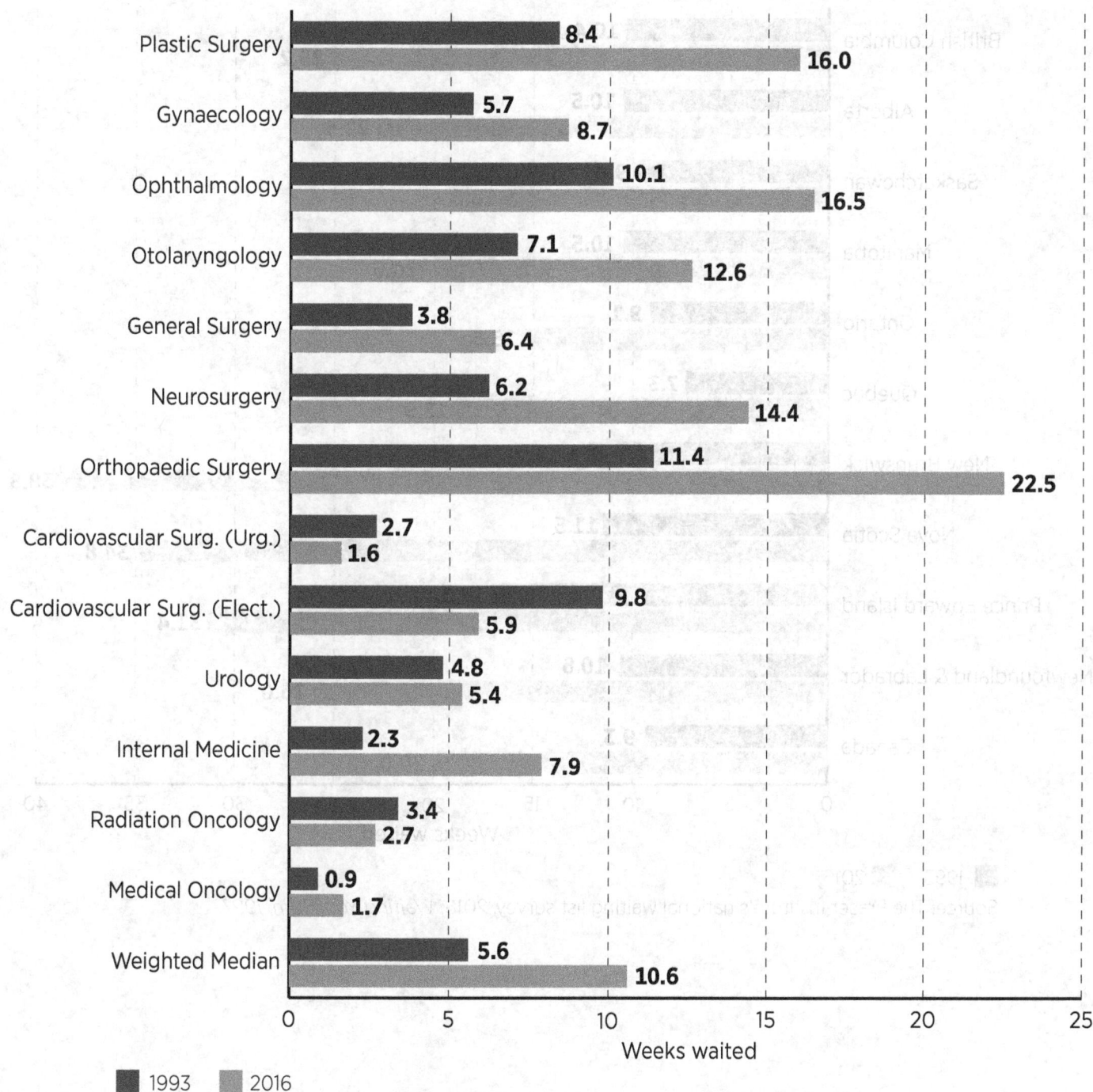

Specialty	1993	2016
Plastic Surgery	8.4	16.0
Gynaecology	5.7	8.7
Ophthalmology	10.1	16.5
Otolaryngology	7.1	12.6
General Surgery	3.8	6.4
Neurosurgery	6.2	14.4
Orthopaedic Surgery	11.4	22.5
Cardiovascular Surg. (Urg.)	2.7	1.6
Cardiovascular Surg. (Elect.)	9.8	5.9
Urology	4.8	5.4
Internal Medicine	2.3	7.9
Radiation Oncology	3.4	2.7
Medical Oncology	0.9	1.7
Weighted Median	5.6	10.6

Weeks waited

■ 1993 ■ 2016

Source: The Fraser Institute's national waiting list survey, 2016; *Waiting Your Turn, 1997.*

Source: © Bacchus Barua and Feixue Ren (2016). Waiting Your Turn: Wait Times for Health Care in Canada, 2016 Report. *Fraser Institute.* *https://www.fraserinstitute.org/studies/waiting-your-turn-wait-times-for-health-care-in-canada-2016. Accessed March 2, 2017.*

Graph 5: Median wait between referral by GP and treatment, by province, 1993 and 2016

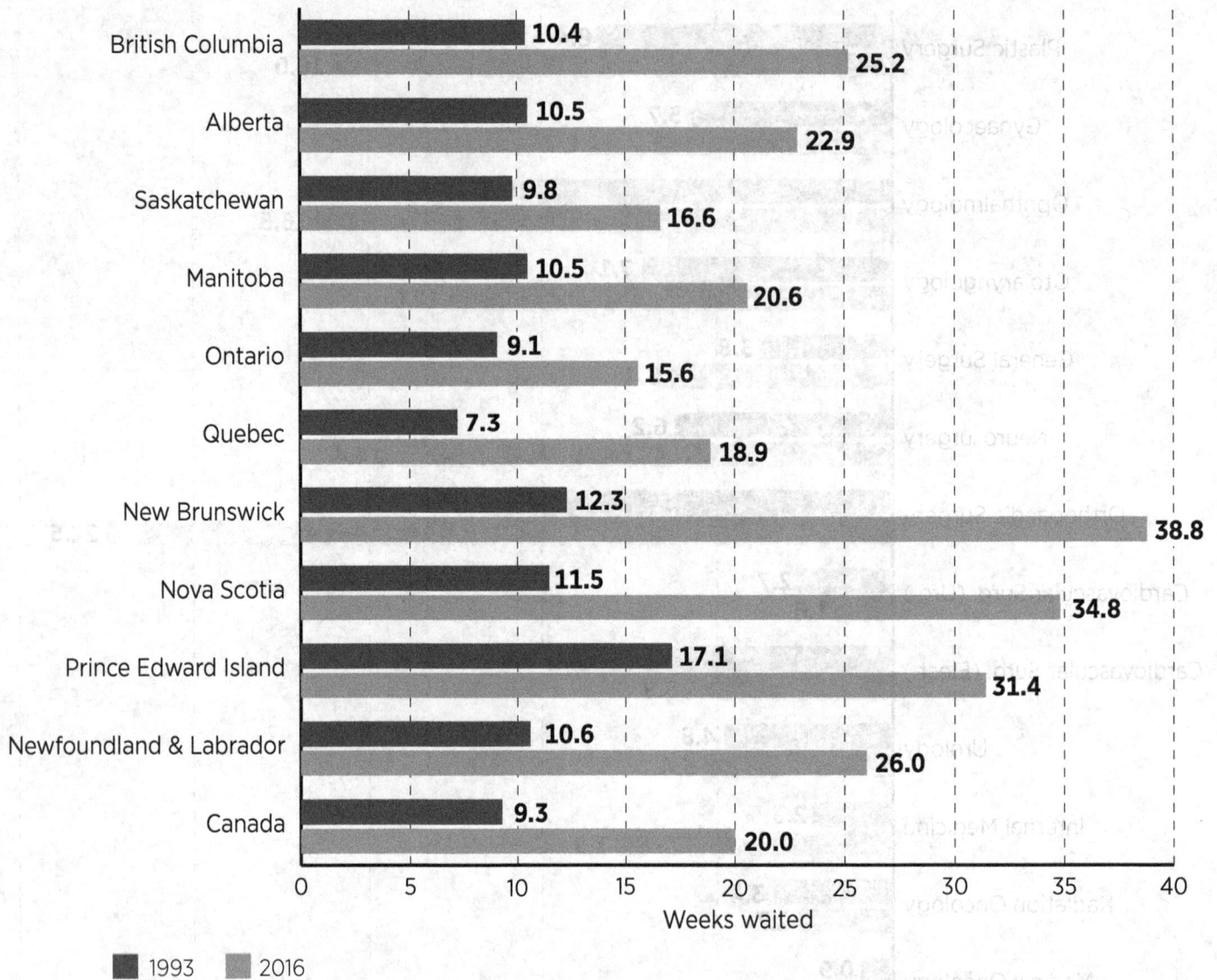

Province	1993	2016
British Columbia	10.4	25.2
Alberta	10.5	22.9
Saskatchewan	9.8	16.6
Manitoba	10.5	20.6
Ontario	9.1	15.6
Quebec	7.3	18.9
New Brunswick	12.3	38.8
Nova Scotia	11.5	34.8
Prince Edward Island	17.1	31.4
Newfoundland & Labrador	10.6	26.0
Canada	9.3	20.0

Weeks waited

■ 1993 ■ 2016

Source: The Fraser Institute's national waiting list survey, 2016; *Waiting Your Turn, 1997.*

Graph 6: Median wait between referral by GP and treatment, by specialty, 1993 and 2016

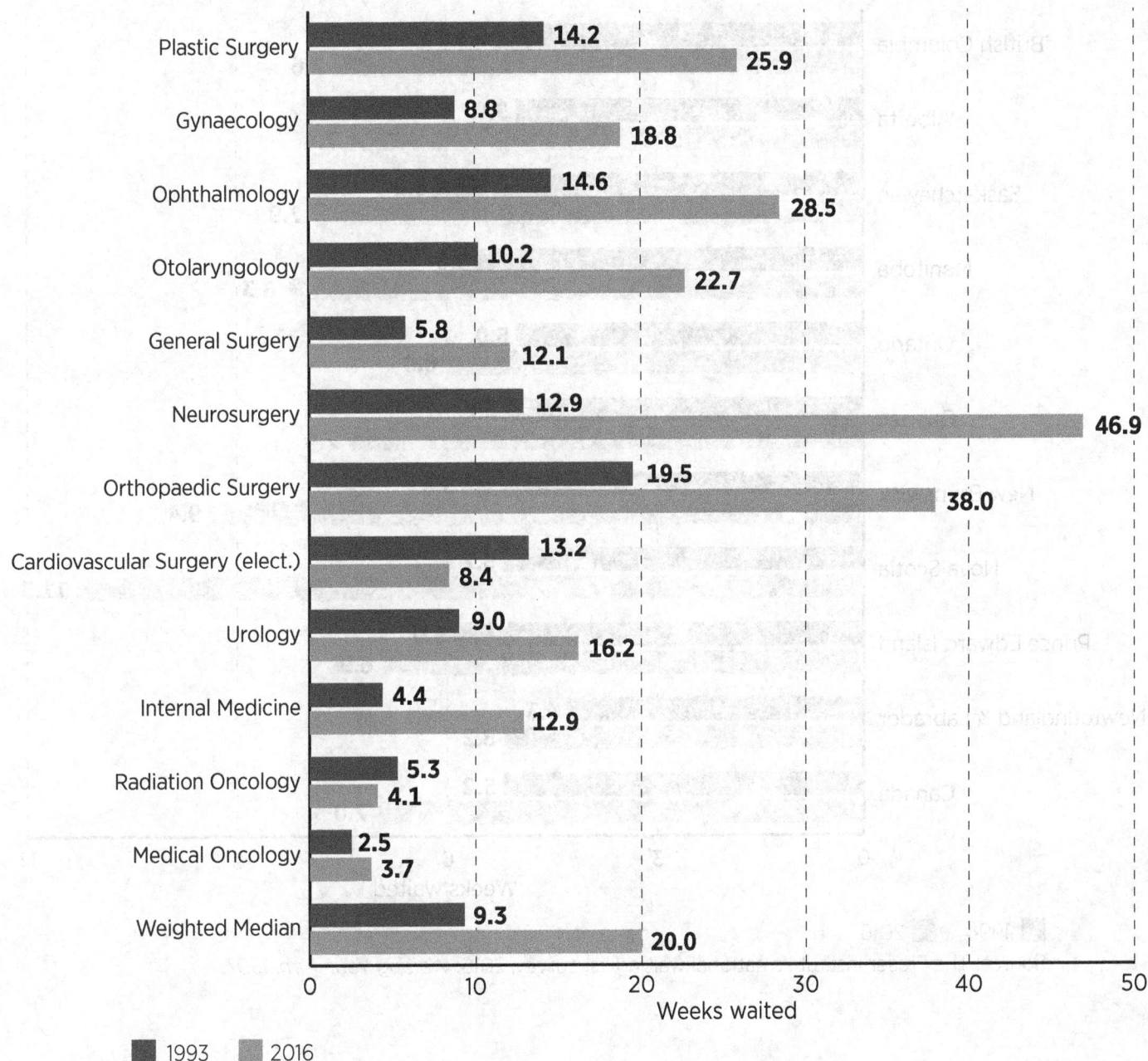

Specialty	1993	2016
Plastic Surgery	14.2	25.9
Gynaecology	8.8	18.8
Ophthalmology	14.6	28.5
Otolaryngology	10.2	22.7
General Surgery	5.8	12.1
Neurosurgery	12.9	46.9
Orthopaedic Surgery	19.5	38.0
Cardiovascular Surgery (elect.)	13.2	8.4
Urology	9.0	16.2
Internal Medicine	4.4	12.9
Radiation Oncology	5.3	4.1
Medical Oncology	2.5	3.7
Weighted Median	9.3	20.0

Weeks waited

■ 1993 ■ 2016

Source: The Fraser Institute's national waiting list survey, 2016; *Waiting Your Turn, 1997.*

Graph 7: Median reasonable wait between appointment with specialist and treatment, by province, 1994 and 2016

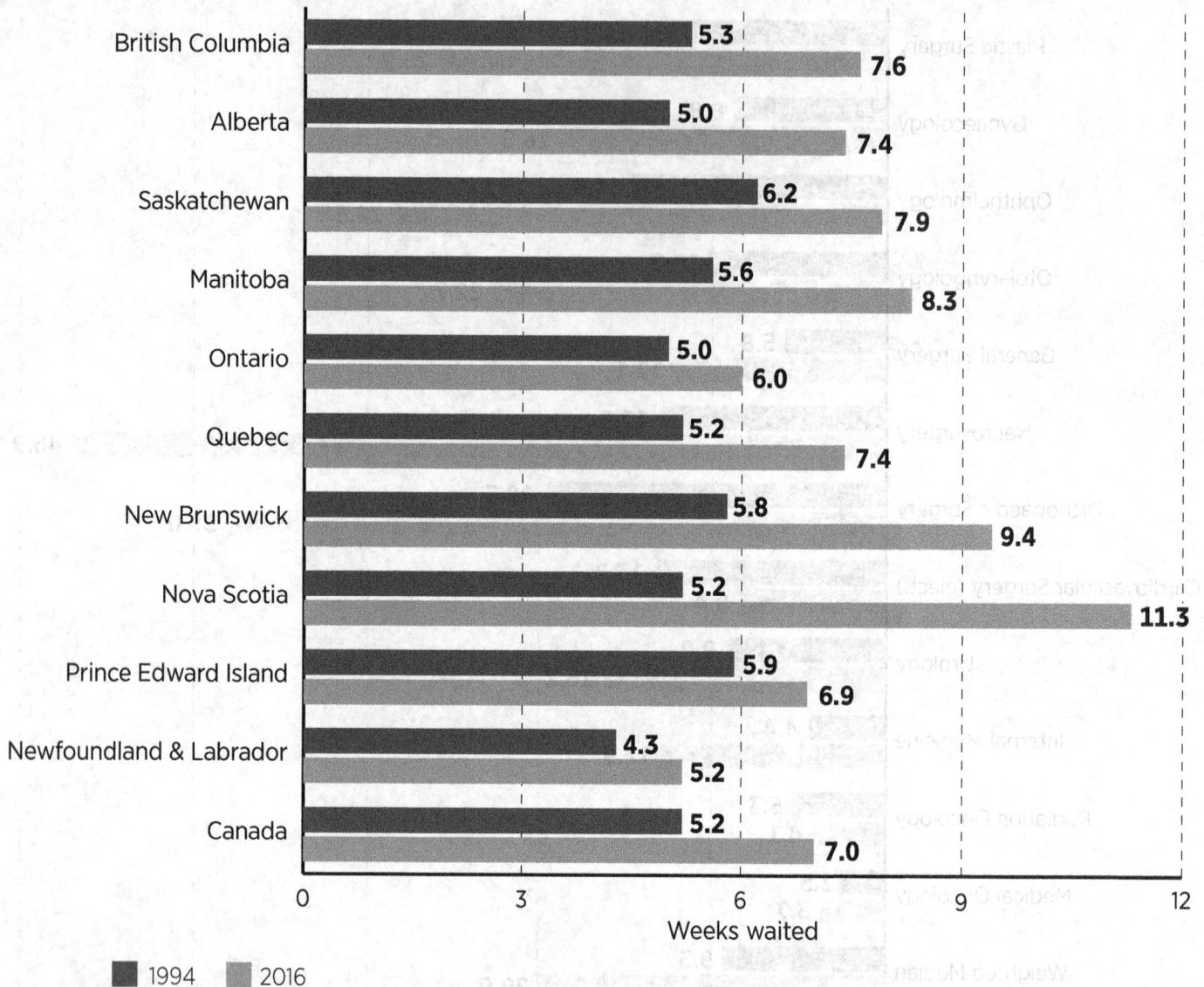

Province	1994	2016
British Columbia	5.3	7.6
Alberta	5.0	7.4
Saskatchewan	6.2	7.9
Manitoba	5.6	8.3
Ontario	5.0	6.0
Quebec	5.2	7.4
New Brunswick	5.8	9.4
Nova Scotia	5.2	11.3
Prince Edward Island	5.9	6.9
Newfoundland & Labrador	4.3	5.2
Canada	5.2	7.0

Weeks waited

■ 1994 ■ 2016

Source: The Fraser Institute's national waiting list survey, 2016; *Waiting Your Turn, 1997.*

Source: © Bacchus Barua and Feixue Ren (2016). Waiting Your Turn: Wait Times for Health Care in Canada, 2016 Report. *Fraser Institute. https://www.fraserinstitute.org/studies/waiting-your-turn-wait-times-for-health-care-in-canada-2016. Accessed March 2, 2017.*

Graph 8: Median reasonable wait between appointment with specialist and treatment, by specialty, 1994 and 2016

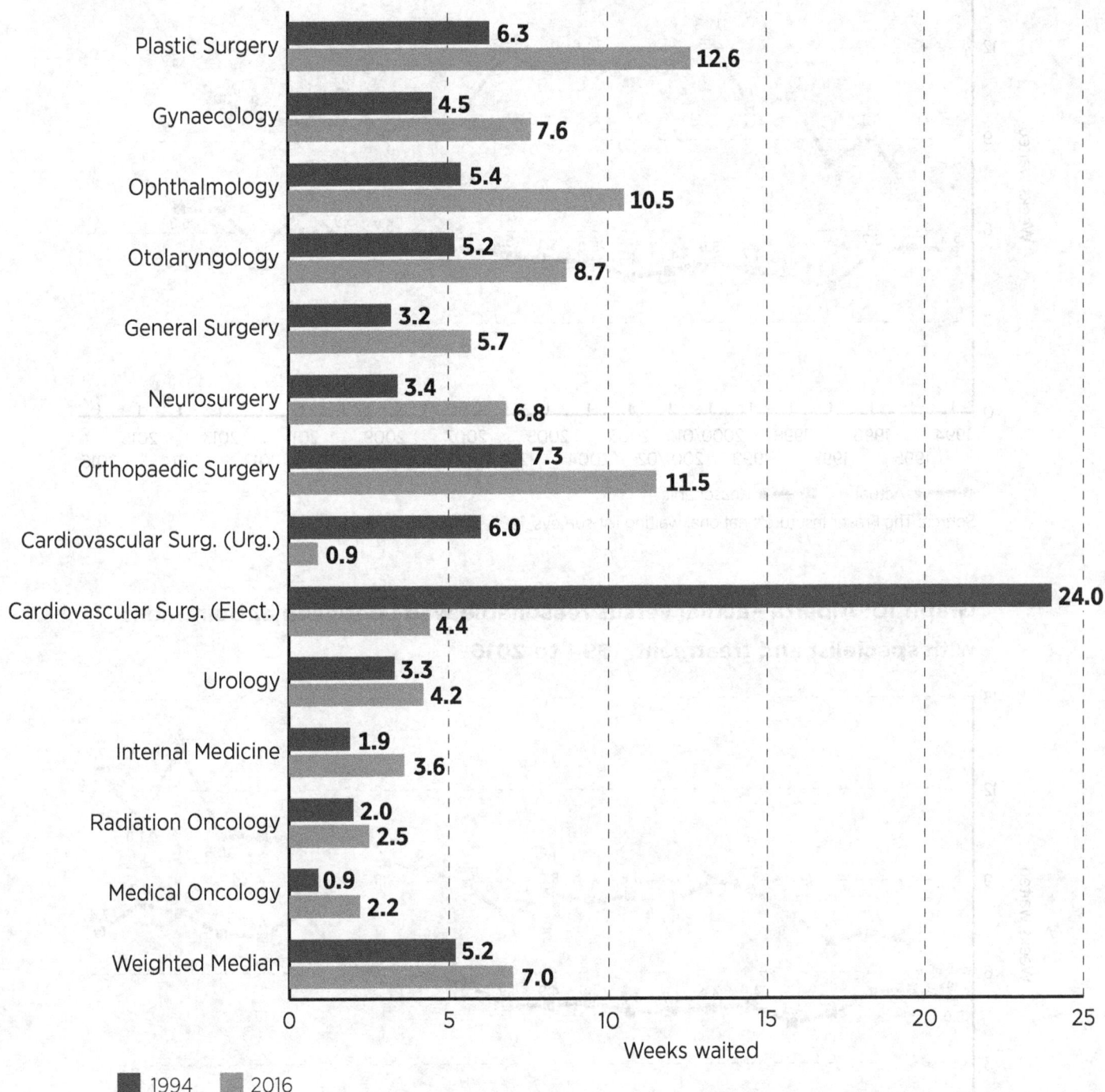

Specialty	1994	2016
Plastic Surgery	6.3	12.6
Gynaecology	4.5	7.6
Ophthalmology	5.4	10.5
Otolaryngology	5.2	8.7
General Surgery	3.2	5.7
Neurosurgery	3.4	6.8
Orthopaedic Surgery	7.3	11.5
Cardiovascular Surg. (Urg.)	6.0	0.9
Cardiovascular Surg. (Elect.)	24.0	4.4
Urology	3.3	4.2
Internal Medicine	1.9	3.6
Radiation Oncology	2.0	2.5
Medical Oncology	0.9	2.2
Weighted Median	5.2	7.0

Weeks waited

■ 1994   ■ 2016

Source: The Fraser Institute's national waiting list survey, 2016; *Waiting Your Turn, 1997*.

Source: © Bacchus Barua and Feixue Ren (2016). Waiting Your Turn: Wait Times for Health Care in Canada, 2016 Report. *Fraser Institute.* *https://www.fraserinstitute.org/studies/waiting-your-turn-wait-times-for-health-care-in-canada-2016. Accessed March 2, 2017.*

Graph 9: British Columbia—actual versus reasonable waits between appointment with specialist and treatment, 1994 to 2016

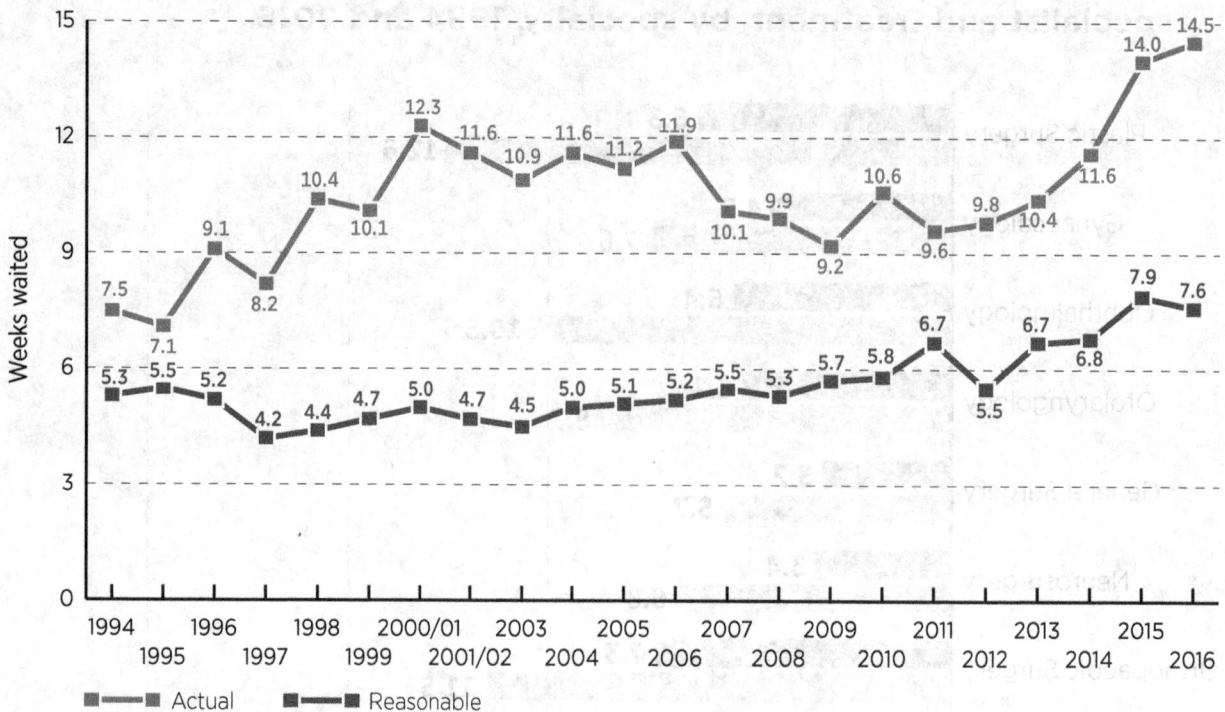

Source: The Fraser Institute's national waiting list surveys, 1995–2016.

Graph 10: Alberta—actual versus reasonable waits between appointment with specialist and treatment, 1994 to 2016

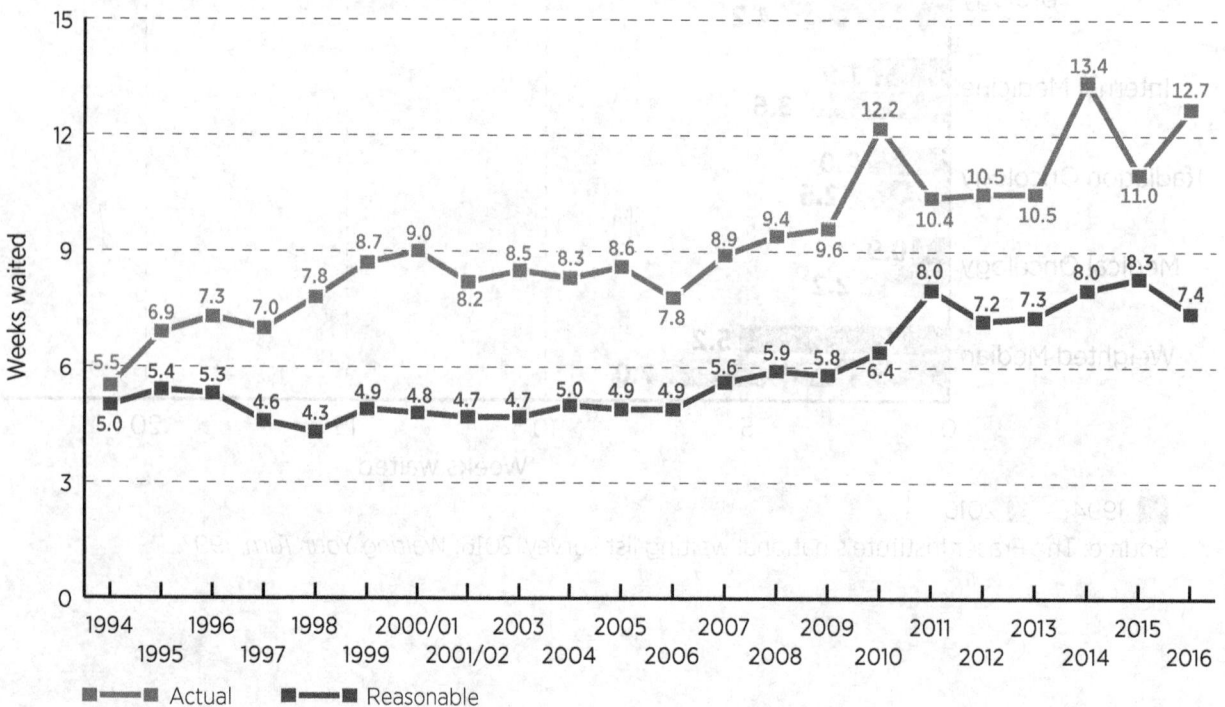

Source: The Fraser Institute's national waiting list surveys, 1995–2016.

Source: © Bacchus Barua and Feixue Ren (2016). Waiting Your Turn: Wait Times for Health Care in Canada, 2016 Report. Fraser Institute. https://www.fraserinstitute.org/studies/waiting-your-turn-wait-times-for-health-care-in-canada-2016. Accessed March 2, 2017.

Graph 11: Saskatchewan—actual versus reasonable waits between appointment with specialist and treatment, 1994 to 2016

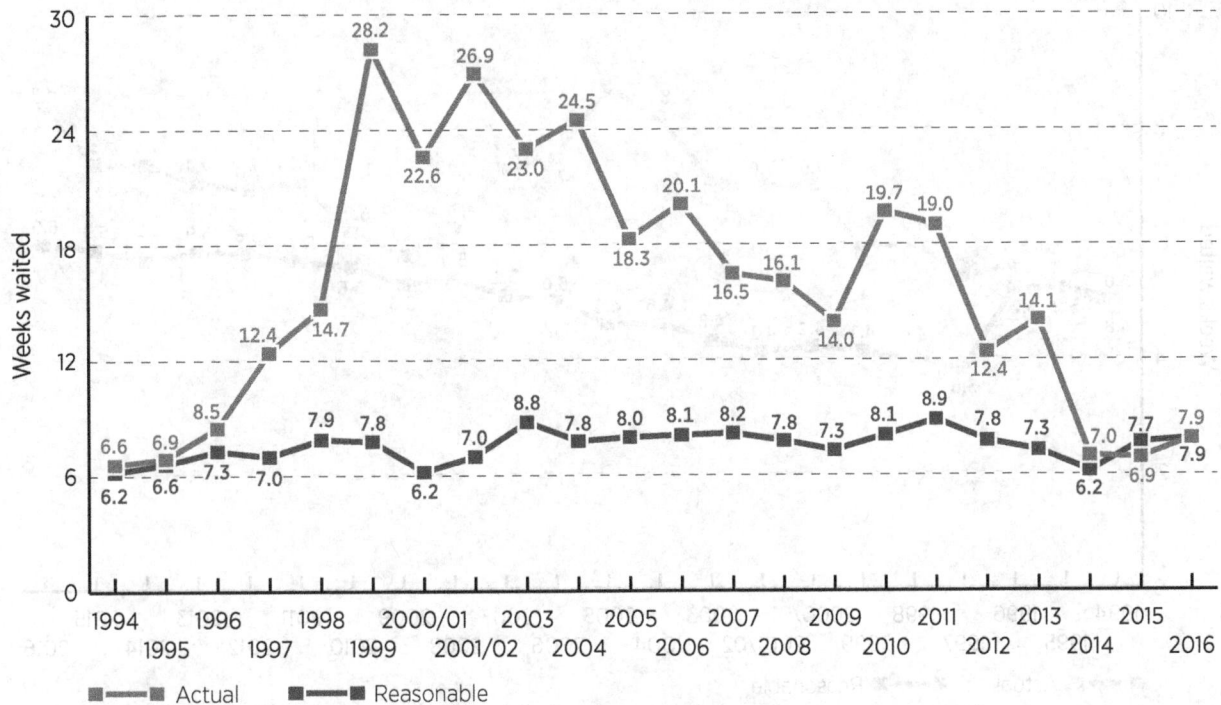

Actual ■——■ Reasonable

Source: The Fraser Institute's national waiting list surveys, 1995–2016.

Graph 12: Manitoba—actual versus reasonable waits between appointment with specialist and treatment, 1994 to 2016

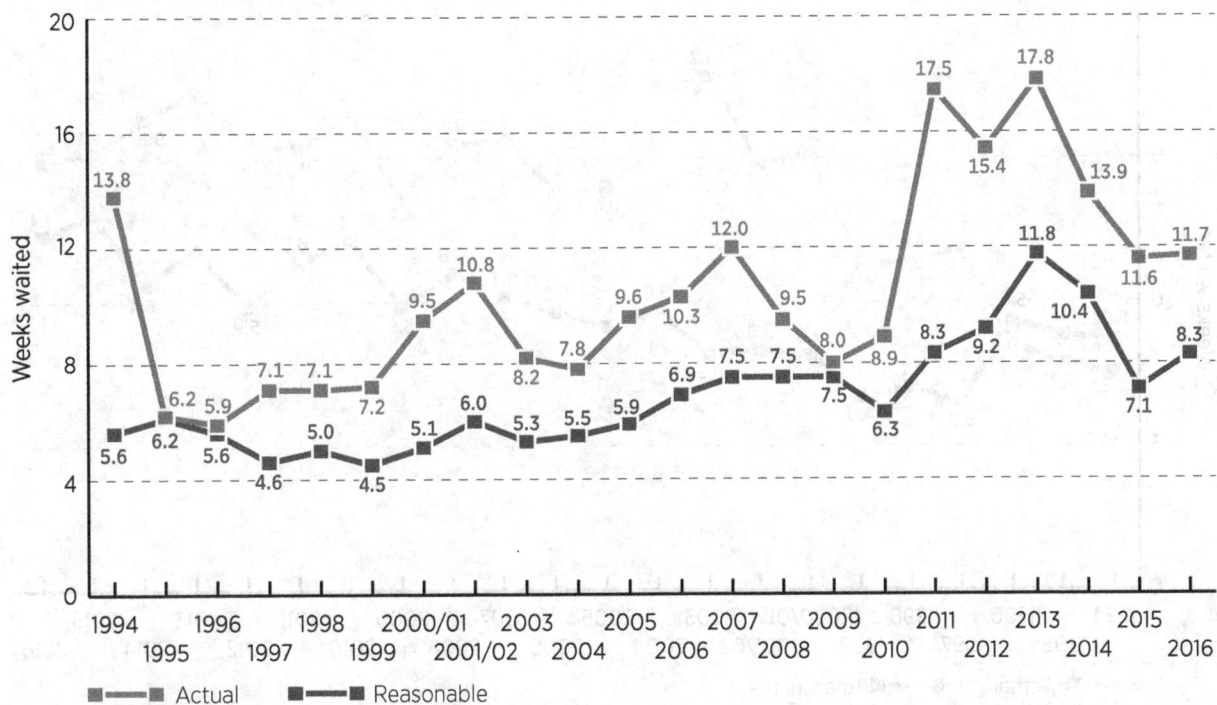

Actual ■——■ Reasonable

Source: The Fraser Institute's national waiting list surveys, 1995–2016.

Source: © Bacchus Barua and Feixue Ren (2016). Waiting Your Turn: Wait Times for Health Care in Canada, 2016 Report. *Fraser Institute.* https://www.fraserinstitute.org/studies/waiting-your-turn-wait-times-for-health-care-in-canada-2016. Accessed March 2, 2017.

Graph 13: Ontario—actual versus reasonable waits between appointment with specialist and treatment, 1994 to 2016

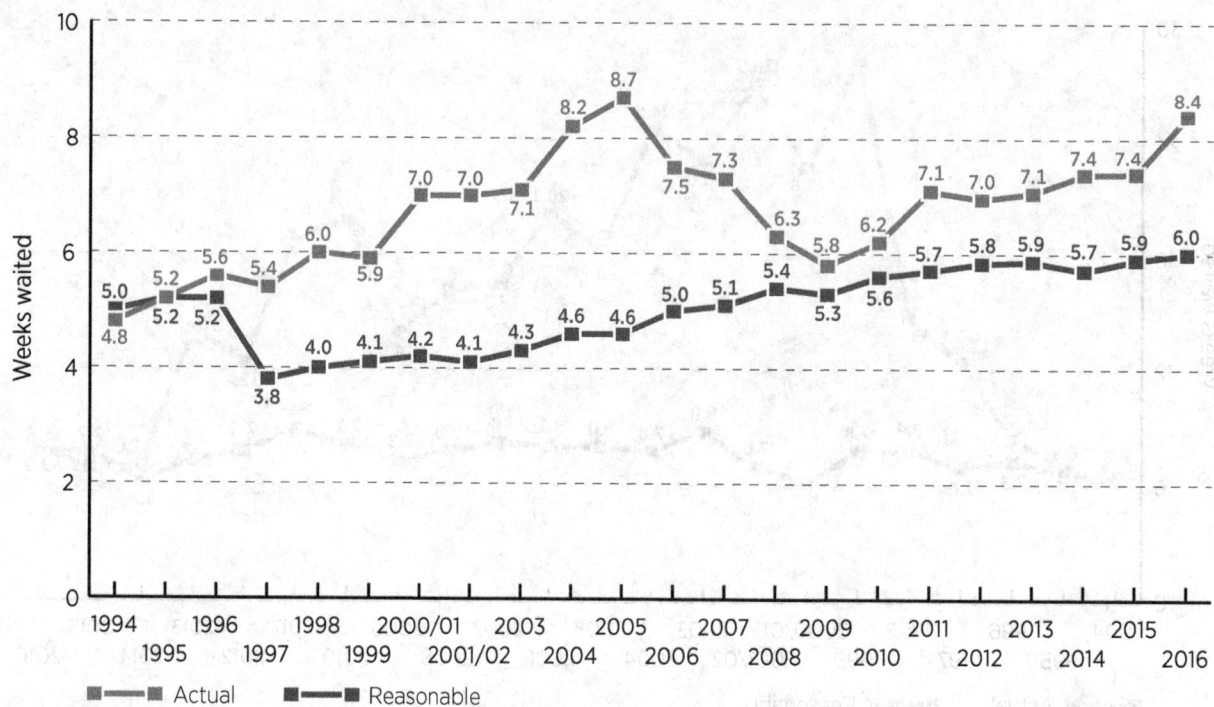

Source: The Fraser Institute's national waiting list surveys, 1995–2016.

Graph 14: Quebec—actual versus reasonable waits between appointment with specialist and treatment, 1994 to 2016

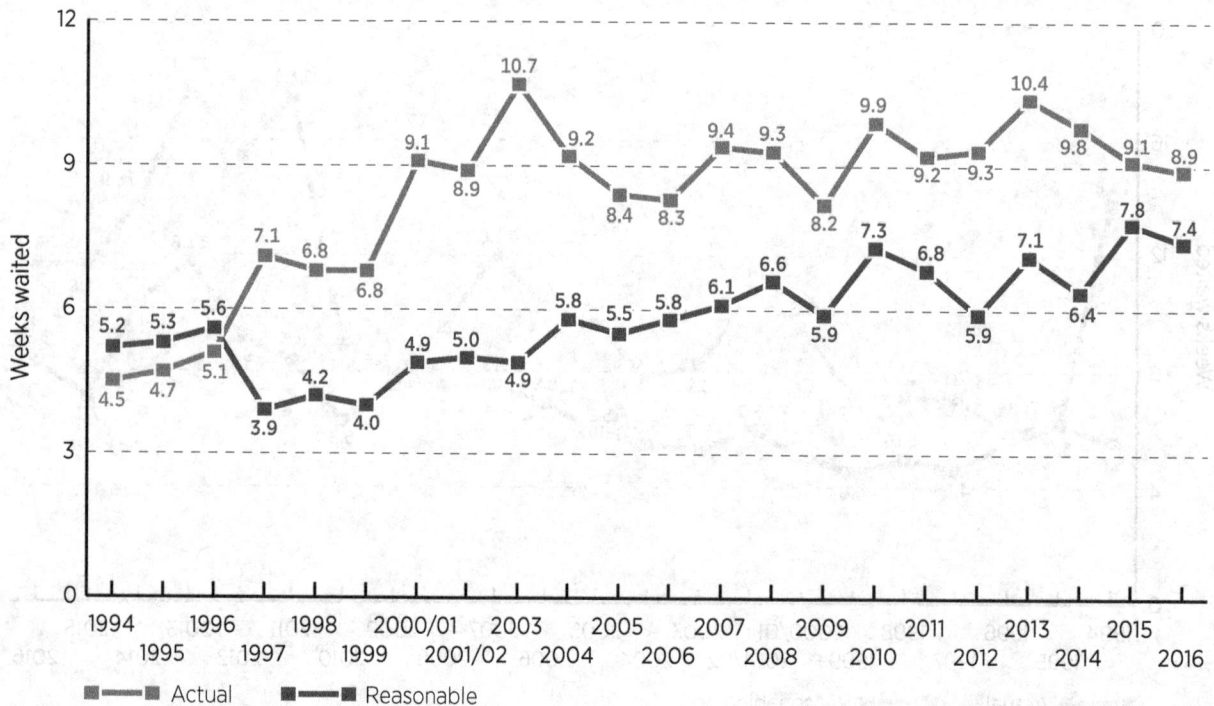

Source: The Fraser Institute's national waiting list surveys, 1995–2016.

Graph 15: New Brunswick—actual versus reasonable waits between appointment with specialist and treatment, 1994 to 2016

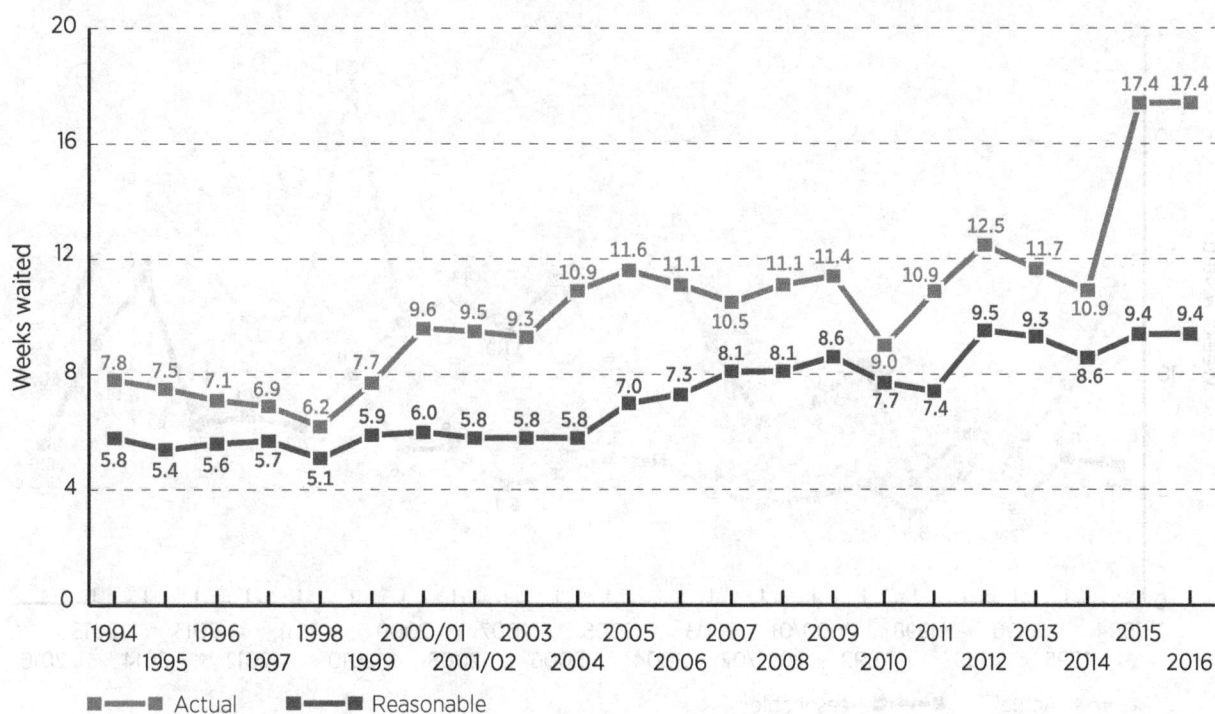

Actual ◼ Reasonable ◼

Source: The Fraser Institute's national waiting list surveys, 1995–2016.

Graph 16: Nova Scotia—actual versus reasonable waits between appointment with specialist and treatment, 1994 to 2016

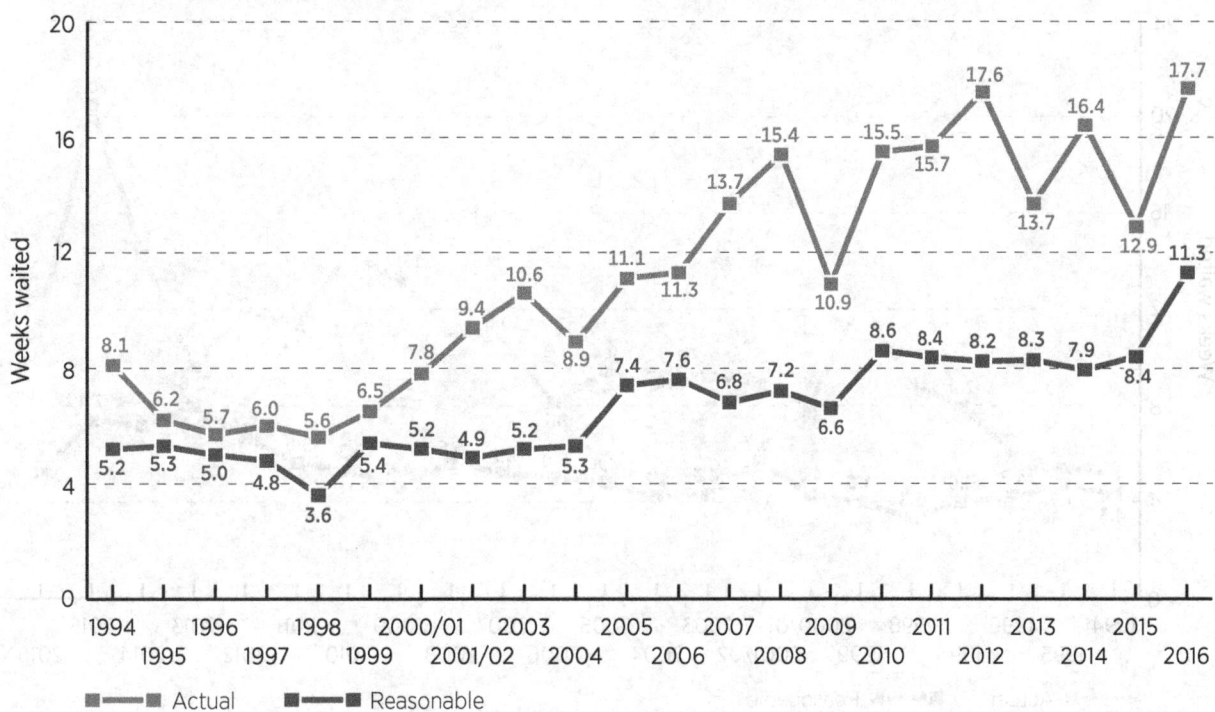

Actual ◼ Reasonable ◼

Source: The Fraser Institute's national waiting list surveys, 1995–2016.

Source: © Bacchus Barua and Feixue Ren (2016). Waiting Your Turn: Wait Times for Health Care in Canada, 2016 Report. Fraser Institute. https://www.fraserinstitute.org/studies/waiting-your-turn-wait-times-for-health-care-in-canada-2016. Accessed March 2, 2017.

Graph 17: Prince Edward Island—actual versus reasonable waits between appointment with specialist and treatment, 1994 to 2016

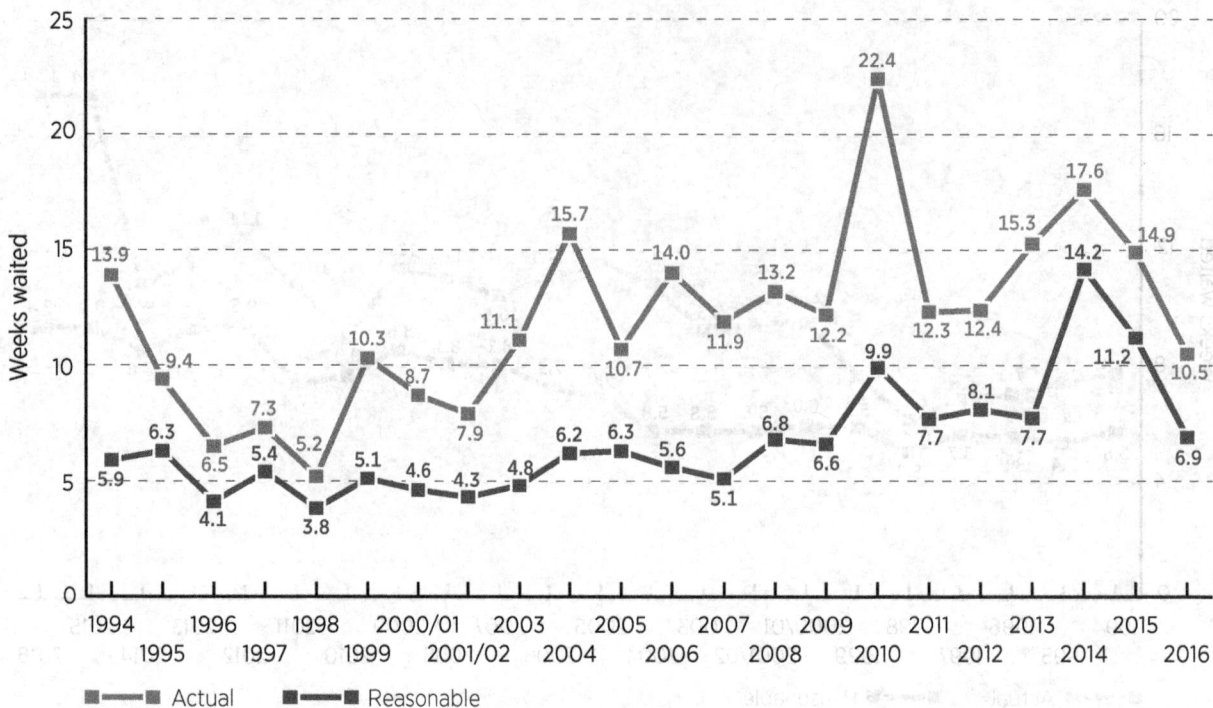

Source: The Fraser Institute's national waiting list surveys, 1995–2016.

Graph 18: Newfoundland & Labrador—actual versus reasonable waits between appointment with specialist and treatment, 1994 to 2016

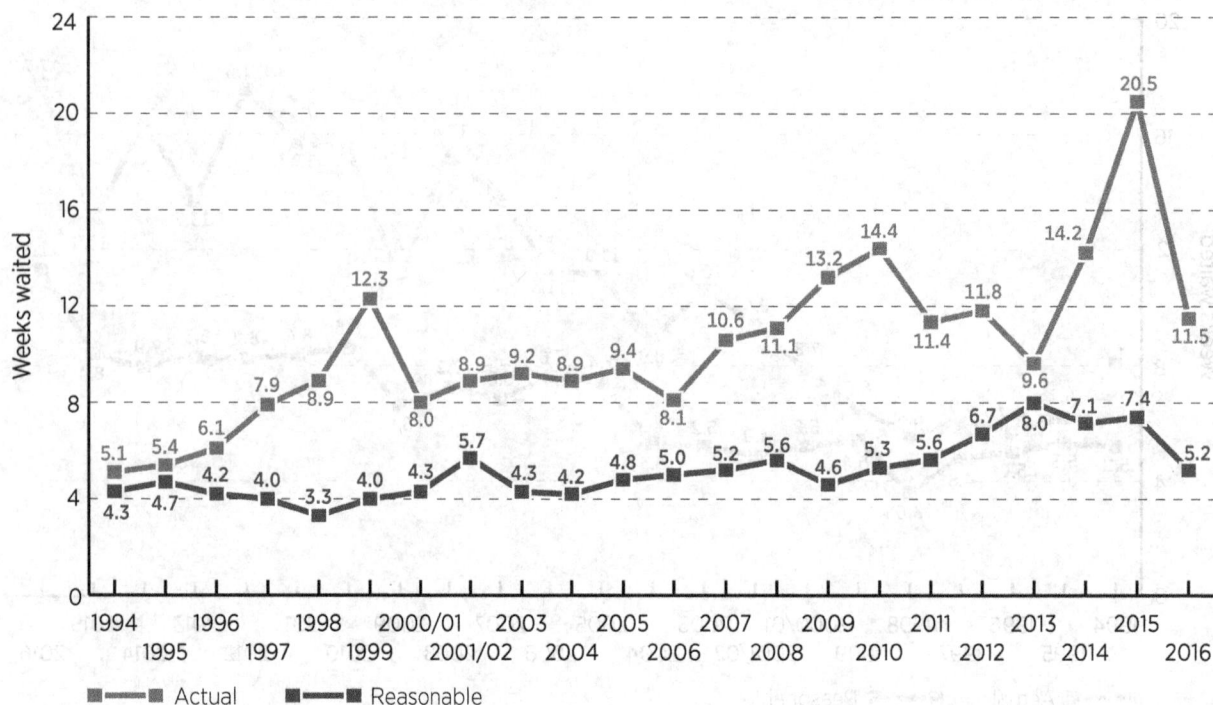

Source: The Fraser Institute's national waiting list surveys, 1995–2016.

Source: © Bacchus Barua and Feixue Ren (2016). Waiting Your Turn: Wait Times for Health Care in Canada, 2016 Report. Fraser Institute. https://www.fraserinstitute.org/studies/waiting-your-turn-wait-times-for-health-care-in-canada-2016. Accessed March 2, 2017.

Graph 19: Canada—actual versus reasonable waits between appointment with specialist and treatment, 1994 to 2016

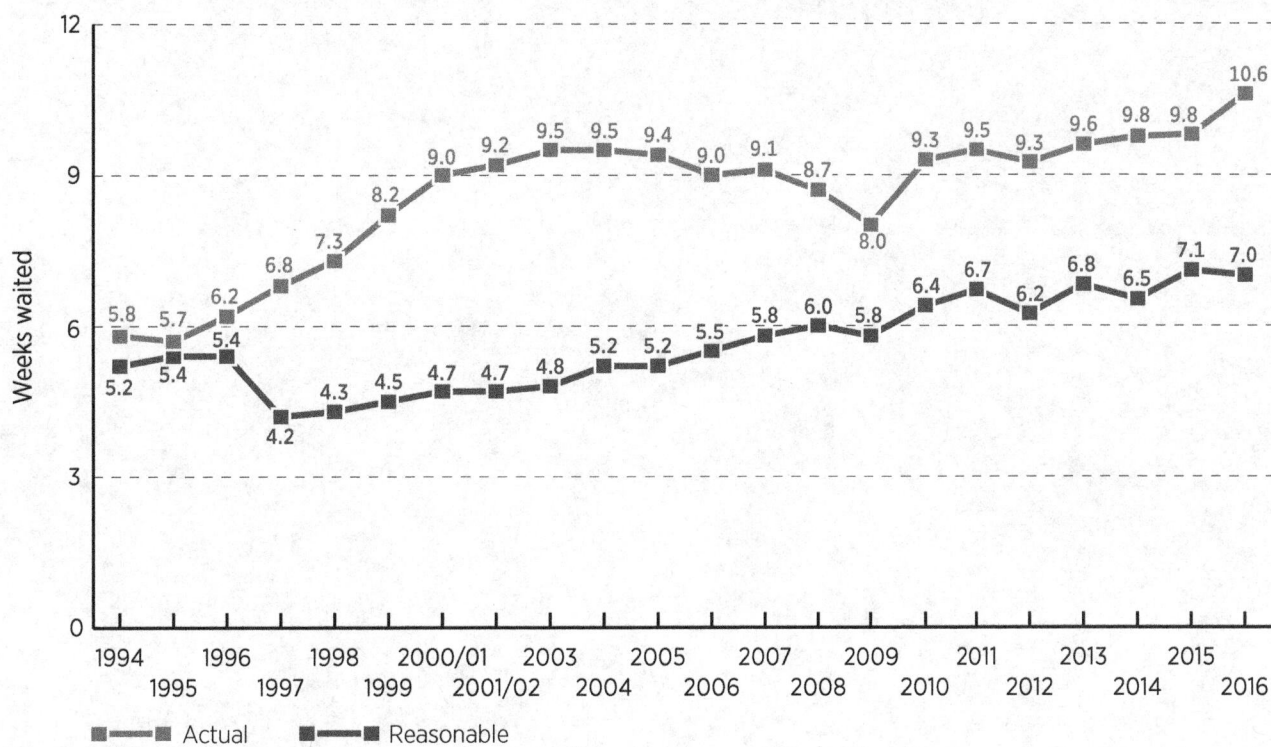

Source: The Fraser Institute's national waiting list surveys, 1995–2016.

Actual — *Reasonable*

Sources for Disease Descriptions

"A Brief History of HIV/AIDS in Canada," Public Health Agency of Canada, last modified September 25, 2011, accessed March 20, 2013, http://www.phac-aspc.gc.ca/aids-sida/info/1-eng.php.

"About Blood Disorders," Canadian Stem Cell Foundation, accessed April 23, 2015, http://stemcellfoundation.ca/en/disease/blood-disorders.

"About Celiac Disease," Canadian Celiac Association, accessed March 20, 2013, http://www.celiac.ca/index.php/about-celiac-disease-2/symptoms-treatment-cd (page no longer available; please see http://www.celiac.ca).

"Achalasia - Esophageal achalasia," PubMed Health, U.S. National Library of Medicine, last modified January 20, 2010, accessed March 6, 2013, http://www.ncbi.nlm.nih.gov/pubmedhealth/PMH0001313 (page no longer available; please see http://www.ncbi.nlm.nih.gov).

"Acne Treatments," *Healthy Living*, Health Canada, last modified December 15, 2006, accessed March 13, 2013, http://www.hc-sc.gc.ca/hl-vs/iyh-vsv/med/acne-eng.php (page no longer available; please see http://www.canada.ca/en/health-canada/services/drugs-medical-devices/acne-treatments.html).

"Addison's disease," Mayo Foundation for Medical Education and Research, last modified December 4, 2012, accessed March 20, 2013, http://www.mayoclinic.com/health/addisons-disease/DS00361

"Addison's disease: Adrenocortical hypofunction; Chronic adrenocortical insufficiency; Primary adrenal insufficiency," PubMed Health, U.S. National Library of Medicine, last modified December 11, 2011, accessed March 20, 2013, http://www.ncbi.nlm.nih.gov/pubmedhealth/PMH0001416 (page no longer available; please see http://www.ncbi.nlm.nih.gov).

ADHD Canada, accessed March 20, 2013, http://www.adhdcanada.com (site discontinued).

"Adjusted disorder," *MedlinePlus*, U.S. National Library of Medicine, last modified July 7, 2012, accessed March 20, 2013, http://www.nlm.nih.gov/medlineplus/ency/article/000932.htm.

"Adjustment disorders," Mayo Foundation for Medical Education and Research, last modified March 17, 2011, accessed March 20, 2013, www.mayoclinic.com/health/adjustment-disorders/DS00584 (page no longer available; please see http://www.mayoclinic.org/diseases-conditions/adjustment-disorders/home/ovc-20310957).

"All About Leprosy," The Leprosy Mission Australia, accessed April 24, 2015, http://www.leprosymission.org.au/TLM/Leprosy.

"Allergies and asthma," Canadian Lung Association, last modified September 24, 2012, accessed March 20, 2013, http://www.lung.ca/diseases-maladies/asthma-asthme/allergies-allergies/index_e.php (page no longer available; please see http://www.lung.ca).

Allergy/Asthma Information Association, accessed March 20, 2013, http://www.aaia.ca.

ALS Canada, accessed March 20, 2013, http://www.als.ca.

ALS Ontario, accessed March 20, 2013, http://alsont.ca (organization no longer exists).

Alzheimer Society of Canada, accessed March 20, 2013, http://www.alzheimer.ca/en.

American Speech-Language-Hearing Association, accessed March 4, 2013, http://www.asha.org.

"Amyotrophic Lateral Sclerosis (ALS) Fact Sheet," National Institute of Neurological Disorders and Stroke, last modified December 20, 2012, accessed March 20, 2013, http://www.ninds.nih.gov/disorders/amyotrophiclateralsclerosis/detail_ALS.htm.

Anderssen, Erin and André Picard, "Raising a child with a mental illness," *The Globe and Mail*, last modified November 22, 2008, accessed March 21, 2013, http://v1.theglobeandmail.com/servlet/story/RTGAM.20081122.wbreakdown2211/BNStory/mentalhealth

"Anti-oxidant supplements ease Gulf War Syndrome," Canadian Veterans Advocacy, last modified March 31, 2012, accessed March 12, 2013, http://canadianveteransadvocacy.com/Board2/index.php?topic=731.0.

"Antisocial personality disorder," Mayo Foundation for Medical Education and Research, last modified October 8, 2010, accessed March 20, 2013, http://www.mayoclinic.com/health/antisocial-personality-disorder/DS00829.

Antony, Martin M., *Specific Phobia*, Anxiety Treatment and Research Centre, accessed March 20, 2013, http://anxiety.stjoes.ca/specificP.htm (page no longer available; please see http://www.stjoes.ca/health-services/mental-health-addiction-services/mental-health-services/anxiety-treatment-research-clinic-atrc/-definitions-and-useful-links/specific-phobia).

Anxiety Disorders Association of Canada, accessed March 20, 2013, http://www.anxietycanada.ca/english/index.php.

"Anxiety Disorders," Centre for Addiction and Mental Health, accessed March 20, 2013, http://www.camh.ca/en/hospital/health_information/a_z_mental_health_and_addiction_information/anxiety_disorders/Pages/Anxiety_Disorders.aspx.

"Appearance Before the Standing Committee on National Defence and Veterans Affairs - Speaking Notes for The Honourable Ronald J. Duhamel," Veterans Affairs Canada, March 29, 2001, accessed March 12, 2013, https://www.veterans.gc.ca/eng/department/press/viewspeech/149 (page no longer available).

Sources for Disease Descriptions

"Arthritis, by sex, and by province and territory," Statistics Canada, last modified June 19, 2012, accessed March 20, 2013, http://www.statcan.gc.ca/tables-tableaux/sum-som/l01/cst01/health52a-eng.htm.

Asthma Society of Canada, *Asthma Facts and Statistics FAQs*, accessed March 20, 2013, http://www.asthma.ca/adults/about/asthma_facts_and_statistics.pdf.

"Ataxia," Mayo Foundation for Medical Education and Research, last modified March 1, 2011, accessed March 20, 2013, http://www.mayoclinic.com/health/ataxia/DS00910.

Autism Society Canada, accessed March 21, 2013, http://www.autismsocietycanada.ca (new site: Autism Canada, http://autismcanada.org).

"Beta Thalassemia (Cooley's Anemia)," Johns Hopkins Medicine Health Library, accessed March 21, 2013, http://www.hopkinsmedicine.org/healthlibrary/conditions/hematology_and_blood_disorders/beta_thalassemia_cooleys_anemia_85,P00081.

Biegstraaten, Marieke, Keith A. Wesnes, Cécile Luzy, Milan Petakov, Mirando Mrsic, Claus Niederau, Pilar Giraldo, et al., "The cognitive profile of type 1 Gaucher disease patients," *Journal of Inherited Metabolic Disease* 35(6): (November 2012): 1093-1099, accessed February 28, 2013. doi: 10.1007/s10545-012-9460-7.

"Birth Defects," KidsHealth, The Nemours Foundation, last modified June 2010, accessed March 25, 2013, http://kidshealth.org/parents/system/ill/birth_defects.html.

"Blindness and Visual Impairment," The Canadian Encyclopedia, accessed March 22, 2013, http://www.thecanadianencyclopedia.com/articles/blindness-and-visual-impairment.

"Blood Disorders," American Society of Hematology, accessed April 23, 2015, http://www.hematology.org/Patients/Blood-Disorders.aspx.

"Blood Disorders," MedlinePlus, accessed April 23, 2015, http://www.nlm.nih.gov/medlineplus/blooddisorders.html.

"Blood, organ and tissue donation," Government of Canada, last modified April 15, 2016, accessed January 24, 2017, http://healthycanadians.gc.ca/diseases-conditions-maladies-affections/donation-contribution-eng.php.

"Borderline personality disorder," Mayo Foundation for Medical Education and Research, last modified August 17, 2012, accessed March 20, 2013, http://www.mayoclinic.com/health/borderline-personality-disorder/DS00442.

Brain Injury Association of Canada, accessed March 4, 2013, http://biac-aclc.ca.

"Brain Injury Fact & Figures," Brain Injury Society of Toronto, accessed March 4, 2013, http://www.bist.ca/brain-injury-fact-figures (page no longer available; please see http://www.bist.ca).

Brain Tumour Foundation of Canada, accessed March 20, 2013, http://www.braintumour.ca.

"Brain Tumours," Neurological Health Charities Canada, accessed March 20, 2013, http://www.mybrainmatters.ca/en/condition/brain-tumours (page no longer available; please see http://www.mybrainmatters.ca).

Brock, G., Ed Moreira Jr., D.B. Glasser and C. Gingell, "Sexual disorders and associated help-seeking behaviors in Canada," PubMed Health, U.S. National Library of Medicine, February 13, 2006, accessed March 22, 2013, http://www.ncbi.nlm.nih.gov/pubmed/16515749.

Brock, Gerald B., Francois Bénard, Richard Casey, Stacy L. Elliot, Jerzy B. Gajewski and Hay C. Lee, "Canadian Male Sexual Health Council Survey to Assess Prevalence and Treatment of Premature Ejaculation in Canada," *The Journal of Sexual Medicine* 6, no. 8 (2009): 2115-2123, doi: 10.1111/j.1743-6109.2009.01362.

Brousseau, Lyn, Marc Hamel, Joel Paris and George Tasca, "A Report on Mental Illnesses in Canada," Health Canada, 2002, accessed March 20, 2013, http://www.cpa.ca/cpasite/userfiles/Documents/Practice_Page/reports_mental_illness_e.pdf (page no longer available; please see http://www.phac-aspc.gc.ca/publicat/miic-mmac/ack-eng.php).

Byrd, Dean A., Ned Stringham, Philip M. Sutton, David Blakeslee, Christopher Rosik, and James E. Phelan, "Gender Identity Disorders in Childhood and Adolescence: A Critical Inquiry and Review of the Kenneth Zucker Research," National Association for Research & Therapy of Homosexuality, March 2007, accessed March 15, 2013, http://www.narth.com/docs/GIDReviewKenZucker.pdf (page no longer available; please see https://www.narth.com).

"Canada launches first gene therapy trial for Fabry disease," Alberta Health Services, last modified January 24, 2013, accessed February 28, 2013, http://www.albertahealthservices.ca/7883.asp (page no longer available; please see http://www.albertahealthservices.ca/news/releases/2013/Page7883.aspx).

Canadian ADHD Resource Alliance, last modified December 17, 2012, accessed March 20, 2013, http://www.caddra.ca.

Canadian AIDS Society, accessed March 20, 2013, http://www.cdnaids.ca.

Canadian Association for Familial Ataxias, *Friedreich's Ataxia (FA) Facts*, accessed March 20, 2013, http://thewalktofightfa.com/documents/Friedreich%20english.pdf (site discontinued).

Canadian Association for Suicide Prevention, accessed March 13, 2013, http://www.suicideprevention.ca.

Canadian Brain Tumour Consortium, accessed March 20, 2013, http://www.cbtc.ca.

Canadian Cancer Society's Advisory Committee on Cancer Statistics, Canadian Cancer Statistics 2016. Toronto, ON: Canadian Cancer Society; 2016. http://www.cancer.ca/~/media/cancer.ca/CW/cancer%20information/cancer%20101/Canadian%20cancer%20statistics/Canadian-Cancer-Statistics-2016-EN.pdf?la=en.

Canadian Cancer Society, accessed April 23, 2015, http://www.cancer.ca.

Canadian Cancer Society, accessed January 23, 2017, http://www.cancer.ca.

Canadian Cancer Society, accessed March 20, 2013, http://www.cancer.ca.

"Canadian Congenital Anomalies Surveillance System (CCASS)," Public Health Agency of Canada, last modified January 3, 2013, accessed March 255, 2013 on the Association of Public Health Epidemiologists in Ontario, http://www.apheo.ca/index.php?pid=202 (page no longer available; please see http://www.phac-aspc.gc.ca/ccasn-rcsac/index-eng.php).

Canadian Congenital Heart Alliance, accessed January 23, 2017, http://www.cchaforlife.org.

Canadian Dermatology Association, accessed March 13, 2013, http://www.dermatology.ca.

Canadian Diabetes Association, accessed February 27, 2013, http://www.diabetes.ca.

Canadian Digestive Health Foundation, accessed February 22, 2013, http://www.cdhf.ca.

Canadian Down Syndrome Society, accessed February 27, 2013, http://www.cdss.ca.

Canadian Down Syndrome Society, accessed January 23, 2017, http://www.cdss.ca.

Canadian Fabry Association, accessed February 28, 2013, http://www.fabrycanada.com.

Canadian Haemoglobinopathy Association, Consensus Statement on the Care of Patients with Sickle Cell Disease in Canada, 2015, accessed January 23, 2017, http://sicklecellanemia.ca/pdf_2016/CANHAEM.pdf.

Canadian Hemophilia Society, accessed April 23, 2015, http://www.hemophilia.ca.

Canadian Institute for the Relief of Pain and Disability, accessed March 25, 2013, http://www.cirpd.org.

Canadian Liver Foundation, accessed March 4, 2013, http://www.liver.ca.

Canadian Mental Health Association, Ontario, accessed March 13, 2013, http://www.ontario.cmha.ca.

"Canadian Multiple Sclerosis Monitoring System," Public Health Agency of Canada, last modifed March 23, 2011, accessed March 5, 2013, http://www.phac-aspc.gc.ca/cd-mc/ms-sp/index-eng.php.

Canadian Sleep Society, accessed March 15, 2013, http://www.canadiansleepsociety.ca.

Canadian Society for the Study of the Aging Male, The Hard Facts, 2010, accessed March 22, 2013, http://www.cssam.com/files/content/VIAG_5205_BetterSexBroch+EHS%20TO_E34.pdf.

Canadian Society of Transplantation, accessed March 13, 2013, http://www.transplant.ca.

"Canadians in Context - Aging Population," Human Resources and Skills Development Canada, last modified March 25, 2013, accessed March 20, 2013, http://www4.hrsdc.gc.ca/.3ndic.1t.4r@-eng.jsp?iid=33 (site discontinued).

"Carpal Tunnel Syndrome Fact Sheet," National Institute of Neurological Disorders and Stroke, last modified March 1, 2013, accessed March 21, 2013, http://www.ninds.nih.gov/disorders/carpal_tunnel/detail_carpal_tunnel.htm.

"Carpal Tunnel Syndrome," Canadian Centre for Occupational Health and Safety, last modified October 15, 2008, accessed March 21, 2013, http://www.ccohs.ca/oshanswers/diseases/carpal.html.

"Cataracts," Mayo Foundation for Medical Education and Research, last modified May 20, 2012, accessed March 22, 2013, http://www.mayoclinic.com/health/cataracts/DS00050.

"Causes of ITP," Nplate, accessed April 23, 2015, http://www.nplate.com/patient/understanding-itp/causes-itp.html.

"Celiac Disease," Canadian Digestive Health Foundation, accessed March 21, 2013, http://www.cdhf.ca/digestive-disorders/celiac.shtml.

"Celiac Disease," Health Canada, last modified August 1, 2012, accessed March 20, 2013, http://www.hc-sc.gc.ca/fn-an/securit/allerg/cel-coe/index-eng.php.

Centre for ADHD Awareness, Canada, accessed March 20, 2013, http://www.caddac.ca.

Centre for Hip Health and Mobility, accessed March 7, 2013, http://www.hiphealth.ca.

"Cerebral Palsy," Cerebralpalsycanada.com, accessed March 20, 2013, http://www.cerebralpalsycanada.com.

"Child and Youth," Mental Health Commission of Canada, accessed March 21, 2013, http://www.mentalhealthcommission.ca/English/Pages/ChildandYouth.aspx (page no longer available; please see http://www.mentalhealthcommission.ca/English/focus-areas/children-and-youth).

"Children and Adolescents with Conduct Disorder," Mental Health Canada, accessed March 21, 2013, http://www.mentalhealthcanada.com/ConditionsandDisordersDetail.asp?lang=e&category=69.

"Chronic fatigue syndrome," Mayo Foundation for Medical Education and Research, last modified June 18, 2011, accessed March 21, 2013, http://www.mayoclinic.com/health/chronic-fatigue-syndrome/DS00395.

"Chronic obstructive pulmonary disease by sex, by province and territory (Number)," Statistics Canada, last modified March 7, 2016, accessed January 24, 2017, http://www.statcan.gc.ca/tables-tableaux/sum-som/l01/cst01/health105a-eng.htm.

"Chronic Respiratory Diseases," Public Health Agency of Canada, last modified February 8, 2013, accessed March 22, 2013, http://www.phac-aspc.gc.ca/cd-mc/crd-mrc/index-eng.php.

Clarke, Anne C.D., *The Care and Treatment of Canada's Multi-Racial Population*, May 28, 2002, access March 5, 2013, http://healthcoalition.ca/wp-content/uploads/2010/05/sickle-cell.pdf (page no longer available).

CNIB, accessed March 22, 2013, http://www.cnib.ca.

"Common Blood Diseases," accessed April 23, 2015, http://www.glutathionediseasecure.com/common-blood-diseases.html.

"Concussion statistics dizzying," McGill University, February 19, 2013, accessed March 4, 2013, http://www.mcgill.ca/newsroom/channels/news/concussion-statistics-dizzying-225078.

"Conduct Disorder," Mental Health America, accessed March 21, 2013, http://www.nmha.org/go/conduct-disorder.

"Congenital Heart Defects Statistics," Heart Defects Society of Windsor and Essex County Inc., last modified July 12, 2012, accessed March 2013, http://www.heartdefectssociety.org/stats.html (page no longer available; please see http://heartdefectssociety.org).

Cooley's Anemia Foundation, accessed March 21, 2013, http://www.thalassemia.org.

"COPD," Canadian Lung Association, last modified November 22, 2012, accessed March 22, 2013, http://www.lung.ca/diseases-maladies/copd-mpoc_e.php.

Cox, D. W., & Templeton, R, "Genetic Diseases," Historica Canada, February 7, 2006, accessed April 28, 2015, http://thecanadianencyclopedia.ca/en/article/genetic-diseases/.

"Crohn's and Colitis Foundation of Canada Reveals Inflammatory Bowel Disease Costs Canadians a Shocking $2.8 Billion a Year," Canada," CNW, last modified November 1, 2012, accessed March 12, 2013, http://www.newswire.ca/en/story/1063207/crohn-s-and-colitis-foundation-of-canada-reveals-inflammatory-bowel-disease-costs-canadians-a-shocking-2-8-billion-a-year.

Crohn's and Colitis Foundation of Canada, accessed February 22, 2013, http://www.ccfc.ca.

Cystic Fibrosis Canada, accessed February 22, 2013, http://www.cysticfibrosis.ca.

Cystic Fibrosis Canada, accessed January 23, 2017, http://www.cysticfibrosis.ca.

"Diabetes, by age group and sex," Statistics Canada, last modified June 19, 2012, accessed February 27, 2013, http://www.statcan.gc.ca/tables-tableaux/sum-som/l01/cst01/health53a-eng.htm.

"Diabetes, by age group and sex," Statistics Canada, last modified March 7, 2016, accessed January 23, 2017, http://www.statcan.gc.ca/tables-tableaux/sum-som/l01/cst01/health53a-eng.htm.

"Diabetes," Public Health Agency of Canada, last modified March 19, 2012, accessed February 27, 2013, http://www.phac-aspc.gc.ca/cd-mc/diabetes-diabete.

"Diabetic retinopathy," Mayo Foundation for Medical Education and Research, last modified March 27, 2012, accessed March 22, 2013, http://www.mayoclinic.com/health/diabetic-retinopathy/DS00447.

"Diagnostic and Statistical Manual of Mental Disorders," Encyclopedia of Mental Disorders, accessed March 21, 2013, http://www.minddisorders.com/Del-Fi/Diagnostic-and-Statistical-Manual-of-Mental-Disorders.html.

"Dissociative disorders," Mayo Foundation for Medical Education and Research, last modified March 3, 2011, accessed March 21, 2013, http://www.mayoclinic.com/health/dissociative-disorders/DS00574 (page no longer available; please see http://www.mayoclinic.org/diseases-conditions/dissociative-disorders/home/ovc-20269555).

"Down Syndrome-Trisomy 21," PubMed Health, U.S. National Library of Medicine, last modified May 16, 2012, accessed February 27, 2013, http://www.ncbi.nlm.nih.gov/pubmedhealth/PMH0001992.

"Drug to treat Female Orgasmic Disorder under speculation," *The Current*, November 21, 2012, http://www.cbc.ca/thecurrent/2012/11/21/drug-to-treat-female-orgasmic-disorder-under-speculation/.

"Dry macular degeneration," Mayo Foundation for Medical Education and Research, last modified November 20, 2012, accessed March 22, 2013, http://www.mayoclinic.com/health/macular-degeneration/DS00284.

"DSM 5th Edition, Status and Issues," GID Reform Advocates, accessed March 15, 2013, http://www.gidreform.org/dsm5.html (site discontinued).

"e-Statistics Report on Transplant, Waiting List and Donor Statistics," Canadian Institute for Health Information, last modified June 30, 2012, accessed March 13, 2013, http://www.cihi.ca/CIHI-ext-portal/internet/en/document/types+of+care/specialized+services/organ+replacements/report_stats2012 (page no longer available; please see https://www.cihi.ca/en/2012-e-statistics-report-on-transplants-waiting-lists-and-donors).

"Early Identification of Speech-Language Delays and Disorders," Let's Talk, No. 32, American Speech-Language-Hearing Association, accessed on LD OnLine, April 29, 2015, http://www.ldonline.org/article/6231.

"Early Warning Signs about Children's Mental Illness Not Evident to Many Canadian Parents," Royal Bank of Canada, last modified October 3, 2011, accessed March 21, 2013, http://www.rbc.com/newsroom/2011/1003-mental-illness-warning.html.

Encyclopedia of Mental Disorders, accessed March 22, 2013, http://www.minddisorders.com.

"Endometriosis: Diagnosis and Treatments," Canadian Women's Health Network, accessed February 22, 2013, http://www.cwhn.ca/node/40781.

Endometriosisinfo.ca, The Society of Obstetricians and Gynaecologists of Canada, accessed February 22, 2013, http://endometriosisinfo.ca.

Epilepsy Canada, accessed March 20, 2013, http://www.epilepsy.ca.

Epilepsy.com, accessed March 20, 2013, http://www.epilepsy.com.

Fabry Community, accessed February 28, 2013, http://www.fabrycommunity.com.

"Facts about Birth Defects," Centers for Disease Control and Prevention, last modified February 24, 2011, accessed March 25, 2013, http://www.cdc.gov/NCBDDD/birthdefects/facts.html.

"Facts at your fingertips," Speech-Language & Audiology Canada, accessed April 29, 2015, http://sac-oac.ca/sites/default/files/resources/May%20Month%20Tips_SLP-EN_proof.pdf.

Farry, Angela and David Baxter, The Incidence and Prevalence of Spinal Cord Injury in Canada, (Rick Hansen Institute, 2010), accessed March 8, 2013, http://www.urbanfutures.com/reports/Report%2080.pdf (page no longer available; please see https://www.ncbi.nlm.nih.gov/pubmed/22555590).

"Fast facts about Chronic Obstructive Pulmonary Disease (COPD) 2011," Public Health Agency of Canada, last modified February 7, 2012, accessed March 22, 2013, http://www.phac-aspc.gc.ca/cd-mc/publications/copd-mpoc/ff-rr-2011-eng.php.

"Fast Facts about Mental Illness," Canadian Mental Health Association, accessed March 21, 2013, http://www.cmha.ca/media/fast-facts-about-mental-illness/#.UUjNJRdJPko.

Favaro, Ava and Elizabeth St. Philip, "CCSVI: Three Years Later," CTV News, November 21, 2012, accessed March 5, 2013, http://www.ctvnews.ca/w5/ccsvi-three-years-later-1.1048091.

Fedoroff, Dr. Paul, and the Mental Health Information Committee of the Children's Hospital of Eastern Ontario, "Gender Identity and Diversity: Information for Parents and Caregivers," Mentalhealth.ca, last modified January 28, 2013, accessed March 15, 2013, http://www.ementalhealth.ca/Ottawa-Carleton/Gender-Identity-and-Diversity-Information-for-Parents-and-Caregivers/index.php?m=article&ID=8888.

Feldman, Mark, "Growth Problems," AboutKidsHealth, last modified March 5, 2010, accessed March 4, 2013, http://www.aboutkidshealth.ca/En/HealthAZ/ConditionsandDiseases/Symptoms/Pages/growthproblems.aspx.

"Female Sexual Dysfunction," MediResource Inc., canada.com, accessed March 22, 2013, http://bodyandhealth.canada.com/condition_info_details.asp?channel_id=0&relation_id=0&disease_id=58&page_no=1.

"Fibromyalgia - Fibromyositis; Fibrositis," PubMed Health, U.S. National Library of Medicine, February 2, 2012, accessed February 27, 2013, http://www.ncbi.nlm.nih.gov/pubmedhealth/PMH0001463.

Flaman, Paul, "Organ and Tissue Transplants: Some Ethical Issues," Topics in Bioethics for Science and Religion Teachers: Readings and Study Guide, ed. by Mervyn A. Lynch and Naomi Stinson, Edmonton Catholic Schools and St. Albert Catholic Schools, (1994), accessed March 13, 2013, http://www.ualberta.ca/~pflaman/organtr.htm.

FM-CFS Canada, last modified November 4, 2011, accessed March 21, 2013, http://www.fmcfs.ca (site discontinued).

Foundation for Prader-Willi Research Canada, accessed March 5, 2013, http://www.fpwr.ca.

Garriguet, Didier, "Bone health: Osteoporosis, calcium and vitamin D," Statistics Canada, last modified July 20, 2011, accessed March 7, 2013, http://www.statcan.gc.ca/pub/82-003-x/2011003/article/11515-eng.htm.

Gaucher Connection, accessed February 28, 2013, http://gaucherconnection.ca.

"Gaucher's disease-Treatments and drugs," Mayo Foundation for Medical Education and Research, last modified July 8, 2011, accessed February 28, 2013, http://www.mayoclinic.com/health/gauchers-disease/DS00972/DSECTION=treatments-and-drugs.

"Gender Identity Disorder Symptoms - Gender Dysphoria," PsychCentral, last modified September 8, 2011, accessed March 15, 2013, http://psychcentral.com/disorders/sx40.htm.

"Gender identity disorder," MedlinePlus, U.S. National Library of Medicine, last modified February 13, 2012, accessed March 15, 2013, http://www.nlm.nih.gov/medlineplus/ency/article/001527.htm.

"Gene Therapy," Health Canada, November 25, 2005, accessed April 28, 2015, http://www.hc-sc.gc.ca/sr-sr/tech/biotech/about-apropos/gen_therap-eng.php.

"Genetic Disorders," MedlinePlus, U.S. National Library of Medicine, accessed April 28, 2015, http://www.nlm.nih.gov/medlineplus/geneticdisorders.html.

"Genetics and Speech Disorders," Speech Buddies Blog, accessed April 29, 2015, https://www.speechbuddy.com/blog/speech-disorders/genetics-and-speech-disorders-the-role-of-family-and-communication-disorders/.

Gilmour, Heather and Kathryn Wilkins, "Migraine," *Health Reports* 12, no. 2, Statistics Canada, accessed March 6, 2013, http://www.statcan.gc.ca/pub/82-003-x/2000002/article/5515-eng.pdf.

"Glaucoma," Mayo Foundation for Medical Education and Research, last modified October 2, 2012, accessed March 22, 2013, http://www.mayoclinic.com/health/glaucoma/DS00283.

"Global leprosy situation, 2012," *Weekly epidemiological record,* pp.317-328, WHO, 2012, accessed April 24, 2015, http://www.who.int/wer/2012/wer8734.pdf?ua=1.

Government of Canada, "Anxiety Disorders," chap. 5 in *The Human Face of Mental Health and Mental Illness in Canada 2006*, accessed from the Mood Disorders Society of Canada, March 20, 2013, http://www.mooddisorderscanada.ca/documents/Consumer%20and%20Family%20Support/Anxiety%20disorders_EN.pdf, 79-86.

Greenberg, Dr. Saul, "Thalassemia," Ontario Association of Pediatricians, last modified February 5, 2009, accessed March 21, 2013, http://www.utoronto.ca/kids/Thalassemia.htm (page no longer available; please see http://www3.sympatico.ca/saulped/Thalassemia.htm).

Grewal, Penny, "The Challenges with Improving Access to Leprosy Treatment," Medicus Mundi Schweiz, April 2002, accessed April 24, 2015, http://www.medicusmundi.ch/de/bulletin/mms-bulletin/zugang-zu-medikamenten/barrieren-erkennen-und-sie-ueberwinden/the-challenges-with-improving-access-to-leprosy-treatment.

"Growth disorders," BioBasics, last modified July 31, 2008, accessed March 4, 2013, http://www.biobasics.gc.ca/english/view.asp?x=760 (site discontinued).

"Guillain-Barré Syndrome Fact Sheet," National Institute of Neurological Disorders and Stroke, published July 2011, accessed March 27, 2017, https://www.ninds.nih.gov/Disorders/Patient-Caregiver-Education/Fact-Sheets/Guillain-Barr%C3%A9-Syndrome-Fact-Sheet.

"Guillain-Barré Syndrome," HealthLinkBC, last modified February 19, 2016, accessed March 27, 2017, https://www.healthlinkbc.ca/health-topics/hw65904.

"Guillain-Barré syndrome," World Health Organization, last modified October 2016, accessed March 27, 2017, http://www.who.int/mediacentre/factsheets/guillain-barre-syndrome/en.

"Gulf War and Health Volume 9: Treatment for Chronic Multisymptom Illness," Institute of Medicine of the National Academies, last modified January 23, 2013, accessed March 12, 2013, http://www.iom.edu/Reports/2013/Gulf-War-and-HealthTreatment-for-Chronic-Multisymptom-Illness/Report-Brief012313.aspx (new site: National Academy of Medicine, https://nam.edu).

"Gulf War Veterans' Medically Unexplained Illnesses," U.S. Department of Veterans Affairs, last modified March 11, 2013, accessed March 12, 2013, http://www.publichealth.va.gov/exposures/gulfwar/medically-unexplained-illness.asp.

"Handout on Health: Osteoarthritis," National Institute of Arthritis and Musculoskeletal and Skin Diseases, last modified July 2010, accessed March 20, 2013, http://www.niams.nih.gov/Health_Info/Osteoarthritis/default.asp.

"Handout on Health: Rheumatoid Arthritis," National Institute of Arthritis and Musculoskeletal and Skin Diseases, last modified April 2009, accessed March 20, 2013, http://www.niams.nih.gov/Health_Info/Rheumatic_Disease/default.asp.

Hart, Stephen D., "Risk Assessment: Sexual Violence and the Role of Paraphilia," Correctional Service Canada, last modified December 18, 2012, accessed March 22, 2013, http://www.csc-scc.gc.ca/text/rsrch/special_reports/shp2007/paraphil10-eng.shtml.

"Head Injuries in Canada: A Decade of Change (1994-1995 to 2003-2004)," Canadian Institute for Health Information, August 2006, accessed March 4, 2013, https://secure.cihi.ca/free_products/ntr_head_injuries_2006_e.pdf.

"Head Injuries," *CBC News*, last modified March 19, 2009, accessed March 4, 2013, http://www.cbc.ca/news/health/story/2009/03/17/f-head-injuries.html.

"Health - Obesity," Human Resources and Skills Development Canada, accessed March 7, 2013, http://www4.hrsdc.gc.ca/.3ndic.1t.4r@-eng.jsp?iid=6 (site discontinued).

Health Canada, "Suicide Prevention, *It's Your Health*, March 2009, accessed March 13, 2013, http://www.hc-sc.gc.ca/hl-vs/iyh-vsv/diseases-maladies/suicide-eng.php.

Health Canada, accessed March 12, 2013, http://www.hc-sc.gc.ca/hl-vs/iyh-vsv/diseases-maladies/index-eng.php.

Heart and Stroke Foundation, accessed January 23, 2017, http://www.heartandstroke.ca.

Heart and Stroke Foundation, accessed March 21, 2013, http://www.heartandstroke.com.

"Hemochromatosis - Iron overload," PubMed Health, U.S. National Library of Medicine, last modified March 4, 2012, accessed March 6, 2013, http://www.ncbi.nlm.nih.gov/pubmedhealth/PMH0001368.

"Hemophilia," Canadian Hemophilia Society, accessed March 4, 2013, http://www.hemophilia.ca/en/educational-material/printed-documents/hemophilia.

"Hepatitis A," Mayo Foundation for Medical Education and Research, last modified September 1, 2011, accessed March 6, 2013, http://www.mayoclinic.com/health/hepatitis-a/DS00397.

"Hepatitis B," Mayo Foundation for Medical Education and Research, last modified September 1, 2011, accessed March 6, 2013, http://www.mayoclinic.com/health/hepatitis-b/DS00398.

"Hepatitis C," Mayo Foundation for Medical Education and Research, last modified May 24, 2011, accessed March 6, 2013, http://www.mayoclinic.com/health/hepatitis-c/DS00097.

"Hepatitis," Health Canada, last modified July 8, 2008, accessed March 6, 2013, http://www.hc-sc.gc.ca/hc-ps/dc-ma/hep-eng.php.

"Hepatitis," Public Health Agency of Canada, last modified April 16, 2012, accessed March 6, 2013, http://www.phac-aspc.gc.ca/hep/index-eng.php.

"Hirschsprung's disease," MedlinePlus, U.S. National Library of Medicine, last modified November 13, 2011, accessed March 6, 2013, http://www.nlm.nih.gov/medlineplus/ency/article/001140.htm.

"HIV & AIDS: Basic Facts," Canadian AIDS Treatment Information Exchange, accessed March 20, 2013, http://www.catie.ca/en/practical-guides/hiv-aids-basic-facts (page no longer available; please see http://www.catie.ca/en/basics).

"HIV and AIDS," Health Canada, last modified May 13, 2011, accessed March 20, 2013, http://www.hc-sc.gc.ca/hc-ps/dc-ma/aids-sida-eng.php.

"HIV/AIDS: It's Your Health," Health Canada and the Public Health Agency of Canada, last modified November 2, 2010, accessed March 20, 2013, http://www.hc-sc.gc.ca/hl-vs/iyh-vsv/diseases-maladies/hiv-vih-eng.php (page no longer available; please see http://www.hc-sc.gc.ca/hc-ps/dc-ma/aids-sida-eng.php).

http://www.cbc.ca/news/health/story/2009/06/17/f-sleep-disorders.html.

http://www.phac-aspc.gc.ca/publicat/2007/lbrdc-vsmrc/index-eng.php#tphp.

"Hunter syndrome," Mayo Clinic, accessed April 14, 2015, http://www.mayoclinic.org/diseases-conditions/hunter-syndrome/basics/definition/con-20026538.

"Hunter syndrome," MedlinePlus, U.S. National Library of Medicine, accessed April 15, 2015, http://www.nlm.nih.gov/medlineplus/ency/article/001203.htm.

HunterPatients.com, Shire, accessed April 15, 2015, http://hunterpatients.com/.

"Huntington disease," Genetics Home Reference, accessed April 23, 2015, http://ghr.nlm.nih.gov/condition/huntington-disease.

Huntington Society of Canada, accessed April 23, 2015, http://www.huntingtonsociety.ca.

"Huntington's disease," Mayo Clinic, July 24, 2014, accessed April 23, 2015, http://www.mayoclinic.org/diseases-conditions/huntingtons-disease/basics/definition/con-20030685.

Hurst, Matt, "Who gets any sleep there days? Sleep patterns of Canadians," *Canadian Social Trends*, Statistics Canada, last modified November 21, 2008, accessed March 15, 2013, http://www.statcan.gc.ca/pub/11-008-x/2008001/article/10553-eng.htm.

"Hydrocephalus," Mayo Foundation for Medical Education and Research, last modified September 13, 2011, accessed March 4, 2013, http://www.mayoclinic.com/health/hydrocephalus/DS00393.

Hypertension Canada, accessed March 4, 2013, http://www.hypertension.ca.

"Hypertension," Public Health Agency of Canada, last modified February 8, 2013, accessed March 4, 2013, http://www.phac-aspc.gc.ca/cd-mc/cvd-mcv/hypertension-eng.php.

"Hypochondria (Hypochondriasis)," Bipolar Central, accessed March 13, 2013, http://www.bipolarcentral.com/otherillnesses/hypochondria.php.

"Hypochondria," Mayo Foundation for Medical Education and Research, last modified November 23, 2010, accessed March 13, 2013, http://www.mayoclinic.com/health/hypochondria/DS00841.

"Impulse Control Disorders and Substance Disorders," Faculty of Science, McMaster University (lecture, 2010), http://www.science.mcmaster.ca/pnb/images/stories/courses/sum2ap3/lecture9_1s.pdf (page no longer available).

"Increased awareness, earlier detection bring relief to challenges of Prader-Willi syndrome," *Endocrine Today*, April 2011, accessed March 5, 2013, http://www.healio.com/endocrinology/pediatric-endocrinology/news/print/endocrine-today/%7Bd761cb1e-43e2-4fd0-9e97-600fc22180b7%7D/increased-awareness-earlier-detection-bring-relief-to-challenges-of-prader-willi-syndrome.

"Infertility and AHR," Assisted Human Reproduction Canada, August 26, 2010, accessed March 6, 2013, http://www.ahrc-pac.gc.ca/v2/patients/infertility-infertilite-eng.php (page no longer available; please see http://www.hc-sc.gc.ca/dhp-mps/brgtherap/legislation/reprod/index-eng.php).

"Infertility," Foundation for Medical Education and Research, last modified September 9, 2011, accessed March 6, 2013, http://www.mayoclinic.com/health/infertility/DS00310.

"Infertility," MediResource Inc., canada.com, accessed March 6, 2013, http://bodyandhealth.canada.com/channel_condition_info_details.asp?disease_id=248&channel_id=2048&relation_id=110053.

"Insomnia," MediResource Inc., canada.com, accessed March 15, 2013, http://bodyandhealth.canada.com/channel_condition_info_details.asp?disease_id=77&channel_id=2045&relation_id=33193.

Johns Hopkins Medicine, accessed April 23, 2015, http://www.hopkinsmedicine.org/healthlibrary/conditions.

Kirkey, Sharon, "Canada Census 2011: Aging population a potential health-care time bomb, *The National Post*, May 29, 2012, http://news.nationalpost.com/2012/05/29/canada-census-2011-aging-population-a-potential-health-care-time-bomb.

Kirkey, Sharon, "Infertility on the rise in Canada: study," *National Post,* last modified February 15, 2012, accessed March 6, 2013, http://news.nationalpost.com/2012/02/15/infertility-on-the-rise-in-canada-study.

Lanes, Andrea, Jennifer L. Kuk, Hala Tamim, "Prevalence and characteristics of Postpartum Depression symptomatology among Canadian women: a cross-sectional study," *BMC Public Health*, 2011, accessed March 22, 2013, http://www.biomedcentral.com/1471-2458/11/302.

Langlois, Kellie A., Andriy V. Samokhvalov, Jürgen Rehm, Selene T. Spence, and Sarah Connor Gorber, "Section B - Anxiety disorders," in *Health State Descriptions for Canadians*, no. 4 (2012), accessed March 20, 2013, http://www.statcan.gc.ca/pub/82-619-m/2012004/sections/sectionb-eng.htm.

Langlois, Kellie A., Andriy V. Samokhvalov, Jürgen Rehm, Selene T. Spence, and Sarah Connor Gorber, "Section C - Childhood conditions," in *Health State Descriptions for Canadians*, no. 4 (2012), accessed March 20, 2013, http://www.statcan.gc.ca/pub/82-619-m/2012004/sections/sectionc-eng.htm.

"Leading causes of death, by sex (Both sexes)," Statistics Canada, last modified December 10, 2015, accessed January 24, 2017, http://www5.statcan.gc.ca/cansim/a26?lang=eng&id=1020561.

"Learning About Cystic Fibrosis," National Genome Research Institute, last modified September 27, 2011, accessed March 22, 2013, http://www.genome.gov/10001213.

"Learning About Tay-Sachs Disease," National Genome Research Institute, last modified March 17, 2011, accessed March 12, 2013, http://www.genome.gov/10001220.

"Leprosy Frequently Asked Questions - American Leprosy Missions," American Leprosy Missions, accessed April 24, 2015, http://www.leprosy.org/leprosy-faqs/.

"Leprosy Today," WHO, accessed April 24, 2015, http://www.who.int/gho/neglected_diseases/leprosy/en/.

"Leprosy," WHO, accessed April 24, 2015, http://www.who.int/gho/neglected_diseases/leprosy/en/.

"Leprosy," WHO, accessed April 24, 2015, http://www.who.int/mediacentre/factsheets/fs101/en.

"Leprosy," World Health Organization, last modified February 2017, accessed March 27, 2017, http://who.int/mediacentre/factsheets/fs101/en.

"Leprosy: MedlinePlus Medical Encyclopedia," U.S National Library of Medicine, accessed April 24, 2015, http://www.nlm.nih.gov/medlineplus/ency/article/001347.htm.

Leukemia & Lymphoma Society of Canada, accessed April 23, 2015, http://www.llscanada.org.

Leung, Wendy, "Psychiatry 'bible' DSM-5 one step closer to publication," *The Globe and Mail*, December 3, 2012, accessed March 21, 2013, http://www.theglobeandmail.com/life/health-and-fitness/health/conditions/psychiatry-bible-dsm-5-one-step-closer-to-publication/article5937980/.

"Life and Breath: Respiratory Disease in Canada (2007)," Public Health Agency of Canada, last modified July 26, 2012, accessed March 22, 2013.

"List of Metabolic Disorders," Botanical-online.com, accessed April 15, 2015, http://www.botanical-online.com/english/metabolicdiseases.htm#listado.

"Living with Myalgic Encephalomyelitis/Chronic Fatigue Syndrome," MediResource Inc., canada.com, accessed March 21, 2013, http://bodyandhealth.canada.com/channel_health_features_details.asp?health_feature_id=367&article_id=1155&channel_id=42&relation_id=10901.

"Lung disease fact sheet," Office on Women's Health, U.S. Department of Health and Human Services, last modified November 29, 2010, accessed March 22, 2013, http://womenshealth.gov/publications/our-publications/fact-sheet/lung-disease.cfm (information now available at http://womenshealth.gov/publications/our-publications/fact-sheet/lung-disease.html).

"Lung disease imposes major costs on Canada's economy," *CNW*, last modified March 15, 2012, accessed March 22, 2013, http://www.newswire.ca/en/story/937597/lung-disease-imposes-major-costs-on-canada-s-economy.

Lupus Canada, accessed March 6, 2013, http://www.lupuscanada.org.

"Lupus," MediResource Inc., canada.com, accessed March 6, 2013, http://bodyandhealth.canada.com/condition_info_details.asp?disease_id=83.

"Lyme Disease Fact Sheet," Public Health Agency of Canada, last modified July 4, 2012, accessed March 12, 2013, http://www.phac-aspc.gc.ca/id-mi/lyme-fs-eng.php.

"Lymphadenitis," New York Times Health Guide, accessed April 27, 2015. http://www.nytimes.com/health/guides/disease/lymphadenitis-and-lymphangitis/overview.html.

"Lymphatic Disease List," Ranker, accessed April 27, 2015, http://www.ranker.com/list/lymphatic-disease-list/diseases-and-medications-info.

"Lymphedema," Lymphedema Association of Ontario, accessed April 27, 2015. https://lymphontario.wildapricot.org/.

"Lymphedema - Treatment of Lymphedema," National Cancer Institute, December 12, 2013, accessed April 27, 2015, http://www.cancer.gov/cancertopics/pdq/supportivecare/lymphedema/Patient/page3.

"Lymphedema," Mayo Clinic, accessed April 27, 2015, http://www.mayoclinic.org/diseases-conditions/lymphedema/basics/definition/con-20025603.

Macon, B. L., & Solan, M., "Blood Cell Disorders," Healthline, May 16, 2012, accessed April 23, 2015, http://www.healthline.com/health/blood-cell-disorders.

"Management of Post-Polio Syndrome," Canadian Abilities Foundation, accessed March 20, 2013, http://abilities.ca/management-of-post-polio-syndrome/.

March of Dimes, accessed March 20, 2013, http://www.marchofdimes.ca.

Marshall, Katherine, and Harold Wynne, "Fighting the odds," *Perspectives on Labour and Income: The Online Edition* 4, no. 12 (December 2003), http://www.statcan.gc.ca/pub/75-001-x/01203/6700-eng.html.

Mayo Clinic, accessed April 23, 2015, http://www.mayoclinic.org.

"Mental illness in children: Know the signs," Mayo Foundation for Medical Education and Research, last modified February 25, 2012, accessed March 21, 2013, http://www.mayoclinic.com/health/mental-illness-in-children/MY01915.

"Migraine," *A.D.A.M. Medical Encyclopedia*, PubMed Health, U.S. National Library of Medicine, last modified December 14, 2011, accessed March 6, 2013, http://www.ncbi.nlm.nih.gov/pubmedhealth/PMH0001728/.

"Migraine," Mayo Foundation for Medical Education and Research, last modified June 4, 2011, accessed March 6, 2013, http://www.mayoclinic.com/health/migraine-headache/DS00120.

Millar, Wayne J., "Chronic Pain," *Health Reports* 7, no. 4 (Spring 1996): 47-53, http://www.statcan.gc.ca/pub/82-003-x/1995004/article/2819-eng.pdf.

"Millions of workers worldwide cannot maintain an active work life due to mental disabilities," iSHN Global, accessed March 20, 2013, http://www.ishnglobal.com/index.php?option=com_content&view=article&id=291:millions-of-workers-worldwide-cannot-maintain-an-active-work-life-due-to-mental-disabilities&catid=37:happening-today (page no longer available; please see http://www.ishn.com).

Money, Deborah and Marc Steben, "Genital Herpes: Gynaecological Aspects," *SOGC Clinical Practice Guideline* no. 206 (April 2008), accessed March 12, 2013, https://sogc.org/wp-content/uploads/2013/01/gui207CPG0804_000.pdf.

"Monogenic Diseases," *Genes and human disease*, World Health Organization, accessed March 12, 2013, http://www.who.int/genomics/public/geneticdiseases/en/index2.html.

Mood Disorders Society of Canada, accessed March 22, 2013, http://www.mooddisorderscanada.ca/.

"Mood disorders, by age group and sex (Percent)," Statistics Canada, last modified March 7, 2016, accessed January 24, 2017, http://www.statcan.gc.ca/tables-tableaux/sum-som/l01/cst01/health113b-eng.htm.

Multiple Sclerosis Society of Canada, accessed January 24, 2017, https://mssociety.ca.

Multiple Sclerosis Society of Canada, accessed March 5, 2013, http://mssociety.ca.

"Multiple sclerosis," Mayo Foundation for Medical Education and Research, last modified December 15, 2012, accessed March 5, 2013, http://www.mayoclinic.com/health/multiple-sclerosis/DS00188 (page no longer available; please see http://www.mayoclinic.org/diseases-conditions/multiple-sclerosis/home/ovc-20131882).

Murphy, Kellie A., Selene T. Spence, Cameron N. McIntosh, Sarah K. Connor Gorber, "Health State Descriptions for Canadians: Musculoskeletal Diseases," Statistics Canada cat. 82-619-MIE, no. 003 (April 2006), http://publications.gc.ca/Collection/Statcan/82-619-MIE/82-619-MIE2006003.pdf.

Muscular Dystrophy Canada, accessed March 5, 2013, http://www.muscle.ca.

"Muscular Dystrophy," MediResource Inc., canada.com accessed March 5, 2013, http://bodyandhealth.canada.com/channel_condition_info_details.asp?channel_id=9&disease_id=91&relation_id=10860.

"Myasthenia Gravis (MG)," Muscular Dystrophy Canada, last modified September 2007, accessed March 4, 2013, http://www.muscle.ca/fileadmin/National/Muscular_Dystrophy/Disorders/425E_Myasthenia_Gravis_2007.pdf (information now available at http://muscle.ca/wp-content/uploads/2012/11/425E_Myasthenia_Gravis_2007.pdf).

Myasthenia Gravis Coalition of Canada, accessed March 4, 2013, http://www.mgcc-ccmg.org/.

"Myasthenia Gravis," MediResource Inc., canada.com accessed March 4, 2013, http://bodyandhealth.canada.com/condition_info_details.asp?disease_id=92.

MyChronicMigraine.ca, accessed March 6, 2013, http://www.mychronicmigraine.ca/.

Myeloma Canada, accessed April 23, 2015, http://www.myelomacanada.ca.

National Association for Down Syndrome, accessed February 27, 2013, http://www.nads.org.

National Ataxia Foundation, accessed March 20, 2013, http://www.ataxia.org.

National Eating Disorder Information Centre, accessed March 15, 2013, http://www.nedic.ca.

National ME/FM Action Network, "Government Data confirms that Canadians with Fibromyalgia are very disadvantaged," Co-Cure, accessed February 27, 2013, http://www.co-cure.org/Data-Can-FM-pdf.pdf (site discontinued).

National Tay-Sachs & Allied Diseases, accessed March 12, 2013, http://www.ntsad.org.

Navaneelan, Tanya, "Suicide rates: An overview," *Health at a Glance*, last modified July 2012, accessed March 13, 2013, http://www.statcan.gc.ca/pub/82-624-x/2012001/article/11696-eng.htm.

Neurofibromatosis Society of Ontario, accessed March 4, 2013, http://www.nfon.ca/.

"New Case Detection," WHO, accessed April 24, 2015, http://www.who.int/lep/situation/new_cases/en/.

"New therapy option approved in Canada for chronic immune thrombocytopenic purpura (ITP)," CNW, January 25, 2011, accessed April 23, 2015, http://www.newswire.ca/en/story/797155/new-therapy-.option-approved-in-canada-for-chronic-immune-thrombocytopenic-purpura-itp (information now available at http://www.newswire.ca/news-releases/new-therapy-option-approved-in-canada-for-chronic-immune-thrombocytopenic-purpura-itp-507501841.html).

NF Canada, accessed March 4, 2013, http://www.nfcanada.ca (site discontinued).

"NINDS Chronic Pain Information Page," National Institute of Neurological Disorders and Stroke, last modified January 10, 2013, accessed March 25, 2013, http://www.ninds.nih.gov/disorders/chronic_pain/chronic_pain.htm.

"NINDS Hydrocephalus Information Page," National Institute of Neurological Disorders and Stroke, last modified February 7, 2013, accessed March 4, 2013, http://www.ninds.nih.gov/disorders/hydrocephalus/hydrocephalus.htm.

"NINDS Neurofibromatosis Information Page," National Institute of Neurological Disorders and Stroke, last modified January 13, 2012, accessed March 4, 2013, http://www.ninds.nih.gov/disorders/neurofibromatosis/neurofibromatosis.htm.

"Number of Alzheimer's patients will triple by 2050: study," *CTVNews.ca*, last modified Feb. 6, 2013, accessed March 20, 2013, http://www.ctvnews.ca/health/number-of-alzheimer-s-patients-will-triple-by-2050-study-1.1145979.

"Obesity in Canada: Snapshot," Public Health Agency of Canada, last modified July 31, 2012, accessed March 7, 2013, http://www.phac-aspc.gc.ca/publicat/2009/oc/index-eng.php.

"Obesity, " Health Canada, December 15, 2006, accessed March 7, 2013, http://www.hc-sc.gc.ca/hl-vs/iyh-vsv/life-vie/obes-eng.php.

"Obesity," MediResource Inc., canada.com accessed March 7, 2013, http://bodyandhealth.canada.com/channel_condition_info_details.asp?channel_id=1055&disease_id=95&relation_id=17519.

Ontario Federation for Cerebral Palsy, accessed March 21, 2013, http://www.ofcp.ca.

Osteogenesis Imperfecta Foundation, accessed March 5, 2013, http://www.oif.org.

"Osteogenesis imperfecta," *A.D.A.M. Medical Encyclopedia*, PubMed Health, U.S. National Library of Medicine, last modified August 2, 2011, accessed March 5, 2013, http://www.ncbi.nlm.nih.gov/pubmedhealth/PMH0002540/.

"Osteogenesis imperfecta," Office of Rare Diseases Research, U.S. Department of Health & Human Services, last modified April 5, 2012, accessed March 5, 2013, https://rarediseases.info.nih.gov/GARD/QnASelected.aspx?diseaseID=1017.

Osteoporosis Canada, accessed March 7, 2013, http://www.osteoporosis.ca.

"Overweight and obese adults (self-reported), 2014," Statistics Canada, last modified November 27, 2015, accessed January 24, 2017, http://www.statcan.gc.ca/pub/82-625-x/2015001/article/14185-eng.htm.

"Overweight and obese youth (self-reported), 2014," Statistics Canada, last modified November 27, 2015, accessed January 24, 2017, http://www.statcan.gc.ca/pub/82-625-x/2015001/article/14186-eng.htm.

"Paget's Disease," MediResource Inc., canada.com accessed March 7, 2013, http://bodyandhealth.canada.com/channel_condition_info_details.asp?disease_id=189&channel_id=10&relation_id=10865.

"Pain Management Health Center," WebMD, LLC, last modified January 20, 2011, accessed March 25, 2013, http://www.webmd.com/pain-management/tc/chronic-pain-topic-overview.

"Panel Concludes Chemicals Caused Gulf War Illnesses - Gulf War Syndrome Caused by Chemical Exposures," Environmental Health Association of Nova Scotia, last modified Spring 2005, accessed March 12, 2013, http://www.environmentalhealth.ca/s05gulfwar.html.

"Paraphilias," MedicineNet, last modified July 30, 2012, accessed March 22, 2013, http://www.medicinenet.com/paraphilia/article.htm.

Park, Jungwee and Sarah Knudson, "Medically unexplained physical symptoms," *Health Reports* 18, no. 1 (February 2007): 43-47, http://www.statcan.gc.ca/pub/82-003-x/2006001/article/sympt/82-003-x2006002-eng.pdf.

Parkinson Society Canada, accessed March 5, 2013, http://www.parkinson.ca.

"Parkinson's Disease," MediResource Inc., canada.com accessed March 5, 2013, http://bodyandhealth.canada.com/channel_condition_info_details.asp?channel_id=2046&disease_id=102&relation_id=33685.

"Parkinson's disease: A primer," CARP, last modified May 4, 2007, accessed March 5, 2013, http://www.carp.ca/2007/05/04/parkinsons-disease-a-primer/.

Payton, Laura, "Veterans of Gulf War, Balkans plead for health aid," *CBC News*, November 9, 2011, http://www.cbc.ca/news/canada/story/2011/11/09/pol-veterans-gulf-war-illness.html.

"Personality Disorders," Canadian Mental Health Association, accessed March 20, 2013, http://edmonton.cmha.ca/mental-health/understanding-mental-illness/personality-disorders/ (page no longer available; please see http://edmonton.cmha.ca/documents/mental-illnesses).

Picard, André, "One in 13 Canadians has serious food allergy," *The Globe and Mail*, last modified August 23, 2012, accessed March 20, 2013, http://www.theglobeandmail.com/life/health-and-fitness/one-in-13-canadians-has-serious-food-allergy/article599131.

"Post-Polio Syndrome," Healthwise, last modified May 12, 2011, accessed March 20, 2013, http://www.healthlinkbc.ca/kb/content/mini/hw184074.html.

"Postpartum Depression," The Canadian Mental Health Association, accessed March 22, 2013, http://www.cmha.ca/mental_health/postpartum-depression/#.UUxzDBdJPko.

"Protein Injection Points to Muscular Dystrophy Treatment," *ScienceDaily*, November 27, 2012, access March 5, 2013, http://www.sciencedaily.com/releases/2012/11/121127094248.htm.

'Psychology Works' Fact Sheet: Tourette Syndrome, Prepared by Dr. B. Duncan McKinlay, Brake Shop Clinic, CPRI, Ministry of Children & Youth Services et al, Canadian Psychological Association, last modified January 2009, accessed March 13, 2013, http://www.cpa.ca/docs/File/Publications/FactSheets/PsychologyWorksFactSheet_TouretteSyndrome.pdf.

Public Health Agency of Canada, "Anxiety Disorders," chap. 4 in *A Report on Mental Illnesses in Canada*, last modified October 03, 2002, accessed March 20, 2013, http://www.phac-aspc.gc.ca/publicat/miic-mmac/chap_4-eng.php.

Public Health Agency of Canada, *The Health of Canada's Young People: a Mental Health Focus*, last modified February 15, 2012, accessed March 20, 2013, http://www.phac-aspc.gc.ca/hp-ps/dca-dea/publications/health-young-people-sante-jeunes-canadiens/index-eng.php.

Public Health Agency of Canada, "The Health of Canadian Children," chap. 3 in *The Chief Public Health Officer's Report on The State of Public Health in Canada 2009*, last modified October 20, 2009, accessed March 21, 2013, http://www.phac-aspc.gc.ca/cphorsphc-respcacsp/2009/fr-rc/cphorsphc-respcacsp06-eng.php.

Public Health Agency of Canada, *Healthy Aging in Canada: A New Vision, A Vital Investment*, accessed March 20, 2013, http://www.phac-aspc.gc.ca/seniors-aines/alt-formats/pdf/publications/public/healthy-sante/vision/vision-eng.pdf.

Public Health Agency of Canada, "Mental Illnesses in Canada: An Overview," chap. 1 in *A Report on Mental Illness in Canada*, last modified January 5, 2012, accessed March 21, 2013, http://www.phac-aspc.gc.ca/publicat/miic-mmac/chap_1-eng.php.

Public Health Agency of Canada, *Report on Sexually Transmitted Infections in Canada*, last modified March 9, 2010, accessed March 12, 2013, http://www.phac-aspc.gc.ca/std-mts/report/sti-its2008/02-eng.php.

Public Health Agency of Canada, "Schizophrenia," chap. 3 in *A Report on Mental Illnesses in Canada*, last modified March 26, 2012, accessed March 13, 2013, http://www.phac-aspc.gc.ca/publicat/miic-mmac/chap_3-eng.php.

Public Health Agency of Canada, *Summary: Estimates of HIV Incidence, Prevalence and Proportion Undiagnosed in Canada, 2014*, November 2015, accessed January 23, 2017, https://www.canada.ca/content/dam/canada/health-canada/migration/healthy-canadians/publications/diseases-conditions-maladies-affections/hiv-aids-estimates-2014-vih-sida-estimations/alt/hiv-aids-estimates-2014-vih-sida-estimations-eng.pdf.

Public Health Agency of Canada, *Tuberculosis in Canada 2014-Pre-release*, last modified March 2016, accessed January 24, 2017, https://www.canada.ca/content/dam/canada/health-canada/migration/healthy-canadians/publications/diseases-conditions-maladies-affections/tuberculosis-2014-tuberculose/alt/tuberculosis-2014-tuberculose-eng.pdf.

Public Safety Canada, "Risk factors associated with conduct disorder," *Research Matters* 7 (July 2012): http://www.publicsafety.gc.ca/cnt/rsrcs/pblctns/cndct-dsrdr/index-en.aspx.

Raynaud's Association, accessed March 7, 2013, http://www.raynauds.org.

"Raynaud's Phenomenon," Canadian Centre for Occupational Health and Safety, last modified October 21, 2008, accessed March 7, 2013, http://www.ccohs.ca/oshanswers/diseases/raynaud.html.

"Raynaud's Phenomenon," Scleroderma Society of Canada, accessed March 7, 2013, http://www.scleroderma.ca/files/Pamphlets/raynaud2.pdf (page no longer available; please see http://www.scleroderma.ca).

Rick Hansen Institute, accessed March 8, 2013, http://www.rickhanseninstitute.org.

"Rickettsial Diseases," BC Centre for Disease Control, last modified May 7, 2012, accessed March 12, 2013, http://www.bccdc.ca/dis-cond/a-z/_r/RickettsialDiseases/default.htm (information now available at http://www.bccdc.ca/health-info/diseases-conditions/rickettsial-diseases).

Rister, Robert, "Hydrocephalus: Water On The Brain," *SteadyHealth.com,* August 23, 2010, accessed March 4, 2013, http://www.steadyhealth.com/articles/Hydrocephalus__Water_on_the_Brain_a1412.html.

Robertson, William C., "Tourette Syndrome and Other Tic Disorders," Medscape Reference, last modified June 15, 2011, accessed March 13, 2013, http://emedicine.medscape.com/article/1182258-overview#aw2aab6b2b5aa.

Royal Bank of Canada, *Silent Families, Suffering Children and Youth*, accessed March 20, 2013, http://www.rbc.com/community-sustainability/_assets-custom/pdf/2012-Childrens-Mental-Health-Parents-Poll-White-Paper.pdf.

Russen, ID, Shiliang Liu, Reg Sauve, KS Joseph and Michael S. Kramer, "Sudden infant death syndrome in Canada," *Chronic Diseases in Canada (CDIC)* 25, no. 1 (2004), accessed March 8, 2013, http://www.phac-aspc.gc.ca/publicat/cdic-mcbc/25-1/a-eng.php.

"Sarcoidosis," Canadian Centre for Occupational Health and Safety, last modified January 2, 2009, accessed March 5, 2013, http://www.ccohs.ca/oshanswers/diseases/sarcoido.html.

"Sarcoidosis," Canadian Lung Association, last modified September 24, 2012, accessed March 5, 2013, http://www.lung.ca/diseases-maladies/a-z/Sarcoidosis-Sarcoidose/index_e.php (page no longer available; please see https://www.lung.ca/lung-health/lung-disease/sarcoidosis-1).

"Sarcoidosis," Quebec Lung Association, last modified October 15, 2012, accessed March 5, 2013, http://www.pq.lung.ca/diseases-maladies/sarcoidosis-sarcoidose/ (page no longer available; please see https://pq.poumon.ca/maladies/sarcoidose/).

Saskatchewan Prevention Institute, *Reducing the Risk of Sudden Infant Death Syndrome (SIDS): What Caregivers Need to Know*, 2011, accessed March 8, 2013, http://www.preventioninstitute.sk.ca/uploads/SIDS%20PowerPoint.pdf (page no longer available; please see http://www.skprevention.ca).

Schizophrenia Society of Canada, accessed March 13, 2013, http://www.schizophrenia.ca.

Scleroderma Society of Canada, accessed March 5, 2013, http://www.scleroderma.ca/.

"Scleroderma," MediResource Inc., canada.com accessed March 5, 2013, http://bodyandhealth.canada.com/condition_info_details.asp?disease_id=198.

Scoliosis Canada, accessed March 5, 2013, http://www.scoliosiscanada.ca/ (site discontinued).

"Scoliosis," Mayo Foundation for Medical Education and Research, last modified February 2, 2012, March 5, 2013, http://www.mayoclinic.com/health/scoliosis/DS00194.

"Scoliosis," MediResource Inc., canada.com accessed March 5, 2013, http://bodyandhealth.canada.com/channel_condition_info_details.asp?disease_id=117&channel_id=9&relation_id=10860.

"Screening and Counselling," Sickle Cell Disease Association of Canada, accessed April 23, 2015, http://www.sicklecelldisease.ca/research-and-testing/screening-counselling (page no longer available; please see http://www.sicklecelldisease.ca/research_testing.php).

"Seasonal allergies: Something to sneeze at," *CBC News*, last modified May 13, 2011, accessed March 20, 2013, http://www.cbc.ca/news/health/story/2010/03/19/f-seasonal-allergies-symptoms.html.

Segal, Jeanne, and Melinda Smith, "Eating Disorder Treatment and Recovery - Help for Anorexia and Bulimia," Helpguide.org, last modified November 2012, accessed March 15, 2013, http://www.helpguide.org/mental/eating_disorder_treatment.htm.

"Sexual Problems in Women," Healthwise, last modified March 29, 2012, accessed March 22, 2013, http://www.healthlinkbc.ca/kb/content/major/uh1854.html#uh1859.

"Sexually Transmitted Infection," MediResource Inc., canada.com accessed March 12, 2013, http://bodyandhealth.canada.com/channel_condition_info_details.asp?disease_id=120&channel_id=1020&relation_id=70907.

"Sickle Cell Anemia," MediResource Inc., canada.com accessed March 5, 2013, http://www.bodyandhealth.canada.com/condition_info_details.asp?disease_id=281.

"Sickle Cell Anemia," New York Times, March 3, 2013, accessed April 23, 2015, http://www.nytimes.com/health/guides/disease/sickle-cell-anemia/overview.html.

Sickle Cell Awareness Group of Ontario, access March 5, 2013, http://sicklecellanemia.ca/.

"Sickle-Cell Anemia," *Diversity and Alberta Health Services*, Alberta Health Services, last modified August 24, 2009, accessed March 5, 2013, http://www.crha-health.ab.ca/programs/diversity/diversity_resources/health_div_pops/black.htm (new site: http://www.albertahealthservices.ca).

Sjögren's Sicety of Canada, accessed March 6, 2013, http://sjogrenscanada.org/.

"Sleep disorders: Roadblocks to a good night's rest," *CBC News*, last modified June 17, 2009, accessed March 15, 2013,

Smith, Dorothy L., and Clifton F. Carbin, "Hearing Loss," *The Canadian Encyclopedia*, accessed March 4, 2013, http://www.thecanadianencyclopedia.com/articles/hearing-loss.

"Speech disorders - children," MedlinePlus, U.S. National Library of Medicine, last modified May 14, 2014, accessed April 29, 2015, http://www.nlm.nih.gov/medlineplus/ency/article/001430.htm.

"Speech Disorders - Children," The New York Times, last modified May 14, 2014, accessed April 29, 2015, http://www.nytimes.com/health/guides/disease/speech-disorders/overview.html.

"Speech Impairment (Adult)," The New York Times, last modified May 28, 2014, accessed April 29, 2015, http://www.nytimes.com/health/guides/symptoms/speech-impairment-adult/overview.html.

"Spina Bifida," CanChild Centre for Childhood Disability Research, accessed January 24, 2017, https://www.canchild.ca/en/diagnoses/spina-bifida.

"Spina bifida," Mayo Foundation for Medical Education and Research, last modified October 4, 2011, accessed March 8, 2013, http://www.mayoclinic.com/health/spina-bifida/DS00417.

"Spina Bifida," MediResource Inc., canada.com accessed March 8, 2013, http://bodyandhealth.canada.com/channel_condition_info_details.asp?disease_id=203&channel_id=9&relation_id=10860.

"Statistics by Country for Addison's Disease," Right Diagnosis, Health Grades Inc., last modified March 1, 2013, accessed March 20, 2013, http://www.rightdiagnosis.com/a/addisons_disease/stats-country.htm.

Statistics Canada, "Arthritis, 2011," *Health Fact Sheets*, last modified June 19, 2012, accessed March 20, 2013, http://www.statcan.gc.ca/pub/82-625-x/2012001/article/11657-eng.htm.

Statistics Canada, "Canada's population estimates: Age and sex, July 1, 2015," *The Daily*, last modified September 29, 2015, accessed January 23, 2017, http://www.statcan.gc.ca/daily-quotidien/150929/dq150929b-eng.htm.

Statistics Canada, "The Canadian Persian Gulf Cohort Study: Detailed Report," Veterans Affairs Canada, November 2, 2005, accessed March 12, 2013, http://www.veterans.gc.ca/pdf/pro_research/gulf-war-linkage-project.pdf.

Statistics Canada, "Deaths from congenital anomalies in Canada, 1974 to 2012," *The Daily*, last modified September 29, 2016, accessed January 23, 2017, http://www.statcan.gc.ca/daily-quotidien/160929/dq160929d-eng.htm.

Statistics Canada, "Diabetes," *Healthy People, Healthy Places*, last modified January 13, 2010, accessed February 27, 2013, http://www.statcan.gc.ca/pub/82-229-x/2009001/status/dia-eng.htm.

Statistics Canada, "Mood disorders, 2009," *Canadian Community Health Survey*, last modified April 29, 2011, accessed March 22, 2013, http://www.statcan.gc.ca/pub/82-625-x/2010002/article/11265-eng.htm.

Statistics Canada, "Population projections: Canada, the provinces and territories, 2013 to 2063," *The Daily*, last modified September 17, 2014, accessed January 23, 2017, http://www.statcan.gc.ca/daily-quotidien/140917/dq140917a-eng.htm.

Statistics Canada, *Profile of disability among adults,* last modified April 4, 2003, accessed April 29, 2015, http://www.statcan.gc.ca/pub/89-577-x/4065022-eng.htm.

Statistics Canada, "Profile of disability among children - Speech difficulties affect a significant number of school-age children," *A profile of disability in Canada,* 2001, last modified April 4, 2003, accessed April 29, 2015, http://www.statcan.gc.ca/pub/89-577-x/4065023-eng.htm#speech_difficulties.

Statistics Canada, "Section F - Personality disorders," *Health State Descriptions for Canadians*, last modified January 31, 2012, accessed March 20, 2013, http://www.statcan.gc.ca/pub/82-619-m/2012004/sections/sectionf-eng.htm.

Statistics Canada, "Section G - Schizophrenia," *Health State Descriptions for Canadians*, last modified January 31, 2012, accessed March 13, 2013, http://www.statcan.gc.ca/pub/82-619-m/2012004/sections/sectiong-eng.htm.

"Statistics," Alzheimer's Foundation for Caregiving in Canada, Inc., accessed March 20, 2013, http://www.alzfdn.ca/AboutAlzheimers/statistics.html (page no longer available; please see http://www.alzfdn.ca/).

"Statistics," Heart and Stroke Foundation, accessed March 4, 2013, http://www.heartandstroke.on.ca/site/c.pvI3IeNWJwE/b.3581729/k.359A/Statistics.htm (page no longer available; please see http://www.heartandstroke.ca).

"Statistics: Liver Disease," Canadian Digestive Health Foundation, accessed March 4, 2013, http://www.cdhf.ca/digestive-disorders/statistics.shtml#liver.

Steege, John F., and Denniz A. Zolnoun. 2009. Evaluation and treatment of dyspareunia. *Obstetrics and gynecology* 113, no. 5: 1124-1136, PubMed Health, U.S. National Library of Medicine, http://www.ncbi.nlm.nih.gov/pubmed/19384129.

"Stroke Stats & Facts," Ontario Stroke Network, accessed January 24, 2017, http://ontariostrokenetwork.ca/information-about-stroke/stroke-stats-and-facts.

Stromswold, Karen, "The Genetics of Speech and Language Impairments," *New England Journal of Medicine* 359 (2008): 2381-2383, 10.1056/NEJMe0807813, http://www.nejm.org/doi/full/10.1056/NEJMe0807813.

"Study discounts Gulf War cancer link," *National Post* (reprinted by Seanbruyea.com), November 4, 2005, http://www.seanbruyea.com/2005/11/study-discounts-gulf-war-cancer-link.

"Study: Insomnia," *The Daily*, November 16, 2005, http://www.statcan.gc.ca/daily-quotidien/051116/dq051116a-eng.htm.

"Sudden Infant Death Syndrome," MediResource Inc., canada.com accessed March 8, 2013, http://bodyandhealth.canada.com/channel_condition_info_details.asp?channel_id=2022&disease_id=118&relation_id=16665.

"Suicide," MediResource Inc., canada.com accessed March 13, 2013, http://bodyandhealth.canada.com/channel_condition_info_details.asp?disease_id=206&channel_id=1053&relation_id=28250.

"Suicides and suicide rate, by sex and by age group (Both sexes no.)," Statistics Canada, last modified December 10, 2015, accessed January 24, 2017, http://www.statcan.gc.ca/tables-tableaux/sum-som/l01/cst01/hlth66a-eng.htm.

"Summary: Estimates of HIV Prevalence and Incidence in Canada, 2011," Centre for Communicable Diseases and Infection Control, Public Health Agency of Canada, last modified November 29, 2012, http://www.phac-aspc.gc.ca/aids-sida/publication/survreport/estimat2011-eng.php (page no longer available; please see https://www.canada.ca/en/public-health/services/publications/diseases-conditions/summary-estimates-hiv-incidence-prevalence-proportion-undiagnosed-canada-2014.html for the 2014 edition of the report).

"Tay-Sachs Disease," Mayo Foundation for Medical Education and Research, accessed March 12, 2013, http://www.mayoclinic.org/tay-sachs-disease/.

Taylor, Paul, "New Hope for Treating Anorexia," *Globe and Mail*, March 7, 2013.

Thalassemia Foundation of Canada, accessed March 21, 2013, http://www.thalassemia.ca.

The Arthritis Society, accessed March 20, 2013, http://www.arthritis.ca.

The Canadian Addison Society, accessed March 20, 2013, http://www.addisonsociety.ca.

The Canadian Foundation for the Study of Infant Deaths, accessed March 8, 2013, http://www.sidscanada.org.

The Endometriosis Network Canada, accessed February 22, 2013, http://www.endometriosisnetwork.ca.

The Hearing Foundation of Canada, accessed March 4, 2013, http://www.thfc.ca (new site: http://www.hearingfoundation.ca).

The International Huntington Association, accessed April 23, 2015, http://www.huntington-assoc.com.

The Kidney Foundation of Canada, accessed March 4, 2013, http://www.kidney.ca.

The National Coalition for Vision Health, accessed March 22, 2013, http://www.visionhealth.ca (site discontinued).

The National Gaucher Foundation of Canada, accessed February 28, 2013, http://www.gauchercanada.ca.

The Sickle Cell Association of Ontario, access March 5, 2013, http://www.sicklecellontario.org (new site: http://sicklecellontario.ca).

The Skin Care Centre, accessed March 13, 2013, http://www.skincarecentre.ca.

"3rd National Symposium on Child & Youth Mental Health," School Based Mental Health and Substance Abuse Consortium, accessed March 21, 2013, http://childyouth.mh.symposium.curriculum.org (site discontinued).

Thyroid Foundation of Canada, accessed January 24, 2017, http://www.thyroid.ca.

Thyroid Foundation of Canada, accessed March 12, 2013, http://www.thyroid.ca.

Tjepkema, Michael, "Insomnia," *Health Reports* 17, no. 1 (November 2005), Statistics Canada, http://www.statcan.gc.ca/ads-annonces/82-003-x/pdf/4225221-eng.pdf (information now available at http://www.statcan.gc.ca/pub/82-003-x/2005001/article/8707-eng.pdf).

Tourette Syndrome Foundation of Canada, accessed March 13, 2013, http://www.tourette.ca.

Transplant Living, accessed March 13, 2013, http://www.transplantliving.org.

"Traumatic brain injury," Mayo Foundation for Medical Education and Research, last modified October 12, 2012, http://www.mayoclinic.com/health/traumatic-brain-injury/DS00552.

"Treatment," The Voice Foundation, accessed April 29, 2015, http://voicefoundation.org/health-science/voice-disorders/overview-of-diagnosis-treatment-prevention/treatment-of-voice-disorders/.

"Trichotillomania in Children and Youth," eMentalHealth.ca, last modified March 2, 2012, accessed March 22, 2013, http://www.ementalhealth.ca/Hamilton/Trichotillomania-in-Children-and-Youth/index.php?m=article&ID=8889.

"Tuberculosis in Canada 2010, Pre-Release," *Tuberculosis Prevention and Control*, last modified April 30, 2012, accessed March 13, 2013, http://www.phac-aspc.gc.ca/tbpc-latb/pubs/tbcan10pre/index-eng.php.

"Tuberculosis," Canadian Lung Association, last modified March 22, 2013, accessed March 23, 2013, http://www.lung.ca/diseases-maladies/tuberculosis-tuberculose_e.php.

Tuberous Sclerosis Canada, accessed March 12, 2013, http://www.tscanada.ca.

"Tuberous sclerosis," Mayo Foundation for Medical Education and Research, last modified November 1, 2011, accessed March 12, 2013, http://www.mayoclinic.com/health/tuberous-sclerosis/DS01032.

Turner Syndrome Society of Canada, accessed March 8, 2013, http://www.turnersyndrome.ca.

"Turner Syndrome," *A.D.A.M. Medical Encyclopedia*, PubMed Health, U.S. National Library of Medicine, last modified March 30, 2012, accessed March 8, 2013, http://www.ncbi.nlm.nih.gov/pubmedhealth/PMH0001417/.

Ubelacker, Sheryl, "1 in 7 couples in Canada seek help to conceive, mostly when woman older: report," *The Canadian Press*, October 17, 2012, accessed on the Calgary Herald March 6, 2013, http://www.calgaryherald.com/health/couples+Canada+seek+help+conceive+mostly+when+woman+older+report/7404028/story.html (page no longer available; please see http://www.huffingtonpost.ca/2012/10/17/1-in-7-couples-in-canada-_n_1974235.html).

Ubelacker, Sheryl, "Leprosy and Other Diseases of Old Still Affect Canadians," *The Canadian Press*, June 25, 2013, accessed on CTVNews April 24, 2015, http://www.ctvnews.ca/health/health-headlines/leprosy-and-other-diseases-of-old-still-affect-canadians-1.1340567.

"Ulcerative Colitis," Canadian Digestive Health, accessed March 12, 2013, http://www.cdhf.ca/digestive-disorders/ulcerative-colitis.shtml.

"Ulcerative Colitis," Crohn's and Colitis Foundation of Canada, accessed March 12, 2013, http://www.ccfc.ca/site/c.ajIRK4NLLhJ0E/b.6349431/k.C04A/Ulcerative_Colitis.htm (new site: Crohn's and Colitis Canada, http://crohnsandcolitis.ca).

"Ulcerative Colitis," MediResource Inc., canada.com accessed March 12, 2013, http://bodyandhealth.canada.com/condition_info_details.asp?disease_id=233.

"Urinary incontinence," Mayo Foundation for Medical Education and Research, last modified June 25, 2011, accessed February 26, 2013, http://www.mayoclinic.com/health/urinary-incontinence/DS00404.

Vaginismus, accessed March 22, 2013, http://www.vaginismus.com.

Ward Health Strategies, "Urinary Incontinence: Burden, Treatment & Options: A Research Paper," *Canadian Continence Foundation*, May 2007, accessed February 26, 2013, http://www.canadiancontinence.ca/pdf/Research_paper_August2007.pdf (page no longer available; the report can be found at http://www.menopauseandu.ca/documents/IncontinenceCanadianPerspectiveContinenceFound.pdf).

Wedro, Benjamin. "Liver Disease," MedicineNet, last modified June 22, 2012, accessed March 4, 2013, http://www.medicinenet.com/liver_disease.

West, Michael, "Canadian Fabry Disease Initiative (CFDI) Enzyme Replacement Therapy (ERT) Study," ClinicalTrials.gov, last modified January 28, 2009, accessed February 28, 2013, http://clinicaltrials.gov/show/NCT00455104.

"What are genetic disorders?" National Human Genome Research Institute, February 27, 2012, accessed April 28, 2015, http://www.genome.gov/19016930.

"What is a growth disorder?," KidsHealth, The Nemours Foundation, last modified June 2011, accessed March 4, 2013, http://kidshealth.org/parent/medical/endocrine/growth_disorder.html.

"What is Asthma?" Canadian Lung Association, last modified September 24, 2012, accessed March 20, 213, http://www.lung.ca/diseases-maladies/asthma-asthme/what-quoi/index_e.php (page no longer available; please see https://www.lung.ca).

"What is gene therapy?" Genetics Home Reference, April 10, 2005, accessed April 28, 2015, http://ghr.nlm.nih.gov/handbook/therapy/genetherapy.

"What is Guillain-Barré syndrome?" Muscular Dystophy Canada, accessed March 27, 2017, http://www.muscle.ca/about-muscular-dystrophy/types-of-neuromuscular-disorders/guillain-barre-syndrome/.

"What Is Hemophilia?" National Heart, Lung, and Blood Institute, last modified July 1, 2011, accessed March 4, 2013, http://www.nhlbi.nih.gov/health/health-topics/topics/hemophilia.

"What is Hunter Syndrome?" Shire, accessed April 17, 2015, http://www.huntersyndrome.info/en-ca/.

"What Is Immune Thrombocytopenia?" National Heart, Lung, and Blood Institute, March 14, 2012, accessed April 23, 2015, http://www.nhlbi.nih.gov/health/health-topics/topics/itp.

"What is Language? What is Speech?" American Speech-Language Hearing Association, accessed April 29, 2015, http://www.asha.org/public/speech/development/language_speech/.

"What Is Leprosy?" Effecthope, accessed April 24, 2015, http://effecthope.org/learn/leprosy (please also see http://www.leprosy.org/leprosy-faqs).

"What Is Sickle Cell Anemia?" National Heart, Lung, and Blood Institute, September 28, 2012, accessed April 23, 2015, http://www.nhlbi.nih.gov/health/health-topics/topics/sca/.

Wilson Disease Association, accessed March 8, 2013, http://www.wilsonsdisease.org.

"Wilson Disease," Canadian Liver Foundation, accessed March 8, 2013, http://www.liver.ca/liver-disease/types/wilsons-disease.aspx.

"Women and Mental Illness," Canadian Mental Health Association, last modified February 3, 2003, accessed March 22, 2013, http://www.ontario.cmha.ca/fact_sheets.asp?cID=3974 (page no longer available; please see http://www.ontario.cmha.ca).

A

Abbotsford Health Protection Office, 591
Abbotsford Home Health Office, 591
Abbotsford Mental Health Office, 242
Abbotsford Public Health Unit, 591
Abbotsford Regional Hospital & Cancer Centre, 591
Abbotsford Social Activity Association, 10
Aberdeen Hospital, 507, 606
Aberdeen House, 247
Ability New Brunswick, 362
Ability Online Support Network, 285
Ability Society of Alberta, 217
Aboriginal Friendship Centre of Calgary, 743
Aboriginal Friendship Centres of Saskatchewan, 743
Aboriginal Health & Community Wellness, 543
Aboriginal Services, 300, 534
Aboriginal Women's Association of Prince Edward Island, 743
AboutFace, 271
Academic Pediatric Association, 295
Académie de Réflexologie du Québec, 737
Acadia Community Health Centre, 575
Access Alliance Multicultural Community Health Centre, 659
Access Counselling & Family Services, 476
ACCESS Downtown, 614
ACCESS NorWest, 614
ACCESS River East, 614
ACCESS Transcona, 614
ACCESS Winnipeg West, 614
Accessible Housing Society, 469
Accessible Media Inc., 158
Acclaim Health, 719
Accreditation Canada, 413
Achilles Canada, 703
Acoustic Neuroma Association of Canada, 68
Action Autonomie, 232
Action Canada for Sexual Health & Rights, 22
Action North Recovery Centre, 379
Action on Smoking & Health, 200
Active Healthy Kids Canada, 272
Active Living Coalition for Older Adults, 2
Acupuncture Canada, 703
Acute & Emergency Services, 553
Acute Care, 89
Addiction & Mental Health Services, 237
Addiction Recovery Centre, 378
Addiction Services, 383
Addiction Services Edmonton, 239
Addiction Services of Thames Valley, 374
Addiction Services Prince Albert, 259
Addictions & Mental Health Ontario, 373
Addictions Foundation of Manitoba, 373
Addictions Recovery Inc., 382
Adlerian Psychology Association of British Columbia, 219
Administration & Finance, 537, 538
Adsum for Women & Children, 290, 475
Adult Children of Alcoholics, 370
Advanced Coronary Treatment (ACT) Foundation of Canada, 174
Advocacy Centre for the Elderly, 6
A.E. MacDonald Ophthalmic Library & William Callahan Reading Room, 410, 507

AERO: Alternative Education Resources for Ontario, 410
Africa Inland Mission International (Canada), 495
African & Caribbean Council on HIV/AIDS in Ontario, 25
African Community Health Services, 476
African Medical & Research Foundation Canada, 724
Africans in Partnership Against AIDS, 34
Aga Khan Foundation Canada, 724
Agassiz Health Protection Office, 591
Agassiz Home Health Office, 591
Agassiz Mental Health Office, 591
Agassiz Public Health Unit, 591
Age & Opportunity Inc., 5
Agincourt Community Services Association, 477
Ahtahkakoop Health Centre, 694
AIDS Action Now, 29
AIDS Coalition of Cape Breton, 29
AIDS Coalition of Nova Scotia, 25, 35
AIDS Committee of Cambridge, Kitchener/Waterloo & Area, 29, 35
AIDS Committee of Durham Region, 29
AIDS Committee of Newfoundland & Labrador, 25
AIDS Committee of North Bay & Area, 30, 35
AIDS Committee of Ottawa, 30
AIDS Committee of Simcoe County, 30
AIDS Committee of Toronto, 30
AIDS Committee of Windsor, 30, 35
AIDS Committee of York Region, 30
The AIDS Foundation of Canada, 22
AIDS Moncton, 29
AIDS New Brunswick, 25, 35
AIDS Niagara, 30
AIDS PEI, 25
AIDS Programs South Saskatchewan, 34, 35
AIDS Saint John, 29
AIDS Saskatoon, 34
AIDS Vancouver, 27, 35
AIDS Vancouver Island, 28, 35
AiMHi - Prince George Association for Community Living, 246
Air Canada Foundation, 703
Airdrie - 209 Centre Avenue West, 237
Airdrie Provincial Building, 237
Airdrie Regional Health Centre, 573
Airspace Action on Smoking & Health, 202
Akausisarvik Mental Health Facility, 252
Al Ritchie Health Action Centre, 696
Al-Anon Family Groups (Canada), Inc., 370
Albert County Health & Wellness Centre, 621
Alberta & Northwest Territories Lung Association, 202
Alberta Aboriginal Women's Society, 741
Alberta Advanced Education, 531
Alberta Aids to Daily Living, 533
Alberta Alliance on Mental Illness & Mental Health, 217
Alberta Amputee Sports & Recreation Association, 755
Alberta Association of Optometrists, 403
Alberta Association of Prosthetists & Orthotists, 455

Alberta Association of Rehabilitation Centres, 217, 444
Alberta Association of the Deaf, 163
Alberta Association on Gerontology, 4
Alberta Cancer Foundation, 84, 713
Alberta Cerebral Palsy Sport Association, 97, 755
Alberta Children's Hospital, 303
Alberta Children's Hospital Foundation, 713
Alberta Children's Hospital Knowledge Centre, 299
Alberta College & Association of Chiropractors, 733
Alberta College of Acupuncture & Traditional Chinese Medicine, 734
Alberta College of Medical Diagnostic & Therapeutic Technologists, 444
Alberta College of Optometrists, 403
Alberta College of Paramedics, 445
Alberta College of Speech-Language Pathologists & Audiologists, 163
Alberta Committee of Citizens with Disabilities, 445
Alberta Continuing Care Association, 4
Alberta Council on Aging, 4
Alberta Cultural Society of the Deaf, 163
Alberta Deaf Sports Association, 163, 755
Alberta Diabetes Foundation, 121
Alberta Easter Seals Society, 714
Alberta Economic Development & Trade, 531
Alberta Gerontological Nurses Association, 4
Alberta Health, 532
Alberta Health Services, 507, 578
Alberta Hospice Palliative Care Association, 728
Alberta Hospital - Ponoka, 157
Alberta Hospital Edmonton, 239
Alberta Institute for Human Nutrition, 558
Alberta Medical Association, 445
Alberta Native Friendship Centres Association, 741
Alberta Neurosurgical Society, 69
Alberta Northern Lights Wheelchair Basketball Society, 755
Alberta Office of the Child & Youth Advocate, 300
Alberta Office of the Public Interest Commissioner, 534
Alberta Psychiatric Association, 218
Alberta Public Health Association, 445
Alberta Reappraising AIDS Society, 24
Alberta Seniors & Housing, 18
Alberta Society of Radiologists, 445
Alberta Sports & Recreation Association for the Blind, 403
Alberta Therapeutic Recreation Association, 755
Alcoholic Beverage Medical Research Foundation, 375
Alcoholics Anonymous (GTA Intergroup), 370
Alcooliques Anonymes du Québec, 374
Alcove Addiction Recovery for Women, 377
Alexandra Hospital, 644
Alexandra Marine & General Hospital, 507, 641
Alexis Creek Health Centre, 591

Indexes

C

Cabinet du Sous-ministre, 551

Calder Health Care Centre, 624

Caledon Community Services, 477

Calgary - 1177-11 Avenue SW, 378

Calgary - 316-7 Avenue SE, 237

Calgary & Area Medical Staff Society, 469

Calgary Alpha House Society, 374

Calgary Association of Self Help, 227

Calgary Association of the Deaf, 168

Calgary Children's Foundation, 288, 718

Calgary Firefighters Burn Treatment Society, 470

Calgary Meals on Wheels, 10

Calgary Seniors' Resource Society, 10

Calgary Sexual Health Centre, 142, 338

Calgary Women's Health Centre, 575

Calgary Youth Addiction Services Centre, 378

Calling Lake Community Health Services, 576

Cambridge Bay Health Centre, 633

Cambridge Memorial Hospital, 16, 508, 637

CAMH Foundation, 720

Campbell River & District Regional Hospital, 592

Campbell River & District United Way, 471

Campbellford Memorial Hospital, 637

Campbellton Regional Hospital, 617

Camperville Health Centre, 608

Camrose Addiction & Mental Health Clinic, 238

Camrose Community Cancer Centre, 89

Camrose Public Health / Rehab, 576

Canada Health Infoway, 414

Canada India Village Aid Association, 725

Canadian Abilities Foundation, 703

Canadian Aboriginal AIDS Network, 22, 740

Canadian Aboriginal Veterans & Serving Members Association, 147

Canadian Academy of Audiology, 158

Canadian Academy of Child & Adolescent Psychiatry, 212

Canadian Academy of Facial Plastic & Reconstructive Surgery, 414

Canadian Academy of Geriatric Psychiatry, 2

Canadian Academy of Psychiatry & the Law, 212

Canadian Addiction Counsellors Certification Federation, 371

The Canadian Addison Society, 1

Canadian ADHD Resource Alliance, 49

Canadian Adult Congenital Heart Network, 114

Canadian Agency for Drugs & Technologies in Health (CADTH), 121

Canadian AIDS Society, 22

Canadian AIDS Treatment Information Exchange (CATIE), 23, 35

Canadian Alliance for Long Term Care, 3

Canadian Alliance of Physiotherapy Regulators, 91

Canadian Alliance on Mental Illness & Mental Health, 212

Canadian Alopecia Areata Foundation, 414

Canadian Amputee Golf Association, 753

Canadian Amputee Sports Association, 753

Canadian Anesthesiologists' Society, 414

Canadian Angelman Syndrome Society, 145

Canadian Apheresis Group, 414

Canadian Art Therapy Association, 415

Canadian Arthritis Network, 44

Canadian Assembly of Narcotics Anonymous, 212

Canadian Association for Child & Play Therapy, 285

Canadian Association for Clinical Microbiology & Infectious Diseases, 415

Canadian Association for Community Living, 415

Canadian Association for Disabled Skiing - National Capital Division, 753, 755, 758

Canadian Association for Educational Psychology, 213

Canadian Association for Enterostomal Therapy, 139

Canadian Association for Health Services & Policy Research, 415

The Canadian Association for HIV Research, 23

Canadian Association for Immunization Research & Evaluation, 416

Canadian Association for Integrative & Energy Therapies, 730

Canadian Association for Medical Education, 416

Canadian Association for Music Therapy, 416

Canadian Association for Neuroscience, 68

Canadian Association for Population Therapeutics, 416

Canadian Association for Sandplay Therapy, 213

Canadian Association for School Health, 416

Canadian Association for Size Acceptance, 274

Canadian Association for Suicide Prevention, 264

Canadian Association for Supported Employment, 213

Canadian Association for the Study of the Liver, 199

Canadian Association for Williams Syndrome, 143

Canadian Association of Acupuncture & Traditional Chinese Medicine, 730

Canadian Association of Ambulatory Care, 416

Canadian Association of Apheresis Nurses, 416

Canadian Association of Bariatric Physicians & Surgeons, 272, 417

Canadian Association of Blue Cross Plans, 417

Canadian Association of Cardio-Pulmonary Technologists, 174

Canadian Association of Cardiovascular Prevention & Rehabilitation, 174

Canadian Association of Centres for the Management of Hereditary Metabolic Diseases, 136

Canadian Association of Child Neurology, 417

Canadian Association of Community Health Centres, 417

Canadian Association of Electroneurophysiology Technologists Inc., 68

Canadian Association of Gastroenterology, 139

Canadian Association of General Surgeons, 418

Canadian Association of Genetic Counsellors, 143

Canadian Association of Hepatology Nurses, 183

Canadian Association of Interventional Cardiology, 174

Canadian Association of Medical Biochemists, 418

Canadian Association of Medical Device Reprocessing, 418

Canadian Association of Medical Oncologists, 76

Canadian Association of Medical Radiation Technologists, 418, 506

Canadian Association of Medical Teams Abroad, 703

The Canadian Association of Naturopathic Doctors, 730

Canadian Association of Nephrology Nurses & Technologists, 194

Canadian Association of Neuropathologists, 418

Canadian Association of Nuclear Medicine, 418

Canadian Association of Nurses in HIV/AIDS Care, 23

Canadian Association of Nurses in Oncology, 76

Canadian Association of Occupational Therapists, 456, 418

Canadian Association of Optometrists, 400

Canadian Association of Paediatric Health Centres, 285

Canadian Association of Paediatric Surgeons, 285

Canadian Association of Pathologists, 419

Canadian Association of Perinatal & Women's Health Nurses, 61

Canadian Association of Pharmacy in Oncology, 76

Canadian Association of Physical Medicine & Rehabilitation, 419

Canadian Association of Physician Assistants, 419

Canadian Association of Physicians of Indian Heritage, 419

Canadian Association of Physicians with Disabilities, 419

Canadian Association of Pregnancy Support Services, 61

Canadian Association of Professionals with Disabilities, 419

Canadian Association of Provincial Cancer Agencies, 76

Canadian Association of Psychosocial Oncology, 77

Canadian Association of Radiation Oncology, 77

Canadian Association of Radiologists, 419

Canadian Association of Research Administrators, 419

Canadian Association of Specialized Kinesiology, 420

Canadian Association of the Deaf, 158, 171

Canadian Association of Thoracic Surgeons, 46

Canadian Association of Transplantation, 393

Canadian Association of Veterans in United Nations Peacekeeping, 147

Canadian Association on Gerontology, 3

Canadian Blind Sports Association Inc., 400

Canadian Blood & Marrow Transplant Group, 65

Indexes

Indexes

Indexes

Indexes

Indexes

Indexes

Indexes

Indexes

Indexes

Indexes

Indexes

Indexes

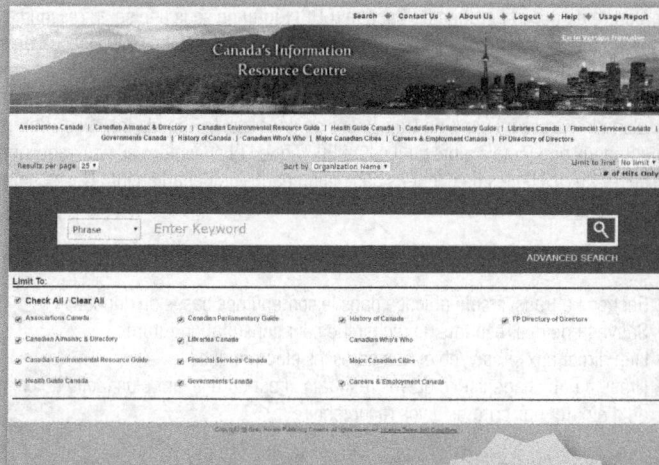

CENTRE DE DOCUMENTATION DU CANADA (CDC)

Consultez en tout temps toutes ces excellentes ressources en ligne grâce au Centre de documentation du Canada (CDC) à
http://circ.greyhouse.ca

Le Centre de documentation du Canada (CDC) regroupe sous une seule ressource en ligne conviviale tout le contenu des ouvrages de référence primés de Grey House Canada. Répertoriant plus de **100 000 entreprises canadiennes, et plus de 140 600 personnes-ressources**, faits et chiffres, il s'agit de la ressource la plus complète en matière de bases de données spécialisées au Canada! Grâce à l'ajout de trois bases de données, le Canada Info Desk Complete est plus avantageux que jamais alors qu'il coûte 50 % que l'abonnement aux ouvrages individuels. Accédez aux 13 bases de données dès maintenant — le Canadian Info Desk Complete vous offre un ensemble complet!

PRINCIPAUX AVANTAGES DU CDC

- Recherche transversale efficace dans le contenu des bases de données
- Sauvegarde des résultats de recherche pour consultation future
- Lien direct aux sites Web et aux adresses électroniques
- Grâce à l'affichage lisible de vos résultats, il est dorénavant plus facile de compiler les résultats ou d'ajouter des critères à vos recherches

CONCEPTION PERSONNALISÉE DE VOS LISTES DE PERSONNES-RESSOURCES!

Le CDC vous permet de définir et d'extraire vos propres listes, et ce, en quelques secondes. Découvrez des clients potentiels, effectuez des recherches par mot-clé, trouvez les participants à une conférence à venir : l'information dont vous avez besoin, au bout de vos doigts.

CHOISISSEZ ENTRE RECHERCHES MOT-CLÉ ET AVANCÉE!

Grâce au CDC, vous pouvez choisir entre une recherche Mot-clé ou Avancée pour localiser l'information avec précision. Vous avez la possibilité d'effectuer des recherches en texte simple ou booléennes puissantes — les recherches sont conçues à l'intention des chercheurs débutants et avancés.

LES PROFILS DU CDC COMPRENNENT :

- Numéros de téléphone, adresses électroniques, numéros de télécopieur et adresses complètes pour toutes les succursales d'un organisme
- Comptes de médias sociaux, comme Twitter et Facebook
- Personnes-ressources clés en fonction des appellations d'emploi
- Budgets, frais d'adhésion, tailles du personnel et plus!

Effectuez des recherches dans le CDC à l'aide de champs uniques ou communs, personnalisés selon vos besoins!

SEULS LES RÉPERTOIRES DE GREY HOUSE VOUS OFFRENT UN CONTENU PARTICULIER QUE VOUS NE TROUVEREZ NULLE PART AILLEURS!

- **Le répertoire des associations du Canada :** sources de financement, activités, publications, congrès, membres, prix, profil de membre
- **Guide parlementaire canadien :** carrières privées et politiques des membres élus, liste complète des comtés et des représentants
- **Guide des ressources environnementales canadiennes :** produits/services/domaines d'expertise, langues de travail, marchés nationaux, type de propriétaire, sources de revenus
- **Services financiers :** type de propriétaire, nombre d'employés, année de la fondation, immobilisations, revenus, symbole au téléscripteur
- **Bibliothèques Canada :** personnel, collections particulières, services, année de la fondation, symbole de bibliothèque national, système régional
- **Gouvernements du Canada :** population municipale
- **Canadian Who's Who :** ville d'origine, publication, formation (diplômes et alma mater), carrière/emploi et employeur
- **Principales villes canadiennes :** données démographiques, ethnicité, immigration, langue, éducation, logement, revenu, main-d'œuvre et transport
- **Guide canadien de la santé :** maladies chroniques et mentales, ressources generales, annexes et statistiques.
- **Carrières et emplois Canada :** associations professionnelles, sites Web d'emplois, employeurs, répertoires par industrie, recruteurs, bourses, conseils sectoriels et emplois d'été
- **Répertoire des administrateurs :** prénom, nom de famille, poste de cadre et d'administrateur, parcours scolaire et professionnel et adresse électronique des cadres supérieurs canadiens; liste des sociétés les plus importantes au Canada et l'information complète des compagnies

Le nouveau CDC facilite la recherche au sein de toutes nos ressources au Canada et procure plus rapidement des résultats plus poussés — des associations au gouvernement en passant par les principales entreprises et les zoos, sans oublier tout un éventail d'organisations! Que vous ayez besoin d'information très détaillée au sujet de votre personne-ressource ou d'une simple adresse électronique, vous pouvez personnaliser votre requête afin qu'elle réponde à vos besoins. Contactez-nous sans tarder pour obtenir un **essai gratuit** ou visitez http://circ.greyhouse.ca

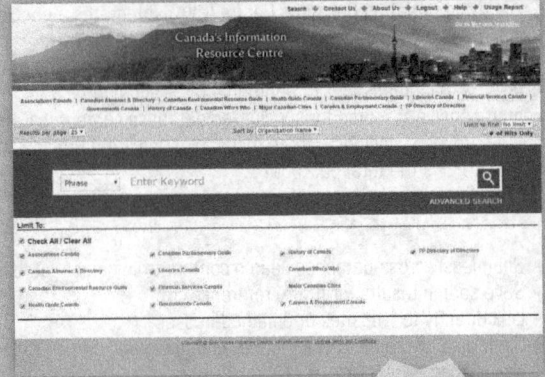

Nouvelle allure, contenu toujours aussi riche!

GREY HOUSE PUBLISHING CANADA
Pour obtenir plus d'information, veuillez contacter Grey House Publishing Canada
par tél. : 1 866 433-4739 ou 416 644-6479 par téléc. : 416 644-1904 | info@greyhouse.ca | www.greyhouse.ca

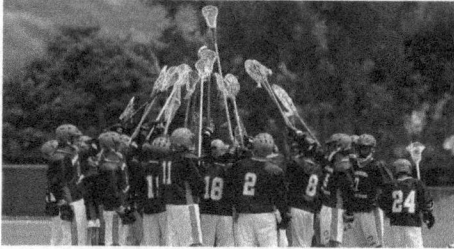

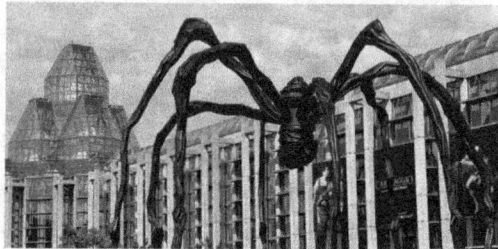

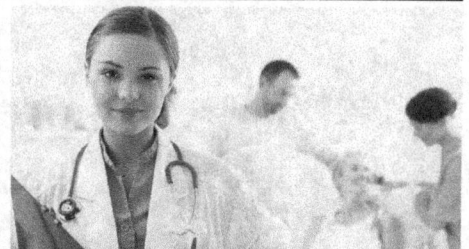

Répertoire et almanach canadien

La ressource de référence au sujet des données et des faits relatifs au Canada

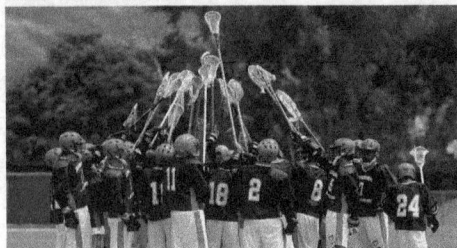

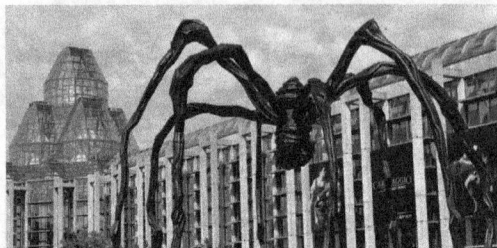

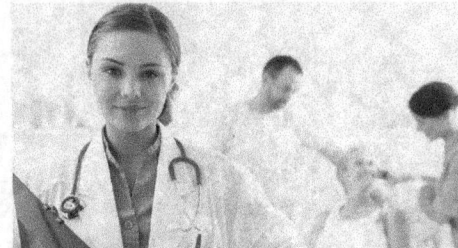

Le *Répertoire et almanach canadien* constitue le guide canadien le plus rigoureux depuis 170 ans. Publié annuellement depuis 1847, il est toujours grandement utilisé dans le monde des affaires, les bureaux gouvernementaux, par les spécialistes de l'information, les chercheurs, les éditeurs ou quiconque est à la recherche d'information actuelle et accessible sur tous les sujets imaginables à propos des gens qui vivent et travaillent au Canada.

À la fois répertoire et guide, le *Répertoire et almanach canadien* dresse le tableau le plus complet du Canada, des caractéristiques physiques jusqu'aux revues économique et commerciale, en passant par les loisirs et les activités récréatives. Il combine des documents textuels, des représentations graphiques, des photographies en couleurs et des listes de répertoires accompagnées de profils détaillés. Autant d'information pointue et organisée de manière à ce qu'elle soit facile à obtenir. Le *Répertoire et almanach canadien* foisonne de renseignements généraux. Il présente des statistiques nationales sur la population, l'emploi, l'IPC, l'importation et l'exportation ainsi que des images des prix nationaux, des symboles canadiens, des drapeaux, des emblèmes et des leaders parlementaires canadiens.

Si vous cherchez des personnes-ressources essentielles un peu partout au Canada, peu importe qu'il s'agisse de projets d'affaires ou d'une question factuelle anecdotique, le Répertoire et almanach canadien vous fournira les pistes dont vous ignoriez l'existence – rapidement et facilement!

TOUTE L'INFORMATION DONT VOUS AUREZ BESOIN, ORGANISÉE EN 17 CATÉGORIES DISTINCTES POUR UNE CONSULTATION FACILE!

Almanach—un aperçu informatif du Canada, notamment l'histoire, la géographie, l'économie et les statistiques essentielles.

Arts et culture—comprends 9 sujets, des galeries aux zoos.

Associations—des milliers d'organisations classées selon 147 sujets différents, de l'actuariat au zoo.

Radiodiffusion—les principales sociétés de radiodiffusion au Canada, les stations radiophoniques et de télévision ainsi que les entreprises de câblodistribution et les diffuseurs thématiques.

Commerce et finance—comptabilité, services bancaires, assurances, principales entreprises et bourses canadiennes.

Éducation—organisé par province et comprend les arrondissements scolaires, les organismes gouvernementaux, les écoles spécialisées et indépendantes, les universités et les établissements techniques.

Gouvernement—s'étend sur trois sections et comprend un guide de référence, des listes fédérales et provinciales, les comtés et arrondissements municipaux ainsi que les cours canadiennes.

Santé—organismes gouvernementaux, hôpitaux, centres de santé communautaires, établissements de soins pour personnes retraitées et de soins de santé mentale.

Sociétés d'avocats—toutes les principales sociétés d'avocats, suivies des sociétés plus petites, classées par province et en ordre alphabétique.

Bibliothèques—la bibliothèque et les archives principales du Canada ainsi que les bibliothèques des ministères, suivis des listes provinciales et des systèmes régionaux.

Édition—livres, magazines et journaux classés par province, y compris leur fréquence et les données relatives à leur diffusion.

Religion—information générale au sujet des groupes religieux et des associations religieuses de 38 dénominations.

Sports—associations de 110 sports distincts; comprend des listes de ligues et d'équipes.

Transport—des listes complètes des principaux modes de transport.

Services publics—associations, organismes gouvernementaux et entreprises de services publics provinciaux.

FORMAT PAPIER OU EN LIGNE—ACCÈS RAPIDE À TOUS LES RENSEIGNEMENTS DONT VOUS AVEZ BESOIN!

Offert sous couverture rigide ou en format électronique grâce au web, le *Répertoire et almanach canadien* offre invariablement un accès instantané aux représentants du gouvernement et aux faits qui font l'objet de vos recherches.

La version imprimée du Répertoire et almanach canadien est vérifiée et mise à jour annuellement. La version en ligne est mise à jour mensuellement. Cette version vous permet de circonscrire la recherche grâce aux champs de l'index comme le nom ou le type d'organisme, le sujet, l'emplacement, le nom ou le titre de la personne-ressource et le code postal.

Les abonnés au service en ligne peuvent générer instantanément leurs propres listes de contacts et les exporter en format feuille de calcul pour une utilisation approfondie – une solution de rechange géniale aux services dispendieux d'un commissionnaire en publipostage.

GREY HOUSE PUBLISHING CANADA

Pour obtenir plus d'information, veuillez contacter Grey House Publishing Canada

par tél. : 1 866 433-4739 ou 416 644-6479 par téléc. : 416 644-1904 | info@greyhouse.ca | www.greyhouse.ca

Associations Canada
Makes Researching Organizations Quick and Easy

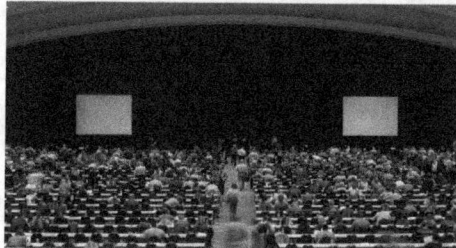

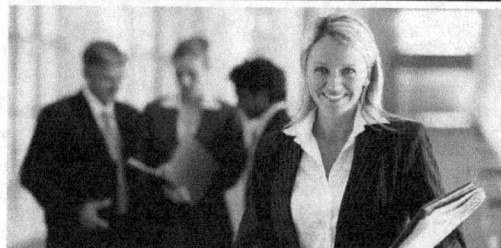

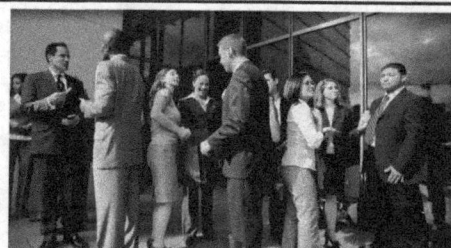

Associations Canada is an easy-to-use compendium, providing detailed indexes, listings and abstracts on over 20,000 local, regional, provincial, national and international organizations (identifying location, budget, founding date, management, scope of activity and funding source—just to name a few).

POWERFUL INDEXES HELP YOU TARGET THE ORGANIZATIONS YOU WANT

There are a number of criteria you can use to target specific organizations. Organized with the user in mind, *Associations Canada* is broken down into a number of indexes to help you find what you're looking for quickly and easily.

- **Subject Index**—listing of Canadian and foreign association headquarters, alphabetically by subject and keyword

- **Acronym Index**—an alphabetical listing of acronyms and corresponding Canadian and foreign associations, in both official languages

- **Budget Index**—Canadian associations, alphabetical within eight budget categories

- **Conferences & Conventions Index**—meetings sponsored by Canadian and foreign associations, listed alphabetically by conference name

- **Executive Name Index**—alphabetical listing of key contacts of Canadian associations, for both headquarters and branches

- **Geographic Index**—listing of headquarters, branch offices, chapters and divisions of Canadian associations, alphabetical within province and city

- **Mailing List Index**—associations that offer mailing lists, alphabetical by subject

- **Registered Charitable Organizations Index**—listing of associations that are registered charities, alphabetical by subject

PRINT OR ONLINE—QUICK AND EASY ACCESS TO ALL THE INFORMATION YOU NEED!

Available in softcover print or electronically via the web, *Associations Canada* provides instant access to the people you need and the facts you want every time. Whereas the print edition is verified and updated annually, ongoing changes are added to the web version on a regular basis. The web version allows you to narrow your search by using index fields such as name or type of organization, subject, location, contact name or title and postal code.

Create your own contact lists! Online subscribers have the option to instantly generate their own contact lists and export them into spreadsheets for further use—a great alternative to high cost list broker services.

ASSOCIATIONS CANADA PROVIDES COMPLETE ACCESS TO THESE HIGHLY LUCRATIVE MARKETS:

Travel & Tourism
- Who's hosting what event...when and where?
- Check on events up to three years in advance

Journalism and Media
- Pure research—What do they do? Who is in charge? What's their budget?
- Check facts and sources in one step

Libraries
- Refer researchers to the most complete Canadian association reference anywhere

Business
- Target your market, research your interests, compile profiles and identify membership lists
- Warm up your cold calls with all the background you need to sell your product or service
- Preview prospects by budget, market interest or geographic location

Association Executives
- Look for strategic alliances with associations of similar interest
- Spot opportunities or conflicts with convention plans

Research & Government
- Scan interest groups or identify charities in your area of concern
- Check websites, publications and speaker availability
- Evaluate mandates, affiliations and scope

GREY HOUSE PUBLISHING CANADA

For more information please contact Grey House Publishing Canada

Tel.: (866) 433-4739 or (416) 644-6479 Fax: (416) 644-1904 | info@greyhouse.ca | www.greyhouse.ca

Associations du Canada

La recherche d'organisations simplifiée

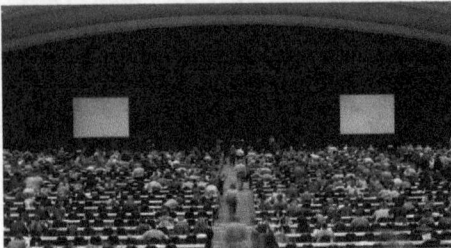

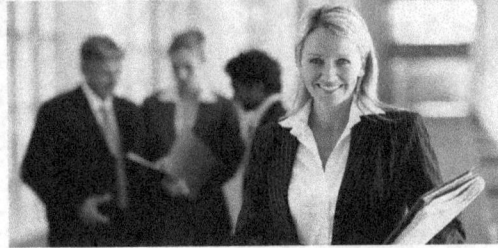

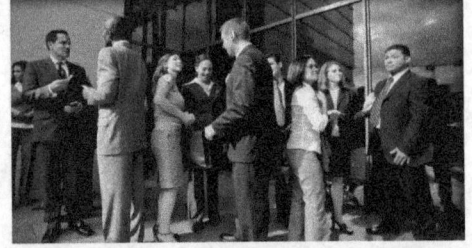

Il s'agit d'un recueil facile d'utilisation qui offre des index, des fiches descriptives et des résumés exhaustifs de plus de 20 000 organismes locaux, régionaux, provinciaux, nationaux et internationaux. Il donne, entre autres, des détails sur leur emplacement, leur budget, leur date de mise sur pied, l'éventail de leurs activités et leurs sources de financement.

En plus d'affecter plus d'un milliard de dollars annuellement aux frais de transport, à la participation à des congrès et à la mise en marché, *Associations du Canada* débourse des millions de dollars dans sa quête pour répondre aux intérêts de ses membres.

DES INDEX PUISSANTS QUI VOUS AIDENT À CIBLER LES ORGANISATIONS VOULUES

Vous pouvez vous servir de plusieurs critères pour cibler des organisations précises. C'est avec l'utilisateur en tête qu'*Associations du Canada* a été divisé en plusieurs index pour vous aider à trouver, rapidement et facilement, ce que vous cherchez.

- **Index des sujets**—liste des sièges sociaux d'associations canadiennes et étrangères; sujets classés en ordre alphabétique et mot-clé.
- **Index des acronymes**—liste alphabétique des acronymes et des associations canadiennes et étrangères équivalentes; présenté dans les deux langues officielles.
- **Index des budgets**—associations canadiennes classées en ordre alphabétique parmi huit catégories de budget.
- **Index des congrès**—rencontres commanditées par des associations canadiennes et étrangères; classées en ordre alphabétique selon le titre de l'événement.
- **Index des directeurs**—liste alphabétique des principales personnes-ressources des associations canadiennes, aux sièges sociaux et aux succursales.
- **Index géographique**—liste des sièges sociaux, des succursales, des sections régionales et des divisions des associations canadiennes; ordre alphabétique au sein des provinces et des villes.
- **Index des listes de distribution**—liste des associations qui offrent des listes de distribution; en ordre alphabétique selon le sujet.
- **Index des œuvres de bienfaisance enregistrées**—liste des associations enregistrées en tant qu'œuvres de bienfaisance; en ordre alphabétique selon le sujet.

OFFERT EN FORMAT PAPIER OU EN LIGNE—UN ACCÈS RAPIDE ET FACILE À TOUS LES RENSEIGNEMENTS DONT VOUS AVEZ BESOIN!

Offert sous couverture souple ou en format électronique grâce au web, *Associations du Canada* donne invariablement un accès instantané aux personnes et aux faits dont vous avez besoin. Si la version imprimée est vérifiée et mise à jour annuellement, des changements continus sont apportés mensuellement à la base de données en ligne. Servez-vous de la version en ligne afin de circonscrire vos recherches grâce à des champs spéciaux de l'index comme le nom de l'organisation ou son type, le sujet, l'emplacement, le nom de la personne-ressource ou son titre et le code postal.

Créez vos propres listes! Les abonnés au service en ligne peuvent générer instantanément leurs propres listes de contacts et les exporter en format feuille de calcul pour une utilisation approfondie – une solution de rechange géniale aux services dispendieux d'un commissionnaire en publipostage.

ASSOCIATIONS DU CANADA OFFRE UN ACCÈS COMPLET À CES MARCHÉS HAUTEMENT LUCRATIFS

Voyage et tourisme
- Renseignez-vous sur les hôtes des événements... sur les dates et les endroits.
- Consultez les événements trois ans au préalable.

Journalisme et médias
- Recherche authentique—quel est leur centre d'activité? Qui est la personne responsable? Quel est leur budget?
- Vérifiez les faits et sources en une seule étape.

Bibliothèques
- Orientez les chercheurs vers la référence la plus complète en ce qui concerne les associations canadiennes.

Commerce
- Ciblez votre marché, faites une recherche selon vos sujets de prédilection, compilez des profils et recensez des listes des membres.
- Préparez votre sollicitation au hasard en obtenant les renseignements dont vous avez besoin pour offrir votre produit ou service.
- Obtenez un aperçu de vos clients potentiels selon les budgets, les intérêts au marché ou l'emplacement géographique.

Directeurs d'associations
- Recherchez des alliances stratégiques avec des associations partageant vos intérêts.
- Repérez des occasions ou des conflits dans le cadre de la planification des congrès.

Recherche et gouvernement
- Parcourez les groupes d'intérêts ou identifiez les organismes de bienfaisance de votre domaine d'intérêt.
- Consultez les sites Web, les publications et vérifiez la disponibilité des conférenciers.
- Évaluez les mandats, les affiliations et le champ d'application.

GREY HOUSE PUBLISHING CANADA Pour obtenir plus d'information, veuillez contacter Grey House Publishing Canada
par tél. : 1 866 433-4739 ou 416 644-6479 par téléc. : 416 644-1904 | info@greyhouse.ca | www.greyhouse.ca

Governments Canada

The Most Complete and Comprehensive Guide to Locating People and Programs in Canada

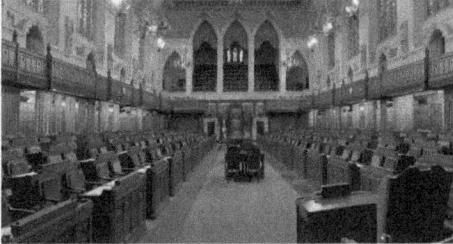

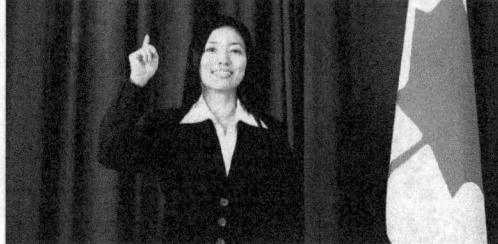

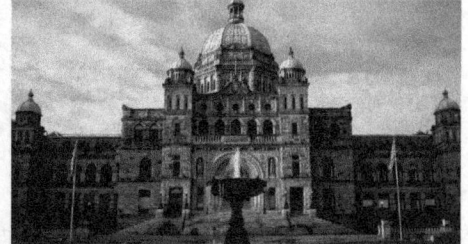

Governments Canada provides regularly updated listings on federal, provincial/territorial and municipal government departments, offices and agencies across Canada. Branch and regional offices are also included, along with all associated agencies, boards, commissions and Crown corporations.

Listings include contact name, full address, telephone and fax numbers, as well as e-mail addresses. You can be sure of our commitment to superior indexing and accuracy.

ACCESS IS PROVIDED TO THE KEY DECISION-MAKERS IN ALL LEVELS OF THE GOVERNMENT INCLUDING:

- Cabinets/ Executive Councils
- Elected Officials
- Governors General/ Lieutenant Governors/ Territorial Commissioners
- Prime Ministers/ Premiers/ Government Leaders
- Auditor General/ Provincial Auditors
- Electoral Officers
- Departments/ Agencies and Administration

GOVERNMENTS CANADA IS AN ESSENTIAL FINDING TOOL FOR:

Lobbyists—Locate the right person for productive conversation on key issues

Lawyers, Accountants and Consultants—Access the most current names and addresses of key contacts in every government office

Librarians—Reduce research time with this all-in-one reference tool

Embassies & Consulates—Find the right referral contact or official from across Canada

Government Employees—Peruse the easy-to-find facts and information on all levels of government

Suppliers to Government—Locate the decision-makers to target your products or services

THESE POWERFUL AND EASY-TO-USE INDEXES WERE DESIGNED TO HELP FIND QUICK AND AUTHORITATIVE RESULTS FOR ANY RESEARCH QUERY.

- **Topical Table of Contents**—a single unified index to all jurisdictions
- **Quick Reference Topics**—a detailed list with references to over 170 topics of interest
- **Highlights of Significant Changes**—a list of highlights of major changes that have recently occurred in government.

- **Contacts**—an invaluable networking and sales tool with over 300 pages of full contact information
- **Website/ Email listings**—organized by government and department or ministry
- **Acronyms**—an alphabetical list of the most commonly used acronyms

GREY HOUSE PUBLISHING CANADA

For more information please contact Grey House Publishing Canada

Tel.: (866)-433-4739 or (416) 644-6479 Fax: (416) 644-1904 | info@greyhouse.ca | www.greyhouse.ca

Gouvernements du Canada

Le guide le plus complet et exhaustif pour trouver des personnes et des programmes au Canada

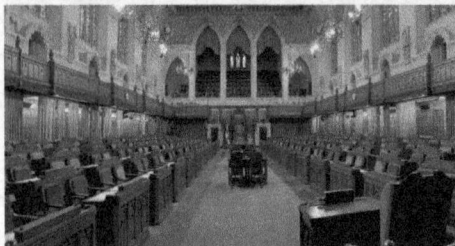

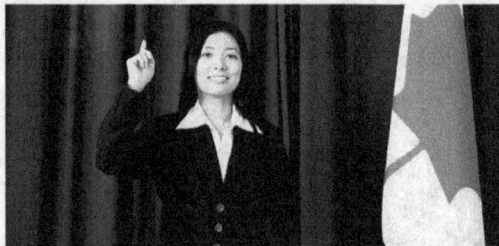

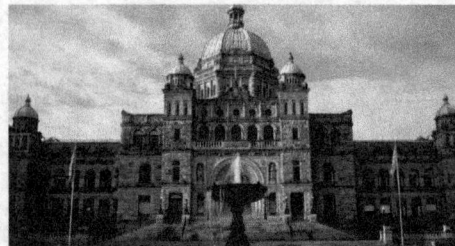

Ce répertoire offre des fiches descriptives mises à jour régulièrement au sujet des ministères fédéraux, provinciaux et territoriaux, des bureaux et des agences du gouvernement de partout au pays. Les directions générales et les bureaux régionaux en font également partie, tout comme les organismes associés, les conseils, les commissions et les sociétés de la Couronne.

Les fiches descriptives comprennent les noms de personnes-ressources, l'adresse complète, les numéros de téléphone et de télécopieur de même que les courriels. Vous pouvez compter sur notre engagement envers la précision et l'indexation de qualité supérieure.

VOUS AVEZ AINSI ACCÈS AUX DÉCIDEURS CLÉS À TOUS LES PALIERS DE GOUVERNEMENT, NOTAMMENT :

- Conseils des ministres/conseils exécutifs
- Représentants élus
- Gouverneur général/lieutenants gouverneurs/commissaires territoriaux
- Premiers ministres/premiers ministres provinciaux/leaders du gouvernement
- Vérificateur général du Canada/vérificateurs provinciaux
- Fonctionnaires électoraux
- Ministères/organismes et administration publique

CES INDEX PUISSANTS ET FACILES D'UTILISATION SONT CONÇUS POUR VOUS AIDER À OBTENIR DES RÉSULTATS RAPIDES ET DIGNES DE FOI, PEU IMPORTE VOTRE RECHERCHE.

- **Table des matières de noms communs**—un seul index unifié pour toutes les juridictions.

- **Guide éclair des sujets**—une liste détaillée accompagnée de références sur plus de 170 sujets d'intérêt.

- **Faits saillants des changements importants**—une liste des principaux changements importants récemment apportés au sein du gouvernement.

- **Personnes-ressources**—un outil irremplaçable de réseautage et de ventes grâce à plus de 300 pages de coordonnées complètes.

- **Listes de sites Web et de courriels**—classées par gouvernement et ministère.

- **Acronymes**—une liste alphabétique des acronymes les plus utilisés.

GOUVERNEMENTS DU CANADA EST L'OUTIL ESSENTIEL DES PROFESSIONNELS POUR TROUVER:

Des groupes de revendication—trouvez les bonnes personnes pour avoir une conversation productive sur des questions-clés.

Des avocats, des comptables et des conseillers—obtenez les noms et les adresses les plus courants des personnes-ressources clés de chaque bureau gouvernemental.

Des bibliothécaires—épargnez du temps de recherche grâce à cet outil de référence complet.

Des ambassades et des consulats—trouvez la bonne personne-ressource ou le bon fonctionnaire en matière de présentation partout au Canada.

Des employés du gouvernement—consultez les faits et renseignements faciles à obtenir à tous les paliers gouvernementaux.

Des fournisseurs du gouvernement—trouvez les décideurs afin de cibler vos produits et services.

GREY HOUSE PUBLISHING CANADA

Pour obtenir plus d'information, veuillez contacter Grey House Publishing Canada

par tél. : 1 866 433-4739 ou 416 644-6479 par téléc. : 416 644-1904 | info@greyhouse.ca | www.greyhouse.ca

Canadian Parliamentary Guide

Your Number One Source for All General Federal Elections Results!

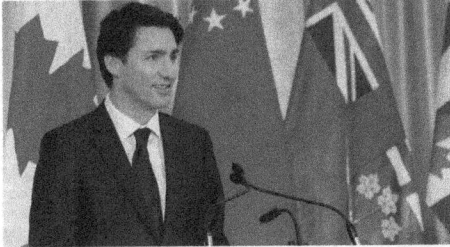
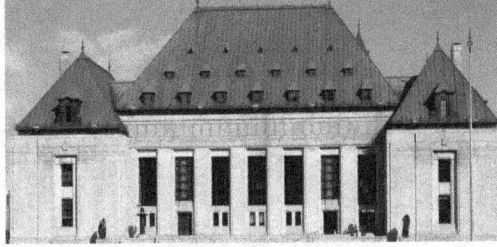
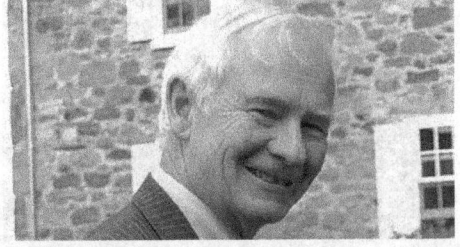

Published annually since before Confederation, the *Canadian Parliamentary Guide* is an indispensable directory, providing biographical information on elected and appointed members in federal and provincial government. Featuring government institutions such as the Governor General's Household, Privy Council and Canadian legislature, this comprehensive collection provides historical and current election results with statistical, provincial and political data.

THE CANADIAN PARLIAMENTARY GUIDE IS BROKEN DOWN INTO FIVE COMPREHENSIVE CATEGORIES

Monarchy—biographical information on Her Majesty Queen Elizabeth II, The Royal Family and the Governor General

Federal Government—a separate chapter for each of the Privy Council, Senate and House of Commons (including a brief description of the institution, its history in both text and chart format and a list of current members), followed by unparalleled biographical sketches*

General Elections

1867–2011

- information is listed alphabetically by province then by riding name

- notes on each riding include: date of establishment, date of abolition, former division and later divisions, followed by election year and successful candidate's name and party

- by-election information follows

2015

- information for the 2015 election is organized in the same manner but also includes information on all the candidates who ran in each riding, their party affiliation and the number of votes won

Provincial and Territorial Governments—Each provincial chapter includes:

- statistical information

- description of Legislative Assembly

- biographical sketch of the Lieutenant Governor or Commissioner

- list of current Cabinet Members

- dates of legislatures since confederation

- current Members and Constituencies

- biographical sketches*

- general election and by-election results, including 2015 general elections in Alberta, Prince Edward Island, Newfoundland & Labrador, and the Northwest Territories.

Courts: Federal—each court chapter includes a description of the court (Supreme, Federal, Federal Court of Appeal, Court Martial Appeal and Tax Court), its history and a list of its judges followed by biographical sketches*

* Biographical sketches follow a concise yet in-depth format:

Personal Data—place of birth, education, family information

Political Career—political career path and services

Private Career—work history, organization memberships, military history

AVAILABLE IN PRINT AND NOW ONLINE!

Available in hardcover print, the *Canadian Parliamentary Guide* is also available electronically via the Web, providing instant access to the government officials you need and the facts you want every time. Use the web version to narrow your search with index fields such as institution, province and name.

Create your own contact lists! Online subscribers can instantly generate their own contact lists and export information into spreadsheets for further use. A great alternative to high cost list broker services!

GREY HOUSE PUBLISHING CANADA

For more information please contact Grey House Publishing Canada

Tel.: (866) 433-4739 or (416) 644-6479 Fax: (416) 644-1904 | info@greyhouse.ca | www.greyhouse.ca

Guide parlementaire canadien

Votre principale source d'information en matière de résultats d'élections fédérales!

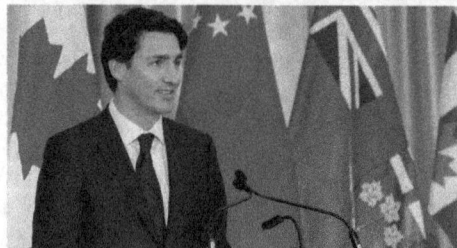

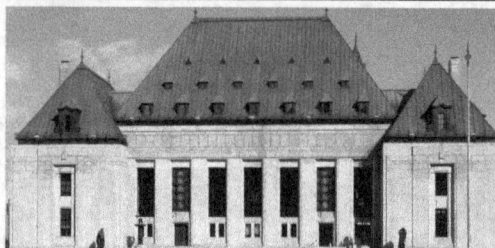

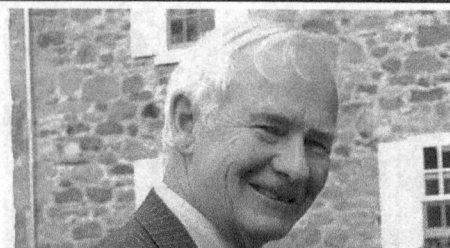

Publié annuellement depuis avant la Confédération, le *Guide parlementaire canadien* est une source fondamentale de notices biographiques des membres élus et nommés aux gouvernements fédéral et provinciaux. Il y est question, notamment, d'établissements gouvernementaux comme la résidence du gouverneur général, le Conseil privé et la législature canadienne. Ce recueil exhaustif présente les résultats historiques et actuels accompagnés de données statistiques, provinciales et politiques.

LE GUIDE PARLEMENTAIRE CANADIEN EST DIVISÉ EN CINQ CATÉGORIES EXHAUSTIVES:

La monarchie—des renseignements biographiques sur Sa Majesté la reine Elizabeth II, la famille royale et le gouverneur général.

Le gouvernement fédéral—un chapitre distinct pour chacun des sujets suivants: Conseil privé, sénat, Chambre des communes (y compris une brève description de l'institution, son historique sous forme de textes et de graphiques et une liste des membres actuels) suivi de notes biographiques sans pareil.*

Les élections fédérales

1867–2011

- Les renseignements sont présentés en ordre alphabétique par province puis par circonscription.

- Les notes de chaque circonscription comprennent : La date d'établissement, la date d'abolition, l'ancienne circonscription, les circonscriptions ultérieures, etc. puis l'année d'élection ainsi que le nom et le parti des candidats élus.

- Viennent ensuite des renseignements sur l'élection partielle.

2015

- Les renseignements de l'élection 2015 sont organisés de la même manière, mais comprennent également de l'information sur tous les candidats qui se sont présentés dans chaque circonscription, leur appartenance politique et le nombre de voix récoltées.

Gouvernements provinciaux et territoriaux—Chaque chapitre portant sur le gouvernement provincial comprend :

- des renseignements statistiques
- une description de l'Assemblée législative
- des notes biographiques sur le lieutenant-gouverneur ou le commissaire
- une liste des ministres actuels
- les dates de périodes législatives depuis la Confédération
- une liste des membres et des circonscriptions
- des notes biographiques*
- les résultats des élections générales et partielles les résultats d'élections générales et partielles, y compris les élections générales de 2015 en Alberta, à l'Île-du-Prince-Édouard, à Terre-Neuve-et-Labrador et aux Territoires du Nord-Ouest.

Cours : fédérale—chaque chapitre comprend : une description de la cour (suprême, fédérale, cour d'appel fédérale, cour d'appel de la cour martiale et cour de l'impôt), son histoire, une liste des juges qui y siègent ainsi que des notes biographiques.*

* Les notes biographiques respectent un format concis, bien qu'approfondi :

Renseignements personnels—lieu de naissance, formation, renseignements familiaux

Carrière politique—cheminement politique et service public

Carrière privée—antécédents professionnels, membre d'organisations, antécédents militaires

OFFERT EN FORMAT PAPIER ET DÉSORMAIS ÉLECTRONIQUE!

Offert sous couverture rigide ou en format électronique grâce au web, le *Guide parlementaire canadien* donne invariablement un accès instantané aux représentants du gouvernement et aux faits qui font l'objet de vos recherches. Servez-vous de la version en ligne afin de circonscrire vos recherches grâce aux champs spéciaux de l'index comme l'institution, la province et le nom.

Créez vos propres listes! Les abonnés au service en ligne peuvent générer instantanément leurs propres listes de contacts et les exporter en format feuille de calcul pour une utilisation approfondie – une solution de rechange géniale aux services dispendieux d'un commissionnaire en publipostage!

Photo de le très honorable Justin Trudeau par Adam Scotti. Photo fournie par le Bureau du Premier ministre © Sa Majesté la Reine du Chef du Canada, 2017.

GREY HOUSE PUBLISHING CANADA

Pour obtenir plus d'information, veuillez contacter Grey House Publishing Canada

par tél. : 1 866 433-4739 ou 416 644-6479 par téléc. : 416 644-1904 | info@greyhouse.ca | www.greyhouse.ca

Directory of Directors

Your Best Source for Hard-to-Find Business Information

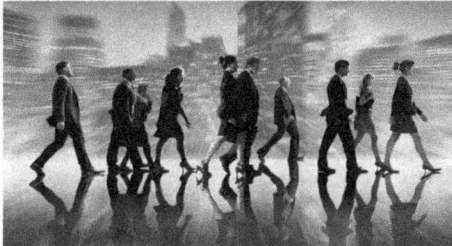

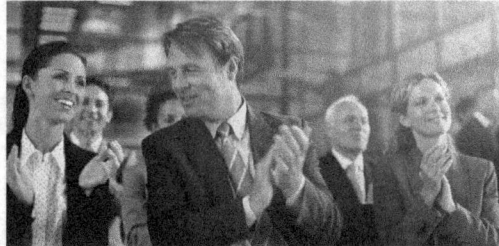

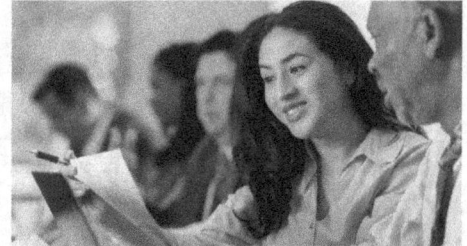

Since 1931, the *Financial Post Directory of Directors* has been recognizing leading Canadian companies and their execs. Today, this title is one of the most comprehensive resources for hard-to-find Canadian business information, allowing readers to access roughly 16,300 executive contacts from Canada's top 1,400 corporations. This prestigious title offers a definitive list of directorships and offices held by noteworthy Canadian business people. It also provides details on leading Canadian companies—publicly traded and privately-owned, including company name, contact information and the names of their executive officers and directors.

ACCESS THE COMPANIES & DIRECTORS YOU NEED IN NO TIME!

The updated 2017 edition of the *Directory of Directors* is jam-packed with information, including:

- **ALL-NEW front matter**: An infographic drawn from data in the book, an excerpt from the Canadian Board Diversity Council's latest Annual Report Card on gender diversity on corporate boards, an excerpt from a survey on board preparedness and crisis oversight by Osler, Hoskin & Harcourt LLP, and rankings from the FP500.

- **Personal listings**: First name, last name, gender, birth date, degrees, schools attended, executive positions and directorships, previous positions held, main business address and more.

- **Company listings**: Boards of directors and executive officers, head office address, phone and fax numbers, toll-free number, web and email addresses.

Powerful indexes enabling researchers to target just the information they need include:

- An **industrial classification index**: List of key Canadian companies, sorted by industry type according to the Global Industry Classification Standard (GICS®).

- A **geographic location index** grouping all companies in the Company Listings section according to the city and province/state of the head office; and

- An **alphabetical list of abbreviations** providing definitions of common abbreviations used for terms, titles, organizations, honours/fellowships and degrees throughout the Directory.

GREY HOUSE PUBLISHING CANADA

For more information please contact Grey House Publishing Canada
Tel.: (866)-433-4739 or (416) 644-6479 Fax: (416) 644-1904 | info@greyhouse.ca | www.greyhouse.ca

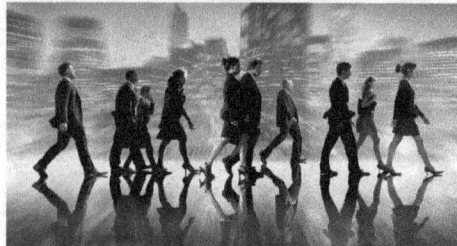

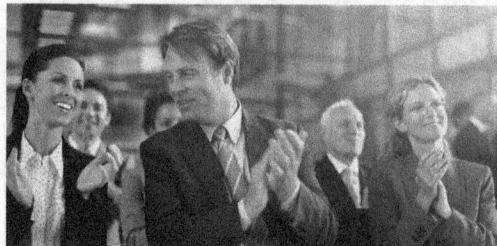

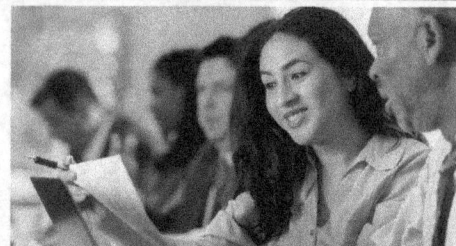

Canadian Who's Who

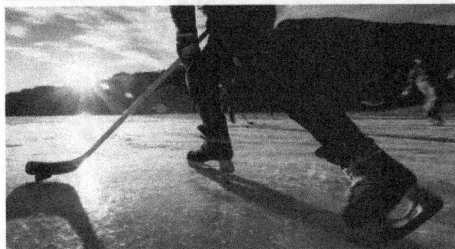

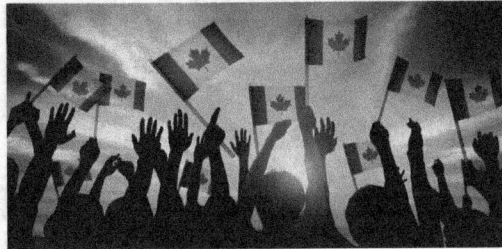

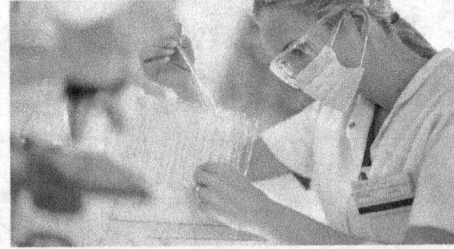

Canadian Who's Who is the only authoritative publication of its kind in Canada, offering access to over 10 000 notable Canadians in all walks of life. Published annually to provide current and accurate information, the familiar bright-red volume is recognized as the standard reference source of contemporary Canadian biography.

Documenting the achievement of Canadians from a wide variety of occupations and professions, *Canadian Who's Who* records the diversity of culture in Canada. These biographies are organized alphabetically and provide detailed information on the accomplishments of notable Canadians, from coast to coast. All who are interested in the achievements of Canada's most influential citizens and their significant contributions to the country and the world beyond should acquire this reference title.

Detailed entries give date and place of birth, education, family details, career information, memberships, creative works, honours, languages, and awards, together with full addresses. Included are outstanding Canadians from business, academia, politics, sports, the arts and sciences, etc.

Every year the publisher invites new individuals to complete questionnaires from which new biographies are compiled. The publisher also gives those already listed in earlier editions an opportunity to update their biographies. Those listed are selected because of the positions they hold in Canadian society, or because of the contributions they have made to Canada.

AVAILABLE ONLINE!

Canadian Who's Who is also available online, through Canada's Information Resource Centre (CIRC). Readers can access this title's in-depth and vital networking content in the format that best suits their needs—in print, by subscription or online.

The print edition of *Canadian Who's Who 2017* contains over 10,000 entries, while the online edition gives users access to 24,000 biographies, including all current listings and 11,000 archived biographies dating back to 1999.

Canadian Who's Who

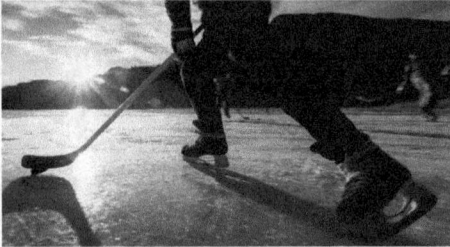

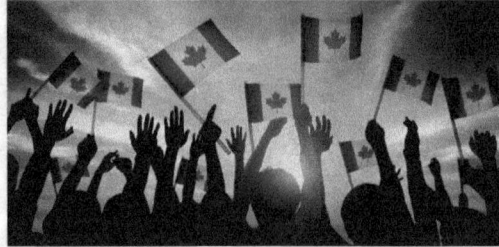

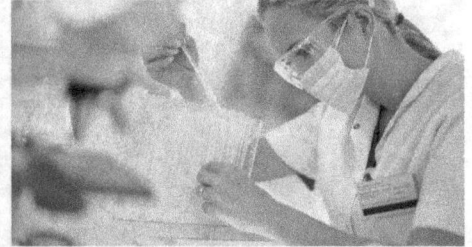

Canadian Who's Who est la seule publication digne de foi de son genre au Canada. Elle donne accès pus de 10 000 dignitaires canadiens de tous les horizons. L'ouvrage annuel rouge vif bien connu, rempli d'information à jour et exacte, est la référence standard en matière de biographies canadiennes contemporaines.

Canadian Who's Who, qui porte sur les réalisations de Canadiens occupant une vaste gamme de postes et de professions, illustre la diversité de la culture canadienne. Ces biographies sont classées en ordre alphabétique et donnent de l'information détaillée sur les réalisations de Canadiens éminents, d'un océan à l'autre. Tous ceux qui s'intéressent aux réalisations des citoyens les plus influents au Canada et à leurs contributions importantes au pays et partout dans le monde doivent se procurer cet ouvrage de référence.

Les entrées détaillées indiquent la date et le lieu de la naissance, traitent de l'éducation, de la famille, de la carrière, des adhésions, des œuvres de création, des distinctions, des langues et des prix - en plus des adresses complètes. Elles comprennent des Canadiens exceptionnels du monde des affaires, des universités, de la politique, des sports, des arts, des sciences et plus encore!

Chaque année, l'éditeur invite de nouvelles personnes à remplir les questionnaires à partir desquels il prépare les nouvelles biographies. Il le remet également aux personnes qui font partie de numéros antérieurs afin de leur permettre d'effectuer une mise à jour. Les personnes retenues le sont en raison des postes qu'elles occupent dans la société canadienne ou de leurs contributions au Canada.

OFFERT EN FORMAT ÉLECTRONIQUE!

Canadian Who's Who est également offert en ligne par l'entremise du Centre de documentation du Canada (CDC). Les lecteurs peuvent accéder au contenu approfondi et essentiel au réseautage de cet ouvrage dans le format qui leur convient le mieux - version imprimée, en ligne ou par abonnement.

L'édition imprimée de *Canadian Who's Who 2017* compte plus de 10 000 entrées tandis qu'en consultant la version en ligne, les utilisateurs ont accès à 24 000 biographies, dont fiches d'actualité et 11 000 biographies archives qui remontent jusqu'à 1999.

GREY HOUSE PUBLISHING CANADA

Pour obtenir plus d'information, veuillez contacter Grey House Publishing Canada
par tél. : 1 866 433-4739 ou 416 644-6479 par téléc. : 416 644-1904 | info@greyhouse.ca | www.greyhouse.ca

Financial Services Canada

Unparalleled Coverage of the Canadian Financial Service Industry

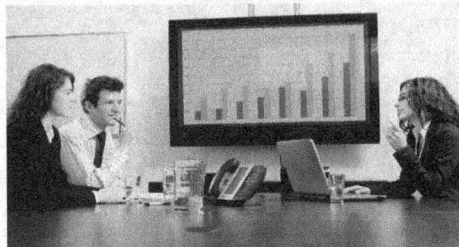

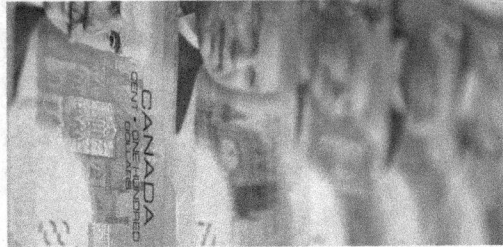

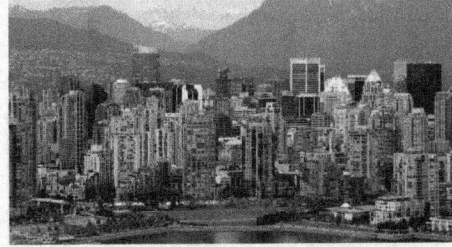

With corporate listings for over 30,000 organizations and hard-to-find business information, *Financial Services Canada* is the most up-to-date source for names and contact numbers of industry professionals, senior executives, portfolio managers, financial advisors, agency bureaucrats and elected representatives.

Financial Services Canada is the definitive resource for detailed listings—providing valuable contact information including: name, title, organization, profile, associated companies, telephone and fax numbers, e-mail and website addresses. Use our online database and refine your search by stock symbol, revenue, year founded, assets, ownership type or number of employees.

POWERFUL INDEXES HELP YOU LOCATE THE CRUCIAL FINANCIAL INFORMATION YOU NEED.

Organized with the user in mind, *Financial Services Canada* contains categorized listings and 4 easy-to-use indexes:

Alphabetic—financial organizations listed in alphabetical sequence by company name

Geographic—financial institutions broken down by town or city

Executive Name—all officers, directors and senior personnel in alphabetical order by surname

Insurance class—lists all companies by insurance type

Reduce the time you spend compiling lists, researching company information and searching for e-mail addresses. Whether you are interested in contacting a finance lawyer regarding international and domestic joint ventures, need to generate a list of foreign banks in Canada or want to contact the Toronto Stock Exchange—*Financial Services Canada* gives you the power to find all the data you need.

PRINT OR ONLINE—QUICK AND EASY ACCESS TO ALL THE INFORMATION YOU NEED!

Available in softcover print or electronically via the web, *Financial Services Canada* provides instant access to the people you need and the facts you want every time.

Financial Services Canada print edition is verified and updated annually. Ongoing changes are added to the web version on a regular basis. The web version allows you to narrow your search by using index fields such as name or type of organization, subject, location, contact name or title and postal code.

Create your own contact lists! Online subscribers have the option to instantly generate their own contact lists and export them into spreadsheets for further use—a great alternative to high cost list broker services.

ACCESS TO CURRENT LISTINGS FOR...

Banks and Depository Institutions
- Domestic and savings banks
- Foreign banks and branches
- Foreign bank representative offices
- Trust companies
- Credit unions

Non-Depository Institutions
- Bond rating companies
- Collection agencies
- Credit card companies
- Financing and loan companies
- Trustees in bankruptcy

Investment Management Firms, including securities and commodities
- Financial planning / investment management companies
- Investment dealers
- Investment fund companies
- Pension/money management companies
- Stock exchanges
- Holding companies

Insurance Companies, including federal and provincial
- Reinsurance companies
- Fraternal benefit societies
- Mutual benefit companies
- Reciprocal exchanges

Accounting and Law
- Accountants
- Actuary consulting firms
- Law firms (specializing in finance)

Major Canadian Companies
- Key financial contacts for public, private and Crown corporations

Associations
- Associations and institutes serving the financial services sector

Financial Technology & Services
- Companies involved in financial software and other technical areas.

Access even more content online:
Government and Publications
- Federal, provincial and territorial contacts
- Leading publications serving the financial services industry

Services financiers au Canada

Une couverture sans pareille de l'industrie des services financiers canadiens

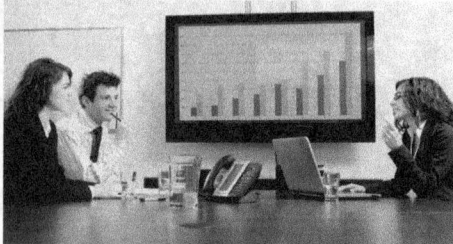

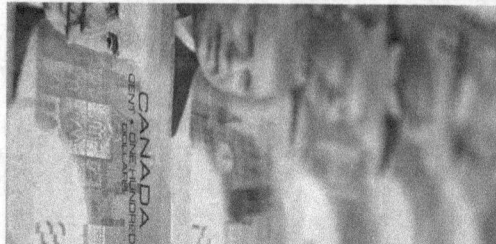

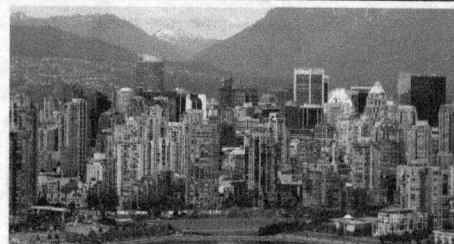

Grâce à plus de 30 000 organisations et renseignements commerciaux rares, *Services financiers du Canada* est la source la plus à jour de noms et de coordonnées de professionnels, de membres de la haute direction, de gestionnaires de portefeuille, de conseillers financiers, de fonctionnaires et de représentants élus de l'industrie.

Services financiers du Canada intègre les plus récentes modifications à l'industrie afin de vous offrir les détails les plus à jour au sujet de chaque entreprise, notamment le nom, le titre, l'organisation, les numéros de téléphone et de télécopieur, le courriel et l'adresse du site Web. Servez-vous de la base de données en ligne et raffinez votre recherche selon le symbole, le revenu, l'année de création, les immobilisations, le type de propriété ou le nombre d'employés.

DES INDEX PUISSANTS VOUS AIDENT À TROUVER LES RENSEIGNEMENTS FINANCIERS ESSENTIELS DONT VOUS AVEZ BESOIN.

C'est avec l'utilisateur en tête que Services financiers au Canada a été conçu; il contient des listes catégorisées et quatre index faciles d'utilisation :

Alphabétique—les organisations financières apparaissent en ordre alphabétique, selon le nom de l'entreprise.

Géographique—les institutions financières sont détaillées par ville.

Nom de directeur—tous les agents, directeurs et cadres supérieurs sont classés en ordre alphabétique, selon leur nom de famille.

Classe d'assurance—toutes les entreprises selon leur type d'assurance.

Passez moins de temps à préparer des listes, à faire des recherches ou à chercher des contacts et des courriels. Que vous soyez intéressé à contacter un avocat en droit des affaires au sujet de projets conjoints internationaux et nationaux, que vous ayez besoin de générer une liste des banques étrangères au Canada ou que vous souhaitiez communiquer avec la Bourse de Toronto, *Services financiers au Canada* vous permet de trouver toutes les données dont vous avez besoin.

OFFERT EN FORMAT PAPIER OU EN LIGNE – UN ACCÈS RAPIDE ET FACILE À TOUS LES RENSEIGNEMENTS DONT VOUS AVEZ BESOIN!

Offert sous couverture rigide ou en format électronique grâce au Web, Services financiers du Canada donne invariablement un accès instantané aux personnes et aux faits dont vous avez besoin. Si la version imprimée est vérifiée et mise à jour annuellement, des changements continus sont apportés mensuellement à la base de données en ligne. Servez-vous de la version en ligne afin de circonscrire vos recherches grâce à des champs spéciaux de l'index comme le nom de l'organisation ou son type, le sujet, l'emplacement, le nom de la personne-ressource ou son titre et le code postal.

Créez vos propres listes! Les abonnés au service en ligne peuvent générer instantanément leurs propres listes de contacts et les exporter en format feuille de calcul pour une utilisation approfondie – une solution de rechange géniale aux services dispendieux d'un commissionnaire en publipostage.

ACCÉDEZ AUX LISTES ACTUELLES...

Banques et institutions de dépôt
- Banques nationales et d'épargne
- Banques étrangères et leurs succursales
- Bureaux des représentants de banques étrangères
- Sociétés de fiducie
- Coopératives d'épargne et de crédit

Établissements financiers
- Entreprises de notation des obligations
- Agences de placement
- Compagnies de carte de crédit
- Sociétés de financement et de prêt
- Syndics de faillite

Sociétés de gestion de placements, y compris les valeurs et marchandises
- Entreprises de planification financière et de gestion des investissements
- Maisons de courtage de valeurs
- Courtiers en épargne collective
- Entreprises de gestion de la pension/de trésorerie
- Bourses
- Sociétés de portefeuille

Compagnies d'assurance, fédérales et provinciales
- Compagnies de réassurance
- Sociétés fraternelles
- Sociétés de secours mutuel
- Échanges selon la formule de réciprocité

Comptabilité et droit
- Comptables
- Cabinets d'actuaires-conseils
- Cabinets d'avocats (spécialisés en finance)

Principales entreprises canadiennes
- Principaux contacts financiers pour les sociétés de capitaux publiques, privées et de la Couronne

Les associations et Technologie et services financiers

Accès à plus de contenu en ligne: Gouvernement et Publications
- Personnes-ressources aux paliers fédéral, provinciaux et territoriaux
- Principales publications qui desservent l'industrie des services financiers

GREY HOUSE PUBLISHING CANADA

Pour obtenir plus d'information, veuillez contacter Grey House Publishing Canada

par tél. : 1 866 433-4739 ou 416 644-6479 par téléc. : 416 644-1904 | info@greyhouse.ca | www.greyhouse.ca

Canadian Environmental Resource Guide

The Only Complete Guide to the Business of Environmental Management

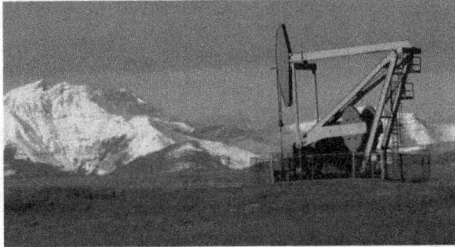

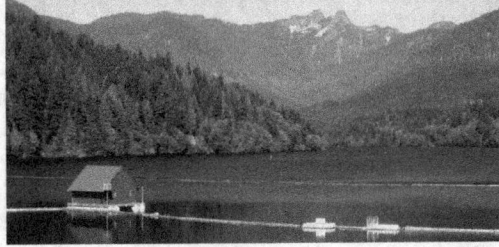

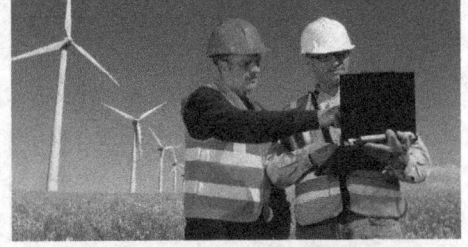

The *Canadian Environmental Resource Guide* provides data on every aspect of the environmental industry in unprecedented detail. It offers one-stop searching for details on government offices and programs, information sources, product and service firms and trade fairs that pertain to the business of environmental management. All information is fully indexed and cross-referenced for easy use. The directory features current information and key contacts in Canada's environmental industry including:

ENVIRONMENTAL UP-DATE

- Information on prominent environmentalists, environmental abbreviations and a summary of recent environmental events

- Updated articles, rankings, statistics and charts on all aspects of the environmental industry

- Trade shows, conferences and seminars for the current year and beyond

ENVIRONMENTAL PRODUCTS & SERVICES

- Comprehensive listings for companies and firms producing and selling products and services in the environmental sector, including markets served, working language and percentage of revenue sources: public and private

- Detailed indexes by subject, geography and ISO

ENVIRONMENTAL GOVERNMENT LISTINGS

- Information on important intergovernmental offices and councils, and listings of environmental trade representatives abroad

- In-depth listings of environmental information at the municipal level, including population and number of households, water and waste treatment, landfill statistics and special by-laws and bans, as well as key environmental contacts for each municipality

Available in softcover print and electronically via the web, the *Canadian Environmental Resource Guide* provides instant access to the people you need and the facts you want every time. The *Canadian Environmental Resource Guide* is verified and updated annually. Ongoing changes are added to the web version on a regular basis.

CANADIAN ENVIRONMENTAL RESOURCE GUIDE OFFERS EVEN MORE CONTENT ONLINE!

Environmental Information Resources—An all-inclusive list of environmental law firms, special libraries and resource centres, educational programs, research centres and foundations and grants

Associations—Thousands of environmental associations, with information on membership, environmental activities, key contacts and more

Government Listings—Every federal and provincial department and agency influencing environmental initiatives and purchasing policies

The web version allows you to narrow your search by using index fields such as name or type of organization, subject, location, contact name or title and postal code.

Create your own contact lists! Online subscribers have the option to instantly generate their own contact lists and export them into spreadsheets for further use—a great alternative to high cost list broker services.

GREY HOUSE PUBLISHING CANADA

For more information please contact Grey House Publishing Canada

Tel.: (866) 433-4739 or (416) 644-6479 Fax: (416) 644-1904 | info@greyhouse.ca | www.greyhouse.ca

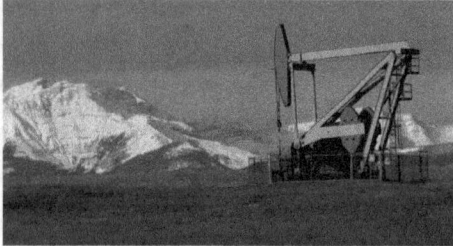

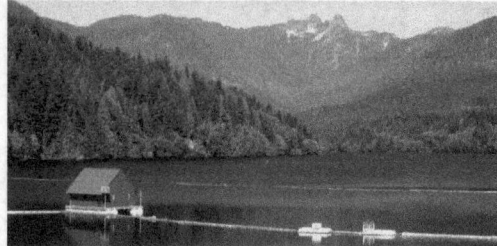

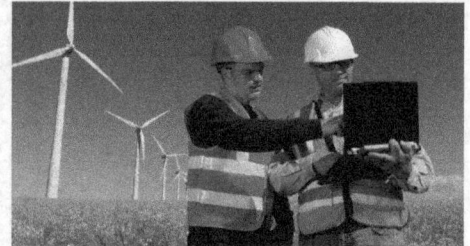

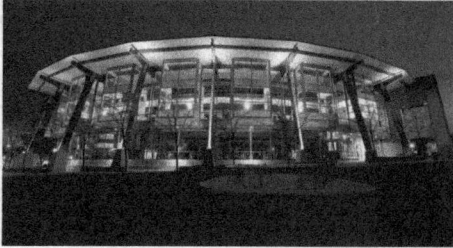

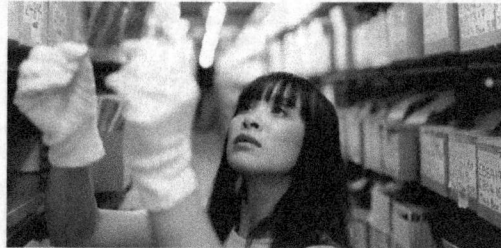

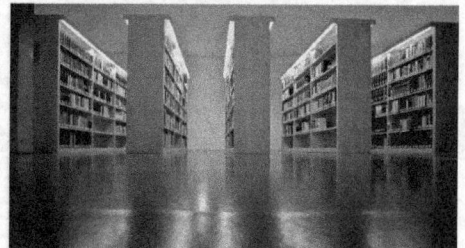

Bibliothèques Canada

Accédez aux renseignements complets et détaillés au sujet des bibliothèques canadiennes

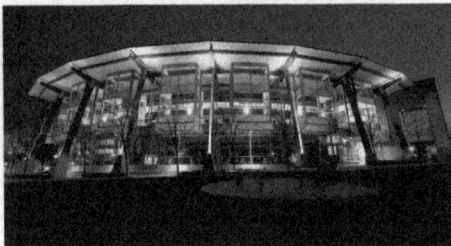

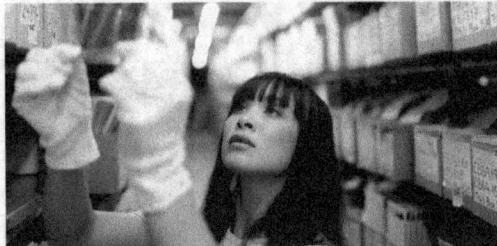

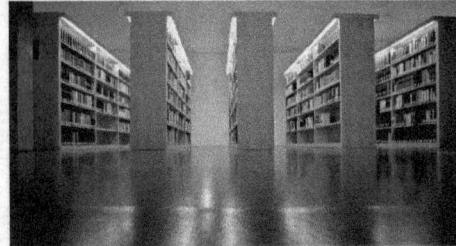

Bibliothèques Canada combine les renseignements les plus à jour provenant du secteur des bibliothèques de partout au Canada, y compris les bibliothèques et leurs succursales, les bibliothèques éducatives, les systèmes régionaux, les centres de ressources, les archives, les périodiques pertinents, les écoles de bibliothéconomie et leurs programmes, les organismes provinciaux et gouvernementaux ainsi que les associations.

Principal répertoire des bibliothèques depuis plus de 30 ans, *Bibliothèques Canada* vous donne accès à près de 10 000 noms et adresses de personnes-ressources pour ces établissements. Il comprend également des détails précieux comme le symbole d'identification de bibliothèque, le nombre de membres du personnel, les systèmes d'exploitation, le type de bibliothèque et le budget attribué aux acquisitions, les heures d'ouverture – autant d'information minutieusement indexée et facile à trouver.

Offert en version imprimée et en ligne, *Bibliothèques Canada* offre des renseignements de qualité, facile d'accès, qui ont été vérifiés et organisés afin de les obtenir facilement. Cinq index conviviaux vous aident dans la navigation du numéro imprimé tandis que la version en ligne vous permet de saisir plusieurs champs d'index pour vous aider à découvrir l'information voulue.

ACCÈS INSTANTANÉ AUX RENSEIGNEMENTS DU DOMAINE DES BIBLIOTHÈQUES CANADIENNES

Conçu pour les éditeurs, les groupes de revendication, les fournisseurs de matériel informatique, les fournisseurs de services Internet et autres groupes qui offrent produits et services aux bibliothèques; les associations qui ont besoin de conserver une liste à jour des ressources bibliothécaires au Canada; les services de recherche, les organismes étudiants et gouvernementaux qui ont besoin d'information au sujet des types de services et de programmes offerts par divers établissements de recherche, *Bibliothèques Canada* vous aide à trouver l'information nécessaire – rapidement et simplement.

LA VERSION EN LIGNE COMPREND DES OPTIONS DE RECHERCHE POUSSÉES...

À partir de l'interface du Centre de documentation du Canada de Grey House Publishing Canada, vous pouvez choisir entre la recherche poussée et rapide pour cibler votre information. Vous pouvez effectuer des recherches par texte simple, conçues à la fois pour les chercheurs débutants et chevronnés, ainsi que des recherches booléennes puissantes. Vous pouvez également restreindre votre recherche à l'aide des champs d'index, comme le nom ou le type d'établissement, le siège social, l'emplacement, l'indicatif régional, le nom de la personne-ressource ou son titre et le code postal. Enregistrez vos recherches pour vous en servir plus tard ou utilisez la fonction de marquage pour afficher, imprimer, envoyer par courriel ou exporter les dossiers sélectionnés.

Les abonnés au service en ligne peuvent générer instantanément leurs propres listes de contacts et les exporter en format feuille de calcul pour une utilisation approfondie – une solution de rechange géniale aux services dispendieux d'un commissionnaire en publipostage.

BIBLIOTHÈQUES CANADA VOUS DONNE TOUS LES RENSEIGNEMENTS ESSENTIELS RELATIFS À CHAQUE ÉTABLISSEMENT :

Leurs nom et adresse, les coordonnées de la personne-ressource, les membres clés du personnel, le nombre de membres du personnel

L'information relative aux collections, le type de bibliothèque, le budget attribué aux acquisitions, le domaine, les collections particulières

Les services aux utilisateurs, le nombre de succursales, les heures d'ouverture, les renseignements relatifs au PEB, les services de photocopie et de microforme, la recherche rémunérée, l'accès à Internet

L'information relative aux systèmes, des détails sur l'accès électronique, les systèmes d'exploitation et ceux en ligne, Internet et le logiciel de messagerie électronique, la connectivité à Internet, l'accès aux ressources électroniques

L'information supplémentaire, y compris les associations, les publications et les systèmes régionaux

Alors que près de 60 % des données sont modifiées annuellement, il est plus important que jamais de posséder la plus récente version de *Bibliothèques Canada*.

GREY HOUSE PUBLISHING CANADA

Pour obtenir plus d'information, veuillez contacter Grey House Publishing Canada

par tél. : 1 866 433-4739 ou 416 644-6479 par téléc. : 416 644-1904 | info@greyhouse.ca | www.greyhouse.ca

Major Canadian Cities
Compared & Ranked

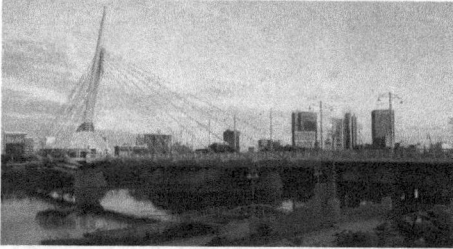

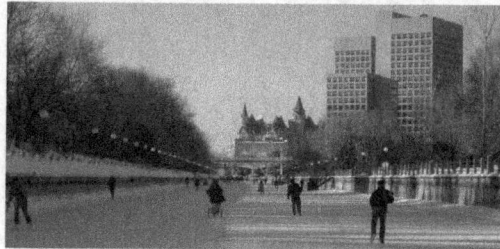

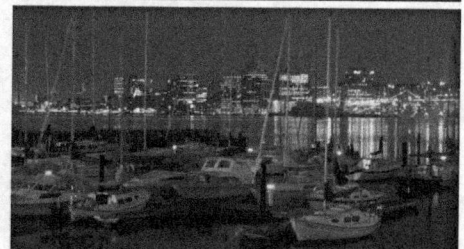

Major Canadian Cities provides the user with numerous ways to rank and compare 50 major cities across Canada. All statistical information is at your fingertips; you can access details about the cities, each with a population of 100,000 or more. On Canada's Information Resource Centre (CIRC), you can instantly rank cities according to your preferences and make your own analytical tables with the data provided. There are hundreds of questions that these ranking tables will answer: Which cities have the youngest population? Where is the economic growth the strongest? Which cities have the best labour statistics?

A city profile for each location offers additional insights into the city to provide a sense of the location, its history, its recreational and cultural activities. Following the profile are rankings showing its uniqueness in the spectrum of cities across Canada: interesting notes about the city and how it ranks amongst the top 50 in different ways, such as most liveable, wealthiest and coldest! These reports are available only from Grey House Publishing Canada and only with your subscription to this exciting new product!

MAJOR CANADIAN CITIES SHOWS YOU THESE STATISTICAL TABLES:

Demographics
- Population Growth
- Age Characteristics
- Male/Female Ratio
- Marital Status

Housing
- Household Type & Size
- Housing Age & Value

Labour
- Labour Force
- Occupation
- Industry
- Place of Work

Ethnicity, Immigration & Language
- Mother Tongue
- Knowledge of Official Languages
- Language Spoken at Home
- Minority Populations
- Education
- Education Attainment

Income
- Median Income
- Median Income After Taxes
- Median Income by Family Type
- Median Income After Taxes by Family Type

Transportation
- Mode of Transportation to Work

GREY HOUSE PUBLISHING CANADA

For more information please contact Grey House Publishing Canada
Tel.: (866) 433-4739 or (416) 644-6479 Fax: (416) 644-1904 | info@greyhouse.ca | www.greyhouse.ca

Principales villes canadiennes

Comparaison et classement

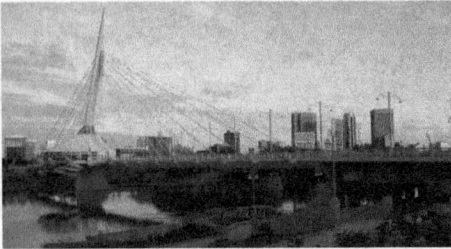

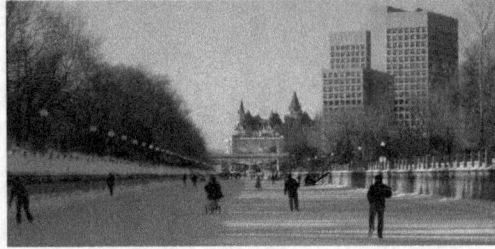

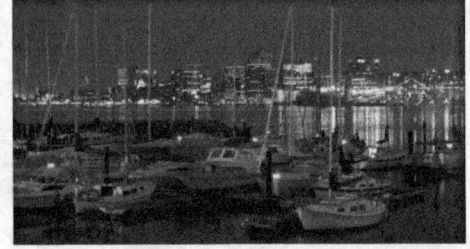

Principales villes canadiennes offre à l'utilisateur de nombreuses manières de classer et de comparer 50 villes principales du Canada. Toute l'information statistique se trouve au bout de vos doigts : vous pouvez obtenir des détails sur les villes, chacune comptant 100 000 habitants ou plus. Dans le Centre de documentation du Canada (CDC), vous pouvez classer instantanément les villes selon vos préférences et créer vos propres tableaux analytiques à l'aide des données fournies. Ces tableaux de classement répondent à des centaines de questions, notamment : quelles villes comptent la population la plus jeune? À quel endroit la croissance économique est-elle la plus forte? Quelles villes présentent les meilleures statistiques en matière de main-d'œuvre?

Un profil de ville offre des renseignements supplémentaires afin de vous donner une idée de son emplacement, de son histoire, de ses activités récréatives et culturelles. Suivent des classements qui démontrent l'unicité de la ville dans un spectre de villes qui se trouvent partout au Canada. Vous trouverez également des remarques intéressantes au sujet de la ville et de son classement parmi les 50 principales villes, par exemple selon celle où il fait le mieux vivre, où se trouvent les plus riches et où il fait le plus froid. Ces rapports sont disponibles uniquement auprès de Grey House Publishing Canada et dans le cadre de votre abonnement à ce nouveau produit emballant!

PRINCIPALES VILLES CANADIENNES COMPREND CES TABLEAUX STATISTIQUES :

Données démographiques

- Croissance de la population
- Caractéristiques relatives à l'âge
- Ratio homme/femme
- État matrimonial

Logement

- Type et taille du logement
- Âge et valeur du logement

Main-d'œuvre

- Population active
- Emploi
- Industrie
- Lieu de travail

Ethnicité, immigration et langue

- Langue maternelle
- Connaissance des langues officielles
- Langue parlée à la maison
- Populations minoritaires
- Formation
- Niveau scolaire

Revenu

- Revenu médian
- Revenu médian après impôts
- Revenu médian par type de famille
- Revenu médian après impôts par type de famille

Transport

- Moyen de transport vers le travail

GREY HOUSE PUBLISHING CANADA

Pour obtenir plus d'information, veuillez contacter Grey House Publishing Canada

par tél. : 1 866 433-4739 ou 416 644-6479 par téléc. : 416 644-1904 | info@greyhouse.ca | www.greyhouse.ca

Mailing List Services

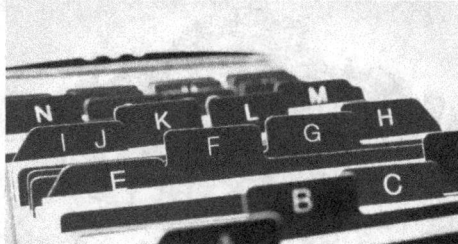

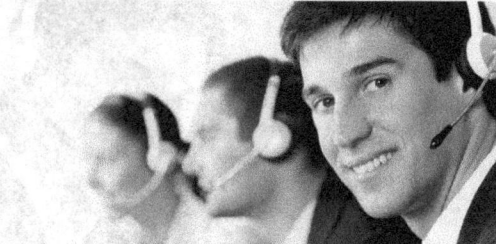

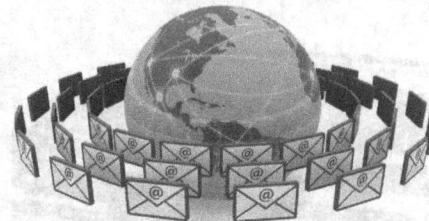

As a boutique provider of mailing lists, Grey House Publishing Canada specializes in the areas below to ensure a high level of accuracy. Our clients return to us time and time again because of the reliability of our information and great customer service. We'll work with you to develop a campaign that provides results. No other list services will work as closely as we do to meet your unique needs.

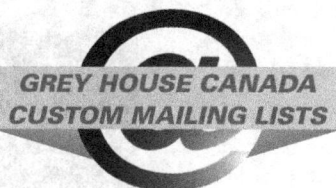

GREY HOUSE CANADA CUSTOM MAILING LISTS

AVAILABILITY

Lists are available on CD, labels and via e-mail. They are provided on a one-time use basis or for a one-year lease. For a quotation on tailor-made lists to suit your needs, inquire using the contact information listed below.

Associations—the most extensive list of Canadian associations available, featuring all professional, trade and business organizations together with not-for-profit groups.

Arts & Culture—the definitive source of key prospects in various Canadian arts and cultural outlets.

Education—the most comprehensive list of educational institutions and organizations in Canada.

Health Care / Hospitals—includes all major medical facilities with chief executives.

Lawyers—key prospects for a number of direct mail offers.

Media—the definitive source of key prospects in various Canadian media outlets, offering the top business managers and/or publishers.

Environmental—a complete profile of the Canadian Environmental scene, constantly revised for the annual Canadian Environmental Resource Guide.

Financial Services—a list of key contacts from the full range of Canada's financial services industry.

Government Key Contacts—a list of key Government contacts, maintained by the Canadian Almanac & Directory, Canada's standard institutional reference for 170 years.

Libraries—the most unique and complete list of government, special and public libraries available.

Major Canadian Companies—listings of Canada's largest private, public and Crown corporations with major key contacts of the top business decision-makers.

GREY HOUSE PUBLISHING CANADA

For more information please contact Grey House Publishing Canada
Tel.: (866) 433-4739 or (416) 644-6479 Fax: (416) 644-1904 | info@greyhouse.ca | www.greyhouse.ca

Services de liste de distribution

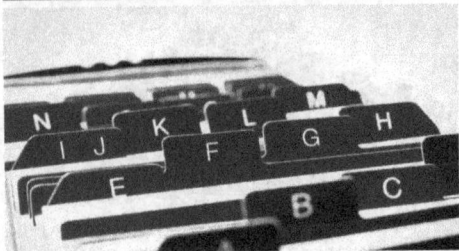

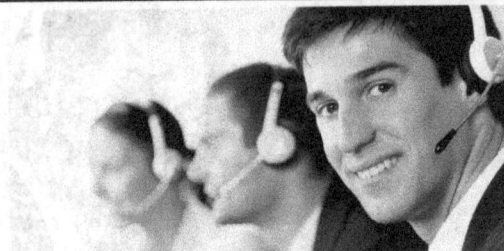

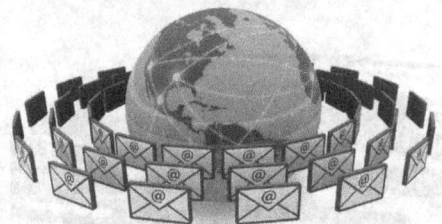

En tant que point de service fournisseur de listes de distribution, Grey House Canada se spécialise dans les domaines ci-dessous pour assurer un degré supérieur de précision. Nos clients nous sont fidèles, car ils souhaitent bénéficier de notre fiabilité et de notre service à la clientèle. Nous collaborerons avec vous pour développer une campagne qui produit des résultats. Aucun autre service de création de listes ne collabore aussi étroitement que nous avec leurs clients pour satisfaire leurs besoins particuliers.

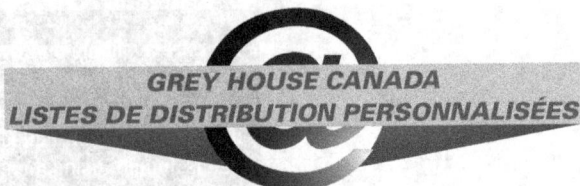

GREY HOUSE CANADA
LISTES DE DISTRIBUTION PERSONNALISÉES

Associations—la liste la plus complète des associations canadiennes qui énumère toutes les associations professionnelles, corporatives et commerciales ainsi que les groupes sans but lucratif.

Arts et culture—la source manifeste des candidats clés des divers vecteurs artistiques et culturels au Canada.

Éducation—la liste la plus complète des établissements et des organismes d'enseignement au Canada.

Soins de santé/hôpitaux—comprend les principaux établissements médicaux et leurs directeurs.

Avocats—les principaux clients potentiels pour nombre d'offres de publipostage direct.

Médias—la source certaine des clients potentiels clés dans divers points de vente de médias canadiens; elle comprend les principaux dirigeants et éditeurs.

Environnement—un profil complet de la scène environnementale canadienne; constamment mis à jour pour le Guide des ressources environnementales canadiennes.

Services financiers—une liste des personnes-ressources clés de tout l'éventail de l'industrie des services financiers du Canada.

Coordonnées gouvernementales clés—une liste des contacts essentiels, entretenue par le Répertoire et almanach canadien, la référence institutionnelle au Canada depuis 170 ans.

Bibliothèques—la liste la plus unique et la plus complète des bibliothèques gouvernementales, spécialisées et publiques disponible.

Principales entreprises canadiennes—une liste des plus grandes sociétés privées, publiques et de la Couronne au Canada, y compris les coordonnées des principaux décideurs du monde des affaires.

DISPONIBILITÉ

Les listes sont offertes sur disque, étiquettes et par courriel. Elles sont fournies sur la base d'une utilisation unique ou d'un abonnement d'un an. Pour obtenir un devis pour une liste personnalisée selon vos besoins, contactez-nous.

GREY HOUSE PUBLISHING CANADA

Pour obtenir plus d'information, veuillez contacter Grey House Publishing Canada
par tél. : 1 866 433-4739 ou 416 644-6479 par téléc. : 416 644-1904 | info@greyhouse.ca | www.greyhouse.ca

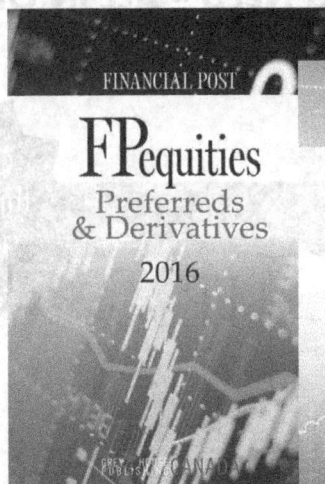

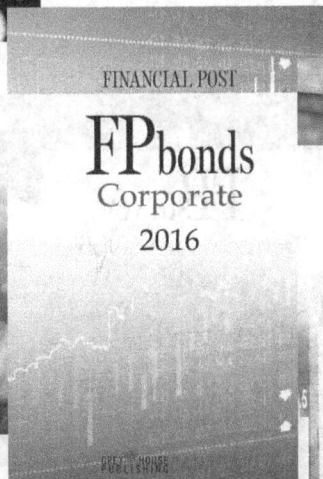

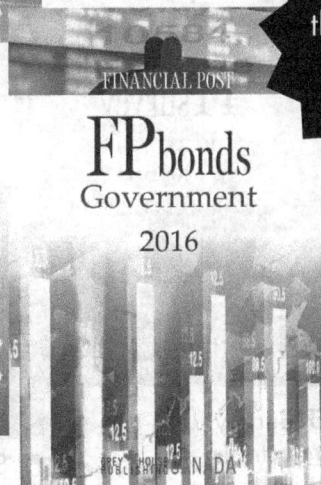

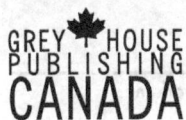

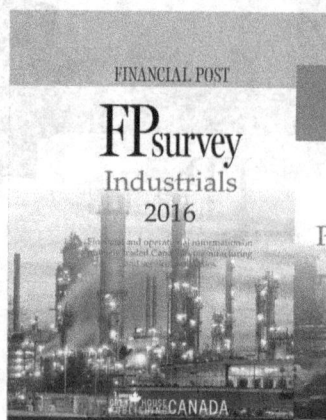

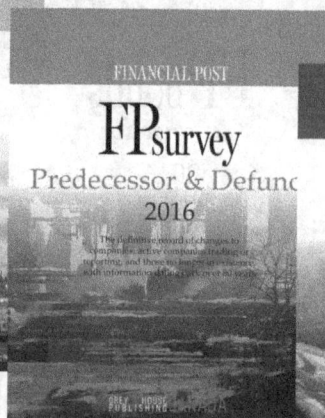

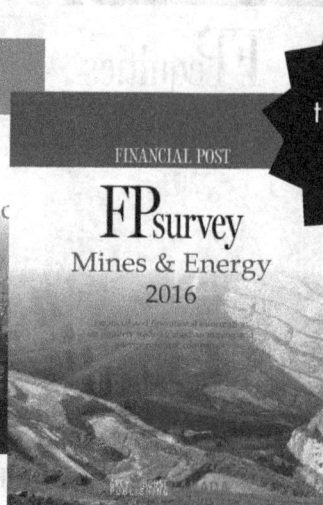

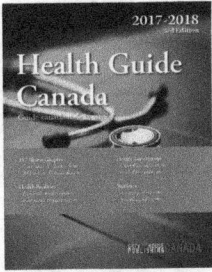

HEALTH GUIDE CANADA
Grey House Publishing Canada
555 Richmond Street West, Suite 512
Toronto, Ontario M5V 3B1

Fax completed forms to: (416) 644-1904
Or email to info@greyhouse.ca

Health Guide Canada is the third edition of a health directory published by Grey House Publishing Canada. It offers a comprehensive overview of 107 chronic and mental illnesses, from Addison's to Wilson's disease. In each chapter you'll find a straightforward medical description, plus a listing of support services and information resources that relate to that condition.

This listing is **FREE**. To ensure a complete and accurate listing in the upcoming edition, simply fill in the questionnaire and return it by **fax, mail or email**. Include any relevant information such as phone, fax or toll free numbers, website and email addresses, and official translations (if applicable).

Please send us this form with any new listings or when current information about an existing listing is changed.
If you have any questions, please call Stuart Paterson at (416) 644-6478 or 1-866-433-4739, ext. 302.
Respond by **Fax**: (416) 644-1904, by **mail** to the address above, or **email** info@greyhouse.ca

Is your organization already listed in this publication? Yes, we're updating existing information_____ No, we're new_____
Completed by: _____Phone:_____Email:_____

ORGANIZATION:

Name: _____

Translated name: _____

Acronym: _____

Street Address: _____

Phone: _____ Toll free: _____

Fax: _____ Email: _____

Website: _____

Social media links: _____

Year founded:_____

Scope of activity: ☐ International ☐ National ☐ Provincial ☐ Local

Mission statement: _____

_____

_____

_____

_____

Number of members: _____

Membership fee: _____

Annual operating budget: ☐ Less than $50,000 ☐ $50,000-99,999 ☐ $100,000-249,000 ☐ $250,000-499,999
☐ $500,000-1,000,000 ☐ $1,500,000-2,999,999 ☐ $3,000,000-4,999,999 ☐ Over $5,000,000

Publications:

Title: _____

Frequency: _____ Price: _____ ISSN: _____

Description: _____

Does your organization have a library/resource centre? ☐ Yes ☐ No

Library/resource centre name:

Chief officers/staff:

Name: _____

Title: _____

Phone: _____ Email: _____

Name: _____

Title: _____

Phone: _____ Email: _____

Name: _____

Title: _____

Phone: _____ Email: _____

Name: _____

Title: _____

Phone: _____ Email: _____

Name: _____

Title: _____

Phone: _____ Email: _____